Davies's Textbook of Adverse Drug Reactions

Davies's Textbook of Adverse Drug Reactions

Fifth Edition

Edited by

D. M. DAVIES, FRCP, FRCP Ed

R. E. FERNER, MD, FRCP

H. DE GLANVILLE, MB, B Chir, DTM&H, DIH

CHAPMAN & HALL MEDICAL
London · Weinheim · New York · Tokyo · Melbourne · Madras

Published by Chapman & Hall, an imprint of Lippincott-Raven Publishers, 2–6 Boundary Row, London SE18HN, UK

Lippincott-Raven Publishers, 227 East Washington Square, Philadelphia, PA 19106-3720, USA

First edition 1977
Second edition 1981
Third edition 1985
Fourth edition 1991
Fifth edition 1998

© 1977, 1981, 1985, 1991 Oxford University Press
© 1998 Lippincott-Raven Publishers

Typeset by Meditext, Weybridge, Surrey
Printed in Great Britain by St Edmundsbury Press Ltd, Bury St Edmunds, Suffolk

ISBN 0 41282480 9

A catalogue record for this book is available from the British Library

Dedicated to the memory of
FRANCIS T. ROBERTS of the United States of America,
LEOPOLD MEYLER of the Netherlands, and
SIR DERRICK DUNLOP of the United Kingdom,
who did so much to remind doctors that drug
therapy could at times be harmful as well as
beneficial.

Foreword to the first edition

by the late Sir Derrick Dunlop, MD, FRCP
First Chairman of the Committee on Safety of Drugs and, later, of the Medicines Commission.

This considerable volume — a tribute principally to the Newcastle Medical School which supplies 22 of its 32 contributors — is the most comprehensive account published of adverse reactions to drugs, and also supplies a very complete bibliography on the subject. Its unsentimental but unavoidably somewhat horrific contents might well give the average reader an aversion to drugs in general, but this would be unjustified. Although modern drugs are formidable agents, if prescribed and used with skill, wisdom, and propriety their benefits far exceed their occasional adverse effects. It is appropriate, therefore, that a foreword to a book on the dangers of drugs should be prefaced by a reminder of the great blessings they have conferred upon society.

Since the beginning of this century the average expectation of life at birth in this and most other European countries has increased by about 25 years. In the early part of the century this improving expectation of longevity was largely the result of better hygiene, housing, and nutrition but during the last 30 or 40 years it has been mostly due to modern medicines (a term taken to include bacteriological products and hormones). Quite apart from their favourable effect on mortality statistics, the relief from suffering resulting from their purely symptomatic uses, and the saving to national economies in diminished morbidity — less time lost from work, fewer and shorter admissions to hospital — is vast but more difficult to compute. It is becoming hard for older physicians to remember and it must be difficult for young ones to imagine what it was like to practise medicine when there was no insulin, vitamin B_{12}, sulphonamides, antibiotics, specifics for tropical diseases, hypotensives, anticoagulants and potent hormones, diuretics and anticonvulsants. Further, few of us would be callous enough to practise medicine without anaesthetics, narcotics, hypnotics, and analgesics.

No revolution, however, no matter how salutary, ever occurs without being harmful to some and the revolution in medicinal therapeutics of the last 50 years is no exception to this rule. Just as the old horse and buggy, though very slow, caused few fatal accidents whereas the modern automobile, though very fast, is a lethal instrument, so the old-fashioned bottle of medicine, elaborately compounded, meticulously bottled, elegantly flavoured, and exquisitely labelled, though relatively ineffective, was also comparatively innocuous whereas modern drugs, like atomic energy, are powerful for good but also for evil. The ill health that may result from their use — 'iatrogenic illness' as it is called or, more optimistically, if a little ironically, 'illness due to medical progress' — has become a new dimension in the aetiology of disease: perhaps up to 10 per cent of patients suffer to a greater or lesser extent from efforts to treat them. Our powers over Nature in this as in other respects have advanced so far that Nature seems to have become retaliatory and to be exacting a massive retribution. A drug that can modify or repress biological processes is invaluable in treatment but if it has this capacity it is bound also to cause adverse effects from time to time. Those who say that nothing but the complete safety of drugs will suffice demand the impossible: a drug without any side-effects is probably an ineffective one. The public who require progress must be prepared for some risk: it has always accepted the not inconsiderable risks of surgery to which some modern drugs are equivalent in efficacy. While shuddering at a death rate of, say, one in 40 000 patients dying as the result of taking a usually valuable remedy (and which surgeon, incidentally, would not be enchanted with such statistics for the most minor operation?) we are much more complacent about the far greater dangers of cigarette smoking, alcoholism, or road accidents. Yet were all drugs invariably prescribed and used properly, and sensible governmental controls were enforced, the dangers would be small, for the majority of their adverse reactions — though by no means all — are due to their well-recognised and predictable side-effects.

The medical profession has not been entirely guiltless in its use of drugs. We must confess that there has been a good deal of excessive, and occasionally ignorant and irresponsible prescribing for which there are many reasons.

Firstly, there are too few doctors in most countries for their increasing populations, so that most are busy and some overworked. Although it takes a long time to elucidate an accurate clinical history, to carry out a careful, physical examination, and to give wise advice, it only takes a moment to write a prescription which often satisfies both patient and doctor that some positive action has been taken. Most excessive prescribing is 'placebo' prescribing for which there is a limited justification — the patient expects some treatment or the doctor wants to give his patient hope. When genuine placebos are prescribed they should be cheap, innocuous, and pharmacologically largely inactive. The old 'tonics' we used to prescribe fulfilled these criteria, but the modern psychotropic drugs do not. The latter have of course changed the whole atmosphere and length of stay in our mental hospitals, have done much to prevent anguish of mind and suicide, and have brought the merciful dispensation of sleep to many in need of it. Nevertheless, they are overprescribed: all the anxieties, frustrations, and disappointments in life do not necessarily demand drug treatment. A good doctor should be a placebo in himself.

Secondly, ignorant prescribing may often be due to inadequate instruction about drugs. In most medical schools pharmacology has traditionally been taught as a pre-clinical subject — a valuable scientific academic discipline, using drugs to illustrate physiological problems — an 'acetylcholine' type of pharmacology, so to speak; but it is impossible at this stage in an undergraduate's career to teach the therapeutic use of drugs: the student is not familiar with pathology, bacteriology, or patients. Fortunately, the relatively new discipline of clinical pharmacology has now been introduced into most medical schools and plays an important part in the undergraduate curriculum and in the continuing education of the postgraduate, instructing them in the therapeutic use of the powerful tools of their trade.

Thirdly, excessive prescribing may be encouraged by the insistent and skillful promotion of drugs by the pharmaceutical industry, some of which, in the past at any rate, has been subject to justifiable criticism. The pharmaceutical industry seems to possess most of the conventional commercial virtues: a high rate of investment; satisfactory labour relations; good quality control; an admirable record of supplying customers during epidemics or individual emergency; generous benefactions to charities and to medical, dental, veterinary, and agricultural research; and a brilliant record of commercial success which in 1975 contributed over £300 million to our export drive. It is therefore a little surprising that few other industries have been subjected to so much adverse

criticism, jealous political antagonism, or stringent bureaucratic controls. It must be confessed that in the creation of this atmosphere the industry itself has not been entirely blameless: in its period of most rapid development from the 1940s till the early 1960s it sometimes got carried away by its success and salesmanship occasionally took precedence over what was best for medicine. It would be idle to deny that commercialism sometimes dictated the marketing of a product before it had been completely investigated or that research workers in industry were occasionally subjected to commercial pressures. Of course, equally, academic research workers are sometimes carried away by their enthusiasms and the medical profession — or any other for that matter — have not always had their actions dictated by motives of pure altruism. In some future Utopia non-profit-making motivations may achieve the same brilliant results without side-effects. Till then we must take the world as we find it and remember that since the October Revolution the state-owned industries in the USSR and its satellites have hardly produced a single new product of real therapeutic importance.

In the old days medicines did not greatly influence the natural history of disease and it was not sufficiently stressed that an account of what drugs a patient had recently been taking should be an invariable and important part of any clinical history. Neglect of drug history taking often persists even in this chemotherapeutic era. Many adverse reactions to drugs exquisitely simulate the signs and symptoms of naturally occurring disorders. Thus complicated, often disagreeable, and expensive investigations are frequently undertaken when a few simple questions about the patient's recent consumption of drugs would have rendered these attempts to elucidate obscure symptoms unnecessary. Further, it is undesirable to anaesthetize or operate on a patient taking certain drugs — corticosteroids for example — without taking precautions; and the danger of giving unsuitable drugs to patients already being given, particularly, monoamine oxidase inhibitors, anticoagulants, or oral hypoglycaemic agents is considerable. When the taking of a drug history has become a routine part of a clinical history a significant advance will have been made in the prevention of adverse reactions to drugs.

Though science does not always lend itself to legislative or regulatory manipulation, modern drugs are such potent weapons that there is a general consensus that the sole responsibility for their production and use can no longer be left entirely to the manufacturer or prescriber. Yet it is difficult to know how far Government should attempt to control their production and prescription without undue interference with the advance of scientific therapeutics, the well-being of the pharmaceutical industry, and the cherished freedom of the doctor, dentist, or veterinary surgeon to prescribe as he thinks best. Inadequate regulation may prejudice public safety but excessive regulation can also be prejudicial in stultifying innovation and delaying the introduction of valuable remedies. The thoughtful legislator must direct his efforts between these two extremes and protect the public from inadequately tested and dangerous drugs, but at the same time permit an orderly progress of research, development, and marketing by the pharmaceutical industry. The operation of controls must be efficient, economical, and expeditious for otherwise the public are denied new and useful drugs. Finally, labelling, while excluding exaggerated and dangerous claims must be sufficiently elastic to permit the physician to exercise his judgement in the use of drugs. Very restrictive or directive types of labelling might result in a so-called learned profession being reduced to signing forms entitling their patients to receive such drugs for such purposes as the regulatory agencies permit.

One of the most urgent tasks confronting us today is to place adverse drug reactions on a sound epidemiological basis. No matter how meticulous the preparatory work of the pharmacologist and clinician may have been before a drug is marketed or how careful a licensing authority may have been in reviewing its protocols, nothing can replace experience of its use in practice over many years. Thus, the computerized collection, tabulation, and analysis of suspected adverse reactions on a national and ultimately on an international scale is of paramount importance and in recent years many countries, including Britain as a pioneer, have established monitoring systems of this nature. Their success depends on the co-operation of the medical profession in reporting suspected adverse reactions, especially to new drugs. It took many decades before the deleterious effects of aspirin on the alimentary canal became apparent and almost as long before it was recognised that the protracted abuse of phenacetin could produce renal papillary necrosis; 35 years elapsed before it became clear that amidopyrine could cause agranulocytosis; and several years before the association of phocomelia with thalidomide became obvious. Had a register of adverse reactions then existed these effects would have become apparent much earlier than was the case. The frequency of even major adverse reactions to drugs is not as yet really well known nor is their cause invariably well understood. A proper understanding of the dangers involved is the first step to their intelligent prevention. This book admirably supplies such an understanding.

Preface

In the first edition of this book, its objectives were described as follows 'In recent years a vast amount has been written about adverse reactions to drugs in a multitude of medical books and journals; yet, paradoxically, this surfeit of information has made it more difficult for clinicians to obtain unambiguous answers to their questions. They now require help to find their way through the jungle of toxicological fact and theory, and it seemed to us that there was a need for a 'map' arranged in the style of an orthodox textbook of medicine and written by doctors able to view the problems posed by adverse reactions in perspective against the background of their own experience.

'Our desire to be comprehensive has been tempered by our wish to produce a book of reasonable size, and we hope that out compromise will satisfy our readers. In a book with so many contributors it is not easy to ensure that each topic is given as much attention as it warrants but no more than it deserves. We have tried very hard to achieve such a balance, and where a section seems disproportionately long it will usually be found that it deals with matters of fundamental importance or with subjects that have been particularly well studied.'

All this remains true of this fifth edition, though some changes have again become necessary. Five new chapters have been added, to make the book more comprehensive. These are entitled 'Regulatory aspects of adverse drug reactions', 'Evaluating the effects of treatment', 'Obstetrical and gynaecological disorders, 'Masking effects of drugs', and 'Medico-legal aspects of adverse drug reactions'; and one chapter, present in the fourth edition — 'Systemic toxicity of topical antiseptics' — has been omitted because the topics discussed in it are now covered in other chapters. To extend the experience needed to edit this wide-ranging exposition on the ill-effects of drugs, Dr R.E. Ferner and Dr H. de Glanville have joined the Editor of earlier editions, to constitute an editorial team. In addition to these changes, all chapters present in the fourth edition have been revised and many have been completely rewritten, some by new authors.

We still believe that our approach — by clinical feature rather than by drug — matches the way the problem usually presents itself to the clinician, but those who wish to discover the full spectrum of adverse reactions to a particular drug or drug group will easily find this information in the Index.

The contributors again express their gratitude to the medical secretaries and librarians who helped them prepare their chapters, and the editors are indebted to Mr R.D.W. Davies, BA for preparing the Index.

May 1998   *D.M.D., R.E.F, H. de G.*

Contents

List of contributors

G. ANSELL, MD, FRCP, FRCR, DMRD, *formerly* Senior Consultant Radiologist, Whiston Hospital, and Lecturer in Radiodiagnosis, University of Liverpool.

C.H. ASHTON, DM, FRCP, Honorary Consultant Psychiatrist, Newcastle City Health Trust; Emeritus Professor of Clinical Psychopharmacology, University of Newcastle upon Tyne.

E-S.K. ASSEM, MB, ChB, Dip Med (Cairo), PhD, FRCP, FRCP Ed, FRCPath, DCH (Cairo), Honorary Consultant Physician (Allergy and Clinical Pharmacology), University College Hospitals Trust; Reader in Immunopharmacology, University College, University of London.

E.E. AZIZ, MB, BCh, MRCP, Senior Registrar in General Medicine and Clinical Pharmacology and Therapeutics, Wolfson Unit of Clinical Pharmacology, University of Newcastle upon Tyne.

D.N. BATEMAN, MSc, MD, FRCP, Consultant Physician, Freeman Hospital; Medical Director, Regional Drug and Therapeutics Centre, Regional Office of the Northern and Yorkshire NHS Executive; Reader in Therapeutics, University of Newcastle upon Tyne.

P.G. BLAIN, BMedSci, MB, BS, PhD, FRCP, C.Biol, FIBiol, MFOM, Honorary Consultant Physician, Newcastle City Health Trust; Professor of Environmental Health, University of Newcastle upon Tyne.

S.M. CALVERT, MB, ChB, MRCOG, Specialist Registrar in Obstetrics and Gynaecology, The General Infirmary at Leeds.

P.J. CAREY, MB, BS, FRCP, FRCPath, Consultant Haematologist, Sunderland Royal Hospital.

M.J.D. CASSIDY, MB, BS, FRCP, Consultant Nephrologist, Nottingham City Hospital.

J. CAVET, BA, MB, BS, MRCP, Specialist Registrar in Haematology, Royal Victoria Infirmary, Newcastle upon Tyne.

J.C.N. CHAN, MD, FRCP, FRCP Ed, FHKAM (Medicine), Associate Professor, Department of Medicine and Therapeutics, Chinese University of Hong Kong.

W.B. CHAN, MB, ChB, Medical Officer, Department of Medicine and Therapeutics, Chinese University of Hong Kong.

C.S. COCKRAM, BSc, MD, FRCP, FRCP Ed, FHKAM (Medicine), Professor of Medicine, Chinese University of Hong Kong.

C.J. DAVIES, MB, BS, FRCA, DRCOG, Senior Registrar in Anaesthesia, St Bartholomew's Hospital, London.

D.M. DAVIES, FRCP, FRCP Ed, Honorary Consultant Physician, Shotley Bridge General Hospital, Co Durham and Emeritus Consultant Physician, Newcastle Health Authority; Founder and Consulting Editor, *Adverse Drug Reaction Bulletin; formerly* Director, Northern Regional Clinical Pharmacology Unit, Newcastle upon Tyne; Professor of Clinical Pharmacology, Chinese University of Hong Kong; Member of the Subcommittee on Safety, Efficacy, and Adverse Reactions, Committee on Safety of Medicines.

M. DAVIS, MD, FRCP, Consultant Physician and Gastroenterologist, Royal United Hospital, Bath.

C. DIAMOND, MB, ChB, FRCS Glas, Emeritus Consultant Ear, Nose, and Throat Surgeon, Freeman Hospital; *formerly* Clinical Lecturer in Ear, Nose, and Throat Studies, University of Newcastle upon Tyne.

J.O. DRIFE, MD, FRCS Ed, FRCOG, Honorary Consultant Obstetrician and Gynaecologist, The General Infirmary at Leeds; Professor of Obstetrics and Gynaecology, University of Leeds.

J.F. DUNNE, BSc, MB, BS, PhD, *formerly* Director, Division of Drugs Management and Policies, World Health Organisation, Geneva.

R.E. FERNER, MSc, MD, FRCP, Consultant Physician, City Hospital, Birmingham; Director, West Midlands Centre for Adverse Drug Reaction Reporting; Editor, *Adverse Drug Reaction Bulletin*.

H. DE GLANVILLE, MB, BChir, DTM&H, DIH, Consulting Editor, *Medicine Digest*, and *The British Journal of Healthcare Computing and Information Management*; *formerly* Lecturer in Public Health, University of Dar-es-Salaam; Medical Director, African Medical and Research Foundation, Nairobi.

R.J. HARRISON, MB, BS, FRCOphth, DTM&H, Consultant Ophthalmologist, Queen's Hospital, Burton upon Trent.

G.H. JACKSON, MA, MD, MRCP, MRCPath, Consultant Haematologist, Royal Victoria Infirmary, Newcastle upon Tyne.

N.P. KEANEY, BSc, MB, BCh, PhD, FRCP, Consultant Physician in General and Respiratory Medicine and Clinical Pharmacology, and Head of Medical Education and Research, Sunderland Royal Hospital and City Hospitals, Sunderland.

M.T. KEARNEY, DM, MRCP, Specialist Registrar in Cardiology, Yorkshire Heart Centre, The General Infirmary at Leeds.

R.J.M. LANE, BSc, MD, FRCP, Consultant Neurologist, West London Neurosciences Centre, Charing Cross Hospital.

D.H. LAWSON, CBE, MD, FRCP Ed, FRCP Glas, FFPM, Vice-President, Royal College of Physicians of Edinburgh; Consultant Physician, Glasgow Royal Infirmary; Visiting Professor of Clinical Pharmacology, University of Strathclyde; Chairman of the Medicines Commission; *formerly* Chairman, Committee on Review of Medicines.

J.S. MALPAS, MB, BS, DPhil, FRCP, FRCR, FRCPCH, FFPM, Emeritus Professor of Oncology, St Bartholomew's Hospital, University of London.

M.L'E. ORME, MA, MD, FRCP, Honorary Consultant Physician, The Royal Liverpool Hospitals Trust; Professor of Clinical Pharmacology, University of Liverpool; Director of Education and Training, North West Regional Office of the NHS Executive.

M. PIRMOHAMED, MB, ChB (Hons), PhD, MRCP, Honorary Consultant Physician, The Royal Liverpool Hospitals Trust; Senior Lecturer in Clinical Pharmacology, University of Liverpool.

S.J. PROCTOR, MB, BS, FRCP, FRCPath, Honorary Consultant Haematologist, Royal Victoria Infirmary; Professor of Haematological Medicine, University of Newcastle upon Tyne.

M.D. RAWLINS, BSc, MD, FRCP, FRCP Ed, FFPM, Honorary Consultant Clinical Pharmacologist, Royal Victoria Infirmary and Freeman Hospital; Professor of Clinical Pharmacology, University of Newcastle upon Tyne; Chairman, Committee on Safety of Medicines.

D.F. ROBERTS, ScD, Emeritus Professor of Human Genetics, University of Newcastle upon Tyne.

P.A. ROUTLEDGE, MD, FRCP, Honorary Consultant Physician, and Medical Director, Welsh Adverse Drug Reactions Scheme and the Therapeutics and Toxicology Centre, Llandough Hospital, Penarth; Professor of Clinical Pharmacology, University of Wales College of Medicine; Member of the External Advisory Board, Committee on Safety of Medicines.

R.A. SEYMOUR, BDS, PhD, FDSRCS, Honorary Consultant in Restorative Dentistry, Royal Victoria Infirmary; Professor of Restorative Dentistry, University of Newcastle upon Tyne.

H.G.M. SHETTY, BSc, MB, BS, FRCP, Consultant Physician, University Hospital of Wales.

A.G. SMITH, MD, FRCP, Consultant Dermatologist, City General Hospital, Stoke-on-Trent.

W.Y. SO, MB, ChB, MRCP, Medical Officer, Department of Medicine and Therapeutics, Chinese University of Hong Kong.

R. SWAMINATHAN, MSc, MB, BS, FRCPath, FRCPA, Honorary Consultant Chemical Pathologist, St Thomas's Hospital; Professor of Chemical Pathology, Guy's and St Thomas's Medical and Dental School, University of London.

C.R. SWANEPOEL, MB, ChB, FRCP Ed, Senior Specialist, Department of Medicine, Groote Schuur Hospital and University of Capetown.

L-B. TAN, BSc, MB, BChir, DPhil, FRCP, FESC, Honorary Consultant Cardiologist, Yorkshire Heart Centre, The General Infirmary at Leeds; Senior Lecturer in Cardiology, University of Leeds.

S.H.L. THOMAS, MD, MRCP, Consultant Physician, Freeman Hospital; Senior Lecturer in Clinical Pharmacology, University of Newcastle upon Tyne.

P.C. WALLER, B.Med.Sci, MD, MPH, FRCP Ed, FFPM, Head of Pharmacovigilance Assessment Group, Post-Licensing Division, Medicines Control Agency, London.

A.C. WOOD, MB BS, MRCP, Senior Registrar in Haematology, Sunderland Royal Hospital.

S.M. WOOD, BSc, MD, FFPM, Director, Post-Licensing Division, Medicines Control Agency, London.

K.W. WOODHOUSE, MD, FRCP, Honorary Consultant Geriatrician, Llandough Hospital, Penarth; Vice-Dean of Medicine and Professor of Geriatric Medicine, University of Wales College of Medicine.

D.J. WRIGHT, MB, ChB, MRCP, Research Registrar in Cardiology, Yorkshire Heart Centre, The General Infirmary at Leeds.

V.T.F. YEUNG, MD, FRCP, FRCP Ed, FHKAM (Medicine), Associate Professor, Department of Medicine and Therapeutics, Chinese University of Hong Kong.

A.H. YOUNG, MB, ChB, PhD, MPhil, MRCPsych, Honorary Consultant Psychiatrist, Newcastle City Health Trust; Senior Lecturer in Neuroscience and Psychiatry, University of Newcastle upon Tyne.

Index compiled by R.D.W. DAVIES, BA.

1. History

Adverse reactions to drugs are as old as Medicine. Some of the earliest writings bear witness to the potential dangers of contemporary medical treatment and the punishments prescribed for incompetent practitioners. The Babylonian *Code of Hammurabi*, of 2200 BC, ordained that a physician who caused a patient's death should lose his hands, and the *Hermetic Books of Thoth* outlined therapeutic paths from which the physician strayed only at his peril.

In the course of medical history many laymen and doctors were to advise caution in therapeutics and to criticize the materia medica and those who used it. Among the first was Homer (*c*. 950 BC), who said of drugs that there were 'many excellent when mingled, and many fatal' (*Odyssey*, IV). Hippocrates (460–370 BC) pleaded 'Do not harm'; Galen (131–201) warned against the dangers of badly written and obscure prescriptions; and Rhazes (860–932) advised 'if simple remedies are effective do not prescribe compound remedies'.

Most of the drugs then in use were of plant or animal origin, but mercury, arsenic, and antimony were also used. The toxic effects of arsenic were well recognized from its deliberate use as a poison, and the dangers of mercurial inunction were also familiar, but toxic properties of antimony attracted less attention.

As time passed, the questionable purity of remedies began to exercise the minds of both civil and professional authorities. In the ninth century, Arabian authorities appointed an official, the *mutasib*, a guardian of public morals whose duties were later to embrace the supervision of the makers of drugs and syrups to ensure the purity of their wares: 'it is necessary that the *mutasib* make them fearful, try them, and warn them against imprisonment. He must caution them with punishment. Their syrups and drugs may be inspected at any time without warning after their shops are closed for the night' (Levey 1963). In the tenth century the school of Salerno, in Italy, was empowered to inspect drugs for adulteration, with dire penalties for transgressors:

'whosoever shall have or sell any poison or noxious drug not useful or necessary to his art, let him be hanged' (Withington 1894).

In 1224 the Hohenstaufen Emperor, Frederick II, ordered the regular inspection of the drugs and mixtures prepared by apothecaries, and pronounced that the life of a purveyor of a poison, a magic elixir, or a love potion would be forfeit if a consumer died; and in the same century the Oath for apothecaries in Basle, Switzerland, included an undertaking to provide for physicians drugs 'of such good quality and of such usefulness that he knows, upon his oath, that it will be good and useful for the confection which the physician is making' (Mez-Mangold 1971). For many years after the foundation of the Royal College of Physicians, in 1518, its Fellows concerned themselves with the quality control of drugs; and the authors of the first *London Pharmacopoeia* (1618) spoke harshly in their preface of 'the very noxious fraud and deceit of those people who are allowed to sell the most filthy concoctions . . . under the name and title of medicaments. . .'. Ironically, they themselves were content to include worms, dried vipers, and fox lung in their catalogue of acceptable remedies. In 1599 a charter granted by James VI of Scotland to what was to become the Royal College of Physicians and Surgeons of Glasgow made provisions for the supervision of the sales of drugs and poisons (Mann 1989).

In the seventeenth century, for the first time, a named drug was proscribed because of its toxicity: members of the Paris Faculty of Physicians were forbidden to use antimony. But the ban could not be maintained after the drug was credited with the cure of an attack of typhoid suffered by Louis XIV in 1657.

Not until 1745, when Sir William Heberden published his *Antitheriaca, Essay on Mithridatium and Theriaca*, was the value of compound remedies and animal extracts seriously questioned. Even so, physicians were very slow in improving their standards of treatment and they long continued to deserve Voltaire's stricture that they 'poured drugs of which they knew little into bodies of which they knew less'.

Perhaps the most elegant and definitive of descriptions of an adverse drug reaction was William Withering's account of digitalis toxicity in 1785: 'The Foxglove, when given in very large and quickly repeated doses, occasions sickness, vomiting, purging, giddiness, confused vision, objects appearing green or yellow, increased secretion of urine with frequent motions to part with it, and sometimes inability to retain it; slow pulse, even as low as 35 in a minute, cold sweats, convulsions, syncope and death'.

At about this time, epidemics of yellow fever in some American states brought to mercury both fame and notoriety. Believing that in this disease 'the gastrointestinal tract was filled with putrid and fermenting biliary substances' and that their expulsion was the key to cure, some physicians advocated large doses of calomel (mercurous chloride) often mixed with other purgatives (Risse 1973). Many patients were apparently unharmed by this heroic therapy, possibly because the vomiting caused by the infection drastically reduced the systemic absorption of the mercury. Others were less fortunate and developed clinical mercurialism with intense salivation; loosening of the teeth; and ulceration, even gangrene, of the mouth and cheeks; and osteomyelitis of the mandible (Risse 1973). Nevertheless, by the next century calomel had become a 'cure-all' in febrile illness, the 'Sampson of the Materia Medica'. But if most doctors had come to view the drug through rose-coloured spectacles, some laymen regarded it (and its prescribers) in a different light:

> Since calomel's become their boast,
> How many patients have they lost,
> How many thousands they make ill,
> Of poison with their calomel.

Some physicians now added their protests. One wrote of 'Calomel considered as a poison' (Mitchell 1844–5), and another, with calomel in mind, commented: 'if the whole materia medica, as it is now used, could be sunk to the bottom of the sea, it would be all the better for mankind — and all the worse for the fishes' (Holmes 1861). Despite such broadsides, calomel remained in favour among physicians for years to come and is believed to have paved the way for such unorthodox (but, at the time, gentler) systems of healing such as homoeopathy, osteopathy, chiropractic, Thompsonianism, and Grahamism.

The nineteenth century saw the appearance in several countries of important new pharmacopœias that for the first time laid down standards of drug purity. In 1848, the first statute was passed to control the quality of drugs in America after quinine imported for the Army was found to have been adulterated.

In the closing years of the nineteenth century and the early years of the twentieth came other innovations. There were formal enquiries into suspected adverse reactions to drugs, the first concerned with sudden deaths during chloroform anæsthesia (McKendrick *et al.* 1880) and the second with jaundice following arsenical treatment of syphilis (Medical Research Council 1922). Then the American Medical Association established the Council on Pharmacy and Chemistry and its publication *New and Nonofficial Remedies*, 'a mighty service for American medicine' (Leake 1929). Next, the American Food, Drug and Insecticide Administration (later the Food and Drug Administration) was established. But much remained to be done. In 1929 Leake drew attention to the inadequacy of existing testing procedures for new drugs: 'many drug firms make the mistake of believing that their chemists can furnish trustworthy pharmacologic opinion. Indeed some eminent chemists impatient with careful pharmacologic technic have ventured to estimate for themselves the clinical possibilities of their own synthetics . . . There is no short cut from the chemical laboratory to the clinic except one that passes too close to the morgue.' His words were prophetic: 107 people died in 1937 as a result of poisoning by an elixir of sulphanilamide containing as a solvent diethylene glycol (Geiling and Cannon 1938). The manufacturers had not troubled to enquire whether the solvent was safe for its purpose; yet the toxic effects of diethylene glycol and closely related compounds were already documented (von Oettingen and Jirouch 1931; Barber 1934). In the wake of the disaster came a Federal Act that forbade the marketing of new drugs until they had been cleared for safety by the Food and Drug Administration.

A major catastrophe of this kind focused attention on the problem of drug toxicity, but awareness and concern were only transient. The profession's threshold of stimulation remained too high and its latent period before reaction too long. It had taken some 47 years to discover that amidopyrine was a potent marrow poison (Wade 1970). Fifteen years had passed before it was appreciated that cinchophen caused jaundice (Worster-Drought 1923) and 11 years more before this fact gained recognition (Wade 1970). Aspirin had been in use for 39 years before it was incriminated as a cause of gastric haemorrhage (Douthwaite 1938) and for another 20 before the news spread adequately (Alvarez and Summerskill 1958). The dangers of chloramphenicol were first appreciated in the early 1950s, yet almost two decades later the Chairman of a US Senate Subcommittee had good cause to complain that warnings of these dangers had gone unheeded (*Journal of the American Medical Association* 1968).

In the 1940s the increasing use of the then relatively new drugs — the sulphonamides, penicillin, and streptomycin — led to a rise in the incidence of a type of indirect, or secondary, adverse drug reaction probably familiar in earlier years only as a complication of the use of morphine or other powerful narcotics in patients with abdominal emergencies or head injuries. This reaction was later labelled 'drug masking' and defined as 'the temporary, more or less complete, suppression of clinical and laboratory signs and symptoms without actual eradication of the basic disease' (Lundsgaard-Hansen 1972). Such reactions were to become commoner when pharmaceutical preparations of corticotrophin and adrenal corticosteroids became available during the following decade. (This subject is discussed more fully in Chapter 32.) In the same period, as the number of powerful new drugs provided by the burgeoning pharmaceutical industry grew apace, another kind of adverse reaction — the interaction of drugs within the body — began to be recognized.

Next, the appearance of a variety of infusion fluids, the use of which was to increase progressively in later years, brought about a resurgence of a third kind of hazard — the *in vitro* drug interaction. This phenomenon had been well known earlier in medical history when the practice of putting many substances into a single medicament (polypharmacy) was commonplace and could result in chemical reactions between constituents which sometimes made the mixture unpalatable, ineffective, or even toxic. Indeed, in the nineteenth and early twentieth centuries instruction on 'incompatibilities' was to be found in contemporary textbooks of pharmacology and therapeutics, such as *Lectures on the Action of Medicines* by Brunton (1897). But polypharmacy of this kind gradually fell into disuse, only to reappear when doctors began to take the convenient but erroneous view that when a formulation of a drug was suitable for intravenous use it could safely be added to an infusion solution; and not infrequently a veritable potpourri of medicaments, one or more possibly incompatible with others or with the infusion fluid, was dripped into a patient's vein, sometimes with serious or even fatal consequences.

Despite the major drug disasters and the great increase in number and variety of other adverse drug reactions during the third and fourth decades of the century, until the 1950s textbooks of medicine devoted comparatively little space to adverse drug reactions, and that only to the ill-effects of one or two drugs. Few medical teachers had much to say on the subject. Epidemiological studies of adverse drug reactions were almost unknown.

Then the climate began to change. In 1952 appeared the first book to concern itself entirely with adverse drug reactions (Meyler 1952). In the same year the Council on Pharmacy and Chemistry of the American Medical Association set up an organization to monitor drug-induced blood dyscrasias. A little while later, the first report of epidemiological studies of adverse drug reactions was published; and in 1960 the Food and Drug Administration began to collect reports of adverse reactions and sponsored new hospital drug-monitoring programmes.

In the winter of 1961 came news of the thalidomide disaster — a sudden upsurge in the number of babies born with the deformities of phocomelia or micromelia. Thalidomide had been prescribed as a 'safe' hypnotic. It had not been tested in animals for teratogenicity, but thousands of babies born to mothers who had taken the drug during pregnancy provided the missing data.

As a result of this horrifying epidemic, many countries established agencies concerned with drug safety such as our own Committee on Safety of Drugs; and later the World Health Organization set up an international bureau to collect and collate information from national drug-monitoring organizations. Such agencies have done much to identify and prevent illness caused by drugs; but they provide no absolute guarantee against outbreaks of novel and quite unpredictable reactions such as those produced by practolol.

Periodicals dealing solely with adverse reactions to drugs, such as *Clin-Alert* in 1962, the *Adverse Drug Reaction Bulletin* in 1966, now began to appear.

In the mid-1960s a somewhat different aspect of drug therapy came under repeated scrutiny. In Britain this had been prompted by the report of the Aitken Committee (1958), set up to examine systems of prescribing, administration, and storage of drugs in hospitals. The Committee concluded that all was not well, and made recommendations for improving matters; and later many physicians, pharmacists, and nurses in several countries made detailed studies of the diverse and complex problems of hospital prescribing and devised new procedures intended to solve them. These various studies and recommendations were reviewed in detail by Haslam (1987). But making recommendations and rules is one thing, getting them accepted and obeyed is another; and years later drug prescribing and administration in hospitals remained far from perfect (Haslam 1988; Davies 1988; Bonati *et al.* 1990). There is ample evidence that errors in drug prescribing, administration, and recording continue to put patients at risk of illness or even death

(Omon *et al.* 1991; LeBelle 1993; Views and Reviews 1996; Television news 1997).

In Great Britain the Medicines Act of 1968 provided new and comprehensive safeguards covering most aspects of drug development, production, and use. The beneficial effects of these measures on drug safety have been supplemented by the wealth of information on rational therapeutics and drug toxicity provided by general and specialized medical journals and books, by the formation of drug and therapeutics committees in many hospitals in this country (George and Hands 1983) and elsewhere, and by teachers of clinical pharmacology and toxicology.

More recently the relatively new (at least in the United Kingdom) schemes for 'medical audit' hold promise of improvements in medical care, both in hospitals (McKee *et al.* 1989; Royal College of Physicians 1989) and general practice (Royal College of General Practitioners 1985; Wilmot 1990); and it is to be hoped that audit protocols will strongly emphasize the importance of the detailed and accurate writing of prescriptions and of records of drug administration.

It is apparent from what has been said here that governments, medical colleges and faculties, editors, research workers, and teachers have done a great deal to improve drug safety. It remains for prescribing doctors, patients, and the pharmaceutical industry to match their efforts. Experienced clinicians with open eyes and an interest in therapeutics know that many powerful and potentially dangerous drugs are used with insufficient thought and caution (Pensabeni-Jasper and Panush 1996) and continue to be given when they might be withdrawn without detriment and, indeed, with benefit to the patient's condition. They would point out that many illnesses are short-lasting and do not require the drug that is often given; that simple and innocuous remedies can provide greater and quicker relief than the more complex remedies usually employed; that the safest drug is not always used when there is a choice; that where one drug would have sufficed, more have often been given (Fincham and Nissenbaum 1991); and that a doctor has sometimes prescribed a drug without knowing what other drugs the patient is taking, or used a mixture not knowing precisely what it contained and the pharmacological actions of its ingredients.

There can be little doubt that much modern medicinal treatment is unnecessary, and the blame for this state of affairs must be shared between doctors, patients, and the pharmaceutical industry. Doctors are probably 'unduly concerned with satisfying the public's "wants" rather than what we think are its "needs"' (Dunlop 1970), and are oversusceptible to the blandishments and misplaced 'generosity' of drug salesmen (*Drug, Disease, Doctor* 1989a). Patients have come to believe that the mildest of symptoms, even the ordinary trials and tribulations of everyday life, must be matched by a drug. The pharmaceutical industry still has grave shortcomings as far as its promotional activities are concerned. These are most blatant in third-world countries with less well-developed or poorly enforced legislation controlling promotion, supply, and use of drugs (Medawar 1989; *Drug, Disease, Doctor* 1989a,b, 1990; Lee 1990; Sarkar 1997), but devious promotional methods are still encountered in countries with stringent drug regulation, such as Britain (*Drug and Therapeutics Bulletin* 1990). Rarely, a pharmaceutical company has concealed from government drug regulatory agencies information about adverse reactions to one of its products (Schonhofer 1991).

We have made considerable progress towards the goal of making drug therapy as safe as is possible, but sadly from time to time we have been reminded by further reports of epidemics of adverse drug reactions of the need for constant vigilance.

In 1954 there were 100 deaths in France from poisoning by Stalinon, an organic compound of tin used in the treatment of boils (Wade 1970). From 1955 onwards interaction of monoamine oxidase inhibitors with some other drugs or with certain foods caused considerable morbidity and several deaths. In the 1960s the contraceptive pill was firmly identified as the cause of a surprising increase in the incidence of thromboembolism in young women. In the 1970s a previously unknown syndrome involving the skin, eyes, and other parts and affecting many patients was found to be due to treatment with the β-adrenoceptor blocking agent practolol. In 1972 an error in pharmaceutical manufacture was to blame for the deaths of 20 French infants from brain damage induced by a dusting powder containing 6% hexachlorophane, a concentration much higher than that intended. Since 1990 a large number of people have suffered serious or fatal illness after taking certain formulations of L-tryptophan. Between 1991 and 1997 in Argentina, Bangladesh, Haiti, India, and Nigeria, many children died from poisoning by medicines containing diethylene glycol as a solvent, replays of the sulphanilamide disaster of 1937 (see above). And there have been disturbing reports of substandard or even bogus drugs being produced in countries in which control of local pharmaceutical manufacture is inadequate or nonexistent (Dunne 1997).

It is unlikely that *complete* safety will ever be attained: we shall only approach that goal when the providers, prescribers, and recipients of therapeutic drugs begin at last to take drug treatment *seriously*.

References

Aitken, J.K. (1958). *Report of the Joint Subcommittee on the Control of Dangerous Drugs and Poisons in Hospitals.* HMSO, London.

Alvarez, A.S. and Summerskill, W.H.J. (1958). Gastrointestinal haemorrhage and salicylates. *Lancet* ii, 920.

Barber, H. (1934). Haemorrhagic nephritis and necrosis of the liver from dioxane poisoning. *Guy's Hosp. Rep.* 84, 267.

Bonati, M., Marchetti, F., Zullini, M.T., *et al.* (1990). Adverse drug reactions in neonatal intensive care units. *Adverse Drug React. Acute Poisoning Rev.* 9, 107.

Brunton, T.L.(1897). *The Action of Medicines*, p. 289. Macmillan, London.

Davies, D.M. (1988). Data provided for the review of Haslam, R. (1988). Drug safety and medication systems in hospitals. *Adverse Drug React. Acute Poisoning Rev.* 3, 133.

Douthwaite, A.H. (1938). Some recent advances in medical diagnosis and treatment. *BMJ* i, 1143.

Drug and Therapeutics Bulletin (1990). Product licences and devious promotion. *Drug Ther. Bull.* 28, 20.

Drug, Disease, Doctor (1989*a*). On physicians' samples and gifts. *Drug, Disease, Doctor* 2, 73.

Drug, Disease, Doctor (1989*b*). Quackery — the ubiquitous game. *Drug, Disease, Doctor* 2, 25.

Drug, Disease, Doctor (1990). Right to information — of doctors? *Drug, Disease, Doctor* 3, 1.

Dunlop, Sir D. (1970). The use and abuse of psychotropic drugs. *Proc. R. Soc. Med.* 63, 1279.

Dunne, J. (1997). Deadly medicines: the cost of substandard drugs. *Medicine Digest* 23 (1), 5.

Fincham, J.E. and Nissenbaum, R.S. (1991). Polypharmacy: a real life example. *J. Pharmacoepidemiology* 2, 79.

Geiling, E.M.K. and Cannon, P.R. (1938). Pathogenic effects of elixir of sulfanilamide (diethylene glycol) poisoning. *JAMA* iii, 919.

George, C.F. and Hands, D.E. (1983). Drug and therapeutics committees and information pharmacy services: the United Kingdom. *World Development* ii, 229.

Haslam, R. (1987). Thesis for the degree of Master of Science, University of Newcastle upon Tyne.

Haslam, R. (1988). Drug safety and medication systems in hospitals. *Adverse Drug React. Acute Poisoning Rev.* 3, 133.

Holmes, O.W. (1861). *Currents and Countercurrents in Medical Science, with other Addresses and Essays*, p. 167. Boston.

Journal of the American Medical Association (1968). Medical News — a report of a U.S. Senate investigation. *JAMA* 203, 54.

Leake, C.D. (1929). The pharmacologic evaluation of new drugs. *JAMA* 93, 1632.

LeBelle, M.J. (1993). Drug names and medication errors — who is responsible? *Canad. Med. Assoc. J.* 149, 941.

Lee, D. (1990). Continued marketing of a useless drug ('Varidase') in Panama. *Lancet* 335, 667.

Levey, M. (1963). Fourteenth century medicine and the Hisba. *Medical History* 7, 176.

Lundsgaard-Hansen, P. (1972) Masking effect of drugs. In *Drug-induced Disease*, Vol. 4 (ed. L. Meyler and H.M. Peck), p. 208. Associated Scientific Publishers, Amsterdam.

McKee, C.M., Lauglo, M., and Lessof, L. (1989). Medical audit: a review. *J. R. Soc. Med.* 82, 474.

McKendrick, J.G., Coats, J., and Newman, D. (1880). Report of the action of anaesthetics. *BMJ* ii 957.

Mann, R.D. (1989). The historical development of medicines regulations. In *International Medicines Regulations* (ed. S.R. Walker and J.P. Griffin), p. 5. Kluwer, London.

Medawar, C. (1989). On our side of the fence. In *Side Effects of Drugs, Annual 13*, p. xix. Elsevier, Amsterdam.

Medical Research Council (1922). Toxic effects following the employment of arsenobenzol preparations. *Special Report Series*, No. 66.

Meyler, L. (1952). *Side Effects of Drugs*. Elsevier, Amsterdam.

Mez-Mangold, L. (1971). *A History of Drugs*, p. 83. F. Hoffmann-La Roche and Co., Basle.

Mitchell, T.D. (1844–5). Calomel considered as a poison. *N. Orleans Med. Surg J.* i, 28.

Omon, D.M., Potyk, R.P., and Koenke, K. (1991). The adverse effect of hospitalization on drug regimens. *Arch. Int. Med.* 151, 1562.

Pensabeni-Jasper, T. and Panush, R.S. (1996). Corticosteroid usage: observations at a community hospital. *Am. J. Med. Sci.* 311, 234.

Risse, G.B. (1973). Calomel and the American Medical Sects during the nineteenth century. *Mayo Clinic Proc.* 48, 57.

Royal College of General Practitioners (1985). *What Sort of Doctor? Report from General Practice 23*. Royal College of General Practitioners, London.

Royal College of Physicians (1989). *Medical Audit — a first Report: What, Why, and How?* Royal College of Physicians of London.

Sarkar, P.K. (1997). What price a glass of water? *Bull. Drug and Health Information* 3, 177.

Schonhofer, P.S. (1991). The nomifensine affair. *Lancet* 338, 1448.

Television news. A child was given 100 times the correct dose of morphine. 'Look North', 27.1.97.

Views and Reviews. (1996). Medication errors — nurses' perspective. *Reactions* 621, 2.

von Oettingen, W.F. and Jirouch E.A. (1931). Pharmacology of ethylene glycol and some of its derivatives. *J. Pharmacol Exp. Ther.* 42, 355.

Wade, O.L. (1970). *Adverse Reactions to Drugs*. Heinemann, London.

Wilmot, J. (1990). Review of medical audit. *J. R. Soc. Med.* 83, 58.

Withering, W. (1785). *An Account of the Foxglove and some of its Medicinal Uses; with Practical Remarks on Dropsy and other Diseases*. Robinson, London.

Withington, E.T. (1894). *Medical History from Earliest Times*, (reprint 1964). The Holland Press, London, *via* Penn, R.G. The state control of medicines: the first 3000 years. *Br. J. Pharmacol.* 8, 293.

Worster-Drought, C. (1923). Atophan poisoning. *BMJ* i. 148.

2. Epidemiology

D. H. LAWSON

Definition

Epidemiology is the study of the distribution and determinants of health-related events in populations and the application of this study to the control of health problems (Last 1983).

Epidemiological studies tend to be grouped into three major categories: (1) the descriptive type, which investigates the occurrence of a specific disease entity within subgroups of the population, paying particular regard to basic characteristics such as age, sex, race, occupation, geographic location, and social class; (2) the analytical type, which usually involves a hypothesis-testing approach to investigating possible associations between disease and a variety of possible causative factors; such studies are usually observational and may involve the techniques of cohort follow-up or case–control analysis; (3) the experimental type of epidemiological study which is usually hypothesis-testing and uses techniques such as randomized controlled clinical trials.

Possible adverse drug reactions have been studied using all three epidemiological strategies. These studies are, however, not easy to conduct, since the definition of an 'adverse drug reaction' is complicated by the fact that the external manifestations of such reactions are not unique. Both humans and animals have a limited number of ways in which they can react to noxious stimuli. Even as clear-cut an event as phocomelia occurring in the offspring of mothers exposed to thalidomide in the early stages of pregnancy is not invariably drug induced. Indeed, there is a magnificent painting by Goya on display in the Prado museum in Madrid that portrays a child suffering from phocomelia — an occurrence which had clearly taken place long before the development of thalidomide.

All major adverse reactions for which drugs have been withdrawn in the recent past — for example, aplastic anaemia (chloramphenicol), Guillain–Barré syndrome (zimeldine), endometrial cancer (unopposed oestrogen replacement therapy), lactic acidosis (phenformin), and acute haemolytic anaemia (nomifensine) — occur naturally in the absence of exposure to drugs. It follows that unless there is a dramatic increase in the observed incidence of such events, as was the case with thalidomide and phocomelia, formal studies are required in order to clarify the drug–disease relationship. While this is true of major events such as have been described, it is also true of minor events such as fatigue, inability to concentrate, nasal congestion, pains in muscles, headaches, skin rash, bizarre dreams, dry mouth, pain in joints, etc, all of which occur naturally in the population. They have been reported, for example, to a varying extent among a sample of 670 healthy university students and hospital staff taking no medications at the time. The observers concluded that the experience with this group indicated the clear need for proper controls in all studies of potential adverse drug reactions (Reidenberg and Lowenthal 1968).

For the practising physician, these observations lead to the conclusion that, while it is easy to decide that a patient has experienced an adverse event, it is not easy to determine the causative noxious stimulant. Similar problems were encountered in the context of the developing understanding of the bacterial aetiology of disease. They were solved by the application of Koch's postulates which should be met before a causative relationship can be accepted between a particular bacterial parasite or disease agent and a disease in question. These are:

1. the agent must be shown to be present in every case of the disease, by isolation in pure culture;
2. the agent must not be found in cases of other diseases;
3. once isolated, the agent must be capable of reproducing the disease in experimental animals;
4. the agent must be recoverable from the experimental disease produced.

Later, Evans (1976) expanded the Koch postulates and applied them more generally to the aetiology of disease. The so-called Evans's postulates are:

1. the prevalence of disease should be significantly higher in those exposed to the hypothesized cause than in controls not so exposed;
2. exposure to the suspected cause should be more frequent amongst those with the disease than in controls without the disease, when all other risk factors are held constant;
3. the incidence of the disease should be significantly higher in those exposed to the purported cause than in those not so exposed, as shown by prospective studies;
3. the disease should follow exposure to the hypothesized causative agent with a distribution of incubation periods in a bell-shaped curve;
5. the spectrum of host responses should follow exposure to the hypothesized agent along a logical biological gradient from mild to severe;
6. a measurable host response following exposure to the hypothesized cause should have a high probability of appearing in those lacking it before exposure, or should increase in magnitude if present before exposure. This response pattern should be infrequent in unexposed persons;
7. experimental reproduction of the disease should occur more frequently in animals or man appropriately exposed to the hypothesized cause than in those not so exposed. This exposure may be deliberate in volunteers, experimentally induced in the laboratory, or may represent a regulation of natural exposure;
8. elimination or modification of the hypothesized cause should decrease the incidence of the disease;
9. prevention or modification of the host response on exposure to the hypothesized cause should decrease or eliminate the disease;
10. all the relationships and findings should make biological and epidemiologic sense.

Clearly, neither Koch's postulates nor the updated Evans's postulates are fulfilled for most hypotheses about drug-related disease. Indeed, in many reports of suspected adverse reactions we know little about pre-exposure status and the stability of this status with time. We often have scant information, poorly described, about the timing and dose of the hypothesized causative agent. The event that was thought to be drug related is often incompletely described. Finally, and understandably, it is very rare for there to be a rechallenge or re-exposure study.

Appreciation of the limitations of these postulates in the everyday world of suspected adverse drug reactions led to a move to develop structures for obtaining reproducible operational identification of adverse drug reactions (Karch and Lasagna 1977; Kramer *et al.* 1979; Hutchinson *et al.* 1979) together with studies to determine the reproducibility of judgements of trained ob-

servers (Blanc *et al.* 1979). Such approaches proved cumbersome in use and have not been widely adopted. Thus the literature on adverse drug reactions is a relatively murky area of substantial subjectivity, where the truth is often difficult to elucidate and supporting data are at best approximations. Because of the evanescent nature of much drug therapy, this difficulty is to be expected, but it must be kept in mind when reviewing individual studies.

Classification of reactions

The Rawlins and Thompson classification of adverse drug reactions into predictable pharmacological reactions (Type A) and unpredictable idiosyncratic reactions (Type B) is now generally accepted to be a helpful way of looking at this problem (Rawlins and Thompson 1977 and see Chapter 5, and is used in this book. Unfortunately, most collected information on adverse reactions ignores this classification or does not provide the necessary detail to allow its derivation. An assumption frequently made by academic pharmacologists is that the pharmacological type of reaction is primarily attributable to inappropriate prescribing and hence intrinsically less 'interesting' or relevant than the idiosyncratic type of reaction, which presents a much greater intellectual challenge. None the less, it is clear from several major studies that pharmacological reactions, whether or not due to inappropriate prescribing, constitute the bulk of adverse drug reactions experienced by the population.

Studies based in medical wards all indicate that unwanted pharmacological actions of drugs are the most common cause of suspected adverse reactions, accounting for approximately 80 per cent of notified drug-related events (Ogilvie and Ruedy 1967; Hurwitz and Wade 1969). The remaining events are most likely to be idiosyncratic or allergic in nature. Hurwitz and Wade (1969) separated pharmacological reactions into those in which an unwanted secondary pharmacological action was the cause of the undesired effect (60 per cent) and those where an excessive effect of the principal pharmacological action was the cause (25 per cent), while the remaining 15 per cent of results were non-pharmacological in nature.

Descriptive studies

Drug use

In a 1979 WHO European Monograph on studies of drug utilization Graham Dukes (1979) began by stating that 'one of the most puzzling features of the world of medicines at the present day is the astonishing and, in some respects, disastrous lack of information about the way in which drugs are used and misused. In most major countries of the world it is still impossible to find out how many medicines are on sale, much less what the turnover of these products might be. Where this basic information is to be found, one is left wondering which physicians are using these products for which patients and why.' Almost 20 years on, similar sentiments are still justified, although the widespead availability of computers in generl practice has improved the situation to some extent. Individual studies have reported wide disparities in drug use between countries and within individual countries, for example, studies on the use of oral anti-diabetic agents saw 10- to 20-fold differences between individual European countries (Bergman 1979; Dukes 1979). Similar studies on variations of psychotropic drug use in Nordic countries have appeared from time to time. Lawson and Jick (1976), in an interesting 'fall-out' from the Boston Collaborative Drug Surveillance Program (BCDSP) medical inpatient studies, reported that the use of drugs in hospitalized patients in the United States was twice that in a matched comparison group in Scotland. The reasons for such differences are not clear, but relate more to physician behaviour than patient need. Perhaps a more striking example of this is the major disparity in the use of intravenous fluids between two hospitals with otherwise virtually identical drug use reported from Glasgow (Lawson 1977).

In a recent multinational post-marketing surveillance study of the angiotensin-converting enzyme inhibitor, ramipril, Lawson and his colleagues (1995) reported widespread differences between countries in co-prescribing habits even in a seemingly coherent cohort of moderate hypertensive subjects. Such differences lead to potential problems in interpreting transnational information derived from spontaneous reporting schemes.

With increasing economic constraints on drug prescribing, health care providers are likely to require much more information on drug-use patterns than heretofore — a development that is to be given every encouragement, being greatly overdue.

Reactions during hospital admission

Reported incidence of adverse drug reactions varies widely, being between 10 and 20 per cent (Seidl et al. 1965; Smith et al. 1966; Hurwitz and Wade 1969). These wide differences reflect variations in the particular definition of adverse reactions used and in the methods used to detect and report suspected reactions; when investigators have relied on others to notify them of suspected reactions the yields have been low, but when they have undertaken a detailed search using independent research workers the yields have been much higher, probably because those from more detailed surveys include milder reactions. Clearly, the available data provide at best only a rough estimate of the overall incidence of adverse drug reactions in hospital.

Most studies so far have concentrated on medical inpatients. There have been a number of small studies looking at surgical inpatients (Armstrong et al. 1976; Danielson et al. 1982), paediatric wards (BCDSP 1972a; Mitchell et al. 1979, 1982), and psychiatric wards (Swett 1974). These reviews tend to record a lower incidence of reactions than are seen in medical inpatients, reflecting the lesser severity of the underlying illness rather than a lower intrinsic toxicity of drugs in these populations.

In an attempt to analyse the situation more rigorously, several workers have reported on the frequency of severe reactions by restricting their analysis to include only reactions of life-threatening severity or those that resulted in death (Armstrong et al. 1976; Porter and Jick 1977). Overall, these workers report a death rate attributable to drug treatment of some 2 per 10 000 surgical patients and 9 per 10 000 medical patients, the drugs most frequently implicated being cardiac glycosides, anticoagulants, and intravenous fluids.

Reactions in outpatients

Few workers have formally studied the overall incidence of adverse effects in outpatients. Mulroy (1973) reported that one in 40 consultations was due to drug-induced disease. Kellaway and his colleagues in Auckland (1973) reported an overall incidence of 32 per cent in 200 patients discharged from hospital who were followed for the ensuing 6 months. Martys (1979) reported that 41 per cent of patients receiving drug treatment developed some type of reaction.

The advent of record-linkage techniques (q.v.) has provided a powerful tool for reviewing adverse effects of individual drugs in the outpatient setting, and because of the large number of patients that can be studied, has given much more powerful assessments of drug safety in the community.

Spontaneous reports to regulatory authorities

Most investigators looking at large series of prospective patients in medical wards report that the commonest adverse reactions recorded were attributable to aspirin and the non-steroidal anti-inflammatory agents, antibiotics, cardiac glycosides, anticoagulants, diuretics, and steroids. Similar conclusions arise from analyses of spontaneous reports to drug regulatory authorities (McQueen 1974; ADRAC 1980; Bem *et al.* 1988). The UK spontaneous report scheme for suspected adverse drug reactions has been an effective, inexpensive, and useful tool to aid regulatory authorities to come to judgements about drug toxicity (Rawlins 1986). There is, however, substantial under-reporting of adverse reactions. Such under-reporting has been studied in general practice (Walker and Lumley 1986; Lumley *et al.* 1986), but not in any detail in hospitals, towards which one might expect the majority of patients with serious adverse reactions to gravitate.

Detailed analysis of cumulative spontaneous reports of adverse reactions is fraught with difficulty (Griffin and Weber 1985, 1986, 1989; Rawlins 1986, 1988*a,b*). The non-steroidal anti-inflammatory agents illustrate this most efficiently. The information available to the UK Committee on Safety of Medicines was analysed in 1986 (CSM 1986). The numbers of suspected serious gastrointestinal reactions to non-steroidal anti-inflammatory agents during 1964–85 were reviewed. The results were considered not only in terms of absolute numbers of reports, but also as the number of reports per million recorded prescriptions. The available data allowed grouping of the non-steroidal agents into three major groups of serious suspected reactions per million prescriptions:

1. ibuprofen, which appeared to have the lowest rate of serious reactions per million prescriptions (13.2). This drug has subsequently become available in pharmacies without prescription;

2. benoxaprofen, fenclofenac, indoprofen, feprazone and the Osmosin formulation of indomethacin, which showed high total reaction 'rates' of between 132 and 555 per million prescriptions. These drugs have been withdrawn from the marketplace;

3. the remaining drugs with rates between 35 and 87 per million prescriptions. These are difficult to separate one from the other and have remained available by prescription.

Of considerable interest are the differences between these reporting rates and the substantially lower rates for the same drugs reported in the United States (Sachs and Bortnichak 1986; Rossi *et al.* 1987). In an analysis of 15 spontaneous reporting schemes for adverse drug reaction monitoring throughout the world, Griffin (1986) clearly showed the wide variability in reporting rates in different countries. Thus, great care should be taken before attempts are made to collate such disparate data

resources and to draw any conclusion. Edwards and his colleagues emphasize this in a review of the World Health Organisation's International Collaborative Programme on Drug Monitoring (Edwards *et al.* 1990). They claim that such a system has strengths as a signal generator or hypotheses-generating system, but has no value as a hypotheses-testing resource. Recently Meyboom and his colleagues in The Netherlands have published an excellent review on the principles of signal detection in pharmacovigilance which is worthy of consultation by all involved in the field (Meyboom *et al.* 1997).

Augmented spontaneous reports of suspected adverse reactions

Several groups have endeavoured to surmount both the under-reporting and the numerous distortions inherent in spontaneous reporting schemes. Notable among these are the augmented spontaneous reporting schemes developed in New Zealand (Coulter and McQueen 1982; Edwards 1987), prescription event monitoring designed by Professor Inman and his group in Southampton (1988), and a number of *ad hoc* studies undertaken by individual drug firms, examples of which would include those of ketotifen (Maclay *et al.* 1984) and captopril (Chalmers *et al.* 1987). In these approaches, detailed studies encouraging reports either of suspected adverse reactions or of events experienced by drug recipients together with feedback, either documentary or via computer terminals, allow a better understanding and quantitation of suspected reactions than has been possible hitherto with spontaneous schemes reporting directly to regulatory authorities.

Analytical studies

Case registries

Case registries first came into vogue as a method of quantitating suspected adverse reactions with the discovery that chloramphenicol could be associated with the development of aplastic anaemia (Yunis 1973). Similar techniques were adopted in the search for a possible aetiological agent in the outbreak of vaginal adenocarcinoma in premenarchal girls noted in the eastern seaboard of the United States (Herbst *et al.* 1971). This technique is of great value where a drug commonly causes an otherwise very rare disease which is clearly defined and not subject to diagnostic confusion. The drug must be in reasonably widespread use and the suspect condition must be virtually non-existent in the absence of the drug.

It is surprising that this technique has not been adopted more extensively since these demonstrations of its potential. For some time now there has been a strong argument for mounting a series of case registries for otherwise rare events that are frequently drug related: examples of these would include acute renal failure, acute hepatic necrosis, Guillain–Barré syndrome, aplastic anaemia, and agranulocytosis (Lawson 1990). The advent of computerisation should render this a relatively inexpensive exercise with great potential for adding to the public body of knowledge about drug safety. Interpretation of such registries is understandably complex and difficult; if, however, up-to-date information is collected, details including possibly drug concentrations in body fluids will greatly assist the process. Moreover, such information, if rigorously collected, could give an early assessment of the magnitude of any public health problem arising from a newly marketed drug.

Cohort studies

In the mid-1980s the United Kingdom Committee on Safety of Medicines reviewed its experience of drug-related problems and concluded that, for new drugs used in the treatment of relatively benign conditions in domiciliary practice, some form of surveillance ought to be in continuous operation for the early years following marketing. In essence, the technique that can most readily address this problem is the cohort study. Several such cohort studies have been undertaken and published, a classic example being that in which some 9928 consecutive cimetidine recipients were reviewed over a period of one year during which time all the diagnoses recorded during episodes of hospital contact, whether inpatient or outpatient, were analysed together with all deaths and the cause of those deaths. Thereafter, the names of patients were noted for future reference by the Central Registry of Deaths and they have now been followed up over a period of 20 years. Such a massive exercise has produced useful data on the patterns of adverse reaction experience with everyday use of H_2-blockers and has been of value in attempting to review the association between H_2-blocker use and upper gastrointestinal tract tumours (Colin-Jones et al. 1983, 1985a,b). These studies are expensive to operate, however, and the facility to undertake them is not widely available. By 1990, a substantial number of this type of observational cohort study had been undertaken and, in reviewing the outcome, the Committee on Safety of Medicines expressed concern at significant methodological problems with them (Waller et al. 1992). Following this, ad hoc studies aimed at hypothesis generation were rarely undertaken

by companies, who came to rely most on record-linkage techniques for postmarketing surveillance (Lawson 1997).

Case–control studies

Case–control studies are of considerable use in testing hypotheses about drug-related disease. The technique is a powerful tool for coming rapidly to a conclusion about suspected adverse drug reactions under certain strict conditions (Sartwell 1974; Jick and Vessey 1979). Used appropriately, this approach can be of great value in studying possible drug-related events in defined populations. Indeed, some investigators have gone so far as to undertake what is called case–control surveillance whereby they investigate a series of well-defined cases in a prospective manner as part of a hospital-based national surveillance programme (Slone et al. 1979). Examples of the type of information available from case–control studies include the associations between cholelithiasis and oral contraceptives (BCDSP 1973), venous thromboembolism and postmenopausal oestrogen therapy (BCDSP 1974), acute pancreatitis and thiazide diuretics (Bourke et al. 1978), upper gastrointestinal bleeding and non- steroidal anti-inflammatory drugs (Langman et al. 1994; Rodriguez and Jick 1994), and many others.

Record-linkage studies

Previously, individually designed cohort studies and case–control studies were conducted as and when required. The availability, however, of powerful computers has led to record-linkage schemes whereby information regarding outcome of hospitalization and drug exposure within hospitals and, latterly, within general practice, is collated and analysed to give us a powerful tool for conducting aetiological research following drug exposure. Finney (1965) foresaw the use of such large databases to generate hypotheses about possible adverse drug effects while avoiding the likelihood of bias contained in physicians' judgements. At the time, however, the necessary computer power was not available. In an early attempt at analysing output from a large data resource, Skegg and Doll (1977) in Oxford reported their ability to identify an increased prevalence of eye and skin problems in practolol recipients when compared with propranolol recipients. These analyses were conducted following the discovery of the practolol syndrome; they confirmed the potential of such large data sources for generating significant information on adverse drug effects. As computer facilities have become more widespread and are able to handle much more information, the possibilities foreseen by Finney in 1965 have become a reality. Foremost amongst such record-linkage studies are those conducted by the Boston Collaborative

Drug Surveillance Program within the Group Health Co-operative Health Maintenance Organisation in Puget Sound (Jick *et al.* 1984; Porter *et al.* 1982). Other studies have been conducted using different data sources within the USA (Strom *et al.* 1985) and Canada (Guess *et al.* 1988). Wayne Ray and his colleagues in Tennessee (1987, 1989) have used Medicaid data to conduct inpatient studies into risk factors for hip fracture, indicating a positive association with long-term psychotropic drug use and a negative association with long-term thiazide diuretic use.

Within the United Kingdom, similar studies were initially developed by the Medicines Evaluation and Monitoring Unit in Dundee (Beardon *et al.* 1989), and more recently came to fruition with the General Practice Research Database belonging to the Department of Health. This linked system covers over 3.5 million individuals enrolled in some 500 general practices and has been in operation for over 10 years (Walley and Mantagni 1997).

Examples of major findings derived from or substantiated by record-linkage schemes include: risks of haematological malignancies associated with medications (Doody *et al.* 1996); risks of hypoglycaemia in relation to human and animal insulins (Jick *et al.* 1990); peptic ulcer disease and corticosteroids (Piper *et al.* 1991); and venous thromboembolism and the newer-generation oral contraceptives (Jick *et al.* 1995).

Risk assessment

Ideally patients and doctors wish to know the benefits they can expect to receive from drug treatment — which are best measured in randomized controlled clinical trials — and the accompanying risks to which they may be subjected. Risk assessments are best made in cohort studies where the background frequency of an event is assessed from a non-exposed control group and compared with the risk in an exposed group. The difference between the two frequencies is the 'attributable risk' or risk directly attributable to the exposure. In a study on a defined population, if one knows the magnitude of the exposure of the study drug in the community, one can then derive the population attributable risk which is of importance to public health planning authorities.

By contrast, in a case–control study the resulting information is provided as a 'relative risk', that is the risk of exposure given disease as compared with the risk of exposure given no disease. Confusion between relative and attributable risks is common and a source of many media scares.

Causality assessment

In observational (non-randomized) studies, the finding of an association between an exposure (e.g. drug treatment) and an event does not necessarily mean that the treatment causes the event. Many other explanations must be considered before a causal interpretation is entertained. Moreover, if the causal interpretation is accepted it may be that the event caused the treatment rather than the treatment causing the event. In any observational study non-causal explanations for association must be regarded as the most likely. These include various types of bias (in data collection and handling) and confounding (in which an intermediate factor is independently linked to the exposure and the event), as well as the widely acknowledged effects of chance (which can readily be assessed by statistical techniques). Before embarking upon major observational studies, investigators unfamiliar with the techniques of epidemiology would be well advised to seek expert advice to assist in study design and planning.

Experimental studies

Most small-scale, randomized, controlled clinical trials do not produce data of major interest to the pharmaco-epidemiologist. Only when one enters the area of large-scale multicentre studies do we see studies of sufficient size to be of potential value. A classic example of this was the use of clofibrate in the secondary prevention of myocardial infarction (Oliver *et al.* 1984). Further studies in this area include such major interventions as the Scandinavian Simvastatin Survival Study Group (1994), the LIPID Study Group (1995) and the West of Scotland Coronary Prevention Study (Shepherd *et al.* 1995). These major interventive studies produce important benefit–risk information to permit rational judgements on long-term use of preventative therapies and as such are of major interest to the epidemiologist. However, it seems likely that this approach will only be conducted in areas such as vascular disease and hormone-replacement therapy, where the potential benefits for the population justify the enormous costs of conducting these studies.

In an attempt to provide information of equivalent value to the major interventional studies at lower cost, the technique of meta-analysis is now being regularly undertaken. This is a method for combining results of groups of (small) studies to derive an overall (summary) estimate of effect. It is applicable both to randomized studies and to observational studies and is likely to be seen more frequently in the future (Prospective Studies Collaboration 1995; Hemminki and McPherson 1997).

Predisposing factors

Race and genetic polymorphism

Recently, considerable interest has been directed towards the role of genetic polymorphism in explaining interindividual variation in susceptibility to adverse drug reactions. Several important genetic polymorphisms have been discovered in the oxidation and acetylation pathways of drug metabolism. Examples include extensive and poor metabolisers of debrisoquine (Mahgoub *et al.* 1977). Poor metabolisers of debrisoquine tend to have reduced first-pass metabolism, increased plasma levels, and exaggerated pharmacological response to this drug, resulting in postural hypotension. By contrast, rapid metabolisers may require considerably higher doses for a standard effect. A little later, it was been shown that nortriptyline and desipramine are metabolised by mechanisms similar to those of debrisoquine (Mellstrom *et al.* 1981), as a result of which the steady-state plasma levels of these drugs are phenotype-dependent (Bertilsson and Aberg-Wistedt 1983). This problem may become most clinically relevant in subjects taking overdoses of these tricyclic antidepressants. Under such circumstances, the serious potential for cardiotoxicity is enhanced in poor metabolisers (Spiker *et al.* 1976).

Acetylator polymorphism is another clinically relevant example of genetic polymorphism. In this case, the drugs particularly affected are procainamide, isoniazid, hydralazine, and phenelzine. There are wide variations in the distributions of rapid acetylators in different races. Rapid acetylators predominate amongst Eskimos and Japanese and slow acetylators amongst Mediterranean Jews. Slow acetylators are more likely to develop peripheral neuropathy due to isoniazid, and lupus erythematosus with procainamide, isoniazid, or hydralazine (Lunde *et al.* 1983). Conversely, fast acetylators may be more susceptible to the toxicity associated with isoniazid (Mitchell *et al.* 1975).

Glucose 6-phosphate dehydrogenase deficiency, which predisposes to some drug-induced haemolytic anaemias, is commoner amongst Africans, Kurdish and Iraqi Jews, some Mediterranean people, and Filipinos, and is relatively infrequent amongst other races.

There is wide interracial variability in the distribution of human lymphocyte antigens (HLA), resulting in racial predisposition to those adverse reactions believed to be associated with HLA phenotype. Several examples of the association of HLA phenotype and adverse drug reaction have been reported, although the mechanisms by which such reactions are mediated have yet to be fully explained. Up till now, particular interest has concentrated in the higher prevalence of toxicity of drugs used in the treatment of rheumatoid arthritis. Whether this observation is a result of more frequent testing of HLA phenotypes in patients with rheumatoid disease is unclear. Veys and others (1978) reported an association with levamisole toxicity and HLA-B27. Bardin and colleagues (1982) reported cases of nephrotoxicity from penicillamine associated with the HLA-DR3 haplotype and Woolley and co-workers (1980) reported associations with toxicity from sodium aurothiomalate and penicillamine in patients with HLA-DR3,DR1.

Racial differences in the incidence of haemolytic anaemia induced by methyldopa have been reported. A positive direct antiglobulin test was found in 15 per cent of Caucasian patients under treatment; but no positive tests were found in 73 Indians and Africans who had been taking methyldopa for at least 3 months (Seedat and Vawda 1968) or in 58 Chinese patients who had received the drugs for at least 9 months (Burns-Cox 1970; Chen and Ooi 1971).

Women in Scandinavia and Chile appear to be particularly susceptible to the cholestatic jaundice induced by oral contraceptives, for reasons that are not clear (Reyes 1982).

Some types of porphyria are aggravated by drugs. These tend to vary in incidence between different races; for instance, acute intermittent porphyria is more frequent in people of Scandinavian, Anglo-Saxon, or German origin than amongst other ethnic groups, while the disease itself is very rare in negroes.

Jick and others (1969) reported that blood group has a significant influence on susceptibility to thromboembolic disease amongst oral contraceptive users, and to digoxin toxicity (BCDSP 1972*b*).

Sex

Several studies have shown that women are more likely to report adverse drug reactions than men. Although this could be explained largely by the greater susceptibility of the female skin and gut to noxious stimuli, women also appear to be more susceptible to the toxic effects of digoxin (Hurwitz and Wade 1969), heparin (Miller 1974), and captopril (Chalmers *et al.* 1987). Agranulocytosis caused by phenylbutazone or chloramphenicol is about three times commoner (D'Arcy and Griffin 1972), and aplastic anaemia due to chloramphenicol is twice as common (Yunis and Bloomberg 1964) in women as in men. Drug-associated lupus erythematosus affects more women than men, as does the spontaneous disease (Lee and Siegal 1968; Batchelor *et al.* 1980).

Age

The elderly

Castleden and Pickles (1988) reviewed the reports of suspected adverse reactions accumulated by the UK Committee on Safety of Medicines during 1965–83. A greater than expected proportion of reports came from elderly subjects. There were 3350 reports concerning individual patients aged 75 years or over, the commonest serious problems affecting the gastrointestinal and haemopoietic systems. As with younger subjects, non-steroidal anti-inflammatory agents accounted for a large proportion of the notified reactions in this age group.

Several cross-sectional studies of the elderly in hospital have indicated they suffer from more adverse reactions than younger patients (Hurwitz 1969; Caranasos *et al.* 1974; Levy *et al.* 1980). None the less, interpretation of such studies is limited by failure to control important age-related variables, including measurements of renal function, hepatic function, plasma protein levels, etc., and the number of medications that a patient was receiving. More recent studies suggest that of the four traditional elements of pharmacokinetics — absorption, distribution, metabolism, and excretion — only absorption appears to be substantially independent of age (Johnson *et al.* 1985). Drug distribution may vary substantially between the young and the old. An age-related increase in body fat may well account for the greater volume of distribution of lipid-soluble medications such as long-acting benzodiazepines, and drug elimination by the kidney may be considerably impaired in elderly subjects owing to age-related decline in renal function, although there is a large interindividual variability in such deterioration (Rowe *et al.* 1976). Coupled with these changes in pharmacokinetic variables, certain pharmacodynamic variables also appear to be affected by age processes. Thus there appears to be an increase in the sensitivity of receptors for many medications in the elderly.

Reidenberg and others (1978) showed an increasing effect in the elderly of a given dose of diazepam despite these subjects having significantly lower plasma levels of the drug at the time. Similar studies have been reported involving other benzodiazepines and opiates (Belville *et al.* 1971; Kaiko 1980). In a classic study using data from the BCDSP, Greenblatt and his colleagues reviewed information from 2542 consecutive flurazepam recipients and showed a strong age and dose effect in relation to the occurrence of undesired drowsiness with this drug (Greenblatt *et al.* 1977). In a large study based on Medicaid prescribing records, Avorn *et al.* (1986) showed that, among a sample of 143 253 recipients, depression (defined as receipt of a tricyclic antidepressant drug) appeared less common in older subjects as compared with younger subjects. This study also showed a higher prevalence of depression among female recipients of β-adrenoceptor blockers when compared with males.

It has been shown that a single dose of digoxin produces a higher plasma concentration and the plasma half-life of the drug is longer than with the same dose in younger people (Ewy *et al.* 1969). This may partly explain the high incidence of digoxin toxicity found in older patients (Ogilvie and Ruedy 1967; Hurwitz and Wade 1969), though potassium depletion induced by powerful modern diuretics in patients taking a poor diet may play a part, as may renal tubular excretory and secretory factors (Hall 1972).

Elderly patients are more likely to bleed during heparin treatment than are younger patients (Walker and Jick 1980). The anticoagulant effect of a single dose of warfarin appears to be greater in the old than in the young (Hewick *et al.* 1975), a finding in keeping with clinical experience. In a review of 321 patients attending a University Hospital, however, Gurwitz and others (1988) failed to show an association between age and bleeding reactions. Similar findings were recorded by Petty and colleagues (1986) in a large retrospective study of patients attending an anticoagulant clinic. Levine and co-workers (1989) surveyed some 171 studies of anticoagulant therapy but were unable to establish any association between age and bleeding, as insufficient information was recorded in many articles reviewed.

It has long been accepted that elderly patients are more sensitive to the effects of powerful analgesics than younger patients; and that they are apt to become confused and disturbed by barbiturates. Possible explanations for these clinical impressions are provided by experiments which show that after a standard single intravenous dose of pethidine the plasma concentration is higher and the half-life of the drug longer in old than in younger subjects (Chan *et al.* 1975); and that the rate of hydroxylation of amylobarbitone is reduced in the elderly (Irvine *et al.* 1974). Elderly patients are particularly prone to cerebral dysfunction when they take nitrazepam in the usual adult dose (Evans and Jarvis 1972).

Experimental studies also suggest that the old may be at greater risk of suffering adverse reactions to phenylbutazone (O'Malley *et al.* 1971) and propranolol (Castleden *et al.* 1975). They are more liable than the young to develop potassium depletion from diuretic therapy, postural hypotension caused by antihypertensive drugs and phenothiazines, urinary retention from anticholinergics and antiparkinsonian drugs, and spontaneous hypothermia associated with treatment with sedatives and tranquillizers (Hall 1972). By contrast, the elderly may be less sensitive to pharmacological effects of propranolol (Vestal *et al.* 1979) and verapamil (Abernethy *et al.* 1986) probably because of impaired secondary responses.

The young

In the neonate, especially when premature, several of the enzymes involved in drug metabolism and elimination are poorly developed, and consequently the risk of adverse reactions to some drugs is increased. The most hazardous drugs in this respect are chloramphenicol, sulphonamides, novobiocin, barbiturates, morphine and its derivatives, and vitamin K and its analogues. In the very young child, chloramphenicol may induce the grey syndrome, characterized by abdominal distension, vomiting, peripheral cyanosis, profound shock, respiratory failure, and death. Sulphonamides, novobiocin, and vitamin K analogues may induce or aggravate kernicterus; and barbiturates, morphine, and other narcotics may cause severe respiratory depression.

Some ototoxic antibiotics (e.g. streptomycin) are eliminated by the kidney more slowly in the young child than in the adult, and toxic effects may occur unless the dose is reduced. The increased sensitivity to digoxin in the first 2 weeks of life may be explained by a similar mechanism (Morselli *et al.* 1983).

The increased sensitivity of the newborn to morphine and its derivatives has been attributed to a poorly developed glucuronidation mechanism, upsets in cholinergic and adrenergic regulation, and the inefficiency of the immature blood–brain barrier. Poorly developed oxidation reactions or inadequate renal function, or both of these, may also account for the poor tolerance of the newborn to some barbiturates (Done and Jung 1970; Gadeke 1972).

Using the data from the UK spontaneous reporting scheme, Bateman and colleagues (1985) showed that extrapyramidal reactions with metoclopramide were reported significantly more often in young adults than expected, the highest rate being seen in young females (190 reports per million prescriptions), and the lowest rate in elderly males (3.5 reports per million prescriptions). This difference is of major clinical importance and appears not to be due to pharmacokinetic abnormalities but rather to different end-organ responses.

End-organ failure

Patients with impaired renal or liver function are at substantially greater than normal risk of developing adverse reactions to drugs eliminated by these organs. Epidemiological techniques have rarely been used in studies in this area, largely because of the complexity of most of the clinical cases surveyed.

Drug formulation

Changes in formulation resulting either in increased bioavailability or in patients being exposed to new excipients may be a cause of epidemics of drug toxicity. Classic examples of this are the development of phenytoin toxicity and of digoxin toxicity following reformulation of old products (Greenblatt *et al.* 1983; Neuvonen 1983). Further details of these incidents are given in a later chapter and the whole question of toxicity arising from excipients in medicines has been well reviewed by Golightly and colleagues (1988*a,b*).

Conclusions

Considering the relatively 'soft' nature of much of the information cited above and the intrinsic difficulty of assessing whether an event is drug related or not, it is hardly surprising that different commentators have come to widely differing conclusions about the overall effect on public health of the hazards of drug therapy. Melmon (1971) from the western USA expressed the view that many lives were lost and much unnecessary hospitalization arose from adverse drug effects. By contrast, Jick (1974), based in Massachusetts but using worldwide data, concluded that drugs were remarkably non-toxic, given their powerful nature and widespread use. Citing information from the BCDSP, he concluded that most adverse reactions were self-limiting and of little consequence to the clinical course of the patient's illness. Serious reactions were uncommon and tended to occur in patients who were ill and suffering from potentially fatal diseases. In his opinion, the main culprits in producing avoidable adverse reactions of major degree were the often uncritical use of intravenous fluids and of electrolyte replacement.

More recently, Inman (1984) made an eloquent plea for investigators in this difficult area to pay some regard to the benefits of drug therapy and its hazards in relation to the expected life-span of the individual recipient. Such an approach is undoubtedly valid and merits more widespread adoption.

The increasing availability of record-linkage schemes covering many millions of patient-years of exposure to medicines means that more accurate assessments can now be made of the hazards of drug therapy. Risks can be established in subsets of the population, for example, the young, the elderly, those with organ failure, those with concomitant drug treatments, and so on. With this information comes the need to use the knowledge wisely. Often those at greatest risks are also those with greatest potential for benefit from the treatment. It is incumbent upon manufacturers, regulators, prescribers, and recipients to use their increased knowledge wisely. Precipitate action to withdraw a medicine because of an identified and quantified risk may be appropriate in some instances; in others the risks of this action may far outweigh the benefits. In an age of increasing litigation, all involved in drug treatment should applaud the availability of systems to improve assessment of risk. Such knowledge must be used appropriately — otherwise the net loss to the public health could far outweigh the gains.

It is clear from the information presented that the use of powerful drugs has increased substantially in the last few decades. With this increase goes a potential for serious adverse reactions. To minimize these risks, prescribers have daily to consider the objectives of their treatment, how long it should continue, which drug they should choose, and how they can estimate the appropriate dose for their patient. Such concerns are important in all subjects, but become particularly clamant where the objective of therapy is not to alleviate symptoms of existing disease, but to prevent the development of complications in patients suffering from asymptomatic abnormalities such as hypertension or hyperlipidaemia. Such individuals are increasingly exposed to powerful medications in order to achieve long-term benefit in the form of reduction in disease progression and consequent prolongation of useful life. Great care must be taken to ensure that the treatment advocated should be as free as possible from risk to health, lest the treatment prove worse than the disease. In order to establish the true risks and benefits of such therapeutic interventions, long-term studies of an epidemiological nature will be required. The technology for such studies is now available.

The population-based large randomized trial is proving valuable, especially in assessing benefits of preventative therapy; it is not without its problems, however, and is no panacea for replacing other methodologies (Charlton *et al.* 1997). The increasing use of record-linkage facilities in the US and Europe is reducing the cost of individual studies and increasing the speed with which results are available. Careful use of the resulting information will lead to greatly improved public health and increasingly rational use of powerful medicines in the coming decade.

Further reading

Hartzema, A.G., Porta, M.S., and Tilson, H.H. (1988). *Pharmacoepidemiology: An Introduction.* Harvey Whitney, Cincinnati.

Inman, W.H.W. (1986). *Monitoring for Drug Safety* (2nd edn). Medical and Technical Press, Lancaster.

Speight, T.M. and Holford, N.H.G. (1997). *Avery's Drug Treatment* (4th edn). ADIS International Press, Auckland.

Strom, B.L. (1989). *Pharmacoepidemiology.* Churchill Livingstone, Edinburgh.

References

Abernethy, D.R., Schwartz, J.B., and Todd, E.L. (1986). Verapamil pharmacokinetics and disposition in young and elderly hypertensive patients. Altered electrocardiographic and hypotensive responses. *Ann. Intern. Med.* 105, 329.

ADRAC (Adverse Drug Reactions Advisory Committee) (1980). ADRAC report for 1980. *Med. J. Aust.* 5, 416.

Armstrong, B., Dinan, B., and Jick, H. (1976). Fatal drug reactions in patients admitted to surgical services. *Am. J. Surg.* 132, 643.

Avorn, J., Everitt, D.E., and Weiss, S. (1986). Increased antidepressant use in patients prescribed beta-blockers. *JAMA* 255, 357.

Bardin, T., Dryll, A., Debeyre, N., *et al.* (1982). HLA system and side effects of gold salts and D-penicillamine treatment of rheumatoid arthritis. *Ann. Rheum. Dis.* 41, 599.

Batchelor, J.R., Welsh, K.I., Mansilla-Tinoco, R., *et al.* (1980). Hydralazine-induced systemic lupus erythematosus: influence of HLA-DR and sex on susceptibility. *Lancet* i, 1107.

Bateman, D.N., Darling, W.M., and Rawlins, M.D. (1985). Extrapyramidal reactions to metoclopramide and prochlorperazine. *Q. J. Med.* 71, 307.

BCDSP (Boston Collaborative Drug Surveillance Program) (1972a). Drug surveillance: problems and challenges. *Pediatr. Clin. North Am.* 19, 117.

BCDSP (Boston Collaborative Drug Surveillance Program) (1972b). Relation between digoxin arrhythmias and ABO blood groups. *Circulation*, 45, 352.

BCDSP (Boston Collaborative Drug Surveillance Program) (1973). Oral contraceptives and venous thromboembolic disease, surgically confirmed gallbladder disease and breast tumours. *Lancet* i, 1399.

BCDSP (Boston Collaborative Drug Surveillance Program) (1974). Surgically confirmed gallbladder disease, venous thromboembolism, and breast tumors in relation to postmenopausal estrogen therapy. *N. Engl. J. Med.* 290, 15.

Beardon, P.H.G., Brown, S.V., and McDevitt, D.G. (1989). Gastrointestinal events in patients prescribed non-steroidal anti-inflammatory drugs: a controlled study using record linkage. *Q. J. Med.* 71, 497.

Belville, J.W., Forrest, W.H., Miller, E., *et al.* (1971). Influence of age on pain relief from analgesics. *JAMA* 217, 1835.

Bem, J.L., Breckenridge, A.M., Mann, R.D., *et al.* (1988). Review of yellow cards (1986): report to the Committee on the Safety of Medicines. *Br. J. Clin. Pharmacol.* 26, 679.

Bergman, U. (1979). International comparisons of drug utilisation: use of antidiabetic drugs in 7 European countries. In *Studies in Drug Utilisation* (ed. U. Bergman, A. Grimsson, A.H.W. Wahba, and B. Westerholm). WHO Regional Publications No. 8. WHO, Copenhagen.

Bertilsson L. and Aberg-Wistedt, A. (1983). The debrisoquine hydroxylation test predicts steady-state plasma levels of desipramine. *Br. J. Clin. Pharmacol.* 15, 388.

Blanc, S., Leuenberger, P., Berger, J.P., *et al.* (1979). Judgement of trained observers on adverse drug reactions. *Clin. Pharmacol. Ther.* 25, 493.

Bourke, J.B., McIllmurray, M.B., Mead, G.M., *et al.* (1978). Drug-associated primary acute pancreatitis. *Lancet* i, 706.

Burns-Cox, C.J. (1970). Negative Coombs test in Chinese on methyldopa. *Lancet* ii, 673.

Caranasos, G.J., Stewart, R.B., and Cluff, L.E. (1974). Drug-induced illness leading to hospitalization. *JAMA* 228, 713.

Castleden, C.M. and Pickles, H. (1988). Suspected adverse drug reactions in elderly patients reported to the Committee on Safety of Medicines. *Br. J. Clin. Pharmacol.* 26, 347.

Castleden, C.M., Kaye, C.M., and Parsons, R.L. (1975). The effect of age on plasma levels of propranolol and practolol in man. *Br. J. Clin. Pharmacol.* 2, 303.

Chalmers, D., Dombey, S.L., and Lawson, D.H. (1987). Post-marketing surveillance of captopril (for hypertension): a preliminary report. *Br. J. Pharmacol.* 24, 343.

Chan, K., Kendall, M.J., Mitchard, M., *et al.* (1975). The effect of ageing on plasma pethidine concentration. *Br. J. Clin. Pharmacol.* 2, 297.

Charlton, B.G, Taylor, P.R.A., and Proctor, S.J. (1997). The PACE (population adjusted clinical epidemiology) strategy: a new approach to multicentred clinical research. *Q. J. Med.* 90, 147.

Chen, B.T.M. and Ooi, B.S. (1971). Negative Coombs test in Chinese on methyldopa. *Lancet* i, 87.

Colin-Jones, D.G., Langman, M.J.S., Lawson, D.H., *et al.* (1983). Postmarketing surveillance of the safety of cimetidine: 12 month mortality report. *BMJ* 286, 1713.

Colin-Jones, D.G., Langman, M.J.S., Lawson, D.H., *et al.* (1985a). Postmarketing surveillance of the safety of cimetidine: 12 month morbidity report. *Q. J. Med.* 54, 253.

Colin-Jones, D.G., Langman, M.J.S., Lawson, D.H., *et al.* (1985b). Postmarketing surveillance of the safety of cimetidine: mortality during second, third and fourth years of follow-up. *BMJ* 291, 1084.

Committee on Safety of Medicines (CSM) Update (1986). Nonsteroidal anti-inflammatory drugs and serious gastrointestinal adverse reactions — 1. *BMJ* 292, 614.

Coulter, D.M. and McQueen, E.G. (1982). Postmarketing surveillance. Achievements and problems in the intensified adverse drug reaction reporting scheme. *N.Z. Family Physician* 1, 13.

Danielson, D.A., Porter, J.B., Dinan, B.J., *et al.* (1982). Drug monitoring of surgical patients. *JAMA* 248, 1482.

D'Arcy, P.F. and Griffin, J.P. (ed.) (1972). *Iatrogenic Diseases*, p. 3. Oxford University Press.

Done, A.K. and Jung, A.L. (1970). Neonatal pharmacology. In *Current Pediatric Therapy*, Vol. 4 (ed. S.S. Gellis and B.M. Kagan), p. 995. Saunders, Philadelphia.

Doody, M.M., Linet, M.S., Glass, A.G., *et al.* (1996). Risks of non-Hodgkin's lymphoma, multiple myeloma and leukaemia associated with common medications. *Epidemiology* 7, 131.

Dukes, M.N.G. (1979). Drug utilisation studies in perspective. In *Studies in Drug Utilisation* (ed. U. Bergman, A. Grimsson, A.H.W. Wahba, and B. Westerholm). WHO Regional Publications No. 8. WHO, Copenhagen.

Edwards, R.I. (1987). Adverse drug reaction monitoring. The practicalities. *Med. Toxicol.* 2, 405.

Edwards, R.I., Lindquist, M., Wiholm, B-E., *et al.* (1990). Quality criteria for early signals of possible adverse drug reactions. *Lancet* 336, 156.

Evans, A.S. (1976). Causation and disease: the Henle–Koch postulates revisited. *Yale J. Biol. Med.* 49, 175.

Evans, J.G. and Jarvis, E.H. (1972). Nitrazepam and the elderly. *BMJ* iv, 487.

Ewy, G.A., Kapadia, G.C., Toa, L., *et al.* (1969). Digoxin metabolism in the elderly. *Circulation* 39, 449.

Finney, D.J. (1965). The design and logic of a monitor of drug use. *J. Chronic Dis.* 18, 77.

Gadeke, R. (1972). Unwanted effects of drugs in the neonate, premature and young child. In *Drug-induced Diseases*, Vol. 4 (ed. L. Meyler and H.M. Peck), p. 585. Associated Scientific Publishers, Amsterdam.

Golightly, L.K., Smolinske, S.S., Bennett, M.C., *et al.* (1988a). Pharmaceutical excipients: adverse effects associated with inactive ingredients in drug products — I. *Med. Toxicol.* 3, 128.

Golightly, L.K., Smolinske, S.S., Bennett, M.C., *et al.* (1988b). Pharmaceutical excipients: adverse effects associated with inactive ingredients in drug products — II. *Med. Toxicol.* 3, 209.

Greenblatt, D.J., Allen, M.D., and Shader, R.I. (1977). Toxicity of high-dose flurazepam in the elderly. *Clin. Pharmacol. Ther.* 21, 355.

Greenblatt, D.J., Smith, T.W., and Koch-Weser, J. (1983). Bioavailability of drugs: the digoxin dilemma. In *Handbook of Clinical Pharmacokinetics* (ed. M. Gibaldi and L.F. Prescott), p. 1. ADIS Health Science Press, Australia.

Griffin, J.P. (1986). Survey of the spontaneous adverse drug reaction reporting schemes in 15 countries. *Br. J. Clin. Pharmacol.* 22, 83.

Griffin, J.P. and Weber, J.C.P. (1985). Voluntary systems of adverse reaction reporting. Part I. *Adverse Drug React. Acute Poisoning Rev.* 4, 213.

Griffin, J.P. and Weber. J.C.P. (1986). Voluntary systems of adverse reaction reporting. Part II. *Adverse Drug React. Acute Poisoning Rev.* 1, 23.

Griffin, J.P. and Weber, J.C.P. (1989). Voluntary systems of adverse reaction reporting. Part III. *Adverse Drug React. Acute Poisoning Rev.* 8, 203.

Guess, H.A., West, R., Strand, L.M., *et al.* (1988). Fatal upper gastrointestinal hemorrhage or perforation among users and nonusers of nonsteroidal anti-inflammatory drugs in Saskatchewan, Canada 1983. *J. Clin. Epidemiol.* 41, 35.

Gurwitz, J.H., Goldberg, R.J., Holden, A., *et al.* (1988). Age-related risks of long-term oral anticoagulant therapy. *Arch. Intern. Med.* 148, 1733.

Hall, M.R.P. (1972). Drugs and the elderly. *BMJ* iii, 582.

Hemminki, E. and McPherson, K. (1997). Impact of postmenopausal hormone therapy on cardiovascular events and cancer: pooled data from clinical trials. *BMJ* 315, 149.

Herbst, A.L., Ulfelder, H., Poskanzer, D.C. (1971). Association of maternal stilboestrol therapy with tumor appearance in young women. *N. Engl. J. Med.* 284, 878.

Hewick, D.S., Moreland, T.A., Shepherd, A.M.M., and Stevenson, I.M. (1975). The effect of age on sensitivity to warfarin sodium. *Br. J. Clin. Pharmacol.* 2, 189P.

Hurwitz, N. (1969). Predisposing factors in adverse reactions to drugs. *BMJ* i, 356.

Hurwitz, N. and Wade, O.L. (1969). Intensive monitoring of adverse reactions to drugs. *BMJ* i, 531.

Hutchison, T.A., Leventhal, J.M., Kramer, M.S., *et al.* (1979). An algorithm for the operational assessment of adverse drug reactions. II. Demonstration of reproducibility and validity. *JAMA* 242, 633.

Inman, W.H.W. (1984). Risks in medical intervention — balancing therapeutic risks and benefits. *P.E.M. News*, 2, 16.

Inman, W.H.W., Rawson, N.S., Wilton, L.V., *et al.* (1988). Postmarketing surveillance of enalapril. I: results of prescription-event monitoring. *BMJ* 297, 826.

Irvine, R.E., Grove, J., Toseland, P.A., *et al.* (1974). The effect of age on the hydroxylation and amylobarbitone sodium in man. *Br. J. Clin. Pharmacol.* i, 41.

Jick, H. (1974). Drugs — remarkably nontoxic. *N. Engl. J. Med.* 291, 824.

Jick, H. and Vessey, M.P. (1979). Case–control studies in the evaluation of drug-induced illness. *Am. J. Epidemiol.* 107, 1.

Jick H., Slone, D., Westerholm, B., *et al.* (1969). Venous thromboembolic disease and ABO blood type: a cooperative study. *Lancet* i, 539.

Jick, H., Madsen, S., Nudelman, P.M., *et al.* (1984). Postmarketing follow-up at Group Health Cooperative of Puget Sound. *Pharmacotherapy* 4, 99.

Jick, H., Hall, G.C., Dean, A.D., *et al.* (1990). A comparison of the risk of hypoglycaemia between users of human and animal insulins. *Pharmacotherapy* 10, 395.

Jick, H., Jick, S.S., Gurewich, V., *et al.* (1995). Risk of idiopathic cardiovascular death and nonfatal venous thromboembolism in women using oral contraceptive with differing progestagen components. *Lancet* 346, 1589.

Johnson, S.L., Mayersohn, M., and Conrad, K.A. (1985). Gastrointestinal absorption as a function of age: xylose absorption in healthy adults. *Clin. Pharmacol. Ther.* 38, 331.

Kaiko, R.F. (1980). Age and morphine analgesia in cancer patients with postoperative pain. *Clin. Pharmacol. Ther.* 28, 823.

Karch, F.E. and Lasagna, L. (1977). Towards the operational identification of adverse drug reactions. *Clin. Pharmacol. Ther.* 21, 247.

Kellaway, G.S.M. (1973). Intensive monitoring for adverse drug effects in patients discharged from acute medical wards. *N.Z. Med. J.* 78, 525.

Kramer, M.S., Leventhal, J.M., Hutchison, T.A., *et al.* (1979). An algorithm for the operational assessment of adverse drug reactions. I. Background description and instructions for use. *JAMA* 242, 623.

Langman, M.J.S., Well, J., Wainwright, P., *et al.* (1996). Risks of bleeding peptic ulcer associated with individual nonsteroidal anti-inflammatory drugs. *Lancet* 343, 1075.

Last, J.M. (1983). *Dictionary of Epidemiology*. Oxford University Press.

Lawson, D.H. (1977). Intravenous fluids in medical inpatients. *Br. J. Clin. Pharmacol.* 4, 299.

Lawson, D.H. (1990). Postmarketing surveillance of drugs. *Proc. R. Coll. Physicians Edinb.* 20, 129.

Lawson, D.H. (1997). Pharmacovigilance in the 1990s. *Br. J. Clin. Pharmacol* 44, 109.

Lawson, D.H. and Jick, H. (1976). Drug prescribing in hospitals: an international comparison. *Am. J. Public Health* 66, 644.

Lawson, D.H., Bridgman, K., de Bock G.H., *et al.* (1995). European postmarketing surveillance of ramipril in hypertension. *Eur. J. Clin. Pharmacol.* 49, 73.

Lee, S.L. and Siegel, M. (1968). Drug-induced systemic lupus erythematosus. In *Drug-induced Diseases*, Vol. 3 (ed. L. Meyler and H.M. Peck), p. 244. Associated Scientific Publishers, Amsterdam.

Levine, M.M., Raskob, R., and Hirsh, J. (1989). Hemorrhagic complications of long-term anticoagulant therapy. *Chest* 95 (suppl.) 265.

Levy, M., Kewitz, H., Altwein, W., *et al.* (1980). Hospital admissions due to adverse drug reactions: a comparative study from Jerusalem and Berlin. *Eur. J. Clin. Pharmacol.* 17, 25.

LIPID Study Group. (1995). Design features and baseline characteristics of the LIPID (Long-term Intervention with Pravastatin in Ischaemic Disease) Study: a randomised trial in patients with previous acute myocardial infarction and/or unstable angina pectoris. *Am. J. Cardiol.* 76, 479.

Lumley, C.E., Walker, S.R., Hall, G.C., *et al.* (1986). The under-reporting of adverse drug reactions seen in general practice. *Pharm. Med.* 1, 205.

Lunde, P.K., Frislid, K., and Hansteen, V. (1983). Disease in acetylator polymorphism. In *Handbook of Clinical Pharmacokinetics* (ed. M. Gibaldi and L.F. Prescott), p. 150. ADIS Health Science Press, Australia.

Maclay, W.P., Crowder, D., Spiro, S., *et al.* (1984).Postmarketing surveillance: practical experience with ketotifen. *Br. Med. J.* 288, 911.

Mahgoub, A., Idle, J.R., Dring, L.G., *et al.* (1977). Polymorphic oxidation of debrisoquine in man. *Lancet* ii, 584.

Martys, C.R. (1979). Adverse reactions to drugs in general practice. *BMJ* ii, 1194.

McQueen, E.G. (1974). New Zealand Committee on adverse drug reactions. *N.Z. J. Med.* 10, 305.

Mellstrom, B., Bertillson, L., Sawe, J., *et al.* (1981). E- and Z-10-hydroxylation of nortriptyline: relationship to polymorphic debrisoquine hydroxylation. *Clin. Pharmacol. Ther.* 30, 189.

Melmon, K.L. (1971). Preventable drug reactions — causes and cures. *N. Engl. J. Med.* 284, 1361.

Meyboom, R.H.B., Egberts, A.C.G., Edwards, I.R., *et al.* (1997). Principles of signal detection in pharmacovigilance. *Drug Safety* 6, 355.

Mitchell, A.A., Goldman, P., Shapiro, S., *et al.* (1979). Drug utilisation and reported adverse reactions in hospitalized children. *Am. J. Epidemiol.* 110, 196.

Mitchell, A.A., Hartz, S.C., Shapiro, S., *et al.* (1982). Patterns of preadmission medication use among hospitalized children. *Pediatr. Pharmacol.* 2, 209.

Mitchell, J.R., Thorgeirsson, U.P., Black, M., *et al.* (1975). Increased incidence of isoniazid hepatitis in rapid acetylators: possible relation to hydralazine metabolites. *Clin. Pharmacol. Exp. Ther.* 18, 70.

Morselli, P.L., Franco-Morselli, R., and Bossi, L. (1983). Clinical pharmacokinetics in newborns and infants: age-related differences and therapeutic implications. In *Handbook of Clinical Pharmacokinetics* (ed. M. Gibaldi and L. F. Prescott), p. 98. ADIS Health Science Press, Australia.

Mulroy, R. (1973). Iatrogenic disease in general practice: its incidence and effects. *BMJ* ii, 407.

Neuvonen, P.J. (1983). Bioavailability of phenytoin: clinical pharmacokinetic and therapeutic implications. In *Handbook of Clinical Pharmacokinetics* (ed. M. Gibaldi and L. F. Prescott), p. 24. ADIS Health Science Press, Australia.

Ogilvie, R.I. and Ruedy, J. (1967). Adverse drug reactions during hospitalisation. *Can. Med. Assoc. J.* 97, 1450.

Oliver, M.F., Heady, J.A., Morris, J.N., *et al.* (1984). WHO cooperative trial on primary prevention of ischaemic heart disease with clofibrate to lower serum cholesterol: final mortality follow-up. Report of the Committee of Principal Investigators. *Lancet* ii, 600.

O'Malley, K., Crooks, J., Duke, E., *et al.* (1971). Effect of age and sex on human drug metabolism. *BMJ* iii, 607.

Petty, D.B., Strom, B.L., Melmon, K.L. (1986). Duration of warfarin anticoagulant therapy and probabilities of recurrent thromboembolism and hemorrhage. *Am. J. Med.* 81, 255.

Piper, J.M., Ray, W.A., Daugherty, J.L., *et al.* (1991). Corticosteroids and peptic ulcer disease: role of non-steroidal anti-inflammatory drugs. *Ann. Intern. Med.* 114, 735.

Porter, J. and Jick, H. (1977). Drug-related deaths among medical inpatients. *JAMA* 237, 879.

Porter, J.B., Hunter, J.R., Danielson, D.A., *et al.* (1982). Oral contraceptives and nonfatal vascular disease: recent experience. *Obstet. Gynecol.* 59, 299.

Prospective Studies Collaboration (1995). Cholesterol, diastolic blood pressure and stroke: 13 000 strokes in 450 000 people in 45 prospective cohorts. *Lancet* 346, 1647.

Rawlins, M.D. (1986). Spontaneous reporting of adverse drug reactions. *Q. J. Med.* 59, 531.

Rawlins, M.D. (1988*a*). Spontaneous reporting of adverse drug reactions. I: The data. *Br. J. Clin. Pharmacol.* 26, 1.

Rawlins, M.D. (1988*b*). Spontaneous reporting of adverse drug reactions. II: Uses. *Br. J. Clin. Pharmacol.* 26, 7.

Rawlins, M.D. and Thompson, J.W. (1977). Pathogenesis of adverse drug reactions. In *Textbook of Adverse Drug Reactions* (ed. D.M. Davies), p. 10. Oxford University Press.

Ray, W.A., Griffin, M.R., Schaffner, W., *et al.* (1987). Psychotropic drug use and the risk of hip fracture. *N. Engl. J. Med.* 316, 363.

Ray, W.A., Griffin, M.R., Downey, W., *et al.* (1989). Long-term use of thiazide diuretics and risk of hip fracture. *Lancet* i, 687.

Reidenberg, M.M. and Lowenthal, D.T. (1968). Adverse non-drug reactions. *N.Engl. J. Med.* 279, 678.

Reidenberg, M.M., Levy, M., Warner, H., *et al.* (1978). Relationship between diazepam dose, plasma level, age and central nervous system depression in adults. *Clin. Pharmacol. Ther.* 23, 371.

Reyes, H. (1982). The enigma of intrahepatic cholestasis of pregnancy: lessons from Chile. *Gastroenterology* 2, 87.

Rodriguez, L.A.G. and Jick, H. (1994). Risks of upper gastro-intestinal bleeding and perforation associated with individual non-steroid anti-inflammatory drugs. *Lancet* 343, 769.

Rossi, A.C., Hsu, J.P., and Faich, G.A. (1987). Ulcerogenicity of piroxicam: an analysis of spontaneously reported data. *BMJ* 294, 147.

Rowe, J.W., Andres, R., Tobin, J.D., *et al.* (1976). The effect of age on creatinine clearance in man: a cross-sectional and longitudinal study. *J. Gerontol.* 31, 155.

Sachs, R.M. and Bortnichak, E.A. (1986). An evaluation of spontaneous adverse drug reactions monitoring systems. *Am. J. Med.* 81 (5B), 49.

Sartwell, P.E. (1974). Retrospective studies: a review for the clinician. *Ann. Intern. Med.* 81, 381.

Scandinavian Simvastatin Survival Study Group. (1994). Randomised trial of cholesterol lowering in 4444 patients with coronary heart disease: The 4S Study. *Lancet* 344, 1383.

Seedat, Y.K. and Vawda, E.I. (1968). The Coombs test and methyldopa. *Lancet* i, 427.

Seidl, L.G., Thornton, G.F., and Cluff, L.E. (1965). Epidemiological studies of adverse drug reactions. *Am. J. Public Health* 65, 1170.

Shepherd, J., Cobbe, S.M., Ford, I., *et al.* (1995). Prevention of coronary heart disease with pravastatin in men with hypercholesterolaemia. *N. Engl. J. Med.* 333, 1301.

Skegg, D.C.G. and Doll, W.R.S. (1977). The frequency of eye complaints and rashes among patients receiving practolol and propranolol. *Lancet* ii, 475.

Slone, D., Shapiro, S., Miettinen, O.S., *et al.* (1979). Drug evaluation after marketing. *Ann. Intern. Med.* 90, 257.

Smith, J.W., Seidl, L.G., and Cluff, L.E. (1966). Studies on the epidemiology of adverse drug reactions. V — Clinical factors influencing susceptibility. *Ann. Intern. Med.* 65, 629.

Spiker, D. G., Weiss, A.N., Chang, S.S., *et al.* (1976). Tricyclic antidepressant overdose: clinical presentation and plasma levels. *Clin. Pharmacol. Ther.* 18, 539.

Strom, B.L., Carson, J.L., Morse, M.L., *et al.* (1985). The computerised on-line Medicaid pharmaceutical analysis and surveillance system: a new resource for postmarketing drug surveillance. *Clin. Pharmacol. Ther.* 38, 359.

Swett, C. (1974). Drowsiness due to chlorpromazine in relation to cigarette smoking. *Arch. Gen. Psychiatry* 31, 211.

Vestal, R.E., Wood, A.J., and Shand, D.G. (1979). Reduced beta-adrenoreceptor sensitivity in the elderly. *Clin. Pharmacol. Ther.* 29, 181.

Veys, E.M., Miclants, H., and Verbruggen, G. (1978). Levamisole induced adverse reactions in HLA-B27 positive rheumatoid arthritis. *Lancet* i, 148.

Walker, A. M. and Jick, H. (1980). Predictors of bleeding during heparin therapy. *JAMA* 244, 1209.

Walker, S.R. and Lumley, C.E. (1986). The attitudes of general practitioners to monitoring and reporting adverse drug reactions. *Pharm. Med.* 1, 195.

Walley, T. and Mantgani, A. (1997). The General Practice Research Database. *Lancet* 350, 1097.

Woolley, P.H., Griffin, J., Panayi, G.S., *et al.* (1980). HLA-DR antigens and toxic reaction to sodium aurothiomalate and D-penicillamine in patients with rheumatoid arthritis. *N. Engl. J. Med.* 303, 300.

Yunis, A.A. (1973). Chloramphenicol-induced bone marrow suppression. *Semin. Hemat.* 10, 225.

Yunis, A.A. and Bloomberg, G.R. (1964). Chloramphenicol toxicity: clinical features and pathogenesis. *Prog. Hematol.* 4, 138.

3. Regulatory aspects of adverse drug reactions

P. C. WALLER and S. M. WOOD

Introduction

This chapter reviews regulatory aspects of adverse drug reactions, focusing on the postmarketing period. During this phase unexpected hazards may be identified and further information gathered about known adverse drug reactions. The process of identifying and responding to risk/benefit issues arising with marketed medicines is known as pharmacovigilance, a responsibility which lies jointly with drug regulatory authorities, pharmaceutical companies, and users of medicines.

Role of regulatory authorities

Historical perspective

The seminal event which led to the development of modern drug regulation was the occurrence in the late 1950s and early 1960s of several thousand cases of a severe form of limb abnormality known as phocomelia, as a consequence of maternal exposure to thalidomide during pregnancy (Burley 1988). Two directly related consequences were the development of spontaneous adverse drug reaction reporting schemes to provide early warnings of such unexpected hazards and legislation to provide regulatory controls on safety, quality, and efficacy of medicines through systems of standards, authorization, pharmacovigilance, and inspection. The systems that have been developed have undoubtedly done much to protect patients and promote public health, and they are continuing to develop in response to scientific progress, technological development, and changes in worldwide markets.

The need for effective pharmacovigilance

Despite the extensive requirements for evidence on quality, efficacy, and safety required to gain a marketing authorization, effective pharmacovigilance remains a high priority for regulatory authorities. Although, the quality and efficacy of a medicine are generally well defined at the time of licensing, conclusions on the adverse effect profiles of medicines from clinical trials are limited by the numbers and selectivity of patients included in such trials, their duration, and the relatively controlled conditions under which they are conducted. Therefore safety in use can only be fully assessed after marketing. It is well recognized that safety hazards may emerge at any time during the life of a product, hence the need continuously to monitor all marketed medicines indefinitely. Spontaneous reporting schemes underpin such monitoring because they are the only practical method currently available of obtaining adverse reaction data for all medicines all the time. However, they have important limitations (see below), and many other sources of information need to be identified and used effectively to monitor the safety of medicines.

Objectives and principles

The objectives of regulatory pharmacovigilance (Waller *et al.* 1996) encompass:

1. long-term monitoring of drug safety in clinical practice to identify previously unrecognized drug safety hazards or changes in the adverse effect profiles;
2. assessment of the risks and benefits of licensed medicines, in order to take action to improve drug safety;
3. provision of information to users to optimize safe and effective use of their medicines; and
4. monitoring the impact of any action taken.

Effective pharmacovigilance is dependent on the availability of information on the clinical effects of medicines in representative populations as used in normal practice. This requires a system for collecting and monitoring suspected adverse drug reactions (ADRs), and processes for reviewing the data to decide whether

further investigation is necessary. All potentially important hazards need to be investigated with a view to
appropriate remedial action based on sound scientific
data. A variety of methods, particularly spontaneous
ADR reporting, provide 'signals' of potential hazards. A
signal is an alert from any available data source that a
drug may be associated with a previously unrecognized
hazard or that a known hazard may be quantitatively or
qualitatively different from existing expectations. Formal pharmaco-epidemiological studies, where available,
are important to confirm or clarify such signals. The
most important outputs of the process are actions which
may be necessary to enable safer use of medicines. These
include, for example, introducing warnings, contraindications, information on adverse effects, or changes to
dosing recommendations. Indications or methods of
supply may be also restricted, although complete withdrawal of a medicine on safety grounds is relatively
unusual. Informing users and explaining the reasons for
the action taken is a critical determinant of the effectiveness of these measures.

Methods used for regulatory pharmacovigilance

Data relating to the safety of marketed medicines are
available from many sources including health professionals, the Marketing Authorization (MA) holder,
other regulatory authorities, worldwide published literature, and academic research institutes. Assessment of
drug safety involves bringing together all the available
information on risks and balancing these against the
benefits. Potentially important safety issues can be
identified at any stage of drug development. In the
postmarketing phase they are particularly likely to be
identified in the first few years after marketing, although
new issues also arise with long-established drugs.

The first stage is the identification of signals of possible
hazards. Regulatory authorities require a proactive and
systematic approach to signal generation. Many signals
are identified but only a minority turn out to require
major action. Judgements have to be made, sometimes
based on limited evidence, as to whether or not there is
an issue in need of attention. There are four key issues
which will determine whether or not a signal should be
investigated further:

1. the *strength* of the signal;
2. whether or not the issue or some aspect of it is *new*;
3. the clinical *importance* as judged by the seriousness of the
   reaction and severity of the cases; and
4. the potential for *preventive* measures by the regulatory
   authority.

When justified through application of thes
signal is investigated by bringing together a
evidence available and, sometimes, by desi
studies to further investigate it. Considerat
an early stage to the possible outcomes and specifically
as to how risks might be minimized.

Spontaneous adverse reaction reporting

Spontaneous suspected adverse reaction reporting
schemes provide the most common source of signals of
drug safety issues for marketed medicines. These collect
individual case reports from health professionals (and, in
some countries, consumers) of adverse events which the
reporter considers *may* be related to the drug or drugs
being taken. In this context there is potential for confusion between the terms 'adverse event' and 'adverse
reaction' which can be avoided by using the term *'suspected adverse reaction'* when referring to a case or series
of cases reported through a spontaneous ADR scheme.
The term 'adverse event' should only be used where all
events are being collected regardless of where or not they
are suspected to be related to a drug. Definitions of these
terms are given in EC legislation (Council Directive
75/319/EEC as amended by 93/39/EEC, Article 29b) and
have also emerged from the International Conference on
Harmonisation (D'Arcy and Harron 1995). These sources
also define what is to be considered serious and expected, criteria which are important determinants of
regulatory reporting requirements for the pharmaceutical industry. In particular, serious reactions have to be
reported to the authorities in the European Community
quickly (within 15 days), and reactions which are both
serious and unexpected have to be reported from any
source worldwide (see below).

There may be several reasons why a reporter suspects
that a drug may have caused an adverse reaction, including the temporal association, a relationship between
discontinuation of the drug and abatement of the possible adverse effect (dechallenge), a recurrence of the
adverse effect with reintroduction of the drug (rechallenge), knowledge of a mechanism, and absence of
alternative explanations for the adverse event. On their
own, none of these reasons (apart from the need for drug
administration to precede the suspected adverse reaction) is essential for suspicion of a causal association, but
the more that apply, the greater suspicion is likely to be.
However, clear-cut causal associations do not invariably
lead to increased reporting since knowledge of a mechanism and the effects of similar drugs may deter
reporting.

In the context of spontaneous reporting, a signal is normally a series of cases of similar suspected adverse reactions reported by health professionals associated with a particular drug. Initially, the key issue is whether or not there is an 'unexpected' number of cases. A single reported case is not usually sufficient to be considered a signal but, in the context of a particular disease which is rare in the general population (e.g. aplastic anaemia, toxic epidermal necrolysis), it is possible to show mathematically that a small number of cases associated with a single drug is unlikely to be a chance phenomenon (Begaud *et al.* 1994) and that this is not greatly dependent on the level of drug exposure. In this situation three cases may be considered a signal and five cases a strong signal. If the event is common in the population likely to be using the drug then clearly a much larger number of cases is needed to raise a signal, although there is no simple formula for determining the precise number. The strength of evidence for the individual cases is then an important consideration. A judgement needs to be made on the evidence available from the individual cases, in particular the quality of the evidence for an association and plausibility of alternative explanations.

The level of drug exposure is not necessarily critical in determining whether or not there is an issue which needs to be investigated further but, in order to put the number of reported cases in context, it is necessary to have an estimate of drug usage (usually prescription data). This enables an approximate assessment of frequency to be made and reporting rates to be calculated. A number of comparative methods are available for using spontaneous reporting data to generate signals. Reporting rates based on usage denominator data (e.g. prescriptions dispensed or defined daily doses [Speirs 1986]) may enable a signal of an increased frequency of a particular ADR in comparison with alternative treatments to be derived. All spontaneous ADR reporting schemes are subject to a variable and unknown degree of underreporting which means that such comparisons are crude. They need to be interpreted carefully, particularly if the drugs being compared have been marketed for different indications or durations, or if there has been significant publicity about the adverse effects of one of the drugs.

The other principal approach for making comparisons between drugs is to use the proportions of all ADRs for a particular drug that are within a particular body system class of reactions (e.g. gastrointestinal or cutaneous) or which are of a particular type (e.g. Stevens–Johnson syndrome). The former is known as profiling (Inman and Weber 1986), a method that has an advantage over reporting rates in that it is independent of the level of usage. The data may be displayed graphically as

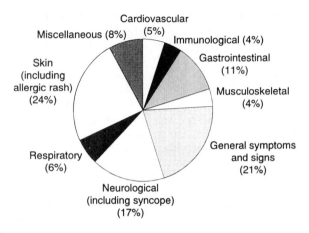

Fig. 3.1
The proportions of 2735 suspected adverse reactions reported in the UK by October 1995 as related to measles and rubella (MR) vaccine, categorized by the body system affected.

adverse reaction profiles, either for individual drugs or products (Fig. 3.1), or to make comparisons (Fig. 3.2). Mathematical use of this proportional approach can also be made by calculating proportional reporting ratios (PRRs) which are akin to odds ratios from a 2×2 table, with the proportion of reactions for a particular drug being divided by the proportion for all drugs within a database (Egberts *et al.* 1997). For example, if 10 per cent of all reactions reported with a new antipsychotic drug were aplastic anaemia but this ADR accounted for only 0.5 per cent of all reactions in the database, the PRR would be 20. In such an example only a small number of cases would be required to make chance an unlikely explanation and to raise a signal. Although

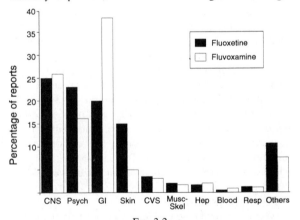

Fig. 3.2
The proportions of suspected adverse reactions reported in the UK by mid-1992 as related to the selective serotonin reuptake inhibitors, fluoxetine, and fluvoxamine, categorized by the body system affected.

PRRs have only recently been used in this context they have important potential for improving signal generation programmes.

Inherent in any spontaneous adverse reaction reporting system is a monitoring process which recognizes the dynamic nature of data. A prerequisite for an effective system is a database in which new reports can be entered speedily, prioritized according to their importance, and from which data can be retrieved and analysed in a variety of ways. The UK's Adverse Drug Reactions On-line Information Tracking or ADROIT database, which was introduced in 1991, provides such facilities (Wood and Coulson 1993). Regular and systematic review of what is new on the database in the context of what was there previously is necessary, most commonly by reviewing individual drugs or products looking for reactions of potential concern. An alternative approach is to bring together all the data for a particular adverse drug reaction and review the drugs which have been suspected of producing the reaction and the numbers of cases.

Spontaneous reporting systems exist throughout the developed world and in many developing countries. The World Health Organisation maintains a database of worldwide spontaneous reporting in Uppsala, Sweden, which holds around one-and-a-half million reports, to which most countries with an established spontaneous reporting scheme supply their data. Drugs are authorized and used differently across the world and, even in neighbouring countries, there are often major differences in clinical practice which may impact on ADR reporting. Whilst it reasonable to review, for example, the number of cases of a possible reaction reported worldwide in the context of worldwide sales data, it should be recognized that differences in clinical practice and patterns of reporting across countries limit this approach.

Spontaneous reporting is a method of collecting a series of cases of suspected adverse drug reactions and it is has the same limitations as any other case series. In particular, the data do not provide definitive information on causality or frequency (Rawlins 1988). Under-reporting is inevitable, variable and usually unquantifiable. It can be partially addressed in various ways, by education and feedback to reporters and by targeting specific factors, for example, serious reactions, new drugs, and specialist groups of reporters. Nevertheless, complete reporting is an unachievable objective which would not necessarily improve the effectiveness and efficiency of these schemes. Most schemes are voluntary and where they have been made compulsory in law there is no evidence that this has led, long-term, to increased reporting, since such legislation has proved unenforceable.

Spontaneous reporting schemes have been proven by experience to be capable of detecting unrecognized drug safety hazards. Examples of drug safety issues for which spontaneous reporting data have been of value are given in the next section. Compared with other methods of studying drug safety the method is relatively simple and cheap to operate, and is applicable to all drugs throughout their marketed life. The effectiveness of a spontaneous reporting scheme is dependent on education and motivation of its reporters, and on having in place the means and procedures for regular screening of the data. It would be unrealistic to expect 100 per cent sensitivity from ADR reporting, and other methods of identifying hazards also need to be used and developed further.

Examples illustrating the value of spontaneous ADR reporting

Spontaneous ADR reporting is of particular value in identifying associations between drugs and rare diseases, such as aplastic anaemia and toxic epidermal necrolysis. Both these conditions are associated with many different drugs and their diagnosis should automatically lead to consideration of possible drug causes. As discussed above, a small number of reported cases may be sufficient to raise a strong signal. In the case of remoxipride, an atypical antipsychotic drug, identification of five cases of aplastic anaemia after use by around 10 000 patients (Committee on Safety of Medicines/Medicines Control Agency 1993) was sufficient to provide clear evidence of an unacceptable risk in comparison to alternatives, and led to the drug being withdrawn.

An unusual and important example of the value of spontaneous ADR reporting is the association between use of high-strength pancreatic enzymes and the development of fibrosing colonopathy in children with cystic fibrosis. The original alert (Smyth et al. 1994) was based on five cases of this previously unrecognized disease, which leads to strictures requiring surgical excision. Subsequently a further eight cases were reported spontaneously in the UK by the time a retrospective search was conducted using a nationwide registry of cases of cystic fibrosis, as part of a confirmatory case–control study (Smyth et al. 1995). Only one new case was identified by the search and thus reporting for this new syndrome with a exclusively drug-induced aetiology was almost complete.

The association of non-steroidal anti-inflammatory drugs (NSAID) with upper gastrointestinal bleeding has been recognized for many years but it was only during the 1980s that substantive epidemiological data emerged, confirming and quantifying this adverse reaction. In the mid-1980s there was concern about the substantial mortality and morbidity associated with these reactions but few data were available comparing the relative toxicity of NSAID. Therefore UK spontaneous ADR data for NSAID were analysed using data from the first 5 years of marketing and prescription data as the denominator (Committee on Safety of Medicines 1986). Such comparisons are crude and need cautious interpretation but there were large differences between NSAID, with almost two orders of magnitude difference in reporting rates for serious gastrointestinal reactions between the highest rate (indoprofen, 555.6 reactions per million prescriptions) and the lowest (ibuprofen 6.6). Two NSAID with particularly high reporting rates of serious gastrointestinal reactions had already been withdrawn from the market (indoprofen and Osmosin) and three others had been withdrawn because of toxicity affecting other organs (benoxaprofen, fenclofenac, and feprazone). Of the 14 NSAID studied which remained on the market, reporting rates for suprofen, based on a small number of cases, were highest. This drug was subsequently withdrawn following identification of an unusual association with flank pain and acute renal failure (Hart et al. 1987). Reporting rates for serious reactions for the other NSAID varied from 13.2 (ibuprofen) to 87.9 per million prescriptions (azapropazone). On the basis of its apparently lesser level of toxicity, sale of ibuprofen without a prescription was permitted in the UK in 1983.

During the late 1980s and early 1990s a series of epidemiological studies examining the relative gastrointestinal toxicity of NSAID were conducted. These have been brought together in a published meta-analysis (Henry et al. 1996). Azapropazone was included in only two of these studies but in both was associated with particularly high relative risks. These studies prompted a further review of UK spontaneous reporting data in which reports from the first 5 years of marketing (during which reporting is known to be high) were excluded. Patterns of relative toxicity seen with spontaneous reporting were similar to those seen in epidemiological studies (Committee on Safety of Medicines/Medicines Control Agency 1994) and led to restrictions on the use of azapropazone.

Experience with NSAID and spontaneous reporting supports the use of cautious comparisons between drugs, providing denominator data are available, new drug reporting bias is taken into account, and there has not been substantial publicity suggesting differential safety during the time period of the analysis. In the case of gastrointestinal reactions, a class effect of all NSAID,

the data gave useful indications of relative toxicity which have been borne out by epidemiological studies. Where a drug in a class produces an effect not seen with the others (e.g. suprofen and flank pain) spontaneous reporting is the most likely method by which it will be detected in the postmarketing period. Another striking example of such a difference is cystitis with tiaprofenic acid, a reaction initially identified in the 1980s, the severity of which (sometimes necessitating cystectomy) was only recognized much later (Crawford et al. 1997).

Use of other methods in the evaluation of drug safety

Formal studies have a particular place in the investigation of signals generated by methods such as spontaneous ADR reporting (hypothesis-testing) although they may also provide the initial evidence producing a drug safety concern. Such studies do not necessarily start with safety as the primary objective but, if they have the potential to provide new safety data, it is important that the emerging evidence is kept under review. In particular, it is vital to maximize the potential of studies which expose large numbers of patients relative to exposure in previous studies. This should be achieved by ensuring that the design and methods facilitate risk assessment (e.g. by including comparator groups and measuring important outcomes). In a randomized double-blind trial, a safety monitoring group with access to the codes but no direct contact with investigators is essential. Such a group is also desirable in open studies. It is important to define in advance the criteria for an adverse effect which would lead to actions such as stopping the study. A more likely result is that a few cases of an unexpected outcome will occur. These need to be evaluated both as individual cases and in the context of the rates of occurrence in the different exposure groups. The advantages of the study design (e.g. control groups, known denominators) and appropriate statistical analysis must be fully utilized in assessing absolute and relative safety.

Most studies investigating the safety of specific medicines are directly sponsored by the manufacturer and are therefore covered by the regulatory guidelines (see below). Those which are not may be identified in the literature or through contact with various organizations which perform such studies, for example, in the UK the Drug Safety Research Unit in Southampton, which conducts prescription-event monitoring (Rawson et al. 1990) and Medicines Monitoring Unit (MEMO) in Tayside (MacDonald and McDevitt 1994), which operates a record linkage database.

Computerised record linkage has been used for drug safety purposes in North America for many years. More recently the UK General Practice Research Database (GPRD) has been extensively used and has been proved to be of considerable value for conducting pharmacoepidemiological studies. By virtue of its size (around four million subjects), representativeness of the whole population and quality of the data (Jick *et al.* 1991) it is an important record linkage database for drug safety studies. Because of the ready availability of data, leading to significant advantages in terms of cost and speed, and the variety of potential applications (Wood and Waller 1996), record linkage is becoming a standard pharmacovigilance tool of comparable value to spontaneous reporting.

Postmarketing regulatory requirements for the pharmaceutical industry

Under both UK and European law, Marketing Authorisation (MA) holders are required to provide information relevant to the safety of licensed medicines to regulatory authorities. The assessment of important safety issues involves close interaction with the MA holder. Where appropriate, manufacturers may be asked to provide safety update reports summarizing all the data available to them on a product or focused on a particular safety issue. The obligations on MA holders are laid down in European Community (EC) Regulation 2309/93 and Directive 75/319, and also in national regulations such as 'The Medicines for Human Use (Marketing Authorizations Etc.) Regulations' (SI 1994/3144) in the UK. Guidance to EC MA holders regarding these obligations has been given in Chapter V of the draft Notice to Applicants (Commission of the European Communities 1994).

Adverse reaction reporting

In the EC, MA holders are required to report serious suspected reactions occurring on EC territory, and serious and unexpected reactions occurring elsewhere, to the relevant authorities within 15 days. Non-serious reactions are submitted by MA holders in a summary form known as line-listings within periodic safety update reports (see below). The criteria for defining whether or not reactions are considered serious and/or unexpected are defined in the EC legislation (Directive 75/319/EEC, Article 29b).

Periodic safety updates

MA holders are required to submit safety updates with a specified format and content (Commission of the European Communities 1996) for all medicines authorized, regardless of the authorization procedure used. The periodicity is 6-monthly for the first 2 years after initial authorization within the EC, annually for the next 3 years, and then 5-yearly. The purpose of periodic safety update reporting is to facilitate regular and systematic screening of worldwide safety data by both pharmaceutical companies and regulatory authorities, and to identify issues needing investigation or action.

Postmarketing studies

Postmarketing studies are not generally regulated by legislation, although in the EC, in exceptional circumstances, they may be a condition of the MA. There are commonly in force voluntary guidelines for postmarketing studies agreed between the regulatory authorities and industry. In the UK these were introduced in the late 1980s (Joint Committee of the ABPI, BMA, CSM, and RCGP 1988) and then revised in 1993 (Medicines Control Agency *et al.* 1994) in response to concerns about the value of the studies that had been conducted (Waller *et al.* 1992). Such guidelines were adopted throughout the EU in the 1994 draft Notice to Applicants. All company-sponsored studies that are relevant to the safety of a marketed medicine are included. The guidelines cover the interactions between regulatory authorities and the MA holder, and specify the information which is to be provided. They also clearly state that such studies should not be conducted for the purposes of promotion.

Risk/benefit evaluation and regulatory action

The purpose of monitoring adverse reactions to medicines is to identify hazards which need further investigation, assessment, or action. This involves searching for supportive data, liaison with MA holders, and detailed review of the evidence. Major issues are subjected to full review leading to the production of an assessment report covering all the relevant information on risks and benefits, including pre- and postmarketing clinical data. In addition, it is sometimes appropriate to include preclinical studies. When major action is taken it is normally based on the advice of an expert committee, such as the Committee on Safety of Medicines. The options for action available are suspension, revocation or variation of the MA(s) and informing users through drug safety bulletins such as the UK's *Current Problems in Pharmacovigilance*.

Various sections of product information may require amendment in response to a drug safety issue, including the following:

Indications	Limiting the indications to particular conditions with the greatest benefits by removal of indications (a) for which the benefits are insufficient to justify use (b) for which use is associated with a greater risk of the ADR.
Dose	Reductions in dose; limitation on duration of treatment (especially for ADRs related to cumulative dose); provision of information on safer administration.
Contraindications	Addition of concomitant diseases and/or medications for which the risks of use are expected to outweigh the benefits.
Drug interactions	Addition of concomitant medications which interact; advice on concurrent prescription and monitoring.
Pregnancy/ lactation	Addition of new information relating to effects on fetus or neonate; revised advice about use in these circumstances based on accumulating experience.
Warnings	Addition of concomitant diseases and/or medication for which the risks of use need to be carefully weighed against the benefits; additional or modified recommendations for pretreatment investigation and for monitoring patients during and after treatment.
Undesirable effects	Addition of newly recognized adverse reactions; improving information about the nature, frequency, and severity of effects already listed.

For urgent new safety issues (usually significant restriction or drug withdrawal on safety grounds) doctors and pharmacists are normally informed through a direct letter either from the regulatory authority or from the responsible MA holder(s). When action has been taken on a particular issue, the effects of action taken are monitored and the issue re-evaluated in the light of any new data which become available.

Communication of drug safety information to users

Provision of information to drug users is essential to support the safe and effective use of medicines. The key requirements for a successful drug safety communication are that it should be specific for the target audience, easily understandable, open and informative, and well balanced, placing the issue in an appropriate context. Proposed communications need to be tested against these requirements by a review process which includes both individuals who are experts in the field and generalists. Communications intended for patients should also be reviewed by lay people.

It is particularly important in any communication about drug safety that essential information is clearly conveyed and not obscured by other less important information. The key facts and recommendations have to be worded unambiguously and placed in a prominently early position, if necessary with use of highlighting.

Information for doctors and pharmacists is routinely provided through the data sheet or the Summary of Product Characteristics (SPC). This is authorized by the regulatory authority on the basis of the available evidence and must be consistent with the MA. Information for patients must also be consistent with the authorization and it is provided routinely to patients through labels and patient information leaflets. In the EC, by virtue of Directive 92/27, these have been a requirement for all newly licensed products from January 1994, and they are being introduced for other medicines over a period of 5 years from that date. The key principles with patient information are that it should, in substance, be the same as the information provided to health professionals but it should be presented in language that a lay audience can understand. Good patient information adds to and reinforces the main issues which should be discussed between health professionals and patients, and does not make statements which could interfere with that relationship.

Ensuring health professionals are informed of important drug safety issues before there is media coverage is a major challenge. In the UK a variety of methods are used including first-class post, electronic networks, and fax cascades. It is also important to ensure that the media are properly informed, and hence direct briefing of the press can be useful, with the aim of encouraging balanced media coverage.

International aspects of regulatory pharmacovigilance

European Community (EC)

The EC has played a role in medicines regulation since Directive 65/65 came into force in 1965. This Directive obliges Member States to put in place a system for authorization of medicines based on safety, quality, and efficacy. At the same time, the UK (which did not enter the EC until 1973) was developing the 1968 Medicines Act, based on the same principles. When UK acceded to the Treaty of Rome, a broad view was taken that the Medicines Act had implemented Directive 65/65 and major change was unnecessary. In the USA the Kefauver–Harris amendment to the Food, Drug, and Cosmetic Act of 1962 expanded the controls of the Food and Drug Administration. All these legislative activities were a consequence of the thalidomide disaster and had protection of public health as their underlying objective. However, EC legislation also has objectives related to a single market for pharmaceuticals, and this has increasingly required regulatory harmonisation. The consequence of this has been the development of the new EC regulatory system which came into force in January 1995 with the establishment of the European Medicines Evaluation Agency (EMEA).

The new framework has three components: a centralised system (restricted to certain products including medicines derived from biotechnology and some new active substances), use of which leads to one NA valid in all Member States; a system of mutual recognition for most other products whereby a national authorization may be recognized in other Member States with identical conditions (or, if not recognized, binding arbitration may be initiated); and authorizations based on existing national procedures. Within these systems pharmacovigilance remains an activity which is based in Member States, with co-ordination at the EMEA for centralised products. The legal basis of the EC system and procedures are defined in amended Directives 65/65 and 75/319 and in Council Regulation 2309/93, the latter being directly effective in Member States and primarily relating to the centralized system. Both this Regulation and Directive 75/319 contain chapters on pharmacovigilance which define the obligations of the Member States and Marketing Authorization (MA) holders. These requirements have been underpinned by guidelines for Member States (Commission of the European Communities 1995) and for MA holders in the draft Notice to Applicants (Commission of the European Communities 1994), which cover adverse reaction reporting requirements, periodic safety update reporting, postauthorization, studies and ongoing risk/benefit evaluation during the postmarketing period. These guidelines are being revised and reissued during 1997–8.

In the EC, decisions relating to pharmacovigilance are taken on a formal basis for products authorized through the centralised and mutual recognition systems. They may be taken formally for products authorized nationally if the matter is deemed to be 'in the interests of the Community' and referred under Article 12 of Directive 75/319/EEC for a binding Opinion by a Member State, MA holder, or the European Commission. In such cases the matter is considered by the Committee for Proprietary Medicinal Products (CPMP), an expert body to which all Member States send two representatives. The CPMP has formed a Pharmacovigilance Working Party which meets to promote the development of common standards and approaches to pharmacovigilance and to consider specific drug safety issues, either as part of a formal procedure or informally at the request of a Member State. In the latter case the products are invariably authorized nationally and the objective is to see if common agreement can be reached on the measures to be taken.

International Conference on Harmonisation

The International Conference on Harmonisation of Technical Requirements for Registration of Pharmaceuticals for Human Use (ICH) is a forum for regulators and industry from the three major worldwide markets, that is, the USA, EC, and Japan, which was created in 1990. The purposes are to promote constructive dialogue between regulators and industry, to identify areas where modifications in technical requirements could lead to more economical use of resources in drug development without compromising safety, and to make recommendations for practical ways of achieving greater harmonisation of regulatory requirements (D'Arcy and Harron 1995). Under the auspices of a Steering Committee, a series of Expert Working Groups (EWGs) and a five-step agreement process have been created, and biennial conferences are held to ensure that the process is transparent. The main focus has so far been on the early phases of drug development but three EWGs are relevant to pharmacovigilance (i.e. Clinical Safety Data Management): Data Elements for Transmission of ADR Reports (E2B); Medical Terminology (M1); and Electronic Standards for Transfer of Information and Data (M2) (D'Arcy and Harron 1995). These three initiatives (E2B, M1, and M2) all relate to the process of communication in pharmacovigilance and reflect its increasingly global nature.

Future directions

In order to promote the safer use of medicines worldwide, regulatory pharmacovigilance must adapt to the changing pharmaceutical marketplace, and harness technological and methodological developments. Developments and improvements to all stages of the process can be anticipated, from signal generation, investigation, and evaluation to communication of the necessary measures to users. In order to meet these aims, continuing development of agreed standards and approaches, and efficient methods of exchanging data, are a high priority.

References

Begaud, B., Moride, Y., Tubert-Bitter, P., *et al.* (1994). False-positives in spontaneous reporting: should we worry about them? *Br. J. Clin. Pharmacol.* 38, 401.

Burley, D.M. (1988). The rise and fall of thalidomide. *Pharm. Med.* 3, 231.

Commission of the European Communities (1994). *Draft Notice to Applicants for marketing authorizations for medicinal products for human use in the European Union* (III/5944/94), p. 75, Brussels.

Commission of the European Communities (1995). *Note for guidance on the procedure for competent authorities on the undertaking of pharmacovigilance* (CPMP/175/95).

Commission of the European Communities (1996). *Note for guidance on clinical safety data management: periodic safety update reports for marketed drugs* (CPMP/ICH/288/95).

Committee on Safety of Medicines (1986). Non- steroidal anti-inflammatory drugs and serious gastrointestinal adverse reactions — 2. *BMJ* 292, 1190.

Committee on Safety of Medicines/Medicines Control Agency (1993). Remoxipride (Roxiam) — aplastic anaemia. *Current Problems in Pharmacovigilance* 19, 9.

Committee on Safety of Medicines/Medicines Control Agency (1994). Relative safety of oral non-aspirin NSAIDs. *Current Problems in Pharmacovigilance* 20, 9.

Crawford, M.L.A., Waller, P.C., and Wood, S.M. (1997). Severe cystitis associated with tiaprofenic acid. *Br. J. Urol.* 79, 578.

D'Arcy, P.F. and Harron, D.W.G. (1995). Background to the Conference. In *Proceedings of the Third International Conference on Harmonisation Yokohama*, p. 1. Queen's University, Belfast.

Egberts, A.C.G., Meyboom, R.H.B., de Koning, F.H.P., *et al.* (1997). Non-puerperal lactation associated with anti-depressant drug use. *Br. J. Clin. Pharmacol.* 44, 277.

Hart, D., Ward, M., and Lifschitz, M.D. (1987). Suprofen-related nephrotoxicity. A distinct clinical syndrome. *Ann. Intern. Med.* 106, 235.

Henry D., Lim, L.L-Y., Garcia Rodriguez, L.A., *et al.* (1996). Variability in risk of gastrointestinal complications with individual non-steroidal anti-inflammatory drugs: results of a collaborative meta-analysis. *BMJ* 312, 1563.

Inman, W.H.W. and Weber, J.C.P. (1986). The United Kingdom. In *Monitoring for Drug Safety* (2nd edn) (ed. W.H.W. Inman), p. 13. MTP Press, Lancaster.

Jick, H., Jick, S.S., and Derby, L.E. (1991). Validation of information recorded on general practitioner based computerised data resource in the United Kingdom. *BMJ* 302, 766.

Joint Committee of ABPI, BMA, CSM and RCGP (1988). Guidelines on post-marketing surveillance. *BMJ* 296, 399.

MacDonald, T.M. and McDevitt, D.G. (1994). The Tayside Medicines Monitoring Unit (MEMO). In *Pharmacoepidemiology* (ed. B.L. Strom), p. 245. John Wiley, Chichester.

Medicines Control Agency, Committee on Safety of Medicines, Royal College of General Practitioners, *et al.* (1994). Guidelines for company-sponsored Safety Assessment of Marketed Medicines (SAMM guidelines). *Br. J. Clin. Pharmacol.* 38, 95.

Rawlins, M.D. (1988). Spontaneous reporting of adverse drug reactions. *Br. J. Clin. Pharmacol.* 26, 1, 7.

Rawson, N.S.B., Pearce, G.L., and Inman W.H.W. (1990). Prescription-event monitoring: methodology and recent progress. *J. Clin. Epidemiol.* 43, 509.

Smyth, R.L., van Velzen, D., Smyth, A.R., *et al.* (1994). Strictures of ascending colon in cystic fibrosis and high-strength pancreatic enzymes. *Lancet* 343, 85.

Smyth, R.L., Ashby, D., O'Hea, U., *et al.* (1995). Fibrosing colonopathy in cystic fibrosis: results of a case–1control study. *Lancet* 346, 1247.

Speirs, C.J. (1986). Prescription-related adverse reaction profiles and their use in risk–benefit analysis. In *Iatrogenic Diseases* (3rd edn) (ed. P.F. D'Arcy and J.P. Griffin), p. 93. Oxford University Press.

Waller, P.C., Wood, S.M., Langman, M.J.S., *et al.* (1992). Review of company post-marketing surveillance studies. *BMJ* 304, 1470.

Waller P.C., Coulson, R.A., and Wood, S.M. (1996). Regulatory pharmacovigilance in the United Kingdom: Current principles and practice. *Pharmacoepidemiology and Drug Safety* 5, 363.

Wood, S.M. and Coulson, R. (1993). Adverse Drug Reactions On-Line Information Tracking (ADROIT). *Pharm. Med.* 7, 203.

Wood, S.M. and Waller, P.C. (1996). Record linkage databases for pharmacovigilance: a UK perspective. In *Databases for Pharmacovigilance* (ed. S.R. Walker), p. 47. Centre for Medicines Research, Carshalton.

4. Evaluating the effects of treatment

J. F. DUNNE

The role of observational research

For more than 50 years the prospective, double-blind comparative trial has served as the basis for determining which drugs qualify for admission into routine medical use, how they should be employed, and which of those available should be preferred in specific circumstances. There is no controversy about the need to resort to controlled clinical experiment for this purpose, but it is important to recognize that these trials provide an indication of what a treatment is capable of achieving, rather than what is achieved when it is used in a routine setting (Black 1996). The aim in designing a clinical trial is to obtain a clear-cut demonstration of drug-induced responses. The strategy is to strip away, as far as is practicable, extraneous sources of variation — both in the selection of patients and in their management — that might confound or independently influence the response to treatment and, in so doing, eliminate sources of bias that could obscure these responses. Any statistically significant difference in selected comparators or end-points between randomized groups of patients allocated to different treatments, it is assumed, can then be attributed with reasonable confidence to differences in the response to these treatments.

These constraints cease to operate when a drug is used in routine practice. It is then inevitably used in a wide assortment of patients and under conditions far removed from those imposed by trial protocols. It will be used in different populations of patients, in different age groups, perhaps at different dosages and for longer periods of time and, inevitably, in patients who are in poor general health, poorly nourished, or who may have other conditions for which they are taking other drugs. Any such factor may influence the response to treatment, sometimes in an adverse manner, in a way that could never have been predicted from the data generated in controlled trials. There is always an underlying reason for an adverse response to treatment, although available knowledge is often inadequate to provide an explanation. In this circumstance, understanding is likely to be advanced only if provision is made to report all such events to an agency with a responsibility to collate them, and to search for common factors and characteristics, and any clustering in time or place, which might provide clues to their causation. These clues provide the basis for further observational research based upon case–control techniques or generation of cohorts designed to examine and to quantify the strength of suspected associations.

These observational studies have a fundamental limitation. They do not provide proof of a cause-and-effect relationship. They are of vital importance, however, in establishing associations between two events (one being the administration of the drug under examination) which are inconsistently related. Whether the association is really determined by the administration of the drug in question or by some confounding factor associated with the patients likely to receive it is not accessible to proof. In the final analysis, causality can only be attributed by inference and plausibility. It is misplaced, however, to regard the information generated by observational studies as in some sense second rate. Experimental and observational studies provide complementary information, and both contributions are essential to safe and effective clinical management. Clinical trials are designed to assess the efficacy of an intervention, albeit in a setting that — in a formal sense — restricts the application of the results to a subgroup of the population of patients likely to benefit from its effect (Hlatky et al. 1988; Ward et al. 1992). Observational studies are designed to investigate events that are infrequently (but apparently) related to treatment, and which could only be studied prospectively under controlled conditions in trials which would often be too large and too extended in time to be practicable. From time to time efforts are made to conduct trials that seek to evaluate drugs under normal conditions of clinical practice, but this has resulted in unsatisfactory compromise (Schwartz 1967).

Because of heightened risk of intrusion of bias, few such studies have gained acceptance for publication in refereed journals.

Generic variation among pharmaceutical preparations

This chapter is concerned with factors that come into play, and may result in adverse effects, only once a drug reaches the marketplace and is used unfettered by the controls imposed during its clinical development. Before considering the biological aspects of the matter, it is important to point out that marketed pharmaceutical products contain an impressive array of excipients, which may differ substantially between generic forms of the same preparation. These excipients serve variously as fillers, binders, stabilizers, preservatives, surface coatings, solvents, emulsifants, dispersants, buffering agents, flavours, and colouring agents. They have a direct effect on the clinical performance of the preparation particularly in so far as they determine the release characteristics of solid dosage forms and depot preparations. Since few materials are totally inert biologically, excipients are implicated from time to time in adverse events, or they are found on routine screening to have potential toxicity which, in some cases, has resulted in restrictive regulatory action. The following examples illustrate the range of the problems that have arisen in recent years.

Chloroform was formerly widely used in pharmaceutical preparations as a solvent, preservative, and flavouring agent as well as for its anaesthetic properties. It was widely excluded from such uses in the late 1970s when positive results were reported from a carcinogenicity screening programme (International Agency on Research in Cancer 1972; National Cancer Institute 1976).

Use of several colourants formerly widely used in solid-dosage forms has been phased out in recent years either by regulatory action or by voluntary agreement of manufacturers, notably because of evidence of carcinogenic activity in animal screens or following reports of serious sensitivity reactions in patients. The most widely used of these — the yellow colouring agent, tartrazine — was withdrawn from many products in the 1980s when it was found to be implicated in development of anaphylactoid reactions in sensitized patients (United Nations 1994).

In 1982 benzyl alcohol was prohibited by the US Food and Drug Administration (FDA) as a preservative in injectable drugs and fluids intended for parenteral administration to neonates. An investigation attributed 16 cases of fatal metabolic acidosis among premature infants to the use of a solution of 0.9 per cent benzyl alcohol in saline which was used to clear intravascular catheters and to reconstitute drugs. Death was preceded by convulsions, and both blood and urine were found to contain high concentrations of benzoic and hippuric acid (United Nations 1994).

Polyoxyethylated castor oil, a non-ionic emulsifying agent used in the preparation of stable injectable liquid preparations of drugs, including anaesthetic agents, was withdrawn in some European countries in the mid-1980s following reports from Italy that it had been associated with cases of severe anaphylactoid reactions, altered blood viscosity, and red cell aggregation (United Nations 1994). It remained in use for the formulation of certain lipophilic drugs, including cyclosporin, for which no viable alternative could be found.

All injectable products containing povidone (polyvinylpyrrolidone with a molecular weight in excess of 12 000), which had been widely used as a stabilizer, were reformulated or withdrawn in Germany in 1983 following reports that large granulomatous lesions had developed at the site of injection, some of which had been mistaken for solid tumours (United Nations 1994). Polyvidone was formerly used as a plasma expander but, because it was shown to be sequestered within the liver and spleen, this use had earlier been abandoned.

Formulation of tablets and capsules that will retain consistent bioavailability throughout their labelled shelf-life can be an exacting task. Variations in particle size of potent substances, including digoxin, has been claimed to cause discernible changes in plasma levels, and deterioration in control of patients with epilepsy has been attributed to switching of formulations of phenytoin (Shorvon 1997). In a formal statement the International Union against Tuberculosis and WHO has warned (1993) that, unless batches of fixed-dose combination antituberculous drugs are consistently demonstrated to be of assured bioavailability, a risk is created not only of treatment failure but also of the emergence of drug-resistant strains of the tubercle bacillus. Substandard products have been reported to be in circulation in some developing countries and their prevalence may be widespread (*Indian Journal of Tuberculosis* 1988). Satisfactory bioavailability is particularly difficult to achieve in products containing rifampicin in combination with isoniazid or isoniazid/pyrazinamide. It has been claimed that not only is it necessary to use materials of the correct specification, but that the order in which they are mixed during the process of formulation can be critical to absorption characteristics (Acocella 1989).

The prevalence of substandard products

A decade ago there would have been little more of consequence to say about shortcomings in marketed drug products. However, in 1988, concern about the prevalence of 'counterfeit, substandard, and spurious products' was first raised in the World Health Assembly. Evidence has since been forthcoming from WHO and other sources that substandard drugs may be responsible for a wide-ranging failure of medical care in less developed regions of the world. A report on the quality of essential drugs on the markets of three countries in equatorial Africa illustrates in a devastating way what can be expected when national drug markets are inadequately controlled (World Health Organization 1995):

– of 26 analysed samples of chloramphenicol, 16 did not conform to specifications. Ten contained too little active ingredient, four contained none, and two tablet formulations failed disintegration testing;
– of 49 samples of trimethoprim/sulfamethoxazole tablets, six contained an insufficient dose and a further six contained neither of the active ingredients;
– eight of 28 samples of ampicillin contained too little of the active ingredient, and one contained none; and
– whereas all but two of 41 samples of quinine met specifications, the remaining two failed seriously. One provided an inadequate dosage. The other contained not quinine but mepacrine.

A similar account of grossly substandard antimalarial products has been reported from the Amazonian region of South America. High rates of relapse and recrudescence of *Plasmodium vivax* malaria were at first attributed to the emergence of strains resistant to primaquine. Subsequently, seven of 15 primaquine products tested between 1994 and 1995 did not comply with pharmacopoeial specifications, and some of these contained less than 20 per cent of the labelled content (Petralanda 1995). The 'enormous variety' of products and batches distributed to rural health posts rendered it impossible to generate reliable data on the reasons for treatment failure, and it was concluded that the situation was not only harming the indigenous population, it was also contributing to the selection of strains of plasmodia resistant to antimalarial drugs in the Americas at large.

The distribution of substandard antimicrobial products, on which these studies were focused, poses a triple threat: treatment failure compromises the health and sometimes the lives of large numbers of patients; the emergence of antibiotic-resistant pathogens is facilitated; and, ultimately, confidence in the health care system is eroded as first doctors and then patients realize that even benign infections are getting out of control.

In one, now notorious incident, the deaths of some 70 children who developed acute renal failure were attributed to a lethal contaminant, diethylene glycol, which was detected in liquid medicines that had been formulated by a local manufacturer (World Health Organization 1996). An investigation undertaken by the US FDA attributed this poisoning to a contaminated drum of glycerin. It is uncertain how the contents of this drum, one of many included in a consignment originating in China, came to be contaminated. En route it was handled by traders and brokers in northern Europe before reaching the manufacturer in Haiti. On the way, it seems that the heading on a certificate of analysis was changed and that stencilling on the drums was altered to indicate, at the stroke of a brush, that the contents — originally described as technical grade — met the specifications of the *United States Pharmacopoeia*. Anyone who assumes that conferring a facelift to a product in transit must be a rare aberration of normal trading practices should know that a term for this intervention is well-recognized in the trade. It is called 'neutralization' (Dunne 1997).

Diethylene glycol is widely used in industry as a solvent and antifreeze. It first intruded into the pharmaceutical arena in 1937, when some 107 children died in New York in a carbon copy of the Haiti incident (Gelling and Cannon 1938). It was this that provided the immediate stimulus to set up the world's first proactive system of drug control in the United States. Since then, the ready availability of diethylene glycol has resulted in identical tragedies being re-enacted in recent years in Argentina, Bangladesh, India, Nigeria, and South Africa (World Health Organization 1996; Bowie and McKenzie 1972; Okuonghae *et al.* 1992; Hanif *et al.* 1995).

It would be misplaced to believe that these incidents are without relevance to countries with highly evolved regulatory authorities. The Australian regulatory authority reports, for instance, that it has recently received a consignment of sulphamethoxazole from India in which the active ingredient was partially replaced by sugar milled to the same particle size and distributed in containers in a way likely to evade detection during routine sampling procedures (World Health Organization 1997a). New initiatives for assuring the quality of imported bulk pharmaceutical ingredients are now high on the agenda in international discussions between regulatory authorities. Counterfeited finished products of varying degrees of sophistication have been of similar concern to regulatory authorities and major pharmaceutical manufacturers for over a decade. Worldwide, some 700 such incidents have been reported to WHO within the past 4 years (World Health Organization 1997a). It is important for both pharmacists and prescribing doctors to be aware that criminality is now deeply ingrained in the international transit and distribution of pharmaceutical products. Whenever inexplicable clustering of an adverse drug-related effect occurs, the immediate response must be to consider whether there is some shortcoming in the quality of the product.

The intrusion of artefact

Observational studies conducted on a scale far greater than could be contemplated in the pre-computer era, have provided a mean of reassessing and re-quantifying some of the hazards known to be associated with long-established drugs. As a consequence of inadequate sampling, massive discrepancies existed in estimates of adverse drug-related haematological events even between neighbouring countries in Europe as recently as the mid-1960s. In Britain the risk of agranulocytosis associated with dipyrone was quoted to be as high as 0.8 per cent per exposure (Huguley 1964). In Sweden the annual incidence rate was calculated as 1:3000 (Böttiger and Westerholm 1975); in Germany as less than 1:10 000 (Arzneimittelkommission der deutschen Ärzteschaft 1965; Gross et al. 1967); and in Finland as less than 1:100 000 (Palva and Mustala 1970; Kantero and Mustala 1972). In many instances these risks are now seen to have been overstated. The International Agranulocytosis and Aplastic Anaemia Study (1986) estimated drug-related risks of agranulocytosis to range (for a variety of different drugs, including dipyrone) from 0.2 to 0.6 per million users during a one-week exposure. Even when the most adverse assumptions were made in interpreting the data (Shapiro 1984), they were judged to be reassuring in comparison with earlier estimates, but they did reveal some new associations. The digitalis glycosides, for instance, overlapped so frequently with other cardiovascular drugs thought to cause blood dyscrasias as to attract suspicion which could only have been generated through formal epidemiological research.

Similar inconsistencies have arisen over death rates attributed to aplastic anaemia. The mortality rate from aplastic anaemia during the early 1980s in Hong Kong — where, it seems, chloramphenicol (generally regarded as a major cause of aplastic anaemia) is prescribed on a scale 10 to 100 times greater than in western Europe (Col and O'Connor 1987) — is estimated to have been no more than 0.4 per 1000 deaths (Kumana et al. 1988). This is less than half the rate estimated by the Department of Health (1987) for the United Kingdom, and substantially lower than published estimates for several other European countries (International Agranulocytosis and Aplastic Anaemia Study 1986). This finding merits further examination given the continued importance of chloramphenicol to the management of serious respiratory infection within most developing countries, and the controversy that its use engenders.

The association of aspirin with Reye's syndrome — characterized by fatty infiltration of the liver and acute non-inflammatory encephalopathy — provides one of the most persuasive examples of the power of modern observational techniques. The association could not have been established prior to the first description of the syndrome in 1963 (Reye et al. 1963). Subsequent uncontrolled observations (Linnemann et al. 1975) and surveillance of cases throughout the United States by the Centers for Disease Control (1985), coupled with the results of two persuasive case–control studies (Halpin et al. 1982; Waldman et al. 1982), provided the basis, in 1982, for issuing the first warning against the use of salicylates in children with influenza and varicella (Centers for Disease Control 1982), and this was followed by a marked decline in the reported incidence of new cases (Centers for Disease Control 1987). Estimates of the incidence of this disease range from 0.3 to 5.6 cases per 100 000 exposed subjects (Johnson et al. 1963; Lichtenstein et al. 1983). The vulnerable subjects are febrile patients under 20 years of age (Centers for Disease Control 1985, 1987). Only a precisely focused observational study undertaken on a national scale could be expected to establish the cause of this rare but often fatal condition. As yet, however, the reason for these cases to be clustered exclusively among younger patients who are treated with aspirin remains unknown.

Variation between patients

An unanticipated serious adverse effect arising in a minority subset of the target population of individuals intended to receive a drug will rarely come to light during preclinical trials. Indeed, such patients may well be excluded from the trial protocol. Particularly if the effect is not closely associated in time with the administration of the product, it may only become apparent (whether by perspicacity or serendipity) through the outcome of a formal epidemiological study.

The evidence on which oestrogenic contraceptives — and subsequently combined oral preparations — were accepted for routine use was directed primarily to efficacy, since at that time no adverse long-term effects were anticipated. By current standards the trials were small in scale, of short duration, and they focused on highly fertile women in their early reproductive years. Only when the relationship between use of these products and thromboembolic disease began to emerge in the early 1960s (Food and Drug Administration 1963, 1966; Cahal 1965) were steps taken to assemble large cohorts of users and control subjects and to retain them under open-ended observation. In due course, estimates obtained from prospective cohort studies in the UK (Mann *et al.* 1975; Mann and Inman 1975; Royal College of General Practitioners 1977; Rosenberg *et al.* 1990) suggested that the excess annual death rate among users rose from about 1:20 000 among women aged between 15 and 34 years to 2:10 000 among those aged 35 to 44 years (a risk some 10-fold greater than that associated with intra-uterine devices) and, most disquieting, to levels as high as 1:700 among women aged 44 to 49 years. These deaths were largely attributable to myocardial infarction in women with other risk factors including obesity, hypertension, diabetes, hypercholesterolaemia, and, not least, cigarette smoking (Mann *et al.* 1975). None the less, the evident danger to older women called the acceptability of these products for routine use into question (Vessey and Doll 1976), resulted in stringent advice to prescribers, and set in train efforts to develop safer products which were to extend over the next two decades. This effort has been rewarded, since recent case–control studies have shown consistently that acute myocardial infarction is extremely rare among non-smoking women under 35 who use second-generation oral contraceptives (Vessey *et al.* 1997; Thorogood *et al.* 1991; Sidney *et al.* 1996; World Health Organization 1997*b*).

Variation in the environment

The benefit of maintaining under surveillance large cohorts of individuals who are treated for long periods with innovative products is now generally recognized. Experience with the antiparasitic drug, ivermectin, in community-based management of onchocerciasis in West Africa indicates the soundness of extending this principle to drugs that are intended for single or intermittent use. Ivermectin, a derivative of a macrocyclic lactone produced by an actinomycete (Campbell 1985), was introduced into human medicine over a decade ago. Trials undertaken in the western African Savannah demonstrated that, for the first time, onchocerciasis could be safely managed by community-based chemotherapy (Pacqué *et al.* 1990). Like diethylcarbamazine (DEC), ivermectin offers no prospect of a radical cure. However, its microfilaricidal action enables sight to be preserved

and pruritus to be relieved by a single oral dose taken once a year (Aziz 1986).

This use of ivermectin now extends into forested areas of west Africa where loiasis co-exists. Through the maintenance of a centralized reporting system on all patients treated with ivermectin, it rapidly became apparent that its use in patients with intense concomitant *Loa loa* microfilaraemia is associated with encephalitic reactions. This was first recognized when several reports of stupor and coma came to light in patients who had received ivermectin within the previous 2 days (World Health Organization 1991; Boussinesq *et al.* 1992). This finding inspired a study of tolerance to ivermectin in over 100 Cameroon volunteers with intense *Loa loa* microfilaraemia (Ducorps 1995). The frequency of acute neurological reactions was found to correlate with the intensity of the initial parasitaemia and with the passage of microfilariae into the cerebrospinal fluid. Above a threshold blood level of 30 000 micrfilariae per millilitre severe signs developed in an unquantified majority of patients. One of these patients developed a stage 2 coma, from which he eventually recovered following three weeks of symptomatic treatment with analgesics, anti-inflammatory and antiallergic agents, and diuretics (Chippaux 1996).

Further concern that ivermectin may have serious neurotoxic potential has recently arisen from an unexpected quarter. For over 5 years ivermectin has been used in developed countries, in the same single oral dose as employed for onchocerciasis in tropical countries, as a highly effective and convenient means of eliminating persistent epidemics of scabies among institutionalized patients (Glazion *et al.* 1993; Meinking *et al.* 1996). However, a pattern of excess deaths noted among 47 residents who received ivermectin in a long-term care facility in Canada has raised concern (Bartkwell and Shields 1997). During a period of 6 months subsequent to treatment with ivermectin, 15 of these 47 patients died, compared with five in an age-matched and sex-matched cohort of untreated residents in the same facility. This difference in mortality rates is highly significant (P<0.0001). Moreover, whereas there was no discernible pattern among the deaths in the control group, 'a sudden change in behaviour with lethargy, anorexia, and listlessness preceded death' in those who had been treated with ivermectin. Some reassurance that ivermectin is not generally hazardous to elderly patients has since been provided from Colombia where, it is said, 'ivermectin has been commonly prescribed for geriatric patients since 1989' (Diazgranados and Costa 1997) but, so far, no factor has been identified to explain the cluster of deaths in Canada.

Drug interaction

There is no evidence that concomitant use of other drugs has contributed to the deaths associated with use of ivermectin in Canada, but two recent events have driven home the need to remain alert to the potential for drug interactions to result in life-threatening adverse events.

For many years deeply entrenched reservations have existed over the use of centrally acting drugs, all of which are modulators of synaptic transmission, in the management of obesity. Cardiovascular toxicity, in particular, has aroused concern. Preparations containing phenyl-propanolamine were withdrawn in Germany and restricted in their use in several other countries in the mid-1980s after they had been associated with hypertensive episodes in susceptible individuals (United Nations 1994). In 1996 additional warning labelling was required in the USA for all products containing this sympatho-mimetic agent following concern that its use may increase risk of haemorrhagic stroke (Food and Drug Administration 1996). Thirty years earlier, preparations containing three anorectic agents — aminorex, cloforex, and chlorphentermine — were withdrawn in Germany (United Nations 1994) after aminorex had been associated with cases of primary pulmonary hypertension — half of which ended fatally — in Austria, Germany, and Switzerland (Gurtner 1990; Fishman 1997).

Within the past few years pulmonary hypertension has re-emerged as a rare but dangerous complication of treatment with the most widely prescribed appetite suppressants, fenfluramine and dexfenfluramine. These substances are structurally related to the amphetamines, but they both enhance release of serotonin from axonal terminals of presynaptic neurones and inhibit its reuptake. They consequently cause substantial depletion of intraneuronal stores of serotonin and release significant quantities into the systemic circulation (McTavish and Heel 1992). Sporadic cases of primary pulmonary hypertension have been associated with their use in the UK, France, Belgium, and the Netherlands (Douglas et al. 1981; McMurray et al. 1986; Pouwels et al. 1990; Brenot et al. 1993; Abenhaim et al. 1996). Almost 100 patients with primary pulmonary hypertension confirmed by cardiac catheterization were identified in these countries between 1992 and 1994 and the condition was shown to be strongly associated with use of these two drugs (Abenhaim et al. 1996).

It was anticipated that, by using smaller doses of these drugs in combination with a non-amphetamine sympathomimetic agent, such hazards might be overcome. A combination of low-dosage fenfluramine and phentermine consequently gained popularity in the United States (National Task Force on the Prevention and Treatment of Obesity 1996). However, very recently, the Mayo Clinic reported that 24 women who had recently developed cardiac valve regurgitation had started taking this combination of drugs within the previous year (Connolly et al. 1997). Eight of these women also had newly diagnosed pulmonary hypertension, and five had required surgery on one or more damaged valves.

Among further reports which were received almost immediately were several that associated valvular lesions with either fenfluramine or dexfenfluramine taken alone (Cannistra et al. 1997; Graham and Green 1997). Within 2 months of the initial alert, fenfluramine and dexfenfluramine had been recalled worldwide. By then, the FDA (1997a) had received over 100 reports of valvular heart disease among patients who had been taking this combination. A similar number of reports of symptomless valve dysfunction had additionally been detected by echocardiography. Within the cohort of exposed patients who were screened, almost one-third had abnormal echocardiograms. This finding is of particular concern because the FDA (1997b) has estimated that some 18 million prescriptions for fenfluramine and phentermine were written in the USA during 1997 alone.

The only other drugs to have been implicated in valvular heart disease are methysergide (Graham et al. 1966; Bana et al. 1974; Misch 1974) and ergotamine (Hauck et al. 1990; Redfield et al. 1992). Although these two compounds are serotonin antagonists, they also possess partial serotonin agonist activity and this is the property which is thought to account for their cardiotoxic effects, and to provide a link with the carcinoid syndrome in which similar valve lesions occur (Pellikka et al. 1993), and which is associated with high circulating levels of serotonin (Rabiolio et al. 1995). Although there is a strong presumption that the cardiotoxic effects of fenfluramine and dexfenfluramine similarly result from high levels of serotonin in the systemic circulation (McTavish and Heel 1992), plasma serotonin concentrations were apparently not measured during the investigations into valvular defects.

The second recent example of the potentially serious consequences of drug interaction is of a metabolic nature (Masheter 1993). Terfenadine, the most widely used of the non-sedating piperidine antihistamines, had been marketed for several years before it became apparent that it had a narrow margin of safety: raised plasma concentrations resulting either from overdosage or impaired hepatic function were found to induce ventricular arrhythmias, apparently by blocking cardiac muscle potassium channels and prolonging the QT interval (Monahan et al. 1990; Woosley et al. 1993). Reports soon followed of arrhythmias and occasional sudden deaths occurring when terfenadine was taken by patients receiving other medicines. Again, these events were associated with raised plasma concentrations of the drug resulting from slowed hepatic inactivation. Hepatic cytochrome P-450 enzymes are involved in the clearance from the blood of about one-third of all drugs currently in use. It has now been shown that this excretory pathway is overwhelmed when terfenadine is taken concurrently with a wide range of other drugs, notably the macrolide antibiotics clarithromycin, oleandomycin, or troleandomycin, and the antifungal agents, ketoconazole or itraconazole; neuroleptics; tricyclic antidepressants; and other drugs liable to disturb electrolyte balance (Honig *et al.* 1992; Honig *et al.* 1993; Nightingale 1997).

A chance observation has shown that even an occasional glass of grapefruit juice can significantly raise plasma concentrations of several drugs, including terfenadine. Grapefruit juice, it seems, transiently inhibits cytochome P-450 enzymes in the intestinal mucosa. In itself, this is a benign effect, but it can be troublesome when it results in increased absorption of substrate drugs (Lown *et al.* 1997). These enzymes had not previously been considered of importance to the pharmacokinetics of orally administered drugs. Having regard to the wide spectrum of activity of the cytochome P-450 enzyme system, it would be surprising if other piperidine antihistamines were not metabolised through the same channels. Many will have a wider margin of safety. However, astemizole has already been associated with cases of ventricular arrhythmia, and case reports held in WHO's international adverse reactions database indicate that disorders of cardiac rate and rhythm, including ventricular disorders, have also been reported in patients taking loratadine, acrivastine, and cetirizine (Lindquist and Edwards 1997).

In the case of terfenadine, the observations of individual clinicians rapidly led to a mechanistic understanding of its hazards. Other cases of apparent drug-related toxicity remain without explanation. It is important that they should not be lost from the record.

Unidentified sources of variation

Insoluble inorganic salts of barium were widely used for many decades in proprietary medicines available over the counter to the public for symptoms of dyspepsia and to promote 'regular' bowel function. In 1972, a patients' association in Western Australia reported that five of its members who had long found bismuth subgallate effective in controlling colostomy function had developed neurological disease (Lowe 1974). Some 25 similar cases were identified in response to a national appeal for further information (Burns *et al.* 1974; Robertson 1974). The clinical characteristics were similar in all cases. General malaise and lack of energy was followed after a period of months or years by failure of memory and power to concentrate. In some cases deterioration had progressed to the extent that patients were bedridden, incontinent, confused, and disoriented. In each case, it was stated, discontinuation of bismuth subgallate resulted in recovery, although in some instances improvement did not become apparent for several months.

It was immediately apparent, however, that this was not a dose-related effect resulting from marginal absorption of bismuth subgallate over prolonged periods of time. Whereas some of the patients had taken these preparations for several years before becoming ill, symptoms had developed in others within a few days of first use. One suggestion was that the illness might result from contamination of some preparations with tellurium, a metal that occurs naturally in association with bismuth, and which had been reported to cause somnolence, restlessness, convulsions, and death (Sollman 1957). Since analysis of samples provided no evidence of such contamination, and in default of any other explanation, all oral preparations of bismuth subgallate were withdrawn from use in Australia in 1974.

Simultaneously with these events in Australia, the first of a series of similar cases was reported from France (Buge *et al.* 1974). More than 100 cases were notified to the Centre Nationale de Pharmacovigilance (1975) within the next year, and in some of these bismuth was detected in both the blood and the urine. In all, some 300 cases were identified in a national survey, of whom 16 had died (Marin-Bouyer 1975). Very few, if any, cases were found to have occurred before 1974, and the majority of cases were reported from northern France, whereas bismuth was more extensively used in the south. The epidemic was brought to an end as soon as all preparations of bismuth were placed on prescription and doctors were warned of their apparent dangers. Two years later, only two possible cases of bismuth toxicity had been reported to the WHO international database of adverse reactions from the 34 participating countries.

Clioquinol, a halogenated 8-hydroxyquinoline, became of interest in the 1930s when it was found to be a useful amoebicide. Following the observation in one report that it appeared to have a broad spectrum of action against other enteropathic protozoa and bacteria, it was first promoted to the public as a treatment for diarrhoea (David *et al.* 1933). As a result of a chance finding, it also became widely used in the management of acrodermatitis enteropathica for 20 years until the drug was shown to be rectifying a selective malabsorption of zinc by forming an absorbable chelate. Some of these children developed optic atrophy (Garcia-Perez *et al.* 1974), but since such patients had formerly not survived, and because very little clioquinol was absorbed, it was thought that this might be a late manifestation of the disease.

Clioquinol had been used for the treatment and prevention of diarrhoea in Japan for 3 decades before subacute myelo-optic neuropathy — prodromal gastrointestinal symptoms, followed by an ascending sensory and motor neuropathy, and, later in some patients, optic nerve atrophy (Tsubaki *et al.* 1965; Kono 1975) — became recognized as a clinical entity in 1964. A few sporadic cases of a disease conforming to this description had been reported over the previous 7 years, but the number of cases increased dramatically from 451 in 1965 to a peak of 2340 in 1969 (Shigematsu *et al.* 1975). A statistical association between the use of clioquinol and the occurrence of subacute myelo-optic neuropathy (SMON) was first reported in 1971 in a series of 171 patients (Tsubaki *et al.* 1971) following the identification of a green deposit on the tongue of some patients, and in the urine and faeces of others, as an iron chelate of clioquinol.

Few new cases of SMON were diagnosed in Japan after September 1970, when all products containing clioquinol were withdrawn from the Japanese market. This established clioquinol as a crucial factor in the development of the disease, but opinions vary on whether this establishes a simple causal relationship (Oakley 1973). No factual evidence has been adduced to explain the rapid and progressive evolution of the epidemic between 1965 and 1969 (Meade 1975); why 15 per cent of the patients had apparently never been exposed to clioquinol (Kuroiwa and Kosaka 1973); why a systematic worldwide search yielded information on less than 100 possible cases of the disease elsewhere, and no indication that Japanese communities living outside Japan were vulnerable (Katahira *et al.* 1976).

A *Lancet* editorial (1980) has suggested that the epidemic neurological illnesses attributed both to bismuth and to clioquinol might be due to increased absorption resulting from an unidentified intestinal infection. Hypotheses, as yet, outstrip the facts. They are of value because they identify possible approaches to further studies. Some, because they are plausible, are held to have substance, but it is important to distinguish between speculation and formal proof.

It is disconcerting when medicines which have apparently long been used with apparent reasonable safety are suddenly and indisputably associated with serious disease. The examples selected in this chapter show how readily subgroups of patients vulnerable to serious drug-related adverse effects can escape detection, and how apparently banal factors such drinking a glass of grapefruit juice, taking two or more drugs together, or treating patients with onchocerciasis in forested areas can place lives at risk. Much remains to be discovered, and the clues can be generated only by astute and thoughtful clinical observation.

References

Abenhaim, L., Moride, Y., Brenot, F., *et al.* (1996). Appetite suppressant drugs and the risk of primary pulmonary hypertension. *N. Engl. J. Med.* 335, 609.

Acocella, G. (1989). Studies of bioavailability of rifampicin in man. *Bull. Int. Union Tuberc. Lung Dis.* 64, 40.

Arzneimittelkommission der deutschen Ärzteschaft (1965). *Deutsches Ärzteblat* 62, 2521.

Aziz, M. (1986). Chemotherapeutic approach to control of onchocerciasis. *Rev. Infect. Dis.* 8, 500.

Bana, D., MacNeal, P., Le Compte, P., *et al.* (1974). Cardiac murmurs and fibrosis associated with methysergide therapy. *Am. Heart J.* 88, 640.

Barkwell, R. and Shields, S. (1997). Déaths associated with ivermectin treatment of scabies. *Lancet* 349, 1144.

Black, N. (1996). Why we need observational studies to evaluate the effectiveness of health care. *BMJ* 312, 1215.

Böttiger, L. and Westerholm, B. (1973). Drug-induced blood dyscrasias in Sweden. *BMJ* iii, 339.

Boussinesq, M., Louis, F., Sam-Abbenyi, A., *et al.* (1992). Description d'un cas d'encéphalopathie après prise orale d'ivermectine. *Rapport commun ORSTOM/OCEAC*, Yaoundé, Cameroun, 26 August 1991.

Bowie, M. and McKenzie, D. (1972). Diethylene glycol poisoning in children. *S. Afr. Med. J.* 46, 931.

Brenot, F., Herve, P., Petitpretz, F., *et al.* (1993). Primary pulmonary hypertension and fenfluramine use. *Br. Heart J.* 70, 537.

Buge, A., Rancurel, G., Poisson, M., *et al.* (1974). Vingt observations d'encéphalopathies aigues avec myoclonies au cours de traitements oraux par sels de bismuth. *Ann. Méd. Interne* 125, 877.

Burns, R., Thomas, D., and Barron, V. (1974). Reversible encephalopathy possibly associated with bismuth subgallate ingestion. *BMJ* i, 220.

Cahal, D. (1965). Safety of oral contraceptives. *BMJ* ii, 1180.

Campbell, W. (1985). Ivermectin: a potent new antiparasitic agent. *Science* 221, 823.

Cannistra, L., Davis, S., and Bauman, A. (1997). Valvular heart disease associated with dexfenfluramine. *N Engl. J. Med.* 337, 636.

Centers for Disease Control (1982). Surgeon General's advisory on the use of salicylates and Reye syndrome. *MMWR Morb. Mortal. Wkly Rep.* 31, 289.

Centers for Disease Control (1985). Reye syndrome: United States, 1984. *MMWR Morb. Mortal. Wkly Rep.* 34, 14.

Centers for Disease Control (1987). Reye syndrome: United States, 1986. *MMWR Morb. Mortal. Wkly Rep.* 36, 691.

Centre Nationale de Pharmacovigilance. (1975). Le bismuth et ses dérivés. *Nouv. Presse Méd.* 25 juin–1 juillet 1975.

Chippaux, J-P., Boussinesq, M., Gardon, J., *et al.* (1996). Severe adverse reaction risks during mass treatment with ivermectin in loiasis-endemic areas. *Parasitology Today* 12, 448.

Col, N. and O'Connor, W. (1987). Estimating worldwide current antibiotic usage: report of task force 1. *Rev. Infect. Dis.* 9 (Suppl. 3), 232.

Connolly, H., Crary, J., McGoon, M., *et al.* (1997) Valvular heart disease associated with fenfluramine/phentermine. *N. Engl. J. Med.* 337, 581.

David, N., Johnstone, H., Reed, A., *et al.* (1933). The treatment of amoebiasis with iodochlorhydroxyquinoline (Vioform NNR). *JAMA* 100, 1658.

Department of Health. *Mortality statistics: Cause: 1981–5.* Series DH2 (ICD No. 284 and deaths from all causes). HMSO, London.

Diazgranados, J. and Costa, J. (1997). Deaths after ivermectin treatment. *Lancet* 349, 1698.

Douglas, J., Munroe, F., Kitchin, A., *et al.* (1981). Pulmonary hypertension and fenfluramine. *BMJ* 283, 881.

Ducorps, M. (1995). Effets secondaires du traitement de la loase hypermicrofilarémique par l'ivermectine. *Bull. Soc. Path. Exot. Filiales* 88, 105.

Dunne, J. (1997). Caveat emptor. *Drugs Quarterly* 1(2), 39.

Fishman, A. (1997). Appetite-suppressant drugs and pulmonary hypertension. *N. Engl. J. Med.* 336, 511.

Food and Drug Administration. (1963). *Final report on Enovid by the ad hoc Committee for the Evaluation of a Possible Etiologic Relation with Thromboembolic Conditions.* FDA, Washington DC.

Food and Drug Administration (1966). Advisory Committee on Obstetrics and Gynecology. *Report on the Oral Contraceptive.* FDA, Washington DC.

Food and Drug Administration (1996). FDA proposes additional warning label on over-the-counter PPA products. *Press Release T96-11.* Bethesda Md, 14 February 1996.

Food and Drug Administration (1997*a*). FDA announces withdrawal of fenfluramine and dexfenfluramine. *HHS News,* US Department of Health and Human Services. 15 September 1997.

Food and Drug Administration (1997*b*). Health advisory on fenfluramine–phentermine for obesity. *HHS News*, US Department of Health and Human Services. 8 July 1997.

Garcia-Perez, A., Castro, C., Franco, A., *et al.* (1974). A case of optic atrophy possibly induced by quinoline in acrodermatitis enteropathica. *Br. J. Dermatol.* 90, 453.

Gelling, E. and Cannon, P. (1938). Pathologic effects of elixir of sulfanilamide (diethylene glycol) poisoning. A clinical and experimental correlation: final report. *JAMA* 111, 919.

Glazion, P., Cartel, J., Alzieu, P., *et al.* (1993). Comparison of ivermectin and benzyl benzoate for treatment of scabies. *Trop. Med. Parasitol.* 44, 331.

Graham, D. and Green, L. (1997). Further cases of valvular heart disease associated with fenfluramine-phentermine. *N. Engl. J. Med.* 337, 635.

Graham, J., Suby, H., Le Compte, P., *et al.* (1966). Fibrotic disorders associated with methysergide treatment for headache. *N. Engl. J. Med.* 274, 359.

Gross, R., Horstmann, H., Vogel, J., *et al.* (1967). Zur Epidemiologie und Klinik der medikamentæs allergischen Agranulozytose. *Med. Welt* 31, 1767.

Gurtner, H. (1990). Aminorex pulmonary hypertension. In *The Pulmonary Circulation: Normal and Abnormal* (ed. A. Fishman), p. 397. University of Pennsylvania Press, Philadelphia.

Halpin, T., Holtzhauer, F., Campbell, R., *et al.* (1982). Reye's syndrome and medication use. *JAMA* 248, 687.

Hanif, M., Mobarak, M., Ronan, A., *et al.* (1995). Fatal renal failure caused by diethylene glycol in paracetamol elixir: the Bangladesh epidemic. *BMJ* 311, 88.

Hauck, A., Edwards, W., Danielson, G., *et al.* (1990). Mitral and aortic valve disease associated with ergotamine therapy for migraine. Report of two cases and review of the literature. *Arch. Pathol. Lab. Med.* 114, 62.

Hlatky, M., Califf, R., Harrell, F., *et al.* (1988). Comparison of predictions based on observational data with the results of randomized controlled trials of coronary artery bypass surgery. *J. Am. Coll. Cardiol.* 11, 237.

Honig, P., Woosley, R., Zamani, K., *et al.* (1992). Changes in the pharmacokinetics and electrocardiographic pharmacodynamics of terfenadine with concomitant administration of erythromycin. *Clin. Pharmacol. Ther.* 52, 231.

Honig, P., Wortham, D., Zamani, K., *et al.* (1993). Terfenadine–ketoconazole interaction: pharmacokinetic and electrocardiographic consequences. *JAMA* 269, 1513.

Huguley, C. (1964). Agranulocytosis caused by dipyrone, a hazardous antipyretic and analgesic. *JAMA* 189, 938.

International Agency on Research in Cancer (1972). Monographs on the evaluation of carcinogenic risk of chemicals in man. 1, 61.

Indian Journal of Tuberculosis (1988). Multi-drug formulations. *Indian J. Tuberc.* 35, 161.

International Agranulocytosis and Aplastic Anaemia Study. (1986). Risks of agranulocytosis and aplastic anaemia: a first report of their relation to drug use with a special relationship to analgesics. *JAMA* 256, 1749.

International Union against Tuberculosis and Lung Disease/ WHO (1993). The promise and reality of fixed-dose combinations with rifampicin. *Tuberc. Lung Dis.* 74, 180.

Johnson, G., Scarletis, T., and Carroll, N. (1963). A study of 16 fatal cases of encephalitis-like disease in North Carolina children. *N. Carolina Med. J.* 24, 464.

Kantero, I., and Mustala, O. (1972). Drug-induced agranulocytosis, with special reference to aminophenazone. 4: children. *Acta Med. Scand.* 192, 327.

Katahira, K., Tejima, R., Kusuhara, S., *et al.* for the SMON Study Group of the Koseisho (1976). An international survey on the recent reports of clioquinol intoxication and the regulations against its use. *Research Report for 1976.* Japanese Ministry of Health, Tokyo.

Kono, R. (1975). Introductory review of subacute myelo-optic neuropathy (SMON) and studies done by the SMON Research Commission. *Jpn J. Med. Sci. Biol.* 28 (Suppl.), 1.

Kumana, C., Li, K., and Chau, P. (1988). World wide variation in chloramphenicol utilization: should it cause concern? *J. Clin. Pharmacol.* 28, 1071.

Kuroiwa, Y. and Kosaka, A. (1973). Survey of SMON cases not taking chinoform. *Report of Study Team for Investigation of SMON in Specific Cases.* Ministry of Health and Welfare, Japan.

Lancet (1980). Idiosyncratic neurotoxicity: clioquinol and bismuth. *Lancet* i, 857.

Lichtenstein, P., Heubi, J., Daugherty, C., *et al.* (1983). Grade 1 Reye's syndrome. A frequent cause of vomiting and liver dysfunction after varicella and upper respiratory tract infection. *N. Engl. J. Med.* 309, 133.

Lindquist, M. and Edwards, R. (1997). Risks of non-sedating antihistamines. *Lancet* 349, 1322.

Linnemann, C., Shea, L., Partin, J., *et al.* (1975). Reye's syndrome: epidemiologic and viral studies, 1963–74. *Am. J. Epidemiol.* 101, 517.

Lowe, D. (1974). Adverse effects of bismuth subgallate. A further report from the Australian Drug Evaluation Committee. *Med. J. Aust.* ii, 664.

Lown, K., Bailey, D., Fontana, R., *et al.* (1997). Grapefruit increases felodipine oral availability in humans by decreasing intestinal CYP3A protein expression. *J. Clin. Invest.* 99, 2545.

Mann, J., and Inman, W. (1975). Oral contraceptives and death from myocardial infarction. *BMJ* ii, 245.

Mann, J., Vessey, M., Thorogood, M., *et al.* (1975). Myocardial infarction in young women with special reference to oral contraceptive practice. *BMJ* ii: 241.

Marin-Bouyer, G. (1975). Intoxications par les sels de bismuth administrés par voie orale. Enquète épidémiologique. *Thérapie* 31, 683.

Masheter, H. (1993). Terfenadine: the first non-sedating antihistamine. *Clin. Rev. Allergy* 11, 5.

McMurray, J., Bloomfield, P., and Miller, H. (1986). Irreversible pulmonary hypertension after treatment with fenfluramine. *BMJ* 293, 51.

McTavish, K. and Heel, R. (1992). Dexfenfluramine: a review of its pharmacological properties and therapeutic potential in obesity. *Drugs* 43, 713.

Meade, T. (1975). Subacute myelo-optic neuropathy and clioquinol: an epidemiological case history for diagnosis. *British Journal of Preventive and Social Medicine* 29, 157.

Meinking, T. Taplin, D., Hermida, J., *et al.* (1996). The treatment of scabies with ivermectin. *N. Engl. J. Med.* 333, 26.

Misch, K. (1974) Development of heart valve lesions during methysergide therapy. *BMJ* ii, 365.

Monahan, B., Ferguson, C., Killeavy, E., *et al.* (1990). Torsades de pointes occurring in association with terfenadine use. *JAMA* 264, 2788.

National Cancer Institute (1976). *Report on the Carcinogenesis Bioassay of Chloroform.* NCI, Washington DC.

National task force on the Prevention and Treatment of Obesity (1996). Long-term pharmacotherapy in the management of obesity. *JAMA* 276, 1907.

Nightingale, S. (1997). FDA proposes to withdraw terfenadine approval. *JAMA* 277, 370.

Oakley, P. (1973). The neurotoxicity of the halogenated hydroxyquinolines. *JAMA* 225, 395.

Okuonghae, H., Ighogboja, I., Lawson, J., *et al.* (1992). Diethylene glycol poisoning in Nigerian children. *Ann. Trop. Paed.* 12, 235.

Pacque, M., Munoz, B., Poetschke, G., *et al.* (1990). Safety of and compliance with community-based ivermectin therapy. *Lancet* 335: 1377.

Palva, I. and Mustala, O. (1970). Drug induced agranulocytosis, with special reference to aminophenazone. 1: adults. *Acta Med. Scand.* 178, 109.

Pellikka, P., Taijik, A., Khanderia, B., *et al.* (1993). Carcinoid heart disease: clinical and echographic spectrum in 74 patients. *Circulation* 87, 1188.

Petralanda, I. (1995) Quality of antimalarial drugs and resistance to *Plasmodium vivax* in Amazonian region. *Lancet* 345, 1433.

Pouwels, H., Smeets, J., Cheriex, E., *et al.* (1990). Pulmonary hypertension and fenfluramine. *Eur. Respir. J.* 3, 606.

Rabiolio, P., Rigolin, V., Wilson, I., *et al.* (1995). Carcinoid heart disease: correlation of high serotonin levels with valvular abnormalities detected by cardiac catheterisation and echocardiography. *Circulation* 92, 790.

Redfield, M., Nicholson, W., Edwards, W., *et al.* (1992). Valve disease associated with ergot alkaloid use: electrogardiographic and pathologic correlations. *Ann. Intern. Med.* 117, 50.

Reye, R., Morgan, G., and Baral, J. (1963). Encephalopathy and fatty degeneration of the viscera: a disease entity in childhood. *Lancet* ii, 749.

Robertson, J. (1974). Mental illness or metal illness? Bismuth subgallate. *Med. J. Aust.* i: 887.

Rosenberg, L., Palmer, J., Lesko, S., *et al.* (1990). Oral contraceptive use and the risk of myocardial infarction. *Am. J. Epidemiol.* 131, 1009.

Royal College of General Practitioners (1977). Oral Contraception Study. Mortality among oral contraceptive users. *Lancet* ii, 727.

Schembre, D. and Boynton, K. (1997). Appetite-suppressant drugs and pulmonary hypertension. *N. Engl. J. Med.* 336, 510.

Schwartz, D. and Lellouch, J. (1967). Explanatory and pragmatic attitudes in clinical trials. *J. Chron. Dis.* 20, 637.

Shapiro, S. (1984). Agranulocytosis and pyrazolone. *Lancet* i, 452.

Shigematsu, I., Yanagawa, H., Yamamoto, S. *et al.* (1975). Epidemiological approach to SMON. *Jpn J. Med. Sci. Biol.* 28 (Suppl.), 23.

Shorvon, S. (1997) quoted in: GPs increasingly favour brand name anticonvulsants. *Pharmaceutical Journal* 259, 320.

Sidney, S., Pettiti, D., Quesenberry, C., *et al.* (1996). Myocardial infarction in users of low-dose oral contraceptives. *Obstet. Gynecol.* 88: 939.

Sollman, T. (1957). *A Manual of Pharmacology* (8th edn). W.B. Saunders, Philadelphia

Thorogood, M., Mann, J., Murphy, M., *et al.* (1991). Is oral contraceptive use still associated with an increased risk of fatal myocardial infarction? *Br. J. Obstet. Gynaecol.* 98, 1245.

Tsubaki, T., Toyokura, Y., and Tsukagoshi, H. (1965). Subacute myelo-optic neuropathy following abdominal symptoms: a clinical and pathological study. *Jpn J. Med.* 4, 181.

Tsubaki, T., Honma, Y, and Hoshi, M. (1971). Neurological syndrome associated with clioquinol. *Lancet* i, 696.

United Nations (1994). Department for Policy Co-ordination and Sustainable Development. *Consolidated list of products whose consumption and/or sale have been banned, withdrawn, severely restricted, or not approved by governments.* 5th issue. United Nations, New York.

Vessey, M. and Doll, R. (1976). Is 'the pill' safe enough to continue using? *Proc. R. Soc. Lond.* Series B. 195, 69.

Vessey, M., McPherson, K., and Johnson, B. (1977). Mortality among women participating in the Oxford/Family Planning Association Contraceptive Study. *Lancet* ii, 731.

Waldman, R., Hall, W., McGee, H., *et al.* (1982). Aspirin as a risk factor in Reye's syndrome. *JAMA* 247, 3089

Ward, L., Fielding, J., Dunn, J., *et al.* (1992). The selection of cases for randomised trials: a registry of concurrent trial and non-trial participants. *Br. J. Cancer* 66, 943.

Woosley, R., Chen, Y., Freiman, J., *et al.* (1993). Mechanism of the cardiotoxic actions of terfenadine. *JAMA* 269, 1535.

World Health Organization (1991). Ivermectin: possible neurotoxicity. *WHO Drug Information* 5, 127.

World Health Organization (1995). La qualité des médicaments sur le marché pharmaceutique africain. *Programme d'Action pour les Médicaments essentiels.* WHO, Geneva.

World Health Organization (1996). Deadly paediatric drugs: diethylene glycol once again. *WHO Drug Information* 10, 84.

World Health Organization (1997a). The dangers of counterfeit and substandard active pharmaceutical ingredients. *WHO Drug Information* 11, 123.

World Health Organization (1997b). Collaborative Study of Cardiovascular Disease and Steroid Hormone Contraception. Acute myocardial infarction and combined oral contraceptives: results of an international multicentre case-control study. *Lancet* 349, 1202.

5. Mechanisms of adverse drug reactions

M. D. RAWLINS and S. H. L. THOMAS

Introduction

The classification of adverse drug reactions and interactions used in previous editions (Rawlins and Thompson 1977) has become widely adopted in the pharmacological and toxicological literature. In this scheme the unwanted effects of drugs are separated into those that represent *augmented* (Type A), but qualitatively normal, pharmacological effects of a particular substance, and those that are qualitatively *bizarre* (Type B) pharmacological effects. It has been suggested that this classification be extended (Grahame-Smith and Aronson 1984, 1992) by adding Type C (long-term effects) and Type D (delayed effects). We do not believe that such additional classes assist in understanding either the mechanisms of adverse drug reactions or their management. Most long-term effects (adaptive changes, rebound phenomena) and delayed effects (carcinogenesis, teratogenesis) are Type A reactions. Nor do we accept that idiosyncrasy (Hoigne 1997), defined as 'abnormal individual sensitivity to a food or drug', is necessarily equivalent to Type B adverse reactions (Rawlins 1997).

Type A (augmented) adverse drug reactions

These reactions are the result of an exaggerated, but otherwise normal, pharmacological action of a drug given in the usual therapeutic doses. Examples include bradycardia with β-adrenoceptor antagonists, haemorrhage with anticoagulants, or drowsiness with benzodiazepine anxiolytics. Type A reactions are predictable from a drug's known pharmacological and toxicological properties. They are usually dose dependent, and their incidence and morbidity are generally relatively high. Their mortality, however, is usually (but not invariably) low.

Type B (bizarre) adverse drug reactions

These reactions are totally aberrant effects that are not to be expected from the known pharmacological actions of a drug when given in the usual therapeutic doses to a patient whose body handles the drug in the normal way. Malignant hyperthermia of anaesthesia, acute porphyria, and many immunological reactions fall into this category. They are usually unpredictable and are not observed during conventional pharmacological and toxicological screening programmes. Type B reactions are often life-threatening or seriously incapacitating.

In individual patients the distinction between Type A and B reactions can usually be made on pharmacological and clinical grounds alone, but in a few instances two separate mechanisms may produce the same effect. Agranulocytosis after chloramphenicol administration, and halothane hepatotoxicity, are probable examples.

Mechanisms of Type A adverse drug reactions

When a group of individuals receive a drug, a spectrum of response is observed. This variability manifests itself either as differing doses required to produce the same effect, or as differing responses to the administration of a defined dose (Smith and Rawlins 1973) and forms the basis of Type A reactions.

Type A reactions are particularly likely to occur with drugs with a low therapeutic index. In some instances a Type A reaction occurs as an exaggeration of the primary pharmacological effect of a drug (the action responsible for its therapeutic action). Examples include bleeding with anticoagulants, hypoglycaemia with antidiabetic agents, and hypotension with antihypertensive drugs. In many instances, however, Type A reactions are the results of a drug's secondary pharmacological properties. An adverse effect may result as a consequence of a drug's primary pharmacological action at some site not associated with its therapeutic actions. Extrapyramidal reactions with classical (dopamine-receptor antagonist) neuroleptic agents, or the delayed carcinogenic effects of cytotoxic drugs and oestrogens, are typical examples. An adverse reaction also may arise from the non-selective nature of the adrenoceptor antagonists, or the gastrointestinal toxicity of non-selective cyclo-oxygenase inhibitors (classical NSAID [non-steroidal anti-inflammatory drugs]), are manifestations of such effects. Thirdly, a Type A reaction may be the result of some pharmacological (or toxicological) property wholly unrelated to, and entirely independent of, the effect that mediates the drug's therapeutic action. Tri-cyclic antidepressants, for example, possess antimuscar-inic ('atropine-like') properties that play no role in their therapeutic actions but which are responsible for the dry mouth, impaired visual accommodation, and difficulty with micturition, that are so frequently noticed by patients receiving these agents. Other examples include the antiandrogenic properties of cimetidine (Soltan *et al.* 1980), and the effects of terodiline (Connolly *et al.* 1991) and terfenadine (Rau *et al.* 1997) on myocardial potass-ium channels, resulting in delayed repolarization (pro-longation of the QT interval) and an increased potential for polymorphic ventricular tachycardia (*torsade de pointes*).

Type A reactions develop in individuals lying at the extremes of dose–response curves for pharmacological and toxicological effects. The reasons why they should occupy this disadvantageous position are threefold: first, the pharmaceutical formulation may predispose some individuals to toxicity; secondly, the way in which some individuals handle drugs is quantitatively abnormal (i.e. a pharmacokinetic change); thirdly, genetic factors or disease may alter the sensitivity of 'target' organs to drugs (i.e. a pharmacodynamic change). In some indi-viduals combinations of these causes may be responsible.

Pharmaceutical causes

Drug quality

In developed countries drug regulatory authorities, and manufacturers' own quality control procedures, ensure that (within certain defined limits) pharmaceutical prod-ucts contain the quantity of 'active' drug that is claimed in the labelling. In less developed countries, however, where drug regulatory requirements may not be so strictly enforced, or where manufacturers are less com-petent, there can be discrepancies between the alleged and actual quantities of the 'active' drug. Excessive amounts will lead to adverse reactions, and insufficient quantities will result in therapeutic failure.

Drug release

The release of active drug from a pharmaceutical prep-aration may vary with particle size, the nature and quantity of excipients used, and the coating materials.

Rapid release of highly irritant drugs may cause local damage to the gastrointestinal tract. Oesophageal ulcer-ation, particularly in patients with motility disorders, has been described in association with NSAID, emepronium bromide, and alendronate. Potassium chloride tablets were accompanied by an unacceptably high incidence of gastrointestinal haemorrhage, perforation, and cicatriz-ation (Boley *et al.* 1965). They were replaced by slow-release preparations, prepared in a wax matrix, to avoid high local (and toxic) concentrations. The large number of reports of gastrointestinal bleeding and perforation with Osmosin (a rate-controlled preparation of indo-methacin also containing, as an excipient, potassium chloride) was also probably due to the high concen-trations of the ingredients on localized areas of the gastrointestinal mucosa (Rawlins and Bateman 1984).

The rate of release may also have an effect on the intensity of the systemic effect of a drug. This is rarely a significant problem with conventional-release phar-maceutical preparations, but controlled-release (de-layed-release) products may cause difficulties. These preparations contain much greater quantities of active drug than conventional-release preparations, in order to achieve a long duration of action. If the integrity of the delaying mechanism is breached, the contents may be released too rapidly, resulting in 'dose-dumping' (Hendeles *et al.* 1985).

Pharmacokinetic causes

Pharmacokinetics is the study of the time course of drug quantities and actions in biological tissues (Dost 1953). It is therefore particularly concerned with the absorp-tion, distribution, and elimination of drugs. Quanti-tative alterations in these processes may give rise to abnormally high concentrations of the drug at its site of action and a correspondingly enhanced biological effect. Such alterations are therefore liable to produce exagger-ated but otherwise predictable pharmacological re-sponses, which are Type A adverse drug reactions. Alternatively, abnormally low drug concentrations may develop and result in therapeutic failure.

Drug absorption

Most drugs are administered orally, and absorption is possible anywhere from the mouth to the anal canal. A few drugs (e.g. levodopa), which are structurally related to naturally occurring dietary substances such as amino acids, are actively absorbed in the small intestines. Most drugs, however, are absorbed by passive diffusion. This occurs with the greatest facility in the jejunum and ileum, where the large mucosal surface area and blood supply promote diffusion of drug molecules across the lipoprotein cell membrane of the enterocytes. Lipid-soluble drugs, which can more readily cross cell membranes, are most readily absorbed. For those drugs that are weak electrolytes, only the non-ionized fraction will dissolve in lipids and be capable of absorption. The absorption of lipid-insoluble drugs is incomplete and frequently variable.

Differences in both the *extent* and *rate* of drug absorption may have profound therapeutic implications. Type A adverse effects can follow changes in either of these.

Extent of absorption

The total amount of drug reaching the general circulation (bioavailability) is obviously dependent on the administered dose. In the case of drugs given by mouth, however, other factors are also important. They include not only the pharmaceutical formulation of the drug, but also the tendency to form complexes with other ingested agents, the motility of the gastrointestinal tract, the absorptive capacity of the gastrointestinal mucosa, and the ability of the gut wall and the liver to destroy drugs before they reach the systemic circulation.

Influence of food　It had been assumed that while food might interfere with the rate of drug absorption, by delaying gastric emptying, it would have little material effect on the extent of absorption (Melander 1978). This is now known to be an oversimplification, for food may influence both the rate and extent of orally administered drugs. With many compounds, effects on the extent of absorption are clinically insignificant. Food, however, enhances the absorption of hydrochlorothiazide, nitrofurantoin, phenytoin, some anthelmintics (albendazole, mebendazole, thiabendazole), and halofantrine (Sjöqvist *et al.* 1997). Concurrent food can also reduce the presystemic hepatic clearance, and increase the bioavailability, of drugs such as propranolol and metoprolol, when given as conventional-release (but not delayed-release) preparations. The mechanism is uncertain. By contrast, the absorption of some antimicrobials (penicillin, rifampicin, isoniazid) is impaired by food.

Influence of other substances (drug interactions)

Charcoal, especially in its activated form, has a pronounced ability to adsorb drugs to its particulate surface. For this reason it is widely used in the treatment of poisoning with a wide range of drugs (Vale and Proudfoot 1992). Cholestyramine, an ion-exchange resin used to bind bile salts in the gut, also binds oral anticoagulants and decreases both plasma drug concentrations and anticoagulant effect (Robinson *et al.* 1971). Cations such as iron, aluminium, and calcium chelate with tetracyc-

lines, and fluoroquinolones (Neuvonen *et al.* 1991) impair their absorption. Oral iron substantially impairs the absorption of penicillamine (Osman *et al.* 1983), levodopa, levodopa/carbidopa combinations, and methyldopa (Campbell *et al.* 1988, 1990).

Gastrointestinal motility　Drug absorption from the stomach is slow compared with that from the small intestine. Changes in gastric emptying rate usually influence the rate rather than the extent of drug absorption (Prescott 1974). Some drugs, such as methyldigoxin, penicillins, and levodopa, are metabolised or inactivated in the stomach, and if emptying is delayed they may be relatively ineffective (Bianchine *et al.* 1971).

Changes in the motility of the small intestine may have important consequences for the extent of drug absorption by altering the time available for equilibration to occur across the gastrointestinal mucosa (Davis 1989). Reduced motility following the administration of propantheline enhances digoxin absorption by allowing the drug to ·remain longer at sites of maximum absorption (Manninen *et al.* 1973).

Gastrointestinal mucosa　Malabsorptive conditions, such as coeliac disease, might be expected to be associated with reduced absorption of drugs given orally. The effects, however, are inconsistent, and vary with the extent of disease as well as with the physico-chemical and pharmacokinetic properties of the drug. Absorption of drugs may be delayed (e.g. amoxycillin), decreased (e.g. thyroxine), increased (e.g. co-trimoxazole), or unchanged (e.g. indomethacin). During remission, however, drug absorption in coeliac disease appears to be normal. Altered absorption of some drugs has been demonstrated in patients with Crohn's disease, acquired immunodeficiency syndrome with gastrointestinal manifestations, and radiation-induced enteropathy but it is difficult to predict in individual patients. Careful monitoring is needed to prevent toxicity or therapeutic failure (Piper *et al.* 1997).

Presystemic elimination of drugs　For many drugs an appreciable fraction of the oral dose never reaches the systemic circulation despite virtually complete absorption from the gastrointestinal lumen. With drugs such as chlorpromazine, cyclosporin, glyceryl trinitrate, lignocaine, ethinyloestradiol, morphine, propranolol, and paracetamol, there is significant metabolism in either the gut wall or the liver before they reach the general circulation. Such presystemic (or 'first-pass') metabolism has several consequences. First, for some drugs (e.g. glyceryl trinitrate), presystemic metabolism is so extensive as to render the oral route ineffective. Secondly, there is substantial individual variation in the extent of presystemic metabolism, which can readily lead to either toxicity or therapeutic failure. Thirdly, presystemic metabolism will be less, and bioavailability greater, in patients with liver disease, thus predisposing them to toxicity. Fourthly, presystemic metabolism is inducible (see below) and can cause a further reduction in systemic bioavailability. Finally, inhibition of presystemic metabolism can result in toxicity. The H_1-antagonist terfenadine normally undergoes virtually complete presystemic metabolism to produce the pharmacologically active metabolite fexofenadine. Inhibition by macrolide antimicrobials, some antifungal agents, or grapefruit juice results in systemic exposure to significant quantities of terfenadine (Rau *et al.* 1997) which (unlike fexofenadine) delays myocardial repolarization and prolongs the electrocardiographic QT interval. This can result (see above) in the development of polymorphic ventricular tachycardia (*torsade de pointes*).

Rate of drug absorption

The speed with which drugs are absorbed after ingestion or injection will determine the plasma concentration–time profile after single drug doses. Delayed absorption will result in a slower rise of plasma drug concentrations, a reduced peak plasma concentration, and a tendency for a more prolonged elimination phase. This may be advantageous if the intention is to produce prolonged pharmacological effects (as with slow-release oral preparations, or depot injections of insulin or corticotrophin). The slower appearance of drug in the circulation, however, may delay the onset and reduce the intensity of drug action. For example, intramuscularly administered phenytoin crystallizes out at its injection site. This results in such a slow rate of absorption that peak plasma concentrations after injection of 1000 mg are rarely more than 2 mg per litre (Karlsson *et al.* 1974); since the therapeutic actions (either anticonvulsant or antiarrhythmic) occur only at concentrations of 10 mg per litre this route of administration is useless. When drugs are administered regularly, delayed absorption results in 'flattening' of plasma drug levels at steady-state during a dosage interval and has no effect on the average concentration during this period. This does not present any particular disadvantage except for those drugs (some antibiotics and cytotoxic agents) for which high peak plasma concentrations are required.

The rate of absorption of orally administered drugs is largely determined by the rate of gastric emptying (Prescott 1974), which is influenced by emotion and pain, by the nature of the gastric contents (volume, composition, and pH), by disease, and by drugs. Thus, ethanol or compounds with anticholinergic activity

(atropine, tricyclic antidepressants, and propantheline) slow gastric emptying (Nimmo *et al.* 1973) and delay absorption, while metoclopramide has the opposite effect.

Drug distribution

Drug molecules that have reached the general circulation are distributed to various tissues and organs. The degree and extent of this will depend (Smith and Rawlins 1973) on regional blood flow, and the facility with which drugs can diffuse across cell membranes (dependent on lipid solubility). In addition, drugs may be sequestered in body fat if they are highly lipid soluble; they may bind to tissue macromolecules; or they may be actively transported across cell membranes or tissue planes.

The extent to which a drug is distributed may be estimated by its distribution volume. This volume relates the amount of drug in the body to its plasma concentration.

$$\text{distribution volume} = \frac{\text{amount of drug in body}}{\text{plasma concentration}}$$

and the greater the extent of distribution, the larger is the volume of distribution. It is important to realize, however, that the volume measured is only *apparent*, and that it does not measure any particular anatomical space except in a few isolated instances.

Regional blood flow

Regional distribution of cardiac output and tissue perfusion rates are obviously important determinants of drug distribution. Our knowledge of the relevance of these processes — particularly in the presence of cardiovascular disease — to the distribution kinetics of particular drugs is scanty. There is increasing evidence, however, that for drugs whose hepatic metabolism is limited largely by liver blood flow (e.g. lignocaine), changes in hepatic perfusion may be extremely important. Thus, in cardiac failure (Thomson *et al.* 1973), after haemorrhage, during infusions of noradrenaline (Benowitz *et al.* 1974), or after β-blockade with propranolol (Ochs *et al.* 1980) or metoprolol (Conrad *et al.* 1983) liver blood flow is decreased and lignocaine clearance is reduced. In heart failure the central volume of distribution is, however, reduced and high drug concentrations may be observed after the administration of loading doses (Shammas and Dickstein 1988).

The changes in regional blood flow that accompany ageing also affect the rate of drug distribution. Liver and renal blood flows are decreased in the elderly (Woodhouse and Wynne 1988; Linderman 1992) leading to reduced rates of elimination of drugs undergoing extensive hepatic metabolism or renal excretion respectively. Moreover, an increased proportion of the cardiac output is distributed to the central nervous system, and this may result in excessive brain tissue concentrations.

Disturbances in drug distribution can also be demonstrated in end-stage renal disease — possibly due to circulatory changes accompanying chronic anaemia. McLeod and others (1976) have shown that in these patients not only is pancuronium elimination reduced (as might be expected), but its distribution volume is increased. These findings explain the clinical observation that patients with renal failure not only develop prolonged neuromuscular blockade following pancuronium but also require larger intravenous doses to produce adequate muscle relaxation.

Plasma protein binding

Many drugs bind loosely (reversibly) to plasma proteins. Acidic drugs bind predominantly to albumin, while basic drugs not only bind to albumin but more especially to the acute phase protein, α_1-acid glycoprotein. The bound drug is biologically inactive but in equilibrium with drug molecules free in plasma water. Only free (unbound) drug is available for distribution extravascularly, for producing biological effects and, in most instances, for elimination either by the kidneys or the liver. For those drugs the extraction ratios of which across these organs are high, however, both free *and* bound molecules may be removed.

Binding of drugs to plasma proteins can alter in a number of circumstances. Decreased binding will occur in patients with hypoalbuminaemia (for acid drugs) irrespective of the cause (e.g. nephrotic syndrome, starvation, liver disease, ageing). Decreased binding is also seen if there is competition for binding sites with endogenous (e.g. bilirubin, free fatty acids) or exogenous (e.g. other drugs) ligands. Increased binding of basic drugs occurs when α_1-acid glycoprotein concentrations rise in association with inflammatory responses (e.g. infections, acute myocardial infarction). Binding to α_1-acid glycoprotein is reduced in individuals with a genetically determined variant form of the protein (Eap *et al.* 1990).

The consequences of altered plasma protein binding are the cause of much confusion (Rawlins 1974; Benet *et al.* 1996; Sjöqvist *et al.* 1997). When highly bound drugs are administered rapidly, and especially after intravenous injection, a decrease in binding will tend to result in elevated free drug concentrations in plasma, and an enhanced pharmacological effect. Such a phenomenon is observed after intravenous diazoxide, a highly protein-bound drug, which produces a greater fall in blood pressure in patients with reduced binding to plasma proteins (Pearson and Breckenridge 1976). When drugs are given more slowly, or on a regular basis, changes in protein binding will have less effect, because the potential for an increase in the free drug concentration will be offset by distribution to other organs, and by increased elimination. At worst, changes in the intensity of drug action will be transient, and in most instances will be without significant effect. Descriptions in the literature of an association between Type A adverse effects and hypoalbuminaemia (Lewis *et al.* 1971; BCDSP 1973; Greenblatt and Koch-Weser 1974) are probably due to alterations in hepatic metabolism. Similarly, the accounts of displacement interactions between warfarin and drugs such as phenylbutazone (Aggeler *et al.* 1967) were due to inhibition of the metabolism of the latter by the former.

Tissue binding

The relatively large apparent volume of distribution of drugs such as nortriptyline (20–50 litres per kg) can only be accounted for by extensive tissue binding. This process is now recognized as an important mechanism for producing some adverse drug reactions.

Tetracyclines chelate with newly formed bone producing a tetracycline–calcium orthophosphate complex. The half-life of tetracycline in bone is of the order of several months (Buyske *et al.* 1960) as compared with a few hours in plasma. Although in adults this is of little clinical consequence, in neonates it may result in a 40 per cent depression of bone growth (Cohlan *et al.* 1963), as well as discolouration and deformation of teeth. Tissue accumulation also appears to be responsible for the pulmonary and hepatic toxicity of drugs such as amiodarone and methotrexate.

Drug elimination

Apart from volatile anaesthetics, drugs are excreted in the urine or bile, or metabolised by the liver to yield metabolites which are then eliminated by the kidneys. Changes in drug elimination rates are probably the most important cause of Type A adverse reactions. Reduced elimination leads to drug accumulation, with toxicity developing as a result of the elevated plasma and tissue levels. Conversely, enhanced elimination rates lead to reduced plasma and tissue drug concentrations, resulting in therapeutic failure.

Renal excretion

Drugs enter the proximal renal tubule by glomerular filtration. In addition, some organic acids are actively transported across the proximal tubular epithelium.

Table 5.1
Some acidic drugs undergoing active tubular secretion

Acetazolamide	Methotrexate
Cephalosporins	Salicylates
Chlorpropamide	Sulphonamides
Cloxacillin	Thiazides
Frusemide	Zidovudine
Indomethacin	

Glomerular filtration produces glomerular fluid drug concentrations identical with those in plasma water. Only unbound drug, therefore, appears in the filtrate and diminished protein binding may enhance renal excretion. Tubular secretory mechanisms also transport only unbound drug from the peritubular capillaries, but in contrast to glomerular filtration they reduce the concentration of drug in plasma water. Bound drug molecules, therefore, dissociate from plasma protein binding sites and so become available for transport. Active tubular secretion (see Table 5.1) is therefore totally independent of protein binding and may result in complete extraction of drugs across the renal vascular bed. Furthermore, interference with tubular secretion may seriously impair drug elimination.

Solute and water reabsorption along the course of the renal tubules will inevitably lead to a concentration gradient across the tubular epithelium. As a result, drugs will tend to diffuse from the nephron into peritubular capillaries, but their ability to cross cell membranes will be dependent upon their lipid solubility. Polar drugs, which are soluble in water (and therefore insoluble in lipid), will be unable to cross this membrane, and their clearances will approach glomerular filtration rate (or renal plasma flow if they undergo active secretion). Drugs that are lipid-soluble, however, will readily cross the tubular epithelium and reach equilibrium with free drug in plasma. Under these circumstances urinary drug concentrations and renal drug clearances will tend to be very low.

Glomerular filtration   Impaired glomerular filtration inevitably leads to reduced elimination of drugs that are undergoing renal excretion. Reduced glomerular filtration occurs in infancy, and in old age (Linderman 1992), as well as in hypovolaemic shock and intrinsic renal disease (Critchley *et al.* 1977). As a result, all these groups of individuals are liable to develop Type A reactions to drugs that are mainly excreted by the kidneys unless appropriate dosage adjustments are made. The absolute necessity for such changes depends on the drug's therapeutic ratio, its particular pharmacokinetic properties, and the degree of impaired glomerular fil-

tration. For only a few drugs (e.g. digoxin, lithium, and aminoglycoside antibiotics) are dosage restrictions necessary when glomerular filtration rates are 50 ml per minute or greater. In patients with more marked impairment of renal function, the doses of many drugs (e.g. angiotensin-converting enzyme inhibitors, β-adrenoceptor antagonists, cephalosporins, and fluoroquinolones) require adjustment. Details of appropriate dosage schedules for patients with impaired renal function can be found in the manufacturer's product prescribing literature. Nomograms for determining dosage schedules, which take into account a patient's renal function, age, and weight, are especially useful for digoxin (Mawer *et al.* 1972) in individuals with stable creatinine clearances.

Active tubular secretion   Some drugs are actively secreted by proximal tubular cells, against a concentration gradient, into the tubular fluid. Separate transport systems exist for acidic (penicillins, frusemide) and basic (amiloride, amphetamine) compounds. Competition between substances sharing the same transport system may reduce their renal clearance.

There is a separate active renal tubular transport system for organic bases, and similar competitive interactions may occur at this site. Thus cimetidine, and to a lesser extent ranitidine, inhibit the renal clearance of procainamide. The tubular secretion of digoxin is inhibited by quinidine (Leakey *et al.* 1980) and amiodarone (Fenster *et al.* 1985).

Tubular reabsorption   Passive tubular reabsorption of drugs may be influenced by urine flow and by the pH of the tubular fluid.

Increases in urine flow rate will decrease the time available for drug in the tubular fluid to equilibrate with free drug in the plasma and interstitial fluid. Moreover, alterations in the solute content of the tubular fluid, which occur following the administration of most diuretics, may effectively reduce the concentration gradient across the tubular epithelium. Consequently, increased urine flow may result in significant increases in the renal clearance of some drugs, and limited use can be made of this in the management of certain types of poisoning. Increased urinary flow rate, as a result of glomerulomegaly and increased kidney size, probably accounts for the enhanced renal elimination of some drugs in patients with cystic fibrosis (Prandota 1988).

The lipid solubility (and therefore the ease with which drugs cross cell membranes) of drugs that are weak electrolytes is dependent upon the pH of the solution in which they are dissolved (Milne *et al.* 1958). The ionized fraction of a weak electrolyte is, for practical purposes, lipid insoluble and so will not undergo passive tubular reabsorption. The non-ionized moiety, however, is lipid soluble and therefore capable of passing across the tubular epithelium. Weak acids (e.g. salicylate) become ionized as pH *increases*, and tubular reabsorption tends to diminish as the tubular fluid becomes more alkaline. Salicylate clearance, which at urinary pH 5 is of the order of 10–20 ml per minute, increases to 150 ml per minute at urinary pH 8. Similarly, the renal clearance of chlorpropamide increases from less than 0.1 ml per min (half-life 68.5 ± 10.5 hours) at a urinary pH of 5, to 15 ml per minute (half-life 49.7 ± 7.4 hours) at a urinary pH of 7. For weak bases (e.g. amphetamine), renal drug clearance increases with *decreasing* urinary pH. The effects of changes in urinary pH on the renal clearance of drugs are not only useful in treating some forms of acute toxicity but they may also account for substantial intraindividual and interindividual variations. Secretion of an alkaline urine may occur as a result of diet (e.g. in vegetarians), or because of other drugs (e.g. antacids, acetazolamide, thiazide diuretics), and an acidic urine is produced by a high-protein diet. In contrast, although drugs such as nortriptyline and propranolol (both weak bases) also undergo pH-dependent excretion, renal elimination plays such a small role in their overall disposal (less than five per cent) that changes in urinary pH can be confidently predicted to be of no clinical significance. Lithium ions undergo active reabsorption, predominantly in the proximal renal tubule, utilizing the same transport system as sodium. Drugs producing a compensatory increase in proximal tubular reabsorption of sodium ions (e.g. thiazide diuretics, metazolone, and frusemide) will increase lithium reabsorption and induce toxicity. NSAID may also facilitate the tubular reabsorption of lithium, giving rise to toxic plasma concentrations (DePaulo *et al.* 1981).

Biliary excretion

Drugs, or their metabolites (especially glucuronides), are likely to be excreted in bile if they are polar and their molecular weight exceeds 400 daltons. Ampicillin and rifampicin, for example, are excreted in high concentrations in bile. The hepatotoxicity of the NSAID benoxaprofen appears to have resulted from the precipitation of its glucuronide conjugate, which accumulates in plasma in patients with renal impairment, within the biliary canaliculi.

Some drugs undergo an enterohepatic recirculation. The drug, or more usually (as with ethinyloestradiol) its glucuronide conjugate, is excreted in the bile and reaches the gastrointestinal tract. The conjugate is hydrolysed by gut bacteria to liberate unchanged drug which is then reabsorbed. It has been suggested that the efficacy of combined oral contraceptives is reduced if a broad-spectrum antibiotic that changes the intestinal flora (e.g. ampicillin) is taken with them, as the enterohepatic recirculation of ethinyloestradiol may then be diminished. Direct evidence for this is, however, slender (Orme *et al.* 1983).

Drug metabolism

Renal excretion is an inefficient means of eliminating lipid soluble drugs because these are extensively reabsorbed in the tubules. During the process of evolution, therefore, pathways have been developed to convert lipid-soluble compounds into lipid-insoluble agents which then undergo excretion by the kidneys. The metabolism of foreign compounds occurs predominantly in the liver, although other organs, including kidney, lung, skin, and gut, have some metabolising capacity. Drug metabolism has traditionally been regarded as a 'detoxification' pathway whereby many drug metabolites are rendered biologically inert. It is apparent, however, that many have pharmacological, therapeutic, or toxicological activity.

In man, drug metabolism can be conveniently divided into two phases (Williams 1967). Phase I (oxidation, reduction, or hydrolysis) exposes functionally reactive groups or adds them to the molecule. Phase II (glucuronidation, sulphation, methylation, acetylation) involves conjugation of the drug at the site of a reactive group produced during Phase I. A typical example of these phases is provided by the metabolism of phenacetin.

Drugs that already have reactive groups (e.g. morphine, paracetamol) undergo Phase II reactions only. Others are sufficiently water soluble after Phase I to be eliminated by renal excretion. Each phase, however, tends to produce metabolites with increasing water solubility and decreasing lipid solubility.

Interindividual differences or alterations in the rate at which drugs are metabolised result in appropriate variations in elimination rates. As with renal excretion, reduced rates of metabolism will give rise to drug accumulation and increase the probability of Type A adverse reactions. Enhanced rates of metabolism may result in therapeutic failure. Some routes of metabolism are subject to wide interindividual differences, even among normal individuals, because of genetic and environmental influences. This particularly applies to oxidation, hydrolysis, and acetylation. Competition for glucuronidation may occur when two drugs metabolised by this pathway are given concurrently.

Microsomal oxidation   Drug oxidation occurs predominantly in the smooth endoplasmic reticulum of

TABLE 5.2
*Major human drug-metabolising cytochrome P450
enzymes and some substrates*

CYP1A2	CYP2C9	CYP2C19
Amitriptyline	Diclofenac	Citalopram
Clozapine	Ibuprofen	Clomipramine
Imipramine	Losartan	Diazepam
Tamoxifen	Phenytoin	Imipramine
Theophylline	*S*-warfarin	Omeprazole
	Tolbutamide	Propranolol

CYP2D6	CYP3A4
Amitriptyline	Codeine
Codeine	Cyclosporin
Clomipramine	Diltiazem
Debrisoquine	Erythromycin
Haloperidol	Lignocaine
Metoprolol	Nifedipine
Paroxetine	Terfenadine
Thoridazine	Verapamil

hepatocytes. It is mediated by a group of enzymes known as the cytochrome P450 superfamily. Currently, 12 families of P450 have been described in mammals of which four (CYP1, CYP2, CYP3, and CYP4) are concerned with drug metabolism. Other P450 families are involved in the synthesis and metabolism of a wide range of endogenous substances include prostanoids, fatty acids, and steroids.

Members of the CYP family are divided into subfamilies depending on the homology of their amino-acid sequences. Subfamilies are depicted by a capital letter, and individual P450 isozymes by a second Arabic numeral. CYP2D6, for example, denotes an isozyme belonging to P450 family 2, subfamily D, and isozyme 6. Table 5.2 shows the main human P450 isozymes involved in drug metabolism. Together they account for about 70 per cent of the total hepatic P450 expression with CYP3A contributing about 30 per cent, CYP2C about 20 per cent and CYP1A2 about 13 per cent of enzyme activity (Shimada *et al.* 1994).

The cytochrome P450 system has important features. There is distinct, but often overlapping, substrate specificity. Debrisoquine has high affinity for 4-hydroxylation by CYP2D6 and is almost entirely metabolised by this enzyme. On the other hand, the hydroxylation of imipramine is also catalysed by CYP2D6 but it is additionally demethylated by CYP1A2, CYP2C19, and (possibly) by CYP3A4. The activities of P450 isozymes also tend to show marked individual variability. Individuals receiving, for example, 300 mg daily of phenytoin achieve steady-state plasma concentrations ranging from 4 to 40 mg per litre (Loeser 1961).

Two of the P450 isozymes, CYP2C19 and CYP2D6, exhibit a genetic polymorphism. Homozygotes for the defective allele or alleles are liable to develop higher plasma drug concentrations at conventional doses, and so are at substantially greater risk of Type A adverse reactions. This is particularly the case with a drug, such as debrisoquine, that is metabolised predominantly by a single P450 isozyme (Mahgoub *et al.* 1977). In this instance, poor metabolisers are likely to develop marked hypotension after single doses. Furthermore, there are marked ethnic differences in the gene frequencies of defective alleles involving CYP2C19 and CYP2D6. Thus, defective oxidation of drugs metabolised by CYP2C19 is observed in 15–25 per cent of Asians but only three per cent of Caucasians. By contrast, defective oxidation involving CYP2D6 is commoner in Caucasians (five per cent) than Asians (one per cent). Oxidative metabolism by other P450 isozymes may exhibit genetic polymorphisms but this has not been confirmed.

Environmental factors influence the activities of P450 isozymes. Reduced catalytic activity has been observed in protein–calorie malnutrition (Walter-Sack and Klotz 1996) and during short-term exposure to relatively high doses of alcohol. The bioflavinoids present in grapefruit, though not orange, juice inhibit CYP3D4 activity and decrease the presystemic metabolism of nifedipine, terfenadine, and cyclosporin (Bailey *et al.* 1994; Rau *et al.* 1997). Drugs metabolised by the same P450 isozyme may competitively inhibit each other's oxidation, leading to increased plasma concentrations and a greater chance of Type A reactions. Erythromycin, cyclosporin, and terfenadine are all metabolised by CYP3A4. Co-medication with erythromycin predisposes to toxicity with cyclosporin or terfenadine. Similarly, many antipsychotics have a high affinity for CYP2D6 and inhibit the metabolism of tricyclic antidepressants (Leonard 1993). A drug may be also be a potent inhibitor of P450 isozymes without being a substrate. Quinidine selectively inhibits CYP2D4; fluvoxamine inhibits CYP1A2; and cimetidine inhibits several different P450s.

Environmental factors can also accelerate the oxidative activity of P450 isozymes by inducing their activity. Heavy cigarette smoking and consumption of charcoal-grilled (broiled) beef induces the activity of CYP1A2. Smokers thus have lower plasma concentrations of theophylline and clozapine than non-smokers. Regular intake of more than 50 g of alcohol daily over weeks or months also induces microsomal oxidation of drugs such as phenytoin and warfarin. A number of drugs are also known to induce P450 isozymes, particularly CYP3A4, as well as glucuronyl transferases (see below). When inducing agents are given to patients receiving a drug (such as warfarin) that undergoes microsomal oxidation, plasma concentrations may be decreased and therapeutic control lost. If, however, the pharmacological effect is mediated by an active metabolite, toxicity may occur (e.g. cyclophosphamide).

Mitochondrial oxidation   Various monoamines (e.g. noradrenaline, tyramine, phenylethylamine, phenylpropanolamine) undergo mitochondrial oxidation. Inhibition of monoamine oxidase (MAO) by inhibitors such as phenelzine and tranylcypromine, which are non-selective and which act irreversibly, can give rise to serious Type A interactions with agents normally undergoing presystemic metabolism by MAO in the liver. Patients taking non-selective MAO inhibitors are therefore liable to develop hypertensive reactions if they consume tyramine (contained in cheese, red wine, etc) or phenylpropanolamine (in proprietary cough and cold medicines). The reversible selective MAO-A inhibitor moclobemide is much less likely give rise to such interactions but sympathomimetic amines should still be avoided (Fitton *et al.* 1992). The interactions between MAO inhibitors and both selective serotonin reuptake inhibitors and pethidine are pharmacodynamic in nature.

Hydrolysis   The neuromuscular-blocking effects of suxamethonium are terminated by hydrolysis of the drug in plasma. Abnormalities of plasma pseudocholinesterase may result in impaired drug elimination and prolonged neuromuscular blockade. Plasma pseudocholinesterase is subject to a rare genetic polymorphism (Smith and Rawlins 1973). Aberrant genes are occasionally encountered, and individuals homozygous for the atypical gene (E_1,E_1) are encountered in one in 2500 of the population (Harris 1964). Such individuals may develop prolonged neuromuscular blockage. Heterozygotes (E_0, E_1) who possess both the usual and atypical gene comprise four per cent of the population; they have normal sensitivities to suxamethonium *in vivo* but can be detected by *in vitro* tests. Phenotypic studies of patients with prolonged neuromuscular blockade after suxamethonium do not always reveal recognizable genetic abnormalities. In some instances these Type A reactions are secondary to liver or renal disease, both of which are associated with impaired plasma pseudocholinesterase activity. Further cases still remain, however, after all these causes have been eliminated (Simpson and Kalow 1966) and may account for 40 per cent of patients with suxamethonium apnoea.

Acetylation   Acetylation is the metabolic pathway by which a number of drugs, including many sulphonamides, dapsone, isoniazid, hydralazine, phenelzine, procainamide, and sulphasalazine, are inactivated. Acetylation is under genetic control and shows a polymorphism: rapid acetylation is autosomally dominant. In the UK about half the population are rapid acetylators, but there are considerable racial differences. The percentage of slow acetylators varies between different populations being around 60 per cent in Europe, 50 per cent in Africa, 15 per cent in Japan and China, and five per cent in the Canadian Inuit (Kalow and Bertilsson 1994).

Slow acetylators eliminate acetylated drugs much less rapidly than other people. Consequently, they are at greater risk from developing Type A adverse reactions. Thus, hydralazine-related systemic lupus erythematosus (Perry *et al.* 1967), isoniazid peripheral neuropathy (Devadatta *et al.* 1960), haematological adverse effects of dapsone (Ellard *et al.* 1974), and adverse effects of sulphasalazine (Schroder and Evans 1972) and procainamide (Woosley *et al.* 1978) occur more frequently in slow acetylators.

Glucuronidation   Several drugs commonly used in clinical practice (e.g. morphine, paracetamol, salicylate, and ethinyloestradiol) are eliminated at least partially as glucuronide conjugates. Not only are these conjugates lipid insoluble, but they are also weak acids and undergo active transport into the renal tubules. There is evidence that, like the cytochrome P450 system, glucuronyl transferases exist in multiple forms with many drugs acting as substrates for more than one isozyme. Glucuronyl transferases are also inducible and the administration of an inducing drug can lead to loss of efficacy of combined oral contraceptive agents.

Effects of sex and age

Although sex has a modest effect on the metabolism of some drugs (Harris *et al.* 1995), these are generally small and without clinical significance. Some of the changes appear to be due to co-medication with combined oral contraceptives, which inhibit the oxidative metabolism of some drugs while inducing glucuronidation (Stoehr *et al.* 1984). Pregnancy, on the other hand, is accompanied by an increase in the rate of microsomal oxidation of some drugs, including metoprolol and phenytoin.

There are, however, important changes in drug metabolism with age. In the neonate, sulphate conjugation is well developed but microsomal oxidation and glucuronidation take place more slowly than in adults. In older children, the oxidative capacity for drugs such as phenytoin and carbamazepine, expressed in body mass, is higher than in adults due to the relatively large size of the liver. At puberty, metabolic rates approach those of adults. Drug metabolism is impaired in the elderly, which is one reason for the susceptibility of older patients to Type A reactions. In fit elderly people, changes in the rates of drug metabolism are mainly due to the age-related decrease in liver blood flow and liver mass (Woodhouse and Wynne 1988). Consequently presystemic metabolism, in particular, is reduced, and the result is greater systemic exposure to those drugs which normally undergo substantial biotransformation in the liver during absorption. In the frail elderly, there appears to be, in addition, a reduction in the intrinsic hepatic drug-metabolising activity, which increases their vulnerability to Type A reactions (Kinirons and Crome 1997).

Effects of disease

Because of the central role of the liver in the drug metabolism, liver disease might be expected to impair drug detoxication and lead to Type A adverse effects. Indeed, there is an increased incidence of adverse reactions to conventional therapeutic doses of many drugs undergoing hepatic metabolism (Naranjo et al. 1978), which is at least partly due to altered rates of elimination. Acute liver damage produces impairment in a variety of pathways of drug metabolism, which broadly parallels the change in prothrombin time. Thus, after acute liver damage from paracetamol poisoning there is a decreased rate of paracetamol metabolism (which provides a prognostic guide to the severity of the poisoning), but also slow metabolism of barbiturates, phenytoin, and antipyrine (Prescott et al. 1971; Prescott 1972). In chronic liver disease there is not only reduced *in vitro* activity of many of the enzymes concerned with drug metabolism (Brodie et al. 1981; Woodhouse et al. 1983) but also shunting of blood, which further reduces hepatic drug clearance. As a consequence, both first-pass hepatic metabolism, and systemic drug clearance (Blaschke 1977) are reduced to an extent which is correlated with the degree of hypoalbuminaemia. The changes do not, however, affect all metabolic pathways in parallel.

Renal disease is associated with alterations in the hepatic clearance of some drugs, although the mechanisms involved are poorly understood and the extent of the problem is ill defined. Thus, phenytoin oxidation is diminished in renal failure, and the conjugation of both metoclopramide (Bateman et al. 1981) and benoxaprofen (Aronoff et al. 1982) is reduced in patients with impaired renal function. The increased risk of adverse effects from metoclopramide in patients with renal disease is probably the result of its reduced elimination.

Toxicity of drug metabolites   Although many products of drug metabolism are biologically inert, it is becoming increasingly apparent that many drug metab-

olites possess important pharmacological and toxicological properties (Garrattini 1985). Thus, the desmethyl metabolites of amitriptyline and imipramine contribute to the actions of their parent compounds. Similarly, carbamazepine epoxide and acetylprocainamide have pharmacological properties that contribute significantly to the overall effects of carbamazepine and procainamide respectively. Some drug metabolites, however, have purely toxic, and no therapeutic, actions. Thus, the methaemoglobinaemia associated with dapsone is due to the formation (by P450 isozymes) of N-hydroxyldapsone, which is co-oxidized with haemoglobin to generate methaemoglobin and nitrosodapsone. Analogously, the urothelial toxicity of cyclophosphamide is mediated by the metabolite acrolein.

The accumulation, in patients with renal disease, of biologically active drug metabolites normally excreted by the kidney may predispose to severe Type A adverse reactions (Verbeeck et al. 1981). Examples include acebutolol (due to its acetyl metabolite), allopurinol (oxypurinol), pethidine (norpethidine), nitroprusside (thiocyanate), and propoxyphene (norpropoxyphene).

A further form of metabolite toxicity, and one which is probably of greatest importance, is mediated by production of highly reactive intermediates. During the course of certain forms of drug metabolism, particularly microsomal oxidation, highly reactive metabolites (peroxides, epoxides, and free radicals) are formed. Various cellular mechanisms for their inactivation are also present, including epoxide hydrolase, superoxide dismutase, and glutathione transferases. Where the rate of formation of reactive metabolites, however, is enhanced (e.g. by increasing the dose, or when the activity of 'activating' enzymes is increased), or the rate of their removal is diminished (e.g. by cellular depletion of glutathione), then severe cellular damage may ensue.

The hepatotoxicity of paracetamol, after overdosage, is also mediated by the formation of a reactive intermediate (Hinson 1980). After therapeutic doses paracetamol is primarily metabolised by glucuronidation and sulphation; only a small proportion is metabolised by P450 isozymes (CYP1A2, CYP2E1 and CYP3A4) to the reactive N-acetyl-p-benzoquinoneimine which, in turn, is detoxified by conjugation with glutathione. In overdosage, however, the glucuronidation and sulphation pathways become saturated, and increasing amounts of the reactive metabolites are formed which may not be adequately detoxified by hepatic glutathione. The reactive benzoquinoneimine metabolite binds covalently to a critical cell protein, and hepatic necrosis occurs. Induction of specific P450 isozymal activity (CYP2E1 in alcoholics and CYP3A4 by anticonvulsants) is associated with more serious liver damage, and a worse prognosis after paracetamol overdosage, due to the increased formation of the reactive metabolite (Bray *et al.* 1992; Zimmerman and Maddrey 1995). The use of precursors of intrahepatic glutathione (methionine and *N*-acetylcysteine), to replenish intracellular stores (Prescott 1996), is thus a highly effective form of treatment after overdosage, provided it is given before irreversible cellular damage has occurred. Renal damage after paracetamol overdosage is also caused by a reactive intermediate, but one that is produced by prostaglandin H synthetase rather than P450 isoenzymes, which are present in only low levels in the regions of the kidney where toxicity occurs.

Pharmacodynamic causes

Many, if not most, Type A adverse drug reactions have a pharmacokinetic basis. Some, however, are undoubtedly due to enhanced sensitivity of target organs or tissues. Moreover, in some individuals, adverse drug reactions derive from a combination of these two.

The reasons why tissues from different individuals should respond differently to drugs are still largely unknown; but evidence is accumulating to show that target organ sensitivity is influenced by the drug receptors themselves, by physiological homoeostatic mechanisms, and by disease.

Drug receptors

Many drugs exert their pharmacological effects by combining with specific receptors (Paton 1970). These receptors may be on cell membranes, or within the cytoplasm or nucleus. Their normal function is to provide the means whereby endogenous extracellular substances may influence intracellular events. There are therefore specific receptors for neurotransmitters (e.g. noradrenaline, dopamine, and acetylcholine), hormones (e.g. glucocorticoids, corticotrophin [ACTH], and sex hormones), vitamins (e.g. vitamins D and K), and lipids (e.g. low-density lipoproteins). Specific receptors appear to be protein molecules and some, though not all, are enzymes. There are two ways in which the target organs of different individuals might respond differently to drugs acting through specific receptors. First, receptors might differ between individuals, some being less 'potent' than others. Secondly, different individuals might have different numbers of receptors in their tissues.

There is little direct evidence to support the first hypothesis. Hereditary warfarin resistance (O'Reilly *et al.* 1964; O'Reilly 1970), however, may be an example.

This disorder, which has now been observed in several families, is manifested by extreme warfarin resistance so that huge doses and very high plasma levels are required to achieve therapeutic anticoagulation. Conversely, these individuals are extremely sensitive to the warfarin-antagonizing actions of vitamin K. These observations are compatible with the hypothesis that affected individuals possess abnormal warfarin–vitamin K receptors, resulting in an increased affinity for vitamin K (Hulse 1996). There are other explanations (such as differences in clotting factor synthesis) that have yet to be excluded. Hereditary warfarin resistance should not be confused with warfarin resistance due to unusually rapid warfarin clearance (Hallak *et al.* 1993).

Indirect estimates have been made of the affinity constants (or pA_2 values) of the β-adrenoceptor antagonists propranolol (McDevitt *et al.* 1976) and labetalol (Sanders *et al.* 1979) in man. Both studies suggested that there may be differences between individuals, and in hypertension, but further work is required to confirm the heterogenicity in man. Reduced sensitivity of cardiac β-receptors to both agonists (isoprenaline) and antagonists (propranolol) has been observed in the elderly. This does not appear to be due to reduced receptor numbers (Elfellah *et al.* 1989), but to reduced agonist binding affinity, receptor efficacy, and activity. This results in a reduced cAMP response to β_2-agonists, as well as to direct adenylate cyclase activators such as forskolin and sodium fluoride (Abrass and Scarpace 1982). The transient pressor response to intravenous clonidine is also lost, probably because of reduced peripheral vascular α_2-adrenergic responsiveness (Ford and James 1994).

The elderly display increased sensitivity to benzodiazepines. This is not purely a pharmacokinetic phenomenon, but the pharmacodynamic mechanism for enhanced sensitivity is unclear. So far, age has not been shown to affect benzodiazepine receptor density or chloride ionophore function. Conversely, the increased sensitivity of the elderly to opiates, which is not due to pharmacokinetic changes, may be due to alterations in opiate receptor density (Stanski and Maitre 1990).

There is now both experimental and clinical evidence to indicate that the number of specific receptors in tissues may vary. Glucocorticoids exert their inhibitory effects on cell growth by combining with specific cytoplasmic protein receptors (Hackney *et al.* 1970). The steroid–receptor complex is then transported into the nucleus where the glucocorticoid combines with a second receptor. Nuclear steroid–receptor complexes modify the control of RNA and protein synthesis, leading to inhibition of cell growth. Cells with diminished amounts of cytoplasmic glucocorticoid receptors are resistant *in vitro* and *in vivo* to the inhibitory effects of steroids. In man, the presence of oestrogen and progestogen receptors in breast tumours appears to determine the *in vivo* response to endocrine therapy (McGuire *et al.* 1977).

Where the receptors for a particular drug are enzymes, qualitative differences may be important mechanisms of altering drug sensitivity. In bacteria, resistance to sulphonamides may be due to the presence of an enzyme with altered affinity for the drug, as shown by Pato and Brown (1963). These workers also showed, however, that certain resistant strains had normal enzymes, and suggested that resistance was due to failure of the drug to enter the cell.

Receptor sensitivity may also be affected by other drugs. The action of specific antagonists and agonists is well known. There is a suggestion, however, that some interactions involve a more subtle mechanism. Although norethandrolone, clofibrate, and thyroxine have no anticoagulant actions by themselves, they all potentiate the anticoagulant effects of warfarin by a mechanism that does not appear to be pharmacokinetic (Schrogie and Solomon 1967). It has been suggested that these drugs all increase the affinity of anticoagulant for its hepatic receptor site (Solomon and Schrogie 1967). Long-term therapy with long-acting β_2-agonists (such as formoterol) causes down-regulation and desensitization of β_2-receptors in the airways. This can be reversed by corticosteroids, which restore the response to β_2-agonists (Tan *et al.* 1996).

Homoeostatic mechanisms

The actions of most drugs occur within the milieu of complex physiological control systems. The magnitude of a drug's effects may be dependent on such physiological factors. For example, intravenous atropine (an acetylcholine antagonist) produces a variable increase in heart rate and some individuals develop tachycardia of 160 beats per minute at a dose which is almost ineffective in others. The magnitude of the observed effect is dependent on the balance between parasympathetic and sympathetic cardiac tone which appears to be under genetic control (Bertler and Smith 1971). The capacity of a homoeostatic reflex to compensate for a drug action may be affected by individual factors or by disease. For example, patients with secondary hyperaldosteronism from, for example, cardiac failure or cirrhosis, are more likely to develop hypokalaemia when treated with diuretics. Similarly, vasodilators are more likely to precipitate postural hypotension in subjects with autonomic neuropathy or those with impaired cardiac function.

Disease

Intercurrent disease may unmask pharmacological effects not apparent in normal individuals. Haemorrhage or perforation of peptic ulcers due to the anti-inflammatory actions of corticosteroids are a typical example. There are many other examples. Bronchoconstriction may be precipitated in patients with obstructive airways disease when given unselective β-adrenoceptor antagonists such as propranolol. Extrapyramidal symptoms are more often precipitated by antidopaminergic drugs in subjects with depleted basal-ganglia dopaminergic transmission, such as the elderly and those with Parkinson's disease. Cardiac failure may be precipitated by negatively inotropic drugs in subjects with impaired left ventricular function, but is unusual in those with normal cardiac function prior to drug exposure. More subtle is the neuromuscular blockade that may be precipitated by streptomycin, neomycin, or kanamycin. These drugs have curare-like actions and reduce the sensitivity of motor end-plates to the depolarizing effects of acetylcholine. Their effects, however, are relatively feeble, and clinically inapparent in normal individuals. In patients already receiving muscle relaxants, or with myasthenia gravis, their pharmacological properties are unmasked and may produce paralysis (Toivakka and Hokkanen 1965).

Altered thyroid function influences the effects of adrenergic agonists and antagonists. In thyrotoxicosis, there is increased sensitivity to adrenergic agonists. This appears to be due to both an increased number of β-receptors and increased receptor efficacy (Wahrenberg *et al.* 1986).

Neoplastic and teratological reasons for abnormal response

The possibility that a drug may be a significant factor in causing teratological or neoplastic changes is well known and these subjects are dealt with in detail in other chapters of this book (see Chapters 7 and 26). These adverse reactions are almost invariably of type A, being dose related and predictable. For example, carcinogenesis may arise from genetic damage which is dose related; this may result in cancer by activation of oncogenes or inactivation of suppressor genes. Similarly, dose-related epigenic drug effects may promote cancer development by, for example, stimulation of cell proliferation, and the aetiology of cancer may be complicated by unpredictable factors, such as the effects of genetic and environmental factors on an individual's ability to metabolise carcinogens, repair DNA damage, or respond to mitogens (Couch 1996). It is also important, however, to consider the possibility that a qualitatively abnormal response to a drug may occur as a result of the presence of some potentially neoplastic or teratological tissue in the organism. A preneoplastic condition may well be transformed into a frankly neoplastic state by the administration of a drug, such as an oestrogen or an androgen, which is given to treat some entirely unrelated condition.

Mechanisms of Type B adverse drug reactions

The distinguishing feature of Type B reactions is that they are aberrant, that is, inexplicable in terms of the normal pharmacology of the drug, and that they form a heterogeneous group. Pathogenetically they are characterized by the existence of some qualitative difference either in the drug, or in the patient, or possibly in both. The cause may be pharmacokinetic or pharmaceutical, or may lie in target organ response.

Pharmaceutical causes

There are three potential sources of Type B adverse reactions due to abnormalities of the drug: firstly, decomposition of the active constituents; secondly, effects of the additives, solubilizers, stabilizers, colourizers, and excipients, commonly incorporated in pharmaceutical preparations; and thirdly, effects from by-products of the active constituents of chemical synthesis. While these are, properly, Type B reactions to the therapeutically active drug they are almost invariably Type A effects of the particular toxic ingredient. Some drugs are chemically stable (e.g. lignocaine), while others are very unstable (e.g. adrenaline). Administration of a decomposed drug is most likely to result in therapeutic failure, particularly if the products are devoid of pharmacological properties. In certain rare instances, however, the decomposition products may be toxic and potentially lethal. Earlier formulations of tetracycline, when stored under warm conditions, change to a brown sticky mass. Degraded formulations of this kind produce a Fanconi-like syndrome (Ehrlich and Stein 1963; Frimpter 1963; Gross 1963) with aminoaciduria, glycosuria, acetonuria, albuminuria, pyuria, elevated plasma α-amino nitrogen, and photosensitivity (Sulkowski and Haserick 1964). Analysis of decomposed capsules showed them to contain 3.5% anhydrotetracycline and 0.5% epiandrotetracycline (Sulkowski and Haserick 1964). Moreover, citric acid, which had been used as a buffering agent for tetracycline preparations, has been shown to increase the degradation process and has therefore been removed; but even in the absence of citric acid, degradation of tetracycline occurs when it is stored at 37°C and 66 per cent relative humidity for 2 months (Walton et al. 1970).

Additives present in pharmaceutical preparations may not be inert. Solvents such as the propylene glycol or ethoxylated castor oil used to dissolve some drugs may themselves have such undesirable effects as hypotension, and anaphylactic reactions, respectively. Colourizers (e.g. tartrazine) and antibacterial agents (e.g. benzoates) may produce immunological reactions.

Manufacturers' controls, and monitoring by national drug regulatory authorities make it most unusual, nowadays, for synthetic by-products to adulterate pharmaceutical preparations. A relatively recent example, however, occurred when a change in the production of L-tryptophan appears to have resulted in the formation of significant quantities of a condensation product (Belongia et al. 1990). This was responsible for the outbreak of a novel and disabling disorder — the eosinophilia–myalgia syndrome — which affected individuals in both the US and the UK (Waller et al. 1991) (see Chapter 18).

Pharmacokinetic causes

Theoretically, abnormalities of absorption, distribution, or elimination might give rise to Type B adverse effects. Both absorption and distribution, however, are predominantly passive processes (see above), and although changes in their kinetics may lead to Type A effects there are no documented Type B reactions that can be attributed to them.

Abnormalities of distribution generally reflect quantitative differences from the norm and therefore predispose to Type A reactions. There is, however, emerging evidence to suggest that the bioactivation of drugs to yield reactive species (as described above) is responsible for a significant proportion of Type B reactions. Binding of such reactive metabolites may result in either direct or immune-mediated toxicity (Pirmohammed et al. 1994). With direct toxicity, metabolite binding to a critical protein interferes with normal cellular function, leading to cellular necrosis. Alternatively, the metabolite acts as a hapten and initiates an immune reaction leading to a hormonal (antibody) or cellular (T-cell) response, or both. The immune response can be directed against the drug (haptenic epitopes), the carrier protein (auto-antigenic determinants), or the neoantigen created by the drug–protein combination (new antigenic determinants). Examples of Type B reactions postulated to occur as a result of bioactivation to yield reactive metabolites include tacrine (hepatotoxicity), clozapine (agranulocytosis), halothane (hepatotoxicity), and carbamazepine (hypersensitivity reactions).

The reasons why only some, and often only a few, individuals develop such Type B reactions, however, remains unclear. Susceptible persons may have overactive specific bioactivation pathways, underactive specific bioinactivation pathways, or immunological characteristics that render them more responsive to haptogenic or neoantigenic stimuli. Understanding these mechanisms is one of the great challenges to contemporary pharmacology and toxicology.

Pharmacodynamic causes

Qualitative abnormalities in the target organ occur for a number of reasons. Such factors as body-weight, age, sex, and route and time of administration all influence the final response of a patient to the dose of a particular drug. In general, changes in one or more of these are likely to produce quantitative and not qualitative differences in the response to drugs. In contrast, the presence of mental or physical illness (or both) may result in qualitative differences as well as a quantitative difference. For example, whereas an antidepressant drug will relieve depression in a patient suffering from this illness, the same drug will have no comparable effect in a mentally normal subject.

Qualitative differences in the response to drugs may be considered as genetic, immunological, or neoplastic and teratogenic.

Genetic causes for abnormal response

In the context of adverse drug reactions the term 'idiosyncrasy' has been used extensively as a label for those bizarre responses that were assumed to be due to some qualitative abnormality in the patient. Until recently, drug 'idiosyncrasies' have tended to form a dustbin for those adverse drug reactions that could not be classified under any other heading. This situation is now changing slowly as their mechanisms become clear, and it has become apparent that many have a genetic basis.

Erythrocyte glucose-6-phosphate dehydrogenase (G6PD) deficiency

Various enzyme deficiencies may affect tissue responses to drugs, and the best known of these is G6PD deficiency. A rare, more severe, sporadic type exists, but the most common forms are endemic inherited defects of intermediate dominance, particularly common in Afro-Americans (10 per cent), black Africans (up to 26 per cent), some Mediterranean races (1 to 7 per cent),

Kurdish and Iraqi Jews (up to 70 per cent), and some Filipinos. Each of these populations has a characteristic profile of deficient G6PD alleles. Many mutations have been sequenced; most involve single amino acid substitutions. It is estimated that 100–400 million individuals in the world are affected by this disorder (Weatherall and Hatton 1987; Mason 1996). G6PD oxidizes glucose-6-phosphate to glucose-6-phosphogluconolactone and reduces NADP to NADPH. In red blood cells this is the only source of NADPH, which is used via glutathione and catalase to reduce peroxidases and other reactive species (Mason 1996). A deficiency of G6PD results in a corresponding deficiency of reduced glutathione, and under these vulnerable conditions oxidizing agents may denature intracellular proteins, including the globin part of the haemoglobin molecule (Frischer and Ahmad 1987; Fletcher et al. 1988). This ultimately leads to haemolysis, accompanied by a rapid fall in haemoglobin concentration, fever, prostration, and the formation of dark urine. Reticulocytosis occurs and Heinz bodies appear in erythrocytes. A large number of commonly used drugs with oxidant properties will cause haemolysis if there is a deficiency of G6PD, and these include 8-aminoquinolines (e.g. primaquine), sulphonamides and sulphones, nitrofurans, analgesics (including aspirin and phenacetin), chloramphenicol, sodium aminosalicylate (PAS), probenecid, quinine, and quinidine (see Marks and Banks 1965; WHO 1967, 1973; Chan et al. 1976; Beutler 1984). Interestingly, slow acetylators of sulphamethazine are particularly susceptible to haemolysis while taking this sulphonamide (Woolhouse and Atu-Taylor 1982).

The prevention and treatment of haemolysis due to G6PD deficiency depends upon a knowledge of the genetic basis of this abnormality. There are two types of G6PD, known as A (abnormal) and B (normal). Since the gene for G6PD is located on the long arm of the X chromosome, G6PD deficiency is an X-linked trait, so that males and homozygous females with the deficiency have a single enzyme-deficient erythrocyte population. Heterozygous females possess two erythrocyte populations, one normal and one G6PD-deficient, with the ratio of the two populations varying from one to 99 per cent. Since only the G6PD-deficient cells are drug-sensitive (and in the typical heterozygous female only about half of the cells are affected), only about one-third of all heterozygous females possess a sufficiently high proportion of G6PD-deficient cells to predispose them to clinically significant haemolysis (WHO 1973).

Apart from intersexual differences in the enzyme, there are striking racial differences, so that whereas the African type (A⁻) is characterized by a mild enzyme deficiency with a mean activity 8.8–20 per cent of normal, the Mediterranean type is characterized by severe deficiency leading to 0 to 4 per cent enzyme activity. Consequently, a potentially haemolytic drug is likely to be much less troublesome in patients with the African than with the Mediterranean type. Much work needs to be done to characterize other racial forms of G6PD deficiency but, as has been pointed out by the WHO Scientific Group on Pharmacogenetics (WHO 1973), the decision to use or to stop treatment with a potentially haemolytic drug must depend upon (a) the type of G6PD deficiency, (b) the sex of the patient, (c) the severity of the disease, (d) the need for the drug, and (e) the availability of alternative agents. Moreover, the degree of haemolysis induced by a particular drug can be accentuated by the presence of additional infection or disease. The detection of G6PD deficiency can be achieved by several different screening methods. The simplest method is to incubate red cells with glucose-6-phosphate, magnesium, and NADP, and then determine NADPH production spectroscopically.

A study in Chinese subjects has shown that, in the absence of oxidant drugs, those with the common G6PD variants (Canton, B(–) Chinese, Hong Kong-Pokfulam) have a compensated haemolytic state, so that in this population chronic haemolytic anaemia due to G6PD deficiency is exceedingly rare (Chan et al. 1976). In spite of this, haemolytic episodes can be provoked by drugs or illness in those with G6PD deficiency. Studies with co-trimoxazole have shown that those Chinese with the same variant of G6PD may nevertheless react differently because of variation in the metabolism of the drug, possibly as the result of coexisting disease that alters hepatic or renal function or some other undefined biochemical or metabolic characteristic (Chan et al. 1976). The list of agents that can provoke this Type B adverse drug reaction due to G6PD deficiency has grown, but reports based only on clinical observation must be accepted with reserve until specific tests such as the ^{51}Cr half-life G6PD erythrocytes (Chan et al. 1976) have been employed to define accurately the haemolytic effects of any drugs that come under suspicion.

Hereditary methaemoglobinaemia

This condition may occur in the presence of mutations affecting the haemoglobin molecule or one of the methaemoglobin reductase enzymes, NADH diaphorase or NADPH diaphorase. Deficiency of NADH diaphorase may be limited to red blood cells (Type I) or may be widespread (Types II and III) and associated with mental retardation. Homozygotes are mildly cyanotic from birth and may be polycythaemic, and have methaemoglobin

concentrations between 15 and 30 per cent. They are exquisitely sensitive to oxidizing agents and develop severe methaemoglobinaemia when exposed. NADPH diaphorase deficiency is very rare. In the event of exposure to oxidizing agents, methaemoglobinaemia responds poorly to methylene blue therapy (Coleman and Coleman 1996). Drugs that are oxidizing agents, nitrites, and all of the drugs listed above as causing haemolysis in the presence of G6PD deficiency can all induce severe methaemoglobinaemia (Cowan and Evans 1964; Cohen et al. 1968). Heterozygotes possess about 50 per cent of the normal enzyme activity and are rarely susceptible to these adverse effects. They have a frequency in the population of one per cent. Neonates express low levels of NADH diaphorase and their blood contains a high proportion of the more unstable haemoglobin F. Thus they are more sensitive to oxidizing agents than older children and there is an inverse relationship between age-dependent erythrocyte activity of the enzyme and prilocaine-induced methaemoglobinaemia (Nilsson et al. 1990). Use of 0.02% chlorhexidine as an incubator disinfectant caused an outbreak of neonatal methaemoglobinaemia, as it decomposes to the oxidizing agent parachloroalinine.

Drug-sensitive haemoglobins

Certain mutations may affect the stability of the haemoglobin molecule. Thus, patients with Hb Zurich and Hb Torino may develop haemolysis in the presence of certain oxidizing drugs. In those patients who are affected, the red cells can be shown to contain denatured haemoglobin present in the form of small inclusion bodies (Heinz bodies). Two small pedigrees have been described with haemoglobin Zurich in which arginine was found to be substituted for histidine at 63rd position of the β-chain of haemoglobin and approximately 150 cases of haemoglobin M in which the haemoglobin is composed of four β-chains (Vesell 1972).

Porphyria

Conditions due to inborn errors that occur at different enzymic sites in the haem biosynthetic pathway cause rare metabolic disorders classified into acute and cutaneous porphyrias (Goldberg and Moore 1980). These conditions are characterized by reduced activity of an enzyme in the haem biosynthesis pathway, resulting in increased substrate formation from release of negative feedback on the rate-limiting enzyme 5-aminolaevulanic acid (ALA) synthase (ALA-S). The most common is acute intermittent porphyria, which is characterized by deficiency of the enzyme porphobilinogen deaminase, which is encoded on chromosome 11. Extensive allelic heterogeneity is recognized, with over 90 separate mutations causing acute intermittent porphyria. Most of these are confined to a few families but one (Trp198Stop) is responsible for the high prevalence of this condition in Sweden. Variegate porphyria, characterized by deficiency in protoporphyrinogen oxidase, is less common and also displays considerable allelic heterogeneity, except in persons of Afrikaans descent, when the mutation ArgSgTryp is often responsible. Hereditary coproporphyria is very rare, and results from deficiency of coproporphyrinogen oxidase (Elder *et al.* 1997). All the conditions are transmitted as autosomal dominants, with the exception of the rare congenital porphyria, which is recessive (Moore and Brodie 1985). The florid clinical condition of acute porphyria can be precipitated by drugs — ethanol and endogenous and exogenous steroid hormones. In contrast, cutaneous hepatic porphyria is most commonly precipitated by ethanol, although oestrogenic steroids have also been implicated. An acquired type may be caused by organic chemicals such as hexachlorobenzene (Cain and Nigogosyan 1963; Kimbrough 1987).

In the acute porphyrias, all patients show similar abdominal and neuropsychiatric disturbances. The most common of these are abdominal pain which is often severe, motor neuropathy, confusion, agitation, and hallucinations. During an acute attack they excrete in their urine large amounts of the porphyria precursors 5-aminolaevulinic acid (ALA) and porphobilinogen (PBG). Earlier experiments failed to demonstrate pharmacological, electroencephalographic, cardiovascular, or behavioural effects of porphyrins (Goldberg *et al.* 1954, 1987) although more recent work has revealed that certain porphyrins can damage membrane proteins and enzymes (Dubbleman *et al.* 1980; Avner *et al.* 1983), which might explain some of the clinical effects. A number of commonly used drugs induce ALA synthase production in the liver, and these agents are usually potent enzyme inducers. Depletion of haem caused by induction of cytochrome P450 may release negative feedback on ALA-S, provoking increased formation of haem precursors such as ALA. Thus, barbiturates, sulphonamides, griseofulvin, oestrogens (including those in oral contraceptives), some anticonvulsants and tranquilizers, possibly general anaesthetics, ethanol, chloroquine, chlorpropamide, and tolbutamide may all precipitate porphyria in susceptible patients (de Matteis 1967; Moore and Brodie 1985). However, attacks may also be precipitated by drugs which are not thought to induce cytochrome P450, such as erythromycin, flucloxacillin, chloramphenicol and nifedipine, and the explanation for this remains elusive.

The sensitivities of patients who are liable to develop acute intermittent porphyria in response to drugs vary widely, with the result that whereas a single dose of a particular drug may trigger off an acute attack in one patient, another may require a number of relatively large doses of the same drug to produce any clinically significant effect.

It requires special studies to determine which drugs are potentially harmful in the different forms of hepatic porphyria and to obtain an estimate of the relative frequencies of the different reactions. In South Africa, Eales (1971) made a study from which he concluded that patients suffering from porphyria variegata should avoid the following drugs: barbiturates, non-barbiturate hypnotics (e.g. glutethimide, meprobamate), pyrazolone compounds (e.g. phenazone), anticonvulsants (e.g. phenytoin), sulphonamides, griseofulvin, synthetic oestrogens and progestogens, and ergot preparations. Other lists of dangerous and 'safe' drugs are also available (*Drug and Therapeutics Bulletin* 1976; Moore and Brodie 1985; and see Chapter 17).

Bleeding disorders

Patients with haemophilia or von Willebrand's disease are particularly sensitive to drugs that influence (albeit weakly) clotting and coagulation mechanisms. In particular, salicylates will prolong the bleeding time of haemophiliacs for several days after a single dose, and this outlasts the presence of detectable levels of aspirin (Weiss *et al.* 1968).

Malignant hyperthermia

Malignant hyperthermia (also known less appropriately as malignant hyperpyrexia) was first described in 1964 (Saidman *et al.* 1964); it can be summarized as a condition in which there is a rapid rise in the body temperature (at least 2°C an hour) occurring without obvious cause during anaesthesia with potent volatile anaesthetics, often in the presence of suxamethonium. Although the early cases were reported from North America, it has since appeared in all parts of the world. The condition affects one in 15 000 children and one in 50 000 adults, and over half the episodes occur in patients aged under 15 years. In addition to the rapid rise of temperature, malignant hyperthermia is characterized by stiffness of the skeletal musculature, hyperventilation, acidosis, hyperkalaemia, and signs of increased activity of the sympathetic nervous system, including tachycardia, vasoconstriction, hypertension, and raised blood glucose concentration. The condition is important because it carries a mortality of the order of 60–70 per cent. There is strong evidence that it is a primary disease of skeletal muscle that is inherited as an autosomal dominant trait. Many of those susceptible to the condition show evidence of myotonia or related muscle disorders (Harriman *et al.* 1973). Recent serological, biochemical, and pedigree studies (McPherson and Taylor 1982; Bender *et al.* 1990; McCarthy *et al.* 1990; MacLennan *et al.* 1990) provide strong evidence of a genetic basis for malignant hyperthermia, showing it to be linked to the q13.1 region of chromosome 19, which codes for the ryanodine receptor, or sarcoplasmic reticulum calcium release gene. In the porcine model of malignant hyperthermia, mutation of this gene causes altered excitation coupling with secondary changes in muscle structure and function (Ben Abraham *et al.* 1997).

In the majority of affected families an elevated serum creatine phosphokinase level can be demonstrated (*The Lancet* 1973; Kelstrup *et al.* 1974). A more accurate prediction can be made, however, by testing specimens from a muscle biopsy *in vitro*, when it is found that those from individuals susceptible to malignant hyperthermia show heightened sensitivity to halothane, caffeine, suxamethonium, potassium chloride, and temperature change (Moulds and Denborough 1974a,b; Melton *et al.* 1989; Allen *et al.* 1990; Hackl *et al.* 1990). It is thus possible to distinguish those members of a family (with a history of malignant hyperthermia) who are not at risk.

When it occurs, it follows the administration of an inhalational general anaesthetic, most commonly halothane, and frequently in combination with suxamethonium; but it has been suggested by Ellis and others (1974) that nitrous oxide may act as a causative factor; and Britt and her co-workers (1974) have incriminated tubocurarine as a possible causative agent. Malignant hyperthermia may also present as heatstroke in subjects with the predisposing myopathy who are exposed to very severe physical stress (Denborough 1982). Several hypotheses have been suggested to explain the mechanism of the condition, but there is overwhelming evidence that the primary *trigger* is an abnormal calcium-induced release of intracellular ionized calcium (Moulds and Denborough 1974a; Ohnishi *et al.* 1986). Once released, it initiates a whole series of secondary changes that lead to the observed clinical changes and that also interact with each other and are thereby self-sustaining (Ording 1989).

It seems likely that fundamental to the condition is some inherited defect of cellular membranes, which would account for many of the other changes observed in malignant hyperthermia both clinically and experimentally. It is possible that there is a link between this disorder and the sudden infant death syndrome (SIDS) because Denborough (1981) found that five of 15 parents whose children died from SIDS had muscles that showed changes indicating susceptibility to malignant hyperthermia. Prevention of malignant hyperthermia is obviously of major importance, and depends on awareness and vigilance by all doctors, especially anaesthetists. Treatment has been greatly facilitated by dantrolene, which inhibits the release of calcium from the sarcoplasmic reticulum and thereby halts the otherwise self-sustaining calcium release mechanisms that result in progressive and potentially fatal damage to susceptible subjects.

Glucocorticoid glaucoma

Since François (1954) first described a glaucoma-like rise in intraocular pressure following prolonged use of cortisone, the effect of glucocorticosteroid eye-drops on intraocular pressure has been studied widely. In a randomly selected population the pressure change shows a trimodal distribution with relative frequencies of 66 per cent, 29 per cent, and five per cent for groups that exhibit low-, intermediate-, and high-pressure changes respectively in response to daily administration of glucocorticoid eye-drops. Family studies established (Armaly 1965, 1966; Schwartz *et al.* 1972) that a two-allele model may explain the phenomenon, with genotypes $p^l p^l$, $p^l p^h$, and $p^h p^h$. The allele p^l is responsible for low pressure and the allele p^h for high pressure, and the individuals with the genotype $p^l p^h$ appear to respond with a continuous rise in intraocular pressure following repeated administration of glucocorticoid eye-drops. On the other hand, a study of the effect of glucocorticoid eye-drops on the intraocular pressure of 63 twins by Schwartz and others (1972) suggested that non-genetic factors may also play a major role in determining variation in the ocular responses to glucocorticoids. The rise in intraocular pressure is usually reversible on stopping the drug, but, after long-term use, patients may be left with irreversible reductions in visual acuity (Butcher *et al.* 1994), although this is probably rare. When administering glucocorticoid eye-drops to patients it is obviously important to be aware of the fact that some individuals may respond with an increase in intraocular pressure which will require withdrawal of the drug. In case of doubt, there is obvious merit in checking intraocular pressure by means of tonometry. It should be noted that glaucoma induced by depot injection of triamcinolone may persist for as long as 10 months after the injection but may resolve promptly after the whitish plaque of residual steroid is removed (Mills *et al.* 1986).

Osteogenesis imperfecta

The production of general anaesthesia with halothane and suxamethonium may lead to a substantial increase of body temperature in patients suffering from osteogenesis imperfecta (Solomons and Myers 1972; Smith 1984). Fortunately, this elevation of body temperature is benign and can be controlled more satisfactorily and readily than in malignant hyperthermia (see above).

Periodic paralysis

This may be associated with several autosomal dominant conditions which are the result of an abnormality of the membrane of skeletal muscle. It is characterized by attacks of flaccid weakness during which either hyperkalaemia (lasting hours) or hypokalaemia (lasting days) may occur. Hyperkalaemic paralysis can be precipitated by the administration of potassium chloride and also by anaesthesia (Egan and Klein 1959; Gross *et al.* 1966; Layzer *et al.* 1967; Pearson and Kalyanaraman 1972). Hypokalaemic paralysis may be precipitated by a number of agents, including insulin, mineralocorticoids (not aldosterone), adrenaline, and ethanol. It has also been noted to follow the administration of ammonium glycyrrhizinate (licorice), and is presumably related to the mineralocorticoid properties of this compound (WHO 1973).

Familial dysautonomia (Riley–Day syndrome)

This condition affects Jewish families who originate from certain areas of Eastern Europe (Brunt and McKusick 1970) and is inherited as an autosomal recessive characteristic that gives rise to a wide variety of neurological disturbances resulting from loss of neurones from the sensory and autonomic nervous systems. The gene for familial dysautonomia has been mapped to chromosome 9 (Blumenfeld *et al.* 1993). These patients produce exaggerated responses to drugs acting on the autonomic nervous system. Thus, the response to the parasympathomimetic drug methacholine is abnormal (Dancis 1968) and disturbances of blood-pressure regulation may develop during general anaesthesia. Patients also exhibit intolerance to halothane and methyoxyflurane (Meridy and Creighton 1971). If affected individuals require general anaesthesia, it is important to reduce the responses of the abnormal autonomic nervous system by prior administration of cholinergic-blocking and adrenergic-blocking agents, such as atropine and propranolol.

Chloramphenicol-induced aplastic anaemia

Chloramphenicol may induce thrombocytopenia, granulocytopenia, or aplastic anaemia, any of which may be dose related and due to the effect of the drug on protein synthesis. In addition, there is a form of aplastic anaemia, induced by chloramphenicol, that appears to be idiosyncratic and which may be due to a genetically determined abnormality of DNA synthesis. Thus, while the other forms of blood dyscrasia, including the non-idiosyncratic form of aplastic anaemia, probably represent a normal and dose-related response of the bone marrow to chloramphenicol, the idiosyncratic form is an entirely separate entity, but like the other forms it calls for immediate withdrawal of the drug.

Cholestatic jaundice induced by oral contraceptives

It is well known that oral contraceptives (especially those with an alkyl substitution at the C_{17} position) may produce cholestatic jaundice. Evidence to date suggests that the familial and racial incidence of cholestatic jaundice following the administration of oral contraceptives may well have a genetic basis (Beeley 1975). It seems likely that oestrogen-induced changes in the composition of membrane lipids may play a major role in the production of cholestasis (Schreiber and Simon 1983). A further possibility is the impairment of sulphation by oestrogens, leading to retention of cholestatic compounds. In pregnant women, those taking oral contraceptives, and controls, hepatic paracetamol sulphation was reduced in those with elevated oestrogens, while platelet sulphotransferase activity was reduced during pregnancy (Davies *et al.* 1994). Further work requires to be carried out in order to clarify the underlying mechanisms.

Chlorpropamide–alcohol flushing (CPAF)

The first reports of facial flushing after ethanol in patients taking chlorpropamide (CPAF) occurred in the 1950s (Whitelock 1959), when it was estimated that it affected 15–30 per cent. A systematic study of 100 Type 2 diabetic patients taking chlorpropamide gave a frequency of 33 per cent (FitzGerald *et al.* 1962). Some authors have, however, suggested that CPAF is less common than previously suggested (Kobberling *et al.* 1980; DeSilva *et al.* 1981). The whole topic has been methodically reviewed by Johnston and others (1984*a,b*), and while there seems little doubt that CPAF exists, there is still uncertainty as to how best to test for it, its mechanism, whether it is inherited, and whether it is associated with certain types of diabetes and with a relative freedom from diabetic vascular complications.

Johnston and others (1984*a*) describe CPAF thus: it consists of a flush of the face, sometimes spreading to the neck, which may be accompanied by injection of the conjunctivae. The flush is visible to observers as well as being felt by the subject. It may be so intense that it gives a burning sensation and, very rarely, a headache. CPAF is not accompanied by sweating or prostration (although in a few patients it is associated with wheezing), but it is often embarrassing. The reaction starts within 10 or 20 minutes of taking alcohol, reaches a peak at 30–40 minutes, and persists for 1–2 hours or more. CPAF is different from the flush due to alcohol alone; patients who have experienced both are in no doubt about the difference.

The original simple challenge test (chlorpropamide 250 mg, then two 40 ml glasses of sherry 12 and 36 hours, respectively, later [Leslie and Pyke 1978; Pyke and Leslie 1978]) is now known to be inadequate, because it has been found that the dose of chlorpropamide influences the frequency of a positive response. A satisfactory test probably requires (1) pretreatment with chlorpropamide 250 mg for 14 days; (2) flush assessment by patient and an observer (85 per cent agreement), (3) measurement of rise of facial skin temperature (significantly greater in 'flushers' in whom it is not simply due to differences in basal temperatures), and (4) the use of thermography, which is a better index of facial skin blood flow than thermometry (Johnston *et al.* 1984*a,b*).

Studies in 12 pairs of identical twins indicated that CPAF is an autosomal dominant inherited trait and is associated with non-insulin-dependent diabetes (especially where there is a strong family history), but not with insulin-dependent diabetes (Leslie and Pyke 1978; Pyke and Leslie 1978). Most of these studies, however, were made with the single-tablet challenge test of patients who were strongly positive flushers, and it is therefore possible that less responsive flushers might show a different pattern of response if they received a prolonged course of chlorpropamide (Johnston *et al.* 1984*a,b*).

The mechanism of CPAF is still not clear, but since flushers seem to be more sensitive than non-flushers to the effect of disulfiram (Antabuse), which inhibits the enzyme acetaldehyde dehydrogenase (ALDH), it seems possible that flushers may metabolise acetaldehyde more slowly than non-flushers. Furthermore, there is evidence that in chlorpropamide–alcohol flushers the increase of plasma acetaldehyde is twice that in non-flushers (Johnston *et al.* 1984*a,b*) and this may be because ALDH is more sensitive to the inhibitory effect of chlorpropamide in flushers (Ohlin *et al.* 1982). The results of more recent work suggest the following:

(1) chlorpropamide is a major determinant of CPAF, which is associated with elevated blood acetaldehyde levels due to the inhibitions of ALDH by chlorpropamide (Groop *et al.* 1984*a,b*);

(2) ALDH activity is increased in Type 2 diabetics and determines CPAF. Furthermore, aldehyde concentration after chlorpropamide with ethanol is higher in patients with CPAF than in those without CPAF (Jerntop *et al.* 1986);

(3) in healthy non-diabetic adults CPAF appears to be a normal phenomenon (Hoskins *et al.* 1987);

(4) CPAF has a different enzymic basis from the ethanol flush reaction of oriental subjects. It seems likely that, in CPAF-positive subjects, ALDH may be particularly susceptible to inhibition by chlorpropamide (Johnston *et al.* 1986);

(5) while CPAF is associated with increased levels of plasma opioid peptides, especially metenkephalin (Leslie *et al.* 1979*a*; Medbak *et al.* 1981; Johnston *et al.* 1984*a*), it seems unlikely that CPAF is *caused* by this effect (Johnston *et al.* 1984*b*);

(6) there appears to be an association between fast acetylator phenotype and CPAF in Type 2, but not Type 1, diabetics; fast acetylators were more frequently CPAF-positive, while slow acetylators were more frequently negative. Furthermore, a linear relationship was found between acetylation rate and the speed of ascent of facial skin temperature after chlorpropamide and ethanol in Type 2 diabetics but not in Type 1 (Bonisolli *et al.* 1985).

Clearly, further studies are required to elucidate these mechanisms and relationships. It is possible that, in the Type B adverse drug reaction, CPAF is associated with a relative freedom from diabetic vascular complications (Leslie *et al.* 1979*b*; Barnett and Pyke 1980; Barnett *et al.* 1981), although not all workers agree with this suggestion (Micossi *et al.* 1982). There are many obvious reasons why every aspect of CPAF should be studied, not only because of the important light it may shed on the pathogenesis of Type 2 diabetes mellitus but also because it should explain the mechanism of this Type B drug reaction and so indicate how it can be avoided.

Immunological reasons for abnormal response

A most important group of qualitatively abnormal responses to drugs are those in which the cause is primarily immunological. In instances where the drug is immunogenic in its own right (e.g. antisera of animal origin) the reaction is obviously a Type A effect. Serum sickness is an example. Most allergic drug reactions, however, are not so obviously Type A responses, and in the absence of known mechanisms they can (perhaps temporarily) be categorized as Type B effects. The mechanisms involved in drug allergy are considered elsewhere in this book (Chapter 27). It seems possible that *human lymphocyte antigens* (HLA) may influence susceptibility to adverse drug reactions and thus could be an important factor in the determination of some Type B reactions. There is evidence that such a mechanism may be involved when patients with rheumatoid arthritis react adversely to levamisole (Schmidt and Mueller-Eckhardt 1977), gold therapy (Latts *et al.* 1980), and penicillamine (Wooley *et al.* 1980); and also in hypertensives who react adversely to hydralazine (Batchelor *et al.* 1980) (see also Chapter 2).

Conclusion

In this chapter we have continued to use a classification of adverse drug reactions that has now enjoyed wide utility for many years. In clinical practice Type A reactions, which are usually dose dependent and pharmacologically predictable, can usually be managed by dose adjustment, by substituting a similar but more selective drug, or by giving additional drugs to antagonize the unwanted effects of the primary agent. By contrast, in patients with Type B reactions, it is normally necessary to withdraw therapy.

References

Abrass, I.B. and Scarpace, P.J. (1982). Caralytic unit of adenylate cyclase: reduced activity in aged human lymphocytes. *J. Clin. Endocrinol. Metab.* 55, 1026.

Acheson, D. (1989). L-tryptophan and eosinophilia–myalgia syndrome in the USA. Department of Health (PL/CMO (89)11), London.

Aggeler, P.M., O'Reilly, R.A., Leong, L., *et al.* (1967). Potentiation of anticoagulant effect of warfarin by phenylbutazone. *N. Engl. J. Med.* 276, 496.

Allen, G.C., Rosenberg, H., and Fletcher, J.E. (1990). Safety of general anesthesia in patients previously tested negative for malignant hyperthermia susceptibility. *Anesthesiology* 72, 619.

Armaly, M.F. (1965). Statistical attributes of the steroid hypertensive response in the clinically normal eye. 1. The demonstration of three levels of response. *Invest. Ophthalmol.* 4, 187.

Armaly, M.F. (1966). The heritable nature of dexamethasone-induced ocular hypertension. *Arch. Ophthalmol.* 75, 32.

Aronoff, G.P., Ozawa, T., Desante, K.A., *et al.* (1982). Benoxaprofen kinetics in renal impairment. *Clin. Pharmacol. Ther.* 32, 190.

Avner, D.L., Larsen, R., and Berenson, M.M. (1983). Inhibition of liver surface membrane Na+, K-adenosine triphosphatase, Mg^2+-adenosine triphosphatase and 5-nucleotidase activities by protoporphyrin. *Gastroenterology* 85, 700.

Bailey, D.G., Arnold, J.M.O., Specer, J.D. (1994). Grapefruit juice and drugs: how significant is the interaction. *Clin. Pharmacokinet.* 26, 91.

Barnett, A.H. and Pyke, D.A. (1980). Chlorpropamide alcohol flushing and large vessel disease in non-insulin dependent diabetics. *BMJ* ii, 261.

Barnett, A.H., Leslie, R.D.G., and Pyke D.A. (1981). Chlorpropamide alcohol flushing and proteinuria in non-insulin-dependent diabetics. *BMJ* 282, 522.

Batchelor, J.R., Welsh, K.I., Mansilla-Tinoco, R., *et al.* (1980). Hydralazine-induced systemic lupus erythematosus: influence of HLA-DR and sex on susceptibility. *Lancet* i, 1107.

Bateman, D.N., Gokal, R., Dodd, T.R.P., *et al.* (1981). The pharmacokinetics of single doses of metoclopramide in renal failure. *Eur. J. Clin. Pharmacol.* 19, 437.

BCDSP (Boston Collaborative Drug Surveillance Program) (1973). Diphenylhydantoin side effects and serum albumin levels. *Clin. Pharmacol. Ther.* 14, 529.

Beeley, L. (1975). Adverse reactions to drugs. *Medicine* 5, 207.

Belongia, E.A., Hedberg, C.W., Gleich, G.J., *et al.* (1990). An investigation of the cause of the eosinophilia–myalgia syndrome associated with tryptophan use. *N. Engl. J. Med.* 323, 357.

Ben Abraham, R., Cahana, A., Krivosic-Horber, R.M. *et al.* (1997). Malignant hyperthermia susceptibility: anesthetic implications and risk stratification. *Q. J. Med.* 90, 13.

Bender, K., Seuff, H., Wienker, T.F., *et al.* (1990). A linkage study of malignant hyperthermia (MH). *Clin. Genet.* 37, 221.

Benet, L.Z., Kroetz, D.L., and Sheiner, L.B. (1996). Pharmacokinetics: the dynamics of drug absorption, distribution and elimination. In *The Pharmacological Basis of Therapeutics* (9th edn) (ed. J.G. Hardman and L.E. Limbird), p. 3. McGraw-Hill, New York.

Benowitz, N., Forsyth, R.P., Melmon, K.L., *et al.* (1974). Lidocaine disposition kinetics in monkey and man. II. Effects of haemorrhage and sympathomimetic drug administration. *Clin. Pharmacol. Ther.* 16, 99.

Bertler, A.A. and Smith, S.E. (1971). Genetic influences in drug responses of the eye and heart. *Clin. Sci.* 40, 403.

Beutler, E. (1984). Sensitivity to drug-induced haemolytic anaemia in glucose-6-phosphate dehydrogenase deficiency. In *Banbury Report 16. Genetic Variability in Responses to Chemical Exposure* (ed. G.S. Omenn and H.V. Gelboin), p. 205. Cold Spring Harbor, New York.

Bianchine, J.F., Calimlin, L.R., Morgan, J.P., *et al.* (1971). Metabolism and absorption of L-3,4-dihydroxyphenylanine in patients with Parkinson's Disease. *Ann. N.Y. Acad. Sci.* 179, 126.

Blaschke, T.F. (1977). Protein binding and kinetics of drugs in liver disease. *Clin. Pharmacokinet.* 2, 32.

Blumenfeld, A., Slaugenhaupt, S.A., Axelrod, F.B., *et al.* (1993). Localization of the gene for familial dysautonomia on chromosome 9 and definition of DNA markers for genetic diagnosis. *Nature Genetics* 4, 160.

Boley, S.J., Allen, A.C., Schultz, L., *et al.* (1965). Potassium-induced lesions of the small bowel. I. Clinical aspects. *JAMA* 193, 997.

Bonisolli, L., Pontiroli, A.E., De-Pasqua, A., *et al.* (1985). Association between chlorpropamide-alcohol flushing and fast acetylator phenotype in type I and type II diabetes. *Acta Diabetol. Lat.* 22, 305.

Boyd, M.R. (1980). Biochemical mechanisms of pulmonary toxicity of furan derivatives. In *Reviews in Biochemical Toxicology,* Vol. 2 (ed. E. Hodgson, J.R. Bond, and R.M. Philpot), p. 71. Elsevier/North-Holland, Amsterdam.

Bray, G.P., Harrison, P.M., O'Grady, J.G., *et al.* (1992). Long-term anticonvulsant therapy worsens outcome in paracetamol-induced fulminant hepatic failure. *Hum. Exp. Toxicol.* 11, 265.

Britt, B.A., Webb, G.E., and LeDuc, C. (1974). Malignant hyperthermia induced by curare. *Can. Anaesth. Soc. J.* 21, 371.

Brodie, M.J., Boobis, A.R., Bulpitt, C.J., *et al.* (1981). Influence of liver disease and environmental factors on hepatic mono-oxygenase activity *in vitro. Eur. J. Clin. Pharmacol.* 20, 39.

Bros, O. (1987). Gastrointestinal mucosal lesions: a drug formulation problem. *Med. Toxicol.* 2, 105.

Brunt, P.W. and McKusick, V.A. (1970). Familial dysautonomia. A report of genetic and clinical studies, with a review of the literature. *Medicine* 49, 343.

Butcher, J.M., Austin, M., McGalliard, J., *et al.* (1994). Bilateral cataracts and glaucoma induced by long term use of steroid eye drops. *BMJ* 309, 43.

Buyske, D.A., Eisner, H.J., and Kelly, R.G. (1960). Concentration and persistence of tetracycline and chlortetracycline in bone. *J. Pharmacol. Exp. Ther.* 130, 150.

Cain, S. and Nigogosyan, G. (1963). Acquired toxic porphyria cutanea tarda due to hexachlorobenzene: Report of 348 cases caused by this fungicide. *JAMA* 183, 88.

Campbell, N.R.C., Paddock, V., and Sundaram, R. (1988). Alteration of methyldopa absorption, metabolism and blood pressure control cases by ferrous sulphate and ferrous gluconate. *Clin. Pharmacol. Ther.* 43, 381.

Campbell, N.R.C., Ranfine, D., Goodridge, A.E. *et al.* (1990). Sinemet–ferrous sulphate interaction in patients with Parkinson's disease. *Br. J. Clin. Pharmacol.* 30, 599.

Chan, T.K., Todd, D., and Tso, S.C. (1976). Drug-induced haemolysis in glucose 6-phosphate dehydrogenase deficiency. *BMJ* ii, 1227.

Cohen, R.J., Sachs, J.R., Wicker, D.J., *et al.* (1968). Methemoglobinemia provoked by malarial chemoprophylaxis in Vietnam. *N. Engl. J. Med.* 279, 1127.

Cohlan, S.Q., Berclander, G., and Tiansic, T. (1963). Growth of inhibition of prematures receiving tetracyclines: a clinical and laboratory investigation. *Am. J. Dis. Child.* 105, 453.

Coleman, M.D. and Coleman, N.A. (1996). Drug-induced methaemoglobinaemia. Tratment issues. *Drug Saf.* 14, 394.

Connolly, M.J., Astrige, P.S., White, E.G., *et al.* (1991). Torsade de pointes, ventricular tachycardia and terodiline. *Lancet* 338, 344.

Conrad, K.A., Byers, J.M., Finley, P.R., *et al.* (1983). Lidocaine elimination effects of metoprolol and propranolol. *Clin. Pharmacol. Ther.* 33, 133.

Couch, D.B. (1996). Carcinogenesis: basic principles. *Drug Chem. Toxicol.* 19 133.

Cowan, W.K. and Evans, D.A.P. (1964). Primaquine and methemoglobin. *Clin. Pharmacol. Ther.* 5, 307.

Critchley, J.A.J., Chan, T.Y.K., and Cumming, A.D. (1977). Renal disease. In *Avery's Drug Treatment* (4th edn) (ed. T.M. Speight and N.H.G. Holford), p. 1067. Adis International, Auckland.

CSM (Committee on Safety of Medicines) (1983). Osmosin (controlled release indomethacin). *Current Problems* No. 11. HMSO, London.

Cunningham, J.L., Leyland, M.J., Delamore, I.W., *et al.* (1974). Acetanilide oxidation in phenylbutazone-associated hypoplastic anaemia. *BMJ* iii, 313.

Dancis, J. (1968). Altered drug response in familial dysautonomia. *Ann. N.Y. Acad. Sci.* 151, 876.

Davidson, H. (1968). *Physiology of the Cerebrospinal Fluid.* Churchill Livingstone, Edinburgh.

Davies, M.H., Ngong, J.M., Yucesoy, M., *et al.* (1994). The adverse influence of pregnancy upon sulphation: a clue to the pathogenesis of intrahepatic cholestasis of pregnancy? *J. Hepatol.* 21, 1127.

Davis, S.S. (1989). Gastrointestinal transit and drug absorption. In *Novel Drug Delivery* (ed. L.F. Prescott and W.S. Nimmo), p. 89. Wiley, Chichester.

de Matteis, F. (1967). Disturbances of liver porphyrin metabolism caused by drugs. *Pharmacol. Rev.* 19, 523.

Denborough, M.A. (1981). Sudden infant death syndrome and malignant hyperpyrexia. *Med. J. Aust.* i, 649.

Denborough, M.A. (1982). Heat stroke and malignant hyperpyrexia. *Med. J. Aust.* i, 204.

DePaulo, J.R., Correa, E.I., and Sapir, D.G. (1981) Renal toxicity of lithium and its implications. *Junior Hospital Medical Journal* 147, 15.

DeSilva, N.E., Tunbridge, W.M.G., and Alberti, K.G.M. (1981). Low incidence of chlorpropramide-alcohol flushing in diet-treated non-insulin-dependent diabetics. *Lancet* i, 128.

Devadatta, S., Gangadharam, P.R.J., Andrews, R.H., *et al.* (1960). Peripheral neuritis due to isoniazid. *Bull. Wld Hlth Org.* 23, 587.

Dost, F.H. (1953). *Der Blutspiegelkinetik der Konzentrationsablaufe in der Kreislauflüssigkeit.* Leipzig.

Drug and Therapeutics Bulletin (1976). Drugs and diet in the hereditary porphyrias. *Drug. Ther. Bull.* 14, 55.

Dubbleman, T.M., De Goeij, A.F., and van Steveninck, J. (1980). Protoporphyria-induced photodynamic effects on transport processes across the membrane of human erythrocytes. *Biophys. Acta* 595, 133.

Eales, L. (1971). Acute porphyria: the precipitating and aggravating factors. Proceedings of the national conference on porphyrin metabolism and porphyria. Cape Town, December 1970. *S. Afr. Lab. Clin. Med.* (special issue) 17, 120.

Eap C.B., Cuendet C., and Baumann, P. (1990). Binding of D-methadone, L-methadone, and DL-methadone to proteins in plasma of healthy volunteers: role of the variants of α_1-acid glycoprotein. *Clin. Pharmacol. Ther.* 47, 338.

Egan, T.J. and Klein, R. (1959). Hyperkalemic familial periodic paralysis. *Pediatrics* 24, 761.

Ehrlich, L.J. and Stein, H.S. (1963). Abnormal urinary findings following administration of achromycin V. *Pediatrics* 31, 697.

Elder, G.H., Hift, R.J., and Meissner, P.N. (1997). The acute porphyrias. *Lancet* 349, 1613.

Elfellah, M.S., Dalling, R., Slater, R.J., *et al.* (1989). β-Adrenoceptors and human skeletal muscle; characterisation of receptor subtype and effect of age. *Br. J. Clin. Pharmacol.* 27, 31.

Ellard, G.A., Gammon, P.T., Savin, L.A., *et al.*(1974). Dapsone acetylation in dermatitis herpetiformis. *Br. J. Dermatol.* 13, 441.

Ellis, F.R., Clarke, I.M.C., Appleyard, T.N., *et al.* (1974). Malignant hyperpyrexia induced by nitrous oxide and treated with dexamethasone. *BMJ* iv, 270.

Fenster, P.E., White, N.W., and Hanson, C.D. (1985). Pharmacokinetic evaluation of the digoxin–amiodarone interaction. *J. Am. Coll. Cardiol.* 108,112.

Fitton, A., Faulds, D., and Goa, K.L. (1992). Moclobemide: a review of its pharmacological properties and therapeutic uses in depressive illness. *Drugs* 43, 561.

FitzGerald, M.G., Gaddie, R., Malins, J.M., *et al.* (1962). Alcohol sensitivity in diabetics receiving chlorpropamide. *Diabetes* 11, 40.

Fletcher K.A., Barton, P.F., and Kelly, J.A. (1988). Studies on the mechanisms of oxidation in the erythrocyte by metabolites of primaquine. *Biochem. Pharmacol.* 37, 2683.

Ford, G.A. and James, O.F.W. (1994). Autonomic blockade in healthy young, healthy and endurance trained elderly persons: haemodynamic responses and effect of cardiac α-adrenergic responsiveness. *Clin. Sci.* 1994: 87: 297.

François, J. (1954). Cortisone et tension oculaire. *Ann. Oculist.* 187, 805.

Frimpter, G.W. (1963). Reversible 'Fanconi syndrome' caused by degraded tetracycline. *JAMA* 184, 111.

Frischer, H. and Ahmad, T. (1987). Consequence of erythrocyte glutathione reductase deficiency. *J. Lab. Clin. Med.* 109, 583.

Garrattini, S. (1985). Active drug metabolites: an overview. *Clin. Pharmacokinet.* 10, 216.

Goldberg, A. and Moore, M.R. (ed.) (1980). The porphyrias. In *Clinics in Haematology*, Vol. 9, p. 225. W.B. Saunders, London.

Goldberg. A., Paton, W.D.M., and Thompson, J.W. (1954). Pharmacology of the porphyrins and porphobilinogen. *Br. J. Pharmacol.* 9, 91.

Goldberg, A., Moore, M.R., McKoll, K.E.L., *et al.* (1987). Porphyria metabolism and the porphyrias. In *Oxford Textbook of Medicine* (ed. D.J. Weatherall, J.G.G. Ledingham, and D.A. Warrell), p. 9.136. Oxford University Press.

Grahame-Smith, D.G. and Aronson, J.K. (1984). *Oxford Textbook of Clinical Pharmacology and Drug Therapy* (1st edn). Oxford University Press.

Grahame-Smith, D.G. and Aronson, J.K. (1992). *Oxford Textbook of Clinical Pharmacology and Drug Therapy* (2nd edn). Oxford University Press.

Greenblatt, D.J. and Koch-Weser, J. (1974). Clinical toxicity of chlordiazepoxide and diazepam in relation to serum albumin concentration: a report from the Boston Collaborative Drug Surveillance Program. *Eur. J. Clin. Pharmacol.* 4, 259.

Groop, L., Eriksson, C.J., Huupponen, R., *et al.* (1984a). Roles of chlorpropamide, alcohol and acetaldehyde in determining the chlorpropamide–alcohol flush. *Diabetologia* 26, 34.

Groop, L., Koskimies, S., and Tolppanen, E.M. (1984b). Characterisation of patients with chlorpropamide–alcohol flush. *Acta Med. Scand.* 215, 141.

Gross, E.G., Dexter, J.D., and Roth, R.G. (1966). Hypokalemic myopathy with myoglobinuria associated with licorice ingestion. *N. Engl. J. Med.* 274, 602.

Gross, J.M. (1963). Fanconi syndrome (adult type) developing secondary to ingestion of outdated tetracycline. *Ann. Intern. Med.* 58, 523.

Hackl, W., Mauritz, W., Schemper, M., *et al.* (1990). Prediction of malignant hyperthermia susceptibility: statistical evaluation of clinical signs. *Br. J. Anaesth.* 64, 411.

Hackney, J.F., Gross, S.R., Aronow, L., *et al.* (1970). Specific glucocorticoid-binding macromolecules from mouse fibroblasts growing *in vitro*. A possible steroid receptor for growth inhibition. *Mol. Pharmacol.* 6, 500.

Hallak, H.O., Wedlund, P.J., Modi, M.W. *et al.* (1993). High clearance of (S)-warfarin in a warfarin-resistant subject. *Br. J. Clin. Pharmacol.* 35, 327.

Harriman, D.G., Summer, D.W., and Ellis, F.R. (1973). Malignant hyperpyrexia myopathy. *Q. J. Med.* 42, 639.

Harris, H. (1964). Enzymes and drug sensitivity. The genetics of serum cholinesterase deficiency in relation to suxamethonium apnoea. *Proc. R. Soc. Med.* 57, 503.

Harris, R.Z., Benet, L.Z., and Schwartz, J.B. (1995). Gender effects in pharmacokinetics and pharmacodynamics. *Drugs* 50, 222.

Hendeles, L., Weinberger, M., Milaretz, G., *et al.* (1985). Food induced 'dose-dumping' from a once a day theophylline product as a cause of theophylline toxicity. *Chest* 87, 758.

Hinson, J.A. (1980). Biochemical toxicology of acetaminophen. In *Reviews in Biochemical Toxicology*, Vol. 2 (ed. E. Hodgson, J.R. Bland, and R.M. Philpot), p. 103. Elsevier/North-Holland, New York.

Hoigne, R. (1997). Should 'idiosyncrasy' be defined as equivalent to Type B adverse drug reactions? *Pharmacoepidemiology and Drug Safety* 6, 213.

Hoskins, P.J., Wiles, P.G., Volkmann, H.P., *et al.* (1987). Chlorpropamide alcohol flushing: a normal response? *Clin. Sci.* 73, 77.

Hulse, M.L. (1996). Warfarin resistance: diagnosis and therapeutic alternatives. *Pharmacotherapy* 16, 1009.

Jerntop, P., Ohlin, H., Sundkvist, G., *et al.* (1986). Effects of chlorpropamide and alcohol on aldehyde dehydrogenase activity and blood acetaldehyde concentration. *Diabetes Res.* 3, 369.

Johnston, C., Wiles, P.G., and Pyke, D.A. (1984a). Chlorpropamide–alcohol flush: the case in favour. *Diabetologia* 26, 1.

Johnston, C., Wiles, P.G., Medbak, S., *et al.* (1984b). The role of endogenous opioids in the chlorpropamide–alcohol flush. *Clin. Endocrinol.* 21, 489.

Johnston, C., Saunders, J.B., Barnett, A.H., *et al.* (1986). Chlorpropamide–alcohol flush reaction and isoenzyme profiles of alcohol dehydrogenase and aldehyde dehydrogenase. *Clin. Sci.* 71, 513.

Kalow, W.I. and Bertilsson, L. (1994). Interethnic factors affecting drug response. *Adv. Drug. Res.* 25, 1.

Karlsson, E., Collste, P., and Rawlins, M.D. (1974). Plasma levels of lidocaine during combined treatment with phenytoin and procainamide. *Eur. J. Clin. Pharmacol.* 7, 455.

Kelstrup, J., Reske-Nielsen, E., Haase, J., *et al.* (1974). Malignant hyperthermia in a family: a clinical and serological investigation of 139 members. *Acta Anaesth. Scand.* 18, 58.

Kimbrough, R.D. (1987). Porphyrins and hepatotoxicity. In *Mechanisms of Chemical-induced Porphyrinopathies* (ed. E.K. Silbergeld and B.A. Fowler), p. 289. The New York Academy of Sciences.

Kinirons, M.T. and Crome, P. (1997). Clinical pharmacokinetic considerations in the elderly: an update. *Clin. Pharmac.* 33, 302.

Kobberling, J., Bengsch, N., Bruggersboer, B., *et al.* (1980). The chlorpropamide–alcohol flush — lack of specificity for non-insulin-dependent diabetes. *Diabetologia* 19, 359.

The Lancet (1973). Prevention of malignant hyperpyrexia. *Lancet* i, 1225.

Latts, J.R., Antel, J.P., Levinson, D.J., *et al.* (1980). Histocompatibility antigens and gold toxicity. *J. Clin. Pharmacol.* 20, 206.

Layzer, R.B., Lovelace, R.E., and Rowland, L.P. (1967). Hyperkalemic periodic paralysis. *Arch. Neurol.* 16, 455.

Leakey, E.B., Reiffel, J.A., Giardina, E.G., *et al.* (1980). The effect of quinidine and other oral antiarrhythmic drugs on serum digoxin: a prospective study. *Am. Int. Med.* 92, 605.

Leonard, M.S. (1993). Genetically determined adverse drug reactions including metabolism. *Drug Safety* 9, 60.

Leslie, R.D.G. and Pyke, D.A. (1978). Chlorpropamide–alcohol flushing: a dominantly inherited trait associated with diabetes. *BMJ* ii, 1519.

Leslie, R.D.G., Pyke, D.A., and Stubbs, W.A. (1979*a*). Sensitivity to enkephalin as a cause of non-insulin-dependent diabetes. *Lancet* i, 341.

Leslie, R.D.G., Barnett, A.H., and Pyke, D.A. (1979*b*). Chlorpropamide–alcohol flushing and diabetic retinopathy. *Lancet* i, 997.

Lewis, G.P., Jusko, W.J., Burke, C.W., *et al.* (1971). Prednisone side effects and serum protein levels. *Lancet* ii, 778.

Linderman, R.D. (1992). Changes in renal function with aging: implications for treatment. *Drugs and Ageing* 2, 423.

Loeser, E.W. (1961). Studies on the metabolism of diphenylhydantoin (Dilantin). *Neurology*, 11, 424.

McCarthy, T.V., Healy, J.M., Haffron, J.J., *et al.* (1990). Localization of the malignant hyperthermia susceptibility locus to human chromosome 19q12–13.2. *Nature* 343, 562.

McDevitt, D.G., Frisk-Holmberg, M., Hollifield, J.W., *et al.* (1976). Plasma binding and the affinity of propranolol for a beta receptor in man. *Clin. Pharmacol. Ther.* 20, 152.

McGuire, W.L., Horwitz, K.D., Pearson, O.H., *et al.* (1977). Current status of estrogen and progesterone receptors in breast cancer. *Cancer* 39, 2934.

MacLennan, D.H., Duff, C., Zorzato, F., *et al.* (1990). Ryanodine receptor gene is a candidate for predisposition to malignant hyperthermia. *Nature* 343, 559.

McLeod, K., Watson, M.K., and Rawlins, M.D. (1976). Pharmacokinetics of pancuronium in normal individuals and in patients with renal failure. *Br. J. Anaesth.* 48, 341.

McPherson, E. and Taylor, C.A. (1982). The genetics of malignant hyperthermia: evidence for heterogeneity. *Am. J. Med. Genet.* 11, 273.

Mahgoub, A., Dring, L.G., Idle, J.R., (1977). Polymorphic hydroxylation of debrisoquine in man. *Lancet*, ii, 584.

Manninen, V., Apajalahti, A., Melin, J., *et al.* (1973). Altered absorption of digoxin in patients given propantheline and metoclopramide. *Lancet* i, 398.

Marks, P.A. and Banks, J. (1965). Drug-induced hemolytic anemias associated with glucose-6-phosphate dehydrogenase deficiency: a generally heterogeneous trait. *Ann. N.Y. Acad. Sci.* 123, 198.

Mason, P.J. (1996). New insights into G6PD deficiency. *Br. J. Haematol.* 94, 585.

Medbak, S., Wass, J.A.H., Clement-Jones, V., *et al.* (1981). Chlorpropamide alcohol flush and circulating metenkephalin: a positive link. *BMJ* 283, 937.

Melander, A. (1978). Influence of food on the bioavailability of drugs. *Clin. Pharmacokinet.* 3, 37.

Melton, A.T., Martucci, R.W., Kien, N.D., *et al.* (1989). Malignant hyperthermia in human-standardization of contracture testing protocol. *Anesth. Analg.* 69, 437.

Meridy, H.W. and Creighton, R.E. (1971). General anaesthesia in eight patients with familial dysautonomia. *Can. Anaesth. Soc. J.* 18, 563.

Micossi, R., Mannucci, P.M., Bozzini, S., *et al.* (1982). Chlorpropamide-alcohol flushing in non-insulin dependent diabetes: prevalence of small and large vessel disease and risk factors for angiopathy. *Acta Diabetol. Lat.* 19, 141.

Mills, D.W., Siebert, L.F., and Climenhaga, M.D. (1986). Depot triamcinolone-induced glaucoma. *Can. J. Ophthalmol.* 21, 150.

Milne, M.D., Scribner, B.H., and Crawford, M.A. (1958). Non-ionic diffusion and the excretion of weak acids and bases. *Am. J. Med.* 24, 709.

Moore, M.R. and Brodie, M.J. (1985). The porphyrias. *Med. Int.* 2, 604.

Moulds, R.F.W. and Denborough, M.A. (1974*a*). Biochemical basis of malignant hyperpyrexia. *BMJ* ii, 241.

Moulds, R.F.W. and Denborough, M.A. (1974*b*). Identification of susceptibility to malignant hyperpyrexia. *BMJ* ii, 245.

Naranjo, C.A., Bristo, U., and Mardonics, R. (1978). Adverse drug reactions in liver cirrhosis. *Eur. J. Clin. Pharmacol.* 13, 429.

Nebert, D.W., Nelson, D.R., Adesnik, M., *et al.* (1989). The P-450 superfamily: updated listing of all gases and recommended nomenclatures for the chromosomal loci. *DNA* 8, 1.

Neuvonen, P.J., Kivisto, K.T., and Lehto, P. (1991). Interference of dairy products with the absorption of ciprofloxacin. *Clin. Pharmacol. Ther.* 50, 498.

Nilsson, A., Engberg, G., Henneberg, S., *et al.* (1990). Inverse relationship between age-dependent erythrocyte activity of methaemoglobin reductase and prilocaine-induced methaemoglobinaemia during infancy. *Br. J. Anaesth.* 64, 72.

Nimmo, J., Heading, R.C., Tothill, P., *et al.* (1973). Pharmacological modification of gastric emptying: effects of propantheline and metoclopramide on paracetamol absorption. *BMJ* i, 587.

Ochs, H.R., Carstens, G., and Greenblatt, D.J. (1980). Reduction in lidocaine clearance during continuous infusions by coadministration of propranolol. *N. Engl. J. Med.* 303, 373.

Ohlin, H., Jerntop, P., Bergstrom, B., *et al.* (1982). Chlorpropamide-alcohol flushing aldehyde dehydrogenase activity and diabetic complications. *BMJ* 285, 838.

Ohnishi, S.T., Waring, A.J., Fang, S-R.G., *et al.* (1986). Abnormal membrane properties of the sarcoplasmic reticulum of pigs susceptible to malignant hyperthermia: Modes of action of halothane, caffeine, dantrolene, and two other drugs. *Arch. Biochem. Biophys.* 247, 294.

O'Reilly, R.A. (1970). The second reported kindred with hereditary resistance to oral anticoagulant drugs. *N. Engl. J. Med.* 282, 1448.

O'Reilly, R.A., Aggeler, P.M., Hoag, M.S., *et al.* (1964). Hereditary transmission of exception resistance to coumarin anticoagulant drugs. The first reported kindred. *N. Engl. J. Med.* 271, 809.

Ording, H. (1989). Pathophysiology of malignant hyperthermia. *Ann. Fr. Anesth. Reanim.* 8, 411.

Orme, M.L'E., Back, D.J., and Breckenridge, A.M. (1983). Clinical pharmacokinetics of oral contraceptive steroids. *Clin. Pharmacokinet.* 8, 95.

Osman, M.A., Patel, R.B., Schuna, A., *et al.* (1983). Reduction in oral penicillamine absorption by food, antacid and ferrous sulphate. *Clin. Pharmacol. Ther.* 33, 465.

Pato, M.L. and Brown, G.M. (1963). Mechanisms of resistance of *Escherichia coli* to sulphonamides. *Arch. Biochem. Biophys.* 103, 443.

Paton, W.D.M. (1970). Receptors as defined by their pharmacological properties. In *Molecular Properties of Drug Receptors* (ed. R. Porter and M. O'Connor). Churchill Livingstone, Edinburgh.

Pearson, C.M. and Kalyanaraman, K. (1972). The periodic paralyses. In *The Metabolic Basis of Inherited Disease* (ed. J.B. Stanburg, J.B. Wyngaarden, and D.S. Fredrickson), p. 1181. McGraw-Hill, New York.

Pearson, R.M. and Breckenridge, A. (1976). Renal function, protein binding and pharmacological response to diazoxide. *Br. J. Clin. Pharmacol.* 3, 169.

Perry, H.M., Sakanoto, A., and Tan, E.M. (1967). Relationship of acetylating enzyme to hydrallazine toxicity. *J. Lab. Clin. Med.* 70, 1020.

Piper, D.W., de Carlo, D.J., Tally, N.J., *et al.* (1997). Gastrointestinal and hepatic disease. In *Avery's Drug Treatment* (4th edn) (ed. T.M. Speight and N.H.G. Holford), p. 933. Adis International, Auckland.

Pirmohamed, M., Kitteringham, N.R. and Park, B.K. (1994). The role of active metabolites in drug toxicity. *Drug Saf.* 11, 114.

Pirmohamed, M., Madden, S., and Park, B.K. (1996). Idiosyncratic drug reactions: metabolic bioactivation as a pathogenic mechanism. *Clin. Pharmacokinet.* 31, 215.

Prandota, J. (1988). Clinical pharmacology of antibiotics and other drugs in cystic fibrosis. *Drugs* 35, 542.

Prescott, L.F. (1972). The modifying effects of physiological variables and diseases upon pharmacokinetics and/or drug response. In *Liver Disease* (Proceedings of the Fifth International Congress on Pharmacology), p. 73. Iuphar, Basle.

Prescott, L.F. (1974). Gastric emptying and drug absorption. *Br. J. Clin. Pharmacol.* 1, 189.

Prescott, L.F. (1996). *Paracetamol (acetaminophen): a Critical Bibliographic Review.* Taylor and Francis, London.

Prescott, L.F., Wright, N., Roscoe, P., *et al.* (1971). Paracetamol half-life and hepatic necrosis in patients with paracetamol overdosage. *Lancet* i, 519.

Pyke, D.A. and Leslie R.D.G. (1978). Chlorpropamide-alcohol flushing: a definition of its relation to non-insulin-dependent diabetes. *BMJ* ii, 1521.

Rau, S.E., Bend, J.R., Arnold, M.O. *et al.* (1997). Grapefruit juice — terfenadine single dose interaction: magnitude, mechanism and relevance. *Clin. Pharmacol. Ther.* 61, 401.

Rawlins, M.D. (1974). Kinetic basis for drug interactions. *Adverse Drug React. Bull.* 46, 152.

Rawlins, M.D. (1997). Commentary: Should idiosyncrasy be defined as equivalent to Type B adverse drug reactions? *Pharmacoepidemiology and Drug Safety* 6, 291.

Rawlins, M.D. and Bateman, D.N. (1984). Contribution of absorption to variation in response to drug. In *Drug Absorption* (ed. L.F. Prescott). Adis Press, Auckland.

Rawlins, M.D. and Thompson, J.W. (1977). Pathogenesis of adverse drug reactions. In *Textbook of Adverse Drug Reactions* (1st edn) (ed. D.M. Davies), p. 44. Oxford University Press.

Robinson, D.S., Benjamin, D.M., and McCormack, J.J. (1971). Interaction of warfarin and nonsystemic gastrointestinal drugs. *Clin. Pharmacol. Ther.* 12, 491.

Saidman, L.J., Havard, E.S., and Eger, E.I. (1964). Hyperthermia during anesthesia. *JAMA* 190, 1029.

Sanders, G.L., Routledge, P.A., Ward, A., *et al.* (1979). Mean steady-state plasma concentrations of labetalol in patients undergoing antihypertensive therapy. *Br. J. Clin. Pharmacol.* 8, 153.

Schmidt, K.L. and Mueller-Eckhardt, C. (1977). Agranulocytosis, levamisole, and HLA-B27. *Lancet* ii, 85.

Schreiber, A.J. and Simon, F.R. (1983). Estrogen-induced cholestasis: pathogenesis and treatment. *Hepatology* 3, 607.

Schroder, H. and Evans, D.A.P. (1972). Acetylator phenotype and adverse effects of sulphasalazine in healthy subjects. *Gut* 13, 278.

Schrogie, J.J. and Solomon, H.M. (1967). The anticoagulant response to bishydroxy-coumarin. II. The effect of D-thyroxine, clofibrate and norethandrolone. *Clin. Pharmacol. Ther.* 8, 70.

Schwartz, J.T., Reuling, F.H., Feinleib, M., *et al.* (1972). Twin heritability study of the effect of corticosteroids on intraocular pressure. *J. Med. Genet.* 9, 137.

Shammas, F.V. and Dickstein, K. (1988). Clinical pharmacokinetics in heart failure: an update. *Clin. Pharmacokinet.* 15, 94.

Shimada, T., Yamazaki, H., Mimura, M. *et al.* (1994). Interindividual variations in human liver cytochrome P450 enzymes involved in the oxidation of drugs, carcinogens and toxic chemicals. *J. Pharmacol. Exp. Ther.* 61, 414.

Simpson, N.E. and Kalow, W. (1966). Pharmacology and biological variation. *Ann. N.Y. Acad. Sci.* 134, 864.

Sjöqvist, F., Borga, O., Dahl, M-L., *et al.* (1997). Fundamentals of clinical pharmacology. In *Avery's Drug Treatment* (4th edn) (ed. T.M. Speight and N.H.G. Holford), p. 1. Adis International, Auckland.

Smith, R. (1984). Osteogenesis imperfecta. *BMJ* 289, 394.

Smith, J.M. and Dodd, T.R.P. (1982). Adverse reactions to pharmaceutical excipients. *Adverse Drug React. Acute Poisoning Rev.* 1, 93.

Smith, S.E. and Rawlins, M.D. (1973). *Variability in Human Drug Response*. Butterworth, London.

Solomon, H.M. and Schrogie, J.J. (1967). Change in receptor site affinity: a proposed explanation for the potentiating effect of D-thyroxine on the anticoagulant response to warfarin. *Clin. Pharmacol. Ther.* 8, 797.

Solomons, C.C. and Myers, D.N. (1972). Hyperthermia of osteogenesis imperfecta and its relationship to malignant hyperthermia. In *International Symposium on Malignant Hyperthermia* (ed. R.A. Gordan, B.A. Britt, and W. Kalow), p. 319. Thomas, Springfield, Illinois.

Soltan, C., Terraza, A., Descomps, B. *et al.* (1980). Cimetidine competition with androgens for binding to human sex skin fibroblasts androgen receptors. *J. Ster. Biochem.* 13, 839.

Stanski, D.R. and Maitre, P.O. (1990). Population pharmacokinetics and pharmacodynamics of thiopental: the effects of age revisited. *Anesthesiology* 72, 412.

Steffensen, G. and Pedersen, S. (1986). Food induced changes in theophylline absorption from a once-a-day theophylline product. *Br. J. Clin. Pharmacol.* 22, 571.

Stoehr, G.B., Krobuth, P.D., Juhl, R.P., *et al.* (1984). Effects of oral contraceptives on triazolam, alprazolam and lorazepam kinetics. *Clin. Pharmacol. Ther.* 36, 683.

Sulkowski, S.R. and Haserick, J.R. (1964). Simulated systemic lupus erythematosus from degraded tetracycline. *JAMA* 189, 152.

Tan, K.S., Grove, A., Cargill, R.I., *et al.* (1996). Effects of inhaled fluticasone propionate and oral prednisolone on lymphocyte beta 2-adrenoceptor function in asthmatic patients. *Chest* 109, 343.

Thomson, P.D., Melmon, K.L., Richardson, J.A., *et al.* (1973). Lidocaine pharmacokinetics in advanced heart failure, liver disease, and renal failure in humans. *Ann. Intern. Med.* 78, 499.

Toivakka, E. and Hokkanen, E. (1965). The aggravating effect of streptomycin on the neuromuscular blockade in myasthenia gravis. *Acta Neurol. Scand.* 41 (Suppl. 13), 275.

Vale, J.A. and Proudfoot, A. (1992). Drug overdosage and poisoning. In *Avery's Drug Treatment* (4th edn) (ed. T.M. Speight and N.H.G. Holford), p. 337. Adis International, Auckland.

Verbeeck, R.K., Branch, R.A., and Wilkinson, G.R. (1981).

Drug metabolites in renal failure: pharmacokinetic and clinical implications. *Clin. Pharmacokinet.* 6, 329.

Vesell, E.S. (1972). Drug therapy: pharmacogenetics. *N. Engl. J. Med.* 287, 904.

Wahrenberg, H., Engfeldt, P., Amer, P., *et al.* (1986). Adrenergic regulation of lipolysis in human adipocytes: findings in hyper- and hypothyroidism. *J. Clin. Endocrinol. Metab.* 63, 631.

Waller, P., Wood, S., Breckenridge, A.M., *et al.* (1991). Eosinophilia–myalgia syndrome associated with prescribed L-tryptophan in the United Kingdom. *Health Trends* 23, 53.

Walter-Sack, I. and Klotz, U. (1996). Influence of diet and nutritional status on drug metabolism. *Clin. Pharmacokinet.* 31, 47.

Walton, V.C., Howlett, M.R., and Seltzer, G.B. (1970). Anhydrotetracycline and 4-epiandrotetracycline in market tetracyclines and aged tetracycline products. *J. Pharmacol. Sci.* 59, 1160.

Weatherall, D.J. and Hatton, C.S.R. (1987). Congenital haemolytic anaemias. *Med. Int.* 2, 1712.

Weiss, H.J., Aledort, L.M., and Kochwa, S. (1968). The effect of salicylates on the hemostatic properties of platelets in man. *J. Clin. Invest.* 47, 2169.

Whitelock, O. (ed.) (1959). Chlorpropamide and diabetes mellitus (Symposium). *Ann. N.Y. Acad. Sci.* 74, 411.

Williams, R.T. (1967). Comparative patterns of drug metabolism. *Fed. Proc. Fedn Am. Soc. Exp. Biol.* 26, 1029.

Woodhouse, K.W.I. and Wynne, H.A. (1988). Age-related changes in liver size and hepatic blood flow: the influence on drug metabolism in the elderly. *Clin. Pharmacokinet.* 15, 287.

Woodhouse, K.W., Williams, F.M., Mutch, E., *et al.* (1983). The effect of alcoholic cirrhosis on the activities of microsomal aldrin epoxidase, 7-ethoxycoumarin *o*-de-ethylase and epoxide hydrolase, and on the concentrations of reduced glutathione in human liver. *Br. J. Clin. Pharmacol.* 15, 667.

Wooley, P.H., Griffin, J., Payani, G.S., *et al.* (1980). HLA-DR antigens and toxic reaction to sodium aurothiomalate and D-penicillamine in patients with rheumatoid arthritis. *N. Engl. J. Med.* 303, 300.

Woolhouse, N.M. and Atu-Taylor, L.C. (1982). Influence of double genetic polymorphism on response to sulfamethazine. *Clin. Pharmacol. Ther.* 31, 377.

Woosley, R.L., Drayer, D.E., Reidenberg, M.M., *et al.* (1978). Effect of acetylator phenotype on the rate at which procainamide induces antinuclear antibodies and the lupus syndrome. *N. Engl. J. Med.* 298, 1157.

WHO (World Health Organization) (1967). Standardisation of procedures for the study of glucose-6-phosphate dehydrogenase. *WHO Tech. Rep. Ser.* 366.

WHO (World Health Organization) (1973). Pharmacogenetics. *WHO Tech. Rep. Ser.* 524.

Zimmerman, H.J. and Maddrey, W.C. (1995). Acetaminophen (paracetamol) hepatotoxicity with regular intake of alcohol: analysis of instances of therapeutic misadventure. *Hepatology* 22, 767.

6. Chromosome damage

D. F. ROBERTS

Clinical cytogenetics — the study of chromosome abnormalities in relation to human pathology — developed following technical advances made between the late 1950s and the early 1970s. That DNA damage inflicted by radiation or chemicals might have cytogenetic effects, and might be detectable in chromosome analysis, had been known for many years, but it was only during the 1980s that the importance of cytogenetic studies in mutagenicity testing gained full recognition. This largely reflected the growing appreciation of the role of chromosome aberration in reproductive loss, congenital malformation, and carcinogenesis. In the last decade, and especially with the arrival of molecular methods which allow the detection of specific DNA and RNA sequences, cytogenetic techniques have been refined and it is possible to be more precise in the location of chromosomal damage (Adinolfi and Crolla 1994).

The nature of chromosome damage

Damage to chromosomes is detected during cell division. In interphase, between mitotic divisions, the chromosomes are long and threadlike, and cannot be individually distinguished under the microscope, though the cell nucleus is very active metabolically. Interphase is divided into three periods, G_1, S, and G_2: in the S (synthesis) period the amount of chromosomal material in the nucleus is doubled, while G_1 and G_2 are periods of metabolic activity and growth. In prophase of mitosis, the chromosomes contract and become more readily visible, and each can be seen to consist of two chromatids. Shortening of the chromosomes continues into metaphase, with sister chromatids still held together at the centromeres; it is in this stage that detailed observation of chromosome morphology and structure can be made. At metaphase, the chromosomes are arranged on the equator of the cell with the spindle structure connecting the centromere of each chromosome to the poles of the cell. The centromeres then divide, separating the sister chromatids, which migrate to opposite poles of the cell under the control of the spindle apparatus. As the two sets of daughter chromosomes separate, the cytoplasm divides. Subsequently, nuclear and cell membranes are formed, and the daughter nuclei pass into the next interphase. Opportunities for exogenous agents to interfere with the chromosomes arise first in interphase during the manufacture of the DNA required for the daughter chromosomes, secondly during prophase, when chromatids condense, and thirdly during anaphase when the sister chromatids separate.

Similarly, in meiosis (the production of gametes) there are opportunities for damage between cell divisions, during replication, and in the separation of chromosomes in each of the two consecutive divisions that are involved in the process.

Substances that cause chromosome damage are termed clastogens (after Shaw 1970).

Chromosome damage may take several forms:

1. gaps: small discontinuities in individual chromatids or in both chromatids of a single chromosome;
2. breaks: involving either a single chromatid, or both chromatids at the same point, and resulting in a deletion and an acentric fragment;
3. chromosome exchanges: translocations, rings, inversions, dicentrics, and other structural alterations;
4. pulverization: extensive destruction of the chromosomes resulting from large numbers of breaks.

In some studies the types of damage are classified as stable — that is, those that are retained over a series of cell divisions (Cs cells), and those that are unstable and disappear relatively rapidly (Cu). Diagrams of the effects of breaks are shown in Figure 6.1, and examples of damage in Figure 6.2.

Chromosome mutagenicity testing

The techniques of experimental examination fall into two categories. The first involves *in vitro* cultures, usually of peripheral blood lymphocytes stimulated to divide by phytohaemagglutinin (PHA). The amounts of damage inflicted on the chromosomes by the addition to such cultures of varying drug concentrations are then compared with control values. Secondly, *in vivo* damage may be examined, using metaphase cells — again, most conveniently blood lymphocytes — from patients undergoing drug therapy, and comparing their levels of chromosome damage with cells from matched controls not exposed to the drug. *In vivo* procedures have frequently been applied to animal studies, but cytogenetic data from such experiments cannot be directly extrapolated to humans because species differ in their drug metabolism both in terms of metabolic rates and by variations in biochemical pathways.

Scoring of gaps, breaks, and other forms of chromatid and chromosome lesions has been well established since the early days of human cytogenetics. The development of reliable chromosome banding techniques in the early 1970s allowed symmetrical chromosome rearrangements (i.e. exchanges that do not alter the shapes of the chromosomes), which were previously undetectable by solid staining, to be recorded. Development of more sophisticated techniques, for example, the sister chromatid exchange (SCE) method, has allowed new approaches to the study of chromosome damage. The SCE method involves incubation of cell cultures for two cycles of DNA replication in the presence of 5-bromodeoxyuridine (BrdU) and differential staining to give the 'harlequin' pattern shown in Figure 6.2. SCE represents rearrangements of material within a given chromosome and, though it has no genotoxic consequences in its own right, provides a very sensitive indicator of genotoxicity, since they may often be induced at mutagen levels too low to produce classical chromosome aberrations. Only 70 per cent of studies show a close correlation

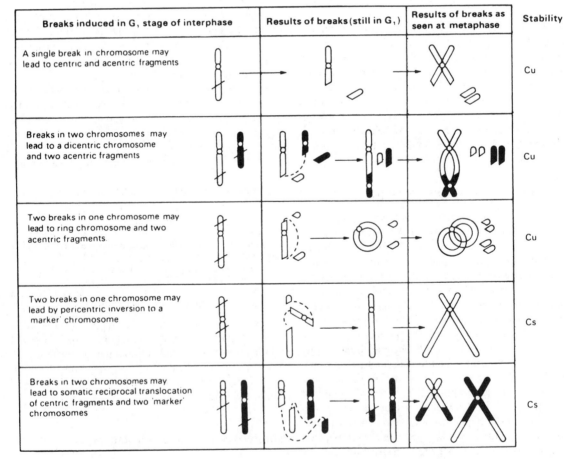

Breaks induced in G, stage of interphase	Results of breaks (still in G₁)	Results of breaks as seen at metaphase	Stability
A single break in chromosome may lead to centric and acentric fragments			Cu
Breaks in two chromosomes may lead to a dicentric chromosome and two acentric fragments			Cu
Two breaks in one chromosome may lead to ring chromosome and two acentric fragments			Cu
Two breaks in one chromosome may lead by pericentric inversion to a 'marker' chromosome			Cs
Breaks in two chromosomes may lead to somatic reciprocal translocation of centric fragments and two 'marker' chromosomes			Cs

FIG. 6.1
Mechanisms of chromosome breakage and rearrangement. (After Stevenson *et al.* 1971.)

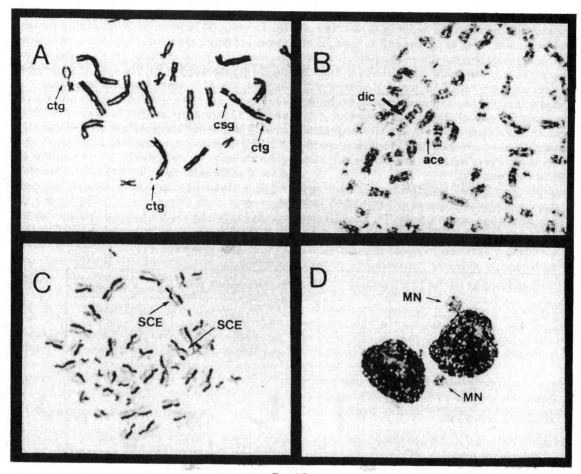

FIG. 6.2

Chromosome damage in human lymphocytes: (a) part of a metaphase cell showing chromosome and chromatid gaps; (b) G-banded preparation showing a dicentric chromosome and an acentric fragment; (c) metaphase cell stained to demonstrate sister chromatid exchanges; (d) micronuclei in a preparation treated with cytochalasin B.

between SCE frequencies and the incidence of classical chromosome abnormalities (Gebhart 1981). Moreover the relationship of SCE to chromosome damage varies according to the drug used (Ferguson and Denny 1995). This suggests that different mechanisms of lesion formation may be involved in the two phenomena, with the implication that SCE techniques should be regarded as a useful addition to and not a replacement for traditional methods of measuring chromosome damage.

'Micronuclei' are useful for scoring *in vivo* damage. These result from the exclusion from daughter nuclei of acentric chromosome fragments (and also of whole chromosomes if the spindle apparatus has been dam-

aged); in interphase, these fragments then appear as small micronuclei separate from the main nucleus (Heddle *et al.* 1983). By the use of cytochalasin B, which allows nuclear division but blocks cytoplasmic separation, cells with micronuclei can be scored rapidly and reliably to give a quantitative index of chromosomal breakage and non-disjunction.

Classical chromosome damage, SCE, and micronuclei all occur spontaneously in normal cells; clastogenicity studies involve screening for excess damage superimposed on this background rate.

The use of DNA or RNA probes has brought a new dimension to studies of chromosome damage, for specific sequences in chromosomes in interphase or metaphase cells can be detected by *in situ* hybridization procedures based on the annealing of probes labelled with the appropriate sequences to their corresponding genomic regions on the chromosomes. After early studies using radio-labelled probes, non-isotopic *in situ* hybridization (NISH) was introduced by Manning *et al.* (1975) using electron microscopy. Today there are several procedures in which the hybridization complexes are more easily visualized, exploiting various fluorochromes, enzymatic reactions, and antibodies to amplify the signals. Each has its advantages. For example, fluorescence *in situ* hybridization (FISH) can show several sequences simultaneously. Such techniques provide much more precise detail, of location of breakpoints or of deleted material, than classical cytogenetic methods, and allow a more rapid scoring of aneuploid cells. They have not yet been widely used in drugdamage studies.

The significance of induced chromosome damage

The significance of induced chromosome damage lies in the role of chromosome aberration in both carcinogenesis and reproduction.

The non-random involvement of chromosome changes in leukaemias and solid tumours, and the elucidation of chromosome rearrangement as a mechanism of oncogene activation, underlie concern about the carcinogenic potential of clastogenic agents. Susceptibility to genetic damage — or inability to repair such damage — is well known as the basis of the 'chromosome fragility syndromes' such as ataxia telangiectasia, Bloom's syndrome, and Fanconi's pancytopenia (Sandberg 1983). Furthermore, a number of studies demonstrate chromosome instability in cells from cancer patients; for example, Brown and colleagues (1985) investigated patients who had two or more primary tumours (and could therefore be regarded as having an inherent susceptibility to cancer) and found elevated levels of chromosome aberrations and SCE in lymphocytes from six of 11 cases. An association between increased rates of *in vivo* lymphocyte chromosome breakage and skin cancer has also been reported (Nordenson *et al.* 1984), while reduced ability to repair bleomycin-generated chromosome damage has been correlated with cancer risk in both a large family affected by high incidences of diverse cancers (Liang *et al.* 1989), and in lymphocytes of 19 patients with testicular cancer who showed elevated levels of chromosome damage compared with controls (Vorechovsky and Zaloudik 1989). Chromosome instability has also been documented in patients with testicular cancer who had not been exposed to chemotherapeutic drugs (van den Berg-de Ruiter *et al.* 1990). Thus, there appear to be strong grounds for concern that agents promoting somatic chromosome mutation may be involved in the initiation of human cancers.

The other main area in which induced chromosome damage may have a significant deleterious effect is in reproduction and embryogenesis. The induction of chromosome mutations in gametes or their precursors may result either in reduced fertility or in chromosomally abnormal offspring. Genetically unbalanced embryos may be either aneuploid as a result of damage to the meiotic spindle, or partially aneuploid as a result of recombination of a structural chromosome abnormality. Such embryos are likely to abort spontaneously and usually show congenital abnormalities if they survive to full-term and birth. Consequently, while the selection inherent in the processes of gametogenesis and in early embryo development probably eliminates the majority of germ cell mutations, the potential hereditary effects of induced chromosome damage are serious.

Genesca and others (1990) compared the incidence of structural chromosome aberration in both lymphocytes and spermatozoa from four treated cancer patients (two after chemotherapy, two after radiotherapy). In all four individuals there were elevated frequencies of cells showing chromosome damage in both tissues when compared with control series. The frequencies of damaged cells were very significantly higher in the spermatozoa than in the lymphocytes; this suggests that extrapolations from studies of somatic cell clastogenicity to potential effects on germ cells may not be straightforward.

The experience of aristolochic acid well illustrates the potential importance of clastogenicity testing of medicinal agents. This drug was in common use for a number of purposes until its abrupt withdrawal from the market in 1981 following evidence of potent carcinogenic effects in experimental rats. About 100 manufacturers of approximately 250 products were affected by the withdrawal of this drug. Abel and Schimmer (1983) subsequently investigated the *in vitro* chromosome-damaging properties of this substance to establish whether cytogenetic studies could have provided advance warning of genotoxic potential. Significant dose-dependent increases in both chromosome damage and SCE were apparent in lymphocyte cultures exposed to aristolochic acid.

Clastogenic compounds have been found in most of the major classes of drugs, including the cytostatic and antineoplastic agents, antibiotics, psychotropic drugs, anticonvulsants, immunosuppressants, and oral contraceptives, and also among drugs in social and illicit use.

The effect of drugs

Antibiotic and antineoplastic drugs

Of the therapeutic drugs, those on which the most investigation has been carried out are the antibiotic and antineoplastic agents, possibly because the action of many of these is directed through the DNA and RNA, and thus is likely to cause chromosome damage. The early studies were succinctly summarized by Sieber and Adamson (1975).

The clastogenic properties of cyclophosphamide have been recognized for many years, induced chromosome damage having been reported both *in vitro* (Urba 1971) and *in vivo* (Schmid and Bauchinger 1973; Dobos *et al.* 1974). The frequency of chromosome aberrations increased exponentially, and sister chromatid exchanges linearly, with dose (Bochkov *et al.* 1986). The damage is thought to result mainly from the DNA crosslinking induced by one of its breakdown products, phosphoramide mustard (Colvin *et al.* 1990), and the DNA binding of another, acrolein (Crook *et al.* 1986), and the single strand DNA breaks it causes. The need to take physiological factors into account in considering genotoxic drug effects is illustrated by the work of Sargent and others (1987). These authors reported statistically significant increases in chromosome breakage in lymphocyte cultures exposed to 0.001–0.00001 μg per ml cyclophosphamide. Whole blood cultures, on the other hand, did not show chromosome instability even at 0.2 μg per ml since binding of the drug to red blood cells prevents activation.

An *in vitro* study by Raposa in 1978 of a range of cytostatic drugs demonstrated increased SCE frequencies after exposure to vincristine, cytarabine, and lycurium at doses too low to produce significant levels of classical chromosome damage. The number of gaps and breaks induced *in vitro* in lymphocyte cultures by treatment with busulphan and triaziquone, however, showed a distinct dependence on dose and on the stage of the cell cycle at the time of treatment (Gebhart 1971).

Lomustine (CCNU), used in melanoma cases, seems to cause prolonged and cumulative increases in SCE levels. In a study by Lambert and colleagues (1979), one patient demonstrated higher lymphocyte SCE frequencies 8 weeks after a second dose of lomustine than were found 6 weeks after the first dose.

Melphalan has been the subject of several investigations. Lambert and others (1984) examined lymphocyte chromosomes from 50 patients with ovarian cancer and found that 5.4 per cent of the cells showed chromosome aberrations, compared with 2.3 per cent in the control group. Since chromosome aberrations were detected in circulating lymphocytes 7–8 years after treatment, this suggests that genetic damage had been inflicted on haematological progenitor cells — an interesting observation in view of the fact that the commonest secondary cancer in melphalan-treated patients is leukaemia. These findings have been strongly supported in a recent study of peripheral blood cells from 14 cancer patients; Mamuris and co-workers (1989) recorded an even more striking elevation in chromosome rearrangements, these being present in 21.5 per cent of patients' cells compared with 1.2 per cent of cells from healthy controls. Chromosomes 5 and 7 were the most frequently involved — these are also the chromosomes most frequently rearranged in secondary leukaemias.

Methotrexate is widely used as a prophylactic measure against CNS involvement in leukaemias. The clastogenic effects of this agent have long been recognized both *in vitro* (e.g. Mondello *et al.* 1984) and *in vivo* (Krogh Jensen and Nyfors 1979).

Dose-dependent clastogenic effects have been reported for cisplatin both in human cells *in vitro* (Srb *et al.* 1986) and in animals *in vivo*. The frequency of micronuclei in cell cultures of skin fibroblasts from healthy children showed that damage following exposure to *cis*-DDP was both dose- and time-dependent (Jirsova and Mandys 1994). The main molecular cause of the damage is the 1 per cent of cisplatin that binds to genomic DNA, for it brings about intrastrand cross-links between two neighbouring guanines or between neighbouring adenine and guanine.

Although most of the anticancer drugs are effective in causing chromosome damage, they vary in their ability to induce sister chromatid exchange. For many alkylating agents, for example, cisplatin, melphalan and mitomycin C, SCE appears at lower drug concentrations and so provides a more sensitive assay than direct measurements of chromosomal aberrations, in contrast to bleomycin and antimetabolites, for example, cytarabine, mercaptopurine, and methotrexate, where chromosome damage is clearly visible but which are less effective inducers of SCE (Ferguson and Denny 1995).

Neocarzinostatin has been shown to be a powerful inducer of chromosome and chromatid aberrations *in vitro*, but relatively poor at inducing SCE (Psaraki and Demopoulos 1988). A dose effect was noted for SCE induction, but only to a maximum of twice the control values.

Unusual forms of chromosome damage, such as 'uncompleted-packing mitotic figures' and 'free chromatin structures', were reported to be induced *in vitro* by the antitumour/antibiotic complex pingyanymycin (Heng *et al.* 1988).

Of the antibiotics used as antineoplastic agents, doxorubicin (adriamycin) — an inhibitor of nucleic acid synthesis — was shown by Neustad (1978) to cause a significant rise in lymphocyte SCE levels *in vitro* (9.6 SCE per cell, after exposure to 1 ng of doxorubicin compared with 4.8 SCE per cell for controls). The chromosome-damaging effect of bleomycin therapy was investigated by Bornstein and others (1971). Chromosomes from bone marrow preparations were screened for aberrations both before, on the last day of, and one month after bleomycin therapy in four carcinoma patients. All post-therapy samples were shown to contain a higher proportion of mitoses with chromosome abnormalities. The effect is specific to early interphase in the cell cycle (Dresp *et al.* 1978), since the main types of aberration after exposure early in the cycle were dicentrics and deletions, but in the G_2 phase were chromatid breaks: the amount of damage was linearly related to dose. This linearity in the G_2 phase was challenged by MacLeod *et al.* (1994) who examined the dose responses in a 5-minute pulse of bleomycin and dispersal of chromatid aberrations (gaps, breaks, exchanges, isochromatid breaks) in cultures of lymphocytes from healthy females. Over a logarithmic range of doses, all types of breaks and the total aberrations increased linearly in the range 6.3 to 100 μg per ml, but were independent of dose below that range. The effect of bleomycin is seen in bone marrow cells and in peripheral lymphocytes in patients, and *in vitro* in human spermatozoa (Kamiguchi *et al.* 1995), and similar spermatozoal damage occurred with daunorubicin, methyl methanesulfonate, and triethylenemelamine. The damage to chromosomes caused by bleomycin is due to its effect on DNA: low concentrations bring about breaks in single-stranded DNA and high concentrations cause breaks in double-stranded DNA (Anderson *et al.* 1995). It inflicts oxidative damage at a specific position in DNA, the C-4' position of deoxyribose, causing lesions predominantly at pyramidines in G-C and G-T sequences (Povirk and Austin 1991). Susceptibility to bleomycin-induced damage is enhanced in cancer patients (Vorechovsky and Zaloudik 1989), and reduced in cultured cells conditioned to a low concentration of bleomycin (Vijaya-laxmi and Burkart 1989) and in those where vitamin C is added to the culture (Anderson *et al.* 1995).

RNA-inhibiting antibiotics, for example, daunorubicin (Sinkus 1972), are clastogenic *in vitro*, while the work of Whang-Peng and others (1969) showed an increase of chromosome aberrations and exchanges in bone marrow metaphases of three out of seven patients receiving daunorubicin treatment.

The aminoglycoside antibiotic doxorubicin, an agent used to treat solid tumours and leukaemia, increases sister chromatid exchanges and chromosome aberrations *in vitro* and *in vivo*, though these disappear rapidly *in vivo* (Neustad 1978).

On the question of possible genotoxic hazards faced by medical staff in handling cytostatic and cytotoxic drugs, results have been mixed and contradictory; for example, Nikula and co-workers (1984) and Sessink *et al.* (1994) reported significantly raised numbers of chromosomally aberrant lymphocytes and of breaks per cell, compared with controls, in hospital staff handling cytostatic agents, but Benhamou and others (1988), found no increase in SCE rates or chromosomal damage in 29 nurses handling these compounds. Such conflicts, apparent in these and over a dozen other studies, may be partly due to variations in the degree and duration of exposure of the subjects. The one prospective study in which chromosome aberrations, SCEs, and micronucleated cells were examined in pharmacists before and after one year of working with cytostatic drugs under careful containment, showed a barely significant increase in mean frequency of SCEs per cell and none in micronuclei or total chromosome aberrations (Roth *et al.* 1994).

A wide range of antibiotics has been assessed for clastogenic potential. Stevenson and Patel (1973*a*) reported an increase of gaps and breaks in lymphocyte cultures of patients treated with chlorambucil. There were similar findings (Palmer *et al.* 1984, 1985) in a group of 10 patients taking the drug for up to 68 months at doses of 2–6 mg per day. A highly significant elevation in SCE levels was noted, the excess correlating with both dose and length of treatment. Follow-up studies suggested that the damage was permanent, or at least very long-lasting.

Ampicillin and carbenicillin were investigated by Jaju and colleagues (1984) in human lymphocyte cultures. Chromosome damage was not observed at therapeutic plasma concentrations, but did appear at higher doses. SCE were not induced by either drug at any concentration tested.

Several antibiotics that inhibit DNA synthesis, such as mitomycin C (Cohen and Shaw 1964), produce chromosome breaks *in vitro*, even at low concentrations. The DNA lesions induced by mitomycin C, 4-nitroquinoline-1-oxide, and ethyl methanesulfonate, persist and elicit SCEs for at least three successive cell cycles (Daza *et al.*

1992). Indeed, the reliable chromosome-damaging action of mitomycin C forms the basis of the cytogenetic diagnosis of Fanconi's pancytopenia — lymphocytes from patients with this chromosome fragility syndrome are less able to repair mitomycin-induced damage *in vitro* than lymphocytes from normal controls.

It is generally considered that the protein inhibitors puromycin, streptomycin, and the tetracyclines have no chromosome-breaking effect (Shaw 1970). The evidence for the genotoxicity of chloramphenicol was reviewed by Rosenkranz (1988). While clastogenic action has been reported in human cells in a number of studies involving both *in vivo* and *in vitro* exposure to chloramphenicol, negative results have been obtained in a number of other test systems for mutagenic potential, and Rosenkranz proposed that the chromosome-damaging properties of this antibiotic do not indicate genuine genotoxicity. Since then, several studies have examined the genotoxicity of chloramphenicol. Martelli *et al.* (1991) concluded that it had only a weak effect at concentrations much higher than those used in human therapy. Sbrana *et al.* (1991) showed that chromosome aberrations only occurred in human lymphocytes exposed to a high level of chloramphenicol during a whole cell cycle, and that exposure only in the G_1 and G_2 phases had no effect. In view of the risks associated with chloramphenicol therapy of human infectious disease, Lafarge-Frayssinet *et al.* (1994) enquired into the effects of its principal metabolites, assessing cytotoxicity in terms of inhibition of DNA synthesis by counting the number of DNA single-strand breaks over a wide range of concentrations. Finding that nitrosochloramphenicol, dehydrochloramphenicol, and dehydrochloramphenicol base induce DNA breaks in human lymphocytes, whereas chloramphenicol itself and three other metabolites are totally devoid of cytotoxic effect except at high concentrations, they concluded that chloramphenicol itself is much less toxic than some of its metabolites and does not present a real problem for human health.

In 1982 the broad-spectrum antibiotic cephaloridine was shown to cause chromosome damage *in vitro* (Jaju *et al.* 1982). A dose effect was reported, and cephaloridine may be considered clastogenic at the upper levels of permissible therapeutic doses.

Immunosuppressants

Several conventional immunosuppressant drugs have been reported to induce chromosomal damage. In 1979, Schuler and others investigated chromosome damage and SCE in patients with chronic renal disease receiving immunosuppressive drugs. Chromosome stability was tested by scoring breaks after exposure of lymphocytes to the alkylating agent lycurium. All treatments were found to produce significantly raised aberration frequencies, and dose effects were noted for all drug regimens except mercaptopurine monotherapy. The greatest clastogenic effects were recorded in patients receiving high doses of cyclophosphamide or chlorambucil, or a combination of vinblastine sulphate, cyclophosphamide, mercaptopurine, and prednisolone.

In vitro, cells from healthy adults cultured with cyclosporin at $1 \mu g$ per ml showed increased SCEs (Yuzawa *et al.* 1986) but Zwanenburg and Cordier (1994) found that at no concentration did cyclosporin increase the frequency of cells with chromosomal aberrations. Yuzawa *et al.* (1987), comparing several drugs, reported that at concentrations of $0.2 g$ per ml inducibility of SCEs per cell was least when treated with cyclosporin, higher with mizoribine, and mercaptopurine, and highest with methotrexate.

For azathioprine, there are contradictory results from various studies of chromosome stability. Apelt and others (1981) demonstrated no significant clastogenic properties *in vitro*, with SCE levels unchanged from control values at all concentrations tested. The *in vivo* study, on the other hand, did reveal a higher incidence of gross chromosome damage compared with controls.

Anticonvulsants

Initial cytogenetic studies of the anticonvulsant drugs phenytoin and ethotoin (e.g. Brogger 1970) suggested that these agents were non-clastogenic *in vivo*, although Muniz and others (1969) were able to induce structural chromosome aberrations in lymphocytes *in vitro* using phenytoin at clinically toxic doses.

Two subsequent studies of women treated with various anticonvulsant drugs and of their children exposed *in utero* (Neuhauser *et al.* 1970; Grosse *et al.* 1972) described increased numbers of metaphases with structural aberrations, but without apparent teratogenic effect. It seems that the fetal abnormalities known to occur after maternal treatment with these and related drugs do not derive directly from gross chromosome damage. A study in 1977 on bone marrow preparations from 22 epileptics suggested that phenytoin is non-clastogenic at therapeutic levels, the mean frequencies of classical chromosome aberrations being 0.5 per cent in patients and 0.4 per cent in the 20 healthy controls (Knuutila *et al.* 1977). These findings appear to differ from those of an *in vitro* study (Garcia Sagredo 1988) of phenytoin, ethosuximide, and phenobarbitone. Lymphocyte cultures were exposed to three drug concentrations ranging from 50 per cent to 300 per cent of therapeutic tissue levels, and significant dose-related increases in chromosome aberrations compared with control values were documented for all cultures.

SCE studies of antiepileptic drugs have produced similarly contradictory results. A trial carried out in 1982 in nine children receiving phenytoin therapy revealed a highly significant increase in mean SCE levels, with controls showing an average of 6.49 SCE per cell and patients 10.3 SCE per cell (Habedank *et al.*1982).

An *in vivo* study following 36 epileptic children for 6 months to 6 years on different anticonvulsant drugs concluded that phenobarbitone, valproic acid, and carbamazepine as long-term monotherapy produced no increase in chromatid or chromosome breakage or SCEs over those in controls (Kitsiou-Tzeli *et al.* 1994). By contrast, investigating sodium valproate, Hu *et al.* (1990) compared 10 epileptic children before and after treatment for 6–7 months; 20 patients treated for 6–52 months with 20 others who had not taken any anticonvulsant over the previous 6 months; and 20 matched healthy children; and *in vitro* cells from healthy children in cultures exposed to different concentrations of valproic acid. The first three comparisons all showed increased frequencies of SCEs per cell with valproic acid treatment, while the *in vitro* study showed an increase in chromatid and chromosome gaps and breaks. In 27 epileptic patients treated with phenytoin, carbamazepine, or valproic acid, the mean level of SCEs per cell (6.77) was significantly higher than in untreated healthy adults (Sardas *et al.* 1994).

Schaumann and colleagues (1985) investigated patients receiving carbamazepine (CBZ) therapy. No significant differences were found in *in vivo* SCE or chromosome damage in lymphocytes between nine patients and their controls. The *in vitro* study, scoring chromosome breaks in blood cultures from six healthy male donors, revealed a strong dose-related response starting at $10 \mu g$ per ml (therapeutic range in serum $4–12 \mu g$ per ml), but no induction of SCE at 5, 10, or $15 \mu g$ per ml. The authors suggested that the negative *in vivo* results are clinically more relevant than the positive *in vitro* result, since the latter arises from the failure of cultured lymphocytes metabolically to clear CBZ.

Psychotropic drugs

Nielsen and others (1968) reported increased damage to chromosomes in 17 patients treated with various psychotropic drugs, in particular, chlorpromazine, perphenazine, and LSD.

The effect of chlorpromazine was confirmed *in vitro* by Kamada and co-workers (1971). Cohen and colleagues (1972), however, investigating perphenazine and chlorpromazine, found no significant differences in chromosome damage between controls and patients before, during, or after 6 weeks of treatment with the two drugs. In accounting for the discrepancies between their findings and those of previous trials, these authors pointed to the lack of established pretreatment damage levels in earlier studies, and to the use of orphenadrine — the clastogenic effect of which had not been investigated — in some patients.

The tranquillizer trifluoperazine was shown by Jenkins (1970) to cause an increase in cells showing chromosome breaks in patients as compared with controls, the percentages being 27.7 and 10.2 respectively. Despite reports in 1969 that lithium might be a chromosome-breaking agent, Garson (1981) found no significant increase in SCE frequencies in 23 psychiatric patients when compared with 19 age-matched controls. Diazepam was found not to have any damaging effect at any concentration or exposure (Staiger 1969). Imipramine showed no increase in chromosome breaks at any concentration in *in vitro* study of cultures from seven donors (Fu and Jarvik 1977).

A significant clastogenic effect was reported for thioridazine (Saxena and Ahuja 1982); chromosome aberration frequencies were significantly elevated in psychiatric patients taking this drug when compared with both psychiatric and normal controls.

Contraceptive agents

Cytogenetic investigations of users of the contraceptive pill have produced controversial results.

Carr (1970) studied spontaneous abortions occurring within 6 months of discontinuing oral contraception and recorded a striking elevation in the incidence of polyploidy, with triploidy occurring four to five times more frequently in fetuses of the post-contraceptive group than in the controls, and a sixfold increase in tetraploidy.

McQuarrie and others (1970) found an increase in chromosome gaps and in the incidence of triploidy in babies born to mothers using oral contraception compared with those born to control mothers. There was no difference, however, in other aneuploidies or frequencies of chromosome breaks between the two groups of babies.

In 1975, a US investigation demonstrated significantly higher levels of chromosome breaks in the lymphocytes of nulligravid women taking the pill (7.8 per cent of metaphases showing breaks) compared with nulligravidae who had never used oral contraceptives (5.5 per cent) (Littlefield *et al.* 1975). These increased breakage frequencies could not, however, be correlated with the duration of contraceptive use. In contrast, Bishun (1976) concluded that the overall findings suggest no increase in chromosomal damage in women who had taken oral contraceptives at normal prescribed dosage for moderately long periods of time before conceiving.

An SCE investigation in 1979 of 15 normal women, 15 women in the third trimester of pregnancy, and 15 pill-users (taking a combined D-norgestrel/ethinyloestradiol preparation for between 6 and 24 months) showed a significantly (75 per cent) increased mean SCE per cell in the women using the oral contraceptives (Murthy and Prema 1979).

No significant induction of either chromosome abnormalities or SCE in lymphocytes *in vitro* was observed in a 1985 study of diethylstilboestrol (DES) and oestradiol carried out by Banduhn and Obe. Micronuclei were noted, but were ascribed by the authors to mitotic spindle disruption rather than chromosome damage. Henderson and Regan (1985) exposed pregnant mice to high doses of diethylstilboestrol dipropionate and then examined maternal bone marrow and fetal liver for clastogenic effects. No increases were apparent in SCE, chromosome breakage, or micronuclei, although the levels of aneuploid and polyploid cells were elevated in both systems. The ability of DES to induce aneuploidy in cultured human cells has been confirmed by De Sario and others (1990). When *in situ* hybridization using a Y chromosome-specific probe labelled radioactively and with biotin was applied in cultures of human peripheral lymphocytes exposed to three concentrations of DES, while both techniques showed an increase of hyperdiploid nuclei, the biotinylated probe was more sensitive and demonstrated that the increase was dose related.

An earlier study compared peripheral lymphocyte chromosome aberrations in 44 women taking hormonal contraception for 7–98 months (mean 38 months) with those in 44 controls who had never used the pill (Pinto 1986). The women using hormonal contraception showed highly significant increases in both the proportions of abnormal cells and in numbers of chromosome aberrations per cell ($P<0.0001$ in both cases).

The antispermatogenic properties of gossypol, and its potential as a male contraceptive agent, have prompted several studies of its effects on human chromosomes. Tsui and colleagues (1983), for example, scored *in vitro* chromosome aberrations, SCE, and micronuclei in blood cultures exposed to gossypol — all with negative results (SCE frequencies did increase with increasing gossypol concentrations, but even at their highest levels

were not significantly greater than in controls). These workers conceded that their results did not rule out effects on spermatogonial chromosomes. *In vitro* culture of seminiferous tubule segments allowed De-yu and others (1988) to study the mutagenic properties — as measured by micronucleus formation — of gossypol in primary spermatocytes at the pachytene-diakinesis stage of meiosis. A small but significant increase in micronucleus formation was observed at subcytotoxic concentrations.

Fertility-enhancing drugs

Increasingly large numbers of couples affected by infertility are undergoing *in vitro* fertilization procedures. Most such techniques rely on the pharmacological induction of ovulation, and the potential adverse effects of the agents used are clearly a matter for concern.

Boué and Boué (1973) produced evidence that the ovulation-inducing drugs human menopausal gonadotrophin and human chorionic gonadotrophin could cause increased chromosome abnormalities in first-trimester abortions if conception occurred during the first two months after treatment. This was corroborated by a prospective study. From patients studied before and after clomiphene therapy, Charles and co-workers (1973) reported increased heteroploidy and chromatid lesions in endometrial tissue.

Bromocriptine, a dopamine agonist used against hyperprolactinaemic infertility, was the subject of cytogenetic investigations by Czeizel and others (1989). They compared peripheral blood lymphocytes from 31 children conceived after bromocriptine administration with those in 31 control children whose mothers had had no fertility problems. No evidence was found of chromosome mutagenic effects, although the study involved merely the recording of loss or gain of whole chromosomes.

Clastogenicity studies of other therapeutic drugs

The clastogenic properties of methotrexate *in vitro* are well established. Melnyk and others (1971) examined lymphocytes, fibroblasts, bone marrow, and testicular tissue from 27 male patients with psoriasis being treated with methotrexate: a significant increase in chromosome damage was found only in the bone marrow cells.

Stevenson and others (1971, 1973*a*,*b*) investigated a number of drugs thought likely to be clastogens. Positive *in vivo* results were obtained for phenylbutazone in lymphocytes from patients with osteoarthrosis, but no damage was recorded in patients taking trimethoprim or sulphamethoxazole.

Isoniazid, an antituberculous agent, has been extensively studied for evidence of chromosome-damaging ability. Early studies (e.g. Obe *et al.* 1973; Bauchinger *et al.* 1978) produced largely negative results. Isoniazid, however, is often used in combination with other drugs, and for at least two of these combinations evidence has emerged for a synergistic chromosome-damaging effect *in vivo*. In one study, chromosome damage in lymphocytes from 10 tuberculous patients receiving a combination of isoniazid and *p*-aminosalicylic acid was compared with that found in control groups of 10 healthy individuals and 10 patients not receiving therapy (Jaju *et al.* 1981); 11.3 per cent more damage — mostly single chromatid gaps and breaks — was recorded in the patients on combination therapy. A significant increase in the frequency of chromatid gaps and breaks was also reported for the isoniazid/thiacetazone combination (Ahuja *et al.* 1981), although the clastogenicity of thiacetazone itself was not determined. Comparison of 15 untreated tuberculosis patients with 15 who had received a combination of isoniazid, rifampicin, and pyrazinamide for 2 months showed no difference in the frequency of SCEs per cell or in the number of chromosome aberrations (chromatid and chromosome breaks, gaps, dicentrics, and acentric fragments) so this combination does not induce chromosome damage (Ekmekci and Sayli 1995).

The clastogenic effects of frusemide, a potent diuretic, were demonstrated by Jameela and others in 1979. Lymphocytes were exposed *in vitro* to three different frusemide concentrations for either 24 or 72 hours. A clear dose response was observed.

Initial studies of the analgesic drug aspirin either failed to demonstrate a chromosome-damaging action (Mauer *et al.* 1970), or showed a weak effect unlikely to be of *in vivo* significance (Loughman 1970). In a study based on long-term fibroblast cultures, however, Meisner and Inhorn (1972) recorded induction of chromosome rearrangements following exposure to 100 and 250 μg per ml. Thus, high concentrations of aspirin at the cellular level appear to be capable of exerting a mutagenic effect.

Cytogenetic effects of paracetamol *in vitro,* first reported by Watanabe (1982) as producing significant increases in chromatid and isochromatid gaps and breaks but not in polyploidy or aneuploidy, were substantiated by Hongslo *et al.* (1991) using therapeutic doses of the drug. There was no increase in the frequency of cells with micronuclei over periods of 1, 3, and 7 days following a dose of 1 g three times in 8 hours administered orally to healthy volunteers (Kocisova and Sram 1990) but there was a slight temporary increase in the number of chromatid breaks per cell 24 hours after the dose (Kocisova *et al.* 1988). A careful evaluation for the International Commission for Protection against Mutagens and Carcinogens (Rannug *et al.* 1995) reported that the increase in chromosome damage seen *in vitro* and sometimes *in vivo* is most probably due to an inhibition of ribonucleotide reductase, for the reactive metabolite(s) of paracetamol binds irreversibly to DNA, causes DNA strand breaks, and inhibits DNA synthesis both for replication and repair.

A strikingly positive clastogenic result was obtained by Gorla and others (1989) in an investigation of nifurtimox, a common treatment for Chagas' disease (trypanosomiasis). Six patients using this drug showed an average 13-fold increase in chromosome aberrations per cell compared with eight untreated patients (23.5 aberrations per 100 cells compared with 1.7 per 100 cells). The authors recommend limiting the use of this agent whenever possible in view of this genotoxic action.

MacKay and colleagues (1988) also reported strongly positive results with clear dosage correlations for the *in vitro* induction of both SCE and micronuclei by sulphasalazine in peripheral blood lymphocytes. It had previously been unclear whether the elevated chromosome damage and SCE reported in patients with inflammatory bowel disease being treated with this agent represented the effects of the disease itself or a by-product of treatment. The results of this *in vitro* study strongly implicated the treatment.

Watson and colleagues (1976) reported elevated frequencies of gaps, dicentrics, and translocations in cultured lymphocytes of diabetic patients undergoing treatment with a sulphonylurea drug. The subsequent demonstration of normal levels of structural chromosome aberrations and of SCE in untreated diabetics (Vormittag 1985) suggests that sulphonylurea drugs may have clastogenic potential.

The antifungal drug griseofulvin *in vitro* enhances the formation of micronuclei to an extent dependent on dose. The strong preponderance of kinetochore positives indicates that the chromosomes failed to segregate properly at mitosis, which is to be expected since the drug affects spindle activity (Kolachana and Smith 1994). The concentrations used *in vitro* in cultured peripheral human lymphocytes suggest that similar effects should be detectable in the blood of patients undergoing therapy. No evidence was obtained for any clastogenic effect of clodronate (a biphosphonate) in 10 patients with Paget's disease: frequencies of chromosome breaks and SCE did not alter significantly between cells examined before the start of therapy and after 2 months of therapy (Borgstrom *et al.* 1987). Finally, the use of feverfew by migraine sufferers appears not to be associated with any risk of chromosome damage, no meaningful differences being noted between SCE levels and chromosome aberrations in 30 patients taking feverfew preparations daily over a period of 11 months and in 30 matched controls (Anderson *et al.* 1988).

Penicillamine, used against rheumatoid arthritis, when tested for *in vitro* clastogenicity in bone marrow metaphases by Jensen and others (1979) produced no increase in either structural chromosome abnormalities or in erythroblast micronuclei. Later work (e.g. Speit and Haupter 1987) has, however, demonstrated induction by this agent of both SCE and chromosome aberrations in cultured mammalian cells.

Drugs in social and illicit use

A very large amount of work on drug clastogenicity has been carried out on the hallucinogenic drugs, particularly LSD. The initial *in vitro* study was carried out by Cohen and others (1967*a,b*). A statistically significant increase in chromosome breaks was found at almost all concentrations and time periods tested. There followed a number of conflicting reports as several groups of workers repeated these experiments with mixed results. More recent work suggests that LSD causes chromosome damage only at concentrations far in excess of realistic tissue levels. Muneer, for example, in 1978, found no significant increase over control values in chromosome aberrations in lymphocytes exposed to LSD.

In parallel with the controversy over results of *in vitro* clastogenicity studies, investigations of *in vivo* chromosome damage in both illicit drug users and patients administered pure LSD for therapeutic purposes also proved contentious. Several groups examined lymphocyte metaphases from illicit LSD users; some found highly significant increases in chromosome abnormalities after relatively little drug exposure, while others could demonstrate no clastogenic effect even in users taking large doses of the drug. It was recognized that these investigations of illicit LSD users were hampered by a number of problems: for example, the accuracy of the information about doses and frequencies of use, the actual amounts of LSD in the compounds consumed, the pattern of multidrug abuse and the poor health and susceptibility to viral infection of the drug users.

In view of these problems, patients on therapeutic LSD were the subject of a number of chromosome studies. An extensive and well-controlled experiment was carried out in 1969 by Tjio and others. The chromosomes of 32 patients were studied before and after they had taken pure LSD; no increase in chromosome break-

age was observed. Bender and Siva Sankar (1968) similarly found no increase over controls in chromosome damage in seven children treated with LSD. On the other hand, Hungerford and colleagues (1968) compared the amounts of chromosome breakage before and after three doses of LSD and also followed up four patients 1–6 months after treatment. The levels before treatment were the same as in controls. In the treated patients there was a transient increase in chromosome breakage which returned to the pretreatment level within 6 months after the final dose.

The chromosomes of children born to LSD users have also been analysed for breaks. Several reports have described individual cases showing elevated chromosome damage, but a study of 41 children born to drug users showed no overall significant increase in chromosomal breakage or rearrangement (Dumars 1971).

The consensus of opinion based on these studies is that high concentrations of LSD do produce chromosome damage *in vitro*, but that at the non-toxic concentrations found in the body there is no significant damage, and while LSD may have a transient and short-term effect on chromosomes *in vivo*, there is no proof that it inflicts long-term damage.

A similar problem of public interest concerns marihuana smoking. There is agreement that the addition of cannabis resin to human lymphocyte cultures does not increase the frequency of chromosomal abnormalities (e.g. Martin *et al.* 1973), but *in vivo* studies have produced both positive and negative findings. A prospective double-blind trial of the cumulative effects of medically supervised marihuana smoking failed to show any measurable effect (Matsuyama *et al.* 1977). Since then, however, evidence has been presented of a strongly positive effect in heroin/marihuana users; Chiesara and others (1983) described an incidence of chromosome anomalies in cells of users of both drugs that was approximately eight times that found in users of marihuana alone, and approximately 21 times that in controls.

No clastogenic hazard was apparent in an *in vivo* study of peyote (mescaline) users carried out by Dorrance and co-workers in 1975, but another habit, the chewing of betel leaf, which is widespread in the tropics, may be deleterious; *in vitro* lymphocyte cultures from healthy donors showed an increase in chromosome damage related to the concentration of leaf extract applied to the culture (Sadasivan *et al.* 1978).

In 1978, Lambert and others reported a significant consumption-related rise in SCE levels in cigarette smokers. This result was not unexpected since benzo(a)-pyrene, the suspected precarcinogen in cigarette smoke, had previously been shown to double SCE levels in human lymphocytes *in vitro*. At the molecular level it has now been shown that benzo(a)pyrene diol epoxide, a major metabolic product, causes mostly covalent modification of guanine residues in DNA, so inducing predominantly transversions and, at low frequency, single base insertions and deletions and frame-shift mutations (Zhu *et al*. 1994). A dose effect was obvious when the smokers were subdivided according to consumption. The cytogenetic observation has been corroborated by other studies; for example, Kao-Shan and others (1987) found significantly elevated SCE levels in both bone marrow and peripheral blood metaphases, and also reported elevated expression of fragile sites at the cancer-associated breakpoints 3p14.2, 11q13.3, 22q12.2, and 11p13–p14.2. Tawn and Cartmell (1989) observed a fourfold increase in dicentric chromosomes in blood preparations from 12 moderate smokers compared to 12 age-matched controls. There was also a statistically significant increase in stable symmetrical aberrations (principally translocations). Since this type of damage is detectable only in banded preparations, the authors emphasize the importance of these techniques in studies of chronic clastogen exposure. The work of Sinues and colleagues (1990) on a series of 53 smokers compared with 41 non-smokers reinforces previous findings of dose-dependent damage.

Interestingly, cytogenetic damage has not been demonstrated in 'passive smokers'. A study of restaurant waiters showed no significant differences between smoking and non-smoking staff in terms of either chromosome aberrations or SCE (Sorsa *et al*. 1989). As part of the same study, these workers also measured SCE levels in cord-blood lymphocytes of newborn babies from 17 smoking and 25 non-smoking mothers. While a clear dose effect was apparent for SCE in the smokers themselves compared with the non-smokers, and while biochemical markers revealed tobacco smoke constituents at very nearly the same levels in maternal and fetal bloods at the time of birth, the SCE frequencies in the cord bloods were significantly lower for both groups. Thus the chromosome damage that has been well documented among active smokers cannot be demonstrated in those passively exposed in these two circumstances.

Ethanol, at realistic tissue concentrations, is probably a low-level mutagen. Alvarez and others (1980) exposed lymphocytes to 0.5 per cent ethanol (approximately half the blood level used to define intoxication in the United States) and recorded a 30 per cent rise in SCE frequency.

Finally, a drug that is in almost universal use in some measure — caffeine. Human lymphocytes in culture from volunteers after a regimen of 800 mg of caffeine daily for one month showed no significant increase in chromosome damage (Weinstein *et al*. 1972); the highest level of caffeine in the plasma was 30 μg per ml. *In vitro*, however, caffeine induced a high frequency of chromatid gaps and breaks. The damage was dose responsive: multiple exposure of lymphocytes to 30 μg per ml was without effect, but exposure to 250–750 μg per ml produced damage.

Caffeine also acts as a co-clastogen; that is, it potentiates the chromosome-damaging properties of other clastogens. Increased frequencies of SCE and gross aberrations (including pulverized metaphases) are found in lymphocytes exposed to mitomycin C and other mutagens when caffeine is also present in the culture medium (Shiraishi *et al*. 1979; Faed and Mourelatos 1978).

Technical problems of measuring chromosome damage

It will be seen from the above that discrepancies between different reports of the damage done to chromosomes by a particular drug are very common. A number of factors contribute to this problem. Of primary concern is the question of controls. The normal controls used in different studies show wide variations in the frequency of chromosome damage, ranging from less than 1 per cent of cells being affected to perhaps 10 per cent. A survey of a large population was published by Bender and others (1988). Chromosome damage and SCE were scored in lymphocytes from 493 subjects and correlations sought with age, race, smoking, and other variables. The only positive associations detected in this study were a strong effect of smoking on SCE levels, and a slight increase with age in the incidence of dicentrics (mean SCE levels in females were also found to be approximately 5 per cent higher than in males, but this simply corresponds to the extra chromosome material involved in the XX constitution compared with the XY). An overall average of eight SCE per cell was apparent in this sample. Schmickel (1967) found a chromosome breakage level of 1.21 per cent in 1569 normal individuals; this seems to correspond to the levels found by the majority of workers.

Variations may be attributable to several factors. First, there may be differences in the criteria on which measurements of damage are based, some workers including chromosome and chromatid gaps, while others exclude this type of aberration from the score of damage, and record only breaks and gross rearrangements.

Secondly, technical aspects of the tissue culture regimen — in particular the composition of the culture medium — can strongly influence the levels of chromosome damage. For example, Morita and colleagues (1989) established that pH changes in the tissue culture medium were capable by themselves of inducing chromosome damage in Chinese hamster ovary cells. This suggests that *in vitro* tests under non-physiological conditions may lead to false-positive results. Differences in the durations of cell culture can also cause discrepancies between different *in vitro* studies of a given drug — the action of the DNA and chromosome repair mechanisms do not allow direct comparisons between, for example, lymphocyte cultures harvested after 48 hours and similar cultures harvested after 72 hours. Differences between individuals in terms of the efficiency of DNA repair may also influence the levels of damage apparent after *in vivo* mutagen exposure — as a result of a number of studies (e.g. Vorechovsky and Zaloudik 1989), a spectrum of chromosomal stability is now envisaged among normal individuals quite apart from the clinically distinct chromosome breakage syndromes.

The findings of Schwartz and others (1990) have some serious implications for the design of SCE studies; while spontaneous SCE levels in their 24 subjects were relatively constant over time, significant variation between different sample days was apparent in the levels induced by bleomycin. This throws into question the validity of single observations of chemically induced SCE.

Another problem in the interpretation of chromosome mutagenicity data is that *in vitro* experiments do not necessarily reflect the condition *in vivo*. The body has complex mechanisms — which may not be available to cells in culture — for disposing of unwanted substances; for example, it was calculated by Loughman and colleagues (1967) that LSD is cleared from the body in about 4 hours. The drug is concentrated in the liver, where the highest concentration (five times that of the blood) will occur after 20 minutes, levelling off at a constant value of 3.5 times that of blood after 2 hours. For a 70 kg adult, a dose of 100 μg LSD would give a maximum concentration of 0.4 ng per g in blood and 1.2 ng per g in the liver. This is equivalent to the lowest of the *in vitro* levels, which produces no damage. The same study, however, found no increase in chromosome damage in a patient who had ingested 4000 μg the day before.

Schneider and Lewis (1982) compared the induction of SCE by four different mutagens in P388 tumour cells grown *in vitro* and *in vivo* in mice. The results showed that certain agents were more effective *in vitro*, while others were more potent *in vivo*, so that caution is necessary in comparing *in vitro* and *in vivo* mutagen screening data.

The most convincing demonstrations of the clastogenic actions of drugs are probably those *in vivo* studies in which the pretreatment levels of chromosome damage and SCE are established and compared with the levels following treatment. The scoring of large numbers of cells (both from the tissue exposed to the drug, and from carefully matched controls) allows greater confidence to be placed in the result, as does the examination of a range of different tissues — lymphocytes, bone marrow, fibroblasts, etc. After *in vivo* exposure, both lymphocytes and fibroblasts require some *in vitro* tissue culture before observation of metaphase cells is feasible. Bone marrow cell populations, on the other hand, are actively proliferating *in vivo* and only a minimal amount of *in vitro* culturing is necessary. For this reason, studies using a bone marrow system probably approximate most closely to the true *in vivo* action of the drug in question.

The detection of chromosome damage thus has implications for both carcinogenesis and teratogenesis, and clastogenicity testing using both SCE techniques and the scoring of major chromosome abnormalities is now established as an important part of drug safety evaluation. It is to be hoped that conflicting and equivocal results will become less common as the methods of cytogenetic analysis continue to improve, and as a degree of standardization emerges in terms of techniques and tissues used and types of damage recorded.

Mechanisms of drug action

The clastogenic drugs investigated exert their breaking effects by several different mechanisms. Those antibiotics which involve DNA inhibition (e.g. mitomycin C, a bifunctional alkylating agent) act by cross-linking the two backbones of the DNA by the formation of a covalent bond with a base. This is also the mechanism of the RNA-inhibiting drugs. Drugs such as cisplatin can cause intrastrand DNA linking as well. The breaking of chromosomes that is observed can also be brought about by the direct scission of the DNA chain, as with some antineoplastic agents (e.g. bleomycin).

Many drugs do not act directly on the DNA molecule but exert an indirect effect. Methotrexate inhibits folic acid, which in turn inhibits inosine production, which inhibits purine synthesis, thus affecting the nucleic acid. It is thought that the anticonvulsant drugs act either in this way or by inhibiting the synthesis of the proteins which are the constituents of the protein matrix. In the majority of drugs, however, the mechanism whereby chromosome damage is brought about remains unclear.

References

Abel, G. and Schimmer, O. (1983). Induction of structural chromosome aberrations and sister chromatid exchanges in human lymphocytes *in vitro* by aristolochic acid. *Hum. Genet.* 64, 131.

Adinolfi, M. and Crolla, J. (1994). Non-isotopic *in situ* hybridisation; clinical cytogenetics and gene mapping applications. *Adv. Hum. Genet.* 22, 187.

Ahuja, Y.R., Jaju, M., and Jaju, M. (1981). Chromosome damaging action of isoniazid and thiacetazone on human lymphocyte cultures *in vivo*. *Hum. Genet.* 57, 321.

Alvarez, M.R., Cimino, L.E., Cory, M.J., *et al.* (1980). Ethanol induction of sister chromatid exchanges in human cells *in vitro*. *Cytogenet. Cell Genet.* 27, 66.

Anderson, D., Jenkinson, P.C., Dewdney, R.S., *et al.* (1988). Chromosomal aberrations and sister chromatid exchanges in lymphocytes and urine mutagenicity of migraine patients: a comparison of chronic feverfew users and matched non-users. *Hum. Toxicol.* 7, 145.

Anderson, D., Basaran, N., Blowers, S.D., *et al.* (1995). The effect of antioxidants on bleomycin treatment in *in vitro* and *in vivo* genotoxicity assays. *Mutat. Res.* 329, 37.

Apelt, F., Kolin-Gerresheim, J., and Bauchinger, M. (1981). Azathioprine, a clastogen in human somatic cells? Analysis of chromosome damage and SCE in lymphocytes after exposure *in vivo* and *in vitro*. *Mutat. Res.* 88, 61.

Banduhn, N. and Obe, G. (1985). Mutagenicity of methyl-2-benzimidazolecarbamate, diethyl-stilbestrol and estradiol: structural chromosome aberrations, sister-chromatid exchanges, C-mitoses, polyploidies and micronuclei. *Mutat. Res.* 156, 199.

Bauchinger, M., Gebhart, E., Fonatsch, Ch., *et al.* (1978). Chromosome analysis in man in the course of chemoprophylaxis against tuberculosis and of antituberculosis chemotherapy with isoniazid. *Hum. Genet.* 42, 31.

Bender, L. and Siva Sankar, D.V. (1968). Chromosome damage not found in leucocytes of children treated with LSD 25. *Science* 159, 749.

Bender, M.A., Preston, R.J., Leonard, R.C., *et al.* (1988). Chromosomal aberration and sister chromatid exchange frequencies in peripheral blood lymphocytes of a large human population sample. II. Extension of age range. *Mutat. Res.* 212, 149.

Benhamou, S., Pot-Deprun, J., Sancho-Garnier, H., *et al.* (1988). Sister chromatid exchanges and chromosomal aberrations in lymphocytes of nurses handling cytostatic agents. *Int. J. Cancer* 41, 350.

Bishun, N.P. (1976). Chromosomes and oral contraceptives. *Proc. R. Soc. Med.* 69, 353.

Bochkov, N.P., Filippova, T.V., Kuzin, S.M., *et al.* (1986). Cytogenetic effects of cyclophosphamide on human lymphocytes *in vivo* and *in vitro*. *Mutat. Res.* 159, 103.

Borgstrom, G.H., Elomaa, I., Blomqvist, C., *et al.* (1987). Cytogenetic investigations of patients on clodronate therapy for Paget's disease of bone. *Bone* 8 (Suppl. 1), 585.

Bornstein, R.S., Hungerford, D.A., Haller, G., *et al.* (1971). Cytogenetic effects of bleomycin therapy in man. *Cancer Res.* 31, 2004.

Boué, J.G. and Boué, A. (1973). Increased frequency of chromosomal anomalies in abortions after induced ovulation. *Lancet* ii, 679.

Brogger, A. (1970). Anticonvulsant drugs and chromosomes. *Lancet* i, 979.

Brown, T., Dawson, A.A., McDonald, I.A., *et al.* (1985). Chromosome damage and sister chromatid exchanges in lymphocyte cultures from patients with two primary cancers. *Cancer Genet. Cytogenet.* 17, 35.

Carr, D.H. (1970). Chromosome studies in selected spontaneous abortions — 1: conception after oral contraceptives. *Can. Med. Assoc. J.* 103, 343.

Charles, D., Turner, J.H., and Redmond, C.J. (1973). The endometrial karyotypic profiles of women after clomiphene citrate therapy. *J. Obstet. Gynaecol. Br. Commonw.* 80, 264.

Chiesara, E., Cutrufello, R., and Rizzi, R. (1983). Chromosome damage in heroin-marijuana and marijuana addicts. *Arch. Toxicol.* 53 (Suppl. 6), 128.

Cohen, M.M. and Shaw, M.W. (1964). Effects of mitomycin C on human chromosomes. *J. Cell Biol.* 23, 386.

Cohen, M.M., Hirschhorn, K., and Frosch, W.A. (1967a). *In vivo* and *in vitro* chromosomal damage induced by LSD 25. *N. Engl. J. Med.* 277, 1043.

Cohen, M.M., Marinello, M.J., and Back, N. (1967b). Chromosomal damage in human leukocytes induced by lysergic acid diethylamide. *Science* 155, 1417.

Cohen, M.M., Lieber, E., and Schwartz, H.N. (1972). *In vivo* cytogenetic effects of perphenazine and chlorpromazine. *BMJ* iii, 21.

Colvin, M. and Chabner, B.A. (1990). Alkylating agents. In *Cancer Chemotherapy: Principles and Practice* (ed. B.A. Chabner and J.M. Collins). Lippincott, Philadelphia.

Crook, T.R., Souhami, R.L., and McLean A.E. (1986). Cytotoxicity, DNA crosslinking, and single strand breaks induced by activated cyclophosphamide and acrolein in human leukemia cells. *Cancer Res.* 46, 5029.

Czeizel, A., Kiss, R., Racz, K., *et al.* (1989). Case–control cytogenetic study in offspring of mothers treated with bromocriptine during early pregnancy. *Mutat. Res.* 210, 23.

Daza, P., Escalza, P., Mateos, S., *et al.* (1992). MMC, 4NQO, and EMS induce long-lived lesions in DNA which result in SCE's during successive cell cycles in human lymphocytes. *Mutat. Res.* 270, 177.

De Sario, A., Vagnarelli, P., and De Carli, L. (1990). Aneuploidy assay on diethylstilbestrol by means of *in situ* hybridization of radioactive and biotinylated DNA probes on interphase nuclei. *Mutat. Res.* 243, 127.

De-yu, L., Lahdetie, J., and Parvinen, M. (1988). Mutagenicity of gossypol analysed by induction of meiotic micro-nuclei *in vitro*. *Mutat. Res.* 208, 69.

Dobos, M., Schuler, D., and Fekete, G. (1974). Cyclophosphamide-induced chromosome aberrations in non-tumorous patients. *Humangenetik* 22, 221.

Dorrance, D., Janiger, O., and Teplitz, L. (1975). Effect of peyote on human chromosomes. *JAMA* 234, 313.

Dresp, J., Schmid, E., and Bauchinger, M. (1978). The cytogenetic effect of bleomycin on human peripheral lymphocytes *in vitro* and *in vivo*. *Mutat. Res.* 56, 341.

Dumars, K.W. (1971). Parental drug usage effect upon chromosomes of progeny. *Pediatrics* 47, 1037.

Ekmekci, A. and Sayli, A. (1995). Cytogenetic study of tuberculosis patients before and after tuberculostatic drug treatment. *Mutat. Res.* 334, 175.

Faed, M.J.W. and Mourelatos, D. (1978). Enhancement by caffeine of SCE frequency in lymphocytes from normal subjects after treatment by mutagens. *Mutat. Res.* 49, 437.

Ferguson, L.R. and Denny, W.A. (1995). Anti-cancer drugs: an underestimated risk or an underutilised resource in mutagenesis. *Mutat. Res.* 331, 1.

Fu, T.K. and Jarvik, L.F. (1977). The *in vitro* effects of imipramine on human chromosomes. *Mutat. Res.* 48, 89.

Garcia Sagredo, J.M. (1988). Effect of anticonvulsants on human chromosomes. 2. *In vitro* studies. *Mutat. Res.* 204, 623.

Garson, O. (1981). Chromosome studies of patients on long-term lithium therapy for psychiatric disorders. *Med. J. Aust.* ii, 37.

Gebhart, E. (1971). Experimental contributions to the problems of achromatic lesions (gaps). *Humangenetik* 13, 98.

Gebhart, E. (1981). Sister chromatid exchange (SCE) and structural chromosome aberration in mutagenicity testing. *Hum. Genet.* 58, 235.

Genesca, A., Barrios, L., Miro, R., *et al.* (1990). Lymphocyte and sperm chromosome studies in cancer-treated men. *Hum. Genet.* 84, 353.

Gorla, N.B., Ledesma, O.S., Barbieri, G.P., *et al.* (1989). Thirteenfold increase of chromosome aberrations non-randomly distributed in chagasic children treated with nifurtimox. *Mutat. Res.* 224, 263.

Grosse, K.P., Schwanitz, G., Rott, H.D., *et al.* (1972). Chromosomenuntersuchungen bei Behandlung mit Anticonvulsiva. *Humangenetik* 16, 209.

Habedank, M., Esser, K.J., Brull, D., *et al.* (1982). Increased sister chromatid exchanges in epileptic children during long-term therapy with phenytoin. *Hum. Genet.* 61, 71.

Heddle, J.A., Hite, M., Kirkhart, B., *et al.* (1983). The induction of micronuclei as a measure of genotoxicity. *Mutat. Res.* 123, 61.

Henderson, L. and Regan, T. (1985). Effects of diethyl stilboestrol dipropionate on SCEs, micronuclei, cytotoxicity, aneuploidy, and cell proliferation in maternal and fetal mouse cells treated *in vivo*. *Mutat. Res.* 144, 27.

Heng, H.Q., Chen, W.Y., and Wang, Y.C. (1988). Effects of pingyanymycin on chromosomes: a possible structural basis for chromosome aberration. *Mutat. Res.* 199, 199.

Hongslo, J.K., Brogger, A., Bjorge, C., *et al.* (1991). Increased frequency of SCE and chromatid breaks in lymphocytes after treatment of human volunteers with therapeutic doses of paracetamol. *Mutat. Res.* 261, 1.

Hu, L., Lu, X., Lu, B., *et al.* (1990). The effect of valproic acid on SCE and chromosome aberrations in epileptic children. *Mutat. Res.* 243, 63.

Hungerford, D.A., Taylor, K.M., Shagass, C., *et al.* (1968). Cytogenetic effects of LSD-25 therapy in man. *JAMA* 206, 2287.

Jaju, M., Jaju, M., and Ahuja, Y.R. (1981). Combined action of isoniazid and para-aminosalicylic acid *in vitro* on human chromosomes in lymphocyte cultures. *Hum. Genet.* 56, 375.

Jaju, M., Jaju, M., and Ahuja Y.R. (1982). Effect of cephaloridine on human chromosomes *in vitro* in lymphocyte cultures. *Mutat. Res.* 101, 57.

Jaju, M., Jaju, M., and Ahuja, Y.R. (1984). Evaluation of genotoxicity of ampicillin and carbenicillin on human lymphocytes *in vitro*: chromosome aberrations, mitotic index, satellite associations of acrocentric chromosomes and sister chromatid exchanges. *Hum. Toxicol.* 3, 173.

Jameela (Miss), Subramanyam, S., and Sadasivan, G. (1979). Clastogenic effects of frusemide on human leukocytes in culture. *Mutat. Res.* 66, 69.

Jenkins, E.C. (1970). Phenothiazines and chromosome damage. *Cytologia* 35, 552.

Jensen, M.K., Rasmussen, G., and Ingeberg S. (1979). Cytogenetic studies in patients treated with penicillamine. *Mutat. Res.* 67, 357.

Jirsova, K. and Mandys, V. (1994). Induction of micronuclei and granular chromatin condensation in human skin fibroblasts influenced by cisplatin (*cis*-DPP) *in vitro*. *Mutat. Res.* 310, 37.

Kamada, N., Brecher, G., and Tjio, J.H. (1971). *In vitro* effects of chlorpromazine and meprobamate on blast transformation and chromosomes. *Proc. Soc. Exp. Biol. Med.* 136, 210.

Kamiguchi, Y., Tateno, H., Iizawa, Y., *et al.* (1995). Chromosome analysis of human spermatozoa exposed to anti-neoplastic agents *in vitro*. *Mutat. Res.* 326, 185.

Kao-Shan, C.S., Fine, R.L., Whang-Peng, J., *et al.* (1987). Increased fragile sites and sister chromatid exchanges in bone marrow and peripheral blood of young cigarette smokers. *Cancer Res.* 47, 6278.

Kitsiou-Tzeli, S., Galla-Voumvouraki, A., Tsezou, A., *et al.* (1994). Cytogenetic studies in children on long-term anti-coagulant therapy. *Acta Pediatrica* 83, 672.

Knuutila, S., Siimes, M., Simell, O., *et al.* (1977). Long-term use of phenytoin: effects on bone marrow chromosomes in man. *Mutat. Res.* 43, 309.

Kocisova, J. and Sram, R.J. (1990). Mutagenicity studies on paracetamol in human volunteers. *Mutat. Res.* 244, 27.

Kocisova, J., Rossner, P., Binkova, B., *et al.* (1988). Cytogenetic analysis of peripheral lymphocytes and lipid peroxidation in plasma. *Mutat. Res.* 209, 161.

Kolachana, P. and Smith, M.T. (1994). Induction of kinetochore-positive micronuclei in human lymphocytes by the antifungal drug griseofulvin. *Mutat. Res.* 322, 151.

Krogh Jensen, M. and Nyfors, A. (1979). Cytogenetic effect of methotrexate on human cells *in vivo*. Comparison between results obtained by chromosome studies on bone marrow cells and blood lymphocytes and by the micronucleus test. *Mutat. Res.* 64, 339.

Lafarge-Frayssinet, C., Robbana-Barnat, S., Frayssinet, C., *et al.* (1994). Cytotoxicity and DNA damaging potency of chloramphenicol and six metabolites. *Mutat. Res.* 320, 207.

Lambert, B., Lindblad, A., Nordenskjold, M., *et al.* (1978). Increased frequency of sister chromatid exchanges in cigarette smokers. *Hereditas* 88, 147.

Lambert, B., Ringborg, U., and Lindblad, A. (1979). Prolonged increase of sister chromatid exchanges in lymphocytes of melanoma patients after CCNU treatment. *Mutat. Res.* 59, 295.

Lambert, B., Holmberg, K., and Einhorn N. (1984). Persist

ence of chromosome rearrangements in peripheral lymphocytes from patients treated with melphalan for ovarian carcinoma. *Hum. Genet.* 67, 94.

Liang, J.C., Pinkel, D.P., Bailey, N.M., *et al.* (1989). Mutagen sensitivity and cancer susceptibility. *Cancer* 64, 1474.

Littlefield, L.G.J., Lewer, W., Miller, F., *et al.* (1975). Chromosome breakage studies in lymphocytes from normal women, pregnant women and women taking oral contraceptives. *Am. J. Obstet. Gynecol.* 121, 976.

Loughman, W.D. (1970). Acetyl salicylic acid and chromosome damage. *Science* 171, 829.

Loughman, W.D., Sargent, T.W., and Israelstam, D.M. (1967). Leukocytes of humans exposed to lysergic acid diethylamide: lack of chromosomal damage. *Science* 158, 508.

MacKay, J.M., Fox, D.P., Brunt, P.W., *et al.* (1988). *In vitro* induction of chromosome damage by sulphasalazine in human lymphocytes. *Mutat. Res.* 222, 27.

MacLeod, R.A.F., Voges, M., Bryant, P.E., *et al.* (1994). Chromatid aberration, dose response and dispersal in human G_2 lymphocytes treated with bleomycin. *Mutat. Res.* 309, 73.

McQuarrie, H.G., Scott, C.D., Ellsworth, H.S., *et al.* (1970). Cytogenetic studies on women using oral contraceptives and their progeny. *Am. J. Obstet. Gynecol.* 108, 659.

Mamuris, Z., Gerbault-Sereau, M., Prieur, M., *et al.* (1989). Chromosomal aberrations in lymphocytes of patients treated with melphalan. *Int. J. Cancer* 43, 80.

Manning, J.E., Hershey, N.D., Brooker, T.R., *et al.* (1975). A new method of *in situ* hybridisation. *Chromosoma* 53, 107.

Martelli, A., Rattiolli, F., Pastorino, G., *et al.* (1991). Genotoxicity testing of chloramphenicol in rodent and human cells. *Mutat. Res.* 260, 65.

Martin, P.A., Thorburn, M.J., and Bryant, J.A. (1973). *In vivo* and *in vitro* studies of cytogenetic effects of *Cannabis sativa* in rats and man. *Teratology* 9, 81.

Matsuyama, S.S., Yen, F.S., Jarvik, L.S., *et al.* (1977). Marijuana exposure *in vivo* and human lymphocyte chromosomes. *Mutat. Res.* 48, 255.

Mauer, I., Weinstein, D., and Solomon, H.M. (1970). Acetylsalicylic acid: no chromosome damage in human leukocytes. *Science* 169, 198.

Meisner, L.F. and Inhorn, S.L. (1972). Chemically induced chromosome changes in human cells *in vitro*. *Acta Cytol.* 16, 41.

Melnyk, J., Duffy, O.M., and Sparkes, R.S. (1971). Human mitotic and meiotic chromosome damage following *in vivo* exposure to methotrexate. *Clin. Genet.* 2, 28.

Mondello, C., Giorgi, R., and Nuzzo, F. (1984). Chromosomal effects of methotrexate on cultured human lymphocytes. *Mutat. Res.* 139, 67.

Morita, T., Watanabe, Y., Takeda, K., *et al.* (1989). Effects of pH in the *in vitro* chromosomal aberration test. *Mutat. Res.* 225, 55.

Muneer, R. (1978). Effects of LSD on human chromosomes. *Mutat. Res.* 51, 403.

Muniz, F.E., Houston, R., Schneider, R., *et al.* (1969). Chromosomal effects of diphenylhydantoin. *Clin. Res.* 17, 28.

Murthy, P.B. and Prema, K. (1979). Sister-chromatid exchanges in oral contraceptive users. *Mutat. Res.* 68, 49.

Neilsen, J., Friedrich, U., and Tsuboi, T. (1968). Chromosome abnormalities and psychotropic drugs. *Nature* 218, 488.

Neuhauser, G., Schwanitz, G., and Rott, H.D. (1970). Zur Frage mutagener und teratogener Wirkung von Antikonvulsiva. *Fortschr. Med.* 88, 819.

Neustad, N.P. (1978). Sister chromatid exchanges and chromosomal aberrations induced in human lymphocytes by the cytostatic drug adriamycin. *Mutat. Res.* 57, 253.

Nikula, E., Kiviniitty, K., Leisti, J., *et al.* (1984). Chromosome aberrations in lymphocytes of nurses handling cytostatic agents. *Scand. J. Work Environ. Health* 10, 71.

Nordenson, I., Beckman, L., Liden, S., *et al.* (1984). Chromosomal aberrations and cancer risk. *Hum. Hered.* 34, 76.

Obe, G., Beek, B., and Radenbach, K.L. (1973). Action of antituberculosis drugs on human leucocyte chromosomes *in vitro*. *Experientia* 29, 1433.

Palmer, R.G., Dore, C.J., and Denman, A.M. (1984). Chlorambucil-induced chromosome damage to human lymphocytes is dose-dependent and cumulative. *Lancet* i, 246.

Palmer, R.G., Dore, C.J., and Denman, A.M. (1985). Chlorambucil-induced chromosome damage to human lymphocytes. *Lancet* ii, 1438.

Pinto, M.R. (1986). Possible effects of hormonal contraceptives on human mitotic chromosomes. *Mutat. Res.* 169, 149.

Povirk, L.F. and Austin, M.J.F. (1991). Genotoxicity of bleomycin. *Mutat. Res.* 257, 127.

Psaraki, K. and Demopoulos, N.A. (1988). Induction of chromosome damage and sister chromatid exchanges in human lymphocyte cultures by the antitumour antibiotic Neocarzinostatin. *Mutat. Res.* 204, 669.

Rannug, U., Holme, J.A., Hongsho, J.K., *et al.* (1995). An evaluation of the genetic toxicity of paracetamol. *Mutat. Res.* 327, 179.

Raposa, T. (1978). Sister chromatid exchange studies for monitoring DNA damage and repair capacity after cytostatics *in vitro* and in lymphocytes of leukaemic patients under cytostatic therapy. *Mutat. Res.* 57, 241.

Riedel, L. and Obe, G. (1984). Mutagenicity of antiepileptic drugs. II. Phenytoin, primidone, and phenobarbital. *Mutat. Res.* 138, 71.

Rosenkranz, H.S. (1988). Chloramphenicol: magic bullet or double-edge sword? *Mutat. Res.* 196, 1.

Roth, S., Norppa, H., Jarventus, H., *et al.* (1991). Analysis of chromosomal aberrations, sister chromatid exchanges and micronuclei in peripheral lymphocytes of pharmacists before and after working with cytostatic drugs. *Mutat. Res.* 325, 157.

Sadasivan, G., Rani, G., and Kumasi, C.K. (1978). Chromosome damaging effect of betel leaf. *Mutat. Res.* 57, 183.

Sandberg, A.A. (1983). *The Chromosomes in Human Cancer and Leukaemia*. Elsevier, New York.

Sardas, S., Ada, M., Karakaya, A.E., *et al.* (1994). Sister chromatid exchanges in epileptic patients on anticonvulsant therapy. *Mutat. Res.* 313, 21.

Sargent, L.M., Roloff, B., and Meisner, L.F. (1987). Mechanisms in cyclophosphamide induction of cytogenetic damage in human lymphocyte cultures. *Cancer Genet. Cytogenet.* 29, 239.

Saxena, R. and Ahuja, Y.R. (1982). Clastogenic effect of the psychotropic drug thioridazine on human chromosomes *in vivo*. *Hum. Genet.* 62, 198.

Sbrana, I., Caretto, S., Rainaldi, G., *et al.* (1991). Induction of chromosomal aberrations and SCE by chloramphenicol. *Mutat. Res.* 248, 145.

Schaumann, B., Satish, J., Barden Johnson, S., *et al.* (1985). Effects of carbamazepine on human chromosomes. *Epilepsia* 26, 346.

Schmickel, R. (1967). Chromosome aberrations in leukocytes exposed *in vitro* to diagnostic levels of X-rays. *Am. J. Hum. Genet.* 19, 1.

Schmid, E. and Bauchinger, M. (1973). Comparison of chromosome damage induced by radiation and cytoxan therapy. *Mutat. Res.* 21, 271.

Schneider, E.L. and Lewis, J. (1982). Comparison of *in vivo* and *in vitro* SCE induction. *Mutat. Res.* 106, 85.

Schuler, D., Dobos, M., Fekete, G., *et al.* (1979). Chromosome mutations and chromosome stability in children treated with different regimes of immunosuppressive drugs. *Hum. Hered.* 29, 100.

Schwartz, S., Astemborski, J.A., Budacz, A.P., *et al.* (1990). Repeated measurement of spontaneous and clastogen-induced sister-chromatid exchange. *Mutat. Res.* 234, 51.

Sessink, P.J.M., Cerna, M., Rossner, P., *et al.* (1994). Urinary cyclophosphamide excretion and chromosomal aberrations in peripheral blood lymphocytes after occupational exposure to antineoplastic agents. *Mutat. Res.* 309, 193.

Shaw, M.W. (1970). Human chromosome damage by chemical agents. *Annu. Rev. Med.* 21, 409.

Shiraishi, Y., Yamamoto, K., and Sandberg, A. (1979). Effects of caffeine on chromosome aberrations and sister chromatid exchanges induced by mitomycin C in BrdU-labelled human chromosomes. *Mutat. Res.* 62, 1 39.

Sieber, S.M. and Adamson, R.H. (1975). Toxicity of antineoplastic agents in man. *Adv. Cancer Res.* 22, 57.

Sinkus, A.G. (1972). Cytogenetic effect of rubomycin C in a culture of human lymphocytes. Chromosomal aberrations at the G_2 stage of the mitotic cycle. *Genetica* (Leningrad) 8, 138.

Sinues, B., Izquierdo, M., and Viguera, J.P. (1990). Chromosome aberrations and urinary thioethers in smokers. *Mutat. Res.* 240, 289.

Sorsa, M., Husgafvel-Pursiainen, K., Jarventus, H., *et al.* (1989). Cytogenetic effects of tobacco smoke exposure among involuntary smokers. *Mutat. Res.* 222, 111.

Speit, G. and Haupter, S. (1987). Cytogenetic effects of penicillamine. *Mutat. Res.* 190, 197.

Srb, V., Kubzova, E., and Kubikova, K. (1986). Chromosome aberration and mitotic activity in human peripheral blood lymphocytes following *in vitro* action of platinum cytostatics *cis*-DDP and EM-Pt. *Neoplasma* 33, 465.

Staiger, G.R. (1969). Studies on the chromosomes of human lymphocytes treated with diazepam *in vitro*. *Mutat. Res.* 10, 635.

Stevenson, A.C., Patel, C.R., Bedford, J., *et al.* (1971). Chromosomal studies in patients taking phenylbutazone. *Ann. Rheum. Dis.* 30, 487.

Stevenson, A.C. and Patel, C.R. (1973*a*). Effects of chlorambucil on human chromosomes. *Mutat. Res.* 18, 333.

Stevenson, A.C., Clarke, G., Patel, C.R., *et al.* (1973*b*). Chromosomal studies *in vivo* and *in vitro* of trimethoprim and sulphamethoxazole. *Mutat. Res.* 17, 255.

Tawn, E.J. and Cartmell, C.L. (1989). The effect of smoking on the frequencies of asymmetrical and symmetrical chromosome exchanges in human lymphocytes. *Mutat. Res.* 224, 151.

Tjio, J.H., Pahnke, W.N., and Kurland, A.A. (1969). LSD and chromosomes. A controlled experiment. *JAMA* 210, 849.

Tsui, Y.C., Creasy, M.R., and Hulten, M.A. (1983). The effect of the male contraceptive agent gossypol on human lymphocytes *in vitro*: traditional chromosome breakage, micronuclei, sister chromatid exchange, and cell kinetics. *J. Med. Genet.* 20, 81.

Urba, M. (1971). Changes in human chromosomes caused by drugs. *Cslka Oftal.* 27, 134.

van den Berg-de Ruiter, E., de Jong, B., Mulder, N.H., *et al.* (1990). Chromosome damage in peripheral blood lymphocytes of patients treated for testicular cancer. *Hum. Genet.* 84, 191.

Vijayalaxmi and Burkart, W. (1989). Resistance and cross-resistance to chromosome damage in human blood lymphocytes adapted to bleomycin. *Mutat. Res.* 211, 1.

Vorechovsky, I. and Zaloudik, J. (1989). Increased breakage of chromosome 1 in lymphocytes of patients with testicular cancer after bleomycin treatment *in vitro*. *Br. J. Cancer* 59, 499.

Vormittag W. (1985). Structural chromosome aberration rates and sister chromatid exchange frequencies in females with type 2 (non-insulin-dependent) diabetes. *Mutat. Res.* 143, 117.

Watanabe, M. (1982). The cytogenetic effects of aspirin and acetaminophen in in vitro human lymphocytes. *Jpn J. Hyg.* 37, 673.

Watson, W.A.F., Petrie, J.C., Galloway, D.B., *et al.* (1976). *In vivo* cytogenetic activity of sulphonylurea drugs in man. *Mutat. Res.* 38, 71.

Weinstein, D., Mauer, I., and Solomon, H.M. (1972). The effect of caffeine on chromosomes of human lymphocytes. *In vivo* and *in vitro* studies. *Mutat. Res.* 16, 391.

Whang-Peng, J., Levanthal, B.G., Adamson, J.W., *et al.* (1969). The effect of daunomycin on human cells *in vivo* and *in vitro*. *Cancer* 23, 113.

Yuzawa, K., Fukao, Y., Iwasaki, Y., *et al.* (1987). Mutagenicity of cyclosporine against human cells. *Transplant. Proc.* 19, 1218.

Yuzawa, K., Kondo, I., Fukao, K., *et al.* (1986). Mutagenicity of cyclosporine. *Transplantation* 42, 61.

Zhu, Y., Dye, S., Stambrook, P.J., *et al.* (1994). Single base deletion induced by benzo(a)pyrene diol epoxide at the adenine phosphoribosyl transferase locus in human fibrosarcoma cell lines. *Mutat. Res.* 321, 73.

Zwanenburg, T.S.B. and Cordier, A. (1994). No cyclosporine induced chromosomal aberrations in human peripheral blood lymphocytes *in vitro*. *Mutat. Res.* 320, 217.

7. Disorders of the fetus and infant

R. E. FERNER

Introduction

Drugs given to the mother can in principle affect the
developing child from the time the egg is fertilized until
the baby is weaned from the breast. Effects on the
chromosomes have already been considered in Chapter 6.
Hardly any information exists to show whether exposure
of the father to drugs could lead to heritable changes in
the genome (Colie 1993).

Cell division, tubular transport, and uterine implantation of the fertilized ovum may be affected. For
example, high-dose oestrogens given shortly after conception result in loss of the conceptus, perhaps by affecting tubular motility, and also by altering the endometrium either directly or by inhibiting luteal function
(*The Lancet* 1983*a*).

The loss rate during the implantation stage (days 0–6
from conception) is probably of the order of 50 per cent
in pregnancies in the general population (Beckman and
Brent 1986), so that it is very hard to know what effect
drug therapy may have on the incidence. The cells are
totipotent at this very early stage of development, and
the outcome of damage is thought to be either loss of the
conceptus or normal continuation of pregnancy (Beck
and Lloyd 1965).

The embryo from the time of implantation until closure of the secondary palate, which marks the end of
organogenesis, is vulnerable to outside agents that can
disturb the programme of development. Cell division,
programmed cell death, and interactions between cells,
as well as cellular nutrition and metabolism, are potentially susceptible to malign external influences. Teratology (from τέϱαϐ, a monster or prodigy) is 'the name
given by Geoffroy de St Hilare to the study or consideration of monsters or anomalies of organization' (*Oxford
English Dictionary*). The possibility that chemical poisons could cause malformations has been recognized for
some years, but only a few scattered observations were

recorded up to 1960 (Willis 1962). After thalidomide was
shown by Lenz and Knapp (1962) to be responsible for
congenital defects, there was heightened awareness of
drugs as potential teratogens, that is, substances whose
presence during embryonic or fetal life can induce abnormal structure or function in the fetus, or the child
after birth.

Fetal health requires normal uterine and placental
function and a normal amnion. Drugs that reduce placental blood flow or cause oligohydramnios can cause
fetal harm. Fetal growth, from the closure of the secondary palate until delivery, can be retarded by the effects of
drugs on cellular nutrition, metabolism, or division.
Drugs that increase or decrease uterine contractility can
cause premature or delayed labour. Neonatal well-being,
which depends on physiological adaptation to the extrauterine world, can also be compromised by drugs given
to the mother before birth or transmitted in the breast
milk after birth.

The first trimester

The susceptibility of the developing embryo and fetus to harm from drugs

The developing embryo is especially vulnerable to harm
because:

1. the embryo contains relatively few differentiated cells, and
   therefore damage to small numbers of cells may have far-
   reaching consequences;
2. cells are dividing rapidly, and so the embryo is intolerant of
   interference with cell division;
3. groups of cells during organogenesis undergo processes,
   including migration, aggregation, cavitation, delamination,
   folding, closure, and fusion, which depend on precise localization in time and space and whose disruption leads to
   abnormal organ formation. Normal embryonic development
   depends on the programmed death (apoptosis) of some

cells. Excessive cell death in regions of programmed cell death may be important (Sulik *et al.* 1988);
4. the metabolizing enzymes of cells in the embryo may differ from those in mature animals. They may not be able to detoxify xenobiotic compounds as effectively, or may more readily transform non-toxic drugs into teratogenic metabolites by bioactivation (Juchau 1989);
5. the immune system does not function during intrauterine development.

The conceptus is also vulnerable, because of the specialized nature of its nutrition, through the metabolically active, vascular placenta. Interruption of nutrition or interference with metabolism can retard intrauterine growth.

Around the time of birth, the major adaptations of heart and lungs to extrauterine life are sensitive to agents (such as opioid analgesics) given to the mother and persisting in the neonatal circulation. (See also Tyl 1988.)

How great a risk do drugs pose to the developing child?

The detection of harm, the association with a particular agent, and the demonstration that this association is causal are all beset with difficulties.

The first suspicion that a drug may cause harm can come from experimental studies in animals, as, for example, with vitamin A (retinoic acid) derivatives (Teelmann 1988). It can come from cohort studies in which the maternal drug exposure and the incidence of malformations in a group of women are analysed, the best example being the Boston Collaborative Perinatal Project (Heinonen *et al.* 1977*b*) in which over 50 000 'mother–infant pairs' were studied and outcomes correlated with some 900 drugs to which they were exposed. Commonly, the earliest warning comes from case reports in which at most a few infants are observed with recognizable abnormalities after the mother has been exposed to a drug in pregnancy. The classical example is the observation (McBride 1961; Lenz and Knapp 1962) of phocomelic infants born to mothers who took thalidomide during the first trimester.

Case–control studies, in which the exposure to a putative causal agent is assessed in affected cases and in a control population matched as closely as possible for relevant factors other than exposure, can also provide helpful information, with the advantage that uncommon conditions can be studied much more effectively than in cohort studies.

Very substantial problems are associated with each method. Animal studies are notoriously difficult to extrapolate to man, as exemplified by the low terato-

genicity of thalidomide in mice and rats. In contrast, cleft palate is easily induced in some strains of mice by administering corticosteroids to the mother, but there is no evidence that corticosteroids cause this defect in man. Cohort studies contain a very low density of information: both exposure to unusual drugs and infants with unusual abnormalities are represented only infrequently, and so the method is insensitive. Since many comparisons are made in a search for possible associations in a study such as the Boston Collaborative Perinatal Project (Heinonen *et al.* 1977*b*), spurious associations will also occur. On average, one in 20 comparisons will show a significant association at $P<0.05$ purely by chance. Cohort studies are not therefore guaranteed to be either specific or sensitive.

The case–control study is retrospective. An association with *prior* exposure is sought *after* the affected case has occurred. This makes it extremely difficult to conduct such a study without bias, in the selection of cases or controls, or in the determination of prior exposure in the two groups. Sackett (1979) has enumerated potential causes of bias in comparative studies. A particular selection bias is introduced by counting only live-born cases and controls (Hook 1982; Khoury *et al.* 1989). The teratogen and the condition with which it is putatively associated may affect prenatal mortality differently, and so the true degree of association can be overestimated or underestimated (Khoury *et al.* 1989). Although more recent studies have been designed to reduce biases, for example, by studying both livebirths and stillbirths (Queisser-Luft *et al.* 1996), they are at best uncertain indicators.

Case reports can claim historical successes (Goldberg and Golbus 1986). The teratogenic effects of thalidomide (Lenz and Knapp 1962), warfarin (Kerber *et al.* 1968), and ethanol (Lemoine *et al.* 1968) were first described in case reports. The more unusual a case, the more likely is it to be described, so very bizarre or rare events are most likely to be detected. This poses a substantial problem, because intuitively the conjunction of two rare events suggests causality. For example, exposure to griseofulvin in the first 3 weeks of pregnancy has been recorded in two cases of conjoined twins (Rosa *et al.* 1987*a*). The chance of this specific event occurring on two occasions is obviously very low indeed. The chance, however, of exposure *in utero* to any one of several thousand chemicals being associated with any one of several thousand anomalies on two occasions, is several million times higher.

The conclusion is that no method can unequivocally demonstrate an association *ab initio*, it can only lead to the hypothesis that an association exists, a hypothesis which can be strengthened by further evidence, for example, from a case–control study designed specifically to examine that hypothesis. Far fewer subjects need be studied to confirm that there is a high probability (say 95 per cent) that a hypothesis is true ($P_\alpha \leq 0.05$) than are needed to refute the same hypothesis with the same degree of certainty ($P_\beta \leq 0.05$). This means that once a hypothesis has been put forward it is more likely to be proved true than false; and so both 'true' and 'unproven' hypotheses remain. Very few drugs have been exonerated after suspicions have been raised. Dicyclomine and the oral contraceptive pill may be rare examples (see below).

Measures of association between exposure to an agent and an adverse effect (for example, congenital anomaly in the offspring) are relative risk (risk ratio) and odds ratio. The relative risk is the ratio of *(the proportion affected in those exposed) : (the proportion affected in those unexposed)*. It therefore requires the complete enumeration of a (large) population, as may be obtained in a cohort study. The odds ratio can be derived from cohort or case–control studies, and is the ratio of *(exposed/unexposed in those affected) : (exposed/unexposed in those unaffected)*. When the proportion affected is small, the odds ratio gives an approximate value for the relative risk (Armitage and Berry 1987). The 95 per cent confidence intervals can be calculated for both ratios. The wider the confidence intervals, the less certain the estimate of risk. They are often so wide as to include unity (no increased risk).

An association does not prove a causal link. The human experience does not constitute a controlled experiment and so the population exposed to the drug often differs systematically from the unexposed population. This would be as true for antituberculous chemotherapy as for antineoplastic therapy. The disease process, rather than the drug, may be the cause of abnormalities in the offspring. This has been postulated for epilepsy and anticonvulsant drugs (Dodson 1989). Clearly, the demonstration that a hypothesized mechanism of action for the suspected teratogen pertains in one or more models strengthens the possibility that it is indeed deleterious, and the observation that an anomaly only occurs in the presence of a given drug and not in a patient with the disease state treated differently implicates it as a noxious agent, at least in the presence of that disease state (as with insomnia and thalidomide). It is salutary to note that none of the many possible mechanisms by which thalidomide is teratogenic has been confirmed (Stephens 1988), and that many drugs are suspected of causing malformations that also occur spontaneously.

Teratogens

Wilson (1977) formulated six general principles of teratogenesis, on which rather stringent criteria for the identification of teratogens can be based. They are summarized as:

1. the susceptibility of a conceptus to teratogenesis depends on its genotype — only certain genotypes are susceptible;
2. the susceptibility to teratogens varies with developmental stage at the time of exposure — organs are particularly sensitive during the critical period of their formation;
3. teratogens act by specific mechanisms — for example, by reducing the availability of a required substrate;
4. abnormal development can lead to death, malformation, growth retardation, or functional disorder;
5. the access of adverse environmental agents to developing tissues depends on the nature of the agents — but, for practical purposes, most drugs of molecular weight <800 can cross the placenta;
6. the observed effects of a teratogen depend on dose.

The molecular actions of teratogens are slowly being elucidated, at least in rodent models (Wells and Winn 1996). Many compounds associated with birth defects are metabolised to reactive intermediates that bind to embryonic proteins or nucleic acids, distort their structure, and alter their function. Cellular mechanisms to repair damage to DNA probably involve the p53 tumour suppressor gene, which mediates apoptosis; rodent species deficient in that gene are more susceptible to teratogens.

Risk, uncertainty, and clinical practice

It is hard to estimate the risk that a given agent is teratogenic in man from survey data, for the reasons described above. This uncertainty colours clinical practice. A drug that could prevent serious harm to the mother (for example, a drug that is an effective prophylactic against malaria) will also potentially prevent harm to the fetus. A drug which is purely for symptomatic relief will not. Where more than one drug exists to treat a particular condition (for example, epilepsy) then their relative safety is of importance. This can be especially hard to determine, as lack of evidence does not prove lack of the potential to cause harm.

The general principle is that since risks of damage to the baby are uncertain and can be high, only drugs that confer clear benefits should ever be prescribed in pregnancy. This principle is only helpful in reducing the risks after pregnancy is diagnosed. Most currently used drugs, with the exception of vitamin A derivatives and cytotoxic drugs, seem unlikely to have a great propensity for causing abnormal babies.

Some reassurance can be derived from the small number of drugs that have clearly been shown to be teratogenic. Even with the most teratogenic drugs, the perceived risk may be greater than the true risk. After first-trimester exposure *in utero* to therapeutic doses of antimetabolite antineoplastic agents, for example, four out of five infants will be normal at birth. A number of reviews (Briggs *et al*. 1994; de Swiet 1995*a*; Koren 1994) provide useful guidance on drug therapy for pregnant women. Schardein's monograph (1993) includes comprehensive reviews of animal studies of teratogens.

The second and third trimesters

Following differentiation of tissues and organs, the fetus becomes progressively less susceptible to teratogenic insult. Drugs given after about the 56th day of gestation (70th day of pregnancy as conventionally calculated) are therefore unlikely to cause congenital defects. Sex hormones are an exception, because of the late development of the reproductive system, and they can cause urogenital defects up to and beyond 12 weeks' gestation. Maternal drug therapy in the second and third trimesters can, however, influence the growth or functional development of formed tissues and organs, or exert toxic effects on fetal tissues. Developing tissues are often more sensitive to drug effects, and adverse effects can occur at doses well within the therapeutic range for the mother. Mechanisms of biotransformation and excretion of many drugs are underdeveloped in the neonate, and drugs given at term may produce postpartum toxicity because maternal elimination can no longer occur.

Many drugs are excreted in breast milk, and some can be absorbed by the neonate in sufficient quantities to produce adverse effects. This aspect has been comprehensively reviewed, with recommendations for advice to breast-feeding mothers (Kauffman *et al*. 1994; Bailey and Ito 1997), and will not be further considered here.

Specific agents

Gastrointestinal drugs

Mineral antacids

The information on antacids is limited. The large prospective study of Heinonen and others (1977*b*) did not consider antacids at all. The retrospective survey by Nelson and Forfar (1971) recorded antacid consumption in 157/1369 women, and found that a greater proportion of women who had abnormal babies had taken antacids (12.4 per cent) than of women who had normal babies (11 per cent). Corresponding figures for the first trimester only were 5.9 per cent vs 2.6 per cent (P<0.01). When self-administered antacids where included, there was still a significant excess of antacid use in the women who were delivered of abnormal babies. No link with any particular antacid was found, and the possibility exists that antacids were taken for gastrointestinal symptoms associated with abnormal pregnancies. There was no significant excess of antacid use, taken over the whole of pregnancy, in women with abnormal babies. A subsequent study (RCGP 1976) failed to show an increased risk. The common symptom of heartburn ('acid reflux') during pregnancy usually occurs during the second and third trimesters, when there is no evidence for increased risk of antacids, though they are best avoided during the first trimester in favour of small meals and loose corsets (Feeney 1982). Antacids are generally considered to be safe in the second and third trimesters, although few specific data are available on their effects on the fetus (Feeney 1982; Lewis *et al*. 1985; *Drug and Therapeutics Bulletin* 1990).

Histamine H₂-antagonists

There are reports of four mothers who took ranitidine during the first trimester and subsequently had normal babies (Cipriani *et al*. 1983; Andrews and Souma 1989).

Cimetidine has been more extensively studied. In a postmarketing surveillance scheme (Jones *et al*. 1985), 20 cimetidine takers and 22 controls became pregnant. Two takers aged 23 had abnormal children: one baby had trisomy 21, and one had no congenital anomalies but had convulsions and died in the neonatal period, probably owing to intrauterine hypoxia. It was doubtful whether either abnormal pregnancy could be imputed to cimetidine. Three cases of women who took cimetidine during the first trimester and had normal babies are recorded (Corazza *et al*. 1982; Meggs *et al*. 1984).

These sparse data do not suggest that H₂-antagonists are major teratogens.

Cimetidine and ranitidine are widely used in obstetric anaesthesia to prevent aspiration of acidic gastric contents during labour and delivery, and appear to cause few adverse effects on the fetus or neonate.

Neonatal Apgar scores and infant progress are reported to be unaffected by cimetidine (McGowan 1979; Ostheimer *et al*. 1982; Hodgkinson *et al*. 1983; McAuley *et al*. 1985). Cimetidine was undetectable in neonatal blood 19 hours after delivery (McGowan 1979), and it does not appear to affect the development of gastric acidity or to increase bacterial colonization of the gastrointestinal tract in the infant (McAuley *et al*. 1985). A case of transient hepatic impairment was, however, reported in an infant exposed to cimetidine in the final month of pregnancy (Glade *et al.* 1980) but there have been no confirmatory reports.

When used peripartum as prophylaxis against Mendelson's syndrome, ranitidine produced no adverse effects on fetal heart rate or rhythm, or on Apgar score and neonatal progress. Plasma levels in the neonate decline rapidly, and are virtually undetectable 12 hours after delivery (Gillet *et al.* 1984; McAuley *et al.* 1984; Boschi *et al.* 1984).

Misoprostol

Misoprostol is a synthetic analogue of prostaglandin E_1 used to prevent gastric ulcers, particularly in patients treated with non-steroidal anti-inflammatory drugs. It can also induce abortion, and is misused for this purpose in Brazil and perhaps elsewhere. Seven cases of severe congenital limb abnormalities in children born after failed attempts at procuring first trimester abortions have been reported (Gonzalez *et al.* 1993). Four of the seven also had cranial nerve lesions (the Möbius sequence). A subsequent case–control study identified 12 children exposed to misoprostol during the first trimester, of whom 4 had major malformations (Castilla and Oriolo 1994). It is likely that high doses of misoprostol during the first trimester interfere with the fetal blood supply.

Antidiarrhoeal agents

There is little information on possible teratogenic effect of this group of drugs. Codeine may produce neonatal effects typical of narcotic analgesics (see below), including respiratory depression, dependence, and withdrawal effects (van Leeuwen *et al.* 1965; Mangurten and Benawra 1980). There are few data on the use of loperamide in pregnancy; only about 0.3 per cent of a standard 2 mg oral dose reaches the systemic circulation (Janssen Pharmaceuticals, personal communication), and pharmacological effects in late pregnancy would appear unlikely.

Laxatives

Senna preparations are generally believed to be safe in the second and third trimesters (Biggs *et al.* 1994; Fagan 1995).

Sulphasalazine and mesalazine (5-aminosalicylic acid)

Inflammatory bowel disease affects young people, and the question often arises whether treatment should continue during pregnancy, particularly if the treatment is prophylactic. Miller (1986) reviewed 10 retrospective series of patients and found no evidence for an increase in congenital abnormalities due to the disease or due to sulphasalazine. However, there has been no controlled trial. There are reports of one case of cleft lip, cleft palate, and hydrocephalus in a baby born to a woman with ulcerative colitis in remission who had taken sulphasalazine throughout pregnancy (Craxi and Pagliarello 1980), of two cases of babies with coarctation and ventricular septal defect (Newman and Correy 1983; Hoo *et al.* 1988), and of a pair of stillborn twins with renal anomalies (Newman and Correy 1983). Three women treated with mesalazine throughout pregnancy had normal children (Habal and Greenberg 1987).

Sulphasalazine is a conjugate of sulphapyridine and mesalazine (5-aminosalicylic acid). It is well absorbed, and since its anti-inflammatory activity is due to the 5-aminosalicylic acid moiety, there is some logic in preferring mesalazine for prophylaxis in pregnant women with ulcerative colitis. The information on both agents is generally reassuring. Sulphasalazine crosses the placenta and reaches a cord-blood concentration about half that in maternal serum (Azad Khan and Truelove 1979). The sulphapyridine component may therefore displace bilirubin from its albumin-binding sites and, in theory, cause kernicterus. Esbjörner and colleagues (1987) found no displacing effect, however, in 15 children whose mothers had taken sulphasalazine throughout pregnancy. They concluded that sulphasalazine could be continued throughout pregnancy without risk of developing kernicterus in the child, although this conclusion may not be valid for premature infants or those with haemolytic disease.

One case of reversible congenital neutropenia has been reported in association with maternal sulphasalazine therapy (Levi *et al.* 1988).

In contrast to the substantial placental transfer of sulphapyridine, 5-aminosalicylic acid (mesalazine) reaches the fetus only in trace amounts (Christensen *et al.* 1987). This pharmacokinetic finding is reassuring, although the safety of mesalazine in pregnancy has yet to be confirmed by clinical studies.

Antihistamine antiemetics

Neither prospective (Heinonen *et al.* 1977*b*) nor retrospective (Nelson and Forfar 1971) studies have demonstrated overall increased malformation rates in women taking chlorpheniramine or promethazine during the first trimester. Meclozine has been suggested to be a human teratogen (Watson 1962), but there were no overall increases in incidence of abnormalities in prospective studies of 1014 (Heinonen *et al.* 1977*b*) and 613 (Milkovich and van den Berg 1976) mothers taking meclozine during the first trimester, nor in a retrospective survey (Nelson and Forfar 1971).

A 'new thalidomide-style drug fear' (de St Jorre 1980*a*) was raised and allegations were made that preparations containing the antihistamine doxylamine (including Debendox in the UK and Bendectin in the US) caused deformities, when the manufacturers were sued by the parents of a boy who was born with Poland's anomaly (unilaterally absent pectoralis major and ipsilateral hand deformity) after his mother had taken Bendectin. Several large trials, all studying cohorts of more than 1000 patients (Bunde and Bowles 1963; Heinonen *et al.* 1977*b*; Newman and Dudgeon 1977; Shapiro *et al.* 1977; Jick *et al.* 1981; Gibson *et al.* 1981; Morelock *et al.* 1982; Smithells and Sheppard 1983; Shiono and Klebonoff 1989) have failed to find an increase in the overall rate of malformations. The 95 per cent confidence limits for relative risk of 0.76 and 1.04 admit of the possibility, however, that doxylamine is a low-grade teratogen, with a risk of a few per cent above background (Orme 1985). Several studies have suggested from subgroup analyses that significant associations might exist between the use of doxylamine and specific teratogenic effects. These have, however, involved different systems: genital tract anomalies (Gibson *et al.* 1981); oesophageal atresia or encephalocoele (Cordero *et al.* 1981); diaphragmatic hernia (Bracken and Berg 1983); pyloric stenosis (Eskanazi and Bracken 1982); congenital heart disease (Rothman *et al.* 1979); microcephaly, cataract, and pulmonary hypoplasia (Shiono and Klebonoff 1989). Since most of the papers report 20–60 subgroup analyses, statistical associations are expected by chance. Case–control studies have specifically failed to find evidence of a significantly increased risk of congenital heart disease (Mitchell *et al.* 1981; Zierler and Rothman 1985), congenital limb defects (Aselton and Jick 1983; McCredie *et al.* 1984), or oral clefts (Mitchell *et al.* 1981). The lack of any consistent evidence of an association with a unique group of malformations is reassuring (Check 1979; Brent 1983; Holmes 1983) and the lack of any observed change in malformation rates after the withdrawal of doxylamine preparations makes it most unlikely that Debendox/Bendectin does cause birth defects. The case of doxylamine shows the difficulty of proving that a small risk does not exist.

Antihistamines with anticholinergic activity might, in theory, cause neonatal anticholinergic effects if used in late pregnancy, but there is little clinical evidence of this to date. What evidence there is suggests that these agents

should be avoided, if possible, in the last few weeks before delivery.

A patient who took clemastine in the last week of pregnancy delivered twins with thrombocytopenia and petechiae (Gadner 1979). Diphenhydramine has been associated with a withdrawal syndrome (restlessness and diarrhoea beginning on the 5th day postpartum) in an infant whose mother had taken 150 mg per day during pregnancy (Parkin 1974). In two early reports, intravenous dimenhydrinate was reported to exert an oxytocic effect on the full-term uterus (Rotter *et al.* 1958; Watt 1961). Kargas and others (1985) reported the unexpected stillbirth at term of a female infant less than 8 hours after her mother had taken a combination of diphenhydramine and temazepam; the authors proposed a synergistic effect.

A neonatal withdrawal syndrome of irritability, poor feeding, and clonic limb movements has also been described in a child whose mother took 600 mg hydroxyzine daily throughout pregnancy (Prenner 1977).

Promethazine is a phenothiazine antihistamine that has been used extensively as an antiemetic in pregnancy, and as an adjunct to obstetric analgesia. Briggs and colleagues (1994, p. 725) have reviewed the adverse effects of this drug in late pregnancy; significant respiratory depression has been reported in small numbers of neonates, but it was not confirmed in larger studies. Transient behavioural and EEG changes have been reported (Borgstedt and Rosen 1986), as has maternal (but not fetal) tachycardia (Riffel *et al.* 1973). Promethazine used in labour has been shown significantly to impair platelet aggregation in the neonate (Corby and Schulman 1971; Whaun *et al.* 1980). The clinical relevance of this finding is unknown, but the potential adverse effects of promethazine in labour have prompted one author to suggest that its use be discontinued, particularly when the fetus is at risk of hypoxia (Hall 1987).

Promotility agents

Metoclopramide is increasingly used to treat nausea and vomiting in late pregnancy, and to prevent gastro-oesophageal reflux during labour and during anaesthesia for Caesarean section. It appears to be well tolerated by both mother and neonate, although it equilibrates rapidly between the mother and fetus. Because it is a centrally acting dopamine antagonist, metoclopramide may affect levels of pituitary hormones, and it is known to cause hyperprolactinaemia and to promote lactation in the puerperium (Kauppila *et al.* 1983). Arvela and colleagues (1983) recorded a mean fetal : maternal ratio of 0.63, and found that metoclopramide increased maternal, but not fetal, plasma prolactin levels. They did, however, find a small but significant increase in TSH concentration in cord blood. Roti and others (1983) reported that metoclopramide had no effect on TSH levels in either maternal or cord blood. In a double-blind placebo-controlled study of metoclopramide in 23 patients undergoing general anaesthesia for Caesarean section, there were no marked differences in Apgar scores, cardiovascular variables, or neurobehavioural scores (Bylsma-Howell *et al.* 1983). Vella and others (1985) compared metoclopramide and promethazine in a double-blind study in 477 mothers in labour; they were equally effective antiemetics and there were no significant differences in neonatal outcome. Neonatal dystonic reactions have not been reported with maternal metoclopramide therapy, although they are theoretically possible. There is little information on the use of domperidone or cisapride during pregnancy.

Anaesthetic drugs

Anaesthetic gases

There is an increased rate of spontaneous abortion in women anaesthetists and theatre nurses (Ad Hoc Committee 1974; Pharoah *et al.* 1977; Vessey and Nunn 1980). Women undergoing general anaesthesia during the first or second trimester also have higher rates of spontaneous abortion than controls (Duncan *et al.* 1986). Nitrous oxide has been particularly implicated (Rowland *et al.* 1992), because it inhibits methionine synthetase, and inactivates vitamin B_{12}. Clearly, unnecessary exposure to anaesthetic agents should be avoided in women who wish to become pregnant or are in the first or second trimester of pregnancy. Reassuring data from 550 pregnancies in which short anaesthetics with N_2O were administered during the first or second trimester (Aldridge and Tunstall 1986; Crawford and Lewis 1986) indicate that the risk is likely to be small. There is no evidence that nitrous oxide is teratogenic in man.

Most inhalational and intravenous anaesthetics are lipid-soluble and easily cross the placenta, depressing the fetal central nervous system (Crawford 1982). Although it has been claimed that such exposure constitutes 'behavioural teratogenesis' (Butcher 1978), there is no evidence that perinatal exposure to CNS depressants produces other than short-term neurobehavioural impairment. The extent of such impairment will depend upon the depth and duration of maternal anaesthesia, and will also be influenced by changes in maternal ventilation, circulation, and uterine perfusion (Bryson 1986; James 1987; Finster 1988). Animal data suggest that deep surgical anaesthesia with halogenated agents

such as isoflurane, halothane, or enflurane can produce significant falls in uterine blood flow, and cause fetal bradycardia and acidosis (Palahniuk and Shnider 1974; Biehl *et al.* 1983*a,b*). The substantial body of clinical evidence suggests, however, that inhalational anaesthetics are unlikely to present a significant risk to the fetus (Konieczko *et al.* 1987).

Intravenous induction agents such as thiopentone also reach the fetus rapidly through the placenta. Thiopentone is detectable in cord blood within seconds of administration, the concentration reaching a peak within 2–3 minutes and then falling exponentially (Kosake *et al.* 1969). If the interval between induction and delivery exceeds about 10 minutes, thiopentone concentrations are well below anaesthetic levels, although respiratory and neurological depression may still be seen in the neonate. With modern techniques, however, the outcomes of Caesarean section under general anaesthesia are similar to those achieved with epidural anaesthesia (Zagorzycki and Brinkman 1982).

Neuromuscular blocking agents

Muscle relaxants such as tubocurarine, gallamine, suxamethonium, pancuronium, and newer agents such as alcuronium, are highly ionized and poorly lipid-soluble. They therefore cross the placenta only to a limited degree and pose little or no hazard to the fetus when used in conventional dosages. Kivalo and Saarikoski (1976) reported a cord : maternal plasma ratio of 0.12 for tubocurarine. A comparable mean fetal : maternal ratio of 0.11 has also been reported for vecuronium, and 0.19 for pancuronium (Dailey *et al.* 1984). Neither drug adversely affected neonatal outcome as assessed by Apgar score. A slightly higher mean fetal : maternal concentration ratio of 0.26 has been reported for alcuronium, but no neonatal adverse effects were evident as judged by Apgar scores (Ho *et al.* 1981).

Local analgesics

Local analgesic agents of the amide group cross the placenta rapidly, although cord : maternal plasma ratios are usually low (e.g. 0.52–0.69 for lignocaine and 0.31–0.44 for bupivacaine) (Pederson *et al.* 1978). Pharmacokinetic data on obstetric analgesia were comprehensively reviewed by Krauer and others (1984).

Agents of the ester group, such as procaine (no longer widely used), are so rapidly hydrolysed by plasma esterase that they present little hazard to the fetus.

Fetal microsomal enzyme system for biotransformation of amide-type local analgesics is immature in the neonate (Zagorzycki and Brinkman 1982), which metabolises these drugs slowly. For example, high levels of lignocaine in the neonate following epidural anaesthesia fall slowly, as the drug is metabolised and excreted in the first few days of life (Kuhnert *et al.* 1979).

Local analgesics can affect the fetus indirectly through changes in utero-placental circulation, or by a direct action on the fetus. Fetal bradycardia, respiratory distress, seizures, and hyperirritability have all been reported (Hill and Stern 1979). Factors contributing to fetal bradycardia include maternal hypotension and fetal hypoxia, leading to metabolic acidosis, and a quinidine-like depressant action on fetal cardiac tissue. Central nervous system toxicity is manifested as respiratory and cardiovascular depression, low Apgar scores, episodes of apnoea, and convulsions (Guillozel 1975; Finster 1976).

Overall, up to 30 per cent of neonates who are exposed to amide-type local analgesics through maternal paracervical or epidural blocks are reported to display recognizable adverse effects at birth (Yaffe and Stern 1976). There are, however, significant pharmacokinetic differences within this group, and bupivacaine appears to be the drug of choice for continuous epidural analgesia in obstetrics (*Drug and Therapeutics Bulletin* 1983), since it has a relatively low fetal : maternal concentration ratio, probably due to extensive protein-binding of the drug in maternal plasma (Ralston and Shnider 1978). It has minimal effects on uterine function (Schellenberg 1977) and, in one study, neonates delivered under bupivacaine epidurals exhibited better muscle tone than those whose mothers had received lignocaine or mepivacaine (Scanlon *et al.* 1974).

The place of newer agents such as ropivacaine is uncertain.

Anti-infective agents

Infections are relatively common during pregnancy, and need to be treated appropriately, but there are few reliable data confirming either the safety or efficacy of anti-infective agents in pregnancy. There is, however, an extensive body of clinical experience (albeit mainly empirical and anecdotal) which indicates that the older-established penicillins such as benzylpenicillin and ampicillin are safe in pregnancy. The treatment of infections in pregnancy has been reviewed by Garland and O'Reilly (1995), Duff (1997), and Edwards (1997).

Anthelmintic agents
Mebendazole

The manufacturers are aware of the outcome of 306 cases when mebendazole was taken during pregnancy, with 26 spontaneous abortions and 17 abnormal babies. Abnormalities included haemangiomata (4 cases), hypospadias

(two cases), and oesophageal atresia and imperforate anus (one case) (T. Simonite, personal communication). There has been no relevant case–control study.

Piperazine

Administration of this drug from day 27 to day 33 after conception and again from day 41 to day 47 was associated with lobster-claw deformities of the hands and feet in the child delivered subsequently (Meyer and Brenner 1988). It is known that differentiation of the limbs occurs in the period 24–36 days after conception. New mutations and sporadic cases of lobster-claw deformity do, however, occur. In the absence of other evidence, it seems unlikely that piperazine is a common cause of lobster-claw deformity. Two other cases, one of anophthalmia and facial cleft and the other of an abnormal foot, have also been reported.

The anthelmintics should, if possible, not be used during the first trimester (Leach 1990).

Piperazine is potentially neurotoxic (Dukes 1980; Leach 1990), although there have been no reports of fetal neonatal neurological effects.

Leach (1990) recommended that anthelminthic agents be avoided during the first trimester. The UK National Teratology Information Service has concluded that neither mebendazole nor piperazine is likely to increase the overall risk of malformation, and women inadvertently exposed to either agent during the first trimester can be reassured (P.R. McElhatton, personal communication).

Antibacterials
Aminoglycosides

Streptomycin and kanamycin, in common with other aminoglycosides, can cause damage to the eighth cranial nerve in treated subjects, and so it is not surprising that ototoxicity has been observed after exposure *in utero* to these antibacterials (Good and Johnston 1971; Jones 1973; Snider *et al.* 1980; Donald and Sellars 1981). Similar considerations presumably apply to gentamicin and the newer aminoglycosides, although no cases have been reported. The incidence of other abnormalities is not apparently increased (Heinonen *et al.* 1977*b*).

Tetracyclines

Cases of discolouration of the cornea (Krejčf and Brettschneider 1983), congenital cataract (Harley *et al.* 1964), limb abnormalities (Carter and Wilson 1962, 1963), and multiple abnormalities (Corcoran and Castles 1977) have been reported after usage of tetracyclines in the first trimester, but prospective trials have shown no significant increase in fetal abnormalities (Elder *et al.*

1971; Heinonen *et al.* 1977*b*). These reports imply that the risks from inadvertently continuing low-dose tetracycline treatment for acne around the time of conception are likely to be small.

Tetracyclines are potent chelating agents and form a complex with calcium that is incorporated in fetal bones and teeth. Calcification of the deciduous teeth begins towards the end of the first trimester, and the yellow-brown discolouration and enamel hypoplasia associated with maternal tetracycline therapy after this stage are now well-recognized (Porter *et al.* 1965; Kutscher *et al.* 1966; Genot *et al.* 1970). Because exchange of calcium does not occur after calcification of teeth is complete, the discolouration is permanent. In later pregnancy, the permanent teeth may be affected. All tetracyclines produce these effects, although Weyman (1965), in a study of 59 children with tetracycline staining of the teeth, showed that the colour varied depending on the drug used; the least objectionable staining (a creamy discolouration) was produced by oxytetracycline.

Tetracyclines are also incorporated into fetal bone, and can cause a reversible retardation of skeletal growth, particularly in premature infants (Cohlan *et al.* 1963; Greene 1976).

Tetracyclines may cause a dose-related acute fatty degeneration of the liver in pregnant women, especially in the presence of impaired renal function, characterized by azotaemia, jaundice, and pancreatitis (Whalley *et al.* 1964; Allen and Brown 1966). While the fetus may not be directly affected, the maternal disorder often leads to fetal morbidity and mortality.

Quinolones

Ciprofloxacin and other quinolone antibacterial agents have been suggested to cause damage to fetal joints in animals (Schulter 1989). A case–control study of 28 women who received norfloxacin failed to detect any increase in fetal malformation rate (Berkovitch *et al.* 1994).

Metronidazole

There is a theoretical risk that metronidazole, by inhibiting aldehyde dehydrogenase, might increase the chances of the fetal alcohol syndrome occurring in the offspring of women who drink during pregnancy (Dunn *et al.* 1979).

Chloramphenicol

The fetus and neonate are deficient in the enzyme system which glucuronidates chloramphenicol. The drug is well known to cause the 'grey baby' syndrome of vomiting, hypothermia, and cardiovascular collapse when given directly to the neonate (Leitman 1979), but there are no reliable reports of this reaction arising from maternal exposure (Gilstrap and Faro 1990). Nevertheless, because of the theoretical risk, and because its haematological toxicity and effects on protein synthesis in dividing cells, chloramphenicol is best avoided throughout pregnancy.

Sulphonamides

Sulphonamides cross the placenta readily, achieving fetal : maternal blood concentration ratios of up to 0.9 (Briggs *et al.* 1994, p. 795). They are highly protein bound and compete with bilirubin for binding sites on plasma albumin, or they may compete with it for immature fetal glucuronyl transferase. In the neonate, when free bilirubin can no longer be cleared via the placenta, jaundice may occur (Dunn 1964), although this appears to be uncommon. Kernicterus is a theoretical possibility, but has not been reported in practice. The risk is likely to be greater in premature infants with immature hepatic function. Sulphonamides may also cause haemolytic anaemia, particularly in individuals deficient in glucose-6-phosphate dehydrogenase (Perkins 1971).

Antifungals

Griseofulvin

Exposure to this drug during early pregnancy had occurred in two cases of conjoined twins reported to a US Food and Drug Administration scheme (Rosa *et al.* 1987*a*). A possible association with spontaneous abortion was also noted. As fission of twins is normally complete by 20 days, only women bearing identical twins and given the drug before 20 days would be susceptible. No cases of griseofulvin exposure were recorded among mothers who gave birth to 39 conjoined twins in Hungary (Métneki and Czeizel 1987) or in 47 cases reported to an international monitoring scheme (Knudsen 1987), but the anomaly is so rare that the US cases should perhaps not be dismissed.

Antimalarials

Quinine

When quinine is taken by women as an abortifacient during the first trimester, and no abortion occurs, then the infant may be delivered with congenital defects of the central nervous system, limbs, face, heart, or other organs (Nishimura and Tanimura 1976). Auditory (Roberts 1870; Taylor 1934) and optic nerve (McKinna 1966) damage can also occur, as might be expected from the toxic effects in adults.

It is much less clear whether therapeutic use in falciparum malaria carries fetal risk, and the disease is so serious that it would not be logical to withhold treatment (*The Lancet* 1983*b,c*).

Chloroquine

There is a suggestion that high doses of chloroquine are ototoxic and retinotoxic (Hart and Naunton 1964), but a comparison of 169 infants exposed to maternal prophylaxis (300 mg per week) and 454 controls failed to find any evidence for a teratogenic effect (Wolfe and Cordero 1985).

Pyrimethamine

This is a folate antagonist and, as with other drugs of this class, it is reported to have caused birth defects — but only in one case of ectopic viscera (Morley *et al.* 1964). It has been suggested that folinic acid should be given concurrently to mothers taking malarial prophylaxis, at least throughout the first trimester (*The Lancet* 1983*c*).

Mefloquine

There are few published data on the use of mefloquine for prophylaxis or treatment during the first trimester. Studies in later pregnancy (Steketee *et al.* 1996; Nosten 1994) suggest that mefloquine is effective in eradicating malarial parasites and reduces the incidence of low-birthweight infants.

Antituberculous drugs

A review of 1939 births from 10 series failed to find evidence for a major teratogenic effect of antituberculous therapy (Snider *et al.* 1980). *p*-Aminosalicylic acid treatment during the first trimester in 43 mothers was associated with congenital defects in five infants (Heinonen *et al.* 1977*b*), a result which may be due to chance.

Rifampicin

This is an enzyme-inducing agent, and therefore increases the rate of metabolism of oral contraceptive hormones, increasing the risk of unwanted pregnancy. In 226 women receiving rifampicin, pregnancy ended in spontaneous abortion or intrauterine death in 10, in neonatal death in 4, and in congenital abnormalities in 9, of whom 4 had limb abnormalities and 3 hydrocephalus or anencephaly (Steen and Stainton-Ellis 1977).

Rifampicin has been associated with two cases of neonatal hypoprothrombinaemia and haemorrhage, caused by maternal vitamin K deficiency (Chouraqui *et al.* 1982).

Isoniazid

Isoniazid may be linked to a number of central nervous system problems, including retardation and convulsions (Lowe 1964; Weinstein and Dalton 1968), but in 85 patients who received isoniazid during the first trimester there were 10 malformations, a non-significant increase (Heinonen *et al.* 1977*b*). Retrospective analysis of a placebo-controlled trial of isoniazid also failed to find a significant difference in fetal outcome (Ludford *et al.* 1973).

Antiretroviral drugs

Vertical transmission of human immunodeficiency virus (HIV) from mother to fetus is an important problem: approximately 7000 infants are born each year to mothers in the United States infected with HIV. Amongst offspring of women who received zidovudine in the first trimester, one child had agenesis of the right kidney and 45 were normal. Two male infants born after exposure to zidovudine in the first trimester were reported to have minor abnormalities; a third infant had polydactyly, and a fourth had features of the fetal alcohol syndrome. Forty-five others were normal (Kumar *et al.* 1994). These authors regarded their data as reassuring. The consensus is in favour of using zidovudine, and possibly other agents (Lindsay and Nesheim 1997; Minkoff and Augenbraun 1997).

Anti-inflammatory agents

Salicylates and other NSAID

The use of NSAID (non-steroidal anti-inflammatory drugs) in pregnancy has been extensively reviewed (Rudolph 1981; Needs and Brooks 1985; Østensen and Husby 1985; Heymann 1986; Brooks and Needs 1989). A case–control study (Zeirler and Rothman 1985) suggested that first-trimester aspirin use might be associated with cardiac defects, though a subsequent case–control study, in which adjustment was made for maternal age, family history, and certain other risk factors (Werler *et al.* 1989), failed to confirm an association.

Two cases of cyclopia in the offspring of women who had taken 3–4 g of salicylate daily during the first trimester (Benawra *et al.* 1980; Agapitos *et al.* 1986) are suggestive of a rare association, which is of theoretical interest. Early in embryogenesis, the forebrain cleaves in the midline and the paired structures of the face are formed. Cleavage defects, often associated with premaxillary agenesis, may be of any degree from cyclopia (no cleavage, single eyeglobe, arhinia) to failure of cleavage of the central incisor teeth. The cerebral anomaly results in a single 'holosphere', and the group of defects is called holoprosencephaly (Yakovlev 1959; Cohen 1982). An autosomal recessive form exists (McKusick 1992). As only the most severe form of cleavage defect has been reported and, as it is extremely rare, salicylates could only be responsible if they blocked the initiating process for midline cleavage in a very unusual, susceptible subgroup. Since congenital cytomegalovirus infection has been linked to cyclopia, it is possible that the salicylates were taken for that infection, which was itself the teratogen. This makes it less likely that salicylate is responsible for cyclopia, but there is a precedent: the plant *Veratrum californium* causes exactly this defect in sheep (Binns *et al.* 1965). It has been suggested (Webster *et al.* 1988) that cyclopia is the extreme form of the facial dysmorphogenesis seen with maternal ethanol abuse or anticonvulsant therapy.

Slone and colleagues (1976) failed to find any evidence of teratogenesis from heavy first trimester exposure to salicylates in 5128 pregnancies compared with 35 418 with no exposure and 9736 with intermediate exposure.

The use of NSAID in late pregnancy, either to treat arthritic disease or to delay premature labour, may be associated with a range of adverse effects.

Prostaglandins are important mediators of fetal function and development. Prostaglandin E_2 produces dilatation of both systemic and pulmonary blood vessels, and is involved in maintaining patency of the ductus arteriosus; prostaglandins may also influence blood flow in various organs, including the kidney. They have a major influence on platelet adhesion and aggregation, and they are also mediators of uterine contraction.

Inhibition of fetal cyclo-oxygenase by NSAID may therefore cause profound circulatory, renal, and haematological effects, and may delay the onset of, and prolong, labour.

Indomethacin has been widely used in the management of threatened premature labour, and its adverse effects are well documented. Manchester and co-workers (1976) reported primary pulmonary hypertension associated with maternal indomethacin therapy, and similar effects have been demonstrated in animal studies (Levin *et al.* 1979). There have been several subsequent reports of this reaction with indomethacin (Truter *et al.* 1986; Demandt *et al.* 1990), naproxen (Wilkinson *et al.* 1979; Wilkinson 1980), and salicylate (Arcilla *et al.* 1969; Perkin *et al.* 1980). The increased pulmonary artery pressure is probably a direct consequence of constriction or premature closure of the fetal ductus arteriosus (Rudolph 1981; Moise *et al.* 1988*a*).

Levin and colleagues (1978) found increased smooth muscle development in the pulmonary vascular bed of infants exposed to NSAID and, in animal models, *in utero* exposure to indomethacin produces similar hypertrophy of pulmonary vascular smooth muscle (Levin *et al.* 1979).

It should be noted, however, that several studies have failed to confirm the association between NSAID and neonatal pulmonary hypertension (Kumor *et al.* 1979; Niebyl *et al.* 1980; Hendricks *et al.* 1990), and at least one study has been challenged (Ovadia 1988) and defended (Moise *et al.* 1988*b*) on methodological grounds. Many variables may influence whether an individual neonate suffers this adverse reaction, including the dose, timing, and duration of exposure to the NSAID, and possible differences in the sensitivity of the ductus arteriosus and pulmonary vasculature to changes in prostaglandin levels. Moreover, all the recorded cases have been associated with use in late pregnancy for threatened premature labour; it is not clear whether the use of an NSAID at an earlier stage of pregnancy for non-obstetric indications carries similar risks. It would be prudent, however, to assume that all cyclo-oxygenase-inhibiting agents have the potential to cause cardiovascular complications, and to avoid them in pregnancy unless there is a clear and specific therapeutic indication.

Prostaglandins are synthesized in the kidney, and NSAID are known occasionally to cause acute renal insufficiency or renal tubular necrosis (see Chapter 14). It is therefore not surprising that renal problems in the neonate have been associated with maternal NSAID therapy. Van der Heijden and others (1988) reported oedema, oliguria, and elevated serum creatinine in five of nine preterm neonates exposed to indomethacin. Simeoni and colleagues (1989) described severe acute renal failure in twins, and transient water and sodium retention with uraemia in a third infant. A case of anuria requiring peritoneal dialysis was associated with indomethacin therapy (Demandt *et al.* 1990).

Several cases of oligohydramnios have been associated with cyclo-oxygenase inhibitors, again in preterm labour (Kirshon 1988; Hickok *et al.* 1989; Goldenberg *et al.* 1989; Wiggins and Elliott 1990; Hendricks *et al.* 1990). Oligohydramnios, growth retardation, and anuria were reported in an infant whose mother had taken 150 mg indomethacin daily for juvenile arthritis, from weeks 27–37 of pregnancy (Cantor *et al.* 1980). A preterm infant developed severe hyponatraemia after fluid retention following the mother's taking an overdose of naproxen 8 hours before delivery (Alun-Jones and Williams 1986).

Neonatal ischaemic brain injury has been described in two pairs of twins exposed to indomethacin *in utero*

(Simeoni *et al.* 1989; Haddad *et al.* 1990). Low urinary prostaglandin E_2 levels were recorded in two of the neonates, and cerebral vasoconstriction induced by indomethacin was postulated.

Aspirin inhibits platelet adhesion and aggregation and therefore impairs haemostasis. Maternal consumption of aspirin in late pregnancy consequently increases the risk of antepartum and postpartum haemorrhage, and of neonatal haemorrhage (Stuart *et al.* 1982). Bleyer and Breckenridge (1970) showed that neonatal haemostasis was sensitive to even small doses of aspirin taken by the mother in late pregnancy. Rumack and colleagues (1981) reported a significantly increased incidence of intracranial haemorrhage in premature infants exposed to aspirin in the last week of pregnancy.

Low-dose aspirin has been used, and without neonatal haemorrhagic complications, in the management of women at risk of pregnancy-induced hypertensive crises and pre-eclampsia (Benigni *et al.* 1989; Schiff *et al.* 1989); and those with migraine (Nelson-Piercy and de Swiet 1996). Garrettson and others (1974) reported the case of a woman who took 6.5 g aspirin per day throughout pregnancy and was then delivered of a healthy female infant who had a plasma salicylate concentration of 250 mg per litre.

Penicillamine

Cutis laxa, that is, abnormally lax skin lacking normal elastic tissue, has been found in several cases where the mother had received penicillamine in pregnancy (Laver and Fairley 1971; Mjølnerød *et al.* 1971; Solomon *et al.* 1977). In two cases (Linares *et al.* 1979; Harpey *et al.* 1983), the defect apparently resolved. This characteristic defect does not occur in the offspring of all women treated with penicillamine, and Lyle (1978) recounts 27 pregnancies: 26 with normal outcome after penicillamine in the first trimester, and one with a 'small ventricular septal defect'.

Cardiovascular drugs

Antiarrhythmic drugs

Amiodarone

The antiarrhythmic drug amiodarone was associated with a large ventricular septal defect in one case where the mother took the drug in the first trimester of pregnancy, but no reported abnormality in 11 others (Ovadia *et al.* 1994; Foster 1994). When taken later in pregnancy, amiodarone can cause congenital hypothyroidism and goitre (Ovadia *et al.* 1994).

Antihypertensive agents

Methyldopa

Methyldopa has been widely used to treat hypertension in pregnancy and most reports indicate that it presents little hazard to the fetus. A large, prospective, controlled study demonstrated the absence of any significant adverse effects, and the developmental progress of infants exposed to methyldopa has been followed up from periods of up to 7½ years (Mutch *et al.* 1977*a,b*; Ounsted *et al.* 1980; Cockburn *et al.* 1982; Redman and Ounsted 1982).

Fetuses exposed to methyldopa for the first time in mid-pregnancy (between 16–20 weeks) were found to have significantly smaller head circumferences at birth, but this did not affect development progress (Redman and Ounsted 1982) and the effect is considered to be of minor clinical significance (Redman 1995).

Methyldopa crosses the placenta freely, and may cause neonatal hypotension (Whitelaw 1981). Two cases of neonatal nasal obstruction have been reported (LeGras *et al.* 1990), and Shimohira and others (1986) described a child with abnormal sleep patterns that were attributed to maternal methyldopa administration. Low concentrations of noradrenaline in cerebrospinal fluid, associated with a marked tremor, were reported in three hypoxic neonates whose mothers had taken methyldopa (Bodis *et al.* 1982).

Minoxidil

Hypertrichosis, which is known to occur in patients taking minoxidil, was observed in the infants of two mothers who took the drug throughout pregnancy, together with other drugs (Kaler *et al.* 1987; Rosa *et al.* 1987*b*). One baby also had other abnormalities, including an omphalocele. In the only other case of intrauterine minoxidil exposure notified to the Food and Drug Administration, the baby died of cyanotic congenital heart disease.

Angiotensin-converting-enzyme (ACE) inhibitors

ACE inhibitors (captopril and enalapril) have been linked with a very rare skull ossification defect in three cases (Duminy and Burger 1981; Mehta and Modi 1989; Cunniff *et al.* 1990) and renal dysgenesis in two cases (Knott *et al.* 1989; Cunniff *et al.* 1990).

The fetal risk from exposure to ACE inhibitors during the first trimester seems small (Anonymous 1997), but exposure during later stages of pregnancy can lead to intrauterine growth retardation, oligohydramnios, and Potter's sequence of hypoplasia of the kidneys and lungs (Guignard *et al.* 1981; Rothberg and Lorenz 1984; Kreft-Jais *et al.* 1988; Schubiger *et al.* 1988; Scott and Purohit

1989; Rosa *et al.* 1989; Cunniff *et al.* 1990; Barr and Cohen 1991). The clinical features are related to fetal hypotension, with a reduction in fetal urine flow, and this can also be manifest as neonatal oliguria, anuria, and renal failure (Barr 1994).

There is general agreement that all ACE inhibitors should be avoided during all stages of pregnancy (Shotan *et al.* 1994). Women who become pregnant whilst taking ACE inhibitors should stop taking them immediately pregnancy is confirmed.

Calcium channel-blocking drugs

A prospective cohort study of the effects of calcium channel-blocking drugs taken by 78 women during the first trimester did not find any significant increase in malformations (Magee *et al.* 1996).

Constantine and others (1987) reported on the use of nifedipine, mainly in combination with atenolol, in 23 pregnant women with severe hypertension. Blood pressure control was good, but there were high rates of Caesarean section, abnormal fetal ECGs, and premature or small-for-dates infants; whether this was due to the hypertension or the medication was uncertain.

Nifedipine is a potent uterine relaxant (Ulmsten *et al.* 1978; Andersson *et al.* 1979; Forman *et al.* 1982) that has been used in the management of preterm labour (Bult-Sarley and Lourwood 1988). Its use to treat hypertension in late pregnancy might therefore be expected to cause delayed or prolonged labour, although no cases have been reported to date.

Diuretics

Thiazides are best avoided in pregnancy. They may aggravate pre-eclampsia by increasing hypovolaemia, possibly precipitating renal failure (Palomaki and Lindheimer 1970). Maternal hypokalaemia (Pritchard and Walley 1961), pancreatitis (Minkowitz *et al.* 1964), and hyperuricaemia may occur, and neonatal thrombocytopenia has been reported (Rodriguez *et al.* 1974).

Metabolic acidosis, hypocalcaemia, and hypomagnesaemia have been described in a preterm infant whose mother was treated with acetazolamide throughout pregnancy (Merlob *et al.* 1990). *In utero* exposure to ethacrynic acid throughout pregnancy has been implicated in a case of neonatal nephrolithiasis (Fischer *et al.* 1988). Ultrasonography at 30 weeks showed polyhydramnios, and massive neonatal diuresis occurred during the first day of life.

β-Adrenoceptor blocking agents

β-Blockers may cause a range of pharmacological (Type A) adverse effects in the second and third trimesters. Many of these reactions may represent the consequences of fetal distress in severely hypertensive, high-risk, pregnancies.

In an early study, intrauterine growth retardation was seen in six of 12 pregnancies in which propranolol was taken by the mother (Pruyn *et al.* 1979). The effect was attributed to impaired uterine blood flow secondary to β-blockade, but severe hypertension is itself known to be associated with placental insufficiency. Atenolol was also associated with low birthweight in a prospective cohort study (Lip *et al.* 1997). A follow-up study of 55 infants who had been exposed to atenolol showed normal development at one year of age (Reynolds *et al.* 1984).

Other adverse effects occasionally reported with β-blockers are respiratory distress (Tunstall 1969), prolonged labour (Habib and McCarthy 1977), bradycardia and hypotension (Woods and Morrell 1982; Brosset *et al.* 1988), and hypoglycaemia (Brosset *et al.* 1988). With the exception of neonatal bradycardia, however, these effects have not been apparent in controlled clinical trials.

Labetalol has both α-blocking and β-blocking activity, together with a direct vasodilator effect. Experience with this antihypertensive agent in pregnancy has been generally favourable, with few reports of clinically significant fetal hypoglycaemia, bradycardia, or respiratory depression. Macpherson and others (1986) made serial measurements of neonatal cardiovascular, metabolic, and thermoregulatory function for the first 72 hours of life in 11 infants exposed to labetalol and in 11 carefully matched controls. The former showed a mild transient hypotension (mean 4.5 mm Hg) which resolved within 24 hours; there were no other significant differences and the authors concluded that labetalol does not cause clinically important sympathetic blockade in the full-term neonate.

A case report (Haraldsson and Geven 1989) suggests that maternal labetalol may be less well tolerated by the premature neonate; an infant born at 33 weeks' gestation had severe bradycardia, diminished femoral pulse, cyanosis, and respiratory depression after delivery by Caesarean section. In a randomized controlled trial against methyldopa in 176 women, however, cardiovascular, metabolic, and respiratory function findings were comparable, including those of a subgroup of 33 infants who were small for gestational age or born before 37 weeks (Plouin *et al.* 1987).

Anticoagulants

Warfarin

Warfarin causes a specific pattern of developmental abnormalities, with nasal hypoplasia and calcific stripping of the epiphyses (chondrodysplasia punctata), in infants exposed during the first trimester. This is called warfarin embryopathy. A similar disorder can occur as an autosomal recessive trait. Two cases of diaphragmatic hernia have been reported in the infants exposed to warfarin *in utero* (Normann and Stray-Pedersen 1989). There is no critical period during organogenesis when exposure to warfarin results in defects: they can be manifest after exposure in the second or third trimester alone. Ginsberg and Hirsh (1988) were able to identify reports of 578 women given oral anticoagulants during pregnancy, of whom 31 had infants with warfarin embryopathy, and 21 suffered 'fetal wastage'. In a prospective study of 72 pregnancies in which warfarin was given during the first 6 weeks of pregnancy, 10 babies had warfarin embryopathy; all occurred in the 35 pregnancies in which warfarin therapy continued into weeks 8–12 (Iturbe-Alessio *et al.* 1986).

In a prospective study of 50 pregnancies in women with artificial heart valves treated with warfarin during the first and second trimesters, there were 18 deaths *in utero* or perinatally, and two cases of warfarin embryopathy (Sareli *et al.* 1989).

Warfarin inhibits the formation of carboxyglutamyl residues from glutamyl residues, and so reduces the binding of calcium to protein; this might explain the abnormal ossification of cartilage which it causes (Hall *et al.* 1980). This hypothesis is supported by the case of a boy with the typical somatotype of warfarin embryopathy who had not been exposed to warfarin *in utero* but who had decreased activities of vitamin-K-dependent coagulation factors (Pauli *et al.* 1987). Abnormal chondrogenesis seems to be a precursor of the abnormal ossification (Barr and Burdi 1976).

Warfarin can cause abnormalities of the central nervous system such as hydrocephaly or microcephaly, optic atrophy, and developmental impairment; there does not appear to be a critical period of exposure (Sherman and Hall 1976; Hall 1976; Holzgreve *et al.* 1976; Warkany 1976; Hall *et al.* 1980). Hall and colleagues (1980), in a review of published cases, concluded that about 3 per cent of liveborn infants exposed to warfarin demonstrated central nervous system abnormalities. The sequelae were more significant and debilitating than those of the embryopathy, and all had been exposed to warfarin in the second or third trimesters, or during both of these.

The microcephaly, optic atrophy, and mental retardation might be due to repeated small intracranial haemorrhages induced by warfarin (Sahul and Hall 1977). Chong and colleagues (1984), however, compared the physical and mental development of 22 children exposed to warfarin during pregnancy with matched controls. There were no significant differences between the exposed children and the controls, or within the study group according to the time of exposure to warfarin; none of the 18 children exposed in the second trimester showed CNS defects. In a study of 30 pregnancies during which the mothers took warfarin from week 13 onwards, there was one case of congenital hydrocephalus, but no case of microcephaly or eye defects (Chen *et al.* 1982). All except the infant with hydrocephalus subsequently showed normal developmental patterns. Central nervous system defects arising from late exposure to warfarin therefore appear to be rare.

Warfarin can cause serious haemorrhagic complications in both mother and fetus towards the end of pregnancy (Villasanta 1965). The fetus and premature neonate have low levels of vitamin K-dependent clotting factors (II, VII, IX, and X) (Bonnar *et al.* 1971; Andrew *et al.* 1981). The fetus may therefore be receiving excessive anticoagulant while the mother's prothrombin time is within the normal range, and fetal or neonatal haemorrhage, sometimes fatal, may ensue. For this reason, a change to heparin is generally recommended in late pregnancy, between weeks 32 and 36, for the remainder of the pregnancy (Hirsh *et al.* 1970; *Drug and Therapeutics Bulletin* 1987; Ginsberg and Hirsh 1988; Ginsberg *et al.* 1989; Oakley 1995).

Heparin

Heparin therapy is occasionally associated with maternal haemorrhage, but it is generally considered to be safe for the fetus, though Hall and others (1980) claimed that the fetal and neonatal morbidity and mortality associated with heparin was as high as with oral anticoagulants. They found that in 135 published cases of heparin exposure there were 19 stillbirths or abortions, 29 premature births (10 fatal), and normal outcomes in only 86.

Ginsberg and Hirsh (1989), in a careful review of the same reports, found that of the pregnancies in which heparin was used, 49 were associated with severe toxaemia, glomerulonephritis, or a history of recurrent abortions. There were 31 (63.3 per cent) adverse outcomes in this group. In an independent review of 186 published studies involving 1325 pregnancies exposed to anticoagulants, Ginsberg and others (1989) found adverse outcomes in 10.5 per cent of cases where heparin was used (after excluding co-morbidity). If prematurity with normal outcome was excluded, the incidence of adverse outcomes was only 3.6 per cent.

This analysis supported the findings of a small controlled trial in which 40 women were randomized to receive heparin or no treatment. There was no increased risk of antenatal or postnatal bleeding in the heparin group, and there was one abortion in each group, although more babies from the heparin group required neonatal intensive care (Howell *et al.* 1983).

Heparin therefore appears to be effective and relatively safe in the prophylaxis and treatment of venous thromboembolic disease in pregnancy and is preferred to warfarin, at least during the first trimester (Ginsberg and Hirsh 1988; Ginsberg *et al.* 1989; Greaves 1993).

Low-molecular-weight heparins may prove to have advantages, including a long duration of action and a lesser tendency to cause thrombocytopenia with prolonged usage (see Chapter 24). Enoxaparin was apparently effective in a small study; no congenital abnormalities were reported (Sturridge *et al.* 1994). Low-dose heparin is ineffective, however, in women with valvular heart disease and, while high-dose heparin may be effective, this has not been demonstrated in controlled clinical trials.

Heparin causes demineralization of bone, and osteoporosis may occur, usually in women treated for 6 months or more. In a study of 20 women given 20 000 units daily, heparin caused a dose-dependent osteopenia, although this was symptomatic in only one case (de Swiet *et al.* 1983). In a more recent study, 12 out of 70 women (17 per cent) given a mean dose of 31 000 units daily exhibited obvious osteopenia on X-rays of the spine and hip. Two suffered multiple fractures of the spine (Dahlman *et al.* 1990).

Drugs acting on the central nervous system

Centrally acting analgesics

There were eight cases of respiratory malformations in the offspring of 563 women who were exposed to codeine during the first trimester, a statistically significant increase (Heinonen *et al.* 1977*b*). Other defects, including congenital heart defects and cleft lip and palate, were more common in babies born to women who took opiates during the first trimester (Saxén 1975; Bracken and Holford 1981).

Fetal exposure to opioid drugs in late pregnancy falls into two main categories: analgesia in labour or for Caesarean section, and abuse by dependent mothers.

The effects of peripartum narcotics on the neonate are well documented. Placental transfer of pethidine and other opioids is rapid and substantial. Pethidine is detectable in amniotic fluid within 30 minutes of a maternal intramuscular injection, and concentrations in cord blood are 80 to 130 per cent of maternal levels (Moore *et al.* 1973; Rothberg *et al.* 1978). The effect on the neonate is characterized by respiratory depression and a low Apgar score (Fishburn 1982), which is likely to be maximal about 3 hours after the intramuscular injection

(Belfrage *et al.* 1981). The respiratory depressant effects can be reversed by naloxone.

Pethidine and its metabolite are only slowly eliminated by the neonate (Kuhnert *et al.* 1980), and neonatal neurobehavioural dysfunction may be evident for 2–3 days (Hodgkinson and Husain 1982). One study has attributed impaired behavioural patterns up to 6 weeks after birth to high cord blood levels of pethidine (Belsey *et al.* 1981). Follow-up studies have not demonstrated any long-term developmental effects from obstetric analgesia. Richards (1981) has reviewed studies in this area.

Narcotic dependency

Drug dependency in pregnant women is an increasing problem (de Swiet 1995*b*), and the incidence of neonatal complications is high. An American study in 830 women dependent on opiates and 400 matched controls found significantly increased risks of meconium staining, anaemia, haemorrhage, multiple pregnancy, prematurity, low birthweight, low Apgar scores, and perinatal mortality. Children of addicts were 5.5 times more likely to be small for gestational age, and the relative risk of perinatal mortality was 2.7 (Ostrea and Chavez 1979).

The fetus may also develop dependence, and a high proportion of infants born to women dependent on narcotics will experience a withdrawal syndrome (de Swiet 1995*b*). The timing of the onset of withdrawal depends upon the rate of elimination of the narcotic; morphine and diamorphine withdrawal symptoms begin with 4–24 hours after delivery, whereas methadone withdrawal may be delayed for up to 1–2 weeks. The withdrawal syndrome is characterized by irritability, hypertonia, tremor, tachypnoea, and sometimes convulsions. It may be fatal, and withdrawal effects can occur *in utero* if the mother stops using narcotics or if narcotic antagonists are given.

The long-term effects of exposure to narcotics *in utero* are poorly understood. The results of follow-up studies are conflicting, and it is often difficult to differentiate the effect of narcotic exposure from that of confounding social and environmental factors (Kaltenbach and Finnegan 1989; Hans 1989). However, studies published to date indicate that prenatal narcotic exposure does not appear to have long-term developmental consequences (Strauss *et al.* 1979; Kaltenbach and Finnegan 1986, 1987).

Antiepileptic drugs

Children born to mothers with epilepsy have an increased risk of congenital malformation (Meadow 1970; Fedrick 1973). Major malformations, and total malformations, were significantly more common in the 305 children born to epileptic mothers in 50 282 mother–child pairs; intellectual development at 8 months and 4 years was slowed and mothers of children with craniofacial anomalies were more likely to have taken anticonvulsants, according to one case–control study (Shapiro *et al.* 1976). A case–control study of 211 pregnant women receiving antiepileptic drugs showed a threefold increase in abnormal outcomes (Waters *et al.* 1994). Craniofacial anomalies and congenital heart disease have been seen with increased frequency in several series (Speidel and Meadow 1972; Millar and Nevin 1973; Niswander and Wertlecki 1973; Nakane *et al.* 1980). Fetal and perinatal loss may also be increased (Speidel and Meadow 1972; Nakane *et al.* 1980; Akhtar and Millac 1987), and birthweight, adjusted for sex and gestational age, may be reduced (Mastroiacovo *et al.* 1988).

All the commonly used antiepileptic drugs have some teratogenic potential (Dodson 1989). Folate deficiency, related to anticonvulsant therapy, may play a pathogenetic role (Hiilesmaa *et al.* 1983; Dansky *et al.* 1987), and there is some experimental evidence in animals that folic acid supplements are protective (Zhu and Zhou 1989).

It is uncertain whether maternal epilepsy itself, independent of drug usage, might predispose to malformations in the fetus (Gaily *et al.* 1989; Keller 1989). Anneggers and others (1974) failed to find malformations in the 26 infants born to mothers with epilepsy 'in remission', or in the 61 babies born to mothers who subsequently developed epilepsy; there was one malformation amongst the 56 offspring of mothers with epilepsy who took no treatment during the first trimester, and 10 in 141 babies whose mothers had taken one or more antiepileptic drug during pregnancy. A Japanese study also found an increased malformation rate in the babies of treated, but not untreated, epileptic mothers (Nakane *et al.* 1980). The probable systematic differences between epileptic women who receive treatment and those who do not, make these studies less useful.

Phenytoin

Phenytoin has been linked to a characteristic (but probably not specific) syndrome, the 'fetal hydantoin syndrome', with dysmorphic features: short nose with broad depressed bridge and inner epicanthic folds; mild hypertelorism; ptosis and strabismus; wide mouth and short webbed neck; cleft lip or palate, or both; and hypoplasia of the nails and distal phalanges. In its most extreme form the cranial anomalies may also include holoprosencephaly (Kotzot *et al.* 1993), and the limb anomalies absence of the hand (Sabry and Farag 1996). The syn-

drome usually includes growth deficiency and developmental delay (Loughnan *et al.* 1973; Hanson and Smith 1977; Hanson 1986). The incidence of recognizable cases is probably 10 per cent of exposed children (Hanson *et al.* 1976).

The mechanism may require a genetically susceptible infant (Phelan *et al.* 1982), and it has been postulated that a genetic defect in the detoxification of a reactive arene oxide metabolite of phenytoin may increase the risk of the syndrome (Strickler *et al.* 1985). The gene for epoxide hydrolase may exist in two allelic forms, one coding for an enzyme of low activity. Buehler and others (1990) predicted the outcome of 19 pregnancies in women taking phenytoin on the basis of the enzyme activity in fetal fibroblast or amniocyte cultures. All four fetuses with epoxide hydrolase activity below 30 per cent developed the fetal hydantoin syndrome, but none of the 15 with activities above 30 per cent did so. (The technique does not work with samples of chorionic villi [Buehler *et al.* 1993]). The similarity of dysmorphic features related to maternal consumption of phenytoin, carbamazepine, primidone, ethanol, or toluene (Hersh *et al.* 1985) may, however, support a direct neurotoxic effect (Dodson 1989).

Sodium valproate

Use of sodium valproate by the mother is associated with a significantly increased risk of spina bifida in the infant, estimated to be 36 times the risk for the non-epileptic mothers and 4 times the risk of epileptic mothers on other therapy (*The Lancet* 1988). Retrospective assessment of risk from cases collected from registers is likely to be inaccurate (*The Lancet* 1988), so the findings are uncertain, but the association has been seen in France (Robert and Guibaud 1982), Italy (Mastroiacovo *et al.* 1983), and Spain (Martínez-Frías *et al.* 1989), and in international studies (Bjerkedal *et al.* 1982; Lindhout and Schmidt 1986). Lumbar spina bifida occurs, but not anencephaly. Sodium valproate causes a characteristic dysmorphic syndrome of epicanthic folds, a flat nasal bridge, a broad nasal base, anteverted nostrils, a shallow philtrum, a thin upper lip, and a thick lower lip (Jäger-Roman *et al.* 1986; Winter *et al.* 1987; Chitayat *et al.* 1988). Both preaxial polydactyly (Buntinx 1992) and preaxial limb reduction deformities (Sharony *et al.* 1993; Ylagan and Budorick 1994) have been described in affected infants. Benzodiazepines may amplify the effects of sodium valproate on the fetus (Laegreid *et al.* 1993).

Other anticonvulsant drugs

Primidone (Rudd and Freedom 1979; Myhre and

Williams 1981; Krauss *et al.* 1984) and carbamazepine (Jones *et al.* 1989), in similar fashion, are associated with a dysmorphic facies, and also fingernail hypoplasia and developmental delay. A severe spinal defect occurred in the fetus of a non-epileptic woman who took a large overdose of carbamazepine at around the time of neural tube closure (Little *et al.* 1993). Troxidone (trimethadione) also probably causes facial dysmorphogenesis, as well as central nervous system malformations, growth retardation, cardiac defects, and renal tract anomalies (German *et al.* 1970; Feldman *et al.* 1977).

There is evidence (Hiilsemaa *et al.* 1983; Lindhout *et al.* 1984; Kaneko *et al.* 1988) that the risks of teratogenesis are several times greater in mothers taking a combination of different antiepileptic drugs than in those treated with one agent. In the Japanese series (Kaneko *et al.* 1988), data were collected prospectively on 172 infants born to mothers who did not themselves have congenital anomalies but who received treatment for epilepsy during the first trimester. The malformation rate was two in 31 infants whose mother took a single agent, but 22 in 141 in those whose mothers received two or more antiepileptic drugs. Lower dosages and more frequent use of single agents to control epilepsy may explain the fall in major malformation rate from 24 per cent in a cohort observed during the years 1971–1984 to 9 per cent in a cohort observed in 1982–1989 (Oguni *et al.* 1992). Whenever possible, therefore, epilepsy in pregnant women should be controlled with a single agent. Carbamazepine or phenytoin may be the best initial choice (Oguni *et al.* 1992).

Psychotropic drugs

Benzodiazepines

Evidence that benzodiazepines are teratogenic comes from retrospective studies showing a higher risk of cleft lip and palate (Safra and Oakley 1975; Saxén and Saxén 1975) and from case reports of babies with dysmorphic features and growth retardation (Laegreid *et al.* 1987, 1989). The dysmorphic features resemble those ascribed to anticonvulsants and ethanol. This evidence has been criticized as insufficient to impute malformation to benzodiazepines (Jick 1988), and a case–control study of 611 infants with cleft lip or palate, or both, failed to demonstrate any increased risk (Rosenberg *et al.* 1983). A report on 64 survivors of pregnancies during which the mother took benzodiazepines identified six children with congenital abnormalities, particularly of the central nervous system; the authors considered that alcohol and substance abuse, rather than benzodiazepine exposure, were likely to explain the high rate of abnormalities

(Bergman *et al.* 1992). Any direct effect of benzodiazepines on malformation rate is small (McElhatton 1994).

Benzodiazepines cross the placenta readily and may produce direct pharmacological effects in the fetus and neonate, or give rise to a perinatal withdrawal syndrome, or produce both of these effects. Diazepam equilibrates between the fetal and maternal circulations within 5–10 minutes, achieving concentrations in the fetal circulation equal to or greater than those in maternal blood (Erkkola *et al.* 1973; Mandelli *et al.* 1975; McAllister 1980). A characteristic 'floppy infant syndrome' may therefore be seen, particularly after high or repeated maternal doses. The symptoms include lethargy and hypotonia, respiratory difficulties, thermoregulatory problems, and feeding difficulties (Cree *et al.* 1973; Rowlatt 1978), and the fetal heart rate may also be affected (Scher *et al.* 1972).

The elimination half-lives of diazepam and its metabolite, desmethyldiazepam, are prolonged in the neonate, and these effects may therefore persist for several days (Mandelli *et al.* 1975). While the neonatal effects of diazepam have been most extensively documented, similar effects are seen with chlordiazepoxide (Stirrat *et al.* 1974), lorazepam (Whitelaw *et al.* 1981), and nitrazepam (Speight 1977) and should be anticipated with any agent in this group.

Published work has focused on the adverse effects of benzodiazepines when used as adjuncts to obstetric analgesia, but chronic maternal exposure to anxiolytic or hypnotic doses is likely to produce similar problems. A neonatal withdrawal syndrome may be seen, particularly if the maternal dosage has been high. The symptoms may take up to 2–3 weeks to appear and resemble those of opiate withdrawal; they include irritability, tremor, hypertonia, hyperactivity, tachypnoea, gastrointestinal disturbances, and vigorous sucking. Cases have been reported with diazepam (Rementeria and Bhatt 1977) and chlordiazepoxide (Athinarayanan *et al.* 1976), and similar effects may occur with any benzodiazepine, particularly those with long elimination half-lives and active metabolites.

Haloperidol

Two case reports have suggested that haloperidol may be linked to limb malformation (Dieulangard *et al.* 1966; Kopelman *et al.* 1975), but none of the mothers of 38 infants with severe limb reduction deformities could recall taking haloperidol (Hanson and Oakley 1975), and no further evidence of the association has emerged.

Withdrawal effects are not normally associated with neuroleptic agents, but Sexson and Barak (1989) have reported a case of withdrawal emergent syndrome, a subtype of tardive dyskinesia, in a neonate whose mother had taken haloperidol throughout pregnancy. The infant developed repeated tongue thrust, abnormal hand posturing, and tremor of all extremities. Most symptoms resolved within a few days, but tongue thrusting continued until 6 months of age.

Phenothiazines

Chronic use of phenothiazines as psychotropic agents during pregnancy, particularly at high doses, may cause pharmacological effects in the fetus and neonate, including hypotonia, lethargy, and hyporeflexia (Hammond and Toseland 1970) and paralytic ileus due to anticholinergic activity (Falterman and Richardson 1980). These effects may be prolonged because of slow elimination of phenothiazines by the neonatal liver.

Third-trimester exposure to antipsychotic agents may also produce extrapyramidal effects in the neonate, characterized by agitation, hypertonicity, tremor, poor sucking and swallowing, and unusual movement patterns. This effect has been reported with chlorpromazine and thioridazine (Hill *et al*. 1966; Levy and Wisniewski 1974) and fluphenazine (O'Connor *et al*. 1981). The symptoms may take several months to resolve, but subsequent infant development appears to be satisfactory (Hill *et al*. 1966).

Antidepressants

There is little information on the safety of older antidepressant drugs. Malformation rates may have been increased by monoamine oxidase inhibitors (Heionen *et al*. 1977*b*) and by unspecified antidepressants (Bracken and Holford 1981). More recent data are generally reassuring (Kuller *et al*. 1996; McElhatton *et al*. 1996).

A study of 228 women taking fluoxetine in pregnancy failed to show any increase in the rate of pregnancy loss or major malformations in comparison with a group of 254 women not taking fluoxetine (Chambers *et al*. 1996). Minor abnormalities were significantly commoner in exposed infants in a subgroup of 250 children examined by the investigators, but details of the abnormalities are not given.

Tricyclic antidepressants are slowly eliminated by the neonate, and may cause a range of adverse effects including tachyarrhythmias, irritability, tremor, urinary retention, tachypnoea, and muscle spasms (Shearer *et al*. 1972; Webster 1973; Prentice and Brown 1989). While many of these symptoms represent direct pharmacological effects, for example, anticholinergic-induced tachycardia and urinary retention, it is clear that a neonatal withdrawal syndrome is sometimes seen, especially after chronic high-dose therapy, and particularly with clomipramine (Ben Musa and Smith 1979; Cowe and Lloyd 1982; Østergaard and Pedersen 1982; Singh *et al*. 1990). Neonatal convulsions were a feature of the two cases reported by Cowe and colleagues (1982) and, in one infant, an intravenous infusion of clompramine was needed for the first 17 days of life to control the convulsions.

Lithium

The possible harm to the fetus from lithium has to be set against the serious effects of mania in the mother. An International Register of Lithium Babies was set up in 1968 to record the outcome in pregnancies in the first trimester of which the mother took lithium (Schou *et al*. 1973; Schou 1976). An apparent increase in the incidence of cardiac defects, particularly of Ebstein's anomaly, has been noted (Nora *et al*. 1974; Weinstein and Goldfield 1975). Ebstein's anomaly, which consists of an abnormal tricuspid valve and right-sided heart defect, was found in four of 11 lithium babies with significant heart defects, out of a total of 180 infants; while in the general population the incidence is about five per 100 000 births. This surprisingly high incidence suggests that many patients with Ebstein's anomaly would have been exposed to lithium *in utero*, but the evidence is against this (Warkany 1988; Källén 1988). A prospective study in 148 women observed one case of Ebstein's anomaly, but no significant increase in the overall rate of congenital abnormalities (Jacobson *et al*. 1992). A meta-analysis suggested a rate of congenital abnormalities of 4–12 per cent in mothers taking lithium, compared with 2–4 per cent in controls (Cohen *et al*. 1994).

Use of lithium in pregnancy may produce severe neonatal toxicity; the features include hypotonia, cyanosis, arrhythmias, cardiomegaly, and diabetes insipidus (Mitzrahi *et al*. 1979; Wilson *et al*. 1983; Morrell *et al*. 1983). In many cases the neonatal toxicity is associated with inadequate control of maternal serum lithium concentrations, although fetal toxicity may occur even if maternal levels are in the normal range. The elimination half-life is greatly prolonged in neonates, values of up to 96 hours having been reported (Mackay *et al*. 1976), as against the usual adult value of about 20 hours. The symptoms of neonatal lithium intoxication may therefore take several weeks to resolve, and two cases of diabetes insipidus persisted for more than 2 months (Rane *et al*. 1978; Mitzrahi *et al*. 1979). Neonatal hypothyroidism has also been reported (Karlsson *et al*. 1975). More recently, two cases of maternal polyhydramnios, thought to be secondary to fetal diabetes insipidus, have been reported (Ang *et al*. 1990; Krause *et al*. 1990).

Antineoplastic agents

Cancer during pregnancy is fortunately rare, and when it occurs the risks of treatment to the fetus are usually of secondary importance. However, 'the risk appears to be significantly lower than is commonly appreciated probably because drug doses, frequency of administration and duration of exposure are important variables' (Doll *et al.* 1988, 1989). Pregnant staff who handle antineoplastic agents may also be at increased risk of abnormal pregnancy (Salevan *et al.* 1985).

Alkylating agents

Briggs and others (1994) recorded six malformed infants in 22 cases where the mother was exposed to busulphan. One of the six had renal tract abnormalities, and similar abnormalities have been reported after chlorambucil (Shotton and Monie 1963) and mustine hydrochloride (mecloethamine) (Mennuti *et al.* 1975). A mother given cyclophosphamide with prednisolone for systemic lupus erythematosus gave birth to a baby with multiple abnormalities, including a dysmorphic facies, dystrophic nails, absent thumbs, and ocular malformations (Kirshon *et al.* 1988). One of twins exposed to cyclophosphamide *in utero* was born with oesophageal atresia, deformity of the right arm, and other anomalies. He developed papillary carcinoma of the thyroid at the age of 12 years, and a neuroblastoma when 14 years old. The other twin was normal (Zemlickis *et al.* 1993). The alkylating agents may also increase the risk of spontaneous abortion (Nicholson 1968). Doll and colleagues (1989) report that the risk of fetal malformations after exposure to alkylating agents in the first trimester is 14 per cent, but there may have been inaccuracies in either the numerator (number of malformations) or the denominator (number of patients), which they obtained from case reports. It has also been suggested that use of single agents, as was previously the practice (Sokal and Lessmann 1960), may be less deleterious than the current clinical practice of giving combination chemotherapy (Garber 1989).

Antimetabolites

The folate antagonist aminopterin was at one time given during the first trimester as an abortifacient. When the pregnancy was continued, the fetus was at risk of severe multiple congenital abnormalities, including anencephaly, meningoencephalocoele, skull ossification defect, low-set ears, and abnormalities of the limbs (Goetsch 1962). Similar abnormalities have been seen after treatment with methotrexate, another folate antagonist (Milunsky *et al.* 1968; Powell and Ekert 1971). Babies with aminopterin embryopathy may achieve 'acceptably normal young-adult status' (Shaw and Rees 1980). Women with rheumatoid arthritis or psoriasis are now sometimes treated with low-dose methotrexate; while there is no evidence of an increased risk of malformations, information is sparse, and fertile women should be asked to use effective contraception whilst taking the drug (Feldkamp and Carey 1993; Tariq and Tariq 1993).

Babies with multiple congenital abnormalities have been born to mothers after fluorouracil (Stephens *et al.* 1980), busulphan, mercaptopurine (Diamond and Anderson 1960), and cytarabine (Wagner *et al.* 1980; Schafer 1981) during the first trimester.

The overall risk ascribed to antimetabolites by Doll and co-workers (1989) was 19 per cent, though this is weighted by the inclusion of aminopterin, which is not used as an antineoplastic agent.

Hormones and endocrine drugs

Drugs used to treat diabetes

Mothers with diabetes have a two-to-threefold increased risk of giving birth to infants with congenital malformations, particularly caudal regression (sacral or vertebral agenesis and hypoplasia or agenesis of the femora), renal tract abnormalities, situs inversus, and cardiac anomalies (Mills *et al.* 1979). These malformations depend on embryological events which occur in the first 6 weeks after conception. The high incidence of malformations makes it substantially more difficult to decide whether antidiabetic drugs are themselves teratogenic, and case reports of malformation in infants of mothers taking sulphonylureas (Soler *et al.* 1976) are difficult to evaluate.

Oral hypoglycaemic agents cross the placenta readily, achieving fetal plasma levels in the adult therapeutic range. They can therefore cause severe and prolonged neonatal hypoglycaemia (Zucker and Simon 1968; Kemball *et al.* 1970); in two cases, exchange transfusion was performed to remove the drug. These agents are therefore generally considered to be contraindicated in pregnancy.

Prostaglandins and prostaglandin analogues

Prostaglandins stimulate the contraction of uterine muscle, and are used as abortifacients, occasionally in the first trimester. Should the abortion fail, there is a risk that the baby will be malformed (Collins and Mahoney 1983). The synthetic prostaglandin analogue misoprostil, used in the treatment of peptic ulceration, is abortifacient (see above).

Sex hormones

Oestrogens and progestogens

The synthetic non-steroidal oestrogen diethylstilboestrol (also known as stilboestrol) was at one time given to women during pregnancy as treatment for threatened spontaneous abortion. If exposure occurred before the ninth week of pregnancy, most female fetuses developed the syndrome of vaginal adenosis, in which the vaginal wall contains histologically demonstrable glandular tissue in addition to the usual vaginal squamous epithelium (Ulfelder 1973, 1976; Herbst 1981). There may also be cervical erosions and malformations of the cervix and upper vagina. The relative prevalence of adenosis in a series of 43 exposed and 159 unexposed female stillbirths and neonates was 18 (95 per cent confidence limits 10–32) (Johnson et al. 1979). Clear-cell adenocarcinoma of the vagina or cervix, which is otherwise extremely rare, is associated with exposure to diethylstilboestrol in utero (Herbst et al. 1971). The cancer occurs between 7 and 29 years of age, in approximately one in 1000 women at risk (Herbst 1981; Melnick et al. 1987). A 7-year prospective study of 718 exposed and 710 control women showed a doubling of the incidence of cervical and vaginal dysplasia; but a history of genital herpes was also substantially more common in the women exposed to diethylstilboestrol (Robboy et al. 1984). A study of 186 cases of genital tract clear-cell adenocarcinoma and 1772 controls showed that a history of vaginal blood loss during pregnancy made only a small difference to the risk of cancer after exposure to diethylstilboestrol, making it clear that it is the drug and not the disease which is responsible for the increased incidence of this cancer (Sharp and Cole 1990). Primary infertility was significantly commoner in women whose mothers had received diethylstilboestrol as part of a double-blind controlled trial than in the daughters of unexposed controls, and the prognosis was poorer (Senekjian et al. 1988). The infertility was related to tubal abnormalities in over 40 per cent of the exposed women but none of the unexposed women.

Men whose mothers had taken diethylstilboestrol from the seventh week of pregnancy were three times more likely to have genital malformations than unexposed men (Wilcox et al. 1995). The majority of malformations were epididymal cysts and hypoplastic testes. The men exposed to diethylstilboestrol were just as fertile as their unexposed control subjects.

Effects on sexual differentiation   Diethylstilboestrol exposure can also cause masculinization of a female fetus (Bongiovanni et al. 1959). Female infants may be born with partial masculinization of the external genitalia after first trimester exposure to synthetic progestogens, ethisterone and norethisterone, for example (Wilkins et al. 1958; Wilkins 1960; Voorhess 1967). Such exposure was common when progestogens were administered for threatened abortion, and as a test for pregnancy. Large doses of progestogens can result in labial ('labioscrotal') fusion before week 13 of gestation, but clitoromegaly subsequently (Grumbach et al. 1959; Grumbach and Ducharme 1960). In male embryos, progestogens administered between weeks 3 and 22 may be feminizing, as shown by hypospadias. The position of the meatus has been correlated with the timing of the progestogen administration (Aarskog 1970, 1979; Goldman 1980).

Female pseudohermaphroditism may also result from maternal treatment during the first trimester with danazol, a derivative of 17-α-ethyltestosterone (Duck and Katayama 1981; Rosa 1984), and testosterone (Resseguie et al. 1985).

Other malformations   Low doses of progestogens are widely used in combination with oestrogens in the oral contraceptive pill, and perhaps as many as 3 per cent of users will inadvertently start or continue the pill in the earliest stages of pregnancy (Gardner et al. 1971). None the less, no definite statement can yet be made about their teratogenicity. There have been suggestions of a syndrome of characteristic anomalies after embryonic exposure to female sex steroids, including the oral contraceptive pill. The acronym VACTERL, standing for vertebral, anorectal, cardiac, tracheo-[o]esophageal, renal, and limb defects, summarizes the clinical features (Nora and Nora 1975). A characteristic facial appearance, and other anomalies, has also been suggested to make up EFESSES, the embryo-fetal exogenous sex steroid exposure syndrome (Lorber et al. 1979). Components of VACTERL — the vertebral anomalies, resulting in neural tube defect (Kasan and Andrews 1980), the cardiac anomalies (Heinonen et al. 1977a), and tracheo-oesophageal atresia (Lammer and Cordero 1986) and limb defects (Janerich et al. 1974; McCredie et al. 1983; Kricker et al. 1986) — have been reported in case–control studies, but each of the positive studies identified only one significant association. There have been several negative studies (Goujard and Rumeau-Rouquette 1977; Savolainen et al. 1981; Cuckle and Wald 1982; Harlap et al. 1985; Katz et al. 1985; Resseguie et al. 1985). It seems unlikely that the risk of any major malformation for children born to women taking oral contraceptives in the first trimester differs by more than a few per cent from the risk of unexposed children (Savolainen et al. 1981; Smithells 1981; WHO

1981). The counsel of perfection is to stop the oral contraceptive for three or four cycles before conceiving.

Clomiphene citrate

This synthetic non-steroidal oestrogen, which stimulates the secretion of gonadotrophins by blocking hypothalamic oestrogen receptors, is used in the induction of ovulation. Neural tube defects, particularly anencephaly and spina bifida, may be more common in infants born after ovulation induction with clomiphene, perhaps by a factor of 2 (Cornel et al. 1989; Vollset 1990). Subfertility may itself be a risk factor for neural tube defect, according to James (1973). A case–control study examined 571 women whose fetus or infant had a neural tube defect, 546 women whose offspring had other abnormalities, and 573 women with normal children (Mills et al. 1990). It found that the odds ratio for maternal use of a fertility drug was 1.3 (95 per cent confidence interval 0.4–4.5) in the group with neural tube defects compared with women whose infants had other abnormalities, and 1.1 (0.56–2.0) when compared with the normal group. Only 24 of the 1680 women questioned had, however, been exposed to a fertility drug at the inception of the index pregnancy.

Corticosteroids

Corticosteroids in pharmacological doses do not appear to be teratogenic in man. Glucocorticoids such as cortisone do cause cleft palate in mice, as explained above. There are a few reports of a baby being born with this common defect after maternal corticosteroid ingestion.

One study has reported an increased incidence (13.9 per cent) of low-birthweight infants in mothers who took 10 mg prednisone daily throughout pregnancy (Reinisch et al. 1978). One case of severe intrauterine growth retardation has been associated with topical use of the potent fluorinated steroid triamcinolone from weeks 12–29 of gestation (Katz et al. 1990).

These findings have not been confirmed by other studies, however. Schatz and others (1975) found no increase in neonatal death or other adverse outcomes in a series of 70 pregnancies in which corticosteroids were used for asthma, apart from a slight excess of prematurity. Children treated in utero with corticosteroids to prevent the respiratory distress syndrome have been followed up extensively, with no evidence of adverse effects on growth, on development, or on neurological function (MacArthur et al. 1982; Collaborative Group on Antenatal Steroid Therapy 1984; Smolders et al. 1990).

There have been occasional reports of neonatal pituitary–adrenal suppression, usually mild and transient, associated with maternal corticosteroid therapy (Grajwer et al. 1977; Ohrlander et al. 1977), but this appears not to be a serious or frequent problem. Corticosteroids are immunosuppressant and long-term therapy with these agents is known to increase the risk of infection in adults (see Chapter 25). There is also evidence of an increased incidence of neonatal infections when steroids are used in the antenatal period (Wong and Taeutsch 1978; Kappy et al. 1979; Smolders et al. 1990).

Antithyroid drugs

Aplasia cutis congenita, the localized absence of skin at birth, as an isolated scalp defect, is rare (Kalb and Grossman 1986; van Dijke et al. 1987). It has occurred in the offspring of women treated with methimazole for hyperthyroidism in pregnancy (Milham and Elledge 1972; Kalb and Grossman 1986). Methimazole is the active metabolite of carbimazole. It has also been suggested that methimazole in animal feed is responsible for an increase in the incidence of aplasia cutis in Spain (Martinez-Frias et al. 1992). Two cases of tracheo-oesophageal fistula have been reported after exposure to methimazole throughout pregnancy (Ramirez et al. 1992).

Thyroid hormones do not cross the placenta, while antithyroid drugs do, so regimens in which the maternal thyroid is completely blocked by antithyroid drugs and the mother given thyroxine should not be used (Cooper 1984). Even doses of antithyroid drugs just sufficient to render the mother euthyroid may result in neonatal hypothyroidism (Cheron et al. 1981). While both propylthiouracil (Cheron et al. 1981) and carbimazole (Sugrue and Drury 1980) may depress fetal thyroid function, the risks are minimal if the lowest possible maintenance dose is used (Burrow 1985). Davis and others (1989) reported on 60 infants whose gestation was complicated by overt maternal thyrotoxicosis. Propylthiouracil was given at doses of 300–800 mg daily, well above recommended maintenance doses in pregnancy (Ramsay 1995), with minimal adverse effects. In a study of 43 infants whose mothers had been taking propylthiouracil or methimazole for Graves' disease, 40 per cent had reduced levels of free T_4 in cord blood, but there were no signs or symptoms of hypothyroidism (Momotani et al. 1986). Long-term follow-up of 25 children exposed in utero to carbimazole showed no developmental or endocrine abnormalities at 3–13 years of age (McCarroll et al. 1976).

Prolonged iodine and iodide ingestion during pregnancy may cause neonatal hypothyroidism and congenital goitre which is sometimes sufficiently large to obstruct the trachea at birth and cause death by asphyxiation (Carswell *et al.* 1970; Mehta *et al.* 1983), and there is a possible association with bilateral cataract (Heinonen *et al.* 1977*b*). Povidone–iodine can be detected in neonatal blood after it has been used for perineal preparation prior to vaginal delivery (Bachrach *et al.* 1984). It was associated with hypothyroidism in the neonate when applied to a maternal surgical wound (Jackson and Sutherland 1981). Ramsay (1995) includes iodinated radiographic contrast media and amiodarone in the list of fetal goitrogens.

Radioactive iodine can be expected to cross the placenta and cause irreversible damage to the fetal thyroid, so pregnancy is an absolute contraindication to its use (Fisher *et al.* 1963; Ramsay 1995).

Drugs used in skin disorders

Vitamin A derivatives

High doses of vitamin A taken during pregnancy are associated with craniofacial and central nervous system malformations (Rothman *et al.* 1995). Vitamin A derivatives such as isotretinoin, etretinate, and acitretin are used in the treatment of several skin disorders.

Isotretinoin (13-*cis*-retinoic acid) is a potent teratogen in man, and causes facial dysmorphism with hypertelorism, microphthalmia, misplaced hair whorls and skull sutures, low-set abnormal ears, and complete cleft palate. Central nervous system anomalies, particularly hydrocephalus and agenesis of the cerebellar vermis; and cardiac malformations, including ventricular septal defect, often accompany the facial dysmorphism (Willhite *et al.* 1986). The risk is estimated at 20 per cent (Lammer *et al.* 1985). Interestingly, thymic hypoplasia may occur, perhaps because of a direct effect of the drug on the thymus (Lammer *et al.* 1985; Cohen *et al.* 1987). Etretinate, another vitamin A derivative, is also teratogenic (Hopf and Mathias 1988). Both drugs are very lipid-soluble and have long half-lives. As a result, maternal plasma etretinate and metabolite concentrations may be measurable many months after treatment ceases (Rinck *et al.* 1989). This implies that the teratogenic effects may also persist, and at least one case of embryopathy with craniofacial and dural anomalies has been reported in a baby conceived one year after the cessation of etretinate treatment (Lammer 1988). A review of six neonates and five aborted fetuses with congenital malformations after exposure to etretinate *in utero* supported the view that women should not conceive during and for 2 years after treatment with oral etretinate or its metabolite acitretin (Geiger 1994). Topical retinoids may also be teratogenic (Camera and Pregliasco 1992; Lipson *et al.* 1993).

Non-therapeutic drugs

Alcohol

Ethanol is teratogenic. Lemoine *et al.* (1968) described 127 cases of infants born to alcoholic parents (and particularly to alcoholic mothers) who showed a characteristic facies, considerable growth retardation, psychomotor perturbations, and an increased incidence of congenital malformations. The craniofacial abnormalities comprised mild to moderate microcephaly with short palpebral fissures, maxillary hypoplasia, a short nose, a smooth philtrum and a thin, smooth upper lip (Jones 1988). The picture is sufficiently characteristic to warrant the name 'fetal alcohol syndrome' (Stratton *et al.* 1996).

The mechanism by which ethanol causes fetal damage is not known, though a number of rather incomplete explanations have been proposed (Hoyseth and Jones 1989). Experiments in rats demonstrate that prenatal and early postnatal exposure to ethanol causes neuronal damage that resembles the damage caused by chronic ethanol administration in adult rats. This seems likely to be due either to disruption of the neural membrane lipids, or to changes in neural cell adhesion molecules, which are important in cell migration during embryogenesis.

The dose of ethanol needed to produce damage, and the period of susceptibility, remain undefined in human pregnancy. Most cases have been diagnosed in the offspring of alcoholic mothers. A prospective study of 650 women, most of whom did not drink heavily, showed a relative risk of low birthweight (<2500 g) of 1.46 (P<0.05, confidence intervals not stated) in drinkers (Day *et al.* 1989). In that study, there was a significant correlation between the consumption of ethanol and other 'abnormal substances', including tobacco and marijuana.

A previous study of 32 870 women had failed to find an increased risk for the offspring of women who took one or two drinks a day during the first trimester (Mills and Graubard 1987). The risks of moderate drinking therefore remain undefined.

In Lemoine's description, 15 infants were born to normal mothers but had alcoholic fathers. Little attention seems to have been paid to this observation in subsequent studies.

Cocaine

Cocaine abuse is associated with an increase in intrauterine death, and possibly with an increased risk of urogenital anomalies, especially in those most heavily exposed (Hutchings 1993).

A case–control study in which women were identified as cocaine users by urine screening in an obstetric hospital found that such women were no more likely to have babies with congenital malformations (Miller *et al.* 1995). It is difficult to know whether screening at the time of childbirth detects women whose children were exposed in the first trimester. Although the babies of cocaine-abusers were small, this may have been because their mothers were twice as likely as non-users to smoke (Miller *et al.* 1995).

Narcotic dependency

Narcotic dependency is discussed above with centrally acting analgesics.

Other abused substances

Tobacco usage has been associated with growth retardation and an increased incidence of intrauterine or neonatal death (Russell *et al.* 1966; Butler *et al.* 1972). This seems likely to be due either to vasoconstriction from nicotine (Manning and Feyerabend 1976) or reduced tissue oxygenation as an effect of carbon monoxide (Longo 1970).

Acknowledgement

I am most grateful to Dr Patricia McElhatton, of the National Teratology Information Service, Royal Victoria Infirmary, Newcaste upon Tyne, for her helpful comments.

References

Aarskog, D. (1970). Clinical and cytogenetic studies in hypospadias. *Acta Paediatr. Scand.* (suppl.) 303, 1.

Aarskog, D. (1979). Current concepts in cancer: Maternal progestins as a possible cause of hypospadias. *N. Engl. J. Med.* 300, 75.

Ad Hoc Committee. (1974). Occupational disease among operating-room personnel: a national study. *Anesthesiology* 41, 321.

Agapitos, M., Georgiou-Theodoropoulou, M., Koutselinis, A., *et al.* (1986). Cyclopia and maternal ingestion of salicylates. *Pediatr. Pathol.* 6, 309.

Akhtar, N. and Millac, P. (1987). Epilepsy and pregnancy: A study of 188 pregnancies in 92 patients. *Br. J. Clin. Pract.* 41, 862.

Aldridge, L.M. and Tunstall, M.E. (1986). Nitrous oxide and the fetus. *Br. J. Anaesth.* 58, 1356.

Allen, E.S. and Brown, W.E. (1966). Hepatic toxicity of tetracycline in pregnancy. *Am. J. Obstet. Gynecol.* 95, 12.

Alun-Jones, E. and Williams, J. (1986). Hyponatremia and fluid retention in a neonate associated with maternal naproxen overdosage. *J. Toxicol. Clin. Toxicol.* 24, 257.

American Academy of Pediatrics, Committee on Drugs. (1989). Transfer of drugs and other chemicals into human milk. *Pediatrics* 84, 924.

Andersson, K.-E., Ingemarsson, I., Ulmsten, U., *et al.* (1979). Inhibition of prostaglandin-induced uterine activity by nifedipine. *Br. J. Obstet. Gynaecol.* 86, 175.

Andrew, M., Bhogal, M., and Karpatkin, M. (1981). Factors XI, XII and prekallikrein in sick and healthy premature infants. *N. Engl. J. Med.* 305, 1130.

Andrews, L.G. and Souma, J.A. (1989). Elevated serum alpha-fetoprotein in a pregnant woman with rheumatoid arthritis. *N. Engl. J. Med.* 321, 262.

Ang, M.S., Thorpe, J.A., and Parisi, V.M. (1990). Maternal lithium therapy and polyhydramnios. *Obstet. Gynecol.* 76, 517.

Annegers, J.F., Elveback, I.R., Hauser, W.A., *et al.* (1974). Do anticonvulsants have a teratogenic effect? *Arch. Neurol.* 31, 364.

Arcilla, R.A., Thilenius, O.G., and Ranniger, K. (1969). Congestive heart failure from suspected ductal closure in utero. *J. Pediatr.* 75, 74.

Armitage, P. and Berry, G. (1987). *Statistical Methods in Medical Research*. Blackwell Scientific, Oxford.

Arvela, P., Jouppila, R., Kauppila, A., *et al.* (1983). Placental transfer and hormonal effects of metoclopramide. *Eur. J. Clin. Pharmacol.* 24, 345.

Aselton, P.J. and Jick, H. (1983). Additional follow-up of congenital limb disorders in relation to Bendectin use. *JAMA* 250, 622.

Athinarayanan, P., Pierog, S.H., Nigam, S.K., *et al.* (1976). Chlordiazepoxide withdrawal in the neonate. *Am. J. Obstet. Gynecol.* 124, 212.

Atkinson, H.C., Begg, E.J., and Darlow, B.A. (1988). Drugs in human milk. Clinical pharmacokinetic considerations. *Clin. Pharmacokinet.* 14, 217.

Azad Khan, A.K. and Truelove, S.C. (1979). Placental and mammary transfer of sulphasalazine. *BMJ* ii, 1553.

Bachrach, L.K., Burrow, G.N., and Gare, D.J. (1984). Maternal–fetal absorption of povidone–iodine. *J. Pediatr.* 104, 158.

Bailey, B. and Ito, S. (1997). Breast-feeding and maternal drug use. *Pediatric Clin. N. Am.* 44, 41.

Barr, M. and Burdi, A.R. (1976). Warfarin-associated embryopathy in a 17-week-old abortus. *Teratology* 14, 129.

Barr, M. (1994) . Teratogen update — angiotensin-converting enzyme-inhibitors. *Teratology* 50, 399.

Barr, M. and Cohen, M.M. (1991). ACE inhibitor fetopathy and hypocalvaria — the kidney skull connection. *Teratology* 44, 485.

Barss, V.A. (1989). Diabetes and pregnancy. *Med. Clin. N. Am.* 73, 685.

Beard, R. and Maresh, M. (1989). Diabetes. In *Medical Disorders in Obstetric Practice* (2nd edn) (ed. M. de Swiet), p. 584. Blackwell Scientific, Oxford.

Beck, F. and Lloyd, J.B. (1965). Embryological principles of teratogenesis. In *Embryopathic Activity of Drugs* (ed. J.M. Robson, F.M. Sullivan, and R.L. Smith), p. 1. Churchill, London.

Beckman, D.A. and Brent, R.L. (1986). Mechanism of known environmental teratogens: drugs and chemicals. *Clin. Perinatol.* 13, 649.

Belfrage, P., Boreus, L.U., Hartvig, P., et al. (1981). Neonatal depression after obstetrical analgesia with pethidine. The role of the injection–delivery time interval and the plasma concentrations of pethidine and norpethidine. *Acta Obstet. Gynecol. Scand.* 60, 43.

Belsey, E.M., Rosenblatt, D.B., Lieberman, B.A., et al. (1981). The influence of maternal analgesia on neonatal behaviour. I. Pethidine. *Br. J. Obstet. Gynaecol.* 88, 398.

Ben Musa, A. and Smith, C.S. (1979). Neonatal effects of maternal clomipramine therapy. *Arch. Dis. Child.* 54, 405.

Benawra, R., Mangurten, H.H., and Duffell, D.R. (1980). Cyclopia and other anomalies following maternal ingestion of salicylates. *J. Pediatr.* 96, 1069.

Benigni, A., Gregorini, G., Frusca, T., et al. (1989). Effect of low-dose aspirin on fetal and maternal generation of thromboxane by platelets in women at risk for pregnancy-induced hypertension. *N. Engl. J. Med.* 321, 357.

Bennett, P.N. (ed.) and members of the WHO Working Group (1988). *Drugs and Human Lactation*. Elsevier, Amsterdam.

Bergman, U., Rosa, F.W., Baum, C., et al. (1992). Effects of exposure to benzodiazepine during fetal life. *Lancet* 340, 694.

Berkovitch, M., Pastuszak, A., Gazarian, M., et al. (1994). Safety of the new quinolones in pregnancy. *Obstet. Gynecol.* 84, 535.

Biehl, D.R., Yarnell, R., Wade, J.G., et al. (1983a). The uptake of isoflurane by the foetal lamb in utero: effect on regional blood flow. *Can. Anaesth. Soc. J.* 30, 581.

Biehl, D., Tweed, W.A., and Cote, J. (1983b). Effect of halothane on cardiac output and regional blood flow in the fetal lamb in utero. *Anesth. Analg.* 62, 489.

Binns, W., James, L.F., and Shupe, J.L. (1965). Embryopathic activity of a poisonous range plant, *Veratrum californicum*. In *Embryopathic Activity of Drugs* (ed. J.M. Robson, F.M. Sullivan, and R.L. Smith), p. 105. Churchill, London.

Bjerkedal, T., Czeizel, A., Goujard, J., et al. (1982). Valproic acid and spina bifida. *Lancet* ii, 1096.

Bleyer, W.A. and Breckenridge, R.T. (1970). The effects of prenatal aspirin on newborn haemostasis. *JAMA* 213, 2049.

Bodis, J., Sulyok, E., Ertl, T., et al. (1982). Methyldopa in pregnancy hypertension and the newborn. *Lancet* ii, 498.

Bongiovanni, A.M., Di George, A.M., and Grumbach, M.M. (1959). Masculinization of the female infant associated with estrogenic therapy alone during gestation. *J. Clin. Endocrinol. Metab.* 19, 1004.

Bonnar, J., McNichol, G.P., and Douglas, A.S. (1971). The blood coagulation and fibrinolytic systems in the newborn and mother at birth. *J. Obstet. Gynaecol. Br. Commonwlth* 78, 355.

Borgstedt, A.D. and Rosen, M.G. (1986). Medication during labor correlated with behavior and EEG of the newborn. *AJDC* 115, 21.

Boschi, S., Di Marco, M.G., Pigna, A., et al. (1984). The effect of ranitidine on gastric pH and volume in patients undergoing Cesarean section: possible relationship to Mendelson's syndrome. *Curr. Ther. Res.* 35, 654.

Bracken, M.B. and Berg, A. (1983). Bendectin (Debendox) congenital diaphragmatic hernia. *Lancet* i, 586.

Bracken, M.B. and Holford, T.R. (1981). Exposure to prescribed drugs in pregnancy and association with congenital malformations. *Obstet. Gynecol.* 58, 336.

Brent, R.L. (1983). The Bendectin saga: another American tragedy. *Teratology* 27, 283.

Briggs, G.G., Freeman, R.K., and Yaffe, S.J. (1994). *Drugs in Pregnancy and Lactation* (4th edn). Williams & Wilkins, Baltimore.

Brooks, P.U. and Needs, C.J. (1989). The use of antirheumatic medication during pregnancy and in puerperium. *Rheum. Dis. Clin. N. Am.* 15, 789.

Brosset, P., Roayette, D., Delhoume, B., et al. (1988). Effets métaboliques et cardiovasculaires chez le nouveau-né des bétabloquants pris par la mère. *Presse Med.* 17, 467.

Bryson, T.H.L. (1986). Anaesthesia during pregnancy. *Clin. Anaesth.* 4, 549.

Buehler, B.A., Delimont, D., van Waes, M., et al. (1990). Prenatal prediction of risk of the fetal hydantoin syndrome. *N. Engl. J. Med.* 322, 1567.

Buehler, B.A., Bick, D., and Delimont, D. (1993). Prenatal prediction of risk of the fetal hydantoin syndrome. *N. Engl. J. Med.* 329, 1660.

Bult-Sarley, J. and Lourwood, D.L. (1988). Nifedipine for preterm labor. *Drug Intell. Clin. Pharm.* 22, 330.

Bunde, C.A. and Bowles, D.M. (1963). A technique for controlled survey of case records. *Curr. Ther. Res.* 5, 245.

Buntinx, I.M. (1992). Preaxial polydactyly in the fetal valproate syndrome. *Eur. J. Pediatr.* 151, 919.

Burrow, G.N. (1985). The management of thyrotoxicosis in pregnancy. *N. Engl. J. Med.* 313, 562.

Butcher, R.E. (1978). Halothane — a behavioral teratogen? *Anesthesiology* 49, 308.

Butler, N.R., Goldstein, H., and Ross, E.M. (1972). Cigarette smoking in pregnancy, its influence on birth weight and perinatal mortality. *BMJ* i, 127.

Bylsma-Howell, M., Riggs, K.W., McMorland, G.H., et al. (1983). Placental transport of metoclopramide: Assessment of maternal and neonatal effects. *Can. Anaesth. Soc. J.* 30, 487.

Camera, G. and Pregliasco, P. (1992). Ear malformation in baby born to mother using tretinoin cream. *Lancet* 339, 687.

Cantor, B., Tyler, T., and Nelson, R.M. (1980). Oligohydramnios and transient neonatal anuria. A possible association with the maternal use of prostaglandin synthetase inhibitors. *J. Reprod. Med.* 24, 220.

Carswell, F., Kerr, M.M., and Hutchison, J.H. (1970). Congenital goitre and hypothyroidism produced by ingestion of iodides. *Lancet* i, 1241.

Carter, M.P. and Wilson, F. (1962). Tetracycline and congenital limb abnormalities. *BMJ* iii, 407.

Carter, M.P. and Wilson, F. (1963). Antibiotics and congenital malformations. *Lancet* i, 1267.

Castilla, E.E. and Orioli, I.M. (1994). Teratogenicity of misoprostol — data from the Latin-American collaborative study of congenital malformations (ECLAMC). *Am. J. Med. Genet.* 51, 161.

Chambers, C.D., Johnson, K.A., Dick, L.M., *et al.* (1996). Birth outcomes in pregnant women taking fluoxetine. *N. Engl. J. Med.* 335, 1010.

Chapman, W.S. (1989). Lithium use during pregnancy. *J. Fla Med. Assoc.* 76, 454.

Check, W.A. (1979). CDC study: no evidence for teratogenicity of Bendectin. *JAMA* 242, 2518

Chen, W.W.C., Chan, C.S., Lee, P.K., *et al.* (1982). Pregnancy in patients with prosthetic valves: an experience with 45 pregnancies. *Q. J. Med.* 203, 358.

Cheron, R.G., Kaplan, M.M., Larsen, P.R., *et al.* (1981). Neonatal thyroid function after propylthiouracil therapy for maternal Graves' disease. *N. Engl. J. Med.* 304, 525.

Chitayat, D., Farrell, K., Anderson, L., *et al.* (1988). Congenital abnormalities in two sibs exposed to valproic acid in utero. *Am. J. Med. Genet.* 31, 369.

Chong, M.B., Harvey, D., and de Swiet, M. (1984). Follow-up study of children whose mothers were treated with warfarin during pregnancy. *Br. J. Obstet. Gynaecol.* 91, 1070.

Chouraqui, J.P., Bessard, G., Favier, M., *et al.* (1982). Haemorrhage due to vitamin K deficiency in pregnant women and newborn babies: relationship with rifampicin in 2 cases. *Thérapie* 37, 447.

Christensen, L.A., Rasmussen, S.N., Hansen, S.H., *et al.* (1987). Salazosulfapyridine and metabolites in fetal and maternal body fluids with special reference to 5-aminosalicylic acid. *Acta Obstet. Gynecol. Scand.* 66, 433.

Cipriani, S., Conti, R., and Vella, G. (1983). Ranitidina in gravidanza. *Clin. Europ.* 22, 86.

Cockburn, J., Moar, V.A., Ounsted, M., *et al.* (1982). Final report of study on hypertension during pregnancy: the effects of specific treatment on the growth and development of the children. *Lancet* i, 647.

Cohen, M.M. (1982). An update on the holoprosencephalic disorders. *J. Pediatr.* 101, 865.

Cohen, M., Rubinstein, A., Li, J.K., *et al.* (1987). Thymic hypoplasia associated with isotretinoin embryopathy. *AJDC* 141, 263.

Cohen, L.S., Friedman, J.M., Jefferson, J.W., *et al.* (1994). A reevaluation of risk of in-utero exposure to lithium. *JAMA* 271, 146.

Cohlan, S.Q., Bevelander, G., and Tiamsie, T. (1963). Growth inhibition of prematures receiving tetracyclines. A clinical and laboratory investigation of tetracycline-induced bone fluorescence. *AJDC* 105, 453.

Colie, C.F. (1993). Male mediated teratogenesis. *Reproductive Toxicology* 7, 3.

Collaborative study on antenatal steroid therapy. (1984). Effects of antenatal dexamethasone administration in the infant: long term follow-up. *J. Pediatr.* 104, 259.

Collins, F.S. and Mahoney, M.J. (1983). Hydrocephalus and abnormal digits after failed first-trimester prostaglandin abortion attempt. *J. Pediatr.* 102, 620.

Constantine, G., Beevers, D.G., Reynolds, A.L., *et al.* (1987). Nifedipine as a second line antihypertensive drug in pregnancy. *Br. J. Obstet. Gynecol.* 94, 1136.

Cooper, D.S. (1984). Antithyroid drugs. *N. Engl. J. Med.* 311, 1353.

Corazza, G.R., Gasbarrini, G., Di Nisio, Q., *et al.* (1982). Cimetidine (Tagamet) in peptic ulcer therapy during pregnancy. *Clin. Trials J.* 19, 91.

Corby, D.G. and Schulman, I. (1971). The effects of antenatal drug administration on aggregation of platelets of newborn infants. *J. Pediatr.* 79, 307.

Corcoran, R. and Castles, J.M. (1977). Tetracycline for acne vulgaris and possible teratogenesis. *BMJ* ii, 807.

Cordero, J.F., Oakley, G.P., Greenberg, F., *et al.* (1981). Is Bendectin a teratogen? *JAMA* 245, 2307.

Cornel, M.C., Ten Kate, L.P., and Te Meerman, G.J. (1989). Ovulation induction, in-vitro fertilisation, and neural tube defects. *Lancet* ii, 1530.

Cowe, L. and Lloyd, D.J. (1982). Neonatal convulsions caused by withdrawal from maternal clomipramine. *BMJ* 184, 1837.

Crawford J.S. (1982). Obstetric analgesia and anaesthesia. *Current Reviews in Obstetrics and Gynaecology* No. 1. Churchill Livingstone, Edinburgh.

Crawford, J.S. and Lewis, M. (1986). Nitrous oxide in early human pregnancy. *Anaesthesia* 41, 900.

Craxi, A. and Pagliarello, F. (1980). Possible embryotoxicity of sulfasalazine. *Arch. Intern. Med.* 140, 1674.

Cree, J.E., Mexer, J., and Hailey, D.M. (1973). Diazepam in labour: its metabolism and effect on the clinical condition and thermogenesis of the newborn. *BMJ* iv, 251.

Cuckle, H.S. and Wald, N.J. (1982). Evidence against oral contraceptives as a cause of neural-tube defects. *Br. J. Obstet. Gynaecol.* 89, 547.

Cunniff, C., Jones, K.L., Phillipson, J., *et al.* (1990). Oligohydramnios sequence and renal tubular malformation associated with maternal enalapril use. *Am. J. Obstet. Gynecol.* 162, 187.

Dahlman, T., Lindvall, N., and Hellgren, M. (1990). Osteopenia in pregnancy during long-term heparin treatment: a radiological study post partum. *Br. J. Obstet. Gynaecol.* 97, 221.

Dailey, P.A., Fisher, D.M., Shnider, S.M., *et al.* (1984). Pharmacokinetics, placental transfer, and neonatal effects of vecuronium and pancuronium administered during caesarean section. *Anesthesiology* 60, 569.

Dansky, L.V., Andermann, E., Rosenblatt, D., *et al.* (1987). Anticonvulsants, folate levels, and pregnancy outcome: A prospective study. *Ann. Neurol.* 21, 176.

Davis, L.E., Lucas, M.J., Hankins, G.D., *et al.* (1989). Thyrotoxicosis complicating pregnancy. *Am. J. Obstet. Gynecol.* 160, 63.

Day, N.L., Jasperse, D., Richardson, G., *et al.* (1989). Prenatal exposure to alcohol: effect on infant growth and morphologic characteristics. *Pediatrics* 84, 536.

de St Jorre, J. (1980). New thalidomide-style drug fear. *Observer*, 20th January.

de Swiet, M. (ed.) (1995a). *Medical Disorders in Obstetric Practice* (3rd edn). Blackwell Scientific, Oxford.

de Swiet, M. (ed.) (1995b). Drug dependence. In *Medical Disorders in Obstetric Practice* (3rd edn), p. 600. Blackwell Scientific, Oxford.

de Swiet, M., Dorrington Ward, P., Fidler, J., *et al.* (1983). Prolonged heparin therapy in pregnancy causes bone demineralization. *Br. J. Obstet. Gynaecol.* 90, 1129.

de Wolf, D., de Schepper, J., Verhaaren, H., *et al.* (1988). Hypothyroid goiter and amiodarone. *Acta Paediatr. Scand.* 77, 616.

Demandt, E., Legius, E., Devlieger, H., *et al.* (1990). Prenatal indomethacin toxicity in one member of monozygous twins; a case report. *Eur. J. Obstet. Gynecol. Reprod. Biol.* 35, 267.

Diamond, J. and Anderson, M.M. (1960). Transplacental transmission of busulfan (Myleran) in a mother with leukemia: production of fetal malformation and cytomegaly. *Pediatrics* 25, 85.

Dieulangard, P., Coignet, J., and Vidal, J.C. (1966). A case of ectro-phocomelia, possibly of drug-induced origin. *Soc. Nat. Gynécol. Obstét. Fr.* (Marseille) 18, 85.

Dodson, W.E. (1989). Deleterious effects of drugs on the developing nervous system. *Clin. Perinatol.* 16, 339.

Doll, D.C., Ringenberg, Q.S., and Yarbro, J.W. (1988). Management of cancer during pregnancy. *Arch. Intern. Med.* 148, 2058.

Doll, D.C., Ringenberg, Q.S., and Yarbro, J.W. (1989). Antineoplastic agents and pregnancy. *Sem. Oncol.* 16, 337.

Donald, P.R. and Sellars, S.L. (1981). Streptomycin ototoxicity in the unborn child. *S. Afr. Med. J.* 60, 316.

Drug and Therapeutics Bulletin (1983). Epidural anaesthesia in obstetrics. *Drug Ther. Bull.* 21, 29.

Drug and Therapeutics Bulletin (1987). Use of anticoagulants in pregnancy. *Drug Ther. Bull.* 25, 1.

Drug and Therapeutics Bulletin (1990). Heartburn in pregnancy. *Drug Ther. Bull.* 28, 11.

Duck, S.C. and Katayama, K.P. (1981). Danazol may cause female pseudohermaphroditism. *Fertil. Steril.* 35, 230.

Duff, P. (1997). Antibiotic selection in obstetric patients. *Infect. Dis. Clin. North Am.* 11, 1.

Dukes, M.N.G. (1980). Anthelmintic drugs. In *Meyler's Side Effects of Drugs* (ed. M.N.G. Dukes), p. 538. Excerpta Medica, Amsterdam.

Duminy, P.C. and Burger, P.du T. (1981). Fetal abnormality associated with the use of captopril during pregnancy. *S. Afr. Med. J.* 80, 805.

Duncan, P.G., Pope, W.D.B., Cohen, M.M., *et al.* (1986). Fetal risk of anesthesia and surgery during pregnancy. *Anesthesiology* 64, 790.

Dunn, P.M. (1964). The possible relationship between the maternal administration of sulphamethoxypyridazine and hyperbilirubinaemia in the newborn. *J. Obstet. Gynecol. Br. Commonwlth* 71, 128.

Dunn, P.M., Stewart-Brown, S., and Peel, R. (1979). Metronidazole and the fetal alcohol syndrome. *Lancet* ii, 144.

Edwards, M.S. (1997). Antibacterial therapy in pregnancy and neonates. *Clin. Perinatol.* 24, 251.

Elder, H.A., Santamarina, B.A.G., Smith, S., *et al.* (1971). The natural history of asymptomatic bacteruria during pregnancy: The effect of tetracycline on the clinical course and the outcome of pregnancy. *Am. J. Obstet. Gynecol.* 111, 441.

Erkkola, R., Kangas, L., and Pekkarinen, A. (1973). The transfer of diazepam across the placenta during labour. *Acta Obstet. Gynecol. Scand.* 52, 167.

Esbjörner, E., Jarnerot, G., and Wranne, L. (1987). Sulphasalazine and sulphapyridine serum levels in children to mothers treated with sulphasalazine during pregnancy and lactation. *Acta Paediatr. Scand.* 76, 137.

Eskenazi, B. and Bracken, M.B. (1982). Maternal dicyclomine-doxylamine-pyridoxine use in pregnancy. *Am. J. Obstet. Gynecol.* 144, 919.

Fagan, E.A. (1995). Disorders of the gastrointestinal tract. In *Medical Disorders in Obstetric Practice* (3rd edn) (ed. M. de Swiet), p. 407. Blackwell Scientific, Oxford.

Falterman, C.G. and Richardson, J. (1980). Small left colon syndrome associated with maternal ingestion of psychotropic drugs. *J. Pediatr.* 97, 308.

Fedrick, J. (1973). Epilepsy and pregnancy: a report from the Oxford record linkage study. *BMJ* ii, 442.

Feeney, J.G. (1982). Heartburn in pregnancy. *BMJ* 284, 1138.

Feldkamp, M. and Carey, J. C. (1993). Clinical teratology counseling and consultation case-report — low-dose methotrexate exposure in the early weeks of pregnancy. *Teratology* 47, 533.

Feldkamp, M., Jones, K.L., Ornoy, A., *et al.* (1997). Postmarketing surveillance for angiotensin-converting enzyme inhibitor use during the first trimester of pregnancy — United States, Canada, and Israel, 1987–1995 [Reprinted from *MMWR* (1997), 46, 240–2]. *JAMA* 277, 1193.

Feldman, G.L., Weaver, D.D., and Lovrien, E.W. (1977). The fetal trimethadione syndrome. *AJDC* 131, 1389.

Finster, M. (1976). Toxicity of local anaesthetics in the foetus and the newborn. *Bull. N.Y. Acad. Med.* 52, 222.

Finster, M. (1988). Surgical anaesthesia for pregnant patient. *Can. J. Anaesth.* 35, 514.

Fischer, A.F., Parker, B.R., and Stevenson, D.K. (1988). Nephrolithiasis following *in utero* diuretic exposure: an unusual case. *Pediatrics* 81, 712.

Fishburn, J.J. (1982). Systemic analgesia during labour. *Clin. Perinatol.* 9, 29.

Fisher, U.D., Voorhess, M.C., and Gardner, L.I. (1963). Congenital hypothyroidism in infant following maternal ^{131}I therapy. *J. Pediatr.* 62, 132.

Forman, A., Gandrup, P., Andersson, K.-E., *et al.* (1982). Effects of nifedipine on oxytocin and prostaglandin $F_{2\alpha}$-induced activity in the postpartum uterus. *Am. J. Obstet. Gynecol.* 144, 665.

Foster, C.J. (1994). Amiodarone in pregnancy. *Am. J. Cardiol.* 74, 307.

Gadner, H. (1979). Purpura bei neugeborenen Zwillingen nach Einnahme eines Antihistaminikums durch die Mutter. *Internist Praxis* 19, 542.

Gaily, E., Granström, M-L., Hiilesmaa, V., *et al.* (1989). Minor anomalies in offspring of epileptic mothers. *J. Pediatr.* 112, 520.

Gallery, E.D.M., Saunders, D.M., Hunyer, S.M., *et al.* (1979). Randomized comparison of methyldopa and oxprenolol for treatment of hypertension in pregnancy. *BMJ* i, 1591.

Garber, J.E. (1989). Long-term follow-up of children exposed in utero to antineoplastic agents. *Sem. Oncol.* 16, 437.

Gardner, L.I., Assemany, S.R., and Neu, R.L. (1971). Syndrome of multiple osseous defects with pretibial dimples. *Lancet* ii, 98.

Garland, S.M. and O'Reilly, M.A. (1995). The risks and benefits of antimicrobial therapy in pregnancy. *Drug Safety* 13, 188.

Garrettson, L.K., Procknal, J.A., and Levy, G. (1974). Fetal acquisition and neonatal elimination of a large amount of salicylate. *Clin. Pharmacol. Ther.* 17, 98.

Geiger, J.M., Baudin, M., and Saurat, J.H. (1994) Teratogenic risk with etretinate and acitretin treatment. *Dermatology* 189, 109.

Genot, M.T., Golan, H.P., Porter, P.J., *et al.* (1970). Effect of administration of tetracycline in pregnancy on the primary dentition of the offspring. *J. Oral Med.* 25, 75.

German, J., Ehlers, K.H., Kowal, A., *et al.* (1970). Possible teratogenicity of trimethadione and paramethadione. *Lancet* ii, 261.

Giamsarellou, H., Kolokythas, E., Petrikkos, G., *et al.* (1989). Pharmacokinetics of three newer quinolones in pregnant and lactating women. *Am. J. Med.* 87, 495.

Gibson, G.T., Colley, D.P., McMichael, A.J., *et al.* (1981). Congenital anomalies in relation to the use of doxylamine/dicyclomine and other antenatal factors. *Med. J. Aust.* i, 410.

Gillet, G.B., Watson, J.D., and Langford, R.M. (1984). Ranitidine and single-dose antacid therapy as prophylaxis against acid aspiration syndrome in obstetric practice. *Anaesthesia* 39, 638.

Ginsberg, J.S. and Hirsh, J. (1988). Optimum use of anticoagulants in pregnancy. *Drugs* 36, 505.

Ginsberg, J.S., Kowalchuk, G., Hirsh, J., *et al.* (1989). Heparin therapy during pregnancy. *Arch. Intern. Med.* 149, 2233.

Glade, G., Saccar, C.L., and Pereira, G.R. (1980). Cimetidine in pregnancy; apparent transient liver impairment in the newborn. *AJDC* 134, 87.

Goetsch, C. (1962). An evaluation of aminopterin as an abortifacient. *Am. J. Obstet. Gynecol.* 83, 1474.

Goldberg, J.D. and Golbus, M.S. (1986). The value of case reports in human teratology. *Am. J. Obstet. Gynecol.* 154, 479.

Goldenberg, R.L., Davis, R.O., and R.C. Baker. (1989). Indomethacin-induced oligohydramnios. *Am. J. Obstet. Gynecol.* 160, 1196.

Goldman, A.S. (1980). Critical periods of prenatal toxicological insults. In *Drug and Chemical Risks to the Fetus and Newborn* (ed. R.H. Schwarz and S.J. Yaffe), p. 26. Alan R. Liss, New York.

Gonzalez, C.H., Vargas, F.R., Perez, A.B., *et al.* (1993). Limb deficiency with or without Möbius sequence in 7 Brazilian children associated with misoprostol use in the first trimester of pregnancy. *Am. J. Med. Genet.* 47, 59.

Good, R. and Johnson, G. (1971). The placental transfer of kanamycin during late pregnancy. *Obstet. Gynecol.* 38, 60.

Goujard, J. and Rumeau-Rouquette, C. (1977). First-trimester exposure to progestagen/oestrogen and congenital malformations. *Lancet* i, 482.

Grajwer, L.A., Lilien, L.D., and Pildes, R.S. (1977). Neonatal subclinical adrenal insufficiency. Result of maternal steroid therapy. *JAMA* 238, 1279.

Greaves, M. (1993). Anticoagulants in pregnancy. *Pharmacol. Ther.* 59, 311.

Greene, G.R. (1976). Tetracyclines in pregnancy. *N. Engl. J. Med.* 295, 512.

Grumbach, M.M. and Ducharme, J.R. (1960). The effects of androgens on fetal sexual development: androgen-induced female pseudohermaphroditism. *Fertil. Steril.* 11, 157.

Grumbach, M.M., Ducharme, J.R., and Moloshok, R.E. (1959). On the fetal masculinizing action of certain oral progestins. *J. Clin. Endocrinol. Metab.* 19, 1369.

Guignard, J-P., Burgener, F., and Calame, A. (1981). Persistent anuria in a neonate: a side-effect of captopril? *Int. J. Pediatr. Nephrol.* 2, 133.

Guillozel, N. (1975). The risk of paracervical anesthesia: intoxication and neurological injury of the newborn. *Pediatrics* 55, 533.

Habal, F.M. and Greenberg, G.R. (1987). Safety of oral 5-aminosalicylic acid in inflammatory bowel disease. *Clinical Controversies in Inflammatory Bowel Diseases. An International Symposium.* Bologna, Sept 9–11.

Habib, A. and McCarthy, J.S. (1977). Effects on the neonate of propranolol administered during pregnancy. *J. Pediatr.* 91, 808.

Haddad, J., Messer, J., Casanova, R., *et al.* (1990). Indomethacin and ischemic brain injury in neonates. *J. Pediatr.* 116, 839.

Hall, J.G. (1976). Warfarin and fetal abnormality. *Lancet* i, 1127.

Hall, J.G., Pauli, R.M., and Wilson, K.M. (1980). Maternal and fetal sequelae of anticoagulation during pregnancy. *Am. J. Med.* 68, 122.

Hall, P.F. (1987). Use of promethazine (Phenergan) in labour. *Can. Med. Assoc. J.* 136, 690.

Hammond, J.E. and Toseland, P.A. (1970). Placental transfer of chlorpromazine. *Arch. Dis. Child.* 45, 139.

Hans, S.L. (1989). Developmental consequences of prenatal exposure to methadone. *Ann. N.Y. Acad. Sci.* 562, 195.

Hanson, J.W. (1986). Teratogen update: fetal hydantoin syndrome. *Teratology* 33, 349.

Hanson, J.W. and Oakley, G.P. (1975). Haloperidol and limb deformity. *JAMA* 231, 26.

Hanson, J.W. and Smith, D.W. (1977). Are hydantoins (phenytoins) human teratogens? *J. Pediatr.* 90, 674.

Hanson, J.W., Myrianthopoulos, N.C., Harvey, M.A.S., *et al.* (1976). Risks to the offspring of women treated with hydantoin anticonvulsants, with emphasis on the fetal hydantoin syndrome. *J. Pediatr.* 89, 662.

Haraldsson, A. and Geven, W. (1989). Severe adverse effects of maternal labetalol in a premature infant. *Acta Paediatr. Scand.* 78, 956.

Harlap, S., Shiono, P.H., and Ramcharan, S. (1985). Congenital abnormalities in the offspring of women who used oral and other contraceptives around the time of conception. *Int. J. Fertil.* 30, 39.

Harley, J.D., Farrar, J.F., Gray, J.B., *et al.* (1964). Aromatic drugs and congenital cataracts. *Lancet* i, 472.

Harpey, J-P., Jaudon, M-C., Clavel, J.-P., *et al.* (1983). Cutis laxa and low serum zinc after antenatal exposure to penicillamine. *Lancet* ii, 858.

Hart, C.W. and Naunton, R.F. (1964). The ototoxicity of chloroquine phosphate. *Arch. Otolaryngol.* 80, 407.

Heinonen, O.P., Slone, D., Monson, R.R., *et al.* (1977a). Cardiovascular birth defects and antenatal exposure to female sex hormones. *N. Engl. J. Med.* 296, 67.

Heinonen, O.P., Slone, D., and Shapiro, S. (1977b). *Birth Defects and Drugs in Pregnancy.* Publishing Sciences Group, Acton, Mass.

Hendricks, S.K., Smith, J.R., Moore, D.E., *et al.* (1990). Oligohydramnios associated with prostaglandin synthetase inhibitors in preterm labour. *Br. J. Obstet. Gynaecol.* 97, 312.

Herbst, A.L. (1981). Diethylstilbestrol and other sex hormones during pregnancy. *Obstet. Gynecol.* (suppl.) 58, 35S.

Herbst, A.L., Ulfelder, H., and Poskanzer, D.C. (1971). Adenocarcinoma of the vagina: association of maternal stilboestrol therapy with tumour appearance in young women. *N. Engl. J. Med.* 284, 878.

Hersh, J.H., Podruch, P.E., Rogers, G., *et al.* (1985). Toluene embryopathy. *J. Pediatr.* 106, 922.

Heymann, M.A. (1986). Non-narcotic analgesics. Use in pregnancy and fetal and perinatal effects. *Drugs* 32 (Suppl. 4), 164.

Hickok, D.E., Hollenbach, K.A., Reilley, S.F., *et al.* (1989). The association between decreased amniotic fluid volume and treatment with nonsteroidal anti-inflammatory agents for preterm labor. *Am. J. Obstet. Gynecol.* 160, 1525.

Hiilesmaa, V.K., Teramo, K., Granström, M-L., *et al.* (1983). Serum folate concentrations during pregnancy in women with epilepsy: relation to antiepileptic drug concentrations, number of seizures, and fetal outcome. *BMJ* 287, 577.

Hill, R.M. and Stern, L. (1979). Drugs in pregnancy: effects on the fetus and newborn. *Drugs* 17, 182.

Hill, R.M., Desmond, M.M., and Kay, J.L. (1966). Extrapyramidal dysfunction in an infant of a schizophrenic mother. *J. Pediatr.* 69, 589.

Hirsh, J., Cade, J.F., and O'Sullivan, E.F. (1970). Clinical experience with anticoagulant therapy during pregnancy. *BMJ* i, 270.

Ho, P.C., Stephens, I.D., and Triggs, E.J. (1981). Caesarean section and placental transfer of alcuronium. *Anaesth. Intens. Care* 9, 113.

Hodgkinson, R. and Husain, F.J. (1982). The duration of effect of maternally administered meperidine on neonatal neurobehaviour. *Anesthesiology* 56, 51.

Hodgkinson, R., Glassenberg, R., Joyce, T.H., *et al.* (1983). Comparison of cimetidine (Tagamet) with antacid for safety and effectiveness in reducing gastric acidity before elective Cesarian section. *Anesthesiology* 59, 86.

Holmes, L.B. (1983). Teratogen update: Bendectin. *Teratology* 27, 277.

Holzgreve, W., Carey, J.C., and Hall, B.D. (1976). Warfarin-induced fetal abnormalities. *Lancet* ii, 914.

Hoo, J.J., Hadro, T.A., and Von Behren, P. (1988). Possible teratogenicity of sulfasalazine. *N. Engl. J. Med.* 318, 1128.

Hook, E.B. (1982). Incidence and prevalence as measures of the frequency of birth defects. *Am. J. Epidemiol.* 116, 743.

Hopf, G. and Mathias, B. (1988). Teratogenicity of isotretinoin and etretinate. *Lancet* ii, 1143.

Howell, R., Fidler, J., and Letsky, E. (1983). The risks of antenatal subcutaneous heparin prophylaxis: a controlled trial. *Br. J. Obstet. Gynaecol.* 90, 1124.

Hoyseth, K.S. and Jones, P.J.H. (1989). Ethanol-induced teratogenesis: characterization, mechanisms and diagnostic approaches. *Life Sci.* 44, 643.

Hutchings, D.E. (1993). The puzzle of cocaine's effects following maternal use during pregnancy — are there reconcilable differences? *Neurotoxicol. Teratol.* 15, 281.

Iturbe-Alessio, I., del Carmen Fonseca, M., Mutchinik, O., *et al.* (1986). Risks of anticoagulant therapy in pregnant women with artificial heart valves. *N. Engl. J. Med.* 315, 1390.

Jackson, H.J. and Sutherland, R.M. (1981). Effect of povidone–iodine on neonatal thyroid function. *Lancet* ii, 992.

Jacobson, S.J., Jones, K., Johnson, K., *et al.* (1992). Prospective multicenter study of pregnancy outcome after lithium exposure during first trimester. *Lancet* 339, 530.

Jäger-Roman, E., Deichl, A., Lakob, S., *et al.* (1986). Fetal growth, major malformations, and minor anomalies in infants born to women receiving valproic acid. *J. Pediatr.* 108, 997.

James, F.M. (1987). Anesthesia for nonobstetric surgery during pregnancy. *Clin. Obstet. Gynecol.* 30, 621.

James, W.H. (1973). Anencephaly, ovulation stimulation, subfertility and illegitimacy. *Lancet* ii, 916.

Janerich, D.T., Piper, J.M., and Glebatis, D.M. (1974). Oral contraceptives and congenital limb-reduction defects. *N. Engl. J. Med.* 291, 697.

Jick, H. (1988). Early pregnancy and benzodiazepines. *J. Clin. Psychopharmacol.* 8, 159.

Jick, H., Holmes, L.B., Hunter, J.R., *et al.* (1981). First-trimester drug use and congenital disorders. *JAMA* 246, 343.

Johnson, L.D., Driscoll, S.G., Hertig, A.T., *et al.* (1979). Vaginal adenosis in stillborns and neonates exposed to diethylstilbestrol and steroidal estrogens and progestins. *J. Am. Coll. Obstet. Gynecol.* 53, 671.

Jones, D.G.C., Langman, M.J.S., Lawson, D.H., *et al.* (1985). Post-marketing surveillance of the safety of cimetidine: twelve month morbidity report. *Q. J. Med.* 54, 253.

Jones, H.C. (1973). Intrauterine ototoxicity. *J. Nat. Med. Assoc.* 65, 201.

Jones, K.L. (1988). Fetal alcohol effects. In *Recognisable Patterns of Human Malformation* (4th edn) (ed. K.L. Jones and D.W. Smith), p. 941. W.B. Saunders, Philadelphia.

Jones, K.L., Lacro, R.V., Johnson, X.A., and Adams, J. (1989). Pattern of malformations in the children of women treated with carbamazepine during pregnancy. *N. Engl. J. Med.* 320, 1661.

Jordheim, O. and Hagen, A.G. (1980). Study of ampicillin levels in maternal serum, umbilical cord serum and amniotic fluid following administration of pivampicillin. *Acta Obstet. Scand.* 59, 315.

Juchau, M.R. (1989). Bioactivation in chemical teratogenesis. *Annu. Rev. Pharmacol. Toxicol.* 29, 165.

Kalb, R.E. and Grossman, M.E. (1986). The association of aplasia cutis congenita with therapy of maternal thyroid disease. *Pediatr. Dermatol.* 3, 327.

Kaler, S.G., Patrinos, M.E., Lambert, G.H., *et al.* (1987). Hypertrichosis and congenital anomalies associated with maternal use of minoxidil. *Pediatrics* 79, 434.

Källén, B. (1988). Comments on teratogen update: Lithium. *Teratology* 38, 597.

Kaltenbach, K. and Finnegan, L.P. (1986). Developmental outcome of infants exposed to methadone *in utero:* a longitudinal study. *Pediatr. Res.* 20, 57.

Kaltenbach, K. and Finnegan, L.P. (1987). Perinatal and developmental outcome of infants exposed to methadone *in utero. Neurotoxicol. Teratol.* 9, 311.

Kaltenbach, K.A. and Finnegan, L.P. (1989). Prenatal narcotic exposure: perinatal and developmental effects. *Neurotoxicology* 10, 597.

Kaneko, S., Otani, K., Fukushima, Y., *et al.* (1988). Teratogenicity of antiepileptic drugs: analysis of possible risk factors. *Epilepsia* 29, 459.

Kappy, K.A., Cetrulo, C.L., Knuppel, R.A., *et al.* (1979). Premature rupture of the membranes; a conservative approach. *Am. J. Obstet. Gynecol.* 134, 655.

Kargas, G.A., Kargas, S.A., Bruyere, H.J., *et al.* (1985). Perinatal mortality due to interaction of diphenhydramine and temazepam. *N. Engl. J. Med.* 313, 1417.

Karlsson, K., Lindstedt, G., Lundberg, P.A., *et al.* (1975). Transplacental lithium poisoning: reversible inhibition of foetal thyroid. *Lancet* i, 1295.

Kasan, P.N. and Andrews, J. (1980). Oral contraception and congenital abnormalities. *Br. J. Obstet. Gynaecol.* 87, 545.

Katz, V.L., Thorp, J.M., and Bowes, W.A. (1990). Severe symmetric intrauterine growth retardation associated with the topical use of triamcinolone. *Am. J. Obstet. Gynecol.* 162, 396.

Katz, Z., Lancet, M., Skornik, J., *et al.* (1985). Teratogenicity of progestogens given during the first trimester of pregnancy. *J. Am. Coll. Obstet. Gynecol.* 65, 775.

Kauffman, R.E., Banner, W., Berlin, C.M., *et al.* (1994). The transfer of drugs and other chemicals into human milk. *Pediatrics* 93, 137.

Kauppila, A., Arvela, P., Koivisto, M., *et al.* (1983). Metoclopramide and breast feeding: transfer into milk and the newborn. *Eur. J. Clin. Pharmacol.* 25, 819.

Keller, D.M. (1989). Teratogenic effects of carbamazepine. *N. Engl. J. Med.* 321, 1480.

Kemball, M.L., McIver, C., Milner, R.D.G., *et al.* (1970). Neonatal hypoglycaemia in infants of diabetic mothers given sulphonylurea drugs in pregnancy. *Arch. Dis. Child.* 45, 696.

Kerber, I.J., Warr, O.S., and Richardson, C. (1968). Pregnancy in a patient with a prosthetic mitral valve. *JAMA* 203, 157.

Khoury, M.J., Flanders, W.D., James, L.M., *et al.* (1989). Human teratogens, prenatal mortality, and selection bias. *Am. J. Epidemiol.* 130, 361.

Kirshon, B. (1988). Prolonged maternal indomethacin therapy associated with oligohydramnios. *Br. J. Obstet. Gynaecol.* 95, 956.

Kirshon, B., Wasserstrum, N., Willis, R., *et al.* (1988). Teratogenic effects of first-trimester cyclophosphamide therapy. *Obstet. Gynecol.* 72, 462.

Kivalo, I. and Saarikoski, S. (1976). Placental transfer of ^{14}C-dimethyl-tubocurarine during caesarean section. *Br. J. Anaesth.* 48, 239.

Knott, P.D., Thorpe, S.S., and Lamont, C.A.R. (1989). Congenital renal dysgenesis possibly due to captopril. *Lancet* i, 451.

Knudsen, L.B. (1987). No association between griseofulvin and conjoined twinning. *Lancet* ii, 1097.

Konieczko, K.M., Chapple, J.C., and Nunn, J.F. (1987). Fetotoxic potential of general anaesthesia in relation to pregnancy. *Br. J. Anaesth.* 59, 449.

Kopelman, A.E., McCullar, F.W., and Heggeness, L. (1975). Limb malformations following maternal use of haloperidol. *JAMA* 231, 62.

Koren, G. (1994). *Fetal–Maternal Toxicology* (2nd edn). Marcel Dekker, New York.

Kosake, Y., Takanashi, T., and Mark, L.C. (1969). Intravenous thiobarbiturate anesthesia for caesarean section. *Anesthesiology* 31, 489.

Kotzot, D., Weigl, J., Huk, W., *et al.* (1993). Hydantoin syndrome with holoprosencephaly — a possible rare teratogenic effect. *Teratology* 48, 15.

Krauer, B., Krauer, F., and Hytten, F. (1984). *Drug Prescribing in Pregnancy*, p. 135. Churchill Livingstone, Edinburgh.

Krause, S., Ebbesen, F., and Lange, A.P. (1990). Polyhydramnios with maternal lithium treatment. *Obstet. Gynecol.* 75, 504.

Krauss, C.M., Holmes, L.B., VanLang, Q.N., *et al.* (1984). Four siblings with similar malformations after exposure to phenytoin and primidone. *J. Pediatr.* 105, 750.

Kreft-Jaïs, C., Plouin P-F., and Tchobrovtsky, C. (1988). Angiotensin converting enzyme inhibitors during pregnancy. *Br. J. Obstet. Gynaecol.* 95, 420.

Krejčf, L. and Brettschneider, I. (1983). Congenital cataract due to tetracycline. *Ophthalmol. Paediatr. Genet.* 3, 59.

Kricker, A., Elliott, J.W., Forrest, J.M., *et al.* (1986). Congenital limb reduction deformities and use of oral contraceptives. *Am. J. Obstet. Gynecol.* 155, 1072.

Kuhnert, B.R., Knapp, D.R., Kuhnert, P.M., *et al.* (1979). Maternal, fetal and neonatal metabolism of lidocaine. *Clin. Pharmacol. Ther.* 26, 213.

Kuhnert, B.R., Kuhnert, P.M., Prochaska, A.L., *et al.* (1980). Meperidine disposition in mother, neonate, and nonpregnant females. *Clin. Pharmacol. Ther.* 27, 486.

Kuller, J.A., Katz, V.L., McMahon, M.J., *et al.* (1996). Pharmacological treatment of psychiatric disease in pregnancy and lactation: fetal and neonatal effects. *Obstet. Gynecol.* 87, 789.

Kumar, R.M., Hughes, P.F., and Khurranna, A. (1994). Zidovudine use in pregnancy — a report on 104 cases and the occurrence of birth defects. *J. Acquir. Immune Defic. Syndr.* 7, 1034.

Kumor, K.M., White, R.D., Blake, D.A., *et al.* (1979). Indomethacin as a treatment for premature labor. Neonatal outcome. *Pediatr. Res.* 13, 370.

Kutscher, A.H., Zegarelli, E.V., Tovell, H.M., *et al.* (1966). Discolouration of deciduous teeth induced by administration of tetracycline antepartum. *Am. J. Obstet. Gynecol.* 96, 291.

Laegreid, L., Olegård, R., Wahlström, J., *et al.* (1987). Abnormalities in children exposed to benzodiazepines *in utero*. *Lancet* i, 108.

Laegreid, L., Olegård, R., Wahlström, J., *et al.* (1989). Teratogenic effects of benzodiazepine use during pregnancy. *J. Pediatrics* 114, 126

Laegreid, L., Conradi, N., Hagberg, G., *et al.* (1992). Psychotropic-drug use in pregnancy and perinatal death. *Acta Obstet. Gynecol. Scand.* 71, 451.

Laegreid, L., Kyllerman, M., Hedner, T., *et al.* (1993). Benzodiazepine amplification of valproate teratogenic effects in children of mothers with absence epilepsy. *Neuropediatrics* 24, 88.

Lammer, E.J. (1988). Embryopathy in infants conceived one year after termination of maternal etretinate. *Lancet* ii, 1080.

Lammer, E.J. and Cordero, J.F. (1986). Exogenous sex hormone exposure and the risk for major malformations. *JAMA* 255, 3128.

Lammer, E.J., Chen, D.T., Hoar, R.M., *et al.* (1985). Retinoic acid embryopathy. *N. Engl. J. Med.* 313, 837.

The Lancet (1983a). Postcoital contraception. *Lancet* i, 855.

The Lancet (1983b). Malaria in pregnancy. *Lancet* ii, 84.

The Lancet (1983c). Pyrimethamine combinations in pregnancy. *Lancet* ii, 1005.

The Lancet (1988). Valproate, spina bifida, and birth defect registries. *Lancet* ii, 1404.

The Lancet (1989). Are ACE inhibitors safe in pregnancy? *Lancet* ii, 482.

Laver, M. and Fairley, X.F. (1971). D-Penicillamine treatment in pregnancy. *Lancet* i, 1019.

Leach, F.N. (1990). Management of threadworm infestation during pregnancy. *Arch. Dis. Child.* 65, 399.

LeGras, M.D., Seifert, B., and Casiro, O. (1990). Neonatal nasal obstruction associated with methyldopa treatment during pregnancy. *AJDC* 144, 143.

Leitman, P.S. (1979). Chloramphenicol and the neonate — 1979 view. *Clin. Perinatol.* 6, 151.

Lemoine, P., Harousseau, H., Borteyru, J-P., *et al.* (1968). Les enfants de parents alcoöliques. Anomalies observées. *Ouest-Med.* 21, 476.

Lenz, W. and Knapp, K. (1962). Die Thalidomidembryopathie. *Dtsch. Med. Wochenschr.* 87, 1232.

Levi, S., Liberman, M., Levi, A., *et al.* (1988). Reversible congenital neutropenia associated with maternal sulphasalazine therapy. *Eur. J. Pediatr.* 148, 174.

Levin, D.L., Fixler, D.E., Morriss, F.C., *et al.* (1978). Morphologic analysis of the pulmonary vascular bed in infants exposed in utero to prostaglandin synthetase inhibitors, *J. Pediatr.* 92, 478.

Levin, D.L., Mills, L. J., and Weinberg, A.G. (1979). Hemodynamic, pulmonary vascular and myocardial abnormalities secondary to pharmacologic constriction of the fetal ductus arteriosus: a possible mechanism for persistent pulmonary hypertension and transient tricuspid insufficiency in the newborn infant. *Circulation* 60, 360.

Levy, W. and Wisniewski, K. (1974). Chlorpromazine causing extrapyramidal dysfunction in newborn infant of psychotic mother. *N.Y. State J. Med.* 74, 684

Lewis, H.L., Weingold, A.B., and the Committee on FDA-related Matters, American College of Gastroenterology. (1985). The use of gastrointestinal drugs during pregnancy and lactation. *Am. J. Gastroenterol.* 80, 912.

Linares, A., Zarranz, J.J., Rodriguez-Alarcon, J., *et al.* (1979). Reversible cutis laxa due to maternal D-penicillamine treatment. *Lancet* ii, 43.

Lindhout, D. and Schmidt, D. (1986). *In utero* exposure to valproate and neural tube defects. *Lancet* i, 1392.

Lindhout, D., Hoppener, J.E.A., and Meinardi, H. (1984). Teratogenicity of antiepileptic drug combinations with special emphasis on epoxidation (of carbamazepine). *Epilepsia* 25, 77.

Lindsay, M.K. and Nesheim, S.R. (1997). Human immunodeficiency virus infection in pregnant women and their newborns. *Clin. Perinatol.* 24, 161.

Lip, G.Y., Beevers, M., Churchill, D. *et al.* (1997). Effect of atenolol on birth weight. *Am. J. Cardiol.* 79, 1436.

Lipson, A.H., Collins, F., and Webster, W.S. (1993). Multiple congenital defects associated with maternal use of topical tretinoin. *Lancet* 341, 1352.

Little, B.B., Santosramos, R., Newell, J.F., *et al.* (1993). Megadose carbamazepine during the period of neural-tube closure. *Obstet. Gynecol.* 82, 705.

Longo, L.D. (1970). Carbon monoxide in the pregnant mother and fetus and its exchange across the placenta. *Ann. N.Y. Acad. Sci.* 174, 313.

Lorber, C.A., Cassidy, S.B., and Engel, E. (1979). Is there an embryo-fetal exogenous sex steroid exposure syndrome (EFESSES)? *Fertil. Steril.* 31, 21.

Loughnan, P.M., Gold, H., and Vance, J.C. (1973). Phenytoin teratogenicity in man. *Lancet* i, 70.

Lowe, C.R. (1964). Congenital defects among children born to women under supervision or treatment for pulmonary tuberculosis. *Br. J. Prev. Soc. Med.* 18, 14.

Ludford, J., Dester, B., and Woolpert, S.F. (1973). Effect of isoniazid on reproduction. *Am. Rev. Respir. Dis.* 108, 1170.

Lyle, W.H. (1978). Penicillamine in pregnancy. *Lancet* i, 606.

McAllister, C.B. (1980). Placental transfer and neonatal effects of diazepam when administered to women just before delivery. *Br. J. Anaesth.* 52, 423.

MacArthur, B.A., Howie, R.N., de Zoete, J.A., *et al.* (1982). School progress and cognitive development of six year old children whose mothers were treated antenatally with betamethasone. *Pediatrics* 70, 99.

McAuley, D.M., Moore, J., Dundee, J.W., *et al.* (1984). Oral ranitidine in labour. *Anaesthesia* 39, 433.

McAuley, D.M., Halliday, H.L., Johnston, J.R., *et al.* (1985). Cimetidine in labour: absence of adverse effect on the high-risk fetus. *Br. J. Obstet. Gynaecol.* 92, 350.

McBride, W.G. (1961). Thalidomide and congenital abnormalities. *Lancet* i, 271.

McCarroll, A.M., Hutchinson, M., McAuley, R., *et al.* (1976). Long-term assessment of children exposed in utero to carbimazole. *Arch. Dis. Child.* 51, 532.

McCredie, J., Kricker, A., Elliott, J., *et al.* (1983). Congenital limb defects and the pill. *Lancet* ii, 623.

McCredie, J., Kricker, A., Elliott, J., *et al.* (1984). The innocent bystander. *Med. J. Aust.* 140, 525.

McElhatton, P.R. (1994). The effects of benzodiazepine use during pregnancy and lactation. *Reproductive Toxicology* 8, 461.

McElhatton, P.R., Garbis, H.M., Elefant, E., *et al.* (1996). The outcome of pregnancy in 689 women exposed to therapeutic doses of antidepressants. A collaborative study of the European Network of Teratology Information Services (ENTIS). *Reproductive Toxicology* 10, 285.

McGowan, W.A.W. (1979). Safety of cimetidine in obstetric patients. *J. R. Soc. Med.* 72, 902.

Mackay, A.V.P., Loose, R., and Glen, A.I.M. (1976). Labour on lithium. *BMJ* i, 878.

McKinna, A.J. (1966). Quinine induced hypoplasia of the optic nerve. *Can. J. Ophthalmol.* 1, 261

McKusick, V.A. (1992). *Mendelian Inheritance in Man* (10th edn). Johns Hopkins University Press, Baltimore.

MacMahon, B. (1981). More on Bendectin. *JAMA* 31, 371.

Macpherson, M., Pipkin, F.B., and Rutter, N. (1986). The effect of maternal labetalol on the newborn infant. *Br. J. Obstet. Gynaecol.* 93, 539.

Magee, L.A., Downar, E., Sermer, M., *et al.* (1995). Pregnancy outcome after gestational exposure to amiodarone in Canada. *Am. J. Obstet. Gynecol.* 172, 1307.

Magee, L.A., Schick, B., Donnenfeld, A.E., *et al.* (1996). The safety of calcium-channel blockers in human pregnancy — a prospective, multicenter cohort study. *Am. J. Obstet. Gynecol.* 174, 823.

Manchester, D., Margolis, H.S., and Sheldon, R.E. (1976). Possible association between maternal indomethacin therapy and primary pulmonary hypertension of the newborn. *Am. J. Obstet. Gynecol.* 126, 467.

Mandelli, M., Morselli, P.L., Nordio, S., *et al.* (1975). Placental transfer of diazepam and its disposition in the newborn. *Clin. Pharmacol. Ther.* 17, 564.

Mangurten, H.H. and Benawra, R. (1980). Neonatal codeine withdrawal in infants of nonaddicted mothers. *Pediatrics* 65, 159.

Manning, F.A. and Feyerabend, C. (1976). Cigarette smoking and fetal breathing movements. *Br. J. Obstet. Gynaecol.* 83, 262.

Martínez-Frías, M.L., Rodriguez-Pinilla, E., and Salvador, J. (1989). Valproate and spina bifida. *Lancet* i, 611.

Martinez-Frías, M.L., Cereijo, A., Rodriguez-Pinilla, E., *et al.* (1992). Methimazole in animal feed and congenital aplasia cutis. *Lancet* 339, 742.

Mastroiacovo, P., Bertollini, R., Morandini, S., *et al.* (1983). Maternal epilepsy, valproate exposure, and birth defects. *Lancet* ii, 1499.

Mastroiacovo, P., Bertollini, R., and Licata, D. (1988). Fetal growth in the offspring of epileptic women: results of an Italian multicentric cohort study. *Acta Neurol. Scand.* 78, 110 .

Meadow, S.R. (1970). Congenital abnormalities and anticonvulsant drugs. *Proc. R. Soc. Med.* 63, 48.

Meggs, W.J., Pescovitz, O.H., Metcalfe, D., *et al.* (1984). Progesterone sensitivity as a cause of recurrent anaphylaxis. *N. Engl. J. Med.* 311, 1236.

Mehta, N. and Modi, N. (1989). ACE inhibitors in pregnancy. *Lancet* ii, 96.

Mehta, P.S., Mehta, S.J., and Vorherr, H. (1983). Congenital iodide goiter and hypothyroidism. *Obstet. Gynecol. Surv.* 38, 237.

Melnick, S., Cole, P., Anderson, D., *et al.* (1987). Rates and risks of diethylstilbestrol-related clear-cell adenocarcinoma of the vagina and cervix. *N. Engl. J. Med.* 316, 514.

Mennuti, M.T., Shepard, T.H., and Mellman, W.J. (1975). Fetal renal malformation following treatment of Hodgkin's disease during pregnancy. *Obstet. Gynecol.* 46, 194.

Merlob, P., Litwin, A., and Mor, N. (1990). Possible association between acetazolamide administration during pregnancy and metabolic disorders in the newborn. *Eur. J. Obstet.* 35, 85.

Métneki, J. and Czeizel, A. (1987). Griseofulvin teratology. *Lancet* i, 1042.

Meyer, H.H. and Brenner, P. (1988). Cleft hand and cleft foot malformation as a possible teratogenic side effect of the anthelmintic piperazine? *Internist* 29, 217.

Milham, S. and Elledge, W. (1972). Maternal methimazole and congenital defects in children. *Teratology* 5, 125.

Milkovich, L. and van den Berg, B. (1976). An evaluation of the teratogenicity of certain antinauseant drugs. *Am. J. Obstet. Gynecol.* 125, 244.

Millar, J.H.D. and Nevin, N.C. (1973). Congenital malformations and anticonvulsant drugs. *Lancet* i, 328.

Miller, J.P. (1986). Inflammatory bowel disease in pregnancy: a review. *J. R. Soc. Med.* 79, 221.

Miller, J.M., Boudreaux, M.C., and Regan, F.A. (1995). A case–control study of cocaine use in pregnancy. *Am. J. Obstet. Gynecol.* 172, 180.

Mills, J.L. and Graubard, B.I. (1987). Is moderate drinking during pregnancy associated with an increased risk for malformations? *Pediatrics* 80, 309.

Mills, J.L., Baker, L., and Goldman, A.S. (1979). Malformations in infants of diabetic mothers occur before the seventh gestational week. *Diabetes* 28, 292.

Mills, J.L., Simpson, J.L., Rhoads, G.G., *et al*. (1990). Risk of neural tube defects in relation to maternal fertility and fertility drug use. *Lancet* 336, 103.

Milunsky, A., Graef, J.W., and Gaynor, M.F. (1968). Methotrexate-induced congenital malformations. *J. Pediatr.* 72, 790.

Minkoff, H. and Augenbraun, M. (1997). Antiretroviral therapy for pregnant women. *Am. J. Obstet. Gynecol.* 176, 478.

Minkowitz, S., Soloway, H., Hall, E.J., *et al*. (1964). Fatal hemorrhagic pancreatitis following chlorothiazide administration in pregnancy. *Obstet. Gynecol.* 24, 337.

Mitchell, A.A., Rosenberg, L., Shapiro, S., *et al*. (1981). Birth defects related to Bendectin use in pregnancy. *JAMA* 245, 2311.

Mitzrahi, E.M., Hobbs, J.F., and Goldsmith, D.I. (1979). Nephrogenic diabetes insipidus in transplacental lithium intoxication. *J. Pediatr.* 94, 493.

Mjølnerød O.K., Dommerud, S.A., and Rasmussen, K. (1971). Congenital connective-tissue defect probably due to D-penicillamine treatment in pregnancy. *Lancet* i, 673.

Moise, K.J. Jr, Huhta, J.C., Sharif, D.S., *et al*. (1988*a*). Indomethacin in the treatment of premature labor. Effects on the fetal ductus arteriosus. *N. Engl. J. Med.* 319, 327.

Moise, K.J. Jr, Huhta, J.C., and Mari, G. (1988*b*). Effects of indomethacin on the fetus. *N. Engl. J. Med.* 319, 1485.

Momotani, N., Noh, J., Oyanagi, H., Ishikawa, N., *et al*. (1986). Antithyroid drug therapy for Graves' disease during pregnancy. *N. Engl. J. Med.* 315, 24.

Moore, J., McNabb, T.G., and McGlynn, J.P. (1973). The placental transfer of pentazocine and pethidine *Br. J. Anaesth.* 45, (suppl.) 798.

Morelock, S., Hingson, R., Kayne, H., *et al*. (1982). Bendectin and fetal development. *Am. J. Obstet. Gynecol.* 142, 209.

Morley, D., Woodland, M., and Cuthbertson, W.F.J. (1964). Controlled trial of pyrimethamine in pregnant women in an African village. *BMJ* i, 667.

Morrell, P., Sutherland, G.R., Buamah, P.K., *et al*. (1983). Lithium toxicity in a neonate. *Arch. Dis. Child.* 58, 539.

Mutch, L.M.M., Moar, V.A., Ounsted, M.K., *et al*. (1977*a*). Hypertension during pregnancy, with and without specific hypotensive treatment. *Early Hum. Dev.* 1, 47.

Mutch, L.M.M., Moar, V.A., Ounsted, M.K., *et al*. (1977*b*). Hypertension during pregnancy, with and without specific hypotensive treatment. II The growth and development of the infant in the first year of life. *Early Hum. Dev.* 1, 59.

Myhre, S.A. and Williams, R. (1981). Teratogenic effects associated with maternal primidone therapy. *J. Pediatr.* 99, 160.

Nakane, Y., Okuma, T., Takahashi, R., *et al*. (1980). Multi-institutional study on the teratogenicity and fetal toxicity of antiepileptic drugs: a report of a collaborative study group in Japan. *Epilepsia* 21, 663.

Needs, C.J. and Brooks, P.M. (1985). Antirheumatic medication in pregnancy. *Br. J. Rheumatol.* 24, 282.

Nelson, M.M. and Forfar, J.O. (1971). Associations between drugs administered during pregnancy and congenital abnormalities of the fetus. *BMJ* i, 523.

Nelson-Piercy, C. and de Swiet, M. (1996). Low dose aspirin may be used for prophylaxis. *BMJ* 313, 691.

Newman, N.M. and Dudgeon, G.I. (1977). A survey of congenital abnormalities and drugs in a private practice. *Aust. N.Z. J. Obstet. Gynecol.* 17, 156.

Newman, N.M. and Correy, J.F. (1983). Possible teratogenicity of sulphasalazine. *Med. J. Aust.* i, 528.

Nicholson, H.O. (1968). Cytotoxic drugs in pregnancy. *J. Obstet. Gynaec. Br. Cwlth* 75, 307.

Niebyl, J.R., Blake, D.A., White, R.D., *et al*. (1980). The inhibition of premature labor with indomethacin. *Am. J. Obstet. Gynecol.* 136, 1014.

Nishimura, H. and Tanimura, T. (1976). *Clinical Aspects of the Teratogenicity of Drugs*. Excerpta Medica, Amsterdam.

Niswander, J.D. and Wertelecki, W. (1973). Congenital malformation among offspring of epileptic women. *Lancet* i, 1062.

Nora, A.H. and Nora, J.J. (1975). A syndrome of multiple congenital anomalies associated with teratogenic exposure. *Arch. Environ. Health* 30, 17.

Nora, J.J., Nora, A.H., and Toews, W.H. (1974). Lithium, Ebstein's anomaly, and other congenital heart defects. *Lancet* ii, 594.

Normann, E.K. and Stray-Pedersen, B. (1989). Warfarin-induced fetal diaphragmatic hernia. *Br. J. Obstet. Gynaecol.* 96, 729.

Nosten, F., Terkuile, F., Maelankiri, L., *et al*. (1994). Mefloquine prophylaxis prevents malaria during pregnancy — a double-blind, placebo-controlled study. *J. Infect. Dis.* 169, 595.

Oakley, C.M. (1995). Anticoagulants in pregnancy. *Br. Heart J.* 74, 107.

O'Connor, M., Johnson, G.H., and James, D.I. (1981). Intrauterine effects of phenothiazines. *Med. J. Aust.* i, 416.

Oguni, M., Dansky, L., Andermann, E., *et al*. (1992). Improved pregnancy outcome in epileptic women in the last decade — relationship to maternal anticonvulsant therapy. *Brain and Development* 14, 371.

Ohrlander, S., Gennser, G., Nilsson, K.O., *et al*. (1977). ACTH test to neonates after administration of corticosteroids during gestation. *Obstet. Gynecol.* 49, 691.

Orme, M.L'E. (1985). Debendox saga. *BMJ* 291, 918.

Østensen, M., and Husby, G. (1985). Antirheumatic drug treatment during pregnancy and lactation. *Scand. J. Rheumatology* 14, 1.

Østergaard, G. and Pedersen, S.E. (1982). Neonatal effects of maternal clomipramine treatment. *Pediatrics*, 69, 233.

Ostheimer, G.W., Morrison, J.A., Lavoie, C., *et al*. (1982). The effect of cimetidine on mother, newborn and neonatal neurobehavior. *Anesthesiology* 57, A405 (abstract).

Ostrea, E.M. and Chavez, C.J. (1979). Perinatal problems (excluding neonatal withdrawal) in maternal drug addiction: a study of 830 cases. *J. Pediatr.* 94, 292.

Ounsted, M.K., Moar, V.A., Good, F.J., *et al.* (1980). Hypertension during pregnancy with and without specific treatment; the children at the age of 4 years. *Br. J. Obstet. Gynaecol.* 87, 19.

Ovadia, M. (1988). Effects of indomethacin on the fetus. *N. Engl. J. Med.* 319, 1484.

Ovadia, M., Brito, M., Hoyer, G. L., *et al.* (1994). Human experience with amiodarone in the embryonic period. *Am. J. Cardiol.* 73, 316.

Palahniuk, R.J. and Shnider, S.M. (1974). Maternal and fetal cardiovascular and acid-base changes during halothane and isoflurane anesthesia in the pregnant ewe. *Anesthesiology* 41, 462.

Palomaki, J.F. and Lindheimer, M.D. (1970). Sodium depletion simulating deterioration in a toxemic pregnancy. *N. Engl. J. Med.* 282, 88.

Parkin, D.E. (1974). Probable Benadryl withdrawal manifestations in a newborn infant. *J. Pediatr.* 85, 580.

Pauli, R.M., Lian, J.B., Mosher, D.F., *et al.* (1987). Association of congenital deficiency of multiple vitamin K-dependent coagulation factors and the phenotype of the warfarin embryopathy: clues to the mechanism of teratogenicity of coumarin derivatives. *Am. J. Hum. Genet.* 41, 566.

Pederson, H., Morishima, H.O., and Finster, M. (1978). Uptake and effects of local anaesthetics in mother and foetus. In *International Anesthesiology Clinics* (Vol. 16), *Regional Anesthesia: Advances and Selected Topics*, p. 73. Little, Brown, Boston.

Perkin, R.M., Levin, D.L., and Clark, R. (1980). Serum salicylate levels and right-to-left ductal shunts in newborn infants with persistent pulmonary hypertension. *J. Pediatr.* 96, 721.

Perkins, R.P. (1971). Hydrops fetalis and stillbirth in a male glucose-6-phosphate dehydrogenase-deficient fetus possibly due to maternal ingestion of sulfisoxazole. *Am. J. Obstet. Gynecol.* 111, 379.

Pharoah, P.O.D., Alberman, E., Doyle, P., *et al.* (1977). Outcome of pregnancy among women in anaesthetic practice. *Lancet* i, 34.

Phelan, M.C., Pellock, J.M., and Nance, W.E. (1982). Discordant expression of fetal hydantoin syndrome in heteropaternal dizygotic twins. *N. Engl. J. Med.* 307, 99.

Plouin, P.F., Bréart, G., Maillard, F., *et al.* (1987). Maternal effects and perinatal safety of labetalol in the treatment of hypertension in pregnancy. Comparison with methyldopa in a randomized trial. *Arch. Mal. Coeur* 80, 952.

Porter, P.J., Sweeney, E.A., Golan, H., *et al.* (1965). Controlled study of the effect of prenatal tetracycline on primary dentition. *Antimicrob. Agents Chemother.* 668.

Powell, H.R. and Ekert, H. (1971). Methotrexate-induced congenital malformations. *Med. J. Aust.* ii, 1076.

Prenner, B.M. (1977). Neonatal withdrawal syndrome associated with hydroxyzine hydrochloride. *AJDC* 131, 529.

Prentice, A. and Brown, R. (1989). Fetal tachyarrhythmia and maternal antidepressant treatment. *BMJ* 298, 190.

Pritchard, J.A. and Walley, P.J. (1961). Severe hypokalemia due to prolonged administration of chlorothiazide during pregnancy. *Am. J. Obstet. Gynecol.* 81, 1241.

Pruyn, S.C., Phelan, J.P., and Buchanan, G.C. (1979). Long-term propranolol therapy in pregnancy: maternal and fetal outcome. *Am. J. Obstet. Gynecol.* 135, 485.

Queisser-Luft, A., Eggers, I., Stolz, G., *et al.* (1996). Serial examination of 20 248 newborn fetuses and infants — correlations between drug exposure and major malformations. *Am. J. Med. Genet.* 63, 268.

Ralston, D.H. and Shnider, S.M. (1978). The fetal and neonatal effects of regional anaesthesia in obstetrics. *Anesthesiology* 48, 34.

Ramirez, A., de los Monteros, A.E., Parra, A., *et al.* (1992). Esophageal atresia and tracheoesophageal fistula in 2 infants born to hyperthyroid women receiving methimazole (Tapazol®) during pregnancy. *Am. J. Med. Genet.* 44, 200.

Ramsay, I. (1995). Thyroid disease. In *Medical Disorders in Obstetric Practice* (3rd edn) (ed. M. de Swiet), p. 459. Blackwell, Oxford.

Ramsay, I., Kaur, S., and Krassas, G. (1983). Thyrotoxicosis in pregnancy: results of treatment by antithyroid drugs combined with T_4. *Clin. Endocrinol.* 18, 75.

Rane, A., Tomson, G., and Bjarke, B. (1978). Effects of maternal lithium therapy in a newborn infant. *J. Pediatr.* 93, 296.

RCGP (Royal College of General Practitioners) Oral Contraceptive Study (1976). The outcome of pregnancy in former oral contraceptive users. *Br. J. Obstet. Gynaecol.* 83, 608.

Redman, C. (1995). Hypertension in pregnancy. In *Medical Disorders in Obstetric Practice* (3rd edn) (ed. M. de Swiet), p. 182. Blackwell, Oxford.

Redman, C.W.G. and Ounsted, M.K. (1982). Safety for the child of drug treatment for hypertension in pregnancy. *Lancet* i, 1237.

Reinisch, J.M., Simon, N.G., Carow, W.G., *et al.* (1978). Prenatal exposure to prednisone in humans and animals retards intrauterine growth. *Science* 202, 436.

Rementeria, J.L. and Bhatt, K. (1977). Withdrawal symptoms in neonates from intrauterine exposure to diazepam. *J. Pediatr.* 90, 123.

Resseguie, L.J., Hick, J.F., Bruen, J.A., *et al.* (1985). Congenital malformations among offspring exposed in utero to progestins, Olmsted County, Minnesota, 1936–1974. *Fertil. Steril.* 43, 514.

Reynolds, B., Butters, L., Evans, J., *et al.* (1984). First year of life after the use of atenolol in pregnancy associated hypertension. *Arch. Dis. Child.* 59, 1061.

Richards, M.P.M. (1981). Effect of analgesics and anaesthetics given in childbirth on child development. *Neuropharmacology* 20, 1259.

Riffel, H.D., Nochimson, D.J., Paul, R.H., *et al.* (1973). Effects of meperidine and promethazine during labor. *Obstet. Gynecol.* 42, 738.

Rinck, G., Gollnick, H., and Orfanos, C.E. (1989). Duration of contraception after etretinate. *Lancet* i, 845.

Robboy, S.J., Noller, K.L., O'Brien, P., *et al.* (1984). Increased incidence of cervical and vaginal dysplasia in 3980 diethylstilbestrol-exposed young women. *JAMA* 252, 2979.

Robert, E. and Guibaud, P. (1982). Maternal valproic acid and congenital neural tube defects. *Lancet* ii, 937.

Roberts, J.B. (1870) quoted in Taylor (1934). Does quinine, given a woman while pregnant, have any effect upon the fetus? *Richmond and Louisville Med. J.* 10, 238.

Rodriguez, S.U., Leiken, S.L., and Hiller, M.C. (1974). Neonatal administration of thiazide drugs. *N. Engl. J. Med.* 270, 881.

Rosa, F.W. (1984). Virilization of the female fetus with maternal danazol exposure. *Am. J. Obstet. Gynecol.* 149, 99.

Rosa, F.W., Hernandez, C., and Carlo, W.A. (1987a). Griseofulvin teratology, including two thoracopagus conjoined twins. *Lancet* i, 171.

Rosa, F.W., Idänpään-Heikkilä, J., and Asanti, R. (1987b). Fetal minoxidil exposure. *Pediatrics* 80, 120.

Rosa, F.W., Bosco, L.A., Graham. C.F., *et al.* (1989). Neonatal anuria with maternal angiotensin-converting enzyme inhibition. *Obstet. Gynecol.* 74, 371.

Rosenberg, L., Mitchell, A.A., Parsells, J.L., *et al.* (1983). Lack of relation of oral clefts to diazepam use during pregnancy. *N. Engl. J. Med.* 309, 1282.

Rothberg, A.D. and Lorenz, R. (1984). Can captopril cause fetal and neonatal renal failure? *Lancet* ii, 482.

Rothberg, R.M., Rieger, C.H.L., and Hill, J.H. (1978). Cord and maternal serum meperidine concentrations and clinical status of the infant. *Biol. Neonate* 3, 80.

Rothman, K.J., Fyler, D.C., Goldblatt, A., *et al.* (1979). Exogenous hormones and other drug exposures of children with congenital heart disease. *Am. J. Epidemiol.* 109, 433.

Rothman, K.J., Moore, L.L., Singer, M.R., *et al.* (1995). Teratogenicity of high vitamin-A intake. *N. Engl. J. Med.* 333, 1369.

Roti, E., Robuschi, G., Emanuele, R., *et al.* (1983). Failure of metoclopramide to affect thyrotropin concentration in the term human fetus. *J. Clin. Endocrinol. Metab.* 56, 1071.

Rotter, C.W., Whitaker, J.L., and Yared, J. (1958). The use of intravenous dramamine to shorten the time of labor and potentiate analgesia. *Am. J. Obstet. Gynecol.* 75, 1101.

Rowland, A.S., Baird, D.D., Weinberg, C.R., *et al.* (1992). Reduced fertility among women employed as dental assistants exposed to high levels of nitrous oxide. *N. Engl. J. Med.* 327, 993.

Rowlatt, R.J. (1978). Effect of maternal diazepam on the newborn. *BMJ* i, 985.

Rubin, P.C., Clark, D.M., Sumner, D.J., *et al.* (1983). Placebo-controlled trial of atenolol in treatment of pregnancy-associated hypertension. *Lancet* i, 431.

Rudd, N.L. and Freedom, R.M. (1979). A possible primidone embryopathy. *J. Pediatr.* 94, 835.

Rudolph, A.M. (1981). The effects of nonsteroidal antiinflammatory compounds on fetal circulation and pulmonary function. *Obstet. Gynecol.* 58, 635.

Rumack, C.M., Guggenheim, M.A., Rumack, B.H., *et al.* (1981). Neonatal intracranial hemorrhage and maternal use of aspirin. *Obstet. Gynecol.* 58, 52S.

Russell, C.S., Taylor, R., and Maddison, R.N. (1966). Some effects of smoking in pregnancy. *J. Obstet. Gynecol. Br. Commonwlth* 73, 742.

Sabry, M.A. and Farag, T.I. (1996). Hand anomalies in fetal-hydantoin syndrome — from nail phalangeal hypoplasia to unilateral acheiria. *Am. J. Med. Genet.* 62, 410.

Sackett, D.L. (1979). Bias in analytic research. *J. Chron. Dis.* 32, 51.

Safra, M.J. and Oakley, G.P. (1975). Association between cleft lip with or without cleft palate and prenatal exposure to diazepam. *Lancet* ii, 478.

Sahul, W.L. and Hall, J.G. (1977). Multiple congenital anomalies associated with oral anticoagulants. *Am. J. Obstet. Gynecol.* 127, 191.

Sareli, P., England, M.J., Berk, M.R., *et al.* (1989). Maternal and fetal sequelae of anticoagulation during pregnancy in patients with mechanical heart valve prostheses. *Am. J. Cardiol.* 63, 1462.

Savolainen, E., Saksela, E., and Saxén, L. (1981). Teratogenic hazards of oral contraceptives analyzed in a national malformation register. *Am. J. Obstet. Gynecol.* 140, 521.

Saxén, I. (1975). Epidemiology of cleft lip and palate. *Br. J. Prev. Soc. Med.* 29, 103.

Saxén, I. and Saxén, L. (1975). Association between maternal intake of diazepam and oral clefts. *Lancet* ii, 498.

Scanlon, J.W., Brown, W.V., Weiss, J.B., *et al.* (1974). Neurobehavioural response of newborn infants after maternal epidural anesthesia. *Anesthesiology* 40, 121.

Schafer, A.I. (1981). Teratogenic effects of antileukemic chemotherapy. *Arch. Intern. Med.* 141, 514.

Schardein, J.L. (1993). *Chemically Induced Birth Defects.* (2nd edn). Marcel Dekker, New York.

Schatz, M., Patterson, R., Zeitz, S., *et al.* (1975). Corticosteroid therapy for the pregnant asthmatic patient. *JAMA* 233, 804.

Schellenberg, J.L. (1977). Uterine activity during lumbar epidural analgesia with bupivacaine. *Am. J. Obstet. Gynecol.* 127, 26.

Scher, J., Hailey, D.M., and Beard, R.W. (1972). The effects of diazepam on the foetus. *J. Obstet. Gynecol. Br. Commonwlth* 79, 635.

Schiff, E., Peleg, E., Goldenberg, M., *et al.* (1989). The use of aspirin to prevent pregnancy-induced hypertension and lower the ratio of thromboxane A_2 to prostacyclin in relatively high risk pregnancies. *N. Engl. J. Med.* 321, 351.

Schluter, G. (1989). Ciprofloxacin; toxicologic evaluation of additional safety data. *Am. J. Med.* 87, 375.

Schou, M. (1976). What happened later to the lithium babies? A follow-up study of children born without malformations. *Acta Psychiatr. Scand.* 54, 193.

Schou, M., Goldfield, M.D., Weinstein, M.R., *et al.* (1973). Lithium and pregnancy — I. Report from the register of lithium babies. *BMJ* ii, 135.

Schubiger, G., Flury, G., and Nussberger, J. (1988). Enalapril for pregnancy-induced hypertension: acute renal failure in a neonate. *Ann. Intern. Med.* 108, 215.

Scott, A.A. and Purohit, D.M. (1989). Neonatal renal failure: a complication of maternal antihypertensive therapy. *Am. J. Obstet. Gynecol.* 160, 1223.

Selevan, S.G., Lindbohm, M-L., Hornung, R.W. *et al.* (1985). A study of occupational exposure to antineoplastic drugs and fetal outcome in nurses. *N. Engl. J. Med.* 313, 1173.

Senekjian, E.K., Potkul, R.K., Frey, K., *et al.* (1988). Infertility among daughters either exposed or not exposed to diethylstilbestrol. *Am. J. Obstet. Gynecol.* 158, 493.

Sexson, W.R. and Barak, Y. (1989). Withdrawal emergent syndrome in an infant associated with maternal haloperidol therapy. *J. Perinatol.* 9, 170.

Shapiro, S., Hartz, S.C., Siskind, V., *et al.* (1976). Anticonvulsants and parental epilepsy in the development of birth defects. *Lancet* i, 272.

Shapiro, S., Heinonen, O.P., Siskind, V., *et al.* (1977). Antenatal exposure to doxylamine succinate and dicyclomine hydrochloride (Bendectin) in relation to congenital malformation, perinatal mortality rate, birth weight and intelligence quotient score. *Am. J. Obstet. Gynecol.* 128, 480.

Sharony, R., Garber, A., Viskochil, D., *et al.* (1993). Preaxial ray reduction defects as part of valproic acid embryofetopathy. *Prenat. Diagn.* 13, 909.

Sharp, G.B. and Cole, P. (1990). Vaginal bleeding and diethylstilbestrol exposure during pregnancy: relationship to genital tract clear cell adenocarcinoma and vaginal adenosis in daughters. *Am. J. Obstet. Gynecol.* 162, 994.

Shaw, E.B. and Rees, E.L. (1980). Fetal damage due to aminopterin ingestion. *AJDC* 134, 1172.

Shearer, W.T., Schreiner, R.L., and Marshall, R.E. (1972). Urinary retention in a neonate secondary to maternal ingestion of nortriptyline. *J. Pediatr.* 81, 570.

Sherman, S. and Hall, B.D. (1976). Warfarin and foetal abnormality. *Lancet* i, 692.

Shimohira, M., Kohyama, J., Kawano, Y., *et al.* (1986). Effect of alpha-methyldopa administration during pregnancy on the development of a child's sleep. *Brain Dev.* 8, 416.

Shiono, P.H. and Klebanoff, M.A. (1989). Bendectin and human congenital malformations. *Teratology* 40, 151.

Shotan, A., Widerhorn, J., Hurst, A., *et al.* (1994). Risks of angiotensin-converting enzyme inhibition during pregnancy — experimental and clinical evidence, potential mechanisms, and recommendations for use. *Am. J. Med.* 96, 451.

Shotton, D. and Monie, I.W. (1963). Possible teratogenic effect of chlorambucil on a human fetus. *JAMA* 186, 74.

Simeoni, U., Messer, J., Weisburd, P., *et al.* (1989). Neonatal renal dysfunction and intrauterine exposure to prostaglandin synthesis inhibitors. *Eur. J. Pediatr.* 148, 371.

Singh, S., Gulati, S., Narang, A., *et al.* (1990). Non-narcotic withdrawal syndrome in a neonate due to maternal clomipramine therapy. *J. Paediatr. Child Health* 26, 110.

Slone, D., Heinonen, O.P., Kaufman, D.W., *et al.* (1976). Aspirin and congenital malformations. *Lancet* i, 1373.

Smith, A.M. (1989). Are ACE inhibitors safe in pregnancy? *Lancet* ii, 750.

Smithells, R.W. (1981). Oral contraceptives and birth defects. *Dev. Med. Child Neurol.* 23, 369.

Smithells, R.W. and Sheppard, S. (1983). Teratogenicity of Debendox and pyrimethamine. *Lancet* ii, 623.

Smolders, de H.H., Neuvel, J., Schmand, B., *et al.* (1990). Physical development and medical history of children who were treated antenatally with corticosteroids to prevent respiratory distress syndrome: a 10- to 12-year follow-up. *Pediatrics* 86, 65.

Snider, D.E., Layde, P.M., Johnson, M.W., *et al.* (1980). Treatment of tuberculosis during pregnancy. *Am. Rev. Respir. Dis.* 122, 65.

Sokal, J.E. and Lessmann, E.M. (1960). Effects of cancer chemotherapeutic agents on the human fetus. *JAMA* 172, 1765.

Soler, N.G., Walsh, C.H., and Malins, J.M. (1976). Congenital malformations in infants of diabetic mothers. *Q. J. Med.* 45, 303.

Solomon, L., Abrams, G., Dinner, M., *et al.* (1977). Neonatal abnormalities associated with D-penicillamine treatment during pregnancy. *N. Engl. J. Med.* 296, 54.

Speidel, B.D. and Meadow, S.R. (1972). Maternal epilepsy and abnormalities of the fetus and newborn. *Lancet* ii, 839.

Speight, A.N.P. (1977). Floppy-infant syndrome and maternal diazepam and/or nitrazepam. *Lancet* ii, 878.

Steen, J.S.M. and Stainton-Ellis, D.M. (1977). Rifampicin in pregnancy. *Lancet* ii, 604.

Steketee, R.W., Wirima, J.J., Hightower, A.W., *et al.* (1996). The effect of malaria and malaria prevention in pregnancy on offspring birth-weight, prematurity, and intrauterine growth retardation in rural Malawi. *Am. J. Trop. Med. Hyg.* 55, 33.

Stephens, J.D., Globus, M.S., Miller, T.R., *et al.*. (1980). Multiple congenital anomalies in a fetus exposed to 5-fluorouracil during the first trimester. *Am. J. Obstet. Gynecol.* 137, 747.

Stephens, T.D. (1988). Proposed mechanisms of action in thalidomide embryopathy. *Teratology* 38, 229.

Stirrat, G.M., Edington, P.T., and Berry, D.J. (1974). Transplacental passage of chlordiazepoxide. *BMJ* ii, 729.

Stratton, K., Howe, C., and Battaglia, F. (eds.) (1996). *Fetal Alcohol Syndrome*. National Academic Press, Washington D.C.

Strauss, M.E., Lessen-Firestone, J.K., Chavez, C.J., *et al.* (1979). Children of methadone treated women at five years of age. *Pharmacol. Biochem. Behav.* (suppl.) 11, 3.

Strickler, S.M., Miller, M.A., Andermann, E., *et al.* (1985). Genetic predisposition to phenytoin-induced birth defects. *Lancet* ii, 746.

Stuart, M.J., Gross, S.J., Eldrad, H., *et al.* (1982). Effects of acetylsalicylic acid ingestion on maternal and neonatal haemostasis. *N. Engl. J. Med.* 307, 909 .

Sturridge, F., Deswiet, H., and Letsky, E. (1994). The use of low-molecular-weight heparin for thromboprophylaxis in pregnancy. *Br. J. Obstet. Gynaecol.* 101, 69.

Sugrue, D. and Drury, M.I. (1980). Hyperthyroidism complicating pregnancy: results of treatment by antithyroid drugs in 77 pregnancies. *Br. J. Obstet. Gynaecol.* 87, 970.

Sulik, K.R., Cook, C.S., and Webster, W.S. (1988). Teratogens and craniofacial malformations: relationships to cell death. *Development* 103 (suppl.), 213.

Tack, E.D. and Perlman, J.M. (1988). Renal failure in sick, hypertensive premature infants receiving captopril therapy. *J. Pediatr.* 112, 805.

Tariq, S. and Tariq, S.M. (1993). Methotrexate in rheumatoid arthritis — can current knowledge and experience justify its use as a first-line disease-modifying agent? *Postgrad. Med. J.* 69, 775.

Taylor, H.M. (1934). Prenatal medication as a possible etiologic factor of deafness in the newborn. *Arch. Otolaryngol.* 20, 790.

Teelmann, K. (1988). Retinoids: toxicology and teratogenicity to date. *Pharmacol. Ther.* 40, 29.

Truter, P.J., Franszen, S., van der Merwe, J.V., *et al.* (1986). Premature closure of the ductus arteriosus causing intrauterine death. *S. Afr. Med. J.* 70, 557.

Tubman, R., Jenkins, J., and Lim, J. (1988). Neonatal hyperthyroxinaemia associated with maternal amiodarone therapy: case report. *Ir. J. Med. Sci.* 157, 243.

Tunstall, M.E. (1969). The effect of propranolol on breathing at birth. *Br. J. Anaesth.* 41, 792.

Tyl, R.W. (1988). Developmental toxicity in toxicologic research and testing. In *Perspectives in Basic and Applied Toxicology* (ed. B. Ballantyne), p. 206. Wright, Bristol.

Ulfelder, H. (1973). Stilboestrol, adenosis, adenocarcinoma. *Am. J. Obstet. Gynecol.* 117, 794.

Ulfelder, H. (1976). DES — Transplacental teratogen — and possibly also carcinogen. *Teratology* 13, 101.

Ulmsten, U., Anderson, K.E., and Forman, A. (1978). Relaxing effects of nifedipine on the non-pregnant uterus in vitro and in vivo. *Obstet. Gynecol.* 52, 436.

van Dijke, C.P., Heydendael, R.J., and de Kleine, M.J. (1987). Methimazole, carbimazole, and congenital skin defects. *Ann. Intern. Med.* 106, 60.

van der Heijden, A.J., Provoost, A.P., Nauta, J., *et al.* (1988). Renal function impairment in preterm neonates related to intrauterine indomethacin exposure. *Pediatr. Res.* 24, 644.

van Leeuwen, G., Guthrie, R., and Stange, F. (1965). Narcotic withdrawal reaction in a newborn infant due to codeine. *Pediatrics* 36, 635.

Vella, L., Francis, D., Houlton, P., *et al.* (1985). Comparison of the antiemetics metoclopramide and promethazine in labour. *BMJ* 290, 1173.

Vessey, M.P. and Nunn, J. F. (1980). Occupational hazards of anaesthesia. *BMJ* 281, 696.

Villasanta, V. (1965). Thromboembolic disease in pregnancy. *Am. J. Obstet. Gynecol.* 93, 142.

Vollset, S.E. (1990). Ovulation induction defects. *Lancet* 335, 178.

Voorhess, M.L. (1967). Masculinization of the female fetus associated with norethindrone-mestranol therapy during pregnancy. *J. Pediatr.* 71, 128.

Wagner, V.M., Hill, J.S., Weaver, D., *et al.* (1980). Congenital abnormalities in baby born to cytarabine treated mother. *Lancet* ii, 98.

Warkany, J. (1976). Warfarin embryopathy. *Teratology* 14, 205.

Warkany, J. (1988). Teratogen update: lithium. *Teratology* 38, 593.

Waters, C.H., Belai, Y., Gott, P. S., *et al.* (1994). Outcomes of pregnancy associated with antiepileptic drugs. *Arch. Neurol.* 51, 250.

Watson, G.I. (1962). Meclozine ('Ancoloxin') and foetal abnormalities. *BMJ* iv, 1446.

Watt, L.O. (1961). Oxytocic effect of dimenhydrinate in obstetrics. *Can. Med. Assoc. J.* 84, 533.

Webster, P.A.C. (1973). Withdrawal symptoms in neonates associated with maternal antidepressant therapy. *Lancet* ii, 318.

Webster, W.S., Lipson, A.H., and Sulik, K.K. (1988). Interference with gastrulation during the third week of pregnancy as a cause of some facial abnormalities and CNS defects. *Am. J. Med. Genet.* 31, 505.

Weinstein, L. and Dalton, A.C. (1968). Host determinants of response to antimicrobial agents (continued). *N. Engl. J. Med.* 279, 524.

Weinstein, M.R. and Goldfield, M.D. (1975). Cardiovascular malformations with lithium use during pregnancy. *Am. J. Psychiatry* 132, 529.

Wells, P.G. and Winn, L.M. (1996). Biochemical toxicology of chemical teratogenesis. *Crit. Rev. Biochem. Mol. Biol.* 31, 1.

Werler, M.M., Mitchell, A.A., and Shapiro, S. (1989). The relation of aspirin use during the first trimester of pregnancy to congenital cardiac defects. *N. Engl. J. Med.* 321, 1639.

Weyman, J. (1965). Tetracyclines and the teeth. *Practitioner* 195, 661.

Whalley, P.J., Adams, R.H., and Combs, B. (1964). Tetracycline toxicity in pregnancy. *JAMA* 189, 357.

Whaun, J.M., Smith, G.R., and Sochor, V.A. (1980). Effect of prenatal drug administration on maternal and neonatal platelet aggregation and PF-4 release. *Haemostasis* 9, 226.

White, A., Andrews, E., Eldridge, R., *et al.* (1994). Birth outcomes following zidovudine therapy in pregnant women [reprinted from *MMWR* (1994) 43, 409]. *JAMA* 272, 17.

Whitelaw, A. (1981). Maternal methyldopa treatment and neonatal blood pressure. *BMJ* 283, 471.

Whitelaw, A.G.L., Gummings, A.J., and McFadyen, I.R. (1981). Effects of maternal lorazepam on the neonate. *BMJ* 282, 1106.

W.H.O. Scientific Group. (1981). *The Effect of Female Sex Hormones on Fetal Development and Infant Health.* WHO, Geneva.

Wiggins, D.A. and Elliott, J.P. (1990). Oligohydramnios in each sac of a triplet gestation caused by Motrin — fulfilling Koch's postulates. *Am. J. Obstet. Gynecol.* 162, 460.

Wilcox, A.J., Baird, D.D., Weinberg, C.R., *et al.* (1995). Fertility in men exposed prenatally to diethylstilboestrol. *N. Engl. J. Med.* 332, 1411.

Wilkins, L. (1960). Masculinization of female fetus due to use of orally given progestins. *JAMA* 172, 1028.

Wilkins, L., Jones, H.W., Holman, G.H., *et al.* (1958). Masculinization of the female fetus associated with administration of oral and intramuscular progestins during gestation: non-adrenal female pseudohermaphrodism. *J. Clin. Endocrinol. Metab.* 18, 559.

Wilkinson, A.R. (1980). Naproxen levels in preterm infants after maternal treatment. *Lancet* ii, 591.

Wilkinson, A.R., Aynsley-Green, A., and Mitchell, M.D. (1979). Persistent pulmonary hypertension and abnormal prostaglandin E levels in preterm infants after maternal treatment with naproxen. *Arch. Dis. Child.* 54, 942.

Willhite, C.C., Hill, R.M., and Irving, D.W. (1986). Isotretinoin-induced craniofacial malformations in humans and hamsters. *J. Craniofac. Genet. Dev. Biol.* (Suppl.) 2, 193.

Willis, R.A. (1962). *The Borderland of Embryology and Pathology* (2nd edn). Butterworths, London.

Wilson, J.G. (1977). Current status of teratology. In *Handbook of Teratology* (ed. J.G. Wilson and F.C. Fraser), p. 47. Plenum Press, New York.

Wilson, N., Forfar, J.C., and Godman, M.J. (1983). Atrial flutter in the newborn resulting from maternal lithium ingestion. *Arch. Dis. Child.* 58, 538.

Winter, R.M., Donnai, D., Burn, J., *et al.* (1987). Fetal valproate syndrome: is there a recognisable phenotype? *J. Med. Genet.* 24, 692.

Wolfe, M.S. and Cordero, J.F. (1985). Safety of chloroquine in chemosuppression of malaria during pregnancy. *BMJ* 290, 1466.

Wong, Y.L. and Taeutsch, H.W. (1978). White blood cell changes and incidence of fever after maternal treatment with glucocorticoids: *Pediatr. Res.* 12, 501.

Woods, D.L. and Morrell, D.F. (1982). Atenolol: side effects in a newborn infant. *BMJ* 285, 691.

Yaffe, S.J. and Stern, L. (1976). Clinical implications of perinatal pharmacology. In *Perinatal Pharmacology and Therapeutics* (ed. B.L. Mirkin), p. 355. Academic Press, New York.

Yakovlev, P.I. (1959). Pathoarchitectonic studies of cerebral malformations. *J. Neuropath. Exp. Neurol.* 18, 22.

Ylagan, L.R. and Budorick, N.E. (1994). Radial ray aplasia in utero — a prenatal finding associated with valproic acid exposure. *J. Ultrasound Med.* 13, 408.

Zagorzycki, M.T. and Brinkman, C.R. III (1982). The effect of general and epidural anesthesia upon neonatal Apgar scores in repeat caesarean section. *Surg. Gynecol. Obstet.* 155, 641.

Zemlickis, D., Lishner, M., Degendorfer, P., *et al.* (1992). Fetal outcome after *in utero* exposure to cancer chemotherapy. *Arch. Intern. Med.* 152, 573.

Zemlickis, D., Lishner, M., Erlich, R., *et al.* (1993). Teratogenicity and carcinogenicity in a twin exposed *in utero* to cyclophosphamide. *Teratogenesis Carcinog. Mutagen.* 13, 139.

Zhu, M-X. and Zhou, S-S. (1989). Reduction of the teratogenic effects of phenytoin by folic acid and a mixture of folic acid, vitamins, and amino acids. *Epilepsia* 30, 246.

Zierler, S. and Rothman, K.J. (1985). Congenital heart disease in relation to maternal use of bendectin and other drugs in early pregnancy. *N. Engl. J. Med.* 313, 347.

Zucker, P. and Simon, G. (1968). Prolonged symptomatic neonatal hypoglycaemia associated with maternal chlorpropamide therapy. *Pediatrics* 42, 824.

8. Cardiac disorders

M. T. KEARNEY, D. J. WRIGHT, and L-B. TAN

Introduction

It is an important truism that cardioactive drugs are used in patients with heart disease. Most adverse drug effects reflect both the properties of the drug concerned and the underlying disease state of the patient. Adverse reactions are frequently predictable on the basis of a drug's known pharmacological actions (Type A adverse reactions — see Chapter 5).

Sometimes it is the disease state which renders the patient susceptible to drug actions that might, in other circumstances, be therapeutic. Furthermore, actions that may be therapeutic in one disease state may be deleterious in another. Thus, drugs with negative inotropic effects may be beneficial in the treatment of ischaemic heart disease, but harmful in patients with reduced cardiac function. Similarly, antiarrhythmic drug therapy may be of value in patients with an established arrhythmia, but arrhythmogenic in others.

Adverse drug reactions on the heart are not confined to drugs primarily used in heart disease. Numerous agents used in the treatment of non-cardiac disorders may exhibit significant cardiotoxicity. For example, in the case of bronchodilator therapy, sympathomimetic effects may cause adverse cardiac effects, while neuroleptic medications may have Class I antiarrhythmic effects responsible for proarrhythmic adverse effects.

There are a myriad of case reports of adverse drug reactions involving the heart. In this chapter we have sought to emphasize the principles and mechanisms underlying these adverse effects, rather than to present an exhaustive catalogue of individual adverse reactions.

Drugs causing tachyarrhythmias

Antiarrhythmic drugs

Antiarrhythmic drug therapy is a two-edged sword, which can cause arrhythmias as well as prevent them. Proarrhythmia (arrhythmogenicity) indicates the capacity of a drug to aggravate an existing arrhythmia, or to provoke a new one, at therapeutic or subtherapeutic concentrations (Zerin and Somberg 1994). Although this definition excludes arrhythmias induced by drug toxicity, we shall discuss some common problems such digoxin toxicity. The proarrhythmic actions of antiarrhythmic drugs are amongst the most serious adverse drug reactions, and may result in life-threatening arrhythmias or death (Ruskin et al. 1983; Cardiac Arrhythmia Suppression Trial Investigators 1989). They arise from a drug's primary pharmacological action. They are, therefore, Type A adverse reactions, though with antiarrhythmic drug therapy an equivalent electrophysiological effect may have an antiarrhythmic action in one patient while having a proarrhythmic action in another.

In view of these different actions, the normal concepts of therapeutic and toxic ranges do not apply. Antiarrhythmic drug therapy is a prescribed risk. With judicious patient selection, the benefits of treatment can outweigh this, but with inadequate patient selection, the converse may apply and risks may exceed benefits. It is, therefore, of particular importance that physicians who prescribe these drugs should be aware of the serious adverse reactions that may arise and of the factors within an individual that may predispose him to increased risk.

Arrhythmogenicity was first described by Selzer and Wray in 1964 when they described quinidine syncope due to ventricular fibrillation occurring during the treatment of chronic atrial fibrillation. Since then a whole array of cardiac and non-cardiac drugs have been implicated in proarrhythmia, and since 1989 numerous studies, notably the Cardiac Arrhythmia Suppression Trial (CAST [Echt et al. 1991]),have more clearly delineated the risks of antiarrhythmic therapy.

Types of arrhythmogenesis

At the simplest level arrhythmogenesis can be divided into two categories, clinical and technical (Campbell 1987). Clinical arrhythmogenesis comprises all pro-arrhythmic effects that are of clinical significance. This includes worsening of an existing arrhythmia, which may accelerate, become more sustained, or become less well-tolerated haemodynamically. The appearance of a new arrhythmia, not seen prior to drug therapy, would also fall into this category. In many cases this new arrhythmia represents the unmasking of a latent susceptibility in a patient with a pre-existing predisposition.

Technical arrhythmogenesis refers to arrhythmogenesis detected by clinical investigations. It comprises an increased frequency of arrhythmias recorded on Holter monitoring or an increased susceptibility to arrhythmia detected by invasive electrophysiological investigation. In both instances the incidence of proarrhythmic events is dependent on the extent of increase in arrhythmia frequency or ease of inducibility which is considered significant. It is generally assumed that cases of technical arrhythmogenesis indicate an increased susceptibility to subsequent arrhythmias that would be of clinical significance. This assumption is, however, unproven, as few investigators would be prepared to take the risk of continuing antiarrhythmic drug therapy to determine whether technical arrhythmogenesis predicts clinical arrhythmogenesis.

Mechanisms of arrhythmogenesis

The electrophysiological actions of antiarrhythmic drugs that cause arrhythmias are the same as those which prevent them. This can be illustrated by considering mechanisms of arrhythmogenesis and the modulation of these mechanisms by antiarrhythmic drug therapy.

There are two basic mechanisms of arrhythmogenesis,

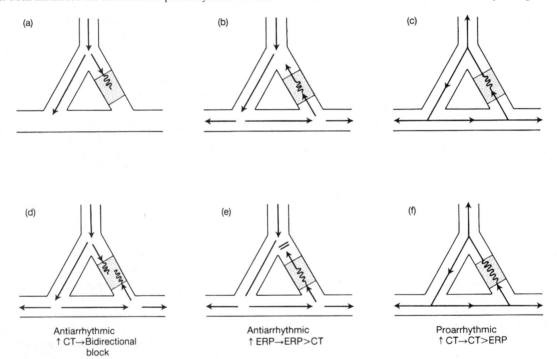

FIG. 8.1

(a)–(c) Mechanism of re-entrant arrhythmias. An impulse propagating anterogradely comes to a bifurcation in the Purkinje system; (a) the impulse is blocked in an area of slow conduction in one limb (shaded area) but continues to conduct through the other limb; (b) the latter impulse then enters the area of slow conduction retrogradely and is able to propagate in that direction; (c) provided the conduction time over the re-entry circuit exceeds the refractory period of the proximal fibres, re-entry can occur.

(d) and (e) Mechanisms of antiarrhythmic effects; (d) a Class II antiarrhythmic agent slows conduction time (CT) resulting in bidirectional block in the area of slow conduction preventing re-entry; (e) a Class III agent prolongs refractoriness so that the effective refractory period (ERP) now exceeds conduction time, preventing re-entry.

(f) Mechanism of proarrhythmic effect. A Class I agent acts on a latent re-entry circuit, which in its native state resembles (e), with refractory period exceeding conduction time. The drug slows conduction further, so that conduction time now exceeds the refractory period, thereby fulfilling criteria for re-entry.

re-entry and abnormal automaticity. Of these, re-entry mechanisms are thought to be more common. Re-entry is easily understood in the case of the Wolff–Parkinson–White syndrome, which involves a well-defined macro-re-entry circuit. In the majority of arrhythmias the re-entry circuit is less clearly defined, involving micro-re-entry within closely adjacent areas of myocardium.

For re-entry to occur there are several requirements (Figs 8.1 a–c). First, there must be an area of unidirectional conduction block. Secondly, there must be a slowing of conduction over the re-entry pathway such that the cycle length of the tachycardia is longer than the longest refractory period at any point over the pathway. Antiarrhythmic drugs can interrupt a re-entry circuit in a number of ways. Firstly, by slowing conduction they can change a zone of unidirectional block into a zone of bidirectional block (Fig. 8.1 d). Secondly, they may prolong refractory periods, such that the longest refractory period exceeds the cycle length of tachycardia, which results in arrhythmia termination (Fig. 8.1 e).

There is, however, another possibility. A patient may have potential re-entry circuits. These fail to fulfil requirements for re-entry in the drug-free state, because the longest refractory period in the pathway exceeds the conduction time over the re-entry pathway. When an antiarrhythmic drug is given, it may create the conditions for re-entry by slowing conduction over the re-entry pathway. The conduction time over the pathway may then exceed the maximum refractory period, resulting in re-entry and the initiation of tachycardia (Fig. 8.1 f).

This principle of potential re-entry circuits is helpful in identifying patients at risk of provocation of arrhythmias by antiarrhythmic agents. Conduction slowing and areas of unidirectional block commonly arise because of fibrosis in the myocardium, resulting from previous infarction. The most common cause of sustained ventricular tachycardia is re-entry at the border zone of an old myocardial infarction. Any patient with previous infarction is therefore at risk from an antiarrhythmic agent facilitating potential re-entry circuits. The likelihood of an antiarrhythmic drug meeting the critical requirements for re-entry will depend on the extent of the area of fibrosis. This is one reason why patients with severe impairment of left ventricular function are at increased risk from therapy with antiarrhythmic drugs (see below).

As regards the second mechanism of arrhythmogenesis, antiarrhythmic drugs can both suppress and increase automaticity (Levine *et al.* 1989). Once again, the electrophysiological mechanisms responsible for pro-arrhythmia are the same as those responsible for antiarrhythmic actions. Antiarrhythmic drugs in Class Ia and Class III of the Vaughan Williams classification prolong action potential duration. They achieve this effect by blocking the outward currents responsible for repolarization. It is now understood that the same effect in some individuals can result in after-depolarizations which can trigger arrhythmias (see below).

Effects of antiarrhythmic therapy on mortality

The Cardiac Arrhythmia Suppression Trial (Echt *et al.* 1991) was the landmark study in antiarrhythmic therapy. This trial randomly assigned patients convalescing from myocardial infarction who had asymptomatic ventricular ectopy to long-term drug therapy or placebo. The assumption was that suppression of ventricular ectopic beats would be beneficial. The mortality rate in patients receiving the active therapy was two to three times greater than in those taking placebo, and there was evidence of increased mortality in subgroups of patients with left ventricular impairment and those at risk of recurrent myocardial ischaemia such as patients with non-Q wave infarction (Akiyama *et al.* 1991). This trial questioned the whole philosophy that treating asymptomatic arrhythmias was desirable or beneficial. Subsequent trials of antiarrhythmic therapy have been as disappointing as CAST I.

Neither moricizine (Green *et al.* 1992) nor quinidine (Morganroth and Goin 1981) improves outcome in patients with ventricular arrhythmia.

The reason for the above findings are unclear. They may be related to the fact that the ability of class I drugs to control arrhythmia is reduced in the presence of increased catecholamine concentrations (Jazayeri *et al.* 1989); furthermore, ischaemia may markedly alter the electrophysiological effects of class I agents (El-Sherif *et al.* 1977).

The failure of class I agents to improve mortality led to the investigation of the potential benefits of class III antiarrhythmic agents. In a population of patients with sustained ventricular tachycardia, *d*-sotalol was more effective than class I anti-arrhythmic agents in suppressing ventricular ectopic activity and preventing the induction of arrhythmia during electrophysiological studies (Mason *et al.* 1993). This study, however, was weakened (Ward and Camm 1993) by failure to include a placebo or conventional β-blocker. Furthermore, the recent Survival with oral *d*-sotalol study (Waldo *et al.* 1995) was terminated early on the advice of the data and safety monitoring committee, as *d*-sotalol led to an excess of deaths in the group of post-infarct patients studied.

While there is some evidence that amiodarone may reduce mortality in patients with heart failure and ventricular ectopy (Pfisterer *et al.* 1992), patients with asymptomatic complex arrhythmias following myocardial infarction (Burkart *et al.* 1990), patients surviving out of hospital cardiac arrest (CASCADE 1993), and patients having sustained a myocardial infarction with frequent or repetitive ventricular ectopics (Cairns *et al.* 1997), there is increasing evidence that implantable defibrillators are more effective than amiodarone in preventing sudden death in patients at high risk for ventricular arrhythmia (Moss *et al.* 1996, and for review see Domanski *et al.* 1997).

Identification of risk

Patient characteristics

A number of patient characteristics that indicate an increased susceptibility to arrhythmogenesis with antiarrhythmic drug therapy have been identified. First and foremost amongst these is the *severity of the rhythm disturbance* requiring treatment. In a series of 1330 patients treated for a mean of 292 days with flecainide, the incidence of proarrythmic events was found to be zero in patients treated for ventricular premature beats, 0.9 per cent in patients treated for non-sustained tachycardia, and 6.6 per cent in patients treated for sustained ventricular tachycardia (Morganroth *et al.* 1986).

Slater and others (1988) found that patients treated for either sustained ventricular tachycardia or ventricular fibrillation were 3.4 times more likely to demonstrate proarrhythmia than patients treated for non-sustained ventricular tachycardia or ventricular premature beats. It is easy to understand why this should be the case. If a patient already has a re-entry circuit responsible for a particular arrhythmia, he may well have other potential re-entry circuits that may be unmasked by the administration of an antiarrhythmic drug.

The second patient characteristic predictive of increased risk is *impaired left ventricular function*. Pratt and others (1989) observed a 15 per cent incidence of life-threatening proarrhythmic complications in patients with an ejection fraction less than 30 per cent, compared with an incidence of two per cent in patients with an ejection fraction greater than 30 per cent. Stanton and others (1989) demonstrated an association between left ventricular regional wall motion abnormalities and arrhythmogenesis. Slater and others (1988) found that patients with an ejection fraction less than 35 per cent were twice as likely to experience proarrhythmia as patients with an ejection fraction greater than 35 per cent.

There are several reasons why impairment of left ventricular function may lead to increased risk. First, increased susceptibility to proarrhythmia may simply be a reflection of an increased extent of fibrosis and an increased number of potential re-entry circuits which may be unmasked by antiarrhythmic drugs. Secondly, antiarrhythmic drugs have been shown to be less effective in suppressing arrhythmias in patients with heart failure (Pratt *et al.* 1989). This decreased efficacy may tilt the risk–balance equation towards risk. Thirdly, most antiarrhythmic drugs themselves have a depressant effect on cardiac function (see below). Fourthly, patients with impaired left ventricular function have increased sympathetic activity and the interaction between sympathetic activation and antiarrhythmic drug therapy may predispose to increased risk. Finally, patients with heart failure are likely to be receiving additional drug treatment for the management of the heart failure, creating the potential for drug interaction. In particular, diuretic-induced hypokalaemia may interact with antiarrhythmic drug therapy.

Structural heart disease   is a further risk factor for proarrhythmic events. This is not an independent risk factor, as most patients with ventricular tachycardia and all patients with impaired left ventricular function will fall into a category of structural heart disease. None the less, it is a useful concept by virtue of exclusion. The risks of a proarrhythmic event in a patient without structural heart disease are relatively low.

There are, therefore, patient characteristics that will identify individuals at increased risk from proarrhythmic complications of antiarrhythmic drug therapy. The risks of arrhythmia aggravation are highest in patients who have already manifested sustained ventricular tachycardia and who have impaired left ventricular function. Knowledge of these predisposing factors is of value in determining the risk of a proarrhythmic event in individual patients. It has been suggested that, in particularly high-risk individuals, the risks of antiarrhythmic drug therapy may become too great for this treatment to be contemplated (Pratt *et al.* 1989). The situation, however, is more complex. As risks increase, potential benefits also increase. It is precisely the patient with malignant ventricular tachyarrhythmias and impaired left ventricular function who most needs successful arrhythmia prevention. Conversely, the patient with ventricular ectopic beats, in whom the risks of antiarrhythmic drug therapy may be remote, stands to benefit least from treatment. There is, therefore, a risk–benefit equation; risks and benefits increase in parallel. Potential benefits and risks need to be assessed individually in every patient in whom antiarrhythmic drug therapy is considered.

Prediction of arrhythmogenicity

Plasma concentrations

Proarrhythmic effects of antiarrhythmic drugs are more

common when drug concentrations exceed the normal therapeutic range. This has been most clearly illustrated in the case of the Class Ic agent flecainide (Morganroth and Horowitz 1984; Nathan *et al*. 1984). The minority of clinical reports of arrhythmogenesis, however, reflect drug toxicity. In the majority of cases arrhythmogenic effects arise within the normal therapeutic range (Velebit *et al*. 1982; Rae *et al*. 1988). Consequently, plasma drug concentrations, although important in detecting toxicity, are of very limited value as a screening test for the prediction of arrhythmogenic effects (Falik *et al*. 1987; Greenberg *et al*. 1987).

12-Lead electrocardiogram

Exaggeration of the normal therapeutic effect of an antiarrhythmic agent may result in changes in the 12-lead ECG that can be used as predictors of toxicity. An example is excessive prolongation of PR and QRS intervals induced by Class Ic agents such as flecainide (Morganroth and Horowitz 1984; Nathan *et al*. 1984). Once again, however, the majority of proarrhythmic effects occur in the normal therapeutic range, without any pronounced ECG changes. Consequently, ECG changes are of limited predictive value and, in general, ECG criteria have not been predictive of proarrhythmia (Slater *et al*. 1988).

Arrhythmogenesis accompanying QT prolongation has been reported with many drugs (see below). QT prolongation is, however, a normal therapeutic effect of Class 1a and Class III antiarrhythmic drugs. The extent of QT prolongation after commencement of quinidine was not found to be predictive of arrhythmogenesis (Etvinsson and Orinius 1980). In general, therefore, QT prolongation has not been found to be a good predictor of arrhythmogenesis.

Dynamic electrocardiography

Holter monitoring can be of value in documenting clinically relevant arrhythmogenesis, as for example when ventricular tachycardia occurs for the first time in the patient receiving antiarrhythmic drug therapy for ventricular ectopic beats. More frequently, however, proarrhythmia is defined on technical grounds on the basis of an increased frequency or complexity of ventricular ectopic beats. The criteria for the recognition of such proarrhythmic events have been defined (Velebit *et al*. 1982) (Table 8.1). Based on these criteria, a proarrhythmic response has been reported to occur in 11 per cent of drug trials.

TABLE 8.1
Criteria for the Holter diagnosis of proarrhythmia

1. Fourfold increase in the hourly frequency of ventricular extrasystoles compared with control recording
2. Tenfold increase in the hourly frequency of repetitive forms (couplets of VT) compared with control recording
3. First occurrence of sustained VT (lasting 1 minute or longer) not present during control studies.

Adapted from Velebit *et al*. (1982)

Invasive electrophysiological testing

Invasive electrophysiological testing has revolutionized the diagnosis and management of a wide range of supraventricular and ventricular tachycardias. Most of these tachycardias are re-entrant in nature and can hence be initiated by critically timed extra stimuli. These extra stimuli provide means of testing drug effects on the underlying re-entrant mechanism, sometimes termed the arrhythmic 'substrate'.

In some cases proarrhythmic effects are clear-cut, such as the appearance of a new sustained ventricular tachycardia when none could be initiated previously (Au *et al*. 1987). In other circumstances, however, the interpretation of electrophysiological findings is dependent on definitions. Rae and associates (1988) have shown that a difference in ease of induction of one extra stimulus is not meaningful, as this can arise from the spontaneous variability in the ease of induction in as many as 15 per cent of patients. In 40 patients in whom well-tolerated ventricular tachycardia was initiated with fewer extra stimuli during drug therapy than at baseline, the drug was continued during follow-up. The recurrence rate of tachycardia was no greater than in patients on regimens in which the number of extra stimuli required for initiation was not reduced. The authors concluded that a reduction in the initiating mode by one extra stimulus is not of sufficient predictive value to be used in clinical practice. In contrast, a difference in ease of induction of two extra stimuli is of value in detecting proarrhythmic effects. Four of five patients in whom this criterion was satisfied experienced sudden death or arrhythmia recurrence during follow-up. The authors suggested four criteria for the diagnosis of proarrhythmia in electrophysiological studies (Table 8.2). Based on these criteria, proarrhythmic effects were detected in eight per cent of drug trials.

TABLE 8.2
Criteria for the diagnosis of proarrhythmia based on electrophysiological testing

1. Conversion of non-sustained to sustained VT
2. Conversion of haemodynamically stable VT to VT requiring cardioversion
3. Reduction by two extrastimuli of the number of extra stimuli required for arrhythmia induction
4. Spontaneous development of VT.

Adapted from Rae *et al.* (1988)

Exercise testing

Exercise testing is of value in detecting proarrhythmic effects of antiarrhythmic drug therapy. One-third of proarrhythmic responses can only be identified on exercise testing (Slater *et al.* 1988). Exercise testing is of particular importance in detecting proarrhythmic effects of Class Ic antiarrhythmic agents. The effects of Ic drugs on conduction are rate dependent: the greater the heart rate the greater the depression of conduction. Increased QRS widening on exercise has been demonstrated with Class Ic agents (Ranger *et al.* 1989). The additional depressant effect on conduction during exercise may contribute to arrhythmogenesis (Anastasiou-Nana *et al.* 1987).

Time of occurrence of proarrhythmic events

Until very recently it was believed that proarrhythmic effects of antiarrhythmic drugs would arise early after starting treatment, within the first few days of commencing therapy. This belief was largely based on experience with quinidine. A small proportion of patients developed *torsade de pointes* within the first few days of commencing therapy (see below). These early arrhythmias on commencing quinidine became recognized as 'quinidine syncope'. Minardo and others (1988) considered 28 patients who developed ventricular fibrillation for the first time after commencing antiarrhythmic drug therapy. The median duration of therapy before the onset of ventricular fibrillation was 3 days. It has consequently been recommended that antiarrhythmic drug therapy should be commenced in hospital.

While there is certainly an increased incidence of proarrhythmia within the first few days of commencing treatment, it has now become clear that proarrhythmic effects are by no means confined to this time. The Cardiac Arrhythmia Suppression Trial (CAST) study randomized patients with an increased frequency of ventricular ectopic beats following myocardial infarction to treatment with flecainide, encainide, or placebo (CAST 1989). An increased mortality was observed in the two active treatment groups in comparison with placebo. This increased mortality was not confined to the first few days after commencing treatment but, rather, continued over weeks and months of treatment. Mortality in the active and placebo groups was still diverging on the premature termination of the study, after a mean treatment period of 10 months.

This finding has shown conclusively that proarrhythmia is not confined to the first few days of treatment. It still seems advisable to begin antiarrhythmic drug therapy in hospital, as there may well be an increased incidence of proarrhythmia in the first days of treatment. Continuing vigilance is, however, also necessary, and an awareness that any arrhythmia may have been caused by treatment rather than reflecting inefficacy of treatment.

Which patients should be treated with antiarrhythmic agents?

There is no doubt that patients with sustained tachyarrhythmias benefit from termination of their arrhythmia. Long-term treatment is however, dependent on an understanding of the underlying pathophysiology. If one does decide to treat with long-term pharmacological therapy one must assess and be able to manage the accompanying risks. A general principle of therapy is applicable: since antiarrhythmic therapy carries finite risks, patients at low risk from arrhythmia (e.g. ectopics) are likely to be worsened by indiscriminate treatment while those at high risk are more likely to benefit from treatment.

Recommendations for the routine screening of a patient commencing antiarrhythmic drug therapy

The empirical use of antiarrhythmic drug therapy, in patients with serious ventricular arrhythmias, is unsatisfactory. Patients should be screened for possible proarrhythmic effects.

There is no single technique or investigation that will detect all possible proarrhythmic effects. As a minimum requirement, a 12-lead ECG, Holter monitoring, and exercise testing should be undertaken. These investigations are relatively easily performed in most hospitals. Invasive electrophysiological testing is also of value, but may be confined to more specialized centres. In patients treated for malignant ventricular arrhythmias, particularly those with impaired left ventricular function, invasive electrophysiological testing is advisable, both to assess the efficacy of drug treatment and to guard against possible proarrhythmic effects. If appropriate means of testing are not available, it is questionable whether antiarrhythmic drug therapy should be commenced at all, as risks may exceed benefits.

Minimizing the risk of proarrhythmia

Before starting therapy, one must bear in mind that, among antiarrhythmic agents, only β-adrenoceptor antagonists have been shown to reduce mortality.

Reversible causes of arrhythmias should be sought. They include concomitant therapy (e.g. digoxin or theophylline), and electrolyte abnormalities such as hypokalaemia, hypocalcaemia, and hypomagnesaemia. Marked prolongation of the QT interval after initiating therapy can identify patients who are at high risk of *torsade de pointes* (Jackman *et al.* 1988). In addition, there are a number of subtleties of the QT interval to be aware of: the QT interval can be quite labile; prolongation may only occur on converting atrial fibrillation to sinus rhythm (Roden *et al.* 1986); and the QT interval may be prolonged after pauses (Jackman *et al.* 1988). Interestingly *torsade de pointes* has been shown to be more common in women (Lehman *et al.* 1996).

Comparison of individual antiarrhythmic agents

With the possible exception of β-blockers, arrhythmia facilitation is a potential property of all antiarrhythmic drugs. Comparison of the relative incidence of proarrhythmic effects with different antiarrhythmic agents is difficult. Inevitably, different drugs have been used in different studies for different indications amongst different patient groups with different definitions of proarrhythmia. These factors alone will account for a varying incidence of proarrhythmic effects.

Consequently, comparisons of the relative incidence of proarrhythmia with different drugs are seldom meaningful. The reported incidence of proarrhythmia with different drugs varies between one and 12 per cent (Stanton *et al.* 1989).

Despite difficulties in comparison, certain patterns of proarrhythmia are emerging (Levine *et al.* 1989). Drugs that prolong the duration of action potentials (Vaughan Williams Class Ia and Class III) have a particular tendency to cause *torsade de pointes*. In contrast, Class Ic agents, whose most marked effect is slowing of conduction, give rise to incessant monomorphic ventricular tachycardia which is difficult or impossible to terminate (Oetgen *et al.* 1983). In addition, this tachyarrhythmia may be seen in overdose with tricyclic antidepressants (Nattel *et al.* 1985) or quinidine (Wetherbee 1952). In each case, it is probable that the differing pattern of proarrhythmia reflects differences in the primary mechanism of antiarrhythmic action.

There is a general belief that the incidence of proarrhythmic effects is lower with amiodarone than with other antiarrhythmic drugs (Mattioni *et al.* 1989). An incidence of four per cent in antiarrhythmic drug trials has been reported (Fogoros *et al.* 1983). It is unclear why this should be the case, in particular why the incidence should be lower than with Class Ia agents, which also prolong action potential duration.

Management of proarrhythmic events

When a proarrhythmic event is suspected, the offending antiarrhythmic drug should be stopped. The possibility of drug or metabolic interactions should be considered, in particular the possibility of hypokalaemia or hypomagnesaemia, which might play a facilitatory role. Drug concentrations should be estimated to determine if the arrhythmia might be due to toxicity. If an arrhythmia is due to a drug, then the arrhythmogenic tendency should resolve as drug concentrations fall. This, however, poses a problem with amiodarone, as the half-life of this drug is measured in months.

If at all possible, addition of other antiarrhythmic drugs should be avoided, as potential drug interactions may further exacerbate the arrhythmia. In some cases, recurrence of arrhythmias can be prevented by ventricular pacing.

Torsade de pointes

The term '*torsade de pointes*' was coined by Dessertenne in 1966 to describe a distinct form of polymorphic ventricular tachycardia in which the QRS complexes appear to 'twist' around the isoelectric line. Over a period of 5–20 beats the amplitude of QRS complexes is seen gradually to increase and subsequently decrease. The pattern is then repeated. This arrhythmia is due to a specific electrophysiological abnormality termed triggered automaticity, which arises as a result of marked prolongation of the cardiac action potential (Roden 1991).

The arrhythmia is important to recognize for a number of reasons. First, it is a serious and potentially fatal condition that is frequently due to drugs or toxins. Secondly, once recognized, it is relatively easily treated. If unrecognized, the arrhythmia can be exacerbated by inappropriate treatment.

The range of drugs that have been reported as causing *torsade de pointes* is extensive (Table 8.3). Antiarrhythmic agents are by far the most commonly reported class of drug associated with the arrhythmia. While any antiarrhythmic drug can cause *torsade*, it is most commonly associated with drugs that prolong action potential duration, that is, Class Ia and Class III agents. Amongst other drugs causing *torsade*, phenothiazines are the next commonest group. Significantly these drugs have electrophysiological properties that are similar to those of group Ia antiarrhythmic agents (see below).

TABLE 8.3
Drugs associated with torsade de pointes

Antiarrhythmic drugs

Group Ia
Disopyramide
Procainamide
Quinidine

Group Ib
Lignocaine*
Mexiletine*

Group Ic
Encainide*

Group III
Amiodarone
Sotalol

Psychotropics
Amitriptyline*
Chlorpromazine*
Doxepin*
Maprotiline*
Thioridazine

Antihypertensives
Diuretics
Ketanserin

Calcium antagonists
Bepridil
Prenylamine

---

* Drugs marked with an asterisk are included on the basis of a
relatively small number of case reports.

Characteristically, when an ECG is available prior to the onset of arrhythmia, this shows QT prolongation. In many cases, giant U waves are evident. Indeed, it seems likely that QT prolongation is due to fusion of the U wave with the T wave. The value of QT prolongation as a predictor of arrhythmia occurrence, however, is unclear. Agents that predispose to *torsade* cause QT prolongation as part of their normal therapeutic action. It has not been possible to establish criteria for pathological degrees of QT prolongation that predict the development of the arrhythmia.

Stratmann and Kennedy (1987) reviewed 197 cases of drug-induced *torsade de pointes* in which information regarding QT intervals before and after drug administration was provided. In 35 per cent of cases QT prolongation was present even before administration of the drug that was implicated. QT prolongation prior to drug administration may, therefore, constitute a risk factor.

The presence of pronounced U waves in many cases of *torsade de pointes* provides a clue to the electrophysiological mechanisms underlying this arrhythmia. Animal studies (Levine *et al.* 1985; Roden and Hoffman 1985) have shown that quinidine may cause after-depolarizations *in vitro*. This action is facilitated by bradycardia and hypokalaemia, conditions known to predispose to *torsade de pointes*. It is possible that the prominent U waves that frequently accompany the arrhythmia are manifestations in the surface ECG of after-depolarizations at the cellular. It is now understood that these after-depolarizations are related to the same mechanisms that are responsible for prolongation of the plateau of the action potential (Sasyniuk *et al.* 1989), prolongation of which is due to inhibition of a slow outward potassium current responsible for repolarization. Inhibition of this outward current, combined with persisting inward current, gives rise to after-depolarizations. These result in accelerated automaticity and this is clinically manifest as polymorphic ventricular tachycardia of the *torsade de pointes* type.

A number of factors predispose to the occurrence of *torsade de pointes* during drug therapy. Hypokalaemia and bradycardia are particularly common contributory factors. A characteristic initiation sequence has been described. Kay and others (1983) reported that a long cycle (the compensatory pause following a premature ventricular contraction) followed by a short cycle (a second early premature ventricular contraction) immediately preceded the onset of arrhythmia in 41 of 44 episodes.

As for other proarrhythmic complications of antiarrhythmic drugs, toxic drug concentrations may be contributory, but the arrhythmia may also arise as an idiosyncratic reaction with drug levels in the normal therapeutic range. This is true of quinidine syncope; drug levels are not predictive of *torsade de pointes* (Selzer and Wray 1964; Bauman *et al.* 1984). With procainamide, by contrast, most cases of *torsade de pointes* are associated with excessive drug levels, which are particularly likely to occur following intravenous administration (Strasberg *et al.* 1981).

Management of torsade de pointes

Once an arrhythmia has been identified as *torsade de pointes*, drug therapy should be critically reviewed to determine the likely cause. Additional contributory factors, particularly hypokalaemia and hypomagnesaemia, should be considered and corrected. Sustained episodes of the arrhythmia causing haemodynamic deterioration should be terminated by DC cardioversion. Further antiarrhythmic drug therapy should be avoided. Once sinus rhythm has been restored, prophylaxis should be initiated against further episodes. As the initiation of episodes is bradycardia-related, this is accomplished by increasing heart rate. One way of achieving this is with an isoprenaline infusion, but this approach is hazardous, as excessive concentrations of catecholamines may exacerbate the arrhythmia. A much safer approach is to insert a temporary pacing wire to maintain heart rate in a target range of 100–120 beats per minute. Ventricular pacing is most commonly used and is the most reliable means of treatment, although in patients with marginal left ventricular function it may be necessary to use atrial pacing to preserve atrioventricular synchrony.

Following recovery, the need for continuing drug therapy should be critically evaluated. If the arrhythmia occurred with therapeutic or subtherapeutic concentrations of the implicated drug, then the drug must not be restarted. If, however, the arrhythmia occurred at markedly toxic levels, the drug could conceivably be restarted at a lower dose. If this option is selected, very careful monitoring of serum levels is necessary to prevent recurrence of toxicity.

In summary, *torsade de pointes* is a particularly distinctive form of ventricular tachycardia. It is a unique arrhythmia in that, in its acquired form, it is always related to drugs or toxins. Metabolic abnormalities frequently play a contributory role. Treatment is to discontinue the offending drug and correct any metabolic disturbance. In addition, temporary pacing is generally necessary to prevent recurrent attacks until aetiological factors have resolved.

Pacing and defibrillation thresholds

Class Ic antiarrhythmic agents cause a rise in pacing threshold, reflecting effects on ventricular conduction. At times this problem may be severe enough to interfere with ventricular capture (Hellestrand *et al*. 1983).

The advent of the automatic implantable cardioverter–defibrillator (AICD) has led to the discovery of a further adverse effect of antiarrhythmic drug therapy. A number of studies have shown that amiodarone therapy raises the threshold for defibrillation. As patients frequently require antiarrhythmic drug therapy concomitantly with an AICD, this is an important and potentially very serious interaction. Fogoros (1984) described a patient who became refractory to AICD cardioversion while taking amiodarone. Two studies have shown that the defibrillation threshold is significantly higher in AICD patients treated with amiodarone (Troup *et al*. 1985; Kelly *et al*. 1988).

For this reason it is advisable to undertake repeated testing of the defibrillation threshold in AICD patients receiving long-term amiodarone therapy. A further study by Daoud and colleagues (1997) showed that amiodarone can increase the energy required to defibrillate ventricular fibrillation by 23 per cent.

Pharmacological causes of proarrythmia

Although the majority of proarrythmic complications of antiarrhythmic drug therapy arise with drug concentrations in the therapeutic range, a proportion of adverse reactions are related to drug toxicity. Pharmacological factors may contribute to these high concentrations.

In a number of reports, antiarrhythmic dosage protocols have been based on pharmacokinetic studies in normal volunteers or stable cardiac patients. These studies do not, however, adequately predict pharmacokinetics in patients with heart failure. This proved to be the case for flecainide. After satisfactory studies in stable cardiac patients, patients with severe disease developed higher than anticipated plasma concentrations of the drug and a high incidence of proarrhythmia (Nathan *et al*. 1984).

Decreased drug clearance may lead to increased plasma concentrations of antiarrhythmic drugs and thus cause exacerbation of arrhythmias. Antiarrhythmics subject to extensive hepatic metabolism are particularly susceptible to interaction with drugs that induce or block hepatic enzymes. For example, cimetidine, which blocks some hepatic enzymes, can cause an increase in plasma concentrations of lignocaine (Feely *et al*. 1982). Similarly, in patients simultaneously receiving phenytoin and quinidine, withdrawal of phenytoin, which induces liver enzymes, has been shown to lead to toxic concentrations of quinidine (Data *et al*. 1976).

Genetic factors may also influence metabolism of antiarrhythmics. The classic example is acetylation of procainamide to N-acetylprocainamide. Patients fall into two phenotypes, slow acetylators and rapid acetylators. N-acetylprocainamide itself prolongs repolarization (Dangman and Hoffman 1981) and has antiarrhythmic and potential proarrhythmic properties. Some cases of *torsade de pointes* induced by procainamide may be due to accumulation of N-acetylprocainamide (Chow *et al*. 1984).

When antiarrhythmic drugs are used in combination, interactions may occur. A marked increase in digoxin concentrations may occur during quinidine (Holt *et al*. 1979) or amiodarone (Fenster *et al*. 1985) administration. Amiodarone has been shown to increase the plasma concentrations of both quinidine and procainamide (Saal *et al*. 1984).

Because of these pharmacokinetic interactions and the possibility of pharmacodynamic interactions, antiarrhythmic drug combinations should only be used with extreme caution.

Digitalis

Plasma concentrations in assessing toxicity

Unlike those caused by other antiarrhythmic agents, digitalis-induced arrhythmias are generally associated with drug toxicity. Therapeutic and toxic ranges, however, overlap: a digitalis concentration therapeutic in one patient may be toxic for another. Although the mean plasma digitalis concentration is elevated in patients with clinical features of toxicity, plasma concentrations are of limited predictive value in individual patients (G.A. Beller *et al*. 1971). Chamberlain and others (1970) found that 21 of 22 patients with signs of toxicity had concentrations above $2\,\mu g$ per litre, but that 21 of 116 patients without signs of toxicity also achieved concentrations in this range.

Because of the limited value of digitalis estimations in diagnosing toxicity, assays should only be undertaken when there is a definite clinical indication. The fact that the patient is taking digitalis is not in itself sufficient justification for an assay, in the absence of other clinical indications. Appropriate indications include suspected toxicity, subtherapeutic clinical response, suspected poor compliance, changing renal function, potential drug interactions, and assessment of the need for continuing treatment (Aronson 1980).

As a generalization, provided the serum potassium is normal, toxicity is unlikely with digoxin concentrations below $2\,\mu g$ per litre, and very likely with values greater than $4\,\mu g$ per litre. It is, however, essential that samples be timed correctly. At least 6 hours should be allowed to elapse between the time of dosing and time of sampling. Samples drawn early after dosing give spuriously high digoxin concentrations and may lead to inappropriate clinical decisions (Gibb *et al*. 1986).

Factors influencing susceptibility to digitalis toxicity

Digoxin is excreted entirely by the kidney. The likelihood of toxicity therefore rises in patients with impaired renal function, particularly the elderly. Just as for other antiarrhythmic agents, the presence of heart disease influences susceptibility to proarrythmic effects. Thus patients with advanced heart disease are more likely to develop toxicity than less ill patients (G.A. Beller *et al*. 1971). Once again, therefore, the dangers of antiarrhythmic drug therapy are greatest in those patients most dependent on treatment.

The interaction of hypokalaemia with digitalis therapy has been recognized for many years. Hypokalaemia and hypomagnesaemia can provoke supraventricular arrhythmias, even in the presence of therapeutic digitalis concentrations (Fisch 1973; Beller *et al*. 1974). As many patients receiving digitalis therapy will also be taking diuretics, there is a considerable potential for drug interaction.

Quinidine (Holt *et al*. 1979) and amiodarone (Fenster *et al*. 1985) increase plasma digitalis concentrations and increase susceptibility to digitalis toxicity (see above).

Features of digitalis toxicity

Digitalis toxicity has both cardiac and non-cardiac manifestations. The gastrointestinal, neurological, visual, and other non-cardiac manifestations of toxicity are discussed elsewhere in this book. Cardiac arrhythmias are common. The reported incidence of arrhythmias varies according to the clinical definition of toxicity. In some studies (e.g. G.A. Beller *et al*. 1971) the presence of arrhythmias has been regarded as an essential prerequisite for the diagnosis of toxicity.

Digitalis toxicity may cause a wide variety of rhythm disturbances (Table 8.4). Digitalis can induce bradyarrhythmias. Increasing degrees of atrioventricular junctional block result from an exaggeration of the drug's normal therapeutic response. Bradycardia accompanying a regularization of ventricular response rate in atrial fibrillation strongly suggests complete heart block, with underlying digitalis toxicity. In patients in sinus rhythm, sinus bradycardia and sinoatrial block may be features of toxicity.

Supraventricular tachycardias are particularly common manifestations of digitalis toxicity. Two arrhythmias are so characteristic as to be pathognomonic — atrial tachycardia with atrioventricular block, and non-paroxysmal atrioventricular nodal tachycardia (Bigger 1985). In atrial tachycardia with atrioventricular block, the ventricular rate is typically slower than in atrial flutter or paroxysmal atrioventricular nodal tachycardia, arrhythmias that would typically be considered in the differential diagnosis. The second pathognomonic arrhythmia is non-paroxysmal atrioventricular nodal tachycardia. The development of a regular tachycardia in a patient whose normal rhythm is atrial fibrillation, is suggestive of this arrhythmia. The ventricular rate is generally relatively slow. The arrhythmia may also be accompanied by atrioventricular dissociation, reflecting digitalis-induced inhibition of antidromic conduction into the atria.

Atrial fibrillation, the commonest indication for digitalis therapy, may itself be provoked by digitalis toxicity. This possibility should be considered when atrial fibrillation occurs in a patient treated with digitalis who was previously in sinus rhythm.

Digitalis may cause frequent or multifocal ventricular ectopic beats. The diagnosis of toxicity is more difficult

TABLE 8.4
Arrhythmias due to digitalis toxicity

Bradycardia
  Sinus bradycardia
  Sinoatrial block
  A–V nodal block
  Marked slowing of ventricular response rate in AF

Supraventricular tachycardias
  Paroxysmal atrial tachycardia with A–V nodal block
  Non-paroxysmal A–V nodal tachycardia

Ventricular rhythms
  Frequent or multifocal ventricular extrasystoles
  Ventricular tachycardia/ventricular fibrillation

than in cases of supraventricular arrhythmias, as many patients requiring digitalis therapy may already have frequent ventricular ectopic activity. The development of bigeminy in a patient with atrial fibrillation is strongly suggestive of digitalis toxicity.

Ventricular tachycardia and ventricular fibrillation are rare manifestations of toxicity. In both cases they indicate severe toxicity, and before the advent of digitalis antibodies carried a poor prognosis.

Management of digitalis toxicity

In patients with suspected digitalis toxicity, primary treatment is, of course, to withdraw the drug. Resolution of toxic effects will take several days, reflecting the long half-life of digitalis preparations. In patients with impaired renal function, resolution will take even longer. Hypokalaemia should be corrected. Magnesium deficiency should also be considered and corrected. A search should be made for concurrent factors that may have contributed to toxicity. Renal impairment due to dehydration from excessive diuretic therapy is a particularly common precipitant. Any additional contributory factors such as dehydration should be corrected.

In most cases of toxicity, these simple measures alone will suffice. In cases of more severe toxicity, complicated by rhythm disturbance, additional measures may be necessary. Drug treatment of digitalis arrhythmias is difficult and best avoided if possible. If treatment is necessary, Class I agents such as lignocaine, procainamide, or phenytoin may be used with caution. Quinidine should be avoided because of its interaction with digitalis. Cardioversion of supraventricular arrhythmias is best avoided, because of risk of precipitating ventricular fibrillation. In general, if arrhythmias are so severe as to necessitate consideration of antiarrhythmic drug therapy, treatment with digoxin immune antibody fragments (Fab) may be preferable.

Digoxin immune antibody fragments are now established as the treatment of choice to achieve rapid reversal of serious digitalis toxicity. They are prepared by injecting sheep with a digitalis–serum albumin complex over several weeks and processing the digitalis-specific antibodies to yield antibody fragments. The fragments are less immunogenic than the whole antibody and are capable of being excreted by the kidneys. The antibody has a greater drug affinity than the tissue receptors, and binds the drug preferentially.

Digoxin immune antibody fragments have proved highly successful in the treatment of digitalis overdosage (Stolshek *et al.* 1988). They are indicated in patients with serious or life-threatening arrhythmias as a result of digitalis toxicity or in patients who have ingested sufficient digitalis to cause concern that such arrhythmias may arise. Antman and others (1990) reported 150 cases of life-threatening digitalis intoxication treated with Fab. Eighty per cent had complete resolution of all signs and symptoms of toxicity, while another 10 per cent showed improvement. Only 10 per cent failed to respond. Signs of toxicity generally resolve within a few hours. Allergic reactions are surprisingly rare. Following treatment, patients may experience hypokalaemia and worsening of heart failure or a rise in ventricular rate, because of withdrawal of the therapeutic effects of digitalis.

Digitalis and mortality

Recent studies have clarified the use of digoxin in heart failure.

The PROVED trial (Uretsky *et al.* 1993) presented data from a withdrawal trial of patients with heart failure taking digoxin. Patients whose digoxin was withdrawn had an increased incidence and earlier onset of heart failure, and reduced exercise capacity. The issue was further clarified by the Digitalis Investigation Group (1997), who showed that digoxin does not reduce overall mortality in patients with heart failure, but reduces hospitalization rates both overall and for worsening heart failure.

The use of digoxin after myocardial infarction remains controversial. Retrospective assessment of the MILIS (Multicentre Investigation of Limitation of Infarct Size) study failed to show any excess mortality associated with digoxin use (Muller *et al.* 1986). On the other hand, Bigger and co-workers (1985) showed a five-fold increase in mortality associated with digoxin use following myocardial infarction. The retrospective nature of these reports limits their value. The patients treated with digoxin after myocardial infarction may have had worse disease and this may be reflected in the worse survival.

However, the results of these studies in patients after a heart attack suggest that digoxin, like other antiarrhythmic agents, should be used with caution.

Positive inotropic agents

Phosphodiesterase inhibitors have been reported to increase the frequency of ventricular extrasystoles (Holmes *et al.* 1985; Anderson *et al.* 1986; Miles *et al.* 1989). A number of trials have now shown that administration of phosphodiesterase inhibitors, while improving symptoms in patients with heart failure lead to an excess mortality (Uretsky *et al.* 1990; Packer *et al.* 1991; Cowley and Skene 1994). Interestingly, the trial carried out by Cowley and Skene (which was terminated early) showed that a group of patients with severe heart failure treated with oral phosphodiesterase inhibitors had a significant improvement in quality of life at the expense of earlier mortality.

The β-agonists have been shown to be similarly detrimental in patients with heart failure. Dobutamine, an intravenous inotrope, increases sinus node automaticity and decreases atrial and AV nodal refractoriness and AV nodal conduction time. Dobutamine also decreases ventricular refractoriness in both healthy and ischaemic myocardium. Dies (1986) reported a double-blind controlled trial of intermittent intravenous dobutamine infusion in patients with heart failure. The drug was administered for 48 hours per week over a 24-week period. The trial was stopped prematurely after recruiting 60 patients. At this time 20 patients had died, of whom 15 had been assigned to, or had crossed over to, dobutamine. These findings did not achieve conventional statistical significance when analysed on either an intention-to-treat or treatment-received basis. Pre-existing ventricular tachycardia was predictive of death in the patients treated with dobutamine. Seven of the 15 deaths occurred during the weekly infusion of the drug. Taken together, these findings suggest the possibility of an increase in life-threatening arrhythmias during the dobutamine infusion. This report raises serious concerns about the possible adverse effects of β-adrenergic stimulation in patients with heart failure.

The partial agonist xamoterol, a β-blocker with intrinsic sympathetic activity, increased mortality in heart failure patients (German and Austrial Xamoterol Study Group; The Xamoterol in Severe Heart Failure Study Group 1990).

In conclusion, positive inotropic agents of differing pharmacological actions (except digoxin) have adverse effects on survival in patients with heart failure, probably by their arrhythmogenicity. However, they may improve symptoms and judgement on their use should be made on an individual patient basis.

β-Blockers

Tachyarrhythmias induced by β-blockers are very rare. *Torsade de pointes* is a well-recognized complication of sotalol treatment (McKibbin *et al.* 1984). This proarrhythmic action, however, is related to the class III antiarrhythmic effects of sotalol rather than to its β-blocker activity. QT prolongation occurs with normal therapeutic doses of this drug. As with other antiarrhythmic agents, *torsade de pointes* may arise in the normal therapeutic range and does not imply drug toxicity.

Calcium antagonists

As a group, the calcium antagonists are relatively free of proarrhythmic actions. There are, however, two exceptions, prenylamine and bepridil, which are known to cause *torsade de pointes* (Leclercq *et al.* 1983; Perelman *et al.* 1987). It seems unlikely the proarrhythmic action is a reflection of calcium channel blockade, since other calcium antagonists do not share this proarrhythmic action. The reason why these two agents differ is uncertain. As far as prenylamine is concerned, a proposed explanation is that the drug may act as a calcium agonist at lower stimulation rates (Bayer *et al.* 1988), increasing transmembrane calcium current. The resultant action potential prolongation would predispose to early afterdepolarizations and *torsade de pointes*. Bepridil is also an unusual calcium antagonist in that it has Class I antiarrhythmic properties (Kane and Winslow 1980). These additional properties may be related to its proarrhythmic potential.

Bronchodilators

In the late 1960s, mortality from asthma showed a sudden rise, in which circumstantial evidence implicated isoprenaline aerosols. Sales of the preparation were higher in countries that experienced increased mortality. In addition, mortality and isoprenaline sales fell in parallel once the problem had been recognized (Inman and Adelstein 1969). While the possibility cannot be excluded that the relationship was coincidental, both factors reflecting a changing pattern of asthma severity, it is widely believed isoprenaline aerosols directly caused the increase in deaths.

There are a number of possible mechanisms whereby an increase in mortality might have arisen. The introduction of inhalers may have given patients a false sense of security and delayed their seeking medical attention. Alternatively, the aerosols themselves may have had a direct toxic effect. In metered-dose aerosols, a β-agonist is combined with fluorinated hydrocarbons, which provide a liquid gas propellant. Excessive inhalation of fluorinated hydrocarbons has been associated with sudden death in solvent abuse (see below). It seems likely, however, that the risk from propellant alone is minimal, unless an aerosol is grossly overused (Dollery *et al.* 1970). The main concern has centred on the possibility that β-agonists may have caused arrhythmias. Patients with severe asthma would be expected to be vulnerable to arrhythmias as a result of hypoxia and endogenous catecholamine stimulation. The addition of exogenous catecholamines might increase this vulnerability. In addition, β-agonists cause hypokalaemia (Smith 1984), a further potential proarrhythmic factor. Hypokalaemia is due to β_2-mediated stimulation of the sodium–potassium exchange pump, which results in increased intracellular potassium uptake (Clausen and Flatman 1980).

Although selective β_2-agonists have a higher selectivity of bronchodilator over chronotropic effects than does isoprenaline, there continues to be concern that even selective β_2-agonists may contribute to arrhythmogenesis. At maximal therapeutic doses, the drugs increase heart rate (Crane *et al.* 1989). An increased frequency of arrhythmias has also been reported (Banner *et al.* 1979; Higgins *et al.* 1987). Fenoterol, in particular, has been noted to cause a more marked tachycardia and hypokalaemic response than salbutamol (Crane *et al.* 1989). This finding is of interest because of an over-representation of fenoterol amongst recent deaths of asthmatics in New Zealand (Sears *et al.* 1987). This observation is subject, however, to a number of interpretations and may simply represent physician preference for a newer drug in patients with more severe disease.

Theophylline similarly has the potential to induce arrhythmias, particularly when serum concentrations achieve toxic levels (Hendeles and Weinberger 1983). Concern has been expressed that combined therapy with theophylline and β_2-agonists may have additive proarrhythmic effects (Wilson *et al.* 1981). There is some evidence that the combination may be proarrhythmic. Laaban and others (1988) undertook Holter recordings during infusions of aminophylline and terbutaline in patients with status asthmaticus. Serious arrhythmias were surprisingly infrequent. Two of 29 patients developed sustained atrial tachycardia, and one developed non-sustained ventricular tachycardia. All the arrhythmias were well tolerated and resolved spontaneously.

The significance of proarrhythmia with bronchodilator therapy remains unresolved. It is generally im-

possible to establish whether patients dying from asthma have had an arrhythmia, since most deaths occur outside hospital. Even if an arrhythmia was established as the cause of death, it would be unclear whether this was related to the severity of an asthmatic attack or to the adverse effects of bronchodilator therapy. While the effects of bronchodilator therapy on mortality in asthma remain controversial, it is increasingly likely that increased use of inhaled bronchodilators is an indication of deteriorating asthma rather than of direct toxicity (Committee on Safety of Medicines 1992; Garret *et al.* 1995).

Diuretics, hypokalaemia, and arrhythmias

The efficacy of diuretic therapy in reducing the incidence of stroke in hypertensive patients is well established (Medical Research Council Working Party 1985). By contrast, diuretic treatment has not proved successful in preventing complications due to coronary heart disease. This paradox has raised the suspicion that unfavourable effects of diuretics in patients with ischaemic heart disease may offset the beneficial effects of pressure reduction.

It is well established that thiazides cause hypokalaemia. In the MRC trial of mild hypertension, mean serum potassium was 3.59 mmol per litre in patients receiving bendrofluazide 5 mg b.d., compared with 4.19 mmol per litre in a placebo group. Almost 50 per cent of patients on diuretics have been reported to have serum potassium values below 3.5 mmol per litre (Morgan and Davidson 1980). Diuretic therapy also causes hypomagnesaemia, which may be an additional contributory factor in the genesis of arrhythmias (Hollifield 1987).

There is no doubt that severe hypokalaemia, with a serum potassium value below 2.5 mmol per litre, can cause arrhythmias (Davidson and Surawicz 1967). It is also clear that hypokalaemia can cause arrhythmias in patients on digitalis therapy and can interact with other drugs to cause *torsade de pointes* (see above). Whether moderate degrees of hypokalaemia, induced by diuretic therapy, cause arrhythmias, however, is controversial.

Many studies have assessed the effects of diuretics on the incidence of ventricular extrasystoles during 24-hour ECG recordings or on exercise testing. Some have found a relationship between diuretic-induced hypokalaemia and arrhythmias, while others have not (for review see Poole-Wilson 1987). The conflicting evidence may reflect the spontaneous variability of arrhythmias on Holter recording and the difficulty that this poses for demonstrating significant change in the incidence of arrhythmias.

Much the largest study was undertaken in conjunction with the Medical Research Council's mild hypertension trial (Medical Research Council Working Party 1983). In this study, patients on thiazide treatment had an increased incidence of ventricular extrasystoles. Although serum potassium correlated with the number of extrasystoles, serum urate correlated equally strongly. The authors concluded that hypokalaemia was a marker of thiazide intake, rather than causally related to the arrhythmias. These conclusions have been questioned (Poole-Wilson 1987). Since serum potassium is very variable and is measured at a single point in time, it is not surprising that the correlation with arrhythmias over a 24-hour period is low.

The balance of evidence favours the view that hypokalaemia induced by thiazides does cause an increased frequency of ventricular extrasystoles. The question then arises, does this matter and do diuretics place patients at risk? It is not possible to answer this question with any certainty. Some of the most suggestive observations are derived from subgroup analysis of the Multiple Risk Factor Intervention Trial (MRFIT). MRFIT (1982) was designed to determine the value of intervention directed at reducing multiple risk factors. The study recruited men with enhanced risk due to smoking, hypercholesterolaemia, or hypertension. Subjects were randomized to special intervention or usual care. Of over 12 000 participants, 8000 had hypertension at entry. Special intervention for these individuals included a programme of stepped drug treatment, starting with a thiazide. In a subgroup of hypertensive men with abnormal ECGs, special intervention was associated with an increased mortality.

Retrospective subgroup analyses are, however, of limited value. They indicate possible effects, which serve to guide further research. It is of particular interest to examine similar subgroups in other studies. Unfortunately, the evidence is conflicting. Analysis of the Oslo Hypertension Study (Holme et al. 1984) supported the MRFIT conclusions. Analysis of the Hypertension Detection and Follow-up Programme study (HDFP 1984) and MRC trial (Miall and Greenberg 1987) failed, however, to show any increase in coronary heart disease mortality in the equivalent subgroup of patients treated with diuretics.

The link between diuretic-induced hypokalaemia and serious arrhythmias therefore remains unproven. To answer this question would require a much larger trial than any that has been conducted hitherto. The need for potassium conservation is therefore controversial. Although it is unproven that hypokalaemia matters, it is equally unproven that it does not. For this reason some

suspicion must remain, so it seems reasonable to avoid hypokalaemia, where possible, through the addition of potassium supplements or the use of potassium-sparing diuretic combinations. It is interesting to note that the only trial hitherto that has demonstrated a reduction in coronary mortality in hypertensive patients was the EWPHE (European Working Party on High Blood Pressure in the Elderly) study, which used a potassium-sparing diuretic combination (hydrochlorothiazide + triamterene) (Amery et al. 1985). This may, of course, be coincidence.

Whatever the direct proarrhythmic effects of hypokalaemia, it is established that hypokalaemia can interact with other drug therapy to cause serious arrhythmias. The interaction of digitalis and hypokalaemia to cause digitalis toxicity is well known (Fisch 1973). Similarly, hypokalaemia is a common accompanying factor in many cases of *torsade de pointes* (Khan et al. 1981). A major interaction between potassium-losing diuretics and the serotonin antagonist ketanserin has been reported (Prevention of Atherosclerotic Complications with Ketanserin Trial Group 1989). A threefold increase in the incidence of sudden death was observed in patients treated with ketanserin who were taking a potassium-losing diuretic at randomization, in comparison with placebo. Ketanserin prolongs the QT interval of the ECG. Zehender and others (1989) reviewed eight patients who developed *torsade de pointes* or ventricular tachycardia during treatment with ketanserin. In most cases predisposing factors, particularly hypokalaemia or diuretic therapy, were evident. It seems possible, therefore, that the excess incidence of sudden death in hypertensive patients on a potassium-losing diuretic treated with ketanserin, is due to the occurrence of *torsade de pointes*. *Torsade de pointes* induced by ketanserin has also been reported in the absence of other predisposing factors (van Camp et al. 1989; Vandermotten et al. 1989).

Thrombolytic therapy

Intravenous thrombolytic therapy is now standard treatment for patients sustaining an acute myocardial infarction (Second International Study of Infarct Survival–ISIS-2 Collaborative Study Group 1988). Reperfusion in animal models of myocardial infarction frequently causes ventricular fibrillation (Jewell et al. 1955). Early fears that thrombolytic therapy for myocardial infarction in man might similarly cause serious ventricular arrhythmias have proved unfounded. Reperfusion arrhythmias do occur, but are generally benign and of no haemodynamic consequence. The most common arrhythmia is accelerated idioventricular rhythm, which occurs in more than 50 per cent of patients with successful reperfusion (Goldberg *et al.* 1983). In addition, ventricular extrasystoles, sinus bradycardia, and atrioventricular block may occur. Ventricular tachycardia and ventricular fibrillation are rare.

Fears are none the less expressed that thrombolytic agents might cause ventricular fibrillation when used outside the coronary care unit. Experience is to the contrary. Simoons and co-workers (1985) reported an incidence of ventricular fibrillation of 14 per cent in patients receiving thrombolytic therapy compared with 23 per cent in a control group. These findings suggest that reduction in infarct size, consequent upon reperfusion, may in fact protect against ventricular fibrillation and more than offset any small incidence of ventricular fibrillation associated with reperfusion.

Antidepressants

Overdose of tricyclic antidepressants frequently results in ECG abnormalities, heart block, and arrhythmias (Pellinen *et al.* 1987). Similar problems can occasionally arise at therapeutic concentrations.

In the therapeutic range, tricyclic antidepressants frequently cause a slight increase in heart rate of up to 10 beats per minute. This effect is mainly due to anticholinergic actions, but in some patients orthostatic hypotension may be a contributory factor. The resulting sinus tachycardia is rarely of clinical consequence although an increase in oxygen consumption may be undesirable in patients with coronary artery disease.

Tricyclic drugs have Class Ia antiarrhythmic properties (Rawling and Fozzard 1978; Weld and Bigger 1980). In patients with heart disease, they have been shown to reduce the frequency of ventricular ectopic beats (Bigger *et al.* 1977; Veith *et al.* 1982). As with other antiarrhythmic agents, however, there is an accompanying proarrhythmic propensity. Fortunately, reports of serious proarrhythmic effects are rare. Amitriptyline and doxepin have been reported to cause *torsade de pointes* (Stratmann and Kennedy 1987).

As regards newer antidepressant drugs, maprotiline, a tetracyclic agent, has similar cardiovascular effects to the tricyclics. Its effects on conduction, and its antiarrhythmic and proarrhythmic properties are similar to those of the tricyclics. Like the tricyclics, it has been reported to cause *torsade de pointes* (Herrmann *et al.* 1983). Some of the newer antidepressant drugs appear to be less cardiotoxic than the tricyclics (Jackson *et al.* 1987; Halper and Mann 1988). The triazolopyridine derivative trazodone, which is unrelated to tricyclic and tetracyclic antidepressant agents, has no anticholinergic effects or depressant effects on conduction. Its proarrhythmic potential is low, although an increase in frequency of ventricular ectopic beats has been described (Janowsky *et al.* 1983). The selective 5-HT re-uptake blocker zimelidine is also considered to have low proarrhythmic potential. *Torsade de pointes* has, however, been reported during overdosage (Liljeqvist and Edvardsson 1989). Mianserin and fluoxetine have been reported to be devoid of proarrhythmic actions (Halper and Mann 1988).

It is important to recognize, when treating arrhythmias due to tricyclic overdose, that tricyclics have Class I antiarrhythmic properties. Treatment with additional Class I antiarrhythmic drugs is likely to be detrimental and these are best avoided.

Phenothiazines

Phenothiazine antipsychotic agents, particularly chlorpromazine and thioridazine, can have significant cardiac sequelae. There is often an increase in heart rate, and QT prolongation and T-wave changes are not uncommon. T-wave changes may persist for up to 2 weeks after cessation of drug therapy (Risch *et al.* 1981). Bundle branch block, complete heart block, and atrial and ventricular tachyarrhythmias are less common but do occur (Risch *et al.* 1981). Sudden death has occurred in patients taking phenothiazines; although the exact cause is unclear it is thought to be due to ventricular tachycardia or complete heart block.

The proarrhythmic properties of phenothiazines are a reason for caution when combining these agents with conventional Class I antiarrhythmic drugs or tricyclic antidepressants. Such combinations are best avoided.

Alcohol

Alcohol is one of the commonest causes of atrial fibrillation, accounting for 15–35 per cent of hospital admissions with new-onset atrial fibrillation (Lowenstein *et al.* 1983; Koskinen *et al.* 1987). Amongst patients aged under 65, it has been reported to account for as many as two-thirds of cases of new-onset atrial fibrillation.

Some of these patients have an overt alcohol-related heart disease (see below). In others, however, there may be no overt chronic heart disease and it seems probable that the arrhythmia is due to acute intoxication. It is well established that alcoholic binges may induce episodes of atrial fibrillation. Attacks cluster at weekends and over holiday periods. Because of this, the arrhythmia has been termed the 'holiday heart syndrome' (Ettinger *et al.* 1978).

clear why acute intoxication with alcohol
use atrial fibrillation. There are a number of
es. These include electrolyte disturbances,
such as hypokalaemia and hypomagnesaemia, which are
often present in heavy drinkers, excess circulating catecholamines, and the effects of acetaldehyde, one of the
metabolic products of alcohol. In addition, alcohol may
have direct electrophysiological effects on the myocardium. Greenspon and Schaal (1983) studied 14 patients
with a history of alcohol-related rhythm disturbances by
invasive electrophysiological testing. In the baseline
state, it was not possible to induce atrial tachyarrhythmias
in any patient. After alcohol intake, repeated electrophysiological testing was able to induce a sustained atrial
tachyarrhythmia in five of 14 patients.

Atrial fibrillation in patients with features of acute
alcohol intoxication is generally of short duration,
patients reverting spontaneously to sinus rhythm within
24 hours (Lowenstein *et al*. 1983). In the absence of
haemodynamic compromise, additional treatment may
not be necessary. Provided there is no overt cardiomyopathy, abstinence will generally prevent arrhythmia recurrence and additional prophylaxis is unnecessary.

Caffeine and methylxanthines

Caffeine has a sympathomimetic effect on the cardiovascular system. Acute caffeine ingestion increases
blood pressure and heart rate (Curtalo and Robinson
1983). Despite the widespread belief that coffee drinking
can cause palpitation, the evidence is equivocal. Electrophysiological studies have shown that caffeine shortens
the refractory period of the right atrium, atrioventricular
node, and right ventricle, and increases the frequency of
sustained tachycardia induced by the extra-stimulus
technique (Dobmeyer *et al*. 1983). A further study has
shown no arrhythmogenic effect of modest coffee intake
(Graboys *et al*. 1989). Sutherland and colleagues (1985)
found that coffee drinking did cause an increase in
arrhythmias, but only in susceptible individuals. The
evidence in relation to more serious ventricular arrhythmias is questionable. Two studies have assessed the
effects of caffeine in susceptible patients. Myers and
others (1987) studied 70 patients during the healing
phase of myocardial infarction, and found no increase in
either the frequency or severity of ventricular arrhythmias. Graboys and colleagues (1989) looked at 50
patients with a history of ventricular tachyarrhythmias
(ventricular tachycardia or fibrillation), and also found
no evidence to support a role for caffeine in arrhythmogenesis. Caffeine toxicity leads to marked sympathetic
activation and is associated with tachyarrhythmias,

hypokalaemia, metabolic acidosis, and hypotension
(Benowitz *et al*. 1982).

In conclusion then, susceptible individuals may experience caffeine-induced arrhythmias. Although caffeine is not contraindicated in patients with heart disease
or a history of arrhythmias, it may be a contributory
factor in arrhythmogenesis.

Theophylline is a common therapy for reversible airways disease. Its most common cardiac effect is a slight
increase in heart rate with minimal effect on blood
pressure. Patients with severe obstructive lung disease or
heart disease are particularly vulnerable to atrial and
ventricular arrhythmias (Van Dellen 1979).

Drug and solvent abuse

The deliberate inhalation of volatile substances to obtain
a 'high' is a relatively common cause of sudden death in
young adolescents: 80 such deaths were recorded in
Britain in 1983 (H.R. Anderson *et al*. 1985). Although
solvent abuse may cause chronic toxicity and cardiomyopathy (McLeod *et al*. 1987), there is extensive
evidence that these deaths are primarily arrhythmic,
induced by acute drug toxicity (Boon 1987). Experimental evidence has shown that volatile substances can sensitize the heart to the action of catecholamines (Shepherd
1989). Sudden death in cases of solvent abuse is often
associated with exercise (Bass 1970), so it has been
suggested that volatile hydrocarbons may sensitize the
heart to the arrhythmogenic effects of adrenergic stimulation (Boon 1987). Although in most instances the
cause of death is not documented, ventricular fibrillation
has been described (Gunn *et al*. 1989).

Cocaine has complex cardiovascular effects (for reviews, see Billman 1990; Isner and Chokshi 1991). Isner
and colleagues (1986) reviewed 26 patients who had
developed cardiovascular problems, directly related to
cocaine. The adverse effects of cocaine in these cases
included ventricular tachycardia, ventricular fibrillation,
acute myocardial infarction, sudden death, or a combination of these events. The authors concluded that
underlying heart disease was not a prerequisite and that
serious cardiovascular events could arise in patients with
normal hearts without predisposing factors. They
further concluded that adverse cardiac consequences
could occur with normal 'recreational' drug concentrations and that adverse effects were not confined to
massive overdosage. Most patients who had experienced
adverse cardiovascular effects took the drug intranasally.
Adverse effects are therefore not confined to parenteral
use of the drug. The effects of cocaine on myocardial
perfusion are discussed below.

Sudden death has also been reported following abuse of the amphetamine analogues MDMA (3,4-methylenedioxymethamphetamine, 'Ecstasy') and MDEA (3,4,-methylenedioxyethamphetamine, 'Eve') (Dowling *et al.* 1987). Serious arrhythmias are well recognized as complicating amphetamine overdose (Benowitz *et al.* 1979) and it seems probable that at least some of these deaths are due to arrhythmias. Underlying heart disease is certainly one factor that predisposes individuals to sudden death while using these drugs. Whether individuals without cardiac disease are also at risk is unclear.

Drugs causing bradyarrhythmias

Drug-induced bradycardias are widely reported. Resultant conduction disturbances include sinus node dysfunction, progressive forms of atrioventricular block, and asystole. The mechanisms underlying these effects may be classified into:

(1) effects that are predictable from knowledge of a drug's electrophysiological properties. Examples of these include all antiarrhythmic agents, β-adrenoceptor antagonists, and calcium antagonists such as verapamil and diltiazem;

(2) indirect effects on cardiac impulse generation and conduction that are secondary to a drug's effects on the patient's metabolic status, including the induction of myocardial ischaemia (Reedy and Zwiren 1983; Richards *et al.* 1985; Martin *et al.* 1987; Nemer *et al.* 1988);

(3) indirect effects on cardiac impulse generation and conduction that are secondary to a drug's effects on haemodynamics. In response to these changes, activation of major reflex arcs, such as the Jarold–von Bezold reflex, occurs (Mark 1983). The efferent limb of this reflex comprises vasodilatation and an increase in vagal tone on the sinus and atrioventricular nodes resulting in significant bradycardia. Cardioinhibition induced through these mechanisms is exemplified by reports concerning nitrate-induced asystole (Rodger and Hyman 1932; Come and Pitt 1976; Lancaster and Fenster 1983);

(4) an idiopathic effect in which the mechanism has yet to be determined.

Unfortunately, in some reports of drug-induced cardiac arrest, the rhythm during the arrest is not given. Many descriptions of drug-induced bradycardias appear in the form of isolated case reports in which essential details that would enable a reasonably firm cause-and-effect relationship to be derived are absent. In many instances, the drug-induced bradycardia occurs when the offending agent is present in toxic doses (Sznajder *et al.* 1984; Brady and Horgan 1988). The compounding effects of pharmacokinetic and pharmacodynamic interactions are often not addressed (Durelli *et al.* 1985; Macnab *et al.* 1987).

The negative chronotropic and dromotropic effects of individual anaesthetic agents, either administered for a local effect or given systemically, are particularly difficult to assess. Many anaesthetic agents have well-defined effects on cardiac cellular electrophysiology, and bradycardia could be predicted from a knowledge of these effects. Serious bradycardia may occur after the induction of general anaesthesia, involving the administration of several drugs. Moreover, the induction of anaesthesia engenders complex changes in cardiovascular reflexes. Bradycardias may reflect a complex interplay between direct drug effects and reflex homoeostatic mechanisms. In the following review, only those agents reported by several authors to cause pathological bradycardias when given in recommended doses and for which a direct, causal relationship seems likely will be discussed.

β-Blockers

As might be expected, β-blockers can cause an excessive bradycardia in some patients. This Type A adverse reaction is due to an excessive therapeutic effect. Often patients will have an underlying predisposition to bradycardia, such as sick sinus syndrome.

Excessive bradycardia may also arise from drug interactions. The interaction with verapamil is particularly well recognized, giving rise to sinus bradycardia and atrioventricular nodal block. Verapamil and β-blockers should not be administered together intravenously. Similarly, patients on oral treatment with one agent should not receive the other intravenously. Problems may also arise occasionally when the drugs are combined orally (Hutchison *et al.* 1984). Excessive bradycardia due to an interaction between oral verapamil and topical β-blockers, administered as eye-drops, has been reported (Pringle and MacEwen 1987).

This interaction is not confined to verapamil. Although the combination of a β-blocker with diltiazem is widely used in the treatment of angina and is in general well tolerated, it may occasionally result in excessive bradycardia. Hassell and Creamer (1989) reported two cases of severe sinus bradycardia induced by the combination of diltiazem with a β-blocker.

Class I antiarrhythmics

It is rare for therapeutic doses of antiarrhythmic drugs to

cause excessive bradycardia. By contrast, toxic doses can result in sinus bradycardia or arrest. When excessive sinus bradycardia does occur in the therapeutic range, this generally reflects pre-existing sinus node disease (Goldberg 1982; Hellestrand et al. 1984). Antiarrhythmic drugs may similarly result in sinoatrial block in patients with pre-existing sinus node dysfunction.

Class I antiarrhythmic drugs, particularly Ic agents (flecainide, encainide, and propafenone), frequently prolong the PR interval and QRS duration in the surface electrocardiogram. It is relatively rare, however, for higher degrees of block to arise within the therapeutic range. Higher degrees of block can arise with toxic drug concentrations, but once again block with therapeutic levels generally reflects pre-existing disease.

Antidepressants

Following the discovery of a causal link between lethal arrhythmias and the use of antidepressant drugs (Coull et al. 1970; Williams and Sherter 1971), especially amitriptyline, which is a member of the tricyclic group, there has been much debate about their safety in patients with cardiac disease (Halper and Mann 1988). Tricyclic agents may prolong the PR, QRS, and QT intervals of the surface ECG. The effects are dose related and are more likely to arise with drug concentrations at the upper end of the therapeutic range (Glassman 1984). These electrocardiographic features are generally without consequence. Higher degrees of heart block are rare unless a patient has pre-existing conduction abnormalities.

Roose and colleagues (1987) conducted a prospective study in 196 patients with depression treated with tricyclic agents (imipramine or nortriptyline) over a period of 9 years; 155 patients had normal electrocardiograms on entry to the study, and the remainder had first-degree block or bundle branch block, or both. Plasma concentrations of the drugs were monitored in approximately half the patients. Nine per cent of those with bundle branch block progressed to second-degree heart block compared with only 0.7 per cent of those with normal cardiograms. In fact, the patient who developed heart block with a previously normal electrocardiogram was later shown to have abnormal His–Purkinje conduction and required permanent pacing. Of 11 patients with first-degree block, none showed progression. These findings are consistent with the known electrophysiological actions of the tricyclics. These drugs act principally on the distal conduction system and hence are a particular risk in patients with bundle branch block.

In his review, Orme (1984) concluded that patients with severe heart disease, defined as heart failure, recent myocardial infarction, or electrocardiographic evidence of bundle branch block or high-degree atrioventricular block should not receive tricyclic agents. These recommendations appear to be well founded. Of the second-generation antidepressants, maprotiline (Hermann et al. 1983) and trazodone (Rausch et al. 1984) have similar effects to the tricyclics on conduction. The tetracyclic agent mianserin appears to be relatively safe in patients with cardiac disease (Burrows et al. 1979). The tachyarrhythmic complications of antidepressants are discussed above.

Carbamazepine

Carbamazepine has been used widely in the treatment of various forms of epilepsy and trigeminal neuralgia. Second and third-degree heart block, which resolved on withdrawing the drug, have been reported (Beermann et al. 1975; Ladefoged and Mogelvang 1982; Boesen et al. 1983; Benassi et al. 1987). Severe bradyarrhythmias generally occur within 7–10 days of commencing therapy. Most of the affected patients are elderly and have pre-existing abnormalities of the resting electrocardiogram. It is likely that carbamazepine unmasks latent conduction system disease. These effects are a consequence of its known Class I effects on mammalian cardiac electrophysiology (Steiner et al. 1970).

Methyldopa

Formal study of the electrophysiological properties of methyldopa has shown that it lengthens the functional and effective refractory periods of the atrioventricular node and significantly prolongs the atrio–His interval during atrial pacing (Gould et al. 1979). The drug has been reported to cause symptomatic sinus bradycardia (Davis et al. 1981), sinus pauses (Scheinmann et al. 1978) and carotid sinus reflex hypersensitivity (Bauerenfiend et al. 1978; Alfino et al. 1981). More recent reports have demonstrated reversible first (Sadjadi et al. 1984), second (Cregler and Mark 1987), and third-degree block (Rosen et al. 1988), respectively.

H₂-antagonists

Asystole and sinus arrest were reported by Cohen and colleagues (1979) in two patients given intravenous cimetidine. In both instances, the bradyarrhythmias occurred within 10 minutes of the injection. They were reinduced on later exposure to the drug by the same route. In later reports, Tordjman and others (1984) and Ishizaki and associates (1987) reported the development of reversible third-degree and first-degree heart block, respectively, in patients given oral cimetidine. Sinus bradycardia and sinus arrest have also been observed with both oral and intravenous cimetidine (Redding *et al.* 1977; Jefferys and Vale 1978).

Bradycardias are not confined to cimetidine. A significant reduction in sinus rate was observed in two patients who were given ranitidine by the oral and intravenous routes by Camarri and colleagues (1982). Interestingly, the bradycardia was abolished after the administration of atropine. Furthermore, it was not reinduced when the same patients were given cimetidine. In another report, asystole occurred after the fifth dose of intravenous ranitidine (Hart 1989) in a young man with no known cardiovascular disease.

The mechanism underlying these rare but dangerous bradycardias is unknown. It has been suggested that they may be manifestations of cardiac ischaemia induced by blockade of the H_2-receptors in the coronary vasculature, which leads to vasoconstriction (Baumann *et al.* 1982). Alternatively, there may be enhancement of parasympathetic tone by inhibition of cholinesterase (Hansen and Bertl 1983).

Drugs causing impairment of cardiac function

Drug effects on cardiac performance

The function of the heart as a pump may be adversely affected by drugs through changes in heart rhythm (as already discussed above) or through interference with the normal physiological contractile processes. Effects on the former have direct consequences on the latter, such as when the rate is too fast or too slow, or the rhythm too irregular, rendering cardiac chamber pumping activity ineffectual. The haemodynamic effects of cardiac arrhythmias have been well known for some time (Resnekov 1970). In addition, conduction defects may compromise cardiac pumping efficacy by inducing asynchronous ventricular contractions (Gibson *et al.* 1988). Asynchronous ventricular contraction induced by drugs is, however, of relatively minor importance in comparison with the ventricular asynchrony which may follow myocardial infarction. This issue will therefore not be discussed further in this chapter.

Drugs can adversely affect the contractile function of the myocardium by direct injury resulting in myocytolysis, which reduces the number of viable myocardial cells, or by direct effects on contractile force (inotropy) or ability to relax (compliance). In addition, drugs may influence contractile function indirectly by causing myocardial ischaemia, by altering preload or afterload, or by causing changes in the interstitial matrix of the myocardium (Caulfield and Bittner 1988). These drug effects may be desirable in certain circumstances but detrimental in others. For instance, β-adrenoceptor blockers and calcium antagonists are known to cause depression of myocardial excitability, conduction, and contraction, and these are put to good use in the treatment of angina, tachyarrhythmias, and hypertrophic obstructive cardiomyopathy, but they can be detrimental in heart failure. Any undesirable cardiac effects caused by these drugs can be regarded as pharmacologically predictable and avoidable by careful dose titration. Similarly, positive inotropic agents are very useful in severe heart failure, but when given to patients with obstructive cardiomyopathy, they can paradoxically induce or worsen the failure. Diuretics and nitrates are widely used in the treatment of patients with acute left ventricular failure following myocardial infarction, but their use in patients with right ventricular infarction may sometimes precipitate shock (due to relative hypovolaemia and hence underfilling of the left ventricle).

Unlike the diagnosis of arrhythmia, in which body surface and intracardiac electrocardiography can detect the abnormality clearly, the diagnosis of myocardial toxicity and depression cannot be made as readily *in vivo*, even with invasive techniques. Interpretation of the published results is therefore necessarily more complicated, and great care must be exercised before one can infer that myocardial toxicity or depression is directly due to the drug under investigation. Because of this, consideration of the methodology employed in studying these drug effects is warranted.

Cardiomyotoxic effects

Methods employed in studying cardiomyotoxic effects

The study of myocardial injury has traditionally relied on histological methods to identify morphological changes in the cellular structures that depict injury. The pattern of changes varies according to the initiating insult, the response to the injury, and the time of observation after the injury. The presence of late changes (e.g. fibrosis) would indicate that irreversible injury has occurred, but it is difficult to be categorical about which early changes signify the reversible or irreversible stages of injury. Furthermore, the sensitivity and specificity of these methods are usually adequate in the identification of large areas of damage, caused by such insults as myocardial infarction, but they may not be sensitive enough to detect single cell deaths, scattered throughout the myocardium. Such low-level changes are more typical of the injuries induced by drugs. Newer techniques, with greater sensitivity and specificity in identifying cell death, are required to study adverse drug reactions on the myocardium (Clark *et al.* 1989).

Many case reports have been published relating particular drugs to the development of cardiomyopathy. It is generally agreed that documentation of such observations is valuable, especially when the same observation is repeatedly made in different cases receiving the same medication. Otherwise, it is often difficult to establish the aetiological role of the drug. This is because of the fact that myocarditis and cardiomyopathy can often occur coincidentally during the course of drug therapy and the diagnosis of these conditions cannot be easily confirmed. It is therefore difficult to prove that a drug has caused a cardiomyopathy. It is equally difficult, however, to prove that a drug is innocent.

Positive inotropic agents

Sympathomimetic agents

By far the most cardiotoxic and the most extensively studied of all sympathomimetic agents is isoprenaline (isoproterenol). Other agents, however, such as adrenaline (epinephrine) and noradrenaline (norepinephrine), which are widely used in intensive care units, have also been shown to cause catecholamine cardiomyopathy. The analogous clinical condition is phaeochromocytoma (Alpert *et al.* 1972; Garcia and Jennings 1972; Cho *et al.* 1987). Whether other commonly used sympathomimetic agents, such as dopamine and dobutamine, can produce similar damage is unknown. The reason may well be that these agents are not as toxic as isoprenaline and noradrenaline. More sensitive methods of detecting small amounts of damage have only recently become available (Benjamin *et al.* 1989).

The characteristic features of the myocardial pathology induced by isoprenaline have been well described (Reichenbach and Benditt 1970; Todd *et al.* 1985*a*). Histological changes (contraction band lesions) can occur as early as 5 minutes after commencement of a high-dose isoprenaline infusion (Todd *et al.* 1985*b*) but these may not constitute irreversible cell damage. The earliest occurrence of cardiomyocyte death was noted 3 hours after subcutaneous injection of isoprenaline (Benjamin *et al.* 1989), and this reaches a peak at about 24 hours. Most of the necrosis occurs in the subendocardial region (Benjamin *et al.* 1989). Unlike isoprenaline, noradrenaline has predominantly vasoconstrictive effects, but the pathological features of myocardial injury are similar to those induced by isoprenaline (Todd *et al.* 1985*b*).

Although catecholamine-induced cardiotoxicity has been known for over 30 years, the mechanisms responsible for the injury have not been fully elucidated. Rona (1985) has suggested that the injurious process is multifactorial, involving a combination of haemodynamic effects (myocardial hypoperfusion — especially in the subendocardial region, tachycardia, increased inotropy), free radical injury via catecholamine oxidative products, microvascular lesions, reperfusion injury, and intracellular calcium overload. The process is often exacerbated in the presence of pre-existing ischaemia secondary to coronary artery disease (Reichenbach and Benditt 1970).

Practical clinical guidelines

The question that arises from the above discussion is therefore whether one should refrain from using sympathomimetic agents to 'flog the tired horse', especially in post-myocardial infarction pump failure. There is an inevitable conflict between the need to 'rest' and preserve the myocardium and the need to stimulate cardiac performance to preserve life. The careful selection of patients who require inotropic support is necessary. Those with adequate cardiac output and systemic arterial pressure should receive vasodilators if support is indicated, rather than positive inotropic agents. Those with markedly impaired cardiac function, such that coronary perfusion pressure is compromised, would benefit from inotropic support, because improvement in coronary perfusion would allay further ischaemic injury. Those with a dilated ventricle may also benefit from inotropic support because a small reduction in ventricular volume may lead to reduction in one major component of myocardial oxygen consumption — the wall tension-related energy requirement (Gibbs *et al.* 1967).

Another practical question is: how long can one safely maintain the patient on catecholamine treatment? Obviously, if the cardiac status is such that inotropic support is no longer necessary, then a catecholamine infusion should be terminated. Not uncommonly, however, one finds that the patient is dependent on the inotropic support. Will the cumulative effect of a prolonged infusion be more detrimental? The answer is that, quite unlike doxorubicin cardiotoxicity, the injury is not proportional to the cumulative dose, provided a steady infusion is maintained. This is because, during prolonged steady infusion, there is gradual desensitization of β-adrenoceptors that renders the cardiac myocyte less susceptible to further catecholamine-induced injury (Tan and Clark 1990). In fact, prolonged infusion of dobutamine has been shown to produce beneficial functional effects (Liang *et al.* 1984). It is not uncommon to see some of the cardiogenic shock patients so treated able to walk out of hospital despite having very limited cardiac reserve. The mechanism of this beneficial effect is presumably peripheral conditioning, similar to that obtained by athletes in the course of exercise-endurance training.

β-Blocker withdrawal

Cardiac events such as unstable angina, acute myocardial infarction or exacerbation of arrhythmia, may follow abrupt β-blocker withdrawal (see below). Such rebound phenomena have been known for more than two decades (Slome 1973; Miller *et al.* 1975). Obviously, not all patients will suffer rebound phenomena on stopping β-blockers, but unfortunately there is no way of predicting which patients are susceptible. The mechanism is thought to be β-adrenoceptor up-regulation with prolonged β-blockade (Glaubiger and Lefkowitz 1977; Heilbrunn *et al.* 1989). Sudden stoppage exposes these extra receptors to unopposed adrenergic stimulation and, in susceptible subjects, it may result in adverse cardiac events which include the cardiomyotoxic effects of endogenous catecholamines.

Other positive inotropic agents

As described above, the mechanism of a drug's ability to generate positive inotropic effects is closely linked to its ability to induce cardiotoxicity. The final common pathway may well be an increase in intracellular calcium, which, in the latter case, is excessive (Fleckenstein 1971; Katz and Reuter 1979; Auffermann *et al.* 1989). Interestingly, calcium excess is also one mode whereby these positive inotropic agents induce arrhythmias (see above). It has been proposed that calcium overload stimulates intracellular phospholipase activity, which in turn causes disintegration of the sarcolemmal membrane, which heralds cell death (Farber *et al.* 1981). It is therefore not surprising that other positive inotropic agents can also induce cardiomyotoxic effects.

Angiotensin has been shown to possess positive inotropic effects (Koch-Weser 1965; Freer *et al.* 1976), and also to cause myocardial necrosis (Gavras *et al.* 1971, 1975; Giacomelli *et al.* 1976; Bhan *et al.* 1982). Both exogenous and endogenous angiotensin II are capable of inducing cardiomyotoxicity (Tan *et al.* 1989).

Digoxin has been used in clinical practice for over 200 years, often as a positive inotropic agent although it is only a weak inotrope. It has a narrow therapeutic range, above which it can increase intracellular calcium (by inhibition of the sodium ATPase pump), but arrhythmogenic effects are more prominent than any cardiomyolytic effects (see above).

Newer non-glycoside and non-catecholaminergic positive inotropic agents, such as the phosphodiesterase inhibitors amrinone, milrinone, and enoximone, have recently been introduced into clinical practice. Direct data on whether they cause cardiac myocyte necrosis is not yet available. Surveys on their effects on mortality in heart failure patients suggest that they may shorten patients' survival (Packer and Leier 1987), but whether this is due to cardiotoxic or proarrhythmic effects of the drugs, or due to the fact that patients receiving these agents are more severely ill, is unknown.

Chemotherapeutic agents

Anthracyclines

Doxorubicin (adriamycin) and daunorubicin (Rubidomycin, Daunomycin) are the best known cardiotoxic antimitotic drugs of the anthracycline antibiotics class. Their antimitotic activity stems from binding to DNA and impairing DNA-polymerase activity and RNA synthesis (Galton 1983). They also interact with cellular enzymes, to generate free radicals which lead to damage of membrane lipids, and bind directly to the cytoskeletal protein spectrin and to cardiolipin, thereby disturbing ion transport. Unfortunately, cardiac myocytes may be susceptible to one or more of these mechanisms of action of the anthracyclines.

Prolonged administration causes cumulative irreversible myocardial damage, culminating in dilated cardiomyopathy, congestive cardiac failure, and cardiogenic shock (Bonadonna and Monfardini 1969; Marmont *et al.* 1969; Kaduk and Seiler 1978). With daunorubicin the incidence of heart failure is dose related, at four per cent in patients receiving cumulative doses up to 550 mg per m^2 and at 14 per cent in those receiving up to 1050 mg per m^2 (von Hoff and Layard 1981; von Hoff *et al.* 1979, 1982; Adams 1982). The risk is higher in children than in adults. Overall, some seven to nine per cent of patients treated with doxorubicin may present with heart failure. This is also dose-related, occurring in three per cent of those receiving a cumulative dose of 400 mg per m^2 and 20 per cent of those receiving 700 mg per m^2 (Adams 1982; von Hoff *et al.* 1982). Moreover, one-fifth of asymptomatic patients had an abnormal resting left ventricular ejection fraction (Dresdale *et al.* 1983). Patients who have received cyclophosphamide or radiotherapy to the chest are more susceptible to anthracycline cardiotoxicity (Minow *et al.* 1977).

The development of heart failure in these patients depends on several factors. The occurrence of toxicity depends on the susceptibility not only of the individual patient but also of the individual myocytes. The reasons for variation in susceptibility are largely unknown. For some reason children are more susceptible. The elderly are also said to be more susceptible, but this may reflect diminished cardiac reserve before treatment in this age-group.

There have been several recommendations on how to institute anthracycline therapy so as to minimize cardiotoxicity (Minow *et al.* 1977; Legha *et al.* 1982). A rational approach is to assess cardiac function with whatever techniques are available locally (as a minimum, an ECG, chest radiograph, and echocardiogram) before treatment, and to repeat the assessment at regular intervals during treatment. Changes indicative of significant cardiac myocyte loss (e.g. loss of R wave amplitude in the ECG, reduced systolic function in the echocardiogram), resulting in onset of compensatory mechanisms (e.g. resting tachycardia, ventricular and atrial dilatation), should indicate that the maximum advisable cumulative dose of anthracycline has been reached, even though the recommended maximum of 550 mg per m^2 may not have been exceeded. By the time patients present with symptoms and signs of heart failure, excessive myocardial damage must have occurred and the prognosis is very poor. Whether more invasive methods of monitoring cardiac effects, such as with regular endomyocardial biopsy (Billingham and Bristow 1984), would provide a more accurate aid in deciding when to discontinue treatment has not been established.

Alcohol

Although ethanol is no longer used in medical practice (except as a disinfectant and a solvent), it is a widely consumed sedative–hypnotic social drug. The syndrome of heart failure is common amongst patients who abuse alcohol. The genesis of the heart failure is multifactorial. Alcohol is a direct myocardial depressant; additionally, alcoholism may precipitate failure due to poor nutritional intake; and finally, alcohol abuse may cause cardiomyopathy, although evidence on this point is surprisingly poor.

There is still no scientifically rigorous evidence to support the hypothesis that alcohol induces dilated cardiomyopathy. To prove that a drug causes cardiomyopathy, it is essential to demonstrate that cardiac myocyte necrosis with its attendant fibrosis follows its administration. This has not been achieved in any animal experimental model with alcohol (Urbano-Marquez *et al.* 1989). The cumulative effect of necrosis eventually leads to the histological pattern of the myocardium seen in patients with dilated cardiomyopathy. The converse is not necessarily true: that is, the presence of histological evidence of dilated cardiomyopathy in a patient who has been abusing alcohol does not necessarily imply that alcohol is the cause. The histological features are indistinguishable from those of primary dilated cardiomyopathy and it is not possible to distinguish the two.

The questions whether those diagnosed as having 'alcoholic cardiomyopathy' would indeed have developed cardiomyopathy without alcohol, whether alcohol hastens the onset of heart failure in susceptible subjects, or whether it causes cardiomyopathy *de novo*, are as yet unsettled. It is worth noting that many long-term alcoholics do not develop dilated cardiomyopathy (Askanas *et al.* 1980; Kino *et al.* 1981; Kelbaek *et al.* 1984).

In vivo and *in vitro* administration of ethanol has been shown to depress myocardial function reversibly (Regan *et al.* 1965; Conway 1968; Nakano and Moere 1972; Timmis *et al.* 1975; Abel 1980; Thomas *et al.* 1980). They are associated with biochemical changes that are also reversible (Sarma *et al.* 1976; Rubin 1979). Alcoholics are notoriously unreliable in providing information about how much they drink (confabulation is not an unusual feature), but Urbano-Marquez and colleagues (1989) have recently claimed success in this attempt and showed dose-related left ventricular dysfunction in a group of alcoholics who have consumed the equivalent of 1200–3500 ml of wine per day for many years. Since alcohol directly depresses myocardial function, a practical point of vital importance is that all patients with dilated cardiomyopathy must abstain from further consumption of alcohol. Some improvement of cardiac function can be expected with abstinence.

There have been many reports of resolution of a cardiomyopathic picture on abstaining (Demakis *et al.* 1974; Kosinski 1989), but equally, in clinical practice, there are many more who remain in congestive heart failure despite abstinence and these cases are not published. Another reason why we need to keep an open mind is that it is not uncommon to see spontaneous normalization of cardiac function in patients with myocarditis (Olinde and Connel 1993). This condition can indeed occur coincidentally in some heavy drinkers, who are inevitably diagnosed as having alcoholic cardiomyopathy. If alcohol were truly toxic and produced histological features of fibrous tissue replacement of myocytes (Urbano-Marquez 1989), such cardiomyopathy would not be expected to resolve completely, unlike myocarditis.

That alcoholism can indirectly precipitate heart failure secondary to poor nutritional intake, resulting in beri-beri heart disease, is well known. In this condition, other manifestations of thiamine deficiency, such as peripheral neuropathy and myopathy, are often present. The treatment is abstinence, vitamin supplementation (including thiamine), and return to normal food intake. The prognosis is good and complete recovery can be expected. No doubt some alcoholics with heart failure may have subclinical levels of malnutrition, and may benefit from vitamin supplementation.

Cocaine

Abuse of cocaine has been associated with many hazards (Cregler and Mark 1986; Isner *et al.* 1986), including death (Mittleman and Wetli 1984; Schachne *et al.* 1984). In a canine model, it has been shown to produce dose-dependent ventricular systolic and diastolic depression (Abel *et al.* 1989). Direct cocaine cardiotoxicity has also been shown by endocardial biopsy (Peng *et al.* 1989). Cocaine is also known as a blocker of the noradrenaline uptake–1 process (Blinks 1966; Iversen 1967). It can therefore potentiate the effects of endogenous catechol-amine and indirectly induce myocardial damage. More recently, Welder and colleagues (1988) have shown that it can induce necrosis directly in cardiac myocytes. The mechanism of this action has not been elucidated.

Myocardial depression

Methods used in studying drug-induced cardiodepression

Just as myotoxicity is often implicated when cardio-myopathy occurs during the use of certain drugs, there are abundant anecdotes of the onset of the syndrome of heart failure associated with drug therapy. This question is compounded by the fact that there is current confusion as to the most appropriate definition of heart failure (Poole Wilson 1989). It should be appreciated that the clinical syndrome of heart failure, as commonly under-stood, does not necessarily arise from myocardial de-pression. It can arise from undue loading of a non-failing heart, for example, with fluid overloading or with excess-ive vasoconstriction. Therefore, when perusing case re-ports that associate the onset of heart failure with drug therapy, caution has to be exercised to note whether the mechanism of failure is indeed myocardial depression, as opposed to contributions from arrhythmia, conduction defects, silent ischaemia per infarction, asynchronous ventricular contraction, heart rate alteration, or unsuit-able preload or afterload. These factors, whether singly or in combination, can precipitate the clinical syndrome of heart failure.

The starting point in gathering information on ino-tropic effects of drugs is usually the study of cardiac muscle strips. Often, due to ease of isolation, atrial muscle is used, and this may behave differently from ventricular muscle. Results in isolated muscle do not necessarily correlate with *in vivo* haemodynamic results (see Procainamide section below). Similarly, *in vivo* animal experimental results cannot be automatically extrapolated and applied to clinical practice, owing to species differences and the greater complexity of clinical conditions. More recently, human cardiac muscle strips have been increasingly used to study drug inotropic effects. *In vitro* effects again, however, may not reflect clinical practice. For example, in a comparative study, nifedipine has been found to be more negatively ino-tropic in isolated human cardiac muscles than either verapamil or diltiazem (see below), which is quite con-trary to clinical experience.

Unlike myotoxic effects of drugs, however, the nega-tive inotropic effects are reversible. Myocardial depress-ant activity, therefore, can be studied by rechallenge under controlled conditions, in order to delineate the various factors influencing ventricular performance. Herein lies another problem: how does one evaluate cardiac function *in vivo*, especially in patients, to deter-mine whether a drug directly depresses myocardial func-tion? The most common methods of studying drug effects on myocardial function in the clinical context have been the use of non-invasive techniques, such as left ventricular ejection fraction, echocardiographic assess-ments, or systolic time intervals (Matos *et al.* 1977; Boudoulas *et al.* 1977a; Trimarco *et al.* 1983). It is well known that ejection fraction and systolic time intervals are highly dependent not only on inotropic states but also on the preload, afterload, heart rate, and the pres-ence of valvular regurgitation. Even the absence of any changes in ejection fraction may be due to balanced effects from negative inotropism and vasodilation. At-tempts to infer that a drug has directly depressed cardiac function because of an observed fall in ejection fraction (e.g. Kowey *et al.* 1982), without measuring effects on peripheral vascular resistance, are methodologically un-justifiable. Therefore, a large number of studies report-ing drug inotropic effects using these methods need to be interpreted with care.

Various indices specific for inotropy have been pro-posed. The proponents of these indices derived them from studies of cardiac muscle mechanics, and made *a priori* claims that they are independent of other factors and solely reflect inotropy. Subsequently, however, when tested in intact hearts, especially in complex clinical cardiological situations, these indices have been found to be dependent on factors other than inotropy. Even the currently most widely accepted index of inotropy, the end-systolic ventricular elastance (E_{max}=end-systolic pressure/volume) has recently been shown to assess the pressure-generating capacity, leaving largely unassessed the flow-generating capacity (Shroff and Motz 1989). Because of these confounding factors, the use of these indices of contractility to identify direct myocardial de-pressant effects of drugs is often inconclusive.

The alternative to indices with *a priori* claims is to control the various factors individually and use analytical methods to arrive at the effects of the drug on a particular factor. For instance, heart rate and rhythm may be controlled by artificially pacing the right atrium. In the absence of changes in the morphology of surface electrocardiogram one can assume invariance of the conduction pattern. Preload can be controlled to some extent using physical means (e.g. by positive or negative lower-body pressure). The direct myocardial effect can then be measured by observing the haemodynamic changes brought about by intracoronary administration of the drug. This method is necessarily invasive and complex. Although it has been used in the study of certain positive inotropic agents (Colucci 1989), it has thus far not been used in the context of studying adverse drug effects on the myocardium. A less invasive and less complex analytical method has been proposed (Tan *et al*. 1987) that can in future be usefully applied to study drug reactions in patient populations, especially those with impaired ventricular function.

Antiarrhythmic agents

Apart from proarrhythmic effects, antiarrhythmic agents are also prone to depress myocardial function. Some, such as disopyramide, β-adrenoceptor blockers, and verapamil, are more prone to precipitate cardiac failure than others. Antiarrhythmic agents that are thought to be least negatively inotropic are lignocaine, mexiletine, tocainide, and oral amiodarone.

Representative drugs from each of the Vaughan Williams classes of antiarrhythmic agent are discussed below. Discussion on the mechanisms by which each drug induces negative inotropism is beyond the scope of this chapter. In general, drugs having direct myocardial depressant activity appear to decrease, by various pathways, the availability of calcium to the contractile elements (Silva Graça and van Zwieten 1972; Schlepper 1989). None of these antiarrhythmic agents is as yet known to induce cardiodepression by alteration in myofilament sensitivity to calcium (Blinks and Endoh 1986; Ruegg 1986).

Class Ia agents

Procainamide   It may come as a surprise to some readers to learn that procainamide at high doses has been shown to exert significant positive inotropic effects on isolated cat right ventricular papillary muscle (Hammermeister *et al*. 1972). This finding was later supported by observations of Williams and Mathew (1984). In the isolated Langendorff rat-heart preparation, however, there were mixed positive and negative inotropic effects of procainamide (Nahas *et al*. 1969).

In contrast, most *in vivo* animal studies have demonstrated a negative inotropic effect (Cote *et al*. 1973, 1975; Lertora *et al*. 1979) with doses above usual therapeutic concentrations. In conscious dogs, O'Rourke and co-workers (1969) did not observe any change in cardiac flow-generating capacity with procainamide infused at therapeutic doses. In a rare experiment, high-dose procainamide was injected into the left coronary artery, and this produced a transient decrease followed by a more sustained increase in left ventricular myocardial force (Folle and Aviado 1966).

The haemodynamic effects of procainamide in man are quite variable. Some studies show vasodilator effects (Burton *et al*. 1976; Block and Winkle 1983) while others show vasoconstriction (Karlsson and Sonnhag 1976) or no change (Miller *et al*. 1973). In most studies, some of them very elegantly performed, insufficient consideration has been given to the peripheral drug effects (e.g. Harrison *et al*. 1963; Jawad-Kanber and Sherrod 1974; Smitherman *et al*. 1979; Geleris *et al*. 1980), rendering the conclusions drawn on the direct inotropic effects of the drug rather questionable (MacAlpin 1975). Collating all the evidence, we may conclude that in man procainamide in therapeutic doses does not exert significant direct inotropic effects on the myocardium.

Quinidine   There is no doubt that, at supratherapeutic doses, quinidine depresses the contraction of isolated cardiac muscle (Hammermeister *et al*. 1972; Tomoda *et al*. 1972). At therapeutic concentrations, however, some claimed that it was negatively inotropic (Hammermeister *et al*. 1972; Tomoda *et al*. 1972), while others disputed this (Kennedy and West 1969; Lameijer and van Zwieten 1974). Studies in intact animals were equally inconclusive, although they all show significant peripheral vasodilatation following intravenous quinidine (Angelakos and Hastings 1960; Folle and Aviado 1966; Walsh and Horwitz 1979). As discussed above, part of the reason for uncertainty is that investigators have found it difficult to separate the inotropic effects, secondary to reflex sympathetic stimulation, from the direct inotropic effects of the drug. One way of circumventing this problem is to study the drug effects in transplanted hearts, and this was done in five patients (Mason *et al*. 1977a). Unfortunately, although there was no change in peripheral vascular resistance, cardiac pump function was thought to be reduced by a decrease in preload, which was presumably secondary to the venodilating effect of quinidine — this leaves the question of direct inotropic effects of intravenous quinidine largely unanswered.

There appears to be a greater consensus on the

myocardial effects of oral quinidine. In dogs, after 2 weeks of oral treatment, there was no obvious fall in blood pressure and myocardial contractility (O'Rourke and Horwitz 1981). Similar results have been reported in human volunteers and patients (Crawford *et al.* 1979). Most significantly, there was no apparent haemodynamic compromise in 652 patients (of whom 35 per cent had heart failure before treatment) treated with oral quinidine in the Boston Collaborative Drug Surveillance Program (Cohen *et al.* 1977).

Disopyramide There is general agreement that of all the Class I antiarrhythmic agents available disopyramide is the most negatively inotropic (Honerjager *et al.* 1986; Bourke *et al.* 1987). This detrimental effect is compounded by its vasoconstrictive effect, which also involves the coronary vasculature (Kötter *et al.* 1980). Studies on isolated cardiac muscle (Mokler and van Arman 1962; Naylor 1976), in intact animals (Walsh and Horwitz 1979), and in man (Jensen *et al.* 1975; Befeler 1975; Willis 1975; Naqvi *et al.* 1979; Leach *et al.* 1980; Thadani *et al.* 1981; Bauman 1981), demonstrated the significant cardiac depressant property of the drug, which may culminate in progressive heart failure (Story *et al.* 1979; Podrid *et al.* 1980).

Class Ib agents

Lignocaine (lidocaine) The *in vitro* effects of lignocaine on isolated muscle strips are uncertain, with reports demonstrating both the presence of negative inotropism (Hammermeister *et al.* 1972; Sheu and Lederer 1985) and its absence (Tomoda *et al.* 1972; Tejerina *et al.* 1983). Evaluation in intact animal hearts showed no significant negative inotropic effects with lignocaine in the dose range used clinically (Lieberman *et al.* 1968; Nahas *et al.* 1969), but it became significantly negatively inotropic at doses above the therapeutic range (Austen and Moran 1965; Nahas *et al.* 1969; Cote *et al.* 1973). Clinical studies have confirmed this finding (Harrison *et al.* 1963; Kötter *et al.* 1980). Even in patients with significant left ventricular dysfunction (Miller *et al.* 1973; Burton *et al.* 1976) lignocaine is relatively free of negative inotropic effects, making it one of the safest antiarrhythmic agents for patients with ventricular arrhythmia. Interestingly, in the last groups of patients, therapeutic doses of lignocaine produced systemic vasoconstriction that may even raise the systemic arterial pressure (Miller *et al.* 1973; Burton *et al.* 1976), without direct myocardial depression.

Mexiletine Studies in animals (Banim *et al.* 1977; Kuhn *et al.* 1977; Pozenel 1977; Carlier 1980; Marshall *et al.* 1981) and man (Campbell *et al.* 1979; Chamberlain *et al.* 1980; Stein *et al.* 1984) have shown that the negative inotropic effect of intravenous and oral mexiletine is minimal and clinical problems are rare.

Tocainide Like mexiletine, tocainide has minimal negative inotropic effects. Few animal studies regarding its direct inotropic effects are available. There is a suggestion of cardiodepression when enormous doses are given (Coltart *et al.* 1974). Two studies in patients undergoing cardiac catheterization showed myocardial depression (Schwartz *et al.* 1979; Ikram 1980). In patients with ischaemic left ventricular dysfunction, however, tocainide produced only a slight and transient rise in peripheral vascular resistance with minimal inotropic changes (Winkle *et al.* 1978; MacMahon *et al.* 1985). During long-term oral treatment with tocainide, only 1.4 per cent of 369 patients developed exacerbation of heart failure (Horn *et al.* 1980).

Class Ic agents

Flecainide Animal studies have demonstrated a direct cardiodepressant effect of flecainide (Hoddess *et al.* 1979; Verdouw *et al.* 1979). Earlier studies on patients with coronary artery disease suggested negative inotropism (Legrand *et al.* 1983; Serruys *et al.* 1983). In a similar group of patients with left ventricular ejection fractions ranging from 20–80 per cent, Josephson and colleagues (1985) demonstrated that flecainide clearly exerted direct myocardial depression. This problem may be compounded by the fact that flecainide clearance from plasma is reduced in heart failure patients (Franciosa *et al.* 1983; Conard and Ober 1984).

Propafenone Pharmacological experiments indicate that propafenone can directly depress myocardial function, partly because it has mild β-blocking and weak calcium antagonist activities (Ledda *et al.* 1981; Dukes and Vaughan Williams 1984; McLeod *et al.* 1984). In patients there are suggestions of negative inotropism (Shen *et al.* 1984; Brodsky *et al.* 1985; Baker *et al.* 1987), although categorical statements about whether the drug causes direct and clinically important cardiodepression must await more rigorous studies.

Class II agents

β-Blockers These agents have been used to treat arrhythmia for over 20 years (Gettes 1970). Their negative inotropic and chronotropic effects are also well known (Epstein *et al.* 1965; Sowton and Hamer 1966; Blinks 1967). Although these effects are desirable when treating, for example, myocardial ischaemia, hypertension, atrial fibrillation, or hypertrophic cardiomyopathy, the danger of inducing cardiac failure should be borne in mind (Conway *et al.* 1968). These type A reactions (excessive myocardial depression and bradycardia) are generally dose dependent, and may be avoided by dose reduction. Indeed, investigators have recently shown that low-dose β-blockade is not only safe but also beneficial in the treatment of dilated cardiomyopathy (J.L. Anderson *et al.* 1985; Engelmeier *et al.* 1985).

Treatment for adverse cardiac reaction to β-blockers depends on the haemodynamic status of the patient. If there is no significant haemodynamic compromise, the patient may be monitored on a coronary care unit until the β-blockade recedes. Bradycardia and conduction defects may be reversed by intravenous atropine (0.6 to 2.4 mg in an adult). If significant haemodynamic compromise occurs, and if the β-blocker is a competitive inhibitor (Blinks 1967; Dollery *et al.* 1969), then careful ECG and haemodynamic monitoring and infusion of an appropriate sympathomimetic agent should be instituted, with dosage titrated against response. High doses (e.g. 200 μg per kg per min of dobutamine) may be required. If there is insufficient response, or the β-blocker is non-competitive, then a phosphodiesterase inhibitor (e.g. milrinone or enoximone) with or without a vasoconstrictor agent may be needed.

β-Adrenoceptor down-regulation

After prolonged infusion of sympathomimetic agents as inotropic support, sudden stopping of the infusion sometimes results in precipitous circulatory collapse. This is secondary to adrenoceptor desensitization and uncoupling (Harden 1983; Karliner *et al.* 1986; Reithmann and Werdan 1989), the consequences of which are similar to β-blockade. It is therefore advisable to tail off the infusion very gradually at a rate commensurate with the resensitization of the adrenoceptors, which may take a day or more (Karliner *et al.* 1986).

Class III agents

Amiodarone   The most important issue surrounding the question 'does amiodarone induce myocardial depression?' is whether it is to the intravenous or the oral form of amiodarone that we are referring. Almost all reports on negative inotropism with amiodarone have been observed in the acute situation using the intravenous preparation of the drug (Singh *et al.* 1976; Installe *et al.* 1981; Schwartz *et al.* 1983). It is not clear how much of this is due to the solvent, polysorbate 80, which is known to be a vasodilator (Breithardt *et al.* 1980) and a cardiodepressant (Gough *et al.* 1982). Like other antiarrhythmic agents, the cardiodepressant activity of amiodarone is dose dependent.

Clinical experience and careful follow-up of large numbers of patients taking oral amiodarone suggest that the oral preparation is devoid of negative inotropic effects (Leak and Eydt 1986; Cleland *et al.* 1987), so much so that if any patient develops heart failure during oral amiodarone therapy, it is important to look for other precipitating factors, such as silent myocardial infarction, before attributing the event to the drug. A haemodynamic study of oral amiodarone in dogs showed marked myocardial depression (Landymore *et al.* 1984), but the daily dose of 15 mg per kg was significantly more than the usual therapeutic dose, and the canine myocardial response may differ from the human. The animal result is also at variance with the results of a double-blind placebo-controlled trial in patients with congestive heart failure, in whom oral amiodarone not only increased the left ventricular ejection fraction but also improved exercise tolerance (Hamer *et al.* 1989).

The reason why acute and chronic antiarrhythmic and haemodynamic effects of amiodarone are different may lie in its mechanisms of action. Although the antiarrhythmic property of amiodarone is usually considered to be Class III (Singh and Vaughan Williams 1970), it has also been shown to have Class II (Charlier 1970) and Class I (Mason *et al.* 1984; Cobbe and Manley 1987) antiarrhythmic activities. The Class I and II effects are apparent with acute treatment, but the manifestation of Class III effects may be delayed (Singh and Vaughan Williams 1970), sometimes becoming obvious only after several weeks of oral treatment. It has been suggested that the mechanism by which amiodarone acts as a Class III agent is through selective inhibition of the effects of T_3 on the myocardium (Singh 1983), perhaps through preferential peripheral conversion of T_4 to reverse-T_3 and inhibition of the binding of T_3 to cell nuclei (Franklyn *et al.* 1985). This explains why chronic treatment with amiodarone is required to convert the myocardium into a 'hypothyroid state' to realize the full benefit of its Class III antiarrhythmic activity. Once this state is reached, lower maintenance doses may be sufficient to achieve the antiarrhythmic goal, and therefore the cardiodepressant effect is minimized.

After prolonged therapy with oral amiodarone, there have been instances when it was difficult to wean patients undergoing cardiac surgery off cardiopulmonary bypass (Gallagher *et al.* 1981; MacKinnon *et al.* 1983), and sustained inotropic support with sympathomimetic agents may be necessary. While part of the explanation may be related to intraoperative loss of myocardium, decreased responsiveness to catecholamines is also contributory. Long-term use of amiodarone results in β-adrenoceptor down-regulation (Brevetti *et al.* 1986). Large doses of sympathomimetic agents, with or without phosphodiesterase inhibitors, may be required. The same treatment regimen described above for stopping inotropic support after prolonged infusion, may be necessary.

Class IV agents

Calcium antagonists Like β-adrenoceptor blockers, calcium antagonists possess negative inotropic and chronotropic effects that may be exploited for therapeutic purposes, but that may equally have detrimental consequences. The cardiodepressant effects of calcium antagonists are secondary to the uncoupling of excitation from contraction, by various mechanisms (Henry 1980; Naylor 1980; Capasso 1985). Their negative inotropic effect may be compounded by a decrease in velocity of myocardial relaxation (Vittone *et al.* 1985) to produce detrimental effects on cardiac function. In isolated cardiac muscle the *in vitro* negative inotropic effect was most marked with nifedipine, compared with verapamil and diltiazem (Henry 1980; Perez *et al.* 1982; Bohm *et al.* 1990), but in clinical practice experience suggests that verapamil is the most cardiodepressant, followed by nifedipine and diltiazem (Colucci 1987; Walsh 1987). It may be that the stronger vasodilator effect of nifedipine causes reflex sympathetic stimulation, obscuring the intrinsic negative inotropic effect that is nevertheless present (Clifton *et al.* 1990).

The treatment of cardiac pump failure induced by calcium antagonists is similar to that of excessive β-blockade, but sometimes an intravenous infusion of calcium may be required (Perkins 1978).

Newer calcium antagonists with a more selectively vasodilator than cardiodepressant action are now available, such as felodipine (Ljung 1985), nicardipine (Pepine 1989), and isradipine (Bohm *et al.* 1990). They may be used in patients who are unlikely to tolerate negative inotropism.

A practical clinical issue worth mentioning concerns the treatment of broad-complex tachycardia. In urgent situations, when no more sophisticated facilities are available, it is sometimes difficult to ascertain whether the tachycardia is ventricular, or supraventricular with aberrant conduction. A common pitfall is to assume the latter diagnosis and give intravenous verapamil. The consequence of this can be disastrous if the diagnosis is wrong, because a patient with ventricular tachycardia does not tolerate the negative inotropic effects of verapamil. In view of the fact that the majority of broad-complex tachycardias are ventricular, if the exact diagnosis is in doubt it is preferable from the point of view of probability and safety, to treat the tachycardia as ventricular and not to use verapamil.

Anaesthetic agents

During surgery there are many factors which can influence cardiac function (e.g. body temperature, level of ventilation and oxygenation, vasodilatation), and consequently it is difficult to isolate the direct effects of a single agent. Some degree of hypotension, for instance, from the cardiodepressant effect of anaesthetic agents, is sometimes considered desirable during surgery. Nevertheless, excessive negative inotropic effects, especially in patients with pre-existing cardiac failure, can become a problem.

Most volatile anaesthetic agents exert cardiodepressant effects. To study their relative potency, one needs to standardize and compare the negative inotropic effects at equivalent levels of anaesthesia. One way of achieving this is by using the same MAC (defined as the minimum alveolar concentration of an anaesthetic required to eliminate movement in response to surgical incision in 50 per cent of subjects). Shimosato and Etsten (1969) found that at equipotent anaesthetic concentrations halothane is about three times more cardiodepressant than cyclopropane, with methoxyflurane, enflurane, and ether (in descending order) lying in between. Paradise and Bibbins (1969) found that chloroform produced the most cardiac depression, with halothane > methoxyflurane > ether in decreasing rank order of depression. Brown and Crout (1971) found the following decreasing order of cardiodepression: enflurane > halothane > methoxyflurane > cyclopropane > ether. Kemmotsu and colleagues (1974) found that halothane, enflurane, isoflurane, and fluroxene showed equivalent cardiodepressant potency, about three to four times that of cyclopropane.

Drugs causing myocardial ischaemia

β-Adrenoceptor blocking agents

Effects of acute withdrawal

There are numerous reports from clinical trials of β-adrenoceptor blocking drugs showing that their abrupt withdrawal from patients with ischaemic heart disease may be associated with an exacerbation of symptoms and may lead to unstable angina, myocardial infarction, and sudden death (Wilson *et al.* 1969; Miller *et al.* 1975; Prichard and Walden 1982; Frishman 1987). Most of the reports have come from studies involving propranolol and most events have occurred during the phase of treatment withdrawal. The mechanisms underlying the syndrome of β-adrenoceptor blocker withdrawal are unknown but are thought to include an increased sensitivity of β-adrenoceptors (see above)

(Boudoulas *et al*. 1977*b*; Nattel *et al*. 1979) and increased myocardial oxygen consumption caused by an increase in heart rate.

Walker and others (1985) studied the effect of abrupt cessation of atenolol therapy in twenty patients using exercise testing and ambulatory S–T-segment monitoring and found no evidence of rebound ischaemia with this long-acting drug although in a similar study Egstrup (1988) found evidence of a significant increase in silent ischaemia. Details of the β-blockers used in this investigation are not presented.

There appears to be evidence supporting the contention that abrupt removal of short-acting drugs such as propranolol may result in withdrawal symptoms in patients with angina. In contrast, withdrawal of long-acting agents such as atenolol does not appear to cause significant rebound angina. Review of the early reports of the β-blocker withdrawal syndrome, however, most of which involved propranolol, indicates that most patients who suffered adverse events had severe or unstable angina. Therefore, patient selection probably had a major influence on the clinical syndrome that was initially described. Drugs with intrinsic sympathomimetic activity, such as pindolol, are not associated with problems of withdrawal. The presence of β-stimulant activity may therefore offset any increase in β-adrenoceptor sensitivity (Molinoff *et al*. 1982).

Effects on plasma lipid profile

Several large, much publicized studies of coronary risk factor intervention have reported a lack of reduction in mortality from coronary heart disease in treated hypertensives. A suggested explanation for this finding is that other coronary risk factors may be affected adversely by antihypertensive treatment (Leren 1987; Lardinois and Neuman 1988). In this regard, the deleterious effects of thiazide diuretics and some β-adrenoceptor antagonists on serum lipids have been examined extensively in recent studies. The effects of β-blockers on lipid metabolism have been reviewed (Kincaid-Smith 1984; Lehtonen 1985; Roberts 1989).

In general, β-blockers without intrinsic sympathomimetic activity tend to increase triglycerides and decrease high-density lipoprotein cholesterol but do not cause significant changes in total or low-density lipoprotein cholesterol concentrations. More specifically, the pooled results of the studies reviewed by van Brummelen (1983) showed that non-selective and β₁-selective agents raised plasma triglycerides by an average of 38 per cent and 21 per cent, respectively, compared with a mean 11 per cent rise for drugs with intrinsic sympathomimetic activity. The mean changes in serum high-density lipo-protein concentrations for the three groups of β-blockers were reductions of 19 per cent and five per cent for the non-selective and β₁-selective agents and an increase of three per cent for those compounds with intrinsic sympathomimetic activity. Sotalol is exceptional in that it causes significant elevations of both total and low-density lipoprotein cholesterol concentrations.

Catecholamines have complex effects on lipid metabolism and the exact mechanism whereby β-blockers affect serum lipid concentrations is unknown. Lipoprotein lipase, tissue lipase, and hepatic lipase are key enzyme systems involved in the catabolism of triglyceride-rich lipoproteins. The inhibition of these enzymes, either directly by β-blockers or by secondary, unopposed α-adrenoceptor stimulation, might account for the observed changes in the plasma lipid subfractions and triglycerides.

Although the adverse effects of β-blockade on plasma lipid profiles are a cause for concern, it must be stressed that there are no published data to confirm the clinical relevance of these effects.

Calcium antagonists

Calcium-channel blockers are a clinically heterogeneous group of drugs with potent cardiovascular effects. They are widely prescribed for patients with hypertension, angina, and arrhythmias. In the last 2 years there has been considerable controversy over the safety of the dihydropyridine calcium-channel antagonists, particularly nifedipine.

In 1995 Furberg and colleagues published a meta-analysis of 16 studies of short-acting nifedipine in moderate to high doses. The meta-analysis showed that high doses of nifedipine (80mg) increase the risk of death, and supported a previous study (Goldbourt *et al*. 1993). However, these data do not apply to all calcium-channel blockers or all formulations of nifedipine. In the 1980s (when all the studies analysed by Furberg and colleagues were carried out), long-acting formulations of nifedipine were not available. These formulations have since been shown to be safe and effective in patients with chronic stable angina (Parmley *et al*. 1992).

Specific receptor sites within calcium channels have been defined for the three major classes and antagonist: the phenylalkamines (e.g. verapamil), the benzothiazepines (e.g. diltiazem), and the dihydropyridines (e.g. nifedipine).

The main adverse effects of the calcium-channel blockers are a reflection of their therapeutic action. The short-acting dihydropyridine, nifedipine, has been shown to cause paradoxical angina (Casolo *et al*. 1989).

The mechanism involves reflex tachycardia secondary to vasodilatation (Stone *et al.* 1983) and increased myocardial oxygen consumption (Jariwalla and Anderson 1978; Rodger and Stewart 1978; Raftos 1980; Feldman *et al.* 1982). It has been suggested that this may be further exacerbated by the 'coronary steal' phenomenon (Boden *et al.* 1985). Paradoxical angina is more likely in patients with impaired left ventricular function and those with proximal coronary stenoses. An important interaction between nifedipine and propranolol, manifesting as deteriorating angina, has been reported (Opie and White 1980). Withdrawal or omission of calcium antagonists in patients with angina may result in worsening symptoms within 48 hours. This rebound phenomenon has been described for nifedipine (Kay *et al.* 1982; Nehring and Camm 1983; Myrhed and Wilholm 1986) and, in isolated reports, for verapamil and diltiazem (Bala Subramamanian *et al.* 1983). The cause of rebound angina is unknown. Bala Subramamanian and others (1983) have proposed that chronic treatment with calcium antagonists may deplete the intracellular pool of calcium ions. Withdrawal of the calcium-channel blockers may be accompanied by an increased flux of calcium ions into vascular smooth muscle cells resulting in an increased tendency to coronary vasospasm. Loaldi and colleagues (1989) compared angiographic, clinical, and electrocardiographic indices in patients with 'mixed' angina, occurring both on effort and at rest, and in patients with Prinzmetal angina. In the first group, 10 of the 22 patients showed evidence of increased ischaemia during treatment with nifedipine, whereas those with Prinzmetal angina had a uniformly favourable response.

What conclusions can be drawn from the data assembled since 1990 regarding calcium-channel blockers? (For a review see Holdright 1997.) Patients with coronary artery disease or hypertension taking short-acting nifedipine should be switched to a long-acting calcium-channel blocker. There is no role for dihydropyridine calcium-channel blockers alone after myocardial infarction, nor in unstable angina.

Nitrates

The benefits of a daily nitrate-free or nitrate-low interval in preventing nitrate tolerance are well established (Cowan 1986; Abrams 1989). Recent studies have suggested, however, that nitrate withdrawal may lead to rebound angina. In occasional patients, overnight removal of nitroglycerin patches has caused an exacerbation of anginal episodes (De Mots and Glasser 1989; Ferrantini *et al.* 1989). The extent to which these results can be extrapolated to other nitrate preparations is uncertain. It is possible that intermittent therapy with nitroglycerin patches is particularly prone to rebound, because of the rapid decline in nitroglycerin concentrations following patch removal. Certainly, previous studies of interval therapy, which have been based on oral preparations of isosorbide dinitrate and isosorbide mononitrate, have failed to find evidence of rebound. Oral preparations and regimens, however, have not undergone such close scrutiny as the patch and it is possible that the problems of nitrate withdrawal may have gone undetected. In view of these concerns, interval therapy should, where possible, be combined with other antianginal treatment, particularly β-blockers, to guard against the possibility of rebound (Cowan 1990).

β_2-Adrenoceptor agonists

β_2-Adrenoceptor agonists are administered intravenously for the inhibition of preterm labour (tocolysis). Ritodrine is used widely in the USA, from where most of the reports of its cardiovascular toxicity originate. Terbutaline and salbutamol are also used for this purpose (Tye *et al.* 1980; Katz *et al.* 1981). Retrosternal pain typical of angina pectoris and associated with electrocardiographic evidence of myocardial ischaemia has been reported by many authors and has been reviewed recently (Benedetti 1983; Ingemarsson *et al.* 1985). Myocardial infarction has been documented in some instances (Benedetti 1983), but in at least one case the patient was known to have coronary artery disease (Bass *et al.* 1979).

In a prospective study to determine the incidence of adverse cardiovascular effects during ritodrine infusion, Schneider and colleagues (1988) reported that eight of their study group of 30 patients developed anginal pain. Certain clinical features were associated with an increased tendency to myocardial ischaemia. These included heart rate in excess of 130 beats per minute, hypokalaemia, hypotension, and anaemia. Anginal pain and the associated electrocardiographic abnormalities were readily reversed by discontinuation of the drug.

The pathophysiology of the myocardial ischaemia is thought to be multifactorial. Tachycardia will reduce the diastolic filling time of the coronary circulation and increase myocardial oxygen consumption. Other contributory factors are listed above. It has been suggested that the placental circulation resembles a large arterio–venous fistula, which reduces aortic diastolic blood pressure, thereby contributing to myocardial insufficiency (Benedetti 1983).

Amphetamines and cocaine

The abuse of the indirect sympathomimetic drugs cocaine and amphetamine has been documented as causing life-threatening cardiac arrhythmias (see above), angina, and myocardial infarction (Cregler and Mark 1986; Isner et al. 1986; Carson et al. 1987). Myocardial infarction may occur either in patients with known coronary artery disease or in those with normal coronary vasculature. Both agents cause an increase in systolic blood pressure and heart rate and thus myocardial oxygen demand. The exact pathophysiology of the coronary occlusion that causes myocardial infarction remains uncertain but it is thought to be a transient focal event. Both cocaine and amphetamine exert indirect pressor effects on the coronary circulation, potentiating the actions of noradrenaline and thereby causing vasospasm (Fiegl 1983). In addition, catecholamines are potent platelet aggregators and may cause thrombosis (Haft et al. 1982). Postmortem studies of the hearts of patients who have died suddenly after taking amphetamines have found histological changes varying from no abnormality through a spectrum that includes arteriolar spasm (Carvey and Reed (1970) and interstitial and endocardial haemorrhage (Orrenius and Maehly 1970).

Dipyridamole

Dipyridamole is a potent coronary vasodilator (Kadatz 1959) that is used both therapeutically and, in conjunction with thallium scintigraphy, in the investigation of ischaemic heart disease. Its actions are mediated by its effects on the coronary and systemic circulations (Marchant et al. 1986). At the cellular level, dipyridamole increases the concentration of adenosine in the arterial wall of resistance vessels (Homback 1987). Although it has been used in the medical management of angina pectoris, it can cause coronary steal and may exacerbate anginal symptoms, particularly in patients with multivessel coronary disease (Feldman et al. 1981; Marchant et al. 1984).

Thyroxine

Previous reports of angina pectoris and myocardial infarction occurring in patients with thyrotoxicosis (Somerville and Levine 1949; Wei et al. 1979; Featherstone and Stewart 1983) have assumed that the ischaemic symptoms have been due to co-existing atheromatous coronary artery disease or coronary spasm (Kotler et al. 1973; Resnekov and Falicov 1977). Additionally, emboli from a fibrillating left atrium and primary in situ coronary thrombosis have been reported. These phenomena are thought to account for the permanent left ventricular segmental wall motion abnormalities that have been described in Graves' disease (Kotler et al. 1973; Proskey

et al. 1977). These reports relate to patients with excessive amounts of endogenous thyroid hormones.

Bergeron and others (1988) have reported the case of a 68-year-old woman who deliberately took an excess of desiccated thyroid (260 mg per day) over a period of time and who presented with clinical thyrotoxicosis and a subendocardial anterior myocardial infarction associated with two large areas of ventricular dyskinesis. Subsequent cardiac catheterization and coronary angiography showed normal coronary artery anatomy and a normal pattern of left ventricular contraction. The authors suggest that coronary spasm with resultant reversible myocardial ischaemia was the most likely pathological mechanism, since all the abnormalities of left ventricular function resolved fully.

Encainide

Barron and Billhardt (1989) have reported a case of a 59-year-old man with dilated cardiomyopathy who developed angina pectoris after receiving 25 mg 8-hourly of the Class Ic antiarrhythmic agent encainide, which had been prescribed for high-grade ventricular ectopy. Previous coronary angiography had shown occlusion of a small diagonal branch of the left anterior descending artery as the only abnormality, although the subject did not have a history of prior angina. The patient complained of typical anginal pain that responded to sublingual nitrates, and dyspnoea, approximately 1–2 hours after each dose, which would equate with the time of peak plasma concentrations (Chase and Sloskey 1987). Encainide was withdrawn but subsequently restarted, when it resulted in identical symptoms. Patients with dilated cardiomyopathy are known to have reduced coronary flow reserve (Pasternac et al. 1982). The authors proposed that encainide might have caused vasoconstriction in the subendocardial vascular bed and thus ischaemia.

Fluorouracil

The antimetabolite fluorouracil has been used for over 30 years as a chemotherapeutic agent. Its adverse gastrointestinal and haematological effects are well known but recent case reports and reviews have indicated that it causes significant cardiotoxicity. This may take the form of myocardial depression (Chaudary et al. 1988) or the induction of angina pectoris (Dent and McColl 1975; Underwood et al. 1983; Blijham et al. 1986; Collins and Weiden 1987; Millward et al. 1988). Fatal myocardial infarction has also been described (Clavel et al. 1988; Ensley et al. 1989).

Collins and Weiden (1987) have estimated that 10 per cent of patients who receive fluorouracil will experience cardiotoxicity and that this is most usual when the drug is given by infusion rather than as an intravenous bolus. Myocardial ischaemia is manifest as anterior wall chest pain typical of angina, usually occurring after the second dose of the drug has been given. The symptoms are accompanied in 80 per cent of cases by significant ECG changes of ischaemia with ST-segment elevation and typical T wave abnormalities. It is probable that in the majority of cases fluorouracil exacerbates underlying heart disease, although it may also induce angina in patients with no previous history of ischaemic heart disease. The mechanism of the drug's cardiotoxicity has not been established. From the clinical observations of the reproducibility of the chest pain and associated ECG abnormalities following the administration of fluoro-uracil, it has been inferred that the drug may cause coronary spasm (Lang-Stevenson *et al.* 1977; Pottage *et al.* 1978; Sanini *et al.* 1981; Labianca *et al.* 1982; Kleinman *et al.* 1987). This seems possible, as several patients who have experienced anginal pain with this drug have been shown to have normal coronary angio-grams (Collins and Weiden 1987).

Vincristine and vinblastine

Mandel and colleagues (1975) described the clinical course of a 58-year-old man with known but stable coronary artery disease who developed myocardial in-farctions after the second and third doses of vincristine. Since this initial report, two other cases of myocardial infarction associated with the administration of vin-cristine (Somers *et al.* 1976; Warden *et al.* 1976) and one case after vinblastine therapy (Lejonc *et al.* 1980) have been published. Coronary angiography was undertaken in one patient and showed a normal coronary vasculature (Warden *et al.* 1976). To account for the changes, the authors speculated that coronary artery spasm had been induced by vincristine, and wondered if previous mantle irradiation might have facilitated this. Vinca alkaloids are toxic to myofibrils: a similar type of injury to vascular smooth muscle cells might induce coronary spasm and result in myocardial ischaemia and necrosis.

In a provocative report, Edwards and colleagues (1979) noted the postmortem findings in two young men who had been treated unsuccessfully with a combination of vinblastine, bleomycin, and cisplatin for testicular teratomas. The subjects had none of the major risk factors for coronary disease. Neither of them had had symptoms of ischaemic heart disease in life and their ECGs were normal. Both, however, had advanced atherosclerotic disease of the major coronary arteries in the absence of atheromatous disease of other major vessels. The authors postulated that this combination of drugs may have accelerated the development of coron-ary atherosclerosis.

Adenosine and ATP

In recent years, considerable research has been under-taken into the physiological and pharmacological effects of the purine nucleoside adenosine and its phosphory-lated derivatives. Adenosine is released from ischaemic cardiac cells into the coronary circulation following the breakdown of adenosine triphosphate (ATP) and aden-osine monophosphate (AMP) (Arch and Newsholme 1978). It is thought to exert protective effects that in-clude local vasodilatation and inhibition of platelet ag-gregation (Edlund *et al.* 1985). Sylven and others (1986, 1987) examined the hypothesis that adenosine causes angina pectoris and have cited evidence to this effect.

The potent negative dromotropic effects of adenosine and ATP on atrioventricular conduction coupled with its lack of significant negative inotropic effects have led to their use, by bolus injection, in the treatment of parox-ysmal tachycardias (Di Marco *et al.* 1983). Several inves-tigators have noted that, shortly after the intravenous administration of these agents, approximately one-third of patients complain of anginal-type chest pain but that this resolves within 60 seconds (Watt and Routledge 1985; Belhasen *et al.* 1988; Rankin *et al.* 1989). There are no concomitant ECG changes of ischaemia and no del-eterious effects have been reported. It has therefore been postulated that adenosine and ATP cause angina by direct sensitization of autonomic nerves (Sylven *et al.* 1989).

Vasopressin

Vasopressin, or antidiuretic hormone, is a potent pressor agent affecting smooth muscle throughout the vascula-ture. The adverse cardiac effects of vasopressin are attributable to the induction of myocardial ischaemia. This is observed both in subjects with normal coronary arteries and those with atheromatous disease. Pressor effects are usually encountered at doses higher than those that cause a maximum antidiuretic effect. Vaso-pressin-induced myocardial infarction and death have been reported. The drug should not be used in patients known to have angina pectoris (B.M. Beller *et al.* 1971; Hays 1985). The synthetic analogue 1-desamino-8-D-arginine vasopressin (DDAVP) has full antidiuretic po-tency, but does not elevate blood pressure or contract smooth muscle. It is therefore more suitable for patients with ischaemic heart disease (Cobb *et al.* 1978).

Ergotamine

Ergotamine is an alkaloid derivative of ergot that is a partial agonist at α-adrenergic and hydroxytryptamine receptors and is used in the treatment of migrainous disorders. It causes vasoconstriction and, in addition to its well-known effects on the peripheral vasculature, may cause angina (Scherf and Schlachman 1948; McNerney and Leedham 1950) and myocardial infarction (Goldfischer 1960; Klein *et al.* 1982; Rall and Schleifer 1985).

Methylxanthines

Theophylline and caffeine are the two most commonly encountered methylxanthines. Both have significant acute effects on the cardiovascular system. In addition, the possibility that coffee drinking may be a risk factor in the pathogenesis of coronary artery disease has been extensively investigated.

The results of earlier studies of coffee consumption and cardiovascular risk are conflicting. This may have been a consequence of suboptimal methodology in study design especially with regard to patient numbers and duration of follow-up (Dawber *et al.* 1974; La Croix *et al.* 1986; Rosenberg *et al.* 1988). Furthermore, some of these studies were retrospective (Jick *et al.* 1973; Klatsky *et al.* 1973). The apparently positive correlation between coffee drinking and cardiovascular morbidity has been attributed mainly to the adverse effects of coffee on serum low-density lipoprotein cholesterol levels.

Reports from Scandinavia indicate that the method of coffee brewing is a significant factor (Bonaa *et al.* 1988). The traditional method of preparation of coffee is by boiling in much of this region. Subjects who made coffee in this way were shown to have higher serum cholesterol concentrations than individuals who drank filtered coffee (Arnesen *et al.* 1984; Aro *et al.* 1987). These findings have been confirmed in a prospective, randomized, cross-over study comparing the effects of the two methods of brewing coffee (Bak and Grobbee 1989). Drinking four to six cups of boiled coffee per day over a 9-week period increased the total serum cholesterol concentration by a mean of 0.48 mmol per litre and the low-density lipoprotein cholesterol concentration by 0.39 mmol per litre from control values. In contrast, there was no significant change in these indices when the subjects consumed the same amount of filtered coffee over an identical period.

Methylxanthines have complex effects on several organ systems and those on the heart and circulation may be particularly significant. Their actions are mediated via several mechanisms including potentiation of the sympathetic nervous system, effects on adenosine and ATP, modulation of the renin–angiotensin system, and stimulation of the brainstem vagal and vasomotor centres (Rall 1985). The effects of methylxanthines on coronary blood flow in humans are controversial. Because of its vasodilator properties, theophylline has been used in the treatment of angina (Russek 1960), but it can also cause myocardial ischaemia (McFadden and Ingram 1988). These reports reflect opposing effects on myocardial oxygen consumption, due to vasodilator properties on the one hand and chronotropic and inotropic effects on the other. The net effect will differ in different individuals and is therefore unpredictable.

The effects of caffeine, administered by drinking coffee, on the exercise tolerance and symptoms in a group of patients with chronic stable angina have been reported (Piters *et al.* 1985). Coffee drinking resulted in a significant increase in the duration of exercise before the onset of angina. The reasons underlying this effect are uncertain but the lack of any deleterious effect is reassuring.

The oral contraceptive pill

Not long after the introduction of the oral contraceptive pill in the early 1960s the cardiovascular risks associated with it became apparent (Stadel 1981). A number of studies described an increased risk of myocardial infarction, systemic hypertension, and thromboembolism in users of the oral contraceptive pill (Dalen and Hickler 1981; Stadel 1981).

In contrast, the use of oestrogen in post-menopausal hormone replacement therapy has been shown to reduce the incidence and mortality of cardiovascular diseases in a number of epidemiological studies (Stampfer *et al.* 1991).

Myocardial ischaemia

Myocardial infarction is rare in premenopausal women is rare, but has been shown to be four times greater in women using high dose oral contraceptive preparations. Women using the oral contraceptive pill who smoke have a 20 times greater risk of myocardial infarction (Barret-Connor and Bush 1991) than do non-smoking non-users. There is a similar multiplicative effect in pill users with other risk factors for ischaemic heart disease.

Why women on the pill have myocardial infarction is unclear. Angiographic data has often shown little or no evidence of atherosclerotic coronary artery disease. It may be that the oral contraceptive pill adversely affects lipid metabolism and leads to hypercoagulability and thrombosis.

Hypertension

Up to five per cent of patients taking an oral contraceptive have mild hypertension; a much smaller group have a more significant rise in blood pressure. Hypertension related to the pill is more likely to occur in women who are older and have a family history of high blood pressure (Dalen and Hickler 1981). Hypertension induced by the pill resolves on stopping taking it (Hodsman *et al.* 1982).

Hormone replacement therapy

In contrast to the relationship between thromboembolic disorders and treatment with the relatively large doses of oestrogens used for oral contraception, there is no good evidence of an association between sex hormone replacement therapy and cardiovascular disease. Indeed, it appears that oestrogens in low dosage exert a protective effect against ischaemic heart disease in postmenopausal women (Ross *et al.* 1981; Bush *et al.* 1983). The postulated mechanism underlying this beneficial effect is an elevation in the concentration of high-density lipoprotein cholesterol, accompanied by a reduction in low-density lipoprotein cholesterol. These changes occur when oestrogens are used in the very low doses appropriate to hormone replacement therapy.

Diuretics

Although neither thiazide nor loop diuretics are known to cause myocardial ischaemia directly, concern has been expressed regarding their effects on circulating lipid concentrations and the possible atherogenic risks (Lasser *et al.* 1984). Increases in both serum triglyceride and low-density lipoprotein cholesterol concentrations with a reduction or no change in high-density lipoprotein cholesterol have been demonstrated following prolonged administration of both types of diuretics (Lant 1985; Weidmann *et al.* 1988). These effects are dose-dependent (Perez-Stable and Caralis 1983). Although the pathogenesis of these changes is unknown they may involve thiazide-induced hyperinsulinaemia (Lardinois and Neuman 1988). As in the case of β-blockers, there is no evidence at present to confirm that the hyperlipidaemia associated with chronic diuretic therapy results in accelerated coronary atherosclerosis.

Drugs and myocardial healing

Corticosteroids and NSAID

The development of a ventricular aneurysm in a patient treated with high-dose corticosteroids for postmyo-cardial infarction (Dressler's) syndrome alerted physicians to the possible deleterious effects of steroids on myocardial healing (Bulkley and Roberts 1974). In a later report, Owensby (1986) described the occurrence of rupture of the right ventricular free wall after insertion of a temporary pacing electrode. Four days after implantation, symptoms and signs of pleuropericarditis were present together with echocardiographic evidence of a small pericardial effusion. The pacing electrode was removed and the effusion resolved over the following 9 days. The patient, however, developed cardiac tamponade 10 weeks later, requiring open drainage of a large pericardial effusion. At operation, perforation of the right ventricular apex was confirmed with evidence of partially organized clot and adhesions, suggesting that the perforation had occurred some time previously. The development of the second effusion was attributed to rupture of the right ventricular apex, the healing of which had been impaired by chronic prednisone therapy (10 mg per day) for steroid-dependent asthma.

More recently, there is a growing amount of evidence to suggest that both corticosteroids and non-steroidal anti-inflammatory drugs (NSAID) impair myocardial repair following myocardial infarction (Delborg *et al.* 1985; Silverman and Pfeifer 1987). In Silverman and Pfeifer's (1987) series of 41 patients with left ventricular free wall rupture, 20 (49 per cent) had received an NSAID. These patients were characterized by being elderly with a mean age of 67 years, and a male preponderance. Few had a history of previous myocardial infarction or congestive cardiac failure and 60 per cent had sustained large transmural anterior infarcts.

Eleven subjects had been given corticosteroids (prednisone, methylprednisone, or dexamethasone) alone, seven had received corticosteroids and an NSAID, and two had had an NSAID only. Indomethacin was the NSAID used in all but one instance. More than half the patients who developed ventricular rupture had received three doses of either type of anti-inflammatory drug and most cases of ventricular rupture occurred within 3 days of commencing therapy. It is possible, however, that the pericarditis for which the anti-inflammatory agents were prescribed was caused by a small extravasation of blood into the pericardial space. This initial leak may have occurred from a limited dehiscence of the ventricle that later extended to a full rupture.

A precursor stage to ventricular rupture is infarct expansion (Hutchins and Bulkley 1978), which begins within hours of the acute ischaemic event. Expansion is characterized by thinning and dilatation of the infarcted area that is not a consequence of further myocardial necrosis. Histologically, there is slippage between the sarcolemmal bundles, and during the healing process fibroblasts enter the myocyte compartment and lay down collagen which connects the disrupted myocytes. There are good experimental and human data to indicate that the administration of anti-inflammatory agents early after myocardial infarction results in enhanced infarct expansion and is a major contributory factor to the formation of ventricular aneurysms (Weisman and Healy 1987).

Infarct expansion ultimately results in ventricular dilatation and complex changes in ventricular architecture and function (Pfeffer and Braunwald 1990). Ventricular dilatation is associated with reduced survival, and clinical studies are in progress to assess the value of various pharmacological agents in preventing infarct expansion. Conversely, the avoidance of drugs that impair myocardial healing after acute infarction is desirable. The most commonly used agents in this regard are corticosteroids and NSAID.

Drugs causing lesions of heart valves

Methysergide and ergotamine

Methysergide and ergotamine are both serotonin (5-hydroxytryptamine) antagonists used in the treatment of migrainous disorders. The cardiotoxic effects of methysergide are rare but were recognized over 30 years ago (Graham et al. 1966; Graham 1967; Bana et al. 1974; Misch 1974). Methysergide therapy is associated with both stenotic and regurgitant lesions of the mitral, aortic, and tricuspid valves, which occur after prolonged therapy. In addition, methysergide may cause myocardial fibrosis (Mason et al. 1977b). Spierings (1988) has reported the development of cardiac murmurs indicative of aortic valve disease in a patient with a history of chronic and excessive ergotamine intake. Hauck and others (1990) described two patients who had taken ergotamine tartrate (Cafergot) chronically for migraine, one of whom developed aortic regurgitation and the other mixed mitral valve disease. Both required valve replacement surgery. Neither subject had a history of rheumatic heart disease nor had they ever been given methysergide. Histological examination of the excised valves showed them to be involved by a proliferative process very similar to that seen in carcinoid heart disease and methysergide-associated valvular disease. Although methysergide and ergotamine are serotonin antagonists they also possess partial agonist activity. It is this property which may account for their cardiotoxic effects and provide a link with the similar pathological processes seen in the carcinoid syndrome.

Fenfluramine and phentermine

Fenfluramine, phentermine, and dexfluramine are sympathomimetic amines which are appetite suppressants, approved in the United States as anorectic agents. A recent study (Connolly et al. 1997) reported heart valve disease within 12 months of starting treatment with fenfluramine–phentermine. These lesions were both left- and right-sided and predominantly regurgitant lesions. Connolly and colleagues pointed out that the histological picture of these valves was virtually indistinguishable from that induced by ergot alkaloids such as ergotamine and methysergide. These drugs have now been withdrawn in both the UK and USA.

Minocycline

Blue-black pigmentation of the aortic and mitral valves in an individual undergoing aortic valve replacement has been reported as a complication of chronic therapy with minocycline (Butler et al. 1985). Minocycline, a tetracycline derivative, had been prescribed at a dose of 200 mg per day for 5 years for chronic sinusitis and had resulted in cutaneous pigmentation. Valve replacement surgery was indicated for stenosis of a congenitally bicuspid aortic valve. At operation both the aortic and mitral valves were pigmented, but there was no evidence of any functional abnormality of the mitral valve. Microscopic examination of the excised aortic valve showed granular pigment distributed both within macrophages and free in the connective tissue and the appearances were identical to those found in the skin biopsies.

Drugs causing pericardial disease

Drugs causing pericardial disease can be classified into those that cause a drug-induced lupus syndrome and those that cause pericarditis as a direct toxic effect. In the latter group there is often evidence of myocarditis (Gold 1967), features of which may dominate the clinical problem (Smith 1966). In some cases of drug-induced lupus syndrome, acute pericarditis may be the first sign of the disease. Hydralazine (Anandadas and Simpson 1986), procainamide (Swarbrick and Gray 1972), and sulphasalazine (Clementz and Dolin 1988; Deboever et al. 1989) have been identified as causes of pericarditis in association with drug-induced lupus.

Pericarditis is a rare but well-documented adverse effect of chemotherapy. It has been described following treatment with anthracyclines (Harrison and Danders 1976; Bristow et al. 1978), actinomycin D (Corder and Flannery 1974), bleomycin (Durkin et al. 1976; Klein

1977), and when cisplatin and fluorouracil are used in combination (Jakubowski and Remeny 1983). Cyclophosphamide (Appelbaum *et al.* 1976; Buja *et al.* 1976; Steinherz *et al.* 1981) and cytarabine (Vaickus and Letendre 1984) may also cause pericarditis when used in high doses. Some authors have suggested that previous radiotherapy to the mediastinum, even if administered several months before chemotherapy is given, may predispose the patients to developing pericarditis but this is far from invariable (Corder and Flannery 1974; Durkin *et al.* 1976).

Pericarditis has been described as an idiosyncratic toxic reaction following the use of minoxidil (Krehlik *et al.* 1985) and of phenylbutazone (Shafar 1965), and as part of penicillin hypersensitivity (Schoenwetter and Silber 1965). Fibrosis of the pericardium is associated with the oculomucocutaneous syndrome induced by practolol and may be seen in the fibrotic reaction seen with methysergide (see above).

An unusual complication of sclerotherapy of oesophageal varices was the accidental leakage of the sclerosant morrhuate sodium into the pericardial cavity after oesophageal perforation, resulting in acute pericarditis. Eight months later the patient presented with cardiac tamponade and constrictive pericarditis requiring operative intervention (Brown and Luchi 1987).

Haemopericardium with or without tamponade is described as a complication of anticoagulant therapy. This may occur spontaneously (Leung *et al.* 1990), or following instrumentation of the heart (Braunwald and Swan 1968). A recently recognized complication of thrombolytic therapy is its inappropriate use in acute aortic dissection that has been misdiagnosed as myocardial infarction (Blankenship and Almquist 1989; Butler *et al.* 1990; Curzen *et al.* 1990), resulting in fatal cardiac tamponade.

References

Abel, F.L. (1980). Direct effects of ethanol on myocardial performance and coronary resistance. *J. Pharmacol. Exp. Ther.* 212, 28.

Abel, F.L., Wilson, S.P., Zhao, R.R., *et al.* (1989). Cocaine depresses the canine myocardium. *Circ. Shock* 28, 309.

Abrams, J. (1989). Interval therapy to avoid nitrate tolerance. Paradise regained? *Am. J. Cardiol.* 64, 931.

Adams, P.C. (1982). Drug-induced heart failure. *Adverse Drug React. Bull.* 92, 336.

Akiyama, T., Pawatan, Y., Greenberg, H., *et al.* (1991). Increased risk of death and cardiac arrest from encainide and flecainide in patients after non-Q wave acute myocardial infarction in the Cardiac Arrhythmia Suppression Trial. *Am. J. Cardiol.* 68, 1551.

Alfino, P.A., Thanavaro, S., Kleiger, R.E., *et al.* (1981). Alpha-methyldopa and carotid sinus hypersensitivity. *N. Engl. J. Med.* 305, 344.

Alpert, L.I., Tanimura, A., and Wertheimer, S. (1972). Cardiomyopathy associated with pheochromocytoma. *Arch. Pathol.* 93, 544.

Amery, A., Birkenhager, W., and Brixko, P. (1985). Mortality and morbidity results from the European working party on high blood pressure in the elderly trial. *Lancet* i, 1349.

Anandadas, J.A. and Simpson, P. (1986). Cardiac tamponade, associated with hydralazine therapy, in a patient with rapid acetylator status. *Br. J. Clin. Pract.* 40, 305.

Anastasiou-Nana, M.I., Anderson, J.L., Stewart, J.R., *et al.* (1987). Occurrence of exercise-induced and spontaneous wide-complex tachycardia during therapy with flecainide for complex ventricular arrhythmias: a probable proarrhythmic effect. *Am. Heart J.* 113, 1071.

Anderson, H.R., MacNair, R.S., and Ramsey, J.D. (1985). Deaths from abuse of volatile substances: a national epidemiological study. *BMJ* 290, 304.

Anderson, J.L., Lutz, J.R., Gilbert, E.M., *et al.* (1985). A randomized trial of low-dose beta-blockade therapy for idiopathic dilated cardiomyopathy. *Am. J. Cardiol.* 55, 471.

Anderson, J.L., Atkins, J.C., Gilbert, E.M., *et al.* (1986). Occurrence of ventricular arrhythmias in patients receiving acute and chronic infusions of milrinone. *Am. Heart J.* 111, 466.

Angelakos, E.T. and Hastings, E.P. (1960). The influence of quinidine and procaine amide on myocardial contractility *in vivo. Am. J. Cardiol.* 5, 791.

Antman, E.M., Wenger, T.L., Butler, V.P., *et al.* (1990). Treatment of 150 cases of life-threatening digitalis intoxication with digoxin-specific Fab antibody fragments. Final report of a multicentre study. *Circulation* 81, 1744.

Appelbaum, V.R., Strauchen, J.A., and Graw, G.R. (1976). Acute lethal carditis caused by high-dose combination chemotherapy. *Ann. Intern. Med.* 85, 339.

Arch, J.R.S. and Newsholme, E.A. (1978). The control of the metabolism of metabolism and hormonal role of adenosine. In *Essays in Biochemistry*, Vol. 14 (ed. P.N. Campbell and W.N. Aldridge), p. 82. Academic Press, New York.

Arnesen, E., Forde, O.H., and Thelle, D.S. (1984). Coffee and serum cholesterol. *BMJ* 288, 1960.

Aro, A., Tuomilheto, J., Kostianinen, E., *et al.* (1987). Boiled coffee increases serum low density lipoprotein concentration. *Metabolism* 36, 1027.

Aronson, J.K. (1980). Indicators for the measurement of plasma digoxin. *Drugs* 26, 230.

Askanas, A., Udoshi, M., and Sadjadi, S.A. (1980). The heart in chronic alcoholism: a noninvasive study. *Am. Heart J.* 99, 9.

Au, P.K., Bhandari, A.K., Bream, R., *et al.* (1987). Proarrhythmic effects of antiarrhythmic drugs during programmed stimulation in patients without ventricular tachycardia. *J. Am. Coll. Cardiol.* 9, 389.

Auffermann, W., Stefenelli, T., Wu, S.T., *et al.* (1989). Influence of positive inotropic agents on intracellular calcium transients. Part 1. Normal rat heart. *Am. Heart J.* 118, 1219.

Austen, W.G. and Moran, J.M. (1965). Cardiac and peripheral vascular effects of lidocaine and procainamide. *Am. J. Cardiol.* 16, 701.

Bak, A.A.A. and Grobbee, D.E. (1989). The effect on serum cholesterol levels of coffee brewed by filtering or boiling. *N. Engl. J. Med.* 321, 1432.

Baker, B.J., Brodsky, M.A., Dinh, H., *et al.* (1987). Hemodynamic effect of propafenone and the experience in patients with congestive heart failure. *J. Electrophysiol.* 1, 527.

Bala Subramanian, V., Bowles, M.J., Khurmi, N.S., *et al.* (1983). Calcium antagonist withdrawal syndrome: objective demonstration with frequency modulated ST segment monitoring. *BMJ* 286, 520.

Bana, D.S., Macneal, P.S., Le Compte, P.M., *et al.* (1974). Cardiac murmurs and fibrosis associated with methysergide therapy. *Am. Heart J.* 88, 640.

Banim, S.O., Da Silva, A., Stone, D., *et al.* (1977). Observations of the haemodynamics of mexiletine. *Postgrad. Med. J.* 53, 74.

Banner, A.S., Sunderrajan, E.V., Agarwac, M.K., *et al.* (1979). Arrhythmogenic effects of orally administered bronchodilators. *Arch. Intern. Med.* 139, 434.

Barret-Connor, E. and Bush, T.L. (1991). Estrogen and coronary heart disease in women. *JAMA* 265, 1861.

Barron, J.T. and Billhardt, R.A. (1989). Angina pectoris with encainide in dilated cardiomyopathy. *Am. Heart J.* 117, 701.

Bass, M. (1970). Sudden sniffing death. *JAMA* 212, 2075.

Bass, O., Friedemann, M., and Kuzil, M. (1979). A case of left myocardial insufficiency after tocolysis by means of beta stimulation. *Schweiz. Med. Wochenschr.* 109, 1427.

Bauernfeind, R., Hall, C., Denes, P., *et al.* (1978). Adverse effects of sympatholytic agents in patients with sinus node dysfunction. *Am. J. Med.* 64, 1013.

Bauman, D.J. (1981). Myocardial depression with disopyramide. *Ann. Intern. Med.* 94, 411.

Bauman, J.L., Bauernfeind, R.A., Hoff, J.V., *et al.* (1984). Torsade de pointes due to quinidine: observations in 31 patients. *Am. Heart J.* 107, 425.

Baumann, G., Loher, U., and Felix, S.B. (1982). Deleterious effects of cimetidine in the presence of histamine on coronary circulation. *Res. Exp. Med.* 180, 209.

Bayer, R., Schwarzmaier, J., and Pernice, R. (1988). Basic mechanisms underlying prenylamine-induced 'torsade de pointes': differences between prenylamine and fenildine due to basic actions of the isomers. *Curr. Med. Res. Opin.* 11, 254.

Beermann, B., Edhag, O., and Vallin, H. (1975). Advanced heart block aggravated by carbamazepine. *Br. Heart J.* 37, 668.

Befeler, B. (1975). The hemodynamic effects of Norpace, Part 1. *Angiology* 26, 99.

Belhasen, B., Glick, A., and Laniado, S. (1988). Comparative clinical and electrophysiological effects of adenosine triphosphate and verapamil on paroxysmal reciprocating junctional tachycardia. *Circulation* 77, 795.

Beller, B.M., Trevino, A., and Urban, E. (1971). Pitressin-induced myocardial injury and depression in a young woman. *Am. J. Med.* 51, 675.

Beller, G.A., Smith, T.W., Abelmann, W.H., *et al.* (1971). Digitalis intoxication. A prospective clinical study with serum level correlations. *N. Engl. J. Med.* 184, 989.

Beller, G.A., Hood, W.B., Smith, T.W., *et al.* (1974). Correlation of serum magnesium levels and cardiac digitalis intoxication. *Am. J. Cardiol.* 33, 225.

Benassi, E., Bo, G.P., Cocito, L., *et al.* (1987). Carbamazepine and cardiac conduction disturbances. *Ann. Neurol.* 22, 280.

Benedetti, T.J. (1983). Maternal complications of parenteral beta-mimetic therapy for preterm labour inhibition. *Am. J. Obstet. Gynecol.* 145, 1.

Benjamin, I.J., Jalil, J.E., Tan, L-B., *et al.* (1989). Isoproterenol-induced myocardial fibrosis in relation to myocyte necrosis. *Circ. Res.* 65, 657.

Benowitz, N.L., Rosenberg, J., and Becker, C.E. (1979). Cardiopulmonary catastrophe in drug-overdosed patients. *Med. Clin. North Am.* 83, 267.

Benowitz, N.L., Osterloh, J., Goldschlager, N., *et al.* (1982). Massive catecholamine release from caffeine poisoning. *JAMA* 248, 1097.

Bergeron, G.A., Goldsmith, R., and Schiller, N.B. (1988). Myocardial infarction, severe reversible ischaemia, and shock following excess thyroid administration in a woman with normal coronary arteries. *Arch. Intern. Med.* 148, 1450.

Bhan, R.D., Giacomelli, F., and Wiener, J. (1982). Adrenergic blockade in angiotensin-induced hypertension. Effect on rat coronary arteries and myocardium. *Am. J. Pathol.* 108, 60.

Bigger, J.T. (1985). Digitalis toxicity. *J. Clin. Pharmacol.* 25, 514.

Bigger, J.T., Fleiss, K.R., Rolnitsky, L.M., *et al.* (1985). Effect of digitalis treatment on survival after acute myocardial infarction. *Am. J. Cardiol.* 55, 623.

Bigger, J.T., Giardina, E.G.C., Perel, J.M., *et al.* (1977). Cardiac antiarrhythmic effect of imipramine hydrochloride. *N. Engl. J. Med.* 196, 206.

Billingham, M.E. and Bristow, M.R. (1984). Evaluation of anthracycline cardiotoxicity: predictive ability and function correlation of endomyocardial biopsy. *Cancer Treat. Symp.* 3, 71.

Billman, G.E. (1990). Mechanisms responsible for the cardiotoxic effects of cocaine. *FASEB J.* 4, 2469.

Blankenship, J.C. and Almquist, A.K. (1989). Cardiovascular complications of thrombolytic therapy in patients with a mistaken diagnosis of acute myocardial infarction. *J. Am. Coll. Cardiol.* 14, 1579.

Blijham, G.H., Fiolet, H.H., van Deijk, W.A., *et al.* (1986). Angina pectoris associated with infusions of 5-FU and vindesine. *Cancer Treat. Rep.* 70, 314.

Blinks, J.R. (1966). Field stimulation as a means of effecting the graded release of autonomic transmitters in isolated heart muscle. *J. Pharmacol. Exp. Ther.* 151, 221.

Blinks, J.R. (1967). Evaluation of the cardiac effects of several beta-adrenergic blocking agents. *Ann. N.Y. Acad. Sci.* 139, 673.

Blinks, J.R. and Endoh, M. (1986). Modification of myofibrillar responsiveness to calcium as an inotropic mechanism. *Circulation* 73 (Suppl. III), 85.

Block, P.J. and Winkle, R.A. (1983). Hemodynamic effects of antiarrhythmic drugs. *Am. J. Cardiol.* 52, 14.

Boden, W.E., Korr, K.S., and Bough, E.W. (1985). Nifedipine-induced hypotension and myocardial ischaemia in refractory angina pectoris. *JAMA* 253, 1131.

Boesen, F., Andersen, E.B., Jensen, E.K., *et al.* (1983). Cardiac conduction disturbances during carbamazepine therapy. *Acta Neurol. Scand.* 68, 49.

Bohm, M., Schwinger, R.H.G., and Erdmann, E. (1990). Different cardiodepressant potency of various calcium antagonists in human myocardium. *Am. J. Cardiol.* 65, 1039.

Bonaa, K., Arnesen, E., Theele, D.S., *et al.* (1988). Coffee and cholesterol: is it all in the brewing? The Tromso study. *BMJ* 297, 1103.

Bonadonna, G. and Monfardini, S. (1969). Cardiac toxicity of daunorubicin. *Lancet* i, 837.

Boon, A. (1987). Solvent abuse and the heart. *BMJ* 794, 722.

Boudoulas, H., Schaal, S.F., Lewis, R.P., *et al.* (1977a). Negative inotropic effects of lidocaine in patients with coronary arterial disease and normal subjects. *Chest* 71, 170.

Boudoulas, H., Lewis, R.P., Kates, R.E., *et al.* (1977b). Hypersensitivity to adrenergic stimulation after propranolol in normal subjects. *Ann. Intern. Med.* 87, 433.

Bourke, J.P., Cowan, J.C., Tansuphaswadikul, S., *et al.* (1987). Antiarrhymic drug effects on left ventricular performance. *Eur. Heart. J.* 8 (Suppl. A), 105.

Brady, H.R. and Horgan, J.H. (1988). Lithium and the heart. Unanswered questions. *Chest* 93, 166.

Braunwald, E. and Swan, H.J.C. (1968). Cooperative study on cardiac catheterization. *Circulation* 37 (Suppl. 1), 1.

Breithardt, G., Seipel, L., and Kuhn, H. (1980). Amiodarone. *Circulation* 61, 213.

Brevetti, G., Chiarello, M., Leone, R., *et al.* (1986). Amiodarone-induced decrease in lymphocyte beta-adrenergic receptor density. *Am. J. Cardiol.* 57, 698.

Bristow, M.R., Thompson, P.D., Martin, R.P., *et al.* (1978). Early anthrocycline cardiotoxicity. *Am. J. Med.* 65, 823.

Brodsky, M.A., Allen, B.J., Abate, D., *et al.* (1985). Propafenone therapy for ventricular tachycardia in the setting of congestive heart failure. *Am. Heart J.* 110, 794.

Brown, B.R. and Crout, J.R. (1971). A comparative study of the effects of five general anesthetics on myocardial contractility. *Anesthesiology* 34, 236.

Brown, D.L. and Luchi, R.J. (1987). Cardiac tamponade and constrictive pericarditis complicating endoscopic sclerotherapy. *Arch. Intern. Med.* 147, 2169.

Buja, L.M., Ferrans, V.J., and Graw, R.G. (1976). Cardiac pathologic findings in patients treated with bone marrow transplantation. *Hum. Pathol.* 7, 17.

Bulkley B.H. and Roberts, W.C. (1974). Steroid therapy during acute myocardial infarction. A cause of delayed healing and of ventricular aneurysm. *Am. J. Med.* 56, 244.

Burrows, G.D., Davies, B., Hamer, A., *et al.* (1979). Effect of mianserin on cardiac conduction. *Med. J. Aust.* ii, 97.

Burton, J.R., Mathew, M.T., and Armstrong, P.W. (1976). Comparative effects of lidocaine and procainamide on acutely impaired hemodynamics. *Am. J. Med.* 61, 215.

Bush, T.L., Cowan, L.D., Barrett-Cooper, E., *et al.* (1983). Estrogen use and all-cause mortality. Preliminary results from the lipids research clinics program follow-up program. *JAMA* 249, 903.

Butler, J., Davies, A.H., and Westaby, S. (1990). Streptokinase in acute aortic dissection. *BMJ* 300, 517.

Butler, J.M., Marks, R., and Sutherland, R. (1985). Cutaneous and cardiac valvular pigmentation with minocycline. *Clin. Exp. Dermatol.* 10, 432.

Cairns, J.A., Connolly, S.J., Roberts, R., *et al.* (1997). Randomised trial of outcome after myocardial infarction in patients with frequent or repetitive premature depolarisations: CAMIAT. Canadian Amiodarone Myocardial Infarction Arrhythmia Trial Investigators. *Lancet* 349, 675.

Camarri, E., Chirone, E., Fanteria, G., *et al.* (1982). Ranitidine-induced bradycardia. *Lancet* ii, 160.

Campbell, N.P.S., Zaidi, S.A., Adgey, A.A.J., *et al.* (1979). Observations on haemodynamic effects of mexiletine. *Br. Heart J.* 41, 182.

Campbell, R.W.F. (1987). Arrhythmogenesis—A European Perspective. *Am. J. Cardiol.* 59, 49E.

Capasso, J.M. (1985). Calcium-induced reversible alterations in excitation-contraction coupling in verapamil-treated rat myocardium. *J. Mol. Cell. Cardiol.* 17, 275.

Carlier, J. (1980). Hemodynamic, electrocardiographic and toxic effects of the intravenous administration of increasing doses of mexiletine in the dog. Comparison with similar effects produced by other antiarrhythmics. *Acta Cardiol.* 25 (Suppl.), 81.

Carson, P., Oldroyd, K., and Phadke, K. (1987). Myocardial infarction due to amphetamine. *BMJ* 294, 1525.

Carvey, R.H. and Reed, D. (1970). Intravenous amphetamine poisoning. Report of three cases. *J. Forensic Sci. Soc.* 10, 109.

Casolo, G.C., Balli, E., Poggesi, L., *et al.* (1989). Increase in number of myocardial ischemic episodes following nifedipine administration in two patients. Detection of silent episodes by Holter monitoring and role of heart rate. *Chest* 95, 541.

CAST (Cardiac Arrhythmia Suppression Trial Investigators) (1989). Increased morbidity due to encainide or flecainide in a randomized trial of arrhythmia suppression after myocardial infarction. *N. Engl. J. Med.* 321, 406.

Caulfield, J.B. and Bittner, V. (1988). Cardiac matrix alterations induced by adriamycin. *Am. J. Pathol.* 133, 298.

Chamberlain, D.A., White, R.J., Howard, M.R., *et al.* (1970). Plasma digoxin concentrations in patients with atrial fibrillation. *BMJ* iii, 429.

Chamberlain, D.A., Jewitt, D.E., Julian, D.G., *et al.* (1980). Oral mexiletine in high-risk patients after myocardial infarction. *Lancet* ii, 1324.

Charlier, R. (1970). Cardiac actions in the dog of a new antagonist of adrenergic excitation which does not produce competitive blockade of adrenoceptors. *Br. J. Pharmacol.* 39, 668.

Chase, S.L. and Sloskey, G.E. (1987). Encainide hydrochloride and flecainide acetate: two Class Ic antiarrhythmic agents. *Clin. Pharm.* 6, 839.

Chaudary, S., Song, S.Y., and Jaski, B.E. (1988). Profound, yet reversible, heart failure secondary to 5-fluorouracil. *Am. J. Med.* 85, 454.

Cho, T., Tanimura, A., and Saito, Y. (1987). Catecholamine-induced cardiopathy accompanied with pheochromocytoma. *Acta Pathol. Jpn* 37, 123.

Chow, M.J., Piergies, A.A., Bowsher, D.J., et al. (1984). Torsades de pointes induced by *N*-acetylprocainamide. *J. Am. Coll. Cardiol.* 4, 621.

Clark, W.A., Tan, L-B., Jalil, J.E., et al. (1989). Assessment of non-ischemic myocardial necrosis with monoclonal antimyosin. *J. Mol. Cell. Cardiol.* 21 (Suppl. II), S156.

Clausen, T. and Flatman, J.A. (1980). Beta-2 adrenoceptors mediate the stimulating effect of adrenaline on active electrogenic Na–K transport in rat soleus muscle. *Br. J. Pharmacol.* 68, 749.

Clavel, M., Simeone, P., and Grivet, B. (1988). Toxicité cardiaque du 5-fluorouracine. Revue de la littérature, cinq nouveau cas. *Presse Méd.* 17, 1675.

Cleland, J.G.F., Dargie, H.J., Findlay, I.N., et al. (1987). Clinical, haemodynamic, and antiarrhythmic effects of long-term treatment with amiodarone of patients in heart failure. *Br. Heart J.* 57, 436.

Clementz, G.L. and Dolin, B.J. (1988). Sulfasalazine-induced lupus erythematosus. *Am. J. Med.* 84, 535.

Clifton, G.D., Booth, D.C., Hobbs, S., et al. (1990). Negative inotropic effect of intravenous nifedipine in coronary artery disease: relation to plasma levels. *Am. Heart J.* 119, 283.

Cobb, W.E., Spare, S., and Reichlin, S. (1978). Neurogenic diabetes insipidus: management with DDAVP. *Ann. Intern. Med.* 88, 183.

Cobbe, S.M. and Manley, B.S. (1987). The influence of ischaemia on the electrophysiological properties of amiodarone in chronically treated rabbit hearts. *Eur. Heart J.* 8, 1241.

Cody, R.J. (1988). Do positive inotropic agents adversely affect the survival of patients with chronic congestive heart failure? *J. Am. Coll. Cardiol.* 12, 559.

Cohen, I.S., Jick, H., and Cohen, S.I. (1977). Adverse reactions to quinidine in hospitalized patients: findings based on data from the Boston Collaborative Drug Surveillance Program. *Prog. Cardiovasc. Dis.* 20, 151.

Cohen, J., Weetman, A.P., Dargie, H.J., et al. (1979). Life-threatening arrhythmias and intravenous cimetidine. *BMJ* ii, 768.

Cohn, J.N. (1989). Inotropic therapy for heart failure. Paradise postponed. *N. Engl. J. Med.* 320, 729.

Cohn, J.N., Archibald, D.G., Ziesche, S., et al. (1986). Effect of vasodilator therapy on mortality in chronic congestive heart failure. Results of a Veterans Administration Co-operative study. *N. Engl. J. Med.* 314, 1547.

Collins, C. and Weiden, P.L. (1987). Cardiotoxicity of 5-fluorouracil. *Cancer Treat. Rep.* 71, 733.

Coltart, D.J., Berndt, T.D., Kernoff, R., et al. (1974). Antiarrhythmic and circulatory effects of Astra W36095. A new lidocaine-like agent. *Am. J. Cardiol.* 34, 35.

Colucci, W.S. (1987). Usefulness of calcium antagonists for congestive heart failure. *Am. J. Cardiol.* 59, 52B.

Colucci, W.S. (1989). Observations on the intracoronary administration of milrinone and dobutamine to patients with congestive heart failure. *Am. J. Cardiol.* 63, 17A.

Come, P.C. and Pitt, B. (1976). Nitroglycerin-induced severe hypotension and bradycardias in patients with acute myocardial infarction. *Circulation* 54, 624.

Conard, G.J. and Ober, R.E. (1984). Metabolism of flecainide. *Am. J. Cardiol.* 53, 41B.

Connolly, H.M., Crary, J.L., McGoon, M.D., et al. (1997) Valulvar heart disease associated with fenfluramine–phentermine. *N Engl. J. Med.* 327. 581.

Conway, N. (1968). Haemodynamic effects of ethyl alcohol in coronary heart disease. *Am. Heart J.* 76, 581.

Conway, N., Seymour, J., and Gelson, A. (1968). Cardiac failure in patients with valvular heart disease after use of propranolol to control atrial fibrillation. *BMJ* ii, 213.

Corder, M.P. and Flannery, E.P. (1974). Possible radiation pericarditis precipitated by actinomycin D. *Oncology* 30, 81.

Cote, P., Harrison, D.C., Basile, J., et al. (1973). Hemodynamic interaction of procainamide and lignocaine after experimental myocardial infarction. *Am. J. Cardiol.* 32, 937.

Cote, P., Schook, J., Harrison, D.C., et al. (1975). Hemodynamic effects of procainamide and quinidine and the influence of beta-blockade before and after experimental myocardial infarction (38935). *Proc. Soc. Exp. Biol. Med.* 149, 958.

Coull, D.C., Crooks, J., Dingwall-Fordyce, I., et al. (1970). Amitriptyline and cardiac disease: risk of sudden death identified by monitoring system. *Lancet* ii, 590.

Cowan, J.C. (1986). Nitrate tolerance. Editorial review. *Int. J. Cardiol.* 12, 1.

Cowan, J.C. (1990). Antianginal drug therapy. *Current Opinion in Cardiology* 5, 453.

Crane, J., Burgess, C., and Beasley, R. (1989). Cardiovascular and hypokalaemic effects of inhaled salbutamol, fenoterol and isoprenaline. *Thorax* 44, 136.

Crawford, M.H., White, D.H., and O'Rourke, R.A. (1979). Effects of oral quinidine on left ventricular performance in normal subjects and patients with congestive cardiomyopathy. *Am. J. Cardiol.* 44, 714.

Cregler, L.L. and Mark, H. (1986). Medical complications of cocaine abuse. *N. Engl. J. Med.* 315, 1495.

Cregler, L.L. and Mark, H. (1987). Second-degree atrioventricular block and alpha-methyldopa: a probable connection. *Mt Sinai J. Med.* 54, 168.

CSM (Committee on Safety of Medicines) (1990). *Current Problems*, No. 28.

CSM (Committee on Safety of Medicines) (1992). *Report of the β Agonist Working Party*. HMSO, London.

Dalen, J.E. and Hickler, R.B. (1981). Oral contraceptives and cardiovascular disease. *Am. Heart J.* 101, 626.

Dangman, K.H. and Hoffman, B.F. (1981). *In vivo* and *in vitro* antiarrhythmic and arrhythmogenic effects of *N*-acetyl procainamide. *J. Pharmacol. Exp. Ther.* 217, 851.

Daoud, E.G., Man, K.C., Horwood, L., *et al.* (1997). Relation between amiodarone and desmethylamiodarone plasma concentrations and ventricular defibrillation energy requirements. *Am. J. Cardiol.* 79, 97.

Data, J.L., Wilkinson, G.R., and Nies, A.S. (1976). Interaction of quinidine with anticonvulsant drugs. *N. Engl. J. Med.* 294, 699.

Davidson, S. and Surawicz, B. (1967). Ectopic beats and atrioventricular conduction disturbances in patients with hypopotassaemia. *Arch. Intern. Med.* 120, 280.

Davis, J.C., Reiffel, J.A., and Bigger, J.T. (1981). Sinus node dysfunction caused by methyldopa and digoxin. *JAMA* 245, 1241.

Dawber, T.R., Kannel, W.B., and Gordon, T. (1974). Coffee and cardiovascular disease: observations from the Framingham Study. *N. Engl. J. Med.* 291, 871.

Deboever, G., Devogelaere, R., and Holvoet, G. (1989). Sulphasalazine-induced lupus-like syndrome with cardiac tamponade in a patient with ulcerative colitis. *Am. J. Gastroenterol.* 84, 85.

Delborg, M., Held, P., Swedberg, K., *et al.* (1985). Rupture of myocardium, occurrence and risk factors. *Br. Heart J.* 54, 11.

Demakis, J.G., Proskey, A., Rahimtoola, S.H., *et al.* (1974). The natural course of alcoholic cardiomyopathy. *Ann. Intern. Med.* 80, 293.

De Mots, H. and Glasser, S.P. (1989). Intermittent transdermal nitroglycerin therapy in the management of chronic stable angina. *J. Am. Coll. Cardiol.* 13, 786.

Dent, R.G. and McColl, I. (1975). 5-Fluorouracil and angina. *Lancet* i, 347.

Dessertenne, F. (1966). La tachycardie ventriculaire à deux foyers opposés variables. *Arch. Méd. Coeur* 59, 263.

Dies, F. (1986). Intermittent dobutamine in ambulatory patients with chronic cardiac failure. *Br. J. Clin. Pract.* (Suppl. 45), 37.

Digitalis Investigation Group. (1997). The effect of digoxin on mortality and morbidity in patients with heart failure. *N. Engl. J. Med.* 336, 525.

Di Marco, J.P., Sellers, T., Berne, R.M., *et al.* (1983). Adenosine: electrophysiological effects and therapeutic use for terminating paroxysmal supraventricular tachycardia. *Circulation* 68, 1254.

Dinwiddie, S.H. (1994). Abuse of inhalants: a review. *Addiction* 89, 925.

Dobmeyer, D.J., Stine, R.A., Leier, C.V., *et al.* (1983). The arrhythmogenic effects of caffeine in human beings. *N. Engl. J. Med.* 308. 814.

Dollery, C.T., Patterson, J.W., and Conolly, M.E. (1969). Clinical pharmacology of beta-receptor-blocking drugs. *Clin. Pharmacol. Ther.* 10, 765.

Dollery, C.T., Draffman, G.H., Davies, D.S., *et al.* (1970). Blood concentrations in man of fluorinated hydrocarbons after inhalation of pressurised aerosols. *Lancet* ii, 1164.

Domanski, M.J., Zipes, D.P., and Schron, E. (1997). Treatment of sudden cardiac death current understandings from randomized trials and future research directions. *Circulation* 95, 2694.

Dowling, G.P., McDonough, E.T., and Bost, R.O. (1987). 'Eve' and 'Ecstasy'. A report of five deaths associated with the use of MDEA and MDMA. *JAMA* 257, 1615.

Dresdale, A., Bonow, R.O., Wesley, T., *et al.* (1983). Prospective evaluation of doxorubicin-induced cardiomyopathy resulting from post-surgical adjuvant treatment of patients with soft tissue sarcomas. *Cancer* 52, 51.

Dukes, I.D. and Vaughan Williams, E.M. (1984). The multiple modes of action of propafenone. *Eur. Heart J.* 5, 115.

Durelli, L., Mutani, R., Sechi, G.P., *et al.* (1985). Cardiac side effects of phenytoin and carbamazepine. A dose-related phenomenon? *Arch. Neurol.* 42, 1067.

Durkin, W.J., Pugh, P.R., and Solomon, J.T. (1976). Treatment of advanced lymphomas with bleomycin (NSC-125066). *Oncology* 33, 140.

Echt, D.S., Liebson, P.R., Mitchell, L.B., *et al.* (1991). Mortality and morbidity in patients receiving ecainide, flecainide, or placebo: the Cardiac Arrhythmia Suppression Trial. *N. Engl. J. Med.* 324. 781.

Edlund, A., Berglund, B., van Dorne, D., *et al.* (1985). Coronary flow regulation in patients with ischaemic heart disease: release of purines and prostacyclin and the effect of inhibitors of prostaglandin formation. *Circulation* 71, 1113.

Edwards, G.S., Lane, M., and Smith, P.E. (1979). Long-term treatment with *cis*-dichlorodiamineplatinum-vinblastine-bleomycin. Possible association with severe coronary artery disease. *Cancer Treat. Rep.* 63, 551.

Egstrup, K. (1988). Transient myocardial ischaemia after abrupt withdrawal of antianginal therapy in chronic stable angina. *Am. J. Cardiol.* 61, 1219.

El-Sherif, N., Scherlag, B.J., Lazzara, R., *et al.* (1977). Reentrant ventricular arrhythmias in the late myocardial infarction period. Mechanism of action of lidocaine. *Circulation* 56, 395.

Engelmeier, R.S., O'Connell, J.B., Walsh, R., *et al.* (1985). Improvement in symptoms and exercise tolerance by metoprolol in patients with dilated cardiomyopathy: a double-blind, randomized, placebo-controlled trial. *Circulation* 72, 536.

Ensley, J.F., Patel, B., Kloner, R., *et al.* (1989). The clinical syndrome of 5-fluorouracil cardiotoxicity. *Invest. New Drugs* 7, 101.

Epstein, S.E., Robinson, B.F., Kahler, R.L., *et al.* (1965). Effects of beta-adrenergic blockade on the cardiac response to maximal and sub-maximal exercise in man. *J. Clin. Invest.* 44, 1745.

Ettinger, P.O., Wu, C.F., and De La Gruz, C. (1978). Arrhythmias and the 'holiday heart'. *Am. Heart J.* 95, 555.

Etvinsson, G. and Orinius, E. (1980). Prodromal ventricular beats produced by a diastolic wave. *Acta Med. Scand.* 208, 445.

Falik, R., Flores, B.T., Shaw, L., *et al.* (1987). Relationship of steady-state serum concentrations of amiodarone and desmethylamiodarone to therapeutic efficacy and adverse effects. *Am. J. Med.* 82, 1102.

Farber, J.L., Chien, K.R., and Mittnacht, S. Jr (1981). The pathogenesis of irreversible cell injury in ischemia. *Am. J. Pathol.* 102, 271.

Featherstone, H.J. and Stewart, D.K. (1983). Angina in thyrotoxicosis: Thyroid-related coronary artery spasm. *Arch. Intern. Med.* 143, 554.

Feely, J., Wilkinson, G.R., McAllister, C.B., *et al.* (1982). Increased toxicity and reduced clearance of lignocaine by cimetidine. *Ann Intern. Med.* 96, 592.

Feldman, R.L., Nichols, W.M., Peppine, C.J., *et al.* (1981). Acute effect of intravenous dipyridamole on regional coronary haemodynamics and metabolism. *Circulation* 64, 333.

Feldman, R.L., Peppine, C.J., Whittle, J., *et al.* (1982). Short- and long-term responses to diltiazem in patients with variant angina. *Am. J. Cardiol.* 49, 554.

Fenster, P.A., White, N.W., and Hanson, C.D. (1985). Pharmacokinetic evaluation of the digoxin-amiodarone interaction. *J. Am. Coll. Cardiol.* 5, 108.

Ferrantini, M., Pirelli, S., Merlini, P., *et al.* (1989). Intermittent transdermal nitroglycerin monotherapy in stable exercise-induced angina: A comparison with continuous schedule. *Eur. Heart J.* 10, 998.

Fiegl, E.O. (1983). Coronary physiology. *Physiol. Rev.* 63, 1.

Fisch, C. (1973). Relation of electrolyte disturbances to cardiac arrhythmias. *Circulation* 47, 409.

Fleckenstein, A. (1971). Specific inhibitors and promoters of calcium action in the excitation-contraction coupling of heart muscle and their role in the prevention or production of myocardial cell lesion. In *Calcium and the Heart* (ed. P. Harris and L. Opie), p. 135. Academic Press, London.

Fogoros, R.N. (1984). Amiodarone-induced refractoriness to cardioversion. *Ann. Intern. Med.* 100, 699.

Fogoros, R.N., Anderson, K.P., Winkle, R.A., *et al.* (1983). Amiodarone: clinical efficacy and toxicity in 96 patients with recurrent, drug refractory arrhythmias. *Circulation* 68, 88.

Folle, L.E. and Aviado, D.M. (1966). The cardiopulmonary effects of quinidine and procainamide. *J. Pharmacol. Exp. Ther.* 154, 92.

Franciosa, J.A., Wilen, M., Weeks, C.E., *et al.* (1983). Pharmacokinetics and hemodynamic effects of flecainide in patients with chronic low output heart failure. *J. Am. Coll. Cardiol.* 1, 699.

Franklyn, J.A., Davis, J.R., Gammage, M.D., *et al.* (1985). Amiodarone and thyroid hormone action. *Clin. Endocrinol.* 22, 257.

Freer, R.J., Pappano, A.J., Peach, M.J., *et al.* (1976). Mechanism for the positive inotropic effect of angiotensin II on isolated cardiac muscle. *Circ. Res.* 39, 178.

Frishman, W.H. (1987). Beta-adrenergic blocker withdrawal. *Am. J. Cardiol.* 59, 26F.

Furberg, C.D., Psaty, B.M., and Meyer, J.V. (1995). Nifedipine: dose related increase in mortality in patients with coronary heart disease. *Circulation* 92, 1326.

Gallagher, J.D., Lieberman, R.W., Meranze, J., *et al.* (1981). Amiodarone-induced complications during coronary artery surgery. *Anesthesiology* 55, 186.

Galton, D.A.G. (1983). Medical aspects of neoplasia. In *Oxford Textbook of Medicine* (ed. D.J. Weatherall, J.G.G. Ledingham, and D.A. Warrell), p. 473. Oxford University Press.

Garcia, R. and Jennings, J.M. (1972). Pheochromocytoma masquerading as a cardiomyopathy. *Am. J. Cardiol.* 29, 568.

Garret, J., Kolbe, J., Richards, G., *et al.* (1995). Nifedipine: dose related increase in mortality in patients with coronary disease. *Circulation* 92, 1326.

Gavras, H., Brown, J.J., MacAdam, R.F., *et al.* (1971). Acute renal failure, tubular necrosis, and myocardial infarction induced in the rabbit by intravenous angiotensin II. *Lancet* ii, 19.

Gavras, H., Kremer, D., Brown, J.J., *et al.* (1975). Angiotensin- and norepinephrine-induced myocardial lesions: experimental and clinical studies in rabbits and man. *Am. Heart J.* 89, 321.

Geleris, P., Boudoulas, H., Schaal, S.F., *et al.* (1980). Effect of procainamide on left ventricular performance in patients with primary myocardial disease. *Eur. J. Clin. Pharmacol.* 18, 311.

German and Austrian Xamoterol Study Group (1988). Double-blind placebo-controlled comparison of digoxin and xamoterol in chronic heart failure. *Lancet* i, 489.

Gettes, L.S. (1970). Beta-adrenergic blocking drugs in the treatment of cardiac arrhythmias. *Cardiovasc. Clin.* 2, 211.

Giacomelli, F., Anversa, P., and Wiener, J. (1976). Effects of angiotensin-induced hypertension on rat coronary arteries and myocardium. *Am. J. Pathol.* 84, 111.

Gibb, I., Cowan, J.C., Parnham, A.J., *et al.* (1986). Use and misuse of a digoxin assay service. *BMJ* 293, 678.

Gibbs, C.L., Mommaerts, W.F.H.M., and Ricchiuti, N.V. (1967). Energetics of cardiac contractions. *J. Physiol. (Lond.)* 191, 25.

Gibson, D.G., Greenbaum, R.A., Pridie, R.B., *et al.* (1988). Correction of left ventricular asynchrony by coronary artery surgery. *Br. Heart J.* 59, 304.

Glassman, A.H. (1984). Cardiovascular effects of tricyclic antidepressants. *Annu. Rev. Med.* 35, 503.

Glaubiger, G. and Lefkowitz, R.J. (1977). Elevated beta-adrenergic receptor number after chronic propranolol treatment. *Biochem. Biophys. Res. Commun.* 78, 720.

Gold, R.G. (1967). Acute non-specific pericarditis. *Postgrad. Med. J.* 43, 534.

Goldberg, D., Reiffel, J.A., Davis, J.C., *et al.* (1982). Electrophysiologic effects of procainamide on sinus node function in patients with and without sinus node disease. *Am. Heart J.* 103, 75.

Goldberg, S., Greenspow, A.S., Urban, P.L., *et al.* (1983). Reperfusion arrhythmia: a marker of extraction of anterograde flow during intracoronary thrombolysis for acute myocardial infarction. *Circulation* 67, 796.

Goldbourt, U., Behar, S., Reicher-Reiss, H., *et al.* for the SPRINT Study group. (1993). Early administration of nifedipine in suspected acute myocardial infarction: the

Second Prevention Reinfarction Israel Nifedipine Trial 2 study. *Arch. Intern. Med.* 153. 345.

Goldfischer, J.D. (1960). Acute myocardial infarction secondary to ergot treatment. *N. Engl. J. Med.* 262, 860.

Gough, W.B., Zeiler, R.H., Barreca, P., *et al.* (1982). Hypotensive action of commercial intravenous amiodarone and polysorbate 80 in dogs. *J. Cardiovasc. Pharmacol.* 4, 375.

Gould, L., Reddy, C.V.R., Singh, B.K., *et al.* (1979). Electrophysiologic properties of methyldopa in man. *Chest* 76, 310.

Graboys, T.B., Blatt, C.M., and Lown, B. (1989). The effect of caffeine on ventricular ectopic activity in patients with malignant ventricular arrhythmia. *Arch. Intern. Med.* 149, 637.

Graham, J.R. (1967). Cardiac and pulmonary fibrosis during methysergide therapy for headache. *Trans. Am. Clin. Climatol. Assoc.* 78, 79.

Graham, J.R., Suby, H.L., Le Compte, P.R., *et al.* (1966). Fibrotic disorders associated with methysergide treatment for headache. *N. Engl. J. Med.* 274, 359.

Greenberg, M.L., Lerman, B.B., Shipe, J.R., *et al.* (1987). Relationship between amiodarone and desmethylamiodarone plasma concentrations and electrophysiological effects efficacy and toxicity. *J. Am. Coll. Cardiol.* 9, 1148.

Greene, H.L., Roden, D.M., Katz, R.J., *et al.* (1992). The Cardiac Arrhythmia Suppression Trial: first CAST . . . then CAST-II. *J. Am. Coll. Cardiol.* 19, 894.

Greenspon, A.J. and Schaal, S.F. (1983). The 'holiday heart': Electrophysiological studies of alcohol effects in alcoholics. *Ann. Intern. Med.* 98, 135.

Gunn, J., Wilson, J., and Mackintosh, A.F. (1989). Butane sniffing causing ventricular fibrillation. *Lancet* i, 617.

Haft, J.I., Kranz, P.D., Albert, F.J., *et al.* (1982). Intravascular platelet aggregation in the heart induced by norepinephrine: microscopic studies. *Circulation* 46, 698.

Halper, J.P. and Mann, J.J. (1988). Cardiovascular effects of antidepressant medications. *Br. J. Psychiatry* 153 (Suppl. 3), 87.

Hamer, A.W.F., Arkles, L.B., and Johns, J.A. (1989). Beneficial effects of low dose amiodarone in patients with congestive cardiac failure: a placebo-controlled trial. *J. Am. Coll. Cardiol.* 14, 1768.

Hammermeister, K.E., Boerth, R.C., and Warbasse, J.R. (1972). The comparative inotropic effects of six clinically used antiarrhythmic agents. *Am. Heart J.* 81, 643.

Hansen, W.D. and Bertl, S. (1983). Inhibition of cholinesterase by ranitidine. *Lancet* i, 235.

Harden, T.K. (1983). Agonist-induced desensitisation of beta-adrenergic receptor linked adenylate cyclase. *Pharmacol. Rev.* 35, 5.

Harrison, D.C., Sprouse, J.H., and Morrow, A.G. (1963). The antiarrhythmic properties of lidocaine and procaine amide. Clinical and physiologic studies of their cardiovascular effects in man. *Circulation* 28, 486.

Harrison, D.T. and Danders, L.A. (1976). Pericarditis in a case of early daunorubicin cardiomyopathy. *Ann. Intern. Med.* 85, 339.

Hart, A. (1989). Cardiac arrest associated with ranitidine. *BMJ* 299, 519.

Hassell, A.B. and Creamer, J.E. (1989). Profound bradycardia after the addition of diltiazem to a beta-blocker. *BMJ* 198, 675.

Hauck, A.J., Edwards, W.D., Danielson, G.K., *et al.* (1990). Mitral and aortic valve disease associated with ergotamine therapy for migraine. Report of two cases and review of the literature. *Arch. Pathol. Lab. Med.* 114, 62.

Hays, R.M. (1985). Agents affecting the renal conservation of water. In *Goodman and Gilman's The Pharmacological Basis of Therapeutics* (7th edn) (ed. A.G. Gilman, L.S. Goodman, T.W. Rall, and F. Murad), p. 908. Macmillan, New York.

HDFP (Hypertension Detection and Follow-up Programme Co-operative Research Group) (1984). The effect of antihypertensive drug treatment on morbidity in the presence of resting electrocardiographic abnormalities at baseline: the HDFP experience. *Circulation* 70, 996.

Hedner T. (1986). Calcium channel blockers: spectrum of side effects and drug interactions. *Acta Pharmacol. Toxicol.* 58 (Suppl. 2), 119.

Heilbrunn, S.M., Shah, P., Bristow, M.R., *et al.* (1989). Increased β-receptor density and improved hemodynamic response to catecholamine stimulation during long-term metoprolol therapy in heart failure. *Circulation* 79, 483.

Held, P.H., Yusuf, S., and Furberg, C.D. (1989). Calcium channel blockers in acute myocardial infarction and unstable angina: an overview. *BMJ* 299, 1187.

Hellestrand, K.J., Burnett, P.J., Milne J.R., *et al.* (1983). Effect of the antiarrhythmic agent flecainide acetate on acute and chronic pacing thresholds. *PACE* 6, 892.

Hellestrand, K., Nathan, A.W., Bexton, R.S., *et al.* (1984). Response of an abnormal sinus node to intravenous flecainide acetate. *PACE* 7, 436.

Hendeles, L. and Weinberger, M. (1983). Theophylline: a 'state of art' review. *Pharmacotherapy* 3, 2.

Hennekens, C.H. and Macmahon B. (1977). Oral contraceptives and myocardial infarction. *N. Engl. J. Med.* 296, 1116.

Henry, P.D. (1980). Comparative pharmacology of calcium antagonists: nifedipine, verapamil and diltiazem. *Am. J. Cardiol.* 46, 1047.

Herrmann, H.C., Kaplan, L.M., and Bierer, B.A. (1983). QT prolongation and torsades de pointes ventricular tachycardia produced by the tetracyclic antidepressant maprotiline. *Am. J. Cardiol.* 51, 904.

Higgins, R.M., Cookson, W.O.C., Lane, D.J., *et al.* (1987). Cardiac arrhythmias caused by nebulised beta-agonist therapy. *Lancet* ii, 863.

Hoddess, A.B., Follansby, W.P., Spear, J.F., *et al.* (1979). Electrophysiologic effects of a new antiarrhythmic agent, flecainide, on the intact canine heart. *J. Cardiovasc. Pharmacol.* 1, 427.

Hodsman, G.P., Robertson, J.I.S., Semple, P.F., *et al.* (1982). Malignant hypertension and oral contraceptives: four cases with two due to the 30μg oestrogen pill. *Eur. Heart J.* 3, 255.

Holdright, D.R. (1997). Calcium-channel antagonists in cardiovascular disease. *Br. J. Hosp. Med.* 57, 552.

Hollifield, T.W. (1987). Magnesium depletion, diuretics and arrhythmias. *Am. J. Med.* 82 (Suppl. 3A), 30.

Holme, I., Helgeland, A., Hjermann, I., *et al.* (1984). Treatment of mild hypertension with diuretics: the importance of ECG abnormalities in the Oslo study and in MRFIT. *JAMA* 251, 1298.

Holmes, J.R., Kubo, S.H., Cody, R.J., *et al.* (1985). Milrinone in congestive heart failure: observations on ambulatory ventricular arrhythmias. *Am. Heart J.* 110, 800.

Holt, D.W., Hayler, A.M., Edmonds, M.E., *et al.* (1979). Clinically significant interaction between digoxin and quinidine. *BMJ* ii, 1401.

Homback, V., Behrenbeck, D.W., Tauchert, M.M., *et al.* (1979). Myocardial metabolism of cyclic 3,5-adenosine monophosphate as influenced by dipyridamole and theophylline in patients with coronary artery disease. *Clin. Cardiol.* 2, 41.

Honerjager, P., Loibl, E., Steidl, I., *et al.* (1986). Negative inotropic effects of tetrodotoxin and seven Class I antiarrhythmic drugs in relation to sodium channel blockade. *Naunyn-Schmiedebergs Arch. Pharmacol.* 332, 184.

Horn, H.R., Hadidian, Z., Johnson, J.L., *et al.* (1980). Safety evaluation of tocainide in the American Emergency Use Program. *Am. Heart J.* 100, 1037.

Huston, J.R. and Bell, G.E. (1966). The effect of thioridazine chloride and chlorpromazine on the electrocardiogram. *JAMA* 198, 16.

Hutchins, G.M. and Bulkley, B.H. (1978). Infarct expansion versus extension: two different complications of acute myocardial infarction. *Am. J. Cardiol.* 41, 1127.

Hutchison, S.T., Lorimer, A.R., Larhdar, A., *et al.* (1984). Beta-blockers and verapamil: a cautionary tale. *BMJ* 289, 659.

Ikram, H. (1980). Hemodynamic and electrophysiologic interactions between antiarrhythmic drugs and beta blockers, with special reference to tocainide. *Am. Heart J.* 100, 1076.

Ingemarsson, I., Arulkumaran, S., and Kottegoda, S.R. (1985). Complications of beta-mimetic therapy in preterm labour. *Aust. N.Z. J. Obstet. Gynaecol.* 25, 182.

Installe, E., Schoevaerdts, J.C., Gadisseux, P., *et al.* (1981). Intravenous amiodarone in the treatment of various arrhythmias following cardiac operations. *J. Thorac. Cardiovasc. Surg.* 81, 302.

Ishizaki, M., Yamada, Y., Kido, T., *et al.* (1987). First-degree atrioventricular block induced by oral cimetidine. *Lancet* i, 225.

ISIS-2 (Second International Study of Infarct Survival): Collaborative group (1982). Randomized trial of intravenous streptokinase, oral aspirin, both or neither among 17,187 cases of suspected acute myocardial infarction ISIS-2. *Lancet* 2, 349.

Isner, J.M. and Chokshi. S.K. (1991). Cardiovascular complications of cocaine. *Curr. Probl. Cardiol.* 16, 95.

Isner, J.M., Estes, N.A., Thompson, P.D., *et al.* (1986). Acute cardiac events temporally related to cocaine abuse. *N. Engl. J. Med.* 315, 1438.

Iversen, L.L. (1967). *The Uptake and Storage of Noradrenaline in Sympathetic Nerves.* Cambridge University Press.

Jackman, W.M., Friday, K.J., and Anderson, J.L. (1988). The long QT syndromes: a critical review, new clinical observations and a unifying hypothesis. *Prog. Cardiovasc. Dis.* 31, 115.

Jackson, W.K., Roose, S.P., and Glassman, A.H. (1987). Cardiovascular toxicity of antidepressant medications. *Psychopathology* 20 (Suppl. 1), 64.

Jakubowski, A.A. and Remeny, N. (1983). Hypotension as a manifestation of cardiotoxicity in three patients receiving cisplatin and 5-fluorouracil. *Cancer* 62, 266.

Janowsky, D., Curtis, G., Zisook, S., *et al.* (1983). Ventricular arrhythmias possibly aggravated by trazodone. *Am. J. Psychiatry* 140, 796.

Jariwalla, A.G. and Anderson, E.G. (1978). Production of ischaemic cardiac pain by nifedipine. *BMJ* i, 1181.

Jawad-Kanber, G. and Sherrod, T.R. (1974). Effect of loading dose of procaine amide on left ventricular performance in man. *Chest* 66, 269.

Jazayeri, M.R., Van Whye, G., and Avitall, B. (1989). Isoproterenol reversal of antiarrhythmic effects in patients with inducible sustained ventricular tachyarrhythmias. *J. Am. Coll. Cardiol.* 14, 705.

Jefferys, D.B. and Vale, J.A. (1978). Cimetidine and bradycardia. *Lancet* i, 828.

Jensen, G., Sigurd, B., and Uhrenholt, A. (1975). Haemodynamic effects of intravenous disopyramide in heart failure. *Eur. J. Clin. Pharmacol.* 8, 167.

Jewell, W.H., Koth, D.R., and Huggins, C.E. (1955). Ventricular fibrillation in dogs after sudden return of flow to the coronary artery. *Surgery* 38, 1050.

Jick, H., Miettinen, D.S., Neff, R.K., *et al.* (1973). Coffee and myocardial infarction. *N. Engl. J. Med.* 289, 63.

Josephson, M.A., Kaul, S., Hopkins, J., *et al.* (1985). Hemodynamic effects of intravenous flecainide relative to the level of ventricular function in patients with coronary artery disease. *Am. Heart J.* 109, 41.

Kadatz, R. (1959). The pharmacology of 2,6-*bis*-(diethanolamino)-4,8-dipiperidinopyrimido (5,4-)-pyrimide, a new compound with coronary dilatory properties. *Arzneim.-Forsch.* 9, 39.

Kaduk, B. and Seiler, G. (1978). Congestive cardiomyopathy after doxorubicin (Adriamycin). *JAMA* 239, 2057.

Kane, K.A. and Winslow, E. (1980). Antidysrhythmic and electrophysiological effects of a new antianginal agent, bepridil. *J. Cardiovasc. Pharmacol.* 2, 193.

Karliner, J.S., Simpson, P.C., Honbo, N., *et al.* (1986). Mechanisms and time course of beta-1 adrenoceptor desensitization in mammalian cardiac myocytes. *Cardiovasc. Res.* 20, 221.

Karlsson, E. and Sonnhag, C. (1976). Haemodynamic effects of procainamide and phenytoin at apparent therapeutic plasma levels. *Eur. J. Clin. Pharmacol.* 10, 305.

Katz, A.M. and Reuter, H. (1979). Cellular calcium and cardiac cell death. *Am. J. Cardiol.* 44, 188.

Katz, M., Robertson, P.A., and Creasy, R.K. (1981). Cardiovascular complications associated with terbutaline treatment for preterm labour. *Am. J. Obstet. Gynecol.* 139, 605.

Kay, G.N., Plumb, V.J., Arciniegas, J.G., *et al.* (1983). Torsade de pointes: the long-short initiating sequence and other clinical features: observations in 32 patients. *J. Am. Coll. Cardiol.* 2, 806.

Kay, R., Blake, J., and Rubin, D. (1982). Possible coronary spasm rebound to abrupt nifedipine withdrawal. *Am. Heart J.* 103, 308.

Kelbaek, H., Eriksen, J., Brynjolf, I., *et al.* (1984). Cardiac performance in patients with asymptomatic alcohol cirrhosis of the liver. *Am. J. Cardiol.* 54, 852.

Kelly, P.A., Cannom, D.W., Garan, H., *et al.* (1988). The automatic implantable cardioverter-defibrillator: efficacy, complications and survival in patients with malignant ventricular arrhythmias. *J. Am. Coll. Cardiol.* 11, 1278.

Kemmotsu, O., Hashimoto, Y., and Shimosato, S. (1974). The effects of fluroxene and enflurane on contractile performance of isolated papillary muscles from failing hearts. *Anesthesiology* 40, 252.

Kennedy, B.L. and West, T.C. (1969). Factors influencing quinidine-induced changes in excitability and contractility. *J. Pharmacol. Exp. Ther.* 168, 47.

Kerin, N.Z. and Somberg, J. (1994). Proarrhythmia: Definition, risk factors, causes, treatment, and controversies. *Am. Heart J.* 128. 575.

Khan, M.M., Logan, K.R., McComb, J.M., *et al.* (1981). Management of recurrent ventricular tachyarrhythmias associated with QT prolongation. *Am. J. Cardiol.* 47, 1301.

Kincaid-Smith, P. (1984). Beta-adrenergic receptor blocking drugs in hypertension. *Am. J. Cardiol.* 53, 12A.

Kino, M., Imamitchi, H., Morigutchi, M., *et al.* (1981). Cardiovascular status in asymptomatic alcoholics, with reference to the level of ethanol consumption. *Br. Heart J.* 46, 545.

Klatsky, A.L., Friedman, G.D., and Siegelaub, A.B. (1973). Coffee drinking prior to acute myocardial infarction: results from the Kaiser-Permanente epidemiological study of myocardial infarction. *JAMA* 226, 540.

Klein, K. (1977). Complications of testicular treatment. *Int. J. Radiat. Oncol. Biol. Phys.* 2, 1049.

Klein, L.S., Simpson, R.J., Stern, R., *et al.* (1982). Myocardial infarction following administration of sublingual ergotamine. *Chest* 82, 375.

Kleinman, N.S., Lehane, D.E., Geyer, C.Y., *et al.* (1987). Prinzmetal's angina during 5-fluorouracil chemotherapy. *Am. J. Med.* 82, 566.

Kloner, R.A., Hale, S., Alker, K., *et al.* (1992). The effects of acute and chronic cocaine use on the heart. *Circulation* 85, 40.

Koch-Weser, J. (1965). Nature of the inotropic action of angiotensin on ventricular myocardium. *Circ. Res.* 16, 230.

Kosinski, R.M. (1989). Alcoholic cardiomyopathy. *N.J. Med.* 86, 773.

Koskinen, P., Kupari, M., Leinonen, H., *et al.* (1987). Alcohol and new onset atrial fibrillation: a case-control study of a current series. *Br. Heart J.* 57, 468.

Kotler, M.N., Michaeides, K.M., Bouchard, R.J., *et al.* (1973). Myocardial infarction associated with thyrotoxicosis. *Arch. Intern. Med.* 132, 732.

Kötter, V., Linderer, T., and Schröder, R. (1980). Effects of disopyramide on systemic and coronary hemodynamics and myocardial metabolism in patients with coronary artery disease: Comparison with lidocaine. *Am. J. Cardiol.* 46, 469.

Kowey, P.R., Friedman, P.L., Podrid, P.J., *et al.* (1982). Use of radionuclide ventriculography for assessment of changes in myocardial performance induced by disopyramide phosphate. *Am. Heart J.* 104, 769.

Krehlik, J.M., Hindson, D.A., Crowley, J.J., *et al.* (1985). Minoxidil-associated pericarditis and fatal cardiac tamponade. *West. J. Med.* 143, 527.

Kuhn, P., Klicpera, M., Kroiss, A., *et al.* (1977). Anti-arrhythmic and haemodynamic effects of mexiletine. *Postgrad. Med. J.* 53, 81.

Laaban, J.P., Iung, B., Chauvet, J.P., *et al.* (1988). Cardiac arrhythmias during the combined use of intravenous aminophylline and terbutaline in status asthmatics. *Chest* 94, 496.

Labianca, R., Beretta, G., Clerici, M., *et al.* (1982). Cardiotoxicity of 5-fluorouracil: a study of 1083 patients. *Tumori* 68, 505.

La Croix, A.Z., Mead, L.A., Liang, K-Y., *et al.* (1986). Coffee consumption and the incidence of coronary heart disease. *N. Engl. J. Med.* 315, 977.

Ladefoged, S.D. and Mogelvang, J.C. (1982). Total atrio-ventricular block with syncope aggravated by carbamazepine. *Acta Med. Scand.* 212, 185.

Lameijer, W. and van Zwieten, P.A. (1974). The interaction between quinidine and propranolol on isolated heart muscle preparations. *Arch. Int. Pharmacodyn.* 209, 10.

Lancaster, L. and Fenster, P.E. (1983). Complete heart block after sublingual nitroglycerin. *Chest* 84, 111.

Landymore, R., Marble, A., Mackinnon, G., *et al.* (1984). Effects of oral amiodarone on left ventricular function in dogs: clinical implications for patients with life-threatening ventricular tachycardia. *Ann. Thorac. Surg.* 37, 141.

Lang-Stevenson, D., Mikhailidis, D.P., and Gillet, D.S. (1977). Cardiotoxicity of 5-fluorouracil. *Lancet* ii, 406.

Lant, A. (1985). Diuretics: clinical pharmacology and therapeutic use. Part I. *Drugs* 29, 57.

Lardinois, C.K. and Neuman, S.L. (1988). The effects of antihypertensive agents on serum lipids and lipoproteins. *Arch. Intern. Med.* 148, 1280.

Lasser, N.L., Ganditis, G., Cutler, J.A., *et al.* (1984). Effect of antihypertensive therapy on serum lipids and lipoproteins in the Multiple Risk Factor Intervention Trial. *Am. J. Med.* 76 (2A), 52.

Leach, A.J., Brown, J.E., and Armstrong, P.W. (1980). Cardiac depression by intravenous disopyramide in patients with left ventricular dysfunction. *Am. J. Med.* 68, 839.

Leak, D. and Eydt, J.N. (1986). Amiodarone for refractory cardiac arrhythmias: 10-year study. Clinical and community studies. *Can. Med. Assoc. J.* 134, 495.

Leclercq, J.F., Ral, S., and Valere P. (1983). Bepridil et torsades de pointes. *Arch. Mal. Coeur* 76, 341.

Ledda, F., Mantelli, L., Manzini, L., *et al.* (1981). Electro-physiological and antiarrhythmic properties of propafenone in isolated preparation. *J. Cardiovasc. Pharmacol.* 3, 1162.

Legha, S.S., Benjamin, R.S., Mackay, B., *et al.* (1982). Reduction of doxorubicin cardiotoxicity by prolonged continuous intravenous infusion. *Ann. Intern. Med.* 96, 133.

Legrand, V., Vandormael, M., Collignon, P., *et al.* (1983). Hemodynamic effects of a new antiarrhythmic agent, flecainide (R-818), in coronary heart disease. *Br. J. Clin. Pharmacol.* 51, 422.

Lehmann, M.H., Hardy, S., Archibald, D., *et al.* (1996). Sex difference in risk of torsade de pointes with *d,l*-sotalol. *Circulation* 94, 2535.

Lehtonen, A. (1985). Effect of beta blockers on blood lipid profile. *Am. Heart J.* 109, 1192.

Lejonc, J.L., Vernant, J.P., Macquin, I., *et al.* (1980). Myocardial infarction following vinblastine treatment. *Lancet* ii, 692.

Leren, P. (1987). Effects of antihypertensive drugs on lipid metabolism. *Clin. Ther.* 9, 326.

Lertora, J.J.L., Glock, D., Stec, G.P., *et al.* (1979). Effects of *N*-acetylprocainamide and procainamide on myocardial contractile force, heart rate and blood pressure (40547). *Proc. Soc. Exp. Biol. Med.* 168, 332.

Leung, W.H., Lau, C.P., Wong, C.K., *et al.* (1990). Fatal cardiac tamponade in systemic lupus erythematosus — a hazard of anticoagulation. *Am. Heart J.* 119, 422.

Levine, J.H., Spear, J.F., Guarnieri, T., *et al.* (1985). Cesium chloride-induced long QT syndrome: demonstration of after depolarisations and triggered activity *in vivo*. *Circulation* 72, 1092.

Levine, J.H., Morganroth, J., and Kadish, A.H. (1989). Mechanisms and risk factors for proarrhythmia with type Ia compared with Ic antiarrhythmic drug therapy. *Circulation* 80, 1049.

Liang, C-S., Sherman, L.G., Doherty, J.U., *et al.* (1984). Sustained improvement of cardiac function in patients with congestive heart failure after short-term infusion of dobutamine. *Circulation* 69, 113.

Lieberman, N.A., Harris, R.S., Katz, R.I., *et al.* (1968). The effects of lidocaine on the electrical and mechanical activity of the heart. *Am. J. Cardiol.* 22, 375.

Liljequist, J-A. and Eduardsson, N. (1989). Torsade de pointes tachycardias induced by overdosage of zimelidine. *J. Cardiovasc. Pharmacol.* 14, 666.

Ljung, B. (1985). Vascular selectivity of felodipine. *Drugs* 29 (Suppl. 2), 46.

Loaldi, A., Fabbiocchi, F., Montorsi, P., *et al.* (1989). Different coronary vasomotor effects of nifedipine and therapeutic correlates in angina with spontaneous and effort components versus Prinzmetal angina. *Am. Heart J.* 117, 315.

Lowenstein, S.R., Gabow, P.A., Cramer, J., *et al.* (1983). The role of alcohol in new-onset atrial fibrillation. *Arch. Intern. Med.* 143, 1882.

MacAlpin, R. (1975). Intravenous procainamide and left ventricular performance. *Chest* 67, 737.

McFadden, E.R. and Ingram, R.H. (1988). Relationship between diseases of the heart and lungs. In *Heart Disease. A Textbook of Cardiovascular Medicine*, Vol. 2 (3rd edn) (ed. E. Braunwald), p. 1879. Saunders, Philadelphia.

McKibbin, J.K., Pocock, W.A., Barlow, J.B., *et al.* (1984). Sotalol, hypokalaemia, syncope and torsade de pointes. *Br. Heart J.* 51, 157.

Mackinnon, G., Landymore, R., and Marble, A. (1983). Myocardial depressant effects of oral amiodarone and their significance in the surgical management of sustained ventricular tachycardia. *Can. J. Surg.* 26, 355.

McLeod, A.A., Stiles, G.L., and Shand, D.G. (1984). Demonstration of beta-adrenoceptor blockade by propafenone hydrochloride: clinical pharmacologic, radioligand binding and adenylate cyclase activation studies. *J. Pharmacol. Exp. Ther.* 228, 461.

McLeod, A.A., Martot, R., Monaghan, M.J., *et al.* (1987). Chronic cardiac toxicity after inhalation of 1,1,1-trichlorethane. *BMJ* 294, 727.

MacMahon, B., Bakshi, M., Branagan, P., *et al.* (1985). Pharmacokinetics and haemodynamic effects of tocainide in patients with acute myocardial infarction complicated by left ventricular failure. *Br. J. Clin. Pharmacol.* 19, 429.

Macnab, A.J., Robinson, J.L., Adderly, R.J., *et al.* (1987). Heart block secondary to erythromycin-induced carbamazepine toxicity. *Pediatrics* 80, 951.

McNerney, J.M. and Leedham, C.L. (1950). Acute coronary insufficiency pattern following intravenous ergotamine studies. *Am. Heart J.* 39, 629.

Magni, G. (1987). Mianserin in the treatment of elderly depressives. *J. Am. Geriatr. Soc.* 35, 707.

Mandel, E.M., Lelinski, N., and Djaldetti, M. (1975). Vincristine induced myocardial infarction. *Cancer* 36, 1979.

Marchant, E., Pichard, A.D., Casenegra, P., *et al.* (1984). Effect of intravenous dipyridamole on regional coronary blood flow with 1-vessel coronary artery disease: evidence against coronary steal. *Am. J. Cardiol.* 53, 718.

Marchant, E., Pichard, A., Rodriguez, J.A., *et al.* (1986). Acute effect of systemic versus intracoronary dipyridamole on coronary circulation. *Am. J. Cardiol.* 57, 1401.

Mark, A.L. (1983). The Bezold–Jarisch reflex revisited: clinical implications of inhibitory reflexes originating in the heart. *J. Am. Coll. Cardiol.* 1, 90.

Marmont, A.M., Damasio, E., and Rossi, F. (1969). Cardiac toxicity of daunorubicin. *Lancet* i, 837.

Marshall, R.J., Muir, A.W., and Winslow, E. (1981). Comparative antidysrhythmic and haemodynamic effects of orally or intravenously administered mexiletine and org 6001 in the anaesthetised rat. *Br. J. Pharmacol.* 74, 381.

Martin, R.R., Lisehora, G.R., Braxton, M., *et al.* (1987). Fatal poisoning from sodium phosphate enema. Case report and experimental study. *JAMA* 257, 2190.

Mason, J.W., Winkle, R.A., Ingels, N.B., *et al.* (1977a). Hemodynamic effects of intravenously administered quinidine on the transplanted human heart. *Am. J. Cardiol.* 40, 99.

Mason, J.W., Billingham, M.E., and Friedman, J.R. (1977b). Methysergide-induced heart disease. A case of multivalvular and myocardial fibrosis. *Circulation* 56, 889.

Mason, J.W., Hondeghem, L.M., and Katzung, B.G. (1984). Block of inactivated sodium channels and of depolarization — induced automatically in guinea pig papillary muscle by amiodarone. *Circ. Res.* 55, 277.

Mason. J.W. (for the electrophysiological study versus electro-cardiographic monitoring investigators) (1993). A comparison of seven antiarrhythmic drugs in patients with ventricular tachyarrhythmias. *N. Engl. J. Med.* 329, 452.

Matos, L., Torok, E., and Hankoczy, J. (1977). Examinations on the inotropic effect of lidocaine. *Ther. Hung.* 25, 36.

Mattioni, T.A., Zheutlin, T.A., Dunnington, C., *et al.* (1989). The proarrhythmic effects of amiodarone. *Prog. Cardiovasc. Dis.* 31, 439.

Medical Research Council Working Party on Mild to Moderate Hypertension (1983). Ventricular extrasystoles during thiazide treatment: substudy of MRC mild hypertension trial. *BMJ* 287, 1249.

Medical Research Council Working Party. (1985). MRC trial of treatment of mild hypertension: principal results. *BMJ* 291, 97.

Miall, W.E. and Greenberg, G. (1987). *Mild Hypertension: Is there Pressure to Treat? An Account of the MRC Trial.* Cambridge University Press.

Miles, W.M., Heger, J.J., Minardo, J.D., *et al.* (1989). The electrophysiological effects of enoximone in patients with preexisting ventricular tachyarrhythmias. *Am. Heart J.* 117, 112.

Miller, R.R., Hilliard, G., Lies, J.E., *et al.* (1973). Hemodynamic effects of procainamide in patients with acute myocardial infarction and comparison with lidocaine. *Am. J. Med.* 55, 161.

Miller, R.R., Olson, H.G., Amsterdam, E.A., *et al.* (1975). Propranolol-withdrawal rebound phenomenon: exacerbation of coronary events after abrupt cessation of antianginal therapy. *N. Engl. J. Med.* 293, 416.

Millward, M.J., Ganju, V., and Buck, M. (1988). Cardiac arrest — a manifestation of 5-fluorouracil. *Aust. N.Z. J. Med.* 18, 693.

Minardo, J.D., Heger, J.J., Miles, W.M., *et al.* (1988). Clinical characteristics of patients with ventricular fibrillation during antiarrhythmic drug therapy. *N. Engl. J. Med.* 319, 257.

Minow, R.A., Benjamin, R.S., Lee, E.T., *et al.* (1977). Adriamycin cardiomyopathy — risk factors. *Cancer* 39, 1397.

Misch, K.A. (1974). Development of heart valve lesions during methysergide therapy. *BMJ* ii, 365.

Mittleman, R.E. and Wetli, C.V. (1984). Death caused by recreational cocaine use. An update. *JAMA* 252, 1889.

Mokler, C.M. and van Arman, C.G. (1962). Pharmacology of a new antiarrhythmic agent, gamma-diisopropylamino-alpha-phenyl-alpha-(2-pyridyl)-butyramide (SC-7031). *J. Pharmacol. Exp. Ther.* 136, 114.

Molinoff, P.B., Aarons, R.D., Nies, A.S., *et al.* (1982). Effects of pindolol and propranolol on β-adrenergic receptors on human lymphocytes. *Br. J. Clin. Pharmacol.* 13, 365S.

Morgan, D.B. and Davidson, C. (1980). Hypokalaemia and diuretics: an analysis of publications. *BMJ* 280, 905.

Morganroth, J. (1987). Risk factors for the development of proarrhythmic events. *Am. J. Cardiol.* 59, 32E.

Morganroth, J. and Horowitz, L.N. (1984). Flecainide: its proarrhythmic effect and expected changes on the surface electrocardiogram. *Am. J. Cardiol.* 53, 89B.

Morganroth. J. and Goin J.E. (1991). Quinidine related mortality in short-to-medium- term treatment of ventricular arrhythmias: a meta analysis. *Circulation* 84, 1977.

Morganroth, J., Anderson, J.L., and Gentzkow, G.D. (1986). Classification by type of ventricular arrhythmia predicts frequency of cardiac events from flecainide. *J. Am. Coll. Cardiol.* 8, 607.

Moss, A., Hall, J., Cannom, D., *et al.* for the Multicentre Automatic Defibrillator Implantation Trial (1996). Improved survival with an implanted defibrillator in patients with coronary disease at high risk for ventricular arrhythmia. *N. Engl. J. Med.* 335, 1933.

MRFIT (Multiple Risk Factor Intervention Trial Research Group) (1982). Multiple risk factor intervention trial. Risk factor changes and mortality results. *JAMA* 248, 1465.

Muller, J.E., Turpi, Z.G., Stone, P.H., *et al.* (1986). Digoxin therapy and mortality after myocardial infarction. Experience in the MILIS study. *N. Engl. J. Med.* 314, 265.

Murphy, E., Jacob, R., and Lieberman, M. (1985). Cytosolic free calcium in chick heart cells. Its role in cell injury. *J. Mol. Cell. Cardiol.* 17, 221.

Myers, M.G., Harris, L., Leenen, F.H.H., *et al.* (1987). Caffeine as a possible cause of ventricular arrhythmias during the healing phase of acute myocardial infarction. *Am. J. Cardiol.* 59, 1024.

Myrhed, M. and Wiholm, B.E. (1986). Nifedipine — a survey of adverse effects. Four years' reporting in Sweden. *Acta Pharmacol. Toxicol. Copenh.* 58 (Suppl. 2), 133.

Nahas, M., Lachapelle, J., and Tremblay, G. (1969). Comparative effect of procainamide and lidocaine on myocardial contractility. *Can. J. Physiol. Pharmacol.* 47, 1038.

Nakano, J. and Moere, S.E. (1972). Effect of different alcohols on the contractile force of the isolated guinea-pig myocardium. *Eur. J. Pharmacol.* 20, 266.

Naqvi, N., Thompson, D.S., Morgan, W.E., *et al.* (1979). Haemodynamic effects of disopyramide in patients after open-heart surgery. *Br. Heart J.* 42, 587.

Nathan, A.W., Hellestrand, K.J., Bexton, R.S., *et al.* (1984). Proarrhythmic effects of the new antiarrhythmic agent flecainide acetate. *Am. Heart J.* 107, 222.

Nattel, S. (1985). Frequency-dependent effects of amitriptyline on ventricular conduction and cardiac rhythm in dogs. *Circulation* 72, 898.

Nattell, S., Rangno, R.E., and Loon, G.V. (1979). Mechanism of propranolol withdrawal phenomena. *Circulation* 59, 1158.

Naylor, W.G. (1976). The pharmacology of disopyramide. *J. Int. Med. Res.* 4, 8.

Naylor, W.G. (1980). Calcium antagonists. *Eur. Heart J.* 1, 225.

Nehring, J. and Camm, A.J. (1983). Calcium antagonist withdrawal syndrome. *BMJ* 286, 1057.

Nemer, W.F., Teba, L., Schiebel, F., *et al.* (1988). Cardiac arrest after acute hyperphosphatemia. *South. Med. J.* 81, 1068.

Oetgen, W.J., Tibbits, P.A., Abt, M.E.O., *et al.* (1983). Clinical and electrophysiologic assessment of oral flecainide acetate for recurrent ventricular tachycardia: evidence for exacerbation of electrical instability. *Am. J. Cardiol.* 52, 746.

Olinde. K.D. and O'Connell. J.B. (1994). Inflammatory heart disease: pathogenesis, clinical manifestations, and treatment of myocarditis. *Annu. Rev. Med.* 45, 481

Opie, L.H. and White, D.A. (1980). Adverse interaction between nifedipine and β-blockade. *BMJ* 281, 1462.

Orme, M.L'E. (1984). Antidepressants and heart disease. *BMJ* 289, 1.

O'Rourke, R.A., Bishop, V.S., Stone, H.L., *et al.* (1969). Lack of effect of procainamide on ventricular function of conscious dogs. *Am. J. Cardiol.* 23, 238.

O'Rourke, R.A. and Horwitz, L.D. (1981). Effect of chronic oral quinidine on left ventricular performance. *Am. Heart J.* 101, 769.

Orrenius, S. and Maehly, A.C. (1970). Lethal amphetamine intoxication. A report of three cases. *J. Legal Med.* 67, 184.

Owensby, D.A. (1986). Corticosteroid therapy and late right ventricular rupture after temporary pacing. *Am. J. Cardiol.* 58, 558.

Packer, M. (1988). Do positive inotropic agents adversely affect the survival of patients with chronic congestive heart failure? Protagonist's viewpoint. *J. Am. Coll. Cardiol.* 12, 562.

Packer, M. and Leier, C.V. (1987). Survival in congestive heart failure during treatment with drugs with positive inotropic actions. *Circulation* 75 (Suppl. IV), 55.

Packer, M., Carver, J.R., Rodeheffer, R.J., *et al.* for the PROMISE Study Research Group (1994). Effect of oral milrinone on mortality in severe chronic heart failure. *N. Engl. J. Med.* 325, 1468.

Pannley, W.W., Nesto, R.W., Singh, B.N., *et al.* and the N-CAP Study Group (1992). Attenuation of the circadian patterns of myocardial ischaemia with nifedipine GITS in patients with chronic stable angina. *J. Am. Coll. Cardiol.* 19, 1380.

Paradise, R.R. and Bibbins, F. (1969). Comparison of the effects of equi-effective concentrations of anesthetics on the force of contraction of isolated perfused rat hearts. *Anesthesiology* 31, 349.

Pasternac, A., Noble, J., Streulens, Y., *et al.* (1982). Pathophysiology of chest pain in patients with cardiomyopathies and normal coronary arteries. *Circulation* 65, 778.

Pellinen, T.J., Farkkilae, M., Heikrila, J., *et al.* (1987). Electrocardiographic and clinical factors of tricyclic antidepressant intoxication. *Ann. Clin. Res.* 19, 12.

Peng, S.K., French, W.J., and Pelikan, P.C.D. (1989). Direct cocaine cardiotoxicity demonstrated by endomyocardial biopsy. *Arch. Pathol. Lab. Med.* 113, 842–5.

Pepine, C. (1989). Nicardipine, a new calcium channel blocker: role for vascular selectivity. *Clin. Cardiol.* 12, 240.

Perelman, M.S., McKenna, W.J., Rowland, E., *et al.* (1987). A comparison of bepridil with amiodarone in the treatment of established atrial fibrillation. *Br. Heart J.* 58, 339.

Perez, J.E., Borda, L., Schuchleib, R., *et al.* (1982). Inotropic and chronotropic effects of vasodilators. *J. Pharmacol. Exp. Ther.* 221, 609.

Perez-Stable, E. and Caralis, P.V. (1983). Thiazide-induced disturbances in carbohydrate, lipid and potassium metabolism. *Am. Heart J.* 106, 245.

Perkins, C.M. (1978). Serious verapamil poisoning: treatment with intravenous calcium gluconate. *BMJ* ii, 1127.

Pfeffer, M.A. and Braunwald, E. (1990). Ventricular remodelling after myocardial infarction. Experimental observations and clinical implications. *Circulation* 81, 1161.

Pfisterer, M. Kiowski, W., Burckhardt, D., *et al.* (1992). Beneficial effect of amiodarone on cardiac mortality in patients with asymptomatic complex ventricular arrhythmias after acute myocardial infarction and preserved but not impaired left ventricular function. *Am. J. Cardiol.* 69, 1399.

Piters, K.M., Colombo, A., Olson, H.G., *et al.* (1985). Effect of coffee on exercise-induced angina pectoris due to coronary artery disease in habitual coffee drinkers. *Am. J. Cardiol.* 55, 277.

Podrid, P.J., Schoeneberger, A., and Lown, B. (1980). Congestive heart failure caused by oral disopyramide. *N. Engl. J. Med.* 302, 614.

Poole-Wilson, P.A. (1987). Diuretics, hypokalaemia and arrhythmias in hypertensive patients: still an unsolved problem. *J. Hypertension* 5 (Suppl. 3), 551.

Poole-Wilson, P.A. (1989). Chronic heart failure: causes, pathophysiology, prognosis, clinical manifestations, investigations. In *Diseases of the Heart* (ed. D.G. Julian, A.J. Camm, K.M. Fox, R.J.C. Hall, and P.A. Poole-Wilson), p. 48. Baillière, London.

Pottage, A., Holt, S., Ludgate, S., *et al.* (1978). Fluorouracil toxicity. *BMJ* i, 547.

Pozenel, H. (1977). Haemodynamic studies on mexiletine, a new antiarrhythmic agent. *Postgrad. Med. J.* 53, 78.

Pratt, C.M., Eaton, C., Francis, M., *et al.* (1989). The inverse relationship between baseline left ventricular ejection fraction and outcome of antiarrhythmic therapy: a dangerous imbalance in the risk-benefit ratio. *Am. Heart J.* 118, 433.

Prevention of Atherosclerotic Complications with Ketanserin Trial Group. (1989). Prevention of atherosclerotic complications: controlled trial of ketanserin. *BMJ* 298, 424.

Prichard, B.N.C. and Walden, R.J. (1982). The syndrome associated with the withdrawal of β-adrenergic receptor blocking drugs. *Br. J. Clin. Pharmacol.* 13 (Suppl. 2), 337S.

Pringle, S.D. and MacEwen, C.J. (1987). Severe bradycardia due to interaction of timolol eye drops and verapamil. *BMJ* 294, 155.

Proskey, A.J., Saksena, F., and Towne, W.D. (1977). Myocardial infarction associated with thyrotoxicosis. *Chest* 72, 109.

Rae, A.P., Kay, H.R., Horowitz, L.N., *et al.* (1988). Proarrhythmic effects of antiarrhythmic drugs in patients with malignant ventricular arrhythmias evaluated by electrophysiological testing. *J. Am. Coll. Cardiol.* 12, 131.

Raftos J. (1980). Verapamil in the long-term treatment of angina pectoris. *Med. J. Aust.* 2, 78.

Rall, T.W. (1985). Central nervous stimulants. The methylxanthines. In *Goodman and Gilman's The Pharmacological Basis of Therapeutics* (7th edn) (ed. A.G. Gilman, L.S. Goodman, T.W. Rall, and F. Murad), p. 589. Macmillan, New York.

Rall, T.W. and Schleifer, L.S. (1985). Oxytocin, prostaglandins, ergot alkaloids, and other drugs; tocolytic agents. In *Goodman and Gilman's The Pharmacological Basis of*

Therapeutics (7th edn) (ed. A.G. Gilman, L.S. Goodman, T.W. Rall, and F. Murad), p. 926. Macmillan, New York.

Ranger, S., Talajie, M., Lemery, R., *et al.* (1989). Amplification of flecainide-induced ventricular conduction slowing by exercise. *Circulation* 79, 1000.

Rankin, A.C., Oldroyd, K.G., and Chong, E. (1989). Value and limitations of adenosine in the diagnosis and treatment of narrow and broad complex tachycardias. *Br. Heart J.* 62, 195.

Rausch, J.L., Pavlinac, D.M., and Newman, P.E. (1984). Complete heart block following a single dose of trazodone. *Am. J. Psych.* 141, 1472.

Rawling, D. and Fozzard, H.A. (1978). Electrophysiological effects of imipramine on cardiac Purkinje fibres. Abstract. *Am. J. Cardiol.* 41, 387.

Rawling, D.A. and Fozzard, H.A. (1979). Effects of imipramine on cellular electrophysiological properties of cardiac Purkinje fibers. *J. Pharmacol. Exp. Ther.* 209, 371.

Redding, P., Devroede, C., and Barbier, P. (1977). Bradycardia after cimetidine. *Lancet* ii, 1227.

Redfield, M.M., Nicholson, W.J., Edwards, W.D., *et al.* (1992). Valve disease associated with ergot alkaloid use: echocardiographic and pathologic correlates. *Ann. Intern. Med.* 117, 50.

Reedy, J.C. and Zwiren, G.T. (1983). Enema-induced hypocalcemia and hyperphosphatemia leading to cardiac arrest during induction of anesthesia in an outpatient surgery center. *Anesthesiology* 59, 578.

Regan, T.J., Weisse, A.B., Moschos, A.B., *et al.* (1965). The myocardial effects of acute and chronic use of ethanol in man. *Trans. Assoc. Am. Physicians* 78, 282.

Reichenbach, D.D. and Benditt, E.P. (1970). Catecholamines and cardiomyopathy: the pathogenesis and potential importance of myofibrillar degeneration. *Hum. Pathol.* 1, 125.

Reithmann, C. and Werdan, K. (1989). Noradrenaline-induced desensitization in cultured heart cells as a model for the defects of the adenylate cyclase system in severe heart failure. *Naunyn-Schmiedebergs Arch. Pharmacol.* 339, 138.

Resnekov, L. (1970). Circulatory effects of cardiac dysrhythmias. *Cardiovasc. Clin.* 2, 49.

Resnekov, L. and Falicov, R.E. (1977). Thyrotoxicosis and lactate-producing angina pectoris with normal coronary arteries. *Br. Heart J.* 39, 1051.

Richards, A., Stather-Dunn, L., and Moodley, J. (1985). Cardiopulmonary arrest after the administration of magnesium sulphate. A case report. *S. Afr. Med J.* 67, 145.

Risch, S.C., Groom, G.P., and Janowski, D.S. (1982). Interfaces of psychopharmacology and cardiology, part 2. *J. Clin. Psychiatry* 42, 47.

Roberts, W.C. 1989. Recent studies on the effects of beta blockers on blood lipid levels. *Am. Heart J.* 117, 709.

Roden, D.M. (1991). The long QT syndrome and torsade de pointes: basic and clinical aspects. In *Cardiac Pacing and Electrophysiology* (3rd edn), p. 265. W.B. Saunders, Philadelphia.

Roden, D.M. and Hoffman, B.F. (1985). Action potential prolongation and induction of abnormal automaticity by low quinidine concentrations in canine Purkinje fibres. Relationship to potassium and cycle length. *Circ. Res.* 56, 857.

Roden, D.M., Woolsey, R.L., and Primm, R.K. (1986). Incidence and clinical features of the quinidine-associated long QT syndrome: implications for patient care. *Am. Heart J.* 111, 1088.

Rodger, C. and Stewart, A. (1978). Side effects of nifedipine. *BMJ* i, 1619.

Rodger, S.H. and Hyman, D. (1932). Harmful effects of nitroglycerin. *Am. J. Med. Sci.* 184, 480.

Rona, G. (1985). Catecholamine cardiotoxicity. *J. Mol. Cell. Cardiol.* 17, 291.

Roose, S.P., Glassman, A.H., Giardina, E.G.V., *et al.* (1987). Tricyclic antidepressants in depressed patients with cardiac conduction disease. *Arch. Gen. Psychiatry* 44, 273.

Rosen, B., Ovsyshcher, I.A., and Zimlichman, R. (1988). Complete atrioventricular block induced by methyldopa. *PACE* 11, 1555.

Rosenberg, L., Palmer, J.R., Kelly, J.P., *et al.* (1988). Coffee drinking and non-fatal myocardial infarction in men under 55 years of age. *Am. J. Epidemiol.* 128, 570.

Ross, R.K., Paginini-Hill, A., Mack, T.M., *et al.* (1981). Menopausal oestrogen therapy and protection from death from ischaemic heart disease. *Lancet* i, 858.

Royal College of General Practitioners' Oral Contraceptive Study. (1981). Further analyses of mortality in oral contraceptive users. *Lancet* i, 541.

Rubin, E. (1979). Alcoholic myopathy in heart and skeletal muscle. *N. Engl. J. Med.* 301, 28.

Ruegg, J.C. (1986). *Calcium in Muscle Activation*. Springer-Verlag, Berlin.

Ruskin, J.N., McGovern, B., Garan, H., *et al.* (1983). Antiarrhythmic drugs: a possible cause of out-of-hospital cardiac arrest. *N. Engl. J. Med.* 309, 1307.

Russek, H.I. (1960). Are the xanthines effective in angina pectoris? *Am. J. Med. Sci.* 239, 877.

Ryan, T.J., Bailey, K.R., McCabe, C.H., *et al.* (1983). The effects of digitalis on survival in high-risk patients with coronary artery disease. The Coronary Artery Surgery Study (CASS). *Circulation* 67, 735.

Saal, A.K., Werner, J.A., Greene, H.L., *et al.* (1984). Effect of amiodarone on serum quinidine and procainamide levels. *Am. J. Cardiol.* 53, 1264.

Sadjadi, S.A., Leghari, R.U., and Berger, A.R. (1984). Prolongation of the PR interval induced by methyldopa. *Am. J. Cardiol.* 54, 675.

Sanini, S., Spaulding, M.B., Masud, A.R.Z., *et al.* (1981). 5-FU cardiotoxicity. *Cancer Treat. Rep.* 65, 1123.

Sarma, J.S., Ikeda, S., Fischer, R., *et al.* (1976). Biochemical and contractile properties of heart muscle after prolonged alcohol administration. *J. Mol. Cell. Cardiol.* 8, 951.

Sasyniuk, B.I., Valdis, M., and Tioy, W. (1989). Recent advances in understanding the mechanisms of drug-induced torsade de pointes arrhythmias. *Am. J. Cardiol.* 64, 29J.

Schachne, J.S., Roberts, B.H., and Thompson, P.D. (1984). Coronary artery spasm and myocardial infarction associated with cocaine usage. *N. Engl. J. Med.* 310, 1665.

Scheinmann, M.M., Strauss, H.C., Evans, G.T., *et al.* (1978). Adverse effect of sympatholytic agent in patient with hypertension and sinus node dysfunction. *Am. J. Med.* 64, 1013.

Scherf, D. and Schlachman, M. (1948). Electrocardiographic and clinical studies on action of ergotamine tartrate and dihydroergotamine 45. *Am. J. Med. Sci.* 216, 673.

Schlepper, M. (1989). Cardiodepressive effects of antiarrhythmic drugs. *Eur. Heart J.* 10 (Suppl. E), 73.

Schneider, P.E., Jonas, E., and Tejani, N. (1988). Detection of cardiac events by continuous electrogram monitoring during ritodrine infusion. *Obstet. Gynecol.* 71, 361.

Schoenwetter, A.M. and Silber, E.N. (1965). Penicillin hypersensitivity, acute pericarditis and eosinophilia. *JAMA* 191, 672.

Schwartz, A., Shen, E., Morady, F., *et al.* (1983). Hemodynamic effects of intravenous amiodarone in patients with depressed left ventricular function and recurrent ventricular tachycardia. *Am. Heart J.* 106, 848.

Schwartz, M., Covino, B., Duce, B., *et al.* (1979). Acute hemodynamic effects of tocainide in patients undergoing cardiac catheterization. *J. Clin. Pharmacol.* 19, 100.

Sears, M.R., Rea, H.H., Fenwick, J., *et al.* (1987). Seventy-five deaths in asthmatics prescribed home nebulisers. *BMJ* 294, 477.

Selzer, A. and Wray, H.W. (1964). Quinidine syncope. Paroxysmal ventricular fibrillation occurring during treatment of chronic atrial arrhythmias. *Circulation* 30, 17.

Serruys, P.W., Vanhaleweyk, G., van den Brand, M., *et al.* (1983). The hemodynamic effect of intravenous flecainide acetate in patients with coronary artery disease. *Br. J. Clin. Pharmacol.* 16, 51.

Shafar, J. (1965). Phenylbutazone-induced pericarditis. *BMJ* ii, 795.

Shen, E.N., Sung, R.J., Morady, F., *et al.* (1984). Electrophysiologic and hemodynamic effects of intravenous propafenone in patients with recurrent ventricular tachycardia. *J. Am. Coll. Cardiol.* 3, 1291.

Shepherd, R.T. (1989). Mechanism of sudden death associated with volatile substance abuse. *Hum. Toxicol.* 8, 287.

Sheu, S-S. and Lederer, W.J. (1985). Lidocaine's negative inotropic and antiarrhythmic actions. Dependence on shortening of action potential duration and reduction of intracellular sodium activity. *Circ. Res.* 57, 578.

Shimosato, S. and Etsten, B.E. (1969). Effects of anesthetic drugs on the heart: a critical review of myocardial contractility and its relationship to haemodynamics. *Clin. Anesthesia* 9, 17.

Shroff, S.G. and Motz, W. (1989). Left ventricular systolic resistance in rats with hypertension and hypertrophy. *Am. J. Physiol.* 257, 386.

Silva Graça, A. and van Zwieten, P.A. (1972). A comparison between the negative inotropic action of various antiarrhythmic drugs and their influence on calcium movements in heart muscle. *J. Pharm. Pharmacol.* 24, 367.

Silverman, H.S. and Pfeifer, M.P. (1987). Relation between use of anti-inflammatory agents and left ventricular free wall rupture during acute myocardial infarction. *Am. J. Cardiol.* 59, 363.

Simoons, M.L., Brand, M., Zwaan, C., *et al.* (1985). Improved survival after early thrombolysis in acute myocardial infarction. *Lancet* ii, 578.

Singh, B.N. (1983). Amiodarone: historical development and pharmacologic profile. *Am. Heart J.* 106, 788.

Singh, B.N. and Vaughan Williams, E.M. (1970). The effect of amiodarone, a new anti-anginal drug, on cardiac muscle. *Br. J. Pharmacol.* 39, 657.

Singh, B.N., Jewitt, D.E., Downey, J.M., *et al.* (1976). Effects of amiodarone and L 8040, novel antianginal and antiarrhythmic drugs, on cardiac and coronary hemodynamic and on cardiac intracellular potentials. *Clin. Exp. Pharmacol. Physiol.* 3, 427.

Slater, W., Lampert, S., Podrid, P.T., *et al.* (1988). Clinical predictors of arrhythmic worsening by antiarrhythmic drugs. *Am. J. Cardiol.* 61, 349.

Slome, R. (1973). Withdrawal of propranolol and myocardial infarction. *Lancet* i, 156.

Smith, S.R. (1984). Metabolic responses to beta-2 stimulants. *J. R. Coll. Phys. Lond.* 18, 190.

Smith, W.G. (1966). Adult heart disease due to the coxsackie virus group B. *Br. Heart J.* 28, 204.

Smitherman, T.C., Gottlich, C.M., Narahara, K.A., *et al.* (1979). Myocardial contractility in patients with ischemic heart disease during long-term administration of quinidine and procainamide. Direct measurement of segmental shortening with radiopaque epicardial markers. *Chest* 76, 552.

Somers, G., Abramov, M., Wittek, M., *et al.* (1976). Myocardial infarction: a complication of vincristine treatment. *Lancet* ii, 690.

Somerville, W. and Levine, S.A. (1949). Angina pectoris and thyrotoxicosis. *Br. Heart J.* 12, 245.

Sowton, E. and Hamer, J. (1966). Hemodynamic changes after beta adrenergic blockade. *Am. J. Cardiol.* 18, 317.

Spierings, E.L.H. (1988). Cardiac murmurs indicative of aortic valve disease with chronic and excessive intake of ergot. *Headache* 28, 278.

Stadel, B.V. (1981). Oral contraceptives and cardiovascular disease. *N. Engl. J. Med.* 305, 612 and 672.

Stampfer, M.J., Colditz, G.A., Willet, W.C., *et al.* (1991). Postmenopausal estrogen therapy and cardiovascular disease. *N. Engl. J. Med.* 325, 756.

Stanton, M.S., Prystowsky, E.N., Fineberg, N.S., *et al.* (1989). Arrhythmogenic effects of antiarrhythmic drugs. A study of 506 patients treated for ventricular tachycardia or fibrillation. *J. Am. Coll. Cardiol.* 14, 209.

Stein, J., Podrid, P., and Lown, B. (1984). Effects of oral mexiletine on left and right ventricular function. *Am. J. Cardiol.* 54, 575.

Steiner, C., Wit, A.L., Weiss, M.B., *et al.* (1970). The antiarrhythmic actions of carbamazepine (Tegretol). *J. Pharmacol. Exp. Ther.* 173, 323.

Steinherz, L.J., Steinherz, P.G., Mangiacasale, D., *et al.* (1981). Cardiac changes with cyclophosphamide. *Med. Pediatr. Oncol.* 9, 417.

Stolshek, B.S., Osterhout, S.K., and Dunham, G. (1988). The role of digoxin-specific antibodies in the treatment of digitalis poisoning. *Med. Toxicol.* 3, 167.

Stone, P.H., Muller, J.E., Turi, Z.G., et al. (1983). Efficacy of nifedipine therapy in patients with refractory angina pectoris: significance of the presence of coronary vasospasm. Am. Heart J. 106, 644.

Story, J.R., Abdulla, A.M., and Frank, M.J. (1979). Cardiogenic shock and disopyramide phosphate. JAMA 242, 654.

Strasberg, B., Sclarovsky, S., Erdberg, A., et al. (1981). Procainamide-induced polymorphous ventricular tachycardia. Am. J. Cardiol. 47, 1309.

Stratmann, H.G. and Kennedy, H.L. (1987). Torsade de pointes associated with drugs and toxins: recognition and management. Am. Heart J. 113, 1471.

Sutherland, D.J., McPherson, D.D., Renton, K.W., et al. (1985). The effect of caffeine on cardiac rate, rhythm and ventricular repolarization. Chest 87, 319.

Swarbrick, E.T. and Gray, I.R. (1972). Systemic lupus erythematosus during treatment with procainamide. Br. Heart J. 34, 288.

Sylven, C., Beermann, B., Jonzon, B., et al. (1986). Angina pectoris-like pain provoked by intravenous adenosine in healthy volunteers. BMJ 293, 227.

Sylven, C., Jonzon, B., Brandt, R., et al. (1987). Adenosine-provoked angina pectoris-like pain — time characteristics, influence of autonomic blockade and naloxone. Eur. Heart J. 8, 738.

Sylven, C., Beerman, B., Lagerquist, B., et al. (1989). Angina pectoris, adenosine and theophylline. Lancet i, 1328.

Sznajder, I., Bentur, Y., and Taitelman, U. (1984). First and second degree atrioventricular block in oxpentifylline overdose. BMJ 288, 26.

Tan, L-B. and Clark, W.A. (1990). Cardioprotective effects of homologous and heterologous beta-adrenergic receptor desensitization. Eur. Heart J 11, 212

Tan, L-B., Murray, R.G., and Littler, W.A. (1987). An analytical method to separate inotropic and vasodilatory drug effects in man. Cardiovasc. Res. 21, 625.

Tan, L-B., Jalil, J.E., Janicki, J.S., et al. (1989). Cardiotoxic effects of angiotensin II. J. Am. Coll. Cardiol. 13, 2A.

Tejerina, T., Barrigon, S., and Tamargo, J. (1983). Comparison of three β-amino anilides: IQB-M-81, lidocaine and tocainide, on isolated rat atria. Eur. J. Pharmacol. 95, 93.

Thadani, U., Manyari, D., Gregor, P., et al. (1981). Hemodynamic effects of disopyramide at rest and during exercise in normal subjects. Cathet. Cardiovasc. Diagn. 7, 27.

Thomas, G., Haider, B., Oldewurtel, H.A., et al. (1980). Progression of myocardial abnormalities in experimental alcoholism. Am. J. Cardiol. 46, 223.

Timmis, G.C., Ramor, R.C., Gordon, S., et al. (1975). The basis for differences in ethanol-induced myocardial depression in normal subjects. Circulation 51, 1144.

Todd, G.L., Baroldi, G., Pieper, G.M., et al. (1985a). Experimental catecholamine-induced myocardial necrosis. I. Morphology, quantification and regional distribution of acute contraction band lesions. J. Mol. Cell. Cardiol. 17, 317.

Todd, G.L., Baroldi, G., Pieper, G.M., et al. (1985b). Experimental catecholamine-induced myocardial necrosis. II. Temporal development of isoproterenol-induced contraction band lesions correlated with ECG, hemodynamic and biochemical changes. J. Mol. Cell. Cardiol. 17, 647.

Tomoda, H., Chuck, L., and Parmley, W.W. (1972). Comparative myocardial depressant effects of lidocaine, ajmaline, propranolol and quinidine. Jpn Circ. J. 36, 433.

Tordjman, T., Korzets, A., Kotas, R., et al. (1984). Complete atrioventricular block and long-term cimetidine therapy. Arch. Intern. Med. 144, 861.

Trimarco, B., Ricciardelli, B., de Luca, N., et al. (1983). Disopyramide, mexiletine and procainamide in the long-term oral treatment of ventricular arrhythmias: antiarrhythmic efficacy and hemodynamic effects. Curr. Ther. Res. 33, 472.

Troup, P.J., Chapman, P.D., Olinger, G.N., et al. (1985). The implanted defibrillator: relation of defibrillating lead configuration and clinical variables to defibrillation threshold. J. Am. Coll. Cardiol. 6, 1315.

Tye, K.H., Deser, K.B., and Benchimol, A. (1980). Angina pectoris associated with terbutaline for premature labor. JAMA 244, 69.

Underwood, D.A., Groppe, C.W., Tsai, A.R., et al. (1983). Coronary insufficiency and 5-fluorouracil therapy. Cleve. Clin. J. Med. 50, 29.

Urbano-Marquez, A., Estruch, R., Navarro-Lopez, F., et al. (1989). The effects of alcoholism on skeletal and cardiac muscle. N. Engl. J. Med. 320, 409.

Uretsky, B.F., Jessup, M., Konstam, M.A., et al. (1990). Multicenter trial of oral enoximone in patients with moderate to moderately severe congestive heart failure. Lack of benefit compared with placebo. Circulation 82, 774.

Uretsky, B.F., Young, J.B., Shahidi, F.E., et al. (1993). Randomized study assessing the effect of digoxin withdrawal in patients with mild to moderate chronic congestive heart failure: results of the PROVED trial. PROVED Investigative Group. J. Am. Coll. Cardiol. 22, 955.

Vaickus, L. and Letendre, L. (1984). Pericarditis induced by high-dose cytarabine therapy. Arch. Intern. Med. 144, 1868.

van Brummelen, P. (1983). The relevance of intrinsic sympathomimetic activity for +-blocker induced changes in plasma lipids. J. Cardiovasc. Pharmacol. 5 (Suppl. 1), S51.

van Camp, G., Dereppe, H., Renard, M., et al. (1989). Ketanserin and syncope. Acta Cardiol. 44, 429.

Van Dellen, R.G. (1979). Theophylline: Practical application of new knowledge. Mayo Clin Proc. 54, 733.

Vandermotten, M., Verhaeghe, R., and De Geest, H. (1989). Ventricular arrhythmias and QT-prolongation during therapy with ketanserin: report of a case. Acta Cardiol. 44, 431.

Veith, R.C., Raskins, M.A., Caldwell, J.H., et al. (1982). Cardiovascular effects of tricyclic antidepressants in depressed patients with chronic heart disease. N. Engl. J. Med. 306, 959.

Velebit, V., Podrid, P., Lown, B., et al. (1982). Aggravation and provocation of ventricular arrhythmias by antiarrhythmic drugs. Circulation 65, 886.

Verdouw, P.D., Deckers, J.W., and Conard, G.J. (1979). Antiarrhythmic and hemodynamic actions of flecainide acetate (R-818) in the ischemic porcine heart. J. Cardiovasc. Pharmacol. 1, 473.

Vittone, L., Cingolani, H.E., and Mattiazzi, R.A. (1985). The link between myocardial contraction and relaxation: the effects of calcium antagonists. *J. Mol. Cell. Cardiol.* 17, 255.

von Hoff, D.D. and Layard, M.W. (1981). Risk factors for development of daunorubicin cardiotoxicity. *Cancer Treat. Rep.* 65 (Suppl. 4), 19.

von Hoff, D.D., Layard, M.W., Basa, P., *et al.* (1979). Risk factors for doxorubicin-induced congestive heart failure. *Ann. Intern. Med.* 91, 710.

von Hoff, D.D., Rozencweig, M., and Piccart, M. (1982). The cardiotoxicity of anticancer agents. *Semin. Oncol.* 9, 23.

Walker, P.R., Marshall, A.J., Farr, S., *et al.* (1985). Abrupt withdrawal of atenolol in patients with severe angina. *Br. Heart J.* 53, 276.

Walsh, R.A. (1987). The effects of calcium-entry blockade on left ventricular systolic and diastolic function. *Circulation* 75 (Suppl. V), 43.

Walsh, R.A. and Horwitz, L.D. (1979). Adverse hemodynamic effects of intravenous disopyramide compared with quinidine in conscious dogs. *Circulation* 60, 1053.

Ward, D.E. and Camm, A.J. (1993). Dangerous ventricular arrhythmias — can we predict drug efficacy? *N. Engl. J. Med.* 329, 498.

Warden, P., Greenwald, E.S., and Grossman, J. (1976). Unusual cardiac reaction to chemotherapy following mediastinal irradiation in a patient with Hodgkin's disease. *Am. J. Med.* 60, 152.

Watt, A.H. and Routledge, P.A. (1985). Adenosine stimulates respiration in man. *Br. J. Clin. Pharm.* 20, 503.

Wei, J.Y., Genecin, A., Greene, H.L., *et al.* (1979). Coronary spasm with ventricular fibrillation during thyrotoxicosis: response to attaining euthyroid state. *Am. J. Cardiol.* 43, 335.

Weidmann, P., Ferrier, C., Saxenhofer, H., *et al.* (1988). Serum lipoproteins during treatment with antihypertensive drugs. *Drugs* 35 (Suppl. 6), 118.

Weisman, H.F. and Healy, B. (1987). Myocardial infarct expansion, infarct extension, and reinfarction: pathophysiologic concepts. *Prog. Cardiovasc. Dis.* 30, 73.

Weld, F.M. and Bigger, J.T. (1980). Electrophysiological effects of imipramine on bovine cardiac Purkinje's and muscle fibres. *Circ. Res.* 46, 167.

Welder, A.A., Smith, M.A., Ramos, K., *et al.* (1988). Cocaine-induced cardiotoxicity *in vitro*. *Toxicology in Vitro* 2, 205.

Williams, J.F. and Mathew, B. (1984). Effect of procainamide on myocardial contractile function and digoxin inotropy. *J. Am. Coll. Cardiol.* 4, 1184.

Wetherbee, D.G., Holzman, D., Brown, M.G. (1952). Ventricular tachycardia following the administration of quinidine. *Am. Heart J.* 43, 89.

Williams, R.B. and Sherter, C. (1971). Cardiac complications of tricyclic antidepressant therapy. *Ann. Intern. Med.* 74, 395.

Willis, P.W. (1975). The hemodynamic effects of Norpace (Part II). *Angiology* 26, 102.

Wilson, J.D., Sutherland, D.C., and Thomas, A.C. (1981). Has the change to beta agonists combined with oral theophylline increased cases of fatal asthma? *Lancet* i, 1235.

Wilson, D.F., Watson, O.F., Peel, J.S., *et al.* (1969). Trasicor in angina pectoris: a double-blind trial. *BMJ* ii, 155.

Winkle, R.A., Anderson, J.L., Peters, F., *et al.* (1978). The hemodynamic effects of intravenous tocainide in patients with heart disease. *Circulation* 57, 787.

Xamoterol in Severe Heart Failure Study Group (1990). Xamoterol in severe heart failure. *Lancet* 336, 1.

Zehender, M., Meinertz, T., Hohnloser, S., *et al.* (1989). Incidence and clinical relevance of QT prolongation caused by the new selective serotonin antagonist ketanserin. *Am. J. Cardiol.* 63, 826.

9. Disorders of the peripheral vascular system

C. J. DAVIES and D. M. DAVIES

Drug-induced hypertension

Sympathomimetic drugs

The use of sympathomimetic drugs such as adrenaline, dobutamine, dopamine, metaraminol, noradrenaline, and phenylephrine by intravenous infusion to correct hypotension can obviously produce an excessive rise in blood pressure unless the dose and the rate of infusion are controlled by careful and continuous monitoring of the arterial pressure. Less likely to be recognized is the danger of systemic hypertension caused by such a drug when it is used for other purposes: as examples, adrenaline given subcutaneously for asthma has caused transient hypertension; a dramatic rise in blood pressure, accompanied by myocardial infarction, has occurred in a patient given the sympathomimetic vasoconstrictor levonordefrin together with mepivacaine for dental anaesthesia (Pearson *et al.* 1987); and the administration of 10% phenylephrine as eye-drops may be followed by systemic hypertension, especially in the neonate (Solosko and Smith 1972; Borromeo-McGrail *et al.* 1973; Matthews *et al.* 1977), and even 2.5% concentrations have had this effect (Lees and Cabal 1981). A significant rise in blood pressure was observed, experimentally, in some healthy young people given a single oral dose of one or other of two phenylpropanolamine-containing preparations, the first marketed as a nasal decongestant and the second as an appetite suppressant. The observers suggested that these drugs should not be available to patients, unless prescribed by a medical practitioner (Horowitz *et al.* 1979). Single doses have even caused hypertension severe enough to warrant admission to hospital (Horowitz *et al.* 1980; McEwen 1983). A severe hypertensive crisis with convulsions occurred in a 13-year-old girl who took a combination of phenylpropanolamine and caffeine daily for 2 weeks for weight reduction (Howrie and Wolfson 1983), and this interaction with coffee has been confirmed in a placebo-controlled study (Lake *et al.* 1989). Another crisis developed in a patient who took indomethacin shortly after phenylpropanolamine (Lee *et al.* 1979), and a third (Gibson and Warrell 1972) in a patient who took phenylpropanolamine after a meal of cheese. These drugs may also induce hypertension by interacting with other drugs (see below).

Antihypertensive drugs

Some of the antihypertensive agents mentioned here are now so little used as to be considered obsolescent, but they are discussed because they may still be prescribed on occasion for those patients who have been treated with them satisfactorily for long periods, in cases unresponsive to more modern drugs, or for disorders other than hypertension. All the drugs dealt with here are currently included in the *British National Formulary*. The most important, in the present context, are the β-adrenoceptor blockers.

Methyldopa, debrisoquine, and bethanidine can cause a rise in blood pressure when administered intravenously, the last two drugs by displacing noradrenaline from nerve endings. Consequently, these antihypertensives are best avoided in the treatment of serious hypertensive crises. Adrenergic-neurone-blocking drugs such as guanethidine, bretylium, bethanidine, and debrisoquine may render the patient unusually sensitive to the pressor effects of noradrenaline (Laurence and Nagle 1961; Muelheims *et al.* 1965), adrenaline, and metaraminol (Stevens 1966). They do this probably by competing with the sympathomimetic drugs for the 'amine pump', which normally helps to terminate the action of catecholamines on receptors by promoting their uptake into nerve endings. Transient hypertension has occurred when these sympathomimetics have been given to patients under treatment with adrenergic-neurone-blocking drugs.

Methyldopa and reserpine may also increase the effect of noradrenaline on the blood pressure, but to a lesser degree that is clinically insignificant (Stockley 1974). A pressor response to labetalol was reported by Crofton and Gabriel (1977), and these authors suggested that intravenous boluses of this drug should be given with caution in patients who are already taking substantial amounts of a β-adrenoceptor blocker, methyldopa, or guanethidine (but see below and under Effect of drugs in the presence of a phaeochromocytoma). Hydralazine has caused a paradoxical rise in blood pressure in a patient with renal artery stenosis, the mechanism being obscure (Webb and White 1980).

Hypertension has also been caused by propranolol (Blum *et al.* 1975) and by acebutolol and sotalol (Gabriel 1976) when the dose of these drugs was increased rapidly. Gabriel (1976) also observed the same response when the dose of guanethidine was increased too quickly. The suggested explanation is that in the presence of high concentrations of circulating catecholamines β-blockade produces unopposed α-adrenoceptor stimulation (Imms *et al.* 1976).

It is now well recognized that the withdrawal of the antihypertensive drug clonidine may lead to a considerable, sometimes fatal, increase in blood pressure due to the massive release of catecholamines from the adrenal medulla (Hunyor *et al.* 1973), producing blood concentrations comparable to those in phaeochromocytoma (Vincent and Pradalier 1993). The rise in blood pressure may begin within a few hours or may be delayed for as long as 17 days (Stelzer *et al.* 1976) and hypertension may occasionally persist for about 2 weeks (Vanholder *et al.* 1977). Reid and others (1977) studied six patients in whom treatment with clonidine in doses of 0.45–5.4 mg daily was abruptly stopped. The blood pressures rose to pretreatment levels within 24–48 hours of withdrawal of the drug and this was accompanied by insomnia, headache, flushing, sweating, and apprehension. Symptoms began 18–24 hours after the last dose of clonidine had been given, and plasma noradrenaline levels and urinary catecholamine excretion increased 24–72 hours after withdrawal. Symptoms were most prominent in patients on higher doses (>1 mg per day) and in those who had previously been receiving other antihypertensive drugs. One patient on a very low dose (0.15 mg per day) had no symptoms and no significant change in blood pressure or catecholamine production after withdrawal. A patient whose oral tablets of clonidine were replaced by skin patches containing the drug developed severe withdrawal hypertension after 6 days (Stewart and Burris 1988), and another patient had a similar reaction when short-term transdermal administration was terminated

(Schmidt and Schuna 1988). Rebound hypertension has also been observed following completion of an epidural infusion of clonidine (Fitzgibbon *et al.* 1996).

As for the treatment of hypertension following the withdrawal of clonidine, the risk involved in using the β-adrenoceptor-blocking drug propranolol has been stressed (Bailey and Neale 1976; Harris 1976) since hypertension may be made worse because of the high concentration of circulating catecholamines, a situation comparable to that present in patients with phaeochromocytoma (see below); but some authors (e.g. Agabiti-Rosei *et al.* 1976; Brown *et al.* 1976) have reported prompt reduction of blood pressure in such cases following the administration of labetalol, a compound which blocks both α-adrenoceptors and β-adrenoceptors, but the fact that this drug has provoked hypertension in the presence of high concentrations of catecholamines (in phaeochromocytoma — see below) should be borne in mind when the drug is used to treat clonidine-withdrawal hypertension.

Slow withdrawal of minoxidil over 4–12 weeks in three children caused rebound hypertension and encephalopathy. The occurrence of rebound hypertension correlated with the total cumulative dose of the drug in mg per kg per week given before withdrawal and the rapidity (4–8 weeks) with which minoxidil was withdrawn, but not with the total duration of therapy, duration at maximum dosage, or the amount of minoxidil in mg per kg on the day prior to withdrawal.

Rebound hypertension did not occur when minoxidil was withdrawn over 12 weeks or if a patient was receiving a small dose (2.5–5 mg per day). Pretreatment with an α-blocker (prazosin) or the discontinuation of the concomitantly administered β-blocker (propranolol) prior to withdrawal seemed to prevent rebound hypertension (Makker and Moorthy 1980). Rebound hypertension has rarely been encountered following the withdrawal of methyldopa (Burden and Alexander 1976; Scott and McDevitt 1976), the withdrawal of propranolol or other β-adrenoceptor blockers, particularly those lacking sympathomimetic activity (Lewis *et al.* 1979), and the ACE inhibitor lisinopril (McAlister and Lewanczuk 1994).

Antagonism of action of antihypertensive drugs

The antihypertensive effect of nifedipine has been reduced by concurrent treatment with rifampicin (Tada *et al.* 1992), and that of guanfacine by amitriptyline (Buckley and Feely 1991). (See also Non-steroidal anti-inflammatory drugs and Antidepressants and antipsychotics below.)

Cyclosporin

Treatment with this immunosuppressive drug, to prevent rejection of transplanted organs or, less commonly, to treat primary autoimmune disorders has caused or aggravated hypertension in many cases. Affected patients have been recipients of transplanted kidneys (Hamilton *et al.* 1982; Canadian Multicentre Transplant Study Group 1983; Ferguson and Sommer 1985; Gordon *et al.* 1985; Krupp *et al.* 1986), lungs (Morrison *et al.* 1993), heart (Hardesty *et al.* 1983; Thompson *et al.* 1986), heart and lungs (Dawkins *et al.* 1985; Burke *et al.* 1986), liver (Malatack *et al.* 1983; Williams *et al.* 1985), or bone marrow (Joss *et al.* 1982); or have been under treatment for rheumatoid arthritis (Berg *et al.* 1986; Dougados and Amor 1987; Weinblatt *et al.* 1987), uveitis, choroiditis, or cicatricial pemphigoid (Palestine *et al.* 1984), severe hypothyroidism (Sennesael *et al.* 1986), or insulin-dependent diabetes mellitus (Ribstein *et al.* 1989). A significant rise in blood pressure has also occurred during short-term, low-dose (5 mg per kg body-weight) treatment for psoriasis (Brown *et al.* (1993).

Hypertension appears to be most severe in cases of heart or heart and lung transplantation and in children (Weidle and Vlasses 1988), is not invariably accompanied by detectable impairment of renal excretory function (Loughran *et al.* 1985; Chapman *et al.* 1987), and cannot be correlated with the dose or serum concentrations of cyclosporin, previous renal disease or hypertension, or concurrent steroid therapy (Weidle and Vlasses 1988).

The precise mechanism by which cyclosporin causes or aggravates hypertension has long remained unclear, but a contribution to its understanding was made by Scherrer and others (1990) who demonstrated a considerable increase in sympathetic neural activity in 14 heart transplant patients, all but two of whom were normotensive before transplantation, when they were treated with cyclosporin. Experiments in animals have produced results that have conflicted with observations made in human subjects as regards the renin–angiotensin–aldosterone system and the production of vasodilatory prostaglandins, and clinical findings have themselves varied in different studies (Weidle and Vlasses 1988).

The subject is of great complexity, and readers should consult reviews by Weidle and Vlasses (1988), *The Lancet* (1988), Schachter (1988), Tao *et al.* (1990), and Scherrer *et al.* (1990) for detailed discussions of this and other aspects of cyclosporin toxicity.

Erythropoietin (Epoetin)

Many patients undergoing repeated haemodialysis for chronic renal failure have suffered a marked increase in blood pressure when given recombinant erythropoietin (EPO) for associated anaemia, this complication being more frequent (Eggert and Stick 1988) and most severe (Raine 1988) in those with pre-existing hypertension, and in four such cases malignant hypertension resistant to additional antihypertensive therapy but responsive to venesection developed (Fahal *et al.* 1991).

The mechanism involved is uncertain. Eggert and Stick (1988) concluded that the increase in blood pressure is due to the rise in haemoglobin concentration under the special circumstances obtaining in renal disease, rather than to some other effect of EPO, since the blood pressure in one of their patients rose regularly after transfusion of erythrocyte concentrates. Involvement of the renin–angiotensin system seems to have been eliminated as a cause, as EPO has caused hypertension in anephric patients (Edmunds and Walls 1988; Tomson *et al.* 1988). The rate of rise of the haematocrit readings correlates with the likelihood of developing hypertension (Wong *et al.* 1990), and Raine (1988) suggested that the sustained dose-dependent rise in haematocrit values leads to a greater whole-blood viscosity, with consequent increase in peripheral resistance, coupled with loss of hypoxic vasodilatation. Martin and Moncada (1988) postulated that the increased quantity of haemoglobin, resulting from EPO therapy, binds to nitric oxide, secreted by endothelial cells, thus negating its powerful vasodilator action, but Vallance and others (1988) opposed this view. Thus the problem awaits further research for its solution.

An unusual case has been reported by Caravaca and others (1997) in which a patient had hypertensive crises when given blood platelet transfusions while receiving EPO, but not when it was withheld.

Ketoconazole

This drug is used mainly for its antifungal properties, but it also inhibits steroid synthesis in the adrenal gland, ovary, and testes by blocking the activity of various enzyme systems and this has led to its use in conditions in which such effects are desirable (e.g. Cushing's syndrome; hyperaldosteronism; precocious puberty; hirsutism; and cancer of the prostate, male breast, and ovary).

A small number of patients have developed hypertension during long-term, high-dose treatment with the drug, and the mechanism is believed to be inhibition of 11β-hydroxylase, resulting in an increase in concentrations of 11-deoxycortisol and deoxycorticosterone (Aabo and De Coster 1987; Leal-Cerro *et al.* 1989), affected patients possibly being unusually sensitive to the mineralocorticoid effect of deoxycorticosterone (Aabo and De Coster 1987).

Non-steroidal anti-inflammatory drugs

Non-steroidal anti-inflammatory drugs (NSAID) can raise the blood pressure in normotensive subjects (Sahloul *et al.* 1990) or untreated hypertensives (Magagna *et al.* 1991) and can also reduce the efficacy of several types of antihypertensive therapy (Sahloul *et al.* 1990; Houston 1991). These drugs vary in their potency in this respect, indomethacin having the greatest effect and sulindac the least. The mechanisms involved are complex but involve prostaglandin production and function and the renin–angiotensin system.

There seems no doubt that the antihypertensive actions of the ACE inhibitors (Ahmad 1991; Morgan and Anderson 1993), β-adrenoceptor antagonists (Schoenfeld *et al.* 1989; Sahloul *et al.* 1990; Abate *et al.* 1991; Houston 1991), and thiazide and related diuretics (Houston 1991) are impaired by NSAID but there is less certainty about α-blockers, calcium antagonists (though felodipine is said not to be affected — Morgan and Anderson 1993), clonidine, methyldopa, and vasodilators (e.g., hydralazine), but one authoritative source of information (*British National Formulary* 1997) claims that all but one of these drugs are less effective when given concurrently with a NSAID, the exception being clonidine, for which no warning of this interaction is given. This subject is also discussed in Chapter 33.

Antidepressants and antipsychotics

Quite apart from their ability to cause hypertension by interacting with other drugs (see below), monoamine oxidase inhibitors and tricyclic compounds can, very occasionally, raise the blood pressure when given alone to normotensive subjects or previously well-controlled hypertensives. The monoamine oxidase inhibitors tranylcypromine (Da Motta and Cordas 1990; Lavin *et al.* 1993) and moclobemide (Coulter and Pillans 1995) have been implicated, as have the tricyclic drugs amitriptyline desipramine, clomipramine, imipramine, and nortriptyline (Hessov 1970, 1971; Buckley and Feeley 1991; Kuekes *et al.* 1992; Louie *et al.* 1992), though the hypertensive effect of imipramine may disappear despite continued treatment (Kuekes *et al.* 1992). Interestingly, although the blood pressure rose in six of 43 patients treated with a tricyclic antidepressant for panic attacks, with or without depression, it did not do so in any of 71 patients with depression alone (Louie *et al.* 1992).

Hypertension has occurred when phenelzine has been given concurrently with fentanyl (Insler *et al.* 1994), and selegeline with fluoxetine (Montastrue *et al.* 1993).

A depressed patient under treatment with selegeline for Parkinson's disease developed hypertension when the selective serotonin reuptake-inhibitor fluoxetine was substituted for amitriptyline as an antidepressive (Suchowersky and de Vries 1990).

When clozapine affects the blood pressure, it usually induces hypotension, but a paradoxical hypertensive reaction has been reported (Ennis and Parker 1997).

Alcohol (ethanol)

Several studies have shown a correlation between alcohol intake and a rise in blood pressure (Criqui *et al.* 1981; Saunders *et al.* 1981; Klatsky *et al.* 1986; Regen 1990). The results of clinical experiments by Grassi and others (1989) suggest that this effect is mediated by activation of the sympathetic nervous system.

Salt

An excessive intake of salt can induce hypertension in susceptible people (Gavras and Gavras 1988). Salt-retaining drugs, particularly licorice and its derivative carbenoxolone, and mineralocorticoids also have this effect (Lai *et al.* 1991).

Drug interactions

In the past there has been uncertainty about the risks of hypertensive crises due to possible interactions between antidepressant drugs and sympathomimetic substances contained in medicines and foods. The confusion has arisen mainly because it has sometimes been too readily assumed that drugs that have some actions in common are pharmacologically identical in all respects, which is not always the case.

This subject is also discussed in Chapter 33.

Monoamine oxidase inhibitor (MAOI) antidepressants

MAOI and directly acting sympathomimetics

The catecholamines adrenaline and noradrenaline are directly acting sympathomimetics, that is, they themselves directly stimulate adrenoceptors. Noradrenaline acts mainly on α-receptors, causing vasoconstriction and a rise in blood pressure, but usually no rise in pulse rate. Adrenaline acts on both α- and β-receptors causing tachycardia in addition to blood pressure changes. Inactivation of noradrenaline released at nerve endings and of injected noradrenaline and adrenaline is achieved mainly by uptake into sympathetic neurones and partly by the enzyme catechol-*o*-methyltransferase. Mono-amine oxidase plays only a very minor part in the process, and that almost exclusively within cells. Conse-quently, on theoretical grounds it can be predicted that MAOI will not potentiate the effects of injected adrena-line and noradrenaline. With noradrenaline, experi-ments in man fulfil this prediction (Horwitz *et al.* 1960; Elis *et al.* 1967; Pettinger and Oates 1968; Barar *et al.* 1971), but with adrenaline they do not, for some actions of this drug are moderately potentiated by certain MAOI (tranylcypromine [Cuthbert and Vere 1971]), though not by others (phenelzine [Barar *et al.* 1971]). The vasoconstrictor felypressin is not potentiated by MAOI. Results of experiments with isoprenaline have been variable.

It is reasonable to conclude that any patient under treatment with an MAOI may safely be given either noradrenaline or felypressin in normal doses; that adrenaline may be given in normal doses if the patient is physically healthy; but that there is a risk involved in giving adrenaline to patients with cardiovascular disease.

In the present state of knowledge, isoprenaline should be given to patients under treatment with MAOI only when its use is absolutely essential.

MAOI and indirectly acting sympathomimetics

Amphetamine and tyramine are indirectly acting sym-pathomimetics, exerting their effect by releasing nor-adrenaline from stores in nerve endings. Ephedrine, metaraminol, phenylpropanolamine, and phenylephrine also have an indirect (as well as a direct) action. The noradrenaline released by nerve impulses is stored in vesicles, but the noradrenaline released by indirectly acting sympathomimetic drugs is 'free' within the cyto-plasm (where its concentration is usually minimal due to the activity of monoamine oxidase). In the presence of MAOI, the concentration of 'free' cytoplasmic nor-adrenaline is markedly increased, so that the effects of indirectly acting sympathomimetic agents are enhanced. Hypertensive crises can therefore occur when an in-directly acting sympathomimetic is taken by a patient under treatment with an MAOI. However, in the case of a patient who was taking one of the newer MAOI, toloxalone, concurrent administration of phenylephrine had no ill effect until terbutaline was added, after which she suffered recurrent attacks of hypertension; blood concentrations of adrenaline and noradrenaline were found to be raised and a phaeochromocytoma was sus-pected but not detected at operation (for intestinal infarction) (Lefebvre *et al.* 1993).

MAOI and food

Hypertensive crises in patients under treatment with MAOI antidepressants were first reported by Ogilvie (1955), who noted attacks of severe headaches associated with palpitations, flushing, sweating, and hypertension in four of 42 patients being treated with iproniazid. These symptoms did not occur in 47 patients treated with isoniazid which, although closely related chemically to iproniazid, is not an MAOI. The cause of this reaction remained obscure until Blackwell (1963) and Womack (1963) identified cheese as a precipitating factor. In the same year, Asatoor and others (1963) identified tyr-amine as the ingredient responsible. They showed that the ingestion of cheese was followed in normal subjects by the excretion of large amounts of *p*-hydroxyphenyl-acetic acid, a metabolic product of tyramine. In patients receiving MAOI, tyramine cannot be broken down and as it is an indirectly acting sympathomimetic agent it has the severe clinical effects described.

Since then a number of other foodstuffs have been identified as possible causes of hypertensive reactions in patients under treatment with MAOI. Yeast extract, which contains both tyramine and histamine, may pro-duce such reactions (Blackwell *et al.* 1965). The oxi-dation of both of these substances is interfered with by the MAOI, and histamine is capable of releasing cate-cholamines from the adrenal medulla, a property of particular importance in patients with phaeochromocy-toma (described below). Whole sliced broad beans, the pods of which contain significant amounts of dopa, may also produce hypertensive crises in patients taking MAOI (Hodge *et al.* 1964; Blomley 1964). Dopa is converted in the body to dopamine, the oxidation of which is impeded by MAOI.

Unfortunately, published lists of proscribed foods are inconsistent, and this has come about because some lists include items damned on the basis of their tyramine content or on the strength of poorly documented case reports. A critical review (Stewart 1976) concluded that a patient should be told to avoid matured cheese; hydro-lysed protein extract (e.g. Marmite, Bovril, but not Bisto); other protein foods that are not fresh or that have been subjected to hydrolysis, fermentation, or 'hang-ing'; alcohol, except in *strict* moderation; broad bean pods; banana skins; raspberries; and any other food that the patient has previously had reason to suspect as a cause of unpleasant symptoms. As far as alcoholic drinks are concerned, Hannah and others (1988) have reas-sessed their risk to patients taking MAOI. They ana-lysed the tyramine content of nine types of beer, 12 of white wine, and 22 of red wine (including 12 of Chianti, which has previously achieved notoriety in this context), and concluded that a half litre of any of these beverages was unlikely to contain enough tyramine to be dangerous. However, cases involving draught (tap) beer have been reported by Tailor and others (1994) and Shulman and colleagues (1997), the former authors pointing out that this type of beer contains a much higher concentration of tyramine than bottled or canned beer. The process by which alcohol-free beer is produced appears to increase the tyramine content, and this type of beverage has interacted with an MAOI to cause attacks of hypertension (Thakore *et al.* 1992).

To this list the depressed gourmet should add caviar (Isaac *et al.* 1977), New Zealand prickly spinach (Comfort 1981), and over-ripe avocado (Generali 1981).

A single case of a hypertensive response to cheese in a patient taking the antihypertensive drug debrisoquine has been reported by Amery and Deloof (1970) who pointed out that this drug had been shown in animal experiments to have monoamine-oxidase-inhibiting properties.

The subject has been examined again in detail by Folks (1983).

Selegeline hydrocholoride is a selective type B monoamine oxidase inhibitor, used mainly as an adjunct to levodopa therapy for Parkinson's disease, though it has also been used as an antidepressant. Because it inhibits only Type B monoamine oxidase (predominant in the striatum of the brain), leaving Type A active in the liver and gut, it has been believed on theoretical grounds not to produce the conditions necessary for the tyramine reaction, but a case has been described in which a patient under treatment with the drug developed transient hypertension and headache when he ate a meal with a high tyramine content (McGrath *et al.* 1989).

Tricyclic antidepressants

Tricyclics and directly acting sympathomimetics

These drugs inhibit the uptake of adrenaline and noradrenaline by nerve endings, so prolonging and intensifying their actions. Svedmyr (1968) observed that the effect of noradrenaline in man was increased ninefold and that of adrenaline threefold by concurrent treatment with a tricyclic antidepressant. Goldman and others (1971) confirmed those findings with noradrenaline, but not with adrenaline which, in their experiments, showed little or no potentiating effect. Felypressin was not potentiated by tricyclic drugs.

Tricyclics and indirectly acting sympathomimetics

It might be supposed that any sympathomimetic with an indirect action would be potentiated by tricyclic drugs because these could interfere with the uptake of cate-

cholamines released by the sympathomimetic. Some sympathomimetics require, however, to be actively transported into the nerve ending before they can release noradrenaline, and tricyclics may prevent this method of uptake, in which case the effect of the sympathomimetic will be diminished rather than potentiated. Inhibition of this kind has been demonstrated (Svedmyr 1968). Nevertheless, it cannot safely be assumed that the effects of all indirectly acting sympathomimetics will be reduced in this way, for some do not require active transport and some have direct actions as well. Furthermore, there is experimental evidence suggesting that some tricyclic compounds may inhibit the metabolism of some indirectly acting sympathomimetics (Stockley 1974).

One may conclude that it is mandatory to avoid giving noradrenaline or adrenaline to patients taking tricyclic antidepressants, and probably best to avoid any sympathomimetic drug in such patients.

A case has been reported in which a patient under treatment with amitriptyline suffered a hypertensive crisis 34 hours after beginning treatment with levodopa, carbidopa, and metoclopramide (Rampton 1977); limited investigations for a phaeochromocytoma (in the presence of which metoclopramide has induced a hypertensive crisis — see below) were negative.

Other interacting drugs

Hypertension has occasionally occurred as a result of interactions between cimetidine and dobutamine (Baraka *et al.* 1992), disulfiram and alcohol (Zapata and Orwin 1992), dihydroergotamine and propranolol (Gandy 1990), phenylpropanolamine and bromocriptine (Chan *et al.* 1994), phenylpropanolamine with methyldopa and oxprenolol (McLaren 1976), and selegeline and fluoxetine (Montastrue *et al.* 1993); in the latter case, high blood concentrations of adrenaline and noradrenaline were detected but no evidence of phaeochromocytoma was found on chest X-rays or an abdominal CT scan.

Hypertensive effects of drugs in the presence of a phaeochromocytoma

Patients with phaeochromocytoma may be given drugs for a variety of reasons: in the unrecognized case for symptoms of the disease or during medical or surgical treatment of some unrelated condition; in the suspected case for diagnostic tests; and in the confirmed case for anaesthesia and adjuvant therapy at operation for removal of the tumour, or for long-term treatment when surgery is impracticable. Many of these drugs are believed to have caused hypertensive crises in these circumstances or thought, on theoretical grounds, to be capable of doing so.

Evaluating published reports is sometimes difficult. This is particularly true of reactions during the induction or maintenance of anaesthesia, because many of the drugs concerned, or closely related compounds, have been given to patients with phaeochromocytoma without ill effects; though it should be noted that in some of these cases drugs other than those suspected of having caused a reaction were administered to the patient concurrently (e.g. barbiturates, other than thiopentone; chloral hydrate; phenoxybenzamine) and these may have modified or prevented the hypertensive effects reported in other patients.

A number of 'explanations' for observed hypertensive crises induced by certain drugs in patients with phaeochromocytoma have been published, but many are simplistic and some conflict with available evidence. For example, in many published articles and in standard textbooks of pharmacology it has been tacitly assumed or even asserted that a number of different drugs release catecholamines either by direct or indirect stimulation via the autonomic nervous system. Thus, the effect of insulin on a phaeochromocytoma has been explained by the response of the sympathetic nervous system to hypoglycaemia, and that of tetraethylammonium to sympathetic discharge provoked by hypotension. These explanations presuppose that chromaffin tumours are innervated, but what little evidence is available on this point suggests that they are not. While literature on every other aspect of phaeochromocytoma is abundant, there is a quite extraordinary dearth of observations, surgical and pathological, on the presence or absence of nerves supplying phaeochromocytomata, and the very few authors who deal with this point state that the tumours do not have a normally developed nerve supply (Robinson and Williams 1956; Coupland 1965; Ratzenhofer 1968). Of course, findings in some phaeochromocytomata cannot confidently be extrapolated to all such tumours, but these pathological observations are supported pharmacologically by the fact that clonidine (which reduces central sympathetic discharge) fails to suppress catecholamine release in patients with phaeochromocytomata but does so in normal subjects — a phenomenon that forms the basis of a diagnostic test for the tumour (Bravo *et al.* 1981). Pentolinium, a ganglion-blocking drug that interrupts preganglionic nervous impulses to sympathetic nerves and the adrenal medulla, would be expected to cause a fall in catecholamine excretion from a phaeochromocytoma if the tumour

were innervated but it fails to do so (Brown *et al.* 1980) and is therefore used in diagnosis.

One can reasonably conclude, therefore, that phaeochromocytomata have no functioning nerve supply and so cannot be stimulated or inhibited by drugs that affect the autonomic nervous system, either directly or indirectly.

Detailed examination of the pharmacological literature shows that the subject is of the greatest complexity (the more so when one takes into consideration the possible differences between man and the animals used in experiments, and the interspecies differences between the animal subjects) and that some drugs are theoretically capable of inducing hypertension in patients with phaeochromocytoma by more than one mechanism.

Postulated mechanisms for hypertensive reactions to drugs in the presence of a phaeochromocytoma are listed in Table 9.1. In Table 9.2 are listed the drugs reported to

TABLE 9.1
Postulated mechanisms for hypertensive crises induced by drugs in the presence of a phaeochromocytoma

A Sudden release of large amounts of catecholamines

  1 From the tumour

    1.1 by direct stimulation of phaeochromocytoma cells
    1.2 by release of histamine, which then stimulates phaeochromocytoma cells (histamine also causes release of catecholamines from nerve endings)
    1.3 by stimulation of phaeochromocytoma cells via the autonomic nerve system*
    1.4 by suppressing levels of endogenous somatostatin, which normally inhibits catecholamine release

  2 From accumulated excessive stores of catecholamines in nerve endings

    2.1 by direct action on nerve endings
    2.2 by indirect action via the autonomic system

B Interference with uptake of circulating catecholamines into nerve endings

C Induction of supersensitivity of catecholamine receptors

D Potentiation of effect of catecholamines on arterioles

E Non-selective β-blockade

F Other possible mechanisms

  1 incomplete β-blockade resulting from inadequate doses of phenoxybenzamine preoperatively
  2 blockade of presynaptic α_2-receptors without effect on α_1-receptors.

---

* This mechanism, postulated by several authors, presupposes that phaeochromocytomata are supplied by functioning nerves, but the surprisingly few relevant histological studies have found no evidence of a normally developed nerve supply to these tumours (see text).

TABLE 9.2

Drugs reported to have caused hypertensive crises in the presence of a phaeochromocytoma or believed on theoretical grounds to be capable of doing so

Drug	Known or postulated mechanism (as classified in Table 9.1)	References to clinical cases, experimental observations, or unsupported statements
β-Adrenoceptor blockers	E	Prichard 1964; Glover and Hutchinson 1964; Ross *et al.* 1967; Briggs *et al.* 1978; Wark and Larkins 1978; Sloand and Thompson 1984; Choi *et al.* 1995; Sheaves *et al.* 1995
Antihistamines	release histamine — see Histamine below	Paton 1957
Antiprotozoal diamidines	release histamine — see Histamine below	Webster 1985
Atropine	D	Swan 1949
Chlorpromazine	releases histamine — see Histamine below	Paton 1957
Corticosteroids	high concentrations produced by corticotrophin stimulation may reach the phaeochromocytoma via glandular veins and stimulate tumour cells — A 1.1	Yard and Kadowitz 1972; Critchley and Ungar 1974; Daggett and Franks 1977
Corticotrophin	increased secretion of corticosteroids — see Corticosteroids above	Ramsay and Langlands 1962; Moorhead *et al.* 1966; Critchley *et al.* 1974
Curare/tubocurarine	release histamine — see Histamine below	Alam *et al.* 1939; Comroe and Dripps 1946; Westgate and van Bergen 1962; Koelle 1970
Dextran	releases histamine — see Histamine below	Lorenz *et al.* 1976
Droperidol	F 1	Maddern *et al.* 1976; Bittar 1979; Sumikawa and Amakata 1977; Oh *et al.* 1978
Ether	A 1.1	Bixby and Troncelliti 1952; Price and Dripps 1970
Gallamine (excessive doses)	releases histamine — see Histamine below	Mushin *et al.* 1949; Sniper 1952
Glucagon	A 1.1	Scian *et al.* 1960; Unger *et al.* 1962; Sarcione *et al.* 1963; Minamori *et al.* 1992
Guanethidine and related compounds*	C	Emmelin and Enström 1961
Histamine	A 1.1 and A 2.1	Burn and Dale 1926; Szczygielski 1932; Siehe 1934; Athos *et al.* 1962; Engelman and Sjoerdsma 1964; Staszewska-Barczak and Vane 1965; Euler 1966; Douglas *et al.* 1967; Douglas 1985;
Insulin	hypoglycaemia — A 2.2 and secretion of glucagon — A 1.1	Goldfein *et al.* 1958; Scian *et al.* 1960; Unger *et al.* 1962; Sarcione *et al.* 1963
Methacholine	hypotension — A 2.2 and (possibly) A 1.1	Volle and Koelle 1970
Metoclopramide/sulpiride	F 2	Corvol *et al.* 1974; Plouin *et al.* 1976; Agabiti-Rosei *et al.* 1977; Spedding 1980; Freestone *et al.* 1996
Monoamine oxidase inhibitors	permit tyramine (see Tyramine below) to enter via gut and liver	Cook and Katritsis 1990
Nicotine (cigarettes, snuff)	A 2.2 and (possibly) A 1.1	Burn *et al.* 1959; Stromblad 1960; Dugan 1967; Cryer *et al.* 1976; McPhaul *et al.* 1984
Octreotide (somatostatin analogue)	? suppresses levels of endogenous somatostatin, which normally reduces catecholamine release from adrenal tissue — A 1.4	Salz *et al.*
Opiates	release antihistamine — see Histamine above	Chaturvedi *et al.* 1974; Lawrence 1978; Fahmy *et al.* 1983
Plasma expanders	release histamine — see Histamine above	Lorenz *et al.* 1976

Table 9.2 continued

Drug	Known or postulated mechanism (as classified in Table 7.1)	References to clinical cases, experimental observations, or unsupported statements
Saralasin	A 1.1 (possibly) directly and by increasing levels of angiotensin II	Feldberg and Lewis 1964; Khairallah *et al.* 1971; Peach 1971; Steele and Lowenstein 1975; Dunn *et al.* 1976; Peach *et al.* 1978
Serotonin-reuptake inhibitors (paroxetine)	serotonin in the vicinity of the phaeochromocytoma — A 1.1	Douglas *et al.* 1967; Seeler *et al.* 1997
Sulpiride — see Metoclopramide		
Suxamethonium	releases histamine — see Histamine above	Smith 1957; Stoner and Urbach 1968
Tetraethylammonium	hypotension — A 2.2 and (possibly) A 1.1	Wilkins *et al.* 1950; Volle and Koelle 1970
Thiopentone	releases histamine — see Histamine above	Lorenz and Doenicke 1978
Tricyclic antidepressants	B	Kaufmann 1974
Trimetaphan	releases histamine — see Histamine above	Volle and Koelle 1970
Tubocurarine —see Curare		
Tyramine	A 2.1	Weiner *et al.* 1962; Engelman and Sjoerdsma 1964
X-ray contrast media	release histamine — see Histamine above	Ansell 1970

* despite the theoretical possibility of such a reaction, no cases have been found in the literature.

have caused hypertensive crises. Also included in this table are a few drugs (e.g. guanethidine and related compounds; monoamine oxidase inhibitors) believed on the strongest theoretical grounds to be capable of inducing hypertension in the presence of a phaeochromocytoma, and about which warnings to this effect have been published; but, interestingly, only a single report involving one of these drugs (the monoamine oxidase inhibitor tranylcypromine [Cook and Katritsis 1990]) has been located by us, and one can only surmise that the pharmacological *milieu* in a patient with phaeochromocytoma, in whom an excess of circulating catecholamines has been present continuously or intermittently for a long period, is unique and quite different from the situation in animal experiments on which predictions of adverse reactions have been based.

The most important drugs in this context are the β-adrenoceptor blockers, because they are routinely used before and during operation for phaeochromocytoma. There is no doubt that non-selective β-adrenoceptor blockers (for a very full discussion of 'selectivity' see Kumana and Marlin 1978) may cause a significant rise in blood pressure in patients with phaeochromocytoma because they abolish the peripheral vasodilator effect of catecholamines while leaving the vasoconstrictor response of α-adrenoceptors unopposed. Consequently, treatment with non-selective β-adrenoceptor-

blocking drugs in phaeochromocytoma should only be started *at the same time as* or *soon after* treatment with an α-adrenoceptor-blocking agent. This was pointed out many years ago by Ross and others (1967), but adverse effects of β-blockers given alone in phaeochromocytoma continued to be reported (Wark and Larkins 1978; Sloand and Thompson 1984; Sheaves *et al.* 1995). The use of labetalol, a drug that blocks both β-adrenoceptors and α-adrenoceptors might seem to be one rational answer to this problem and, indeed, it has been used successfully for this purpose (Agabiti-Rosei *et al.* 1976). However, cases in which the drug provoked a hypertensive crisis have been reported by Sheaves and others (1995) and by Briggs and colleagues (1978); in the latter case the predominant catecholamine secreted by the tumour was adrenaline.

Another drug that has been tried with the aim of preventing hypertensive crises during anaesthesia and operation when removing phaeochromocytomata is the somatostatin analogue octreotide. The theoretical basis for its use is that as endogenous somatostatin inhibits secretion of catecholamines from the adrenal gland, and most phaeochromocytomata contain a large number of somatostatin receptors, administration of a somatostatin analogue might reduce catecholamine output from the tumour. However, instead of having the predicted effect the intravenous infusion of octreotide induced a

TABLE 9.3
*Drugs (other than those discussed in the text) reported
to have caused hypertension*

ACTH (corticotrophin)	*
Amphotericin B	Dukes and Perfect 1990; Omizo *et al.* 1993; Katz and Cohn 1994; Le *et al.* 1996
Analgesics (abuse)	Prescott 1972; Küster and Ritz 1989
Anticholinesterase (eye-drops)	Nelemans 1972
Bromocriptine	Makadassi *et al.* 1996
Carbamazepine	Killian and Fromm 1968
Chlorpropamide	Schmitt and Moore 1993
Ciprofloxacin (in an infant)	Atasoy *et al.* 1995
Cisplatin	İçli *et al.* 1993
Clomethiazole	Laurenson and Davis 1985
Clozapine	George and Winther 1996
Corticosteroids	*
Corticosteroid withdrawal (in children)	Sanders *et al.* 1992
Dimercaprol	Brown and Kulkarni 1967
Dinoprost	Veber *et al.* 1992
Disulfiram	Supprian 1969
Docetaxel	Schrijvers *et al.* 1993
Doxorubicin	Paterson 1978
Ergometrine	Browning 1974
Fat emulsions	Schindel 1972
Fluorescein (angiography)	McAllister 1981
Fluorometholone	Schroeder and Weeth 1967
Glyceryl trinitrate	Carmeli *et al.* 1994
Indigo carmine (renal function tests)	Wu and Johnson 1969
Ketamine	Knox *et al.* 1970; Murphy 1993
Levodopa	*Drug and Therapeutics Bulletin* 1969
Lithium	Meltzer and Sealey 1990
Mesna	Gilleece and Davies 1991
Muromonab-CT3	Spieker *et al.* 1991
Nalorphine	Otteni *et al.* 1969
Naloxone	Tanaka 1974; Gremse *et al.* 1986; Schoenfeld *et al.* 1987
Nifedipine	Ben-Noun 1991
Nitroglycerin	Carmeli *et al.* 1994
Oral contraceptives	*
Paclitaxel	Solimando *et al.* 1996
Pentazocine (large doses)	Brown 1969
Phentolamine	Marriott 1957
Promethazine (intravenously)	Adelman *et al.* 1959
Prostaglandins	Veber *et al.* 1992
Pyrazinamide	Goldberg *et al.* 1997
Scopolamine	Keshtan *et al.* 1992
Sex hormones	*
Sorbitol	Winter *et al.* 1973
Sulpiride	Mayer and Montgomery 1989
Tacrine	Allain *et al.* 1996
Tolazoline	Nickerson 1970

* The number of reported cases is too great for references to
be listed here.

hypertensive crisis. The authors were unable to offer a satisfactory explanation of this paradoxical response, though they did suggest the possibility that octreotide (which mainly stimulates type II somatostatin receptors) suppressed levels of endogenous somatostatin (which stimulates at least five types of somatostatin receptors) with the overall effect of increasing catecholamine secretion by the tumour.

At the present time the most satisfactory alternative to combined treatment with α- and β-adrenoceptor-blocking drugs appears to be the calcium channel-blocking drug nicardipine (Proye *et al.* 1989).

The subject of adverse reactions to drugs in the presence of a phaeochromocytoma has been reviewed in greater detail elsewhere (Davies 1987).

Other drugs causing hypertension

A wide variety of other drugs have occasionally caused hypertension, in some cases by mechanisms that at the moment are not entirely clear. They are listed in Table 9.3.

Peripheral vasoconstriction

Some drugs cause vasoconstriction; when this is of moderate degree the patient may experience coldness of the extremities which can at times mimic Raynaud's phenomenon (see below); when it is more severe it may produce intermittent claudication; and when intense it may cause tissue necrosis, particularly when the patient already has atheromatous narrowing of the arteries.

Drugs used for their vasoconstrictor effects

It is to be expected that drugs, such as metaraminol and noradrenaline, used for their vasoconstrictor effect (once popular in the treatment of shock) will at times cause ischaemia of peripheral tissues. Such complications appear, however, to be uncommon when the drugs are given intravenously unless there is leakage into the tissues surrounding the point of entry of the injection or infusion, when tissue necrosis may occur.

Dihydroergotamine has been used in combination with lignocaine and low-dose heparin to prevent post-operative thromboembolism, because of its action in constricting capacitance vessels thus promoting venous return; but unfortunately this form of treatment has occasionally been complicated by severe arterial spasm, sometimes resulting in gangrene (*SADRAC Bulletin* 1989).

Drugs used for migraine

Some of the drugs used in the treatment of migraine have vasoconstrictor properties which at times may be harmful. Thus, ergotamine has caused peripheral ischaemia, rarely resulting in gangrene, even when doses have not been excessive.

There have been several reports of peripheral ischaemia in patients under treatment with either ergotamine or dihydroergotamine when they were also given one of the macrolide antibiotics — erythromycin (Lagier *et al.* 1979), clarithromycin (Horowitz *et al.* 1996), or troleandomycin. It has been suggested that in such cases the antibiotic may simply have inhibited the hepatic enzymes involved in the metabolism of the ergot alkaloid (Hayton 1969; Bacourt and Couffinhal 1978; Franco *et al.* 1978; Vayssairat *et al.* 1978). Methysergide has caused ischaemic pain (Leyton 1964) and coldness in the limbs, and even arterial occlusion (Raw and Gaylis 1976; Ameli *et al.* 1977).

Drugs used for other purposes

Ergometrine given intramuscularly has caused peripheral gangrene on rare occasions (Valentine *et al.* 1977).

Dopamine, used in the treatment of shock or acute cardiac failure may cause peripheral vasoconstriction and even tissue necrosis if the dose is excessive (Alexander *et al.* 1975; Julka and Nora 1976; Maggi *et al.* 1982). The presence of disseminated intravascular coagulation has been suspected as a contributory cause of dopamine-induced peripheral gangrene (Kaul *et al.* 1997).

Bromocriptine, a dopaminergic-receptor stimulant that has been used to inhibit the secretion of prolactin, to reduce circulating growth hormone levels, and to treat some cases of Parkinson's disease, may at times cause troublesome peripheral vasoconstriction (Sachdev *et al.* 1975; Wass *et al.* 1976; Wass *et al.* 1977).

Vasopressin, given by infusion in the treatment of portal hypertension, has caused cutaneous gangrene, even though there was no evidence of subcutaneous extravasation in several of the cases (Anderson and Johnston 1983). This treatment has also caused ischaemia of the scrotum in two patients (Chang *et al.* 1989).

Ischaemia of one leg followed treatment with dexfenfluramine and minocycline, given together for obesity and acne respectively (Prate and Spreux 1992).

An injection of an allergen mixture for allergic rhinitis was thought to have been responsible for ischaemia of the fingers in a patient who had had anaphylactic reactions to this treatment previously (Cabrera *et al.* 1993).

Excessive use of the nasal decongestant fenoxazoline has resulted in digital ischaemia and gangrene (Hauet *et al.* 1996).

β-Adrenoceptor blocking agents may induce vasoconstriction. This is usually mild and produces only coldness of the extremities but it has caused intermittent claudication in previously asymptomatic patients (Rodger *et al.* 1976) and even peripheral gangrene in rare instances (Vale and Jeffereys 1978). It has been suggested that the dominance of α-adrenergic sympathetic activity, resulting from β-adrenoceptor blockade, produces disturbances of the peripheral haemodynamics by eliminating the capacity of the blood vessels in muscle to respond to β_2-mediated vasodilatation (Dukes 1979).

Drugs causing vasoconstriction only by local irritation

A variety of drugs that have no significant vasoconstrictor effects when given by mouth or by intravenous injection (without leakage from the site of injection) may cause intense arterial spasm, sometimes resulting in gangrene, if accidentally injected into or very near to an artery or if they reach an artery by spread from the site of an intramuscular or intravenous injection (e.g. barbiturates [Mindham 1975]; benzylpenicillin [Friederszick 1949]; diazepam [Wing-Tin *et al.* 1994]; diphenhydramine [Ramsdell 1989]; flucloxacillin [McGrath 1992]; phenytoin [Sentenie *et al.* 1992]; promazine [Bounameaux *et al.* 1990]).

Methylmethacrylate used in joint replacement surgery has caused severe damage to arteries with which it has come into contact (Hirsh *et al.* 1976).

Raynaud's phenomenon

Cases of drug-induced vascular disorders which the observers considered to have had features suggestive of Raynaud's phenomenon have been reported, but not all of these reports make it clear why they were so labelled and were not merely examples of simple drug-induced vasospasm. The drugs involved in these cases are various β-adrenoceptor blockers, including timolol eye-drops (Meuche *et al.* 1990), antineoplastic agents given singly or in combination (Werquin 1987; Anderson *et al.* 1988; Shall *et al.* 1988; Kampman *et al.* 1989; Epstein 1991; Heier 1991; De Pablo *et al.* 1992; Von Gunten *et al.* 1993; Arslan *et al.* 1994; Goffin *et al.* 1994; Bachmeyer *et al.* 1996; Creutzig *et al.* 1996; Peschere *et al.* 1996), bromocriptine (Quagliarello and Barakat 1987; Zenore *et al.* 1996), cyclosporin (Deray *et al.* 1986; Davenport 1993), fentanyl with propofol (Bedford and Lockey 1995), fluoxetine (Rudnick 1997), fluvoxamine (Bell *et al.* 1996), gemfibrozil (Smith and Hurst 1993), pergolide (Monk *et al.* 1984), and thiothixene (McCance-Katz 1991).

Acrocyanosis and erythromelalgia

Acrocyanosis is characterized by blueness and coldness of the hands and feet, sometimes accompanied by sweating of the affected parts, differing from Raynaud's disease in that it is not episodic. Erythromelalgia is a condition in which there is an unpleasant burning discomfort in the distal parts of the upper or lower limbs, with or without associated discolouration of the parts involved. In some cases described in the literature no clear distinction is made between the two conditions.

Acrocyanosis is usually idiopathic, but cases with somewhat similar features have been attributed to imipramine (Anderson and Morris 1988) and fluoxetine (Gunzberger and Martinez 1992).

True erythromelalgia is probably due to thrombocythaemia, with intravenous activation of platelets leading to thromboses and arteriolar inflammation (Drenth 1989). A syndrome superficially resembling the disease has been associated with treatment with nifedipine (Brodmerkel 1983; Fisher and Padnick 1983) and nicardipine (Levesque *et al.* 1989); in the latter case a platelet count was made and was normal. An erythromelalgia-like condition has also been attributed to treatment with anticancer and immunosupressant drugs, given singly or in combination (Shall *et al.* 1988; Kampmann *et al.* 1989; Portal *et al.* 1994); bromocriptine (Eisler *et al.* 1981); influenza vaccine (Confino *et al.* 1997); pergolide (Monk *et al.* 1984); and verapamil (Drenth *et al.* 1992).

Drug-induced hypotension

Introduction

Drug-induced hypotension is difficult to categorize clearly and neatly, because the ways in which this adverse reaction may be produced are diverse and more than one mechanism may operate in an individual reaction; and because published reports often provide too little information to enable one to do more than guess at the mechanism or mechanisms involved in the cases described. Furthermore, it is possible that some of the hypotensive reactions that have been attributed to injected drugs were due not to the drugs themselves but to a vasovagal response to anxiety in a nervous patient.

It should be noted that as the number of published reports of drug-induced hypotension is so large, references will not be given when the reaction is now firmly established as a complication of treatment with a widely used drug, but they will be provided when the reaction is considered to be an unusual response to the drug concerned.

Mechanisms

Drug-induced hypotension can be mediated by a fall in cardiac output due to direct myocardial depression or to reduced venous return (caused by either venodilatation or hypovolaemia), by a reduction in peripheral vascular resistance, or by a combination of these effects.

Reduced peripheral vascular resistance and venous dilatation

Hypotension due to reduction in peripheral vascular resistance can result from the effects of drugs on the neurological control of the vascular bed; from a direct effect on blood vessels by either the drug itself or by chemical mediators released by its action; or as a consequence of depletion of substances which normally help to maintain adequate vascular tone.

Antihypertensive drugs

Many antihypertensive drugs have an effect on the neurological control of the blood vessels. Some — the thiazides and hydralazine — appear to act principally by a direct effect on the vascular smooth muscle. The β-adrenoceptor blocking drugs have multiple and complex actions that still have not yet been completely elucidated. Irrespective of the site or sites of their primary action, however, in most cases their final effect is to reduce peripheral vascular resistance; and clearly all drugs with a very potent action of this kind can at times cause an excessive fall in blood pressure that may inconvenience or harm the patient. Such hypotension may occur acutely either during or soon after the giving of a drug or, when related to the posture of the patient, at any time during the period of action of the drug. Hypotension caused by drugs may also be of gradual onset and sustained, but it may still be acutely aggravated by changes in posture in some cases. Whether or not posture precipitates or aggravates drug-induced hypotension depends on the way in which a drug affects the control of peripheral resistance; when vascular reflexes are not greatly impaired then postural hypotension is not to be expected, but when they are lost then postural hypotension may be very severe.

Almost all antihypertensive drugs can at times cause severe hypotension (which may have very serious consequences, particularly in severe or malignant hypertension [*British Medical Journal* 1979]). This occurs most commonly during treatment with those agents that interfere with efferent sympathetic outflow; thus, the adrenergic-neurone blockers (e.g. bethanidine, bretylium, debrisoquine, guanethidine), and α-adrenoceptor blockers (e.g. prazosin) are particularly likely to cause postural hypotension. Most cases of severe postural hypotension caused by prazosin have occurred at the beginning of treatment (Bendall *et al*. 1975; Bloom *et al*. 1975; Committee on Safety of Medicines 1975; Curtis and Bateman 1975; Gabriel *et al*. 1975; Seedat *et al*. 1975; Turner 1976) and appear to be the result of α-blockade (Bateman *et al*. 1979), but tolerance develops rapidly (Graham *et al*. 1976).

This 'first-dose hypotension' is dose related and usually occurs while the patient is standing, most often in those with depletion of extracellular fluid. It is characterized by a sudden change from tachycardia to bradycardia accompanied by a fall in blood pressure severe enough to cause syncope. The mechanism involved is said to be activation of the Bezold–Jarisch cardiovascular depressor reflex (Semple *et al*. 1988).

Other antihypertensive drugs that may have the first-dose effect are the other α-adrenoceptor blockers, indoramin (Gould *et al*. 1981) and terazosin (Sperzel *et al*. 1986); the 5-hydroxytryptamine antagonist ketanserin, which also has some α-blocking activity (Waller *et al*. 1987); angiotensin-converting-enzyme inhibitors (also used for heart failure) (Hodsman *et al*. 1983; Cleland *et al*. 1985; Wieland and Stäubli 1988; Russell and Jones 1989; Mullen 1990; Mets *et al*. 1992; Parish and Miller 1992; Maclean *et al*. 1993; Bagger 1997); nifedipine (Bertel 1987; Wachter 1987; Goswami and Gurtoo 1993; Impey 1993); and some β-adrenoceptor blockers — acebutolol (Tirlapur *et al*. 1986) and atenolol (Kholeif and Isles 1989). The cases described by the latter authors were examples of the hyponatraemic–hypotensive syndrome — malignant hypertension accompanied by hyponatraemia and hyperkalaemia.

The thiazides, methyldopa, hydralazine, clonidine, and the β-adrenoceptor blockers appear to be less likely to cause severe postural hypotension, though clonidine has caused a severe hypotensive reaction when used as a diagnostic test in a patient with phaeochromocytoma (Given *et al*. 1983).

Drugs used for other purposes may also have this effect (see below). Saralasin, a drug given intravenously to detect angiotensin-mediated hypertension, may at times cause severe hypotension (Pettinger and Keeton 1975; Fagard *et al*. 1976) (this drug has also caused a hypertensive crisis in the presence of phaeochromocytoma — see earlier). The α-adrenoceptor blockers benzodioxane and phentolamine were once widely used in tests for suspected phaeochromocytoma, with the object of reducing the blood pressure significantly, though not excessively, if the test proved positive. Unfortunately catastrophic hypotension occurred on occasion (Green and Grimsley 1953; Bierman and Partridge 1951) and was sometimes fatal (Emanuel *et al*. 1956; Roland 1959) and this was one reason why these tests fell into disuse. Haemorrhagic necrosis of phaeochromocytoma has been attributed to the use of such drugs, in particular phentolamine. The mechanism is unknown, but it is suggested that the lowering of the systolic blood pressure may cause the already precarious blood supply within the tumour to become inadequate or, alternatively, that the α-adrenoceptor blockers produce vasodilatation within the tumour, flooding an already necrotic area with blood and initiating a progressive interstitial haemorrhage within the tumour, ending in either haemorrhagic necrosis of the whole tumour or rupture of the capsule with retroperitoneal haematoma formation (Van Way *et al*. 1976).

Vasodilator drugs

Although all those antihypertensive drugs that reduce peripheral resistance could reasonably be called 'vasodilators', this term is more usually used for drugs commonly used for vasospastic disorders, such as Raynaud's phenomenon; for angina pectoris (see below); or (less rationally) for peripheral ischaemia caused by atheromatous narrowing of arteries. Some of these drugs act purely as α-adrenoceptor blocking agents; some act directly on vascular smooth muscle; a few have both these effects; and others enhance β-adrenergic activity. Many drugs of this kind (which include thymoxamine, tolazoline, azapetine, inositol nicotinate, bemethan, kallidinogenase, nicotinyl tartate, isoxsuprine, and glyceryl trinitrate — including the ointment [van Reempts and Van Overmaire 1990]) may occasionally cause significant hypotension.

It is worth emphasizing that it is now accepted that glyceryl trinitrate, still regarded by some as a specific 'coronary artery vasodilator', produces its beneficial effect mainly by dilating the peripheral veins, causing an acute fall in venous return, a fall in cardiac output (reducing the cardiac workload), and systemic hypotension; first-dose hypotension (described earlier) has also been caused by this and other vasodilator organic nitrates (Semple *et al*. 1988). This hypotensive effect does not, however, usually cause symptoms unless aggravated by the hypotensive effect of a drug given concurrently. Thus, one of our patients who had been under treatment with glyceryl trinitrate for several years without any ill effect developed syncopal attacks that were attributed to epilepsy of late onset until it was realized that attacks had coincided with the taking of a glyceryl trinitrate tablet and had begun when the patient had started treatment with chlorpromazine (which also has a hypotensive effect), given for anxiety. A synergistic action of this kind may also be encountered when other combinations of drugs with hypotensive effects are used.

Vancomycin and erythromycin

Among the antibiotics, vancomycin appears to have a peculiar propensity to cause hypotension, sometimes severe, when given by intravenous infusion. When patients undergoing cardiac surgery were given either cefazolin alone or combined with vancomycin during or after operation, 50 per cent of those given vancomycin (at an infusion rate three times higher than recommended by the manufacturer) in addition to cefazolin, developed severe hypotension compared with just over 14 per cent of those given cefazolin alone (Romanelli *et al.* 1993). This reaction is more likely when the infusion solution is too concentrated or administered too quickly, and it appears to be due to histamine release (Newfield and Roizen 1979), direct myocardial depression (Cohen *et al.* 1970), peripheral vasodilatation (Cohen *et al.* 1970), or a combination of these effects. Histamine release is probably responsible for the erythematous rash that has been an early feature of some of these cases (Lacouture *et al.* 1987; Best *et al.* 1989).

Fatal cardiac arrest has also followed intravenous administration of vancomycin in a 2-year-old girl after an operation (Mayhew and Deutsch 1985).

In rare instances, erythromycin, given orally or intravenously, has caused hypotension (Dan and Fiegl 1993; Brown 1995).

Verapamil

A number of cases of hypotension caused by verapamil have been reported, and several studies have shown that the fall in blood pressure can be prevented by pretreatment with calcium salts (Jameson and Hargarten 1992; Kuhn and Schriger 1992) or reversed by these salts after it has occurred (Lee and Cohan 1995). Patients with arrhythmias other than atrial fibrillation and with a low pretreatment systolic blood pressure appear to be at the greatest risk of this complication (Burke *et al.* 1993).

Endogenous vasodilator substances

Acute hypotension is one of the features of anaphylactic and anaphylactic-like reactions induced by drugs, when it is due to the effect on the blood vessels of one or more of a number of mediators, including histamine (see Chapter 27). Some drugs (e.g. dextrans, opiates) release histamine by a non-immunological mechanism, and such an action may be responsible for the hypotension that sometimes complicates the administration of radiographic contrast media (see Chapters 27 and 28).

Drugs used during anaesthesia

Almost all intravenously administered inducing agents and anaesthetic gases may cause hypotension by depressing the vasomotor centre. Some neuromuscular blocking agents can also cause a fall in blood pressure — probably by reducing venous return. Hypotension is a well-recognized feature of spinal or epidural anaesthesia.

Hypotension is a well-recognized hazard of general anaesthesia in patients taking MAOI, and for this reason it is usually recommended that the drug be stopped for a period before operation, and some have believed 2 weeks to be adequate. However, Sprung and others (1996) have reported a case in which severe hypotension occurred during operation even though treatment with the MAOI tranylcypromine had been discontinued 20 days before surgery.

Sedatives, tranquillizers, and antipsychotics

Many of these drugs can cause a fall in blood pressure, principally by an action on the vasomotor centre. When these drugs are given by mouth in normal therapeutic doses, the hypotensive response is minimal and usually of little clinical significance (though a case of very severe orthostatic hypotension has occurred after 5 days of treatment with clozapine [Bredbacka *et al.* 1993], and thioridazine has also caused hypotension in an elderly patient [Cowen and Meythaler 1994]), but when administered by intravenous (or even intramuscular) injection the hypotensive effect is greater and can be severe if the injection is given too rapidly; chlorpromazine is particularly hazardous in this respect. This effect can be particularly pronounced in the elderly in whom cardiovascular reflex control may already be compromised. Great care should be taken with dosage. Clozapine-induced hypotension has been successfully treated, without stopping the drug, by giving moclobemide and the meat extract Bovril (Taylor *et al.* 1995) or fludrocortisone (Testani 1994) concurrently.

Antidepressants

Antidepressants of the MAOI group or the tricyclic group may cause significant hypotension, particularly related to posture, in some patients. The mechanisms involved are complex and incompletely understood, but a decrease in peripheral vascular resistance, principally due to an effect on the vasomotor centre, is probably involved to some degree. In one remarkable case (Ferguson 1994) the tricyclic drug imipramine induced severe hypotension and cardiogenic shock in a patient with a phaeochromocytoma, instead of the hypertensive crisis that would be expected (see Table 9.2). Constantino and others (1993) made the interesting observation that patients unable to tolerate tricyclic antidepressants because of orthostatic hypotension, were able to do so after they had received electroconvulsive therapy, and suggested that a drug–disease interaction might be a significant factor in tricyclic-induced hypotension.

Opiates

These drugs can reduce blood pressure by inducing histamine release, reduced sympathetic drive, and vagal stimulation; the result of these effects is usually not clinically significant, but codeine phosphate is well known to cause severe hypotension if given intravenously to children, and Parke and others (1992) have reported three cases of life-threatening hypotension in adults given the drug by this route, while Chambers and Baggoley (1992) described the same complication, fatal in two cases, in elderly patients treated with morphine (7–15 mg), with or without frusemide, for acute pulmonary oedema, and advise caution with dosage when giving the drug before admission to hospital.

Oxytocin

Oxytocin is known to have a hypotensive effect, but usually this is mild and not clinically significant. Bolus injections, however, have caused a precipitous fall in blood pressure (*Journal of the American Medical Association* 1974).

Levodopa

Paradoxically, levodopa, a precursor of noradrenaline, is a well-recognized cause of troublesome postural hypotension (Calne *et al.* 1970; Hoehn 1975). It has been suggested that this effect is due to its breakdown to dopamine which is taken up by nerve endings and then released 'diluting' the effect of noradrenaline released concurrently (Burn 1970), and this hypothesis led to the use of propranolol to prevent levodopa-induced postural hypotension with the object of antagonizing the effect of the dopamine on peripheral resistance vessels, a treatment claimed to have been successful (Duvoison 1970). Shanks (1970) disputed these theories, however, and neither the reaction nor the prophylactic effect of propranolol can be said to have been satisfactorily explained.

Diuretics

Loop diuretics, such as frusemide, may induce first-dose hypotension, discussed above, when given intravenously (Semple *et al.* 1988).

Prostaglandins

Dinoprost (prostaglandin $F_{2\alpha}$) and dinoprostone (prostaglandin E_2), prostaglandins used in obstetrics, have caused alarming, and sometimes fatal hypotension when injected into the myometrium (Douglas *et al.* 1989; Kilpatrick and Thorburn 1990; Marcus *et al.* 1997), extra-amniotically (Wein *et al.* 1989), or into the uterine cavity (Partridge *et al.* 1988). Such events may also be due to the first-dose effect (Semple *et al.* 1988).

Hypotension in peripheral neuropathy

Hypotension, particularly postural hypotension, may complicate drug-induced polyneuropathy, probably due to impairment of neurological control of peripheral vascular resistance and, when there is muscular paralysis, a fall in venous return.

Hypovolaemia

Hypovolaemia occurs in acute haemorrhage induced by drugs. It also complicates iatrogenic sodium and water depletion caused by diuretics, and is a feature of acute adrenal insufficiency which may occur in patients during adrenal corticosteroid therapy or following withdrawal of such therapy; during treatment with aminoglutethimide and metyrapone; or, very rarely, as a result of haemorrhage into the adrenals in patients taking anticoagulants (see Chapter 15). Hypovolaemia is also the mechanism by which hypotension is produced in drug-induced ketoacidosis and lactic acidosis (see Chapter 16).

Mixed or obscure mechanisms

A large number of isolated reports have attributed hypotensive reactions to a wide variety of drugs, particularly when given parenterally. The pharmacological mechanisms involved are at the moment incompletely understood. The drugs involved are listed in Table 9.4.

Drug interactions causing hypotension

Severe hypotension has occurred in patients taking enalapril when clozapine was given concurrently (Aronowitz *et al.* 1994), when patients under treatment with enalapril were given stable plasma protein solution (McKenzie 1990; Young, 1990), and pergolide was taken concurrently with lisinopril (Kando *et al.* 1990).

TABLE 9.4
*Drugs (other than those discussed in the text) reported
to have caused hypotension*

Acetylcholine (intraocular injection)	Erickson and Yousuf 1991
Acrylic bone cement	Newens and Volz 1972; Peebles *et al.* 1972; *The Lancet* 1974
Aprotinin	Böhrer *et al.* 1990
Atropine and propanidid	Clarke 1969
BCG injections (intralesional in melanoma)	Cohen *et al.* 1991
Bromocriptine	Linch *et al.* 1978
Cimetidine	Mahon and Kolton 1978
Deferrioxamine (intravenously)	Bentur *et al.* 1991
Disulfiram with general anaesthesia	Diaz and Hill 1979
Dobutamine (stress electrocardiography)	Marcovitz *et al.* 1993
Doxacuronium chloride	Reich 1989
Ethamsylate	Watson 1972; Langdon 1977
Etoposide	Cerosimo *et al.* 1989; Tester *et al.* 1990
Fibrinolytics (alteplase, anistreplase, streptokinase)	Brenot *et al.* 1991; Tisdale *et al.* 1992
Indigo carmine (prostatectomy)	Shir and Raja 1993
Interferon alpha-2a (intravenously)	Hanson and Leggette 1997
Interleukin-2	Lissoni *et al.* 1990
Interleukin-2 with interferon alfa 2b	Allaouchiche *et al.* 1990
Iodised oil (lymphography)	Lossef and Barth 1993
Iopamidol (CT scan)	Lucas *et al.* 1992
Lignocaine (retrobulbar block)	Cardan *et al.* 1987
Metoclopramide	Park 1978; Pegg 1980
Muromonab-CT3	Turner and Holman 1993
Netilmicin (slow intravenous infusion)	Rygnestad 1997
Pentagastrin	McCloy and Baron 1977
Pentamidine	Western *et al.* 1976; Siddiqui and Ford 1995
Phenoperidine with propranolol	Woods 1978
Podophyllin	Montaldi *et al.* 1974
Protamine sulphate	Fadali *et al.* 1974; Weiss *et al.* 1990
Salbutamol	Ng and Sen 1974
Simvastatin	French and White 1989
Soap enema	Egdell and Johnson 1973
Terbutaline (subcutaneous) (in patients with autonomic dysfunction)	Pingleton *et al.* 1982
Teniposide	McLeod *et al.* 1991
Thiothixene	Burnett *et al.* 1975
Trazodone	Spivak *et al.* 1987
Viloxazine	Pinder *et al.* 1977
Vitamin K_1	Loeliger 1975
Zidovudine	Loke *et al.* 1990

Aortic dissection and aneurysm

The need for accuracy in the diagnosis of acute myocardial infarction before employing thrombolytic therapy has been stressed by Curzen and others (1990) and Butler and colleagues (1990), who have reported cases in which extension of aortic dissection was attributed to streptokinase given for presumed myocardial infarction.

Very prolonged treatment (15–20 years) with adrenal corticosteroids was suspected as the cause of abdominal aortic aneurysm in five women, aged between 43 and 75 years (Sato *et al.* 1995).

Thromboembolic disease

Members of several different therapeutic groups of drugs have been recognized as causes of thromboembolic disease. In some cases, genetic abnormalities of haemostatic mechanisms appear to have predisposed affected patients to this complication; in others, acquired immunological disturbances seem to have played a part (see below).

Oral contraceptives

It is now well established that women taking oral contraceptives are more at risk of venous thrombosis than are women who do not take these drugs, and the same is true of those given an oestrogen alone or in combination with a progestogen as hormone replacement therapy (Committee on Safety of Medicines 1996) or for some other purpose (Werder *et al.* 1990). Some affected patients have been found to have deficiencies of clotting-inhibitor factors: protein C (Girolami *et al.* 1992; Roger *et al.* 1992), protein S (Villa *et al.* 1996), or antithrombin III (Girolami *et al.* 1993); and cases have been reported in which antiphospholipid antibodies were detected (Girolami *et al.* 1996).

In a case of venous thrombosis in which the patient was taking a combination of cyproterone and ethinyloestradiol, antibodies to cyproterone were found and were believed to have played some part in inducing the condition (Leroy *et al.* 1990). Other abnormalities relating to blood coagulation have been investigated by Bokarewa and others (1995). As far as oral contraceptives are concerned, the risk of their causing thromboembolic disease appears to be increased by cigarette smoking, obesity, and a past or family history of thromboembolism.

The commonest sites for thrombosis are the veins of the lower legs, and the disorder may remain localized, ascend to involve other veins, including the vena cava, portal vein, and renal veins, or may give rise to emboli that may lodge in branches of the pulmonary artery or (in the rare case of paradoxical embolism) pass through an atrial or ventricular septal defect to reach a systemic artery. Thrombi may also form within arteries, leading to intermittent claudication (van Vroonhoven 1977), or cerebral, coronary, or mesenteric thrombosis.

Heparin and other antithrombotic drugs

Paradoxically, when heparin is used for preventing or treating thromboembolism it may sometimes cause venous or arterial thrombus formation as part of the 'thrombocytopenia and thrombosis' syndrome. First observed in animals (Copley and Robb 1942; Fidlar and Jaques 1948; Quick et al. 1948), it was subsequently recognized in human patients (Rhodes et al. 1973) and soon confirmed by a large number of case reports too numerous to list here. At least two types of heparin-induced thrombocytopenia have been described (Barber et al. 1987). One is common (incidence perhaps as high as 30 per cent), mild, of rapid onset (2nd–4th day), is not usually associated with haemorrhage or thrombosis, and therefore unlikely to be fatal, and is thought to be due to temporary sequestration of platelets (Gollub and Ulin 1962). Another is more severe; of delayed onset (7th–10th day), unless the patient has received heparin previously, in which case it may occur earlier; is accompanied by recurrent thrombotic episodes, with a mortality as high as 29 per cent (Barber et al. 1987); and appears to be associated with a heparin-dependent IgG antibody that is not directed against heparin but which induces synthesis of thromboxane and aggregation of platelets (Chong et al. 1982; Sandler et al. 1985). In both forms thrombocytopenia persists for as long as heparin is continued, but in the severe form thrombotic episodes may occur for a while after the platelet count has returned to normal. Treatments that have been suggested (in addition to withholding heparin) are oral anticoagulants or aspirin with dipyridamole (Kelton and Hirch 1980; Silver et al. 1983); danaparoid (Boon et al. 1994); immunoglobulin G (Prull et al. 1992); or streptokinase, sometimes in very low doses (Ferrari et al. 1996) by intravenous or intra-arterial injection (Fiessinger et al. 1984). Transfusions of platelet concentrate have failed to raise the platelet count to normal (Babcock et al. 1976).

Thrombosis associated with heparin therapy in the presence of a normal platelet count was studied by Hach-Wunderle and others (1994). In five affected patients, platelet-activating autoantibodies directed against heparin were detected (cf. findings of Chong and others — see above). After heparin was withheld and anticoagulation was continued using the heparinoid Orgaran

(after negative tests for heparin autoantibody cross-reactivity), there were no further thromboses, and in three of the patients the platelet count rose, suggesting that the 'normal' platelet count during heparin therapy had, in fact, been a relative thrombocytopenia.

Thrombosis with thrombocytopenia has also been attributed to the antiemetic drug ondansetron (see below under Anticancer drugs and immunosuppressants).

Thrombolytic therapy for acute myocardial infarction, with such drugs as streptokinase, anistreplase, and alteplase, carries the risk of disintegration of pre-existing clot with consequent embolization, sometimes recurrent (Yasaka et al. 1994), but Stafford and others (1989), who have reported such complications, concluded that the risks are outweighed by the potential benefits, a view with which some others concur (*Drug and Therapeutics Bulletin* 1990).

These drugs have also been responsible for cholesterol-crystal embolism, which appears to arise from atherosclerotic lesions in the aorta or other large arteries when the soft lipid cores become exposed and crystals of cholesterol break off and enter the circulation. A clue to the nature of the emboli is provided by livedo reticularis which appears in some of the cases, and widespread ecchymoses are also seen occasionally. The organs and tissue affected depend on the site of the atheromatous plaque from which the crystals originate. In some reported cases the diagnosis has been confirmed by biopsy or postmortem examination (Queen et al. 1990; Beutler et al. 1991; Dupin et al. 1992; Mendia et al. 1992; Gupta et al. 1993; Pochmaliki et al. 1993; Balestra et al. 1994; Ben-Chitrit et al. 1994; Diethelm et al. 1994; Aggarwal and Tjahja 1996; Blankenship 1996). By comparison, cholesterol embolism caused by the combination of heparin and a coumarin anticoagulant appears to be rare (Caux et al. 1991).

A most unusual type of embolism is that caused by oxygen, in one case released from hydrogen peroxide used to irrigate an open hemithorax following pulmonary lobectomy (Konrad et al. 1997).

Other substances forming emboli are discussed in Chapter 10.

Antituberculous therapy — rifampicin

A retrospective study comparing 7542 tuberculous patients with 252 controls with non-tuberculous lung abscesses was undertaken to determine whether there is an association between antituberculous therapy and venous thrombosis (White 1989). A significantly greater number of the patients given rifampicin (2.7 per cent of 4391) than of patients not having the drug (0.5 per cent), or controls (0.4 per cent) developed venous thrombosis.

The relative risk of venous thrombosis in patients treated with rifampicin was estimated to be 4.74, but the author concluded that the benefit of the drug in this disease outweighs its risks. He suggests that concurrent low-dose heparin therapy might be a useful prophylactic against this complication.

Anticancer drugs and immunosuppressants

Venous thrombosis is a not infrequent complication of treatment with anticancer drugs either given singly (fluorouracil — Gradishar *et al.* 1991; tamoxifen — Desmukh *et al.* 1995; McDonald *et al.* 1995; Weitz *et al.* 1997) or in combinations (Hall *et al.* 1988; Levine *et al.* 1988; Milne *et al.* 1988; Castaman *et al.* 1990; Clarke *et al.* 1990; Durand *et al.* 1993; Theodossiou *et al.* 1994; Cutuli *et al.* 1995; Williams and Foster 1995; Pritchard *et al.* 1996), and include the retinoids when used for promyelocytic leukaemia (Runde *et al.* 1991; Forjas De Lacerdo *et al.* 1993; Marinakis *et al.* 1993), interferon alfa given for hairy cell leukaemia, and interferons alfa and gamma used to treat chronic myeloid leukaemia or multiple myeloma (Reid *et al.* 1992). Some of these drugs have also been blamed for arterial occlusion, sometimes leading to gangrene (Garstin *et al.* 1990; Conti and Scher 1992; Fertakos and Mintzer 1992; Molloy *et al.* 1995; Mathews *et al.* 1997). In a retrospective review of thrombosis accompanied by thrombocytopenia in patients who had received anticancer drugs, it was found that this complication had occurred only in those who had also been given the antiemetic drug ondansetron concurrently (Coates *et al.* 1992).

Immunosuppressive therapy has also been associated with both venous and arterial thrombosis in recipients of kidney or heart transplants, sometimes in the grafts themselves and sometimes elsewhere. The drugs involved were combinations of cyclosporin with prednisone (Marti *et al.* 1991; Kronenberg *et al.* 1993), and cyclosporin with azathioprine and prednisone (Kronenberg *et al.* 1993), the latter combination being more thrombogenic than the former and the incidence being greater in diabetics and increasing with age in non-diabetics; and muromonab–CT3 (OKT3) alone (Abramowicz *et al.* 1992; Gomez *et al.* 1992) or combined with high-dose methyl prednisolone (Abramowicz *et al.* 1994).

ACE inhibitors

A case of renal artery thrombosis following enalapril in a patient with atheroma of the artery has been reported (Main and Wilkinson 1989); in another case, thrombosis occurred in the renal artery supplying a transplanted kidney, when the patient was given captopril for renovascular hypertension (Dussol *et al.* 1994).

Other drugs

Other drugs suspected of having caused venous or arterial thrombosis include carbamazepine (Komori *et al.* 1994), dihydroergotamine (Iaquinto *et al.*1991), diuretics (Green *et al.* 1988), erythropoietin (Aunsholt *et al.* 1992; Taylor *et al.* 1992), factor VIIa (Schulman *et al.* 1991), filgastrim (Kawachi *et al.* 1996), foscarnet (Calligaro *et al.* 1994), paroxetine with zotepine (Pantel *et al.* 1997), ovarian stimulants (Kligman *et al.* 1993), vasopressin (Hod *et al.* 1992), and X-ray contrast media (Esplugas *et al.* 1993). In one case involving high-dose corticosteroids, antiphospholipid antibodies were detected in the patient's blood (Davies and Triplett 1990). Thromboembolism arising from thrombosis of varicose veins induced by sclerosant therapy appears to be very rare, but a suspected case in which the sclerosant polidocanol was used has been reported (*SADRAC Bulletin* 1997).

Vascular leak syndrome

This disorder is a common adverse effect of the antineoplastic drug aldesleukin (recombinant interleukin-2). It appears to result from capillary damage, though the precise mechanism is as yet uncertain. It is characterized by peripheral oedema, sometimes accompanied by ascites, pleural effusion, and pulmonary oedema; and hypotension, impaired renal function, oliguria, and respiratory failure may ensue (Siegel and Puri 1991; Vial and Descoles 1992).

Thrombotic thrombocytopenic purpura

This rare disease is characterized pathologically by obstruction of the microcirculation by clumps of platelets, accompanied by haemolytic anaemia and thrombocytopenia in the peripheral blood. Thrombosis in major blood vessels is rarely if ever found. Clinical features include fever, neurological damage and psychiatric disturbances, renal failure, and purpura, sometimes with severe haemorrhage in the gastrointestinal tract and elsewhere.

In most cases the aetiology is unknown but in a few an adverse drug reaction has been suspected as the cause. The drugs involved are cyclosporin (Dzick *et al.* 1987), the antithrombotic agent defibrotide (Perotti *et al.* 1995), the H$_2$-receptor antagonist famotidine (Kallal and Lee

1996), levonorgestrel contraceptive implants (Frazer *et al.* 1996), and the antiplatelet drug ticlopidine (Page *et al.* 1991; Ellie *et al.* 1992).

Vasculitis

Arteritis

Inflammatory changes in arteries may occur as a result of an adverse reaction to a drug, and although such changes are usually considered to be manifestations of a hypersensitivity reaction this has not been established beyond doubt. The subject is discussed in more detail in Chapter 27.

Polyarteritis nodosa

The aetiology of the naturally occurring disease is unknown, but a seemingly identical condition has sometimes been attributed to an adverse drug reaction involving an immunological mechanism. The subject is discussed in Chapter 27.

Phlebitis

Inflammatory changes in veins may be produced by drugs injected intravenously, or may be part of a widespread reaction of which arteritis may also be a feature; and an interesting case has been described in which phlebitis initially caused by an injection of diazepam recurred when the patient was later treated with penicillamine given orally (Brandstetter *et al.* 1981).

Cutaneous vasculitis

Lesions resulting from this disorder are described in Chapter 19.

Types of reactions

Of the adverse reactions affecting the peripheral vascular system, almost all of those in which the mechanism is known or suspected appear to be of Type A, though the reactions to intravenous radiographic contrast media and anaphylactic reactions are of Type B (see Chapter 5).

References

Aabo, K. and De Coster, R. (1987). Hypertension during high-dose ketoconazole treatment: a probable mineralocorticoid effect. *Lancet* ii, 637.

Abate, M.A., Neely, J.L., Layne, R.D., *et al.* (1991). Interaction of indomethacin and sulindac with labetalol. *Br. J. Clin. Pharmacol.* 31, 363.

Abramowicz, D., Pradier, O., Marchant, A., *et al.* (1992). Induction of thromboses within renal grafts by high-dose prophylactic CD3. *Lancet* 339, 777.

Abramowicz, D., Pradier, O., De Pauw, L., *et al.* (1994). High dose glucocorticosteroids increase the procoagulant effects of OKT3. *Kidney Int.* 46, 1596.

Adelman, M.H., Jacobson, E., Lief, A., *et al.* (1959). Promethazine hydrochloride in surgery and obstetrics. *JAMA* 169, 73.

Agabiti-Rosei, E., Alicandri, C.L., and Corea, L. (1977). Hypertensive crisis in patients with phaeochromocytoma given metoclopramide. *Lancet* i, 600.

Agabiti-Rosei, E., Brown, J.J., Lever, A.F., *et al.* (1976). Treatment of phaeochromocytoma and of clonidine withdrawal with labetalol. *Br. J. Clin. Pharmacol.* 3 (suppl. 3), 809.

Aggarwal, K. and Tjahja, I.E. (1996). Atheroembolic disease following administration of tissue plasminogen activator (TPA). *Clin. Cardiol.* 19, 906.

Ahmad, S. (1991). Indomethacin–enalapril interaction: an alert. *South. Med. J.* 84, 411.

Alam, M., Anrep, G.V., Barsoum, G.S., *et al.* (1939). Liberation of histamine from the skeletal muscle. *J. Physiol.* (Lond.) 95,148.

Alexander, C.S., Sako, Y., and Mikulic, E. (1975). Pedal gangrene associated with the use of dopamine. *N. Engl. J. Med.* 293, 591.

Allain, H. Maruelle, L., Beneton, C., *et al.* (1996). Acute episodes of high blood pressure induced by tacrine. *Presse Méd.* 25, 1388.

Allaouchiche, B., Mercatello, A., Tognet, E., *et al.* (1990). Prospective effects of norepinephrine infusion in acute renal failure induced by interleukin-2 therapy. *Nephron* 55, 438.

Ameli, F.M., Nathanson, M., and Elkan, I. (1977). Methysergide therapy causing vascular insufficiency of the upper limb. *Can. J. Surg.* 20, 158.

Amery, A. and Deloof, W. (1970). Cheese reaction during debrisoquine treatment. *Lancet* ii, 613.

Anderson, J.R. and Johnston, G.W. (1983). Development of cutaneous gangrene during continuous peripheral infusion of vasopressin. *BMJ* 287, 1657.

Anderson, L.B., Thestrup-Pedersen, K., and Sell, A. (1988). Nifedipine treatment of Raynaud's phenomenon secondary to chemotherapy. *Dermatologica* 177, 19.

Anderson, R.P. and Morris B.A.P. (1988). Acrocyanosis due to imipramine. *Arch. Dis. Child.* 63, 204.

Ansell, G. (1970). Adverse reactions to contrast agents; scope of problem. *Invest. Radiol.* 5, 374.

Aronowitz, J.S., Chakos, M.H., Safferman, A.Z., *et al.* (1994). Syncope associated with the combination of clozapine and enalapril. *J. Clin. Psychopharmacol.* 14, 429.

Arslan, M.. Ozyillkan, E., Kayhan, B., *et al.* (1994). Raynaud's phenomenon associated with alpha-interferon therapy. *J. Intern. Med.* 235, 503.

Asatoor, A.M., Levi, A.J., and Milne, M.D. (1963). Tranylcypromine and cheese. *Lancet* ii, 733.

Atasoy, H., Erdem, G. Ceyhan, M., *et al.* (1995). Hypertension associated with ciprofloxacin use in an infant. *Ann. Pharmacother.* 29, 2049.

Athos, W.J., McHugh, B.P., Fineberg, S.E., *et al.* (1962). The effect of guanethidine on the adrenal medulla. *J. Pharmacol. Exp. Ther.* 137, 229.

Aunsholt, N.A., Ahibom, G., Steffenson, G., *et al.* (1992). Fibrinolytic capacity in haemodialysis patients treated with recombinant human eythropoetin. *Nephron* 62, 284.

Babcock, R.B., Dumper, C.W., and Scharfman, W.B. (1976). Heparin-induced immune thrombocytopenia. *N. Engl. J. Med.* 295, 237.

Bachmeyer, C., Farge, D., Gluckman, E., *et al.* (1996). Raynaud's phenomenon and digital necrosis induced hy interferon-alpha. *Br. J. Dermatol.* 135, 481.

Bacourt, F. and Couffinhal, J.H.C. (1978). Ischémie des membres par association déhydroergotamine triacétyloléandomycine. Nouvelle observation. *Nouv. Presse Méd.* 7, 1561.

Bagger, J.P. (1997). Adverse event with first-dose perindopril in congestive heart failure. *Lancet* 349, 1671.

Bailey, R.R. and Neale, T.J. (1976). Rapid clonidine withdrawal with blood pressure overshoot exaggerated by beta-blockade. *BMJ* i, 943.

Balestra, B., Radaelli, A., and Noseda, G. (1994). Cholesterol embolism: a heavy price to pay after fibrinolysis. *Schweiz. Med. Wochenschr.* 124, 2046.

Baraka, A., Nauphal, M., and Arab, W. (1992). Cimetidine-dobutamine interaction? *Anaesthesia* 47, 965.

Barar, F.S.K., Boakes, A.J., Benedikter, L.B., *et al.* (1971). Interactions between catecholamines and tricyclic and monoamine oxidase inhibitor antidepressive agents in man. *Br. J. Pharmacol.* 43, 472P.

Barber, F.A., Burton, W.C., and Guyer, R. (1987). The heparin-induced thrombocytopenia and thrombosis syndrome. Report of a case. *J. Bone Joint Surg.* 68-A, 935.

Bateman, D.N., Hobbs, D.C., Twomey, T.M. *et al.* (1979). Prazosin, pharmokinetics and concentration effect. *Eur. J. Clin. Pharmacol.* 16, 177.

Bedford, N.M. and Lockey, D.J. (1995). Raynaud's syndrome following intravenous induction of anaesthesia. *Anaesthesia* 50, 248.

Bell, C., Coupland. M., and Creamer, P. (1996). Digital infarction in a patient with Raynaud's phenomenon associated with treatment with a specific serotonin receptor inhibitor: a case report. *Angiology* 47, 901.

Ben-Chitrit, S., Korzets, Z., Hershkovitz, R., *et al.* (1994). Cholesterol embolisation syndrome following thrombolytic therapy with streptokinase and tissue plasminogen activator. *Nephrol. Dial. Transplant.* 9, 428.

Ben-Noun, L. (1991). Unresponsiveness to nifedipine treatment. *Ann. Pharmacother.* 75, 99.

Bendall, M.J., Baloch, K.H., and Wilson, P.R. (1975). Side effects due to treatment of hypertension with prazosin. *BMJ* ii, 727.

Bentur, Y., McGuigan, M., and Koren, G. (1991). Deferoxamine (desferrioxamine): new toxicities for an old drug. *Drug Safety* 6, 37.

Berg, K.J., Forre, O., Bjerkhoel, F., *et al.* (1986). Side-effects of cyclosporin A treatment in patients with rheumatoid arthritis. *Kidney Int.* 29, 1180.

Bertel, O. (1987). Symptomatic hypotension induced by nifedipine. *Arch. Intern. Med.* 147, 1683.

Best, C.J., Ewart, M., and Summer, E. (1989). Perioperative complications following the use of vancomycin in children: a report of two cases. *Br. J. Anaesth.* 62, 576.

Beutler, J.J., Sulzer, H.A., and van Straten, R. (1991). Cholesterol embolism after intravenous anisoylated plasminogen-streptokinase activator complex. *Neth. J. Med.* 39, 373.

Bierman, H.R. and Partridge, J.W. (1951). Untoward reactions to tests for epinephrine-secreting tumours (pheochromocytoma). *N. Engl. J. Med.* 244, 582.

Bittar, D.A. (1979). Innovar-induced hypertensive crisis in patients with pheochromocytoma. *Anesthesiology* 50, 366.

Bixby, E.W. and Troncelliti, M.V. (1952). Anesthesia in operation for pheochromocytoma (abstract from correspondence). *JAMA* 148, 1443.

Blackwell, B. (1963). Tranylcypromine. *Lancet* ii, 414.

Blackwell, B., Marley, E., and Mabbit, L.A. (1965). Effects of yeast extract after monoamine oxidase inhibitors. *Lancet* i, 940.

Blankenship, J.C. (1996). Cholesterol embolisation after thrombolytic therapy. *Drug Safety* 14, 78.

Blomley, D.J. (1964). Monoamine oxidase inhibitors. *Lancet* ii, 1181.

Bloom, D.S., Rosendorff, C., and Kramer, R. (1975). Clinical evaluation of prazosin as the sole agent for the treatment of hypertension. A double-blind cross-over study with methyldopa. *Curr. Ther. Res.* 18, 144.

Blum, I., Atsmon, A., Steiner, M., *et al.* (1975). Paradoxical rise in blood pressure during propranolol treatment. *BMJ* iv, 623.

Böhrer, H., Bach, A., Fleischer, F., *et al.* (1990). Adverse haemodynamic effects of high-dose aprotinin in a paediatric cardiac patient. *Anaesthesia* 45, 853.

Bokarewa, H.I., Falk, G., Sten-Linder, H., *et al.* (1995). Thrombotic risk factors and oral contraceptives. *J. Lab. Clin. Med.* 126, 294.

Boon, D.M.S., Michiels, J.J., Stibbe, J., *et al.* (1994). Heparin-induced thrombocytopenia and antithrombotic therapy. *Lancet* 344, 1296.

Borromeo-McGrail, V., Bordiuk, J.M., and Keitel, H. (1973). Systemic hypertension following ocular administration of 10% phenylephrine in the neonate. *Pediatrics* 51, 1032.

Bounameaux, H., Schneider, P.A., Huber-Sauteur, E., *et al.* (1990). Severe ischaemia of the hand following intra-arterial promazine injection: effects of vasodilatation, anticoagulation, and local thrombolysis with tissue-type plasminogen activator. *Vasa* 19, 68.

Brandstetter, R.D., Gotz, V.P., Mar, D.D., *et al.* (1981). Exacerbation of diazepam-induced phlebitis by oral penicillamine. *BMJ* 283, 525.

Bravo, E.L., Tarazi, R.C., Fouad, F.M. *et al.* (1981). Clonidine-suppression test. A useful aid in the diagnosis of pheochromocytoma. *N. Engl. J. Med.* 305, 623.

Bredbacka, P-E., Paukkala, E., Kinnunen, E., *et al.* (1993). Can severe cardiorespiratory dysfunction induced by clozapine be predicted? *Int. Clin. Psychopharmacol.* 8, 205.

Brenot, F., Pacouret, G., Meyer, G., *et al.* (1991). Adverse reactions with anistreplase. *Lancet* 338, 114.

Briggs, R.S.J., Birtwell, A.J., and Pohl, J.E.F. (1978). Hypertensive response to labetalol in phaeochromocytoma. *Lancet* i, 1045.

British Medical Journal (1979). Dangerous antihypertension treatment. *BMJ* ii, 228.

British National Formulary No. 33. (1997). List of drug interactions. British Medical Association and Royal Pharmaceutical Society of Great Britain, London.

Brodmerkel, G.J. Jr (1983). Nifedipine and erythromelalgia. *Ann. Intern. Med.* 99, 415.

Broughan, T.A., Kottke-Marchantt, K., and Vogt, D.P. (1996). The white clot syndrome in hepatic transplantation. *Transplantation* 61, 982.

Brown, A.L., Wilkinson, R., Thomas, T.H., *et al.* (1993). The effect of short-term low-dose cyclosporin on renal function and blood pressure in patients with psoriasis. *Br. J. Dermatol.* 128, 550.

Brown, A.S. (1969). Pentazocine, a potent analgesic: evaluation for anaesthetic use. *Proc. R. Soc. Med.* 62, 805.

Brown, G.R. (1995). Erythromycin-induced hypotension. *Ann. Pharmacother.* 29, 934.

Brown, J.J., Robertson, A.S., Agabiti-Rosei, E., *et al.* (1976). Emergency treatment of hypertensive crisis following clonidine withdrawal. *BMJ* i, 1341.

Brown, J.R. and Kulkarni, M.V. (1967). A review of the toxicity and metabolism of mercury and its compounds. *Med. Serv. J. Can.* 23, 786.

Brown, M.J., Lewis, P.J., and Dollery, C.T. (1980). Diagnosis of small phaeochromocytomas. *Lancet* i, 1185.

Browning, D.J. (1974). Serious side effects of ergometrine and its use in routine obstetric practice. *Med. J. Aust.* 1, 957.

Buckley, M. and Feely, J. (1991). Antagonism of antihypertensive effect of guanfacine by tricyclic antidepressants. *Lancet* 337, 1173.

Burden, A.X.C. and Alexander, C.P.T. (1976). Hypertension after acute methyldopa withdrawal. *BMJ* i, 1056.

Burke, C.M., Theodore, J., Baldwin, J.C., *et al.* (1986). Twenty-eight cases of human heart-lung transplantation. *Lancet* i, 517.

Burke, T.G., Garaets, D.R., and Ferguson, D.W. (1993). Hypotension associated with intravenous verapamil administration for urgent therapy of arrhythmias. *Pharmacotherapy* 13, 269.

Burn, J.H. (1970). Hypotension caused by L-dopa. *BMJ* i, 629.

Burn, J.H. and Dale H.H. (1926). The vasodilator action of histamine and its physiological significance. *J. Physiol.* (Lond.) 61, 185.

Burn, J.H., Leach, E.H., Rand, M.J., *et al.* (1959). Peripheral effects of nicotine and acetylcholine resembling those of sympathetic stimulation. *J. Physiol.* (Lond.) 148, 332.

Burnett, G.B., Little, S.R., Graham, N., *et al.* (1975). The assessment of thiothixene in chronic schizophrenia. A double-blind controlled trial. *Dis. Nerv. Syst.* 36, 625.

Butler, J., Davies, A.H., and Westaby, S. (1990). Streptokinase in acute aortic dissection. *BMJ* 300, 517.

Cabrera, G.E., Citera, G., Gutiérrez, M., *et al.* (1993). Digital vasculitis following allergic desensitization treatment. *J. Rheumatol.* 20, 1970.

Calligaro, K.D., Stern, J., and DeLaurentis, D.A. (1994). Foscarnet: a possible cause of ulnar artery thrombosis in a patient with AIDS. *J. Vasc. Surg.* 20, 1007.

Calne, D.B., Brennan, J., Spiers, A.S.D., *et al.* (1970). Hypotension caused by L-dopa. *BMJ* i, 474.

Canadian Multicentre Transplant Study Group (1983). A randomized clinical trial of cyclosporine in cadaveric renal transplantation. *N. Engl. J. Med.* 309, 809.

Caravaca, F., Fernández, A., Barquilla, J.F., *et al.* (1997). Hypertensive crises following platelet transfusions in a patient on erythropoietin therapy. *Nephrol. Dial. Transplant.* 12, 815.

Cardan, E., Pop, R., and Neghutiu, S. (1987). Prolonged haemodynamic disturbance following attempted retrobulbar block. *Anaesthesia* 42, 668.

Carmeli, Y., Rosenheck, S., and Bursztyn, M. (1994). Paradoxic glyceryl trinitrate induced hypertension. *Chest* 105, 1621.

Castaman, G., Rodeghiero, F., and Dini, E. (1990). Thrombotic complications during L-asparaginase treatment for acute lymphatic leukaemia. *Haematologica* 75, 567.

Caux, F., Chosidow, O., Weshler, J., *et al.* (1991). Cholesterol crystal emboli after anticoagulant therapy. *Presse Méd.* 20, 1949.

Cerosimo, R.J., Calarese, P., and Karp, D.D. (1989). Acute hypotensive reaction to etoposide with successful rechallenge: case report and review of the literature. *Ann. Pharmacotherapy* 23, 876.

Chambers, J.A. and Baggoley, C.J. (1992). Pulmonary oedema — prehospital treatment. Caution with morphine dosage. *Med. J. Aust.* 157, 326.

Chan, J.C.N., Critchley, J.A.J., and Cockram, C.S. (1994). Postpartum hypertension, bromocriptine and phenylpropanolamine. *Drug Invest.* 8, 254.

Chang, F-Y., Cheng, J-T., Lai, K-H., *et al.* (1989). Scrotal ischaemia after intravenous vasopressin therapy for hemorrhagic esophageal varices. *NY State J. Med.* 89, 583.

Chapman, J.R., Marcen, R., Arias, M., *et al.* (1987). Hypertension after renal transplantation. A comparison of cyclosporin and conventional immunosuppression. *Transplantation* 43, 860.

Chaturvedi, N.C., Walsh, M.J., Boyle, D., *et al.* (1974). Diamorphine-induced attack of paroxysmal hypertension in phaeochromocytoma. *BMJ* ii, 538.

Choi, K.L., Wat, M.S., Ip, T.P., *et al.* (1995). Phaeochromocy-toma associated with myasthenia gravis precipitated by pro-pranolol treatment. *Aust. N.Z. J. Med.* 25, 257.

Chong, B.H., Pitney, W.R., and Castaldi, P.A. (1982). Hep-arin-induced thrombocytopenia. Association of thrombotic complications with heparin-dependent IgG antibody that induces thromboxane synthesis and platelet aggregation. *Lancet* ii, 1246.

Clarke, C.S., Otridge, B.W. and Carney, D.N. (1990). Throm-boembolism. A complication of weekly chemotherapy in the treatment of non-Hodgkin's lymphoma. *Cancer* 66, 2027.

Clarke, R.S.J. (1969). Hypotensive reaction after propanidid. *BMJ* iv, 369.

Cleland, J.G.F., Dargie, H.J., McAlpine, H., *et al.* (1985). Severe hypotension after first dose of enalapril in heart failure. *BMJ* 291, 1309.

Close, A.S., Frackleton, W.H., and Cory, R.C. (1956). Cu-taneous necrosis due to nor-epinephrine: mechanism and prevention. *Clin. Res. Proc.* 4, 241.

Coates, A.S., Childs, A., Cox, K., *et al.* (1992). Severe vascular effects with thrombocytopenia and renal failure following emetogenic chemotherapy and ondansetron. *Ann. Oncol.* 3, 719.

Cohen, L.S., Weschler, A.S., and Mitchell, J.H. (1970). De-pression of cardiac function by streptomycin and other antimicrobial agents. *Am. J. Cardiol.* 26, 505.

Cohen, M.H., Elin, R.J., and Cohen, B.J. (1991). Hypotension and disseminated intravascular coagulation following intra-lesional bacillus Calmette-Guérin therapy for locally meta-static melanoma. *Cancer Immunol. Immunother.* 32, 315.

Comfort, A. (1981). Hypertensive reactions to New Zealand prickly spinach in woman taking phenelzine. *Lancet* ii, 472.

Committee on Safety of Medicines (1975). Prazosin and loss of consciousness. The present position. *Curr. Prob.* I.

Committee on Safety of Medicines (1996). Risk of venous thrombosis with hormone replacement tharapy. *Current Problems in Pharmacovigilance* 22, 9.

Comroe, J.H. Jr and Dripps, R.D. (1946). The histamine-like action of curare and tubocurarine injected intracutaneously and intra-arterially in man. *Anesthesiology* 7, 260.

Confino, I., Passwell, J.H., and Padeh, S. (1997). Erythro-melalgia following influenza vaccine in a child. *Clin. Exp. Rheumatol.* 15, 111.

Constantino, E.A., Roose, S.P., and Woodring, S. (1993) . Tricyclic-induced orthostatic hypotension. Significant dif-ference in depressed and non-depressed states. *Pharmaco-psychiatry* 26, 125.

Conti, J.A. and Scher, H.I. (1992). Acute arterial thrombosis after escalated-dose methotrexate, vinblastine, doxo-rubicin, and cisplatin chemotherapy with recombinant gra-nulocyte colony-stimulating factor. A possible new recombinant granulocyte colony-stimulating factor toxicity. *Cancer* 70, 2699.

Cook, R.F. and Katritsis, D. (1990). Hypertensive crisis pre-cipitated by a monoamine oxidase inhibitor in a patient with phaeochromocytoma. *BMJ* 300, 614.

Copley, A.L. and Robb, T.P. (1942). Studies on platelets. III. The effect of heparin *in vivo* on the platelet count in mice and dogs. *Am. J. Clin. Pathol.* 12, 563.

Corvol, P., Bisseliches, F., and Alexandre, J.M. (1974) Pous-sées hypertensives déclenchées par le sulpiride. *Sem. Hop. Paris* 50, 1265.

Coulter, D.N. and Pillans, P.I. (1995). Hypertension with moclobemide. *Lancet* 346, 1032.

Coupland, R.E. (1965). *The Natural History of the Chromaffin Cell.* Longman, London.

Cowen, T.D. and Meythaler, J.M. (1994). Hypotensive effects of thioridazine in an elderly patient with traumatic brain damage. *Brain Inj.* 8, 735.

Creutzig, A., Caspary, L., and Freund, M. (1996). The Raynaud phenomenon and interferon therapy. *Ann. Intern. Med.* 125, 423.

Criqui, M.H., Wallace, R.B., Mishkel, M., *et al.* (1981). Al-cohol consumption and blood pressure: the Lipid Research Clinics Prevalence Study. *Hypertension* 3, 557.

Critchley, J.A.J. and Ungar, A. (1974). Do the anterior pit-uitary and adrenal cortex participate in the reflex response of the adrenal medulla to arterial hypoxia? *J. Physiol.* (Lond.) 239, 16.

Critchley, J.A.J., West, C.P., and Waite, J. (1974). Dangers of corticotrophin in phaeochromocytoma. *Lancet* ii, 782.

Crofton, M. and Gabriel, R. (1977). Pressor response after intravenous labetalol. *BMJ* ii, 737.

Cryer, P.E., Haymond, N.W., Santiago, J.V., *et al.* (1976). Norepinephrine and epinephrine release and adrenergic mediation of smoking-associated hemodynamic and meta-bolic events. *N. Engl. J. Med.* 195, 573.

Curtis, J.R. and Bateman, F.J.A. (1975). Use of prazosin in the management of hypertension in patients with chronic renal failure and in renal transplant recipients. *BMJ* iv, 432.

Curzen, N.P., Clarke, B., and Gray, H.H. (1990). Intravenous thrombolysis for suspected myocardial infarction: a caution-ary note. *BMJ* 300, 513.

Cuthbert, M.F. and Vere, D.W. (1971). Potentiation of the cardiovascular effects of some catecholamines by a mono-amine oxidase inhibitor. *Br. J. Pharmacol.* 43, 471P.

Cutuli, B., Petit, J.C., and Schumacher, C. (1995). Throm-boembolic accidents in postmenopausal patients treated by tamoxifen as adjuvant treatment: frequency, risk factors, and prevention. *Bull. Cancer* 82, 51.

Da Motta, T. and Cordas, T.A. (1990). Autoinduction of hypertensive reactions by tranylcypromine. *J. Clin. Psycho-pharmacol.* 10, 232.

Daggett, P. and Franks, S. (1977). Steroid responsiveness in a phaeochromocytoma. *BMJ* i, 84.

Dan, M. and Fiegl, D. (1993). Erythromycin-associated hypo-tension. *Pediatr. Infect. Dis. J.* 12, 692.

Davenport. A. (1993). The effect of renal transplantation and treatment with cyclosporin on the prevalence of Raynaud's phenomenon. *Clin. Transplant.* 7, 4.

Davies, G.E. and Triplett, D.A. (1990). Corticosteroid-associated blue toe syndrome: role of phospholipid anti-bodies. *Ann. Intern. Med.* 113, 893.

Davies, D.M. (1987). Phaeochromocytoma and adverse drug reactions. *Adverse Drug React. Acute Poisoning Rev.* 6, 91.

Dawkins, K.D., Jamieson, S.W., Hunt, S.A. *et al.* (1985). Long-term results, hemodynamics, and complications after combined heart-lung transportation. *Circulation* 71, 919.

De Pablo, P., Aguillar, A., Gallego, M.A., *et al.* (1992). Raynaud's phenomenon and intralesional bleomycin. *Acta Derm. Venereol.* (Stockh.) 72, 465.

Deray, G., Hoang, P., Achour, L., *et al.* (1986). Cyclosporin and Raynaud's phenomenon. *Lancet* ii, 1092.

Deshmukh, N. and Tripathi, S.P. (1995). Thrombosis of tibial arteries in a patient receiving tamoxifen therapy. *Cancer* 76, 1006.

Diaz, J.H. and Hill, G.E. (1979). Hypotension with anesthesia in disulfiram-treated patients. *Anesthesiology* 51, 366.

Diethelm, A., Vorburger, C., Anabitarte, M., *et al.* (1994). Cholesterol crystal embolization as a complication of fibrinolytic treatment of acute myocardial infarction. *Schweiz. Med. Wochenschr.* 124, 1437.

Dougados, M. and Amor, B. (1987). Cyclosporin in rheumatoid arthritis: preliminary clinical results of an open trial. *Arthritis Rheum.* 30, 83.

Douglas, M.J., Farquarson, D.F., Ross, P.L.E., *et al.* (1989). Cardiovascular collapse following an overdose of prostaglandin F$_2$ alpha: a case report. *Can. J. Anaesth.* 36, 466.

Douglas, W.W. (1985). Autocoids: Histamine and 5-hydroxytryptamine (serotonin) and their antagonists. In *Goodman and Gilman's The Physiological Basis of Therapeutics* (7th edn) (ed. A.G. Gilman, L.S. Goodman, T.W. Rall, and F. Murad), p. 609. Macmillan, New York.

Douglas, W.W., Kanno, T., and Sampson, S.R. (1967). Effects of acetylcholine and other medullary secretogogues and antagonists on the membrane potential of adrenal chromaffin cells: analysis employing techniques of tissue culture. *J. Physiol.* (Lond.) 188, 107.

Drenth, J.P.H. (1989). Erythromelalgia induced by nicardipine. *BMJ* 298, 1582.

Drenth, J.P.H., Michiels, J.J., Van Joost. T., *et al.* (1992). Verapamil-induced secondary erythromelalgia. *Br. J. Dermatol.* 127, 292.

Drug and Therapeutics Bulletin (1969). L-Dopa for Parkinsonism. *Drug Ther. Bull.* 7, 59.

Drug and Therapeutics Bulletin (1990). Thrombolytic therapy and pre-existing clots. *Drug Ther. Bull.* 28, 44.

Dugan, W.M. (1967). Pheochromocytoma and smoking. *Arch. Intern. Med.* 120, 365.

Dukes, C.S. and Perfect, J.R. (1990). Amphotericin-B induced malignant hypertensive episodes. *J. Infect. Dis.* 161, 588.

Dukes, M.N.G. (1979). Antianginal and beta-adrenoceptor blocking drugs. In *Side Effects of Drugs Annual*, Vol. 3 (ed. M.N.G. Dukes), p. 164. Excerpta Medica, Amsterdam.

Dunn, F.G., De Carvalho, J.G.R., Kem, D.C., *et al.* (1976). Pheochromocytoma crisis induced by saralasin. Relation of angiotensin analogue to catecholamine release. *N. Engl. J. Med.* 295, 605.

Dupin, N., Chosidow, O., Pockmaliki, G., *et al.* (1992). Cholesterol crystals emboli after fibrinolytic treatment. *Ann. Dermatol. Venereol.* 119, 842.

Durand, J.M., Quiles, N., Kaplanski, G., *et al.* (1993). Thrombosis and recombinant interferon-alpha. *Am. J. Med.* 95, 115.

Dussol, B., Nicolino, F., Brunet, P., *et al.* (1994). Acute transplant artery thrombosis induced by angiotensin-converting inhibitor in a patient with renovascular hypertension. *Nephron* 66, 102.

Duvoison, R.V. (1970). Hypotension caused by L-dopa. *BMJ* ii, 47.

Dzik, W.H., Georgi, B.A., Khettry, V., *et al.* (1987). Cyclosporin-associated thrombotic thrombocytopenic purpura following liver transplantation: successful treatment with plasma exchange. *Transplantation* 44, 570.

Edmunds, M.E. and Walls, J. (1988). Blood pressure and erythropoietin. *Lancet* i, 352.

Egdell, R.W. and Johnson, W.D. (1973). Postpartum hypotension and erythema: an adverse reaction to soap enema. *Am. J. Obstet. Gynecol.* 117, 1146.

Eggert, P. and Stick, C. (1988). Blood pressure increase after erythrocyte transfusion in end-stage renal disease. *Lancet* i, 1343.

Eisler, T., Hall, R.P., Kalavar, K.A.R., *et al.* (1981). Erythromelalgia-like eruption in parkinsonian patients treated with bromocriptine. *Neurology* 31, 1368.

Elis, J., Laurence, D.R., Hattie, H., *et al.* (1967). Modification by monoamine oxidase inhibitors of the effect of some sympathomimetics on blood pressure. *BMJ* ii, 75.

Ellie, B., Durrieu, C., Besse, P., *et al.* (1992). Thrombotic thrombocytopenic purpura associated with ticlopidine. *Stroke* 23, 922.

Emanuel, D.A., Rowe, G.G., Musser, M.J., *et al.* (1956). Prolonged hypotension with fatal termination after phentolamine (Regitine) methanesulfonate test. *JAMA* 161, 436.

Emmelin, N. and Engstrøm, J. (1961). Supersensitivity of salivary glands following treatment with bretylium or guanethidine. *Br. J. Pharmacol. Chemother.* 16, 315.

Engelman, K. and Sjoerdsma, A. (1964). A new test for pheochromocytoma: pressor responsiveness to tyramine. *JAMA* 189, 81.

Ennis, L.M. and Parker, R.M. (1997). Paradoxical hypertension associated with clozapine. *Med. J. Aust.* 166, 278.

Epstein, E. (1991). Intralesional bleomycin and Raynaud's phenomenon. *J. Am. Acad. Dermatol.* 24. 785.

Erickson, S.R. and Yousuf, M.J. (1991). Hypotension and bradycardia possibly associated with intraocular injection of acetylcholine. *Ann. Pharmacother.* 25, 1178.

Esplugas, E., Cequier, A., Jara, P., *et al.* (1993). Contrast media influence on thrombotic risk during coronary angiography. *Sem. Thromb. Hemost.* 19 (suppl. 1), 192.

Euler, U.S. von. (1966). Relationship between histamine and the autonomic nervous system. In *Histamine: Its Chemistry, Metabolism and Physiological and Pharmacological Actions* (ed. M. Rocha e Silva). Part 1. *Handbuch der experimentellen Pharmakologie*, Vol. 18, p. 318. Springer-Verlag, Berlin.

Fadali, M.A., Ledbetter, B.S., Papacostas, C.A., *et al.* (1974). Mechanism responsible for the cardiovascular depressant effect of protamine sulphate. *Ann. Surg.* 180, 232.

Fagard, R., Amery, A., and Timmermans, U. (1976). Severe hypotension during infusion of saralasin. *Lancet* i, 1136.

Fahal, I.H., Yaqoob, M., and Ahmad, R. (1991). Phlebotomy for erythropoietin-associated malignant hypertension. *Lancet* 337, 1227.

Fahmy, N.R., Sunder, N., and Sojer, N.A. (1983). Role of histamine in the haemodynamic and plasma catecholamine responses of morphine. *Clin. Pharmacol. Ther.* 33, 615.

Feldberg, W. and Lewis, J. (1964). The action of peptides on the adrenal medulla and release of adrenaline by bradykines and angiotensin II. *J. Physiol.* (Lond.) 171, 98.

Ferguson, K.L. (1994). Imipramine-provoked paradoxical pheochromocytoma crisis: a case of cardiogenic shock. *Am. J. Emergency Med.* 12, 190.

Ferguson, R.M. and Sommer, B.G. (1985). Cyclosporine in renal transplantation: a single institutional experience. *Am. J. Kidney Dis.* 5, 296.

Ferrari, E., Morand, P., and Baudouy, M. (1996). Treatment of the heparin-induced thrombosis–thrombocytopenia syndrome by very low dose streptokinase. *Heart* 76, 185.

Fertakos, R.J. and Mintzer, D.M. (1992). Digital gangrene following chemotherapy for Aids-related Kaposi's sarcoma. *Am. J. Med.* 93, 581.

Fidlar, E. and Jaques, L.B. (1948). The effect of commercial heparin on the platelet count. *J. Lab. Clin. Med.* 33, 1410.

Fiessinger, J.N., Aiach, M., Roncato, M., *et al.* (1984). Critical ischemia during herapin-induced thrombocytopenia: treatment by intra-arterial streptokinase. *Thromb. Res.* 33, 235.

Fisher, J.R. and Padnick, G. (1983). Nifedipine and erythromelalgia. *Ann. Intern. Med.* 98, 671.

Fitzgibbon, D.R., Rapp, S.E., Butler, S.H., *et al.* (1996). Rebound hypertension and withdrawal associated with discontinuation of an infusion of epidural clonidine. *Anesthesiology* 84. 729.

Folks, D.G. (1983). Monoamine oxidase inhibitors: reappraisal of dietary considerations. *J. Clin. Psychopharmacol.* 3, 249.

Forjas De Lacerda, J., Alves Do Carmo, J., Lurdes Guerra, M., *et al.* (1993). Multiple thrombosis in acute promyelocytic leukaemia after tretinoin. *Lancet* 342, 114.

Franco, A., Bourlard, P., Massot, C., *et al.* (1978). Ergotisme aigu par association dihydroergotamine–triacétyloléandomycine. *Nouv. Presse Méd.* 7, 205.

Fraser, J.L., Millenson, M., Malynn, E.R., *et al.* (1996). Possible association between the Norplant contraceptive system and thrombotic thrombocytopenic purpura. *Obstet. Gynecol.* 87. 860.

Freestone, S., Duffield, J., Lee, M.R., *et al.* (1996). Pressor effect of metoclopramide in phaeochromocytoma. *Postgrad. Med. J.* 72, 188.

French, J. and White, H. (1989). Transient symptomatic hypotension in a patient on simvastatin. *Lancet* ii, 807.

Friederszick, F.K. (1949). Embolien während intramuskulärer Penicillin Behandlung. *Klin. Wochenschr.* 27, 173.

Gabriel, R. (1976). Paradoxical rise in blood pressure during propranolol treatment. *BMJ* i, 219.

Gabriel, R., Meek, D., and Mamtora, H. (1975). Adverse reactions to prazosin. *BMJ* iv, 41.

Gandy, W. (1990). Dihydroergotamine interaction with propranolol. *Ann. Emergency Med.* 19, 221.

Garstin, I.W., Cooper, G.G., and Hood, J.M. (1990). Arterial thrombosis after treatment with bleomycin and cisplatin. *BMJ* 300, 1018.

Gavras, H. and Gavras, I. (1988). Salt-induced hypertension: the interactive role of vasopressin and of the sympathetic nervous system. *J. Hypertension* 7, 601.

Generali, J.A. (1981). Hypertensive crisis resulting from avocados and a MAO inhibitor. *Drug Intell. Clin. Pharmacol.* 15, 904.

George, T.P. and Winther, L.C. (1996). Hypertension after initiation of clozapine. *Am. J. Psychiatry* 153, 1368.

Gibson, G.J. and Warrell, D.A. (1972). Hypertensive crises and phenylpropanolamine. *Lancet* ii, 492.

Gilleece, M.H. and Davies, J.M. (1991). Mesna therapy and hypertension. *Ann. Pharmacother.* 25, 867.

Girolami, A., Simioni, P., Sartori, M.T., *et al.* (1992). Oral contraceptives caused thrombosis in a monovular twin with protein C deficiency, while the other, without medication, remained asymptomatic. *Blood Coagul. Fibrinolysis* 3, 119.

Girolami, A., Zanardi, S., Simioni, P., *et al.* (1993). Are oral contraceptives a more important risk factor than pregnancy in women with congenital antithrombin III deficiency? *Blood Coagul. Fibrinolysis* 4, 841.

Girolami, A, Zanon, E., Zanardi, S., *et al.* (1996). Thromboembolic disease developing during oral contraceptive therapy in young females with antiphospholipid antibodies. *Blood Coagul. Fibrinolysis* 7, 497.

Given, B.D., Taylor, T., Lilly, L.S., *et al.* (1983). Symptomatic hypotension following the clonidine suppression test for pheochromocytoma. *Arch. Intern. Med.* 143, 2195.

Glover, W.E. and Hutchinson, J.J. (1964). The effect of a beta-receptor antagonist (propranolol) on the cardiovascular response to intravenous infusion of noradrenaline in man. *J. Physiol.* (Lond.) 177, 59P.

Goffin, E., Angangco, R., Shapiro, L.M., *et al.* (1994). Digital gangrene following chemotherapy. *Am. J. Med.* 96, 57.

Goldberg, J., Moreno, F., and Barbara, J. (1997). Acute hypertension as an adverse effect of pyrazinamide. *JAMA* 177, 1356.

Goldfien, A., Zileli, M.S., Despointes, L.H., *et al.* (1958). The effect of hypoglycaemia on the adrenal secretion of epinephrine and norepinephrine in the dog. *Endocrinology* 62, 749.

Goldman, V., Astrøm, A., and Evers, H. (1971). The effect of a tricyclic antidepressant on the cardiovascular effects of local anaesthetic solutions containing different vasoconstrictors. *Anaesthesia* 26, 91.

Gollub, S. and Ulin, A.W. (1962). Heparin-induced thrombocytopenia in man. *J. Lab. Clin. Med.* 59, 430.

Gómez, E., Aguardo, S., Gago, E., *et al.* (1992). Main graft vessels thromboses due to conventional-dose OKT3 in renal transplantation. *Lancet* 339, 1612.

Gordon, R.D., Iwatsuki, S., Shaw, B.W., *et al.* (1985). Cyclosporine–steroid combination therapy in 84 cadaveric renal transplants. *Am. J. Kidney Dis.* 5, 307.

Goswani, R. and Gurtoo, A. (1993). Hypertension and hyperparathyroidism — narrowed therapeutic safety with nifedipine. *Postgrad. Med. J.* 69, 752.

Gould, B.A., Mann, S., Davies, A., *et al.* (1981). Indoramin: 24-hour profile of intra-arterial ambulatory blood pressure: a double-blind placebo-controlled crossover study. *Br. J. Clin. Pharmacol.* 12, 675.

Gradishar, W., Vokes, E., Schilsky, R., *et al.* (1991). Vascular events in patients receiving high-dose infusional 5-fluorouracil-based chemotherapy: the University of Chicago experience. *Med. Pediatr. Oncol.* 19, 8.

Graham, R.M., Thornell, I.R., Gain, J.M., *et al.* (1976). Prazosin: the first dose phenomenon. *BMJ* ii, 1293.

Grassi, G.M., Somers, V.K., Renk, W.S., *et al.* (1989). Effects of alcohol on blood pressure and sympathetic nerve activity in normotensive humans: a preliminary report. *J. Hypertension* 7 (suppl. 6), S20.

Green, H.D. and Grimsley, W.T. (1953). Effect of Regitine (c-7337) in patients, particularly those with peripheral vascular disease. *Circulation* 7, 487.

Green, S.T., Ng, J.P., and Callaghan, M. (1988). Metolazone and axillary vein thrombosis. *Scott. Med. J.* 33, 211.

Gremse, D.A., Artman, M., and Boerth, R.C. (1986). Hypertension associated with naloxone treatment for clonidine poisoning. *Pediatrics* 108, 776.

Gunzberger, D.M. and Martinez, D. (1992). Adverse vascular effects associated with fluoxetine. *Am. J. Psychiatry* 149, 1751.

Gupta, B.K., Spinowitz, B.S., Charytan, C., *et al.* (1993). Cholesterol crystal embolization-associated renal failure after therapy with recombinant tissue-type plasminogen activator. *Am. J. Kidney Dis.* 21, 659.

Hach-Wunderle, V., Kainer, K., Krug, B., *et al.* (1994). Heparin-assaciated thrombosis despite normal platelet counts. *Lancet* 344, 46.

Hall, M.R., Richards, M.A., and Harper, P.G. (1988). Thromboembolic events during combination chemotherapy for germ-cell malignancy. *Lancet* ii, 1259.

Hamilton, D.V., Carmichael, D.J.S., Evans, D.B., *et al.* (1982). Hypertension in renal transplant recipients on cyclosporine A and corticosteroids and azathioprine. *Transplant Proc.* 14, 597.

Hannah, P., Glover, V., and Sandler, M. (1988). Tyramine in wine and beer. *Lancet* i, 879.

Hanson, D.S. and Leggette, C.T. (1997). Severe hypotension following inadvertent intravenous administration of interferon alfa-2a. *Ann. Pharmacother.* 31, 371.

Hardesty, R.L., Griffith, B.P., Debski, R.F., *et al.* (1983). Experience with cyclosporine in cardiac transplantation. *Transplant Proc.* 15 (suppl. 1), 2553.

Harris, A.L. (1976). Clonidine withdrawal and blockade. *Lancet* i, 596.

Hauet, T., Ramassamy, A., Badia, P., *et al.* (1996). Digital ischaemia associated with fluoxazoline intoxication. Case report and review of the literature. *Rev. Med. Interne* 17, 66.

Hayton, A.C. (1969). Precipitation of acute ergotism by triacetyloleandomycin. *N.Z. Med. J.* 69, 42.

Heier, M.S., Nilsen, T., Graver, V., *et al.* (1991). Raynaud's phenomenon after combination chemotherapy of testicular cancer, measured by laser Doppler flowmetry. A pilot study. *Br. J. Cancer* 63, 550.

Hessov, I. (1970). Hypertension during imipramine treatment. *Lancet* i, 84.

Hessov, I. (1971). Hypertension during chlorimipramine therapy. *BMJ* i, 406.

Hirsh, S.A., Robertson, H., and Gorniowsky, M. (1976). Arterial occlusion secondary to methylmethacrylate use. *Arch. Surg.* 111, 204.

Hod, G., Halevy, A., Scapa, E., *et al.* (1992). Mesenteric vein thrombosis — a possible late complication of endoscopic sclerotherapy. *J. Clin. Gastroenterol.* 15, 269.

Hodge, J.V., Nye, E.R., and Emerson, G.W. (1964). Monoamine-oxidase inhibitors, broad beans, and hypertension. *Lancet* i, 1108.

Hodsman, G.P., Isles, C.G., Murray, G.D., *et al.* (1983). Factors related to the first-dose hypotensive effect of captopril: prediction and treatment. *BMJ* 286, 832.

Hoehn, M.M. (1975). Levo-dopa-induced postural hypotension. *Arch. Neurol.* 32, 50.

Horowitz, J.D., McNeill, J.J., Sweet, B., *et al.* (1979). Hypertension and postural hypotension induced by phenylpropanolamine (Trimolets). *Med. J. Aust.* i, 175.

Horowitz, J.D., Lang, W.J., Howes, L.G., *et al.* (1980). Hypertensive response induced by phenylpropanolamine in anorectic and decongestant preparations. *Lancet* i, 60.

Horrowitz, R.S., Dart, R.C., and Gomez, R.F. (1996). Clinical ergotism with lingual ischemia induced by clarithromycin–ergotamine interaction. *Arch. Intern. Med.* 156, 456.

Horwitz, D., Goldberg, L.I., and Sjoerdsma, A. (1960). Increased blood pressure responses to dopamine and norepinephrine produced by monoamine oxidase inhibitors in man. *J. Lab. Clin. Med.* 56, 747.

Houston, M.C. (1991). Non-steroidal anti-inflammatory drugs and antihypertensives. *Am. J. Med.* 9 (suppl. 5A), 42.

Howrie, D.L. and Wolfson, J.H. (1983). Phenylpropanolamine-induced hypertensive seizures. *J. Pediatrics* 102, 143.

Hunyor, S.N., Hansson, L., Harrison, T.S., *et al.* (1973). Effects of withdrawal: possible mechanisms and suggestions for management. *BMJ* ii, 209.

Iaquinto, G., Ambrosone, L., and Rotiroti, D. (1991). A case of portal thrombosis arising after treatment with dihydroergotamine. *Ital. J. Gastroenterol.* 23, 219.

Içli, F., Karaouz, H., Dinçol, D., *et al.* (1993). Severe vascular toxicity associated with cisplatin-based chemotherapy. *Cancer* 72, 587.

Imms, F.J., Neame, R.L.B., and Powis, D.A. (1976). Paradoxical rise in blood pressure during propranolol treatment. *BMJ* i, 218.

Impey, L. (1993). Severe hypotension and fetal distress following sublingual administration of nifedipine to a patient with severe pregnancy-induced hypertension at 33 weeks. *Br. J. Obstet. Gynaecol.* 100, 959.

Insler, S.R., Kraenzler, E.J., Licina, M.G., *et al.* (1994). Cardiac surgery in a patient taking monoamine oxidase inhibitors: an adverse fentanyl reaction. *Anesth. Analg.* 78, 593.

Isaac, T., Mitchell, B., and Grahame-Smith, D.G. (1977). Monoamine oxidase inhibitors and caviar. *Lancet* ii, 816.

Jameson, S.J. and Hargarten, S.W. (1992). Calcium pretreatment to prevent verapamil-induced hypotension in patients with SVT. *Ann. Emergency Med.* 21, 84.

Joss, D.V., Barrett, S.J., Kendra, J.R., *et al.* (1982). Hypertension and convulsions in children receiving cyclosporin A. *Lancet* i, 906.

Journal of the American Medical Association (1974). Medical News — A warning about oxytocin in bolus form. *JAMA* 230, 1373.

Julka, N.K. and Nora, J.R. (1976). Gangrene aggravation after use of dopamine. *JAMA* 235, 2812.

Kallal, S.M. and Lee, M. (1996). Thrombotic thrombocytopenic purpura associated with histamine H_2-receptor antagonist therapy. *West. J. Med.* 164, 446.

Kampmann, K.K., Graves, T., and Rogers, S.D. (1989). Acral erythema secondary to high-dose cytosine arabinoside with pain worsened by cyclosporin infusion. *Cancer* 63, 2482.

Kando, J.C., Keck, P.E., and Wood, P.A. (1990). Pergolide-induced hypotension. *Ann. Pharmacotherapy* 24, 543.

Kashtan, H.I., Heyneker, T.J., and Morell, R.C. (1992). Atypical response to scopolamine in a patient with type IV hereditary sensory and autonomic neuropathy. *Anesthesiology* 76, 140.

Katz, B.Z. and Cohn, R.A. (1994). Amphotericin B and hypertension. *Pediatr. Infect. Dis. J.* 113, 839.

Kaufmann, J.S. (1974). Pheochromocytoma and tricyclic antidepressants. *JAMA* 229, 1282.

Kaul, S., Sarela, A.I., Supe, A.N., *et al.* (1997). Gangrene complicating dopamine therapy. *J. R. Soc. Med.* 90, 80.

Kawachi, Y., Watanabe, A., Uchidat, T., *et al.* (1996). Acute arterial thrombosis due to platelet aggregation in a patient receiving granulocyte-stimulating factor. *Br. J. Haematol.* 94, 413.

Kelton, J.G. and Hirsh, J. (1980). Bleeding associated with antithrombotic therapy. *Sem. Hematol.* 17, 259.

Khairallah, P.A., Davila, D., and Papanicolaou, N. (1971). Effects of angiotensin infusion on catecholamine uptake and reactivity in blood vessels. *Circ. Res.* 28 (suppl. 2), 96.

Kholeif, M. and Isles, C. (1989). Profound hypotension after atenolol in severe hypertension. *BMJ* 298, 161.

Killian, J.M. and Fromm, G.A. (1968). Carbamazepine in the treatment of neuralgia. Use and side effects. *Arch. Neurol.* 19, 129.

Kilpatrick, A.W.A. and Thorburn, J. (1990). Severe hypotension due to intramyometrial injection of prostaglandin E2. *Anaesthesia* 45, 848.

Klatsky, A.L., Friedman, G.D., and Armstrong, M.A. (1986). The relationship between alcoholic beverage use and other traits to blood pressure: a new Kaiser Permanente Study. *Circulation* 73, 628.

Kligman, I., Noyes, N., and Benadiva, C.A. (1993). Massive deep vein thrombosis in a patient with antithrombin III deficiency undergoing ovarian stimulation for in-vitro fertilization. *Fertil. Steril.* 63, 673.

Knox, J.W.D., Bovill, J.G., Clark, R.S.J., *et al.* (1970). Clinical studies of induction agents, XXXVI: Ketamine. *Br. J. Anaesth.* 42, 875.

Koelle, G.B. (1970). Neuromuscular blocking agents. In *The Pharmacological Basis of Therapeutics* (5th edn) (ed. L.S. Goodman and A. Gilman), p. 612. Collier Macmillan, London.

Komori, K., Naito, H., Ito, T., *et al.* (1994). A case of thrombophlebitis and SIADH possibly associated with long-term carbamazepine treatment. *Shinyaku to Rinsho* 43, 1195.

Konrad, C., Schüpfer, G., and Wietlisbach, M. (1997). Pulmonary embolism and hydrogen peroxide. *Can. J. Anaesth.* 44, 338.

Kronenberg, F., Lhotta, K., Joannidis, M., *et al.* (1993). Thromboembolic complications in renal allograft recipients: triple-drug therapy in comparison with cyclosporine A–prednisone. *Clin. Transplant.* 7, 339.

Krupp, P., Gulich, A., and Timonen, P. (1986). Treatment with cyclosporine combination therapy. *Transplant Proc.* 18, 991.

Kuekes, E.D., Wigg, C., Bryant, S., *et al.* (1992). Hypertension is a risk in adolescents treated with imipramine. *J. Child Adolescent Psychopharmacol.* 2, 241.

Kuhn, M. and Schriger, D.L. (1992). Low-dose calcium pretreatment to prevent verapamil-induced hypotension. *Am. Heart J.* 124, 231.

Kumana, C.P. and Marlin, G.E. (1978). Selectivity of beta-adrenoceptor agonists. In *Recent Advances in Clinical Pharmacology* (ed. P. Turner and D.G. Shand), p. 31. Churchill, Edinburgh.

Küster, G. and Ritz, E. (1989). Analgesic abuse and hypertension. *Lancet* ii, 1105.

Lacouture, P.G., Epstein, M.F., and Mitchell, A.A. (1987). Vancomycin-associated shock and rash in infants. *J. Pediatr.* 111, 615.

Lagier, G., Castot, A., Ribonlet, G., *et al.* (1979). Un cas d'ergotisme mineur semblant en rapport avec une potentialisation de l'ergotamine par l'éthylsuccinate d'erythromycine. *Thérapie* 34, 515.

Lai, K.N., Richards, A.M., and Nicholls, M.G. (1991). Drug-induced hypertension. *Adverse Drug React. Acute Toxicol. Rev.* 10, 1.

Lake, C.R., Zalaga, G., Bray, J., *et al.* (1989). Transient hypertension after two phenylpropanolamine diet aids and the effects of caffeine: a placebo-controlled follow-up study. *Am. J. Med.* 86, 427.

The Lancet (1974). Acrylic cement and the cardiovascular system. *Lancet* ii, 1002.

The Lancet (1988). Cyclosporin hypertension. *Lancet* ii, 1234.

Langdon, L. (1977). Transient hypotension following intravenous ethamsylate (Dicynene). *BMJ* i, 1472.

Laurence, D.A. and Nagle, R.E. (1961). The interaction of bretylium with pressor agents. *Lancet* i, 593.

Laurenson, V.G. and Davis, F.M. (1985). An adverse reaction to clomethiazole. *Anaesth. Intens. Care* 13, 438.

Lavin, M.R., Mendelowitz, A., Kronig, M.H., *et al.* (1993). Spontaneous hypertensive reactions with monoamine oxidase inhibitors. *Biol. Psychiatry* 3, 146.

Lawrence, C.A. (1978). Pethidine-induced hypertension in phaeochromocytoma. *Br. Med J.* i, 149.

Le, Y., Rana, K.Z., and Dudley, M.N. (1996). Amphotericin-B-associated hypertension. *Ann. Pharmacother.* 30, 765.

Leal-Cerro, A., Garcia-Luna, P.P., Villar, J., *et al.* (1989). Arterial hypertension as a complication of prolonged ketoconazole treatment. *J. Hypertension* 7 (suppl. 6), S 212.

Lee, D.W. and Cohan, B. (1995). Refractory cardiogenic shock and complete heart block after verapamil SR and metoprolol treatment: a case report. *Angiology* 46, 517.

Lee, K.Y., Beilin, L.J., and Vandongen, R. (1979). Severe hypertension after ingestion of an appetite suppressant (phenylpropanolamine) with indomethacin. *Lancet* i, 1110.

Lees, B.J. and Cabal, L.A. (1981). Increased blood pressure following pupillary dilatation with 2.5% phenylephrine hydrochloride in preterm infants. *Pediatrics* 68, 231.

Lefebvre, H., Richard, R., Noblet, C., *et al.* (1993). Life-threatening pseudophaeochromocytoma after toloxalone, terbutaline, and phenylephrine. *Lancet* 341, 555.

Leroy, O., Beuscart, C., Senneville, E., *et al.* (1990). Deep venous thrombosis and antibodies to cyproterone. *Lancet* 336, 509.

Levesque, H., Moore, L.M., and Courtois, H. (1989). Erythromelalgia induced by nicardipine. *BMJ* 298, 1252.

Levine, M.N., Gent, M., Hirsh, J., *et al.* (1988). The thrombogenic effect of anticancer drug therapy in women with stage II breast cancer. *N. Engl. J. Med.* 318, 404.

Lewis, M.J., Ross, P.J., and Henderson, A.H. (1979). Rebound effect after stopping beta-blockers. *BMJ* ii, 606.

Leyton, N. (1964). Methysergide in the prophylaxis of migraine. *Lancet* i, 830.

Linch, D.C., Swan, K.M., Muttlemann, M.F., *et al.* (1978). Bromocriptine-induced postural hypotension in acromegaly. *Lancet* ii, 321.

Lissoni, P., Barni, S., Cattaneo, C., *et al.* (1990). Evaulation of the cardiovascular toxicity related to cancer immunotherapy with interleukin-2 by monitoring atrial natriuretic peptide secretion: a case report. *Tumori* 76, 603.

Loeliger, E.A. (1975). Drugs affecting blood clotting and fibrinolysis. In *Meyler's Side Effects of Drugs* (ed. M.N.G. Dukes), p. 777. Excerpta Medica, Amsterdam.

Loke, R.H.T., Murray-Lyon, I.M., and Carter, G.D. (1990). Postural hypotension related to zidovudine in a patient infected with HIV. *BMJ* 300, 163.

Lorenz, W. and Doenicke, A. (1978). Anaphylactoid reactions and histamine release by intravenous drugs used in surgery and anaesthesia. In *Adverse Response to Intravenous Drugs* (ed. J. Watkins and A.M. Ward), p. 83. Academic Press, London.

Lorenz, W., Doenicke, A., Messmer, H.-J., *et al.* (1976). Histamine release in human subjects by modified gelatin (Haemaccel) and dextran: an explanation for anaphylactoid reactions observed under clinical conditions. *Br. J. Anaesth.* 48, 151.

Lossef, S.V. and Barth, K.H. (1993). Severe delayed hypotension after lymphangiography with iodised oil: case report. *AJR* 161, 417.

Loughran, T.P., Deeg, H.J., Dahlberg, S., *et al.* (1985). Incidence of hypertension after bone marrow transplantation among 112 patients randomized to either cyclosporin or methotrexate as graft-versus-host disease prophylaxis. *Br. J. Haematol.* 59, 547.

Louie, A.K., Louie, E.K., and Lannon, R.A. (1992). Systemic hypertension associated with tricyclic antidepressant treatment in patients with panic disorder. *Am. J. Cardiol.* 70, 1306.

Lucas, L.M., Colley, C.A., and Gordon, G.H. (1992). Case report: multisystem failure following intravenous iopamidol. *Clin. Radiol.* 45, 276.

McAlister, F.A. and Lewanczuk, R. (1994). Hypertensive crisis after discontinuation of ACE inhibitor. *Lancet* 344, 1502.

McAllister, R.G. Jr (1981). Hypertensive crisis and myocardial infarction after fluorescein angiography. *South. Med. J.* 74, 504.

McCance-Katz, E.F. (1991). New onset Raynaud's phenomenon in a schizophrenic patient. *J. Clin. Psychiatry* 52, 89.

McCloy, R.F. and Baron, J.H. (1977). Acute reaction to pentagastrin. *Lancet* i, 548.

McDonald, C., Alexander, F.E., and Whyte, B.W. (1995). Scottish Cancer Trials Breast Group. Cardiac and vascular morbidity in women receiving adjuvant tamoxifen for breast cancer in a randomised trial. *BMJ* 311, 977.

McEwen, J. (1983). Phenylpropanolamine-associated hypertension after the use of over-the-counter appetite suppressant product. *Med. J. Aust.* ii, 71.

McGrath, P. (1992). Accidental intra-arterial flucloxacillin: management using guanethidine. *Anaesth. Intens. Care* 20, 517.

McGrath, P.J., Stewart, J.W., and Quitkin, F.M. (1989). A possible L-deprenyl-induced hypertensive reaction. *J. Psychopharmacol.* 9, 310.

McKenzie, A.J. (1990). Possible interaction between SPPS and enalapril. *Anaesth. Intens. Care* 18, 124.

McLaren, E.H. (1976). Severe hypertension produced by interaction of phenylpropanolamine with methyldopa and oxprenolol. *BMJ* ii, 283.

Maclean, D., Maton, S.M., Bibby, A.J., *et al.* (1993). Incidence of first-dose hypotension with quinaloprin in patients with mild to moderate hypertension. *Br. J. Clin. Pract.* 47, 234.

McLeod, H.L., Baker, D.K., Jr, Pui, C-H., *et al.* (1991). Somnolence, hypotension and metabolic acidosis following high-dose teniposide treatment in children with leukaemia. *Cancer Chemother. Pharmacol.* 29, 150.

McPhaul, M., Punzi, H.A., Sandy, A., *et al.* (1984). Snuff-induced hypertension in pheochromocytoma. *JAMA* 252, 2860.

Maddern, P.J., Davis, N.L., and McGlew, I. (1976). Case report: pheochromocytoma. Aspects of management. *Anaesth. Intens. Care* 4, 156.

Magagna, A., Abdel-Haq, B., Favilla, S., *et al.* (1991). Indomethacin raises blood pressure in untreated essential hypertensives: a double-blind randomly allocated study versus placebo. *J. Hypertens.* 9 (suppl. 6), 242.

Maggi, J.D., Angelots, J., and Scott, J.P. (1982). Gangrene in a neonate following dopamine therapy. *J. Pediatr.* 100, 323.

Mahon, W.A. and Kolton, N. (1978). Hypotension after intravenous cimetidine. *Lancet* i, 828.

Main, J. and Wilkinson, R. (1989). Early renal artery occlusion after enalapril in atheromatous renal artery stenosis. *BMJ* 229, 394.

Makadassi, R., de Cagny, B., Lobjoie, E., *et al.* (1996). Convulsions, hypertension and acute renal failure in postpartum: role of bromocriptine. *Nephron* 72, 732.

Makker, S.P. and Moorthy, B. (1980). Rebound hypertension following minoxidil withdrawal. *J. Pediatr.* 96, 762.

Malatack, J.J., Zitelli, B.J., and Gartner, J.C. (1983). Pediatric liver transplantation under therapy with cyclosporin A and steroids. *Transplant Proc.* 15, 1292.

Marcus, M.A.E., Vertommen, J.D., and Van Aken, H., *et al.* (1997). Prostaglandin-induced ventricular fibrillation during cesarian section. *Int. J. Obstet. Anaesth.* 6, 130.

Marinakis, T., Papadimitriou, C.A., Koufos, C., *et al.* (1993). A recently recognized entity associated with the treatment of promyelocytic leukaemia. *Haematologica* 78, 192.

Markovitz, P.A., Bach, D.S., Mathias, W., *et al.* (1993). Paradoxical hypotension during dobutamine stress electrocardiography: clinical and diagnostic implications. *J. Am. Coll. Cardiol.* 21, 1080.

Marriott, H.J.L. (1957). An alarming pressor reaction to Regitine. *Ann. Intern. Med.* 44, 1001.

Marti, V., Moya, C., Fontcuberta, J., *et al.* (1991). Pulmonary thromboembolism during imnunosuppressive therapy with cyclosporin in a patient with heart transplantation. *Med. Clin.* (Barc.) 96, 197.

Martin, J. and Moncada, S. (1988). Blood pressure, erythropoietin, and nitric oxide. *Lancet* i, 644.

Mathews, J., Goel, R., Evans, W.K., *et al.* (1997). Arterial occlusion in a patient with peripheral vascular disease treated with platinum-based regimens for lung cancer. *Cancer Chemother. Pharmacol.* 40, 19.

Matthews, T.G., Wilczek, Z.N., and Shennan, A.T. (1977). Eye-drop induced hypertension. *Lancet* ii, 827.

Mayer, R.D. and Montgomery, S.A. (1989). Acute hypertensive episode induced by sulpiride. *Hum. Psychopharmacol. Clin. Exp.* 4, 149.

Mayhew, J.F. and Deutsch, S. (1985). Cardiac arrest following administration of vancomycin. *Can. Anaesth. Soc. J.* 32, 65.

Meltzer, J.I. and Sealey, J. (1990). Malignant hypertension during chronic lithium therapy: a new syndrome and cause of a false positive captopril test. *J. Hypertens.* 3, 73A.

Mendia, R., D'Aloya, G., Cavaliere, G., *et al.* (1992). Does thrombolysis produce cholesterol embolisation? *Lancet* 339, 562.

Mets, T., De Bock, V., and Praet, J.P. (1992). First-dose hypotension, ACE inhibitors and heart failure in the elderly. *Lancet* 339, 1481.

Meuche, C., Heidrich, H., and Blickman, H. (1990). Raynaud's syndrome following the use of eyedrops containing timolol. *Fortschr. Ophthalmol.* 87, 45.

Milne, A., Talbot, S., and Bevan, D. (1988). Thromboses during cytotoxic chemotherapy. *BMJ* 297, 624.

Minamori, Y., Yammoto, M., Tanaka, A., *et al.* (1992). Hazard of glucagon test in diabetic patients: hypertensive crisis in asymptomatic pheochromocytoma. *Diabetes Care* 15, 1437.

Mindham, R.H.S. (1975). Hypnotics and sedatives. In *Meyler's Side Effects of Drugs* (ed. M.N.G. Dukes), p. 67. Excerpta Medica, Amsterdam.

Molloy, R.G., Welch, G.C., Drury, J.K., *et al.* (1995). Arterial thrombosis after chemotherapy with cisplatin, vincristine, and methotrexate. *Br. J. Clin. Pract.* 49, 50.

Monk. B.E., Parkes, J.D., and Du Vivier, A. (1984). Erythromelalgia following pergolide administration. *Br. J. Dermatol.* 111, 97.

Montaldi, D.H., Giambrone, J.P., Courey, N.G., *et al.* (1974). Podophyllin poisoning associated with the treatment of condylomata acuminata: a case report. *Am. J. Obstet. Gynecol.* 119, 1130.

Montastrue, J.L., Chamontin, B., Senard, J.M., *et al.* (1993). Pseudophaeochromocytoma in parkinsonian patient treated with fluoxetine plus selegiline. *Lancet* 341, 555.

Moorhead, E.L.II., Caldwell, J.R., Kelly, A.R., *et al.* (1966). The diagnosis of pheochromocytoma: analysis of 26 cases. *JAMA* 196, 1107.

Morgan, T. and Anderson, A. (1993). Interaction of indomethacin with felodipine. *J. Hypertension* 11 (suppl. 5), S338.

Morrison, R.J., Short, H.D., Noon, G.P., *et al.* (1993). Hypertension after lung transplantation. *J. Heart Lung Transplant.* 12, 92B.

Muelheims, G.H., Entrup, R.W., Paiewonsky, D., *et al.* (1965). Increased sensitivity of the heart to catecholamine-induced arrhythmias following guanethidine. *Clin. Pharmacol. Ther.* 6, 757.

Mullen, P.J. (1990). Unexpected first-dose hypotensive reaction to enalapril. *Postgrad. Med. J.* 66, 1087.

Murphy, J.L., Jr. (1993). Hypertension and pulmonary oedema associated with ketamine administration in a patient with a history of substance abuse. *Can. J. Anaesth.* 40, 160.

Mushin, W.W., Wien, R., Mason, D.F.J., *et al.* (1949). Curare-like actions of tri(diethylaminoethoxy)-benzine triethyliodide. *Lancet* i, 726.

Nelemans, F.A. (1972). Cholinomimetic drugs and anticholinesterases. In *Side Effects of Drugs*, Vol. 7 (ed. L. Meyler and A. Herxheimer), p. 240. Excerpta Medica, Amsterdam.

Newens, A.F. and Volz, R.G. (1972). Severe hypotension during prosthetic hip surgery with acrylic bone cement. *Anesthesiology* 36, 298.

Newfield, P. and Roizen, M.F. (1979). Hazards of rapid administration of vancomycin. *Ann. Intern. Med.* 91, 581.

Ng, K.H. and Sen, D.K. (1974). Hypotension with intravenous salbutamol in premature labour. *BMJ* iii, 211.

Nickerson, M. (1970). Drugs inhibiting adrenergic nerves and structures innervated by them. In *The Pharmacological Basis of Therapeutics* (ed. L.S. Goodman and A. Gilman), p. 560. Collier Macmillan, London.

Ogilvie, C.M. (1955). The treatment of pulmonary tuberculosis with iproniazid (1-isonicotinyl-2-isopropyl hydrazine) and isoniazid (isonicotinyl hydrazine). *Q. J. Med.* 24, 175.

Oh, T.E., Turner, C.W., Ilett, K.F., *et al.* (1978). Mechanism of the hypertensive effects of droperidol in phaeochromocytoma. *Anaesth. Intens. Care* 6, 322.

Omizo, M.K.N., Bryant, R.E., and Loveless, M.O. (1993). Amphotericin B-induced malignant hypertension. *Clin. Infect. Dis.* 17, 817.

Otteni, J.C., Sauvage, M.R., and Gauthier-Lafaye, J.P. (1969). Effets cardiovasculaires de la pentazocine. *Anaesth. Anal. Réanim.* 26, 271.

Page, Y., Tardy, B., Zeni, F., *et al.* (1991). Thrombotic thrombocytopenic purpura related to ticlopidine. *Lancet* 337, 774.

Palestine, A.G., Nussenblatt, B.B., and Chan, C.C (1984). Side-effects of systemic cyclosporine in a patient *not* undergoing transplantation. *Am. J. Med.* 77, 652.

Pantel, J., Schröder, J., Eysenbach, K., *et al.* (1997). Two cases of deep vein thrombosis associated with a combined paroxetine and zotepine therapy. *Pharmacopsychiatry* 30, 109.

Parish, R.C. and Miller, L.J. (1992). Adverse effects of angiotensin converting enzyme (ACE) inhibitors. An update. *Drug Safety* 7, 14.

Park, G.R. (1978). Hypotension following intravenous administration of metoclopramide during hypotensive anaesthesia for intracranial aneurysm. *Br. J. Anaesth.* 50, 1268.

Parke, T.J., Nandi, P.R., Bird, K.J., *et al.* (1992). Profound hypotension following intravenous codeine phosphate. Three case reports and some recommendations. *Anaesthesia* 47, 852.

Partridge, B.L., Key, T., and Reisner, L.S. (1988). Life-threatening effects of intravascular absorbtion of PGF₂ during therapeutic termination of pregnancy. *Anesth. Analg.* (Cleveland) 67, 111.

Paterson, A.H.G. (1978). Hypertensive reaction to adriamycin. *Cancer Treat. Rep.* 62, 1269.

Paton, W.D.M. (1957). Histamine release by compounds of simple chemical structure. *Pharmacol. Rev.* 9, 269.

Peach, M.J. (1971). Adrenal medullary stimulation induced by angiotensin, angiotensin II, and analogues. *Circ. Res.* 28 (Suppl. 2), 107.

Peach, M.J., Cline, W.H.J., and Watts, D.T. (1978). Release of adrenal catecholamines by angiotensin II. *Circ. Res.* 35, 592.

Pearson, A.C., Labovitz, A.J., and Kern, M.J. (1987). Accelerated hypertension complicated by myocardial infarction after use of a local anesthetic/vasoconstrictor preparation. *Am. Heart J.* 114, 662.

Peebles, D.J., Ellis, R.H., Stride, S.D.K., *et al.* (1972). Cardiovascular effects of methylmethacrylate cement. *BMJ* i, 349.

Pegg, M.S. (1980). Hypotension following metoclopramide injection. *Anaesthesia*, 35, 615.

Perotti, C., Toretta, L., Costamagna, L., *et al.* (1995). Thrombotic thrombocytopenic purpura after defibrotide therapy. *Haematologica* 79, 569.

Peschère, M., Zulman, G.B., Vogel, J-J., *et al.* (1996). Fingertip necrosis during chemotherapy with bleomycin, vin-cristine, and methotrexate for HIV-related Kaposi's sarcoma. *Br. J. Dermatol.* 134, 378.

Pettinger, W.A. and Keeton, K. (1975). Hypotension during angiotensin blockade with saralasin. *Lancet*, i, 1387.

Pettinger, W.A. and Oates, J.A. (1968). Supersensitivity to tyramine during monoamine oxidase inhibition in man; mechanism at the level of adrenergic neuron. *Clin. Pharmacol. Ther.* 9, 341.

Pinder, R.M., Brogden, R.N., Speight, T.M., *et al.* (1977). Voloxazine: a review of its pharmacological properties and therapeutic efficacy in depressive illness. *Drugs* 13, 401.

Pingleton, S.K., Schwartz, O., Szymanski, D., *et al.* (1982). Hypotension associated with terbutaline in acute quadriplegia. *Am. Rev. Resp. Dis.* 126, 723.

Plouin, P.F., Menard, J., and Corvol, P. (1976). Hypertensive crises in patient with phaeochromocytoma given metoclopramide. *Lancet* ii, 1357.

Pochmalaki, G., Meunier, P., Feldman, L., *et al.* (1993). Cholesterol embolisation after thrombolysis. *Arch. Mal. Coeur* 86, 263.

Portal, I., Cardenal, F., and Garcia-del-Muro, X. (1994). Etoposide-related acral erythema. *Cancer Chemother. Pharmacol.* 34, 181.

Prate, B. and Spreux, A. (1992). Subacute ischaemia of the left lower leg during dexfenfluramine and minocycline therapy. *Thérapie* 47, 438.

Prescott, L.F. (1972). Antipyretic analgesics and drugs used in rheumatic diseases and gout. In *Side Effects of Drugs*, Vol. 7 (ed. L. Meyler and A. Herxheimer), p. 156. Excerpta Medica, Amsterdam.

Price, H.L. and Dripps, R.D. (1970). General anaesthetics. In *The Pharmacological Basis of Therapeutics* (ed. L.S. Goodman and A. Gilman), p. 81. Collier Macmillan, London.

Prichard, B.N.C. (1964). Some cardiovascular actions of adrenergic beta-receptor blocking drugs in man. *Pharmacologist* 6, 166.

Pritchard, K.I., Paterson, A.H.G., and Paul, N.A. (1996). Increased thromboembolic complications with concurrent tamoxifen and chemotherapy in a randomized trial of adjuvant therapy for women with breast cancer. *J. Clin. Oncol.* 14, 2731.

Proye, C., Thevenin, D., Cecat, P., *et al.* (1989). Exclusive use of calcium channel blockers in preoperative and intraoperative control of pheochromocytoma: hemodynamic and free catecholamines assays in ten consecutive patients. *Surgery* 106, 1149.

Prull, A., Nechwatal, R., Riedel, H., *et al.* (1992). Treatment of heparin-induced thrombocytopenia and thrombosis with immunoglobulin. *Dtsch. Med. Wochenschr.* 117, 1838.

Quagliarello, J. and Barakat, R. (1987). Raynaud's phenomenon in infertile women treated with bromocriptine. *Fertil. Steril.* 48, 877.

Queen, H., Biem, H.J., Moe, G.W., *et al.* (1990). Development of cholesterol embolization syndrome after intravenous streptokinase for acute myocardial infarction. *Am. J. Cardiol.* 65, 1042.

Quick, A.J., Schanberge, J.N., and Stefanini, M. (1948). The effect of heparin on platelets *in vivo*. *J. Lab. Clin. Med.* 33, 1424.

Raine, A.E.G. (1988). Hypertension, blood viscosity and cardiovascular morbidity in renal failure: implications of erythropoietin therapy. *Lancet* i, 97.

Rampton, D.S. (1977). Hypertensive crisis in a patient given Sinemet, metoclopramide, and amitriptyline. *BMJ* ii, 607.

Ramsay, I.D. and Langlands, J.H.M. (1962). Phaeochromocytoma with hypotension and polycythaemia. *Lancet* ii, 126.

Ramsdell, W.M. (1989). Severe reaction to diphenhydramine. *Am. Acad. Dermatol.* 21, 1318.

Ratzenhofer, M. Personal communication to Winkler, H. and Smith, A.D. (1968). Catecholamines in phaeochromocytoma: normal storage but abnormal release? *Lancet* i, 793.

Raw, K. and Gaylis, H. (1976). Acute arterial spasm of the lower extremities after methysergide therapy. *S. Afr. Med. J.* 50, 1999.

Regen, T.J. (1990). Alcohol and the cardiovascular system. *JAMA* 264, 377.

Reich, D.L. (1989). Transient systemic arterial hypotension and cutaneous flushing in response to doxacuronium chloride. *Anesthesiology* 71, 783.

Reid, J.L., Wing, L.N.H., Dargie, H.J., *et al.* (1977). Clonidine withdrawal in hypertension. Changes in blood pressure and plasma and urinary noradrenaline. *Lancet* i, 1171.

Reid, T.J. III, Lombardo, F.A., Redmond, J. III, *et al.* (1992). Digital vasculitis associated with interferon therapy. *Am. J. Med.* 92, 702.

Rhodes, G.R., Dixon, R.H., and Silver, D. (1973). Heparin-induced thrombocytopenia with thrombotic and hemorrhagic manifestations. *Surg. Gynecol. Obstet.* 136, 409.

Ribstein, J., Rodier, M., and Mimran, A. (1989). Effect of cylosporin on blood pressure and renal function of recent type 1 diabetes mellitus. *J. Hypertension* 7 (suppl. 6), S198.

Robinson, M.J. and Williams, A. (1956). Clinical and pathological details of two cases of phaeochromocytoma in childhood. *Arch. Dis. Child.* 31, 69.

Rodger, J.C., Sheldon, C.O., Lerski, R.A., *et al.* (1976). Intermittent claudication complicating beta-blockade. *BMJ* i, 1125.

Roger, N., Pedrol, E., Casademont, J., *et al.* (1992). Protein C deficiency as a cause of deep vein thrombosis undergoing oral contraceptive treatment. *Med. Clin.* (Barc.) 98, 119.

Roland, C.B. (1959). Pheochromocytoma in pregnancy. Report of a fatal reaction to phentolamine (Regitine) methanesulfonate. *JAMA* 171, 1806.

Romanelli, V.A., Howie, M.B., Myerowitz, P.D., *et al.* (1993). Intraoperative and postoperative effects of vancomycin administration in cardiac surgery patients: a prospective, double-blind, randomized trial. *Crit. Care. Med.* 21, 1124.

Ross, E.J., Prichard, B.N.C., Kaufman, L., *et al.* (1967). Preoperative and operative management of patients with phaeochromocytoma. *BMJ* i, 191.

Rudnick, A. (1997). Fluoxetine-induced Raynaud's phenomenon. *Biol. Psychiatry* 41, 1218.

Runde, V., Aul, C., Heyll, A., *et al.* (1991). All-trans retinoic acid — not only a differentiating agent, but also an inducer of thromboembolic events in patients with acute promyelocytic leukaemia. *Onkologie* 14 (suppl. 2), 134.

Russell, R.M. and Jones, R.M. (1989). Postoperative hypotension associated with enalapril. *Anaesthesia* 44, 837.

Rygnestad, T. (1997). Severe hypotension associated with netilmicin treatment. *BMJ* 315, 31.

SADRAC Bulletin (1989). Dihydroergotamine + lidocaine — vasospasm. *Bulletin from the Swedish Adverse Drug Reactions Advisory Committee* 54, 1.

SADRAC Bulletin (1997). Polidocanol-embolism. *Bulletin from the Swedish Adverse Drug Reactions Advisory Committee* 65, 2.

Sachdev, Y., Gomez-Pan, A., Tunbridge, W.M.G., *et al.* (1975). Bromocriptine therapy in acromegaly. *Lancet* ii, 1164.

Sahloul, M.Z., al-Kiek, R., Ivanovich, P., *et al.* (1990). Non-steroidal anti-inflammatory drugs and antihypertensives. Cooperative malfeasance. *Nephron* 56, 345.

Salz, L.B., Tiersten, A., Hassan, B.N., *et al.* (1995). Acute hypertensive crisis following octreotide administration in a patient with malignant phaeochromocytoma. *Oncology Reports* 2, 1129.

Sanders, B.P., Portman, R.J., Ramey, R.A., *et al.* (1992). Hypertension during reduction of long-term steroid therapy in young subjects with asthma. *J. Allergy Clin. Immunol.* 89, 816.

Sandler, R.M., Seifer, D.B., Morgan, K., *et al.* (1985). Heparin-induced thrombocytopenia and thrombosis. Detection and specificity of a platelet-aggregation IgG. *Am. J. Clin. Pathol.* 83, 760.

Sarcione, E.J., Back, N., Sokal, J.E., *et al.* (1963). Elevation of plasma epinephrine levels produced by glucagon *in vivo*. *Endocrinology* 72, 523.

Sato, O., Takagi, A., Miyata, T., *et al.* (1995). Aortic aneurysm in patients with autoimmune disorders treated with corticosteroids. *Eur. J. Endovasc. Surg.* 10, 366.

Saunders, J.B., Beevers, D.G., and Paton, A. (1981). Alcohol-induced hypertension. *Lancet* ii, 856.

Schachter, M. (1988). Cyclosporine A and hypertension. *J. Hypertension* 6, 511.

Scherrer, U., Vissing, S.F., Morgan, B.J., *et al.* (1990). Cyclosporine-induced sympathetic activation and hypertension after heart transplantation. *N. Engl. J. Med.* 323, 693.

Schindel, L. (1972). Intravenous infusion solutions and emulsions. In *Side Effects of Drugs* (ed. L. Meyler and A. Herxheimer), p. 479. Excerpta Medica, Amsterdam.

Schmidt, G.R. and Schuna, A.A. (1988). Rebound hypertension after discontinuation of transdermal clonidine. *Clin. Pharm.* 7, 772.

Schmitt, J.K. and Moore, J.R. (1993). Hypertension secondary to chlorpropamide with amelioration by changing to insulin. *Am. J. Hypertens.* 6, 317.

Schoenfeld, A., Friedman, S., Bod, N., *et al.* (1989) Antagonism of antihypertensive drug therapy in pregnancy by indomethacin? *Am. J. Obstet.* 161, 204.

Schoenfeld, A., Friedman, S., Stein, L.B., *et al.* (1987). Severe hypertension reaction after naloxone injection during labor. *Arch. Gynecol.* 240, 45.

Schrijvers, D. Wanders, J., Dirix, L., *et al.* (1993). Coping with toxicities of docetaxel (Taxotere TM). *Ann. Oncol.* 4, 610.

Schroeder, J.M. and Weeth, J.B. (1967). Phase II evaluation of fluorometholone (NSC-33001). *Cancer Chemother. Abstr.* 51, 525.

Schulman, S., Johnsson, R., and Lindmarker, P. (1991). Thrombotic complications after substitution with a factor VII concentration. *Thromb. Haemost.* 66, 619.

Scian, L.F., Westerman, C.D., Verdesca, A.S., *et al.* (1960). Adrenocortical and medullary effects of glucagon in dogs. *Am. J. Physiol.* 199, 867.

Scott, J.N. and McDevitt, B.G. (1976). Rebound hypertension after acute methyldopa withdrawal. *BMJ* ii, 367.

Seedat, Y.K., Bhoola, R., and Rampono, J.G. (1975). Prazosin in treatment of hypertension. *BMJ* ii, 305.

Seeler, H.A.J., de Meijer, P.H.E., and Meinclers, A.E. (1997). Serotonin reuptake-inhibitor unmasks a pheochromocytoma. *Ann. Intern. Med.* 126, 333.

Semple, P.F., Thoren, P., and Lever, A.F. (1988). Vasovagal reactions to cardiovascular drugs: the first dose effect. *J. Hypertension* 6, 601.

Sennesael, J., Dupont, A.G., Verbeeler, D.L., *et al.* (1986). Hypertension and cyclosporine. *Ann. Intern. Med.* 104, 729.

Sentenie, J.B., Tuinbreijer, W.E., Kreis, R.W., *et al.* (1992). Digital gangrene after accidental intra-arterial injection of phenytoin (Epanutin R$_m$). *Eur. J. Surg.* 158, 315.

Shall, L., Lucas G.S., Whittaker, J.A., *et al.* (1988). Painful red hands: a side effect of leukaemia therapy. *Br. J. Dermatol.* 119, 249.

Shanks, R.G. (1970). Hypotension caused by L-dopa. *BMJ* iii, 403.

Shaub, R.O. (1960). Ischemic necrosis due to administration of metaraminol. *JAMA* 172, 154.

Sheaves, R., Chew, S.L., and Grossman, A.B. (1995). The dangers of unopposed beta-adrenergic blockade in phaeochromocytoma. *Postgrad. Med. J.* 71, 58.

Shir, Y. and Raja, S.N. (1993). Indigo carmine-induced severe hypotension in patients undergoing radical prostatectomy. *Anesthesiology* 79, 378.

Shulman, K.I., Tailor, S.A.N., Walker, S.E., *et al.* (1997). Tap (draught) beer and monoamine oxidase inhibitor dietary restrictions. *Can. J. Psychiatry* 42, 310.

Siddiqui, M.A. and Ford, P.A. (1995). Acute severe autonomic insufficiency during pentamidine therapy. *South. Med. J.* 88, 1087.

Siegel, J.P., Puri, R.K. (1991). Interleukin-2 toxicity. *J. Clin. Oncol.* 9, 694.

Siehe, H.J. (1934). Die Reaktion des denervierten Nebennierenmarkes auf humorale Sekretionsweise. *Arch. Ges. Physiol.* 234, 204.

Silver, D., Kapsch, D.N., and Tsoi, E.K.M. (1983). Heparin-induced thrombocytopenia, thrombosis, and hemorrhage. *Ann. Surg.* 198, 301.

Sloand, E.M. and Thompson, B.T. (1984). Propranolol induced pulmonary edema and shock in a patient with pheochromocytoma. *Arch. Intern. Med.* 144, 173.

Smith, G.W. and Hurst, N.P. (1993). Vasculitis, Raynaud's phenomenon and polyarthritis associated with gemfihrozil therapy. *Br. J. Rheumatol.* 32, 84.

Smith, N.L. (1957). Histamine release by suxamethonium. *Anaesthesia* 12, 293.

Sniper, W. (1952). The estimation and comparison of histamine release by muscle relaxants. *Br. J. Anaesth.* 24, 232

Solimando, D.A., Jr, Phillips, E.T., Weiss, R.B., *et al.* (1996). Hypertensive reactions associated with paclitaxel. *Cancer Invest.* 14, 340.

Solosko, D. and Smith, R.B. (1972). Hypertension following 10 per cent phenylephrine ophthalmic. *Anesthesiology* 36, 187.

Spedding, M. (1980). Effects of metoclopramide and isoprenaline on the rat vas deferens: interaction with adrenoceptors. *Br. J. Pharmacol.* 71, 113.

Sperzel, W.D., Glassman, H.N., Jordan D.C., *et al.* (1986). Overall safety of terazosin as an antihypertensive agent. *Am. J. Med.* 80 (suppl. 5B), 77.

Spieker. C., Barenbrock, M., Wieneke, R., *et al.* (1991). Acute hypertension after renal allograft rejection therapy with OCT3. *Int. J. Med. Res.* 19, 419.

Spivak, B., Radvan, M., and Shine, M. (1987). Postural hypotension with syncope possibly precipitated by trazodone. *Am. J. Psychiatry* 144, 1512.

Sprung, J., Distel, D., Bloomfield, E.L., *et al.* (1996). Cardiovascular collapse during anaesthesia in a patient with preoperatively discontinued chronic MAO inhibitor therapy. *J. Clin. Anaesth.* 8, 662.

Stafford, P.J., Strachan, C.J.L., Vincent, R., *et al.* (1989). Multiple microemboli after disintegration of clot during thrombolysis for acute myocardial infarction. *BMJ* 299, 1310.

Staszewska-Barczak, J. and Vane, J.R. (1965). The release of catecholamines from the adrenal medulla by histamine. *Br. J. Pharmacol.* 24, 728.

Steele, J.M. Jr, and Lowenstein, J. (1975). Differential effects of angiotensin II analogue on pressor and adrenal receptors in the rabbit. *Circ. Res.* 35, 592.

Stelzer, F.T., Stubenbord, J.J., Sreenivasan, V., *et al.* (1976). Late toxicity of clonidine withdrawal. *N. Engl. J. Med.* 294, 1182.

Stevens, F.R.T. (1966). A danger of sympathomimetic drugs. *Med. J. Aust.* ii, 576.

Stewart, M. (1976). MAOIs and food — fact and fiction. *Adverse Drug React. Bull.* 58, 196.

Stewart, M. and Burris, J.F. (1988). Clonidine: rebound hypertension. *Drug Intell. Clin. Pharm.* 22, 573.

Stockley, I. (1974). *Drug Interactions and their Mechanisms.* The Pharmaceutical Press, London.

Stoner, T.R. and Urbach, K.F. (1968). Cardiac arrhythmias associated with succinylcholine in a patient with pheochromocytoma. *Anesthesiology* 19, 1228.

Stromblad, B.C.R. (1960). Effect of denervation and of cocaine on action of sympathetic amines. *Br. J. Pharmacol.* 15, 328.

Suchowersky, O. and Devries, J. (1990). Possible interactions between Deprenyl and Prozac. *Can. J. Neurol. Sci.* 17, 352.

Sumikawa, K. and Amakata, Y. (1977). The pressor effect of droperidol on a patient with pheochromocytoma. *Anesthesiology* 46, 359.

Supprian, U. (1969). Ueber einen Fall von Antabus-intoxikation. *Nervenarzt* 40, 276.

Svedmyr, N. (1968). The influence of a tricyclic antidepressant agent (protriptyline) on some of the circulatory effects of noradrenaline and adrenaline in man. *Life Sci.* 7, 77.

Swan, H.J.C. (1949). Effects of noradrenaline in the human circulation. *Lancet* ii, 508.

Szczygielski, J. (1932). Die adrenalinabsondernde Wirkung des Histamins und ihre Beinflussung durch Nikotin. *Naunyn Schmiedebergs Arch. Exp. Pathol. Pharmakol.* 166, 319.

Tada, Y., Tsuda, Y., Otsuka, T., *et al.* (1992). Case report: nifedepine–rifampicin interaction attenuates the blood pressure in a patient with essential hypertension. *Am. J. Med. Sci.* 303, 25.

Tailor, S.A.N., Shulma, N.K.I., Walker, S.E., *et al.* (1994). Hypertensive episode associated with phenelzine and tap beer — a re-analysis of the role of pressor amines in beer. *J. Clin. Psychopharmacol.* 14, 5.

Tanaka, G.Y. (1974). Hypertensive reaction to naloxone. *JAMA* 228, 25.

Tao, P.K., Nicholls, M.G., and Lai, K.N. (1990). The complications of newer transplant antirejection drugs: treatment with cyclosporin A, OKT3, and FK 506. *Adverse Drug React. Acute Poisoning Rev.* 9, 123.

Taylor, D., Reveley, A., and Faivre, F. (1995). Clozapine-induced hypotension treated with moclobemide and Bovril. *Br. J. Psychiatry* 167, 409.

Taylor, J.E., McLaren, M., Henderson, I.S., *et al.* (1992). Prothrombotic effect of epoetin therapy and epoetin withdrawal in haemodialysis patients. *Nephrol. Dial. Transplant.* 7, 1158.

Testani, M., Jr. (1994). Clozapine-induced orthostatic hypotension treated with fludrocortisone. *J. Clin. Psychiatry* 55, 497.

Tester, W.J., Cohn, J.B., Fleekop, P.D., *et al.* (1990). Successful rechallenge to etoposide after an acute vasomotor response. *J. Clin. Oncol.* 8, 1600.

Thakore, R.E., Dinan, T.G., Kelleher, M., *et al.* (1992). Alcohol-free beer and the irreversible monoamine oxidase inhibitors. *Int. Clin. Psychopharmacol.* 7, 59.

Theodossiou, C., Kroog, C., Ettinghausen, S., *et al.* (1994). Acute arterial thrombosis in a patient with breast cancer after treatment with fluorouracil, leucovorin, cyclophosphamide, and interleukin-3. *Cancer* 74, 2808.

Thompson, M.E., Shapiro, A.P., Johnsen, A.M., *et al.* (1986). The contrasting effects of cyclosporin A and azathioprine on arterial blood pressure and renal function following cardiac transplantation. *Int. J. Cardiol.* 11, 219.

Tirlapur, V.G., Evans, P.J., and Jones, M.K. (1986). Shock syndrome after acebutolol. *Br. J.Clin. Pract.* 40, 33.

Tisdale, J.E., Colucci, R.D., Ujhelyi, M.R., *et al.* (1992). Evaluation and comparison of the adverse effects of streptokinase and alteplase. *Pharmacotherapy* 12, 440.

Tomson, C.R.V., Venning, M.C., and Ward, M.K. (1988). Blood pressure and erythropoietin. *Lancet* i, 351.

Turner, A.S. (1976). Prazosin in hypertension. *BMJ* ii, 1257.

Turner, M.C. and Holman, J.M., Jr. (1993). Late reactions during initial OKT3 treatment. *Clin. Transplant.* 7, 1.

Unger, R.H., Eisentraut, A.M., McCall, M.S., *et al.* (1962). Measurement of endogenous glucagon in plasma and the influence of blood glucose concentrations upon its secretion. *J. Clin. Invest.* 41, 682.

Vale, J.A. and Jeffereys, D.B. (1978). Peripheral gangrene complicating beta-blockade. *Lancet* i, 1216.

Valentine, B.H., Martin, M.A., and Phillips, N.V. (1977). Collapse during operation following intravenous ergotamine. *Br. J. Anaesth.* 49, 81.

Vallance, P., Benjamin, N., and Collier, J. (1988). Erythropoietin, haemoglobin, and hypertensive crises. *Lancet* i, 1107.

van Reempts, P. and Van Overmeir, B. (1990). Topical use of nitroglycerin in neonates. *J. Pediatr.* 116, 155.

van Vroonhoven, T.J.M. (1977). Intermittent claudication in premenopausal women. *J. Cardiovasc. Surg.* 18, 291.

van Way, C.W., Faraci, R.P., Cleveland, H.C., *et al.* (1976). Hemorrhagic necrosis of pheochromocytoma associated with phentolamine administration. *Ann. Surg.* 184, 26.

Vanholder, R., Carpenter, R.J., Schurgers, M., *et al.* (1977). Rebound phenomenon during gradual withdrawal of clonidine. *BMJ* i, 1138.

Vayssairat, M., Fiessinger, J.N., Becquemin, M.H., *et al.* (1978). Association déhydroergotamine et triacétyloleandomycine. Rôle dans une necrose digitale iatrogène. *Nouv. Presse Méd.* 7, 2077.

Veber, B., Gauté, M., Michel-Cherqui, M., *et al.* (1992). Severe hypertension during postpartum haemorrhage after I.V. administration of prostaglandin E$_2$. *Br. J. Anaesth.* 68, 623.

Vial, T. and Descoles, J.L. (1992). Clinical toxicity of interleukin-2. *Drug Safety* 7, 417.

Villa, P., Aznar, J., Mira, Y., *et al.* (1996). Third generation oral contraceptives and low free protein S as a risk for thrombosis. *Lancet* 347, 397.

Vincent, D. and Pradalier, A. (1993). Pheochromocytoma-like catecholamine levels induced by clonidine cessation. *Eur. J. Med.* 2, 313.

Volle, R.L. and Koelle, G.B. (1970). Ganglionic stimulating and blocking agents. In *The Pharmacological Basis of Therapeutics* (ed. L. S. Goodman and A. Gilman), pp. 596, 598. Collier Macmillan, London.

Von Gunten, C.F., Roth E.L., and Von Roem, J.H. (1993). Raynaud phenomenon in three patients with acquired immunodeficiency syndrome-related Kaposi sarcoma treated with bleomycin. *Cancer* 72, 2004.

Wachter, R.M. (1987). Symptomatic hypertension induced by nifedipine in the acute treatment of severe hypertension. *Arch. Intern. Med.* 147, 556.

Waller, P.C., Cameron, H.A., and Ramsay, L.E. (1987). Profound hypotension after the first dose of ketanserin. *Postgrad. Med. J.* 63, 305.

Wark, J.D. and Larkins, R.G. (1978). Pulmonary oedema after propranolol therapy in two cases of phaeochromocytoma. *BMJ* i, 1395.

Wass, J.A.H., Thorner, M.O., and Besser, G.M. (1976). Digitalis vasospasm with bromocriptine. *Lancet* i, 1135.

Wass, J.A. H., Thorner, M.O., Morris, D.V. *et al.* (1977). Long-term treatment of acromegaly with bromocriptine. *BMJ* i, 875.

Watson, B. (1972). Transient hypotension following intravenous ethamsylate (Dicynene). *BMJ* i, 1664.

Webb, D.G. and White J.P. (1980). Hypertension after taking hydralazine. *BMJ* 280, 1582.

Webster, L.T. (1985). Drugs used in the chemotherapy of protozoal infections. In *Goodman and Gilman's The Pharmacological Basis of Therapeutics* (7th edn) (ed. A.G. Gilman, L.S. Goodman, T.W. Rall, and F. Murad), p. 1062. Macmillan, New York.

Weidle, P.J. and Vlasses, P.H. (1988). Systemic hypertension associated with cyclosporine: a review. *Drug Intell. Clin. Pharm.* 22, 443.

Wein, P., Robertson, B., and Ratten, G.J. (1989). Cardiorespiratory collapse and pulmonary oedema due to intravascular absorption of prostaglandin $F_{2\alpha}$ administered intra-amniotically for midtrimester termination of pregnancy. *Aust. N.Z. J. Obstet. Gynaecol.* 29, 261.

Weinblatt, M.E., Coblyn, J.S., Fraser, P.A. *et al.* (1987). Cyclosporin A treatment of refractory rheumatoid arthritis. *Arthritis Rheum.* 30, 11.

Weiner, N., Draskoczy, P.R., and Burack, W.R. (1962). Ability of tyramine to liberate catecholamines *in vivo*. *J. Pharmacol. Exp. Ther.* 137, 47.

Weiss, M.E., Chatham, F., Kagey-Sobotka, A. *et al.* (1990). Serial immunological investigation in a patient who had a life-threatening reaction to intravenous protamine. *Clin. Exper. Allergy* 20, 713.

Weitz, I.C., Israel, V.K., and Lieberman, H.A. (1997). Tamoxifen-associated venous thrombosis and activated protein C resistance due to factor V Leiden. *Cancer* 79, 2024.

Werder, E.A., Waibel, P., Sege, D., *et al.* (1990). Severe thrombosis during oestrogen treatment of tall stature. *Eur. J. Pediatr.* 149, 389.

Werquin, S., Kacet, S., Caron, J. *et al.* (1987). Raynaud's phenomenon and finger necrosis after treatment of an ovarian seminoma with bleomycin, vinblastine, and 5-fluorouracil. *Ann. Cardiol. Angiol.* 36, 409.

Western, K.A., Perera, D.R., and Schultz, M.G. (1976). Pentamidine isethionate in the treatment of *Pneumocystis carinii* pneumonia. *Ann. Intern. Med.* 73, 695.

Westgate, H.D. and van Bergen, F.H. (1962). Changes in histamine blood levels following D-tubocurarine. *Can. Anesth. Soc. J.* 9, 497.

White, N.W. (1989). Venous thrombosis and rifampicin. *Lancet* ii, 434.

Wieland, T. and Stäubli, M. (1988). Serious complications of enalapril therapy with cardiac failure. *Schweiz. Med. Wochenschr.* 118, 1789.

Wilkins, R.W., Geer, W.E.R., and Culbertson, J.W. (1950). Extensive laboratory studies of a patient with pheochromocytoma before and after successful operation. *Arch. Intern. Med.* 86, 51.

Williams, P. and Foster, M.E. (1995). Deep vein thrombosis related to formestane. *Breast* 4, 71.

Williams, R., Blackburn, A., Neuberger, J., *et al.* (1985). Long-term use of cyclosporin in liver grafting. *Q. J. Med.* 57, 897.

Wing-Tin, L.N., Elalaoui, M.Y., and Akula, E. (1994). Arterial spasm after administration of diazepam. *Br. J. Anaesth.* 72, 139.

Winter, S., Frankle, H., Ribot, S., *et al.* (1973). Sorbitol-induced coma in uremic patients undergoing peritoneal dialysis. *J. Newark Beth Israel Med. Center* 23, 175.

Womack, A.M. (1963). Tranylcypromine. *Lancet* ii, 463.

Wong, K.C., Li, P.K.T., Lui, S.F., *et al.* (1990). *Adverse Drug React. Acute Poisoning Rev.* 9, 183.

Woods, K.L. (1978). Hypotensive effect of propranolol and phenoperidine in tetanus. *BMJ* ii, 1164.

Wu, C.C. and Johnson, A.J. (1969). The vasopressor effects of indigo carmine. *Henry Ford Hosp. Med. J.* 17, 131.

Yard, A.C. and Kadowitz, P.J. (1972). Studies on the mechanism of hydrocortisone potentiation of vasoconstrictor response to epinephrine in the anaesthetized animal. *Eur. J. Pharmacol.* 20, 1.

Yasaka, M., Yamaguchi, T., Yonehara, T., *et al.* (1994). Recurrent embolization during intravenous administration of tissue plasminogen activator in acute cardioembolic stroke. *Angiology* 45, 481.

Young, K. (1990). Enalapril and SPPS. *Anaesth. Intensive Care* 18, 583.

Zapata, E. and Orwin, A. (1992). Severe hypertension and bronchospasm during disulfiram–ethanol test reaction. *BMJ* 305, 870.

Zenore, T., Durieu, I., Nagnoug F., *et al.* (1996). Raynaud's phenomenon associated with bromocriptine. *Rev. Med. Interne* 17, 948.

10. Respiratory disorders

N. P. KEANEY

Introduction

Pulmonary damage caused by undesired effects of drugs is being recognized with increasing frequency in clinical practice. The manner in which the lung responds to a toxic insult is limited and drugs in a particular category are very likely to induce the same adverse drug reaction (ADR). The symptoms and signs and the radiological and laboratory features, are mainly non-specific. An adverse drug reaction may therefore be readily confused with an exacerbation of a continuing disease process. This is especially true if the onset is subacute or chronic, and great vigilance is necessary if the correct diagnosis is to be made. A recent development is a continuously updated list of drugs that may injure the respiratory system on a Web page at:

http://www.pneumotox.com/lungdrug

(Foucher *et al.* 1997). Thus suspicion about an ADR can be readily confirmed for new drugs and a tentative diagnosis made. Rechallenge is not usually undertaken to confirm a diagnosis of pulmonary adverse reactions — surprisingly in view of the widespread clinical use of challenge testing in the assessment of occupational asthma and extrinsic allergic alveolitis, for example, in pigeon fanciers.

In some instances the ADR is due to a known pharmacological effect of the drug (Type A reaction) and in others it is the result of totally aberrant and unpredictable effects (Type B reaction). In many, the underlying mechanism is obscure, but usually it is possible to identify the level in the respiratory tract at which the disorder is arising. Only the pulmonary vasculature, bronchi and lower airways, lung parenchyma, pleural space, mediastinum, and central ventilatory control and respiratory muscles will be discussed here; the upper airways and nose are discussed in Chapter 22.

Pulmonary vasculature

Pulmonary arteries

Pulmonary thromboembolism

Pharmacoepidemiological investigation was firmly established as a methodology in the 1960s with the convincing demonstration that the incidence of thromboembolic disease necessitating hospitalization was nine times higher in women who had taken oral contraceptives than in those who had not (Vessey and Doll 1968). The strong possibility of an association with the dose of oestrogen in combined preparations was subsequently shown (Inman *et al.* 1970), and Lehrman (1976), not surprisingly, found an increased risk of thromboembolism in transsexual males treated with high doses of oral oestrogen. More recently, Vessey and colleagues (1986) have confirmed the thromboembolic risk of oral contraceptives in a large prospective study of 17 000 married women, aged 25–39 years, in whom 105 episodes of venous thromboembolism occurred, 71 postoperatively. The incidence of certain or probable deep venous thrombosis or pulmonary embolism was 0.43 per thousand woman-years in users and 0.06 in non-users of oral contraceptives. The prevalence of postoperative problems was high, but the risk was confined to current users. Sue-Ling and Hughes (1988) believed the risk of pregnancy did not warrant discontinuing a combined oral contraceptive preoperatively but a progestogen-only pill is undoubtedly safer. Hormone-replacement therapy (HRT) has recently come under scrutiny and three papers were reviewed in a *Lancet* editorial by Vandenbroucke and Helmerhorst (1996); the relative risk of venous thrombosis ranged from 2.1 to 6.9 and was related to the daily dose of oestrogen. The absolute risk was low at one extra case per 5000 users per year at an odds ratio of 3.5.

Other forms of embolism

Pulmonary embolization of particulate matter may occur during intravenous therapy and incorrect techniques may result in part of a cannula being sheared off. Intravenous illicit substance abuse may cause pulmonary thrombosis or granulomatous vasculitis or infections, for example, a staphylococcal abscess. Self-administration of crushed tablets is especially dangerous because of particulate fillers, which impact in pulmonary arterioles, and episodes with clinical features of pulmonary embolism may occur (Ali and Banks 1973). Progression to severe pulmonary hypertension and death may follow (Wendt *et al.* 1964). Foreign body granulomatosis due to corn starch (Hahn *et al.* 1969) or microcrystalline cellulose (Tomashefski *et al.* 1981) or talc (Heffner *et al.* 1990) is well recognized. Lysis and embolization of a right atrial clot infected with the cutaneous fungus *Malassezia furfur* followed urokinase administration, necessitating left pneumonectomy because of multiple pulmonary infarcts that had become infected with the fungus (Hassall *et al.* 1983). *M. furfur* pulmonary vasculitis has been reported following parenteral feeding with Intralipid (Redline and Dahms 1981) — the accumulation of lipid in pulmonary capillaries (well documented in neonates and infants) becoming the focus of the infection with this highly lipophilic fungus.

Perfusion lung scans utilize embolized particles, for example, macroaggregated albumin labelled with the radioisotope ^{99m}technetium. The investigation has a remarkable safety record and is only risky in patients with severe pulmonary hypertension (Dworkin *et al.* 1966; Child *et al.* 1975).

Pulmonary hypertension

From 1967 to 1969 an increase in the incidence of pulmonary hypertension occurred. It was particularly noted in Switzerland and seems to have been confined to those countries in which the appetite-suppressant aminorex fumarate was marketed (Follath *et al.* 1971; Kay *et al.* 1971). The syndrome was characterized by progressive dyspnoea, cardiac failure, effort syncope, and sometimes sudden death. The evidence implicating aminorex fumarate is circumstantial but strong. Animal experiments failed, however, to reproduce the syndrome, even in primates. Pulmonary hypertension has been reported in association with other anorectics including amphetamines (Malmquist *et al.* 1970), fenfluramine (McMurray *et al.* 1986), and dexfenfluramine (Abenhaim *et al.* 1996). It may follow use of an oral contraceptive (Kleiger *et al.* 1976) and, as mentioned above, may complicate intravenous substance abuse. In September 1997 the marketing of fenfluramine and dexfenfluramine was suspended voluntarily in Europe and North America because of a report (Connolly *et al.* 1997) of development of anomalies of cardiac valves in 30 per cent of 292 obese patients using these drugs, particularly in combination with phentermine.

The eosinophilia–myalgia syndrome due to L-tryptophan: pulmonary hypertension

In 1989 a new syndrome typified by eosinophilia and myalgia was attributed to tryptophan used either as a health food supplement or as an antidepressant. It involves the skin, fascia, and muscle but breathlessness and cough are frequent (Medsger 1990). Surprisingly, even with severe respiratory distress the chest radiograph shows normal lung fields. A rapid response to steroid therapy in 4 days with normalization of hypoxaemia and pulmonary hypertension and the other clinical features was reported by MacLennan and Steward (1990). A number of cases were reported and a particular manufacturer was linked epidemiologically to many cases in the USA. Subsequently L-tryptophan was withdrawn from both the nutritional and pharmaceutical markets internationally. This disorder is discussed in greater detail in Chapter 18. The Spanish toxic oil syndrome caused by ingestion of adulterated cooking oil has many similarities (Bolster and Silver 1994).

Pulmonary vasculitis

The current views about the classification of vasculitis are usefully reviewed by Lie (1994). Drug hypersensitivity-related vasculitis is placed with other secondary vasculitides. The clinical features depend on the size of the blood vessels involved and whether immune-complexes or necrosis occurs. Polyarteritis nodosa affects predominantly medium-sized vessels, is usually idiopathic and its diagnosis can be difficult in the absence of systemic manifestations. Not surprisingly, therefore, a number of drugs were proposed as aetiological agents, for example, gold salts, iodides, penicillin, phenytoin, and sulphonamides (Symmers 1958).

Diffuse intrapulmonary haemorrhage (DIH)

Involvement of small vessels — arterioles, capillaries, and venules — by the vasculitic inflammatory process may occur with or without medium vessels being affected. Capillaritis is associated with diffuse (alveolar) haemorrhage. This phenomenon is best recognized in Goodpasture's syndrome, in which circulating antibodies to glomerular basement membrane (anti-GBM) can be detected, and glomerulonephritis (GN) is usual. Three fatal cases of DIH with GN due to penicillamine given for Wilson's disease have been described (Sternlieb *et al.* 1975). It has also occurred with penicillamine given for rheumatoid arthritis (Turner Warwick 1981) but, as anti-GBM was absent in the six patients in whom it was estimated, it is inappropriate to call the reaction Goodpasture's syndrome. DIH, with or without GN, seems a more accurate description. This type of response has been reported with aminoglutethimide (Rodman *et al.* 1986); cocaine smoking (Murray *et al.* 1988); nitrofurantoin (Bucknall *et al.* 1987); febarbamate — a tranquillizer (Gali *et al.* 1986); and amphotericin (Haber *et al.* 1986). An interaction between amphotericin and leucocyte infusion in patients with leukaemia was reported by Wright and colleagues (1981). Fourteen of 22 patients receiving these therapies developed haemoptysis, and the chest X-rays showed widespread pulmonary infiltrates. Open lung biopsy in four showed DIH. Five of the 14 affected patients died from respiratory failure.

In DIH, haemoptysis is usual and may be profuse, and the decrease in haemoglobin level is proportional to the degree of pulmonary infiltration. The onset may be rapid and the clinical and radiological findings have been mistaken for left ventricular failure; the absence of cardiomegaly in DIH may be a helpful differentiating feature. At bronchoscopy, blood is seen throughout the bronchial tree and bronchoalveolar lavage will show haemosiderin-laden macrophages, as will transbronchial biopsy. Alveolar haemorrhage may also be seen on transbronchial biopsy but video-assisted thoracoscopic lung biopsy or autopsy will show widespread bleeding into alveoli and alveolar walls. Very often the appearances obscure evidence of a pulmonary vasculitis. Smith (1990) has suggested that a capillaritis is the underlying pathological process in drug-related DIH, in contrast to the other diseases in which it has been described, for example, polyarteritis nodosa, rheumatoid arthritis (in the absence of penicillamine), Wegener's granulomatosis (positive antineutrophil cytoplasmic antibody), and a miscellany of other conditions, both infective and idiopathic. In view of the potential seriousness of DIH it is not surprising that rechallenge is rarely attempted, but Gali and colleagues (1986) reported eosinophilia and a skin rash when their patient was re-exposed to febarbamate.

Alveolar haemorrhage is not an inevitable consequence of pulmonary vasculitis. Two patients with a hypersensitivity reaction to phenytoin, manifesting as fever, breathlessness, hypoxaemia, maculopapular rash, lymphadenopathy, and bilateral pulmonary infiltrate on chest X-ray, were diagnosed as having hypersensitivity pneumonitis on transbronchial lung biopsy (TBB). Open lung biopsy, however, revealed histological evidence of a vasculitis (Michael and Rudin 1981). TBB are usually very small and are unlikely to sample vessels of sufficient size to detect vasculitis. The modern approach to this problem is to proceed to a diagnostic thoracoscopic biopsy.

Drug-related systemic lupus erythematosus (D-RSLE)

Pleuropulmonary manifestations are common in acute SLE, whether drug-induced or idiopathic. Cough, breathlessness, and pleuritic pain are usual presenting symptoms and radiologically there may be patchy pulmonary infiltrates or a pleural reaction, or both of these. A small-lung syndrome is of unclear cause but does not seem to be due to pulmonary fibrosis. Withdrawal of the drug responsible and administration of corticosteroids usually results in complete resolution. A confounding feature, however, is the propensity with which patients with SLE react to drugs rather frequently. Procainamide is the most frequent cause of D-RSLE and a review of 17 cases (Byrd and Schanzer 1969) found that onset of SLE varied from 1–35 weeks from the start of treatment with this drug. Seven patients had pleurisy, sometimes with an effusion, but only one developed a pulmonary infiltrate. Hydralazine and isoniazid are also well recognized as causes of D-RSLE. A number of other drugs have been implicated and the subject is discussed further in Chapter 18.

Pulmonary capillaries: pulmonary oedema

Intravenous fluids

Excessive intravenous infusion of fluid is the most frequent cause of iatrogenic pulmonary oedema. Blood and plasma-expanding agents are a threat to patients with inadequate cardiac reserves, especially in the presence of renal impairment. In the presence of severe renal failure even solutions of glucose in water may be dangerous.

Adult respiratory distress syndrome (ARDS)

In severely ill patients, injury to the alveolar–capillary membrane can occur, and so pulmonary oedema may follow replacement of major blood loss by electrolyte solutions. Activation of neutrophils, which become sequestered in the pulmonary circulation and adhere to the pulmonary capillary endothelium, has been proposed as the general mechanism underlying ARDS. Increasing leakiness of the basement membrane, an intra-alveolar exudate, and an inflammatory cell infiltrate ensue. With continued damage to the capillary endothelium extravasation of a proteinaceous fluid into the alveolar walls and alveoli results in stiff lungs and impaired gas exchange. Profound hypoxaemia follows and when associated with multiple organ failure a mortality rate of 80 per cent is common. Incorporation of the exudate into the alveolar wall results in its organization and subsequent fibrosis, unless the insult is single and of short duration. This condition is called the adult respiratory distress syndrome but when it is drug induced the term non-cardiogenic pulmonary oedema has been used. Measurement of pulmonary arterial wedge pressure may help in the diagnosis of ARDS.

Narcotics and intravenous abuse

Many cases of non-cardiogenic pulmonary oedema as a complication of heroin (diamorphine) abuse were encountered 20–25 years ago in the USA (Steinberg and Karliner 1968; Frand *et al.* 1972). The condition was also described with methadone (Schaaf *et al.* 1973), of which as little as 60 mg orally was found to precipitate pulmonary oedema (Zyroff *et al.* 1974). With narcotics the problem is exacerbated by the possibility of continuing reactions to impurities in 'street' heroin injected by addicts, but it is well established that pulmonary oedema can be caused by pharmaceutically pure diamorphine. The syndrome is not like anaphylaxis, as the onset is commonly delayed, for more than 24 hours in some instances. The severity is variable, ranging from a few basal crackles to typical 'butterfly' infiltrative radiological changes, from mild dyspnoea to overwhelming respiratory failure with severe hypoxaemia necessitating mechanical ventilation. Improvement of clinical and blood gas states takes 1–2 days, and radiological changes clear after 1–4 days. Recovery of pulmonary function may be delayed for many days and may be incomplete.

When a stuporose patient maintains a constant posture, unilateral oedema may occur, as was first described in 1880 by Osler. The mechanism of the oedema is not clear. The condition has been thought to be analogous to neurogenic pulmonary oedema, seen sometimes with raised intracranial pressure. Neither coma nor severe hypoxaemia are, however, prerequisites. Evidence of increased membrane permeability has been found in narcotic-related pulmonary oedema, in which oedema fluid with a higher protein content can be collected from the airways than in oedema due to raised pulmonary venous pressure in left ventricular failure (Katz *et al.* 1972). Intriguingly, naloxone has been reported to cause pulmonary oedema (Flacke *et al.* 1977; Schwartz and Koenigsberg 1987). Other reports implicate codeine (Sklar and Timms 1977) and dextropropoxyphene overdose (Bogartz and Miller 1971; Young 1972). Intravenous injection (illicit) of the sedative ethchlorvynol

has caused non-cardiogenic pulmonary oedema (Glauser *et al.* 1976), and a similar problem arose in a 28-year-old woman who smoked crystals of methylamphetamine (Nestor *et al.* 1989).

Other drugs

A reaction to hydrochlorothiazide, giving the appearances of pulmonary oedema in hypertensive patients without impaired left ventricular function, has been described in a number of patients (Steinberg 1968; Beaudry and Laplante 1973). Acute breathlessness, hypoxaemia, basal crackles, and radiological changes occurred within 45 minutes of ingestion. The response could be repeated on challenge with a single tablet. Administration of salicylates in high dosage may cause pulmonary oedema. This was initially described during treatment of rheumatic carditis but has generally been due to overdosage (self-poisoning); one such patient was found to have a normal pulmonary wedge pressure (Hrnicek *et al.* 1974). Overdose of colchicine led to a fatal outcome in which pulmonary oedema was a feature (Hill *et al.* 1975). Fatal ARDS developing 4 days after overdosage with amitriptyline has been described (Marshall and Moore 1973). Parenteral administration of β-adrenoceptor agonists, for example, terbutaline (Stubblefield 1978) or ritodrine (Elliott *et al.* 1978; Gentili *et al.* 1988), may cause pulmonary oedema. The mechanism is unclear, but a hyperdynamic circulation as in late pregnancy and premature labour seem to be predisposing factors. Adrenaline has produced fulminating pulmonary oedema when given during anaesthesia (Ersoz and Finestone 1971; Woldorf and Pastore 1972).

Intravenous urography has, rarely, caused pulmonary oedema (Cameron 1974; Chiu and Gambach 1974). Maxwell (1974) reported pulmonary oedema within 2 minutes of a second intravenous injection of cyclophosphamide and a female patient with lymphangitis carcinomatosa developed fatal ARDS 2 hours after intravenous chemotherapy with a combination of vinblastine and mitomycin (Ballen and Weiss 1988) (other reactions to this combination are also discussed under Hypersensitivity pneumonitis). ARDS has also been reported after vinblastine alone (Israel and Olson 1987).

Biliary infusion of mono-octanoin to dissolve gallstones has been reported by Hine and co-workers (1988) to have caused pulmonary oedema in four individuals. They calculated a minimal incidence of 1 in 1000 cases. In a renal transplant recipient, Dean and colleagues (1987) reported ARDS following infusion of antilymphocytic globulin. Four litres of fluid had been given as well. Antithymocyte globulin led to ARDS after cardiac transplantation (Murdock *et al.* 1987).

Pulmonary oedema occurring during blood transfusion is very likely to be attributed to circulatory overload, but some episodes occur in circumstances that preclude this explanation and sometimes the reaction is seen as part of a general anaphylactoid response. Antibodies to transfused IgA appear to underlie a proportion of reactions to otherwise compatible blood. Respiratory distress, overt pulmonary oedema, and even death may follow (Leikola et al. 1973; Pineda and Tazwell 1975). Reese and others (1975) have reported an adverse pulmonary reaction to cryoprecipitate in a haemophiliac in whom none of the above mechanisms seem applicable and who, in addition, had no antiplatelet or lymphocytotoxic antibodies. Pulmonary oedema following intravenous infusion of fresh frozen plasma, ascribed to an allergic reaction on the basis of systemic vasodilatation and a normal pulmonary capillary wedge pressure, has been described (O'Connor et al. 1981).

Pulmonary veins

Pulmonary veno-occlusive disease has been reported in three patients with malignancies who received cytotoxic chemotherapy (Lombard et al. 1987). One patient developed progressive breathlessness 10 years after MOPP (twice), COPP (four times), and radiotherapy for Hodgkin's disease. At autopsy there were multiple thromboemboli in the pulmonary arteries and in large and small pulmonary veins. No primary source of embolism was found. In two other patients with brain tumours, radiotherapy was followed by 6 months of treatment with carmustine. Four months later dyspnoea developed, progressing to death from respiratory failure within 6 weeks. At postmortem examination, occlusive lesions were found in small pulmonary veins in both patients. The role of chemotherapy or radiotherapy in these cases is obscure, but the pathogenesis in the first case is clearly different from that in the other two. Joselson and Warnock (1983) also described this complication of cytotoxic chemotherapy.

Bronchi and lower airways

Foreign bodies

The true incidence of the inhalation of tablets and capsules is probably grossly underestimated, because most modern formulations are designed with rapid dissolution characteristics. Sustained-release preparations may possess wax matrices and persistence of these after inhalation of a salbutamol 'Spandet' and a terbutaline 'SA' tablet has been reported (Coppack et al. 1984). Considering the frailty of some recipients, especially the elderly, it is surprising that tablets and capsules are not incriminated as inhaled foreign bodies more frequently.

Drug effects upon the sputum

Patients may perceive their sputum to have become more tenacious following effective antibiotic therapy, which eliminates purulence. Atropine and other drugs with anticholinergic properties, for example, tricyclic antidepressants, may cause unpleasant stickiness of bronchial secretions. Part of the clinical problem is due to drying of the mouth or pharynx, or both, so that sputum is more difficult to expectorate. In this regard, concern has arisen about the use of the quaternary atropine derivative ipratropium in patients with airflow obstruction due to chronic bronchitis. Because of its quaternary nature, however, little of the drug is distributed systemically, and bronchial mucus is not altered by it in vitro (Francis et al. 1975).

Aspiration of oily medications from nose drops or oral medication may give rise to lipoid pneumonia, and sputum may contain globules of oil.

Haemoptysis

This symptom may complicate thrombocytopenia due to cytotoxic drugs. Usually the blood produced appears only as streaks and is perhaps due to pharyngeal or laryngeal trauma, especially when there is ulceration. More dramatic haemoptysis may complicate intrapulmonary bleeding related to treatment with anticoagulants (Reussi et al. 1969; R.S. Bone et al. 1976), particularly where there are pulmonary infarcts or lung cysts (Kent 1965). (See also Pulmonary vasculitis — diffuse intrapulmonary haemorrhage).

Bronchial mucosa

Early clinical reports of the successful use of steroid aerosols in the long-term treatment of asthma commonly contained guarded reference to the theoretical possibility of atrophic changes, analogous to those produced in the skin by high doses of topical steroid preparations, developing in the bronchial wall. Histological studies of bronchial mucosa obtained by bronchoscopy (Andersson and Smidt 1974; Thiringer et al. 1975) have failed, however, to reveal any changes after over a year of

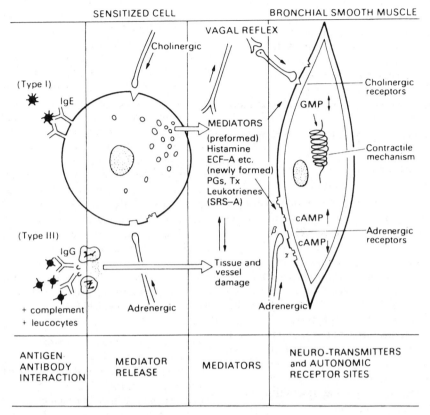

SENSITIZED CELL   BRONCHIAL SMOOTH MUSCLE

FIG. 10.1
The controlling factors in muscular tone. The action of drugs to cause airways obstruction may be at any of the four stages.

continuous treatment and, after many years of very widespread long-term use of the preparations, there is no clinical evidence of such an effect. Infection with *Candida albicans* appears to be limited to the oropharynx and larynx, presumably because 80–90 per cent of inhaled particles are deposited at these sites.

Airflow obstruction

The calibre of small airways is dependent to a considerable extent upon the tone of bronchial smooth muscle. In normal individuals, changes in calibre are minor and barely appreciable; in the presence of chronic airflow obstruction, however, small differences can be important. In asthma, very large alterations of bronchial calibre can occur, owing partly to contraction of bronchial smooth muscle but also contributed to by mucosal oedema of airways and intraluminal inflammatory mucus. A multitude of humoral factors can influence bronchial tone either directly or via vagal cholinergic reflexes.

Allergic reactions (Type I hypersensitivity — immediate) (Gell and Coombs 1968) are characterized by IgE-linked release of pharmacologically active mediators from mast cells. This release may be modulated by physical, neural, humoral, and pharmacological factors. Non-specific release of mediators can also be effected, for example, by quaternary compounds or by surface-active agents. The mediators, some of which are preformed (e.g. histamine, eosinophilic chemotactic factor of anaphylaxis, various peptides), and others synthesized *de novo* (e.g. from the membrane-bound phospholipid arachidonic acid), determine the degree of bronchoconstriction and inflammation characteristic of local anaphylaxis in the airways. Immediate reactions may be followed hours later by delayed responses (Type III hypersensitivity), the effect of which can last hours to days. Drugs causing reversible airflow obstruction act through the mechanisms outlined above and the model shown in Figure 10.1 provides a basis for the following classification of these drug reactions (see Chapter 5) into Type B (1) and Type A (2–5):

1. drugs that are antigenic;
2a. drugs that directly release mediators;
2b. drugs that affect the synthesis of mediators;
3a. drugs that stimulate reflex bronchoconstriction;
3b. drugs that are mediators or related to mediators;
3c. drugs that inhibit mediator breakdown;
4. drugs that act as agonists or antagonists at autonomic receptor sites;
5. drugs that alter the disposition or metabolism of antiasthmatic drugs.

1. Drugs that are antigenic

Allergens used in tests and desensitization

Testing for allergy inevitably requires the administration of allergens topically or otherwise. Intradermal injection of such materials occasionally provokes dangerous asthmatic attacks that may be immediate or delayed. Such reactions are very much less frequent with the much smaller quantity of allergen introduced when skin prick testing is utilized, but in patients with eczema even this method can cause anaphylaxis. Courses of desensitizing injections used for the prophylaxis of hay fever may have to be curtailed because of the production of unacceptable asthma following each injection. The guidelines for the management of asthma produced by the British Thoracic Society (*British Medical Journal* 1990) advise against any attempts at desensitization.

Inhalation challenge testing using aerosols containing the suspected allergen has become more widely used in recent times, both for diagnosis and for the assessment of novel experimental antiallergic compounds. The dose–response methodology avoids the risk of immediate severe bronchospasm, but delayed reactions may occasionally be serious.

Drugs containing animal protein

Nasal insufflation of pituitary extract of porcine or bovine origin may induce asthma and parenchymal pulmonary reactions (Pepys 1969). A powdered pancreatic extract used by patients with cystic fibrosis may be inhaled while being added to food and Sakula (1977) has reported rhinitis and asthma in patients and relatives attributable to this cause. Enteric-coated tablets are not the preferred formulation.

Antibiotics

Anaphylaxis can follow administration of a variety of drugs, and asthma is a frequent accompaniment of such reactions. Penicillins are the most frequent cause of drug-induced anaphylaxis, and there is almost always a history of previous treatment with a course of penicillin which has usually been trouble-free. Dalgaard (1965) investigated 20 deaths due to penicillin in Denmark and found that 18 of the patients had previously received penicillin (six with reactions, usually rashes). Of significance was the high incidence of a pre-existing allergic tendency, mostly asthma, in 11 of the dead. Similar findings have been reported in 151 fatal reactions (Idsøe *et al.* 1968). Penicillin sensitivity is complex and is due in some individuals to impurities. Prick and patch tests are unfortunately rather unreliable and deaths have resulted from intradermal tests of penicillin. This topic is discussed in greater detail in Chapter 27.

Cross-reactions to cephalosporins in some patients allergic to penicillin have been a concern in view of the structural similarities but sensitivity to cephalosporins is not an inevitable consequence of penicillin sensitivity (Rahal *et al.* 1968), and the second- and third-generation cephalosporins have, by and large, been free from cross-reactions. Other antibiotics reported to have caused asthma are demeclocycline erythromycin, nitrofurantoin, griseofulvin, neomycin, streptomycin, and chloramphenicol, but such reactions are rare when compared with those due to penicillin.

Dextran

Anaphylactic reactions to parenterally administered preparations of iron–dextran have been reported (Becker *et al.* 1966; Wallerstein 1968). Similar reactions can occur with intravenous solutions of dextran used in the treatment of hypovolaemia The incidence is higher with the larger molecular-weight dextran 70 than with dextran 40 (Laxenaire *et al.* 1976a).

Other drugs have been reported to cause asthma in individual patients, for example, maprotiline (Dubovsky and Freed 1988), 8-methoxypsoralen (Ramsey and Marks 1988), and metoclopramide on two occasions in the same patient (Chung *et al.* 1985).

2a. Drugs that directly release mediators

Iodine-containing contrast media

Anaphylaxis occurring with these agents has an incidence of 1 in 14 000 and is accompanied in 12 per cent of cases by severe airflow obstruction (Ansell 1970). The reactions are particularly likely to affect allergic individuals and the induced asthma may last for days. Small intravenous doses have been used to test 204 patients with a history of previous reactions, and the value of subsequent protection with an antihistamine is described by Yocum and others (1978). In those with only a vague history of previous hypersensitivity and negative pretests (untreated with an antihistamine), the incidence of reactions was five per cent. Amongst those with a clear history of a previous reaction but negative pretests, about 20 per cent had a second reaction, but this figure could be reduced to about four per cent by pretreatment with chlorpheniramine. Two-thirds of those with a positive pretest went on to have a second reaction despite pretreatment with chlorpheniramine. Pretreatment with corticosteroid drugs appears to offer some protection (Zweiman *et al.* 1975; Lasser *et al.* 1977); the dose may have to be moderately high. Mild bronchoconstriction (a mean decrease of 7.5 per cent in FEV_1) was observed in most patients receiving a high-osmolality agent, sodium iothalamate; allergic subjects were more likely to react (Dawson *et al.* 1983). The time-course of the reaction (onset after 4–5 minutes; recovery within 30 minutes) is compatible with mediator release, but whether a similar mechanism can be invoked for severe bronchospasm is unknown. Cough during pulmonary angiography is much more common with a high-osmolality agent (Smith *et al.* 1987).

Intravenous anaesthetic agents

Induction of anaesthesia can cause anaphylaxis, and cross-reactions occur — raising the possibility that a non-allergic mechanism is responsible. The reaction is usually rapid in onset but occasionally delayed for up to an hour (Laxenaire *et al.* 1976*b*). Death may ensue from circulatory failure or apparently complete airflow obstruction. A muscle relaxant is almost always given as well, and the relative importance of the two drugs is uncertain. The combination of thiopentone and suxamethonium is by far and away the most frequent cause of bronchoconstrictive reactions (Vignon *et al.* 1976), but it is unclear whether there is an explanation for this other than that this combination is that most often used. Clarke and others (1975, 1977) found that about a quarter of those reacting to thiopentone were atopic and that previous exposure to thiopentone carried only a very slight increase in risk of an adverse reaction. A more clear-cut case for mediator release has been made for the poorly soluble steroid drugs alphaxalone and alphadolone (Althesin), which require a surface-active agent, polyoxyethylated castor oil (Cremophor EL) so that an adequate dose can be accommodated in a minimal volume (Jago and Restall 1978; CSM 1979).

Muscle relaxants

Anaphylaxis and marked bronchoconstriction may follow the intravenous administration of tubocurarine (Comroe and Dripps 1946), suxamethonium (Eustace 1967), pancuronium (Heath 1973), vecuronium (O'Callaghan *et al.* 1986), and atracurium and alcuronium (Beemer *et al.* 1988). The reaction is almost certainly due to histamine release by these quaternary ammonium compounds, a

process demonstrable *in vitro* and by intradermal testing (Heath 1973).

Other drugs

Morphine administered parenterally is regularly found to cause bronchospasm and it can be shown to release histamine when given intradermally. Hydrocortisone as the sodium phosphate salt (Partridge and Gibson 1978) or the sodium succinate salt (Kounis 1976) may cause acute anaphylactic reactions. It seems unlikely that an endogenous corticosteroid would give rise to true allergy, and as the reaction is immediate and not delayed for many hours, a mechanism involving phospholipase A_2 is excluded. There is clinical evidence of systemic histamine release in such patients; and also with methylprednisolone (Mendelson *et al.* 1974). Quaternary preservatives such as benzalkonium are sometimes present in aerosol preparations (see below — ipratropium, beclomethasone) and probably act by causing mediator release rather than by an irritant action because, even when given by injection as in a hepatitis B vaccine, thiomersal has caused asthma and urticaria (Lohiya 1987).

2b. Drugs that affect the synthesis of mediators

Aspirin and other non-steroidal anti-inflammatory drugs (NSAID)

Asthma usually develops in sensitive individuals about 30 minutes after ingestion of aspirin; it may be accompanied by flushing and rhinorrhoea. The severity of the reaction varies and does not seem to be proportional to the pre-existing airflow obstruction, as near-fatal attacks occur in patients with minimal or long-quiescent asthma. It is extremely important, therefore, that attention is paid to any patient acknowledging a previous history of 'allergy' to aspirin. Partial attacks involving rhinorrhea, angioedema, or urticaria, alone or in any combination, may occur. The phenomenon is particularly associated with late-onset intrinsic asthma and is often accompanied by nasal polyposis. The syndrome was first delineated by Samter and Beers (1967) and its incidence is estimated at one in 10 asthmatics (McDonald *et al.* 1972). Some patients may be unaware of their sensitivity, and eight per cent of one group of patients developing some degree of bronchospasm after aspirin challenge gave no such history (Spector *et al.* 1979).

Patients with aspirin sensitivity are almost invariably cross-reactive to NSAID (and to the colouring agent tartrazine [E102]). Numerous reports in the literature are to be found describing individuals who have reacted, sometimes fatally, to particular NSAID, for example, indomethacin, phenylbutazone, mefenamic acid, flufenamic acid, diclofenac, or naproxen. The structural heterogenicity of these compounds argues against an immune mechanism. There is some evidence, however, for a common property, namely inhibition of the synthesis of prostanoids derived from arachidonic acid via cyclo-oxygenase (COX) activity. This inhibition was thought to result in an imbalance between the bronchoconstrictor prostaglandins (F, A, B, and D_2) and those that are bronchodilator (PGE series and epoprostenol). Arachidonic acid, released from membrane-bound phospholipid, is also available for conversion to the products of 5-lipoxygenase activity, of which the most important are the leukotrienes. A shunting of arachidonic acid from prostanoid to leukotriene (LT) synthesis is an alternative explanation for asthma induced by aspirin. To test this theory Nasser and colleagues (1994) utilized an inhibitor of 5-lipoxygenase, ZD2138, and showed that this compound protected against aspirin-induced bronchoconstriction (20 per cent vs five per cent fall in FEV_1). This was associated with a 74 per cent inhibition of the rise in urinary excretion of LTE_4 at 6 hours after aspirin ingestion and a 72 per cent reduction *ex vivo* of LTB_4 at 12 hours. This group has recently shown that mast cell degranulation may be an early event in aspirin-induced asthma (Nasser *et al.* 1996) and previously sodium cromoglycate has been shown to be protective in this condition (Martelli and Usandivaras 1977). Two isoenzymes of COX exist: COX-1 is constitutive and COX-2 is inducible by inflammatory cytokines, and Mitchell and Belvisi (1997) hypothesize that a novel series of products, the 15-epilipoxins, is involved because aspirin modifies COX-2 so that 15-HETE (hydroxyeicosatetraenoic acid), a substrate for 5-lipoxygenase is produced. It is of interest that just giving a LT-receptor antagonist may not be as effective as inhibition of 5-lipoxygenase at preventing aspirin-induced asthma.

A genetic predisposition seems likely — familial clustering (Miller 1971; von Maur *et al.* 1974) and an increased prevalence of the HLA-DQw2 antigen have been found (Mullarkey *et al.* 1986) — but modulation of bronchial reactivity also seems probable, as Spector and colleagues (1979) in their challenge studies found negative tests in about one-third of those reporting previous aspirin sensitivity. The story is further complicated by occasional asthmatic reactions to paracetamol (acetaminophen), an analgesic without anti-inflammatory activity which inhibits intracerebral cyclo-oxygenase. Szczeklik and Gryglewski (1983) reported reactions to paracetamol and phenacetin in four per cent of aspirin-sensitive patients. It is of interest that some asthmatic patients are improved by aspirin (*British Medical Journal* 1973).

Opiate derivatives such as codeine and dihydrocodeine are safe analgesics to use in patients of this group.

3a. Drugs that stimulate reflex bronchoconstriction

All therapeutic aerosols may reflexly trigger vagally mediated bronchoconstriction, preventable by prior administration of atropine or a bronchodilator. The effect is mediated by a non-specific physical or irritant action, for example, inhalation of sodium cromoglycate as a dry powder formulation may cause coughing and wheezing (Morrison Smith 1975). Beclomethasone dipropionate, even as a pressurized aerosol, not uncommonly initiates mild wheezing. There is indirect evidence against this being a specific hypersensitivity, as patients may respond to the propellant alone (Bryant and Pepys 1976; Shim and Williams 1987). It has become routine to recommend taking a bronchodilator before inhaling a steroid. Some surprise was caused when the anticholinergic drug ipratropium bromide was reported to cause bronchoconstriction in three patients using a metered-dose pressurized aerosol (Connolly 1982). Other workers reported bronchoconstriction when the drug was administered by nebulization (Howarth 1983; Patel and Tullet 1983). Altounyan showed that nebulized hypotonic solutions cause bronchoconstriction in asthmatics with hyperreactive airways (Schoeffed *et al.* 1981), and the manufacturers of ipratropium now market the drug in isotonic saline. Removal of the preservatives EDTA and benzalkonium has also been material in reducing the incidence of adverse reactions (Rafferty *et al.* 1988). Both ipratropium and benzalkonium are quaternary ammonium compounds (see above — Direct release of mediators), and benzalkonium has been proposed (Beasley *et al.* 1986) as the reason why an infant developed severe wheeze soon after receiving nebulized beclomethasone (Clark 1986). Unit-dose vials are to be encouraged; as they are sterile, no preservative is needed and cross-infection is less likely (Barclay *et al.* 1990).

Metabisulphite (E223) is used widely in food and drink as a preservative/antioxidant. It was also present in some bronchodilator aerosols; the bronchospasm it causes is likely to be due to the generation of sulphur dioxide (Meeker and Wiedemann 1990). Evidence against the degranulation of mast cells in the reaction has been reported by Sprenger and colleagues (1989) who challenged patients sensitive to metabisulphite; the circulating neutrophil chemotactic factor activity did not increase, in contrast to an increase observed following antigen challenge (Nagy *et al.* 1982). The phenomenon of metabisulphite sensitivity can be observed occasionally in hospital inpatients recovering from acute severe asthma, whose peak flow charts will show a dip at an unexpected time (e.g. afternoon). Examination of the labels on bottles (e.g. of Lucozade) on their bedside lockers will reveal the ingredients and appropriate advice can be given. Bronchial reactions to nebulized acetylcysteine (once used as a mucolytic aerosol in cystic fibrosis) usually occur in asthmatic subjects and seem to be related to the concentration of acetylcysteine used (Council on Drugs 1964). Aerosolized antibiotics regularly cause tightness in the chest in patients with cystic fibrosis in whom colistin is used for chronic *Pseudomonas* colonization. Symptoms were not attributable to pentamidine used in AIDS for the prophylaxis of *Pneumocystis carinii* pneumonia (Smith *et al.* 1988).

3b. Drugs that are mediators orrelated to mediators

Bronchial provocation tests with histamine may cause unexpectedly severe bronchospasm in asthmatic patients with marked bronchial hyperreactivity. Prostaglandin $F_{2\alpha}$ is bronchoconstrictive and severe asthma has been reported during its infusion to induce a therapeutic abortion in a patient with chronic eczema (Fishburn *et al.* 1972).

3c. Drugs that inhibit mediator breakdown

Anticholinesterases

Acetylcholine released from cholinergic nerves is rapidly hydrolysed by local acetylcholinesterase and exerts no activity remote from the site of release. The anticholinesterase neostigmine markedly increases local concentrations of acetylcholine, and is given to reverse the action of long-acting competitive antagonist muscle relaxants, such as tubocurarine and pancuronium, used during anaesthesia and surgery. Atropine is usually used concomitantly with neostigmine to prevent the predictable bronchospasm and bradycardia. Interestingly, Pratt (1988) reported three patients in whom the short-acting anticholinergic glycopyrronium did not prevent neostigmine inducing bronchospasm. Pyridostigmine and neostigmine are used in myasthenia gravis and may aggravate asthma. Ecothiopate, a long-acting anticholinesterase used in eye-drops for glaucoma, was reported to exacerbate airflow obstruction in a patient with emphysema (Fratto 1979).

Angiotensin-converting-enzyme inhibitors (ACEI)

ACEI (e.g. captopril, enalapril) prevent the enzymatic activation of the peptide angiotensin I to angiotensin II. ACEI also inactivate bradykinin and possibly other vasoactive peptides. Cough as an adverse effect of these drugs has been related to persistence of such peptides, and the incidence of this adverse reaction has varied from 0.2 per cent of 13 295 hypertensive patients taking part in postmarketing surveillance of captopril (Chalmers *et al.* 1987) to one to three per cent of individuals involved in prescription-event monitoring of a large

population taking enalapril (Inman 1986; Inman *et al.* 1988). The cough is characteristically dry and unproductive and usually recurs when alternative ACEI are substituted. There seems to be a dose effect in some individuals. Experimental studies have shown that the cough reflex can be stimulated by capsaicin, a partial agonist at substance P receptors on non-myelinated sensory (C) nerve fibres, and sensitivity to capsaicin is increased by administration of an ACEI to patients known to have cough induced by the drug (Fuller and Choudry 1987). This is a complex area involving the modulatory interaction of many mediators, and, interestingly, the NSAID sulindac has been shown to prevent the induction of cough by ACEI (Nicholis and Gilchrist 1987). The new class of antihypertensive drugs, angiotensin antagonists, of which losartan is the first to the marketplace, can be substituted for ACEI. There is little evidence that ACEI aggravate asthma but Popa (1987) described a man whose FEV_1 fell when challenged with captopril but not when challenged with propranolol. More systematic investigation has shown an increase in bronchial hyperreactivity in symptomatic patients rechallenged with ACE inhibitors (Bucknall *et al.* 1988). In contrast, withdrawing captopril did not improve bronchial hyperreactivity in another study (Kaufman *et al.* 1989). Asthma seems to be a very much less likely adverse effect with ACEI than cough.

4. Drugs that act as agonists or antagonists at autonomic receptor sites

Cholinergic agonists

Carbachol and related drugs are sometimes given to increase the contractility of the bladder and may induce bronchoconstriction (Fig. 10.1). Aggravation of asthma has been reported with pilocarpine eye-drops for glaucoma (Bruchhausen *et al.* 1969) and with deanol for severe dyskinesia (Nesse and Carroll 1976). Methacholine used in bronchial provocation testing can occasionally cause unexpectedly severe bronchoconstriction even in individuals not regarded as asthmatic (Stenton *et al.* 1990).

β-Adrenoceptor agonists

Atypical responses to inhaled isoprenaline have been ascribed to overuse of this bronchodilator aerosol (Keighley 1966; Patterson *et al.* 1968). Two factors are relevant: dosage and selectivity. Isoprenaline is a nonselective β-adrenoceptor agonist which is rapidly inactivated by catechol-*o*-methyltransferase (COMT) and has to be administered in high dosage to ensure an adequate duration of action. Undesirable systemic effects were frequently associated with high peak blood levels of isoprenaline. Of the modern β-agonist bronchodilators only the short-acting rimiterol is a substrate for COMT. The duration of action of the others is therefore longer, and smaller doses (in terms of relative potency) need to be inhaled. β_2-Adrenoceptor selectivity is an incidental advantage which followed from the molecular design required for COMT resistance. When the distributional selectivity achieved by administering these drugs by inhalation, rather than by the oral or parenteral routes, is considered, β_2-selectivity is a relatively less important attribute than COMT resistance.

Lowering of arterial oxygen tension

Adrenergic and xanthine bronchodilators are also vasodilators and their administration will increase ventilation/perfusion (V/Q) mismatching and thereby lower arterial PO_2 in normal and asthmatic individuals. The observed changes are usually small and if nebulized bronchodilators are driven by oxygen then any changes will be clinically insignificant. The effect of intravenous salbutamol has been compared with that of the drug when inhaled and found to cause more V/Q imbalance in acute severe asthma (Ballester *et al.* 1989). In contrast, in chronic obstructive pulmonary disease (COPD) the rise in cardiac output with intravenous salbutamol can counterbalance the effect of pulmonary vasodilatation, and in hypoxic patients with chronic bronchitis the net effect can be no change in PO_2. Indeed, the manufacturers of pirbuterol have claimed that pulmonary vasodilatation is a positive advantage rather than an adverse effect!

Tolerance at β-adrenoceptors

Sudden death in asthma: role of pressurized aerosols

Between 1959 and 1966 the mortality from asthma increased dramatically in the UK (Speizer *et al.* 1968a), and overuse of isoprenaline inhalers was thought to be responsible (Speizer *et al.* 1968b; Fraser *et al.* 1971). Subsequently, caution was advised in the use of bronchodilator aerosols and the mortality from asthma declined to previous levels (Inman and Adelstein 1969). Inhaled prophylactic antiasthmatic therapy with sodium cromoglycate and beclomethasone became the norm in the early 1970s and was undoubtedly a very significant development. Nevertheless, even at that time unacceptable deaths from asthma occurred and it seems that some patients, their families, and their doctors (both in the community and in hospital) are rather poor at recognizing the severity of an attack of acute asthma and at instituting early treatment with corticosteroids in sufficiently high doses (Ormerod and Stableforth 1980).

Unfortunately, a small number of asthmatic deaths are due to severe immediate reactions and seem to be unavoidable.

The mechanisms whereby isoprenaline might cause death have been widely discussed. Hypoxaemia is minor, as mentioned above. Such high doses could lead to the development of tolerance to β-adrenoceptor agonists during long-term therapy and to a need to increase dosage further and risk toxicity, for example, cardiac stimulation and possibly fatal arrhythmia. Tolerance to the cardiac chronotropic effects of adrenergic agonists is well recognized. The observation that normal airways can become resistant to salbutamol (Holgate *et al.* 1977) could not be confirmed by Keaney and colleagues (1980; and unpublished observations), but numbers were small in all these studies. Resistance of asthmatic airways to oral adrenergic bronchodilators has been found (Bhatan and Davis 1975; Larsson *et al.* 1977). An insight into possible mechanisms of tolerance has come from study of genetic polymorphisms of the β_2-adrenoceptor. In a series of three studies Lipworth found evidence to suggest that tolerance to the long-acting β-adrenoceptor agonist formoterol could develop in asthmatic patients. Subsequent analysis of the genotypes of subsets of patients from these studies showed that there was significant correlation of a tendency to bronchodilator desensitization with particular genotypes (Tan *et al.* 1997). Further work is required to confirm these fascinating results.

Role of nebulized bronchodilators

In the light of the above discussion, there was a sense of *déjà vu* when the report of Jackson and colleagues (1982) appeared identifying an increase in mortality from asthma in New Zealand not seen in other countries. Again it was probable that inadequate education of patients underlay the phenomenon (Clarke and Newman 1984). A new factor to be considered in the patients in New Zealand was excessive reliance on domiciliary aerosol treatment using nebulizers to deliver higher doses of bronchodilators. In a subsequent survey of 271 deaths from asthma between 1981 and 1983 in New Zealand, 75 individuals had home nebulizers (Sears *et al.* 1987). Poor patient compliance (36 per cent), delay in seeking help (35 per cent), and inadequate treatment or assessment (36 per cent) were identified in these patients; 81 per cent of deaths occurred 'during a witnessed attack of severe asthma unresponsive to usual treatment', which included nebulized high-dose β-agonists in two-thirds of cases. Of some concern was the observation that 45 per cent of patients with fatal asthma used fenoterol (49 per cent salbutamol) in their nebulizer, whereas the ratio of sales of fenoterol to those of salbutamol (in 20 ml units) was 13 800 to 35 000. The use of fenoterol in New Zealand was five times higher than in other countries and Crane and colleagues (1989) blamed fenoterol for the excess of asthma deaths. This conclusion has been disputed (Buist *et al.* 1989; O'Donnell *et al.* 1989) on the basis of inadequate assessment of the severity of the final attack. This criticism has been rejected as irrelevant and an extended analysis using different controls added further support to the hypothesis that inhaled fenoterol is associated with an increased risk of death in patients with severe asthma (Pearce *et al.* 1990*a*). The odds ratio of death from asthma was 1.99 (95 per cent confidence interval [CI] 1.12–3.55) in patients given fenoterol and rose to 9.82 (95 per cent CI 2.23–43.4) for the group defined by admission for asthma in the previous year and by having had an oral corticosteroid prescribed at the time of admission. An alternative hypothesis that risk for death from asthma may simply be associated with a propensity for doctors to prescribe fenoterol (Spitzer and Buist 1990) has been rejected (Pearce *et al.* 1990*b*). When fenoterol was removed from the New Zealand market in 1990 the mortality from asthma declined immediately and hospital admissions halved (Sears, M.R. personal communication). Recent evidence suggests that while frequent use of β_2-adrenoceptor agonists for symptomatic relief is appropriate and safe, regular scheduled programmes of inhaled bronchodilator therapy may be deleterious in terms of decreasing the protective effect against bronchoconstriction, despite substantially shifting the dose response curve to the right (Sears 1995). The effect of bronchodilator drugs in masking the severity of asthma, so that treatment with inhaled or systemic corticosteroids is delayed, is a theme of much concern to respiratory physicians. New inhaled bronchodilators, such as salmeterol, have a duration of action of up to 12 hours and may in time raise issues similar to those involving isoprenaline in the 1960s and fenoterol in the 1980s.

β-Adrenoceptor antagonists

This group of drugs will prevent adrenergic bronchodilators from exerting their therapeutic action. Asthmatic patients, however, are additionally susceptible to β-blockers, and even the small systemic concentrations that follow topical application of a β-blocker in eye drops for glaucoma, for example, timolol (Shoene *et al.* 1981), can provoke severe asthma. Timolol, like propranolol, is a non-selective β-blocker, but even highly cardioselective practolol may provoke bronchospasm (Macdonald

and McNeill 1968). Interestingly, propranolol has no effect on airway resistance in normal subjects (McNeill 1964) even in overdose (Frishman *et al.* 1979). The mechanism by which β-blockers cause bronchospasm in asthmatics is far from clear. It is not simply due to interference with the action of circulating adrenaline or released noradrenaline on bronchial smooth muscle, because both anticholinergic drugs (Ind *et al.* 1989) and sodium cromoglycate (Koeter *et al.* 1982) prevent propranolol from inducing bronchoconstriction.

A β-blocking action may not be an obvious attribute of a drug marketed for treating mild cardiac failure, but xamoterol is an example of such a product which acts as a partial agonist at cardiac β-receptors and would be expected to aggravate asthma (Waller 1990). Propafenone, used for treating cardiac arrhythmias, is primarily a Class 1c agent with some β-blocking activity and it can precipitate asthma (Veale *et al.* 1990).

5. Drugs that affect the disposition or metabolism of antiasthmatic drugs

Induction of microsomal enzymes utilizing cytochrome P-450 increases the clearance of drugs that undergo oxidative metabolism, (e.g. prednisolone). Anticonvulsants such as carbamazepine, phenytoin, and phenobarbitone, and the antituberculous antibiotic rifampicin are the most commonly used drugs that cause enzyme induction. Asthma control was found to deteriorate in three patients on maintenance corticosteroid therapy following administration of phenobarbitone (Brooks *et al.* 1972). Evidence of increased steroid metabolism was observed, the elimination half-life of ingested dexamethasone being reduced.

Irreversible airflow obstruction

Bronchiolitis obliterans has been described in patients with rheumatoid arthritis and ulcerative colitis. Its occurrence in patients with these diseases has been attributed to penicillamine in rheumatoid disease (Scott *et al.* 1981) and to sulphasalazine in ulcerative colitis (Williams *et al.* 1982).

Lung parenchyma

The arrangement of topics in this section is arbitrary. Most approaches to classifying drug-related parenchymal damage have been pharmacopoeial in nature, which obviously necessitates much repetition. In order to keepthis to a minimum, parenchymal injury has been grouped into: (i) acute and (ii) subacute or chronic reactions. An alternative description would be of (i) reversible pneumonitis and (ii) fibrotic pulmonary disease. Inevitably some cases will overlap either with another category, or with ARDS, and attention will be drawn to this when appropriate. The clinical features of acute pneumonitis and pulmonary fibrosis are presented in general terms for each topic rather than with each drug mentioned; first, however, parenchymal complications of aspiration are discussed.

Inhalation

Sedative drugs, especially opiates, which obtund pharyngeal and laryngeal reflexes, permit inhalation of food, secretions, or vomitus, leading to the subsequent development of pneumonitis. Local anaesthesia of the glottis may also be followed by aspiration. Fatal respiratory failure has been caused by inhalation of activated charcoal, given to patients suffering from drug overdoses with lowered consciousness, when vomiting occurred (Rau *et al.* 1988). Liquid paraffin or oily nasal drops may lead to lipoid pneumonia from unrecognized aspiration. The clinical features are usually mild (Volk *et al.* 1951), and the diagnosis is confirmed by identifying globules of oil in sputum or lung biopsy material (Weill *et al.* 1964). Inhalation of a capsule of cyclosporin, giving rise to a peripheral pulmonary mass, and the finding of the vehicle in which cyclosporin is dissolved on transthoracic fine-needle aspiration (Gould *et al.* 1990), have been mentioned earlier.

Drug-related infection of the lungs

Drugs may cause pneumonia (i) by being contaminated and inhaled (Barclay *et al.* 1990); (ii) by permitting aspiration of infected material (e.g. opiates); (iii) by suppressing host defences to pathogens (e.g. cytotoxic chemotherapy, high-dose corticosteroids); or (iv) by altering respiratory flora (e.g. alkalinization of gastric juice with antacids or cimetidine was associated with colonization of stomach and trachea by the same bacteria and a high incidence [60 per cent] of pneumonia in an intensive care unit) (DuMoulin *et al.* 1982), and Freeman (1980) has stated that prophylactic broad-spectrum antibiotics alter tracheal flora and cause increased mortality after cardiac surgery.

Opportunistic infections

Patients can become immunosuppressed for a number of reasons and with a severity that varies, as does their susceptibility to different types of infection. Thus, even low-dosage corticosteroid therapy can reactivate pulmonary tuberculosis, but such an individual, like the patient being treated for leukaemia who still has preserved immunoglobulin levels and an adequate neutrophil count, should not be regarded as immunodeficient. In general hospital clinical practice, cytotoxic chemotherapy is the most usual reason for immunodeficiency and the diagnostic approach to the problem of diffuse pulmonary infiltration in the immunocompromised host has been recently reviewed by Rosenow (1990). The presentation, physical examination, and chest X-ray are rarely diagnostic, and bronchoscopy with bronchial lavage and transbronchial biopsy may be needed to establish the cause. Rosenow describes the experience at the Mayo Clinic, where 75 per cent of immunocompromised patients with diffuse pulmonary disease have an opportunistic infection, sometimes with more than one unusual organism. Further investigation with open lung biopsy attributed the diffuse infiltration to adverse drug effects in 15 per cent of the total, and the remaining 10 per cent of cases were due to recurrence of underlying disease, idiopathic fibrosis (? from radiotherapy), or unrelated disease. The use of cyclosporin A as an immunosuppressant agent has considerably reduced the problem of nosocomial infection in transplant patients. Nevertheless, cytomegalovirus and *Pneumocystis carinii* infections remain the most frequent problems; invasive aspergillosis and candidiasis are rather more difficult to diagnose without open lung biopsy. Drug-related infections are discussed further in Chapter 25.

Acute diffuse hypersensitivity pneumonitis

Drug-related hypersensitivity pneumonitis, with or without pulmonary eosinophilia, is characterized by a variety of radiological shadows evident on the chest X-ray, accompanied by eosinophilia in the blood in many instances. More recently, eosinophilia or lymphocytosis, or both, in fluid obtained by bronchoalveolar lavage have been identified. The radiological shadowing may be of segmental appearance or irregularly fan-shaped, of medium density, and often of peripheral distribution. Occasionally a micronodular appearance is found. Pleural effusions are common. Gas transfer is impaired and airflow obstruction may occur. Symptoms are of cough, breathlessness, and occasionally wheezing. The prognosis with this type of reaction is good, principally because the acute presentation usually results in immediate withdrawal of the offending drug. Corticosteroid therapy speeds resolution and complete recovery is possible.

Antibacterial drugs

The first case of drug-related eosinophilia to be reported was due to penicillin (Reichlin *et al.* 1953). Acute pneumonitis due to ampicillin, with an eosinophilic alveolitis on transbronchial biopsy has also been reported (Poe *et al.* 1980). Oral sulphonamides (Feigenberg *et al.* 1967) and the sulphonamide derivatives chlorpropamide (Bell 1964) and sulphasalazine (Sigvaldson and Sorensen 1983) may also cause hypersensitivity pneumonitis/pulmonary eosinophilia; nowadays sulphonamide derivatives are most frequently associated with this syndrome. Eosinophilia is not universal in pneumonitis due to sulphasalazine. Typically, symptoms develop 2–5 months after the start of treatment. Occasionally the course of the pulmonary complication is fulminating, as in the case reported by Davis and MacFarlane (1974) in which pulmonary fibrosis was found at autopsy, even though the patient had been given steroid therapy prior to and, in higher dosage, during the month of the illness. Metronidazole was administered on two occasions to a patient who developed hypersensitivity pneumonitis both times (Kristenson and Fryden 1988). Cephalexin (Smith and Weinstein 1987), tetracycline (Ho *et al.* 1979), nalidixic acid (Dan *et al.* 1986), may also give rise to an allergic pulmonary reaction.

The acute eosinophilic response to nitrofurantoin may become persistent (Vaughan-Jones and Goldman 1968), and the case reported by Magee and colleagues (1986) was of acute onset after 7 days' treatment. An open lung biopsy showed granulomata with giant cells, and re-challenge was positive. Subacute and chronic reactions to nitrofurantoin are discussed further below.

Non-steroidal anti-inflammatory drugs

With the high prescription rate for this group of drugs, some of which are available over the counter to the public, it is surprising that pulmonary eosinophilia is not more frequently reported. The mode of action of NSAID involves inhibition of cyclo-oxygenase activity. Arachidonic acid is diverted to the synthesis of the products of lipoxygenase, many of which, like the leukotrienes, have eosinophilic chemotactic activity. Weber and Essigman (1986) briefly reviewed the literature regarding pulmonary alveolitis and NSAID. They also documented information obtained by the Committee on Safety of Medicines from the yellow-card reporting system. This adverse drug reactions register had recorded 29 reports of diffuse pneumonitis attributed to treatment with NSAID involving indomethacin, azapropazone, benoxaprofen, piroxicam, diclofenac, and ibuprofen. A

positive rechallenge had been identified with indomethacin, and there was a cross-reaction between azapropazone and piroxicam. Only 12 of the 29 patients had rheumatoid arthritis (four being seropositive), and patients with osteoarthritis are also susceptible (11 in this series). Stromberg and others (1987) reported six cases of acute pulmonary infiltrates due to tolfenamic acid from Finland. Three occurred early in the course of treatment and three were delayed; the changes resolved in all cases when the drug was discontinued. Rechallenge was positive in three of the patients. Two chronic fibrotic reactions were also identified. Two similar reactions to fenbufen (Chuck *et al.* 1987; Swinburn 1988), three to azapropazone (Albazzad *et al.* 1986), and one to fenoprofen (Barbadi *et al.* 1986) have been described.

More recently an American perspective (Goodwin and Glenny 1992) details a case attributed to naproxen and presents data from the FDA ADR Spontaneous Reporting Program from 1982 to 1989 which identified 21 cases of pneumonitis with eosinophilia, one case of allergic pneumonitis, and six cases of interstitial pneumonitis associated with naproxen. In the USA over this period the prescription rate for ibuprofen was twice that for naproxen, yet only nine cases of hypersensitivity pneumonitis due to the former were reported to the FDA.

Cytotoxic drugs

Acute pulmonary reactions are relatively infrequent with cytotoxic drugs. Methotrexate accounts for most reports. Although the majority of the reported pulmonary complications of treatment with this folic acid antimetabolite have developed after many weeks of treatment, pulmonary reactions have been reported as early as 12 days after commencement. The reaction is not generally regarded as dose related because the total dose received has varied from 40–6500 mg, but there may be a more subtle relationship with frequency of doses. There is a much higher incidence of pneumonitis in patients receiving daily methotrexate injections (Nesbit *et al.* 1976). Pulmonary reactions had not been reported in patients receiving less than 20 mg weekly until low-dose methotrexate (10 mg weekly) became established as a third-line treatment for rheumatoid arthritis. Of 23 cases of acute pneumonitis on low-dosage methotrexate, three were fatal and the prevalence has been established at four per cent (Searles and McKendry 1987; Green *et al.* 1988; Ridley *et al.* 1988; Zitnik and Cooper 1990). The main features in evolution of the pulmonary reactions to methotrexate have been described in three excellent reviews of the subject (Whitcomb *et al.* 1972; Nesbit *et al.* 1976; Sostman *et al.* 1976). Typically cough, fever, dyspnoea, and sometimes cyanosis are accompanied by diffuse pulmonary mottling evident on the chest X-ray. Other radiographic changes include alveolar filling pattern, especially in the lower zones, pleural effusion, and hilar lymphadenopathy (Everts *et al.* 1973). Occasionally, symptoms precede the radiological changes; in patients with leukaemia the disease is almost always in remission when the pulmonary complications develop. Eosinophilia is present in about half of the reported cases. Lung biopsies have revealed non-specific features resembling the changes seen in lung disease associated with other antineoplastic drugs with aggregates of inflammatory cells, including eosinophils, plasma cells, and lymphocytes in the interstitial tissue and, to a lesser extent, within alveolar spaces.

In some cases symptoms and signs of pneumonitis have resolved spontaneously despite continuation of methotrexate treatment, usually with longer persistence of the X-ray changes. Resolution despite continued treatment is not a feature of other pulmonary reactions associated with eosinophilia (e.g. due to sulphasalazine). Rapid resolution of the pulmonary reaction is reported after administration of corticosteroid drugs. Of four deaths secondary to the pulmonary effects of methotrexate in higher dosage in one series, three were in individuals who did not receive corticosteroid treatment; the fourth was treated with a corticosteroid but succumbed to infection (Sostman *et al.* 1977). The pulmonary reaction to methotrexate can develop despite the concurrent administration of corticosteroid treatment. Relapse of pneumonitis on reintroduction of methotrexate has been recorded once (Goldman and Moschella 1971). Daunorubicin has been employed in the treatment of three cases (Pasquinucci *et al.* 1971) but spontaneous recovery was the probable reason for improvement (Cooper *et al.* 1986).

Procarbazine has been the subject of a number of reports of an allergic pneumonitis with prominent eosinophilia. Pleural effusions are common. The reaction may subside within a few days on withdrawal of the drug (Dohner *et al.* 1972; Lokich and Moloney 1972). Not surprisingly, steroids have been shown to be beneficial in this allergic reaction (Lewis 1984). Usually other drugs have been given, but prompt relapse has occurred on challenge with procarbazine (Jones *et al.* 1972; Ecker *et al.* 1978).

Azathioprine has been associated with an acute restrictive pulmonary reaction causing impairment of gas transfer and radiological signs of basal atelectasis or infiltration (Rubin *et al.* 1972; Weisenberger 1978; Carmichael *et al.* 1983). Withdrawal of the drug resulted in disappearance of the radiological abnormalities. There has been a single report of a similar reaction to mercaptopurine, the active metabolite of azathioprine (Sostman *et al.* 1977).

Mitomycin is an alkylating antibiotic and more than 50 cases of pulmonary toxicity associated with it have been recorded (Fielding *et al.* 1978; Gunstream *et al.* 1983; Twohig and Matthay 1990). There may be a fulminant fatal interstitial pneumonitis (Andrews *et al.* 1979). An incidence of approximately five per cent in a large series was reported by Buzdar and co-workers (1980), and interaction with *Vinca* alkaloids markedly increases the frequency of pneumonitis; for example Ozols and colleagues (1983) found this adverse reaction in five of 13 women (39 per cent) treated with mitomycin and vinblastine (with progesterone) for recurrence of ovarian carcinoma; two died of respiratory failure. Mitomycin alone occasionally causes a rapidly progressive interstitial pneumonitis, and an excellent response to corticosteroid therapy is to be expected (Buzdar *et al.* 1980). Despite the high incidence of the reaction there is little evidence to explain its pathogenesis. I have managed a patient with steroid-responsive mitomycin-related diffuse pneumonitis who developed fatal thrombotic thrombocytopenic purpura (TTP) some months later. Mitomycin was the only cytotoxic drug given, and at autopsy there was minimal recurrence of colonic carcinoma a year after colectomy.

A syndrome of renal insufficiency, thrombocytopenia, and microangiopathic haemolytic anaemia, very often aggravated by infusion of blood or blood products, has been linked with mitomycin, and some 40 patients with this problem (also labelled haemolytic–uraemic syndrome) have been described (Twohig and Matthay 1990). This mitomycin-related syndrome differs from idiopathic TTP in that neurological complications seem to be less prevalent. TTP is thought to be due to a defect in the capillary endothelium that affects its ability to release von Willebrand factor multimers enzymatically, and in experimental animals mitomycin injected into a platelet-free renal artery has caused local changes characteristic of TTP. The occurrence of pneumonitis and TTP in the same patient may be coincidental but the propensity for patients with the mitomycin-related TTP to develop non-cardiogenic pulmonary oedema argues for some relationship to pulmonary toxicity.

With bleomycin a chronic pulmonary fibrosis is recognized and this is discussed below, but there have been a couple of reports involving six patients with hypersensitivity pneumonitis and pulmonary eosinophilia due to bleomycin (Holyoye *et al.* 1978; Yousem *et al.* 1985).

Other drugs

Diffuse alveolitis has been attributed to penicillamine used in the treatment of rheumatoid arthritis (Eastmond 1976; Camus et al. 1982). Scott and colleagues (1981) described a syndrome of sudden onset of dyspnoea, crackles, and bilateral diffuse pulmonary shadowing on the chest X-ray beginning 5–16 weeks after the start of treatment in six patients who were being given gold injections. They also reviewed the literature, finding that of a total of 20 pulmonary reactions to gold, nine had resolved. Gold treatment had been discontinued in all and six had received corticosteroid therapy. The total dose of sodium aurothiomalate given ranged from 350–1000 mg. IgE levels rose after gold injection and an immune basis for the reaction is certain (Zitik and Cooper 1990) especially as Partenen and others (1987) showed that all but three of 17 patients with rheumatoid arthritis and gold-induced pneumonitis expressed at least one of two high-risk major histocompatibility-complex patterns. Lung biopsies have been taken in a number of cases and the histological changes are of septal thickening with infiltration by lymphocytes, plasma cells, and eosinophils (Autran et al. 1978), but the cellular reaction in one case was so dense as to resemble adenocarcinoma (James et al. 1978). In a further case the appearances were those of fibrosing alveolitis (Geddes and Brostoff 1976). Symptoms in this case recurred when gold was reintroduced and resolved completely when treatment stopped. This pattern seems fairly typical of other case reports. Impairment of pulmonary function may, however, prove to be permanent (Daymond and Griffiths 1980; Scott et al. 1981).

Pepys (1969) described pulmonary eosinophilia induced by pituitary snuff, and a similar reaction to inhaled cromoglycate has been described in two cases (Lobel et al. 1972; Repo and Nieminen 1976) is of uncertain origin as pulmonary eosinophilia occurs spontaneously in patients with asthma.

Intravesical BCG has been used for immunotherapy of recurrent transitional cell carcinoma, and three cases of hypersensitivity pneumonitis due to this method of treatment have been reported by Israel-Biet and colleagues (1987). An acute onset after multiple (3–8) treatments was characterized by lymphocytosis on bronchial alveolar lavage, with an increase in T_4/T_8 ratios compared with the patient's own circulating lymphocyte and control values. The chest X-ray showed no abnormality in one patient whereas bilateral micronodular shadowing was observed in the first two patients with the syndrome.

Individual cases of hypersensitivity pneumonitis have been reported with mephenesin (Rodman et al. 1958),

imipramine (Wilson et al. 1963), phenytoin (Bayer 1976), metformin (Klapholz et al. 1986), and nomifensine (Patel et al. 1988).

Pulmonary oxygen toxicity

High concentrations of oxygen are toxic to the alveoli and pulmonary capillaries. Proliferative changes may develop in the walls of capillaries within a few hours of exposure to 100 per cent oxygen at atmospheric pressure. Normal subjects breathing pure oxygen at this pressure developed substernal distress which becomes unbearable after 48–72 hours (Dolezal 1962). Bronchoscopic studies have shown reduced mucus velocity, and tracheitis developing during the first 6 hours (Sackner et al. 1975). Reduction in vital capacity and arterial desaturation accompany the exposure (Comroe et al. 1945; Ernsting 1961), but normality is restored within 48 hours. Shorter periods of exposure, up to 12 hours, do not appear to affect gas exchange or pulmonary circulation in normal subjects (van de Water et al. 1970). Patients undergoing intermittent positive pressure ventilation are prone to develop obscure pulmonary collapse and radiological shadowing; there are many potential causes of this, but the use of a high concentration of inspired oxygen is probably important in some cases. Indirect evidence of the effect of oxygen has been provided at autopsy studies, and Nash and co-workers (1967) demonstrated a relationship between alveolar haemorrhage, thickening of the alveolar walls, and hyaline membrane formation, and the concentration of inspired oxygen employed before death. Understanding of the pathogenesis of ARDS, however, has led to a realization that oxygen toxicity is of less significance than previously thought. Molecular and clinical aspects of oxygen toxicity have been reviewed by Jackson (1990). A fraction of the oxygen consumed in aerobic metabolism is converted to superoxide and thence to hydrogen peroxide. The capacity of the normal scavenging mechanisms (e.g. superoxide dismutase [glutathione peroxidase], catalase, and the non-enzymatic antioxidants β-carotene, α-tocopherol, ascorbate, cysteine) may in some clinical circumstances be overwhelmed. Autocatalytic destructive peroxidation of membrane lipids then follows. In animal experiments, synthesis of surfactant is also impaired by hyperoxia. In man, the dose–duration response relationship between oxygen and toxicity is broad and inspired oxygen fractions below 0.45 are unlikely to be harmful except after an exceedingly long exposure (Frank 1979). Short breaks in the exposure greatly improve tolerance. Jackson (1990) has outlined toxic interactions between oxygen and various therapies (e.g. radiotherapy or bleomycin) with or without prophylactic corticosteroid therapy.

Drug-induced pulmonary fibrosis

Ganglion-blocking agents

Unexplained breathlessness and widespread radiological shadowing that were not due to pulmonary oedema occurred in three of 54 patients being treated with the quaternary ganglion-blocker hexamethonium for severe hypertension (Doniach *et al*. 1954). This was the first instance of a report of drug-induced pulmonary fibrosis, and the histological features were further detailed by Heard (1962). The appearances were those of bronchiectasis and widespread fibrosis of the lungs with distortion and destruction of alveoli. A thorough postmortem study by Perry and colleagues (1957) found 'fibrinous pneumonitis' only in those patients who had received hexamethonium. Other ganglion-blockers, mecamylamine and pentolinium, were also found to be associated with the development of pulmonary fibrosis (Hildeen *et al*. 1958; Rokseth and Storstein 1960). While the above account is only of historical interest nowadays, it emphasizes the unexpected in pulmonary toxicology.

Cytotoxic drugs

That cytotoxic chemotherapy can cause chronic parenchymal lung damage is perhaps not surprising, and in this therapeutic area bleomycin has become a model drug in animal experimentation. Cytotoxic pulmonary toxicity has been recently reviewed very comprehensively by Jules-Elysee and White (1990), Twohig and Matthay (1990), Smith (1990), and Cooper and Matthay (1987), while Cooper and colleagues (1986) have given more detail about proposed mechanisms of toxicity. In general the factors predisposing to cytotoxic lung damage include (i) total cumulative dose; (ii) the age of the patient; (iii) prior or concurrent radiotherapy; (iv) (mainly subsequent) oxygen therapy; and (v) concomitant cytotoxic drug administration. Total cumulative dose seems to be important for bleomycin, busulphan, and carmustine. Older patients may be more sensitive to bleomycin toxicity. Synergistic toxicity between radiotherapy and bleomycin, busulphan, and mitomycin has been demonstrated. Postoperative oxygen therapy, for example, has been associated with enhanced bleomycin pulmonary toxicity, as have multidrug regimens that include carmustine, mitomycin (especially with vinblastine), cyclophosphamide, bleomycin, and methotrexate.

Chronic pneumonitis/pulmonary fibrosis is the most common clinical presentation — a pattern associated with virtually all categories of cytotoxic drugs (except for procarbazine, with which only hypersensitivity has been described). The symptoms are of malaise, unproductive cough, and breathlessness progressing over several weeks or months. On examination there are usually crackles on auscultation of the chest. The chest X-ray is the principal screening test for detecting pulmonary fibrosis, although it is limited in sensitivity and specificity. The clinical application of diagnostic radiology in evaluating drug-induced pulmonary disease has been reviewed by Taylor (1990). Interstitial pulmonary fibrosis may present radiologically with a reticular or nodular pattern, or both, with many agents. Pleural effusions are uncommon in these reactions. Computed tomography is more sensitive in detecting bleomycin toxicity, the evolution of which can be studied as it progresses from an initially pleural-based to a basal reticulonodular pattern. Magnetic resonance imaging has not yet proved of value. It is very likely that monitoring of carbon monoxide transfer factor or vital capacity would detect changes earlier. In another context, the lesson from lung transplantation is that repeated transbronchial biopsy is the most sensitive technique available for detecting the early stages of the parenchymal reaction of rejection.

Diagnosis may be difficult if there has been previous radiotherapy and if opportunistic infection or progression of the primary disease cannot be excluded. By and large an invasive diagnostic effort will reduce uncertainty for both clinician and patient (Rosenow 1990). Rechallenge is seldom needed, as alternative therapy is almost always available. Transbronchial and open lung biopsies show typical features of damage to Type I pneumocytes with consequent proliferation of the cuboidal Type II pneumocytes that line part or all of the alveoli. Active reparative pneumocytes will also be affected by the cytotoxic drug initiating the damage, and the cytological consequences of interfering with synthesis of DNA will be apparent. These include large hyperchromatic nuclei, bizarre chromatin patterns, cell giantism, etc. Epithelial atypia is evident on cytological examination of sputum.

Bleomycin

Pulmonary toxicity with bleomycin was noted in the initial clinical studies and preclinical animal toxicology. The susceptibility of the lung partially relates to the high ambient PO_2, as bleomycin generates superoxide and also interacts with oxygen therapy and radiotherapy in augmenting pulmonary toxicity in man and experimental animals. Occasionally, as discussed earlier, acute hypersensitivity pneumonitis can develop, but the chronic reaction is much more frequent and is dose related with patients varying in their susceptibility. Salem (1971) evaluated 56 patients aged 16–83 years by chest X-ray, lung biopsy, and pulmonary function testing, and found frank or suspected pulmonary fibrosis in 41 per cent of the 34 patients who were given a cumulative dose of more than 200 mg bleomycin per m^2 compared with 22 per cent of those given a lower dose. The older patients were more susceptible and 16 of the 19 reactions occurred in the 40 patients over 50 years of age. This influence of age seemed to be independent of a cumulative dose effect. Whether it related to renal dysfunction is unclear; bleomycin is excreted unchanged in urine but a proportion is inactivated enzymatically by a hydrolase. These early findings have been confirmed (Cooper *et al.* 1986) especially with regard to age and there seems to be a threshold at 450–500 units (450–500 mg) above which pulmonary toxicity is probable. There are well-documented cases of pulmonary fibrosis at lower doses, however, particularly in association with other risk factors. One patient of Salem (1971) had severe fibrotic changes at autopsy after 140 mg per m^2. The smallest reported dose associated with a pulmonary reaction was 60 units of bleomycin, which caused ARDS and alveolar fibroblast proliferation at autopsy in a patient with renal impairment (McLeod *et al.* 1987), and Iacovino and colleagues (1976) reported two fatal instances of interstitial pneumonitis in younger men given 105 and 165 units of bleomycin, respectively. A reversible reaction after 180 mg (15 mg weekly) has been described (Brown *et al.* 1978). Asymptomatic reactions without radiological changes have been detected by pulmonary function testing. This approach gave an overall incidence of pulmonary toxicity of between 33 per cent and 71 per cent (Pascual *et al.* 1973; Yagoda *et al.* 1972).

In younger age-groups, Lucraft and co-workers (1982) described 38 patients with testicular teratoma who received four doses of 90 mg of bleomycin and in whom the carbon monoxide transfer factor fell by 10 per cent after the first dose but not thereafter. An abnormal gallium scan, which reverted to normal after corticosteroid treatment, was seen in one patient whose lungs at autopsy were histologically normal (Rubery and Coakley 1980). Gallium is preferentially taken up by neutrophils, and the above report is of interest in view of the experimental finding that bleomycin can acutely increase the neutrophil count in fluid obtained by bronchoalveolar lavage in dogs (Fahey *et al.* 1982). A clinical correlate may be the increase in the percentage of neutrophils in the lavage fluid seen in four patients with bleomycin toxicity (Cooper *et al.* 1986). An increase in neutrophils is also found, however, in end-stage idiopathic pulmonary fibrosis and has been recognized as indicating a poor prognosis with little likelihood of a response to corticosteroid therapy. Another factor to be considered is whether bleomycin has been used in the past in a given patient. All previous regimens containing bleomycin should be included in calculating the total dose, as no period between doses adequate to abolish a possible increased risk of pulmonary dysfunction due to previous administration has yet been established (Cooper *et al.* 1986).

Alkylating agents

For many, busulphan lung is the archetype of drug-induced pulmonary toxicity, but other alkylating agents in common use, such as cyclophosphamide, chlorambucil, and melphalan, are also toxic to the lung.

Busulphan The incidence of pulmonary toxicity with this drug is four per cent (Cooper *et al.* 1986), but autopsy studies have shown subclinical damage in about half the cases. It is of interest that busulphan is chemically related to hexamethonium (see above). Almost always treatment will have been in progress for many months or even many years before symptoms develop, and there seems to be a threshold cumulative dose of 500 mg below which pulmonary toxicity has not occurred unless radiotherapy or other cytotoxic chemotherapy has been exhibited. The onset of toxicity is insidious. Fever is usual and is accompanied by cough and dyspnoea. The early histological features include proteinaceous alveolar oedema and dysplastic Type II pneumocytes, while advanced cases may have 'honeycomb lung' with alveoli replaced by masses of fibrous tissue (Heard and Cooke 1968). The condition is irreversible, and mean survival after diagnosis has been 5 months (Cooper *et al.* 1986). Pleural effusion has occurred in two cases. A complicating feature of pulmonary fibrosis due to busulphan has been the development of alveolar cell carcinoma (Min and Györkey 1968; Rosenow 1972). Busulphan should be withdrawn. There have been anecdotal reports of response to corticosteroid therapy, but awareness of the cumulative dose risk and monitoring of lung function at this threshold may help avoid clinical toxicity.

Chlorambucil and melphalan There have been fewer reports of pulmonary toxicity with these drugs but the clinical features are similar to other cases of drug-induced pulmonary fibrosis and the prognosis is poor (Twohig and Matthay 1990). One patient with chlorambucil toxicity, however, had a restrictive pulmonary defect (low transfer factor), a scattered interstitial mononuclear infiltrate on lung biopsy, and a dramatic response to withdrawal of the drug and corticosteroid therapy (Cole *et al.* 1978). Of seven patients reported with melphalan pulmonary toxicity, five died from progressive fibrosis (Major *et al.* 1980; Cooper *et al.* 1986). One patient who received 592 mg of melphalan over 8 months, even though the diagnosis of myeloma had not been established, developed a cough, progressive dyspnoea, and had a carbon monoxide transfer factor 30 per cent of the predicted value (Goucher *et al.* 1980). There was interstitial lung disease on an open lung biopsy. Corticosteroids were given but symptoms failed to improve despite radiological clearing. Westerfield and others (1980) described a patient whose recovery seemed complete. Major and colleagues (1980) reported one death, of a pharmacist who treated himself with melphalan apparently because myeloma had been mentioned to him in the differential diagnosis of his illness.

Cyclophosphamide   This drug is very widely used as a cytotoxic agent and, in lower dosage, as an immunosuppressant, yet Cooper and colleagues (1986) found only 20 cases of cyclophosphamide-induced pulmonary fibrosis recorded in the literature, in eight of which the patients had also received vincristine. Its rarity makes it a diagnosis of exclusion, which may be difficult without lung biopsy, particularly in patients with systemic or pulmonary vasculitis or granulomatosis. Fever, cough, and progressive breathlessness are common. Interstitial pneumonitis has occurred after prolonged cyclophosphamide treatment for Hodgkin's disease (Topilow *et al.* 1973), whereas Patel and colleagues (1976) reported pulmonary fibrosis on open lung biopsy in a 72-year-old woman in whom the infiltrates cleared completely when cyclophosphamide (given concurrently with vincristine and prednisolone) was stopped and continuous treatment with high-dose prednisolone was instituted. Immunosuppressant doses have also caused two fatal pulmonary reactions (Burke *et al.* 1982). One patient had rapidly progressive glomerulonephritis (GN) and was given 100 mg per day for 7 weeks and the other had refractory nephrotic syndrome and received 200 mg per day for 13 weeks. Mark and colleagues (1978) also reported a patient with GN who developed a restrictive ventilatory defect with an 'extensive intra-alveolar histiocytic infiltrate and septal thickening'. Improvement after withdrawal of cyclophosphamide was slow in spite of the administration of prednisolone.

Carmustine   The nitrosoureas are particularly used as single agents in the treatment of intracranial tumours, and Twohig and Matthay (1990) identified more than 80 reports of pulmonary toxicity, the majority of which occurred with carmustine (BCNU). The first case was reported in 1976, more than 10 years after the introduction of this drug. A possible explanation for the delay is the variable survival of patients and also the slow development of the pulmonary fibrosis, which shows all the usual histological features of cytological dysplasia; uniquely, however, the fibroblast proliferation is not accompanied by an obvious degree of inflammatory cell infiltrate (Weiss *et al.* 1981). Indeed, many cases of pulmonary toxicity developed quite late, for example, 3–4 years after treatment, and Cooper and others (1986) stated the incidence of this complication to be 20–30 per cent, while the mortality rate has varied from 45–55 per cent in different series. A recent report calls for a complete reappraisal of this brief summary of the scope of the problem, however. O'Driscoll and colleagues (1990) examined a cohort of survivors of carmustine chemotherapy in childhood. Of 31 children (aged 2–16 years) given carmustine for brain tumours, only 17 survived, and six of these died subsequently from pulmonary fibrosis, two within 3 years of treatment and four from 8–13 years after treatment. Eight of the remaining patients were available to be studied, 10–17 years after treatment. The findings were cough and dyspnoea in four, and in six an abnormal chest X-ray with upper zone fibrotic changes with unique computed tomographic appearances; for the group, vital capacity was 54 per cent, and transfer factor ranged from 28–78 per cent, of the predicted values, whereas the transfer coefficient (K_{CO}) ranged from 93–151 per cent. Bronchoalveolar lavage showed an increase in the percentage of macrophages containing fibronectin. Transbronchial biopsy showed interstitial fibrosis and elastosis. The recognition of an active pulmonary fibrotic process up to 17 years after treatment with carmustine emphasizes the need to follow up these patients and consider single lung transplantation as the pulmonary fibrosis progresses.

Nitrofurantoin

Pulmonary reactions to this drug are among the most frequently reported adverse effects on the lungs. A spectrum of reactions is seen in which acute, subacute, and chronic forms may be distinguished (Hailey *et al.* 1969; Sovijarvi *et al.* 1977). The acute reaction is discussed with other examples of hypersensitivity pneumonitis. Subacute reactions develop after about 4 weeks of continuous treatment, and fever and intense breathlessness occur. Eosinophilia is not universal and a raised antinuclear antibody can sometimes be detected (Selroos and Edgren 1975). Chronic reactions are of insidious onset and are associated with long-term prophylactic treatment lasting more than 6 months. Withdrawal of nitrofurantoin is the principal therapeutic approach. The majority of reactions are not severe, but persistent damage is common with the chronic reaction, in which lung biopsy will show vascular sclerosis with fibrosis and thickening of alveolar septa, together with interstitial inflammation. Interestingly, desquamative pneumonitis has been described with nitrofurantoin (R.D. Bone *et al.* 1976), and this type of reaction can be expected to respond reasonably satisfactorily to corticosteroid therapy with more complete resolution than if the drug were merely withdrawn.

Amiodarone

Amiodarone has several antiarrhythmic actions and unusual pharmacokinetics. This latter feature is attributable to the lipid solubility of the drug and its metabolites. Accumulation in the tissues and a broad spectrum of adverse reactions ensue. A recent meta-analysis of prophylactic amiodarone after myocardial infarction and in congestive heart failure (Amiodarone Trials Meta-Analysis Investigators, 1997) reviewed 13 trials (nine randomly controlled, and four open studies published from 1987 to 1997) and concluded that amiodarone reduced total mortality by 13 per cent in the 6553 patients. The excess risk of pulmonary toxicity, defined as 'lung infiltrates', was 1.1 per cent (1.6–0.5 per cent [in controls]; odds ratio 3.1, P = 0.0003). Higher doses of amiodarone are required for the management of resistant ventricular and supraventricular arrhythmias and the first report of amiodarone pulmonary toxicity was by Rotmensch and colleagues (1980). They described a 50-year-old man who developed lassitude and tachypnoea after one month of amiodarone in a dose of 400 mg daily. The chest X-ray showed diffuse pulmonary shadowing; FVC was 46 per cent of the predicted value; PaO_2 was 6.0 kPa, and pulmonary hypertension was found with a normal wedge pressure. Amiodarone was discontinued; prednisolone 60 mg per day was started; and within 2 weeks there was complete resolution. Many descriptions of individual cases and series followed but in most the speed of onset and resolution were not as rapid as this. Kennedy (1990) identifies two main clinical patterns.

More common is a subacute presentation with cough and increased breathlessness, sometimes with weight loss. A chest radiograph will show diffuse interstitial infiltrates bilaterally. The other mode of presentation resembles that of the first patient described above and is a more acute illness. This group of patients are pyrexial and have chest X-ray changes with a more alveolar distribution of opacification. Pleural effusions are unusual but have been described (Sobol and Rakita 1982; Gonzales-Rothi *et al.* 1987). Eosinophilia is not a feature. Confluent opacities, which may be peripheral, apical, or pleurally based, have been described (March-

linski *et al.* 1982; Gefter *et al.* 1983). Monitoring of the CO transfer factor as a method of early detection of amiodarone pulmonary toxicity was advocated in the third edition of this book. Kennedy (1990) has reviewed the evidence that has been presented in the interim and concludes that patients should have pulmonary function testing when they are in a stable condition before or soon after starting amiodarone. He states that testing should be repeated whenever the clinical picture suggests the possibility of pulmonary toxicity. A fall of 15–20 per cent in transfer factor is a certain predictor of amiodarone toxicity. Lesser degrees of impairment are not significant, especially if the patient is asymptomatic.

The histological features of pulmonary toxicity due to amiodarone are typical of this whole group of chronic fibrotic reactions with one exception, that is, the intra-alveolar accumulation of 'foamy' macrophages, which can also be detected after bronchoalveolar lavage. They are a marker of amiodarone accumulation and are present in patients who do not have pulmonary toxicity (Myers *et al.* 1987). Electron microscopy has shown that the 'foamy' appearance is due to dense lamellar cytoplasmic inclusions containing phospholipid (with amiodarone and desethylamiodarone). This phospholipidosis is probably central to the aetiology of amiodarone pulmonary toxicity and occurs because of the unique pharmacokinetic properties of the drug and its metabolite. They each have a huge volume of distribution (5000 litres) and this requires a very long elimination half-life ($t_{1/2}$) that is biphasic, representing clearance from well-diffused and poorly diffused tissues; values for $t_{1/2}$ of 45–60 days are quoted (Martin 1990). It will be apparent therefore that stopping the drug in a patient with toxicity will not result in rapid clearing of the affected tissue or organ, particularly if the drug has accumulated significantly following administration for a prolonged period.

Both the parent drug and its major metabolite, desethylamiodarone, are concentrated in the lung up to 1000-fold compared with serum levels. Given this accumulation a direct toxic effect would be considered a likely mechanism, particularly as part of the damage seems to occur much more frequently in patients receiving higher doses (Marchlinski *et al.* 1982; Suarez *et al.* 1983; Gefter *et al.* 1983). Daily doses of amiodarone greater than 400 mg are associated with a 5–7 per cent incidence of interstitial pneumonitis.

There are, however, two populations of patients, those with and those without evidence of inflammation and immunological reaction and it may be that these people also have different histological appearances on lung biopsy; for example, Myers and colleagues (1987) found 'organizing pneumonia' in a quarter of their patients with amiodarone toxicity. This type of histological picture is expected to respond to corticosteroid therapy, as did a patient who had features of fibrosing alveolitis associated with chronic amiodarone administration who continued to deteriorate when the drug was stopped (Butland and Millard 1984). One patient reported by Adams and colleagues (1986), however, developed frank toxicity despite receiving corticosteroid treatment incidentally. They also found that reduction or withdrawal of steroids was associated with clinical deterioration in two patients and with a decline in pulmonary function tests in four others. These were patients who received doses of 400–600 mg daily for 8 months or so and in whom the steroid therapy was reduced before one would expect clearance of amiodarone from tissues. In other patients improvement following reduction of the dose was greater than when steroids were given. Nevertheless, Kennedy (1990) recommends treating patients with amiodarone pulmonary toxicity with corticosteroids; a typical regimen consists of an initial dose of 40–60 mg with subsequent tapering based on the severity of the illness and the clinical response. Treatment continues for 4–6 months with close clinical follow-up. Some patients require continuous steroid therapy with the low, almost physiological, dose of 10 mg of prednisolone on alternate days. Given the life-threatening ventricular arrhythmias for which amiodarone therapy is usually instituted, it is understandable that doctors are reluctant to reduce the dose once a stable clinical situation has been achieved. Nevertheless, this would seem to be the best prophylactic means of reducing the incidence of amiodarone pulmonary toxicity.

Other drugs

Virtually all drug reactions that cause an acute hypersensitivity pneumonitis may lead to persistent sequelae, especially when the cause of the reaction is not recognized and the offending agent is not discontinued. This is likely if the onset is insidious or if respiratory disease is a recognized complicating feature of the underlying disease.

The antiarrhythmic drug tocainide has occasionally been associated with the development of pulmonary fibrosis, and a recent report described the computed tomographic appearances (Stein et al. 1988).

Other parenchymal problems

Carcinoma of the lung has been mentioned above in relation to busulphan lung, and theoretically it may complicate any chronic pulmonary fibrosis (cf. 'scar cancer' in healed fibrotic pulmonary tuberculosis). Pulmonary nodules have been described in patients receiving chemotherapy with cisplatin, bleomycin, and vinblastine (CBV) for germ-cell tumours (Zucker et al. 1987), and Trump and others (1988) saw new basal nodules on computed tomography after CBV in 11 patients with intrathoracic tumours. All of the patients recovered. Talcott and colleagues (1987) found cavitating granulomas on open lung biopsy following CBV. In 2.8 per cent of patients receiving an infusion of bleomycin, acute chest pain, which in some instances was thought to be due to myocardial ischaemia, developed; in others there was a pleuritic element. Six of the 10 patients had pulmonary metastases and pain developed on the second or third day of therapy. The pain recurred in two of seven patients. There were no long-term sequelae, and White and colleagues (1987) concluded that continuing the therapy was safe. An unusual consequence of intravenous drug abuse has been the development of severe bullous emphysema due to methylphenidate (Sherman et al. 1987), and this may follow other granulomatous reactions to other intravenous illicit substance abuse (Heffner et al. 1990).

Drugs affecting the pleura

Pleural space

Pleural effusion may complicate heart failure and the nephrotic syndrome and may be provoked by excessive intravenous infusion of colloid. Peritoneal dialysis has been associated with recurrent pleural effusions, presumably due to the passage of dialysis fluid through developmental transdiaphragmatic communications (Holm et al. 1971). Pleural effusions complicating ARDS may not be apparent if the chest X-ray is taken in the supine position. They may also occasionally occur as part of an acute or chronic parenchymal reaction to a drug, for example, with nitrofurantoin (Robinson 1964) or amiodarone (Sobol and Rakita 1982). Gonadotrophin has caused acute ascites and hydrothorax (Mrouch and Kase 1967).

Methysergide

Pleural thickening, fibrosis, and effusion can be produced by this drug. As a rule the patient has been taking the treatment for several months before the onset of the reaction is made apparent by the development of pleural pain, breathlessness, fever, and malaise. Examination may reveal signs of an effusion with a loud pleural rub. The chest X-ray usually shows a uniform hazy shadowing over the lower lung fields. A restrictive ventilatory defect is generally present. Occasionally there is nodular thickening of the pleura, which suggests tumour formation. Although the pleural lesion is usually described as fibrosis, improvement in symptoms and in the radiological appearance has been reported after cessation of treatment, and Kok-Jensen and Lindeneg (1970) found persisting severe disability in only two out of 12 cases in which treatment had been withdrawn because of pleuropulmonary complications. The mechanism underlying the development of the pleural changes is quite unknown and withdrawal of the drug is the only measure required to bring about improvement. Pulmonary mediastinal fibrosis and retroperitoneal fibrosis also occur with this drug.

Bromocriptine

Bromocriptine, like methysergide, is an ergot derivative and is used as a dopaminergic agonist in Parkinson's disease, particularly where 'on–off' phenomena occur with levodopa. Therapy therefore tends to be long-term, and Rinne (1981) drew attention to pleuropulmonary fibrosis with pleural effusion in seven of 123 parkinsonian patients being treated with bromocriptine. Five of the seven were also receiving levodopa. The manufacturer's cumulative experience from 1974 to 1981 amounted to 4000 patient-years and only a single report was on file (Krupp 1981); in the same correspondence LeWitt and Calne (1981) reported one patient. It is only with subsequent case reports and series and longer term treatment that convincing circumstantial evidence has accumulated of a very real problem in a minority of patients taking bromocriptine.

Of 441 reports to the Committee on Safety of Medicines since 1971 mentioning bromocriptine, two are for pleural fibrosis and two for pulmonary fibrosis, but McElvaney and others (1988) found seven patients with pleuropulmonary fibrosis which they attributed to bromocriptine, in a survey based in British Columbia. The dose-range was 22–50 mg per day and all were men who were over 55 years of age and heavy cigarette smokers. The onset of symptoms occurred 9 months to 4 years after starting treatment. The patients complained of dyspnoea, pleuritic pain, and an unproductive cough. The chest X-ray showed unilateral or bilateral pleural thickening and basal pulmonary fibrosis. Lung function was impaired with reduced static and dynamic lung volumes, and the CO transfer factor was reduced in proportion to the change in lung volume, that is, the diffusion coefficient (K_{CO}) was normal or raised. Open pleural biopsy in two patients revealed an exudative effusion with eosinophilia and pleural fibrosis with

occasional inflammatory cells. No cause other than bromocriptine was found after investigation and clinical benefit followed cessation of therapy in five patients. In two patients bromocriptine was continued and one deteriorated.

Tornling and colleagues (1986) described four cases (three of them non-smokers) aged 61–65 years who developed their reactions 2–3 years after starting bromocriptine, the eventual doses being 20–50 mg per day. Corticosteroid therapy was used with some improvement but most benefit was seen after withdrawal of bromocriptine. I have managed a patient in whom symptoms began 7 years after the start of treatment with marked clinical improvement on stopping bromocriptine, especially with regard to his breathlessness and cough that had been productive of mucoid sputum. His sense of well-being improved and weight gain was substantial, but radiological changes have been minor after 4 months. Having regard to this patient's late development of the reaction, one must suspect that many more cases of pleuropulmonary fibrosis will develop as time elapses and the duration of therapy increases. It is not surprising therefore that retroperitoneal fibrosis has also occurred with bromocriptine therapy (Bowler *et al.* 1986; Herzog *et al.* 1989), and Ward and others (1987) reported patients with both retroperitoneal and pleuropulmonary fibrosis. McElvaney and colleagues (1988) also described pleuropulmonary fibrosis in a patient treated with another ergot derivative, mesulergine, with clinical benefit following its withdrawal. The occurrence of progressive pulmonary fibrosis in patients taking methysergide, ergotamine, LSD, or bromocriptine seems to be dose related. One theory of the aetiology suggests that antagonism at serotonin (5-HT) receptors is important, but further clarification is awaited, especially with regard to activity of these drugs at different 5-HT receptor subtypes.

Pleural fibrosis and effusion have been observed as a complication of practolol therapy (Hall *et al.* 1978).

Haemothorax

Haemothorax has occurred in patients on anticoagulant therapy who have fallen and fractured ribs (Hamaker *et al.* 1969; Diamond and Fell 1973) or who have developed haemorrhagic pulmonary infarction following pulmonary embolism (Simon *et al.* 1969; Millard 1971).

Pneumothorax and pneumomediastinum

Pneumothorax has been reported to complicate the chemotherapy of germ-cell tumours with pulmonary metastases (Schulman *et al.* 1979). Abusers of illicit substances may indulge in extraordinary measures to increase their 'high' (Heffner *et al.* 1990). As peripheral veins become thrombosed, jugular and subclavian access may be attempted, which may result in laceration of the apex of the lung and pneumothorax. Use of the inhalational route can be accompanied by attempts to maximize absorption from alveolar surfaces. A Valsalva manoeuvre after maximal inspiration is reasonably safe but abusers who get a partner to augment their total lung capacity may suffer barotrauma. Alkaloidal cocaine seems to be particularly associated with pneumomediastinum.

Respiratory muscles and their central nervous control

Drug-induced neuromuscular disorders

This subject is discussed in detail in Chapter 20 and there is little that applies exclusively to respiratory muscles. Prolonged apnoea after the administration of suxamethonium, due to pseudocholinesterase deficiency, is well recognized. The aminoglycoside antibiotics may also aggravate neuromuscular blockade, especially in the presence of renal impairment or myasthenia gravis. Neomycin is probably the most dangerous of the drugs in this regard. Spinal anaesthesia, accidentally produced by local anaesthetic agents, may cause dangerous respiratory depression, especially if the cervical spinal cord is affected.

An interesting reaction to levodopa in postencephalitic parkinsonism has been recognized (Granerus *et al.* 1974; De Keyser and Vincken 1985). Within 2 hours of taking levodopa, the rate and depth of respiration become irregular and symptomatic dyspnoea arises. The phenomenon is dose related.

Tiapride, a substituted benzamide, effective in dyskinesia induced by levodopa, normalized the spirogram in one patient, who became free of dyspnoea (De Keyser and Vincken 1985). Hyperventilation is a well-recognized effect of salicylate overdose; the effect is sometimes quite striking and may be associated with tetany.

Depression of central ventilatory control

All sedative and anaesthetic agents are capable of depressing ventilation even in normal individuals, particularly if given in sufficiently high dosage. Patients with hepatic failure are particularly prone to respiratory depression when treated with agents that are largely detoxicated in the liver, for example, benzodiazepines; and patients with renal failure are vulnerable to morphine, as morphine-6-glucuronide has sedative activity and depends on renal excretion. Elderly individuals often show a surprising susceptibility to sedatives. Respiratory depression by drugs administered in standard doses is perhaps most often seen in patients with chronic bronchitis, long-standing airflow obstruction, and chronic compensated Type II respiratory failure. There is probably no drug capable of producing sedation with complete safety in such individuals. In severe asthma with exhaustion and retention of carbon dioxide, sedative drugs are particularly dangerous, and mechanical ventilation is the required treatment in this circumstance. Dangerous respiratory depression is most likely to arise from postoperative analgesia and during the intravenous sedation that is now commonly used to cover minor surgery, dental procedures, endoscopy, and various types of needle biopsy. Narcotic addiction in mothers has been associated with a fourfold increase in the sudden infant death. The defect in the chemical control of breathing persists in babies for several weeks, long after methadone, for example, has been cleared from their blood (Shannon and Kelly 1982).

Oxygen in respiratory failure with airflow obstruction

Patients with chronic respiratory failure and those who gradually develop respiratory failure are commonly insensitive to the ventilatory stimulus of carbon dioxide. During an acute infective exacerbation, worsening airflow obstruction causes further retention of carbon dioxide, and under these circumstances hypoxaemia is the main stimulus to breathing. If oxygen is administered, this hypoxic drive is removed and ventilation diminishes further, leading to still greater accumulation of carbon dioxide. Carbon dioxide exerts a narcotic effect at high partial pressures and stupor resulting from this will result in a failure to cough up secretions, leading in turn to further deterioration in ventilatory status and the likelihood of the development of bronchopneumonia. This sequence of events is now widely understood. Problems may be minimized by serial measurement of arterial blood gases and only giving sufficient oxygen to avoid progressive elevation of P_{CO_2}. Administration of an infusion of doxapram may be useful in the short term to stimulate ventilation and so permit adequate oxygen therapy. If deterioration occurs despite this therapy, mechanical ventilation may be necessary, especially in patients with bronchopneumonia.

References

Abenhaim, L., Moride, Y., Brenot, F. *et al.* (1996). Appetite suppressant drugs and the risk of primary pulmonary hypertension. *N. Engl. J. Med.* 335, 609.

Adams, P.G., Gibson, G.J., Morley, A.R., *et al.* (1986). Amiodarone pulmonary toxicity: Clinical and subclinical features. *Q. J. Med.* 59, 449.

Albazzaz, M.K., Harvey, J.E., Hoffman, J.N., *et al.* (1986). Alveolitis and haemolytic anaemia induced by azapropazone. *BMJ* 293, 1537.

Ali, N. and Banks, T. (1973). Pentazocine addiction causing bacterial endocarditis and pulmonary embolism. *Chest* 64, 762.

Amiodarone Trial Meta-analysis Investigators (1997). Effect of prophylactic amiodarone on mortality after acute myocardial infarction: meta-analysis of individual data from 6500 patients in randomised trials. *Lancet* 350, 1417.

Andersson, L. and Smidt, C.M. (1974). An investigation of the bronchial mucous membrane after long-term treatment with beclomethasone diproprionate (Becotide). *Acta Allergol.* 29, 354.

Andrews, A.T., Bowman, H.S., Patel, S.B., *et al.* (1979). Mitomycin and interstitial pneumonitis. *Ann. Intern. Med.* 90, 127.

Ansell, G. Adverse reactions to contrast agents — scope of problem. *Invest. Radiol.* 5, 374.

Autran, P., Garbe, L., Pommier De Santi, P., *et al.* (1978). Un cas d'accident rare de la chrysothérapie: une miliare pulmonaire allergique. *Rev. Fr. Mal. Respir.* 6, 183.

Ballen, K.K. and Weiss, S.T. (1988). Fatal acute respiratory failure following vinblastine and mitomycin administration for breast cancer. *Am. J. Med. Sci.* 295, 558.

Ballester, E., Reyes, A., Roca, J., *et al.* (1989). Ventilation–perfusion mismatching in acute severe asthma: effects of salbutamol and 100% oxygen. *Thorax* 44, 258.

Barbadi, F., Quenzer, F., and Rapp, K. (1986). Pulmonary sensitivity to Nalfon. *Ann. Allergy* 57, 205.

Barclay, K., Keaney, M.G.L., Glew, E., *et al.* (1990). Multiresistant *Haemophilus influenzae*. *Lancet* 335, 549.

Bayer, A.S. (1976). Dilantin toxicity, miliary pulmonary infiltrates and hypoxemia. *Ann. Intern. Med.* 85, 475.

Beasley, R., Rafferty, P., and Holgate, S. (1986). Benzalkonium chloride and bronchoconstriction. *Lancet* ii, 127.

Beaudry, C. and Laplante, L. (1973). Severe allergic pneumonitis from hydrochlorothiazide. *Ann. Intern. Med.* 78, 251.

Becker, C.E., MacGregor, R.R., Walker, K.S., *et al.* (1966). Fatal anaphylaxis after intramuscular iron dextran. *Ann. Intern. Med.* 65, 745.

Beemer, G.H., Dennis, W.L., Platt, P.R., *et al.* (1988). Adverse reactions to atracurium and alcuronium. *Br. J. Anaesth.* 61, 680.

Bell, R.J.M. (1964). Pulmonary infiltration with eosinophils caused by chlorpropamide. *Lancet* i, 1249.

Belongia, E.A., Hedberg, C.W., Gleich, G.J., *et al.* (1990). An investigation of the cause of eosinophilia–myalgia syndrome associated with tryptophan use. *N. Engl. J. Med.* 323, 357.

Bertelsen, K. and Dalgaard, J.B. (1965). Death from penicillin; cases from Denmark with autopsies. *Nord. Med.* 73, 173.

Bhatia, SP.P. and Davies, H.J. (1975). Evaluation of tolerance after continuous oral administration of salbutamol to asthmatic patients. *Br. J. Clin. Pharmacol.* 2, 463.

Bogartz, L.J. and Miller, W.C. (1971). Pulmonary oedema associated with proproxyphene intoxication. *JAMA* 215, 259.

Bolster, M.B. and Silver, R.M. (1994). Eosinophilia–myalgia syndrome, toxic oil syndrome, and diffuse fasciitis with eosinophilia. *Curr. Opin. Rheumatol.* 6, 642.

Bone, R.D., Wolfe, J., Sobonya, R.E., *et al.* (1976). Desquamative interstitial pneumonia following chronic nitrofurantoin therapy. *Am. J. Med.* 60, 677.

Bone, R.S., Jay, S.J., Reynolds, R.C., *et al.* (1976). Massive pulmonary haemorrhage: a rare complication of heparin therapy. *Am. J. Med. Sci.* 272, 197.

Bowler, J.V., Ormerod, I.E., and Legg, N.J. (1986). Retroperitoneal fibrosis and bromocriptine. *Lancet* ii, 466.

British Medical Journal (1973). Analgesics and asthma. *BMJ* iii, 419.

British Medical Journal (1990). Guidelines for the management of asthma in adults. *BMJ* 301, 651.

Brooks, S.M., Werk, E.E., Ackerman, S.J., *et al.* (1972). Adverse effects of phenobarbital on corticosteroid metabolism in patients with bronchial asthma. *N. Engl. J. Med.* 286, 1125.

Brown, W.G., Hassan, F.M., and Barbee, R.A. (1978). Reversibility of severe bleomycin induced pneumonitis. *JAMA* 239, 2012.

Bruchhausen, D., Haschem, J., and Dardene, M.U. (1969). Effect of pilocarpine administered into the conjunctival sac on airway obstruction in asthmatics. *German Medical Monthly* 14, 587.

Bryant, D.H. and Pepys, J. (1976). Bronchial reactions to aerosol inhalant vehicle (beclomethasone dipropionate). *BMJ* i, 1319.

Bucknall, C.E., Adamson, M.R., and Banham, S.W. (1987). Non fatal pulmonary haemorrhage associated with nitrofurantoin. *Thorax* 42, 475.

Bucknall, C.E., Neilly, J.B., Carter, R., *et al.* (1988). Bronchial hyperreactivity in patients who cough after receiving angiotensin converting enzyme inhibitors. *BMJ* 296, 86.

Buist, A.S., Burney, P.G.J., and Feinstein, A.R. (1989). Fenoterol and fatal asthma. *Lancet* i, 1071.

Burke, D.A., Stoddart, J.C., Ward, M.K., *et al.* (1982). Fatal pulmonary fibrosis occurring during treatment with cyclophosphamide. *BMJ* 285, 696.

Butland, R.J.A. and Millard, F.J.C. (1984). Fibrosing alveolitis associated with amiodarone. *Eur. J. Respir. Dis.* 65, 616.

Buzdar, A.U., Legha, S.S., Luna, M.A., *et al.* (1980). Pulmonary toxicity of mitomycin. *Cancer* 45, 236.

Byrd, R.B. and Schanzer, B. (1969). Pulmonary sequelae in procainamide-induced lupus-like syndrome. *Dis. Chest* 55, 170.

Cameron, J.D. (1974). Pulmonary oedema following drip-infusion urography. Case report. *Radiology* 111, 89.

Camus, P., Reybet-Degat, O., Justrabo, E., et al. (1982). D-penicillamine-induced severe pneumonitis. *Chest* 81, 376.

Carmichael, D.J.S., Hamilton, D.V., Evans, D.B., et al. (1983). Interstitial pneumonitis associated with azathioprine in a renal transplant patient. *Thorax* 38, 951.

Chalmers, D., Dombey, S.L., and Lawson, D.H. (1987). Post marketing surveillance of captopril (for hypertension): a preliminary report. *Br. J. Clin. Pharmacol.* 24, 343.

Child, J.S., Wolfe, J.B., Tashkin, D., et al. (1975). Fatal lung scan in case of pulmonary hypertension due to obliterative pulmonary vascular disease. *Chest* 67, 308.

Chiu, C.L. and Gambach, R.R. (1974). Hypaque pulmonary oedema, a case report. *Radiology* 111, 91.

Chuck, A.J., Wilcox, M., and Bossingham, D.H. (1987). Fenbufen-associated pneumonitis. *Br. J. Rheumatol.* 26, 475.

Chung, M.M., Chetty, K.G., and Jerome, D. (1985). Metoclopramide and asthma. *Ann. Intern. Med.* 103, 809.

Clark, R.J. (1986). Aggravation of asthma by beclomethasone in a thirty-month-old boy. *Lancet* ii, 574.

Clarke, R.S.J., Dundee, J.W., Garrett, R.T., et al. (1975). Adverse reactions to intravenous anaesthetics. A survey of 100 reports. *Br. J. Anaesth.* 47, 575.

Clarke, R.S.J., Fee, J.P.H., and Dundee, J.W. (1977). Factors predisposing to hypersensitivity-reactions to intravenous anaesthetics. *Proc. R. Soc. Med.* 79, 782.

Clarke, S.W. and Newman, S.P. (1984). Therapeutic aerosols 2 — Drugs available by the inhaled route. *Thorax* 39, 1.

Cohen, A.J., King, T.E. Jr, and Downey, G.P. (1994). Rapidly progressive bronchiolitis obliterans with organising pneumonia. *Crit. Care Med.* 149, 1670.

Cole, S.R., Myers, T.J., and Klatsky, A.U. (1978). Pulmonary disease with chlorambucil therapy. *Cancer* 41, 455.

Comroe, J.H. Jr and Dripps, R.D. (1946). The histamine like action of curare and tubocurarine injected intra-cutaneously and intra-arterially in man. *Anaesthesiology* 7, 260.

Comroe, J.H. Jr, Dumke, P.R., and Deming, M. (1945). Oxygen toxicity. The effect of inhalation of high concentrations of oxygen for twenty-four hours on normal man at sea level and at a simulated altitude of 18,000 feet. *JAMA* 128, 710.

Connolly, H.M., Crary, J.L., McGoon, M.D., et al. (1997). Valvular heart disease associated with fenfluramine–phentermine. *N. Engl. J. Med.* 337, 581.

Connolly, K. (1982). Adverse reaction to ipratropium bromide. *BMJ* 285, 934.

Cooper, J.A.D. Jr and Matthay, R.A. (1987). Drug induced pulmonary disease. *Disease-a-Month* 33, 61.

Cooper, J.A.D. Jr, White, D.A., and Matthay, R.A. (1986). Drug induced pulmonary disease Part 1: Cytotoxic drugs. *Am. Rev. Respir. Dis.* 133, 321.

Coppack, S.W., Gillett, M.K., and Snashall, P.D. (1984). Inappropriately inhaled bronchodilators. *Thorax* 39, 472.

Council on Drugs. (1964). A mucolytic agent; acetylcysteine (Mucomyst). *JAMA* 190, 147.

Crane, J., Pearce, N., Flatt, A., et al. (1989). Prescribed fenoterol and death from asthma in New Zealand. 1981–1983: case–control study. *Lancet* i, 917.

CSM (Committee on Safety of Medicines) (1979). Alphaxalone/Alphadalone. *Current Problems* No. 4. HMSO, London.

Dalgaard, J.B. and Bertelsen, K. (1965). Penicillin dodsfald. 16 secerede danske tilfaelde. *Nord. Med.* 73, 173.

Dan, M., Aderka, D., Topilsky, M., et al. (1986). Hypersensitivity pneumonitis induced by nalidixic acid. *Arch. Intern. Med.* 146, 1423.

Davis, D. and Macfarlane, A. (1974). Fibrosing alveolitis and treatment with sulphasalazine. *Gut* 15, 185.

Dawson, P., Pitfield, J., and Brittan, J. (1983). Contrast media and bronchospasm: a study with iopamidol. *Clin. Radiol.* 34, 227.

Daymond, T.J. and Griffiths, I.D. (1980). Pulmonary disease due to gold in rheumatoid arthritis. *Rheumatol. Rehab.* 19, 120.

Dean, N.C., Amend, W.C., and Matthay, M.A. (1987). Adult respiratory distress syndrome related to antilymphocyte globulin therapy. *Chest* 91, 619.

De Keyser, J. and Vincken, W. (1985). L-dopa-induced respiratory disturbance in Parkinson's disease suppressed by tiapride. *Neurology* 35, 235.

Diamond, M.T. and Fell, S.C. (1973). Anticoagulant induced massive hemothorax. *N.Y. State J. Med.* 73, 691.

Dohner, V.A., Ward, H.P., and Standord, R.E. (1972). Alveolitis during procarbazine, vincristine and cyclophosphamide therapy. *Chest* 62, 636.

Dolezal, V. (1962). Some humoral changes in man produced by continuous oxygen inhalations at normal barometric pressure. *Riv. Med. Aeronaut. Spaz.* 25, 219.

Doniach, I., Morrison, B., and Steiner, R.E. (1954). Lung changes during hexamethonium therapy for hypertension. *Br. Heart J.* 16, 101.

Douglas, A.S., Eagles, J.M., and Mowat, N.A.G. (1990). Eosinophilia–myalgia syndrome associated with tryptophan. *BMJ* 301, 387.

Dubovsky, S.L. and Freed, C. (1988). Exercise-induced bronchospasm caused by maprotiline. *Psychosomatics* 29, 104.

Du Moulin, G.C., Patterson, D.G., Hedley Whyte, J., et al. (1982). Aspiration of gastric bacteria in antacid treated patients; a frequent cause of post-operative colonisation of the airway. *Lancet* i, 242.

Dworkin, H.J., Smith, J.R., and Bull, F.E. (1966). A reaction following administration of macroaggregated albumin (MAA) for a lung scan. *AJR* 98, 427.

Eastmond, C.J. (1976). Diffuse alveolitis as a complication of penicillamine treatment for rheumatoid arthritis. *BMJ* i, 1506.

Ecker, M.D., Jay, B., and Keohand, M.F. (1978). Procarbazine lung. *AJR* 131, 527.

Elliott, H.R., Abdulla, V., and Hayes, P.J. (1978). Pulmonary oedema associated with ritodrine infusion and betamethasone administration in premature labour. *BMJ* ii, 799.

Ernsting, J. (1961). The effect of breathing high concentrations of oxygen upon the diffusing capacity of the lung in man. *J. Physiol.* (Lond.) 155, 51P.

Ersoz, N. and Finestone, S.C. (1971). Adrenaline induced pulmonary oedema and its treatment: a report of two cases. *Br. J. Anaesth.* 43, 709.

Eustace, B.R. (1967). Suxamethonium-induced bronchospasm. *Anaesthesia* 22, 638.

Everts, C.S., Westcott, J.L., and Bragg, D.G. (1973). Methotrexate therapy and pulmonary disease. *Radiology* 107, 539.

Fahey, P.J., Utell, M.J., Mayewski, R.J., *et al.* (1982). Early diagnosis of bleomycin pulmonary toxicity using B.A.L. in dogs. *Am. Rev. Respir. Dis.* 126, 126.

Fiegenberg, D.S., Weiss, H., and Krishman, H. (1967). Migratory pneumonia with eosinophilia associated with sulphonamide administration. *Arch. Intern. Med.* 120, 85.

Fielding, J.W.I., Stockley, R.A., and Brookes, V.S. (1978). Interstitial lung disease in a patient treated with 5-fluorouracil–mitomycin C. *BMJ* ii, 602.

Fishburne. J.I. Jr, Brenner, W.E., Bracksma, *et al.* (1972). Bronchospasm complicating intravenous prostaglandin F for therapeutic abortion. *Obstet. Gynecol.* 39, 892.

Flacke, J.W., Flacke, W.E., and Williams, G.D. (1977). Acute pulmonary edema following naloxone reversal of high-dose morphine anaesthesia. *Anesthesiology* 47, 376.

Follath, F., Burkhart, F., and Schweitzer, W. (1971). Drug induced pulmonary hypertension? *BMJ* i, 265.

Fouchet, P., Biour, M., Blayac, J.P. *et al.* (1997). Drugs that may injure the respiratory system. *Therapie* J. 10, 265.

Francis, R.A., Thomson, M.L., Pavia, D., *et al.* (1975). The effect of Sch 1000 MDI on the mucociliary clearance and lung function of healthy volunteers. *Postgrad. Med. J.* 51 (Suppl. 7), 110.

Frand, U.I., Shim, C.S., and Williams, M.H. (1972). Heroin induced pulmonary oedema; sequential studies of pulmonary function. *Ann. Intern. Med.* 77, 29.

Frank, L. (1979). The lung and oxygen toxicity. *Arch. Intern. Med.* 139, 347.

Fraser, P.M., Speizer, F.E., Waters, S.D.M., *et al.* (1971). The circumstances preceding death from asthma in young people in 1968–1969. *Br. J. Dis. Chest* 65, 71.

Fratto, C. (1979). Provocation of bronchospasm by eye drops. *Ann. Intern. Med.* 88, 362.

Freeman, R. (1980). Short term adverse effects of antibiotic prophylaxis for open heart surgery. *Thorax* 35, 941.

Frishman, W., Jacob, H., Eesenber, E., *et al.* (1979). Clinical pharmacology of the new beta-adrenergic blocking drugs. Part 8. Self poisoning with beta-adrenoceptor blocking agents: recognition and management. *Am. Heart J.* 98, 798.

Fuller, R.W. and Choudry, N.B. (1987). Increased cough reflex associated with angiotensin converting enzyme inhibitor cough. *BMJ* 295, 1025.

Gali, J.M., Vilanova, J.L., and Mayers, M. (1986). Pulmonary haemorrhage and eosinophilia due to febarbamate. *Respiration* 49, 231.

Geddes, D.M. and Brostoff, J. (1976). Pulmonary fibrosis associated with hypersensitivity to gold salts. *BMJ* i, 1444.

Gefter, W.B., Epstein, D.M., Pietra, G.G., *et al.* (1983). Lung diseases caused by amiodarone, a new antiarrhythmic agent. *Radiology* 147, 339.

Gentili, D.R., Kelly, K.M., Benjamin, E., *et al.* (1988). Ritodrine associated pulmonary oedema. *N.Y. State J. Med.* 88, 326.

Glauser, F.L., Smith, W.R., Caldwell, A., *et al.* (1976). Ethchlorvynol (Placidyl)-induced pulmonary oedema. *Ann. Intern. Med.* 84, 46.

Goldman, G.C. and Moschella, S.L. (1971). Severe pneumonitis occurring during methotrexate therapy. *Arch. Dermatol.* 103, 194.

Gonzalez-Rothi, R.J., Hannan, S.E., Hood, I., *et al.* (1987). Amiodarone pulmonary toxicity presenting as bilateral exudative pleural effusions. *Chest* 92, 179.

Goodwin, S.D. and Glenny, R.W. (1992). Nonsteroidal anti-inflammatory drug-associated pulmonary infiltrates with eosinophilia. *Arch. Intern. Med.* 152, 1521.

Goucher, G., Rowland, V., and Hawkins, J. (1980). Melphalan-induced pulmonary interstitial fibrosis. *Chest* 77, 805.

Gould, F.K., McGregor, C.G., Freeeman, R., *et al.* (1990). Respiratory complications following cardiac surgery. The role of microbiology in its evaluation. *Anaesthesia* 40, 1061.

Granerus, A.K., Jagenburg, R., Nilson, N.J., *et al.* (1974). Respiratory of disturbance during L-dopa treatment of Parkinson's syndrome. *Acta Med. Scand.* 195, 39.

Green, L., Shatner, A., and Birkinstat, H. (1988). Severe reversible interstitial pneumonitis induced by low dose methotrexate; report of a case and review of the literature. *J. Rheumatol.* 15, 110.

Gunstream, S.R., Seidenfeld, J.J., Sobonya, R.E., *et al.* (1983). Mitomycin-associated lung disease. *Cancer Treat. Rep.* 67, 301.

Haber, R.H., Oddone, E.Z., Gurbels, P.A., *et al.* (1986). Acute pulmonary decompensation due to amphotericin B in the absence of granulocyte transfusions. *N. Engl. J. Med.* 315, 836.

Hahn, H.H., Schweid, A.I.D., and Beaty, H.N. (1969). Complications of injecting dissolved methylphenidate tablets. *Arch. Intern. Med.* 123, 656.

Hailey, F.J., Glasscock, H.W. Jr, and Hewitt, W.F. (1969). Pleuropneumonic reactions to nitrofurantoin. *N. Engl. J. Med.* 281, 1087.

Hall, D.R., Morrison, J.B., and Edwards, F.R. (1978). Pleural fibrosis after practolol therapy. *Thorax* 33, 822.

Hamaker, W.R., Buchman, R.J., Cox, W.A., *et al.* (1969). Hemothorax: a complication of anticoagulant therapy. *Ann. Thorac. Surg.* 8, 564.

Hassall, E., Vich, T., and Ament, M.E. (1983). Pulmonary embolus and *Malassezia* pulmonary infection related to urokinase therapy. *J. Pediatr.* 102, 722.

Heard, B.E. (1962). Fibrous healing of old iatrogenic pulmonary oedema (hexamethonium lung). *J. Pathol. Bacteriol.* 83, 159.

Heard, B.E. and Cooke, R.A. (1968). Busulphan lung. *Thorax* 23, 187.

Heath, M.L. (1973). Bronchospasm in an asthmatic patient following pancuronium. *Anaesthesia* 28, 437.

Heffner, J.E., Harkey, R.A., and Schabel, S.I. (1990). Pulmonary reactions from illicit substance abuse. *Clin. Chest Med.* 11, 151.

Herzog, H., Minne, H., and Ziegler, R. (1989). Retroperitoneal fibrosis in a patient with macroprolactinoma treated with bromocriptine. *BMJ* 298, 1315.

Hildeen, T., Krogsgaard, A.R., and Vimtrup, B.J. (1958). Fatal pulmonary changes during the medical treatment of malignant hypertension. *Lancet* ii, 830.

Hill, R.N., Spragg, R.G., Wedel, M.K., *et al.* (1975). Adult respiratory distress syndrome associated with colchicine intoxication. *Ann. Intern. Med.* 83, 523.

Hine, L.K., Arrowsmith, J.B., and Gallo-Torres, H.E. (1988). Mono-octanoin-associated pulmonary edema. *Am. J. Gastroenterol.* 83, 1128.

Ho, D., Tashkin, D.P., Bein, M., *et al.* (1979). Pulmonary infiltrates with eosinophilia associated with tetracycline. *Chest* 76, 33.

Holgate, S.T., Baldwin, C.J., and Tattersfield, A.E. (1977). Beta-adrenergic agonist resistance in normal human airways. *Lancet* ii, 375.

Holm, J., Leiden, B., and Lindquist, B. (1971). Unilateral pleural effusion — a rare complication of peritoneal dialysis. *Scand. J. Urol. Nephrol.* 5, 84.

Holyoye, P.Y., Luna, M., Mackay, B., *et al.* (1978). Bleomycin hypersensitivity pneumonitis. *Ann. Intern. Med.* 88, 47.

Howarth, P.H. (1983). Bronchoconstriction in response to ipratropium bromide. *BMJ* 286, 1825.

Hrnicek, G., Skelton, J., and Miller, W.C. (1974). Pulmonary oedema and salicylate intoxication. *JAMA* 230, 866.

Iacovino, J.R., Leitner, J., Abbas, A.K., *et al.* (1976). Fatal pulmonary reaction from low doses of bleomycin. An idiosyncratic tissue response. *JAMA* 235, 125.

Idsøe, O. and Wang, K.Y. (1958). Penicillin-sensitivity reactions in Taiwan. *Bull. WHO* 18, 323.

Idsøe, O., Guthe, T., Wilcox, R.R., *et al.* (1968). Nature and extent of penicillin side-reactions with particular reference to fatalities from anaphylactic shock. *Bull. WHO* 38, 159.

Ind, P.W., Dixon, C.M.S., Fuller, R.W., *et al.* (1989). Anticholinergic blockade of beta-blocker-induced bronchoconstriction. *Am. Rev. Respir. Dis.* 139, 1390.

Inman, W.H.W. (1986). Enalapril-induced cough. *Lancet* ii, 1218.

Inman, W.H.W. and Adelstein, A. M. (1969). Rise and fall of asthma mortality in England and Wales in relation to use of pressurised aerosols. *Lancet* ii, 279.

Inman, W.H.W., Vessey, M.P., Westerholm, B., *et al.* (1970). Thromboembolic disease and the steroidal content of oral contraception. A report to the Committee on Safety of Drugs. *BMJ* ii, 203.

Inman, W.H.W., Rawson, N.S.B., Wilton, L.V., *et al.* (1988). Post marketing surveillance of enalapril. 1: Results of prescription–event monitoring. *BMJ* 297, 826.

Israel, R.H. and Olson, J.P. (1978). Pulmonary edema associated with intravenous vinblastine. *JAMA* 240, 1585.

Israel-Biet, D., Venet, A., Sandron, J., *et al.* (1987). Pulmonary complications of intravesical Bacille Calmette-Guérin immunotherapy. *Am. Rev. Respir. Dis.* 135, 763.

Jackson, R.M. (1990). Molecular pharmacologic and clinical aspects of oxygen-induced lung injury. *Clin. Chest Med.* 11, 73.

Jackson, R.T., Beaglehole, R., Rea, H.H., *et al.* (1982). Mortality from asthma: a new epidemic in New Zealand. *BMJ* 285, 771.

Jago, R.H. and Restall, J. (1978). Sensitivity testing for Althesin. *Anaesthesia* 33, 644.

James, D.W., Winster, W.F., and Hamilton, E.B.D. (1978). Gold lung. *BMJ* i, 1523.

Jones, S.E., Moore, M., Blank, N., *et al.* (1972). Hypersensitivity to procarbazine (Matulane) manifested by fever and pleuropulmonary reaction. *Cancer* 29, 498.

Joselson, R. and Warnock, M. (1983). Pulmonary venoocclusive disease after chemotherapy. *Hum. Pathol.* 14, 88.

Jules-Elysée, K. and White, D.A. (1990). Bleomycin-induced pulmonary toxicity. *Clin. Chest Med.* 11, 1.

Katz, S., Aberman, A., Frand, U.I., *et al.* (1972). Heroin pulmonary oedema. Evidence for increased pulmonary capillary permeability. *Am. Rev. Respir. Dis.* 106, 472.

Kaufman, J., Casanova, J.E., Riedl, P., *et al.* (1989). Bronchial hyperreactivity and cough due to angiotensin-converting enzyme inhibitors. *Chest* 95, 544.

Kay, J.J. (1974). The aminorex controversy. *Thorax* 29, 266.

Kay, J.M., Smith, P., and Heath, D. (1971). Aminorex and the pulmonary circulation. *Thorax* 26, 262.

Keaney, N.P., Churton, S., and Stretton, T.B. (1980). Failure to demonstrate tolerance to inhaled salbutamol in volunteers. In *Proceedings of the First World Conference in Clinical Pharmacology and Therapeutics* (ed. P. Turner), p. 165. Macmillan, London.

Keighley, J.F. (1966). Iatrogenic asthma associated with adrenergic aerosols. *Ann. Intern. Med.* 65, 985.

Kennedy, J.I. Jr (1990). Clinical aspects of amiodarone pulmonary toxicity. *Clin. Chest Med.* 11, 119.

Kent, D.G. (1965). Bleeding into pulmonary cyst associated with anticoagulant therapy. *Am. Rev. Respir. Dis.* 92, 108.

Klapholz. L., Leitersdorf, E., and Weinrauch, L. (1986). Pneumonitis and leucocytoclastic vasculitis due to metformin. *BMJ* 293, 483.

Kleiger, R.E., Boxer, M., Ingham, R.E., *et al.* (1976). Pulmonary hypertension in patients using oral contraceptives. *Chest* 69, 143.

Koeter, G.H., Menrs, H., Manchy, J.G.R., *et al.* (1982). Protective effect of disodium cromoglycate on propranolol challenge. *Allergy* 37, 587.

Kok-Jensen, A. and Lindeneg, O. (1970). Pleurisy and fibrosis of the pleura during methysergide treatment of hemicrania. *Scand. J. Respir. Dis.* 51, 218.

Kounis, N.G. (1976). Untoward reactions to corticosteroids: intolerance to hydrocortisone. *Ann. Allergy* 36, 203.

Kristenson, M. and Fryden, A. (1988). Pneumonitis caused by metronidazole. *JAMA* 260, 184.

Krupp, P. (1981). Pleuropulmonary changes during longer term bromocriptine treatment for Parkinson's disease. *Lancet* i, 44.

Larsson, S., Svedmyr, N., and Thiringer, G. (1977). Lack of bronchial beta adrenoceptor resistance in asthmatics during long term treatment with terbutaline. *J. Allergy Clin. Immunol.* 59, 93.

Lasser, E.C., Lang, J., Sorak, M., *et al.* (1977). Steroids: theoretical and experimental basis for utilization in prevention of contrast media reactions. *Radiology* 125, 1.

Laxenaire, M.C., Jacob, F., and Noel, P. (1976*a*). Accidents anaphylactoïdes liées à l'emploi de dextran de poids moléculaire 40,000. *Ann. Anesth. Fr.* 17, 101.

Laxenaire, M.C., Monteret-Vautrin, D.A., Moeller, R., *et al.* (1976*b*). Accidents anaphylactoïdes liées à l'emploi de produits anesthésiques et adjuvants à propos de 18 cas. *Ann. Anesth. Fr.* 17, 85.

Lehrman, K.L. (1976). Pulmonary embolism in a transexual man taking diethylstilbestrol. *JAMA* 235, 532.

Leikola, J., Koistinen, J., Lehtinen, J., *et al.* (1973). IgA-induced anaphylactic transfusion reactions: a report of four cases. *Blood* 42, 111.

Lewis, L.D. (1984). Procarbazine associated alveolitis. *Thorax* 39, 206.

LeWitt, P.A. and Calne, D.B. (1981). Pleuropulmonary changes during long-term bromocriptine treatment for Parkinson's disease. *Lancet* i, 44.

Lie, J.T. (1994). Nomenclature and classification of vasculitis: plus ça change, plus c'est la même chose. *Arthritis Rheum.* 37, 182.

Lobel, H., Machtey, I., and Eldror, M.Y. (1972). Pulmonary infiltrates with eosinophilia in asthmatic patient treated with disodium cromoglycate. *Lancet* ii, 1032.

Lohiya, G. (1987). Asthma and urticaria after hepatitis B. vaccination. *West. Med. J.* 147, 341.

Lokich, J.J. and Moloney, W.C. (1972). Allergic reaction to procarbazine. *Clin. Pharmacol. Ther.* 13, 573.

Lombard, C.M., Chung, A., and Winokur, S. (1987). Pulmonary veno-occlusive disease following therapy for malignant neoplasms. *Chest* 92, 871.

Lucraft, H.H., Wilkinson, P.M., Stretton, T.B., *et al.* (1982). Role of pulmonary function tests in the prevention of bleomycin pulmonary toxicity during chemotherapy for metastatic testicular teratoma. *Eur. J. Cancer Clin. Oncol.* 18, 133.

Macdonald, A.G. and McNeill, R.S. (1968). A comparison of the effect on airway resistance of a new beta-blocking drug ICI 50172 and propranolol. *Br. J. Anaesth.* 40, 508.

MacDonald, J.R., Mathison, D.A., and Stevenson, D.D. (1972). Aspirin intolerance in asthma. *J. Allergy Clin. Immunol.* 50, 198.

McElvaney, N.G., Wilcox, P.G., Churg, A., *et al.* (1988). Pleuropulmonary disease during bromocriptine treatment for Parkinson's disease. *Arch. Intern. Med.* 148, 2231.

MacLennan, A.C. and Stewart, D.G. (1990). Eosinophilia-myalgia syndrome associated with tryptophan. *BMJ* 301, 387.

McLeod, B.E., Lawrence, H.J., Smith, D.W. *et al.* (1987). Fatal belomycin toxicity from a low cumulative dose in a patient with renal insufficiency. *Cancer* 60, 2617.

McMurray, J., Bloomfield, P., and Miller, H.C. (1986). Irreversible pulmonary hypertension after treatment with fenfluramine. *BMJ* 292, 239.

McNeill, R.S. (1964). Effect of a beta-adrenergic blocking agent, propranolol, on asthmatics. *Lancet* ii, 1101.

Magee F., Wright, J.L., Chan, W., *et al.* (1986). Two unusual pathological reactions to nitrofurantoin: case reports. *Histopathology* 10, 701.

Major, P.P., Laurin, S., and Bettez, P. (1980). Pulmonary fibrosis following therapy with melphalan: a report of two cases. *Can. Med. Assoc. J.* 123, 197.

Malmquist, J., Trell, E., Torp, A., *et al.* (1970). A case of drug induced (?) pulmonary hypertension. *Acta Med. Scand.* 188, 265.

Marchlinski, F.E., Gansler, T.S., Waxman, H.L., *et al.* (1982). Amiodarone pulmonary toxicity. *Ann. Intern. Med.* 97, 839.

Mark, G.J. Lehimgar-Zadeh, A., and Ragsdale, B.D. (1978). Cyclophosphamide pneumonitis. *Thorax* 33, 89.

Marshall, A. and Moore, K. (1973). Pulmonary disease after amitriptyline overdosage. *BMJ* i, 716.

Marshall, A.J., Eltringham, W.K., Barritt, D.W., *et al.* (1977). Respiratory disease associated with practolol. *Lancet* ii, 1254.

Martelli, N.A. and Usandivaras, G. (1977). Inhibition of aspirin-induced bronchoconstriction by sodium cromoglycate inhalation. *Thorax* 32, 684.

Martin, W.J. (1990). Mechanisms of amiodarone pulmonary toxicity. *Clin. Chest Med.* ii, 131.

Maxwell, I. (1974). Reversible pulmonary edema following cyclophosphamide therapy. *JAMA* 229, 137.

Medsger, T.A. Jr (1990). Tryptophan-induced eosinophilia–myalgia syndrome. *N. Engl. J. Med.* 322, 926.

Meeker, D.P. and Wiedemann, H.P. (1990). Drug-induced bronchospasm. *Clin. Chest Med.* 11, 163.

Mendelson, L.M., Meltzer, E.O., and Hamburger, R.N. (1974). Anaphylaxis-like reactions to corticosteroid therapy. *J. Allergy Clin. Immunol.* 54, 125.

Michael, J.R. and Rudin, M.L. (1981). Acute pulmonary disease caused by phenytoin. *Ann. Intern. Med.* 95, 452.

Millard, C.E. (1971). Massive hemothorax complicating heparin therapy for pulmonary infarction. *Chest* 59, 235.

Miller, F.E. (1971). Aspirin-induced bronchial asthma in sisters. *Ann. Allergy* 29, 263.

Min, K.W. and Györkey, F. (1968). Interstitial pulmonary fibrosis, atypical epithelial changes and bronchiolar cell carcinoma following busulphan therapy. *Cancer* 22, 1027.

Morrison Smith, J. (1975). The value and safety of disodium cromoglycate. *Allergol. Immunopathol.* 3, 29.

Mrouch, A. and Kase, N. (1967). Acute ascites and hydrothorax after gonadotrophin therapy. *Obstet. Gynecol.* 30, 346.

Mullarkey, M.F., Thomas, P.S., Hansen, J.A. *et al.* (1986). Association of aspirin-sensitive asthma with HLA-DQW2. *Am. Rev. Respir. Dis.* 133, 261.

Murdock, D.K., Lawless, C.E., Collins, E., *et al.* (1987). ARDS following equine ATG therapy. *Chest* 92, 578.

Murray, R.J., Albin, R.J., Mergner, W., *et al.* (1988). Diffuse alveolar haemorrhage temporally related to cocaine smoking. *Chest* 93, 427.

Myers, J.L., Kennedy, J.I., and Plumb, V.J. (1987). Amiodarone lung: pathologic findings in clinically toxic patients. *Hum. Pathol.* 18, 349.

Nagy, L., Lee, T.H., and Kay, A.B. (1982). Neutrophil chemotactic activity in antigen-induced late asthmatic reactions. *N. Engl. J. Med.* 306, 497.

Nash, G., Blennerhasset, J.H., and Pontoppidan. H. (1967). Pulmonary lesions associated with oxygen therapy and artificial ventilation. *N. Engl. J. Med.* 276, 368.

Nesbit, M., Krivit, W., Heyn, R., *et al.* (1976). Acute and chronic effects of methotrexate on hepatic, pulmonary and skeletal systems. *Cancer* 37, 1048.

Nesse, R. and Carroll. J. (1976). Cholinergic side-effects associated with deanol. *Lancet* ii, 50.

Nestor, T.A., Tamamoto, W.I., Kam, T.H., *et al.* (1989). Acute pulmonary oedema caused by crystalline methamphetamine. *Lancet* ii, 1277.

Nicholis, M.G. and Gilchrist, N.L. (1987). Sulindac and cough induced by converting enzyme inhibitors. *Lancet* i, 21.

O'Callaghan, A.C., Scadding, G., and Watkins, J. (1986). Bronchospasm following the use of vecuronium. *Anaesthesia* 41, 940.

O'Connor, P.C., Erskine, J.G., and Pringle, T.H. (1981). Pulmonary oedema after transfusion with fresh frozen plasma. *BMJ* 282, 379.

O'Donnell, T.V., Holst, P.E., Rea, H.H., *et al.* (1989). Fenoterol and fatal asthma. *Lancet* i, 1070.

O'Driscoll, B.R., Hasleton, P.S., Taylor, P.M. *et al.* (1990). Active lung fibrosis up to 17 years after chemotherapy with carmustine (BCNU) in childhood. *N. Engl. J. Med.* 323, 378.

Ormerod, L.P. and Stableforth, D.E. (1980). Asthma mortality in Birmingham 1975–7. *BMJ* 280, 687.

Ozols, R.F., Hogan, W.M., Ostchega, Y., *et al.* (1983). M.V.P. (mitomycin, vinblastine and progesterone): a second line regimen in ovarian cancer with a high incidence of pulmonary toxicity. *Cancer Treat. Rep.* 67, 721.

Partenen, J., Van Assendelft, A.H., Koskimies, S., *et al.* (1987). Patients with rheumatoid arthritis and gold induced pneumonitis express two high-risk major histocompatibility complex patterns. *Chest* 92, 277.

Partridge, M.B. and Gibson, G.J. (1978). Adverse bronchial reactions to intravenous hydrocortisone in two aspirin-sensitive asthmatic patients. *BMJ* i, 1521.

Pascual, R.S., Mosher, M.B., Sikand, R.A., *et al.* (1973). Effects of bleomycin on pulmonary function in man. *Am. Rev. Respir. Dis.* 108, 211.

Pasquinucci, G., Ferrar, P., and Castellari, R. (1971). Daunorubicin treatment of methotrexate pneumonia. *JAMA* 216, 2017.

Patel, A.R., Shah,P.C., Rhee, H.L., *et al.* (1976). Cyclophos-Poephamide therapy and interstitial pulmonary fibrosis. *Cancer* 38, 1542.

Patel, H., Keshavan, M.S., and Pitts, K.E. (1988). Adverse lung reactions to nomifensine: a posthumous note. *Clin. Neuropharmacol.* 10, 190.

Patel, K.R. and Tullett, W.M. (1983). Bronchoconstriction in response of ipratropium bromide. *BMJ* 286, 1318.

Paterson, J.W., Conolly, M.E., Davies, D.S., *et al.* (1968). Isoprenaline resistance and the use of pressurised aerosols in asthma. *Lancet* ii, 426.

Pearce, N., Grainger, J., Atkinson, M., *et al.* (1990*a*). Case control study of prescribed fenoterol and death from asthma in New Zealand. *Thorax* 45, 170.

Pearce, N., Crane, J., Burgess, C., *et al.* (1990*b*). Case-control study of prescribed fenoterol and death from asthma in New Zealand, 1977–81: authors' reply. *Thorax* 45, 745.

Pepys, J. (1969). *Hypersensitivity Diseases of the Lungs due to Fungi and Organic Dusts*, p. 112. Karger, Basle.

Perry, H.M., O'Neil, R.M., and Thomas, W.A. (1957). Pulmonary disease following chronic chemical ganglionic blockade. *Am. J. Med.* 22, 37.

Pineda, A.A. and Taswell, H.F. (1975). Transfusion reactions associated with anti-IgA antibodies: report of four cases and review of the literature. *Transfusion* 15, 10.

Poe, R.H., Condemi, J.J., Weinstein, S.S., *et al.* (1980). Adult respiratory distress syndrome related to ampicillin sensitivity. *Chest* 77, 449.

Popa, V. (1987). Captopril-related (and induced?) asthma. *Am. Rev. Respir. Dis.* 136, 999.

Pratt, P.C. (1974). Pathology of pulmonary oxygen toxicity. *Am. Rev. Respir. Dis.* 110 (Suppl.), 51.

Rafferty, P., Beasley, R., and Holgate, S.T. (1988). Comparison of the efficacy of preservative free ipratropium bromide and Atrovent nebuliser solution. *Thorax* 43, 446.

Rahal, J.J., Meyers, B.R., and Weinstein, L. (1968). Treatment of bacterial endocarditis with cephalothin. *N. Engl. J. Med.* 279, 1305.

Ramsey, B. and Marks, J.M. (1988). Bronchoconstriction due to 8-methoxypsoralen. *Br. J. Dermatol.* 119, 83.

Rau, N.R., Nagaraj, M.V., Prakash, P.S., *et al.* (1988). Fatal pulmonary aspiration of oral activated charcoal. *BMJ* 297, 918.

Redline, R.W. and Dahms, B.B. (1981). *Malassezia* pulmonary vasculitis in an infant on long-term Intralipid therapy. *N. Engl. J. Med.* 305, 1395.

Reese, E.P. Jr, McCullough, J.J., and Craddock, P.R. (1975). An adverse pulmonary reaction to cryoprecipitate in a haemophiliac. *Transfusion* 15, 583.

Reichlin, S., Loveless, M.H., and Kane, E.G. (1953). Loeffler's syndrome following penicillin therapy. *Ann. Intern. Med.* 38, 113.

Repo, U.K. and Nieminen, P. (1976). Pulmonary infiltrates with eosinophilia and urinary symptoms during disodium cromoglycate treatment. A case report. *Scand. J. Respir. Dis.* 57, 1.

Reussi, C., Schiavi, J.E., Altman, R., *et al.* (1969). Unusual complications in the course of anticoagulant therapy. *JAMA* 46, 460.

Ridley, M.G., Wolfe, C.S., and Mathews, J.A. (1988). Life threatening acute pneumonitis during low dose methotrexate treatment for rheumatoid arthritis: a case report and review of the literature. *Ann. Rheum. Dis.* 47, 784.

Rinne, U.K. (1981). Pleuropulmonary changes during long-term bromocriptine treatment for Parkinson's disease. *Lancet* i, 44.

Robinson, B.R. (1964). Pleuropulmonary reaction to nitrofurantoin. *JAMA* 189, 239.

Rodman, D.M., Hanley, M., and Parsons, P. (1986). Aminoglutethimide, alveolar damage and haemorrhage. *Ann. Intern. Med.* 105, 633.

Rodman, T., Fraimow, W., and Myerson, R.M. (1958). Loeffler's syndrome: report of a case associated with administration of mephenesin carbamate (Tolseram). *Ann. Intern. Med.* 48, 668.

Rokseth, R. and Storstein, O. (1960). Pulmonary complication during mecamylamine therapy. *Acta Med. Scand.* 167, 23.

Rosenow, E.C. (1972). The spectrum of drug-induced pulmonary disease. *Ann. Intern. Med.* 77, 977.

Rosenow, E.C. (1990). Diffuse pulmonary infiltrates in the immunocompromised host. *Clin. Chest Med.* ii, 55.

Rotmensch, H.H., Liron, M., Tupilski, M., *et al.* (1980). Possible association of pneumonia with amiodarone. *Am. Heart J.* 100, 412.

Rubery, E.D. and Coakley, A.J. (1980). Early detection of lung toxicity after bleomycin therapy. *Cancer Treat. Rep.* 64, 732.

Rubin, G., Baume, P., and Vandenberg, R. (1972). Azathioprine and acute restrictive lung disease. *Aust. N.Z. J. Med.* ii, 272.

Sackner, M.A., Lauda, J., Zapafa, A., *et al.* (1975). Pulmonary effects of oxygen breathing: a 6 hour study in normal men. *Ann. Intern. Med.* 82, 40.

Sakula, A. (1977). Bronchial asthma due to allergy to pancreatic extract: a hazard in the treatment of cystic disease. *Br. J. Dis. Chest* 71, 295.

Salem, P.A. (1971). Pulmonary changes and bleomycin. *Cancer Bull.* 23, 68.

Samter, M. and Beers, R.F. (1967). Concerning the nature of intolerance to aspirin. *J. Allergy* 40, 281.

Schoeffed, R.E., Anderson, S.A., and Altounyan, R.E.C. (1981). Bronchial hyperreactivity in response to inhalation of ultrasonically nebulised solutions of distilled water and saline. *BMJ* 283, 1285.

Schoene, R.B., Martin, T.R., Charan, N.B., *et al.* (1981). Timolol-induced bronchospasm in asthmatic bronchitis. *JAMA* 206, 130.

Schulman, P., Cheng, E., Cvitkovic, E., *et al.* (1979). Spontaneous pneumothorax as a result of intensive cytotoxic chemotherapy. *Chest* 75, 194.

Schwartz, J.A. and Koenigsberg, M.D. (1987). Naloxone-induced pulmonary edema. *Ann. Emerg. Med.* 16, 1294.

Scott, D.L., Bradby, G.V., Altman, T.J., *et al.* (1981). Relationship of gold and penicillamine therapy to diffuse interstitial lung disease. *Ann. Rheum. Dis.* 40, 136.

Searles, G. and McKendry, R.J.R. (1987). Methotrexate pneumonitis in rheumatoid arthritis: potential risk factors. Four case reports and a review of the literature. *J. Rheumatol.* 14, 1164.

Sears, M.R. (1995). Changing patterns in asthma morbidity and mortality. *J. Invest. Allergol. Clin. Immunol.* 5, 66.

Sears, M.R., Rea, H.H., Fenwick, J., *et al.* (1987). Seventy five deaths in asthmatics prescribed home nebulisers. *BMJ* 294, 477.

Selroos, O. and Edgren, J. (1975). Lupus-like syndrome associated with pulmonary reaction to nitrofurantoin. *Acta Med. Scand.* 197, 125.

Shannon, D.C. and Kelly, D.H. (1982). SIDS and near-SIDS. *N. Engl. J. Med.* 306, 959.

Sherman, C.B., Hudson, L.D., and Pierson, D.J. (1987). Severe precocious emphysema in intravenous methylphenidate (Ritalin) abusers. *Chest* 92, 1085.

Shim, C. and Williams, M.H. Jr (1987). Cough and wheezing from beclomethasone aerosol. *Chest* 91, 207.

Sigvaldson, A. and Sorenson, S. (1983). Interstitial pneumonia due to sulphasalazine. *Eur. J. Respir. Dis.* 64, 229.

Simon, H.B., Daggett, W., and De Sanctis, R.W. (1969). Hemothorax as a complication of anticoagulant therapy in the presence of pulmonary infarction. *JAMA* 208, 1830.

Sklar, J. and Timms, R.M. (1977). Codeine-induced pulmonary edema. *Chest* 72, 230.

Smith, D.C., Lois, J.F., Gomes, A.S., *et al.* (1987). Pulmonary arteriography: Comparison of cough stimulation effects of diatrizoate and ioxaglate. *Radiology* 162, 617.

Smith, D.E., Herd, D., and Gazzard, B.G. (1988). Reversible bronchoconstriction with nebulised pentamidine. *Lancet* ii, 905.

Smith, G.J.W. (1990). The histopathology of pulmonary reactions to drugs. *Clin. Chest Med.* 11, 95.

Smith, J.H. and Weinstein, V.F. (1987). Cephalexin associated pulmonary infiltration with circulating eosinophilia. *BMJ* 294, 776.

Sobol, S.M. and Rakita, I. (1982). Pneumonitis and pulmonary fibrosis associated with amiodarone treatment: a possible complication of a new antiarrhythmic drug. *Circulation* 65, 819.

Sostman, H.D., Matthay, R.A., Putman, C.E., *et al.* (1976). Methotrexate-induced pneumonitis. *Medicine* (Baltimore) 55, 371.

Sostman, H.D., Matthay, R.A., and Putman, C.E. (1977). Cytotoxic drug-induced disease. *Am. J. Med.* 62, 608.

Sovijarvi, A.R.A., Lemola, M., Stenius, B., *et al.* (1977). Nitrofurantoin-induced acute, subacute and chronic pulmonary reactions. A report of 66 cases. *Scand. J. Respir. Dis.* 58, 41.

Spector, S.L., Wangarrd, C.H., and Farr, R.S. (1979). Aspirin and concomitant idiosyncrasies in adult and asthmatic patients. *J. Allergy Clin. Immunol.* 64, 500.

Speizer, F.E., Doll, R., and Heaf, P. (1968a). Observations on recent increase in mortality from asthma. *BMJ* i, 335.

Speizer, F.E., Doll, R., Heaf, P., and Strang, L.B. (1968b). Investigation into use of drugs preceding death from asthma. *BMJ* i, 339.

Spitzer, W.O. and Buist, A.S. (1990). Case-control study of prescribed fenoterol and death from asthma in New Zealand. *Thorax* 45, 645.

Sprenger, J.D., Altman, L.C., Marshall, S.G., *et al.* (1989). Studies of neutrophil chemotactic factor of anaphylaxis in metabisulphite sensitivity. *Ann. Allergy* 62, 117.

Stein, M.G., Demarco, T., Gamsu, G., *et al.* (1988). Computed tomography: pathologic correlation in lung disease due to tocainide. *Am. Rev. Respir. Dis.* 137, 458.

Steinberg, A.D. (1968). Pulmonary oedema following ingestion of hydrochlorothiazide. *JAMA* 204, 825.

Steinberg, A.D. and Karliner, J.S. (1968). The clinical spectrum of heroin pulmonary edema. *Arch. Intern. Med.* 122, 122.

Stenton, S.C., Duddridge, M., Walters, E.H., *et al.* (1990). An unusual response to methacholine. *Thorax* 45, 819.

Sternlieb, L., Bennett, B., and Scheinberg, I.H. (1975). D-penicillamine-induced Goodpasture's syndrome in Wilson's disease. *Ann. Intern. Med.* 82, 673.

Stromberg, C., Palva, E., Alhova, E. *et al.* (1987). Pulmonary infiltration induced by tolfenamic acid. *Lancet* ii, 685.

Stubblefield, P.G. (1978). Pulmonary oedema occurring after therapy with dexamethasone and terbutaline for premature labour: a case report. *Am. J. Obstet. Gynecol.* 132, 341.

Suarez, L.D., Poderoso, J.J., Elsner, B., *et al.* (1983). Subacute pneumopathy during amiodarone therapy. *Chest* 83, 566.

Sue-ling, H. and Hughes, L.E. (1988). Should the pill be stopped preoperatively? *BMJ* 296, 447.

Swinburn, C.R. (1988). Pulmonary infiltrations and lymphadenopathy in association with fenbufen. *Hum. Toxicol.* 7, 35.

Symmers, W. St. C. (1958). The occurrence of so-called collagen diseases, and of other diseases systemically affecting the connective tissues as a manifestation of sensitivity to drugs. In *Sensitivity Reactions to Drugs* (ed. M.L. Rosenheim and R. Moulton), p. 209. Blackwell, Oxford.

Szczeklik, A. and Gryglewski, R.J. (1983). Asthma and anti-inflammatory drugs. Mechanism and clinical patterns. *Drugs* 25, 533.

Szczeklik, A. and Nizankowska, E. (1978). Asthma relieved by aspirin and by other cyclo-oxygenase inhibitors. *Thorax* 33, 664.

Talcott, J.A., Gernick, M.B., Stomper, P.C., *et al.* (1987). Cavitary lung nodules associated with combination chemotherapy containing bleomycin. *J. Urol.* 138, 619.

Tan, S., Hall, I.P., Dewar, J., *et al.* (1997). Association between β_2-adrenoceptor polymorphism and susceptibility to bronchodilator desensitisation in moderately severe stable asthmatics. *Lancet*, 350, 995.

Taylor, C.R. (1990). Diagnostic imaging techniques in the evaluation of drug induced pulmonary disease. *Clin. Chest Med.* 11, 87.

Thiringer, G., Eriksson, N., Nalmberg, R., *et al.* (1975). Bronchoscopic biopsies of bronchial mucosa before and after beclomethasone dipropionate therapy. *Postgrad. Med. J.* 51 (Suppl. 4), 30.

Tomashefski, J.F. Jr, Hirsch, C.S., and Jolly, P.N. (1981). Microcrystalline cellulose pulmonary embolism and granulomatosis. A complication of illicit intravenous injections of pentazocine tablets. *Arch. Pathol. Lab. Med.* 105, 89.

Topilow, A.A., Rothenberg. S.P., and Cottrell, T.S. (1973). Interstitial pneumonia after prolonged treatment with cyclophosphamide. *Am. Rev. Respir. Dis.* 108, 114.

Tornling, G., Unge, G., Axelsson, G., *et al.* (1986). Pleuropulmonary reactions in patients on bromocriptine treatment. *Eur. J. Respir. Dis.* 68, 35.

Trump, D.L., Bartel, E., and Pozniak, M. (1988). Nodular pneumonitis after chemotherapy for germ cell tumours. *Ann. Intern. Med.* 109, 431.

Turner-Warwick, M.E.H. (1981). Adverse reactions affecting the lung: possible association with D-penicillamine. *J. Rheumatol.* 8, 166.

Twohig, K.J. and Matthay, R.A. (1990). Pulmonary effects of cytotoxic agents other than bleomycin. *Clin. Chest Med.* 11, 31.

Vanderbroucke, J.P. and Helmerhorst, F.M. (1996). Risk of venous thrombosis with hormone-replacement therapy. *Lancet* 348, 972.

van de Water, J.M., Kagey, K.S., Miller, I.T., *et al.* (1970). Response of lung to 6 to 12 hours of 100 per cent oxygen inhalation in normal men. *N. Engl. J. Med.* 283, 621.

Vaughan-Jones, R. and Goldman, L. (1968). Persistent eosinophilia after nitrofurantoin. *Lancet* i, 306.

Veale, D., McComb, J.M., and Gibson, G.J. (1990). Propafenone. *Lancet* 335, 979.

Vessey, M.P. and Doll, R. (1968). Investigation of relation between use of oral contraceptives and thromboembolic disease. *BMJ* ii, 199.

Vessey, M.P., Mant, D., Smith, A., *et al.* (1986). Oral contraceptives and venous thromboembolism: findings in a large prospective study. *BMJ* 292, 526.

Vignon, H., Gay, R., and Laxenaire, M.C. (1976). Observations cliniques d'accidents anaphylactoïdes per et post anesthétiques. Résultat d'enquête a posteriori. *Ann. Anesth. Fr.* 17, 117.

von Maur, K., Adkinson, N.F., van Metre, T.E., *et al.* (1974). Aspirin intolerance in a family. *J. Allergy Clin. Immunol.* 54, 380.

Waller, D.G. (1990). β-adrenoceptor partial agonists: a renaissance in cardiovascular therapy? *Br. J. Clin. Pharmacol.* 30, 157.

Wallerstein, R.A. (1968). Intravenous iron–dextran complex. *Blood* 32, 690.

Ward, C.D., Thompson, J., and Humby, M.D. (1987). Pleuropulmonary and retroperitoneal fibrosis associated with bromocriptine treatment. *J. Neurol. Neurosurg. Psychiatry* 50, 1706.

Weber, J.C.P. and Essigman, W.K. (1986). Pulmonary alveolitis and NSAIDs — fact or fiction? *Br. J. Rheumatol.* 25, 5.

Weill, H., Ferrans, V.J., and Gray, R.M. (1964). Early lipoid pneumonia: roentgenologic anatomic and physiologic characteristics. *Am. J. Med.* 36, 370.

Weisenberger, D.D. (1978). Interstitial pneumonitis associated with azathioprine therapy. *Am. J. Clin. Pathol.* 69, 181.

Weiss, R.B., Poster, D.S., and Penta, J.S. (1981). The nitrosoureas and pulmonary toxicity. *Cancer Treat. Rev.* 8, 111.

Westerfield, B.T., Michalski, J.P., McCombs, C., *et al.* (1980). Reversible melphalan-induced lung damage. *Am. J. Med.* 68, 767.

Whitcomb, M.E., Schwarz, M.I., and Tormey, D.C. (1972). Methotrexate pneumonitis: case report and review of the literature. *Thorax* 27, 636.

White, D.A., Schwartzberg, L.S., Kris, M.G., *et al.* (1987). Acute chest pain during bleomycin infusion. *Cancer* 59, 1582.

Williams, T., Eidns, L., and Thomas, P. (1982). Fibrosing alveolitis, bronchiolitis obliterans and sulfasalazine therapy. *Chest* 81, 766.

Wilson, I.C., Gambill, J.M., and Sandifer, M.G. (1963). Loeffler's syndrome occurring during imipramine therapy. *Am. J. Psychiatry* 119, 892.

Woldorf, N.M. and Pastore, P.N. (1972). Extreme epinephrine sensitivity with a general anaesthesia. *Arch. Otolaryngol.* 96, 272.

Wright, D.G., Robichard, K.J., Pizzo, P.A., *et al.* (1981). Lethal pulmonary reactions associated with the combined use of amphotericin B and leukocyte transfusions. *N. Engl. J. Med.* 304, 1185.

Yagoda, A., Mukherji, B., Young, C., *et al.* (1972). Bleomycin and antitumour antibiotic: clinical experience in 274 patients. *Ann. Intern. Med.* 77, 861.

Yocum, M.W., Heller, A.M., and Abels, R.I. (1978). Efficacy of intravenous pretesting and antihistamine prophylaxis in radiocontrast media-sensitive patients. *J. Allergy Clin. Immunol.* 62, 309.

Young, D.J. (1972). Propoxyphene suicides: report of nine cases. *Arch. Intern. Med.* 129, 62.

Yousem, S.A., Lifson, J.D., and Colby, T.V. (1985). Chemotherapy induced eosinophilic pneumonia: relation to bleomycin. *Chest* 88, 103.

Zitnik, R.J. and Cooper, J.A.D. (1990). Pulmonary disease due to antirheumatic agents. *Clin. Chest Med.* 11, 139.

Zucker, P.K., Khoun, N.F., and Rosenshein, N.B. (1987). Bleomycin-induced pulmonary nodules: a variant of bleomycin pulmonary toxicity. *Gynecol. Oncol.* 28, 284.

Zweiman, B., Mishkin, M.M., and Hildreth, E.A. (1975). An approach to the performance of contrast studies in contrast material reactive persons. *Ann. Intern. Med.* 83, 159.

Zyroff, J., Slovis, T.L., and Nagler, J. (1974). Pulmonary edema induced by methadone. *Radiology* 112, 567.

11. Oral and dental disorders

R. A. SEYMOUR

Introduction

Many drugs have been implicated as causes of adverse reactions affecting the mouth and associated structures. These are discussed in this chapter under the following categories: (1) oral mucosa and tongue; (2) periodontal tissues; (3) dental structures; (4) salivary glands; (5) cleft lip and palate; (6) muscular and neurological disorders; (7) taste disturbances, and halitosis; (8) drug-induced oral infections; (9) facial oedema; and (10) blood dyscrasias. The vast majority of adverse drug reactions that affect the mouth and associated structures are of the Type B (see Chapter 5).

Oral mucosa and tongue

The effects of drugs on the oral mucosa can be manifested in a variety of ways including hypersensitivity reactions, oral ulceration, lichenoid eruptions, and oral systemic lupus erythematosus (SLE). In addition, systemic drug therapy can cause erythema multiforme and SLE.

Hypersensitivity reactions

The main type of hypersensitivity reaction that affects the oral mucosa is Type IV (Coombs and Gell 1968), a delayed reaction mediated by sensitized T lymphocytes; reactions of this type can be classified as 'stomatitis medicamentosa' (fixed drug eruption) when due to a systemic medication, and as 'stomatitis venenata' when due to contact hypersensitivity.

Stomatitis medicamentosa (fixed drug eruption)

Oral manifestations of drug hypersensitivity are considerably less common than skin reactions. The lesions vary greatly in appearance, from areas of erythema to areas of ulceration. In the early phase of the reaction,

vesicles or bullae which quickly break down may be found on the palate, lips, or tongue. A fixed drug eruption is one that appears at the same site each time a particular drug is administered. The eruption may be a solitary lesion, particularly at the first attack, but after repeated attacks new lesions may appear together with lesions involving the original site. The time elapsing between ingestion of the drug and the appearance of the lesion varies from a few hours to 24 hours. Drugs that have been involved in fixed drug eruptions include salicylates, meprobamate, sulphonamides, dapsone, oxyphenbutazone, and tetracyclines (Seymour et al. 1996). The last-named group only rarely (Murray and Defco 1982) affect the oral mucosa though they not infrequently cause fixed drug eruptions of the skin.

Stomatitis with erythematous, bullous, or ulcerative lesions, in the absence of skin involvement, has been reported as an adverse reaction to barbiturates (Kennett 1968), phenindione (Hollman and Wong 1964), indomethacin (Guggenheimer and Ismail 1975), and penicillamine (Lam 1980; Eisenberg et al. 1981). Gold therapy causes adverse reactions in 30 per cent; 3.3 per cent develop a stomatitis and glossitis (Gordon et al. 1975). It may also cause widespread oral ulceration, which on healing may leave appearances suggestive of lichen planus. Sjögren's syndrome has been considered a contraindication to gold therapy, but in this survey reactions were not more common in patients with the syndrome than in those without. Adverse reactions to lignocaine are rare, but a fixed drug eruption has occurred in a 7-year-old atopic child exposed to 2.2 ml of Xylonor 2% special (a solution containing lignocaine hydrochloride, noradrenaline, adrenaline, and saline) (Curley and Baxter 1987).

The mechanism involved in a fixed drug eruption is uncertain, but a humoral agent has been detected in serum during an exacerbation. An intradermal injection of the patient's serum produced an inflammatory response in previously affected areas of skin (Wyatt et al. 1972). Ultrastructure studies from lesions of fixed drug eruptions have demonstrated features similar to those in other bullous reactions (e.g. erythema multiforme and toxic epidermal necrolysis). Dyskeratotic bodies, indicative of severe epidermal injury, have been found in the epidermis (De Dobbeleer and Achten 1977).

Stomatitis venenata (contact stomatitis)

Contact hypersensitivity implies a local reaction of the mucosa after repeated contact with one of many causative agents. Common allergens in contact stomatitis include antibiotics, mouthwashes, toothpastes, topical anaesthetics, cosmetics, food additives, antiseptic lozenges, various dental alloys, and chewing gum. The interval between contact with the allergen and the development of hypersensitivity may vary from days to years. The stomatitis may show erythematous lesions and there may be mucosal oedema. The patient may complain of a burning sensation in the mouth together with xerostomia.

Allergic reactions to amalgam are rare, and when they occur are probably due to the mercury contained in the amalgam (Duxbury et al. 1982). In such cases, the intraoral reactions consist of mucosal swelling accompanied by a burning sensation and blister formation (James et al. 1985) (see also Amalgam and Lichenoid eruptions).

The constituents of various dentifrices are commonly implicated as a cause of contact sensitivity. Plasma cell gingivitis or contact stomatitis has also been attributed to toothpaste containing cinnamonaldehyde (Thyne et al. 1989; Lamey et al. 1990), formalin (CSM 1984); and herbal toothpaste (MacLeod and Ellis 1989).

A condition termed 'atypical gingivostomatitis' has been described (Perry et al. 1973). Affected patients complained of a 'burning mouth' and were found to have gingivitis, glossitis, and angular cheilitis. Histological findings in these cases included considerable plasma cell infiltration of the gingival tissues. Symptoms and signs abated in all patients when they avoided chewing gum and dentifrices, but recurred in most of them when they started using these substances again.

Stainless steel wires, extensively used in dentistry, in orthodontics, in oral surgery, and in prosthodontics, caused a reaction following wiring of the jaws of one patient (Schriver et al. 1976), and the reaction appeared to be due to the nickel in the alloy; and because of the escalating costs of precious metals there is an increasing use of nickel–chromium alloys in dentistry; those commonly available have a nickel content of 60–80% by weight, and adverse reactions to such alloys are likely to increase (Basker 1981). A further case of a Type IV cell-mediated reaction to the nickel content of orthodontic wire has been described (Dunlop et al. 1989). Again, symptoms resolved when the wires were removed. Nickel hypersensitivity has also been implicated in causing severe alveolar bone loss after placement of porcelain fused to metal crowns (Bruce et al. 1995) with a high nickel content. A local hypersensitivity reaction was accompanied by severe localized bone loss in the area where the crowns were fitted. Beryllium is also sometimes used as a

constituent in dental alloys for crown and bridge restorations. When used in such alloys, beryllium tends to migrate to the surface because of its small atomic radius, and its negative charge makes it react with water (saliva), forming beryllium hydroxide. Two cases of a beryllium-induced contact gingivostomatitis have been reported (Haberman et al. 1993).

Recent concern over the use of mercury has renewed interest in the use of palladium as a substitute in dental alloys, but this is not without unwanted effects, including hypersensitivity reactions such as allergic contact dermatitis, and it is therefore questionable whether it is a suitable alternative to amalgam. Palladium and platinum are also incorporated into dental alloys for use in crown and bridgework, and the problem of contact stomatitis due to both these metals has been highlighted (Koch and Baum 1996).

Isolated — incidence estimated to be 1:1000 by Churgin and Payne (1981) — cases of a localized allergic response to Scutan, an ethylene imine temporary crown material, have been reported. The response is usually due to the unpolymerized material.

Topically applied iodoform, chlorhexidine, or stannous fluoride are frequently used in dentistry, and may cause contact stomatitis (Yaacob and Jalil 1986; Maurice et al. 1988; Razak and Latifah 1988).

Hydroquinone is often mixed with acrylic monomer to prevent its spontaneous polymerization and can be incorporated into acrylic prostheses, although at a concentration of less than 0.1%. Other components of acrylic are often implicated as causing an allergic contact stomatitis, but contact stomatitis due to hydroquinone itself can also occur (Torres et al. 1993). Patients 'allergic' to acrylic, should also be tested for hydroquinone. If positive, a new prosthesis should be constructed using a different monomer.

Lipsticks and lip-liners containing various constituents are used extensively as cosmetics. Allergic contact cheilitis, although rare, has been attributed to castor oil, oxybenzone, and mandelic acid in lipsticks (Fisher 1991; Aguirre et al. 1992, 1994) and to para-tertiary butylphenol in a lip-liner (Angelini et al. 1993).

Flavoured lipsalves have become increasingly popular over recent years. Case reports have implicated the various flavouring agents (i.e. strawberry and vanilla) in causing an allergic contact cheilitis (Ferguson and Beck 1995; Taylor et al. 1996).

Several food additives have now been recognized as causing either a contact stomatitis or cheilitis (Lewis et al. 1995). Those identified include menthol, peppermint oil, dodecyl gallate, butylated hydroxyanisole, and octyl gallate. Dietary investigations and patch testing are now standard investigations for patients presenting with sore mouths and swelling of the lips.

The burning mouth syndrome is a fairly common condition. The pathogenesis is uncertain, but it may be due to psychogenic factors; hormonal withdrawal; folate, iron, or pyridoxine deficiency; or local hypersensitivity reactions to the materials utilized in dental prostheses. In a retrospective study on 22 patients with burning mouth syndrome, six patients (all of whom wore dentures) showed positive contact allergy to constituents of the acrylic-based denture materials, in particular, N-dimethyl-4-toluidine, 4-tolyldiethanolamine, benzoylperoxide, and oligotriacrylate (Dutree-Meulenberg *et al.* 1992). Obviously, patients wearing dental prostheses presenting with burning mouth syndrome should be patch tested for the various constituents of dental acrylic.

Three cases of 'scalded mouth' caused by the angiotensin-converting-enzyme inhibitor captopril have been reported (Vlasses *et al.* 1982). These cases were not accompanied by an eosinophilia or by fever. Further cases, caused by lisinopril (Savino and Haushalter 1992) and enalapril (Brown *et al.* 1997), have been described. The mechanism of ACE-inhibitor 'scalded mouth' is uncertain, but it may be a subclinical manifestation of lichen planus (see later).

Erythema multiforme (Stevens–Johnson syndrome)

Erythema multiforme, which when severe is termed the Stevens–Johnson syndrome, is a mucocutaneous disorder characterized by various clinical types of lesion including bullae, vesicles, papules, macules, and wheals. The mucous membranes (oral, ocular, genital) are commonly involved, and at times the lesions are restricted to these membranes. The aetiology of the disorder varies from hypersensitivity to foods and drugs to allergy secondary to viral, bacterial, or fungal infections. It has been estimated that drug therapy is the alleged trigger mechanism in four per cent of cases (Lozada and Silverman 1978), but in the Stevens–Johnson syndrome drug association increases to 80 per cent (Cameron *et al.* 1966). Drugs which have been frequently implicated in erythema multiforme are barbiturates, penicillin, and long-acting sulphonamides (Cameron *et al.* 1966). Less often suspected have been phenylbutazone, chlorpropamide (Tullett 1966; Kanefsky and Medoff 1980), phenytoin (Watts 1962), meprobamate, carbamazepine (Coombes 1965), salicylates, clindamycin (Fulghum and Catalano 1973), rifampicin (Nyirenda and Gill 1977), sulindac (Levitt and Pearson 1980), minoxidil (Di Santis and Flanagan 1981), ethambutol (Pegram *et al.* 1981), ampicillin (Konstantinidis *et al.* 1985), phenothiazines (Rees 1985), and doxycycline (Lewis-Jones *et al.* 1988). Erythema multiforme has also been attributed to the use of iodine-containing mouthwashes (Tal and Dekel 1986). Rubin (1977) reported a case of Stevens–Johnson syndrome following the use of 30% sulphacetamide eyedrops, the patient having been sensitized by previous sulphamethoxazole therapy. The Stevens–Johnson syndrome has also been caused by slow-release theophylline (Brook *et al.* 1989) and an antimalarial combination of chloroquine and sulphadoxine–pyrimethamine (Ortel *et al.* 1989).

The oral lesions of erythema multiforme should disappear within 14 days of stopping the offending drug. The Stevens–Johnson syndrome is much more serious, and potentially fatal. Local lesions are treated with topical steroids, but most cases require systemic steroid therapy and medical management.

Oral ulceration

Local irritants

A number of chemicals used by dental surgeons can cause 'burns' of the oral mucosa if injudiciously applied — for example, trichloroacetic acid used in the treatment of pericoronitis. However, drugs used for other purposes may cause local irritation of the mouth; such drugs are discussed below.

Aspirin

Aspirin (acetylsalicylic acid) is a weak organic acid. Some patients attempt to relieve toothache by placing an aspirin tablet against the offending tooth. There is no evidence that this practice has any benefit in the management of toothache, and the corrosive action of the acidic aspirin may result in a fairly large area of ulceration. Surprisingly, the alarming appearance which can be produced is not matched by equal discomfort. Aspirin has also been incorporated into chewing gum and use of this has been associated with oral ulceration (Claman 1967).

Other drugs

Other drugs considered to have caused oral ulceration are toothache solutions containing menthol, phenol, clove oil, camphor, and chloroform in varying proportions (Feaver 1982); hydrogen peroxide, occasionally used in certain periodontal procedures (though its suitability for this purpose has been questioned [Rees and Orth 1986], particularly at a concentration of 3%) and in the management of acute necrotizing ulcerative gingivitis; potassium chloride tablets which can also damage tooth enamel, especially if sucked (McAvoy 1974); isoprenaline tablets placed sublingually (Brown and Botas 1973); pancreatin powder or tablets, if held in the mouth before swallowing (Derby 1970); ergotamine tartrate, which has also caused necrosis of the tongue (Wolpaw *et al.* 1973; Vazquez-Doval *et al.* 1994) in the presence of temporal arteritis, possibly by triggering spasm in partially thrombosed arteries; cocaine, possibly by inducing intense vasoconstriction, in abusers who have applied it topically to test its purity (Dello-Russo and Temple 1982; Parry *et al.* 1996); paraquat, entering the mouth accidentally (Dobson and Smith 1987); lithium (Nathan 1995), which has also caused geographical tongue; and tetracyclines (Nordt 1996), especially doxycycline, perhaps because of their low pH (2.3) in solution.

Anticancer drugs given systemically may also cause oral ulceration (Bottomley 1977), either by a primary action or by inducing leucopenia. Non-steroidal anti-inflammatory drugs (NSAID) are other culprits, particularly phenylbutazone (Sperling 1969), indomethacin, and ibuprofen (Guggenheim and Ismail 1975), though naproxen (secondarily to leucopenia) (Kaziro 1980), and flurbiprofen (Healy and Thornhill 1995) have also been implicated. NSAID-induced oral ulceration may be due to a vasculitic process rather than to a direct effect on prostaglandin synthesis. Finally, the antimalarial proguanil has caused oral ulceration severe enough to require withdrawal of the drug (Daniels 1986).

Vesiculo-bullous lesions

Drug-induced vesiculo-bullous lesions affecting the orofacial region are rare. Corticosteroids may predispose the oral mucosa to bulla formation. Patients using steroid inhalers for more than 5 years are more prone to the development of oral blistering (High and Main 1989). The authors conclude that such use of corticosteroid inhalers may be one causal factor in the development of angina bullosa.

The mechanism of inhaled steroid-induced vesiculo-bullous lesions remains uncertain but the reaction may be the consequence of a direct irritant effect. Alternatively, it may simply represent activation of a latent or subclinical viral infection in susceptible individuals, due to decreased local resistance (Pillans 1994).

Naproxen has also been implicated in the development of a bullous photodermatitis, with lesions affecting the hands and lips and is possibly dose dependent (Rivers and Barneston 1989); and penicillamine has caused pemphigus-like mucosal lesions (Eisenberg *et al.* 1981).

Lupus erythematosus

Lupus erythematosus exists in two clinical forms; systemic lupus erythematosus (SLE), which affects various tissues and organs, and chronic discoid lupus erythematosus, which is basically a mucocutaneous disorder. The causes of the condition are unknown, but genetic factors may play a part in the aetiology of the former. It is now recognized that some cases of SLE are induced or precipitated by drugs. A characteristic immunological feature of the condition is the presence of antibodies to double-stranded DNA, although in the drug-related disease antibodies to DNA may be absent or low. The oral mucosa is involved in about 20 per cent of patients with SLE, and females are more often affected than males. The oral lesions may vary from erythematosus areas to aphthae-like ulcerations or lesions resembling lichen planus. Drug-related SLE is discussed in detail in Chapter 18.

Lichenoid eruptions

The term lichenoid drug eruptions can be used in two senses. Firstly, drug eruptions similar to or identical with lichen planus; and secondly, drug eruptions that do not necessarily look like lichen planus clinically, but which have histological features very like this condition. β-Adrenoceptor blocking agents (e.g. propranolol, atenolol) are examples of drugs which cause lichenoid eruptions of the latter category.

Lichenoid eruptions, with white ulcerated sloughs on the lips, occurred after 8 months of treatment with chlorpropamide, resolved when the drug was withdrawn, and recurred when the drug was given again later, though not when the dose was kept below 250 mg daily (Dinsdale *et al.* 1968).

Of 75 patients with oral lichen planus, 20 were taking NSAID (diflunisal, fenclofenac, flurbiprofen, or ibuprofen) when first seen, and an eruption caused by oral indomethacin, which subsided when the drug was withheld but reappeared when it was given again as a suppository, was also encountered (Hamburger and Potts 1983). Fenclofenac was also suspected in another case (Ferguson *et al.* 1984). Potts and others (1987) found that patients with oral lichen planus used significantly more NSAID in than did control patients with other mucosal lesions.

Methyldopa is another drug that occasionally produces lesions of the oral mucosa resembling those of lichen planus. Hay and Reade (1978) described 17 patients, who presented over a period of 8 years, with oral lesions which were attributed to the drug.

Five cases representative of the sample were described in some detail. The patients had been referred for the management of painful and persistent ulceration of the oral mucosa. The lesions in the mouth resembled erosive lichen planus or benign mucous membrane pemphigoid. The tongue and buccal mucosa were involved in most cases. Biopsies were taken from eight of the patients, and the results varied: some histological features were strongly suggestive of lichen planus, whereas other features suggested a benign mucous membrane pemphigoid (which was excluded in some doubtful instances by immunofluorescent investigations). The mechanism whereby methyldopa causes lichenoid reactions is uncertain. The patients in this series showed complete healing with relief of symptoms only on withdrawal of the drug. In some cases, the process of resolution took many months. One patient was further challenged with the drug and eruptions recurred. This finding may indicate a hypersensitivity type of reaction.

The authors of this useful review stressed the problem of diagnosis when a drug-induced disorder mimics a natural disease. An interesting observation in this study was the preponderance of females affected by drug-induced problems of the oral mucous membranes. There has been much discussion over the role of amalgam restorations and oral lichen planus. It has been suggested that a contact hypersensitivity reaction to mercury released during corrosion of silver amalgam restorations is a causative factor in oral lichenoid reactions. Such a hypothesis has been considered to be supported by the finding that hypersensitivity to mercury has been found among 16–62 per cent of patients who present with oral lichen planus, compared with 2–4 per cent in a normal population (James et al. 1987). Furthermore, replacing amalgam restorations with alternative filling material has produced resolution of the oral lichenoid reactions (Laine et al. 1992). The pathogenesis of oral lichen planus is multifactorial and the evidence suggests that mercury may be causative in some patients. However, epicutaneous patch testing to mercury is not particularly useful in identifying such patients (Ostman et al. 1996).

Other drugs that can cause lichenoid eruptions are amiphenazole (Dinsdale and Walker 1966); chloroquine; mepacrine; gold (Russell et al. 1996); arsenical compounds; bismuth; practolol (Felix et al. 1974), which has also caused recurrent ulceration of the oral and nasal mucosa (Wright 1975); and lithium carbonate (Hogan et al. 1985; Menni et al. 1997), which may produce this condition by an effect on T-cell function.

Unlike true lichen planus, which may last for 20 years or more, drug-induced lichenoid eruptions disappear once the drug has been stopped. It has been suggested that drugs associated with lichenoid reactions act as agents uncovering the latent disease of lichen planus, or amplify a previous disorder, rather than inducing the disease de novo (Lacey et al. 1983).

Discolouration of oral mucosa and teeth

Discolouration of the tissues may be produced by direct contact with a drug or may follow the absorption of a drug after systemic administration. In the past, staining of the oral mucosa was often due to treatment involving metals such as silver, bismuth, gold, lead, mercury, zinc, and copper. Most of these are now rarely used therapeutically, and if staining is found it may be a result of the person's occupation. For example, lead poisoning is an occupational hazard and chronic poisoning from ingestion, inhalation, or skin absorption of lead will produce a bluish line around the gingival margins. Cases of lead poisoning (from inadvertently eating 'old paint') tend to occur in children and the mentally retarded. Dentists working with such patients should be aware of the oral manifestations of lead poisoning (Lockhart 1981).

Stannous fluoride toothpastes sometimes produce blackish or greenish extrinsic stains on the teeth.

This staining may be due to the combination of stannous ions with sulphides (released by bacterial action in the mouth) which produces insoluble stannous sulphide. Animal experiments suggest that the low pH of stannous fluoride causes denaturation of the pellicle protein with subsequent exposure of the sulphydryl groups. The latter forms stannous sulphide with the stannous ions present in the preparation (Ellingsen et al. 1982).

Discolouration of the oral mucosa is often associated with the antimalarial drugs, with chloroquine producing a bluish-grey pigmentation of the hard palate and gingiva and mepacrine a yellowish mucosal pigmentation (Giansanti et al. 1971; Veraldi et al. 1992). The mechanism and localization (i.e. always in the palate) of quinoline-induced pigmentation is uncertain. Light and electron microscopy studies show that the pigment is either melanin or iron (Tuffanelli et al. 1963; Giansanti et al. 1971). Pigment is found in the epithelium and the macrophages of the underlying connective tissues (Watson and MacDonald 1974). The authors suggest that the pathological pigment originated from the epithelial melanocytes, because they observed active melanocytes and compound melanosomes in keratocytes.

Other drugs that cause discolouration of the oral mucosa were reviewed by Vogel and Deasy (1977). They include phenothiazines (long-term therapy), especially chlorpromazine, which cause a bluish-grey discolouration of the oral mucosa. The incidence of the discolouration is less than one per cent, and it is suggested that the cause is an accumulation of a metabolite in the tissues. Pigmentation of the oral mucosa can also be caused by the use of oral contraceptives, and cessation of the drug does not produce complete regression of pigmentation.

Oral contraceptives and hormone replacement therapy (HRT) appear to have a stimulating effect on the secretion of pituitary melanocyte-stimulating hormone, which cause discoloration. A further case report of epithelial melanosis of the gingival tissues from the use of the oral contraceptive supports this hypothesis (Hertz et al. 1980). HRT has also been reported to cause oral pigmentation (Perusse and Morency 1991). Oral pigmentation in the case described was of a melanotic type and resolved when the patient was taken off therapy. Oestrogen derivatives that are a constituent of HRT can induce increased production of β-melano-stimulating hormone and adrenocorticotrophic hormone, triggered by lowering of the free plasma cortisol concentration associated with the medication. Oestrogens are well known to induce high levels of cortisol-binding globulin, which contribute to decreased bioavailability of the free portion of plasma cortisol. In turn, by inhibiting feedback of the anterior hypophysis, this oestrogen-induced lowering of free plasma cortisol produces a hypersecretion of ACTH and β-melano-stimulating hormone. The latter may cause the increased oral pigmentation.

A bluish-grey band of pigmentation at the attached and free gingival junction has been reported to occur after systemic minocycline therapy (Bechner et al. 1986; Siller et al. 1994). In this case, the gingival discolouration arose from the underlying bone. When the gingival tissues were separated from the bone, they assumed their normal colour. The underlying bone, however, was grey, which suggests an interaction between the drug and bone during its formation. Minocycline has also been implicated in causing hyperpigmentation of the lips (Chu et al. 1994), and tongue (Meyerson et al. 1995; Katz et al. 1995). The lip lesion was described as a blue-brown discolouration of the lower lip following long-term therapy for acne. Biopsy of the lip reported 'post-inflammatory pigmentary alteration with a small focus of vascular interface dermatitis'. This description would suggest a fixed drug eruption as opposed to a drug-induced increase in melanin production. In the two tongue reports, black pigmentation of the tongue occurred in patients treated with minocycline for dermatological conditions. Black discolouration of the tongue (see below) is usually due to the 'black hairy' phenomenon characterized by hypertrophy of the filiform papillae. With minocycline, the black pigmentation may arise as a result of the deposition of either minocycline-metabolite complexes, and/or granules containing melanin, iron, or calcium in the submucosa of the lingual tissues.

Pigmented lesions of the tongue (dark macular patches) are reported to occur in heroin addicts who inhale the smoke (Westerhof et al. 1983). Histologically, the lesions are packed with melanocytes. The mechanism of these changes is uncertain. A similar lesion secondary to methyldopa therapy has been described (Brody and Cohen 1986). Although biopsy material was not available, the authors suggested that the darkening of the tongue might be due to a breakdown of methyldopa or its metabolites on exposure to air. The pigment produced is most likely to be melanin, a product of dopa metabolism.

Staining of the teeth, restorations, dentures, and the dorsum of the tongue is the most common problem associated with use of chlorhexidine; it does not appear to be related to solution concentration (Rebstein 1978). Discolouration also occurs on the dorsum of the tongue when chlorhexidine is used as a mouth rinse, but does not occur when the compound is used as a dentifrice or a gel. Various studies have shown that the incidence of staining can be reduced if chlorhexidine mouthwash is used only at night (Addy et al. 1982); if the mouthwash is used with an oxidizing agent, such as 1% peroxymono-sulphate solution (Eriksen et al. 1983) or with stannous fluoride (Ellingsen et al. 1982).

Staining from chlorhexidine shows marked inter-individual variation and patients have been identified as 'stainers' and 'non-stainers' (Solheim et al. 1980). This variation may be related to individual plaque control, for it has been demonstrated that a close correlation exists between plaque preventative capability and discolouration after chlorhexidine rinses (Solheim et al. 1980). This finding may indicate that the primary site for discolouration is the acquired pellicle and not the constituents of bacterial plaque. Three possible mechanisms for chlorhexidine-induced staining have been suggested (Eriksen et al. 1983): non-enzymic browning reactions (Maillard reactions), formation of pigmented metal sulphides, and dietary factors.

Maillard reactions

The Maillard reaction is a non-enzymic browning reaction involving carbohydrates, peptides, and proteins as substrates. These substrates undergo a series of condensation and polymerization reactions resulting in the formation of brown pigmented compounds known as melanoids. Reactions are catalysed by a high pH and excess of amino acids, and also by chlorhexidine (Nordbo 1979). The glycoprotein of the acquired pellicle may also provide a substrate for the Maillard reaction.

Formation of the metal sulphides

The proteins of the acquired pellicle are joined by disulphide bridges. When pellicle proteins are denatured, the disulphide bridges are split, yielding free sulphydryl groups. The latter can react with iron or tin ions in food substances to form pigmented metal sulphides. Chlorhexidine will denature pellicle protein (Hjeljord et al. 1973), thus facilitating the formation of pigmented ferric (brown) and stannous (yellow) sulphides.

Dietary factors

Many food substances contain aldehydes and ketones, which may react with chlorhexidine to form coloured products and stain tooth surfaces. It has also been shown that chlorhexidine-induced tooth staining is related to the consumption of tea, coffee, and red wine (Addy et al. 1979). The latter contains high levels of tannins, which are strong denaturants.

Although staining of the teeth is a troublesome unwanted effect associated with use of chlorhexidine, the stain can be readily removed with a mild abrasive and a dental handpiece.

Black hairy tongue

The most common discolouration of the tongue is a condition known as black hairy tongue. This results from hypertrophy of the filiform papillae, which may grow to half-an-inch in length. The condition is usually asymptomatic, although the lengthened papillae may be a nuisance. The colour is usually black, but may be one of various shades of brown. Usually the filiform papillae are maintained at a functional length by normal physiological wear, but if the environment of the mouth is altered, the rate of desquamation of the filiform papillae may be reduced. The exact mechanism by which this condition is produced is unknown. Penicillin lozenges, oral penicillins, and other topical antimicrobials have caused black hairy tongue, as has sodium perborate used in mouthwashes. There is no really effective treatment for this condition.

Periodontal tissues

Systemic drug therapy can have an adverse effect on the periodontal tissues. The most common example is drug-induced gingival overgrowth. Drugs most frequently implicated in this condition include phenytoin, cyclosporin, calcium-channel blockers, and oral contraceptives. Isolated case reports have indicated that gingival changes may also occur with sodium valproate, erythromycin (see later), trimethoprim–sulfamethoxazole (Caron et al. 1997), vigabatrin (Katz et al. 1997), and phenobarbitone (Gregoriou et al. 1996). Additionally, certain types of systemic drug therapy can affect the inflammatory and immunological response of the periodontal tissues to bacterial plaque. Such drugs include immunosuppressives, corticosteroids, and NSAID. Patients on these drugs show a reduced response of their periodontal tissues to bacterial plaque (Seymour and Heasman 1988), hence this cannot be considered as an adverse effect. This subject is also discussed in Chapter 22.

Drug-induced gingival hyperplasia (overgrowth)

Phenytoin

It is now well established that phenytoin therapy is associated with gingival overgrowth. Many studies reporting this unwanted effect have been reviewed by Hassell (1981). The incidence of phenytoin-induced gingival overgrowth is approximately 50 per cent (Angelopoulos and Goaz 1972), but it is higher in both teenagers (Kapur et al. 1973) and institutionalized epileptics (Hassell et al. 1984). Phenytoin-induced gingival overgrowth does not appear to be related to sex or race (Hassell 1981).

Gingival overgrowth usually becomes apparent during the first 3 months after starting phenytoin (Dummett 1954) and is most rapid in the first year (Aas 1963). Clinically the condition begins as a diffuse swelling of the interdental papillae, which

may then coalesce (Angelopoulos 1975). The gingival tissues can have a nodular appearance, but the colour (which ranges from coral pink to a deep bluish-red) depends upon the amount of inflammatory infiltrate present in the tissues (Esterberg and White 1945). In severe cases the clinical crowns may be covered (Dolin 1951). The incidence and severity of the condition is greatest on the labial aspects of the upper and lower anterior teeth (Esterberg and White 1945; Angelopoulos and Goaz 1972).

It has been reported that patients receiving phenytoin have less bone loss than those taking sodium valproate (Seymour et al. 1985). Thus patients on phenytoin appear to have a degree of 'resistance' to further periodontal destruction. This finding may also be attributable to the action of phenytoin on the immune system. Phenytoin-induced mucosal changes have also been reported in the edentulous patient (Dreyer and Thomas 1978; McCord et al. 1992). In these case reports, irritation of the oral mucosa by the denture and subsequent candidal infection may have been a significant predisposing factor.

Phenytoin pharmacokinetics and gingival overgrowth

The relationship between the incidence and severity of the gingival changes and pharmacokinetic variables of phenytoin remains a contentious issue. Early studies demonstrated a correlation between the daily dose of phenytoin and the extent of gingival overgrowth (Panuska et al. 1961; Klar 1973) but others contest this view (Dolin 1951; Angelopoulos and Goaz 1972; Kapur et al. 1973). Similarly, some investigators have reported a significant relationship between plasma levels of phenytoin and the severity of gingival overgrowth (Kapur et al. 1973; Little et al. 1975; Addy et al. 1983), whereas others have found no relationship (Hassell et al. 1984; Dahllof and Modeer 1986). In the latter two studies, the patients were taking only phenytoin, whereas several of the patients in the other investigations were taking several anticonvulsant drugs. Drugs such as sodium valproate, carbamazepine, and phenobarbitone alter the pharmacokinetics of phenytoin. It has been demonstrated that polypharmacy in epilepsy causes a significant increase in the prevalence of the abnormality (Maguire et al. 1986).

There appears to be no discernible relationship between the plasma pharmacokinetics of phenytoin and the incidence and severity of gingival overgrowth. Obviously some baseline concentration (or dosage) of the drug is required for overgrowth to take place. Perhaps the local tissue concentrations of the drug may be more relevant in determining the gingival response.

Oral hygiene and phenytoin-induced gingival overgrowth

Any change in gingival contour will impede mechanical plaque removal and allow plaque to accumulate at the gingival margin and in the interproximal spaces. Such accumulations cause inflammatory changes in the tissues that further distort the gingival contour. Cross-sectional studies have tended to show a significant relationship between the extent of gingival hyperplasia and plaque accumulation. These studies suffer from the 'chicken or egg' dilemma in terms of separating cause and effect. Longitudinal studies have reported a positive relationship between oral hygiene and the severity of phenytoin-induced gingival changes (Steinberg and Steinberg 1982; Addy *et al.* 1983).

It has also been clearly demonstrated that a plaque control programme prevents or reduces the severity of gingival overgrowth when starting phenytoin therapy (Philstrom *et al.* 1980; Modeer and Dahllof 1987). Similarly, use of the antiplaque agent chlorhexidine as a 0.2% (w/v) mouthrinse is of value in preventing the condition, especially after surgery (O'Neil and Figures 1982). These studies further emphasize the role of bacterial plaque in the pathogenesis of this undesirable effect.

Cyclosporin

Cyclosporin is a selective immunosuppressant acting mainly on the T-cell response. The drug is widely used in transplant surgery, to prevent graft rejection.

It is now well recognized that one of the unwanted effects of cyclosporin therapy is gingival overgrowth. Early studies evaluating the use of cyclosporin in transplant surgery reported 'gingival overgrowth' as one of the unwanted effects associated with the drug (Calne *et al.* 1981; Starzl *et al.* 1981) and many further case reports have appeared in the dental literature (Rateitschak-Pluss *et al.* 1983; Wysocki *et al.* 1983; Adams and Davies 1984; Bennett and Christian 1985; Rostock *et al.* 1986).

The condition occurs in about 30 per cent of patients taking the drug (Wysocki *et al.* 1983; Seymour *et al.* 1987). The incidence is higher in children (Daley and Wysocki 1984) and slightly higher in female patients (Tyldesley and Rotter 1984), but appears to be lower in bone marrow than in renal transplant patients (Beveridge 1983). As with phenytoin, gingival changes have also been described in an edentulous patient (Thomason *et al.* 1994).

Cyclosporin pharmacokinetics and gingival overgrowth

The relationship between cyclosporin dosage, pharmacokinetics, and duration of therapy with the incidence and severity of gingival overgrowth remains a contentious issue. Most of the early studies reported no relationship between dose and gingival overgrowth (Daley *et al.* 1986; Phillips *et al.* 1986; McGaw *et al.* 1987). However, many of these patients were on high doses of cyclosporin compared with the titrated dosages in current use.

Few studies have investigated the relationship between plasma or total blood concentrations of cyclosporin and gingival overgrowth. Plasma concentrations of cyclosporin have been reported to be more closely related to the gingival changes in kidney transplant patients than various periodontal variables (Seymour and Jacobs 1992). Others have reported that whole-blood concentrations of cyclosporin show no correlation with the incidence and severity of cyclosporin-induced gingival overgrowth (McGaw *et al.* 1987; Schulz *et al.* 1990). Obviously, some 'baseline concentration' of cyclosporin is necessary for overgrowth to occur in the 'responder patient'. These levels may vary markedly from patient to patient.

Cyclosporin is also secreted in saliva, but the concentrations do not appear to correlate with those in plasma (Phillips *et al.* 1986). Salivary concentrations appear to relate to gingival overgrowth severity (Daley *et al.* 1986). However, only eight patients were evaluated for this correlation and this may limit the significance of the finding.

Oral hygiene and cyclosporin-induced gingival overgrowth

The role of bacterial plaque and gingival inflammation in the pathogenesis of cyclosporin-induced gingival overgrowth remains uncertain. Some cross-sectional studies show a relationship between overgrowth and both plaque scores and gingival inflammation (Tyldesley and Rotter 1984; McGaw *et al.* 1987), whereas others have failed to substantiate this finding (Seymour *et al.* 1987; Schulz *et al.* 1990). The argument about whether plaque and gingival inflammation are the cause or the result of the gingival overgrowth is obviously as applicable with cyclosporin as with phenytoin.

Attention to oral hygiene improved the gingival condition of renal transplant patients medicated with cyclosporin (Seymour and Smith 1991). However, this measure alone failed to prevent the development of gingival overgrowth.

Calcium-channel blockers

These drugs are used extensively in the management of cardiovascular disorders. In particular, they are used in the control of angina, hypertension, and cardiac arrhythmias. The dihydropyridines, especially nifedipine, are the most frequently cited agents. However, this may be a reflection on the widespread use of these particular drugs. It has been estimated that between 10 and 15 per cent of dentate patients medicated with nifedipine experience clinical signs of gingival overgrowth (Barak *et al.* 1987; Barclay *et al.* 1992). These studies were based on a hospital population, thus they do not represent a random sample.

The influence of factors such as age, nifedipine dose, duration of medication, plaque levels, gingival inflammation, and the extent of periodontal destruction on the development and severity of nifedipine-induced gingival overgrowth is not known. The sequestration of nifedipine in the crevicular fluid of patients with significant hypertrophy has been demonstrated (Ellis *et al.* 1992). Crevicular fluid is a transudate derived from serum, production of which is directly related to the level of inflammation present in the gingival tissue. The fluid can be collected on filter papers or in micropipettes at the gingival margin. Since crevicular fluid is 'locally' produced, drug concentrations may be a reflection of tissue activity. Although the sequestration of nifedipine in crevicular fluid is of interest, it has not been established whether it is important in the development and severity of gingival overgrowth. Nifedipine is frequently prescribed to organ transplant patients to reduce the nephrotoxic effects of cyclosporin (Freehally *et al.* 1987). Since both drugs cause gingival overgrowth, they appear to have an additive effect on the gingival tissues (Slavin and Taylor 1987; King *et al.* 1993; Thomason *et al.* 1993). Approximately 50 per cent of transplant patients experience clinically significant overgrowth when treated with the combination of cyclosporin and nifedipine (Thomason *et al.* 1993). This compares with a figure of 30 per cent for cyclosporin alone.

Gingival overgrowth has also been reported following chronic usage of felodipine (Lombardi *et al.* 1991), nitrendipine (Brown *et al.* 1990), and amlodipine (Ellis *et al.* 1993). In this last report, significant sequestration of amlodipine was observed in the crevicular fluid of the 'responder' patients (cf. nifedipine).

A few cases of gingival overgrowth associated with verapamil have been reported in the literature (Cucchi *et al.* 1985; Smith and Glenert 1987; Pernu *et al.* 1989). It has recently been estimated that four per cent of patients taking verapamil may experience gingival overgrowth (Miller and Damm 1992).

The various cases of the disorder do not share any common clinical or demographic features that may indicate any underlying causal factor. Gingival fibroblasts have been cultured from one of the patients with gingival overgrowth (Pernu *et al.* 1989). Cell culture showed that the proliferation rate and protein and collagen production from these fibroblasts were markedly lower than from control cells obtained from healthy gingiva. Incubation of normal gingival fibroblasts in the presence of verapamil showed reduced protein and collagen synthesis. These findings suggest that verapamil affects the proliferation of selected fibroblast subpopulations and alters the balance between regeneration and degradation.

Again, only a few cases of gingival overgrowth associated with diltiazem have been reported (Colvard *et al.* 1986; Giustiniani *et al.* 1987; Bowman *et al.* 1988). The histological appearance of the gingival tissues is similar to that observed with nifedipine.

Other drugs

Gingival overgrowth (hyperplasia) has been described in association with chronic sodium valproate treatment (Syrjanen and Syrjanen 1979; Behari 1991). Both reports concerned children, and on change of anticonvulsant therapy to carbamazepine the gingival lesions resolved. The pathogenesis of sodium valproate-induced gingival overgrowth remains uncertain. A single case report described gingival hyperplasia in a 6-year-old child following use of erythromycin syrup (Valsecchi and Cainelli 1992). The gingival changes showed all the classic signs of the more conventional drug-induced gingival overgrowths, and resolved on cessation of the drug. The patient was rechallenged with erythromycin and the changes recurred. The mechanism of erythromycin-induced gingival overgrowth remains uncertain.

Pathogenesis of drug-induced gingival hyperplasia

An appraisal of the various investigations into the pathogenesis of drug-induced gingival overgrowth supports the hypothesis that it is multifactorial. When all the evidence is considered, there appear to be three significant factors important in the expression of these gingival changes, notably drug variables, plaque-induced inflammatory changes in the gingival tissues, and genetic factors. The last determines the heterogeneity of the gingival fibroblast. Genetic factors could also influence drug metabolism, pharmacokinetics, and pharmacodynamics. The many inflammatory changes that occur within the gingival tissues appear to orchestrate the interaction between drug and fibroblast and the subsequent activity of this cell. Alternatively, the various inducing drugs can influence directly the inflammatory response, by either affecting the nature of the cellular infiltrate or the release of the various cytokines, prostaglandins, or growth factors. All three factors can influence the control of the collagen matrix by affecting the synthesis and release of matrix metalloproteinases and tissue inhibitors of metalloproteinase. It is likely that the activity of these effector molecules will prove to be significant in the pathogenesis of drug-induced gingival overgrowth, and these mechanisms warrant further investigation.

Phenytoin was the first drug implicated in causing gingival overgrowth. When other drugs were implicated in the gingival changes, attention was directed to identification of a possible unifying hypothesis. All three drugs have different pharmacological properties, but all influence the Ca^{2+}/Na^+ flux (Messing *et al.* 1985; Gelfand *et al.* 1986; Gelfand *et al.* 1987). An *in vitro* study has shown that phenytoin, verapamil, and nifedipine all inhibited Ca^{2+} uptake of gingival fibroblasts. The inhibition of the $Ca2^+$ uptake correlated with the rate of fibroblast proliferation in fibroblast proliferation rate (Fujii and Kobayashi 1990). Thus, the action of the various implicated drugs on Ca^{2+}/Na^+ flux may prove to be the key to providing a unifying hypothesis which links three dissimilar drugs with a common unwanted effect.

Treatment of drug-induced gingival overgrowth

The treatment and prevention of the disorder remains unsatisfactory. For some patients, a change in drug therapy can be considered, but this is dependent upon co-operation with the patient's physician. For the organ transplant patient there is little or no scope for the withdrawal of cyclosporin, and repeated gingival surgery remains the main treatment option. Drug-induced gingival overgrowth is disfiguring, and can interfere with both mastication and speech. A thorough understanding of the pathogenesis of this unwanted effect is essential if we are to devise appropriate regimens for its prevention and treatment.

Gingival and periodontal changes caused by oral contraceptives

The effects of oral contraceptives upon gingival and periodontal tissues are well documented. Several case reports have described a hyperplastic oedematous gingivitis following the use of oral contraceptives, which resolves when the drugs are withdrawn (Lynn 1967: Kaufman 1969; Sperber 1969; Chevallier 1970). This response appears to be a secondary reaction to the presence of local irritants, especially dental plaque. The maintenance of adequate plaque control is conducive to gingival health despite continued administration of oral contraceptives (Pearlman 1974). These reports have been confirmed by the results of studies that have shown clearly that hormonal contraceptives are associated with an increase in severity of gingival inflammation (El Ashiry et al. 1970; Das et al. 1971). However, Knight and Wade (1974) failed to demonstrate significant differences in either plaque or gingivitis levels between a group of females taking oral contraceptives over a period of 1½ years and age-matched controls. Subjects receiving the hormones for more than 18 months, however, exhibited greater periodontal destruction than either of the two previous groups and it was suggested that this was due to an altered host resistance seen in the long-term hormone group.

The effects of oestrogen and progesterone on the oral mucosa and periodontal tissues have been extensively studied. Oestrogen causes an increase in the acid mucopolysaccharide content of connective tissue in human oral mucosa (Schiff and Burn 1961). Progesterone increases the permeability of the gingival vasculature of rabbits by causing endothelial cell dysfunction and reversible gap formation (Mohamed et al. 1974).

Gingival exudate levels are also raised in females taking oral contraceptives (Lindhe and Bjorn 1967). The influence of the contraceptive was most marked during the menstrual phase when the production of ovarian oestrogen and progesterone is minimal (Lindhe et al. 1969). Sex hormones appear to have a more marked effect upon gingival exudate levels in the presence of a chronic gingivitis (Lindhe et al. 1968a; Hugoson 1970). This effect may result from an increased vascularization of the chronically inflamed tissues (Lindhe and Branemark 1968) and an increase in the permeability of the gingival vessels (Lindhe et al. 1968b). These findings indicate that oestrogen and progesterone affect primarily the vascular response of irritated tissues, without necessarily aggravating the components of the classical inflammatory reaction.

The implication that oestrogens and progesterone are causal in producing or modifying the gingival response to dental plaque is dependent upon the demonstration of these hormones and their metabolic products within the tissues. There is now substantial evidence to suggest that oestrogen receptors do exist in gingival tissues (Bashirelahi et al. 1977), and that the gingival tissues metabolise the sex hormones (El Attar 1974; El Attar and Hugoson 1974; Ojanotko and Harri 1978; Vittek et al. 1979). Chronically inflamed gingival tissue is twice as active as healthy tissue in metabolising progesterone and the chemical nature of progesterone metabolites also differs between healthy and diseased tissues (El Attar 1971; El Attar et al. 1973; Harri and Ojanotko 1978). The metabolite 5-pregnanedione is a product of the conversion of progesterone in normal gingival tissue, whereas its isomer, 6-pregnanedione, is a metabolite in chronically inflamed tissue. In both instances, however, the major active metabolite of progesterone is 20-hydroxyprogesterone, which is increased fourfold in inflamed tissues (El Attar et al. 1973). This evidence suggests that the accumulation of metabolic products of the naturally occurring sex hormones is an important factor in the pathogenesis of chronic gingivitis. A positive correlation has been found between plasma levels of progesterone and its metabolites with the degree of gingival inflammation (Vittek et al. 1979). Although these biochemical analyses have been undertaken on naturally occurring hormones circulating at elevated levels in the pregnant state, no evidence is available to suggest that circumstances are any different in patients taking oral contraceptives.

When there is an increase in circulating sex hormones, either through pregnancy or from taking the oral contraceptive, the patient's gingival tissues are more susceptible to plaque-induced inflammatory changes, including the development of the so-called pregnancy epulis. It is therefore essential that such patients maintain optimal plaque control to reduce the risk of further periodontal damage.

Dental structures

Systemic drug therapy can affect the dental structures, although this is mainly an indirect effect mediated by a drug-induced alteration in the oral environment. The best example of this indirect effect is xerostomia and dental caries. Also considered in this section is the problem of sugar-based medicines and dental caries.

Xerostomia and dental caries

Prolonged treatment with a drug which reduces salivary flow can increase the risk of dental caries. However, xerostomia and dental caries appear to be a particular problem in patients treated with lithium and tricyclic antidepressants.

Lithium

Dental caries is reported to be a complication of lithium treatment (Gillis 1978). Rugg-Gunn (1979), in a review on lithium and dental caries, pointed to extensive surveys on natives of New Guinea (Schamschula et al. 1978) in which inverse correlations were found between caries experience and lithium levels in dental enamel, plaque, and saliva. No relation was found between caries experience and total lithium levels in the soil. This would suggest a possible cariostatic effect of lithium, and Rugg-Gunn (1979) also postulated that the high caries increment reported was more likely to be due to impaired salivary secretion. Mason and colleagues (1979) suggested that there were good reasons why patients on lithium therapy could have a high prevalence of dental caries, whether salivary gland function is impaired or not. Patients on lithium therapy can develop nephrogenic diabetes insipidus. As a consequence, they become dehydrated and drink excessively. They may complain of dryness of the mouth and this may be accounted for in three ways — it may be an effect of the drug directly on salivary gland function, or be secondary to the dehydration, or it may be related to the depressive illness.

Tricyclic antidepressants

Most psychoactive drugs, especially the tricyclic antidepressants and the phenothiazines, have significant anticholinergic properties. This commonly results in dryness of the mouth, which occasionally contributes to carious destruction of the teeth (Bassuk and Schoonover 1978). The tricyclics cause a marked decrease in salivary secretion during the first week of therapy, but then secretion gradually improves.

A number of factors may be involved in the problem of tricyclic-induced dental caries; the depressed patient may have a lower than normal rate of salivary flow; the drug or drugs used in the treatment of the depression may cause a dryness of the mouth which, in the case of the tricyclics, may be severe. There is a clear relationship between salivary flow and the incidence of tooth decay. Because of the dryness of the mouth, the patient may eat a lot of sweets to try and ameliorate the condition. This in itself may contribute to the further carious destruction of the teeth.

Tricyclic antidepressants are sometimes used in children for the treatment of enuresis. It has been shown that children receiving such treatment also have a high incidence of dental caries (von Knorring and Wahlin 1986), though only if the treatment lasts longer than 1 month. The authors suggest that a drug-induced hyposecretion of saliva is the main cause. However, they also suggest that enuretic children wake up more in the night and often take some sucrose-containing drink or snack. It is thus not surprising that enuretic children receiving treatment with antidepressants have a higher caries incidence than normal children (von Knorring and Wahlin 1986). They suggest that physicians prescribing a tricyclic drug for a child should arrange for optimal caries prophylaxis at the start.

Sugar-based medicines and dental disease

Sugars (sucrose, glucose, and fructose) are widely used in the formulation of liquid medicines. It is now well established that long-term use of such medicines in children is associated with increased caries (Roberts and Roberts 1979; Hobson 1985; Kenny and Somaya 1989; Maguire 1994), and the term 'medication caries' has been used to describe this condition (Hobson 1985). Plaque pH studies have looked at acid production from the fermentation by plaque bacteria of a number of liquid oral medicines, including cough medicines and penicillin syrups (Feigal and Jensen 1982; Imfeld 1983; Rekola 1989). These studies have shown that medicines sweetened with sucrose cause a prolonged pH depression. The effects of this are more pronounced if sweetened medicines are given at night when reduced salivary flow decreases resistance to caries (Lagerlof and Dawes 1985).

Sugar has many advantages as a constituent of medicines. It is cheap, non-toxic, and soluble. In liquid form, sugars provide important diluent, preservative, and viscosity-modifying properties. These, together with the sweetening properties of sugars, improving palatability and compliance with the medicine, make the replacement of sugars with non-sugar-based alternatives difficult. In addition, sugar beet as the raw product enjoys a well-protected position as a commodity produced in the European Community (EC), supported by a large farming lobby. This has restricted progress in the campaign for the sugar-free option as, at present, manufacturers can claim EC export subsidies and production refunds on finished medicinal products containing sucrose, reducing the cost of sucrose by 30–40 per cent (Bond and Fields 1990). As a result, the cost of replacing sucrose with a more expensive non-sugar alternative, both in raw costs and reformulated terms, has restricted the availability of sugar-free medicines. In 1984, of 210 liquid and syrup medicines available in the UK (National Pharmaceutical Association [NPA] 1984) 161 (77 per cent) were sugar-based, and nearly 100 per cent of paediatric preparations contained sugar (Hobson 1985). Various recommendations were put forward in 1985 to try and reduce the use of sugar in paediatric medicines and encourage the pharmaceutical industry to produce sugar-free liquid preparations. By 1986 the number of preparations listed by the NPA had increased to 298, of which 103 (35 per cent) were sugar-free (National Pharmaceutical Association 1986). By the late 1980s some progress had been made in widening the availability of sugar-free alternatives to sugar-based medicines (Hobson and Fuller 1987), but this small improvement had mainly occurred in high-profile 'over-the-counter' products such as minor analgesics, cough suppressants, and antitussives, most of which are taken on a short-term basis.

The COMA report published in 1989 (Department of Health 1989) looked at dietary sugars and human disease, and considered the impact of sugars in medicines in relation to dental caries. One recommendation stated that: 'An increasing number of liquid medicines are available in sugar-free formulations. When medicines are needed, particularly long-term, sugar-free formulations should be selected by parents and medical practitioners. The panel recommends that government should seek the means to reduce the use of sugared liquid medicines.'

In quantity terms, over 60 per cent of prescriptions dispensed for potential long-term use in children are sugar based (Maguire and Rugg-Gunn 1994a). Children taking these medicines are most likely to be suffering from epilepsy, cystic fibrosis, chronic renal failure, chronic constipation, and asthma (Maguire and Rugg-Gunn 1994b), and the detrimental effects of sugar-based medicines on the dental health of these children are very relevant when certain dental procedures can carry greatly increased morbidity in medically compromised children.

Educational campaigns involving parents of young children, pharmacists, health visitors, and doctors have been undertaken in the North West Region of England (Mackie et al. 1993; Bentley et al. 1994) to facilitate a change to sugar-free medication. These have had some success, but reaching doctors with the sugar-free medicine health message has been difficult.

This aspect of sugar in medicines and dental disease was reinforced recently in the COMA report on weaning and the weaning diet (Department of Health 1994), in which attention was drawn to the availability of sugar-free formulations of proprietary paediatric medicines, but the lack of sugar-free generic preparations. It encouraged the trend to eliminate unnecessary sugars from all medicines and recommended that all paediatric medicines should be sugar-free.

β-Adrenoceptor blockers

A recent study (Breuer et al. 1996) has reported on the dental findings of patients on long-term β-blocker therapy. Patients taking these drugs exhibit reduced dental calculus formation, but a higher incidence of root surface caries and cervical restorations. These findings would suggest that β-blockers decrease the rate of mineralization in the oral cavity, but since they do not appear to alter stimulated salivary pH or flow rate, or phosphate and ionic or total calcium concentrations, their effect on the mineralization process must be attributed to other mechanisms. Two hypotheses appear plausible: changes in salivary mineralization rates caused by either direct physico-chemical effects of the secreted β-blocker in the saliva, or by alterations in the salivary protein/glycoprotein composition, enzymes, and oral bacterial flora owing to systemic pharmacological effects of the drugs.

Other agents affecting dental structures

Phenytoin

The anticonvulsant drug phenytoin is reported to cause abnormalities in the roots of teeth (Girgis et al. 1980). Defects include shortening of the root, root resorption, and an increased deposition of cementum. The mechanism of phenytoin-induced root abnormalities is uncertain, but it may be related to the inhibition of vitamin D

metabolism or parathyroid hormone production by the drug (Harris and Goldhaber 1974; Robinson et al. 1978).

Local anaesthetic agents

Local anaesthetic agents such as lignocaine and prilocaine are cytotoxic to the enamel organ and will interfere with amelogenesis (Hammarstrom 1970). It has been suggested that the pressures used during intraligamentary injections can force anaesthetic agents into any underlying tooth germs that may be present (Brannstrom et al. 1982). The possibility of damage to permanent successor teeth following intraligamentary injections of local anaesthetics in the primary dentition was investigated in an animal model by Brannstrom et al. (1984). These workers found that the injection of prilocaine and lignocaine via the periodontal ligament of primary teeth produced enamel hypoplasia in the permanent dentition.

Tetracycline staining of the teeth

The possible effects of tetracyclines on developing teeth have been well documented over the years. Immediately after absorption tetracyclines are built into the calcifying tissues and this becomes a permanent feature in the teeth. Weyman (1965), in a clinical investigation of 59 children with tetracycline staining of the teeth, showed a colour difference depending on the drug or drugs used. It appeared that chlortetracycline produced a grey-brown discolouration; yellow staining of varying intensity occurred in patients who had taken tetracycline, oxytetracycline, or demethylchlortetracycline. The third type, a brownish-yellow discolouration, was of mixed origin. The degree of staining was variable, sometimes it was hardly noticeable, and the least objectionable staining was produced by oxytetracycline. This discolouration only occurs during the formative period of the crowns of the teeth. If at all possible, the use of tetracyclines should be avoided at this time.

Fluoride

Enamel mottling is commoner in children who live in areas where the water-supply fluoride level is optimal than in children in low-fluoride areas (Milsom and Mitropoulis 1990). It has been suggested that this might be a consequence of an additive effect of fluoride from toothpaste, as it is possible for young children to obtain the recommended daily intake of fluoride from toothpaste alone (Rock 1994).

Antineoplastic agents

Increased sensitivity of the teeth and gingivae may occasionally be caused by antineoplastic drugs (Bottomley et al. 1977).

This apart, chemotherapeutic agents used in the treatment of childhood malignancy can interfere with formation of the dental tissues. Such drugs can disrupt the development of the enamel organ and produce a number of dental abnormalities, including failure of the tooth to develop, microdontia, hypoplasia, enamel opacities, constrictions and thinning of the root, and arrested root development (Maguire *et al.* 1987*a*,*b*; Welbury 1987). It appears that although dental development may be influenced by anticancer drugs in childhood, the incidence of dental caries and periodontal disease is not affected (Maguire *et al.* 1987*b*). In addition to these effects on the teeth, it should be remembered that current treatment with antineoplastic drugs may produce oral ulceration, increase the incidence of oral infections, and increase the risk of haemorrhage.

Radiotherapy

Radiotherapy for the treatment of orofacial malignancy in children may also affect dental development. Root formation can be impaired if irradiation takes place before apical closure occurs (McGinnis *et al.* 1985).

Doxapram

This respiratory stimulant has been shown to cause premature appearance of tooth buds (Tay-Uyboco *et al.* 1991).

Smoking

Maternal smoking is known to affect birth weight; the effect on the dentition, however, is not so dramatic. It has been reported that there are minor reductions (two to three per cent) in crown size of the deciduous dentition of children born to mothers who smoke. This effect appears to vary between races and sexes (Heikkinen *et al.* 1992).

Ciprofloxacin

A retrospective study evaluated the effect of ciprofloxacin on skeletal and tooth development after it had been administered to infants and neonates (Lumbiganon *et al.* 1991). In two of 10 patients followed up, a greenish discolouration of the teeth was observed. The staining appeared to be intrinsic since it could not be removed by mechanical means. The mechanism of such staining is uncertain, but it is recommended that ciprofloxacin should be given to newborn infants only in exceptional circumstances.

Salivary glands

The salivary glands are under control of the autonomic nervous system, mainly the parasympathetic division. Stimulation of the parasympathetic nerves causes glandular secretion. Because of their innervation, salivary gland function can be affected by a variety of drugs which can produce xerostomia or ptyalism. Certain systemic drug therapy can also produce pain and swelling of the salivary glands.

Xerostomia

Xerostomia (dryness of the mouth) can be caused by many drugs, and can be very troublesome to the patient. It can also cause a problem in denture retention, and dentists should be aware that drugs can be the cause. The only effective treatment is to stop the drug, but this action is rarely necessary. Drugs that can cause dryness of the mouth by their parasympatholytic activity include the following:

1. drugs competing with acetylcholine in parasympathetic (and sympathetic) ganglia, such as now obsolete ganglion-blocking antihypertensive drugs like pentolinium, mecamylamine, and pempidine;

2. drugs that compete with acetylcholine release at the parasympathetic effector junction. Most of the drugs that cause xerostomia do so in this way. They include atropine and atropine-like antispasmodics (e.g. poldine and propantheline bromide); tricyclic antidepressants (e.g. amitriptyline), and tetracyclic antidepressants (e.g. maprotiline hydrochloride); many antiparkinsonian drugs, such as benzhexol, benztropine mesylate, and orphenadrine; antihistamine drugs (H_1-blockers), some of which are phenothiazines. Somewhat weaker anticholinergic activity is exhibited by the phenothiazine derivatives, but this activity is sufficient to cause dryness of the mouth. Clonidine, used for hypertension and for migraine, frequently produces xerostomia. Selective antimuscarinic drugs, such as the antisecretory drug pirenzepine, are also associated with xerostomia;

3. drugs acting on the sympathetic effector function. Salivary flow is probably influenced to some extent by sympathetic as well as parasympathetic activity. Drugs acting at the sympathetic neuro-effector junction, such as amphetamine, may very slightly reduce salivary flow. A high incidence of caries has been observed in amphetamine abusers (Digugno *et al.* 1981). These authors suggest that this is due to both the reduced salivary flow rate and to a decrease in salivary calcium and phosphate concentration caused by this drug.

A number of other drugs, of which levodopa is one, have been reported to cause dryness of the mouth, and some of these have central actions. Antineoplastic drugs occasionally cause dryness of the mouth. Serotonin antagonists (e.g. ondansetron), which are used as antiemetics during chemotherapy, and thiabendazole can also cause dry mouth.

Ptyalism

Salivary secretion is increased by drugs that have a

cholinergic effect, either by acting directly on parasympathetic receptors (e.g. pilocarpine) or by acting as cholinesterase inhibitors and so preventing the destruction of acetylcholine by cholinesterase (e.g. neostigmine).

Salivary secretion tends to be increased by mercurial salts, iodides, and bromides (drugs that are little used in modern therapeutics). Ketamine, an intravenous anaesthetic agent, may cause severe salivation. It has been suggested that all patients who are to receive ketamine should be premedicated with atropine (Davies 1972). Clozapine-induced nocturnal sialorrhoea is a well recognized unwanted effect of this drug that can cause distressing choking (Pearlman 1994). The problem is particularly pertinent when the drug is used in the treatment of Parkinson's disease, since the latter is often accompanied by impaired swallowing. The mechanism of sialorrhoea due to clozapine is uncertain, since the anticholinergic properties of the drug might be expected to decrease salivary flow. Other drugs (now rarely used) that occasionally cause excessive salivation include the antileprotic drug ethionamide and the anthelminthic niridazole.

Pain and swelling affecting the salivary glands

Drugs that have been suspected of causing swelling and/or pain in the parotid or submandibular salivary glands are phenylbutazone and oxyphenbutazone (Gross 1969; Chen *et al.* 1977; Speed and Spelman 1982) and naproxen (Knulst *et al.* 1995); methyldopa (Mardt *et al.* 1974), clonidine (Onesti *et al.* 1971), bethanidine (Klein 1972), and bretylium; nifedipine (Bosch *et al.* 1986); phenytoin (Brandenburg *et al.* 1992); nitrofurantoin (Pellinen and Kalske 1982) and doxycycline (Pan and Quintela 1991); chlormethiazole (Bosch *et al.* 1994); cimetidine, famotidine, and ranitidine (Tomasko 1985); and chlorhexidine mouth washes. Iodine, which apart from its use in the preoperative preparation for thyroidectomy, is employed mainly in the form of radiographic contrast media (see also Chapter 28), can also affect the salivary glands, but with contrast media (Inbur and Bourne 1972; Kohri *et al.* 1977) such reactions are rare (Tucker and Di Bagno 1956). Ritodrine used during pregnancy has caused salivary gland enlargement with hypersecretion of amylase (Minakami *et al.* 1992). Haemorrhage into the submandibular glands, presenting as a sublingual swelling, has occurred in a patient having anticoagulant therapy with warfarin (De Castro *et al.* 1970).

Sjögren's syndrome includes parotid swelling, and the histamine (H_2)-receptor antagonists cimetidine, famotidine, and ranitidine have been reported to aggravate the disease (Tomasko 1988). The condition is quite common in rheumatoid arthritis, for which NSAID are frequently used, so that salivary gland swelling could be part of the disease rather than a complication of its treatment. However, parotid enlargement in Sjögren's syndrome occurs relatively late in the course of rheumatoid arthritis, hence its sudden appearance in the early stages of the disease may well indicate an adverse reaction to an anti-inflammatory drug.

Mechanisms in the drug-associated salivary gland disorders

The cases attributed to phenylbutazone, oxyphenbutazone, nitrofurantoin, and methyldopa had features suggesting an allergic reaction; iodine 'mumps' could be explained by the ability of salivary glands to concentrate iodine (up to 100 times the plasma levels (Talner *et al.* 1971), the high concentration having a local inflammatory action. Ritodrine may have produced its effect stimulation of β-adrenoceptors in the salivary glands. The ways in which the other drugs produced their adverse effects are obscure.

Cleft lip and palate

A few drugs have been firmly implicated, and many others suspected, as causes of cleft lip and palate and other teratogenic abnormalities. They are discussed in detail in Chapter 7.

Muscular and neurological disorders

Some drugs can cause extrapyramidal disorders characterized by muscular dyskinesia and dystonia, and in some cases a parkinsonian syndrome. These conditions are discussed in detail in Chapter 20, but their effects on the muscles of facial expression and mastication and of the neck will also be dealt with here.

Drug-induced extrapyramidal disturbances, which can be acute or chronic (tardive), include facial grimacing and distortions, protruding and rolling of the tongue, chewing movements, torticollis, retrocollis, opisthotonus, oculogyric crises, and other involuntary movements. Dislocation of the jaw may occur in some cases (Kraak 1967; Bradshaw 1969; Smith 1973; Wood 1978). In drug-induced parkinsonism there is often a mask-like facies, increased salivation, dysphagia, and dysarthria. In the commoner type of movement disorders, which usually occur in young adults, the onset is acute and the symptoms and signs regress quickly when the offending drug is withdrawn. In tardive dyskinesia, which is less common (Schicle *et al.* 1975) and which affects the elderly, particularly women, who have taken antipsychotic drugs for many years, the onset of the abnormalities is delayed, sometimes for many years;

they may be irreversible (Walton 1971), though in most instances gradual improvement follows drug withdrawal.

The drugs that have been associated with these disorders are predominantly the phenothiazines (e.g. chlorpromazine, fluphenazine, prochlorperazine, trifluoperazine) and the butyrophenones (e.g. benperidol, droperidol, haloperidol, trifluoperidol), but other drugs have been implicated, including carbamazepine, diazoxide, levodopa, metoclopramide, reserpine, and tricyclic antidepressants.

Facial pain and tardive dyskinesia

According to Bassett and others (1986), tardive dyskinesia is an uncommon and sometimes unrecognized cause of orofacial pain. Describing two patients who had been taking antipsychotic drugs the authors stated that the presenting complaints and symptoms are quite characteristic of this disorder. They also pointed out that tardive dyskinesia is a painless syndrome in itself, but secondary orofacial pain can result from chronic mild trauma between a denture-bearing mucosa and dentures, which occurs with the abnormal movement. However, not all involuntary movements in a patient taking an antipsychotic drug are necessarily indicative of a tardive dyskinesia. Many elderly people have a mild degree of involuntary dystonic-type movements. Ill-fitting dentures may also produce oral muscular activity (Sutcher et al. 1971). However, if the patient has clearly observable facial movements and has also a history of taking antipsychotic drugs, it is not unreasonable to think of drug-induced tardive dyskinesia. There is no really satisfactory treatment for the condition other than cessation of drug therapy when, in many instances, it slowly improves. The management of such patients is for the supervising physician to undertake. The dental surgeon should be aware that such drug reactions exist and refer the patient when they are recognized. It is, of course, important to ensure that all dental work is satisfactory and that ill-fitting dentures are not adding to the problem, or the cause of the trouble. Facial pain has also been reported following use of a controlled-release theophylline preparation (Townend 1989). The mechanism of this unwanted effect is uncertain.

Meige's syndrome

The blepharospasm–oromandibular dystonia syndrome (Meige's syndrome) has been related to long-term combination therapy with levodopa and carbidopa (Weiner and Nausieda 1982). The syndrome has also been associated with the overuse of a self-prescribed nasal decongestant spray containing 0.5% phenylephrine hydrochloride, 0.2% chlorpheniramine maleate, and benzalkonium chloride (Dristan) (Powers 1982).

Neuropathy

Many drugs are capable of causing a toxic neuritis of branches of the trigeminal nerves (Kay 1972). Drugs reported to have caused sensations of numbness, tingling, or burning in the face or mouth include the carbonic anhydrase inhibitor acetazolamide; the antimicrobial drugs streptomycin, colistin, polymyxin B, isoniazid, nalidixic acid, nitrofurantoin, and pentamidine; several of the antidepressant drugs of the monoamine oxidase inhibitor group (e.g. phenelzine), and of the tricyclic group (e.g. amitriptyline); the β-adrenoceptor-blocking agent propranolol; the oral antidiabetic compounds tolbutamide and chlorpropamide; gonadotrophin-releasing-hormone analogues; the migraine remedy ergotamine; the antihypertensive drug hydralazine; and nicotinic acid in large doses.

Taste disturbance

Many drugs induce abnormalities of taste by processes not yet properly understood. The alteration in taste may be simply a blunting or decreased sensitivity in taste perception (hypogeusia), a total loss of the ability to taste (ageusia), or a distortion in perception of the correct taste of a substance, for example, sour for sweet (dysgeusia).

Penicillamine

Sulphydryl compounds, especially penicillamine, are a common cause of taste disturbance. Penicillamine is used to chelate copper in Wilson's disease (hepatocellular degeneration). It is also used to treat rheumatoid arthritis, in which its mode of action is unknown. In many patients, penicillamine causes partial or total loss of taste (Henkin et al. 1967). A decrease in taste acuity was reported to occur in 23 of 73 patients given penicillamine for conditions other than Wilson's disease (Scheinberg 1968). The incidence of taste disturbances in patients treated with penicillamine for Wilson's disease was much lower. About 25 per cent of patients with rheumatoid arthritis receiving penicillamine treatment experience taste disturbances (Jaffe 1968). It seems that there is a marked difference in the frequency of this unfortunate effect between patients being treated for Wilson's disease and those being treated for other conditions. It seems apparent that the loss of taste that may occur is directly related to the copper depletion that commonly follows the use of the drug. Penicillamine produces a negative copper balance, which is unlikely to occur in Wilson's disease where there is an elevated total body copper. However, administration of copper salts does not prevent the effect, and taste abnormalities occur with other sulphydryl compounds which are not copper-chelating agents (Jaffe 1983).

It has also been suggested that penicillamine-induced taste disturbances are due to a direct effect of the drug on the receptor cells (Lyle 1974). Furthermore, taste disturbances have been found to be dose related (Day *et al.* 1974). If the dose of penicillamine is below 900 mg daily, there is a 25 per cent incidence of taste disturbance in patients with Wilson's disease. The incidence increases to 50 per cent when the daily dose exceeds 900 mg. It would appear that taste disturbance is reversible within a period of 8–10 weeks, whether or not penicillamine is discontinued (Jaffe 1986).

Angiotensin-converting-enzyme (ACE) inhibitors

Captopril appears to be the ACE inhibitor most frequently implicated in causing taste disturbances (dysgeusia), with some two to four per cent of patients reporting this unwanted effect (Henkin 1989). Impaired salty taste is the most frequent complaint. The extent of captopril-induced dysgeusia seems to be related to dose and renal function and can be compounded by smoking. Taste disturbances tend to be self-limiting and reversible in 2–3 months even if the drug is continued. However, it may cause patients to lose weight, which is certainly a reason for them to stop or request a change of treatment.

It has been suggested that the sulphydryl group on the captopril molecule is the cause of the taste disturbance (see above). However, other ACE inhibitors that do not contain an active sulphydryl group also cause taste disturbances; thus an alternative mechanism may be responsible. Low plasma zinc concentrations are also associated with a reduction in taste discrimination and activity. Captopril binds to the zinc site of the converting enzyme (a metalloenzyme), and can also inhibit the zinc metalloenzyme gustin, which is intimately involved in taste (Neil-Dwyer and Marus 1989). While an interaction between captopril and the zinc metalloenzyme may cause the taste disturbance, ACE inhibitors have no effect on plasma zinc concentrations or intraerythrocyte zinc levels.

Other drugs

Drugs reported as having caused disorders of taste,

usually in the form of diminished taste acuity, include aspirin, clofibrate, carbimazole, ethambutol, ethionamide, gold salts, griseofulvin, imipramine, levodopa, lincomycin, lithium carbonate, phenindione, and prothionamide (Rollin 1978; Guerrier and Uziel 1979). Systemic griseofulvin can render certain foods profoundly tasteless, the effect gradually worsening for as long as the patient takes the drug. Furthermore, the effect may take some months to disappear after the drug is withdrawn (Griffiths 1976). A metallic taste may be an unpleasant feature of treatment with the biguanide antidiabetic drug metformin. Similarly, a metallic taste is not uncommon in patients treated with metronidazole.

The subject of taste disorders is also discussed in Chapter 22.

Halitosis

One or two instances of drug-induced halitosis have been reported. Bauman (1975) reported that several patients taking the sublingual form of isosorbide dinitrate had complained of 'bad breath'. This problem appeared with the onset of therapy, was reversible after discontinuing the drug, and recurred when therapy was resumed. Disulfiram is also reported to cause a slightly unpleasant breath odour (O'Reilly and Motley 1977). This is attributed to a metabolic product of the drug.

Oral infections induced or aggravated by drugs

Many types of systemic drug therapy can alter the oral flora and therefore predispose the mouth to bacterial and fungal infection. Drugs that have been implicated in this problem include corticosteroids, antimicrobials, anticancer drugs, immunosuppressive agents, and oral contraceptives. This subject is discussed fully in Chapter 25.

Alveolar osteitis (dry sockets)

The use of oral contraceptives has been associated with a significant increase in the frequency of dry sockets (alveolar osteitis) after removal of impacted lower third molars (Catellani *et al.* 1980). The probability of dry sockets increases with the oestrogen dose in the oral contraceptive. The authors suggest that dry sockets can be minimized by carrying out the extractions during days 23–28 of the tablet cycle.

Facial oedema

Facial oedema is often a manifestation of drug-induced

hypersensitivity reactions. It has also been associated with administration of mianserin (Leibovitch *et al.* 1987), and has followed excessive use of an adrenaline bronchodilator (Loria and Wedner 1989).

It is now recognized that ACE inhibitors are a significant cause of angioedema (Israeli and Hall 1992). The precise mechanism whereby this group of drugs causes angioedema remains uncertain. The most plausible explanation is that angioedema arises as a consequence of an alteration in bradykinin metabolism in susceptible patients. Any area of the body may be involved, but most commonly it affects the face and mucous membranes, tongue, lips, and larynx. In severe cases, it can result in serious acute respiratory distress, airway obstruction, and death. It has been estimated that the prevalence of this unwanted effect is in the range of 0.1–0.2 per cent (Thompson and Fable 1990). In most cases, symptoms are usually mild and relatively short-lived and this may imply that the true incidence of angioedema is greater than the prevalence data indicates. Captopril, lisinopril, and enalapril are the ACE inhibitors most frequently implicated in angioedema, but this may be a reflection on their widespread use. Most case reports suggest that angioedema usually occurs within hours or at most weeks after starting the ACE inhibitor, and reverses within hours of stopping (Israeli and Hall 1992). However, it can develop after long-term therapy (Chin and Buchan 1990). Droperidol, an intravenous anaesthetic agent, has been implicated in causing rapid swelling and local cyanosis of the tongue within 5 minutes of administration (Clark 1993). The swelling responded to promethazine 25 mg intravenously, which suggests a vascular mechanism as opposed to being oedematous. Intravenous clindamycin has caused swelling of both nasal passages and lips (Segars and Threlkeld 1993). Hypersensitivity reactions to clindamycin are rare and the reaction observed might have been caused by one of the ingredients (e.g. benzyl alcohol) in the intravenous preparation.

Drug-induced blood dyscrasias

As the dental surgeon may be the first person to see a patient with a blood dyscrasia, he should be familiar with the manifestations of these disorders. The oral signs of many of the blood disorders are similar to lesions occurring as a result of infection, and diagnosis on clinical grounds alone is not possible. Nevertheless, there are pointers that should alert the dental surgeon to the possibility of a blood disorder, drug-induced or otherwise. The following signs and symptoms should arouse suspicion (Weiss 1973), unexplained spontaneous mu-cosal bleeding, numerous oral petechiae, excessive post-extraction haemorrhage, pallor of the oral mucosa, unresponsive oral infections, prolonged atrophy of lingual papillae, sore tongue or mouth without local irritation, unexplained bruising, and ulcerated mucosa accompanied by pyrexia.

The drugs causing blood dyscrasias and bleeding disorders are discussed in Chapter 24, but it should be mentioned here that lingual haematoma has followed the use of streptokinase (Williams *et al.* 1994) and sublingual (Cohen and Warman 1989) and submandibular (De Castro *et al.* 1970) haemorrhage has been caused by warfarin.

Drugs of abuse

The widespread abuse of cocaine has an impact on dental practice. One example is post-extraction haemorrhage in the early postoperative period after third-molar surgery, which arose from cocaine snorting by an addict (Johnson and Brown 1993). It was thought that the adrenergic effects of cocaine on heart rate and blood pressure increased the propensity to post-extraction haemorrhage.

References

Aas, E. (1963). Hyperplasia gingivae diphenylhydantoinea. *Acta Odontol. Scand.* 21 (Suppl. 34), 1.

Aberer, W., Holub, H., Strohal, R., *et al.* (1993). Palladium in dental alloys — the dermatologists' responsibility to warn? *Contact Dermatitis* 28, 163.

Adams, D. and Davies G. (1984). Gingival hyperplasia associated with cyclosporin. A report of two cases. *Br. Dent. J.* 157, 89.

Addy, M., Prayitno, S., Taylor, L., *et al.* (1979). An in vitro study of the role of dietary factors in the aetiology of tooth staining associated with the use of chlorhexidine. *J. Periodont. Res.* 14, 403.

Addy, M., Moran, J., Davies, *et al.* (1982). The effect of single morning and evening rinses of chlorhexidine on the development of tooth staining and plaque accumulation. A blind crossover trial. *J. Clin. Periodontol.* 9, 134.

Addy, V., McElay, J.C., Eyre, G., *et al.* (1983). Risk factors in phenytoin-induced gingival overgrowth. *J. Periodontol.* 54, 373.

use of chlorhexidine. *J. Periodont. Res.* 14, 403.

Aguirre, A., Izu, R., Gardeazabal, J., *et al.* (1992). Allergic contact cheilitis from a lipstick containing oxybenzone. *Contact Dermatitis* 27, 267.

Aguirre, A., Manzano, D., Izu, R., *et al.* (1994). Allergic contact cheilitis from mandelic acid. *Contact Dermatitis* 31, 133.

Angelini, E., Marinaro, C., Carrozzo, A.M., *et al.* (1993). Allergic contact dermatitis of the lip margins from paratertiary-butylphenol in a lip liner. *Contact Dermatitis* 28, 146.

Angelopoulos, A.P. (1975). Diphenylhydantoin gingival hyperplasia. A clinicopathological review. 1. Incidence, clinical features and histopathology. *J. Can. Dent. Assoc.* 41, 103.

Angelopoulos, A.P. and Goaz, P.W. (1972). Incidence of diphenylhydantoin gingival hyperplasia. *Oral Surg.* 34, 898.

Backman, N., Holm, A.K., Hanstrom, L., *et al.* (1989). Folate treatment of diphenylhydantoin-induced gingival hyperplasia. *Scand. J. Dent. Res.* 97, 222.

Barclay, S., Thomason, J.M., Idel, J.R., *et al.* (1992). The incidence and severity of nifedipine-induced gingival overgrowth. *J. Clin. Periodontol.* 19, 311.

Bashirelahi, N., Organ, R., and Bergquist, J.J. (1977). Steroid binding protein in human gingiva. *J. Dent. Res.* 56, 125.

Basker, R. M. (1981). Nickel sensitivity — some dental implications. *Br. Dent. J.* 151, 414.

Bassett, A., Remick, R.A., and Blasberg, B. (1986). Tardive dyskinesia: an unrecognised cause of orofacial pain. *Oral Surg.* 61, 570.

Bassuk, E. and Schoonover, S. (1978). Rampant dental caries in the treatment of depression. *J. Clin. Psychiatry* 39, 163.

Bauman, D. (1975). Halitosis from isosorbide dinitrate. *JAMA* 234, 482.

Beehner, M., Houston, G.D., and Young, J. D. (1986). Oral pigmentation secondary to minocycline therapy. *J. Oral Maxillofac. Surg.* 44, 582.

Behari, M. (1991). Gingival hyperplasia due to sodium valproate. *J. Neurol. Neurosurg. Psychiatry* 54, 279.

Bennett, J.A. and Christian, J.M. (1985). Cyclosporin-induced gingival hyperplasia: case report and literature review. *J. Am. Dent. Assoc.* 111, 272.

Bentley, E., Mackie, I.C., Fuller, S., *et al.* (1994). Smile for sugar-free medicines — a dental health education campaign. *Journal of the Institute of Health Education* 32, 36.

Beveridge, T. (1983). Cyclosporin A: clinical results. *Transplant. Proc.* 15, 433.

Bond. S. and Fields, C.D. (1991). Formulating sugar-free oral liquid medicines. In *Sugarless — the Way Forward* (ed. A. Rugg-Gunn), p. 154. Elsevier Applied Science, London.

Bosch, X., Campistol, J.M., Botey, A., *et al.* (1986). Nifedipine-induced parotitis. *Lancet* ii, 467.

Bosch, X., Sans, M., Martinez-Orozco, F., *et al.* (1994). Parotitis induced by chlormethiazole. *BMJ* 309, 1620.

Bottomley, W.K., Perlin, E., and Ross, G.R. (1977). Antineoplastic agents and their oral manifestations. *Oral Surg.* 44, 527.

Bowman, J., Levy, B.A., and Grubb, R.V. (1988). Gingival overgrowth induced by diltiazem. *Oral Surg.* 65, 183.

Bradshaw, R.B. (1969). Perphenazine dystonia presenting as recurrent dislocation of the jaw. *J. Laryngol. Otol.* 83, 79.

Brandenburg, A.H., Smits, M.G., Voorbrood, B.S., *et al.* (1992). Submandibular salivary gland hypertrophy induced by phenytoin. *Epilepsia* 34, 151.

Brannstrom, H., Nordenvall, K.-J., and Hedstrom, K.G. (1982). Periodontal tissue changes after intraligamentary anaesthesia. *J. Dent. Child.* 49, 417.

Brannstrom, H., Lindskog, S., and Nordenvall, K-J. (1984). Enamel hypoplasia in permanent teeth induced by periodontal ligament anesthesia of primary teeth. *J. Am. Dent. Assoc.* 109, 735.

Breuer, M.M., Mboya, S.A., Moroi, H., *et al.* (1996). Effect of selected beta-blockers on supragingival calculus formation. *J. Periodontol.* 67, 428.

Brody, H. and Cohen, M. (1986). Black tongue secondary to methyldopa therapy. *Cutis* 38, 187.

Brook, U., Singer, L., and Fried, D. (1989). Development of severe Stevens–Johnson syndrome after administration of slow-release theophylline. *Pediatr. Dermatol.* 6, 126.

Brown, R.D. and Bolas, G. (1973). Isoprenaline ulceration of the tongue: a case report. *Br. Dent. J.* 134, 336.

Brown, R.S., Sein, P., Corio, R., *et al.* (1990). Nitrendipine-induced gingival hyperplasia. *Oral Surg.* 70, 593.

Brown, R.S., Krakow, A.M., Douglas, T., *et al.* (1997). 'Scalded mouth syndrome' caused by angiotensin converting enzyme inhibitors. *Oral Surg.* 83, 665.

Bruce, G.J. and Hall, W.B. (1995). Nickel hypersensitivity-related periodontitis. *Compendium* 16, 178.

Calne, R.Y., Rolles, K., and White, D.J.G., *et al.* (1981). Cyclosporin A in clinical organ grafting. *Transplant. Proc.* 13, 349.

Cameron, A.J., Baron, J.H., and Priestley, B.L. (1966). Erythema multiforme, drugs and ulcerative colitis. *BMJ* ii, 1174.

Caron, F., Meurice, J.G., Dore, P., *et al.* (1997). Gingival hyperplasia: a new side effect associated with trimethoprim-sulphamethoxazole (TML-SMX) treatment in pulmonary nocardosis. *Therapie* 52, 73.

Catellani, J.E., Harvey, S., Erikson, S.H., *et al.* (1980). Effect of oral contraceptive cycle on dry socket. *J. Am. Dent. Assoc.* 101, 777.

Chen, J.H., Ottolenghi, P., and Distenfeld, A. (1977). Oxyphenbutazone-induced sialadenitis. *JAMA* 238, 1399.

Chevallier, M.E. (1970). Mouth manifestations and oral contraceptives. *Rev. Odontol. Stomatol.* 28, 96.

Chin, M.L. and Buchan, D.A. (1990). Severe angioedema after long-term use of an angiotensin converting enzyme inhibitor. *Ann. Intern. Med.* 112, 312.

Chu, P., Van, S.L., Yen, T.S., *et al.* (1994). Minocycline hyperpigmentation localised to the lips: an unusual fixed drug reaction? *J. Am. Acad. Dermatol.* 30, 802.

Churgin, L.S. and Payne, J.C. (1981). Sensitised tissue response to an ethylene imine derivative transitional crown material. *J. Prosthet. Dent.* 46, 179.

Claman, H.N. (1967). Mouth ulcers associated with prolonged chewing of gum containing aspirin. *JAMA* 202, 651.

Clark, R. (1993). Tongue-swelling with droperidol. *Anaesth. Intens. Care* 21, 898.

Cohen, A. and Warman, S.P. (1989). Upper airway obstruction secondary to warfarin-induced sublingual hematoma. *Arch. Otolaryngol Head Neck Surg.* 115, 718.

Colvard, M., Bishop, J., Weissman, D., *et al.* (1986). Cardiazem-induced gingival hyperplasia: a report of two cases. *Periodont. Case Report.* 8, 67.

Committee for the Safety of Medicines (1984). Macleans Sensitive Teeth Formula Toothpaste. *Newsletter,* 13 July.

Coombes, B. W. (1965). Stevens-Johnson syndrome associated with carbamazepine ('Tegretol'). *Med. J. Aust.* 1, 895.

Coombs, R.R.A. and Gell, P.G.H. (1968). Classification of allergice reactions responsible for clinical hypersensitivity and disease, In *Clinical Aspects of Immunology* (ed. P.H. Gell and R.R.A. Coombs), p. 575. Blackwell, Oxford.

Cucchi, G., Giustiniani, S., and Robustelli, F. (1985). Gingival hyperplasia caused by verapamil. *Ital. J. Cardiol.* 15, 556.

Curley, R. and Baxter, P.W. (1987). An unusual cutaneous reaction to lignocaine. *Br. Dent. J.* 162, 113.

Dahllof, G. and Modeer, T. (1986). The effect of a plaque control programme on the development of phenytoin-induced gingival overgrowth. *J. Clin. Periodontol.* 13, 845.

Daley, T.D. and Wysocki, G.P. (1984). Cyclosporin therapy, its significance to the periodontist. *J. Periodontol.* 55, 708.

Daley, T.D.. Wysocki, G.P., and Day, C. (1986). Clinical and pharmacological correlations in cyclosporin-induced gingival hyperplasia. *Oral Surg.* 62, 417.

Daniels, A.M. (1986). Mouth ulceration associated with proguanil. *Lancet* i, 269.

Darby, C.W. (1970). Pancreatic extracts. *BMJ* ii, 299.

Das, A.K., Bhowmick, S., and Dutta, A. (1971). Oral contraceptives and periodontal disease. *J. Ind. Dent. Assoc.* 43, 155.

Davies, C.K. (1972). Problems with ketamine anaesthesia. *BMJ* iv, 178.

Day, A. T., Golding, J.R., Lee, P.N., *et al.* (1974). Penicillamine in rheumatoid disease: a long-term study. *BMJ* i, 180.

De Castro, C.M., Hall, R.J., and Glasser, S.P. (1970). Salivary gland haemorrhage — an unusual complication of coumarin anticoagulation. *Am. Heart J.* 80, 675.

De Dobbeleer, G. and Achten, G. (1977). Fixed drug eruption: ultrastructural study of dyskeratotic cells. *Br. J. Dermatol.* 96, 239.

Dello-Russo, N.M. and Temple, H.V. (1982). Cocaine effects on the gingiva. *J. Am. Dent. Assoc.* 104, 13.

Department of Health (1989). Committee on Medical Aspects of Food Policy. *Diet, Sugar and Human Disease.* (No. 37), p. 16, 41. HMSO, London.

Department of Health (1994). Committee on Medical Aspects of Food Policy. Report of Working Group on the Weaning Diet. *Weaning and the Weaning Diet*, (No. 145), p. 76. HMSO, London.

Digugno, F., Perec, C.J., and Tocci, A.A. (1981). Salivary secretion and dental caries experience in drug addicts. *Arch. Oral Biol.* 26, 363.

Dinsdale, R.C.W. and Walker, A.E. (1966). Amiphenazole sensitivity with oral ulceration. *Br. Dent. J.* 121. 460.

Dinsdale, R.C.W., Ormerod, T.P., and Walker, A.E. (1968). Lichenoid eruption due to chlorpropamide. *BMJ* i, 100.

Di Santis, D.J. and Flanagan, T. (1981). Minoxidil-induced Stevens–Johnson syndrome. *Arch. Intern. Med.* 141, 1515.

Dobson, R. and Smith, A.C. (1987). Effect of paraquat on the oral mucosa. *Br. Dent. J.* 163, 160.

Dolin, H. (1951). Dilantin hyperplasia. *Milit. Surg.* 109, 134.

Dreyer, W. and Thomas, C. (1978). Diphenylhydantoin-induced hyperplasia of the masticatory mucosa in an edentulous epileptic patient. *Oral Surg.* 45, 701.

Dummett, C.O. (1954). Oral tissue reactions from Dilantin medication in the control of epileptic seizures. *J. Periodontol.* 25, 112.

Dunlap, C., Vincent, S.K., and Barker, B.F. (1989). Allergic reaction to orthodontic wire: report of a case. *J. Am. Dent. Assoc.* 118, 449.

Dutree-Meulenberg, R., Lozel, M.M., and van Joost, T. (1992). Burning mouth syndrome: a possible etiologic role for local contact hypersensitivity. *J. Am. Acad. Dermatol.* 26, 935.

Duxbury, A. J., Watts, D. C., and Eade, R. J. (1982). Allergy to dental amalgam. *Br. Dent. J.* 152, 344.

El-Ashiry, G. M., El-Kafrawy, A. H., Nasr, M. F., *et al.* (1970). Comparative study of the influence of pregnancy and oral contraceptives on the gingivae. *Oral Surg.* 30, 472.

El-Attar, T.M.A. (1971). Metabolism of progesterone-in vitro in human gingiva with periodontitis. *J. Periodontol.* 42. 72 1.

El-Attar, T.M.A. (1974). The in vitro conversion of male sex steroid 1,2 -^{3}H-androstenedione in normal and inflamed human gingiva. *Arch. Oral Biol.* 19, 1185.

El-Attar, T.M.A. and Hugoson, A. (1974). Comparative metabolism of female sex steroids in normal and chronically inflamed gingiva of the dog. *J. Periodont. Res.* 9, 284.

El-Attar, T.M.A., Roth, G.D., and Hugoson, A. (1973). Comparative metabolism of 4-^{14}C-progesterone in normal and chronically inflamed human gingival tissue. *J. Periodont. Res.* 8, 79.

Ellingsen, J.E., Eriksen, H.M., and Rolla, G. (1982). Extrinsic staining caused by stannous fluoride. *Scand. J. Dent. Res.* 90, 9.

Ellis, J.S., Seymour, R.A., Monkman, S.C., *et al.* (1992). Gingival sequestration of nifedipine in nifedipine-induced gingival overgrowth. *Lancet* 339, 1382.

Ellis, J.S., Seymour, R.A., Thomason, J.M., *et al.* (1993). Amlodipine-induced gingival overgrowth and sequestration in crevicular fluid. *Lancet* 341, 1102.

Eriksen, H.M., Solheim, H., and Nordbo, H. (1983). Chemical plaque control and prevention of extrinsic tooth discolouration in vivo. *Acta Odontol. Scand.* 41, 87.

Esterberg, H.L. and White, P.M. (1945). Sodium dilantin gingival hyperplasia. *J. Am. Dent. Assoc.* 32, 16.

Fawcett, L.B., Buck, S.J., Beckman, D.A., *et al.* (1996). Is there a no-effect dose for corticosteroid-induced cleft palate? The contribution of endogenous corticosterone to the incidence of cleft palate in mice. *Pediatr. Res.* 39, 856.

Feaver, F. (1982). Action called for sale of toothache solutions. *Br. Dent. J.* 152, 3.

Feigal, R.J. and Jensen, M.E. (1982). The cariogenic potential of liquid medications: a concern for the handicapped patient. *Spec. Care Dent.* 2, 20.

Felix, R.H., Ive, F.A., and Dahl, M.G.C. (1974). Cutaneous and ocular reactions to practolol. *BMJ* iv, 321.

Ferguson, J.E. and Beck, M.H. (1995). Contact sensitivity to a vanilla lip salve. *Contact Dermatitis* 33, 352.

Ferguson, M.M., Wiesenfeld, D., and MacDonald, D.G. (1984). Oral mucosal lichenoid eruption due to fenclofenac. *J. Oral. Med.* 39, 39.

Fisher, A. (1991). Allergic cheilitis due to castor oil in lipsticks. *Cutis* 47, 389.

Freehally, J., Walls, J., Mistry, N., *et al.* 1987). Does nifedipine ameliorate cyclosporin A nephrotoxicity? *BMJ* 295, 295.

Fugii, A. and Kobayashi, S. (1990). Nifedipine inhibits calcium uptake of nifedipine sensitive gingival fibroblasts. *J. Dent. Res.* 67, 332.

Fulghum, D.D. and Catalano, P.M. (1973). Stevens–Johnson syndrome from clindamycin. A case report. *JAMA* 223, 318.

Gelfand, E.W., Cheung, R.K., Grinstein, S., *et al.* (1986). Characterisation of the role of calcium influx in mitogen-induced triggering and human T-cells. Identification of calcium-dependent and calcium-independent signals. *Eur. J. Immunol.* 16, 907.

Gelfand, E.W., Cheung, R.K., and Mills, G.B. (1987). The cyclosporine inhibits lymphocyte activation at more than one site. *J. Immunol.* 138, 1115.

Giansanti, J.S., Tillery, D.E., and Olansky, S. (1971). Oral mucosal pigmentation resulting from anti-malarial therapy. *Oral Surg.* 31, 66.

Gillis, A. (1978). Lithium carbonate and dental caries. *BMJ* ii, 1717.

Girgis, S.S., Staple, P.H., Miller, W.A., *et al.* (1980). Dental root abnormalities and gingival overgrowth in epileptic patients receiving anticonvulsant therapy. *J. Periodontol.* 51, 474.

Giustiniani, S., Della-Cuna, F. R., and Marien, M. (1987). Hyperplastic gingivitis during diltiazem therapy. *Int. J. Cardiol.* 15, 247.

Gordon, M.H., Tiger, L.H., and Ehrlich, M.D. (1975). Gold reactions are not more common in Sjogren's syndrome. *Ann. Intern. Med.* 82, 47.

Gregoriou, A.P., Schneider, P.E., and Shaw, P.R. (1996). Phenobarbital-induced gingival overgrowth? Report of two cases and complications in management. *ASDC J. Dent. Child.* 63, 408.

Griffiths, I.P. (1976). Abnormalities of smell and taste. *Practitioner* 217, 907.

Gross, L. (1969). Oxyphenbutazone-induced parotitis. *Ann. Intern. Med.* 70, 1229.

Guerrier, Y. and Uziel, A. (1979). Clinical aspects of taste disorders. *Acta Otolaryngol.* 87, 232.

Guggenheimer, J. and Ismail, Y.H. (1975). Oral ulcerations associated with indomethacin therapy: report of 3 cases. *J. Am. Dent. Assoc.* 90, 632.

Haberman, A., Pratt, M., and Storrs, F. J. (1993). Contact dermatitis from beryllium in dental alloys. *Contact Dermatitis* 28, 157.

Hamburger, J. and Potts, A.J.C. (1983). Non-steroidal anti-inflammatory drugs and oral lichenoid reactions. *BMJ* 287, 1258.

Hammarstrom, L. (1970). Specific uptake of some drugs in ameloblasts and developing enamel. *Acta Odontol. Scand.* 28, 187 .

Harri, M.-P. and Ojanotko, A.O. (1978). Progesterone metabolism in healthy and inflamed female gingiva. *J. Steroid Biochem.* 9, 826.

Harris, M. and Goldhaber, P. (1974). Root abnormalities in epileptics and the inhibition of parathyroid hormone-induced bone resorption by diphenylhydantoin in tissue cultures. *Arch. Oral Biol.* 19, 981.

Hassell, T. M., O'Donnell, J., Pearlman, J., *et al.* (1984). Phenytoin-induced gingival overgrowth in institutionalised epileptics. *J. Clin. Periodontol.* 11, 242.

Hay, K.D. and Reade, P.C. (1978). Methyldopa as a cause of oral mucous membrane reactions. *Br. Dent. J.* 145, 195.

Healy, C.M. and Thornhill, M.H. (1995). An association between recurrent oro-genital ulceration and non-steroidal anti-inflammatory drugs. *J. Oral. Pathol. Med.* 24, 46.

Heikkinen, T., Alvesalo. L., Osborne, R.H., *et al.* (1992). Maternal smoking and tooth formation in the foetus. 1. Tooth crown size in the deciduous dentition. *Early Hum. Dev.* 30, 49.

Henkin, R.I. (1989). Converting enzyme inhibitors in the treatment of hypertension. *N. Engl. J. Med.* 320, 1750.

Henkin, R.I., Keiser, H.R., Jaffe, I.A., *et al.* (1967). Decreased taste sensitivity after D-penicillamine reversed by copper administration. *Lancet* ii, 1268.

Hertz, R.S., Beckstead, P.C., and Brown, W.J. (1980). Epithelial melanosis of the gingiva possibly resulting from the use of oral contraceptives. *J. Am. Dent. Assoc.* 100, 713.

High, A. and Main, D.M.G. (1989). Angina bullosa haemorrhagica: a complication of long-term steroid inhaler use. *Br. Dent. J.* 165, 176.

Hjeljord, L.G., Sonju, T., and Rolla, G. (1973). Chlorhexidine-protein interactions. *J. Periodont. Res.* 8 (Suppl. 12), 11.

Hobson, P. (1985). Sugar based medicines and dental disease. *Community Dent. Health* 2, 57.

Hobson, P. and Fuller, S. (1987). Sugar-based medicines and dental disease progress report. *Community Dent. Health* 4. 169.

Hogan, D.J., Burgess, W.R., Epstein, J.D., *et al.* (1985). Lichenoid stomatitis associated with lithium carbonate. *J. Am. Acad. Dermatol.* 13, 243.

Hollman, A. and Wong, H.O. (1964). Phenindione sensitivity. *BMJ* ii, 730.

Hugoson, A. (1970). Gingival inflammation and female sex hormones. *J. Periodontol. Res.* (Suppl. 5) 1, 76.

Imbur, D.J. and Bourne, R.B. (1972). Iodine mumps following excretory urography. *J. Urol.* 108, 629.

Imfeld, T. (1983). Identification of low caries risk dietary components. In *Monographs in Oral Science* (ed. H. Meyers). Karger, Basel.

Israeli, Z.H. and Hall, W.D. (1992). Cough and angioneurotic oedema associated with ACE inhibitor therapy. A review of the literature and pathophysiology. *Ann. Intern. Med.* 117, 234.

Jaffe, I.A. (1968). Effects of penicillamine on the kidney and on taste. *Postgrad. Med. J.* 44 (Suppl.), 15.

Jaffe, I.A. (1983). Thiol compounds with penicillamine-like activity and possible mode of action in rheumatoid arthritis. *Clin. Pharmacol. Ther.* 3, 555.

Jaffe, I.A. (1986). Adverse effects profile of sulphydryl compounds in man. *Am. J. Med.* 80, 471.

James, J., Ferguson, M.M., and Forsyth, A. (1985). Mercury allergy as a cause of burning mouth. *Br. Dent. J.* 159, 287.

James, J., Ferguson, M.M., Forsyth, A., *et al.* (1987). Oral lichenoid reactions related to mercury sensitivity. *Br. J. Oral Maxillofac. Surg.* 25, 474.

Johnson, C. and Brown, R.S. (1993). How cocaine abuse affects post-extraction bleeding. *J. Am. Dent. Assoc.* 124, 60.

Kanefsky, T.M. and Medoff, S.I. (1980). Stevens–Johnson syndrome and neutropenia with chlorpropamide. *Arch. Intern. Med.* 140, 1543.

Kapur, R.N., Girgis, S., Little, T.M., *et al.* (1973). Diphenylhydantoin-induced gingival hyperplasia; its relationship to dose and serum levels. *Dev. Med. Child Neurol.* 15, 483.

Katz, J., Marmary, Y., and Azaz, B. (1986). Iodine mumps following parotid sialography. *J. Oral Med.* 41, 149.

Katz, J., Barak, S., Shemer, J., *et al.* (1995). Black tongue associated with minocycline therapy. *Arch. Dermatol.* 131, 620.

Katz, J., Giuol, N., Chaushu, G., *et al.* (1997). Vigabatrin-induced gingival overgrowth. *J. Clin. Periodontol.* 24, 180.

Kaufman, A.Y. (1969). An oral contraceptive as an aetiological factor in producing hyperplastic gingivitis and a neoplasm of the pregnancy tumour type. *Oral Surg.* 28, 666.

Kaziro, G.S. (1980). Oral ulceration and neutropenia associated with naproxen. *Aust. Dent. J.* 25, 333.

Kennett, S. (1968). Stomatitis medicamentosa due to barbiturates. *Oral Surg.* 25, 351.

Kenny, D. and Somaya, P. (1989). Sugar load of oral liquid medications on chronically ill children. *J. Canad. Dent. Assoc.* 55. 43.

King, G., Fullinfaw, R., and Higgins, T.J. (1993). Gingival hyperplasia in renal allograft recipients receiving cyclosporin A and calcium antagonists. *J. Clin. Periodont.* 20, 286.

Klar, L.A. (1973). Gingival hyperplasia during dilantin therapy: a survey of 312 patients. *J. Public Health Dent.* 33, 180.

Klein, F. (1972). Hypotensive drugs. In *Side Effects of Drugs* Vol. 7 (ed. L. Meyler and A. Herxheimer), p. 298. Associated Scientific Publishers, Amsterdam.

Knight, G.M. and Wade, A.B. (1974). The effects of hormonal contraceptives on the human periodontium. *J. Periodont. Res.* 9, 18.

Knulst, A.C., Stengs, C.J.M., Baart de la Faille, H., *et al.* (1995). Salivary gland swelling following naproxen therapy. *Br. J. Dermatol.* 133, 647.

Kohri, K., Miyoshi, S., Nagahara, A., *et al.* (1977). Bilateral parotid enlargement ('iodine mumps') following excretory urography. *Radiology* 122, 654.

Konstantinidis, A.B., Markopoulos, A. and Trigonides, G. (1985). Ampicillin-induced erythema multiforme. *J. Oral. Med.* 40, 168.

Kraak, J.G. (1967). A drug-initiated dislocation of the temporomandibular joint: report of a case. *J. Am. Dent. Assoc.* 74, 1247.

Lacey, M., Reade, P.C., and Hay, K.D. (1983). Lichen planus: theory of pathogenesis. *Oral Surg.* 56, 521.

Lagerlof, F. and Dawes, C. (1985). Effect of sucrose as a gustatory stimulus on the flow rates of parotid and whole saliva. *Caries Res.* 19, 206.

Laine, J., Kalimo, K., Forsell, H., *et al.* (1992). Resolution of oral lichenoid lesions after replacement of amalgam restorations in patients allergic to mercury compounds. *Br. J. Dermatol.* 126, 10.

Lam, P.P. (1980). Severe stomatitis caused by penicillamine. *Br. Dent. J.* 149, 180.

Lamey, P-J., Rees, T.D., and Forsyth, A. (1990). Sensitivity reaction to the cinnamonaldehyde component of toothpaste. *Br. Dent. J.* 168, 115.

Leibovitch, G., Maaravi, I., and Shaley, O. (1987). Severe facial oedema and glossitis associated with mianserin. *Lancet* ii, 871.

Levitt, L. and Pearson, R.W. (1980). Sulindac-induced Stevens–Johnson syndrome. *JAMA* 243, 1262.

Lewis, F.M., Shah, M., and Gawkrodger, D.J. (1995). Contact sensitivity to food additives can cause oral and perioral symptoms. *Contact Dermatitis* 33, 429.

Lewis-Jones, M., Evans, S., and Thompson, C.M. (1988). Erythema multiforme occurring in association with lupus erythematosus during therapy with doxycycline. *Clin. Exp. Dermatol.* 13, 245.

Lindhe, J. and Bjorn, A.L. (1967). Influence of hormonal contraceptives on the gingiva of women. *J. Periodont. Res.* 2, 1.

Lindhe, J. and Branemark, P.I. (1968). The effect of sex hormones on vascularisation of granulation tissue. *J. Periodont. Res.* 3, 6.

Lindhe, J., Attstrom, R., and Bjorn, A.L. (1968a). Influence of sex hormones on gingival exudation in dogs with chronic gingivitis. *J. Periodont. Res.* 3, 279.

Lindhe, J., Birch, J., and Branemark, P.I. (1968b). Vascular proliferation in pseudopregnant rabbits. *J. Periodont. Res.* 3. 13.

Lindhe, J., Attstrom, R., and Bjorn, A.L. (1969). The influence of progestogen and gingival exudation during menstrual cycles. *J. Periodont. Res.* 4, 97.

Little, T.M., Girgis, S.S. and Masotti, R.E. (1975). Diphenyl-hydantoin-induced gingival hyperplasia: its response to changes in drug dosage. *Dev. Med. Child Neurol.* 17, 421.

Lockhart, P.B. (1981). Gingival pigmentation as the sole presenting sign of chronic lead poisoning. *Oral Surg.* 52, 143.

Lombardi, T., Fiore-Donno, G., Belser, U., *et al.* (1991). Felodipine-induced gingival hyperplasia: a clinical and histologic study. *J. Oral Pathol. Med.* 20, 89.

Loria, R. and Wedner, J.H. (1989). Facial swelling secondary to inhaled bronchodilator abuse: catecholamine-induced sialadenosis. *Ann. Allergy* 62, 289.

Lozada, F. and Silverman, S. (1978). Erythema multiforme. Clinical characteristics and natural history in 50 patients. *Oral Surg.* 46, 628.

Lumbiganon, P., Pengsaa, K., and Sockpranee, T. (1991). Ciprofloxacin in neonates and its possible adverse effect on the teeth. *Pediatr. Infect. Dis. J.* 10, 619.

Lyle, W.H. (1974). Penicillamine and zinc. *Lancet* ii, 1140.

Lynn. B.D. (1967). 'The pill' as an etiological agent in hypertrophic gingivitis. *Oral Surg.* 24, 333.

Mcallan, L.H. and Adkins, K.F. (1986). Drug-induced palatal pigmentation. *Aust. Dent. J.* 31, 1.

McAvoy, B.R. (1974). Mouth ulceration and slow-release potassium tablets. *BMJ* iv, 164.

McCord, J., Sloan, P., Quayle, A.A., *et al.* (1992). Phenytoin hyperplasia occurring under complete dentures: a clinical report. *J. Prosthet. Dent.* 68, 569.

McGaw, T., Lam, S., and Coates, J. (1987). Cyclosporin-induced gingival overgrowth: correlation with dental plaque scores, gingivitis scores and cyclosporin levels in serum and saliva. *Oral Surg.* 64, 293.

McGinnis, J.P., Hopkins, K.P., Thompson, E.I., *et al.* (1985). Tooth root growth impairment after mantle radiation in long-term survivors of Hodgkin's disease. *J. Am. Dent. Assoc.* 111, 584.

Mackie. I., Worthington, H.V., and Hobson, P. (1993). An investigation into sugar containing and sugar-free over-the-counter medicines stocked and recommended by pharmacists in the North Western Region of England. *Br. Dent. J.* 175, 93.

MacLeod, R. and Ellis, J.S. (1989). Plasma cell gingivitis related to the use of herbal toothpaste. *Br. Dent. J.* 166, 375.

Maguire, A. (1994). Problems areas in liquid oral medication. In *Sugarless — The Way Forward* (ed. A. Rugg-Gunn), p. 43. Elsevier Applied Science, London.

Maguire, A. and Rugg-Gunn, A.J. (1994*a*). Consumption of prescribed and over-the-counter (OTC) liquid oral medicines (LOMS) in Great Britain and the Northern Region of England, with special regard to sugar content. *Public Health* 108, 121.

Maguire, A. and Rugg-Gunn, A.J. (1994*b*). Long-term use of liquid oral medicines in paediatrics. *Int. J. Pediatr. Dent.* 4, 93.

Maguire, A., Murray, J.J., Craft, A.W., *et al.* (1987*a*). Radiological features of the long-term effects from treatment of malignant disease in childhood. *Br. Dent. J.* 162, 99.

Maguire, A., Craft, A.W., Evans, R.G., *et al.* (1987*b*). The long-term effects of treatment on the dental condition of children surviving malignant disease. *Cancer* 60, 2 5 70.

Maguire, J.. Greenwood, R., Lewis, D., *et al.* (1986). Phenytoin-induced gingival overgrowth is dependent upon comedication. *J. Dent. Res.* 65, 249.

Mardh, P.A., Belfrage, I., and Naversten, E. (1974). Sialadenitis following treatment with alpha-methyldopa. *Acta Med. Scand.* 195, 333.

Mason, D.K., Ferguson, M.M., and Mason, W.N. (1979). Lithium treatment and dental caries. *Br. Dent. J.* 146, 136.

Maurice, P., Hopper, C., Punnia-Moorthy, A., *et al.* (1988). Allergic contact stomatitis and cheilitis from lodoform used in a dental dressing. *Contact Dermatitis* 8, 114.

Menni, S., Barbareschi, G., Fargetti, I., *et al.* (1995). Eruptions lichénoides de la muqueuse buccale induites par le carbonate de lithium. *Ann. Dermatol. Venereol.* 122, 91.

Messing, R.O., Carpenter, C.L., and Greenberg, D.A. (1985). Mechanism of calcium channel inhibition by phenytoin: comparison with classic calcium channel antagonists. *J. Pharmacol. Exp. Ther.* 235, 407.

Meyerson, M.A., Cohen, P.R., and Hymes, S.R. (1995). Lingual hyperpigmentation associated with minocycline therapy. *Oral Surg.* 79, 180.

Miller. C. and Damm, D.D. (1992). Incidence of verapamil-induced gingival hyperplasia in a dental population. *J. Periodontol.* 63, 453.

Milsom, K. and Mitropoulis, C.M. (1990). Enamel defects in 8-year-old children in fluoridated and non-fluoridated parts of Cheshire. *Caries Res.* 24, 286.

Minakami, H., Takahashi, T., Izumi, A., *et al.* (1992). Enlargement of the salivary gland after ritodrine treatment in pregnant women. *BMJ* 304, 668.

Modeer, T. and Dahliof, G. (1987). Development of phenytoin induced gingival overgrowth in non-institutionalised epileptic children subject to different plaque programs. *Acta Odontol. Scand.* 45, 81.

Mohamed, A.M., Waterhouse, J.P., and Friederici, H.H.R. (1974). The microvasculature of the rabbit gingiva as affected by progesterone: an ultrastructural study. *J. Periodontol.* 45, 50.

Murray, J.J. and Welbury, R.R. (1987). The long-term effects of treatment on the dental condition of children surviving malignant disease. *Cancer* 60, 2570.

Murray, V.K. and Defco, C.P. (1982). Intra-oral fixed drug eruptions following tetracycline administration. *J. Periodontol.* 53, 267.

Nathan, K.I. (1995). Development of mucosal ulcerations with lithium carbonate therapy. *Am. J. Psychiatry* 152, 956.

National Pharmaceutical Association (1984*a*). *Notes for Proprietors — Sugar Content of Medicines.*

National Pharmaceutical Association (1984*b*). *Notes for Proprietors — Sugar Content of Medicines.*

National Pharmaceutical Association (1986). *Notes for Proprietors — Sugar Content of Medicines.*

Neil-Dwyer, G. and Marus, A. (1989). ACE-inhibitors in hypertension, assessment of taste and smell function in clinical trials. *J. Hum. Hypertens.* 3, 169.

Nordbo, H. (1979). Ability of chlorhexidine and benzalkonium chloride to catalyse browning reactions in vitro. *J. Dent. Res.* 58, 1429.

Nordt, S.P. (1996). Tetracycline-induced oral mucosal ulcerations. *Ann. Pharmacother.* 30, 547.

Nyirenda, R. and Gill, G.V. (1977). Stevens–Johnson syndrome due to rifampicin. *BMJ* ii, 1189.

O'Brien, W.M. and Bagby, G.F. (1985). Rare adverse reactions to NSAIDS. *J. Rheumatol.* 12, 562.

Ojanotko, A.O. and Harri, M.P. (1978). Testosterone metabolism in chronically inflamed male gingival tissue. *J. Steroid Biochem.* 9, 825.

O'Neil, T. and Figures, K.H. (1982). The effects of chlorhexidine and mechanical methods of plaque control on recurrence of gingival hyperplasia in young patients taking phenytoin. *Br. Dent. J.* 152, 130.

Onesti, G., Bock, K.D., Heimsoth, V., *et al.* (1971). Clonidine: a new antihypertensive agent. *Am. J. Cardiol.* 28, 74.

O'Reilly, R.A. and Motley, C.H. (1977). Breath odour after disulfiram. *JAMA* 238, 2600.

Ortel, B., Sivayathorn, A., and Honigsinann, H. (1989). An unusual combination of phototoxicity and Stevens–Johnson syndrome due to antimalarial therapy. *Dermatology* 178, 39.

Ostmann, P.-O., Anneroth, G., Skoglund, A., *et al.* (1996). Amalgam-associated oral lichenoid reactions; clinical and histologic changes after removal of amalgam fillings. *Oral Surg.* 81, 459.

Pan, V.C. and Quintela, G.A. (1991). Doxycycline-induced parotitis. *Postgrad. Med. J.* 67, 313.

Panuska, H.J., Gorlin, R.J., Bearman, J.E., *et al.* (1961). The effect of anticonvulsant drugs upon the gingiva — a series of analysis of 1048 patients. Part 1. *J. Periodontol.* 31, 15.

Parry, J., Porter, S. and Scully, C. (1996). Mucosal lesions due to oral cocaine use. *Br. Dent. J.* 182, 462.

Pearlman, C. (1994). Clozapine, nocturnal sialorrhea and choking. *J. Clin. Psychopharmacol.* 14, 283.

Pearlman, B.A. (1974). An oral contraceptive drug and gingival enlargement: the relationship between local and systemic factors. *J. Clin. Periodontol.* 1, 47.

Pegram, P.S., Mountz, J.D., and O'Bar, P.R. (1981). Ethambutol-induced toxic epidermal necrolysis. *Arch. Intern. Med.* 141, 1677.

Pellinen, T.J. and Kalske, J. (1982). Nitrofurantoin-induced parotitis. *BMJ* 285, 34.

Pernu, H., Olkarinen, K., and Hietanen, J. (1989). Verapamil-induced gingival overgrowth: a clinical, histologic and biochemical approach. *J. Oral. Med. Pathol.* 18, 422.

Perry, H.O., Deffner, N.F., and Sheridan, P.J. (1973). Atypical gingivostomatitis — nineteen cases. *Arch. Dermatol.* 107, 872.

Perusse, R. and Morency, R. (1991). Oral pigmentation induced by Premarin. *Cutis* 48, 61.

Phillips, B., Shen, S., and Lesko, L. (1986). Levels of cyclosporin-A in human parotid fluid and whole saliva. *J. Dent. Res.* 65, 353.

Philstrom, B., Carson, J.F., Smith, Q.T., *et al.* (1980). Prevention of phenytoin associated gingival enlargement — a 15-month longitudinal study. *J. Periodontol.* 51, 311.

Pillans, P. (1994). Mouth blistering and ulceration associated with inhaled steroids [letter]. *Respir. Med.* 88, 159.

Potts, A., Hamburger, J., and Scully, C. (1987). The medication of patients with oral lichen planus and the association of non-steroidal anti-inflammatory drugs. *Oral Surg.* 64, 541.

Powers, J.M. (1982). Decongestant-induced blepharospasm and orofacial dystonia. *JAMA* 247, 3244.

Rateitschak-Pluss, E.M., Hefti, A., Lortscher, R., *et al.* (1983). Initial observations that cyclosporin-A induces gingival enlargement in man. *J. Clin. Periodontol.* 10, 237.

Razak, I. and Latifah, R.J. (1988). Unusual hypersensitivity reaction to stannous fluoride. *Ann. Dent.* 43, 37.

Rebstein, F. (1978). Plak-out and Broxojet 3007. Clinical study. *Oral Surg. Oral Med. Oral Path.* 88, 1155.

Rees, T.D. (1985). Phenothiazine: another possible aetiological agent in erythema multiforme. *J. Periodontol.* 56, 480.

Rees, T. and Orth, C.F. (1986). Oral ulcerations with the use of hydrogen peroxide. *J. Periodontol.* 57, 689.

Rekola, M. (1989). In vivo acid production from medicines in syrup form. *Caries Research* 23, 412.

Rivers, J. and Barneston, S.C.R. (1989). Naproxen-induced bullous photodermatitis. *Med. J. Aust.* 151, 167.

Roberts, J.F. and Roberts, G.J. (1979). Relation between medicines sweetened with sucrose and dental disease. *BMJ* ii. 14.

Robinson, P.B., Rowe, D.J.F., and Harris, M. (1978). The effects of diphenylhydantoin and vitamin D deficiency on developing teeth in the rat. *Arch. Oral Biol.* 23. 137.

Rock, W. (1994). Young children and fluoride toothpaste. *Br. Dent. J.* 177, 17.

Rollin, H. (1978). Drug related gustatory disorders. *Ann. Otol. Rhinol. Laryngol.* 87, 1.

Rubin, Z. (1977). Ophthalmic-sulphonamide-induced Stevens–Johnson syndrome. *Arch. Dermatol.* 113, 235.

Rugg-Gunn, A.J. (1979). Lithium treatment and dental caries. *Br. Dent. J.* 146, 136.

Russell, M.A., King, L.E., and Boyd, A.S. (1996). Lichen planus after consumption of a gold-containing liquor. *N. Engl. J. Med.* 334, 603.

Savino, L. and Haushalter, H.M. (1992). Lisinopril-induced 'scalded mouth syndrome'. *Ann. Pharmacother.* 26, 1381.

Schamschula, R.G., Atkins, B.L., Barnes, D. E., *et al.* (1978). WHO study of dental caries aetiology in Papua, New Guinea. WHO, Geneva.

Scheinberg, I.H. (1968). Toxicity of penicillamine. *Postgrad. Med. J.* 44 (Suppl. 1), 1.

Schiele, B.C., Gallant, D., Simpson, G., *et al.* (1973). A persistent neurological syndrome associated with anti-psychotic drug use. *Ann. Intern. Med.* 79, 99.

Schiff, M. and Burn, H.F. (1961). The effect of intravenous estrogens on ground substance. *Arch. Otolaryngol.* 71, 765.

Schriver, W.V.R., Shereff, R.H., Domnitz, J.M., *et al.* (1976). Allergic response to stainless steel wire. *Oral Surg.* 42, 578.

Schulz, A. *et al.* (1990). Cyclosporin-induzierte Gingivahyperplasia bei Patienten mit Nierentransplantaten. *Dtsch. Zahnärztl. Z.* 45, 414.

Segars, L. and Threlkeld, K.R. (1993). Clindamycin-induced lip and nasal passage swelling. *Ann. Pharmacother.* 27, 885.

Seymour, R.A. (1996). Adverse drug reactions affecting the mouth and associated structures. In *Adverse Drug Reactions in Dentistry* (ed. R.A. Seymour, J.G. Meechan, and J.G. Walton), p. 89. Oxford University Press.

Seymour, R.A. and Heasman, P.A. (1988). Drugs and the periodontium. A review. *J. Clin. Periodontol.* 15, 1.

Seymour, R.A. and Jacobs, D.J. (1992). Cyclosporin and the gingival tissues. *J. Clin. Periodontol.* 19, 1.

Seymour, R.A. and Smith, D.G. (1991). The effect of a plaque control programme on the incidence and severity of cyclosporin-induced gingival changes. *J. Clin. Periodontol.* 18, 107.

Seymour, R.A., Smith, D.G., and Rogers, S.R. (1987). The comparative effects of azathioprine and cyclosporin on some gingival health parameters of renal transplant patients. *J. Clin. Periodontol.* 14, 610.

Seymour, R.A., Thomason, J.M., and Nolan, A. (1997). Oral lesions in organ transplant patients. *J. Oral. Pathol. Med.* 26, 297.

Siller, G., Todd, M.A., and Savage, N.W. (1994). Minocycline-induced oral pigmentation. *J. Am. Acad. Dermatol.* 30, 350.

Slavin, J. and Taylor, J. (1987). Cyclosporin, nifedipine and gingival hyperplasia. *Lancet* ii, 739.

Smith, A.J. (1973). Perphenazine side-effects presenting in oral surgical practice. *Br. J. Oral Surg.* 10, 349.

Smith, M. and Glenert, U. (1987). Gingivhyperplasi forarsaget af behandling med verapamil. *Tandlaegebladet* 91, 849.

Solheim, H., Eriksen, H.M., and Nodbo, H. (1980). Chemical plaque control and extrinsic discolouration of teeth. *Acta Odontol. Scand.* 38, 359.

Speed, B.R. and Spelman, D.W. (1982). Sialadenitis and systemic reaction associated with phenylbutazone. *Aust. N.Z. J. Med.* 12, 261.

Sperber, G.H. (1969). Oral contraceptive hypertrophic gingivitis. *J. Dent. Assoc. S. Afr.* 24, 37.

Sperling, J.L. (1969). Adverse reactions with long-term use of phenylbutazone and oxyphenbutazone. *Lancet* ii, 535.

Starzl, T.E., Klintmalm, G.B.G., Porter, K.A., *et al.* (1981). Liver transplantation with use of cyclosporin A and predisone. *N. Engl. J. Med.* 395, 266.

Steinberg, S. and Steinberg, A.D. (1982). Phenytoin-induced gingival overgrowth in severely retarded children. *J. Periodontol.* 53, 429.

Sutcher, H.D., Underwood, R.B., Beatty, R.A., *et al.* (1971). Orofacial dyskinesia: a dental dimension. *JAMA* 216, 1459.

Syrjanen, S. and Syrjanen, K. (1979). Hyperplastic gingivitis in a child receiving sodium valproate. *Proc. Finn. Dent. Assoc.* 75, 95.

Tal, H. and Dekel, A. (1986). Oral mouthwash and erythema multiforme. *J. Oral. Med.* 41, 147.

Talner, L.B., Lang, S.H., Brasch, R.C., *et al.* (1971). Elevated salivary iodine and salivary gland enlargement due to iodinated contrast media. *AJR* 112, 380.

Taylor, A.E.M., Lever, L., and Lawrence, C.M. (1996). Allergic contact dermatitis from strawberry lipsalve. *Contact Dermatitis* 34, 142.

Tay-Uyboco, J., Kwiatkowsky, K., Cates, D.B., *et al.* (1991). Clinical and physiological responses to prolonged nasogastric administration of doxapram for apnoea of prematurity. *Biol. Neonate* 59, 190.

Thomason, J.M, Seymour, R.A., and Rice, N. (1993). The prevalence and severity of cyclosporin and nifedipine-induced gingival overgrowth. *J. Clin. Periodontol.* 20, 37.

Thomason, J.M., Seymour, R.A., and Soames, J.V. (1994). Severe mucosal hyperplasia of the edentulous maxilla associated with immunosuppressant therapy. *J. Prosthet. Dent.* 72, 1.

Thompson, T. and Frable, A.S. (1993). Drug-induced life-threatening angioedema revisited. *Laryngoscope* 103, 10.

Thyne, G., Young, D.W., and Ferguson, M.M. (1989). Contact stomatitis caused by toothpaste. *N.Z. Dent. J.* 85, 124.

Tomasko, M. (1988). Recurrent parotitis with H2 receptor antagonist in a patient with Sjögren's syndrome. *Am. J. Med.* 85, 271.

Torres, V., Mano-Azul, A.C., Correla, T., *et al.* (1993). Allergic contact cheilitis and stomatitis from hydroquinane in an acrylic dental prosthesis. *Contact Dermatitis* 29, 102.

Townend, J. (1989). Myofacial pain from theophylline. *Br. Dent. J.* 168, 438.

Tucker, A.S. and Di Bagno, G. (1956). Intravenous urography, a comparative study of Neo-Ipax and Urokon. *Am. J. Radiol.* 75. 855.

Tuffanelli, D., Abrahams, R.K., and Dubois, E.I. (1963). Pigmentation from antimalarial therapy: its possible relationship to ocular lesions. *Arch. Dermatol.* 88, 419.

Tullet, G.L. (1966). Fatal case of toxic erythema after chlorpropamide (Diabinese). *BMJ* i, 148.

Tyldesley, W.R. and Rotter, E. (1984). Gingival hyperplasia induced by cyclosporin. *Br. Dent. J.* 157, 305.

Valsecchi, R. and Cainelli, T. (1992). Gingival hyperplasia induced by erythromycin [letter]. *Acta Dermatol. Venereol.* (Stockh) 72, 157.

Vazquez-Doval. J., Martinex-Vila, E., Legarda, I., *et al.* (1994). Tongue necrosis secondary to ergotamine tartrate in a patient with temporal arteritis [letter]. *Arch. Dermatol.* 130, 261.

Veraldi, S., Schianchi-Veraldi, R., and Scarabelli, G. (1992). Pigmentation of the gums following hydroxychloroquine therapy. *Cutis* 49, 281.

Vittek, J., Rappaport, S.C., Gordon, G.G., *et al.* (1979). Concentration of circulating hormones and metabolism of androgens by human gingiva. *J. Periodontol.* 50, 254.

Vlasses, P.H., Rotmensch, H.H., Ferguson, R.K., *et al.* (1982). 'Scalded mouth' caused by angiotensin-converting enzyme inhibitors. *BMJ* 284, 1672.

Vogel, R.I. and Deasy, M.J. (1977). Extrinsic discoloration of the oral mucosa. *J. Oral. Med.* 32, 14.

von Knorring, A. and Wahlin, Y.B. (1986). Tricyclic antidepressants and dental caries in children. *Neuropsychobiology* 15, 143.

Walton, J.N. (ed.) (1971). Treatment in neurology, an outline. In *Essentials of Neurology* (3rd edn), p. 428. Pitman Medical, London.

Watson, I.B. and MacDonald, D.G. (1974). Amodiaquine-induced oral pigmentation — a light and electron-microscopic study. *J. Oral Pathol.* 3, 16.

Watts, J.C. (1962). Fatal case of erythema multiforme exudativum (Stevens–Johnson syndrome) following therapy with Dilantin. *Pediatrics* 30, 592.

Weiner, W.I. and Nausieda, P.A. (1982). Meige's syndrome during long-term dopaminergic therapy in Parkinson's disease. *Arch. Neurol.* 39, 451.

Weiss, J.I. (1973). Thrombocytopenic purpura: the dentist's responsibility. *J. Am. Dent. Assoc.* 87, 165.

Welbury, R. (1987). Chemotherapy and childhood cancer: Dental implications. *Dental Update* 16, 3.

Westerhof, W., Wolters, E.Ch., Brookbakker, J.T.W., *et al.* (1983). Pigmented lesions of the tongue in heroin addicts — fixed drug eruption. *Br. J. Dermatol.* 109, 605.

Weyman, J. (1965). Tetracyclines and the teeth. *Practitioner.* 195, 661.

Williams, P.J., Jani, P., and McGlashan, J. (1994). Lingual haematoma following treatment with streptokinase. *Anaesthesia* 49, 417.

Wolpaw, J., Brottem, J.L. and Martin, H.L. (1973). Tongue necrosis attributed to ergotamine in temporal arteries. *JAMA* 225, 514.

Wood, G.D. (1978). An adverse reaction to metoclopramide therapy. *Br. J. Oral Surg.* 15, 278.

Wright, P. (1975). Untoward effects associated with practolol administration: oculomucocutaneous syndrome. *BMJ* i, 595.

Wyatt, E., Greaves, M.W., and Sondergaard, J. (1972). Fixed drug eruption (phenolphthalein): evidence for a blood-borne mediator. *Arch. Dermatol.* 106, 671.

Wysocki, G.P., Gretzinger, H.A., Laupaus, A., *et al.* (1983). Fibrous hyperplasia of the gingiva: a side effect of cyclosporin A therapy. *Oral Surg.* 55, 274.

Yaacob, M. and Jalil, R. (1986). An unusual hypersensitivity reaction to chlorhexidine. *J. Oral Med.* 41, 145.

12. Gastrointestinal disorders

D. N. BATEMAN and E. E. AZIZ

Introduction

The gastrointestinal tract is a common site of adverse drug reactions, no doubt owing to the fact that most drug administration is by this route. Hurwitz and Wade (1969) reported nearly 30 years ago that the gut was the target site in between 20 and 40 per cent of well-documented adverse reactions in hospitals. Adverse reaction surveillance in the UK by 'yellow card' reporting continues to show that the gastrointestinal tract is prominent amongst organs reported as being involved, but this may reflect high reporting of adverse reactions to certain commonly used drugs, for example, non-steroidal inflammatory agents. It is important to note that gastrointestinal adverse effects are a common cause of non-compliance in general practice (Martys 1979).

When addressing the issue of drug-induced gastrointestinal disorders, it should be borne in mind that virtually all drugs may cause disturbance of gastrointestinal function in some patients. It is important, therefore, to differentiate adverse reactions that involve a pathological change from those that do not, particularly when the symptoms are, for example, nausea and vomiting or change in bowel habit.

Non-specific symptoms of this type have a psychological component, and it has been suggested that, as for some other adverse drug reactions, these are more likely to occur in women (Stewart and Cluff 1974).

Glossitis and stomatitis

These disorders are discussed in Chapters 11 and 22.

Oesophagus

Drug-induced changes in the oesophagus result from three principal causes: changes in motility, changes in mucosal integrity, and infection secondary to drugs. Additionally, drugs may obstruct the oesophagus by forming a mass of congealed material, as in the case reported by Hart in which sucralfate prevented swallowing because it had formed such an obstruction (Hart *et al.* 1989). Such an occurrence is most likely to be seen in drug overdose. The oesophagus may be a site at which a systemic adverse reaction is manifest, but examples are very uncommon.

Oesophageal motility

The tone of the lower oesophageal sphincter, and oesophageal motility are both important in swallowing and in ensuring that gastric acid is kept from the lower oesophagus. Drugs that impair the sphincter, such as opiates and anticholinergics, are therefore to be expected to produce symptoms secondary to reflux of acid from the stomach.

Oesophageal spasm ('nutcracker oesophagus') has been caused by propranolol in therapeutic dosage (Bassoth *et al.* 1987) and in overdose (Panos *et al.* 1986). The presumed mechanism of this effect is β-adrenergic blockade. Interestingly, nifedipine, which reduces the amplitude of oesophageal contractions, was a successful substitute for propranolol in the management of hypertension in the case reported by Bassoth, mentioned above. Nifedipine itself is often associated with upper abdominal pain, which may be due in part to effects on oesophageal motility, or on the lower oesophageal sphincter.

Chlormethiazole has been reported to cause dysphagia associated in one case with considerable (13 kg) weight loss (Dewis *et al.* 1982).

Oesophageal motility is often abnormal in the elderly, and this may result in gelatin-coated preparations disintegrating within the oesophagus (Perkins *et al.* 1994) and thus causing mucosal damage.

Ulceration and stricture

Oesophageal ulceration, with the possibility of resultant stricture, is recognized to occur with certain drug forms. Thus, doxycycline capsules (Al-Dujaili *et al.* 1983; van Klingeren 1983) seem particularly likely to cause this problem. Heller and colleagues (1982) reviewed 76 patients with benign oesophageal stricture and found more of them (22) had taken non-steroidal anti-inflammatory drugs (NSAID) than had members of a control group (10), but also found that emepromium bromide and potassium chloride were likely to be factors in six other patients. The latter two drugs are recognized causes of oesophageal ulceration (Al-Dujaili *et al.* 1983), and other case reports suggest that NSAID also cause oesophageal ulceration; this, however, may be more likely in patients with pre-existing oesophageal disease (Coates *et al.* 1986).

Ulcers of the oesophagus have been attributed to treatment with antibiotics other than doxycycline, including tetracycline (Crowson *et al.* 1976), clindamycin (Sutton and Gosnold 1977), and phenoxymethylpenicillin tablets (Suissa *et al.* 1987). Ulceration of the oesophagus has also complicated treatment with clorazepate (Maroy and Moullot 1986). One common feature of many of these reports is the suggestion that posture may have been inappropriate, or that insufficient liquid was taken with the tablet to ensure its passage into the stomach. This was a suggested mechanism for oesophageal stricture associated with swallowing a single 800 mg ibuprofen tablet without water (Levine *et al.* 1994). Experimental studies have shown that abnormal transit of tablets may be quite common and may occur in up to 22 per cent of swallowing (Hey *et al.* 1982). Tablets should therefore be taken with the patient upright and with an adequate amount of fluid. Small, heavier tablets tend to pass more readily into the stomach. In one case report, hiccups were believed to have caused impaired motility, leading to oesophageal injury by co-trimoxazole tablets (Seibert and Al-Kawas 1986).

Infection

Fungal infection of the oesophagus with *Candida* species is a well-recognized complication of broad-spectrum antibiotics. In one case, a child receiving erythromycin developed vomiting and haematemesis that was attributed to this complication (Hachiya *et al.* 1982). This type of infection is discussed further in Chapter 25.

Oesophageal injury in systemic disease

Rarely, oesophageal damage may result from other causes. Thus submucosal haematoma, causing retrosternal pain and haematemesis in a patient with polycythaemia rubra vera, was ascribed to the bleeding tendency caused by aspirin administration (Chapman *et al.* 1986). Oesophageal varices attributable to hepatic damage by busulphan and thioguanine, given to patients for treatment for chronic myeloid leukaemia, were reported by Key and colleagues (1987).

Nausea and vomiting

These are very common adverse reactions, and it is likely that most drugs will cause them under appropriate conditions. In practice, it is therefore necessary to differentiate drugs which almost always cause nausea and vomiting (as do, for example, many cytotoxic drugs) from those that rarely do so. In addition, nausea and vomiting may be useful guides to toxicity from drugs for which plasma concentrations relate to pharmacological effects and when these symptoms are features of early toxicity. Examples are digitalis and theophylline (Mucklow 1978).

The pathophysiology of nausea and vomiting is poorly understood. In the brain the vestibular apparatus, the vomiting centre, the nucleus of the tractus solitarius, and higher centres are all possible sites of drug effects (Peroutka and Snyder 1982). That higher centres are important in inducing nausea is clear from the phenomenon of anticipatory vomiting seen in some patients receiving cytotoxic chemotherapy. The mechanisms by which cytotoxic drugs produce nausea and vomiting remain unclear (Harris 1982), but work on antiemetics for cancer chemotherapy suggests that for some cytotoxic drugs, particularly the highly emetic drug cisplatin, 5-hydroxytryptamine (5-HT) receptors are important, since ondansetron and other 5-HT$_3$-receptor antagonists are very effective in the management of vomiting induced by cancer chemotherapy. SSRI antidepressants, which block 5-HT uptake, are prone to cause nausea as an adverse effect.

In animals, irritants that are instilled into the stomach can induce nausea and vomiting. Whether direct gastric irritation in man is a common cause of nausea and vomiting is unclear. Certainly, reflex pathways exist to carry stimuli from the gut to the relevant central centres in the nucleus of the tractus solitarius.

Most drugs that cause nausea and vomiting, including digitalis glycosides, opiates, oestrogens, and levodopa, all probably act on the chemoreceptor trigger zone, which is in the floor of the fourth ventricle and outside the blood–brain barrier. Tolerance develops to the nausea produced by some drugs, and this is seen with dopamine agonists, such as levodopa or bromocriptine (Wass *et al.* 1977), opiates, and oestrogens.

Nausea associated with the salts of potassium and iron is sometimes attributed to direct gastric irritation. The mechanisms by which antibiotics produce nausea are unclear, though erythromycin has effects on gut motility (Janssens *et al.* 1990), acting as a motilin agonist. As such it has been investigated as a therapeutic tool in diabetic gastroparesis and following gastric surgery (Burt *et al.* 1996). Exactly how this ties in with the nausea that seems to be associated more commonly with enteric-coated tablets (Carter *et al.* 1987) is unclear. Stang (1986) has suggested a possible association between erythromycin use and hypertrophic pyloric stenosis in a baby.

Stomach and duodenum

Altered gastric emptying

Drugs may either increase or reduce the rate of gastric emptying. Drugs that delay gastric emptying include those possessing anticholinergic activity, and opiates. Delay in gastric emptying may produce a sensation of fullness or nausea, but will also delay, and may impair, the absorption of concurrently administered compounds (Nimmo 1979). This effect needs to be remembered in patients receiving drugs with a narrow therapeutic index. Thus morphine has been shown to reduce the efficacy of mexilitine as an antiarrhythmic in patients following myocardial infarction (Pottage *et al.* 1978).

Drugs that increase gastric emptying, including metoclopramide, domperidone, and cisapride, may increase the absorption rate of other drugs. This may be particularly relevant for drugs producing central nervous sedative effects, including antihistamines, benzodiazepines, or alcohol. The sedative effects are more pronounced when these drugs are absorbed more quickly.

Drugs may occasionally form congealed masses (bezoars) in the stomach, and examples reported in the literature include potassium chloride (Antonescu 1989) and sustained-release theophylline tablets in overdosage. Smith (1987) reported the formation of bezoars in four of 11 patients admitted with an overdose of sustained-release theophylline tablets.

Peptic ulceration

Non-steroidal anti-inflammatory drugs

Non-steroidal anti-inflammatory drugs (NSAID) all inhibit the cyclo-oxygenase enzyme. The adverse effects have been documented since 1938, when Douthwaite and Lintot reported on the gastroscopic changes seen with aspirin (Douthwaite and Lintot 1938). Over the following 60 years the toxicity profile of NSAID has become much more clear. All of the currently used NSAID have a propensity to cause upper gastrointestinal (GI) toxicity in animal models. The discovery of two differen types of cyclo-oxygenase (Cox^1 and Cox^2) has led to the possibility that drugs that are selective inhibitors of Cox^2 would avoid the risk of GI toxicity inherent in the drugs at present available. At the time of writing, however, it is too early to know whether this new development will result in a safer group of drugs which are equally effective in reducing symptoms in arthritis.

NSAID all seem to cause GI mucosal damage in animals and man. It is, however, difficult to relate this mucosal damage directly with the incidence of peptic ulceration, of which the more serious complications are acute bleeding and perforation. What is clear is that these complications are more frequent in patients receiving more than one non-steroidal agent at a time. Thus Caruso and Bianchi Porro (1980) found that 10 per cent of patients taking more than one NSAID had frank peptic ulceration.

Information on the relative toxicity of different NSAID has been accumulating over the past decades. The sources of this information have included spontaneous adverse reaction reporting systems, such as the 'yellow card scheme' in the UK, case–control studies, and larger cohort studies based on large computer databases in general practice.

These data all seem to point in the same direction. They suggest there is a difference in risk of acute GI haemorrhage or perforation with different agents. At low doses (below 1500 mg) the risk of upper GI complications with ibuprofen is of the order of 2–3 times normal (Garcia Rodrigues and Jick 1994) whereas with piroxicam in the same study it was 18 (95 per cent confidence limits 8.2–39.6). These results are essentially similar to those found in studies conducted in Australia, Spain, the USA, and the UK (Bateman 1996). The studies have also confirmed that paracetamol, about which in the past there has been debate, is not associated with an increased risk of GI haemorrhage. In the case of aspirin it is clear that the effect is dose related and that doses of the order of 75 mg a day, as used in cardiovascular prophylaxis, are safest, the risk rising with increasing dose above this level.

Other drugs

A number of other agents have been associated with gastric damage. Bhasin and Singh (1988) reported four patients who developed haemorrhagic gastric erosions while being treated with chloroquine for malaria. A case of chronic gastritis associated with gold has been reported (Benfield *et al.* 1986). The largest survey of drug adverse effects on the upper gastrointestinal tract was reported by the Boston Collaborative Drug Surveillance Program (Jick 1981). Major gastrointestinal bleeding was reported in 4.5 per cent of patients receiving ethacrynic acid in this survey as compared with 1.2 per cent for heparin, 0.5 per cent for corticosteroids, and 0.2 per cent for warfarin. There was an apparent summation effect when ethacrynic acid and steroids were combined, in that two out of 22 patients exposed to this combination developed gastrointestinal bleeding. Whether the ethacrynic acid is actually responsible for gastrointestinal bleeding has been debated, and Dargie and Dollery (1975) have suggested that the ethacrynic acid was started in some patients after bleeding had occurred.

When taken in overdose, theophylline and steroids have been reported to cause gastric perforation (Guss *et al.* 1986). This might be due to the increased acid production induced by theophylline and to the presence of corticosteroids.

The issue of corticosteroids and gastric ulceration remains controversial. As noted above, Jick (1981) reported an apparent increase in gastrointestinal haemorrhage in patients receiving steroids. One problem is that corticosteroids may mask the symptoms of ulceration. An evaluation of data on 3064 patients in 71 clinical trials suggested a higher incidence of peptic ulcer disease (1.8 per cent) in patients receiving steroids than in controls (0.8 per cent). The incidence seemed to vary directly with the dose of steroids (Messer *et al.* 1983). Gastrointestinal haemorrhage was also more frequent in steroid-treated patients than in controls. Other workers have criticized this study on methodological grounds (Conn and Poynard 1984) but clinicians continue to report series of patients in whom steroid therapy seems to be a contributory factor in peptic ulceration. Thus, Dayton and colleagues (1987) reported that 25 out of 151 patients with perforated peptic ulcer had received corticosteroids within a week of the perforation. Voskuyl and colleagues (1993) examined serious upper GI events in 2315 patients with possible or definite rheumatoid arthritis. They found that corticosteroids were an indepedent risk factor in their model, as was a history of previous peptic ulceration, and age over 60 years.

Potassium salts, particularly if given in a wax-matrix formulation (McMahon *et al.* 1982), are associated with gastrointestinal lesions visible on gastroscopy. Delay in gastric emptying by an anticholinergic drug increases the effect of the potassium salt. Despite these data, a large prospective study from the Boston Collaborative Drug Surveillance Program did not associate potassium use and upper gastrointestinal bleeding in a group of 15 791 patients (Aselton and Jick 1983).

Rarely, very dramatic adverse effects on the stomach occur, such as the case of gastric rupture and death in a child who was given ipecacuanha syrup for treatment of poisoning (Knight and Doucet 1987), or the case reported by Ananth and colleagues (1988) in which lithium resulted in vomiting sufficient to cause a Mallory–Weiss tear.

Small intestine

Disordered motility

Drugs possessing anticholinergic or opiate activity will reduce small bowel motility, as well as gastric motility. On occasions this suppression of activity may be sufficient to cause a paralytic ileus, and this has been reported with tricyclic antidepressants (Burkitt and Sutcliffe 1961; Gander and Devlin 1963; McNeill 1966; Clarke 1971) as well as with atropine (Beatson 1982). In patients suffering from poisoning with this type of drug, a clinical condition that simulates acute intestinal obstruction may occur (Figiel and Figiel 1973). Drug-induced neuropathy can also effect the nerve supply to the gut, so producing a syndrome similar to paralytic ileus; this has been associated with vincristine (Mannes *et al.* 1976). Very rarely, obstruction of the small bowel lumen may occur from bezoar formation (Burruss *et al.* 1986).

Increased motility throughout the small bowel may result in diarrhoea, although clinically it is often difficult to tell whether the effects are principally on the large bowel or the small bowel. Thus, gold salts have been associated with diarrhoea and eosinophilia (Michet *et al.* 1987) and with terminal ileitis (Geltner *et al.* 1986), the latter case being of interest since the patient appeared to respond to chelation of the gold with dimercaprol. Purgatives increase the loss of duodenal mucosal cells and increase protein loss into the gut. In some patients this may be severe enough to present as steatorrhoea (Langman 1982). A patient has been described in whom diarrhoea and abdominal pain were associated with small intestinal biopsy changes that were attributed to sulindac (Freeman 1986).

Ulceration, haemorrhage, and infection

The small bowel is a site at which slow-release formulations have been demonstrated to cause local lesions, occasionally leading to stricture. Thus, potassium tablets are well recognized to cause this problem (Boley *et al.* 1965; Davies and Brightmore 1970). Lofgren and colleagues (1982) have described a case in which the use of slow-release potassium chloride was associated with jejunal perforation, and Brower (1986) reported this complication in a patient with Crohn's disease. Iron tablets have caused gangrene of a Meckel's diverticulum (Alaily 1974). Osmotic-pump delivery systems seem at particular risk of causing local ulceration or perforation of the small bowel, and for this reason a preparation of indomethacin (Osmosin) was withdrawn from the United Kingdom market (CSM 1983).

The vascular supply of the bowel may be damaged in a number of ways. Mesenteric venous thrombosis has been associated with oral contraceptive use (Greig 1989), and abuse of cocaine has resulted in gangrene in both an adult (Mizrahi *et al.* 1989) and in a neonate whose mother had taken the drug (Telsey *et al.* 1988). Mesenteric infarction may also result from the use of vasoconstrictor drugs, particularly in patients whose splanchnic circulation is already compromised (Brown *et al.* 1959; Alves *et al.* 1979). Mesenteric arterial occlusion has been reported in association with the oral contraceptive pill and may affect either the large or small bowel (Brennan *et al.* 1968; Kilpatrick *et al.* 1968; Cotton and Lea Thomas 1971; Nothmann *et al.* 1973). This adverse effect is likely to be associated with the use of oral contraceptives with higher oestrogen contents.

Jejunal haematomata have been reported in association with warfarin (Aziz Khan *et al.* 1982), and haemorrhagic necrosis of the small intestine has also been attributed to digitalis glycosides (Gazes *et al.* 1961; Muggia 1967), although this may have been in part due in these patients to poor intestinal blood flow secondary to heart failure.

Ulceration and stricture of the small bowel have been reported with normal formulations of NSAID (Madhok *et al.* 1986; Saverymuttu *et al.* 1986). NSAID have also been associated with multiple strictures (Kwo and Tremaine 1995). Gold, which one of the patients described by Madhok and colleagues (1986) was also receiving, may cause a panenteritis (Roe *et al.* 1972). Ischaemic damage to the small bowel has also been associated with vasculitis attributed to lithium therapy (Cannon 1982).

Flucytosine was reported to cause erosive enteritis affecting the small bowel of patients treated for *Cryptococcus neoformans* infections (White and Traube 1982). Omeprazole, which is very effective in reducing acid production in the stomach, may increase the risk of enteric infection and two authors have suggested this as a potential problem (Neal *et al.* 1996; Schapira *et al.* 1996),

the former reporting a patient in whom this problem seemed to have occurred. The subject is discussed further in Chapter 25.

Malabsorption

Drug-induced malabsorption may occur because of an interaction between drugs and particular nutrients. Examples include chelation of tetracycline and calcium ions (Kuwin and Finland 1961), cholestyramine and iron (Thomas *et al.* 1972), and cholestyramine and vitamin B_{12} (Coronato and Glass 1973). Cholestyramine also binds to bile salts and in this way causes steatorrhoea and malabsorption of fat-soluble vitamins (Zurier *et al.* 1965). This subject is discussed further in Chapters 25 and 33.

A single drug may also cause either specific malabsorption syndromes or a generalized malabsorption state. Thus, drugs that alter mitotic activity of the small intestinal wall may cause malabsorption, and well-established examples of drugs that do this are colchicine (Race *et al.* 1970) and methotrexate (Trier 1962; Stebbins and Pearson 1967). Many cytotoxic drugs will impair gut cell division and cause malabsorption, thus mild steatorrhoea is quite common. Jejunal mucosal changes and steatorrhoea have also been associated with allopurinol (Chen *et al.* 1982), methyldopa (Schneerson and Gazzard 1977), and phenindione (Juel-Jensen 1959).

Some antibiotics have been associated with malabsorption, including neomycin, which in addition to binding bile salts (Hardison and Rosenberg 1969) probably also interferes with protein synthesis within the enterocyte causing damage to the brush border as shown by changes in disaccharidases (Reiner and Patterson 1966). Large doses of neomycin produce partial villous atrophy (Jacobson *et al.* 1960; Dobbins *et al.* 1968). Tetracyclines, in addition to impairing the absorption of calcium, as mentioned above, may also cause steatorrhoea (Mitchell *et al.* 1982) and impair iron absorption (Greenberger *et al.* 1967). Malabsorption has also been demonstrated following treatment with kanamycin, polymyxin, or bacitracin (Steiner *et al.* 1961; Powell *et al.* 1962; Faloon *et al.* 1966).

Mefenamic acid causes a malabsorption syndrome and diarrhoea, associated in some patients with colitis (Hall *et al.* 1983). Of the adverse reaction reports to this drug received by the Committee on Safety of Medicines between 1963 and 1989, 18 per cent were for diarrhoea and colitis.

Cathartics may result in mild steatorrhoea, presumably due to intestinal hurry, particularly if taken in large amounts (Heizer *et al.* 1968).

Specific nutritional deficiencies affecting folate and B_{12} metabolism have been associated with drug therapy. Anticonvulsants have been reported to cause a fall in red cell and serum folate in a high proportion of patients receiving these agents (Reynolds 1968). Some workers have suggested that these drugs impair folate absorption (Benn *et al.* 1971; Gerson *et al.* 1972). Other workers have suggested the principal problem in these patients is poor diet (Rose and Johnson 1978), or the enzyme-inducing effects of the anticonvulsants on folate metabolism (Labadarios *et al.* 1978).

Absorption of vitamin B_{12}, as mentioned above, is inhibited by neomycin and cholestyramine. Sodium aminosalicylate (PAS) interferes with the ileal transport of vitamin B_{12}, perhaps by inhibiting a folate-dependent enzyme system (Palva *et al.* 1966). Folic acid therapy seems to protect against this particular malabsorption syndrome (Paaby and Nervin 1966). Colchicine also seems capable of producing reversible impairment of vitamin B_{12} absorption (Webb *et al.* 1968), and the biguanides metformin and phenformin seem to impair it by an effect on mucosal transport (Berchtold *et al.* 1971; Tomkin *et al.* 1971; Tomkin 1973). Biguanides also have other effects on the brush border, including reduction in disaccharidase activity (Berchtold *et al.* 1971). An alteration in the pH of the ileal contents has been suggested as a cause of the impairment of the absorption of B_{12} seen with potassium chloride therapy (Palva *et al.* 1972), and one case of megaloblastic anaemia attributed to this cause has been reported (Salokannel *et al.* 1970).

Colon

Antimicrobial-associated colitis

Diarrhoea occurs in up to 30 per cent of individuals treated by antimicrobial agents (Beaugerie 1996). Most such cases can be classified into two categories: diarrhoea associated with *Clostridium difficile* infection, and cases in which no pathophysiological mechanism is recognized. *Cl. difficile* intestinal infection results in a wide spectrum of disease, ranging from mild antimicrobial-associated diarrhoea to life-threatening pseudomembranous colitis. *Cl. difficile* accounts for 15–25 per cent of cases of antimicrobial-associated diarrhoea and for almost all cases of antimicrobial-associated pseudomembranous colitis (Barbut and Petit 1996).

Pseudomembranous colitis

Pseudomembranous colitis is a rare but potentially severe complication of antimicrobial treatment, which is characterized by the proliferation of the bacterium *Cl. difficile* in the colon. It generally occurs after more than 4 days of treatment. It may be associated with diarrhoea, abdominal pain, fever, and vomiting. Complications include hypokalaemia, renal failure, and hypoproteinaemia. Pseudomembranes are usually found between the rectum and left angle of the colon. Recovery usually takes place after one week of oral metronidazole or vancomycin, or both of these. Cytotoxin detection in the stool remains the single best routine laboratory test for diagnosis. *Cl. difficile* is carried in the gastrointestinal tract of less than three per cent of the normal adult population but can be isolated fom the faeces of 50–70 per cent of asymptomatic neonates (Barbut and Petit 1996).

Pseudomembranous colitis may occur in the immunocompromised chronic colitic patient without prior history of antimicrobial use (Chen and Woods 1996). The presentation can be that of pseudomembranous panenteritis and septicaemia. In immunocompromised patients with *Cl. difficile* colitis there is no statistically significant difference in relapse rates between those treated with vancomycin or metronidazole (Schweitzer *et al.* 1996). A few case reports have, however, linked metronidazole with the development of pseudomembranous colitis, and at least one case report linked albendazole, which is an antimicrobial that is chemically related to metronidazole, with pseudomembranous colitis in a patient with AIDS and intestinal microsporidiosis (Shah *et al.* 1996).

There have been reports of *Cl. difficile*-associated diarrhoea after chemotherapy in cancer patients who had not received any antimicrobial agents before the onset of diarrhoea (Sriuranpong and Voravud 1995).

The pathogenesis of pseudomembranous colitis relies on the disruption of the normal bacterial flora of the colon, colonization with *Cl. difficile*, and the release of toxins that cause mucosal inflammation and damage. Clindamycin is reputed to be notorious for inducing *Cl. difficile* colitis, but in current practice broad-spectrum penicillins and cephalosporins are the agents most frequently implicated (Devenyi 1995). There have been reports of pseudomembranous colitis following clarithromycin therapy to treat *Helicobacter pylori* infection and duodenal ulceration (Teare *et al.* 1995).

High incidences of nosocomial *Cl. difficile*-associated diarrhoea do not necessarily indicate clonal epidemics. Numerous strains of *Cl. difficile* may be found even among clustered cases of diarrhoea (Samore *et al.* 1994).

Risk factors for *Cl. difficile*-associated diarrhoea include antimicrobial therapy, advanced age, immunodeficiency, antineoplastic agents, antacid use, use of a nasogastric tube, intensive care, and prolonged hospital stay. It has been suggested that pseudomembranous colitis may be more common in patients with abnormally slow bowel motility (Schulze-Delrieu 1983) and that some antimicrobial agents can reduce colonic motility and plasma concentrations achieved clinically (Lees and Percy 1981). Although most cases of pseudomembranous colitis can be effectively treated medically, surgical intervention is indicated when signs of peritonitis occur (Morris *et al.* 1994).

Other types of antimicrobial-associated colitis

There has been a case report of isolation of vancomyin-dependent *Enterococcus faecium* from stool following oral vancomycin therapy (Dever *et al.* 1995). It has been suggested that this organism might have evolved from a vancomycin-resistant, vancomycin-independent *E. faecium* in the presence of high concentrations of vancomycin in the intestine.

Ischaemic colitis

Ischaemia of the colon has been reported as a complication of treatment with various drugs. Lambert and colleagues (1982) reported a patient who had received vasopressin for variceal haemorrhage and developed this syndrome. They felt that underlying atherosclerosis may have been a factor. Vasculitis has been associated with clindamycin therapy (Sweeny and Sheehan 1979), affecting the small vessels of the entire bowel wall. Colonic ischaemia has been attributed to treatment with cisplatin and fluorouracil for malignant disease, though the patient involved had also received radiation, another risk factor (Zilling and Ahren 1989). Ischaemic colitis has also been associated with hormonal therapy (with oral contraceptive steroids in particular [Schneiderman and Cello 1986]) and with danazol (Miyata *et al.* 1988).

Other causes of colitis

NSAID, particularly mefenamic acid (Hall *et al.* 1983) but also fenbufen (Bunney 1989), flufenamic acid, naproxen, and ibuprofen (Ravi *et al.* 1986), have been reported to cause colitis. Penicillamine (Houghton *et al.* 1989) and gold (Kirkham *et al.* 1989) have also both been associated with colitis in patients suffering from rheumatoid arthritis.

Colitis has been reported in one patient in association with jaundice induced by methyldopa (Bonkowsky and Brisbane 1976), and Graham and co-workers (1981) have reported six cases of colitis with methyldopa which were positive on rechallenge. Martin and colleagues

(1987) reported a patient in whom proctocolitis was associated with treatment with isotretinoin; they also commented on the fact that the manufacturers of this drug had data suggesting there might be other cases in which a similar association existed.

Other colonic disorders

Ulceration, bleeding, and perforation

Some authors suggest that NSAID may have precipitated a relapse of ulcerative colitis (Rampton and Sladen 1981), severe colonic bleeding (Schwartz 1981), or acute perforation of colonic diverticula (Coutrot *et al.* 1978).

Colonic strictures have also been reported, in one case leading to large-bowel obstruction (Robinson *et al.* 1995).

Colonic cancer

The anthroquinone purgative danthron has been reported to cause tumours in animals, and a single case report has suggested such an association in an 18-year-old woman (Patel *et al.* 1989). There is also a report of colonic carcinoma after chemotherapy in a patient with Hodgkin's disease (Aggarwal *et al.* 1989).

Increased gastrin levels are found in patients taking proton-pump inhibitors. Some colonic cancers have gastrin receptors, but the significance of these observations is not clear. To date there is no evidence these drugs are associated with cancer in man.

Diarrhoea due to other causes

Diarrhoea may be due to drug effects on the small bowel, as mentioned above. It may be difficult to be precise about the particular site of action in an individual patient. Chronic diarrhoea can occur as a feature of purgative abuse (Cummings 1974), and this is particularly common in the United Kingdom where many elderly patients take purgatives regularly. Anthraquinones, such as senna, produce damage to the myenteric plexus of the large bowel in chronic use, and this may result in constipation for which the patient takes further doses of purgatives. The amount of watery diarrhoea produced by cathartics may be sufficient to cause electrolyte disturbance or weight loss.

Antacid salts, particularly magnesium, will produce osmotic diarrhoea, which is believed to be due to the presence of the poorly absorbed osmotically active compound in the gut lumen.

Digitalis overdose causes diarrhoea, and a number of other drugs acting on the cardiovascular system have been associated with diarrhoea. These include, particularly, the adrenergic-neurone blocking antihypertensives (e.g. guanethidine and debrisoquine) and, more rarely, methyldopa and β-adrenoceptor blocking agents (Bulpitt and Dollery 1973; Robinson and Burtner 1981).

Diarrhoea associated with bacterial overgrowth secondary to high-dose corticosteroids has been reported (Denison and Wallerstedt 1989). Chenodeoxycholic acid causes diarrhoea in a dose-related manner (Dowling 1977).

Diarrhoea in breast-fed infants

Single case reports associate the use of sulphasalazine or mesalazine with diarrhoea in the breast-fed infants of mothers receiving these drugs, suggesting excretion into breast milk (Branski et al. 1986; Nelis 1989).

Constipation

Constipation is commonly associated with drugs that delay gastrointestinal motility, such as opiates, antiparkinsonian drugs, or anticholinergics. Occasionally, this form of constipation may be particularly severe, and a case in which stercoral perforation of the bowel occurred in a patient receiving amitriptyline has been reported (Cass 1978). Faecal impaction has been caused by charcoal when used to treat a patient who had taken an amitriptyline overdose (Anderson and Ware 1987); such patients should therefore be given osmotic purgatives routinely.

Aluminium hydroxide and calcium carbonate antacids are constipating and iron salts are also a frequent cause of this complaint. Faecal impaction has been reported in an infant of low birth-weight who was given cholestyramine (Merten and Grossman 1980), and Swift and Thayer (1987) reported a case of constipation associated with lithium in a patient who had scleroderma.

Proctitis

Proctitis is associated with the local application of irritant drugs in the form of suppositories. The NSAID indomethacin and phenylbutazone have both been reported to have caused proctitis and rectal ulceration (Cheli and Ciancamerla 1974; Levy and Gaspar 1975). Ergot suppositories have been associated with anal ulcers (Weinert and Grussenderf 1980). An unusual case of alcohol-induced proctitis, due to self-administration of whisky per rectum, was reported by Bhalotra (1988). The rare complication of rectovaginal fistula in a patient with granulocytopenia secondary to amidopyrine was

reported by Garre and colleagues (1976). Later, Hobbin and Champion (1986) reported a fistula between the vulva and the rectum associated with indomethacin suppositories, on this occasion presumably due to local damage to the rectal mucosa.

Anal burning has been associated with peppermint oil capsules (Weston 1987) and perineal irritation is well documented to occur after intravenous injection of dexamethasone (Baharav et al. 1986).

Pancreatitis

Although drug-induced pancreatic dysfunction is rarer than many other gastrointestinal adverse reactions, it is being increasingly recognized as a complication of treatment with a wide range of drugs. The mechanisms by which drugs produce pancreatic damage are not always clear. On occasions, however, it is obvious that a clear precipitant can be identified, as in the example of ergotamine-induced ischaemic pancreatitis reported after overdose of the drug (Deviere et al. 1987).

The largest group of drugs to be associated with pancreatitis is the sulphonamide antibacterials and the chemically related diuretics. Block and colleagues (1970) described haemorrhagic pancreatitis associated with sulphamethizole and sulphasalazine. Many diuretics are derived from sulphonamides and pancreatitis has been associated with most of this group including chlorothiazide (Johnston and Cornish 1959; Cornish et al. 1961), chlorthalidone (Jones and Caldwell 1962), and frusemide (Wilson et al. 1967; Buchanan and Cane 1977). Drug-induced pancreatitis secondary to diuretics can be very severe and occasionally fatal (Eckhauser et al. 1987). Epidemiological studies suggest that thiazide diuretics are the drugs most commonly implicated in patients presenting with acute pancreatitis (Bourke et al. 1978; Pickleman et al. 1979). Kristensen and colleagues (1980) suggested that frusemide induced a rise of serum isoamylases in patients receiving the drug. This study is difficult to interpret, since frusemide could have an effect on the renal clearance of the enzyme.

The pancreatic dysfunction associated with sulphasalazine, which can be demonstrated on rechallenge (Suryapranata et al. 1986), was originally believed to be due to the sulphonamide component of the drug. Interestingly, later reports suggested that mesalazine (5-aminosalicylate), which is also used for treating ulcerative colitis, could cause pancreatitis (Deprez et al. 1989; Sachedina et al. 1989). This raises the possibility that the salicylate component of sulphasalazine was the agent responsible for pancreatic dysfunction in some of the earlier cases. Certainly, patients who are switched from sulphasalazine to a newer agent because of pancreatic dysfunction still need careful monitoring.

A number of other anti-infective agents have been associated with the pancreatitis. Pentamidine, which is structurally related to the biguanides (which have been implicated in pancreatitis in isolated cases [Bourke *et al.* 1978]), may cause diabetes, and has also been associated with acute pancreatitis (Murphy and Josephs 1981). The opportunistic infections that occur in patients suffering from AIDS have meant that pentamidine is being more widely used. A case with potentially fatal pancreatitis was reported by Zuger and colleagues (1986) following intravenous pentamidine, and more recently Herer and colleagues (1989) reported two cases of abnormalities of serum amylase and lipase, compatible with pancreatitis, a diagnosis supported in one by CAT-scanning, associated with pentamidine administration by aerosol. Again, both patients were HIV-positive. A complicated case of pancreatitis, occurring in a patient who had undergone cadaver renal transplantation and developed *Nocardia* infection, has been described by Antonow (1986); in this patient initial administration of co-trimoxazole with subsequent rechallenge caused pancreatitis. This is perhaps not surprising in view of the fact that sulphonamides are known to cause pancreatic dysfunction. Other antibacterials associated with pancreatic dysfunction include metronidazole (in a case which was positive on a rechallenge [Celifarco *et al.* 1989]), and erythromycin, occurring at both standard therapeutic doses (Hawksworth 1989) and in overdose (Gumaste 1989). Nitrofurantoin has also been associated with pancreatitis, positive on rechallenge (Nelis 1983).

NSAID have been associated with pancreatic dysfunction. Sulindac caused pancreatitis on rechallenge (Siefkin 1980; Lilly 1981), and a case has been described in which pancreatitis was associated with cholangitis in a patient who developed a high eosinophil count associated with the drug (Lerche *et al.* 1987). The authors considered that the bile duct injury was likely to have been caused by a hypersensitivity (allergic) reaction. In this patient rechallenge was positive, and the eosinophilic response was noted on more than one occasion. Haye (1986) has reported a case in which piroxicam was associated with clinical pancreatitis. A patient who developed pancreatitis while receiving mefenamic acid (van Walraven *et al.* 1982) was not rechallenged.

The anticonvulsant drugs sodium valproate and carbamazepine are also associated with pancreatic dysfunction. The evidence is far stronger with sodium valproate (CSM 1981; Parker *et al.* 1981; Ng 1982), and some deaths have been caused by this agent (Murphy and Lyon 1981; Williams *et al.* 1983). Soman and Swenson (1985) reported a case of pancreatitis induced by carbamazepine in an elderly lady of 73. They also noted that three other possible cases had been reported to the manufacturers of the drug.

The oral contraceptive pill has been associated with pancreatitis, and this is usually attributed to alteration in circulating lipids. Patients with existing hyperlipidaemias, particularly those of Types IV and V in the Frederickson classification, seem to be particularly at risk. Parker (1983) has suggested that it is unlikely that patients with normal blood lipids are at risk of pancreatitis until they are aged over 40 years.

A number of cytotoxic agents used in the management of malignant disease, or as immunosuppressants, have been noted to cause pancreatic dysfunction. In one large study colaspase (asparaginase) caused acute pancreatitis in 2.5 per cent of 1400 patients treated (Greenstein *et al.* 1979), and azathioprine has also been associated with pancreatitis (Nakashima and Howard 1977). Since cytotoxic agents are often used in combination, it may be difficult to establish the true culprit. Thus, Puckett and colleagues (1982) reported a case of pancreatitis associated with a combination of cyclophosphamide with doxorubicin and vincristine. Didanosine used in the treatment of AIDS is associated with a high frequency of pancreatitis in clinical use, though this was not so in its original clinical trials. In one retrospective survey 12 (23.5 per cent) of 51 patients on treatment developed clinical pancreatitis and over 60 per cent had elevated transaminases (Maxson *et al.* 1992).

In two cases of pancreatitis suspected to have been caused by methyldopa (van der Heide *et al.* 1981; Ramsay *et al.* 1982) the diagnosis was supported by recurrence on rechallenge. Claims of an association between β-adrenoceptor blocking drugs and pancreatitis (Durrington and Cairns 1982) were not supported by such evidence.

It has been suggested that cimetidine prolongs the rise in serum amylase concentration when used in the management of pancreatitis, but whether this is due to increased pancreatic damage is uncertain (*British Medical Journal* 1981). A patient in whom pancreatic dysfunction was associated with taking cimetidine was reported by Nott and De Sousa (1989), but in view of its very widespread use cimetidine seems to carry a very low risk of causing pancreatic damage.

Pancreatic damage may also be a rare complication of therapy with gold, and cases associated with both intramuscular and oral administration of gold have been reported (Eisemann *et al.* 1989). Pancreatitis following administration of lovastatin, positive on rechallenge, has been reported from Germany in a patient with Gilbert's syndrome (Pluhar 1989). A case report from Canada noted overdose of amoxapine and procyclidine causing pancreatitis (Jeffries and Masson 1985). The fact that pancreatic dysfunction is associated with gallstones is relevant to the observation that the incidence of pancreatitis was increased in the treated group in the clofibrate study organized by the World Health Organization (ROCPI 1980), as clofibrate is known to cause gallstones.

More difficult is the issue of steroids and pancreatitis. Large doses of steroids have been reported to cause pancreatitis (Riemenschneider *et al.* 1968), and a high incidence of focal necrosis in the pancreas has been reported at autopsy in patients who had been treated with steroids (David *et al.* 1970). Steinberg and Lewis (1981) re-evaluated the evidence associating steroids and pancreatitis and noted that while there were many anecdotal reports of an association there were no consistent secretory or histological changes that could be attributed to the drugs. There were no rechallenge studies and their conclusions were that steroids probably did not cause this condition. Two-thirds of the reports identified by these authors involved children. Overall, it seems that steroids are not likely to be a significant contributory cause of pancreatitis in adults.

Peritonitis

Sclerosing peritonitis

This condition was recognized before the introduction of β-adrenergic antagonists (Meyboom 1975), but a large number of cases have been caused by treatment with one member of this group of drugs, practolol (Brown *et al.* 1974; Dunstone and Ive 1975; Hensen *et al.* 1975; Minton *et al.* 1975). There have been occasional reports of this disorder in association with treatment with other β-blockers, including oxprenolol (Kennedy and Ducrow 1977), timolol (Baxter-Smith *et al.* 1978), and metoprolol (Clark and Terris 1983); but detailed review by Castle (1985) has thrown doubt on the suggestion of a causal relationship in such cases.

Other types of peritonitis

Granulomatous peritonitis following surgery, as a result of the glove starch, is also well recognized and on occasions may be very severe, as in the case reported by Michowitz and Stavorovsky (1983), of a 52-year-old man who developed intestinal obstruction secondary to a mass of adhesions. Reports of this complication have included other unusual presentations, as in the case of gastric outflow obstruction described by Steiner and

colleagues (1996). Pathological changes are associated with a variety of dusting powders (Ellis 1994).

A case of infective peritonitis associated with methylprednisolone pulse therapy has been reported in a woman receiving this drug for rheumatoid arthritis (Oto *et al.* 1983).

Infective peritonitis may also complicate treatment of renal failure with peritoneal dialysis; it may then be fungal or bacterial.

Retroperitoneal fibrosis

This disorder is discussed in detail in Chapter 18.

Type A and Type B reactions

Most adverse effects of drugs on the gut represent Type A reactions. For other effects, for example pancreatitis, the mechanisms of the adverse reactions are not well understood and these reactions probably come into the category of Type B events.

References

Aggarwal, P., Sharma, S.K., Wali, J.P., *et al.* (1989). Colonic carcinoma after chemotherapy of Hodgkin's disease. *J. Clin. Gastroenterol.* 1, 340.

Alaily, A.B. (1974). Gangrene of Meckel's diverticulum in pregnancy due to iron tablet. *BMJ* i, 103.

Al-Dujaili, M., Salole, E.G., and Florence, A.T. (1983). Drug formulation and oesophageal injury. *Adverse Drug React. Acute Poisoning Rev.* 2, 235.

Alves, M., Patel, V., Douglas, E., *et al.* (1979). Gastric infarction, a complication of selective vasopressin infusion. *Am. J. Dig. Dis.* 24, 409.

Ananth, J., Savodnik, I., and Yang, H. (1988). Lithium-associated Mallory–Weiss syndrome. *J. Clin. Psychiatry* 49, 412.

Anderson, I.M. and Ware, C. (1987). Syrup of ipecacuanha. *BMJ* 294, 578.

Antonescu, C.G. (1989). Potassium chloride and gastric outlet obstruction. *Ann. Intern. Med.* 111, 855.

Antonow, D.R. (1986). Acute pancreatitis associated with trimethoprim-sulphamethoxazole. *Ann. Intern. Med.* 104, 363.

Aselton, P.J. and Jick, H. (1983). Short-term follow-up study of wax matrix potassium chloride in relation to gastrointestinal bleeding. *Lancet* i, 184.

Aziz Khan, R., Piepgrass, W., and Wilhelm, M.C. (1982). Anticoagulant-induced haematomas of the small intestine. *South. Med. J.* 75, 242.

Baharav, E., Harpaz, D., Mittelman, M., *et al.* (1986). Dexamethasone-induced perineal irritation. *N. Engl. J. Med.* 314, 515.

Barbut, F. and Petit, J.C. (1996). Epidemiology of *Clostridium difficile* nosocomial infections. *Presse Méd.* 25, 385.

Bassoth, G., Gaburri, M., Pelli, M.A., *et al.* (1987). Oesophageal pain exacerbated by propranolol. *BMJ* 294, 1655.

Bateman, D.N. (1996). Re-evaluation of gut toxicity of NSAIDs. In *NSAIDs: COX-2 Enzyme Inhibitors* (ed. J. Vane, J. Botting, and J. Botting), p. 189. Kluwer Academic Publishers, Dordrecht.

Baxter-Smith, D.C., Monypenny, I.J., and Dorricott, N.J. (1978). Sclerosing peritonitis in patients on timolol. *Lancet* ii, 149.

Beaugerie, L. (1996). Diarrhoea caused by antibiotic therapy. *Revue du Praticien* 46, 171.

Benn, A., Swan, C.H.J., Cooke, W.T., *et al.* (1971). Effect of intraluminal pH on the absorption of pteroylmonoglutamic acid. *BMJ* i, 148.

Berchtold, P., Dahlqvist, A., Gustafson, A., *et al.* (1971). Effects of a biguanide (metformin) on vitamin B_{12} and folic acid absorption and intestinal enzyme activities. *Scand. J. Gastroenterol.* 6, 751.

Bhalotra, R. (1988). Alcohol-induced proctitis in a human. *J. Clin. Gastroenterol.* 10, 592.

Bhasin, D.K. and Singh, R. (1988). Chloroquine phosphate induced gastroduodenitis. *Gastrointest. Endosc.* 34, 488.

Block, M.B., Genant, H.K., and Kirsner, J.B. (1970). Pancreatitis as an adverse reaction to salicylazasulfapyridine. *N. Engl. J. Med.* 282, 380.

Boley, S.J., Allen, A.C., Schultz, L., *et al.* (1965). Potassium-induced lesions of the small bowel. I. Clinical aspects. *JAMA* 193, 997.

Bonkowsky, H.L. and Brisbane, J. (1976). Colitis and hepatitis caused by methyldopa. *JAMA* 236, 1602.

Bourke, J.B., McIllmurray, M.B., Mead, G.M., *et al.* (1978). Drug associated primary acute pancreatitis. *Lancet.* i, 706.

Branski, D., Kerem, E., Gross-Kieselstein, E., *et al.* (1986). Bloody diarrhoea — a possible complication of sulfasalazine transferred through human breast milk. *J. Pediatr. Gastroenterol. Nutr.* 5, 316.

Brennan, M.F., Clarke, A.M., and Macbeth, W.A.A. (1968). Infarction of the midgut associated with oral contraceptives. *N. Engl. J. Med.* 279, 1213.

British Medical Journal (1981). Non-ulcer uses of cimetidine. *BMJ* 283, 89.

Brower, R.A. (1986). Jejunal perforation possibly induced by slow-release potassium in a patient with Crohn's disease. *Dig. Dis. Sci.* 31, 1387.

Brown, P., Baddeley, H., Read, A.E., *et al.* (1974). Sclerosing peritonitis, an unusual reaction to a beta-adrenergic-blocking drug (practolol). *Lancet* ii, 1477.

Brown, R.B., Rice, B.H., and Szakacs, J.E. (1959). Intestinal bleeding and perforation complicating treatment with vasoconstrictors. *Ann. Surg.* 150, 790.

Bulpitt, C.J. and Dollery, C.T. (1973). Side-effects of hypotensive agents evaluated by a self-administered questionnaire. *BMJ* iii, 485.

Bunney, R.G. (1989). Non-steroidal anti-inflammatory drugs and the bowel. *Lancet,* ii, 1047.

Burkitt, E.A. and Sutcliffe, C.K. (1961). Paralytic ileus after amitriptyline, *BMJ* ii, 1648.

Burruss, G.L., van Voarst, S.J., Crawford, A.J., *et al.* (1986). Small bowel obstruction from an antacid bezoar: a ranitidine antacid interaction. *South. Med. J.* 79, 917.

Burt, M., Scott, A., Williard, W.C., *et al.* (1996). Erythromycin stimulates gastric emptying after esophagectomy with gastric replacement: a randomized clinical trial. *J. Thorac. Cardiovasc. Surg.* 111, 649.

Cannon, S.R. (1982). Intestinal vasculitis and lithium carbonate-associated diarrhoea. *Postgrad. Med. J.* 58, 445.

Carter, B.L., Woodhead, J.C., Cole, K.S., *et al.* (1987). Gastrointestinal side-effects of erythromycin preparations. *Drug Intell. Clin. Pharm.* 21, 734.

Caruso, I. and Bianchi Porro, G. (1980). Gastroscopic evaluation of anti-inflammatory agents. *BMJ* i, 75.

Cass, A.J. (1978). Stercoral perforation: case of drug-induced impaction. *BMJ* ii, 932.

Castle, W.M. (1985). Drugs and fibrotic reactions — Part I. *Adverse Drug React. Bull.* 113, 422.

Celifarco, A., Warschauer, C., and Burakoff, R. (1989). Metronidazole-induced pancreatitis. *Am. J. Gastroenterol.* 84, 958.

Chapman, C.S., Swart, S.S., and Wood, J.K. (1986). Oesophageal apoplexy associated with aspirin ingestion in polycythaemia rubra vera. *Clin. Lab. Haem.* 8, 265.

Cheli, R. and Ciancamerla, G. (1974). Proctiti emorragiche da medicamenti locali. *Minerva Gastroenterol.* 20, 56.

Chen, B., Shapira, J., Ravid, M., *et al.* (1982). Steatorrhoea induced by allopurinol. *BMJ* 284, 1914.

Chen, F.C. and Woods, R. (1996). Pseudomembranous panenteritis and septicaemia in a patient with ulcerative colitis. *Aust. N.Z. J. Surg.* 66, 565.

Clark, C.V. and Terris, R. (1983). Sclerosing peritonitis associated with metoprolol. *Lancet* i, 937.

Clarke, I.M.C. (1971). Adynamic ileus and amitriptyline. *BMJ* ii, 531.

Coates, A.G., Nostrant, T.T., Wilson, J.A.P., *et al.* (1986). Esophagitis caused by non-steroidal anti-inflammatory medication: case reports and reviews of the literature on pill-induced esophageal injury. *South. Med. J.* 79, 1094.

Conn, H.O. and Poynard, T. (1984). Adrenocorticosteroid therapy and peptic ulcer disease. *N. Engl. J. Med.* 310, 201.

Cornish, A.L., McClellan, J.T., and Johnston, D.H. (1961). Effects of chlorothiazide on the pancreas. *N. Engl. J. Med.* 265, 673.

Coronato, A. and Glass, G.B.J. (1973). Depression of the intestinal uptake of radio-vitamin B_{12} by cholestyramine. *Proc. Soc. Exp. Biol. Med.* 142, 1341.

Cotton, P.B. and Lea Thomas, M. (1971). Ischaemic colitis and the contraceptive pill. *BMJ* iii, 27.

Coutrot, S., Roland, D., Barbier, J., *et al.* (1978). Acute perforation of colonic diverticula associated with short-term indomethacin. *Lancet* ii, 1055.

Crowson, T.D., Head, L.H., and Ferrante, W.A. (1976). Esophageal ulcers associated with tetracycline therapy. *JAMA* 235, 2747.

CSM (Committee on Safety of Medicines) (1981). Sodium valproate (Epilim). *Current Problems No. 6.* HMSO, London.

CSM (Committee on Safety of Medicines) (1983). Osmosin (controlled-release indomethacin). *Current Problems No. 11.* HMSO, London.

Cummings, J.H. (1974). Laxative abuse. *Gut* 15, 758.

Dargie, H.J. and Dollery C.T. (1975). Adverse reactions to diuretic drugs. In *Meyler's Side Effects of Drugs*, Vol. 8 (ed. M.N.G. Dukes), p. 483. Excerpta Medica, Amsterdam.

David, D.S., Grieco, M.H., and Cushman, P. (1970). Adrenal glucocorticoids after twenty years. A review of their clinically relevant consequences. *J. Chron. Dis.* 22, 637.

Davies, D.R. and Brightmore, T. (1970). Idiopathic and drug-induced ulceration of the small intestine. *Br. J. Surg.* 57, 134.

Dayton, M.T., Kleckner, S.C., and Brown, D.K. (1987). Peptic ulcer perforation associated with steroid use. *Arch. Surg.* 122, 376.

Denison, H. and Wallerstedt, S. (1989). Bacterial overgrowth after high-dose corticosteroid treatment. *Scand. J. Gastroenterol.* 24, 561.

Deprez, P., Descamps, Ch., and Fiasse, R. (1989). Pancreatitis induced by 5-aminosalicylic acid. *Lancet* ii, 445.

Devenyi, A.G. (1995). Antibiotic-induced colitis. *Semin. Paediatr. Surg.* 4, 215.

Dever, L.L., Smith, S.M., Handwerger, S., *et al.* (1995). Vancomycin-dependent *Enterococcus faecium* isolated from stool following oral vancomycin therapy. *J. Clin. Microbiol.* 33, 2770.

Deviere, J., Reuse, D., and Askenasi, R. (1987). Ischaemic pancreatitis and hepatitis secondary to ergotamine poisoning. *Clin. Gastroenterol.* 9, 350.

Dewis, P., Local, F., Anderson, D.C., *et al.* (1982). Reversible oesophageal dysphagia and long-term ingestion of chlormethiazole. *BMJ* 284, 705.

Dobbins, W.O., Herrero, B.A., and Mansbach, C.M. (1968). Morphologic alterations associated with neomycin induced malabsorption. *Am. J. Med. Sci.* 255, 63.

Douthwaite, A.H. and Lintott, G.A.M. (1938). Gastroscopic observation of the effect of aspirin and certain other substances on the stomach. *Lancet* ii, 1222.

Dowling, R.H. (1977). Chenodeoxycholic acid therapy of gallstones. In *Clinics in Gastroenterology, 6. Bile acids* (ed. G. Paumgartner), p. 141. W.B. Saunders, London.

Dunstone, G.H. and Ive, F.A. (1975). Sclerosing peritonitis and practolol. *Lancet* i, 275.

Durrington, P.N. and Cairns, S.A. (1982). Acute pancreatitis: a complication of beta-blockade. *BMJ* 284, 1016.

Eckhauser, M.L., Dokler, M.A., and Imbembo, A.L. (1987). Diuretic-associated pancreatitis: a collective review and illustrative cases. *Am. J. Gastroenterol.* 82, 865.

Eisemann, A.D., Becker, N.J., Miner, P.B., *et al.* (1989). Pancreatitis and gold treatment of rheumatoid arthritis. *Ann. Intern. Med.* 111, 860.

Ellis, H. (1994). Pathological changes produced by surgical dusting powders. *Ann. R. Coll. Surg. Engl.* 76, 5.

Faloon, W.W., Paes, I.C., Woolfolk, D., *et al.* (1966). Effect of neomycin and kanamycin upon intestinal malabsorption. *Ann. N.Y. Acad. Sci.* 132, 879.

Figiel, L.S. and Figiel, S.J. (1973). Diphenoxylate hydrochloride intoxication simulating intestinal obstruction. *Am. J. Gastroenterol.* 59, 267.

Freeman, H.J. (1986). Sulindac associated small bowel lesion. *J. Clin. Gastroenterol.* 8, 569.

Gander, D.R. and Devlin, H.B. (1963). Ileus after amitriptyline. *BMJ* i, 1160.

Garcia Rodriguez, L.A. and Jick, H. (1994). Risk of upper gastrointestinal bleeding and perforation associated with individual non-steroidal anti-inflammatory drugs. *Lancet* 343, 769.

Garre, M., Campion, J.P., Bouget, J., *et al.* (1976). Nécrose du rectum au cours d'une granulopénie due à l'amidopyrine. *Nouv. Presse Méd.* 5, 2633.

Gazes, P.C., Holmes, C.R., Moseley, V., *et al.* (1961). Acute haemorrhage and necrosis of the intestines associated with digitalization. *Circulation* 23, 358.

Geltner, D., Sternfield, M., Becker, S.A., *et al.* (1986). Gold-induced ileitis. *J. Clin. Gastroenterol.* 8, 184.

Gerson, C.D., Hepner, G.W., Browns, N., *et al.* (1972). Inhibition by diphenylhydantoin of folic acid absorption in man. *Gastroenterology* 63, 246.

Graham, C.F., Gallagher, K., and Jones, J.K. (1981). Acute colitis with methyldopa. *N. Engl. J. Med.* 304, 1044.

Greenberger, N.J., Ruppert, R.D., and Cuppage, F.E. (1967). Inhibition of intestinal iron transport induced by tetracycline. *Gastroenterology* 53, 590.

Greenstein, R., Nogeire, C., Ohnuma, T., *et al.* (1979). Management of asparaginase-induced hemorrhagic pancreatitis complicated by pseudocyst. *Cancer* 43, 718.

Greig, J.D. (1989). Oral contraceptives and intestinal ischaemia. *J.R. Coll. Gen. Pract.* 39, 76.

Gumaste, V.V. (1989). Erythromycin induced pancreatitis. *Am. J. Med.* 86, Part 1, 725.

Guss, C., Schneider, A.T., and Chiaramonte, L.T. (1986). Perforated gastric ulcer in an asthmatic treated with theophylline and steroids: Case report and literature review. *Ann. Allergy* 56, 237.

Hachiya, K.A., Kobayashi, R.H., and Antonson, D.L. (1982). Candida esophagitis following antibiotic usage. *Pediatr. Infect. Dis.* 1, 168.

Hall, R.I., Petty, A.H., Cobden, I., *et al.* (1983). Enteritis and colitis associated with mefenamic acid. *BMJ* 287, 1182.

Hardison, W.G.M. and Rosenberg, I.H. (1969). The effect of neomycin on bile salt metabolism and fat digestion in man. *J. Lab. Clin. Med.* 74, 564.

Harris, A.L. (1982). Cytotoxic-therapy-induced vomiting is mediated via enkephalin pathways. *Lancet* i, 714.

Hart, R.S., Levin, B., and Gholson, C.F. (1989). Esophageal obstruction caused by sucralfate impaction. *Gastrointest. Endosc.* 35, 474.

Hawksworth, C.R.E. (1989). Acute pancreatitis associated with infusion of erythromycin lactobionate. *BMJ* 298, 190.

Haye, O.L. (1986). Piroxicam and pancreatitis. *Ann. Intern. Med.* 104, 895.

Heizer, W.D., Warshaw, A.L., Waldmann, T.A., *et al.* (1968). Protein-losing gastroenteropathy and malabsorption associated with factitious diarrhoea. *Ann. Intern. Med.* 68, 839.

Heller, S.R., Fellows, I.W., Ogilvie, A.L., *et al.* (1982). Non-steroidal anti-inflammatory drugs and benign oesophageal stricture. *BMJ* 285, 167.

Hensen, A., Rhemrev, P.E.R., and Kapteyn, J.T.L. (1975). Sclerosing peritonitis and practolol. *Lancet* i, 275.

Herer, B., Chinet, T., Labrune, S., *et al.* (1989). Pancreatitis associated with pentamidine by aerosol. *BMJ* 298, 605.

Hey, H., Jorgensen, F., Sorensen, K., *et al.* (1982). Oesophageal transit of six commonly used tablets and capsules. *BMJ* 285, 1717.

Hobbin, E. and Champion, G. (1986). Indomethacin suppositories. *J. Am. Geriatr. Soc.* 34, 325.

Houghton, A.D., Nadel, S., and Stringer, M.D. (1989). Penicillamine-associated total colitis. *Hepatogastroenterology* 36, 198.

Hurwitz, N. and Wade, O.L. (1969). Intensive hospital monitoring of adverse reactions to drugs. *BMJ* i, 531.

Jacobson, E.D., Prior, J.R., and Faloon, W.W. (1960). Malabsorptive syndrome induced by neomycin: morphologic alterations in the jejunal mucosa. *J. Lab. Clin Med.* 56, 245.

Jeffries, J.J. and Masson, J. (1985). Pancreatitis following overdose with amoxapine and procyclidine. *J. Psychiatry* 30, 546.

Johnston, D.H. and Cornish, A.L. (1959). Acute pancreatitis in patients receiving chlorothiazide. *JAMA* 170, 2054.

Jones, M.P. and Caldwell, J.R. (1962). Acute hemorrhagic pancreatitis associated with administration of chlorthalidone. *N. Engl. J. Med.* 267, 1029.

Juel-Jensen, B.E. (1959). Sensitivity to phenindione. Report of a case of severe diarrhoea. *BMJ* ii, 173.

Kennedy, S.C. and Ducrow, M. (1977). Fibrinous peritonitis. *BMJ* i, 1598.

Key, N.S., Emerson, P.M., Allan, N.C., *et al.* (1987). Oesophageal varices associated with busulphan-thioguanine combination therapy for chronic myeloid leukaemia. *Lancet* ii, 1050.

Kilpatrick, Z.M., Silverman, J.F., Betancourt, E., *et al.* (1968). Vascular occlusion of the colon and oral contraceptives. *N. Engl. J. Med.* 278, 438.

Kirkham, B., Wedderburn, L., and Macfarlane, D.G. (1989). Gold-induced colitis. *Br. J. Rheumatol.* 28, 272.

Knight, K.M. and Doucet, J.H. (1987). Gastric rupture and death caused by ipecac syrup. *South. Med. J.* 80, 786.

Kristensen, B., Skov, J., and Pertslund, N.A. (1980). Frusemide-induced increase in serum iso-amylases. *BMJ* ii, 978.

Kuwin, C.M. and Finland, D.M. (1961). Clinical pharmacology of the tetracycline antibiotics. *Clin. Pharm. Ther.* 2, 51.

Kwo, P.Y. and Tremain, W.J. (1995). Non-steroidal anti-inflammatory drug-induced enteropathy: case discussion and review of the literature. *Mayo Clin. Proc.* 70, 55.

Labadarios, D., Dickerson, J.W.T., Parke, E.B., *et al.* (1978). The effects of chronic drug administration on hepatic enzyme induction and folate metabolism. *Br. J. Clin. Pharmacol.* 5, 167.

Lambert, M., de Peyer, R., and Muller, A.F. (1982). Reversible ischemic colitis after intravenous vasopressin therapy. *JAMA* 247, 666.

Langman, M.J.S. (1982). Gastrointestinal drugs. In *Side Effects of Drugs, Annual 6* (ed. M.N.G. Dukes), p. 315. Excerpta Medica, Amsterdam.

Lees, G.M. and Percy, W.M. (1981). Antibiotic-associated colitis: an in vitro investigation of the effects of antibiotics on intestinal motility. *Br. J. Clin. Pharmacol.* 73. 535.

Lerche, A., Vyberg, M., and Kirkegaard, E. (1987). Acute cholangitis and pancreatitis associated with sulindac (Clinoril). *Histopathology* 11, 647.

Levine, M.S., Borislow, S.M., Rubesin, S.E., *et al.* (1994). Esophageal stricture caused by a Morin tablet (ibuprofen). *Abdominal Imaging* 19, 6.

Levy, N. and Gaspar, E. (1975). Rectal bleeding and indomethacin suppositories. *Lancet* i, 577.

Lilly, E.L. (1981). Pancreatitis after administration of sulindac. *JAMA* 246, 2680.

Lofgren, R.P., Rothe, P.R., and Carlson, G.J. (1982). Jejunal perforation associated with slow release potassium chloride therapy. *South. Med. J.* 75, 1154.

McMahon, F.G., Ryan, J.R., Akdamar, K., *et al.* (1982). Upper gastrointestinal lesions after potassium chloride supplements: a controlled clinical trial. *Lancet* ii, 1059.

McNeill, D.C. (1966). Adynamic ileus and nortriptyline. *BMJ* i, 1360.

Madhok, R., MacKenzie, J.A., Lee, R.D., *et al.* (1986). Small bowel ulceration in patients receiving non-steroidal anti-inflammatory drugs for rheumatoid arthritis. *Q. J. Med.* 58, 53.

Mannes, P., Derriks, R., Moens, R., *et al.* (1976). Multidisciplinary curative treatment for disseminated carcinoma of the breast. *Cancer Treat. Rep.* 60, 85.

Maroy, B. and Moullot, P. (1986). Oesophageal burn due to chlorazepate dipotassium (Tranxene). *Gastrointest. Endosc.* 32, 240.

Martin, P., Manley, P.N., Depew, W.T., *et al.* (1987). Isotretinoin-associated proctosigmoiditis. *Gastroenterology* 93, 606.

Martys, C.R. (1979). Adverse reactions to drugs in general practice. *BMJ* ii, 1194.

Maxson, C.J.I., Greenfield, S.M., and Turner, J.L. (1992). Acute pancreatitis as a common complication of 2′,3′-dideoxyinosine therapy in the acquired immunodeficiency syndrome. *Am. J. Gastroenterol.* 87, 708.

Merten, D.F. and Grossman, H. (1980). Intestinal obstruction associated with cholestyramine therapy. *AJR* 134, 827.

Messer, J., Reitman, D., Sacks, H.S., *et al.* (1983). Association of adrenocorticosteroid therapy and peptic-ulcer disease. *N. Engl. J. Med.* 309, 21.

Meyboom, R.H.B. (1975). Practolol and sclerosing peritonitis. *Lancet* i, 334.

Michet, C.J., Pakela, J., and Luthra, H. (1987). Auranofin-associated colitis and eosinophilia. *Mayo Clin. Proc.* 62, 142.

Michowitz, M. and Stavorovsky, M. (1983). Granulomatous peritonitis caused by glove starch. *Postgrad. Med. J.* 59, 593.

Minton, M., Newland, A., Knowles, G., *et al.* (1975). Sclerosing peritonitis and practolol. *Lancet* i, 276.

Mitchell, T.H., Stamp, T.C.B., and Jenkins, M.V. (1982). Steatorrhoea after tetracycline. *BMJ* 285, 780.

Miyata, T., Tamechika, Y., and Torisu, M. (1988). Ischaemic colitis in a 33-year-old woman on danazol treatment for endometriosis. *Am. J. Gastroenterol.* 83, 1420.

Mizrahi, S., Laor, D., and Stamler, B. (1989). Intestinal ischaemia induced by cocaine abuse. *Arch. Surg.* 123, 394.

Morris, L.L., Villalba, M.R., and Glover, J.L. (1994). Management of pseudomembranous colitis. *Am. Surg.* 60, 548.

Mucklow, J.C. (1978). Plasma drug concentrations in the prevention and diagnosis of adverse drug reactions. *Adverse Drug React. Bull.* 73, 260.

Muggia, F.M. (1967). Haemorrhagic necrosis of the intestine: its occurrence with digitalis intoxication. *Am. J. Med. Sci.* 253, 263.

Murphy, S.A. and Josephs, A.S. (1981). Acute pancreatitis associated with pentamidine therapy. *Arch. Intern. Med.* 141, 56.

Murphy, M.J. and Lyon, L.W. (1981). Valproic acid associated pancreatitis in an adult. *Lancet* i, 41.

Nakashima, Y. and Howard, J.M. (1977). Drug induced acute pancreatitis. *Surg. Gynecol. Obstet.* 145, 105.

Neal, K.R., Scott, H.M., Slack, R.C.B., *et al.* (1996). Omeprazole as a risk factor for campylobacter gastroenteritis: case–control study. *BMJ* 312, 414.

Nelis, G.F. (1983). Nitrofurantoin-induced pancreatitis: Report of a case. *Gastroenterology* 84, 1032.

Nelis, G.G. (1989). Diarrhoea due to 5-aminosalicylic acid in breast milk. *Lancet* i, 383.

Ng, J.Y.K. (1982). Acute pancreatitis and sodium valproate. *Med. J. Aust.* ii, 362.

Nimmo W. S. (1979). Gastric emptying and drug absorption. In *Drug Absorption* (ed. L.F. Prescott and W.S. Nimmo), p. 11. Adis Press, Auckland.

Nothmann, B.J., Chittinand. S., and Schuster, M.M. (1973). Reversible mesenteric vascular occlusion associated with oral contraceptives. *Am. J. Dig. Dis.* 18, 361.

Nott, D.M. and De Sousa, B.A. (1989). Suspected cimetidine-induced acute pancreatitis. *Br. J. Clin. Pract.* 43, 264.

Oto, A., Oktay, A., and Sozen, T. (1983). Methylprednisolone pulse therapy and peritonitis. *Ann. Intern. Med.* 99, 282.

Paaby, P. and Nervin, E. (1966). The absorption of vitamin B_{12} during treatment with para-aminosalicyclic acid. *Acta Med. Scand.* 180, 561.

Palva, I.P., Heinivaara, O., and Mattila, M. (1966). Drug-induced malabsorption of vitamin B_{12}. 3. Interference of PAS and folic acid in the absorption of vitamin B_{12}. *Scand. J. Haematol.* 3, 149.

Palva, I.P., Salokannel, S.J., Timonen, T., *et al.* (1972). Drug-induced malabsorption of vitamin B_{12} during treatment with slow-release potassium chloride. *Acta Med. Scand.* 191, 335.

Panos, R.J., Tso, E., Barish, R.A., *et al.* (1986). Esophageal spasm following propranolol overdose relieved by glucagon. *Am. J. Emerg. Med.* 4, 227.

Parker, P.H., Helinek, G.L., Ghishan, F.K., *et al.* (1981).

Recurrent pancreatitis induced by valproic acid: A case report and review of the literature. *Gastroenterology* 80, 826.

Parker, W.A. (1983). Estrogen-induced pancreatitis. *Clin. Pharm.* 2, 75.

Patel, P.M., Selby, P.J., Deacon, J., *et al.* (1989). Anthraquinone laxatives and human cancer: an association in one case. *Postgrad. Med. J.* 65, 216.

Perkins, A.C., Wilson, C.G., Blackshaw, P.E., *et al.* (1994). Impaired oesophageal transit of capsule versus tablet formulations in the elderly. *Gut* 35, 1363.

Peroutka, S.J., and Snyder, S.H. (1982). Antiemetics: neurotransmitter receptor-binding predicts therapeutic actions. *Lancet* i, 658.

Pickleman J., Straus, F.H., and Paloyan, E. (1979). Pancreatitis associated with thiazide administration. *Arch. Surg.* 114, 1013.

Pluhar, W. (1989). A case of possibly lovastatin-induced pancreatitis in conjunction with Gilbert's syndrome. *Wien. Klin. Wochenschr.* 101, 551.

Pottage, A., Campbell, R.W.F., Achuff, S.C., *et al.* (1978). The absorption of oral mexiletine in coronary care patients. *Eur. J. Clin. Pharmacol.* 13, 393.

Powell, R.C., Nunes, W.T., Harding, R.S., *et al.* (1962). The influence of non-absorbable antibiotics on serum lipids and the excretion of neutral sterols and bile acids. *Am. J. Clin. Nutr.* 11, 156.

Puckett, J.B., Butler, W.M., and McFarland, J.A. (1982). Pancreatitis and cancer chemotherapy. *Ann. Intern. Med.* 97, 453.

Race, T.F., Paes, I.C., and Faloon, W.W. (1970). Intestinal malabsorption induced by oral colchicine. Comparison with neomycin and cathartic agents. *Am. J. Med. Sci.* 259, 32.

Rampton, D.S. and Sladen, G.E. (1981). Relapse of ulcerative proctocolitis during treatment with non-steroidal anti-inflammatory drugs. *Postgrad. Med. J.* 57, 297.

Ramsay, L.E., Wakefield, V.A., and Harris, E.E. (1982). Methyldopa-induced chronic pancreatitis. *Practitioner* 226, 1166.

Ravi, S., Keat, A.C., and Keat, E.C.B. (1986). Colitis caused by non-steroidal anti-inflammatory drugs. *Postgrad. Med. J.* 62, 773.

Reiner, E. and Patterson, M. (1966). The effect of neomycin on disaccharidase activity of the small bowel. *Clin. Res.* 14, 49.

Reynolds, E.H. (1968). Mental effects of anticonvulsants and folic acid metabolism. *Brain* 91, 197.

Riemenschneider, T.A., Wilson, J.E., and Vernier, R.L. (1968). Glucocorticoid-induced pancreatitis in children. *Pediatrics* 41, 428.

Robinson, H.M., Wheatley, T., and Leach, I.H. (1995). Non-steroidal anti-inflammatory drug-induced colonic stricture. An unusual cause of bowel obstruction and perforation. *Dig. Dis. Sci.* 40, 315.

Robinson, J.D. and Burtner, D.E. (1981). Severe diarrhoea secondary to propranolol. *Drug Intell. Clin. Pharm.* 15, 49.

ROCPI (Report of the Committee of Principal Investigators) (1980). WHO co-operative trial on primary prevention of ischaemic heart disease using clofibrate to lower serum cholesterol: mortality follow-up. *Lancet* ii, 379.

Roe, M., Sears, A.D., and Arndt, J.H. (1972). Gold reaction panenteritis. A case report with radiodiagnostic findings. *Radiology* 104, 59.

Rose, M. and Johnson, I. (1978). Reinterpretation of the haematological effects of anticonvulsant treatment. *Lancet* i, 1349.

Sachedina, B., Saibil, F., Cohen, L.B., *et al.* (1989). Acute pancreatitis due to 5-aminosalicylate. *Ann. Intern. Med.* 110, 490.

Salokannel, S.J., Palva, I.P., and Takkunen, J.T. (1970). Malabsorption of vitamin B_{12} during treatment with slow-release potassium chloride. *Acta Med. Scand.* 187, 431.

Samore, M.H., Bettin, K.M., DeGirolami, P.C., *et al.* (1994). Wide diversity of *Clostridium difficile* types at a tertiary referral hospital. *J. Infect. Dis.* 170, 615.

Saverymuttu, S.H., Thomas, A., Grundy, A., *et al.* (1986). Ileal stricturing after long-term indomethacin treatment. *Postgrad. Med. J.* 62, 967.

Schapira, M., Roquet, M.E., Henrion, J., *et al.* (1996). Severe nontyphoidal salmonellosis probably in relation with omeprazole treatment: report of 2 cases. *Acta Gastroenterol. Belg.* 59, 168.

Schneerson, J.M. and Gazzard, B.G. (1977). Reversible malabsorption syndrome caused by methyldopa. *Br. Med J.* ii, 1456.

Schneiderman, D.J. and Cello, J.P. (1986). Intestinal ischaemia and infarction associated with oral contraceptives. *West. J. Med.* 145, 350.

Schulze-Delrieu, K. (1983). Pseudomembranous colitis and the neuromuscular actions of antibiotics. *Gastroenterology* 85, 1221.

Schwartz, H.A. (1981). Lower gastrointestinal side-effects of non-steroidal anti-inflammatory drugs. *J. Rheumatol.* 8, 952.

Schweitzer, M.A., Sweiss, I., Silver, D.L., *et al.* (1996). The clinical spectrum of *Clostridium difficile* colitis in immunocompromised patients. *Am. Surg.* 62, 603.

Seibert, D. and Al-Kawas, F. (1986). Trimethoprim–sulfamethoxazole, hiccups, and oesophageal ulcers. *Ann. Intern. Med* 105, 976.

Shah, V., Marino, C., and Altice, F.L. (1996). Albendazole-induced pseudomembranous colitis. *Am. J. Gastroenterol.* 91, 1453.

Siefkin, A.D. (1980). Sulindac and pancreatitis. *Ann. Intern. Med.* 93, 932.

Smith, W.D.F. (1987). Endoscopic removal of a pharmacobezoar of slow-release theophylline. *BMJ* 294, 125.

Soman, M. and Swenson, D. (1985). A possible case of carbamazepine-induced pancreatitis. *Drug. Intell. Clin. Pharm.* 19, 925.

Sriuranpong, V. and Voravud, N. (1995). Antineoplastic-associated colitis in Chulalongkorn University Hospital. *J. Med. Assoc. Thai.* 78, 424.

Stang, H. (1986). Pyloric stenosis revisited in St Paul. *Minn. Med.* 69, 661.

Stebbins, P.L. and Pearson, C.C. (1967). Methotrexate in treatment of psoriasis: case report of a severe reaction secondary to induced malabsorption. *Bull. Mason Clin.* 21, 20.

Steinberg, W.M. and Lewis, J.H. (1981). Steroid-induced pancreatitis: does it really exist? *Gastroenterology* 81, 799.

Steiner, A., Howard, E., and Akgun S. (1961). Effect of antibiotics on the serum cholesterol concentration of patients with atherosclerosis. *Circulation* 24, 729.

Steiner, Z., Mogliner, J., and Bahar, Y. (1996). Gastric outlet obstruction due to starch granuloma. *Eur. J. Pediatr. Surg.* 6, 364.

Stewart, R.B. and Cluff, L.E. (1974). Gastrointestinal manifestations of adverse drug reactions. *Am. J. Dig. Dis.* 19, 1.

Suissa, A., Parason, M., Lachter, J., *et al.* (1987). Penicillin VK-induced esophageal ulcerations. *Am. J. Gastroenterol.* 82, 482.

Suryapranata, H. and De Vries, H. (1986). Pancreatitis associated with sulphasalazine. *BMJ* 292, 732.

Sutton, D.R. and Gosnold, J.K. (1977). Oesophageal ulceration due to clindamycin. *BMJ* i, 1598.

Sweeney, E.C. and Sheehan, J.P. (1979). Clindamycin-associated colonic vasculitis. *BMJ* ii, 1188.

Swift, R.M. and Thayer, W. (1987). Increased obstipation in a patient with scleroderma following therapy with lithium. *J. Clin. Psychopharm.* 7, 358.

Teare, J.P., Booth, J.C., Brown, J.L., *et al.* (1995). Pseudomembranous colitis following clarithromycin therapy. *Eur. J. Gastroenterol. Hepatol.* 7, 275.

Telsey, A.M., Merrit, T.A., and Dixon, S.D. (1988). Cocaine exposure in a term neonate. *Clin. Pediatr.* 27, 547.

Thomas, F.B., Salaburey, D., and Greenberger, N.J. (1972). Inhibition of iron absorption by cholestyramine. *Am. J. Dig. Dis.* 17, 263.

Tomkin, G.H. (1973). Malabsorption of vitamin B_{12} in diabetic patients treated wtih phenformin: a comparison with metformin. *BMJ* iii, 673.

Tomkin G.H., Hadden, D.R., Weaver, J.A., *et al.* (1971). Vitamin B_{12} status of patients on long-term metformin therapy. *BMJ* ii, 685.

Trier, J.S. (1962). Morphologic alterations induced by methotrexate in the mucosa of the human proximal intestine. I. Serial observations by light microscopy. *Gastroenterology* 42, 297.

van der Heide, H., Ten Haaft, M.A., and Stricker, B.H. (1981). Pancreatitis caused by methyldopa. *BMJ* 282, 1930.

van Klingeren, B. (1983). Penicillins, cephalosporins and tetracyclines. In *Side Effects of Drugs Annual 7* (ed. M.N.G. Dukes), p. 71. Excerpta Medica, Amsterdam.

van Walraven, A.A., Edels, M., and Fong, S. (1982). Pancreatitis caused by mefenamic acid. *Can. Med. Assoc. J.* 126, 894.

Voskuyl, A.E., Van de Laar, M.A., Moens, H.J., *et al.* (1993). Extra-articular manifestations of rheumatoid arthritis: risk factors for serious gastrointestinal events. *Ann. Rheum. Dis.* 52, 771.

Wass, J.A.H., Thorner, M.O., Morris, D.V., *et al.* (1977). Long-term treatment of acromegaly with bromocriptine. *BMJ* i, 875.

Webb, D.I., Chodos, R.B., Mahar, C.Q., *et al.* (1968). Mechanism of vitamin B_{12} malabsorption in patients receiving colchicine. *N. Engl. J. Med.* 279, 845.

Weinert, V. and Grussenderf, E.I. (1980). Anokutaner Ergotismus gangraenosus. *Hautarzt* 31, 668.

Weston, C.F. (1987). Anal burning and peppermint oil. *Postgrad. Med. J.* 63, 717.

White, C.A. and Traube, J. (1982). Ulcerating enteritis associated with flucytosine therapy. *Gastroenterology* 83, 1127.

Williams, L.H.P., Reynolds, R.P., and Emery, J.L. (1983). Pancreatitis during sodium valproate treatment. *Arch. Dis. Child.* 58, 543.

Wilson, A.E., Mehra, S.K., Gomersal, C.R., *et al.* (1967). Acute pancreatitis associated with frusemide therapy. *Lancet* i, 105.

Wingate, D.L. (1990). Potent acid reduction and risk of enteric infection. *Lancet* i, 222.

Zilling, T.L. and Ahren, B. (1989). Ischaemic pancolitis. A serious complication of chemotherapy in a previously irradiated patient. *Acta Chir. Scand.* 155, 77.

Zuger, A., Wolf, B.Z., El-Sadr, W., *et al.* (1986). Pentamidine-associated fatal acute pancreatitis. *JAMA* 256, 2383.

Zurier, R.B., Hashim, S.A., and van Itallie, T.B. (1965). Effect of medium chain triglyceride on cholestyramine induced steatorrhoea in man. *Gastroenterology* 49, 490.

13. Hepatic disorders

M. DAVIS

Introduction

The liver is a major target for damage by therapeutic agents. In a large Danish survey, liver damage accounted for five per cent of total adverse drug reactions reported, but 15 per cent of those that were fatal (Friis and Andreasen 1992). It is estimated that about two per cent of all cases of jaundice in hospital patients are drug induced, and in the elderly the frequency may be up to 20 per cent (Schenker and Bay 1994). Up to 15 per cent of cases of fulminant hepatic failure are due to an adverse drug reaction (Williams 1996).

Spectrum of hepatotoxicity from drugs

The spectrum of liver lesions produced by drugs is broad, and encompasses the whole range of abnormalities produced by other causes (Table 13.1). The severity of reactions varies from minor abnormalities in liver function tests in otherwise asymptomatic individuals to full-blown liver damage with all its clinical manifestations. Clinically it is convenient to classify these reactions according to whether they are:

Dose-dependent: arising in any individual who ingests a sufficient quantity of the drug, the commonest example encountered in clinical practice being acute hepatocellular necrosis from paracetamol overdose; or

Dose-independent: arising as a rare complication of therapeutic doses of drugs. Although the frequency of such reactions for any given agent is low they account for the vast majority of hepatic drug reactions encountered in clinical practice.

With increased understanding of the mechanisms of hepatotoxic drug reactions the distinction between dose-dependent and dose-independent mechanisms has become less clear-cut (see below).

TABLE 13.1
Spectrum of hepatic abnormalities from drugs

Acute parenchymal/cholestatic
Hepatic necrosis
Cholestatic hepatitis
Pure cholestasis
Fatty infiltration
Granulomatous infiltration

Chronic parenchymal
Active chronic hepatitis
Hepatic fibrosis and cirrhosis
Hepatic phospholipidosis

Chronic cholestasis
Vanishing bile duct syndrome
Sclerosing cholangitis
Gallstones

Vascular
Budd–Chiari syndrome
Veno-occlusive disease
Sinusoidal lesions – dilatation
                  – peliosis hepatis
                  – perisinusoidal fibrosis
                  – non-cirrhotic portal hypertension
                  – nodular regenerative hyperplasia

Liver tumours
Adenoma
Focal nodular hyperplasia
Hepatocellular carcinoma
Angiosarcoma
Cholangiocarcinoma

Drug metabolism and mechanisms of toxicity

Most therapeutic agents are non-polar, lipid-soluble compounds that cannot readily be eliminated from the body because they are avidly absorbed across renal tubular and bile ductular epithelium. The drug metabolising system converts these substances to polar, water-soluble derivatives that can be excreted efficiently in urine and bile. Some endogenous compounds

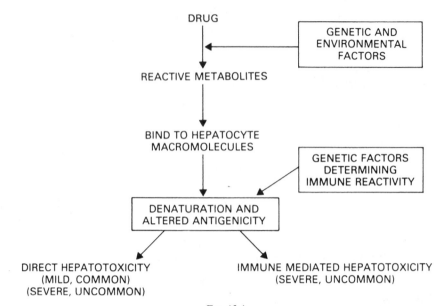

Fig. 13.1
Postulated relationship between direct toxicity and immunological mechanisms in the pathogenesis of adverse hepatic drug reactions.

(e.g. bilirubin and bile acids) are also handled in this way. Drug-metabolising enzymes are found in many tissues of the body but because of its size the liver is quantitatively the most important.

Phase I metabolism and cytochrome P-450 isoenzymes

Drug metabolism takes place in two stages. The first is Phase I metabolism, which involves the creation of a polar group by reactions such as oxidation, reduction, or demethylation. Generally these lead to inactivation of the drug, although sometimes the products of Phase I reactions are more biologically active than the parent compound. Some drugs are converted to chemically reactive metabolites, a process important in the pathogenesis of certain forms of drug-induced liver injury.

The most important site for Phase I reactions is the smooth endoplasmic reticulum of the hepatocyte, corresponding to the microsomal fraction on biochemical cell fractionation. These reactions are mediated by cytochrome P-450-containing mixed function oxidases, so called because they catalyse the biotransformation of a wide variety of substrates. It used to be thought that the substrate specificity of these enzymes was low, but broad. It is now known that cytochrome P-450 exists in multiple isoenzyme forms. Each of these has its own characteristics in terms of specificity for substrates and factors which regulate activity, including genetic factors and response to enzyme inducers and inhibitors (Wrighton and Stevens 1992). The phenotype of an individual, with regard to the quantity and

type of P-450 isoenzymes expressed in the liver, will determine the rate at which a particular compound is metabolised, and the pathway down which this occurs.

A nomenclature has been developed that groups the various P-450 enzymes into families and subfamilies. There are four cytochrome P-450 (CYP) families involved in drug metabolism and members of each of these families share over 40 per cent of their aminoacid sequences in common. Within each family, subfamilies share 70 per cent or more of their aminoacid sequences in common and each subfamily is denoted by a letter, prefixed by a number to denote the family. Individual enzymes in a subfamily are then numbered sequentially (e.g. CYP1A2 is the second member of subfamily 1 of family A) (Wrighton and Stevens 1992; Park *et al.* 1995).

Experimental studies have now identified the isoenzymes responsible for formation of reactive metabolites of many hepatotoxic drugs. This, together with a developing knowledge of factors that modulate activities of these different isoenzymes, is improving our understanding of these reactions. There are considerable differences between mammalian species with respect to the substrate specificity and regulation of P-450 isoenzymes, and it has become clear that extrapolation of data in this area from experimental animal models to man has little or no relevance (Wrighton and Stevens 1992).

Phase II metabolism

The second stage of drug metabolism, Phase II metabolism, involves conjugation of the Phase I metabolite with a variety of substrates, notably glucuronide, sulphate, and glutathione. The resulting polar conjugate is then eliminated in urine or bile; the latter route assumes greater importance as the molecular weight of the conjugate increases over a threshold value of approximately 300.

Although Phase II reactions are generally considered to result in detoxification of drugs, they can in some situations be associated with hepatotoxicity. This applies particularly to some non-steroidal anti-inflammatory drugs (NSAID, q.v.), whose glucuronide conjugates are often chemically unstable, with the potential to break down to derivatives that can cause liver damage.

Mechanisms of hepatotoxicity and determinants of susceptibility

Most hepatotoxic drug metabolites are formed by Phase I metabolism. Normally these highly chemically reactive products are formed in tiny quantities only, and are rapidly detoxified, but if their rate of formation exceeds the liver's capacity for detoxification they will accumulate. Often liver damage is associated with tight binding of such reactive drug metabolites to liver cell components. This is the basis for the mechanism of hepatic damage following paracetamol overdose (q.v.), where the routes for safe biotransformation of the drug become overwhelmed, and metabolism changes to favour production of a hepatotoxic derivative.

Some drugs associated with dose-independent hepatotoxicity also exert their deleterious effects through metabolites (e.g. isoniazid, halothane, chlorpromazine, and tacrine [q.v.]). Symptomatic liver injury from dose-independent reactions is rare (0.1 per cent or less) but the incidence of minor hepatic dysfunction is sometimes 10 per cent or more. The severity of liver involvement might reflect the extent to which a drug is metabolised through hepatotoxic pathways, perhaps regulated by an individual's P-450 isoenzyme profile. This process has been termed metabolic idiosyncrasy.

There is some evidence that susceptibility to liver damage via metabolic idiosyncrasy is governed by both environmental and genetic factors, which regulate the balance between hepatotoxic and non-hepatotoxic pathways of drug metabolism (Fig. 13.1). Thus, the frequency and severity of hepatic damage from isoniazid is greater in patients treated concomitantly with the enzyme-inducing drug rifampicin, which increases the rate of formation of a hepatotoxic isoniazid metabolite (q.v.). In addition, inherited individual differences in capacity for drug acetylation also appear, at least partially, to determine susceptibility to liver damage from isoniazid, whereas variations in hydroxylation capacity may be important in determining susceptibility to other reactions (e.g. perhexiline, chlorpromazine [q.v.]). An environmental manipulation such as chronic alcohol abuse, which increases the rate of formation of a reactive paracetamol metabolite, while impairing safe detoxification through glucuronide and glutathione conjugation, can cause the drug to be hepatotoxic even at therapeutic doses (q.v.).

The activity of some cytochrome P-450 enzymes can be assessed indirectly by use of marker substances that are metabolised exclusively by these isoenzymes. Use of such 'metabolic probes' includes caffeine for CYP1A2, debrisoquine for CYP2D6, and lignocaine for CYP3A4 (Fontana and Watkins 1995). Unfortunately, as yet, application of such technology has not been helpful in predicting patients at risk from hepatic drug reactions. This is probably because additional factors, so far unidentified, are likely to determine whether or not a reactive metabolite will produce liver damage.

It is not known how binding of reactive drug metabolites leads to liver damage, and some of the theories are discussed in the section on paracetamol.

A number of other factors determine susceptibility to liver damage from drugs. The elderly are particularly susceptible to hepatic reactions from NSAID (q.v.). Impaired renal function, leading to accumulation of glucuronide conjugates of NSAIDs may be important, because these conjugates have the potential to degrade to toxic derivatives. The increased susceptibility of old people to cholestatic reactions from flucloxacillin and co-amoxiclav (amoxycillin and clavulanic acid), however, has not been explained. Similarly, patients with AIDS appear to be particularly prone to cholestatic reactions from some antibiotics, especially co-trimoxazole, and the reason for this is not known. Certain drug combinations appear to act synergistically to produce hepatotoxic reactions. Apart from effects of enzyme induction referred to above (e.g. potentiation of isoniazid hepatotoxicity by rifampicin), there are other reactions for which mechanisms remain to be elucidated. These include chronic cholestatic reactions from various drugs when taken together, and the synergistic hepatotoxicity of certain combinations of anticancer agents.

Some drug reactions are accompanied by manifestations suggesting the involvement of a hypersensitivity reaction (e.g. fever, arthralgia, and eosinophilia). There is evidence that some of these (e.g. halothane hepatitis) involve an immunological attack directed against drug-metabolite-altered liver membrane proteins (Fig. 13.1). This is discussed further in the section on Halothane.

Type A or Type B?

Dose-dependent reactions, notably hepatocellular necrosis following overdose of paracetamol, arise as a result of exaggeration of normal properties of the drugs. These reactions can be classified as Type A.

Dose-independent reactions require the interaction of a host susceptibility factor for the reaction to appear, and these reactions can be classified as Type B.

Diagnosis and management of hepatic drug reactions

Diagnosis of dose-dependent liver damage, notably hepatic necrosis from paracetamol overdose, is usually evident, but in occasional cases diagnosis can present a problem when a clear history of drug ingestion is not available, as for instance when a patient is admitted confused or unconscious in liver failure. Dose-independent reactions are often difficult to pinpoint. The spectrum of histological liver injury is broad and the liver has a limited capacity to react to injurious stimuli, so the lesions produced by drugs are often indistinguishable from those due to other causes.

For drug-induced liver injury to be diagnosed the timing of the reaction in relation to start of treatment must be compatible, and it should resolve on drug withdrawal (Benichou 1990). Recommended criteria are summarized in Tables 13.2 and 13.3. Otherwise diagnosis of these reactions is largely by exclusion of other causes. A thorough history and a high index of suspicion are probably the most important aids to diagnosis. Specific enquiry should be made about use of alternative medicines and recreational drugs, because many are hepatotoxic and patients very often will not vouchsafe that they are taking them.

Acute drug-induced hepatitis sometimes resembles acute viral hepatitis; at times so closely that it is often impossible to differentiate it from that condition. Investigations should include serological testing for hepatitis A, B, and C viruses as well as other agents including infectious mononucleosis and cytomegalovirus.

Predominantly cholestatic drug-induced liver lesions have to be differentiated from other forms of obstructive jaundice, particularly extrahepatic biliary obstruction due to stones or carcinoma, and ultrasound and endoscopic cholangiography are helpful in this respect. This is especially the case when recovery after withdrawal of the drug is slow, or in some cases of cholestatic hepatitis where abdominal pain, fever and jaundice can closely mimic ascending cholangitis. Chronic drug-induced cholestasis (q.v.) can be difficult to differentiate from primary biliary cirrhosis.

Many systemic diseases are accompanied by abnormalities of hepatic function, and it is important to differentiate them from reactions to drugs given to treat these conditions.

Marked cholestatic jaundice may accompany severe sepsis and can also complicate the postoperative recovery of patients undergoing surgery for major trauma, who have usually received multiple blood transfusions. Differentiation from hepatocellular injury is based on the demonstration of normal transaminase levels, but cholestatic reactions to therapeutic agents, for example parenteral nutrition, can be difficult to diagnose in this situation. Severe prolonged hypotension can lead to hepatocellular necrosis, and patients with cardiac failure may become jaundiced, with elevations in serum transaminases from hepatic congestion as well as myocardial injury. Intrahepatic cholestasis can sometimes occur in lymphoma in the absence of mechanical obstruction, and gross elevations in hepatic alkaline phosphatase often accompany diffuse infiltrative lesions of the liver, be they neoplastic, infective, or granulomatous.

Other conditions associated with abnormal liver function include inflammatory bowel disease, which is associated with a spectrum of lesions mainly involving the biliary system, manifested by elevations in hepatic alkaline phosphatase. Similarly, rheumatoid arthritis, SLE and polyarteritis nodosa can be complicated by a variety of liver abnormalities that could wrongfully be ascribed to drugs used in their treatment.

There are no histological features specific for drug-induced liver lesions. On liver biopsy, a heavy eosinophilic infiltrate or the presence of granulomata arouses suspicion of a hepatic drug reaction. Marked fatty change is not usually a feature of viral hepatitis, but it can occur in drug-induced hepatitis.

Identifying the agent responsible, especially if the patient is receiving several drugs, can pose problems. If

TABLE 13.2
Diagnosis of hepatotoxic reactions
Onset of symptoms in relation to duration of exposure

	Suggestive	Compatible	Incompatible
Hepatocellular			
Onset from starting drug	5–90 days	<5 or >90 days	started after reaction
Onset after drug discontinued		<15 days	>15 days unless slowly metabolised
Cholestatic			
Onset from starting drug	5–90 days	<5 or >90 days	started after reaction
Onset after drug discontinued		< 1 month	> 1 month

(From Benichou 1990)

alternatives are available, they should be substituted. Occasionally, if no such alternative exists, it may be necessary to resort to diagnostic challenge, but this should not be undertaken lightly because it may precipitate a severe reaction. This is particularly so in cases of acute hepatocellular damage caused by hypersensitivity, and challenge should be avoided in this situation. The mortality from hepatic drug reactions that are clinically manifest (i.e. with jaundice) is approximately 10 per cent, while deaths from cholestatic reactions are less common, and challenge is probably safer. Diagnostic challenge should be carried out under inpatient supervision, starting with subtherapeutic doses of the drug. A patient should never be subjected to this procedure until liver function test abnormalities from the suspected reaction have returned completely to normal. A doubling of transaminase or alkaline phosphatase levels following drug readministration is considered a positive challenge (Benichou 1990).

Monitoring liver function tests during drug therapy

Monitoring liver function tests in the first few weeks of therapy with drugs known to cause hepatic damage by metabolic idiosyncrasy (e.g. pyrazinamide, isoniazid) can give early warning of an impending severe reaction, and timely withdrawal will avoid a potentially life-threatening illness. It is also advisable in patients taking drugs known to lead insidiously to chronic liver disease, although these tests often do not reflect the severity of hepatic disruption (e.g. methotrexate, dantrolene). Monitoring is not helpful in predicting a hypersensitivity reaction. Minor abnormalities (AST less than twice normal) are often self-limiting and progress can be monitored, while elevations greater than threefold should be an indication for drug withdrawal, even if the patient is asymptomatic. This is discussed further in the section on Antituberculous drugs.

Acute parenchymal and cholestatic liver disease

Acute parenchymal liver disease from dose-dependent drug reactions is manifested by acute necrosis of centrilobular hepatocytes. This is further discussed in the section on Paracetamol.

Acute hepatocellular damage from dose-independent reactions can present with a wide spectrum of changes, from mild, asymptomatic elevations in serum transaminases to a severe hepatitic illness with jaundice. Some drugs (salicylates, valproic acid) cause an illness identical to Reye's syndrome, with encephalopathy and microvesicular fatty infiltration of the liver. Minor abnormalities in liver function tests are sometimes self-limiting and resolve with continued drug administration, while in other cases they progress to symptomatic hepatitis. The reasons for such differences in natural history are largely unknown. Hepatitis from some drugs often occurs in the context of a hypersensitivity reaction, with prominent fever, skin rashes, arthralgia, and eosinophilia, while for other agents such features are rarely if ever seen.

Cholestatic reactions from drugs are divided into those in which cholestasis is the only abnormality, with little or no inflammatory component (canalicular cholestasis, pure cholestasis), and those in which there is an associated inflammatory element in portal tracts and hepatocytes (hepatocanalicular cholestasis, cholestatic hepatitis). Pure cholestasis is characteristically associated with synthetic oestrogens and androgens, and can also complicate treatment with rifampicin and fusidic acid, where jaundice is due to competition between bilirubin and the drugs for excretion into the bile. The majority of cholestatic drug reactions fall into the cholestatic hepatitis category, and they are often associated with manifestations of hypersensitivity. Cholestatic hepatitis from some drugs can be accompanied by prominent systemic symptoms, including abdominal pain and fever, which can mimic ascending cholangitis. These

TABLE 13.3
Diagnosis of hepatotoxic reactions
Changes in liver function tests after drug withdrawal

	Suggestive	*Compatible*	*Incompatible*
Hepatocellular			
Decrease in ALT > 50 per cent	<8 days	<1 month	decrease < 50 per cent
Cholestatic			
Decrease in alkaline phosphatase and/or bilirubin	>50 per cent within 6 months	<5 per cent within 6 months	no change

(From Benichou 1990)

drugs include benorylate, captopril, erythromycin, and ranitidine (q.v.)

Analgesics and anti-inflammatory drugs

Paracetamol

Overdose with the analgesic paracetamol is the most important cause of acute toxic hepatitis in the United Kingdom and its popularity as a means of attempted suicide has spread to other parts of the world. Its mechanism of hepatotoxicity has been extensively studied and this has lead to the development of specific therapies.

Clinical features

These are now well known. The patient usually becomes nauseated and vomits in the early stages after overdose, and this is followed by a period of apparent recovery until signs of hepatic necrosis supervene 48–72 hours after ingestion of tablets. Early loss of consciousness is not seen unless the patient has taken a mixed overdose with a sedative, or a combined preparation (co-proxamol) containing paracetamol and the narcotic analgesic propoxyphene.

Hepatic damage almost invariably accompanies the ingestion of 15 g or more, and although the degree of liver damage produced by paracetamol is dose-related in experimental animals (Mitchell *et al.* 1973*a*), there appears to be considerable variation in susceptibility amongst humans (Davis *et al.* 1976). Individuals who abuse alcohol are particularly at risk (see below).

The spectrum of liver injury is wide, ranging from a mild transient hepatitis to fulminant hepatic failure. This severe complication has a very high mortality and should only be treated in a specialist unit. The likelihood of progression to fulminant hepatic failure can be predicted from the INR and other biochemical parameters early in the course of the illness so that patients at risk can be transferred to a specialist unit without delay (Canalese *et al.* 1981; Harrison *et al.* 1990). Late transfer, once hepatic encephalopathy has supervened, is associated with a high mortality from cerebral oedema and coning (Canalese *et al.* 1981). The prognosis of severely affected cases has been greatly improved by liver transplantation, provided the patient is transferred at a sufficiently early stage (Mutimer *et al.* 1994).

The characteristic liver lesion is necrosis of centrilobular hepatocytes. In those who progress to fulminant hepatic failure wide areas of confluent necrosis are seen, often with survival of only a few hepatocytes in the periportal areas (Portmann *et al.* 1975).

Mechanisms

Following therapeutic doses of paracetamol, the majority of the drug is rapidly metabolised to glucuronide and sulphate conjugates, with a small proportion being converted by the cytochrome P-450 isoenzyme CYP3A4 to a highly chemically reactive metabolite of the drug, probably *N*-acetyl-*p*-benzoquinoneimine (NAPQI) (Corcoran *et al.* 1980; Thummel *et al.* 1993). Normally this is a very minor route of metabolism for paracetamol, and such NAPQI as is produced is rapidly detoxified by reduced glutathione (GSH) within liver cells (Fig. 13.2). The resulting glutathione conjugate is further metabolised to yield cysteine and mercapturate conjugates which are excreted in the urine.

Following overdose with paracetamol, pathways for glucuronidation and sulphation of the drug become saturated (Jollow *et al.* 1974; Davis *et al.* 1976; Howie *et al.* 1977). In consequence, metabolism of the drug is diverted towards formation of the NAPQI metabolite; at higher concentrations of paracetamol this reaction is probably catalysed by other P-450 isoenzymes, namely CYP2E1 and CYP1A2 (Raucy *et al.* 1989). Depletion of hepatocellular GSH occurs because hepatic synthesis of this nucleophile cannot keep pace with increased requirements for conjugation (Mitchell *et al.* 1973*b*; Lauterburg and Mitchell 1981*b*), a situation exacerbated by suppression

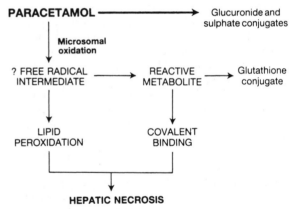

FIG. 13.2
Pathways of paracetamol metabolism
in relation to hepatotoxicity

of glutathione synthesis in the first few hours after ingestion of hepatotoxic quantities of paracetamol (Lauterburg and Mitchell 1982). In consequence the reactive paracetamol metabolite is free to bind to thiol groups in hepatocyte proteins (Jollow *et al.* 1973; Potter *et al.* 1973).

Covalent binding and liver cell necrosis Because covalent binding and hepatic necrosis are closely correlated, it has been inferred that the two events are causally related and that liver damage is due to alkylation of vital macromolecules within the hepatocyte (Yamada 1983). Direct proof is lacking, however, and challenges to the theory have come from studies showing dissociation between hepatic injury and covalent binding, particularly under the influence of certain protective agents

(Labadarios *et al.* 1977; Sakaida *et al.* 1995). Other potential mechanisms must, therefore be considered; probably several are involved.

Lipid peroxidation   Peroxidative damage by chemicals arises from their metabolism by cytochrome P-450-dependent, mixed-function oxidases to free radicals. Free radicals contain an unpaired electron, which makes them highly unstable and chemically reactive. Donation of this electron to oxygen leads to formation of highly reactive superoxide, and when a free radical comes into proximity to unsaturated lipids, as in cell membranes, it initiates a self-perpetuating peroxidative decomposition, with disruption of membrane structure and function (Slater 1984; Poli 1993).

Paracetamol is metabolised to a free radical, which can produce lipid peroxidation *in vitro* and *in vivo* in experimental animals (Rosen *et al.* 1983; Mason and Fischer 1986). It has been postulated that this compound is the precursor of the reactive metabolite NAPQI (Rosen *et al.* 1983).

Hepatic reduced glutathione is important in protecting against peroxidative damage (Kretzschmar 1996); it acts as a cofactor for the enzyme glutathione peroxidase, which reduces lipid hydroperoxides and hydrogen peroxide produced from oxygen free radicals. As a result, glutathione becomes oxidized, and a decrease in the ratio of reduced to oxidized glutathione (GSH : GSSG) is a marker of oxidative stress. Evidence for such a process in response to paracetamol has been obtained by some but not by others (Rosen *et al.* 1983; Lauterburg *et al.* 1984*b*; Smith *et al.* 1984; Jaeschke 1990).

Iron is an important cofactor for generation of lipid peroxides. The iron chelator desferrioxamine protects against liver injury from paracetamol in the experimental situation, which provides further support for the lipid peroxidation hypothesis (Ito *et al.* 1994; Sakaida *et al.* 1995).

Other factors   Paracetamol leads to increased permeability of the inner mitochondrial membrane and inhibits respiration in this organelle (Harris and Hamrick 1993; Donnelly *et al.* 1994). This toxic effect on mitochondria could be due to alkylation or peroxidation by NAPQI and related metabolites, or to increases in intracellular calcium which accompany covalent binding of paracetamol metabolites (Corcoran *et al.* 1988). Treatment of rats with the calcium-channel inhibitor diltiazem protects against liver damage (Deakin *et al.* 1991; Satorres *et al.* 1995).

Electron microscope studies have demonstrated that, following exposure to hepatotoxic doses of paracetamol, abnormal weak areas appear in the hepatocyte membrane; *in vivo* these are manifested as endocytic vacuoles, resulting from invagination of the affected areas of membrane by vascular pressure (Walker *et al.* 1983). In association with these changes, pores appear in the sinusoidal epithelium, allowing leakage of plasma and, later, erythrocytes (Walker *et al.* 1980; Walker *et al.* 1985). Studies using a vascular casting technique have shown profound abnormalities with congestive changes in the centrilobular microvasculature as early as five hours after administration of the drug (Lim *et al.* 1995). Such congestion could contribute to cell death by causing hypoxia, particularly in the centrilobular area where oxygen supply is normally lowest. Prostaglandins, including the prostaglandin E1 analogue misoprostol, exert a protective effect (Lim *et al.* 1995).

Non-parenchymal cells within the liver may also contribute to hepatocyte injury by releasing a range of cytotoxic and pro-inflammatory mediators including free radicals and cytokines (Laskin and Pilaro 1986; Laskin *et al.* 1986). Pretreatment of rats with inhibitors of Kupffer cell function protects against paracetamol hepatotoxicity without apparently influencing the metabolic activation of the drug to the toxic intermediate (Laskin and Pilaro 1986; Goldin *et al.* 1996).

Susceptibility to liver damage from paracetamol

Susceptibility to liver damage from paracetamol is governed mainly by a balance between the capacity for formation of the reactive NAPQI metabolite and capacity for its detoxification with glutathione. Alternative pathways for paracetamol metabolism (glucuronide and sulphate conjugation) are also theoretically important since they may determine how much of the drug is available for metabolic activation.

Experimental studies in animals have shown that the threshold for hepatotoxicity from paracetamol is lowered by pretreatment with enzyme-inducing agents (Mitchell *et al.* 1973*a*). There is good evidence that patients with enzyme induction by chronic alcohol abuse, and also possibly those taking enzyme-inducing anticonvulsants, are particularly susceptible (Bray *et al.* 1991; Bray *et al.* 1992). Conversely, cimetidine, a potent inhibitor of microsomal enzymes, protects against paracetamol-induced hepatic necrosis in experimental animals by inhibiting metabolic activation of the drug (Mitchell *et al.* 1981, 1984). Acute dosing with ethanol (as opposed to chronic consumption) exerts a protective effect via the same mechanism (Sato and Lieber 1981; Sato *et al.* 1981). Neither has found its way into clinical practice for treatment of paracetamol overdose. Pharmacokinetic studies in humans have shown that cimetidine must be given before paracetamol if it is to decrease metabolic activation of paracetamol, which is clearly inappropriate to the clinical situation (Mitchell *et al.* 1984; Vendemiale *et al.* 1987). Acute ingestion of alcohol in volunteers decreased urinary excretion of cysteine and mercapturic acid conjugates of paracetamol, and therefore by inference, formation of its reactive metabolite (Critchley *et al.* 1983). However, very large quantities were needed: the equivalent of approximately eight pints of beer or half a bottle of spirits for a 70 kg human over an 8-hour period.

Measures to enhance glucuronide conjugation of paracetamol protect against liver damage (Hazelton *et al.* 1986), while there is evidence from animal studies that Gunn rats, which have congenital jaundice due to defective glucuronide conjugation, are more susceptible than normal animals to liver damage from paracetamol (Morais and Wells 1989). Human studies in patients with Gilbert's syndrome indicate that they are also potentially at risk because they metabolise less of the drug by glucuronide conjugation and more via the reactive metabolite (Morais *et al.* 1992).

Starvation could also predispose to paracetamol hepatotoxicity by inhibiting glucuronide conjugation through a reduced supply of UDP-glucuronic acid, but a far more important mechanism is via depletion of hepatocellular stores of glutathione (Lauterburg and Mitchell 1981a; Whitcomb and Block 1994). Glutathione depletion also occurs in association with heavy alcohol intake (Lauterburg et al. 1984a; Lauterburg and Velez 1988), and is an important mechanism predisposing chronic alcohol abusers to liver damage from paracetamol (see below).

Young children are probably less susceptible to hepatic damage from paracetamol than adults. This may partly be due to a relative immaturity of microsomal enzymes catalysing formation of the reactive metabolite (Hart and Timbrell 1979), and partly because they have a greater capacity for sulphate conjugation of the drug (Lieh et al. 1984).

Liver damage from therapeutic doses of paracetamol

Alcohol abuse   Chronic alcohol abuse increases susceptibility to liver damage from overdoses of paracetamol and there is now good evidence that heavy drinkers run the risk of hepatotoxicity from the drug even when taken in therapeutic doses (Zimmerman and Maddrey 1995). Ethanol when taken chronically induces the activity of microsomal CYP2E1, which is one of the isoenzymes catalysing the formation of the reactive NAPQI metabolite (Raucy et al. 1989; Perrot et al. 1989). Increased formation of the metabolite is also thought to occur as a result of malnutrition, which decreases glucuronide conjugation of the drug and diverts more of its metabolism via this pathway. Not only is more reactive metabolite formed but also detoxification is impaired in alcohol abusers because tissue glutathione stores are often depleted (Lauterburg and Velez 1988).

The histological lesion, centrilobular necrosis, is identical to that seen after overdose. Hepatic damage is usually seen within the first week of taking the drug, although longer durations have been recorded. In the largest series of patients with this complication 40 per cent had taken less than 4 g per day of the drug and only seven per cent had taken over 15 g, which is the generally accepted threshold limit for hepatotoxicity (Zimmerman and Maddrey 1995).

Extremely high levels of serum transaminases are characteristic, with figures ranging from 3000 to 48 000 IU per litre in more than 90 per cent of cases. Levels in viral hepatitis are usually much more modest (less than 2000 IU per litre) and transaminase levels of over 500 IU per litre in alcoholic hepatitis are virtually unknown.

The mortality from the condition has been reported at 20 per cent. Individuals who drink more than 60 g per day of alcohol should take no more than 2 g of paracetamol a day (Zimmerman and Maddrey 1995). Use of a combined paracetamol–methionine preparation (co-methiamol) should be considered in this and the other high-risk situations listed below, although their effectiveness has not been tested clinically.

Concomitant antituberculous therapy   Reports in the literature of hepatic necrosis complicating therapeutic doses of paracetamol in patients receiving antituberculous therapy indicate that the drug should be used with caution in this group of patients (Murphy et al. 1990; Moulding et al. 1991; Nolan et al.

1994). Isoniazid induces the isoenzyme CYP2E1 and it is presumably by this mechanism that the hepatotoxicity of paracetamol is enhanced (Zand et al. 1993; Nicod et al. 1997).

Other groups potentially at risk   Although there is no direct evidence in the literature, it would seem sensible to use paracetamol with caution in individuals taking enzyme-inducing anticonvulsants and also those with malnutrition, including eating disorders, where low glutathione stores could put them at risk.

Patients with HIV infection may be particularly vulnerable, and a case report (Shriner and Goetz 1992) describes acute hepatocellular necrosis in such a patient after 3.3 g paracetamol taken over 36 hours. The patient was also being treated with zidovudine and it was postulated that this drug enhanced paracetamol toxicity by inhibiting its glucuronidation; low reserves of hepatic glutathione associated with malnutrition could also have contributed. A single report (Kwan et al. 1995) describes the development of abnormal liver function tests in a healthy volunteer during the course of a pharmacokinetic study of warfarin and paracetamol in a daily dose of 4 g. No risk factors could be identified.

Two case reports (Johnson and Tolman 1977; Bonkowsky et al. 1978) have implicated paracetamol in doses of 3–4 g per day as a cause of active chronic hepatitis. A recent report describes chronic granulomatous liver disease progressing to cirrhosis attributed to therapeutic doses of paracetamol; each time the drug was taken liver function tests deteriorated (Lindgren et al. 1997). The same authors also report a case of pure cholestasis with no parenchymal injury, occurring after 4 g paracetamol daily for a week; the patient made a full recovery after about 5 months.

Therapy for paracetamol overdose

Treatments for paracetamol overdose are centred on administration of compounds which boost hepatocellular stores of glutathione (Davis 1986). The compounds used clinically are N-acetylcysteine and methionine (Vale and Proudfoot 1995). The former is preferred because its conversion to glutathione *in vivo* involves fewer enzymatic stages than methionine, and also it can be given intravenously, which is an advantage in patients who usually have nausea and vomiting. A combined preparation of paracetamol with methionine (co-methiamol) has been marketed with the aim of ensuring that glutathione stores keep pace with requirements for detoxification of the reactive paracetamol metabolite. It is not widely used because of its cost, but it should be considered in high-risk patients (see above).

Other glutathione precursors, particularly cysteamine (Prescott et al. 1976) have been used in the past but have now been discontinued because of unpleasant adverse effects. Other compounds, such as S-adenosyl methionine are protective in experimental animals but have not as yet found their way into clinical use (Bray et al. 1992).

A number of other compounds including vitamin E and ascorbic acid have been shown to exert some protective effect in experimental animals (Davis 1986). Propylthiouracil is also effective experimentally; hypothyroidism impairs oxidative

TABLE 13.4
Dosage schedules for methionine and N-acetylcysteine

Methionine	2.5g orally 4 hourly for 16 hours
N-*acetylcysteine*	*intravenously:* 150 mg per kg in 5% dextrose over 15 minutes Followed by 50 mg per kg in 5% dextrose over 4 hours Followed by 100 mg per kg in 5% dextrose over 16 hours *orally:* Loading dose of 140 mg per kg Followed by 70 mg per kg 4-hourly for 68 hours (total of 17 doses)

drug metabolism but the effect of propylthiouracil is greater than would be expected from its effect on the thyroid alone. It is thought that it may act as a surrogate glutathione by conjugating with the reactive metabolite (Yamada and Kaplowitz 1980).

Clinical use of protective agents

A high proportion of patients presenting after a paracetamol overdose will not have absorbed enough of the drug to put them at risk, but clinical history is unreliable and the prognosis cannot be predicted from clinical features because the onset of liver damage is delayed. A useful guide to the outcome can be obtained from an estimate of the plasma concentration of the drug at a known time after overdose (Vale and Proudfoot 1995). Development of these so-called 'treatment lines' was based on early clinical studies of untreated patients before effective therapies were available. The nomogram most commonly in use in the United Kingdom is the so called 'two hundred line'; patients with plasma levels above a line joining the plasma concentration of 200 mg per litre at 4 hours and 30 mg per litre at 15 hours on a semilogarithmic plot have a high risk of developing significant liver damage, and should be treated with protective agents. Chronic alcohol abusers are particularly susceptible and it has been recommended that the line be lowered in this group of patients to 100 mg per litre at 4 hours and 15 mg per litre at 15 hours. Other groups of patients who should also probably be treated as at high risk include those taking enzyme-inducing drugs such as anticonvulsants and antituberculous agents, and also those with eating disorders, since starvation puts them at risk by depleting hepatic glutathione levels.

Treatment regimens with methionine and acetylcysteine are shown in Table 13.4.

Since its introduction as a protective agent in 1979, occasional adverse effects of *N*-acetylcysteine have been reported (Mant *et al.* 1984). The commonest of these has been an urticarial rash with occasional angioedema, bronchospasm, and hypotension. Reactions usually start 20–60 minutes after starting the infusion and are readily controlled by stopping the drug and giving symptomatic treatment with antihistamines. Similar but more severe reactions, which can be fatal, have accompanied accidental overdose with the compound as a result of incorrect dosage calculations.

The conventionally held view is that protective agents are only effective in preventing liver disease from paracetamol if given within the first 10–15 hours after overdose. This correlates with the results of experimental studies showing little efficacy once paracetamol metabolites have become covalently bound within the liver. However, it has been shown that acetylcysteine can be beneficial even if administration is delayed for between 15–30 hours after overdose, with a lower mortality and a lower rate of progression to grade 3 and 4 encephalopathy (Keays *et al.* 1991). This is almost certainly mediated by a beneficial effect of acetylcysteine on circulatory haemodynamics rather than any effect on paracetamol metabolism (Harrison *et al.* 1991).

Dextropropoxyphene

Cholestatic hepatitis is a rare but well-documented complication of dextropropoxyphene. It characteristically presents with jaundice, abdominal pain, and rigors and may be mistaken for gallstone disease (Bassendine *et al.* 1986; Rosenberg *et al.* 1993).

Non-steroidal anti-inflammatory drugs

Although symptomatic liver damage from NSAID is uncommon (estimated incidence between 0.001–0.05 per cent) (Walker 1997) these reactions are clinically important because of the very widespread use of these drugs. Minor elevations in serum transaminases in otherwise asymptomatic patients are much more common (up to 15 per cent), the frequency differing according to the individual agent (Boelsterli *et al.* 1995).

The pattern of liver injury is variable, depending on the drug. Thus indomethacin and diclofenac cause hepatocellular necrosis (Banks *et al.* 1995), whereas sulindac produces a more cholestatic reaction with or without hepatitis (Tarazi *et al.* 1993). The clinical features are also different for the various drugs; sulindac-induced liver injury is associated with manifestations of hypersensitivity, whereas reactions from diclofenac generally are not.

Diclofenac

Minor elevations in serum transaminases (less than three times normal) are seen in 15 per cent of patients taking diclofenac (Helfgott *et al.* 1990). More severe liver lesions are much less frequent, probably of the order of 0.01 per cent. In a recent analysis of 180 cases reported to the United States Food and Drug Administration there was a predominance of females (79 per cent, which was disproportionate in relation to the user population), and the elderly (71 per cent at 60 years of age or older).

There was also predominance (77 per cent) of patients with osteoarthritis (Banks *et al.* 1995).

Most cases present within 3 months of starting treatment, although longer latent intervals have been described. Typically patients present with anorexia, nausea, abdominal pain, and jaundice. Features of hypersensitivity are uncommon although they have been reported.

The pattern of liver injury is usually acute hepatocellular necrosis or cholestatic hepatitis. Histologically there is necrosis of centrilobular hepatocytes with some periportal inflammation. Occasional cases of active chronic hepatitis have been described (Purcell *et al.* 1991; Scully *et al.* 1993; Banks *et al.* 1995).

Mechanisms   The mechanism of diclofenac hepatotoxicity is not known but is probably metabolic idiosyncrasy. The drug is toxic to hepatocytes *in vitro* and inhibition of its metabolism has a protective effect (Schmitz *et al.* 1992). While diclofenac, in common with many NSAID, forms reactive derivatives via oxidative metabolism, the relevance of these to hepatotoxicity in man is controversial. More attention has focused on pathways for glucuronide conjugation of these drugs (Boelsterli *et al.* 1995). Acyl glucuronides are frequently unstable under physiological conditions, and can convert to reactive metabolites with the potential to bind to liver cell proteins. Such binding has been demonstrated with diclofenac in isolated hepatocytes and the process can be inhibited by inclusion of a specific UDP-glucuronyl transferase inhibitor (Kretz-Rommel and Boelsterli 1993).

Glucuronide conjugates of NSAID are excreted primarily in the urine and their elimination will therefore be reduced if renal function is impaired. Accumulation of glucuronide conjugates could increase the potential for toxicity and this may explain the increased susceptibility of the elderly (Boelsterli *et al.* 1995).

A few cases of diclofenac hepatitis associated with features of hypersensitivity have been reported, and to explain these a mechanism involving immune sensitization to diclofenac metabolite-altered liver antigens has been proposed (Banks *et al.* 1995).

Sulindac

Of the currently available NSAID, sulindac has the highest propensity to cause hepatotoxicity (Walker 1997). In a retrospective survey of general practice prescriptions for NSAID in the UK involving over 600 000 patients the incidence of acute liver injury from sulindac was 25 times greater than for the overall NSAID group (Garcia *et al.* 1994). Analysis of reports of NSAID-induced liver injury submitted to the FDA supports this; although sulindac accounted for only 10 per cent of all NSAID prescriptions it was listed in 25 per cent of reports of hepatotoxicity (Tarazi *et al.* 1993).

The clinical presentation of sulindac hepatotoxicity is generally associated with manifestations of hypersensitivity, with associated fever and rash and sometimes the Stevens–Johnson syndrome (Klein and Khan 1983). Prompt relapse on rechallenge with the drug is characteristic. In a recent series the female-to-male ratio was 3.5 to 1, and the pattern of liver injury was pure cholestasis or cholestatic hepatitis in two-thirds. Eosinophilia and other features of hypersensitivity were more common in patients with these histological changes. Onset of illness is usually in less than 8 weeks and sometimes within 4 weeks of starting therapy (Tarazi *et al.* 1993).

Piroxicam

Minor elevations in serum transaminases have been recorded in one to two per cent of individuals. More severe hepatic injury appears to be rare and no accurate estimate of its frequency is available (Jick *et al.* 1992). Acute hepatic necrosis (Lee *et al.* 1986; Planas *et al.* 1990) and cholestatic hepatitis (Hepps *et al.* 1991) have been described and some cases have been fatal.

Naproxen

Hepatotoxicity from naproxen is rare. The pattern may be cholestatic or hepatocellular (Bass 1974; Andrejak *et al.* 1987; Manoukian and Carson 1996). Jaundice occurs 1–12 weeks after starting treatment. The mechanism is unknown although clinical features of hypersensitivity in one case suggested the involvement of immune mechanisms.

Ibuprofen

Liver damage from ibuprofen is rare with only sporadic reports in the literature (Royer *et al.* 1984; Friis and Andreasen 1992). Liver injury usually develops within 3 weeks of starting treatment and hepatic damage is often associated with features of hypersensitivity and sometimes with the Stevens–Johnson syndrome (Sternlieb and Robinson 1978). Most of the reported liver lesions were acute hepatocellular necrosis, but cholestasis has also been reported. This includes one case of severe chronic cholestasis associated with 'ductopenia' (vanishing bile duct syndrome) after 3 weeks treatment (Alam Ferrell *et al.* 1996).

Indomethacin

Liver injury from indomethacin is rare and no estimates of its frequency are available. Less than 5 per cent of reported adverse effects of the drug have involved hepatic damage (Lewis 1984).

Liver injury occurs between 1 and 7 months of starting

treatment. Hepatocellular necrosis, cholestasis, and microvesicular steatosis have been described (Boelsterli *et al.* 1995).

Etodolac

Etodolac is one of the newer NSAID and has been considered relatively safe with only a small incidence of a reversible rise in transaminases or bilirubin. Recently, however, a case of fulminant hepatic failure complicating treatment with this drug has been reported (Mabee *et al.* 1995).

Nabumetone

This recently introduced NSAID is a pro-drug with a reportedly low incidence of gastrointestinal adverse effects. Data on hepatic toxicity are scanty; premarketing testing in the USA revealed transaminase abnormalities in 0.7 per cent of 1677 patients (Bernhard 1992).

Tolmetin

Elevated serum transaminase levels have been reported in up to five per cent of patients receiving this drug (O'Brien 1983). A case of multisystem failure associated with microvesicular steatosis of the liver has been reported in a 15-year-old girl with Still's disease; blood levels of the drug at autopsy were 20 times the normal therapeutic level (Shaw and Anderson 1991).

Clometacin

This analgesic is widely used in France, and, in contrast to other NSAID, the commonest pattern of liver injury is active chronic hepatitis (Pessayre *et al.* 1981). Liver disease becomes apparent after a latent period of 6 months to several years; it regresses on withdrawal of the drug but progresses to cirrhosis if it is continued.

Females are characteristically affected more frequently than males; in one study the female predominance was 29 to one (Islam *et al.* 1989). The clinical syndrome resembles autoimmune active chronic hepatitis with high levels of immunoglobulins and antinuclear antibodies. Manifestations of hypersensitivity with skin rash and eosinophilia are also sometimes found.

Salicylates

Elevations in serum transaminases have been reported in up to two-thirds of patients receiving high doses of salicylates for connective tissue disorders (Prescott 1980). Patients with rheumatoid arthritis and SLE appear to be the most susceptible, with a reported incidence in the range of 20–70 per cent (Zimmerman 1981). Low serum albumin levels appear to be a risk factor (Gitlin 1980). Most patients have been young, and females are affected more than males; recovery is prompt

if the drug is stopped and clinically most patients are asymptomatic, although symptomatic liver injury has been reported (Benson 1983).

Liver biopsies show mild acute hepatocellular injury with focal necrosis. Liver injury is dose dependent and is rarely seen with circulating levels of the drug below 150 mg per litre (Zimmerman 1981).

The mechanism of the hepatotoxicity is not known. The drug exerts dose-dependent toxicity on isolated hepatocytes at concentrations within the therapeutic range (Tolman *et al.* 1978).

Reye's syndrome from aspirin

This condition is characterized by acute microvesicular hepatic steatosis and hyperammonaemia in infants and young children; it leads to fulminant hepatic failure, which is frequently fatal. Numerous aetiologies have been proposed but salicylates and the anticonvulsant valproic acid (q.v.) have been causally incriminated.

Reye's syndrome associated with aspirin is most commonly associated with use of the drug in the prodromal phases of viral infections, although it has also been reported in children taking it for connective tissue disorders (Sillanpaa *et al.* 1975; Daum *et al.* 1976). Case–control studies have shown a sevenfold increase in risk from Reye's syndrome from aspirin in a dose of 15 mg per kg per day (Pinsky *et al.* 1988). This effectively means that there is no safe dose for children in the prodrome of viral infections, and the use of paediatric aspirin preparations for this purpose has now been discontinued.

Gold salts

These preparations have been associated with cholestatic jaundice in a number of reports. Jaundice generally appears after a second or subsequent dose and there is usually associated eosinophilia, skin rashes, lymphadenopathy, and other manifestations of hypersensitivity (Pessayre *et al.* 1979; Smith 1986; Hansen *et al.* 1991). The liver lesion characteristically improves on withdrawal of the drug although this improvement may be slow.

Patients with HLA DR3 are particularly prone to all types of adverse effects from gold salts (skin rashes, proteinuria, and liver damage), while the lowest frequency of adverse effects was seen in patients with DR7 (Gran *et al.* 1983). However, the HLA type does not predict the organ targeted by the adverse reaction.

Penicillamine

Cholestasis or cholestatic hepatitis from penicillamine is usually accompanied by manifestations of hypersensitivity (Devogelaer *et al.* 1985; Gefel *et al.* 1985; Kumar *et al.* 1985). While the liver lesion usually improves promptly on withdrawal of therapy, prolonged intra-hepatic cholestasis has been described (Jacobs *et al.* 1994).

Allopurinol

Hepatic necrosis from allopurinol occurs as part of a generalized hypersensitivity syndrome (Al Kawas *et al.* 1981). Typical patients are middle-aged men with poor renal function taking high doses of the drug (Arellano and Sacristan 1993). Deaths from fulminant hepatic failure have been reported (Butler *et al.* 1977). Granu-lomatous hepatitis has also been described (Medline *et al.* 1978; Swank *et al.* 1978; Stricker *et al.* 1989). Fibrin-ring granulomata, usually only seen in association with Q fever, have been described in one report (Vanderstigel *et al.* 1986) but others have not confirmed this association (Stricker *et al.* 1989).

Anaesthetic agents

Halothane

Although halothane is now little used, studies on liver damage from the drug have provided valuable infor-mation on the mechanisms of hepatic drug reactions, particularly immunological aspects.

Exposure to halothane may be complicated by a wide spectrum of liver injury (Benjamin *et al.* 1985). Minor, transient elevations in serum transaminases have been documented by screening studies in up to 20 per cent of patients repeatedly anaesthetized with this agent (Trowell *et al.* 1975; Wright *et al.* 1975). At the other end of the spectrum is severe hepatocellular necrosis leading to fulminant hepatic failure with a high mortality. This complication is so rare that accurate estimates of its frequency cannot be made; the incidence probably lies between one in 22 000 and one in 35 000 halothane anaesthetics (National Halothane Study 1966)

The clinical course is characteristic (Neuberger and Williams 1984). Sometimes the reactions begin with fever, and unexplained postoperative fever may have been recorded after previous anaesthetics. Eosinophilia is seen in a variable proportion of cases and microsomal antibodies appear transiently more frequently than in acute viral hepatitis.

Severe hepatic damage is more common in patients who have been exposed to halothane on more than one occasion, particularly if the interval between exposures is short (National Halothane Study 1966; Mushin *et al.* 1971; Inman and Mushin 1974). Current advice is to avoid halothane if it has been used within 3 months, or if there is a history of previous reactions, particularly fever or jaundice (CSM 1997). However, halothane hepatitis has been reported following re-exposure to the drug after an interval of many years (Lee *et al.* 1988; Martin *et al.* 1992) and many anaesthetists now do not use it at all in adults.

It used to be thought that children did not develop this complication but there are a few well-documented cases in the world literature (Kenna *et al.* 1987a). In contrast to the adult cases, however, the number of reports implicat-ing children is extremely small.

Hepatitis is also a rare but well-documented compli-cation of occupational exposure to halothane in an-aesthetists and laboratory workers. The characteristic story is of recurrent episodes of hepatitis, each corres-ponding to a return to work and exposure to the drug (Klatskin and Kimberg 1969; Keiding *et al.* 1984; Suther-land and Smith 1992).

Mechanisms

Halothane hepatotoxicity has been extensively studied and there is evidence that both direct hepatotoxicity and immune mechanisms are involved. Both involve the production of chemically reactive halothane metabolites produced by different metabolic pathways (Fig. 13.3).

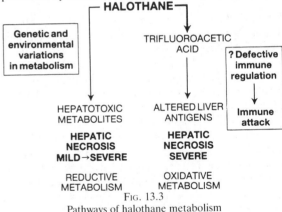

Fig. 13.3
Pathways of halothane metabolism in relation to hepatotoxicity

Direct toxicity   Experimental studies have demon-strated that halothane is directly hepatotoxic to a num-ber of animal species. In rat, mouse, and guinea-pig models the drug can produce dose-related necrosis of centrilobular hepatocytes. This is associated with tight covalent binding of a reactive halothane metabolite to microsomal proteins in the centrilobular region (van Dyke and Gandolfi 1974; van Dyke and Wood 1975). The first animal model for direct halothane hepatotox-icity was in the rat, and for hepatic damage to occur it was necessary to stimulate the reductive pathway of halothane metabolism preferentially (Brown and Sipes 1977). This involves removal of one of the fluorine atoms from the halothane molecule with the formation of a reactive difluoro intermediate. In this rat model, hepatic damage was not seen when halothane metabolism occurred via the oxidative pathway, which is the major route for biotransformation of the drug (Jee *et al.* 1980).

The guinea-pig is particularly susceptible to halothane-induced liver damage and is now the preferred species for its study (Lind *et al.* 1994; Lind and Gandolfi 1997). Hepatic necrosis occurs after exposure to subanaesthetic doses of the drug. Hepatic glutathione exerts a protective effect and diminishes intrahepatic binding of reactive halothane metabolites (Lind *et al.* 1990). In contrast to the rat model, hepatotoxicity of halothane in the guinea-pig is associated exclusively with oxidative metabolism of the drug (Lind *et al.* 1989). Administration of dimethyl sulphoxide (DMSO) protects against liver damage even when its administration is delayed. DMSO does not effect the generation or binding of halothane metabolites and its mode of action is not known.

The relevance of these studies to the clinical situation in man is not known. Both oxidative and reductive metabolism of halothane occurs in humans, although the former pathway greatly predominates (Sharp *et al.* 1979). It is tempting to speculate that individual differences in the generation of hepatotoxic halothane metabolites could form the basis for individual susceptibility to liver damage from the drug. However, as yet there are no studies to confirm or refute this hypothesis.

Immune mechanisms   Many clinical features of halothane hepatitis suggest that immune mechanisms are involved, and there is now a body of experimental evidence in support of this. A number of studies have demonstrated that patients with severe hepatic necrosis from halothane have humoral and cell-mediated immunity directed against hepatocyte components which have been altered by a halothane metabolite (Vergani *et al.* 1980; Kenna *et al.* 1987c). Evidence for such sensitization is not seen simply as a result of acute liver damage or halothane anaesthesia *per se* and does not occur in patients with only minor damage from the drug.

There is now considerable evidence that liver antigens become altered by metabolites produced by the oxidative pathway of halothane metabolism (Vergani *et al.* 1980). This pathway is catalysed by the microsomal mixed-function oxidase CYP2E1 with formation of trifluoroacetic acid (TFA), the major metabolite of halothane (Kharasch *et al.* 1996). A reactive precursor of TFA binds to liver membrane proteins, and the TFA-altered products would have the potential to stimulate an immune reaction if they appeared immunologically 'foreign' (Martin *et al.* 1993; Smith *et al.* 1993; Kitteringham *et al.* 1995). To be accessible to the immune system such altered determinants would have to be expressed on the cell surface membrane, and studies with isolated hepatocytes have shown this to be the case (Ilyin *et al.* 1994).

TFA–liver protein adducts are created in all individuals exposed to halothane, yet only those who develop severe halothane hepatitis have antibodies to them (Kenna *et al.* 1987b; Kenna *et al.* 1988; Sakaguchi *et al.* 1994). This implies that the majority of individuals are immunologically tolerant of these altered antigens, perhaps as a result of prior exposure to an endogenous compound with a similar configuration (Frey *et al.* 1995; Gut *et al.* 1995).

Enflurane

A review of 24 cases of suspected enflurane hepatitis suggested a limited potential for the drug to produce liver damage with centrilobular necrosis (Lewis *et al.* 1983b). In a subsequent more detailed study of 88 patients there were sufficient data to incriminate enflurane in only 15 cases, so it is a very rare event (Eger *et al.* 1986). Its frequency has been estimated to be in the region of one in 800 000 exposures to the drug. Isolated case reports continue to appear, and apparent cross-sensitization with halothane has also been described (Sigurdsson *et al.* 1985; Schneider 1996; Reeves 1997).

Enflurane is metabolised to TFA derivatives which, like those from halothane, can lead to the generation of altered antigens. These react with antibodies directed against halothane-metabolite-altered liver components (Christ *et al.* 1988a,b; Laster *et al.* 1997).

Isoflurane

Although isoflurane can produce hepatic necrosis in rats (van Dyke 1982), there is little evidence that it causes liver damage in man. Occasional case reports suggest that it can lead to hepatitis, although very rarely (Carrigan and Straughen 1987; Sinha *et al.* 1996). Metabolism in humans is extremely limited and in experimental animals the drug has far less capacity than either halothane or enflurane to produce altered liver proteins. An expert committee reviewed 45 cases of suspected isoflurane hepatitis but could not positively exclude alternative aetiologies in any of them (Stoelting *et al.* 1987).

Antibiotics

Erythromycin

Jaundice due to cholestatic hepatitis from erythromycin is most frequently associated with the estolate preparation (Braun 1969; Ginsburg 1986), although well-documented cases have been reported complicating treatment with erythromycin ethylsuccinate, erythromycin propionate, and the intravenous lactobionate formulation (Pessayre et al. 1976; Bachman et al. 1982; Keeffe et al. 1982; Gholson and Warren 1990). The latter, unusually, led to fulminant hepatic failure. Epidemiological studies in the United Kingdom and USA have provided widely differing estimates of the frequency of symptomatic liver reactions to erythromycin preparations, from 0.2 to 14 per 100 000 prescriptions in current users of erythromycin preparations (Carson et al. 1993; Derby et al. 1993b; Perez and Garcia 1993). Asymptomatic abnormalities in liver function tests occur more frequently, in up to 15 per cent.

Jaundice usually appears on day 7–14 of treatment and is frequently accompanied by severe colicky abdominal pain, which may mimic ascending cholangitis. Histologically the predominant abnormality is cholestasis, but hepatocellular necrosis is almost invariably present in varying degree (Zafrani et al. 1979).

Pseudotumours of the liver simulating malignancy have been reported in a patient taking erythromycin estolate. Histologically, eosinophilic infiltration and necrosis were the only abnormalities, and when the drug was stopped the abnormalities resolved (Rigauts et al. 1988).

A high (60 per cent) incidence of eosinophilia and a prompt relapse of hepatitis on rechallenge with the drug are consistent with an allergic basis for erythromycin-induced liver injury. Erythromycin is metabolised to unstable derivatives with the capacity to bind to hepatic proteins, and these could form the target for an immunological attack (Pessayre et al. 1985). On the other hand, a direct toxic potential for the drug has been shown by its capacity to produce a dose-related impairment of bile flow and BSP clearance in isolated rat liver preparations (Kendler et al. 1972). In addition, toxic effects can be seen in isolated hepatocytes incubated with therapeutic concentrations of erythromycin estolate, while much higher concentrations of other erythromycin preparations are needed to produce the same effect (Zimmerman et al. 1973).

Cross-hepatotoxicity between erythromycin and amoxycillin clavulanic acid has been reported (Horsmans and Geubel 1994).

A case of prolonged cholestasis caused by erythromycin in a patient already taking chlorpropramide has been described (Geubel et al. 1988). Histologically there was disappearance of small intrahepatic bile ducts. Since both erythromycin and chlorpropramide can produce cholestasis it has been suggested that by giving the two drugs together this effect was potentiated.

Penicillin

Hepatic damage from penicillin itself is extremely uncommon and occurs as part of a generalized hypersensitivity reaction. In contrast, liver damage from semi-synthetic penicillins is well documented.

Flucloxacillin

Flucloxacillin usually produces cholestasis with little or no hepatitis (Eckstein et al. 1993), although acute hepatocellular necrosis has also been reported. The reaction may not appear until after the antibiotic has been stopped (Miros et al. 1990). A worrying feature is the high proportion of patients who develop a chronic cholestatic syndrome with loss of small interlobular bile ducts (Turner et al. 1989; Davies et al. 1994).

The frequency of the complication has been calculated at between one in 11 000 to one in 30 000 prescriptions (Olsson et al. 1992; Devereaux et al. 1995). Increasing age and a prolonged duration of flucloxacillin treatment are risk factors for the development of liver damage from flucloxacillin. Fairley and colleagues calculated that patients aged over 55 years are 18.61 times more likely to develop this complication than those under the age of the 30, while the odds ratio for patients given the drug for over 14 days was 7.13 compared with those treated for a shorter period of time (Fairley et al. 1993). It has been recommended that flucloxacillin should not be prescribed for longer than one week unless *Staphylococcus aureus* has been identified as a pathogen.

The related drugs cloxacillin and oxacillin can produce a similar clinical picture with cholestatic hepatitis (Olsson et al. 1992).

Amoxycillin–clavulanic acid

Amoxycillin has little or no potential to cause liver damage but there are now several reports of jaundice when the drug is combined with clavulanic acid (co-amoxiclav, Augmentin) (Verhamme et al. 1989; Larrey et al. 1992a; Habior et al. 1994). The clavulanic acid rather than the penicillin moiety appears to be responsible for the reaction.

Co-amoxiclav-induced hepatic damage is manifested as a cholestatic hepatitis with lesions of the interlobular bile ducts (Hautekeete *et al.* 1995*a*; Ryley *et al.* 1995), and onset may be delayed for up to 4 weeks after stopping the drug. There may be associated signs of hypersensitivity. While the majority of patients affected make a complete recovery within 4 months, a few may progress to a chronic cholestatic syndrome with loss of small interlobular bile ducts (Ryley *et al.* 1995). Granulomatous hepatitis has also been described (Silvain *et al.* 1992).

The frequency of liver damage from co-amoxiclav has been calculated at between 1–1.7 in 10 000 (Larrey *et al.* 1992*a*; Garcia *et al.* 1996). Risk factors are increasing age and male sex (Thomson *et al.* 1995). Patients over the age of 55 years are 16 times more likely to develop liver damage from co-amoxiclav than those under the age of 30, and the complication occurs two to four times more frequently in men than women. In contrast to flucloxacillin jaundice, duration of treatment does not appear to be a risk factor.

A very similar pattern of liver injury has been reported complicating treatment with ticarcillin–clavulanic acid (Sweet and Jones 1995).

Cephalosporins

Liver damage from cephalosporins is extremely rare but occasional cases have been reported complicating use of first-generation drugs. Minor reversible abnormalities in liver function tests can occur in up to seven per cent of patients treated with third-generation agents but no cases of symptomatic hepatitis have to date been reported (Westphal *et al.* 1994).

Sulphonamides

Hepatic damage complicating treatment with sulphonamides occurs with an estimated frequency of 0.6 per cent, although minor abnormalities in liver function tests in asymptomatic patients can occur in up to 10 per cent (Westphal *et al.* 1994). Acute hepatic necrosis, cholestasis, or cholestatic hepatitis can be seen (VanOmmen 1974; Weinstein and Weinstein 1974).

The mechanisms underlying this reaction are not known. The frequent association of liver damage with manifestations of hypersensitivity suggests the involvement of immune mechanisms. It has also been shown that sulphonamides can undergo metabolic activation to produce cell damaging reactive metabolites (Shear *et al.* 1986). Sulphonamide reactions of all types are more common in slow acetylators of the drug (Rieder *et al.* 1991).

Co-trimoxazole and trimethoprim

Cholestatic jaundice is a rare complication of co-trimox-azole therapy and is often associated with manifestations of hypersensitivity (Berg and Daniel 1987). In one reported case there was prolonged cholestasis and associated phospholipid infiltration of hepatocytes (Munoz *et al.* 1990). Co-trimoxazole is one of the causes of chronic cholestasis with the 'vanishing bile duct' syndrome (Yao *et al.* 1997)

The estimated frequency is around five per 10 000 (Jick and Derby 1995), but is substantially higher amongst patients with AIDS (Wofsy 1987; Medina *et al.* 1990).

Occasional cases of cholestatic jaundice from trimethoprim have been reported (Tanner 1986; Singh and Singh 1991; Vial *et al.* 1997). Lindgren and colleagues surveyed all adverse hepatic reaction to trimethoprim over a 10-year period and estimated the incidence at 1 in 1.36 million defined daily doses of the drug (Lindgren and Olsson 1994).

Fluoroquinolones

The related fluoroquinolones ciprofloxacin, ofloxacin, and pefloxacin can lead to minor abnormalities in serum transaminases in otherwise asymptomatic patients. Severe hepatic dysfunction is uncommon (Jick *et al.* 1993; Jick 1997). Ciprofloxacin can rarely cause an acute cholestatic hepatitis, and a case of acute hepatic necrosis from ofloxacin has been reported. Both drugs can also cause cholestasis with no associated inflammatory component (Grassmick *et al.* 1992; Sherman and Beizer 1994; Hautekeete *et al.* 1995*c*; Labowitz and Silverman 1997).

Tetracyclines

Hepatic damage from oral tetracyclines is not a clinical problem but liver damage from intravenously administered preparations is well documented. Now that these are seldom, if ever used, the problem is largely of historical interest. Most of the reported cases were in pregnant women given large doses for pyelonephritis (Whalley *et al.* 1974). Tetracycline is excreted predominantly in the urine and its plasma clearance is impaired in patients with renal failure.

The histological lesion is identical with the acute fatty liver of pregnancy, with central and midzonal necrosis and prominent infiltration with fine intracytoplasmic fat droplets (Davis and Kaufman 1966). Hepatic encephalopathy and death from fulminant hepatic failure were common. An identical lesion can be reproduced in animals. The fatty infiltration appears to be caused by impaired mitochondrial respiration (Fromenty and Pessayre 1995).

Minocycline

Minocycline, a member of the tetracycline group, can also cause liver damage, sometimes leading to fulminant hepatic failure (Davies and Kersey 1989; Min *et al.* 1992), but the pattern is different from that seen with tetracycline itself. Skin rashes and eosinophilia are frequent accompaniments, and in one reported case fatty infiltration was macrovesicular (Burette *et al.* 1984). Acute hepatocellular necrosis, and sometimes active chronic hepatitis are also increasingly being reported, often in association with a lupus-like syndrome (Gough *et al.* 1996; Malcolm *et al.* 1996; Golstein *et al.* 1997).

Nitrofurantoin

Cholestatic hepatitis, usually accompanied by systemic features of hypersensitivity, generally appears between 1–5 weeks after starting nitrofurantoin (Bhagwat and Warren 1969; Engel *et al.* 1975; Mulberg and Bell 1993). Hepatic damage accompanied by neurotoxicity from the drug has been reported, as has granulomatous hepatitis (Sippel and Agger 1981). One unusual case reported the development of cholestatic hepatitis in a teenager after drinking milk from a cow that was being treated with this drug (Berry *et al.* 1984).

Nitrofurantoin has also been reported as the cause of a condition resembling autoimmune active chronic hepatitis, with elevated IgG and antinuclear and anti-smooth-muscle antibodies (Black *et al.* 1980; Yeong *et al.* 1990). Most patients have been female and the disease appeared after at least 6 months of treatment with the drug; sometimes it had been taken for years. The liver lesion can regress if the drug is stopped but progresses to cirrhosis if it is continued (Sharp *et al.* 1980).

Fusidic acid

This antibiotic competes with conjugated bilirubin at the biliary canaliculus for excretion into the bile. Its use in patients with severe sepsis can be complicated by deep jaundice (Humble *et al.* 1980; Kutty *et al.* 1987); other liver function tests are disturbed little or not at all. The reaction probably reflects an accentuation by the drug of the tendency to cholestasis produced by sepsis.

Antifungal agents

Ketoconazole

Ketoconazole can produce asymptomatic abnormalities in liver function tests in 5–10 per cent of individuals receiving it, although in a recent study of patients with fungal infection of the nails the incidence was 17.5 per cent (Chien *et al.* 1997). In the same series the incidence of clinically manifest hepatitis was just under 3 per cent, elderly patients being the most affected. Females are affected twice as frequently as males and the timing of onset of liver injury is very variable, between 2 and 26 weeks after starting treatment. Jaundice is usually hepatocellular in nature, and occasionally fulminant hepatic failure may ensue (Stricker *et al.* 1986; van Parys *et al.* 1987). Cholestatic lesions have also been described and recovery from these can be slow (Benson *et al.* 1988). Signs of hypersensitivity do not accompany liver damage from ketoconazole and the drug has been shown to be directly hepatotoxic in animals (Stricker *et al.* 1986).

Fluconazole

Abnormalities in liver function tests associated with fluconazole resolve when it is withdrawn. One study questioned the relationship of such abnormalities to liver injury because liver biopsies from two patients taking the drug showed no evidence of hepatic damage (Trujillo *et al.* 1994). There is increasing evidence that patients with HIV are particularly prone to hepatic damage from fluconazole and a case of fatal hepatic necrosis has been described (Jacobson *et al.* 1994; Guillaume *et al.* 1996).

Thiabendazole

Thiabendazole may cause cholestasis (Davidson *et al.* 1988), sometimes accompanied by the sicca syndrome (Fink *et al.* 1979). Chronic cholestasis from the drug has been reported (Roy *et al.* 1989).

Niclofolan

Niclofolan, used for the treatment of fascioliasis, may also cause cholestatic jaundice (Reshef *et al.* 1982).

Antituberculous drugs

All of these compounds, with the exception of streptomycin and possibily ethambutol, cycloserine, and capreomycin are liable to produce liver damage. Current guidelines for the treatment of pulmonary tuberculosis specify three potentially hepatotoxic drugs: rifampicin, isoniazid, and pyrazinamide for 2 months followed by 4 months of rifampicin and isoniazid (Joint Tuberculosis Committee 1990). The incidence of tuberculosis has been increasing since 1987, exposing a greater number of patients to the risks of liver damage.

Isoniazid

Serum transaminase concentrations rise in 10–20 per

cent of asymptomatic patients receiving chemoprophylaxis with isoniazid (Scharer and Smith 1969; Bailey *et al.* 1974; Byrd *et al.* 1977). These abnormalities generally appear within the first 2 months of therapy and often revert spontaneously to normal despite continuing the drug (Bailey *et al.* 1973). In contrast, symptomatic jaundice is much less common in patients taking this drug, with reported incidences of 0.5–3 per cent (Garibaldi *et al.* 1972; Maddrey 1981; Derby *et al.* 1993a). Most reported cases of symptomatic isoniazid-related hepatitis have developed within the first 3 months of starting treatment, although there are a few well-documented cases appearing at 4 and 5 months (Maddrey and Boitnott 1973). Concomitant treatment with other antituberculous drugs, particularly rifampicin, increases the frequency of liver damage, with estimated incidences of 2.7–10 per cent (Parthasarathy *et al.* 1986; Steele *et al.* 1991). The onset of hepatitis is also accelerated by concomitant rifampicin therapy with symptoms developing as early as 10 days after starting treatment (Pessayre *et al.* 1977).

Clinical features are very similar to those of acute viral hepatitis, and 'flu-like symptoms with non-specific gastrointestinal upset are common in the early stages of the illness. They should be taken seriously, because the reported mortality is in the region of 13 per cent. Symptoms starting more than 2 months after onset of treatment carry a poor prognosis (Black *et al.* 1975). Manifestations of hypersensitivity are infrequent.

Isoniazid usually causes acute hepatitis, but active chronic hepatitis has also been reported (Maddrey and Boitnott 1979).

Mechanisms

Susceptibility to isoniazid hepatotoxicity is age related and until recently there were few reports of this complication in patients under the age of 35 (Farer *et al.* 1977; Maddrey 1981; Van den Brande *et al.* 1995; Hwang *et al.* 1997). However, there is evidence that this pattern is changing, and an increasing number of young people are being affected (Ozick *et al.* 1995). Risk factors include HIV infection, alcohol abuse (Gronhagen-Riska *et al.* 1978), and malnutrition (Singh *et al.* 1995). The role of infection with the hepatitis B virus in this respect is controversial (Wu *et al.* 1990; Hwang *et al.* 1997).

The mechanism appears to be metabolic idiosyncrasy. The initial and rate-limiting step in detoxification of isoniazid involves its acetylation, with subsequent hydrolysis and liberation of isonicotinic acid and acetylhydrazine (Fig. 13.4). This derivative subsequently undergoes further acetylation to form diacetylhydrazine. Liver damage is mediated via a highly chemically reactive hydrazine metabolite of isoniazid, and early studies suggested that it was derived exclusively from acetyl-hydrazine (Mitchell and Jollow 1975; Nelson *et al.* 1976). Since the rate of isoniazid acetylation is genetically determined, it was

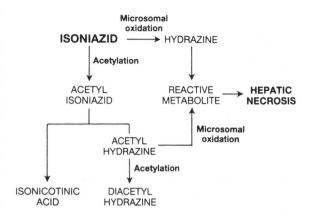

Fig. 13.4
Pathways of isoniazid metabolism
in relation to hepatotoxicity

proposed that individuals with the rapid acetylator phenotype would be more at risk of developing liver damage, since a greater proportion of the drug would be available for conversion to the toxic metabolite (Mitchell *et al.* 1975). However, pharmacokinetic studies in rapid acetylators showed that while they converted a greater proportion of isoniazid to acetylhydrazine, any propensity for accumulation of this potentially hepatotoxic precursor was offset by an increased rate of detoxification by conversion to diacetyl isoniazid (Timbrell *et al.* 1978). It was subsequently shown that the hydrazine derivative could be produced from the parent molecule without the need for prior acetylation (Lauterburg *et al.* 1985b). This shifted the emphasis from rapid to slow acetylation status as being an important factor predisposing to liver damage from the drug. Indeed, accumulation of hydrazine and its oxidation (by inference, to a toxic metabolite) is greater in slow than in rapid acetylators (Beever *et al.* 1982; Lauterburg *et al.* 1985a,b).

Determination of acetylator status is of limited value in predicting hepatotoxicity from isoniazid (Gurumurthy *et al.* 1984; Singh *et al.* 1995; Hwang *et al.* 1997), and there are other determinants of susceptibility. Probably the most important is concomitant therapy with rifampicin, which is a potent enzyme-inducing agent that stimulates the rate of hydrazine formation by microsomal oxidases from both isoniazid and acetylisoniazid. Pharmacokinetic and epidemiological studies suggest that the former pathway (i.e. conversion of isoniazid to hydrazine) is the more important (Gangadharam 1986; Kukongviriyapan and Stacey 1991). The incidence of hepatic dysfunction in both slow and fast acetylators of isoniazid receiving this drug in combination with rifampicin was approximately 3.5 per cent, in contrast with frequencies of 1.4 per cent and 0.5 per cent in slow and fast acetylators respectively receiving isoniazid alone (Gurumurthy *et al.* 1984).

There are well-documented clinical reports of liver damage in patients taking isoniazid together with therapeutic doses of paracetamol (see under Paracetamol).

Pyrazinamide

Hepatic reactions to pyrazinamide appear to be dose related, with a 60 per cent incidence in patients taking 60 mg per kg daily compared with two per cent in those receiving 20–40 mg per kg (Fouquet *et al.* 1965; East African/British Medical Research Council 1973). However, even the lower doses now used can cause hepatitis (al Sarraf *et al.* 1996). Patients developing fulminant hepatic failure from antituberculous regimens containing pyrazinamide appear to have a particularly bad prognosis; in a study by Durand and colleagues (1995) seven out of nine patients died, compared with one out of nine patients who had received isoniazid and rifampicin alone 1995.

Sodium aminosalicylate

Hypersensitivity reactions to this drug with fever, rashes, and lymphadenopathy occur in up to five per cent of patients, and in 40 per cent of these serum transaminases become elevated (Simpson and Walker 1960). If the drug is not withdrawn at an early stage a florid hepatitis with a reported mortality of 21 per cent may develop.

Rifampicin

Unconjugated hyperbilirubinaemia is not uncommon during the first 1–2 weeks of therapy with rifampicin; the drug competes with bilirubin for uptake into the hepatocyte. There is often an accompanying rise in the conjugated fraction, due to competition with the drug itself for excretion into the bile (Capelle *et al.* 1972). These abnormalities usually clear within the first 2–3 weeks of treatment, reflecting the potent enzyme-inducing properties of rifampicin. If jaundice persists, underlying liver disease should be suspected (McConnell *et al.* 1981).

The intrinsic hepatotoxicity of rifampicin appears to be low, although occasional cases of centrilobular necrosis have been described (Westphal *et al.* 1994). Its major involvement in hepatotoxic drug reactions is by potentiating liver injury caused by other compounds, particularly isoniazid (q.v.).

Ethionamide

Ethionamide and the related drug prothionamide produce elevations in serum transaminases in about 10 per cent of patients. Studies in patients treated with the drug for leprosy suggest that it is particularly hepatotoxic in combination with rifampicin (Cartel *et al.* 1983), and the incidence of liver damage can be reduced by administering rifampicin twice weekly instead of daily (Pattyn *et al.* 1984).

Management of abnormal liver function tests in patients on antituberculous therapy

Although symptomatic liver disease is almost invariably preceded by prodromal symptoms, recent studies have drawn attention to the fact that these are generally ignored (Mitchell *et al.* 1995; Thompson *et al.* 1995). Thompson and colleagues (1995) have suggested the following protocol:

— liver function tests should be measured in all patients before starting treatment and every 2 weeks for the first 8 weeks. Thereafter, monitoring can be reduced to 4-weekly intervals for as long as the patient is on treatment. For isolated elevations in transaminases to less than three times the upper limit of normal, liver function tests should be monitored weekly and if levels rise above this limit isoniazid should be withdrawn. Hyperbilirubinaemia in association with raised transaminases is an indication for stopping isoniazid. Isolated hyperbilirubinaemia in patients on rifampicin does not denote hepatotoxicity (see above); it is usually self-limiting, but if it does not resolve within two weeks the drug should probably be withdrawn and another agent substituted. All medications should be stopped promptly if there are any systemic symptoms;

— following withdrawal of isoniazid, liver function tests should be performed weekly;

— if there is no resolution, all other drugs should be stopped. If liver function tests return to normal after withdrawal of isoniazid, other agents may be substituted, and some clinicians advocate reintroduction of drugs even after symptomatic liver damage, but this is controversial (Thompson *et al.* 1995; Dossing *et al.* 1996;). Reintroduction of isoniazid without rifampicin, on the basis that it will be less hepatotoxic on its own, is an alternative strategy (Askgaard *et al.* 1995).

Antiviral drugs

Zidovudine and other antiretroviral agents

Zidovudine can produce a syndrome of microvesicular steatosis with lactic acidosis. Most patients affected have been young women with HIV infections (Gradon *et al.* 1992; Olano *et al.* 1995; Ragni *et al.* 1995). The reactions may be caused by inhibition of mitochondrial respiration (Schwartz 1995), and the liver lesion can be reproduced experimentally in animals (Corcuera *et al.* 1996).

The drug may potentiate liver injury from therapeutic doses of paracetamol (see under Paracetamol).

Didanosine, which is also used for treatment of retroviral infection, has been associated with fulminant hepatic failure from acute hepatocellular necrosis (Lai *et al.*

1991; Lacaille *et al.* 1995). Hepatotoxicity from zalcita-bine has also been described (Henry *et al.* 1996).

Interferons

Abnormal liver function tests characteristically ac-company successful clearance of hepatitis B virus by use of these agents and the abnormalities are related to destruction of virus-infected liver cells rather than to the drug used itself (Alexander *et al.* 1987). However, abnor-malities in liver function, which have been thought to be due to hepatotoxicity from interferons, have sometimes limited therapy (Berris and Feinman 1991; Shimizu *et al.* 1994).

Fialuridine

This drug held great promise for the treatment of chronic hepatitis B. Early studies showed it to be safe in the short term but a longer-term study had to be abruptly termi-nated because of progressive hepatic dysfunction with lactic acidosis (McKenzie *et al.* 1995). Liver histology showed marked microvesicular and macrovesicular steatosis and cholestatis (Kleiner *et al.* 1997). On elec-tron microscopy there was disruption of mitochondria with accumulation of small fat droplets. Inhibition of mitochondrial respiration by the drug is the postulated mechanism for this reaction (Schwartz 1995).

Anticonvulsants

Phenytoin

Acute hepatocellular necrosis is a well-documented complication of treatment with phenytoin, and is fre-quently accompanied by manifestations of allergy, with rashes, lymphadenopathy, and eosinophilia (Olsson and Zettergren 1988; Smythe and Umstead 1989). The com-plication can occur at any age, and has been reported in infancy (Roberts *et al.* 1990). In 80 per cent of cases symptoms appear within the first 6 weeks of treatment.

Although acute hepatic necrosis or lobular hepatitis are the commonest histological abnormalities, chole-static (Taylor *et al.* 1984) and granulomatous hepatitis (Cook *et al.* 1981) have also been documented.

The associated clinical features strongly suggest in-volvement of immune mechanisms. Circulating anti-bodies to phenytoin have been described in association with hepatic damage (Kleckner *et al.* 1975), and cell-mediated immunity to the drug has also been demon-strated in a patient who developed an allergic reaction with hepatic necrosis (Kahn *et al.* 1984). Sensitization to phenobarbitone was also demonstrated in the latter case.

Phenytoin is metabolised to a chemically reactive epoxide derivative and it has been suggested that indi-viduals deficient in the enzyme epoxide hydrolase might be at risk from hepatitis from the drug (Pantarotto *et al.* 1982; Moustafa *et al.* 1983). Lymphocytes from patients with this deficiency were particularly susceptible to lysis by epoxide phenytoin metabolites, which had been gen-erated *in vitro* by a mouse hepatic microsomal system (Spielberg *et al.* 1981; Spielberg 1986).

Phenobarbitone

Acute hepatitis is a rare complication of treatment with phenobarbitone, and generally occurs as part of a gen-eralized hypersensitivity illness (Godwin *et al.* 1967; Mockli *et al.* 1989). Usually the reaction is seen within 8 weeks of starting treatment. A case has been reported in an 8-month-old infant, in which *in vitro* challenge of the patient's lymphocytes with cytochrome P-450-generated phenobarbitone metabolites showed extensive cyto-toxicity (Roberts *et al.* 1990).

Carbamazepine

Carbamazepine is structurally similar to the tricyclic antidepressants. Mild to moderate elevations in liver enzymes have been observed in up to 22 per cent of patients within the first 6–8 weeks of treatment (Zimmer-man 1978*a*; Askmark and Wiholm 1990). Hepatic nec-rosis, granulomatous infiltration, and cholestasis have been described (Levander 1980; Hadzic *et al.* 1990; La Spina *et al.* 1994; Kong 1996). The latter can progress to chronic cholestasis with 'vanishing bile duct' syndrome (Forbes *et al.* 1992; de Galocsy *et al.* 1994). Hepatic damage from carbamazepine is frequently associated with allergic manifestations suggesting an immunologi-cal aetiology. Hepatic necrosis has been described after carbamazepine overdose (Luke *et al.* 1986), suggesting that the drug has a direct hepatotoxic potential as well.

Sodium valproate

Abnormalities in serum transaminases complicate use of sodium valproate in 11 per cent of patients receiving the drug (Powell-Jackson *et al.* 1984). A much less common complication closely resembles Reye's syndrome with microvesicular fatty infiltration of the liver and hyperam-monaemia leading to coma, with a high mortality (Suchy *et al.* 1979; Ware and Millward 1980). In severely affected cases liver transplantation offers a prospect of survival. Fatty infiltration of the liver is often associated with some degree of centrilobular necrosis. The cause of this is not known.

Reye's syndrome induced by sodium valproate usually occurs in the first 6 months of therapy (Scheffner *et al.*

1988), and is particularly common in epileptic children under the age of two. Concomitant therapy with other anticonvulsant drugs greatly increases the risk (which rises to one in 500 compared with one in 37 000 receiving valproate alone), and developmental delay and concomitant metabolic disorders are additional risk factors (Powell-Jackson *et al.* 1984; Dreifuss *et al.* 1987). Recognition of these has led to a decline in the incidence of valproate-induced Reye's syndrome from one in 10 000 in 1978–84 to one in 49 000 in 1985–86 (Dreifuss *et al.* 1989) and subsequently (Bryant and Dreifuss 1996).

Mechanisms

The bulk of evidence indicates that sodium valproate acts as a mitochondrial poison via its metabolites 4-en-valproic acid and 2,4-diene-valproic acid (Fromenty and Pessayre 1995). These metabolites inhibit mitochondrial β-oxidation and lead to depletion of acetyl CoA and carnitine (Coulter 1991; Krahenbuhl *et al.* 1995). The latter is important for metabolism of long-chain fatty acids and for regulation of mitochondrial acetyl CoA. Metabolic studies in children and young adults receiving valproic acid have shown that levels of the putative hepatotoxic metabolite 4-en-valproic acid increase with decreasing age, with concomitant therapy with other anticonvulsants (Kondo *et al.* 1992), and with dose (Anderson *et al.* 1992). This fits with the epidemiological data and the experimental observation that generation of 4-en-valproic acid is mediated by a microsomal P-450 isoenzyme, which is inducible by phenobarbitone (Rettie *et al.* 1987). However, although differences from the usual pattern of valproic acid metabolism occur in patients with liver damage from the drug, there is no pattern which will predict susceptibility to this complication (Fisher *et al.* 1992).

In a recent study Bohles and colleagues (1996) found high blood ammonia levels in 35 per cent of 69 patients. Carnitine levels were subnormal and supplementation with this nutrient was associated with a fall in ammonia levels. None of these patients was symptomatic and the link between these findings and full-blown Reye's syndrome remains to be established. Ishikura and colleagues describe a child with sodium valproate overdose in whom levels of 4-en-valproic acid decreased after carnitine therapy; no hepatic damage occurred; and a beneficial effect of carnitine administration was inferred (Ishikura *et al.* 1996).

Genetic factors may be important in determining susceptibility. Appleton described two children with Reye's syndrome from valproate; siblings of both subsequently developed the illness without having taken the drug (Appleton *et al.* 1990).

Newer antiepileptic drugs

Acute hepatocellular necrosis may complicate treatment with felbamate, and deaths from fulminant hepatic failure have been reported (Schmidt and Kramer 1994; O'Neil *et al.* 1996). The estimated incidence is one in 8000 patient exposures.

Vigabatrin and lamotrigine have not to date been associated with hepatic toxicity (Schmidt and Kramer 1994).

Antidepressants

Tricyclic and tetracyclic antidepressants

While clinically manifest liver damage from tricyclic antidepressants is rare, more minor degrees of hepatic dysfunction, manifested by abnormalities in biochemical liver function tests in otherwise asymptomatic patients, are far more common (Pessayre and Larrey 1988). These abnormalities are often transient. Estimates of the incidence of this complication vary widely; figures of up to 10 per cent have been cited for amitriptyline, while for imipramine and desipramine incidences of up to 24.7 per cent and 8.7 per cent respectively have been quoted (Hoge and Biederman 1987).

Precise estimates of the incidence of severe hepatic damage from tricyclic antidepressants are difficult to obtain. A figure of 0.5–1.0 per cent is widely quoted, from a paper published in 1965 (Klerman and Cole 1997). As might be predicted from their close structural similarities, cross-hepatotoxic reactions between different members of the group can occur (Kennedy 1983; Larrey *et al.* 1986), and also between tricyclic agents and phenothiazines (Larrey *et al.* 1986; Remy *et al.* 1995).

Amitriptyline

Both acute hepatic necrosis and a predominantly cholestatic lesion have been reported with this drug (Anderson and Henrikson 1978; Danan *et al.* 1984). Daily doses have ranged between 25–150 mg with onset of symptoms 25 days to 10 months after starting therapy. Prominent pyrexia and eosinophilia have been present in some cases. A prolonged cholestatic illness with loss of small, interlobular bile ducts has also been reported as a complication of amitriptyline therapy (Larrey *et al.* 1988a).

Imipramine

Imipramine can produce acute hepatitis, often with a pronounced cholestatic component (Weaver *et al.* 1977; Moskovitz *et al.* 1982). As with amitriptyline, high fever and eosinophilia are often present. Chronic cholestasis with hepatic fibrosis has also been described (Horst *et al.* 1980).

Desipramine

This drug is the demethylated derivative of imipramine, to which the latter is metabolised *in vivo*. It has been implicated in the pathogenesis of acute hepatic necrosis in three reported cases (Price *et al.* 1983; Morrow *et al.*

1989). Doses of between 125–150 mg had been taken for up to 3 weeks before onset of symptoms. One patient had previously received imipramine, but it had been discontinued because of a rash; when desipramine was substituted the rash did not resolve and fatal hepatic necrosis supervened a few days later.

Amineptine

This tricyclic depressant is widely used in a number of countries, including France, where it accounts for 80 per cent of hepatitis caused by antidepressant drugs. Both hepatic necrosis and pure cholestasis have been described (Pessayre and Larrey 1988; Sebastian *et al.* 1994; Lazaros *et al.* 1996). Liver damage characteristically occurs within 3 months of starting therapy and is often associated with fever and eosinophilia. A quite different liver lesion, with prominent infiltration of liver cells by microvesicular fat droplets resembling alcoholic fatty liver, has also been described in association with this drug. The lesion can be reproduced in mice, and is due to inhibition of mitochondrial β-oxidation (Le Dinh *et al.* 1988). The large number of cases of liver damage reported suggests that amineptine may have a greater potential to produce liver injury than the other tricyclic drugs.

Maprotiline

Two case reports have implicated maprotiline in the pathogenesis of acute hepatitis; in one patient, who was asymptomatic, the condition was detected on screening (Moldawsky 1984; Aleem and Lingam 1987). The latent intervals were long (4 years and 288 days respectively), and although abnormalities resolved when the drug was discontinued, intercurrent acute hepatitis C could equally well have been the cause.

Dothiepin

A mixed cholestatic/hepatocellular pattern of injury has been reported with this drug, but the reaction is obviously rare (Stricker and Spoelstra 1985).

Lofepramine

Reports of cholestatic and hepatocellular injury have been described (CSM 1988). All occurred within 8 weeks of starting treatment and subsided on withdrawal of the drug. Nine patients developed jaundice. It has been recommended that liver function tests should be monitored in the first 12 weeks of treatment with this drug (Kelly *et al.* 1993).

Mianserin

Mianserin has been reported as causing both cholestasis and hepatocellular necrosis, with one case relapsing on reintroduction of the drug (Goldstraw *et al.* 1983; Otani *et al.* 1989).

Trazodone

Cholestasis and cholestatic hepatitis have both been reported complicating trazodone therapy. The reaction appeared after a latent period of 2 weeks to 5 months and regressed on drug withdrawal (Sheikh and Nies 1983; Longstreth and Hershman 1985). Fatal acute hepatocellular necrosis has been described (Hull *et al.* 1994), and a case of active chronic hepatitis has also been reported (Beck *et al.* 1993).

Monoamine oxidase inhibitors

Iproniazid was withdrawn from clinical use in Great Britain and the United States because of its propensity to cause liver damage, but it is still used in some countries. The usual picture is one of hepatic necrosis, generally occurring in the first 3 months of treatment (Gollini *et al.* 1992; Rosenblum *et al.* 1997).

Phenelzine can also produce hepatic necrosis (Zimmerman and Ishak 1987). Cross-toxicity has been described with different monoamine-oxidase inhibitors, which are chemically related. The overall incidence of hepatotoxicity is probably higher than with the tricyclic drugs, having been estimated at approximately one per cent.

Serotonin-specific reuptake inhibitors

There are isolated reports of acute hepatitis, and also cholestasis complicating treatment with fluoxetine (Friedenberg and Rothstein 1996; Dollow 1996; Cosme *et al.* 1996).

A single case report describes hepatitis in a patient treated for severe depression with paroxetine (Helmchen *et al.* 1996).

Sedatives, tranquillizers, and other drugs affecting the central nervous system

Chlorpromazine

The estimated incidence of hepatic damage from chlorpromazine lies between 0.1–0.5 per cent. A survey of GP prescriptions in the United Kingdom identified a cohort of 10502 users of chlorpromazine, 14 of whom had illnesses compatible with drug-induced liver disease, giving a frequency of 1.3 per 1000 users (Derby *et al.* 1993). Abnormal liver function tests without jaundice are much more common and may be seen in a quarter or more of patients treated with phenothiazines (Zimmerman 1978b).

Jaundice usually appears in the second to fourth week of treatment and the onset may be acute, with fever and abdominal pain, or insidious. Signs of hypersensitivity with fever and eosinophilia are seen in up to 70 per cent of subjects and associated skin rashes occur in up to five per cent (Zimmerman 1978b).

Serum alkaline phosphatase concentrations are characteristically markedly elevated while transaminase elevations are more modest. Typically, the histological picture is one of cholestasis with relatively little hepatocellular injury. A portal inflammatory infiltrate is also characteristic, with eosinophils in up to 50 per cent of cases. Neutrophil infiltration between portal areas and lobules is seen in approximately 25 per cent of cases (Ishak and Irey 1972).

Symptoms generally regress on drug withdrawal and two-thirds of patients will have recovered after 8 weeks. The remaining third may have a more prolonged course (see below under Chronic cholestasis).

Other phenothiazines have been reported to cause jaundice; these include fluphenazine (Holt 1984), haloperidol (Dincsoy and Saelinger 1982), prochlorperazine (Lok and Ng 1988), and thioridazine (Weiden and Buckner 1973). Cross-sensitivity between chlorpromazine and other phenothiazines has been observed.

Mechanisms

Chlorpromazine and its metabolites can produce abnormalities in the hepatic cytoskeleton and impair bile secretion (Elias and Boyer 1979; Ros et al. 1979). The latter is associated with the disruption of cell membranes and impaired activities of the hepatocyte membrane enzymes Na^+/K^+ ATPase and Mg^{++} ATPase, both of which are involved in secretion of bile. The extent of these toxic effects can be modified by metabolism of the drug. The dihydroxy metabolite of chlorpromazine impairs bile secretion at concentrations in which the parent compound has no effect, and is 100 times more potent an inhibitor of hepatocyte membrane Na^+/K^+ ATPase (Kendler et al. 1972). In contrast, the sulphoxide metabolite does not produce these effects. Those individuals who are poor metabolisers of chlorpromazine to the sulphoxide derivative or extensive metabolisers to the dihydroxy metabolite, or both, might thus be more susceptible to cholestatic liver damage from chlorpromazine. Watson and colleagues tested this hypothesis in 12 patients after recovery from chlorpromazine jaundice and found all of them to be poor sulphoxidators (Watson et al. 1988). This contrasted with a frequency of 22 per cent in normal controls and 23.8 per cent in liver disease controls. In contrast, hydroxylation capacity was high in all patients, giving support to this hypothesis.

Dantrolene

Dantrolene sodium, an agent chemically related to phenytoin and used in the treatment of spasticity, was associated with a 1.8 per cent incidence of abnormal liver function tests in one large series, in which one-third of the patients became jaundiced (Utili et al. 1977). Chan (1990) examined case reports on all adverse hepatic drug reactions associated with dantrolene which had been reported to the manufacturer over a one-year period. Symptomatic liver disease with jaundice was found in 36 of the 122 cases, and 26 died. Histologically the liver lesions may show acute hepatic necrosis, a non-specific portal tract infiltrate, or chronic active hepatitis with or without cirrhosis. Chronic active hepatitis accounted for 68 per cent of all liver lesions from which biopsy material was available.

Signs of liver damage do not generally appear until after at least 2 months of therapy. The cases reviewed by Utili and colleagues had all been taking doses in excess of 200 mg daily, but three of the four patients in another report had taken 150 mg per day or less (Wilkinson et al. 1979). In another series, the mean dantrolene dose was significantly higher in fatal than non-fatal cases (582 and 263 mg per day respectively) (Chan 1990).

The mechanism of the hepatotoxicity is not known. Features of hypersensitivity are generally absent, although rechallenge with a therapeutic dose of the drug can result in a prompt relapse and liver damage (Utili et al. 1977). Metabolic studies have indicated that dantrolene is metabolised by hepatic mixed-function oxidases to a chemically reactive intermediate which is detoxified by glutathione conjugation (Arnold et al. 1983).

Chronic liver disease associated with dantrolene may show few clinical symptoms, and routine monitoring of liver function tests has been recommended to prevent insidious progression to cirrhosis.

Benzodiazepines

Hepatic injury from this group of drugs is very uncommon. Occurrences of cholestasis or cholestatic hepatitis have been reported from chlordiazepoxide (Lo et al. 1967), diazepam (Tedesco and Mills 1982), and flurazepam (Reynolds et al. 1981). The onset of liver disease occurs from a few days to several weeks after starting treatment and signs of hypersensitivity may be present.

Barbiturates

Liver injury from this group of drugs is uncommon. When it occurs, it usually does so in the context of a generalized hypersensitivity reaction with fever, skin rashes, lymphadanopathy, splenomegaly, and eosinophilia. Onset is usually within 2 months of starting treatment and resolution can be slow. Both acute hepatocellular necrosis and cholestasis can occur (Shapiro et al. 1980; Kahn et al. 1984; Mockli et al. 1989; Roberts et al. 1990).

Tacrine

This reversible choline esterase inhibitor can lead to modest improvements in cognitive defects in patients with Alzheimer's disease, but causes abnormal serum transaminase concentrations (Beermann 1993). Symptomatic hepatitis is rare, and histological data on tacrine-induced liver damage are limited, but centrilobular necrosis and granulomatous hepatitis have both been reported (Ames *et al*. 1990; Hammel *et al*. 1990). Watkins and colleagues analysed data from multicentre trials of tacrine involving a total of 2446 patients. They found ALT levels greater than the upper limit of normal on at least one occasion in 49 per cent, greater than three times normal in 25 per cent, and greater than 20 times normal in two per cent (Watkins *et al*. 1994). The elevated ALT levels were generally asymptomatic and were mostly seen within 12 weeks of starting treatment. Women were more frequently affected than men. Abnormalities resolved promptly on discontinuing the drug. Of 145 patients who were rechallenged, in 88 per cent it was possible to resume long-term therapy with the drug. No deaths occurred. Weekly monitoring of liver function has been recommended in patients taking the drug (Woo and Lantz 1995).

Tacrine is metabolised to chemically reactive metabolites generated by the cytochrome P-450 isoenzyme CYP1A2 (Woolf *et al*. 1993). Caffeine is also metabolised by this enzyme, but studies using the caffeine breath test to identify patients at risk from liver damage have been disappointing (Fontana *et al*. 1996).

Recent studies have shown that tacrine increases mitochondrial respiration, leading to energy wastage and decreases in levels of ATP (Berson *et al*. 1996). These effects were observed using levels of the drug comparable to those used clinically, and it has been postulated that they might be involved in the pathogenesis of liver injury.

Cardiovascular drugs

Methyldopa

Approximately five per cent of patients taking methyldopa develop abnormal liver function tests, although most remain asymptomatic and the abnormalities may resolve despite continuing the drug. The incidence of symptomatic liver disease is probably less than one per cent. The pattern varies widely: there may be acute hepatic necrosis, which can be massive, leading to fulminant hepatic failure (Toghill *et al*. 1974). This tends to be seen after short-term therapy; in those taking the drug for longer periods, prominent fatty infiltration and fi-

brosis are seen (Arranto and Sotaniemi 1981*a,b*). Cholestatic jaundice has also been described (Rao 1986; Moses *et al*. 1989), as has granulomatous infiltration (Bezahler 1982; Mirada *et al*. 1991).

Some patients develop an illness indistinguishable from autoimmune active chronic hepatitis with hyperglobulinaemia and autoantibodies (Maddrey 1980). It usually develops after several months of methyldopa therapy, particularly if it is continued after the onset of signs of hepatocellular dysfunction. In one reported case there was progression from acute to chronic liver damage after the drug had been stopped. A generalized systemic illness with fever and hepatic dysfunction has been attributed to methyldopa. The illness resolved on withdrawal of the drug (Stanley and Mijch 1986).

In vitro studies have demonstrated that methyldopa is converted by microsomal enzymes to an unstable metabolite which binds to its site of formation (Dybing *et al*. 1976; Dybing and Nelson 1978). A direct toxic effect of the drug could form the basis for the high incidence of mild hepatic injury revealed by monitoring liver function tests during drug administration. An immunological basis for the reaction is suggested by the demonstration of antibodies, directed against methyldopa-metabolite-altered liver cell membrane antigens, in patients with hepatitis from the drug (Mackay 1985; Neuberger *et al*. 1985).

β-Adrenoreceptor blockers

Hepatic reactions from this group of drugs are extremely rare but occasional cases have been reported, particularly with labetalol. The commonest liver lesion is acute hepatocellular necrosis, and fatalities have been reported (Douglas *et al*. 1989; Clark *et al*. 1990; Stumpf 1991). Onset of symptoms can be from 3 weeks to 6 months after starting therapy. Labetalol can also cause active chronic hepatitis (Clark *et al*. 1990).

Isolated reports of centrilobular hepatic necrosis complicating metoprolol therapy, with relapse on rechallenge have appeared (Larrey *et al*. 1988*b*). Metabolism of this drug is retarded in individuals with poor hydroxylator status, but hepatotoxicity from metoprolol is not associated with this phenotype (Lennard 1989). Hepatitis from acebutolol is accompanied by pyrexia, and some cases have relapsed promptly on rechallenge (Tanner *et al*. 1989). A mild cholestatic reaction has been reported with atenolol (Schwartz *et al*. 1989).

Angiotensin-converting-enzyme (ACE) inhibitors

Liver damage from this group of drugs is rare. Most descriptions of captopril-induced liver injury have emphasized the strongly cholestatic features (Crantock *et al.* 1991), although a mixed hepatocellular/cholestatic picture and predominant hepatocellular necrosis have also been reported (Rahmat *et al.* 1985). The illness may mimic ascending cholangitis. Onset of liver damage can vary from one week to 20 months from starting treatment although most reactions occur within 3 months (Crantock *et al.* 1991; Hagley 1991). Recovery is usually complete but may be slow.

A similar clinical picture may be seen with enalapril (Todd *et al.* 1990). Acute hepatitis from lisinopril occurred in one patient after 2 weeks of treatment but the drug was continued and the patient progressed to fulminant hepatitis (Larrey *et al.* 1990). Chronic hepatitis from the drug has also been described (Droste and de Vries 1995). Cross-hepatotoxicity between different ACE inhibitors can occur, so they should all be avoided if a patient develops hepatitis after one of them (Hagley *et al.* 1992, 1993).

The mechanism for these reactions is not known. Enalapril is directly hepatotoxic to rats via a reactive metabolite formed by a microsomal mixed-function oxidase of the CYP3A subfamily. Glutathione exerts a protective effect (Jurima and Huang 1992).

Calcium-channel inhibitors

Liver injury from this group of compounds is extremely uncommon. Isolated instances of jaundice from hepatic necrosis or cholestatic hepatitis have been described in association with diltiazem (Traverse *et al.* 1994), verapamil (Hare and Horowitz 1986; Burgunder *et al.* 1988), and nifedipine (Richter and Schwandt 1987). A lesion resembling alcoholic hepatitis, with steatosis and Mallory bodies, has been described in one case (Babany *et al.* 1989). Diltiazem may produce a granulomatous hepatitis (Sarachek *et al.* 1985; Toft *et al.* 1991).

Quinidine

Hepatic necrosis associated with this drug is usually accompanied by manifestations of hypersensitivity with rashes, fever, and eosinophilia. The liver lesion is predominantly hepatitic with a variable element of cholestasis (Herman and Bassan 1975; Knobler *et al.* 1986). Granulomatous infiltration can also occur (Bramlet *et al.* 1980). Relapse of the liver lesion on rechallenge is characteristic. This is an extremely rare complication.

Although hypersensitivity reactions to the chemically related compound quinine are not uncommon, liver damage is very rare. Cholestatic hepatitis with granulomatous infiltration and other features of hypersensitivity has been described (Punukollu *et al.* 1990).

Procainamide

Intrahepatic cholestasis (Ahn and Tow 1990; Chuang *et al.* 1993) and a granulomatous hepatitis (Rotmensch *et al.* 1978) have both been reported in association with procainamide, but the complication is extremely rare.

Amiodarone

Mild elevations in serum transaminases occur in 25 per cent of patients receiving amiodarone; these may resolve despite continued treatment (Geneve *et al.* 1989; Rothenberg *et al.* 1994). Acute hepatic necrosis, sometimes leading to fulminant hepatic failure is a rare occurrence, usually associated with intravenous loading with the drug (Kalantzis *et al.* 1991; Morelli *et al.* 1991).

Chronic liver disease from amiodarone is discussed below in the section on Chronic liver disease.

Diuretics

Frusemide is a dose-related hepatotoxin in mice, liver damage being mediated via covalent binding of a chemically reactive metabolite of the drug, but there is no evidence that it produces liver damage in man (McMurtry and Mitchell 1977). Prolonged use of frusemide in infants, particularly those undergoing total parenteral nutrition (TPN), leads to gallstone formation (Whitington and Black 1980; Callahan *et al.* 1982). Randall and colleagues found a 21 per cent incidence in those receiving TPN and frusemide compared with two per cent in those on TPN alone (Randall *et al.* 1992).

Hepatitis has been described as an extremely rare complication of ethacrynic acid administration (Datey *et al.* 1967).

Tienilic acid was withdrawn from use in the USA because of its high propensity to cause hepatic reactions (one in 800 patients), usually acute hepatocellular necrosis (FDA 1980). There is usually associated evidence of hypersensitivity with eosinophilia and liver–kidney microsomal antibodies (LKM2 antibodies) (Homberg *et al.* 1984). This antibody is directed against the cytochrome P-450 isoenzyme CYP2C9, which catalyses biotransformation of the drug (Beaune *et al.* 1987). Sensitization to drug-altered liver membrane components has also been described (Neuberger and Williams 1989).

Anticoagulants

A few cases of cholestatic jaundice from warfarin have been described (Jones *et al.* 1980; Adler *et al.* 1986; Chaudhry and Oelsner 1995). Acute hepatitis and cholestatic hepatitis have both been reported in the early literature associated with generalized hypersensitivity reactions to phenindione (Portal and Emanuel 1961; Perkins 1962).

Mild abnormalities in liver function tests are not uncommon during heparin therapy and the pattern may be either hepatocellular or cholestatic. Symptomatic liver disease with jaundice has not been reported.

Streptokinase

Transient abnormalities in hepatic function during streptokinase treatment are uncommon, and jaundice induced by the compound is extremely rare (Mager et al. 1991). The occurrence of transient abnormalities in liver function tests in two brothers treated with streptokinase and heparin after myocardial infarction led to the suggestion that genetic factors might predispose to this complication (Pipek et al. 1994).

Liver haematomas, which can rupture, have been reported as rare complications of streptokinase therapy (Willis and Bailey 1984; Skakun and Shman 1986).

Antiplatelet drugs

Cholestatic hepatitis from ticlopidine has been described in a few reports (Grimm and Litynski 1994; Cassidy et al. 1995). In some cases this has been prolonged in spite of withdrawal of the drug (Nurhussein 1993; Naschitz et al. 1995). A case of granulomatous hepatitis has also been described (Ruiz et al. 1995).

Antithyroid drugs

Propylthiouracil

Abnormal liver function tests were seen in 28 per cent of 54 patients screened during treatment with propylthiouracil (Liaw et al. 1993). Infection with hepatitis viruses was excluded. Liver biopsy in three patients showed mild perivenular focal necrosis or ill-defined granulomata. All cases occurred within the first 2 months of treatment and resolved after discontinuation of the drug, or in some cases after reduction of dosage.

Severe hepatocellular necrosis from propylthiouracil is uncommon but fatalities from fulminant hepatic failure have been described (Hanson 1984; Garty et al. 1985; Deidiker and deMello 1996; Ozenirler et al. 1996). Cholestatic jaundice is an uncommon complication of propylthiouracil therapy (Seidman et al. 1986).

Carbimazole and methimazole

Carbimazole produces a predominantly cholestatic pattern of liver injury with a variable amount of hepatic necrosis (Blom et al. 1985; Vitug and Goldman 1985; Ozenne et al. 1989). It is usually seen within 4 weeks of starting the drug and on stopping the drug the liver lesion recedes, although this may take some months. Fatal cases have been reported (Epeirier et al. 1996).

Cholestatic jaundice due to methimazole is rare (Schmidt et al. 1986; Arab et al. 1995). A case mimicking sclerosing cholangitis has been reported (Schwab et al. 1996), and granulomatous hepatitis has also been described (Di Gregorio et al. 1990).

Oral antidiabetic drugs

Chlorpropramide

This drug is reported to cause cholestatic hepatitis in 0.5 per cent of recipients (Schneider et al. 1984). Prolonged cholestasis with disappearance of interlobular bile ducts has been described in a patient receiving chlorpropramide and erythromycin; a metabolic interaction between the two drugs has been postulated as the mechanism (Geubel et al. 1988). Cholestatic jaundice has been reported after overdose with chlorpropramide (Frier and Stewart 1977).

Tolbutamide

This antidiabetic agent may cause hepatic damage similar to that caused by chlorpropramide, but it does so less commonly (Tygstrup 1978). Cross-toxicity between tolbutamide and chlorpropramide can occur, but glibenclamide can be given safely in this situation (Rumboldt and Bota 1984).

Tolazamide

Cholestatic jaundice from tolazamide is a rare event (Bridges and Pittman 1980). It generally resolves on withdrawal of the drug, but one case of chronic liver disease has been described (Nakao et al. 1985).

Hormonal agents

Oral contraceptives and anabolic steroids

Jaundice from this class of compound is mainly associated with a 17-α-substituted-19-nor (no radical) configuration. Substitution in the 17-α position with an alkyl or other group greatly increases the cholestatic potential (Schreiber and Simon 1983). Jaundice has also been described in association with unsubstituted steroids, particularly if these are used in high doses (Garrigues et al. 1986; Foitl et al. 1989; Fedorkow et al. 1989).

Oral contraceptives

Published figures for the incidence of jaundice from oral contraceptives (approximately one in 10 000 in Europe and North America but 1 in 4000 in Scandinavia and Chile) reflects use of the older preparations (Schaffner 1966). The incidence is probably now much lower with the almost universal adoption of low-oestrogen formulations.

Symptoms and signs of liver damage usually occur within 4 weeks of starting the tablets, with anorexia, malaise, pruritus, and jaundice; hepatic damage developing after the third month of usage is unlikely to be due to oral contraceptives (Metreau et al. 1972). Systemic manifestations of hypersensitivity do not occur. Alkaline phosphatase levels are only modestly raised and may be normal and, although transaminase elevation is not generally striking, severe hepatic necrosis has been reported (Dooner et al. 1971). Recovery is usually prompt on discontinuing medication. The contraceptive pill may precipitate symptoms of active chronic hepatitis and primary biliary cirrhosis by aggravating cholestasis.

Mechanisms

Constitutional factors may be important in determining whether or not jaundice will develop, for it is especially prevalent in women with a personal or family history of idiopathic recurrent cholestasis in pregnancy (Dalen and Westerholm 1974; Schreiber and Simon 1983). This explains the more frequent occurrence of jaundice in women taking oral contraceptives in Scandinavia and Chile, where the incidence of cholestasis in pregnancy is high. Individuals with Dubin–Johnson syndrome or benign recurrent cholestasis may also be particularly susceptible (Lindberg 1992).

The pathophysiology of oestrogen-induced cholestasis is not clear, but animal studies have shown that ethinyloestradiol inhibits bile flow and also the biliary excretion of bilirubin and bile salts. This may be due to inhibition of the activity of hepatocyte membrane Na^+/K^+ ATPase, or to changes in membrane fluidity and permeability (King and Blitzer 1990).

Anabolic steroids

Pure cholestasis with little or no parenchymal involvement is said to occur in one to two per cent of all patients taking orally active anabolic steroids, notably methyltestosterone and norethandrolone. Use of oxymetholone, a 17-substituted non-virilizing androgen, in the treatment of aplastic anaemia is associated with a high incidence of abnormal liver function tests, and cholestasis may be aggravated by cyclosporin, another cholestatic agent (Wood and Yin 1994).

Clinically, jaundice due to anabolic steroids usually appears in the first few weeks of taking them, preceded by symptoms of malaise, anorexia, nausea, and pruritus. Serum alkaline phosphatase is raised in two-thirds of cases but, in contrast with drugs causing cholestatic hepatitis, values are rarely over three times normal.

Cholestatic reactions to danazol have been reported (Silva et al. 1989; Alvaro et al. 1996). On electron microscopy, biliary canaliculi are very dilated; the changes are more severe than with other anabolic steroids. A beneficial effect of S-adenosyl methionine on severe danazol-induced cholestasis has been reported (Bray et al. 1993). (See also under Liver tumours and Vascular lesions.)

Oestrogen and androgen antagonists

Tamoxifen

This oestrogen antagonist can produce a wide spectrum of liver lesions including hepatocellular necrosis (Ching et al. 1992), cholestasis (Blackburn et al. 1984), peliosis hepatis (Loomus et al. 1983), and non-alcoholic steatohepatitis (NASH) (Pinto et al. 1995). The latter condition is histologically identical to alcoholic hepatitis with fatty infiltration, lobular inflammation and hepatocyte degeneration with or without fibrosis (Sheth et al. 1997). It has been associated with a wide variety of conditions. NASH should be suspected if sustained rises in transaminases are seen; these are usually modest. Liver biopsy is needed to confirm the diagnosis and if it is present tamoxifen should be withdrawn to avoid progression to cirrhosis.

Tamoxifen casues cancer in rats by damaging DNA through formation of adducts (Williams et al. 1993). This has led to concerns that it might exert a similar effect in humans (Jordan 1995). Current evidence, based on epidemiological studies, suggests that it does not and, experimentally, tamoxifen has less of a damaging effect on DNA in human than rat liver (Carlson 1997; Wogan 1997).

Cyproterone acetate

Acute hepatitis is a rare complication of treatment with this androgen antagonist but fatal cases have been reported (Blake et al. 1990; Parys et al. 1991; Murphy and Collins 1996). Isolated cases of hepatocellular carcinoma associated with use of cyproterone have been reported (Kattan et al. 1994; Watanabe et al. 1994). However, a multicentre surveillance study of long-term use of this drug in 2506 patients did not reveal a single case of this neoplasm (Rabe et al. 1996).

Flutamide

Fourfold or greater increases in transaminases were seen in 0.36 per cent of 1091 patients treated with flutamide, a non-steroidal androgen antagonist (Gomez *et al.* 1992). In a recent study the drug had to be withdrawn because of abnormalities in liver function tests in 14 of 65 patients, although significant toxicity was noted in only four of these (S.A. Rosenthal *et al.* 1996). The incidence of symptomatic liver damage in another study was estimated at around 0.03 per cent (Wysowski and Fourcroy 1996). Symptomatic liver damage may present either as acute hepatocellular necrosis, which may be fatal, or as a cholestatic hepatitis. Liver injury develops between 13 and 210 days after starting treatment, and liver function tests should be monitored during flutamide therapy. Experimental studies have shown that flutamide is converted to a hepatotoxic metabolite which inhibits mitochondrial respiration in isolated liver cells (Fau *et al.* 1994).

Lipid-lowering agents

Nicotinic acid (niacin)

Liver damage from nicotinic acid can present as acute hepatocellular necrosis (Clementz and Holmes 1987), cholestasis (Patel and Taylor 1994), or as chronic liver disease with portal fibrosis (Sugerman and Clark 1974; Einstein *et al.* 1975). It usually complicates long-term therapy, and with standard preparations is rarely seen with doses less than 3 g per day (Winter and Boyer 1973).

In contrast, use of sustained-release preparations is associated with a very much higher frequency of hepatotoxicity (Etchason *et al.* 1991). Usually abnormalities develop in the first 2 months of treatment (Mullin *et al.* 1989). Kenney and colleagues found evidence of hepatic dysfunction with serum transaminase levels exceeding three times the upper limit of normal in 52 per cent of patients taking slow-release preparations (Kenney *et al.* 1994). The incidence of hepatic abnormality in those on standard formulations was zero. In another study the incidence of liver injury, defined by somewhat stricter criteria, was just under five per cent (Gray *et al.* 1994). Dose for dose, sustained-release niacin is more effective in lowering blood cholesterol levels than the standard preparation but is also more hepatotoxic; abnormal liver tests occur with daily doses as low as 1 g. Risk factors, apart from level of dosage, include pre-existing liver disease, heavy alcohol intake, and diabetes. Liver abnormalities usually subside within a few weeks of discontinuing the drug but fulminant hepatic failure has been reported (Mullin *et al.* 1989). It has been recommended that doses be reduced by 50–70 per cent if a standard preparation is changed to a slow-release formulation. Liver function tests should be monitored within 6 weeks of any dose increment and 3-monthly for the duration of therapy (Gray *et al.* 1994).

Niacin preparations are available 'over-the-counter' without prescription, so there is considerable potential for hepatotoxic reactions from their unsupervised use, when doses exceeding those recommended may commonly be taken.

HMG-CoA-reductase inhibitors

Simvastatin, pravastatin, lovastatin, and fluvastatin can all produce minor elevations in serum transaminase levels in up to two per cent of patients (Walker 1992), although in one study the incidence was higher at around five per cent (Ballare *et al.* 1992). Symptomatic liver disease is uncommon but acute cholestatic hepatitis caused by simvastatin has been reported (Ballare *et al.* 1991).

Clofibrate

Clofibrate and related drugs (gemfibrozil, bezofibrate, and fenofibrate) have not been associated with significant hepatotoxicity, although a single case of cholestatic hepatitis with granulomatous infiltration has been reported with clofibrate (Pierce and Chesler 1978).

Gastrointestinal drugs

Histamine H₂-receptor antagonists

Liver abnormalities occur in less than one per cent of patients treated with the currently available H_2- receptor antagonists, the most frequent abnormality being mild elevations of transaminases (Smallwood *et al.* 1995). There are isolated reports of hepatitis with centrilobular necrosis from cimetidine (Schwartz *et al.* 1986), which has also been implicated in the pathogenesis, relapse, or both, of active chronic hepatitis (Boyd *et al.* 1989). Garcia and colleagues have estimated the risk of acute liver injury from cimetidine at around one in 5000 users (Garcia *et al.* 1997). The incidence with other H_2-receptor antagonists appears to be lower.

A few clinical reports implicate ranitidine as the cause of a predominantly cholestatic hepatitis, which can sometimes resemble ascending cholangitis with prominent fever and rigors (Hiesse *et al.* 1985; Souza 1986; Devuyst *et al.* 1993). Eosinophilic infiltration within the liver and a response to rechallenge in some cases suggest that immunological mechanisms are involved in the pathogenesis.

Acute hepatitis is a rare complication of famotidine therapy (Ament *et al.* 1994) and cross-hepatotoxicity with cimetidine has been described (Hashimoto *et al.* 1994). A case of subacute hepatic necrosis from nizatidine with progression to cirrhosis has been reported (Chey *et al.* 199).

1998 [handwritten]

Proton-pump inhibitors

There is a small incidence of mild abnormalities in liver function tests (less than one per cent) from both omeprazole and lansoprazole (Arnold 1994).

Sulphasalazine

Severe hepatocellular necrosis has been described as part of a generalized hypersensitivity reaction to sulphasalazine (Ribe *et al.* 1986; Marinos *et al.* 1992). Cholestatic hepatitis may also occur, again usually in association with other manifestations of hypersensitivity (Mitrane *et al.* 1986). It can complicate use of the drug for either ulcerative colitis or rheumatoid arthritis. Onset of liver damage may be delayed; one case report described it in a patient who had taken the drug without problems for 15 years (Lennard and Farndon 1983). Neurotoxicity can be seen in association with the hepatotoxic reaction (Schoonjans *et al.* 1993). Fulminant hepatic failure has been described and one report suggests that N-acetylcysteine may have ameliorated hepatic damage (Gabay *et al.* 1993).

Liver damage from sulphasalazine is generally considered to be due to the sulphonamide moiety. However, hepatic reactions to sulphasalazine and 5-aminosalicylic acid have occurred in the same patient, indicating a causative role for the salicylate moiety (Burke *et al.* 1987). Cholestasis complicating 5-aminosalicylic acid therapy in a patient with Crohn's disease has been described (Stoschus *et al.* 1997).

Chenodeoxycholic acid and ursodeoxycholic acid

About one-third of patients treated with chenodeoxycholic acid (CDCA) show dose-related rises in serum transaminases (Schoenfield and Lachin 1981). These are asymptomatic, seldom exceed three times the upper limit of normal, are usually manifest in the first 3 months of treatment, and tend to resolve despite continuing the drug. In the National Co-operative Gallstone study, electron microscopy of baseline liver biopsies showed some features of intrahepatic cholestasis, which became more prevalent after 9 and 24 months, and in four patients symptomatic liver disease developed (Phillips *et al.* 1983).

Most orally administered CDCA is ultimately converted to lithocholic acid by enteric bacteria; lithocholic acid is hepatotoxic in those animal species that are unable to sulphate and excrete it (Gadacz *et al.* 1976). In man, however, sulphation and excretion are highly efficient, although in one study a low measured lithocholic acid 'sulphation fraction' was associated with CDCA-induced hypertransaminasaemia (Marks *et al.* 1981).

Ursodeoxycholic acid appears to have little or no potential for hepatotoxicity in man or experimentally in isolated liver cells (Miyazaki *et al.* 1984).

Disulfiram

An acute hepatitic reaction can occasionally complicate disulfiram therapy in alcoholics. The reaction, which may be fatal, usually occurs within 2–8 weeks of starting therapy and is characterized by marked elevation in transaminases, unlike the picture seen with alcoholic liver disease (Cereda *et al.* 1989; Forns *et al.* 1994). Many of the fatal cases have occurred because early evidence of liver damage was ignored. Fortnightly monitoring of liver function tests has been recommended for the first 3 months of treatment and 3-monthly thereafter (Wright *et al.* 1988).

Oxyphenisatin

This laxative has now been withdrawn from many countries because of its high propensity to cause active chronic hepatitis when taken for a prolonged period (Maddrey and Boitnott 1977). In single doses it is safe, and is still used for bowel preparation for radiological procedures.

Immunosuppressive agents

Azathioprine and mercaptopurine

Hepatotoxicity from mercaptopurine is generally not seen until the daily dose exceeds 2 mg per kg. Either a cholestatic or a hepatocellular pattern of injury may be seen (Einhorn and Davidson 1964).

Azathioprine can occasionally produce pure cholestasis or a cholestatic hepatitis (DePinho *et al.* 1984; Cooper *et al.* 1986; Perini *et al.* 1990; Horsmans *et al.* 1991). Carriage of hepatitis B or C viruses seems to predispose to this complication in renal transplant recipients (Pol *et al.* 1996). Liver damage from azathioprine can sometimes be associated with a hypersensitivity syndrome (Jeurissen *et al.* 1990). The drug differs from mercaptopurine in having an imidazole side-chain, which undergoes hydrolysis *in vivo* with liberation of mercaptopurine. Rechallenge studies in a patient with a hypersensitivity syndrome complicated by jaundice after azathioprine, showed that the former was due to the imidazole side-chain, and the jaundice to the mercaptopurine moiety (Davis *et al.* 1980). (See also under Vascular lesions of the liver.)

Cyclosporin

Cyclosporin can produce cholestasis (Mason 1989; Bluhm *et al.* 1992), and this adverse effect appears to be related to higher blood levels of cyclosporin; it is usually reversible by dose reduction (Lindholm and Kahan 1993). Similar abnormalities are seen in patients with inflammatory bowel disease treated with cyclosporin, and the drug may be particularly toxic in patients receiving total parenteral nutrition (Lorber *et al.* 1987; Actis *et al.* 1995; Moore *et al.* 1995).

Cyclosporin inhibits bile flow and inhibits conjugation of bile acids in experimental animals (Le Thai *et al.* 1988; Roman *et al.* 1989; Coleman *et al.* 1995; Vessey and Kelley 1995). Experimentally, abnormalities of bile flow can be improved by ursodeoxycholic acid (Queneau *et al.* 1994) and by *S*-adenosyl methionine (Fernandez *et al.* 1995).

Cyclosporin may also cause gallstones or biliary sludge; in one series this complication was seen in 2.4 per cent of transplant patients treated with this drug whereas it did not occur in patients immunosuppressed with azathioprine and prednisolone (Lorber *et al.* 1987).

Tacrolimus

Liver abnormalities from this immunosuppressive agent have been reported in five of 50 liver transplant recipients (Fisher *et al.* 1995). Raised transaminases reflected congestive changes, with sinusoidal dilatation and dropout of perivenular hepatocytes. Abnormalities resolved rapidly on withdrawal of the drug.

Anticancer drugs

Antimetabolites

Cytarabine

Reversible abnormalities in liver function tests have been recorded in 24 of 27 leukaemic patients treated with this drug by intravenous infusion (Perry 1992). Liver damage is usually not accompanied by symptoms or signs but occasional cases of cholestatic jaundice complicating high dosages of the drug have been reported (George *et al.* 1984).

Fluorouracil

Hepatic damage from fluorouracil is very uncommon but its derivative floxuridine can produce an acute hepatitis, which is dose related and which is reversible on cessation of treatment (Shepard *et al.* 1985; Doria *et al.* 1986). The drug can also produce bile-duct strictures resembling those seen in primary sclerosing cholangitis when it is infused into the common hepatic artery for treatment of hepatic metastases from colorectal carcinoma (Bolton and Bowen 1986; Dikengil *et al.* 1986). It generally develops several months after the start of chemotherapy.

In some patients the bile-duct strictures appear to be reversible but in most cases they persist, and may progress, despite cessation of treatment (Kemeny *et al.* 1985; Shepard *et al.* 1985). Cirrhosis can develop (Pettavel *et al.* 1986). Strictures typically involve the upper part of the common bile duct and the confluence of the right and left hepatic ducts, sparing the distal common bile duct (Dikengil *et al.* 1986). This differs from the situation often seen in primary sclerosing cholangitis, in which the distal common bile duct is often involved. The pathogenesis is unknown but ischaemic damage to the upper part of the common bile duct is a possible explanation.

Fluorouracil combined with levamisole improves survival in colonic carcinoma, but nearly 40 per cent of patients treated with this regimen showed liver enzyme abnormalities, compared with 16 per cent of those treated with levamisole alone. Abnormalities were mild and resolved on cessation of treatment (Moertel *et al.* 1993).

Tegafur

This drug is converted to fluorouracil by hepatic microsomal enzymes. It can cause minor abnormalities in liver function tests, and also more severe hepatic dysfunction in patients with pre-existing liver disease, in whom it may lead to death from hepatic decompensation (Lee and Farrell 1997).

Chronic hepatitis has been reported with tegafur and tamoxifen, using doses of both drugs that on their own would not be expected to produce liver damage (Maruyama *et al.* 1995). A similar clinical and histological picture has been reported for tegafur and uracil, suggesting that synergistic hepatotoxicity can also occur with these two compounds (Kobayashi *et al.* 1995).

Methotrexate

See under Chronic parenchymal liver disease.

Alkylating agents

Hepatic necrosis from alkylating agents is extremely uncommon, although there are rare reports of hepatitis from busulphan (Morris and Guthrie 1988) and cyclophosphamide (Aubrey 1970; Snyder *et al.* 1993). Progression to cirrhosis has been described.

Streptozotocin, carmustine (BCNU), and lomustine (CCNU) are all associated with abnormalities in liver function tests in up to two-thirds of patients treated with these agents. The abnormalities are generally mild and do not give rise to symptoms (Perry 1992). (See also under Vascular lesions of the liver.)

Antitumour antibiotics

Bleomycin, mitozantrone, and mitomycin have a low potential for hepatotoxicity and although transient elevations in liver enzymes may be seen during treatment these rarely cause problems. Mithramycin, in contrast, leads to transaminase elevations in almost all patients treated with it (Perry 1992). The effect is dose related and the complication is very much less common when mithramycin is used in lower doses for correction of hypercalcaemia (Green and Donehower 1984).

Other agents

Hepatic necrosis has been reported from etoposide, and this complication usually arises after high-dose therapy (Johnson *et al.* 1983). Cisplatin has been associated with hepatic steatosis, cholestasis, and hepatocellular necrosis (Patt *et al.* 1986; Cersosimo 1993), although it is generally used in combination with other drugs, which makes its role in causing liver injury difficult to assess.

Colaspase can lead to fatty infiltration of the liver; this has been found at autopsy in up to 47 per cent of patients treated with it (Haskell *et al.* 1969).

Total parenteral nutrition

Abnormal liver function tests are seen in approximately 25 per cent of patients in the first 2 weeks of TPN. Transaminase elevations are the first to appear, often within one week, while evidence of cholestasis with elevations in bilirubin and alkaline phosphatase are not normally seen until 2–4 weeks after starting TPN (Leaseburge *et al.* 1992). Abnormalities are usually more marked in children (Fleming 1994).

Fatty infiltration of centrilobular and mid-zonal hepatocytes is the earliest liver lesion to be seen. Bile duct proliferation with periportal inflammation and centrilobular cholestasis may develop after about 3 weeks of TPN; this may lead to fibrosis and cirrhosis if TPN is continued (Stanko *et al.* 1987; Mullick *et al.* 1994). In contrast, abnormalities usually resolve if it is withdrawn although recovery may be slow. Cholestatic liver disease complicating TPN is particularly common in infants (Moss *et al.* 1993).

Mechanisms

There are numerous theories for the aetiology of this complication, and undoubtedly many factors contribute.

Excessive calories

Fatty liver is more common with regimens using dextrose as the primary calorie source (Keim 1987), but it will occur with an excessive intake of calories whatever their origin (Chang and Silvis 1974; Lindor *et al.* 1979; Keim 1987; Campos *et al.* 1990). Replacement of dextrose by lipid to provide up to one-third of calories leads to a decrease in the incidence of fatty infiltration but the problem increases again with higher quantities of fat, so daily administration should not exceed 1 g per kg (McDonald *et al.* 1973; Freund 1991).

Choline deficiency

Choline is essential for the synthesis of LDL (low-density lipoprotein) to transport fat out of hepatocytes. Deficiency of this nutrient has been described in patients on TPN (Buchman *et al.* 1992). Administration of choline or lecithin leads to improvement as judged by liver density on CT scan (Buchman *et al.* 1995).

Carnitine deficiency

Carnitine is required for fatty acid oxidation, and deficiency of this nutrient is another suggested cause of fatty infiltration. Urinary carnitine excretion increases in the postoperative period (Tanphaichitr and Lerdvuthisopon 1981). Two case reports describe carnitine deficiency in patients on TPN; abnormal liver tests improved after supplementation (Worthley *et al.* 1983; Palombo *et al.* 1987). However, a larger survey of patients on home TPN found no benefit (Bowyer *et al.* 1988).

Essential fatty acid deficiency

Essential fatty acid deficiency leads to hepatic steatosis (Keim and Mares 1984; Kaminski *et al.* 1984), but this is unlikely to be an important cause of this complication with modern feeding regimens, which contain abundant lipid.

Intestinal bacteria

An adverse effect of intestinal bacteria, with increased formation of the hepatotoxic bile acid lithocholic acid, has also been postulated (Fouin *et al.* 1982). Improvement was demonstrated after administration of metronidazole (Capron *et al.* 1983; Lambert and Thomas 1985).

Tumour necrosis factor

Tumour necrosis factor mediates cholestasis from endotoxin and also leads to fatty infiltration of the liver (Whiting *et al.* 1995). Treatment of rats with an anti-TNF antibody protects against these changes (Pappo *et al.* 1995), and a similar beneficial effect results from administration of polymyxin (Pappo *et al.* 1992), which is associated with a marked reduction in output of TNF from peritoneal macrophages. These promising lines of research require clinical follow-up.

Manganese

Manganese levels are frequently elevated during parenteral

nutrition, particularly in association with cholestasis (Reynolds *et al.* 1994). It has been difficult to unravel whether cholestasis is caused by high levels of manganese or vice versa. A recent study in children showing improvement in cholestasis after manganese withdrawal suggests that it may have a causative role (Fell *et al.* 1996).

Management of TPN-associated liver abnormalities

Minor abnormalities may resolve with continued treatment but close monitoring is essential and, if they progress, TPN should be stopped. This can pose a major therapeutic dilemma in a patient with intestinal failure who is totally dependent on parenteral feeding. Ursodeoxycholic acid improves TPN-associated cholestasis in experimental animals (Duerksen *et al.* 1996) and there is some evidence that it is of clinical benefit (Spagnuolo *et al.* 1996). *S*-adenosyl methionine is also helpful in experimental animals (Belli *et al.* 1994), but has not been tried clinically. Currently neither these, nor other potential treatments discussed above, have any proven clinical value.

Gallstones and biliary sludge

Patients on TPN have an increased risk of gallstones and biliary sludge (Bower *et al.* 1990; Fleming 1994). In one series, all patients receiving TPN for 6 weeks or more had ultrasound evidence of biliary sludge and 42 per cent developed gallstones (Gafa *et al.* 1987). This occurs in children as well as in adults and is frequently complicated by cholecystitis (Matos *et al.* 1987; Rescorla and Grosfeld 1992). Acalculous cholecystitis can also occur in patients on TPN. If cholecystitis develops, early cholecystectomy should be carried out to avoid further complications (Roslyn *et al.* 1984).

Gall-bladder contractility is reduced in patients on TPN and this is probably the most important cause of the problem (Roslyn *et al.* 1983a,b; Gafa *et al.* 1987). This effect can be reversed by enteral feeding, and wherever possible patients on TPN should be given some food by mouth because this reduces the frequency of symptomatic gall-bladder disease, and possibly also hepatic dysfunction.

Recreational drugs

'Ecstasy'

Use of 'Ecstasy' (3,4-methylenedioxyamphetamine) may be complicated by acute hepatocellular necrosis leading in some cases to fulminant hepatic failure (Dykhuizen *et al.* 1995). Some, but not all, of these cases have had other complications of use of the drug, including hyperpyrexia and dehydration. The picture in less severe cases resembles an acute viral hepatitis (Fidler *et al.* 1996). Patients may present with symptoms some months after becoming regular users of 'Ecstasy'.

MDA is the abbreviation for methylenedioxyamphetamine, and also for methylene dianiline, a hepatotoxic compound used as a hardener for epoxy resins. An outbreak of acute cholestatic hepatitis occurred after a party at which drinks were adulterated with the latter substance, which had been acquired in the mistaken belief that it was 'Ecstasy'. Fortunately all those affected made a complete recovery (Tillmann *et al.* 1997). Methylene dianiline has previously been involved in an epidemic of jaundice when, in 1965, it involved 84 individuals who had eaten bread which had been made with flour contaminated with this compound (Kopelman *et al.* 1966).

Cocaine

Abuse of cocaine can lead to hepatic damage with centrilobular necrosis (Perino *et al.* 1987; Porter *et al.* 1988). In one series of 39 patients with acute cocaine intoxication there was biochemical evidence of liver injury in 59 per cent (Silva *et al.* 1991).

Cocaine is directly hepatotoxic in mice where it produces an identical histological pattern of liver injury to that seen in man. Lipid peroxidation and mitochondrial injury are both seen (Teaf *et al.* 1984; Devi and Chan 1997). Toxicity is associated with the production of a reactive metabolite of cocaine and the cytochrome P-450 isoenzyme CYP3A plays a central role (Le Duc *et al.* 1993; Pellinen *et al.* 1994). Continued regular use of cocaine could theoretically enhance susceptibility to hepatotoxicity, because experimental daily administration of the drug leads to stimulation of its own metabolism via CYP3A (Pasanen *et al.* 1995). Chronic alcohol ingestion and protein malnutrition also potentiate cocaine hepatotoxicity in experimental animals (Boyer and Petersen 1990; Odeleye *et al.* 1992).

Vitamins and herbal medicines

There is an increasing interest in alternative therapies throughout the western world; in a national survey in the USA one in three respondents had used at least one unconventional therapy in the previous year (Eisenberg *et al.* 1993). Some of these include use of vitamins in large doses, or herbal preparations, in the mistaken belief that because they are 'natural' they are not toxic. The preparations themselves, because they are not sold as drugs, are not subject to the same rigorous standardization and safety testing as conventional therapeutic agents. The contents are often mislabelled on the packets (Huxtable 1992) and many preparations are adulterated by western medicines and toxic heavy metals (Keen *et al.* 1994).

Patients taking herbal preparations usually do so without the knowledge of their doctors. Specific enquiry about their use should always be made in patients presenting with liver disease.

Vitamin A

This is discussed above under Chronic parenchymal liver disease.

Nicotinic acid

This is discussed above under Lipid-lowering drugs.

Pyrrolizidine alkaloids

These are discussed under Vascular lesions.

Germander

Extracts from the blossoms of germander (*Teucrium chamaedrys*) have been used for centuries as antiseptics and to aid slimming. Acute hepatitis may complicate their use, usually after about 2 months (Larrey *et al.* 1992*b*). The liver lesion usually resolves after stopping the preparation, but with continued use active chronic hepatitis and cirrhosis have been reported (Dao *et al.* 1993). Most cases of germander-associated hepatitis have been in young or middle-aged women using the preparation for weight reduction. An epidemic of hepatitis associated with its use in France led to its being banned there.

Extracts of germander are directly toxic to hepatocytes; the damage is mediated via metabolic activation of its constituent furano diterpenoids to reactive metabolites by the cytochrome P-450 isoenzyme CYP3A (Loeper *et al.* 1994; Lekehal *et al.* 1996). Glutathione exerts a protective effect; weight-reducing diets would be expected to enhance hepatotoxicity by depleting liver glutathione stores. Some cases of active chronic hepatitis have resembled autoimmune active chronic hepatitis, suggesting that immune mechanisms may also be involved in these cases (Ben *et al.* 1993).

Chaparral

Chaparral is prepared from the leaves of the creosote bush (*Larrea tridentata*) and is thought to have anti-inflammatory and antiviral properties; it is used particularly by patients infected with HIV (Kassler *et al.* 1991). Its active ingredient is nordihydroguaiaretic acid, an antioxidant which inhibits cyclo-oxygenase and lipoxygenase pathways (Shappell *et al.* 1990). It can produce acute hepatocellular necrosis (Katz and Saibil 1990), cholestatic hepatitis, or chronic hepatitis with cirrhosis (Gordon *et al.* 1995; Sheikh *et al.* 1997). Clinical presentation may be from 3–52 weeks after starting the preparation. The liver lesion usually resolves after the preparation is discontinued (Sheikh *et al.* 1997). In one reported case cholestatic hepatitis was associated with marked narrowing of the biliary tree on ERCP (Alderman *et al.* 1994).

Jin Bu Huan

Jin Bu Huan is a Chinese herbal medication marketed for its analgesic, sedative, and antispasmodic properties. Accidental ingestion in young children can result in coma with respiratory depression. In adults it can produce acute hepatitis up to 6 months after starting to take the preparation (Woolf *et al.* 1994; Horowitz *et al.* 1996). Liver damage resolves after stopping the preparation but relapses promptly when it is reintroduced.

The active ingredient in *Jin Bu Huan*, L-tetrahydropalmitine, is a potent CNS depressant and this probably explains its toxic effect in children. However, the component responsible for hepatic damage is not known.

Pennyroyal

Pennyroyal is prepared from the leaves of either *Mentha pulegium* or *Hedeoma pulegoides*. It is used to flavour other herbal preparations, and has been used since Roman times to induce abortion and bring on menstruation. It is well known as a hepatotoxin, producing acute centrilobular necrosis which, in severely affected cases, may lead to death from fulminant hepatic failure (Anderson *et al.* 1996).

The liver damage is thought to be mediated by one of its constituents, pulegone; this is metabolised to a reactive derivative which binds to liver cell proteins. This process is associated with depletion of hepatocellular glutathione and treatment with *N*-acetylcysteine has been recommended.

Other herbal preparations

Cases of hepatitis from mistletoe (*Viscum album*), used to treat asthma, have been reported but the preparation used was a mixture of mistletoe and skullcap (*Scutellaria*) (Harvey and Colin-Jones 1981). The latter preparation, and also valerian (*Valeriana officinalis*), used for nervous tension, has also been reported to cause hepatitis (MacGregor *et al.* 1989). However, in most cases the preparations used have contained several different herbs and, furthermore, the actual ingredients have not necessarily been those stated on the label (Huxtable 1992).

The glue thistle (*Atractylis gummifera*) grows wild around the Mediterranean coastline, and extracts from its root have been used as an antipyretic, emetic, and purgative. The glue-like substance secreted by the plant is also used by children as chewing gum. Several cases of acute hepatocellular necrosis complicated by early hypoglycaemia have been reported (Georgiou *et al.* 1988). The condition is frequently fatal. Toxicity appears to be due to inhibition of mitochondrial oxidative phosphorylation by its constituents gummiferin and potassium atractylate (Hedili *et al.* 1989).

Seatone is derived from an extract of the New Zealand green-lipped mussel, and its use has been advocated in rheumatoid arthritis (Gibson and Gibson 1981). A granulomatous hepatitis presenting with severe abdominal pain has been reported after taking the compound for 3 weeks (Ahern *et al.* 1980).

The herbal preparation *syo-saiko-to* is frequently given to patients with liver disease but can itself produce acute hepatocellular injury (Itoh *et al.* 1995). A number of other reports of hepatotoxicity from Chinese herbal preparations have appeared, usually when they have been given for skin conditions. Identification of the toxin responsible is hampered by the large number of different plants in these preparations, and also the fact that they are frequently adulterated by other compounds, including western medicines and toxic heavy metals (Keen *et al.* 1994).

A case of autoimmune active chronic hepatitis, apparently triggered by *Da Chai Hu Tang*, a Japanese herbal preparation, has recently been reported (Kamiyama *et al.* 1997).

Granulomatous liver disease

Granulomatous infiltration of the liver can be caused by a number of drugs (Table 13.5), sometimes without other hepatic abnormalities but more commonly accompanying an acute hepatitic or cholestatic reaction to a drug. In a survey of 95 cases of granulomatous liver disease approximately one-third were thought to be due to drugs (McMaster and Hennigar 1981). Some of these reactions are accompanied by a generalized granulomatous reaction throughout the body (e.g. penicillin and some of the sulphonamides), whereas other reactions involve the liver exclusively.

Diagnosis of a drug-induced granulomatous liver lesion depends on exclusion of other causes, because there are no features that are particularly specific for these lesions when they are produced by drugs. They are generally situated in the periportal areas and, with the exception of lesions induced by gold, do not contain particulate material. The concomitant presence of other liver lesions, particularly focal hepatocyte necrosis,

TABLE 13.5
Drug-induced granulomatous liver disease

Antimicrobials

Co-amoxiclav (amoxycillin/ clavulanic acid)	(Silvain *et al.* 1992)
Isoniazid	(McMaster and Hennigar 1981)
Nitrofurantoin	(Alcalde *et al.* 1994)
Penicillin	(McMaster and Hennigar 1981)
Sulphonamides	(Callen and Soderstrom 1978)

Anticonvulsants

Carbamazepine	(Levander 1980; Swinburn *et al.* 1986)
Phenytoin	(Mullick and Ishak 1980)

Analgesic/anti-inflammatory

Aspirin	(McMaster and Hennigar 1981)
Gold	(Harats *et al.* 1985)
Paracetamol	(Lindgren *et al.* 1997)
Phenylbutazone	(Ishak *et al.* 1977; Benjamin *et al.* 1981)

Cardiovascular

Diltiazem	(Sarachek *et al.* 1985)
Disopyramide	(Koch *et al.* 1985)
Hydralazine	(Jori and Peschile 1973)
Methyldopa	(McMaster and Hennigar 1981; Bezahler 1982)
Procainamide	(McMaster and Hennigar 1981)
Quinidine	(Bramlet *et al.* 1980)
Ticlopidine	(Ruiz *et al.* 1995)

Oral hypoglycaemics

Chlorpropamide	(Saw *et al.* 1996)
Glyburide	(Rigberg *et al.* 1976)
Tolbutamide	(Bloodworth and Hamwel 1961)

Miscellaneous

Allupurinol	(Stricker *et al.* 1989)
Chlorpromazine	(Ben *et al.* 1990)
Halothane	(Shah and Brandt 1983)
Oral contraceptives	(Malatjalian and Graham 1982)
Seatone	(Ahero *et al.* 1980)
Sulphasalazine	(Callen and Soderstrom 1978; Namlas *et al.* 1981)

cholestasis, and eosinophilic infiltration, are pointers to a drug-induced aetiology.

Chronic parenchymal liver disease

Active chronic hepatitis

Active chronic hepatitis (Table 13.6) can be produced by many drugs, all of which can also cause acute hepatitis (Maddrey 1980). Some of these reactions are indistinguishable from autoimmune active chronic hepatitis, with hyperglobulinaemia and autoantibodies (e.g. methyldopa, nitrofurantoin, clometacin). Active chronic

TABLE 13.6
Drug-induced active chronic hepatitis

Analgesic/anti-inflammatory

Diclofenac	(Mazeika and Ford 1989; Scully *et al.* 1993)
Paracetamol	(Johnson and Tolman 1977; Bonkowsky *et al.* 1978)

CNS

Benzarone	(Hautekeete *et al.* 1995)
Dantrolene	(Chan 1990)
Phenytoin	(Beck*et al.* 1993)
Trazodone	(Beck 1993)

Antimicrobials

Isoniazid	(Black *et al.* 1975)
Minocycline	(Malcolm *et al.* 1996)
Nitrofurantoin	(Burgert *et al.* 1995)

Anticancer

Tegafur + uracil	(Kobayashi 1995)
Tegafur + tamoxifen	(Maruyama *et al.* 1995)

Herbal

Germander	(Ben *et al.* 1993)
Chaparral	(Gordon *et al.* 1995)
Da Chai Hu Tang	(Kamiyama *et al.* 1997)

Miscellaneous

Cimetidine	(Boyd *et al.* 19891)
Etretinate	(Weiss *et al.* 1985; Sanchez *et al.* 1993)
Labetalol	(Clark *et al.* 1990)
Lisinopril	(Droste and de Vries 1995)
Oxyphenisatin	(Maddrey 1980)
Papaverine	(Poncin *et al.* 1986)
Propylthiouracil	(Maggiore *et al.* 1989)

hepatitis associated with other drugs (e.g. isoniazid) is not usually associated with manifestations of autoimmunity. The reactions are discussed in more detail above under the individual drugs.

It is very important to take a careful drug history from all patients presenting with active chronic hepatitis. If the offending agent is withdrawn liver damage resolves, albeit slowly, over a period of weeks. Conversely, if the drug is continued liver damage progresses even if the patient is treated with steroids and/or immunosuppressive agents.

Phospholipidosis and alcoholic hepatitis-like liver lesions

Amiodarone

The characteristic liver lesion associated with amiodarone is infiltration of liver cells with phospholipid droplets. Identical liver lesions are seen with two other antianginal/antiarrhythmic drugs, perhexiline maleate and diethylaminoethoxyhexoestrol. These three drugs are all amphiphilic, and can enter lysosomes, where they become trapped, due to the acidic environment within these organelles, and form stable complexes with phospholipids. These can be demonstrated histochemically and by electron microscopy and are similar to those seen with the congenital lipid storage diseases such as Tay–Sachs disease. The abnormalities are usually asymptomatic but progression, for reasons unknown, can occur to an alcoholic-hepatitis-like lesion with polymorphonuclear cell infiltrates and Mallory bodies; fibrosis and cirrhosis can ensue (Lewis 1990).

Liver injury from amiodarone appears to be dose related, and other manifestations of amiodarone toxicity, including corneal deposits, pulmonary fibrosis, neuropathy, and thyroid dysfunction may be associated. Progression to cirrhosis can occur if the drug is not withdrawn (Rigas *et al.* 1986; Lewis *et al.* 1990). Provided this stage has not been reached the liver abnormality regresses on withdrawal of the drug, but this can take many months; presumably this reflects the slow rate at which intracellular drug-phospholipid complexes can be mobilized.

It is not known whether the phospholipid inclusions are important in the pathogenesis of alcoholic-hepatitis-like lesions. A morphological study of patients receiving the drug in doses of 200–400 mg per day for 4 months to 15 years, suggests that they are not (Guigui *et al.* 1988). Lysosomal phospholipid inclusions were found in the livers of all patients receiving the drug, regardless of whether or not there was other evidence of liver damage. It is not known why some patients go on to develop progressive liver damage; in one analysis cardiac function as measured by left ventricular ejection fraction was more impaired in those who developed hepatic adverse effects than in those who did not (Tisdale *et al.* 1995). In another study (Pollak *et al.* 1990), patients with hepatic or pulmonary abnormalities, or both, had received higher doses of amiodarone than those without complications, and the ratio of blood levels of amiodarone to levels of its main metabolite desethylamiodarone was higher. They also had higher pretreatment transaminase levels.

Liver function tests should be monitored regularly in patients taking amiodarone. They are rarely severely disturbed even when there is progressive liver disease; jaundice is exceptional and transaminase elevations seldom rise over three times normal. If transaminase levels are sustained over twice normal, serious consideration should be given to liver biopsy; there is no currently available non-invasive technique for assessing the severity of the underlying liver lesion.

Diethylaminoethoxyhexoestrol

The first reports of hepatic damage from this coronary vasodilator emanated from Japan; in affected patients abnormal phospholipid storage was also noted in lungs, myocardium, and spleen. Clinically, patients presented with hepatomegaly, pyrexia, oedema, and weight loss, and some cases progressed to cirrhosis with a fatal outcome (Thaler 1988).

Perhexilene maleate

Liver damage from perhexilene appears after several months or even years of treatment and may be associated with other clinical manifestations of toxicity, including peripheral neuropathy due to an accumulation of drug-phospholipid complexes. Cirrhosis can ensue (Satz *et al.* 1991). The drug is metabolised by hydroxylation and individuals with poor hydroxylator phenotype are particularly predisposed to both hepatic and neurological complications from this drug (Morgan *et al.* 1984).

Hepatic fibrosis and cirrhosis

Methotrexate

This antimetabolite, which acts by inhibition of dihydrofolate reductase, has a well-established potential for hepatotoxicity. The early liver lesion comprises patchy hepatocellular necrosis with infiltration by large fat droplets and inflammation, which is predominantly periportal in distribution (Lewis and Schiff 1988). Collagen deposition in the space of Disse and lysosomal abnormalities can be seen on electron microscopy in all patients receiving the drug, even if light microscopic appearances are normal (Bjorkman *et al.* 1988). Progression of collagen deposition results in macroscopic fibrosis in periportal areas and ultimately cirrhosis can develop (Nyfors and Poulsen 1977; Zachariae *et al.* 1980; Ashton *et al.* 1982). These abnormalities rarely result in symptoms and biochemical liver function tests usually show little or no abnormality (Zachariae and Sogaard 1987; Shergy *et al.* 1988). Serial histological studies have shown that cirrhosis induced by methotrexate does not progress in an aggressive fashion even if the drug is continued, although complications, particularly with portal hypertension, continue to develop insidiously even if liver function tests are normal (Zachariae *et al.* 1996).

Development of methotrexate-induced liver damage is dose related and the high (up to 25 per cent) incidence of hepatic fibrosis and cirrhosis reported in early studies reflected the use of high daily doses of the drug (up to 50 mg per week) (Dahl *et al.* 1971; Nyfors 1977) . There is also good evidence that daily dosing is more hepatotoxic than giving the same cumulative amount in weekly doses (Dahl *et al.* 1972). Current therapeutic regimens for psoriasis and rheumatoid arthritis employ 15 mg of methotrexate per week or less, and with such doses the incidence of liver damage is minimal (Lewis and Schiff 1988).

In addition to total dose and dosing regimen, other factors seem to be important in determining liver susceptibility to injury from methotrexate. These include underlying liver disease, alcohol abuse, and the combination of obesity and diabetes mellitus (Lewis and Schiff 1988). In most reports, serious liver injury has been seen with cumulative doses in excess of 1.5–2 g (Tobias and Auerbach 1973; Themido *et al.* 1992), and there is some evidence that patients with psoriasis may be more susceptible to this complication than those with rheumatoid disease. This may be because the prevalence of alcohol abuse is higher in psoriatic patients than those with rheumatoid arthritis. In most of the studies quoted, however, patients with the latter condition had received lower cumulative doses of methotrexate than those with psoriasis.

The recommendations of the American College of Gastroenterology (Lewis and Schiff 1988) are that patients with psoriasis should undergo a liver biopsy before methotrexate is started; the presence of significant liver disease, particularly if the patient is actively drinking or has previously received hepatotoxic drugs (e.g. vitamin A) are relative contraindications. Biochemical liver function tests are not a particularly sensitive guide to the degree of underlying liver damage but nevertheless it is recommended that these be monitored at 3-6 monthly intervals, with a repeat liver biopsy after each 1.5 g cumulative dose.

Recommendations for patients with rheumatoid arthritis are considerably more relaxed. This is because abnormalities in liver function tests provide a much more sensitive guide to the underlying liver lesion (Kremer *et al.* 1996). No case of clinically significant liver disease has been reported in a patient treated with methotrexate for rheumatoid arthritis when liver function tests were consistently normal on regular monitoring. In the light of these findings the American College of Rheumatology has recommended that pretreatment liver biopsy should be carried out only in patients with a history of excessive alcohol consumption, persistently abnormal baseline transaminases, or chronic hepatitis B or C (Kremer *et al.* 1994).

It has also been suggested that patients with insulin-dependent diabetes should be included in this high-risk category (Erickson *et al.* 1995). In other patients pre-treatment liver function tests and hepatitis viral serology should be obtained and liver function tests monitored at 4–8 week intervals. Liver biopsy is recommended if serum transaminases are above the upper limit of normal in more than 50 per cent of estimations over a 12-month period. When liver enzyme abnormalities persist the dose of methotrexate should be decreased, followed by temporary discontinuation if the liver enzymes remain abnormal.

An audit of these guidelines (Erickson *et al.* 1995) concluded that they were clinically useful and resulted in considerable cost savings by avoiding liver biopsies. The guidelines were, however, based on patients in their first 5 years of treatment, and whether they would be applicable over longer periods of treatment will need to be established.

Hepatic ultrasound scanning may be useful in monitoring; a normal scan excludes pathological changes whereas, if it is abnormal, biopsy is needed to differentiate fatty change from fibrosis and cirrhosis. Serial estimations of procollagen peptide as an index of fibrogenesis appear to be helpful, in that liver disease is very unlikely if levels remain low (Boffa *et al.* 1996). Dynamic hepatic scintigraphy is also useful in pinpointing patients progressing to fibrosis who require further investigation with liver biopsy (van Dooren *et al.* 1996).

Vitamin A

The recommended daily intake for this vitamin is 5000 IU for adult males and 4000 IU for non-pregnant adult females (Roenigk 1988). Ninety per cent of vitamin A is stored in the liver in Ito cells, which are modified fibroblasts lining the sinusoids. Supplements of vitamin A have been used in the treatment of psoriasis, in which the skin lesion bears some resemblance to that seen in vitamin A deficiency. Other less defined indications for vitamin A supplements include the prophylaxis of cancer and arthritis, and preparations containing this compound are readily available 'over-the-counter' so it is easy to exceed the recommended daily doses by a factor of 10 or more (Olson 1983; Inkeles *et al.* 1986; Minuk *et al.* 1988). It is at this level (around 50 000 IU per day for 2 years or more) that toxic symptoms may occur (Leo and Lieber 1988; Fallon and Boyer 1990). Cumulative dose appears to be important; in one series the smallest continuous daily consumption leading to cirrhosis was 25 000 IU over 6 years, whereas higher daily doses (100 000 IU or more) taken over two-and-a-half years resulted in similar histological changes (Geubel *et al.* 1991). Patients with renal failure may be more suscep-

tible and there is a report of such a patient on dialysis who developed toxicity after supplementation with approximately 4000 IU per day (Shmunes 1974). Protein malnutrition may exacerbate hepatotoxicity from vitamin A by preventing its mobilization from the liver (Weber *et al.* 1982).

Clinical manifestations of vitamin A toxicity include general malaise and weakness, alopecia, muscle wasting, pruritus, exfoliative dermatitis, and liver damage. The early liver lesion consist of fatty infiltration with large vesicles in Ito cells; subsequently perisinusoidal fibrosis with accumulation of collagen within the space of Disse may develop (Zafrani *et al.* 1984). This appears to occur as a result of Ito cells being transformed into fibroblasts with increased collagen production (Kent *et al.* 1976), a sequence of events which is also associated with alcohol-induced perisinusoidal fibrosis. Indeed, there is evidence that alcohol and vitamin A act synergistically to produce this lesion in experimental animals (Leo and Lieber 1983). Continuation of vitamin A eventually leads to cirrhosis (Jacques *et al.* 1979), whereas if it is stopped the liver lesion slowly regresses (Guarascio *et al.* 1983; Oren and Ilan 1992). Cases of non-cirrhotic portal hypertension have also been described due to obstruction of portal venules (Guarascio *et al.* 1983).

Etretinate

This is an analogue of retinoic acid but it does not accumulate in the liver in significant amounts. It has been shown to be effective in the treatment of psoriasis. Because of the problems with vitamin A, its effect on the liver has been carefully studied. Asymptomatic alterations in liver function tests have been described (Thirumoorthy and Shupack 1988) and also more severe reactions, including acute hepatocellular necrosis (van-Voorst *et al.* 1984; Fallon and Boyer 1990), cholestatic hepatitis (Weiss *et al.* 1984; Khouri *et al.* 1987; Kano *et al.* 1994), and active chronic hepatitis (Weiss *et al.* 1985; Sanchez *et al.* 1993). The presence of eosinophilia in one case and the prompt relapse on rechallenge in another suggest a hypersensitivity reaction to the drug.

Chronic cholestasis

A syndrome that clinically and histologically resembles primary biliary cirrhosis (PBC) occurs in association with a number of drugs, all of which have been shown to produce acute cholestasis (Table 13.7). Antimitochondrial antibodies are usually absent. Histologically there is disappearance of small (less than 0.03 mm diameter)

TABLE 13.7
Drug-induced chronic cholestasis
(Vanishing bile duct syndrome)

Antimicrobials

Amoxycillin	(Davies *et al* .1994)
Clindamycin	(Altraif *et al.* 1994)
Co-amoxiclav	(Ryley *et al.* 1995)
(amoxycillin + clavulanic acid)	
Co-trimoxazole	(Kowdley *et al.* 1992; Altraif *et al.* 1994; Muller *et al.* 1996)
Erythromycin +chlorpropamide	(Geubel *et al.* 1988)
Flucloxacillin	(Turner *et al.* 1989; Miros *et al.* 1990; Davies *et al.* 1994)
Tetracyclines	(Hunt and Washington 1994)
Thiabendazole	(Manivel *et al.* 1987; Roy *et al.* 1989)

CNS

Amitriptyline	(Larrey *et al.* 1988*a*)
Carbamazepine	(Forbes *et al.* 1992; de Galocsy *et al.* 1994)
Chlorpromazine	(Moradpour *et al.* 1994)
Chlorpromazine + valproic acid	(Bach *et al.* 1989)
Cyproheptadine	(Larrey *et al.* 1987)
Imipramine	(Horst *et al.* 1980)
Prochlorperazine	(O'Brien *et al.* 1996)

intrahepatic bile ducts (vanishing bile duct syndrome). The drugs most frequently implicated have been the phenothiazines, in particular chlorpromazine, and several antibiotics (Vial *et al.* 1997).

The syndrome may be manifested as chronic cholestatic jaundice with its attendant complications or just as persistently abnormal liver function tests (predominantly alkaline phosphatase) with no symptoms or signs. In either situation liver function usually returns to normal although this may take several years. In some cases abnormalities can be permanent, albeit subclinical, as for imipramine. In others the disease may progress, as with thiabendazole; one patient required liver transplantation (Roy *et al.* 1989). Prolonged cholestasis with progressive liver disease has been reported from a combination of chlorpropramide and erythromycin and chlorpromazine and valproic acid. Mutual potentiation of the affects of two hepatotoxic drugs was presumably involved but the mechanisms have not been identified. Altraif and colleagues described the syndrome following treatment with clindamycin; a second biopsy after clinical improvement showed resolution of cholestasis but persistence of duct paucity. Three years later treatment with ampicillin caused another episode of cholestatic hepatitis and duct paucity on rebiopsy, suggesting cross-

reactivity between clindamycin and ampicillin (Altraif *et al.* 1994).

Other biliary abnormalities

Chemotherapy with floxuridine (q.v.), administered into the hepatic artery, can cause abnormalities of the biliary tree very similar to sclerosing cholangitis.

Vascular lesions

Budd–Chiari syndrome

Several case reports have suggested an association between use of oral contraceptives and hepatic vein thrombosis (Lewis *et al.* 1983*a*; Maddrey 1987). Valla and colleagues (1986), in a case–control study of 33 women with Budd–Chiari syndrome, identified a relative risk of 2.37 for this complication in users of oral contraceptives. This figure is very close to that for other vascular complications from these compounds.

Veno-occlusive disease

Veno-occlusive disease (VOD) is characterized by non-thrombotic concentric narrowing of the lumen of central hepatic veins by connective tissue. It occurs in the absence of obstruction of large hepatic veins. Severe centrilobular congestion and necrosis reflect the venous blockage. Presentation may be acute with right upper quadrant pain, ascites, and, in the most severely affected cases, hepatic failure. This progresses to cirrhosis in those who survive. Alternatively, cirrhosis may develop insidiously over a number of years and present with its complications, including hepatocellular carcinoma.

Pyrrolizidine alkaloids

These alkaloids are present in numerous plant species but hepatotoxicity in man most commonly results from consumption of plants or extracts of plants belonging to the families Heliotropium, Crotalaria, Senecio, and Symphytum (comfrey). Veno-occlusive disease (VOD) is the main liver lesion produced by this group of compounds (Valla and Benhamou 1988).

Poisoning may present as an epidemic if it is due to contamination of food by alkaloid-containing plants (Tandon *et al.* 1978). Sporadic cases are generally due to inadvertent self-poisoning from consumption of alkaloid-containing plant extracts with alleged health-giving properties. Infusions or tablets containing comfrey are particularly frequently implicated in this respect (Ridker et al. 1985; Ridker and McDermott 1989; Couet et al. 1996). A fatal case of VOD has been described in a baby whose mother took herbal tea containing comfrey throughout pregnancy. The mother, however, suffered no ill-effects (Roulet et al. 1988).

Immunosuppressive and antineoplastic drugs

Numerous reports clearly implicate azathioprine and the chemically related drug mercaptopurine as a cause of VOD (Katzkal et al. 1986; Haboubi et al. 1988; Liano et al. 1989). Most patients affected have been renal transplant recipients receiving corticosteroids, and there has been a striking predominance of males. The onset is typically delayed for at least 6 months after starting the drug and may be much later than this. The mode of presentation is different from that in other causes of VOD, with prominent jaundice and histological features of both cholestasis and centrilobular necrosis. Sinusoidal and perivenular fibrosis, peliosis hepatis, and nodular regenerative hyperplasia (see below) can sometimes be seen as associated pathological lesions; it is possible that they are aetiologically linked (Wanless et al. 1980).

Rapid deterioration with death from hepatic failure and complications of portal hypertension may occur, or the disease may take a more prolonged course. Mortality is high but partial regression of the lesion after withdrawal of the drug, particularly in the less fulminant cases, has been reported (Adler et al. 1987; Kohli et al. 1996).

Conditioning for bone marrow transplantation

Radiation damage to the liver is a common cause of VOD and is a dose-related phenomenon, rarely being seen with doses below 30 Gy unless the patient is receiving concomitant chemotherapy (Fajardo and Colby 1980), when doses as little as 10 Gy may be sufficient to produce this complication. Damage is usually localized to the section of the liver that has been exposed and usually manifests itself within 2–5 weeks of irradiation. Anticoagulation has been proposed for prophylaxis.

High-dose chemotherapy with busulphan or cyclophosphamide for bone marrow transplantation is complicated by VOD of the liver in approximately 25 per cent of patients (Styler et al. 1996). For busulphan the pharmacokinetics of the drug can be used to predict the likelihood of this complication, and monitoring busulphan plasma levels can allow adjustments of drug dosage to minimize the risk of this complication (Dix et al. 1996). There is evidence that heparin prophylaxis may reduce the incidence of this complication (Rosenthal et al. 1996a).

Thioguanine

This drug is chemically related to azathioprine and mercaptopurine. It has been implicated as a cause of VOD but since it has generally been used in association with other antineoplastic agents this has often been difficult to prove, although liver histology may revert to normal when the drug is withdrawn (D'Cruz et al. 1983; Kao and Rosenblate 1993; Bonkovsky et al. 1996).

Dacarbazine

Patients receiving this drug for melanoma seem particularly prone to develop injury to small- and medium-sized hepatic veins. The reported incidence is between one and three per cent. The vascular lesion induced by dacarbazine differs from classical VOD in that it is thrombotic (Greenstone et al. 1981; Ceci et al. 1988; Marsh 1989).

Other antineoplastic drugs

Other drugs implicated include doxorubicin (adriamycin), vincristine, carmustine (Ware and Millward 1980), and mitomycin.

A combination of cyclophosphamide and busulphan appears to be a potentially potent cause of this complication (Morgan et al. 1991; Kasai et al. 1992; Styler et al. 1996). Other toxic combinations include dactinomycin with vincristine (Green et al. 1988, 1990); methotrexate with busulphan and cyclophosphamide (Essell et al. 1992); carmustine with cyclophosphamide and carboplatin (Ware and Millward 1980; Jones et al. 1990); doxorubicin with mitomycin (Craft and Pembrey 1987); vincristine with actinomycin D and cyclophosphamide (Kanwar et al. 1995; Ortega et al. 1997).

Mechanism of VOD

Both dacarbazine and azathioprine are directly hepatotoxic to sinusoidal endothelial cells in culture, and glutathione exerts a protective effect (De Leve 1994; De Leve et al. 1996b). Cyclophosphamide, in contrast, is not toxic but a metabolite, as yet unidentified, is (De Leve et al. 1996a). For dacarbazine, the occurrence of eosinophilic infiltration in the liver and other organs, and the fact that the reaction often occurs during a second course of treatment after the first has been well tolerated, are pointers to a hypersensitivity mechanism (McClay et al. 1987).

Oestrogens

Although oestrogens can produce the Budd–Chiari syndrome, their role in producing VOD is controversial. In an interesting study, Setchell and colleagues (1987) found a high incidence of VOD amongst cheetahs in a zoo where there was also a high frequency of reproductive failure amongst this species. The latter was eventually traced to the fact that the animals' feeds contained plant-based oestrogens. When this was remedied, procreation resumed and there was resolution of the hepatic abnormalities. Based on these observations, the authors suggested that oestrogens were the cause of VOD, although it has been pointed out that other dietary factors may also have been involved. Synthetic oestrogens have also been implicated.

Hepatic sinusoidal dilatation and peliosis hepatis

Dilatation of hepatic sinusoids has most frequently been associated with use of oral contraceptives. It is usually asymptomatic, but very rarely it may be associated with right upper quadrant pain with jaundice and elevations in transaminases and alkaline phosphatase. The condition regresses after drug withdrawal (Weinberger *et al.* 1985).

Peliosis hepatis is characterized by dilated blood filled cysts, bordered by hepatocytes. It has been reported in women taking oral contraceptives and it may represent an exaggerated form of the sinusoidal dilatation described above (Kerlin *et al.* 1983). In most cases, however, the vascular lesion has been adjacent to a liver tumour and could well have been caused by localized venous obstruction.

Sinusoidal dilatation and peliosis hepatis, in the absence of other liver lesions, have been demonstrated in the livers of female-to-male transsexuals receiving orally active anabolic steroids (Westaby *et al.* 1977). This suggests that these compounds, which are chemically related to the synthetic steroids in oral contraceptives, have a true potential to produce these lesions. Other reports implicating these drugs have generally centred on patients with conditions such as rheumatoid arthritis or Hodgkin's disease, and the vascular abnormality could have been caused by the disease or its complications rather than by the anabolic steroids (Naeim *et al.* 1973; Bagheri and Boyer 1974).

Azathioprine-associated peliosis hepatis has been reported mainly in renal transplant recipients, in whom it may occur alone or in combination with other abnormalities (Haboubi *et al.* 1988). Portal hypertension with oesophageal varices and ascites can occur in association (Gerlag *et al.* 1985).

Nodular regenerative hyperplasia

Azathioprine therapy may also be complicated by nodular regenerative hyperplasia; in this condition there are nodules of apparently regenerating hepatocytes scattered throughout the parenchyma. Intervening areas of atrophy are often seen, implying that the condition arises secondary to localized hepatocyte injury. It may be complicated by portal hypertension, presumably due to pressure effects. It has mainly been described in renal transplant recipients treated with azathioprine or mercaptopurine but may also occur in patients with rheumatoid arthritis and haematological disorders (Wanless *et al.* 1980; Haboubi *et al.* 1988; Stromeyer and Ishak 1997).

Other vascular complications

Hepatic infarction has been described in association with use of oral contraceptives (Jacobs 1984). This may be related to intimal hyperplasia; these agents produce such changes in blood vessels elsewhere in the body, and they also occur in pregnancy.

Along with other thrombotic complications of oral contraceptives, thrombosis of the portal vein has been the subject of a few case reports (Capron *et al.* 1981).

Spontaneous rupture of the liver, an extremely rare complication of pregnancy, has been described following use of oestrogens and oral contraceptives (Frederick *et al.* 1974), and also in a pregnant cocaine abuser (Moen *et al.* 1993).

Liver tumours

Adenoma

Oral contraceptives

Since the first report, in 1973, of hepatic adenomata in long-term users of oral contraceptives (Baum *et al.* 1997), a large number of publications confirming this association have appeared (Christopherson and Mays 1977*a*; Mays and Christopherson 1984). The upsurge in the numbers of this previously extremely rare tumour indicated that its association with oral contraceptives was more than a matter of chance. Hormone dependence was further suggested by its occasional appearance in pregnancy and the puerperium when levels of gonadal steroids are high (Christopherson *et al.* 1977*b*), and the association of a virtually identical picture with synthetic anabolic steroids (see below).

A characteristic feature of these tumours is their extreme vascularity. Histologically they contain collections of dilated thin-walled blood vessels resembling peliosis hepatis. As a result of this extreme vascularity, haemorrhage into the tumour or rupture with haemoperitoneum are common modes of presentation (Kerlin *et al.* 1983; Mays and Christopherson 1984). In many cases, however, tumours may present as an asymptomatic abdominal mass or with episodes of upper abdominal pain, probably due to small haemorrhages into the tumour. They frequently go misdiagnosed for years (Neuberger *et al.* 1980).

Management

The behaviour of hepatic adenomata induced by oral contraceptives is unpredictable, which makes it difficult to give dogmatic guidelines on management. Progression is likely if oral contraceptives are not discontinued, but in many cases regression of the lesion has been reported if the pill is stopped, although this is not invariable (Edmondson *et al.* 1977; Steinbrecher *et al.* 1981; Buhler *et al.* 1982; Nagorney 1995). In others, progression to hepatocellular carcinoma has been described (Davis *et al.* 1975; Gordon *et al.* 1986; Tao 1991; Foster and Berman 1994; Perret *et al.* 1996).

If tumour resection is not carried out the patient should be carefully monitored with serial ultrasound or CT scans of the liver.

Anabolic steroids

As with the lesion induced by oral contraceptives, these tumours are highly vascular with areas of peliosis hepatis, and can rupture spontaneously (Westaby et al. 1977; Paradinas *et al.* 1977; Westaby *et al.* 1983; Touraine *et al.* 1993). Athletes who use anabolic steroids in short bursts do not appear to develop this complication, but one who took them for 3 years presented with a ruptured tumour (Creagh *et al.* 1988).

These liver lesions have mostly been associated with 17-alkylated preparations, but multiple adenomata have been described in a renal transplant recipient who had been taking testosterone enanthate, which is not a 17-alkylated compound (Carrasco *et al.* 1984). Hepatic adenomas have been reported from danazol taken for periods of 6 months to 2 years (Middleton *et al.* 1989; Fermand *et al.* 1990; Kahn *et al.* 1991).

Focal nodular hyperplasia

This lesion has also frequently been reported as complicating long-term use of oral contraceptives (Scott *et al.* 1984; Hagay *et al.* 1988). Many of these abnormalities are discovered incidentally but they may present with rupture and haemoperitoneum (Kerlin *et al.* 1983; Mays and Christopherson 1984).

Whether or not this lesion is aetiologically related to oral contraceptives is controversial, but overall epidemiological evidence is against it (Klatskin 1977; Mays and Christopherson 1984). It can occur in both sexes, and at any age, and the overall incidence has not altered with the introduction of oral contraceptives, as it has for adenoma. It is, however, highly likely that oral contraceptives increase the vascularity of these lesions, and predispose to the haemorrhage and rupture which bring them to clinical attention (Mathieu *et al.* 1989). Similar considerations apply to the association of this lesion with anabolic steroids.

Hepatocellular carcinoma

Oral contraceptives

Several studies have shown increases in relative risk of hepatocellular carcinoma from continuous use of oral contraceptives for periods of 5 years or more (Forman *et al.* 1986; Neuberger *et al.* 1986; La Vecchia *et al.* 1989). However, epidemiological studies have failed to show an overall increase in incidence of this neoplasm amongst women over a time period when use of oral contraceptives was increasing (Mant and Vessey 1995; Waetjen and Grimes 1996). The overall role of these compounds in the pathogenesis of hepatocellular carcinoma must therefore be small.

Hepatocellular carcinomas associated with oral contraceptives tend to present more frequently with rupture, haemorrhage, and pain, and survival is longer (Hromas *et al.* 1985). Some are histologically identical to fibrolamellar hepatoma, which is characteristically seen in young people and has a better prognosis. Circulating levels of alphafetoprotein are usually not elevated, although it has been suggested that this marker may be useful for detecting malignant transformation of adenomata (Foster and Berman 1994).

Anabolic steroids

All reported cases of hepatocellular carcinoma from anabolic steroids have been associated with 17-alpha-alkylated steroids for the treatment of bone marrow aplasia, the correction of impotence, or for the maintenance of secondary sexual characteristics in female-to-male transsexuals (Westaby *et al.* 1977; Coombes *et al.* 1978). In general, the doses taken have been high. It appears that patients with Fanconi's anaemia are especially susceptible, developing liver tumours after a shorter period than patients taking androgens for other reasons.

The majority of androgen-related tumours have been described as histologically indistinguishable from primary hepatocellular carcinoma. The tumours tend to be less aggressive, however, although this is not always the case (Gleeson *et al.* 1991). Regression has been reported following androgen withdrawal (Farrell *et al.* 1975). Elevated serum levels of alphafetoprotein are not seen with these neoplasms.

These tumours are frequently highly vascular and the surrounding liver parenchyma may be infiltrated with dilated blood-filled cysts characteristic of peliosis hepatis. These may rupture either into the liver parenchyma or the peritoneal cavity (Paradinas *et al.* 1977).

Hepatocellular carcinoma has also been demonstrated as a complication of treatment with danazol for 2–4 years (Buamah 1985; Weill *et al.* 1988).

Liver tumours following thorotrast

Thorotrast, a colloidal suspension of thorium dioxide, was used as a radiological contrast medium between the late 1920s and mid-1950s. It accumulates in the reticuloendothelial system, particularly in the liver, and since thorium is radioactive with a half-life of approximately 400 years the local radiation dose can be substantial. This is reflected in a high incidence of malignancies, particularly involving the liver, reported at various intervals after exposure. The characteristic tumour associated with thorotrast is angiosarcoma, but cholangiocarcinoma and hepatocellular carcinoma have also been reported (Imai *et al.* 1988; Ito *et al.* 1988). Because of the long latent period between exposure and presentation, cases are still being reported (Weber *et al.* 1995; Lee *et al.* 1996; Srinivasan and Dean 1997), and it is predicted that this will continue into the second decade of the 21st century.

Other hepatobiliary malignancies

A retrospective survey of 83 patients with biliary carcinoma showed that a much higher number than expected had been taking methyldopa (Broden and Bengtsson 1980). The explanation for this is unclear.

Concerns that use of enzyme-inducing anticonvulsants and benzodiazepines might predispose to hepatobiliary malignancy have not been confirmed in two epidemiological studies (Rosenberg *et al.* 1995; Olsen *et al.* 1995).

References

Actis, G.C., Debernardi, V.W., Lagget, M., *et al.* (1995). Hepatotoxicity of intravenous cyclosporin A in patients with acute ulcerative colitis on total parenteral nutrition. *Liver* 15, 320.

Adler, E., Benjamin, S.B., and Zimmerman, H.J. (1986). Cholestatic hepatic injury related to warfarin exposure. *Arch. Intern. Med.* 146, 1837.

Adler, M., Delhaye, M., Deprez, C., *et al.* (1987). Hepatic vascular disease after kidney transplantation: report of two cases and review of the literature. *Nephrol. Dial. Transplant.* 2, 183.

Ahern, M.J., Milazzo, S.C., and Dymock, R. (1980). Granulomatous hepatitis and Seatone. *Med. J. Aust.* 2, 151.

Ahn, C.S. and Tow, D.E. (1990). Intrahepatic cholestasis due to hypersensitivity reaction to procainamide. *Arch. Intern. Med.* 150, 2589.

Al Kawas, F.H., Seeff, L.B., Berendson, R.A., *et al.* (1981). Allopurinol hepatotoxicity. Report of two cases and review of the literature. *Ann. Intern. Med.* 95, 588.

Al Sarraf KA, Michielsen, P.P., Hauben, E.I., *et al.* (1996). Hepatotoxicity after a short course of low-dose pyrazinamide. *Acta Gastroenterol. Belg.* 59, 251.

Alam, I., Ferrell, L.D., and Bass, N.M. (1996). Vanishing bile duct syndrome temporally associated with ibuprofen use. *Am. J. Gastroenterol.* 91, 1626.

Alcalde, M., Garcia, D.M., Najarro, F., *et al.* (1994). Hepatitis toxica y autoinmune tipo I-like y anemia hiporregenerativa por bendazaco [Toxic and autoimmune type I-like hepatitis and hyporegenerative anemia caused by bendazac]. *Rev. Esp. Enferm. Dig.* 85, 404.

Alderman, S., Kailas, S., Goldfarb, S., *et al.* (1994). Cholestatic hepatitis after ingestion of chaparral leaf: confirmation by endoscopic retrograde cholangiopancreatography and liver biopsy. *J. Clin. Gastroenterol.* 19, 242.

Aleem, A. and Lingam, V. (1987). Hepatotoxicity following treatment with maprotiline. *J. Clin. Psychopharmacol.* 7, 54.

Alexander, G.J.M., Brahm, J., Fagan, E.A., *et al.* (1987). Loss of HbsAg with interferon therapy in chronic hepatitis B virus infection. *Lancet* ii, 66.

Altraif, I., Lilly, L., Wanless, I.R., *et al.* (1994). Cholestatic liver disease with ductopenia (vanishing bile duct syndrome) after administration of clindamycin and trimethoprim-sulfamethoxazole. *Am. J. Gastroenterol.* 89, 1230.

Alvaro, D., Piat, C., Francia, C., *et al.* (1996). Ultrastructural features of danazol-induced cholestasis: a case study. *Ultrastruct. Pathol.* 20, 491.

Ament, P.W., Roth, J.D., and Fox, C.J. (1994). Famotidine-induced mixed hepatocellular jaundice. *Ann. Pharmacother.* 28, 40.

Ames, D.J., Bhathal, P.S., Davies, B.M., *et al.* (1990). Heterogeneity of adverse hepatic reactions to tetrahydroaminoacridine. *Aust. N.Z. J. Med.* 20, 193.

Anderson, B.N. and Henrikson, I.R. (1978). Jaundice and eosinophilia associated with amitriptyline. *J. Clin. Psychiatry* 39, 730.

Anderson, G.D., Acheampong, A.A., Wilensky, A.J., *et al.* (1992). Effect of valproate dose on formation of hepatotoxic metabolites. *Epilepsia* 33, 736.

Anderson, I.B., Mullen, W.H., Meeker, J.E., *et al.* (1996). Pennyroyal toxicity: measurement of toxic metabolite levels in two cases and review of the literature. *Ann. Intern. Med.* 124, 726.

Andrejak, M., Davion, T., Gineston, J.L., *et al.* (1987). Cross hepatotoxicity between non-steroidal anti-inflammatory drugs. *BMJ* (Clin.Res. Ed.) 295, 180.

Appleton, R.E., Farrell, K., Applegarth, D.A., *et al.* (1990). The high incidence of valproate hepatotoxicity in infants may relate to familial metabolic defects. *Can. J. Neurol. Sci.* 17, 145.

Arab, D.M., Malatjalian, D.A., and Rittmaster, R.S. (1995). Severe cholestatic jaundice in uncomplicated hyperthyroidism treated with methimazole. *J. Clin. Endocrinol. Metab.* 80, 1083.

Arellano, F. and Sacristan, J.A. (1993). Allopurinol hypersensitivity syndrome: a review. *Ann. Pharmacother.* 27, 337.

Arnold T.H., J., Epps, J.M., Cook, H.R., *et al.* (1983). Dantrolene sodium: urinary metabolites and hepatotoxicity. *Res. Commun. Chem. Pathol. Pharmacol.* 39, 381.

Arnold, R. (1994). Safety of proton pump inhibitors — an overview. *Aliment. Pharmacol. Ther.* 8 (Suppl. 1), 65.

Arranto, A.J. and Sotaniemi, E.A. (1981*a*). Histologic follow-up of alpha-methyldopa-induced liver injury. *J. Scand. Gastroenterol.* 16, 865.

Arranto, A.J. and Sotaniemi, E.A. (1981*b*). Morphologic alterations in patients with alpha-methyldopa-induced liver damage after short- and long-term exposure. *J. Scand. Gastroenterol.* 16, 853.

Ashton, R.E., Millward, S.G., and White, J.E. (1982). Complications in methotrexate treatment of psoriasis with particular reference to liver fibrosis. *J. Invest. Dermatol.* 79, 229.

Askgaard, D.S., Wilcke, T., and Dossing, M. (1995). Hepatotoxicity caused by the combined action of isoniazid and rifampicin. *Thorax* 50, 213.

Askmark, H. and Wiholm, B.E. (1990). Epidemiology of adverse reactions to carbamazepine as seen in a spontaneous reporting system. *Acta Neurol. Scand.* 81, 131.

Aubrey, D.A. (1970). Massive hepatic necrosis after cyclophosphamide. *BMJ* 3, 588.

Babany, G., Uzzan, F., Larrey, D., *et al.* (1989). Alcoholic-like liver lesions induced by nifedipine. *J. Hepatol.* 9, 252.

Bach, N., Thung, S.N., Schaffner, F., *et al.* (1989). Exaggerated cholestasis and hepatic fibrosis following simultaneous administration of chlorpromazine and sodium valproate. *Dig. Dis. Sci.* 34, 1303.

Bachman, B.A., Boyd, W.P., Jr, and Brady, P.G. (1982). Erythromycin ethylsuccinate-induced cholestasis. *Am. J. Gastroenterol.* 77, 397.

Bagheri, S.A. and Boyer, J.L. (1974). Peliosis hepatis associated with androgenic-anabolic steroid therapy. A severe form of hepatic injury. *Ann. Intern. Med.* 81, 610.

Bailey, W.C., Taylor, S.L., Dascomb, H.E., *et al.* (1973). Disturbed hepatic function during isoniazid chemoprophylaxis. *Am. Rev. Respir. Dis.* 107, 523.

Bailey, W.C., Weill, H., de Roen, T.A., *et al.* (1974). The effect of isoniazid on transaminase levels. *Ann. Intern. Med.* 81, 200.

Ballare, M., Campanini, M., Catania, E., *et al.* (1991). Acute cholestatic hepatitis during simvastatin administration. *Recenti Prog. Med.* 82, 233.

Ballare, M., Campanini, M., Airoldi, G., *et al.* (1992). Hepatotoxicity of hydroxy-methyl-glutaryl-coenzyme A reductase inhibitors. *Minerva Gastroenterol. Dietol.* 38, 41.

Banks, A.T., Zimmerman, H.J., Ishak, K.G., *et al.* (1995). Diclofenac-associated hepatotoxicity: analysis of 180 cases reported to the Food and Drug Administration as adverse reactions. *Hepatology* 22, 820.

Bass, B.H. (1974). Jaundice associated with naproxen. *Lancet* i, 998.

Bassendine, M.F., Woodhouse, K.W., Bennett, M., *et al.* (1986). Dextropropoxyphene induced hepatotoxicity mimicking biliary tract disease. *Gut* 27, 444.

Baum, J.K., Holtz, F., Bookstein, J.J., *et al.* (1997). Possible association between benign hepatomas and oral contraceptives. *Lancet* 926.

Beaune, P., Dansette, P.M., Mansuy, D., *et al.* (1987). Human anti-endoplasmic reticulum antibodies appearing in a drug-induced hepatitis are directed against a human liver cytochrome P-450 that hydroxylates the drug. *Proc. Natl. Acad. Sci. USA* 84, 551.

Beck, P.L., Bridges, R.J., Demetrick, D.J., *et al.* (1993). Chronic active hepatitis associated with trazodone therapy. *Ann. Intern. Med.* 118, 791.

Beermann, B. (1993). Side effects of long acting cholinesterase inhibitors. *Acta Neurol. Scand.* 149 (Suppl.), 53.

Beever, I.W., Blair, I.A., and Brodie, M.J. (1982). Circulating hydrazine during treatment with isoniazid/rifampicin in man. *Br. J. Clin. Pharmacol.* 13, 599.

Belli, D.C., Fournier, L.A., Lepage, G., *et al.* (1994). S-adenosylmethionine prevents total parenteral nutrition-induced cholestasis in the rat. *J. Hepatol.* 21, 18.

Ben, Y.A., Bloom, A., Lijovetzky, G., *et al.* (1990). Chlorpromazine-induced liver and bone marrow granulomas associated with agranulocytosis. *Isr. J. Med. Sci.* 26, 449.

Ben, Y.M., Mavier, P., Metreau, J.M., *et al.* (1993). Hépatite chronique active et cirrhose induites par la germandrée petit-chêne. Trois cas. *Gastroenterol. Clin. Biol.* 17, 959.

Benichou, C. (1990). Criteria of drug-induced liver disorders. Report of an international consensus meeting. *J. Hepatol.* 11, 272.

Benjamin, S.B., Ishak, K.G., Zimmerman, H.J., *et al.* (1981). Phenylbutazone liver injury: a clinical-pathologic survey of 23 cases and review of the literature. *Hepatology* 1, 255.

Benjamin, S.B., Goodman, Z.D., Ishak, K.G., *et al.* (1985). The morphologic spectrum of halothane-induced hepatic injury: analysis of 77 cases. *Hepatology* 5, 1163.

Benson, G.D. (1983). Hepatotoxicity following the therapeutic use of antipyretic analgesics. *Am. J. Med.* 75, 85.

Benson, G.D., Anderson, P.K., Combes, B., *et al.* (1988). Prolonged jaundice following ketoconazole-induced hepatic injury. *Dig. Dis. Sci.* 33, 240.

Berg, P.A. and Daniel, P.T. (1987). Co-trimoxazole-induced hepatic injury — an analysis of cases with hypersensitivity-like reactions. *Infection* 15 (Suppl. 5), S259.

Bernhard, G.C. (1992). Worldwide safety experience with nabumetone. *J. Rheumatol.* 19 (Suppl), 84.

Berris, B. and Feinman, S.V. (1991). Thyroid dysfunction and liver injury following alpha-interferon treatment of chronic viral hepatitis. *Dig. Dis. Sci.* 36, 1657.

Berry, W.R., Warren, G.H., and Reichen, J. (1984). Nitrofurantoin-induced cholestatic hepatitis from cow's milk in a teenaged boy. *West. J. Med.* 140, 278.

Berson, A., Renault, S., Letteron, P., *et al.* (1996). Uncoupling of rat and human mitochondria: a possible explanation for tacrine-induced liver dysfunction. *Gastroenterology* 110, 1878.

Bezahler, G.H. (1982). Fatal methyldopa-associated granulomatous hepatitis and myocarditis. *Am. J. Med. Sci.* 283, 41.

Bhagwat, A.G. and Warren, R.E. (1969). Hepatic reaction to nitrofurantoin. *Lancet* ii, 1369.

Bjorkman, D.J., Hammond, E.H., Lee, R.G., *et al.* (1988). Hepatic ultrastructure after methotrexate therapy for rheumatoid arthritis. *Arthritis Rheum.* 31, 1465.

Black, M., Mitchell, J.R., Zimmerman, H.J., *et al.* (1975). Isoniazid-associated hepatitis in 114 patients. *Gastroenterology* 69, 289.

Black, M., Rabin, L., and Schatz, N. (1980). Nitrofurantoin-induced chronic active hepatitis. *Ann. Intern. Med.* 92, 62.

Blackburn, A.M., Amiel, S.A., Millis, R.R., *et al.* (1984). Tamoxifen and liver damage. *BMJ* (Clin. Res. Ed.) 289, 288.

Blake, J.C., Sawyerr, A.M., Dooley, J.S., *et al.* (1990). Severe hepatitis caused by cyproterone acetate. *Gut* 31, 556.

Blom, H., Stolk, J., Schreuder, H.B., *et al.* (1985). A case of carbimazole-induced intrahepatic cholestasis. An immune-mediated reaction? *Arch. Intern. Med.* 145, 1513.

Bloodworth, J.M.B. and Hamwei, G.J. (1961). Histopathologic lesions associated with sulfonylurea administration. *Diabetes* 10, 90.

Bluhm, R.E., Rodgers, W.H., Black, D.L., *et al.* (1992). Cholestasis in transplant patients — what is the role of cyclosporin? *Aliment. Pharmacol. Ther.* 6, 207.

Boelsterli, U.A., Zimmerman, H.J., and Kretz-Rommel, A. (1995). Idiosyncratic liver toxicity of nonsteroidal anti-inflammatory drugs: molecular mechanisms and pathology. *Crit. Rev. Toxicol.* 25, 207.

Boffa, M.J., Smith, A., Chalmers, R.J., *et al.* (1996). Serum type III procollagen aminopeptide for assessing liver damage in methotrexate-treated psoriatic patients. *Br. J. Dermatol.* 135, 538.

Bohles, H., Sewell, A.C., and Wenzel, D. (1996). The effect of carnitine supplementation in valproate-induced hyperammonaemia. *Acta Paediatr.* 85, 446.

Bolton, J.S. and Bowen, J.C. (1986). Biliary sclerosis associated with hepatic artery infusion of floxuridine. *Surgery* 99, 119.

Bonkovsky, H.L., Mudge, G.H., and McMurtry, R.J. (1978). Chronic hepatic inflammation and fibrosis due to low doses of paracetamol. *Lancet* i, 1016.

Bonkovsky, H.L., Banner, B.F., Lambrecht, R.W., *et al.* (1996). Iron in liver diseases other than hemochromatosis. *Semin. Liver Dis.* 16, 65.

Bower, R., Mrdeza, M.A., and Block, G.E. (1990). Association of cholecystitis and parenteral nutrition. *Nutrition* 6, 125.

Bowyer, B.A., Miles, J.M., Haymond, M.W., *et al.* (1988). L-carnitine therapy in home parenteral nutrition patients with abnormal liver tests and low plasma carnitine concentrations. *Gastroenterology* 94, 434.

Boyd, P.T., Lepre, F., and Dickey, J.D. (1989). Chronic active hepatitis associated with cimetidine. *BMJ* 298, 324.

Boyer, C.S. and Petersen, D.R. (1990). Potentiation of cocaine-mediated hepatotoxicity by acute and chronic ethanol. *Alcohol Clin. Exp. Res.* 14, 28.

Bramlet, D.A., Posalaky, Z., and Olson, R. (1980). Granulomatous hepatitis as a manifestation of quinidine hypersensitivity. *Arch. Intern. Med.* 140, 395.

Braun, P. (1969). Hepatotoxicity of erythromycin. *J. Infect. Dis.* 119, 300.

Bray, G.P., Harrison, P.M., and O'Grady, J.G. (1992). Long-term anticonvulsant therapy worsens outcome in paracetamol-induced fulminant hepatic failure. *Hum. Exp. Toxicol.* 11, 265.

Bray, G.P., Mowat, C., Muir, D.F., *et al.* (1991). The effect of chronic alcohol intake on prognosis and outcome in paracetamol overdose. *Hum. Exp. Toxicol.* 10, 435.

Bray, G.P., Tredger, J.M., and Williams, R. (1992). *S*-adenosylmethionine protects against paracetamol hepatotoxicity in two mouse models. *Hepatology* 15, 297.

Bray, G.P., Tredger, J.M., and Williams, R. (1993). Resolution of danazol-induced cholestasis with *S*-adenosylmethionine. *Postgrad. Med. J.* 69, 237.

Bridges, M.E. and Pittman, F.E. (1980). Tolazamide-induced cholestasis. *South. Med. J.* 73, 1072.

Broden, G. and Bengtsson, L. (1980). Biliary carcinoma associated with methyldopa therapy. *Acta Chir. Scand.* Suppl. 500 (Suppl.), 7.

Brown, B.R. and Sipes, G. (1977). Biotransformation and hepatotoxicity of halothane. *Biochem. Pharmacol.* 26, 2091.

Bryant, A.E. and Dreifuss, F.E. (1996). Valproic acid hepatic fatalities. III. U.S. experience since 1986. *Neurology* 46, 465.

Buamah, P.K. (1985). An apparent danazol-induced primary hepatocellular carcinoma: case report. *J. Surg. Oncol.* 28, 114.

Buchman, A.L., Dubin, M., Jenden, D., *et al.* (1992). Lecithin increases plasma free choline and decreases hepatic steatosis in long-term total parenteral nutrition patients. *Gastroenterology* 102, 1363.

Buchman, A.L., Dubin, M.D., Moukarzel, A.A., *et al.* (1995). Choline deficiency: a cause of hepatic steatosis during parenteral nutrition that can be reversed with intravenous choline supplementation. *Hepatology* 22, 1399.

Buhler, H., Pirovino, M., Akobiantz, A., *et al.* (1982). Regression of liver cell adenoma. A follow-up study of three consecutive patients after discontinuation of oral contraceptive use. *Gastroenterology* 82, 775.

Burette, A., Finet, C., Prigogine, T., *et al.* (1984). Acute hepatic injury associated with minocycline. *Arch. Intern. Med.* 144, 1491.

Burgert, S.J., Burke, J.P., and Box, T.D. (1995). Reversible nitrofurantoin-induced chronic active hepatitis and hepatic cirrhosis in a patient awaiting liver transplantation. *Transplantation* 59, 448.

Burgunder, J.M., Abernethy, D.R., and Lauterburg, B.H. (1988). Liver injury due to verapamil. *Hepatogastroenterology* 35, 169.

Burke, D.A., Manning, A.P., Williamson, J.M., *et al.* (1987). Adverse reactions to sulphasalazine and 5-amino salicylic acid in the same patient. *Aliment. Pharmacol. Ther.* 1, 201.

Butler, R.C., Shah, S.M., Grunow, W.A., *et al.* (1977). Massive hepatic necrosis in a patient receiving allopurinol. *JAMA* 237, 473.

Byrd, R.B., Horn, B.R., Griggs, G.A., *et al.* (1977). Isoniazid chemoprophylaxis. Association with detection and incidence of liver toxicity. *Arch. Intern. Med.* 137, 1130.

Callahan, J., Haller, J.O., Cacciarelli, A.A., *et al.* (1982). Cholelithiasis in infants: association with total parenteral nutrition and furosemide. *Radiology* 143, 437.

Callen, J.P. and Soderstrom, R.M. (1978). Granulomatous hepatitis associated with salicylazosulfapyridine therapy. *South. Med. J.* 71, 1159.

Campos, A.C., Oler, A., Meguid, M.M., *et al.* (1990). Liver biochemical and histological changes with graded amounts of total parenteral nutrition. *Arch. Surg.* 125, 447.

Canalese, J., Gimson, A.E., Davis, M., *et al.* (1981). Factors contributing to mortality in paracetamol-induced hepatic failure. *BMJ* (Clin. Res. Ed.) 282, 199.

Capelle, P., Dhumeaux, D., Mora, M., *et al.* (1972). Effect of rifampicin on liver function in man. *Gut* 13, 366.

Capron, J.P., Lemay, J.L., Muir, J.F., *et al.* (1981). Portal vein thrombosis and fatal pulmonary thromboembolism associated with oral contraceptive treatment. *J. Clin. Gastroenterol.* 3, 295.

Capron, J.P., Gineston, J.L., Herve, M.A., *et al.* (1983). Metronidazole in prevention of cholestasis associated with total parenteral nutrition. *Lancet* i, 446.

Carlson, R.W. (1997). Scientific review of tamoxifen. Overview from a medical oncologist. *Semin. Oncol.* 24, S1.

Carrasco, D., Pallardo, L., Prieto, M., *et al.* (1984). Hepatic adenomata and androgen treatment. *Ann. Intern. Med.* 100, 316.

Carrigan, T.W. and Straughen, W.J. (1987). A report of hepatic necrosis and death following isoflurane anesthesia. *Anesthesiology* 67, 581.

Carson, J.L., Strom, B.L., Duff, A., *et al.* (1993). Acute liver disease associated with erythromycins, sulfonamides, and tetracyclines. *Ann. Intern. Med.* 119, 576.

Cartel, J.L., Millan, J., Guelpa, L.C., *et al.* (1983). Hepatitis in leprosy patients treated by a daily combination of dapsone, rifampin, and a thioamide. *Int. J. Lepr. Other Mycobact. Dis.* 51, 461.

Cassidy, L.J., Schuster, B.G., and Halparin, L.S. (1995). Probable ticlopidine-induced cholestatic hepatitis. *Ann. Pharmacother.* 29, 30.

Ceci, G., Bella, M., Melissari, M., *et al.* (1988). Fatal hepatic vascular toxicity of DTIC. Is it really a rare event? *Cancer* 61, 1988.

Cereda, J.M., Bernuau, J., Degott, C., *et al.* (1989). Fatal liver failure due to disulfiram. *J. Clin. Gastroenterol.* 11, 98.

Cersosimo, R.J. (1993). Hepatotoxicity associated with cisplatin chemotherapy. *Ann. Pharmacother.* 27, 438.

Chan, C.H. (1990). Dantrolene sodium and hepatic injury. *Neurology* 40, 1427.

Chang, S. and Silvis, S.E. (1974). Fatty liver produced by hyperalimentation of rats. *Am. J. Gastroenterol.* 62, 410.

Chaudhry, S. and Oelsner, D. (1995). Cholestatic reaction to warfarin. *Am. J. Gastroenterol.* 90, 853.

Chey, W.D., Kochman, M.L., Traber, P.G., *et al.* (199). Possible nizatidine-induced subfulminant hepatic failure. *J. Clin. Gastroenterol.* 20, 164.

Chien, R.N., Yang, L.J., Lin, P.Y., *et al.* (1997). Hepatic injury during ketoconazole therapy in patients with onychomycosis: a controlled cohort study. *Hepatology* 25, 103.

Ching, C.K., Smith, P.G., and Long, R.G. (1992). Tamoxifen-associated hepatocellular damage and agranulocytosis. *Lancet* 339, 940.

Christ, D.D., Kenna, J.G., Kammerer, W., *et al.* (1988*a*). Enflurane metabolism produces covalently bound liver adducts recognized by antibodies from patients with halothane hepatitis. *Anesthesiology* 69, 833.

Christ, D.D., Satoh, H., Kenna, J.G., *et al.* (1988*b*). Potential metabolic basis for enflurane hepatitis and the apparent cross-sensitization between enflurane and halothane. *Drug Metab. Dispos.* 16, 135.

Christopherson, W.M. and Mays, E.T. (1977*a*). Liver tumors and contraceptive steroids: experience with the first one hundred registry patients. *J. Natl Cancer Inst.* 58, 167.

Christopherson, W.M., Mays, E.T., and Barrows, G. (1977*b*). A clinicopathologic study of steroid-related liver tumors. *Am. J. Surg. Pathol.* 1, 31.

Chuang, L.C., Tunier, A.P., Akhtar, N., *et al.* (1993). Possible case of procainamide-induced intrahepatic cholestatic jaundice. *Ann. Pharmacother.* 27, 434.

Clark, J.A., Zimmerman, H.J., and Tanner, L.A. (1990). Labetalol hepatotoxicity. *Ann. Intern. Med.* 113, 210. [published erratum appears in *Ann. Intern. Med.* (1990) 113, 485].

Clementz, G.L. and Holmes, A.W. (1987). Nicotinic acid-induced fulminant hepatic failure. *J. Clin. Gastroenterol.* 9, 582.

Coleman, R., Wilton, J.C., Stone, V., *et al.* (1995). Hepatobiliary function and toxicity in vitro using isolated hepatocyte couplets. *Gen. Pharmacol.* 26, 1445.

CSM (Committee on Safety of Medicines) (1988). Lofepramine (Gamamil) and abnormal tests of liver function. *Current Problems* No. 23. HMSO, London.

Committee on Safety of Medicines (1997). Reminder: Hepatotoxicity with halothane. *Current Problems* No. 23 (May). HMSO, London.

Cook, I.F., Shilkin, K.B., and Reed, W.D. (1981). Phenytoin induced granulomatous hepatitis. *Aust. N.Z. J. Med.* 11, 539.

Coombes, G.B., Reiser, J., Paradinas, F.J., *et al.* (1978). An androgen-associated hepatic adenoma in a trans-sexual. *Br. J. Surg.* 65, 869.

Cooper, C., Cotton, D.W., Minihane, N., *et al.* (1986). Azathioprine hypersensitivity manifesting as acute focal hepatocellular necrosis. *J. R. Soc. Med.* 79, 171.

Corcoran, G.B., Mitchell, J.R., Vaishnav, Y.N., *et al.* (1980). Evidence that acetaminophen and *N*-hydroxyacetaminophen form a common arylating intermediate, *N*-acetyl-*p*-benzoquinoneimine. *Mol. Pharmacol.* 18, 536.

Corcoran, G.B., Bauer, J.A., and Lau, T.W. (1988). Immediate rise in intracellular calcium and glycogen phosphorylase a activities upon acetaminophen covalent binding leading to hepatotoxicity in mice. *Toxicology* 50, 157.

Corcuera, T., Alonso, M.J., Picazo, A., *et al.* (1996). Hepatic morphological alterations induced by zidovudine (ZDV) in an experimental model. *Pathol. Res. Pract.* 192, 182.

Cosme, A., Barrio, J., Lobo, C., *et al.* (1996). Acute cholestasis by fluoxetine. *Am. J. Gastroenterol.* 91, 2449.

Couet, C.E., Crews, C., and Hanley, A.B. (1996). Analysis, separation, and bioassay of pyrrolizidine alkaloids from comfrey (*Symphytum officinale*). *Natural Toxins* 4, 163.

Coulter, D.L. (1991). Carnitine, valproate, and toxicity. *J. Child Neurol.* 6, 7.

Craft, P.S. and Pembrey, R.G. (1987). Veno-occlusive disease of the liver following chemotherapy with mitomycin C and doxorubicin. *Aust. N.Z. J. Med.* 17, 449.

Crantock, L., Prentice, R., and Powell, L. (1991). Cholestatic jaundice associated with captopril therapy. *J. Gastroenterol. Hepatol.* 6, 528.

Creagh T.M., Rubin, A., and Evans, D.J. (1988). Hepatic tumours induced by anabolic steroids in an athlete. *J. Clin. Pathol.* 41, 441.

Critchley, J.A., Dyson, E.H., Scott, A.W., *et al.* (1983). Is there a place for cimetidine or ethanol in the treatment of paracetamol poisoning? *Lancet* i, 1375.

D'Cruz, C.A., Wimmer, R.S., Harcke, H.T., *et al.* (1983). Veno-occlusive disease of the liver in children following chemotherapy for acute myelocytic leukemia. *Cancer* 52, 1803.

Dahl, M.G., Gregory, M.M., and Scheuer, P.J. (1971). Liver damage due to methotrexate in patients with psoriasis. *BMJ* 1, 625.

Dahl, M.G., Gregory, M.M., and Scheuer, P.J. (1972). Methotrexate hepatotoxicity in psoriasis — comparison of different dose regimens. *BMJ* 1, 654.

Dalen, E. and Westerholm, B. (1974). Occurrence of hepatic impairment in women jaundiced by oral contraceptives and in their mothers and sisters. *Acta Med. Scand.* 195, 459.

Danan, G., Bernuau, J., Moullot, X., *et al.* (1984). Amitriptyline-induced fulminant hepatitis. *Digestion* 30, 179.

Dao, T., Peytier, A., Galateau, F., *et al.* (1993). Hépatite chronique cirrhogène à la germandrée petit-chêne *Gastroenterol. Clin. Biol.* 17, 609.

Datey, K.K., Deshmukh, S.N., Dalvey, C.P., *et al.* (1967). Hepatocellular damage with ethacrynic acid. *BMJ* iii, 152.

Daum, F., Zucker, P., and Cohen, M.I. (1976). Acute liver failure and encephalopathy (Reye's syndrome?) during salicylate therapy. *Acta Paediatr. Scand.* 65, 747.

Davidson, R.N., Weir, W.R., Kaye, G.L., *et al.* (1988). Intrahepatic cholestasis after thiabendazole. *Trans. R. Soc. Trop. Med. Hyg.* 82, 620.

Davies, M.G. and Kersey, P.J. (1989). Acute hepatitis and exfoliative dermatitis associated with minocycline. *BMJ* 298, 1523.

Davies, M.H., Harrison, R.F., Elias, E., *et al.* (1994). Antibiotic-associated acute vanishing bile duct syndrome: a pattern associated with severe, prolonged, intrahepatic cholestasis. *J. Hepatol.* 20, 112.

Davis, J.S. and Kaufman, R.H. (1966). Tetracycline toxicity: a clinicopathologic study with special reference to liver damage and its relationship to pregnancy. *Am. J. Obstet. Gynecol.* 95, 523.

Davis, M. (1986). Protective agents for acetaminophen overdose. *Semin. Liver Dis.* 6, 138.

Davis, M., Portmann, B., Searle, M., *et al.* (1975). Histological evidence of carcinoma in a hepatic tumour associated with oral contraceptives. *BMJ* 4, 496.

Davis, M., Simmons, C.J., Harrison, N.G., *et al.* (1976). Paracetamol overdose in man: relationship between pattern of urinary metabolites and severity of liver damage. *Q. J. Med.* 45, 181.

Davis, M., Eddleston, A.L., and Williams, R. (1980). Hypersensitivity and jaundice due to azathioprine. *Postgrad. Med. J.* 56, 274.

de Galocsy, C., Horsmans, Y., Rahier, J., *et al.* (1994). Vanishing bile duct syndrome occurring after carbamazepine administration: a second case report. *J. Clin. Gastroenterol.* 19, 269.

De Leve, L.D. (1994). Dacarbazine toxicity in murine liver cells: a model of hepatic endothelial injury and glutathione defense. *J. Pharmacol. Exp. Ther.* 268, 1261.

De Leve, L.D., Wang, X., and Huybrechts, M.M. (1996a). Cellular target of cyclophosphamide toxicity in the murine liver: role of glutathione and site of metabolic activation. *Hepatology* 24, 830.

De Leve, L.D., Wang, X., Kuhlenkamp, J.F., *et al.* (1996b). Toxicity of azathioprine and monocrotaline in murine sinusoidal endothelial cells and hepatocytes: the role of glutathione and relevance to hepatic venoocclusive disease. *Hepatology* 23, 589.

Deakin, C.D., Gove, C.D., Fagan, E.A., *et al.* (1991). Delayed calcium channel blockade with diltiazem reduces paracetamol hepatotoxicity in mice. *Hum. Exp. Toxicol.* 10, 119.

Deidiker, R. and deMello, D.E. (1996). Propylthiouracil-induced fulminant hepatitis: case report and review of the literature. *Pediatr. Pathol. Lab. Med.* 16, 845.

DePinho, R.A., Goldberg, C.S., and Lefkowitch, J.H. (1984). Azathioprine and the liver. Evidence favoring idiosyncratic, mixed cholestatic-hepatocellular injury in humans. *Gastroenterology* 86, 162.

Derby, L.E., Gutthann, S.P., Jick, H., *et al.* (1993*a*). Liver disorders in patients receiving chlorpromazine or isoniazid. *Pharmacotherapy*. 13, 353.

Derby, L.E., Jick, H., Henry, D.A., *et al.* (1993*b*). Erythromycin-associated cholestatic hepatitis. *Med. J. Aust.* 158, 600.

Devereaux, B.M., Crawford, D.H., Purcell, P., *et al.* (1995). Flucloxacillin associated cholestatic hepatitis. An Australian and Swedish epidemic? *Eur. J. Clin. Pharmacol.* 49, 81.

Devi, B.G. and Chan, A.W. (1997). Impairment of mitochondrial respiration and electron transport chain enzymes during cocaine-induced hepatic injury. *Life Sci.* 60, 849.

Devogelaer, J.P., Huaux, J.P., Coche, E., *et al.* (1985). A case of cholestatic hepatitis associated with D-penicillamine therapy for rheumatoid arthritis. *Int. J. Clin. Pharmacol. Res.* 5, 35.

Devuyst, O., Lefebvre, C., Geubel, A., *et al.* (1993). Acute cholestatic hepatitis with rash and hypereosinophilia associated with ranitidine treatment. *Acta Clin. Belg.* 48, 109.

Di Gregorio, C., Ghini, F., and Rivasi, F. (1990). Granulomatous hepatitis in a patient receiving methimazole. *Ital. J. Gastroenterol.* 22, 75.

Dikengil, A., Siskind, B.N., Morse, S.S., *et al.* (1986). Sclerosing cholangitis from intraarterial floxuridine. *J. Clin. Gastroenterol.* 8, 690.

Dincsoy, H.P. and Saelinger, D.A. (1982). Haloperidol-induced chronic cholestatic liver disease. *Gastroenterology* 83, 694.

Dix, S.P., Wingard, J.R., Mullins, R.E., *et al.* (1996). Association of busulfan area under the curve with veno-occlusive disease following BMT. *Bone Marrow Transplant.* 17, 225.

Dollow, S. (1996). Antidepressant-associated fatal intrahepatic cholestasis. *Lancet* 347, 1268.

Donnelly, P.J., Walker, R.M., and Racz, W.J. (1994). Inhibition of mitochondrial respiration in vivo is an early event in acetaminophen-induced hepatotoxicity. *Arch. Toxicol.* 68, 110.

Dooner, H.P., Hoyl, C., Aliaga, C., *et al.* (1971). Jaundice and oral contraceptives. *Acta Hepatosplenol.* 18, 84.

Doria M.I., J., Shepard, K.V., Levin, B., *et al.* (1986). Liver pathology following hepatic arterial infusion chemotherapy. Hepatic toxicity with FUDR. *Cancer* 58, 855.

Dossing, M., Wilcke, J.T., Askgaard, D.S., *et al.* (1996). Liver injury during antituberculosis treatment: an 11-year study. *Tuber. Lung Dis.* 77, 335.

Douglas, D.D., Yang, R.D., Jensen, P., *et al.* (1989). Fatal labetalol-induced hepatic injury. *Am. J. Med.* 87, 235.

Dreifuss, F.E., Santilis, N., Langer, D.H., *et al.* (1987). Valproic acid fatalities: a retrospective review. *Neurology* 37, 379.

Dreifuss, F.E., Langer, D.H., Moline, K.A., *et al.* (1989). Valproic acid hepatic fatalities. II. US experience since 1984. *Neurology* 39, 201.

Droste, H.T. and de Vries, R.F. (1995). Chronic hepatitis caused by lisinopril. *Neth. J. Med.* 46, 95.

Duerksen, D.R., Van, A.J., Gramlich, L., *et al.* (1996). Intravenous ursodeoxycholic acid reduces cholestasis in parenterally fed newborn piglets. *Gastroenterology* 111, 1111.

Durand, F., Bernuau, J., Pessayre, D., *et al.* (1995). Deleterious effect of pyrazinamide on the outcome of patients with fulminant or subfulminant liver failure during antituberculous treatment including isoniazid. *Hepatology* 21, 929.

Dybing, E. and Nelson, S.D. (1978). Metabolic activation of methyldopa and other catechols. *Arch. Toxicol.* Suppl. 117.

Dybing, E., Nelson, S.D., Mitchell, J.R., *et al.* (1976). Oxidation of alpha-methyldopa and other catechols by cytochrome P-450-generated superoxide anion: possible mechanism of methyldopa hepatitis. *Mol. Pharmacol.* 12, 911.

Dykhuizen, R.S., Brunt, P.W., Atkinson, P., *et al.* (1995). Ecstasy-induced hepatitis mimicking acute viral hepatitis. *Gut* 36, 939.

East African/British Medical Research Council (1973). Retreatment Investigation Second Report. Streptomycin plus PAS plus pyrazinamide in the retreatment of pulmonary tuberculosis in East Africa. *Tubercle* 54, 283.

Eckstein, R.P., Dowsett, J.F., and Lunzer, M.R. (1993). Flucloxacillin induced liver disease: histopathological findings at biopsy and autopsy. *Pathology* 25, 223.

Edmondson, H.A., Reynolds, T.B., Henderson, B., *et al.* (1977). Regression of liver cell adenomas associated with oral contraceptives. *Ann. Intern. Med.* 86, 180.

Eger, E.I., Smuckler, E.A., Ferrell, L.D., *et al.* (1986). Is enflurane hepatotoxic? *Anesth. Analg.* 65, 21.

Einhorn, M. and Davidson, I. (1964). Hepatotoxicity of mercaptopurine. *JAMA* 188, 802.

Einstein, N., Baker, A., Galper, J., *et al.* (1975). Jaundice due to nicotinic acid therapy. *Am. J. Dig. Dis.* 20, 282.

Eisenberg, D.M., Kessler, R.C., Foster, C., *et al.* (1993). Unconventional medicine in the United States: prevalence, costs, and patterns of use. *N. Engl. J. Med.* 328, 246.

Elias, E. and Boyer, J.L. (1979). Chlorpromazine and its metabolites after polymerisation and gelation of actin. *Science* 206, 1404.

Engel, J.J., Vogt, T.R., and Wilson, D.E. (1975). Cholestatic hepatitis after administration of furan derivatives. *Arch. Intern. Med.* 135, 733.

Epeirier, J.M., Pageaux, G.P., Coste, V., *et al.* (1996). Fulminant hepatitis after carbimazole and propranolol administration. *Eur. J. Gastroenterol. Hepatol.* 8, 287.

Erickson, A.R., Reddy, V., Vogelgesang, S.A., *et al.* (1995). Usefulness of the American College of Rheumatology recommendations for liver biopsy in methotrexate-treated rheumatoid arthritis patients. *Arthritis Rheum.* 38, 1115.

Essell, J.H., Thompson, J.M., Harman, G.S., *et al.* (1992). Marked increase in veno-occlusive disease of the liver associated with methotrexate use for graft-versus-host disease prophylaxis in patients receiving busulfan/cyclophosphamide. *Blood* 79, 2784.

Etchason, J.A., Miller, T.D., Squires, R.W., *et al.* (1991). Niacin-induced hepatitis: a potential side effect with low-dose time-release niacin. *Mayo Clin. Proc.* 66, 23.

Fairley, C.K., McNeil, J.J., Desmond, P., *et al.* (1993). Risk factors for development of flucloxacillin associated jaundice *BMJ* 306, 233 [published erratum appears in *BMJ* (1993) 307, 1179].

Fajardo, L.F. and Colby, T.B. (1980). Pathogenesis of veno-occlusive liver disease after radiation. *Arch. Path. Lab. Med.* 104, 584.

Fallon, M.B. and Boyer, J.L. (1990). Hepatic toxicity of vitamin A and synthetic retinoids. *J. Gastroenterol. Hepatol.* 5, 334.

Farer, L.S., Glassroth, J.L., and Snider, D.E., Jr. (1977). Isoniazid related hepatotoxicity. *Ann. Intern. Med.* 86, 114.

Farrell, G.C., Joshua, D.E., Uren, R.F., *et al.* (1975). Androgen-induced hepatoma. *Lancet* i, 430.

Fau, D., Eugene, C., Berson, A., *et al.* (1994). Toxicity of the antiandrogen flutamide in isolated rat hepatocytes. *J. Pharmacol. Exp. Ther.* 269, 954.

FDA (Federal Drug Administration) (1980). Ticrynafen recalled. *FDA Drug Bull.* 10, 3.

Fedorkow, D.M., Corenblum, B., and Shaffer, E.A. (1989). Cholestasis induced by oestrogen after liver transplantation. *BMJ* 299, 1080.

Fell, J.M., Reynolds, A.P., Meadows, N., *et al.* (1996). Manganese toxicity in children receiving long-term parenteral nutrition. *Lancet* 347, 1218.

Fermand, J.P., Levy, Y., Bouscary, D., *et al.* (1990). Danazol-induced hepatocellular adenoma. *Am. J. Med.* 88, 529.

Fernandez, E., Galan, A.I., Moran, D., *et al.* (1995). Reversal of cyclosporine A-induced alterations in biliary secretion by *S*-adenosyl-L-methionine in rats. *J. Pharmacol. Exp. Ther.* 275, 442.

Fidler, H., Dhillon, A., Gertner, D., *et al.* (1996). Chronic ecstasy (3,4-methylenedioxymetamphetamine) abuse: a recurrent and unpredictable cause of severe acute hepatitis. *J. Hepatol.* 25, 563.

Fink, A.I., MacKay, C.J., and Cutler, S.S. (1979). Sicca complex and cholangiostatic jaundice in two members of a family probably caused by thiabendazole. *Ophthalmology* 86, 1892.

Fisher, A., Mor, E., Hytiroglou, P., *et al.* (1995). FK506 hepatotoxicity in liver allograft recipients. *Transplantation* 59, 1631.

Fisher, E., Siemes, H., Pund, R., *et al.* (1992). Valproate metabolites in serum and urine during antiepileptic therapy in children with infantile spasms: abnormal metabolite pattern associated with reversible hepatotoxicity. *Epilepsia* 33, 165.

Fleming, C.R. (1994). Hepatobiliary complications in adults receiving nutrition support. *Dig. Dis.* 12, 191.

Foitl, D.R., Hyman, G., and Lefkowitch, J.H. (1989). Jaundice and intrahepatic cholestasis following high-dose megestrol acetate for breast cancer. *Cancer* 63, 438.

Fontana, R.J. and Watkins, P.B. (1995). Genetic predisposition to drug-induced liver disease. *Gastroenterol. Clin. North Am.* 24, 811.

Fontana, R.J., Turgeon, T.F., Woolf, T.F., *et al.* (1996). The caffeine breath test does not identify patients susceptible to tacrine hepatotoxicity. *Hepatology* 23, 1430.

Forbes, G.M., Jeffrey, G.P., Shilkin, K.B., *et al.* (1992). Carbamazepine hepatotoxicity: another cause of the vanishing bile duct syndrome. *Gastroenterology* 102, 1385.

Forman, D., Vincent, T.J., and Doll, R. (1986). Cancer of the liver and the use of oral contraceptives. *BMJ* 292, 1357.

Forns, X., Caballeria, J., Bruguera, M., *et al.* (1994). Disulfiram-induced hepatitis. Report of four cases and review of the literature. *J. Hepatol.* 21, 853.

Foster, J.H. and Berman, M.M. (1994). The malignant transformation of liver cell adenomas. *Arch. Surg.* 129, 712.

Fouin, F.H., Quernec, L., Erlinger, S., *et al.* (1982). Hepatic alterations during total parenteral nutrition in patients with inflammatory bowel disease: a possible consequence of lithocholate toxicity. *Gastroenterology* 83, 932.

Fouquet, J., Teyssier, I., Bacle, Y., *et al.* (1965). L'action antibactillaire, l'usage thérapeutique et les dangers du pyrazinamide. *Rev. Tuberc. Pneumol. Paris* 29, 930.

Frederick, W.C., Howard, R.G., and Spatola, S. (1974). Spontaneous rupture of the liver in patient using contraceptive pills. *Arch. Surg.* 108, 93.

Freund, H.R. (1991). Abnormalities of liver function and hepatic damage associated with total parenteral nutrition. *Nutrition.* 7, 1.

Frey, N., Christen, U., Jeno, P., *et al.* (1995). The lipoic acid containing components of the 2-oxoacid dehydrogenase complexes mimic trifluoroacetylated proteins and are autoantigens associated with halothane hepatitis. *Chem. Res. Toxicol.* 8, 736.

Friedenberg, F.K. and Rothstein, K.D. (1996). Hepatitis secondary to fluoxetine treatment. *Am. J. Psychiatry* 153, 580.

Frier, B.M. and Stewart, W.K. (1977). Cholestatic jaundice following chlorpropamide self-poisoning. *Clin. Toxicol.* 11, 13.

Friis, H. and Andreasen, P.B. (1992). Drug-induced hepatic injury: an analysis of 1100 cases reported to the Danish Committee on Adverse Drug Reactions between 1978 and 1987. *J. Intern. Med.* 232, 133.

Fromenty, B. and Pessayre, D. (1995). Inhibition of mitochondrial beta-oxidation as a mechanism of hepatotoxicity. *Pharmacol. Ther.* 67, 101.

Gabay, C., De, B.M., and Palazzo, E. (1993). Sulphasalazine-related life-threatening side effects: is *N*-acetylcysteine of therapeutic value? *Clin. Exp. Rheumatol.* 11, 417.

Gadacz, T., Allan, R.N., Macke, E., *et al.* (1976). *Gastroenterology* 70, 1125.

Gafa, M., Sarli, L., Miselli, A., *et al.* (1987). Sludge and microlithiasis of the biliary tract after total gastrectomy and postoperative total parenteral nutrition. *Surg. Gynecol. Obstet.* 165, 413.

Gangadharam, P.R. (1986). Isoniazid, rifampin, and hepatotoxicity. *Am. Rev. Respir. Dis.* 133, 963.

Garcia, R.L., Williams, R., Derby, L.E., *et al.* (1994). Acute liver injury associated with nonsteroidal anti-inflammatory drugs and the role of risk factors. *Arch. Intern. Med.* 154, 311.

Garcia, R.L., Stricker, B.H., and Zimmerman, H.J. (1996). Risk of acute liver injury associated with the combination of amoxicillin and clavulanic acid. *Arch. Intern. Med.* 156, 1327.

Garcia, R.L., Wallander, M.A., and Stricker, B.H. (1997). The risk of acute liver injury associated with cimetidine and other acid-suppressing anti-ulcer drugs. *Br. J. Clin. Pharmacol.* 43, 183.

Garibaldi, R.A., Drusin, R.E., Ferbee, S.H., *et al.* (1972). Isoniazid-associated hepatitis. *Am. Rev. Respir. Dis.* 106, 357.

Garrigues, G.V., Berenguer, L.J., Ponce, G.J., *et al.* (1986). A non-C17-alkylated steroid and long-term cholestasis. *Ann. Intern. Med.* 104, 135.

Garty, B.Z., Kauli, R., Ben, A.J., *et al.* (1985). Hepatitis associated with propylthiouracil treatment. *Drug Intell. Clin. Pharm.* 19, 740.

Gefel, D., Harats, N., Lijovetsky, G., *et al.* (1985). Cholestatic jaundice associated with D-penicillamine therapy. *Scand. J. Rheumatol.* 14, 303.

Geneve, J., Zafrani, E.S., and Dhumeaux, D. (1989). Amiodarone-induced liver disease. *J. Hepatol.* 9, 130.

George, C.B., Mansour, R.P., Redmond, J., *et al.* (1984). Hepatic dysfunction and jaundice following high-dose cytosine arabinoside. *Cancer* 54, 2360.

Georgiou, M., Sianidou, L., Hatzis, T., *et al.* (1988). Hepatotoxicity due to *Atractylis gummifera-L. Clin. Toxicol.* 26, 487.

Gerlag, P.G., Lobatto, S., Driessen, W.M., *et al.* (1985). Hepatic sinusoidal dilatation with portal hypertension during azathioprine treatment after kidney transplantation. *J. Hepatol.* 1, 339.

Geubel, A.P., Nakad, A., Rahier, J., *et al.* (1988). Prolonged cholestasis and disappearance of interlobular bile ducts following chlorpropamide and erythromycin ethylsuccinate. Case of drug interaction? *Liver* 8, 350.

Geubel, A.P., De, G.C., Alves, N., *et al.* (1991). Liver damage caused by therapeutic vitamin A administration: estimate of dose-related toxicity in 41 cases. *Gastroenterology* 100, 1701.

Gholson, C.F. and Warren, G.H. (1990). Fulminant hepatic failure associated with intravenous erythromycin lactobionate. *Arch. Intern. Med.* 150, 215.

Gibson, R.G. and Gibson, S.L. (1981). Seatone in arthritis. *BMJ* 282, 1785.

Ginsburg, C.M. (1986). A prospective study on the incidence of liver function abnormalities in children receiving erythromycin estolate, erythromycin ethylsuccinate or penicillin V for treatment of pneumonia. *Pediatr. Infect. Dis.* 5, 151.

Gitlin, N. (1980). Salicylate hepatotoxicity: the potential role of hypoalbuminemia. *J. Clin. Gastroenterol.* 2, 281.

Gleeson, D., Newbould, M.J., Taylor, P., *et al.* (1991). Androgen associated hepatocellular carcinoma with an aggressive course. *Gut* 32, 1084.

Godwin, E.L., Rees, K.R., and Varcoe, J.S. (1967). Nuclear RNA synthesis in rat liver during the early stages of chemical carcinogenesis. *Br. J. Cancer* 21, 166.

Goldin, R.D., Ratnayaka, I.D., Breach, C.S., *et al.* (1996). Role of macrophages in acetaminophen (paracetamol)-induced hepatotoxicity. *J. Pathol.* 179, 432.

Goldstraw, P.W., Hanna, N., and Moyes, H.C. (1983). Mianserin and jaundice. *N.Z. Med. J.* 96, 985.

Gollini, C., Dallari, R., Cervi, F., *et al.* (1992). Epatite acuta da iproniazide. *Recenti Prog. Med.* 83, 354.

Golstein, P.E., Deviere, J., and Cremer, M. (1997). Acute hepatitis and drug-related lupus induced by minocycline treatment. *Am. J. Gastroenterol.* 92, 143.

Gomez, J.L., Dupont, A., Cusan, L., *et al.* (1992). Incidence of liver toxicity associated with the use of flutamide in prostate cancer patients. *Am. J. Med.* 92, 465.

Gordon, D.W., Rosenthal, G., Hart, J., *et al.* (1995). Chaparral ingestion. The broadening spectrum of liver injury caused by herbal medications. *JAMA* 273, 489.

Gordon, S.C., Reddy, K.R., Livingstone, A.S., *et al.* (1986). Resolution of a contraceptive-steroid-induced hepatic adenoma with subsequent evolution into hepatocellular carcinoma. *Ann. Intern. Med.* 105, 547.

Gough, A., Chapman, S., Wagstaff, K., *et al.* (1996). Minocycline induced autoimmune hepatitis and systemic lupus erythematosus-like syndrome. *BMJ* 312, 169.

Gradon, J.D., Chapnick, E.K., and Sepkowitz, D.V. (1992). Zidovudine-induced hepatitis. *J. Intern. Med.* 231, 317.

Gran, J.T., Husby, G., and Thorsby, E. (1983). HLA DR antigens and gold toxicity. *Ann. Rheum. Dis.* 42, 63.

Grassmick, B.K., Lehr, V.T., and Sundareson, A.S. (1992). Fulminant hepatic failure possibly related to ciprofloxacin. *Ann. Pharmacother.* 26, 636.

Gray, D.R., Morgan, T., Chretien, S.D., *et al.* (1994). Efficacy and safety of controlled-release niacin in dyslipoproteinemic veterans. *Ann. Intern. Med.* 121, 252.

Green, D.M., Finklestein, J.Z., Norkool, P., *et al.* (1988). Severe hepatic toxicity after treatment with single-dose dactinomycin and vincristine. A report of the National Wilms' Tumor Study. *Cancer* 62, 270.

Green, D.M., Norkool, P., Breslow, N.E., *et al.* (1990). Severe hepatic toxicity after treatment with vincristine and dactinomycin using single-dose or divided-dose schedules: a report from the National Wilms' Tumor Study. *J. Clin. Oncol.* 8, 1525.

Green, L. and Donehower, R.C. (1984). Hepatic toxicity of low doses of mithramycin in hypercalcemia. *Cancer Treat. Rep.* 68, 1379.

Greenstone, M.A., Dowd, P.M., Mikhailidis, D.P., *et al.* (1981). Hepatic vascular lesions associated with dacarbazine treatment. *BMJ* 282, 1744.

Grimm, I.S. and Litynski, J.J. (1994). Severe cholestasis associated with ticlopidine. *Am. J. Gastroenterol.* 89, 279.

Gronhagen-Riska, C., Hellstrom, P.E., and Froseth, B. (1978). Predisposing factors in hepatitis induced by isoniazid-rifampicin treatment for tuberculosis. *Am. Rev. Respir. Dis.* 118, 461.

Guarascio, P., Portmann, B., Visco, G., *et al.* (1983). Liver damage with reversible portal hypertension from vitamin A intoxication: demonstration of Ito cells. *J. Clin. Pathol.* 36, 769.

Guigui, B., Perrot, S., Berry, J.P., *et al.* (1988). Amiodarone-induced hepatic phospholipidosis: a morphological alteration independent of pseudoalcoholic liver disease. *Hepatology* 8, 1063.

Guillaume, M.P., De, P.C., and Cogan, E. (1996). Subacute mitochondrial liver disease in a patient with AIDS: possible relationship to prolonged fluconazole administration. *Am. J. Gastroenterol.* 91, 165.

Gurumurthy, P., Krishnamurthy, M.S., Nazareth, O., *et al.* (1984). Lack of relationship between hepatic toxicity and acetylator phenotype in three thousand South Indian patients during treatment with isoniazid for tuberculosis. *Am. Rev. Respir. Dis.* 129, 58.

Gut, J., Christen, U., Frey, N., *et al.* (1995). Molecular mimicry in halothane hepatitis: biochemical and structural characterization of lipoylated autoantigens. *Toxicology* 97, 199.

Habior, A., Walewska, Z.B., and Butruk, E. (1994). Hepatocellular–cholestatic liver injury due to amoxycillin–clavulanic acid combination. *Clin. Investig.* 72, 616.

Haboubi, N.Y., Ali, H.H., Whitwell, H.L., *et al.* (1988). Role of endothelial cell injury in the spectrum of azathioprine-induced liver disease after renal transplant: light microscopy and ultrastructural observations. *Am. J. Gastroenterol.* 83, 256.

Hadzic, N., Portmann, B., Davies, E.T., *et al.* (1990). Acute liver failure induced by carbamazepine. *Arch. Dis. Child.* 65, 315.

Hagay, Z.J., Leiberman, R.J., Katz, M., *et al.* (1988). Oral contraceptives and focal nodular hyperplasia of the liver. *Arch. Gynecol. Obstet.* 243, 231.

Hagley, M.T. (1991). Captopril-induced cholestatic jaundice. *South. Med. J.* 84, 100.

Hagley, M.T., Benak, R.L., and Hulisz, D.T. (1992). Suspected cross-reactivity of enalapril- and captopril-induced hepatotoxicity. *Ann. Pharmacother.* 26, 780.

Hagley, M.T., Hulisz, D.T., and Burns, C.M. (1993). Hepatotoxicity associated with angiotensin-converting enzyme inhibitors. *Ann. Pharmacother.* 27, 228.

Hammel, P., Larrey, D., Bernuau, J., *et al.* (1990). Acute hepatitis after tetrahydroaminoacridine administration for Alzheimer's disease. *J. Clin. Gastroenterol.* 12, 329.

Hansen, R.M., Varma, R.R., and Hanson, G.A. (1991). Gold induced hepatitis and pure red cell aplasia. Complete recovery after corticosteroid and *N*-acetylcysteine therapy. *J. Rheumatol.* 18, 1251.

Hanson, J.S. (1984). Propylthiouracil and hepatitis. Two cases and a review of the literature. *Arch. Intern. Med.* 144, 994.

Harats, N., Ehrenfeld, M., Shalit, M., *et al.* (1985). Gold-induced granulomatous hepatitis. *Isr. J. Med. Sci.* 21, 753.

Hare, D.L. and Horowitz, J.D. (1986). Verapamil hepatotoxicity: a hypersensitivity reaction. *Am. Heart J.* 111, 610.

Harris, S.R. and Hamrick, M.E. (1993). Antagonism of acetaminophen hepatotoxicity by phospholipase A2 inhibitors. *Res. Commun. Chem. Pathol. Pharmacol.* 79, 23.

Harrison, P.M., O'Grady, J.G., Keays, R.T., *et al.* (1990). Serial prothrombin time as prognostic indicator in paracetamol induced fulminant hepatic failure. *BMJ* 301, 964.

Harrison, P.M., Wendon, J.A., Gimson, A.E., *et al.* (1991). Improvement by acetylcysteine of hemodynamics and oxygen transport in fulminant hepatic failure. *N. Engl. J. Med.* 324, 1852.

Hart, J.G. and Timbrell, J.A. (1979). The effect of age on paracetamol hepatotoxicity in mice. *Biochem. Pharmacol.* 28, 3015.

Harvey, J. and Colin-Jones, J.D. (1981). Mistletoe hepatitis. *BMJ* (Clin.Res.Ed.) 282, 186.

Hashimoto, F., Davis, R.L., and Egli, D. (1994). Hepatitis following treatments with famotidine and then cimetidine. *Ann. Pharmacother.* 28, 37.

Haskell, C.M., Canellos, G.P., Leventhal, B.G., *et al.* (1969). L-asparaginase: therapeutic and toxic effects in patients with neoplastic disease. *N. Engl. J. Med.* 281, 1028.

Hautekeete, M.L., Brenard, R., Horsmans, Y., *et al.* (1995a). Liver injury related to amoxycillin-clavulanic acid: inter-lobular bile-duct lesions and extrahepatic manifestations. *J. Hepatol.* 22, 71.

Hautekeete, M.L., Henrion, J., Naegels, S., *et al.* (1995b). Severe hepatotoxicity related to benzarone: a report of three cases with two fatalities. *Liver* 15, 25.

Hautekeete, M.L., Kockx, M.M., Naegels, S., *et al.* (1995c). Cholestatic hepatitis related to quinolones: a report of two cases. *J. Hepatol.* 23, 759.

Hazelton, G.A., Hjelle, J.J., and Klaassen, C.D. (1986). Effects of butylated hydroxyanisole on acetaminophen hepatotoxicity and glucuronidation in vivo. *Toxicol. Appl. Pharmacol.* 83, 474.

Hedili, A., Warnet, J.M., Thevenin, M., *et al.* (1989). Biochemical investigation of atractylis gummifera-L hepatotoxicity in the rat. *Arch. Toxicol.* 13 (Suppl.), 312.

Helfgott, S.M., Sandberg, C.J., Zakim, D., *et al.* (1990). Diclofenac-associated hepatotoxicity. *JAMA* 264, 2660.

Helmchen, C., Boerner, R.J., Meyendorf, R., *et al.* (1996). Reversible hepatotoxicity of paroxetine in a patient with major depression. *Pharmacopsychiatry* 29, 223.

Henry, K., Acosta, E.P., and Jochimsen, E. (1996). Hepatotoxicity and rash associated with zidovudine and zalcitabine chemoprophylaxis. *Ann. Intern. Med.* 124, 855.

Hepps, K.S., Maliha, G.M., Estrada, R., *et al.* (1991). Severe cholestatic jaundice associated with piroxicam. *Gastroenterology* 101, 1737.

Herman, J.E. and Bassan, H.M. (1975). Liver injury due to quinidine. *JAMA* 234, 310.

Hiesse, C., Cantarovich, M., Santelli, C., *et al.* (1985). Ranitidine hepatotoxicity in renal transplant patient. *Lancet* i, 1280.

Hoge, S.K. and Biederman, J. (1987). Liver function tests during treatment with desipramine in children and adolescents. *J. Clin. Psychopharmacol.* 7, 87.

Holt, R.J. (1984). Fluphenazine decanoate-induced cholestatic jaundice and thrombocytopenia. *Pharmacotherapy* 4, 227.

Homberg, J.C., Andre, C., and Abuaf, N. (1984). A new anti-liver-kidney microsome antibody (anti-LKM2) in tienilic acid-induced hepatitis. *Clin. Exp. Immunol.* 55, 561.

Horowitz, R.S., Feldhaus, K., Dart, R.C., *et al.* (1996). The clinical spectrum of Jin Bu Huan toxicity. *Arch. Intern. Med.* 156, 899.

Horsmans, Y. and Geubel, A.P. (1994). Amoxycillin-clavulanic acid-erythromycin cross-liver toxicity: a case report. *J. Hepatol.* 21, 911.

Horsmans, Y., Rahier, J., and Geubel, A.P. (1991). Reversible cholestasis with bile duct injury following azathioprine therapy. A case report. *Liver* 11, 89.

Horst, D.A., Grace, N.D., and Lecompte, P.M. (1980). Prolonged cholestasis and progressive hepatic fibrosis following imipramine therapy. *Gastroenterology* 79, 550.

Howie, D., Adriaenssens, P.I., and Prescott, L.F. (1977). Paracetamol metabolism following overdosage: application of high performance liquid chromatography. *J. Pharm. Pharmacol.* 29, 235.

Hromas, R.A., Srigley, J., and Murray, J.L. (1985). Clinical and pathological comparison of young adult women with hepatocellular carcinoma with and without exposure to oral contraceptives. *Am. J. Gastroenterol.* 80, 479.

Hull, M., Jones, R., and Bendall, M. (1994). Fatal hepatic necrosis associated with trazodone and neuroleptic drugs. *BMJ* 309, 378.

Humble, M.W., Eykin, S.J., and Phillips (1980). Staphylococcal bacteraemia, fusidic acid and jaundice. *BMJ* 280, 1495.

Hunt, C.M. and Washington, K. (1994). Tetracycline-induced bile duct paucity and prolonged cholestasis. *Gastroenterology* 107, 1844.

Huxtable, R.J. (1992). The myth of benificent nature: the risks of herbal preparations. *Ann. Intern. Med.* 117, 165.

Hwang, S.J., Wu, J.C., Lee, C.N., et al. (1997). A prospective clinical study of isoniazid-rifampicin-pyrazinamide-induced liver injury in an area endemic for hepatitis B. *J. Gastroenterol. Hepatol.* 12, 87.

Ilyin, G.P., Rissel, M., Malledant, Y., et al. (1994). Human hepatocytes express trifluoroacetylated neoantigens after in vitro exposure to halothane. *Biochem. Pharmacol.* 48, 561.

Imai, H., Kiyosawa, K., Nakamura, M., et al. (1988). A case of cholangiocarcinoma detected after follow-up for seven years for thorotrast deposition. *Gastroenterol. Jpn* 23, 570.

Inkeles, S.B., Connor, W.E., and Illingworth, D.R. (1986). Hepatic and dermatologic manifestations of chronic hypervitaminosis A in adults. Report of two cases. *Am. J. Med.* 80, 491.

Inman, W.H. and Mushin, W.W. (1974). Jaundice after repeated exposure to halothane: an analysis of reports to the Committee on Safety of Medicines. *BMJ* i, 5.

Ishak, K.G. and Irey, N.S. (1972). Hepatic injury associated with the phenothiazines. Clinicopathologic and follow up study of 36 patients. *Arch. Pathol.* 93, 283.

Ishak, K.G., Kirchner, J.P., and Dhar, J.K. (1977). Granulomas and cholestatic–hepatocellular injury associated with phenylbutazone. Report of two cases. *Am. J. Dig. Dis.* 22, 611.

Ishikura, H., Matsuo, N., Matsubara, M., et al. (1996). Valproic acid overdose and L-carnitine therapy. *J. Anal. Toxicol.* 20, 55.

Islam, S., Mekhloufi, F., Paul, J.M., et al. (1989). Characteristics of clometacin-induced hepatitis with special reference to the presence of anti-actin cable antibodies. *Autoimmunity* 2, 213.

Ito, Y., Kojiro, M., Nakashima, T., et al. (1988). Pathomorphologic characteristics of 102 cases of thorotrast-related hepatocellular carcinoma, cholangiocarcinoma, and hepatic angiosarcoma. *Cancer* 62, 1153.

Ito, Y., Suzuki, Y., Ogonuki, H., et al. (1994). Role of iron and glutathione redox cycle in acetaminophen-induced cytotoxicity in cultured rat hepatocytes. *Dig. Dis. Sci.* 39, 1257.

Itoh, S., Marutani, K., Nishijima, T., et al. (1995). Liver injuries induced by herbal medicine, syo-saiko-to (xiao-chai-hu-tang). *Dig. Dis. Sci.* 40, 1845.

Jacobs, J.W., van der Weide, F., and Kruijsen, M.W. (1994). Fatal cholestatic hepatitis caused by D-penicillamine. *Br. J. Rheumatol.* 33, 770.

Jacobs, M.B. (1984). Hepatic infarction related to oral contraceptive use. *Arch. Intern. Med.* 144, 642.

Jacobson, M.A., Hanks, D.K., and Ferrell, L.D. (1994). Fatal acute hepatic necrosis due to fluconazole. *Am. J. Med.* 96, 188.

Jacques, E.A., Buschmann, R.J., and Layden, T.J. (1979). The histopathologic progression of Vitamin A induced hepatic injury. *Gastroenterology* 76, 599.

Jaeschke, H. (1990). Glutathione disulfide formation and oxidant stress during acetaminophen-induced hepatotoxicity in mice in vivo: the protective effect of allopurinol. *J. Pharmacol. Exp. Ther.* 255, 935.

Jee, R.C., Sipes, I.G., Gandolfi, A.J., et al. (1980). Factors influencing halothane hepatotoxicity in the rat hypoxic model. *Toxicol. Appl. Pharmacol.* 52, 267.

Jeurissen, M.E., Boerbooms, A.M., van de Putte, L.B., et al. (1990). Azathioprine induced fever, chills, rash, and hepatotoxicity in rheumatoid arthritis. *Ann. Rheum. Dis.* 49, 25.

Jick, H. and Derby, L.E. (1995). A large population-based follow-up study of trimethoprim-sulfamethoxazole, trimethoprim, and cephalexin for uncommon serious drug toxicity. *Pharmacotherapy* 15, 428.

Jick, H., Derby, L.E., Garcia, R.L., et al. (1992). Liver disease associated with diclofenac, naproxen, and piroxicam. *Pharmacotherapy* 12, 207.

Jick, S. (1997). Ciprofloxacin safety in a pediatric population. *Pediatr. Infect. Dis. J.* 16, 130.

Jick, S.S., Jick, H., and Dean, A.D. (1993). A follow-up safety study of ciprofloxacin users. *Pharmacotherapy.* 13, 461.

Johnson, D.H., Greco, F.A., and Wolff, S.N. (1983). Etoposide-induced hepatic injury: a potential complication of high-dose therapy. *Cancer Treat. Rep.* 67, 1023.

Johnson, G.K. and Tolman, K.G. (1977). Chronic liver disease and acetaminophen. *Ann. Intern. Med.* 87, 302.

Joint Tuberculosis Committee (1990). Chemotherapy and management of tuberculosis. *Thorax* 45, 403.

Jollow, D.J., Mitchell, J.R., Potter, W.Z., et al. (1973). Acetaminophen-induced hepatic necrosis. II. Role of covalent binding in vivo. *J. Pharmacol. Exp. Ther.* 187, 195.

Jollow, D.J., Thorgeirsson, S.S., Potter, W.Z., et al. (1974). Acetaminophen-induced hepatic necrosis. VI. Metabolic disposition of toxic and nontoxic doses of acetaminophen. *Pharmacology* 12, 251.

Jones, D.B., Makepeace, M.C., and Smith, P.M. (1980). Jaundice following warfarin therapy. *Postgrad. Med. J.* 56, 671.

Jones, R.B., Shpall, E.J., Ross, M., et al. (1990). High-dose carboplatin, cyclophosphamide, and BCNU with autologous bone marrow support: excessive hepatic toxicity. *Cancer Chemother. Pharmacol.* 26, 155.

Jordan, V.C. (1995). Tamoxifen and tumorigenicity: a predictable concern. *J. Natl Cancer Inst.* 87, 623.

Jori, G.P. and Peschile, C. (1973). Hydralazine disease associated with transient granulomas in the liver. A case report. *Gastroenterology* 64, 1163.

Jurima, R.M. and Huang, H.S. (1992). Enalapril hepatotoxicity in the rat. Effects of modulators of cytochrome P450 and glutathione. *Biochem. Pharmacol.* 44, 1803.

Kahn, H.D., Faguet, G.B., Agee, J.F., *et al.* (1984). Drug-induced liver injury. In vitro demonstration of hypersensitivity to both phenytoin and phenobarbital. *Arch. Intern. Med.* 144, 1677.

Kahn, H., Manzarbeitia, C., Theise, N., *et al.* (1991). Danazol-induced hepatocellular adenomas. A case report and review of the literature. *Arch. Pathol. Lab. Med.* 115, 1054.

Kalantzis, N., Gabriel, P., Mouzas, J., *et al.* (1991). Acute amiodarone-induced hepatitis. *Hepatogastroenterology* 38, 71.

Kaminski, D.L., Adams, A., and Jellinek, M. (1984). The effect of hyperalimentation on hepatic lipid content and lipogenic enzyme activity in rats and man. *Surgery* 88, 93.

Kamiyama, T., Nouchi, T., Kojima, S., *et al.* (1997). Autoimmune hepatitis triggered by administration of an herbal medicine. *Am. J. Gastroenterol.* 92, 703.

Kano, Y., Fukuda, M., Shiohara, T., *et al.* (1994). Cholestatic hepatitis occurring shortly after etretinate therapy. *J. Am. Acad. Dermatol.* 31, 133.

Kanwar, V.S., Albuquerque, M.L., Ribeiro, R.C., *et al.* (1995). Veno-occlusive disease of the liver after chemotherapy for rhabdomyosarcoma: case report with a review of the literature. *Med. Pediatr. Oncol.* 24, 334.

Kao, N.L. and Rosenblate, H.J. (1993). 6-Thioguanine therapy for psoriasis causing toxic hepatic venoocclusive disease. *J. Am. Acad. Dermatol.* 28, 1017.

Kasai, M., Kiyama, Y., Watanabe, M., *et al.* (1992). Toxicity of high-dose busulfan and cyclophosphamide as a preparative regimen for bone marrow transplantation. *Transplant. Proc.* 24, 1529.

Kassler, W.J., Blanc, P., and Greenblatt, R. (1991). The use of medicinal herbs by HIV infected patients. *Arch. Intern. Med.* 151, 2281.

Kattan, J., Spatz, A., Culine, S., *et al.* (1994). Hepatocellular carcinoma during hormonotherapy for prostatic cancer. *Am. J. Clin. Oncol.* 17, 390.

Katz, M. and Saibil, F. (1990). Herbal hepatitis: subacute hepatic necrosis secondary to chaparral leaf. *J. Clin. Gastroenterol.* 12, 203.

Katzka, D.A., Saul, S.H., Jorkasky, D., *et al.* (1986). Azathioprine and hepatic venocclusive disease in renal transplant patients. *Gastroenterology* 90, 446.

Keays, R., Harrison, P.M., Wendon, J.A., *et al.* (1991). Intravenous acetylcysteine in paracetamol induced fulminant hepatic failure: a prospective controlled trial. *BMJ* 303, 1026.

Keeffe, E.B., Reis, T.C., and Berland, J.E. (1982). Hepatotoxicity to both erythromycin estolate and erythromycin ethylsuccinate. *Dig. Dis. Sci.* 27, 701.

Keen, R.W., Deacon, A.C., Delves, H.T., *et al.* (1994). Indian herbal remedies for diabetes as a cause of lead poisoning. *Postgrad. Med. J.* 70, 113.

Keiding, S., Dossing, M., and Hardt, F. (1984). A nurse with liver injury associated with occupational exposure to halothane in a recovery unit. *Dan. Med. Bull.* 31, 255.

Keim, N.L. (1987). Nutritional effectors of hepatic steatosis induced by parenteral nutrition in the rat. *JPEN* 11, 18.

Keim, N.L. and Mares, P.J. (1984). Development of hepatic steatosis and essential fatty acid deficiency in rats with hypercaloric, fat-free parenteral nutrition. *J. Nutr.* 114, 1807.

Kelly, C., Roche, S., Naguib, M., *et al.* (1993). A prospective evaluation of the hepatotoxicity of lofepramine in the elderly. *Int. Clin. Psychopharmacol.* 8, 83.

Kemeny, M.M., Battifora, H.A., Blayney, D.W., *et al.* (1985). Sclerosing cholangitis after continuous hepatic artery infusion of FUDR. *Ann. Surg.* 202, 176.

Kendler, J., Anuras, S., Laborda, O., *et al.* (1972). Perfusion of the isolated rat liver with erythromycin estolate and other derivatives. *Proc. Soc. Exp. Biol. Med.* 139, 1272.

Kenna, J.G., Neuberger, J., Mieli, V.G., *et al.* (1987a). Halothane hepatitis in children. *BMJ* 294, 1209.

Kenna, J.G., Neuberger, J., and Williams, R. (1987b). Identification by immunoblotting of three halothane-induced liver microsomal polypeptide antigens recognized by antibodies in sera from patients with halothane-associated hepatitis. *J. Pharmacol. Exp. Ther.* 242, 733.

Kenna, J.G., Neuberger, J., and Williams, R. (1987c). Specific antibodies to halothane-induced liver antigens in halothane-associated hepatitis. *Br. J. Anaesth.* 59, 1286.

Kenna, J.G., Neuberger, J., and Williams, R. (1988). Evidence for expression in human liver of halothane-induced neoantigens recognized by antibodies in sera from patients with halothane hepatitis. *Hepatology* 8, 1635.

Kennedy, P. (1983). Liver cross-sensitivity to antipsychotic drugs. *Br. J. Psychiatry* 143, 312.

Kenney, J.M., Proctor, J.D., Harris, S., *et al.* (1994). A comparison of the efficacy and toxic effects of sustained- vs immediate-release niacin in hypercholesterolemic patients. *JAMA* 271, 672.

Kent, G., Gay, S., Inouye, T., *et al.* (1976). Vitamin A containing lipocytes and formation of type III collagen in liver injury. *Proc. Natl. Acad. Sci. USA* 73, 3719.

Kerlin, P., Davis, G.L., McGill, D.B., *et al.* (1983). Hepatic adenoma and focal nodular hyperplasia: clinical, pathologic, and radiologic features. *Gastroenterology* 84, 994.

Kharasch, E.D., Hankins, D., Mautz, D., *et al.* (1996). Identification of the enzyme responsible for oxidative halothane metabolism: implications for prevention of halothane hepatitis. *Lancet* 347, 1367.

Khouri, M.R., Saul, S.H., Dlugosz, A.A., *et al.* (1987). Hepatocanalicular injury associated with vitamin A derivative etretinate. An idiosyncratic hypersensitivity reaction. *Dig. Dis. Sci.* 32, 1207.

King, P.D. and Blitzer, B.L. (1990). Drug-induced cholestasis: pathogenesis and clinical features. *Semin. Liver Dis.* 10, 316.

Kitteringham, N.R., Kenna, J.G., and Park, B.K. (1995). Detection of autoantibodies directed against human hepatic endoplasmic reticulum in sera from patients with halothane-associated hepatitis. *Br. J. Clin. Pharmacol.* 40, 379.

Klatskin, G. (1977). Hepatic tumors: possible relationship to use of oral contraceptives. *Gastroenterology* 73, 386.

Klatskin, G. and Kimberg, D.V. (1969). Recurrent hepatitis attributable to halothane sensitization in an anesthetist. *N. Engl. J. Med.* 280, 515.

Kleckner, H.B., Yakulis, U., and Heller, P. (1975). Severe sensitivity to diphenylhydantoin with circulating antibodies to the drug. *Ann. Intern. Med.* 83, 522.

Klein, S.M. and Khan, M.A. (1983). Hepatitis, toxic epidermal necrolysis and pancreatitis in association with sulindac therapy. *J. Rheumatol.* 10, 512.

Kleiner, D.E., Gaffey, M.J., Sallie, R., *et al.* (1997). Histopathologic changes associated with fialuridine hepatotoxicity. *Mod. Pathol.* 10, 192.

Klerman, G.L. and Cole, J.O. (1997). Clinical pharmacology of imipramine and related antidepressant compounds. *Pharmacol. Rev.* 17, 101.

Knobler, H., Levi, I.S., Gavish, D., *et al.* (1986). Quinidine induced hepatitis. *Arch. Intern. Med.* 146, 526.

Kobayashi, F., Ikeda, T., Sakamoto, N., *et al.* (1995). Severe chronic active hepatitis induced by UFTR containing tegafur and uracil. *Dig. Dis. Sci.* 40, 2434.

Koch, H.K., Gropp, A., and Oehlert, W. (1985). Drug-induced liver injury in liver biopsies of the years 1981 and 1983, their prevalence and type of presentation. *Pathol. Res. Pract.* 179, 469.

Kohli, H.S., Jain, D., Sud, K., *et al.* (1996). Azathioprine-induced hepatic veno-occlusive disease in a renal transplant recipient: histological regression following azathioprine withdrawal. *Nephrol. Dial. Transplant.* 11, 1671.

Kondo, T., Kaneko, S., Otani, K., *et al.* (1992). Associations between risk factors for valproate hepatotoxicity and altered valproate metabolism. *Epilepsia* 33, 172.

Kong, K.H. (1996). Carbamazepine-induced hepatitis in a patient with cervical myelopathy. *Arch. Phys. Med. Rehabil.* 77, 305.

Kopelman, H., Scheuer, P.J., and Williams, R. (1966). The liver lesion in Epping jaundice. *Q.J. Med.* 35, 553.

Kowdley, K.V., Keeffe, E.B., and Fawaz, K.A. (1992). Prolonged cholestasis due to trimethoprim sulfamethoxazole. *Gastroenterology* 102, 2148.

Krahenbuhl, S., Mang, G., Kupferschmidt, H., *et al.* (1995). Plasma and hepatic carnitine and coenzyme A pools in a patient with fatal, valproate induced hepatotoxicity. *Gut* 37, 140.

Kremer, J.M., Alarcon, G.S., Lightfoot, R.W., Jr, *et al.* (1994). Methotrexate for rheumatoid arthritis. Suggested guidelines for monitoring liver toxicity. American College of Rheumatology. *Arthritis Rheum.* 37, 316.

Kremer, J.M., Furst, D.E., Weinblatt, M.E., *et al.* (1996). Significant changes in serum AST across hepatic histological biopsy grades: prospective analysis of 3 cohorts receiving methotrexate therapy for rheumatoid arthritis. *J. Rheumatol.* 23, 459.

Kretz-Rommel, A. and Boelsterli, U.A. (1993). Diclofenac covalent protein binding is dependent on acylglucuronide formation and is inversely related to acute cell injury in cultured rat hepatocytes. *Toxicol. Appl. Pharmacol.* 120, 155.

Kretzschmar, M. (1996). Regulation of hepatic glutathione metabolism and its role in hepatotoxicity. *Exp. Toxicol. Pathol.* 48, 439.

Kukongviriyapan, V. and Stacey, N.H. (1991). Chemical-induced interference with hepatocellular transport. Role in cholestasis. *Chem. Biol. Interact.* 77, 245.

Kumar, A., Bhat, A., Gupta, D.K., *et al.* (1985). D-penicillamine-induced acute hypersensitivity pneumonitis and cholestatic hepatitis in a patient with rheumatoid arthritis. *Clin. Exp. Rheumatol.* 3, 337.

Kutty, K.P., Nath, I.V., Kothandaraman, K.R., *et al.* (1987). Fusidic acid-induced hyperbilirubinemia. *Dig. Dis. Sci.* 32, 933.

Kwan, D., Bartle, W.R., and Walker, S.E. (1995). Abnormal serum transaminases following therapeutic doses of acetaminophen in the absence of known risk factors. *Dig. Dis. Sci.* 40, 1951.

La Spina, I., Secchi, P., Grampa, G., *et al.* (1994). Acute cholangitis induced by carbamazepine. *Epilepsia* 35, 1029.

La Vecchia, C., Negri, E., and Parazzini, F. (1989). Oral contraceptives and primary liver cancer. *Br. J. Cancer* 59, 460.

Labadarios, D., Davis, M., Portmann, B., *et al.* (1977). Paracetamol-induced hepatic necrosis in the mouse — relationship between covalent binding, hepatic glutathione depletion and the protective effect of alpha-mercaptopropionylglycine. *Biochem. Pharmacol.* 26, 31.

Labowitz, J.K. and Silverman, W.B. (1997). Cholestatic jaundice induced by ciprofloxacin. *Dig. Dis. Sci.* 42, 192.

Lacaille, F., Ortigao, M.B., Debre, M., *et al.* (1995). Hepatic toxicity associated with 2'-3' dideoxyinosine in children with AIDS. *J. Pediatr. Gastroenterol. Nutr.* 20, 287.

Lai, K.K., Gang, D.L., Zawacki, J.K., *et al.* (1991). Fulminant hepatic failure associated with 2',3'-dideoxyinosine (ddI). *Ann. Intern. Med.* 115, 283.

Lambert, J.R. and Thomas, S.M. (1985). Metronidazole prevention of serum liver enzyme abnormalities during total parenteral nutrition. *JPEN* 9, 501.

Larrey, D., Rueff, B., Pessayre, D., *et al.* (1986). Cross hepatotoxicity between tricyclic antidepressants. *Gut* 27, 726.

Larrey, D., Geneve, J., Pessayre, D., *et al.* (1987). Prolonged cholestasis after cyproheptadine-induced acute hepatitis. *J. Clin. Gastroenterol.* 9, 102.

Larrey, D., Amoyhal, G., Pessayre, D. *et al.* (1988a). Amitriptyline-induced prolonged cholestasis. *Gastroenterology* 94, 200.

Larrey, D., Henrion, J., Heller, F., *et al.* (1988b). Metoprolol-induced hepatitis: rechallenge and drug oxidation phenotyping. *Ann. Intern. Med.* 108, 67.

Larrey, D., Babany, G., Bernuau, J., *et al.* (1990). Fulminant hepatitis after lisinopril administration. *Gastroenterology* 99, 1832.

Larrey, D., Vial, T., Micaleff, A., *et al.* (1992a). Hepatitis associated with amoxycillin-clavulanic acid combination report of 15 cases. *Gut* 33, 368.

Larrey, D., Vial, T., Pauwels, A., *et al.* (1992b). Hepatitis after germander (*Teucrium chamaedrys*) administration: another instance of herbal medicine hepatotoxicity. *Ann. Intern. Med.* 117, 129.

Laskin, D.L. and Pilaro, A.M. (1986). Potential role of activated macrophages in acetaminophen hepatotoxicity. I. Isolation and characterization of activated macrophages from rat liver. *Toxicol. Appl. Pharmacol.* 86, 204.

Laskin, D.L., Pilaro, A.M., and Ji, S. (1986). Potential role of activated macrophages in acetaminophen hepatotoxicity. II. Mechanism of macrophage accumulation and activation. *Toxicol. Appl. Pharmacol.* 86, 216.

Lauterburg, B.H. and Mitchell, J.R. (1981a). In vivo regulation of hepatic glutathione synthesis: effects of food deprivation or glutathione depletion by electrophilic compounds. *Adv. Exp. Med. Biol.* 136 Pt A, 453.

Lauterburg, B.H. and Mitchell, J.R. (1981b). Regulation of hepatic glutathione turnover in rats in vivo and evidence for kinetic homogeneity of the hepatic glutathione pool. *J. Clin. Invest.* 67, 1415.

Lauterburg, B.H. and Mitchell, J.R. (1982). Toxic doses of acetaminophen suppress hepatic glutathione synthesis in rats. *Hepatology* 2, 8.

Lauterburg, B.H., Smith, C.V., Hughes, H., et al. (1984). Biliary excretion of glutathione and glutathione disulfide in the rat. Regulation and response to oxidative stress. *J. Clin. Invest.* 73, 124.

Lauterburg, B.H., Smith, C.V., Todd, E.L., et al. (1985a). Oxidation of hydrazine metabolites formed from isoniazid. *Clin. Pharmacol. Ther.* 38, 566.

Lauterburg, B.H., Smith, C.V., Todd, E.L., et al. (1985b). Pharmacokinetics of the toxic hydrazino metabolites formed from isoniazid in humans. *J. Pharmacol. Exp. Ther.* 235, 566.

Lauterburg, B.H. and Velez, M.E. (1988). Glutathione deficiency in alcoholics: risk factor for paracetamol hepatotoxicity. *Gut* 29, 1153.

Lazaros, G.A., Stavrinos, C., Papatheodoridis, G.V., et al. (1996). Amineptine induced liver injury. Report of two cases and brief review of the literature. *Hepatogastroenterology* 43, 1015.

Le Dinh, T., Freneaux, E., Labbe, G., et al. (1988). Amineptine, a tricyclic antidepressant, inhibits the mitochondrial oxidation of fatty acids and produces microvesicular steatosis of the liver in mice. *J. Pharmacol. Exp. Ther.* 247, 745.

Le Duc, B.W., Sinclair, P.R., Shuster, L., et al. (1993). Norcocaine and N-hydroxynorcocaine formation in human liver microsomes: role of cytochrome P450 3A4. *Pharmacology* 46, 294.

Le Thai, B., Dumont, M., Michel, A., et al. (1988). Cholestatic effect of cyclosporine in the rat. An inhibition of bile acid secretion. *Transplantation* 46, 510.

Leaseburge, L.A., Winn, N.J., and Schloerb, P.R. (1992). Liver test alterations with total parenteral nutrition and nutritional status. *JPEN* 16, 348.

Lee, A.U. and Farrell, G.C. (1997). Drug-induced liver disease. *Curr. Opin. Gastroenterol.* 13, 199.

Lee, F.I., Tharakan, J., Vasudev, K.S., et al. (1996). Malignant hepatic tumours associated with previous exposure to Thorotrast: four cases. *Eur. J. Gastroenterol. Hepatol.* 8, 1121.

Lee, S.C., Yamamoto, G., Chueh, C.H., et al. (1988). Unexplained hepatitis following reexposure to halothane at 10-year interval. *Ma. Tsui. Hsueh. Tsa. Chi.* 26, 329.

Lee, S.M., O'Brien, C.J., Williams, R., et al. (1986). Subacute hepatic necrosis induced by piroxicam. *BMJ* 293, 540.

Lekehal, M., Pessayre, D., Lereau, J.M., et al. (1996). Hepatotoxicity of the herbal medicine germander: metabolic activation of its furano deterpenoids by cytochrome P450 3A depletes cytoskeleton-associated protein thiols and forms plasma membrane blebs in rat hepatocytes. *Hepatology* 24, 212.

Lennard, M.S. (1989). Metoprolol-induced hepatitis: is the rate of oxidation related to drug-induced hepatotoxicity? *Hepatology* 9, 163.

Lennard, T.W. and Farndon, J.R. (1983). Sulphasalazine hepatotoxicity after 15 years' successful treatment for ulcerative colitis. *BMJ* 287, 96.

Leo, M.A. and Lieber, C.S. (1983). Hepatic fibrosis after longterm administration of ethanol and moderate vitamin A supplementation in the rat. *Hepatology* 3, 1.

Leo, M.A. and Lieber, C.S. (1988). Hypervitaminosis A: a lover's lament. *Gastroenterology* 8, 412.

Levander, H.G. (1980). Granulomatous hepatitis in a patient receiving carbamazepine. *Acta Med. Scand.* 208, 333.

Lewis, J.H. (1984). Hepatic toxicity of nonsteroidal anti-inflammatory drugs. *Clin. Pharm.* 3, 128.

Lewis, J.H. and Schiff, E. (1988). Methotrexate-induced chronic liver injury: guidelines for detection and prevention. The ACG Committee on FDA-related matters. American College of Gastroenterology. *Am. J. Gastroenterol.* 83, 1337.

Lewis, J.H., Tice, H.L., and Zimmerman, H.J. (1983a). Budd–Chiari syndrome associated with oral contraceptive steroids. Review of treatment of 47 cases. *Dig. Dis. Sci.* 28, 673.

Lewis, J.H., Zimmerman, H.J., Ishak, K.G., et al. (1983b). Enflurane hepatotoxicity. A clinicopathologic study of 24 cases. *Ann. Intern. Med.* 98, 984.

Lewis, J.H., Mullick, F., Ishak, K.G., et al. (1990). Histopathologic analysis of suspected amiodarone hepatotoxicity. *Hum. Pathol.* 21, 59.

Liano, F., Moreno, A., Matesanz, R., et al. (1989). Venoocclusive hepatic disease of the liver in renal transplantation: is azathioprine the cause?. *Nephron* 51, 509.

Liaw, Y.F., Huang, M.J., Fan, K.D., et al. (1993). Hepatic injury during propylthiouracil therapy in patients with hyperthyroidism. A cohort study. *Ann. Intern. Med.* 118, 424.

Lieh, L.M., Sarnaik, A.P., Newton, J.F., et al. (1984). Metabolism and pharmacokinetics of acetaminophen in a severely poisoned young child. *J. Pediatr.* 105, 125.

Lim, S.P., Andrews, F.J., and O'Brien, P.E. (1995). Acetaminophen-induced microvascular injury in the rat liver: protection with misoprostol. *Hepatology* 22, 1776.

Lind, R.C. and Gandolfi, A.J. (1997). Late dimethyl sulfoxide administration provides a protective action against chemically induced injury in both the liver and the kidney. *Toxicol. Appl. Pharmacol.* 142, 201.

Lind, R.C., Gandolfi, A.J., and Hall, P.D. (1989). The role of oxidative biotransformation of halothane in the guinea pig model of halothane-associated hepatotoxicity. *Anesthesiology* 70, 649.

Lind, R.C., Gandolfi, A.J., and Hall, P.D. (1990). Covalent binding of oxidative biotransformation intermediates is associated with halothane hepatotoxicity in guinea pigs. *Anesthesiology* 73, 1208.

Lind, R.C., Gandolfi, A.J., and Hall, P.M. (1994). A model for fatal halothane hepatitis in the guinea pig. *Anesthesiology* 81, 478.

Lindberg, M.C. (1992). Hepatobiliary complications of oral contraceptives. *J. Gen. Intern. Med.* 7, 199.

Lindgren, A. and Olsson, R. (1994). Liver reactions from trimethoprim. *J. Intern. Med.*. 236, 281.

Lindgren, A., Aldenborg, F., Norkrans, G., *et al.* (1997). Paracetamol-induced cholestatic and granulomatous liver injuries. *J. Intern. Med.*. 241, 435.

Lindholm, A. and Kahan, B.D. (1993). Influence of cyclosporine pharmacokinetics, trough concentrations, and AUC monitoring on outcome after kidney transplantation. *Clin. Pharmacol. Ther.* 54, 205.

Lindor, K.D., Fleming, C.R., Abrams, A., *et al.* (1979). Liver function values in adults receiving total parenteral nutrition. *JAMA* 241, 2398.

Lo, K.J., Eastwood, I.R., and Eidelman, S. (1967). Cholestatic jaundice associated with chlordiazepoxide hydrochloride (Librium) therapy. Report of a case and review of the literature. *Am. J. Dig. Dis.* 12, 845.

Loeper, J., Descatoire, V., Letteron, P., *et al.* (1994). Hepatotoxicity of germander in mice. *Gastroenterology* 106, 464.

Lok, A.S. and Ng, I.O. (1988). Prochlorperazine-induced chronic cholestasis. *J. Hepatol.* 6, 369.

Longstreth, G.F. and Hershman, J. (1985). Trazodone-induced hepatotoxicity and leukonychia. *J. Am. Acad. Dermatol.* 13, 149.

Loomus, G.N., Aneja, P., and Bota, R.A. (1983). A case of peliosis hepatis in association with tamoxifen therapy. *Am. J. Clin. Pathol.* 80, 881.

Lorber, M.I., Van, B.C., Flechner, S.M., *et al.* (1987). Hepatobiliary and pancreatic complications of cyclosporine therapy in 466 renal transplant recipients. *Transplantation* 43, 35.

Luke, D.R., Rocci, M.L., Jr, Schaible, D.H., *et al.* (1986). Acute hepatotoxicity after excessively high doses of carbamazepine on two occasions. *Pharmacotherapy* 6, 108.

Mabee, C.L., Mabee, S.W., Baker, P.B., *et al.* (1995). Fulminant hepatic failure associated with etodolac use. *Am. J. Gastroenterol.* 90, 659.

McClay, E., Lusch, C.J., and Mastrangelo, M.J. (1987). Allergy-induced hepatic toxicity associated with dacarbazine. *Cancer Treat. Rep.* 71, 219.

McConnell, J.B., Powell, J.P., Davis, M., *et al.* (1981). Use of liver function tests as predictors of rifampicin metabolism in cirrhosis. *Q. J. Med.* 50, 77.

McDonald, A.T.J., Phillips, M.J., and Jeejeebhoy, K.N. (1973). Reversal of fatty liver by intralipid in patients on total parenteral nutrition. *Gastroenterology* 64, 885.

MacGregor, F.B., Abernethy, V.E., Dahabra, S., *et al.* (1989). Hepatotoxicity of herbal remedies. *BMJ* 299, 1156.

Mackay, I.R. (1985). Induction by drugs of hepatitis and autoantibodies to cell organelles: significance and interpretation. *Hepatology* 5, 904.

McKenzie, R., Fried, M.W., Sallie, R., *et al.* (1995). Hepatic failure and lactic acidosis due to fialuridine (FIAU), an investigational nucleoside analogue for chronic hepatitis B. *N. Engl. J. Med.* 333, 1099.

McMaster, K.R. and Hennigar, G.R. (1981). Drug-induced granulomatous hepatitis. *Lab. Invest.* 44, 61.

McMurtry, R.J. and Mitchell, J.R. (1977). Renal and hepatic necrosis after metabolic activation of 2-substituted furans and thiophenes, including furosemide and cephaloridine. *Toxicol. Appl. Pharmacol.* 42, 285.

Maddrey, W.C. (1980). Drug-related acute and chronic hepatitis. *Clin. Gastroenterol.* 9, 213.

Maddrey, W.C. (1981). Isoniazid-induced liver disease. *Semin. Liver Dis.* 1, 129.

Maddrey, W.C. (1987). Hepatic vein thrombosis (Budd–Chiari syndrome):possible association with oral contraceptives. *Semin. Liver Dis.* 7, 32.

Maddrey, W.C. and Boitnott, J.K. (1973). Isoniazid hepatitis. *Ann. Intern. Med.* 79, 791.

Maddrey, W.C. and Boitnott, J.K. (1977). Drug-induced chronic liver disease. *Gastroenterology* 72, 1348.

Maddrey, W.C. and Boitnott, J.K. (1979). Drug-induced chronic hepatitis and cirrhosis. *Prog. Liver Dis.* 6, 595.

Mager, A., Birnbaum, Y., and Zlotikamien, B. (1991). Streptokinase-induced jaundice in patients with acute myocardial infarction. *Am. Heart J.* 121, 1543.

Maggiore, G., Larizza, D., Lorini, R., *et al.* (1989). Propylthiouracil hepatotoxicity mimicking autoimmune chronic active hepatitis in a girl. *J. Pediatr. Gastroenterol. Nutr.* 8, 547.

Malatjalian, D.A. and Graham, C.H. (1982). Liver adenoma with granulomas. The appearance of granulomas in oral contraceptive-related hepatocellular adenoma and in the surrounding nontumorous liver. *Arch. Pathol. Lab. Med.* 106, 244.

Malcolm, A., Heap, T.R., Eckstein, R.P., *et al.* (1996). Minocycline-induced liver injury. *Am. J. Gastroenterol.* 91, 1641.

Manivel, J.C., Bloomer, J.R., and Snover, D.C. (1987). Progressive bile duct injury after thiabendazole administration. *Gastroenterology* 93, 245.

Manoukian, A.V. and Carson, J.L. (1996). Nonsteroidal antiinflammatory drug-induced hepatic disorders. Incidence and prevention. *Drug Saf.* 15, 64.

Mant, J.W. and Vessey, M.P. (1995). Trends in mortality from primary liver cancer in England and Wales 1975–92: influence of oral contraceptives. *Br. J. Cancer* 72, 800.

Mant, T.G., Tempowski, J.H., Volans, G.N., *et al.* (1984). Adverse effects of acetylcysteine and the effects of overdose. *BMJ* 289, 217.

Marinos, G., Riley, J., Painter, D.M., *et al.* (1992). Sulfasalazine-induced fulminant hepatic failure. *J. Clin. Gastroenterol.* 14, 132.

Marks, J.W., Sue, S.O., Perlman, B.J., *et al.* (1981). Sulfation of chenodeoxycholic acid-induced elevations in patients with gallstones. *J. Clin. Invest.* 68, 1190.

Marsh, J.C. (1989). Hepatic vascular toxicity of dacarbazine (DTIC): not a rare complication. *Hepatology* 9, 790.

Martin, J.L., Dubbink, D.A., Plevak, D.J., *et al.* (1992). Halothane hepatitis 28 years after primary exposure. *Anesth. Analg.* 74, 605.

Martin, J.L., Kenna, J.G., Martin, B.M., *et al.* (1993). Halothane hepatitis patients have serum antibodies that react with protein disulfide isomerase. *Hepatology* 18, 858.

Maruyama, S., Hirayama, C., Abe, J., *et al.* (1995). Chronic active hepatitis and liver cirrhosis in association with combined tamoxifen/tegafur adjuvant therapy. *Dig. Dis. Sci.* 40, 2602.

Mason, J. (1989). Pharmacology of cyclosporin (Sandimmune)VII: pathophysiology and toxicology of cyclosporin in humans and animals. *Pharmacol. Rev.* 42, 423.

Mason, R.P. and Fischer, V. (1986). Free radicals of acetaminophen: their subsequent reactions and toxicological significance. *Fed. Proc.* 45, 2493.

Mathieu, D., Zafrani, E.S., Anglade, M.C., *et al.* (1989). Association of focal nodular hyperplasia and hepatic hemangioma. *Gastroenterology* 97, 154.

Matos, C., Avni, E.F., Van, G.D., *et al.* (1987). Total parenteral nutrition (TPN) and gallbladder diseases in neonates. Sonographic assessment. *J. Ultrasound. Med.* 6, 243.

Mays, E.T. and Christopherson, W. (1984). Hepatic tumors induced by sex steroids. *Semin. Liver Dis.* 4, 147.

Mazeika, P.K. and Ford, M.J. (1989). Chronic active hepatitis associated with diclofenac sodium therapy. *Br. J. Clin. Pract.* 43, 125.

Medina, I., Mills, J., Leoung, G., *et al.* (1990). Oral therapy for *Pneumocystis carinii* pneumonia in the acquired immunodeficiency syndrome. A controlled trial of trimethoprimsulfamethoxazole versus trimethoprim-dapsone. *N. Engl. J. Med.* 323, 776.

Medline, A., Cohen, L.B., Tobe, B.A., *et al.* (1978). Liver granulomas and allopurinol. *BMJ* i, 1320.

Metreau, J.M., Dhumeaux, D., and Berthelot, P. (1972). Oral contraceptives and the liver. *Digestion* 7, 318.

Middleton, C., McCaughan, G.W., Painter, D.M., *et al.* (1989). Danazol and hepatic neoplasia: a case report. *Aust. N.Z. J. Med.* 19, 733.

Min, D.I., Burke, P.A., Lewis, W.D., *et al.* (1992). Acute hepatic failure associated with oral minocycline: a case report. *Pharmacotherapy* 12, 68.

Minuk, G.Y., Kelly, J.K., and Hwang, W.S. (1988). Vitamin A hepatotoxicity in multiple family members. *Hepatology* 8, 272.

Mirada, C.A., Monteagudo, J.M., Sole, V.J., *et al.* (1991). Methyldopa-induced granulomatous hepatitis. *DICP* 25, 1269.

Miros, M., Kerlin, P., Walker, N., *et al.* (1990). Flucloxacillin induced delayed cholestatic hepatitis. *Aust. N.Z. J. Med.* 20, 251.

Mitchell, I., Wendon, J., Fitt, S., *et al.* (1995). Antituberculous therapy and acute liver failure. *Lancet* 345, 555.

Mitchell, J.R. and Jollow, D.J. (1975). Metabolic activation of drugs to toxic substances. *Gastroenterology* 68, 392.

Mitchell, J.R., Jollow, D.J., Potter, W.Z., *et al.* (1973a). Acetaminophen-induced hepatic necrosis. I. Role of drug metabolism. *J. Pharmacol. Exp. Ther.* 187, 185.

Mitchell, J.R., Jollow, D.J., Potter, W.Z., *et al.* (1973b). Acetaminophen-induced hepatic necrosis. IV. Protective role of glutathione. *J. Pharmacol. Exp. Ther.* 187, 211.

Mitchell, J.R., Thorgeirsson, U.P., Black, M., *et al.* (1975). Increased incidence of isoniazid hepatitits in rapid acetylators: possible relation to hydranize metabolites. *Clin. Pharmacol. Ther.* 18, 70.

Mitchell, M.C., Schenker, S., Avant, G.R., *et al.* (1981). Cimetidine protects against acetaminophen hepatotoxicity in rats. *Gastroenterology* 81, 1052.

Mitchell, M.C., Schenker, S., and Speeg, K.V., Jr. (1984). Selective inhibition of acetaminophen oxidation and toxicity by cimetidine and other histamine H2-receptor antagonists in vivo and in vitro in the rat and in man. *J. Clin. Invest.* 73, 383.

Mitrane, M.P., Singh, A., and Seibold, J.R. (1986). Cholestasis and fatal agranulocytosis complicating sulfasalazine therapy: case report and review of the literature. *J. Rheumatol.* 13, 969.

Miyazaki, K., Nakayama, F., and Koga, A. (1984). Effect of chenodeoxycholic acid and ursodeoxycholic acid on isolated adult human hepatocytes. *Dig. Dis. Sci.* 79, 1123.

Mockli, G., Crowley, M., Stern, R., *et al.* (1989). Massive hepatic necrosis in a child after administration of phenobarbital. *Am. J. Gastroenterol.* 84, 820.

Moen, M.D., Caliendo, M.J., Marshall, W., *et al.* (1993). Hepatic rupture in pregnancy associated with cocaine use. *Obstet. Gynecol.* 82, 687.

Moertel, C.G., Fleming, T.R., MacDonald, J.S., *et al.* (1993). Hepatic toxicity associated with fluorouracil plus levamisole adjuvant therapy. *J. Clin. Oncol.* 11, 2386.

Moldawsky, R.J. (1984). Hepatotoxicity associated with maprotiline therapy: case report. *J. Clin. Psychiatry* 45, 178.

Moore, R.A., Greenberg, E., and Tangen, L. (1995). Cyclosporine-induced worsening of hepatic dysfunction in a patient with Crohn's disease and enterocutaneous fistula. *South. Med. J.* 88, 843.

Moradpour, D., Altorfer, J., Flury, R., *et al.* (1994). Chlorpromazine-induced vanishing bile duct syndrome leading to biliary cirrhosis. *Hepatology* 20, 1437.

Morais, S.M. and Wells, P.G. (1989). Enhanced acetaminophen toxicity in rats with bilirubin glucuronyl transferase deficiency. *Hepatology* 10, 163.

Morais, S.M., Uetrecht, J.P., and Wells, P.G. (1992). Decreased glucuronidation and increased bioactivation of acetaminophen in Gilbert's syndrome. *Gastroenterology* 102, 577.

Morelli, S., Guido, V., De, M.P., *et al.* (1991). Early hepatitis during intravenous amiodarone administration. *Cardiology* 78, 291.

Morgan, M.Y., Reshef, R., Shah, R.R., *et al.* (1984). Impaired oxidation of debrisoquine in patients with perhexiline liver injury. *Gut* 25, 1057.

Morgan, M., Dodds, A., Atkinson, K., *et al.* (1991). The toxicity of busulphan and cyclophosphamide as the preparative regimen for bone marrow transplantation. *Br. J. Haematol.* 77, 529.

Morris, L.E. and Guthrie, T.H.J. (1988). Busulfan-induced hepatitis. *Am. J. Gastroenterol.* 83, 682.

Morrow, P.L., Hardin, N.J., and Bonadies, J. (1989). Hypersensitivity myocarditis and hepatitis associated with imipramine and its metabolite, desipramine. *J. Forensic Sci.* 34, 1016.

Moses, A., Zahger, D., and Amir, G. (1989). Cholestatic liver injury after prolonged exposure to methyldopa. *Digestion* 42, 57.

Moskovitz, R., DeVane, C.L., Harris, R., *et al.* (1982). Toxic hepatitis and single daily dosage imipramine therapy. *J. Clin. Psychiatry* 43, 165.

Moss, R.L., Das, J.B., and Raffensperger, J.G. (1993). Total parenteral nutrition-associated cholestasis: clinical and histopathologic correlation. *J. Pediatr. Surg.* 28, 1270.

Moulding, T.S., Redeker, A.G., and Kanel, G.C. (1991). Acetaminophen, isoniazid, and hepatic toxicity. *Ann. Intern. Med.* 114, 431.

Moustafa, M.A., Claesen, M., Adline, J., *et al.* (1983). EWvidence for an arene-3,4-oxide as a metabolic intermediate in the *meta-* and *para*-hydroxylation of phenytoin in the dog. *Drug Metab. Dispos.* 11, 574.

Mulberg, A.E. and Bell, L.M. (1993). Fatal cholestatic hepatitis and multisystem failure associated with nitrofurantoin. *J. Pediatr. Gastroenterol. Nutr.* 17, 307.

Muller, A.F., Toghill, P.J., and Smith, P. (1996). 'Relapse' of chronic active hepatitis — not always what it seems. *Postgrad. Med. J.* 72, 431.

Mullick, F.G. and Ishak, K.G. (1980). Hepatic injury associated with diphenylhydantoin therapy. A clinicopathologic study of 20 cases. *Am. J. Clin. Pathol.* 74, 442.

Mullick, F.G., Moran, C.A., and Ishak, K.G. (1994). Total parenteral nutrition: a histopathologic analysis of the liver changes in 20 children. *Mod. Pathol.* 7, 190.

Mullin, G.E., Greenson, J.K., and Mitchell, M.C. (1989). Fulminant hepatic failure after ingestion of sustained-release nicotinic acid. *Ann. Intern. Med.* 111, 253.

Munoz, S.J., Martinez, H.A., and Maddrey, W.C. (1990). Intrahepatic cholestasis and phospholipidosis associated with the use of trimethoprim–sulfamethoxazole. *Hepatology* 12, 342.

Murphy, B.J. and Collins, B.J. (1996). Severe hepatitis and liver failure induced by cyproterone acetate. *Aust. N.Z. J. Med.* 26, 724.

Murphy, R., Swartz, R., and Watkins, P.B. (1990). Severe acetaminophen toxicity in a patient receiving isoniazid. *Ann. Intern. Med.* 113, 799 [published erratum appears in *Ann. Intern. Med.* (1991) 114, 253].

Mushin, W.W., Rosen, M., and Jones, E.V. (1971). Posthalothane jaundice in relation to previous administration of halothane. *BMJ* 3, 18.

Mutimer, D.J., Ayres, R.C.S., Neuberger, J.M., *et al.* (1994). Serious paracetamol poisoning and the results of liver transplantation. *Gut* 35, 809.

Naeim, F., Copper, P.H., and Semion, A.A. (1973). Peliosis hepatis. Possible etiologic role of anabolic steroids. *Arch. Pathol.* 95, 284.

Nagorney, D.M. (1995). Benign hepatic tumors: focal nodular hyperplasia and hepatocellular adenoma. *World J. Surg.* 19, 13.

Nakao, N.L., Gelb, A.M., Stenger, R.J., *et al.* (1985). A case of chronic liver disease due to tolazamide. *Gastroenterology* 89, 192.

Namias, A., Bhalotra, R., and Donowitz, M. (1981). Reversible sulfasalazine-induced granulomatous hepatitis. *J. Clin. Gastroenterol.* 3, 193.

Naschitz, J.E., Khamessi, R., Elias, N., *et al.* (1995). Ticlopidine-induced prolonged cholestasis. *J. Toxicol. Clin. Toxicol.* 33, 379.

National Halothane Study (1966). Summary of the National Halothane Study. Possible association between halothane anesthesia and postoperative hepatic necrosis. Report by Subcommittee on the National Halothane Study of the Committee on Anesthesia, National Academy of Sciences, National Research Council. *JAMA* 197, 775.

Nelson, S.D., Mitchell, J.R., Timbrell, J.A., *et al.* (1976). Isoniazid and iproniazid: activation of metabolites to toxic intermediates in man and rat. *Science* 193, 901.

Neuberger, J. and Williams, R. (1984). Halothane anaesthesia and liver damage. *BMJ* 289, 1136.

Neuberger, J. and Williams, R. (1989). Immune mechanisms in tienilic acid associated hepatotoxicity. *Gut* 30, 515.

Neuberger, J., Portmann, B., Nunnerley, H.B., *et al.* (1980). Oral-contraceptive-associated liver tumours: occurrence of malignancy and difficulties in diagnosis. *Lancet* i, 273.

Neuberger, J., Kenna, J.G., Nouri, A.K., *et al.* (1985). Antibody mediated hepatocyte injury in methyldopa induced hepatotoxicity. *Gut* 26, 1233.

Neuberger, J., Forman, D., Doll, R., *et al.* (1986). Oral contraceptives and hepatocellular carcinoma. *BMJ* 292, 1355.

Nicod, L., Viollon, C., Regnier, A., *et al.* (1997). Rifampicin and isoniazid increase acetaminophen and isoniazid cytotoxicity in human HepG2 hepatoma cells. *Hum. Exp. Toxicol.* 16, 28.

Njoku, D., Laster, M.J., Gong, D.H., *et al.* (1997). Biotransformation of halothane, enflurane, isoflurane, and desflurane to trifluoroacetylated liver proteins: association between protein acylation and hepatic injury. *Anesth. Analg.* 84, 173.

Nolan, C.M., Sandblom, R.E., Thummel, K.E., *et al.* (1994). Hepatotoxicity associated with acetaminophen usage in patients receiving multiple drug therapy for tuberculosis. *Chest* 105, 408.

Nurhussein, M.A. (1993). Ticlopidine-induced prolonged cholestasis. *J. Am. Geriatr. Soc.* 41, 1371.

Nyfors, A. (1977). Liver biopsies from psoriatics related to methotrexate therapy. 3. Findings in post-methotrexate liver biopsies from 160 psoriatics. *Acta Pathol. Microbiol. Scand. A.* 85, 511.

Nyfors, A. and Poulsen, H. (1977). Morphogenesis of fibrosis and cirrhosis in methotrexate-treated patients with psoriasis. *Am. J. Surg. Pathol.* 1, 235.

O'Brien, C.B., Shields, D.S., Saul, S.H., *et al.* (1996). Drug-induced vanishing bile duct syndrome: response to ursodiol. *Am. J. Gastroenterol.* 91, 1456.

O'Brien, W.M. (1983). Longterm efficacy and safety of tolmetin sodium in treatment of geriatric patients with rheumatoid arthritis and osteoarthritis. *J. Clin. Pharmacol.* 23, 309.

O'Neil, M.G., Perdun, C.S., Wilson, M.B., *et al.* (1996). Felbamate-associated fatal acute hepatic necrosis. *Neurology* 46, 1457.

Odeleye, O.E., Lopez, M.C., Smith, B.T., *et al.* (1992). Cocaine hepatotoxicity during protein undernutrition of retrovirally infected mice. *Can. J. Physiol. Pharmacol.* 70, 338.

Olano, J.P., Borucki, M.J., Wen, J.W., *et al.* (1995). Massive hepatic steatosis and lactic acidosis in a patient with AIDS who was receiving zidovudine. *Clin. Infect. Dis.* 21, 973.

Olsen, J.H., Schulgen, G., Boice, J.D., Jr, *et al.* (1995). Antiepileptic treatment and risk for hepatobiliary cancer and malignant lymphoma. *Cancer Res.* 55, 294.

Olson, J.A. (1983). Adverse effects of large doses of vitamin A and retinoids. *Semin. Oncol.* 10, 290.

Olsson, R. and Zettergren, L. (1988). Anticonvulsant-induced liver damage. *Am. J. Gastroenterol.* 83, 576.

Olsson, R., Wiholm, B.E., Sand, C., *et al.* (1992). Liver damage from flucloxacillin, cloxacillin and dicloxacillin. *J. Hepatol.* 15, 154.

Oren, R. and Ilan, Y. (1992). Reversible hepatic injury induced by long-term vitamin A ingestion. *Am. J. Med.* 93, 703.

Ortega, J.A., Donaldson, S.S., Ivy, S.P., *et al.* (1997). Venoocclusive disease of the liver after chemotherapy with vincristine, actinomycin D, and cyclophosphamide for the treatment of rhabdomyosarcoma. A report of the Intergroup Rhabdomyosarcoma Study Group, Childrens Cancer Group, the Pediatric Oncology Group, and the Pediatric Intergroup Statistical Center. *Cancer* 79, 2435.

Otani, K., Kaneko, S., Tasaki, H., *et al.* (1989). Hepatic injury caused by mianserin. *BMJ* 299, 519.

Ozenirler, S., Tuncer, C., Boztepe, U., *et al.* (1996). Propylthiouracil-induced hepatic damage. *Ann. Pharmacother.* 30, 960.

Ozenne, G., Manchon, N.D., Doucet, J., *et al.* (1989). Carbimazole-induced acute cholestatic hepatitis. *J. Clin. Gastroenterol.* 11, 95.

Ozick, L.A., Jacob, L., Comer, G.M., *et al.* (1995). Hepatotoxicity from isoniazid and rifampicin in inner-city AIDS patients. *Am. J. Gastroenterol.* 90, 1978.

Palombo, J.D., Schnure, F., Bistrian, B.R., *et al.* (1987). Improvement of liver function tests by administration of L-carnitine to a carnitine deficient patient receiving home parenteral nutrition. *JPEN* 11, 88.

Pantarotto, C., Arboix, M., Sezzana, P., *et al.* (1982). Studies on 5,5-diphenylhydantoin irreversible binding to rat liver microsomal proteins. *Biochem. Pharmacol.* 31, 1501.

Pappo, I., Bercovier, H., Berry, E.M., *et al.* (1992). Polymyxin B reduces total parenteral nutrition-associated hepatic steatosis by its antibacterial activity and by blocking deleterious effects of lipopolysaccharide. *JPEN* 16, 529.

Pappo, I., Bercovier, H., Berry, E., *et al.* (1995). Antitumor necrosis factor antibodies reduce hepatic steatosis during total parenteral nutrition and bowel rest in the rat. *JPEN* 19, 80.

Paradinas, F.J., Bull, T.B., Westaby, D., *et al.* (1977). Hyperplasia and prolapse of hepatocytes into hepatic veins during long-term methyltestosterone therapy: possible relationships of these changes to the development of peliosis hepatis and liver tumours. *Histopathology* 1, 225.

Park, B.K., Pirmohamed, M., and Kitteringham, N.R. (1995). The role of cytochrome P450 enzymes in hepatic and extrahepatic human drug toxicity. *Pharmacol. Ther.* 68, 385.

Parthasarathy, R., Sarma, G.R., Janardhanam, B., *et al.* (1986). Hepatic toxicity in South Indian patients during treatment of tuberculosis with short-course regimens containing isoniazid, rifampicin and pyrazinamide. *Tubercle* 67, 99.

Parys, B.T., Hamid, S., and Thomson, R.G. (1991). Severe hepatocellular dysfunction following cyproterone acetate therapy. *Br. J. Urol.* 67, 312.

Pasanen, M., Pellinen, P., Stenback, F., *et al.* (1995). The role of CYP enzymes in cocaine-induced liver damage. *Arch. Toxicol.* 69, 287.

Patel, S.D. and Taylor, H.C. (1994). Intrahepatic cholestasis during nicotinic acid therapy. *Cleve. Clin. J. Med.* 61, 70.

Patt, Y.Z., Boddie, A.W., Jr, Charnsangavej, C., *et al.* (1986). Hepatic arterial infusion with floxuridine and cisplatin: overriding importance of antitumor effect versus degree of tumor burden as determinants of survival among patients with colorectal cancer. *J. Clin. Oncol.* 4, 1356.

Pattyn, S.R., Janssens, L., Bourland, J., *et al.* (1984). Hepatotoxicity of the combination of rifampin-ethionamide in the treatment of multibacillary leprosy. *Int. J. Lepr. Other Mycobact. Dis.* 52, 1.

Pellinen, P., Stenback, F., Raunio, H., *et al.* (1994). Modification of hepatic cytochrome P450 profile by cocaine-induced hepatotoxicity in DBA/2 mouse. *Eur. J. Pharmacol.* 292, 57.

Perez, G.S. and Garcia, R.L. (1993). The increased risk of hospitalizations for acute liver injury in a population with exposure to multiple drugs. *Epidemiology* 4, 496.

Perini, G.P., Bonadiman, C., Fraccaroli, G.P., *et al.* (1990). Azathioprine-related cholestatic jaundice in heart transplant patients. *J. Heart Transplant.* 9, 577.

Perino, L.E., Warren, G.H., and Levine, J.S. (1987). Cocaineinduced hepatotoxicity in humans. *Gastroenterology* 93, 176.

Perkins, L. (1962). Phenindione jaundice. *Lancet* i, 125.

Perret, A.G., Mosnier, J.F., Porcheron, J., *et al.* (1996). Role of oral contraceptives in the growth of a multilobular adenoma associated with a hepatocellular carcinoma in a young woman. *J. Hepatol.* 25, 976.

Perrot, N., Nalpas, B., Yang, C.S., *et al.* (1989). Modulation of cytochrome P450 isozymes in human liver, by ethanol and drug intake. *Eur. J. Clin. Invest.* 19, 549.

Perry, M.C. (1992). Chemotherapeutic agents and hepatotoxicity. *Semin. Oncol.* 19, 551.

Pessayre, D. and Larrey, D. (1988). Acute and chronic drug-induced hepatitis. *Baillière's Clin. Gastroenterol.* 2, 385.

Pessayre, D., Marie, C., and Benhamou, J.P. (1976). Hépatite due au propionate d'érythromycine. *Arch. Fr. Mal. App. Dig.* 65, 405.

Pessayre, D., Bentata, M., and Degott, C. (1977). Isoniazid-rifampicin fulminant hepatitis. *Gastroenterology* 72, 284.

Pessayre, D., Feldmann, G., Degott, C., et al. (1979). Gold salt-induced cholestasis. *Digestion* 19, 56.

Pessayre, D., Degos, F., Feldmann, G., et al. (1981). Chronic active hepatitis and giant multinucleated hepatocytes in adults treated with clometacin. *Digestion* 22, 66.

Pessayre, D., Larrey, D., Funck, B.C., et al. (1985). Drug interactions and hepatitis produced by some macrolide antibiotics. *J. Antimicrob. Chemother.* 16 (Suppl. A), 181.

Pettavel, J., Gardiol, D., Bergier, N., et al. (1986). Fatal liver cirrhosis associated with long-term arterial infusion of floxuridine. *Lancet* ii, 1162.

Phillips, M.J., Fisher, R.L., Anderson, D.W., et al. (1983). Ultrastructural evidence of intrahepatic cholestasis before and after chenodeoxycholic acid therapy in patients with cholelithiasis: The National Co-operative Gallstone Study. *Hepatology* 3, 209.

Pierce, E.H. and Chesler, D.L. (1978). Possible association of granulomatous hepatitis with clofibrate therapy. *N. Engl. J. Med.* 299, 314.

Pinsky, P.F., Hurwitz, E.S., and Schonberger, L.B. (1988). Reye's Syndrome and aspirin: Evidence for a dose-related effect. *JAMA* 260, 657.

Pinto, H.C., Baptista, A., Camilo, M.E., et al. (1995). Tamoxifen-associated steatohepatitis — report of three cases. *J. Hepatol.* 23, 95.

Pipek, R., Avizohar, O., and Levy, Y. (1994). Transient hepatic dysfunction in two brothers receiving heparin and streptokinase: a genetic predisposition? *Int. J. Cardiol.* 46, 299.

Planas, R., De, L.R., Quer, J.C., et al. (1990). Fatal submassive necrosis of the liver associated with piroxicam. *Am. J. Gastroenterol.* 85, 468.

Pol, S., Cavalcanti, R., Carnot, F., et al. (1996). Azathioprine hepatitis in kidney transplant recipients. A predisposing role of chronic viral hepatitis. *Transplantation* 61, 1774.

Poli, G. (1993). Liver damage due to free radicals. *Br. Med. Bull.* 49, 604.

Pollak, P.T., Sharma, A.D., and Carruthers, S.G. (1990). Relation of amiodarone hepatic and pulmonary toxicity to serum drug concentrations and superoxide dismutase activity. *Am. J. Cardiol.* 65, 1185.

Poncin, E., Silvain, C., Touchard, G., et al. (1986). Papaverine-induced chronic liver disease. *Gastroenterology* 90, 1051.

Portal, R.W. and Emanuel, R.W. (1961). Phenindione hepatitis complicating anticoagulant therapy. *BMJ* ii, 1318.

Porter, J.M., Sussman, M.S., and Rosen, G.M. (1988). Cocaine-induced hepatotoxicity. *Hepatology* 8, 1713.

Portmann, B., Talbot, I.C., Day, D.W., et al. (1975). Histopathological changes in the liver following a paracetamol overdose: correlation with clinical and biochemical parameters. *J. Pathol.* 117, 169.

Potter, W.Z., Davis, D.C., Mitchell, J.R., et al. (1973). Acetaminophen-induced hepatic necrosis. 3. Cytochrome P-450-mediated covalent binding in vitro. *J. Pharmacol. Exp. Ther.* 187, 203.

Powell-Jackson, P.R., Tredger, J.M., and Williams, R. (1984). Hepatotoxicity of sodium valproate: a review. *Gut* 25, 673.

Prescott, L.F. (1980). Hepatotoxicity of mild analgesics. *Br. J. Clin. Pharmacol.* 10 (Suppl. 2), 373S.

Prescott, L.F., Sutherland, G.R., Park, J., et al. (1976). Cysteamine, methionine, and penicillamine in the treatment of paracetamol poisoning. *Lancet* ii, 109.

Price, L.H., Nelson, J.C., and Waltrip, R.W. (1983). Desipramine-associated hepatitis. *J. Clin. Psychopharmacol.* 3, 243.

Punukollu, R.C., Kumar, S., and Mullen, K.D. (1990). Quinine hepatotoxicity. An underrecognized or rare phenomenon? *Arch. Intern. Med.* 150, 1112.

Purcell, P., Henry, D., and Melville, G. (1991). Diclofenac hepatitis. *Gut* 32, 1381.

Queneau, P.E., Bertault, P.P., Guitaoui, M., et al. (1994). Improvement of cyclosporin A-induced cholestasis by tauroursodeoxycholate in a long-term study in the rat. *Dig. Dis. Sci.* 39, 1581.

Rabe, T., Feldmann, K., Heinemann, L., et al. (1996). Cyproterone acetate: is it hepato- or genotoxic? *Drug Saf.* 14, 25.

Ragni, M.V., Amato, D.A., LoFaro, M.L., et al. (1995). Randomized study of didanosine monotherapy and combination therapy with zidovudine in hemophilic and non-hemophilic subjects with asymptomatic human immunodeficiency virus-1 infection. AIDS Clinical Trial Groups. *Blood* 85, 2337.

Rahmat, J., Gelfand, R.L., Gelfand, M.C., et al. (1985). Captopril-associated cholestatic jaundice. *Ann. Intern. Med.* 102, 56.

Randall, L.H., Shaddy, R.E., Sturtevant, J.E., et al. (1992). Cholelithiasis in infants receiving furosemide: a prospective study of the incidence and one-year follow-up. *J. Perinatol.* 12, 107.

Rao, K.V. (1986). Cholestatic jaundice associated with methyldopa. *Minn. Med.* 69, 720.

Raucy, J.L., Lasker, J.M., Lieber, C.S., et al. (1989). Acetaminophen activation by human liver cytochromes P-450IIE1 and P-4501A2. *Arch. Biochem. Biophys.* 271, 270.

Reeves, M. (1997). Acute hepatitis following enflurane anaesthesia. *Anaesth. Intensive Care* 25, 80.

Remy, A.J., Larrey, D., Pageaux, G.P., et al. (1995). Cross hepatotoxicity between tricyclic antidepressants and phenothiazines. *Eur. J. Gastroenterol. Hepatol.* 7, 373.

Rescorla, F.J. and Grosfeld, J.L. (1992). Cholecystitis and cholelithiasis in children. *Semin. Pediatr. Surg.* 1, 98.

Reshef, R., Lok, A.S., and Sherlock, S. (1982). Cholestatic jaundice in fascioliasis treated with niclofolan. *BMJ (Clin. Res. Ed.)* 285, 1243.

Rettie, A.E., Rettenmeier, A.W., Howald, W.N., et al. (1987). Cytochrome P-450-catalyzed formation of delta 4-VPA, a toxic metabolite of valproic acid. *Science* 235, 890.

Reynolds, R., Lloyd, D.A., and Slinger, R.P. (1981). Cholestatic jaundice induced by flurazepam hydrochloride. *Can. Med. Assoc. J.* 124, 893.

Reynolds, A.P., Kiely, E., and Meadows, N. (1994). Manganese in long term paediatric parenteral nutrition. *Arch. Dis. Child.* 71, 527.

Ribe, J., Benkov, K.J., Thung, S.N., *et al.* (1986). Fatal massive hepatic necrosis: a probable hypersensitivity reaction to sulfasalazine. *Am. J. Gastroenterol.* 81, 205.

Richter, W.O. and Schwandt, P. (1987). Serious side effect of nifedipine. *Arch. Intern. Med.* 147, 1852.

Ridker, P.M. and McDermott, W.V. (1989). Comfrey herb tea and hepatic veno-occlusive disease. *Lancet* i, 657.

Ridker, P.M., Ohkuma, S., McDermott, W.V., *et al.* (1985). Hepatic venocclusive disease associated with the consumption of pyrrolizidine-containing dietary supplements. *Gastroenterology* 88, 1050.

Rieder, M.J., Shear, N.H., Kanee, A., *et al.* (1991). Prominence of slow acetylator phenotype among patients with sulfonamide hypersensitivity reactions. *Clin. Pharmacol. Ther.* 49, 13.

Rigas, B., Rosenfeld, L.E., Barwick, K.W., *et al.* (1986). Amiodarone hepatotoxicity. A clinicopathologic study of five patients. *Ann. Intern. Med.* 104, 348.

Rigauts, H.D., Selleslag, D.L., Van, E.P., *et al.* (1988). Erythromycin-induced hepatitis: simulator of malignancy. *Radiology* 169, 661.

Rigberg, L.A., Robison, M.J., and Espiritu, C.R. (1976). Chlorpropamide-induced granulomas. A probable hypersensitivity reaction in liver and bone marrow. *JAMA* 235, 409.

Roberts, E.A., Spielberg, S.P., Goldbach, M., *et al.* (1990). Phenobarbital hepatotoxicity in an 8-month-old infant. *J. Hepatol.* 10, 235.

Roenigk, H.H.J. (1988). Liver toxicity of retinoid therapy. *J. Am. Acad. Dermatol.* 19, 199.

Roman, I.D., Monte, M.J., Esteller, A., *et al.* (1989). Cholestasis in the rat by means of intravenous administration of cyclosporine vehicle, Cremophor EL. *Transplantation* 48, 554.

Ros, E., Small, D.M., and Carey, M.C. (1979). Effects of chlorpromazine hydrochloride on bile salt synthesis, bile formation and biliary lipid secretion in the rhesus monkey: a model for chlorpromazine-induced cholestasis. *Eur. J. Clin. Invest.* 9, 29.

Rosen, G.M., Singletary, W.V.J., Rauckman, E.J., *et al.* (1983). Acetaminophen hepatotoxicity. An alternative mechanism. *Biochem. Pharmacol.* 32, 2053.

Rosenberg, W.M., Ryley, N.G., Trowell, J.M., *et al.* (1993). Dextropropoxyphene induced hepatotoxicity: a report of nine cases. *J. Hepatol.* 19, 470.

Rosenberg, L., Palmer, J.R., Zauber, A.G., *et al.* (1995). Relation of benzodiazepine use to the risk of selected cancers: breast, large bowel, malignant melanoma, lung, endometrium, ovary, non-Hodgkin's lymphoma, testis, Hodgkin's disease, thyroid, and liver. *Am. J. Epidemiol.* 141, 1153.

Rosenblum, L.E., Korn, R.J., and Zimmerman, H.J. (1997). Hepatocellular jaundice as a complication of iproniazid therapy. *Arch. Intern. Med.* 105, 583.

Rosenthal, J., Sender, L., Secola, R., *et al.* (1996). Phase II trial of heparin prophylaxis for veno-occlusive disease of the liver in children undergoing bone marrow transplantation. *Bone Marrow Transplant.* 18, 185.

Rosenthal, S.A., Linstadt, D.E., Leibenhaut, M.H., *et al.* (1996). Flutamide-associated liver toxicity during treatment with total androgen suppression and radiation therapy for prostate cancer. *Radiology* 199, 451.

Roslyn, J.J., Berquist, W.E., Pitt, H.A., *et al.* (1983a). Increased risk of gallstones in children receiving total parenteral nutrition. *Pediatrics* 71, 784.

Roslyn, J.J., Pitt, H.A., Mann, L.L., *et al.* (1983b). Gallbladder disease in patients on long-term parenteral nutrition. *Gastroenterology* 84, 148.

Roslyn, J.J., Pitt, H.A., Mann, L., *et al.* (1984). Parenteral nutrition-induced gallbladder disease: a reason for early cholecystectomy. *Am. J. Surg.* 148, 58.

Rothenberg, F., Franklin, J.O., and DeMaio, S.J. (1994). Use, value, and toxicity of amiodarone. *Heart Dis. Stroke* 3, 19.

Rotmensch, H.H., Yust, I., Siegman, I.Y., *et al.* (1978). Granulomatous hepatitis: a hypersensitivity response to procainamide. *Ann. Intern. Med.* 89, 646.

Roulet, M., Laurini, R., Rivier, L., *et al.* (1988). Hepatic veno-occlusive disease in newborn infant of a woman drinking herbal tea. *J. Pediatr.* 112, 433.

Roy, A.K., Mahoney, H.C., and Levine, R.A. (1993). Phenytoin-induced chronic hepatitis. *Dig. Dis. Sci.* 38, 740.

Roy, M.A., Nugent, F.W., and Aretz, H.T. (1989). Micronodular cirrhosis after thiabendazole. *Dig. Dis. Sci.* 34, 938.

Royer, G.L., Seckman, C.E., and Welshman, I.R. (1984). Safety profile: fifteen years of clinical experience with ibuprofen. *Am. J. Med.* 77, 25.

Ruiz, V.P., Zafon, C., Segarra, A., *et al.* (1995). Ticlopidine-induced granulomatous hepatitis. *Ann. Pharmacother.* 29, 633.

Rumboldt, Z. and Bota, B. (1984). Favorable effects of glibenclamide in a patient exhibiting idiosyncratic hepatotoxic reactions to both chlorpropamide and tolbutamide. *Acta Diabetol. Lat.* 21, 387.

Ryley, N.G., Fleming, K.A., and Chapman, R.W. (1995). Focal destructive cholangiopathy associated with amoxycillin/clavulanic acid (Augmentin). *J. Hepatol.* 23, 278.

Sakaguchi, Y., Inaba, S., Irita, K., *et al.* (1994). Absence of anti-trifluoroacetate antibody after halothane anaesthesia in patients exhibiting no or mild liver damage. *Can. J. Anaesth.* 41, 398.

Sakaida, I., Kayano, K., Wasaki, S., *et al.* (1995). Protection against acetaminophen-induced liver injury in vivo by an iron chelator, desferrioxamine. *J. Scand. Gastroenterol.* 30, 61.

Sanchez, M.R., Ross, B., Rotterdam, H., *et al.* (1993). Retinoid hepatitis. *J. Am. Acad. Dermatol.* 28, 853.

Sarachek, N.S., London, R.L., and Matulewicz, T.J. (1985). Diltiazem and granulomatous hepatitis. *Gastroenterology* 88, 1260.

Sato, C. and Lieber, C.S. (1981). Mechanism of the preventive effect of ethanol on acetaminophen-induced hepatoxicity. *J. Pharmacol. Exp. Ther.* 218, 811.

Sato, C., Nakano, M., and Lieber, C.S. (1981). Prevention of acetaminophen-induced hepatotoxicity by acute ethanol administration in the rat: comparison with carbon tetra-chloride-induced hepatoxicity. *J. Pharmacol. Exp. Ther.* 218, 805.

Satorres, J., Perez-Mateo, M., Mayol, M.J., *et al.* (1995). Protective effect of diltiazem against acetaminophen hepatotoxicity in mice. *Liver* 15, 16.

Satz, N., Tauber, M., Streuli, R., *et al.* (1991). Perhexiline maleate-induced hepatitis. *Hepatogastroenterology* 38, 314.

Saw, D., Pitman, E., Maung, M., *et al.* (1996). Granulomatous hepatitis associated with glyburide. *Dig. Dis. Sci.* 41, 322.

Schaffner, F. (1966). The effect of oral contraceptives on the liver. *JAMA* 198, 1019.

Scharer, L. and Smith, J.P. (1969). Serum transaminase elevations and other hepatic abnormalities in patients receiving isoniazid. *Ann. Intern. Med.* 71, 1113.

Scheffner, D., Konig, S., Rauterberg, R.I., *et al.* (1988). Fatal liver failure in 16 children with valproate therapy. *Epilepsia* 29, 530.

Schenker, S. and Bay, M. (1994). Drug disposition and hepatotoxicity in the elderly. *J. Clin. Gastroenterol.* 18, 232.

Schmidt, D. and Kramer, G. (1994). The new anticonvulsant drugs. Implications for avoidance of adverse effects. *Drug Saf.* 11, 422.

Schmidt, G., Borsch, G., Muller, K.M., *et al.* (1986). Methimazole-associated cholestatic liver injury: case report and brief literature review. *Hepatogastroenterology* 33, 244.

Schmitz, G., Stauffert, I., Sippel, H., *et al.* (1992). Toxicity of diclofenac to isolated hepatocytes. *J. Hepatol.* 14, 408.

Schneider, H.L., Hornbach, K.D., Kniaz, J.L., *et al.* (1984). Chlorpropamide hepatotoxicity: report of a case and review of the literature. *Am. J. Gastroenterol.* 79, 721.

Schneider, M. (1996). Fatal hepatic necrosis following cardiac surgery and enflurane anaesthesia. *Anaesth. Intensive Care* 24, 289.

Schoenfield, L.J. and Lachin, J.M. (1981). Chenodiol (chenodeoxycholic acid) for dissolution of gallstones: the National Cooperative Gallstone Study. A controlled trial of efficacy and safety. *Ann. Intern. Med.* 95, 257.

Schoonjans, R., Mast, A., Van den, Abeele, A.G., *et al.* (1993). Sulfasalazine-associated encephalopathy in a patient with Crohn's disease. *Am. J. Gastroenterol.* 88, 1759.

Schreiber, A.J. and Simon, F.R. (1983). Estrogen-induced cholestasis: clues to pathogenesis and treatment. *Hepatology* 3, 607.

Schwab, G.P., Wetscher, G.J., Vogl, W., *et al.* (1996). Methimazole-induced cholestatic liver injury, mimicking sclerosing cholangitis. *Langenbecks. Arch. Chir.* 381, 225.

Schwartz, J.T., Gyorkey, F., and Graham, D.Y. (1986). Cimetidine hepatitis. *J. Clin. Gastroenterol.* 8, 681.

Schwartz, M.N. (1995). Mitochondrial toxicity — new adverse drug effects. *N. Engl. J. Med.* 333, 1146.

Schwartz, M.S., Frank, M.S., Yanoff, A., *et al.* (1989). Atenolol-associated cholestasis. *Am. J. Gastroenterol.* 84, 1084.

Scott, L.D., Katz, A.R., Duke, J.H., *et al.* (1984). Oral contraceptives, pregnancy, and focal nodular hyperplasia of the liver. *JAMA* 251, 1461.

Scully, L.J., Clarke, D., and Barr, R.J. (1993). Diclofenac induced hepatitis. 3 cases with features of autoimmune chronic active hepatitis. *Dig. Dis. Sci.* 38, 744.

Sebastian, D.J., Simon, M.M., and Uribarrena, E.R. (1994). Hepatic and pancreatic injury associated with amineptine therapy. *J. Clin. Gastroenterol.* 18, 168.

Seidman, D.S., Livni, E., Ilie, B., *et al.* (1986). Propylthiouracil-induced cholestatic jaundice. *J. Toxicol. Clin. Toxicol.* 24, 353.

Setchell, K.D.R., Gosselin, S.J., Welsh, M.B., *et al.* (1987). Dietary estrogens — a probable cause of infertility and liver disease in captive cheetahs. *Gastroenterology* 93, 225.

Shah, I.A. and Brandt, H. (1983). Halothane-associated granulomatous hepatitis. *Digestion* 28, 245.

Shapiro, P.A., Antonioli, D.A., and Peppercorn, M.A. (1980). Barbiturate-induced submassive hepatic necrosis. Report of a case and review of the literature. *Am. J. Gastroenterol.* 74, 270.

Shappell, S.B., Taylor, A.A., Hughes, H., *et al.* (1990). Comparison of antioxidant and nonantioxidant lipoxygenase inhibitors on neutrophil function. Implications for pathogenesis of myocardial reperfusion injury. *J. Pharmacol. Exp. Ther.* 252, 531.

Sharp, J.H., Trudell, J.R., and Cohen, E.N. (1979). Volatile metabolites and decomposition products of halothane in man. *Anesthesiology* 50, 2.

Sharp, J.R., Ishak, K.G., and Zimmerman, H.J. (1980). Chronic active hepatitis and severe hepatic necrosis associated with nitrofurantoin. *Ann. Intern. Med.* 92, 14.

Shaw, G.R. and Anderson, W.R. (1991). Multisystem failure and hepatic microvesicular fatty metamorphosis associated with tolmetin ingestion. *Arch. Pathol. Lab. Med.* 115, 818.

Shear, N.H., Spielberg, S.P., Grant, D.M., *et al.* (1986). Differences in metabolism of sulfonamides predisposing to idiosyncratic toxicity. *Ann. Intern. Med.* 105, 179.

Sheikh, K.H. and Nies, A.S. (1983). Trazodone and intrahepatic cholestasis. *Ann. Intern. Med.* 99, 572.

Sheikh, N.M., Philen, R.M., and Love, L.A. (1997). Chaparral-associated hepatotoxicity. *Arch. Intern. Med.* 157, 913.

Shepard, K.V., Levin, B., Karl, R.C., *et al.* (1985). Therapy for metastatic colorectal cancer with hepatic artery infusion chemotherapy using a subcutaneous implanted pump. *J. Clin. Oncol.* 3, 161.

Shergy, W.J., Polisson, R.P., Caldwell, D.S., *et al.* (1988). Methotrexate-associated hepatotoxicity: retrospective analysis of 210 patients with rheumatoid arthritis. *Am. J. Med.* 85, 771.

Sherman, O. and Beizer, J.L. (1994). Possible ciprofloxacin-induced acute cholestatic jaundice. *Ann. Pharmacother.* 28, 1162.

Sheth, S.G., Gordon, F.D., and Chopra, S. (1997). Non-alcoholic steatohepatitis. *Ann. Intern. Med.* 126, 137.

Shimizu, Y., Joho, S., and Watanabe, A. (1994). Hepatic injury after interferon-alpha therapy for chronic hepatitis C. *Ann. Intern. Med.* 121, 723.

Shmunes, E. (1974). Hypervitaminosis A in a patient with alopecia receiving renal dialysis. *Arch. Dermatol.* 115, 882.

Shriner, K. and Goetz, M.B. (1992). Severe hepatotoxicity in a patient receiving both acetaminophen and zidovudine. *Am. J. Med.* 93, 94.

Sigurdsson, J., Hreidarsson, A.B., and Thjodleifsson, B. (1985). Enflurane hepatitis. A report of a case with a previous history of halothane hepatitis. *Acta Anaesthesiol. Scand.* 29, 495.

Sillanpaa, M., Makela, A.L., and Koivikko, A. (1975). Acute liver failure and encephalopathy (Reye's syndrome?) during salicylate therapy. *Acta Paediatr. Scand.* 64, 877.

Silva, M.O., Reddy, K.R., McDonald, T., *et al.* (1989). Danazol-induced cholestasis. *Am. J. Gastroenterol.* 84, 426.

Silva, M.O., Roth, D., Reddy, K.R., *et al.* (1991). Hepatic dysfunction accompanying acute cocaine intoxication. *J. Hepatol.* 12, 312.

Silvain, C., Fort, E., Levillain, P., *et al.* (1992). Granulomatous hepatitis due to combination of amoxicillin and clavulanic acid. *Dig. Dis. Sci.* 37, 150.

Simpson, D.G. and Walker, J.H. (1960). Hypersensitivity to para-aminosalicylic acid. *Am. J. Med.* 29, 297.

Singh, J., Arora, A., Garg, P.K., *et al.* (1995). Antituberculosis treatment-induced hepatotoxicity: role of predictive factors. *Postgrad. Med. J.* 71, 359.

Singh, J., Garg, P.K., and Tandon, R.K. (1996). Hepatotoxicity due to antituberculosis therapy. Clinical profile and reintroduction of therapy. *J. Clin. Gastroenterol.* 22, 211.

Singh, U.K. and Singh, V.K. (1991). Cholestatic jaundice caused by trimethoprim. *Indian J. Pediatr.* 58, 373.

Sinha, A., Clatch, R.J., Stuck, G., *et al.* (1996). Isoflurane hepatotoxicity: a case report and review of the literature. *Am. J. Gastroenterol.* 91, 2406.

Sippel, P.J. and Agger, W.A. (1981). Nitrofurantoin-induced granulomatous hepatitis. *Urology* 18, 177.

Skakun, N.P. and Shman (1986). Effektivnost antioksidantov pri porazhenii pecheni izoniazidom. *Farmakol. Toksikol.* 49, 86.

Slater, T.F. (1984). Free-radical mechanisms in tissue injury. *Biochem. J.* 222, 1.

Smallwood, R.A., Berlin, R.G., Castagnoli, N., *et al.* (1995). Safety of acid-suppressing drugs. *Dig. Dis. Sci.* 40 (Suppl.), 57S.

Smith, C.V., Hughes, H., and Mitchell, J.R. (1984). Free radicals in vivo. Covalent binding to lipids. *Mol. Pharmacol.* 26, 112.

Smith, G.C., Kenna, J.G., Harrison, D.J., *et al.* (1993). Auto-antibodies to hepatic microsomal carboxylesterase in halothane hepatitis. *Lancet* 342, 963.

Smith, M.D. (1986). Hepatitis and neutropenia secondary to gold thiomalate therapy for rheumatoid arthritis. *Aust. N.Z. J. Med.* 16, 72.

Smythe, M.A. and Umstead, G.S. (1989). Phenytoin hepatotoxicity: a review of the literature. *DICP* 23, 13.

Snyder, L.S., Heigh, R.I., and Anderson, M.L. (1993). Cyclophosphamide-induced hepatotoxicity in a patient with Wegener's granulomatosis. *Mayo Clin. Proc.* 68, 1203.

Souza, L.M. (1986). Ranitidine and hepatic injury. *Ann. Intern. Med.* 105, 140.

Spagnuolo, M.I., Iorio, R., Vegnente, A., *et al.* (1996). Urso-deoxycholic acid for treatment of cholestasis in children on long-term total parenteral nutrition: a pilot study. *Gastroenterology* 111, 716.

Spielberg, S.P. (1986). In vitro analysis of idiosyncratic drug reactions. *Clin. Biochem.* 19, 142.

Spielberg, S.P., Gordon, G.B., Blake, D.A., *et al.* (1981). Predisposition to phenytoin hepatotoxicity assessed in vitro. *N. Engl. J. Med.* 305, 722.

Srinivasan, R. and Dean, H.A. (1997). Thorotrast and the liver revisited. *J. Toxicol. Clin. Toxicol.* 35, 199.

Stanko, R.T., Nathan, G., Mendelow, H., *et al.* (1987). Development of hepatic cholestasis and fibrosis in patients with massive loss of intestine supported by parenteral nutrition. *Gastroenterology* 92, 197.

Stanley, P. and Mijch, A. (1986). Methyldopa: an often overlooked cause of fever and transient hepatocellular dysfunction. *Med. J. Aust.* 144, 603.

Steele, M.A., Burk, R.F., and DesPrez, R.M. (1991). Toxic hepatitis with isoniazid and rifampin. A meta-analysis. *Chest* 99, 465.

Steinbrecher, U.P., Lisbona, R., Huang, S.N., *et al.* (1981). Complete regression of hepatocellular adenoma after withdrawal of oral contraceptives. *Dig. Dis. Sci.* 26, 1045.

Sternlieb, P. and Robinson, R.M. (1978). Stevens–Johnson syndrome plus toxic hepatitis due to ibuprofen. *N.Y. State J. Med.* 78, 1239.

Stoelting, R.K., Blitt, C.D., Cohen, P.J., *et al.* (1987). Hepatic dysfunction after isoflurane anesthesia. *Anesth. Analg.* 66, 147.

Stoschus, B., Meybehm, M., Spengler, U., *et al.* (1997). Cholestasis associated with mesalazine therapy in a patient with Crohn's disease. *J. Hepatol.* 26, 425.

Stricker, B.H. and Spoelstra, P. (1985) *Drug-induced Hepatic Injury.* Elsevier, Amsterdam.

Stricker, B.H., Blok, A.P., Bronkhorst, F.B., *et al.* (1986). Ketoconazole-associated hepatic injury. A clinicopathological study of 55 cases. *J. Hepatol.* 3, 399.

Stricker, B.H., Blok, A.P., Babany, G., *et al.* (1989). Fibrin ring granulomas and allopurinol. *Gastroenterology* 96, 1199.

Stromeyer, F.W. and Ishak, K.G. (1997). Nodular transformation (nodular 'regenerative' hyperplasia) of the liver. *Hum. Pathol.* 12, 60.

Stumpf, J.L. (1991). Fatal hepatotoxicity induced by hydralazine or labetalol. *Pharmacotherapy* 11, 415.

Styler, M.J., Crilley, P., Biggs, J., *et al.* (1996). Hepatic dysfunction following busulfan and cyclophosphamide myeloablation: a retrospective, multicenter analysis. *Bone Marrow Transplant.* 18, 171.

Suchy, F.J., Balistreri, W.F., Buchino, J.J., *et al.* (1979). Acute hepatic failure associated with the use of sodium valproate. *N. Engl. J. Med.* 300, 962.

Sugerman, A.A. and Clark, C.G. (1974). Jaundice following the administration of niacin. *JAMA* 228, 202.

Sutherland, D.E. and Smith, W.A. (1992). Chemical hepatitis associated with occupational exposure to halothane in a research laboratory. *Vet. Hum. Toxicol.* 34, 423.

Swank, L.A., Chejfec, G., and Nemchausky, B.A. (1978). Allopurinol-induced granulomatous hepatitis with cholangitis and a sarcoid-like reaction. *Arch. Intern. Med.* 138, 997.

Sweet, J.M. and Jones, M.P. (1995). Intrahepatic cholestasis due to ticarcillin-clavulanate. *Am. J. Gastroenterol.* 90, 675.

Swinburn, B.A., Croxson, M.S., Miller, M.V., *et al.* (1986). Carbamazepine induced granulomatous hepatitis. *N.Z. Med. J.* 99, 167.

Tandon, H.D., Tandon, B.N., and Mattocks, A.R. (1978). An epidemic of veno-occlusive disease of the liver in Afghanistan. Pathologic features. *Am. J. Gastroenterol.* 70, 607.

Tanner, A.R. (1986). Hepatic cholestasis induced by trimethoprim. *BMJ* (Clin. Res. Ed.) 293, 1072.

Tanner, L.A., Bosco, L.A., and Zimmerman, H.J. (1989). Hepatic toxicity after acebutolol therapy. *Ann. Intern. Med.* 111, 533.

Tanphaichitr, V. and Lerdvuthisopon, N. (1981). Urinary carnitine excretion in surgical patients on total parenteral nutrition. *JPEN* 5, 505.

Tao, L.C. (1991). Oral contraceptive-associated liver cell adenoma and hepatocellular carcinoma. Cytomorphology and mechanism of malignant transformation. *Cancer* 68, 341.

Tarazi, E.M., Harter, J.G., Zimmerman, H.J., *et al.* (1993). Sulindac-associated hepatic injury: analysis of 91 cases reported to the Food and Drug Administration. *Gastroenterology* 104, 569.

Taylor, J.W., Stein, M.N., Murphy, M.J., *et al.* (1984). Cholestatic liver dysfunction after long-term phenytoin therapy. *Arch. Neurol.* 41, 500.

Teaf, C.M., Freeman, R.W., and Harbison, R.D. (1984). Cocaine-induced hepatotoxicity: lipid peroxidation as a possible mechanism. *Drug Chem. Toxicol.* 7, 383.

Tedesco, F.J. and Mills, L.R. (1982). Diazepam (Valium) hepatitis. *Dig. Dis. Sci.* 27, 470.

Thaler, H. (1988). Fatty change. *Baillière's Clin. Gastroenterol.* 2, 453.

Themido, R., Loureiro, M., Pecegueiro, M., *et al.* (1992). Methotrexate hepatotoxicity in psoriatic patients submitted to long-term therapy. *Acta Derm. Venereol.* 72, 361.

Thirumoorthy, T. and Shupack, J.L. (1988). Adverse hepatic reactions associated with etretinate in patients with psoriasis — analysis of 22 cases. *Ann. Acad. Med. Singapore* 17, 477.

Thompson, N.P., Caplin, M.E., Hamilton, M.I., *et al.* (1995). Anti-tuberculosis medication and the liver: dangers and recommendations in management. *Eur. Respir. J.* 8, 1384.

Thomson, J.A., Fairley, C.K., Ugoni, A.M., *et al.* (1995). Risk factors for the development of amoxycillin-clavulanic acid associated jaundice. *Med. J. Aust.* 162, 638.

Thummel, K.E., Lee, C.A., Kunze, K.L., *et al.* (1993). Oxidation of acetaminophen to *N*-acetyl-*p*-benzoquinoneimine by human CYP3A4. *Biochem. Pharmacol.* 45, 1563.

Tillmann, H.L., van Pelt, F.N., Martz, W., *et al.* (1997). Accidental intoxication with methylene dianiline p,p′-diaminodiphenylmethane: acute liver damage after presumed ecstasy consumption. *J. Toxicol. Clin. Toxicol.* 35, 35.

Timbrell, J.A., Wright, J.M., and Baillie, T.A. (1978). Monoacetylhydrazine as a metabolite of isoniazid in man. *Clin. Pharmacol. Ther.* 22, 602.

Tisdale, J.E., Follin, S.L., Ordelova, A., *et al.* (1995). Risk factors for the development of specific noncardiovascular adverse effects associated with amiodarone. *J. Clin. Pharmacol.* 35, 351.

Tobias, H. and Auerbach, R. (1973). Hepatotoxicity of long-term methotrexate therapy for psoriasis. *Arch. Intern. Med.* 132, 391.

Todd, P., Levison, D., and Farthing, M.J. (1990). Enalapril-related cholestatic jaundice. *J. R. Soc. Med.* 83, 271.

Toft, E., Vyberg, M., and Therkelsen, K. (1991). Diltiazem-induced granulomatous hepatitis. *Histopathology* 18, 474.

Toghill, P.J., Smith, P.G., Benton, P., *et al.* (1974). Proceedings: Liver damage in patients taking methyldopa. *Gut* 15, 342.

Tolman, K.G., Peterson, P., Gray, P., *et al.* (1978). Hepatotoxicity of salicylates in monolayer cell cultures. *Gastroenterology* 74, 205.

Touraine, R.L., Bertrand, Y., Foray, P., *et al.* (1993). Hepatic tumours during androgen therapy in Fanconi anaemia. *Eur. J. Pediatr.* 152, 691.

Traverse, J.H., Swenson, L.J., and McBride, J.W. (1994). Acute hepatic injury after treatment with diltiazem. *Am. Heart J.* 127, 1636.

Trowell, J., Peto, R., and Smith, A.C. (1975). Controlled trial of repeated halothane anaesthetics in patients with carcinoma of the uterine cervix treated with radium. *Lancet* i, 821.

Trujillo, M.A., Galgiani, J.N., and Sampliner, R.E. (1994). Evaluation of hepatic injury arising during fluconazole therapy. *Arch. Intern. Med.* 154, 102.

Turner, I.B., Eckstein, R.P., Riley, J.W., *et al.* (1989). Prolonged hepatic cholestasis after flucloxacillin therapy. *Med. J. Aust.* 151, 701.

Tygstrup, N. (1978). Clinical aspects of drug-induced hepatitis. *Arch. Toxicol.* Suppl. 125.

Utili, R., Boitnott, J.K., and Zimmerman, H.J. (1977). Dantrolene associated hepatic injury. Incidence and character. *Gastroenterology* 62, 610.

Vale, J.A. and Proudfoot, A.T. (1995). Paracetamol (acetaminophen) poisoning. *Lancet* 346, 547.

Valla, D. and Benhamou, J.P. (1988). Drug-induced vascular and sinusoidal lesions of the liver. *Baillière's Clin. Gastroenterol.* 2, 481.

Valla, D., Lee, M.G., Poynard, T., *et al.* (1986). Risk of hepatic vein thrombosis in relation to recent use of oral contraceptives. A case–control study. *Gastroenterology* 90, 807.

van-Voorst, V.P., Houthoff, H.J., Eggink, H.F., *et al.* (1984). Etretinate (Tigason) hepatitis in 2 patients. *Dermatologica* 168, 41.

Van den Brande, P., Van Steenbergen, W., Vervoort, G., *et al.* (1995). Aging and hepatotoxicity of isoniazid and rifampicin in pulmonary tuberculosis. *Am. J. Respir. Crit. Care Med.* 152, 1705.

van Dooren, G.R., Kuijpers, A.L., Buijs, W.C., *et al.* (1996). The value of dynamic hepatic scintigraphy and serum aminoterminal propeptide of type III procollagen for early detection of methotrexate-induced hepatic damage in psoriasis patients. *Br. J. Dermatol.* 134, 481.

van Dyke, R. (1982). Hepatic centrilobular necrosis in rats after exposure to halothane, enflurane, or isoflurane. *Anesth. Analg.* 61, 812.

van Dyke, R.A. and Gandolfi, A.J. (1974). Studies on irreversible binding of radioactivity from (14C)-halothane to rat hepatic microsomal lipids and protein. *Drug Metab. Dispos.* 2, 469.

van Dyke, R.A. and Wood, C.L. (1975). In vitro studies on irreversible binding of halothane metabolite to microsomes. *Drug Metab. Dispos.* 3, 51.

van Parys, G., Evenepoel, C., Van Damme, B., *et al.* (1987). Ketoconazole-induced hepatitis: a case with a definite cause–effect relationship. *Liver* 7, 27.

Vanderstigel, M., Zafrani, E.S., Lejonc, J.L., *et al.* (1986). Allopurinol hypersensitivity syndrome as a cause of hepatic fibrin ring granulomas. *Gastroenterology* 90, 188.

VanOmmen, R.A. (1974). Untoward effects of antimicrobial agents on major organ systems. *Med. Clin. North Am.* 58, 465.

Vendemiale, G., Altomare, E., Trizio, T., *et al.* (1987). Effect of acute and chronic cimetidine administration on acetaminophen metabolism in humans. *Am. J. Gastroenterol.* 82, 1031.

Vergani, D., Mieli, V.G., Alberti, A., *et al.* (1980). Antibodies to the surface of halothane-altered rabbit hepatocytes in patients with severe halothane-associated hepatitis. *N. Engl. J. Med.* 303, 66.

Verhamme, M., Ramboer, C., van de Bruaene, P., *et al.* (1989). Cholestatic hepatitis due to an amoxycillin/clavulanic acid preparation. *J. Hepatol.* 9, 260.

Vessey, D.A. and Kelley, M. (1995). Inhibition of bile acid conjugation by cyclosporin A. *Biochim. Biophys. Acta* 1242, 49.

Vial, T., Biour, M., Descotes, J., *et al.* (1997). Antibiotic-associated hepatitis: update from 1990. *Ann. Pharmacother.* 31, 204.

Vitug, A.C. and Goldman, J.M. (1985). Hepatotoxicity from antithyroid drugs. *Horm. Res.* 21, 229.

Waetjen, L.E. and Grimes, D.A. (1996). Oral contraceptives and primary liver cancer: temporal trends in three countries. *Obstet. Gynecol.* 88, 945.

Walker, A.M. (1997). Quantitative studies of the risk of serious hepatic injury in persons using nonsteroidal antiinflammatory drugs. *Arthritis Rheum.* 40, 201.

Walker, J.F. (1992). Worldwide experience with simvastatin/lovastatin. *Eur. Heart J.* 13 (Suppl. B), 21.

Walker, R.M., Racz, W.J., and McElligott, T.F. (1980). Acetaminophen-induced hepatotoxicity in mice. *Lab.Invest.* 42, 181.

Walker, R.M., Racz, W.J., and McElligott, T.F. (1983). Scanning electron microscopic examination of acetaminophen-induced hepatotoxicity and congestion in mice. *Am. J. Pathol.* 113, 321.

Walker, R.M., Racz, W.J., and McElligott, T.F. (1985). Acetaminophen induced hepatotoxic congestion in mice. *Hepatology* 5, 233.

Wanless, I.R., Godwin, T.A., Allen, F., *et al.* (1980). Nodular regenerative disorders of the liver in haematologic disorders: a possible response to obliterative portal venopathy. A morphometric study of nine cases with an hypothesis on the pathogenesis. *Medicine (Baltimore)* 59, 367.

Ware, S. and Millward, S.G. (1980). Acute liver disease associated with sodium valproate. *Lancet* ii, 1110.

Watanabe, S., Yamasaki, S., Tanae, A., *et al.* (1994). Three cases of hepatocellular carcinoma among cyproterone users. Ad hoc Committee on Androcur Users. *Lancet* 344, 1567.

Watkins, P.B., Zimmerman, H.J., Knapp, M.J., *et al.* (1994). Hepatotoxic effects of tacrine administration in patients with Alzheimer's disease. *JAMA* 271, 992.

Watson, R.G., Olomu, A., Clements, D., *et al.* (1988). A proposed mechanism for chlorpromazine jaundice — defective hepatic sulphoxidation combined with rapid hydroxylation. *J. Hepatol.* 7, 72.

Weaver, G.A., Pavlinac, D., and Davis, J.S. (1977). Hepatic sensitivity to imipramine. *Dig. Dis.* 22, 551.

Weber, E., Laarbaui, F., Michel, L., *et al.* (1995). Abdominal pain: do not forget Thorotrast! *Postgrad. Med. J.* 71, 367.

Weber, F.L.J., Mitchell, G.E.J., Powell, D.E., *et al.* (1982). Reversible hepatotoxicity associated with hepatic vitamin A accumulation in a protein-deficient patient. *Gastroenterology* 82, 118.

Weiden, P.L. and Buckner, C.D. (1973). Thioridazine toxicity. Agranulocytosis and hepatitis with encephalopathy. *JAMA* 224, 518.

Weill, B.J., Menkes, C.J., Cormier, C., *et al.* (1988). Hepatocellular carcinoma after danazol therapy. *J. Rheumatol.* 15, 1447.

Weinberger, M., Garty, M., Cohen, M., *et al.* (1985). Ultrasonography in the diagnosis and follow up of hepatic sinusoidal dilatation. *Arch. Intern. Med.* 145, 927.

Weinstein, L. and Weinstein, A.J. (1974). The pathophysiology and pathoanatomy of reactions to antimicrobial agents. *Adv. Intern. Med.* 19, 109.

Weiss, V.C., West, D.P., Ackerman, R., *et al.* (1984). Hepatotoxic reactions in a patient treated with etretinate. *Arch. Dermatol.* 120, 104.

Weiss, V.C., Layden, T., Spinowitz, A., *et al.* (1985). Chronic active hepatitis associated with etretinate therapy. *Br. J. Dermatol.* 112, 591.

Westaby, D., Ogle, S.J., Paradinas, F.J., *et al.* (1977). Liver damage from long-term methyltestosterone. *Lancet* ii, 262.

Westaby, D., Portmann, B., and Williams, R. (1983). Androgen related primary hepatic tumors in non-Fanconi patients. *Cancer* 51, 1947.

Westphal, J.F., Vetter, D., and Brogard, J.M. (1994). Hepatic side-effects of antibiotics. *J. Antimicrob. Chemother.* 33, 387.

Whalley, P.J., Martin, F.G., Adams, R.H., *et al.* (1974). Tetracycline toxicity in pregnancy. *JAMA* 189, 357.

Whitcomb, D.C. and Block, G.D. (1994). Association of acetaminophen hepatotoxicity with fasting and ethanol use. *JAMA* 272, 1845.

Whiting, J.F., Green, R.M., Rosenbluth, A.B., *et al.* (1995). Tumor necrosis factor-alpha decreases hepatocyte bile salt uptake and mediates endotoxin-induced cholestasis. *Hepatology* 22, 1273.

Whitington, P.F. and Black, D.D. (1980). Cholelithiasis in premature infants treated with parenteral nutrition and furosemide. *J. Pediatr.* 97, 647.

Wilkinson, S.P., Portmann, B., and Williams, R. (1979). Hepatitis from dantrolene sodium. *Gut* 20, 33.

Williams, G.M., Iatropoulos, M.J., Djordjevic, M.V., *et al.* (1993). The tri-phenylethylene drug tamoxifen is a strong liver carcinogen in the rat. *Carcinogenesis* 14, 315.

Williams, R. (1996). Classification, etiology, and considerations of outcome in acute liver failure. *Semin. Liver Dis.* 16, 343.

Willis, S.M. and Bailey, S.R. (1984). Streptokinase-induced subcapsular hematoma of the liver. *Arch. Intern. Med.* 144, 2084.

Winter, S.L. and Boyer, J.L. (1973). Hepatic toxicity from large doses of vitamin B3 (nicotinamide). *N. Engl. J. Med.* 289, 1180.

Wofsy, C.B. (1987). Use of trimethoprim-sulfamethoxazole in the treatment of *Pneumocystis carinii* pneumonitis in patients with acquired immunodeficiency syndrome. *Rev. Infect. Dis.* 9 (Suppl. 2), S184.

Wogan, G.N. (1997). Review of the toxicology of tamoxifen. *Semin. Oncol.* 24, S1.

Woo, J.K. and Lantz, M.S. (1995). Alzheimer's disease: how to give and monitor tacrine therapy. *Geriatrics* 50, 50.

Wood, P. and Yin, J.A. (1994). Oxymetholone hepatotoxicity enhanced by concomitant use of cyclosporin A in a bone marrow transplant patient. *Clin. Lab. Haematol.* 16, 201.

Woolf, G.M., Petrovic, L.M., Rojter, S.E., *et al.* (1994). Acute hepatitis associated with the Chinese herbal product *jin bu huan*. *Ann. Intern. Med.* 121, 729.

Woolf, T.F., Pool, W.F., Bjorge, S.M., *et al.* (1993). Bioactivation and irreversible binding of the cognition activator tacrine using human and rat liver microsomal preparations: species differences. *Drug Metab. Dispos.* 21, 874.

Worthley, L.I., Fishlock, R.C., and Snoswell, A.M. (1983). Carnitine deficiency with hyperbilirubinemia, generalized skeletal muscle weakness and reactive hypoglycemia in a patient on long-term total parenteral nutrition: treatment with intravenous L-carnitine. *JPEN* 7, 176.

Wright, C., Vafier, J.A., and Lake, C.R. (1988). Disulfiram-induced fulminating hepatitis: guidelines for liver-panel monitoring. *J. Clin. Psychiatry* 49, 430.

Wright, R., Eade, O.E., Chisholm, M., *et al.* (1975). Controlled prospective study of the effect on liver function of multiple exposures to halothane. *Lancet* i, 817.

Wrighton, S.A. and Stevens, J.C. (1992). The human hepatic cytochromes P450 involved in drug metabolism. *Crit. Rev. Toxicol.* 22, 1.

Wu, J.C., Lee, S.D., Yeh, P.F., *et al.* (1990). Isoniazid-

rifampin-induced hepatitis in hepatitis B carriers. *Gastroenterology* 98, 502.

Wysowski, D.K. and Fourcroy, J.L. (1996). Flutamide hepatotoxicity. *J. Urol.* 155, 209.

Yamada, T. (1983). Covalent binding theory for acetaminophen hepatotoxicity. *Gastroenterology* 85, 202.

Yamada, T. and Kaplowitz, N. (1980). Propylthiouracil: a substrate for the glutathione S-transferases that compete with glutathione. *J. Biol. Chem.* 255, 3508.

Yao, F., Behling, C.A., Saab, S., *et al.* (1997). Trimethoprim-sulfamethoxazole-induced vanishing bile duct syndrome. *Am. J. Gastroenterol.* 92, 167.

Yeong, M.L., Swinburn, B., Kennedy, M., *et al.* (1990). Hepatic veno-occlusive disease associated with comfrey ingestion. *J. Gastroenterol. Hepatol.* 5, 211.

Zachariae, H., Kragballe, K., and Sogaard, H. (1980). Methotrexate induced liver cirrhosis. Studies including serial liver biopsies during continued treatment. *Br. J. Dermatol.* 102, 407.

Zachariae, H. and Sogaard, H. (1987). Methotrexate-induced liver cirrhosis. A follow-up. *Dermatologica* 175, 178.

Zachariae, H., Sogaard, H., and Heickendorff, L. (1996). Methotrexate-induced liver cirrhosis. Clinical, histological and serological studies — a further 10-year follow-up. *Dermatology* 192, 343.

Zafrani, E.S., Ishak, K.G., and Rudzki, C. (1979). Cholestatic and hepatocellular injury associated with erythromycin esters: report of nine cases. *Dig. Dis. Sci.* 24, 385.

Zafrani, E.S., Bernuau, J., and Feldman, G. (1984). Peliosis-like ultrastructural changes of the hepatic sinusoids in human chronic hypervitaminosis A: report of three cases. *Hum. Pathol.* 15, 1166.

Zand, R., Nelson, S.D., and Slattery, J.T. (1993). Inhibition and induction of cytochrome P4502E1-catalyzed oxidation by isoniazid in humans. *Clin. Pharmacol. Ther.* 54, 142.

Zimmerman, H.J. (1978a). Drug-induced liver disease. *Drugs* 16, 25.

Zimmerman, H. J. (1978b) *Hepatotoxicity: the Adverse Effects of Drugs and other Chemicals on the Liver.* Appleton Century Crofts, New York.

Zimmerman, H.J. (1981). Effects of aspirin and acetaminophen on the liver. *Arch. Intern. Med.* 141, 333.

Zimmerman, H.J. and Ishak, K.G. (1987). The hepatic injury of monoamine oxidase inhibitors. *J. Clin. Psychopharmacol.* 7, 211.

Zimmerman, H.J. and Maddrey, W.C. (1995). Acetaminophen (paracetamol) hepatotoxicity with regular intake of alcohol: analysis of instances of therapeutic misadventure. *Hepatology* 22, 767.

Zimmerman, H.J., Kendler, J., and Libber, E. (1973). Studies on the in vitro cytotoxicity of erythromycin estolate. *Proc. Soc. Exp. Biol. Med.* 144, 759.

14. Renal disorders

C. R. SWANEPOEL and M. J. D. CASSIDY

Introduction

In health the kidneys receive 25 per cent of the cardiac output. They are able to filter, concentrate, metabolise, and eliminate many different drugs and are particularly vulnerable to drug toxicity. Pacifici and colleagues (1989) provide a review of drug metabolising enzymes in the human kidney. Drug toxicity may occur through a variety of mechanisms, including direct and indirect biochemical effects as well as immunological effects. Pre-existing renal disease will potentiate the effects of renally metabolised and excreted drugs and will necessitate a change in drug dosage to avoid both renal and systemic toxicity; this problem is not addressed in this chapter.

The spectrum of drug-induced renal damage as we will discuss it is tabulated in Table 14.1. Many drugs are capable of causing a variety of renal defects that may occur in isolation or in combination and are thus beyond the confines of artificial tabulation. These drugs are discussed in the sections we think they fit into best; for example, the aminoglycosides are discussed in the section on acute tubular necrosis (ATN), though before producing ATN they cause changes in tubular function. With other drugs such as the non-steroidal anti-inflammatory agents (NSAID) renal damage may take several forms; space is therefore given to these drugs in several sections, that is, in functional renal impairment, glomerulonephritis, and acute interstitial nephritis (AIN). Good reviews of the renal syndromes associated with the use of NSAID are provided by Clive and Stoff (1984) and more recently in an editorial comment by Pugliese and Cinotti (1997). Johnson and colleagues (1994) give a valuable and balanced update, also describing interactions between NSAID and co-prescribed drugs which result in significant adverse effects.

Functional renal impairment

Under this heading we include those drugs that may acutely reduce glomerular filtration rate (GFR) by

TABLE 14.1
The spectrum of drug-induced renal disease

1. Functional renal impairment
   affecting glomerular filtration
   affecting tubular secretion, reabsorption, or
   concentration
2. Acute renal failure
   tubular damage (acute tubular necrosis, osmotic
   nephrosis)
   vascular damage (acute vasculitis, haemolytic–
   uraemic syndrome)
   glomerular damage (rapidly progressive nephritis)
   interstitial damage (acute interstitial nephritis)
   obstruction (acute tubular blockage, retroperitoneal
   fibrosis, ureteric blockage, and acute retention)
3. Glomerulonephritis
   nephrotic syndrome
   lupus nephritis
4. Crystalluria, renal calculi, and calcium nephropathy
5. Chronic interstitial nephritis and papillary necrosis
   (analgesic nephropathy; Chinese herbs nephropathy)
6. Miscellaneous
   haematuria
   incontinence
   drugs affecting tests of renal function

affecting the normal physiological mechanisms controlling glomerular filtration; we will also discuss those drugs that interfere with tubular function but which are not necessarily associated with structural change.

Glomerular effects

The NSAID have little effect on GFR in normal subjects but in salt-depleted patients, in those with congestive cardiac failure or cirrhosis, and in those with pre-existing renal failure GFR may fall significantly (Clive and Stoff 1984; Delaney and Segel 1985; Pugliese and Cinotti 1997). Others at risk include premature infants, patients with systemic lupus erythematosus, and the elderly (Zipser and Henrich 1986). During exercise, in healthy individuals, the ingestion of indomethacin reduces renal blood flow and GFR when compared with controls (Walker *et al.* 1994). Renal failure can be precipitated by the concomitant use of an NSAID and a diuretic (Lynn *et al.* 1985); triamterene appears to be a specific culprit (Weinberg *et al.* 1985) and it should not be used in combination with an NSAID.

The capacity to suppress renal prostaglandins (and thus exert this type of functional effect) varies with different NSAID. This varying adverse-effect profile may be explained on the basis of the NSAID inhibition of two different isoenzymes with cyclo-oxygenase activity, COX-1 (prostaglandin endoperoxide H synthase-1; PGHS-1) and COX-2 (prostaglandin endoperoxide H synthase-2; PGHS-2). For example, those agents which preferentially inhibit the COX-2 enzyme (and in so doing have been defined as having a low COX ratio), will treat inflammation effectively and cause less harm to the stomach and kidneys. Churchill and others (1995) examined the selectivity of the various NSAID against human recombinant COX-2 and COX-1 and noted that diclofenac had a much lower COX ratio (i.e. is less toxic to stomach and kidneys) than indomethacin and ibuprofen. O'Brien (1986) previously reported on the favourable adverse-effect profile of diclofenac. The NSAID with the lowest COX ratio in the Churchill study was meloxicam. Large clinical studies are needed, however, to define the exact therapeutic role of these COX-2 inhibitors (Pugliese and Cinotti 1997).

The commonest adverse effects of NSAID related to the kidney are hyperkalaemia, increased sodium retention, oedema, and a fall in GFR. Patients specifically at risk are diabetics, those with pre-existing renal disease, and patients receiving β-blockers, potassium-sparing diuretics, or angiotensin-converting-enzyme (ACE) inhibitors (Zipser and Henrich 1986; Seelig *et al.* 1990; Matzke and Frye 1997). A combination of dehydration, an NSAID, and an ACE inhibitor is particularly hazardous as the under-perfused glomerulus normally relies on angiotensin II to maintain a pressure gradient across the glomerulus by its constrictor effect on mesangial cells and efferent arterioles (Blythe 1983).

Acute azotaemia may be due to other drugs that may functionally reduce GFR. In an illustrative case described by Reid and Muther (1987), acute oliguria developed in a patient with congestive cardiac failure and pneumonia who was given a nitroprusside infusion; the renal failure was rapidly reversible on tapering and discontinuing the infusion. They postulate a renal 'steal' with preferential dilatation of vascular beds as a cause.

Hypotension and renal impairment of a functional nature have also been described during infusion of atrial natriuretic factor in patients with liver cirrhosis with ascites (Ferrier *et al.* 1989).

The metabolites of the tetracyclines (with the exception of doxycycline which is metabolised by the liver) build up in renal failure and lead to vomiting and dehydration; this is in addition to their antianabolic effect, which causes a rise in blood urea, further aggravates the uraemic state, and can precipitate dialysis in some patients. Rarely, tetracyclines (minocycline) have been associated with interstitial nephritis (Walker *et al.* 1979; Wilkinson *et al.* 1989) and, as mentioned above, demeclocycline can cause nephrogenic diabetes insipidus.

Interleukin 2 may also cause prerenal renal failure (Christiansen *et al.* 1988). By stimulating release of other cytokines, which cause endothelial cells to leak fluid, it can cause hypovolaemia and hypotension; as interleukin 2 also inhibits the release of renal prostaglandins, the normal compensatory mechanism for hypovolaemia is impaired and prerenal renal failure ensues (Hamblin 1990). As expected, the use of indomethacin compounds the problem. The effect on GFR can be partially reversed by noradrenaline (Allaouchiche *et al.* 1990).

The normal physiological mechanisms that autoregulate renal blood flow may be lost in the severely ill patient; in the intensive care unit, where urine output is measured hourly, it is well recognized that drugs which reduce blood pressure often reduce urine flow. With regard to the use of antihypertensive drugs in the clinic, β-blockers cause a mild reduction in GFR (Warren 1976), the relatively cardioselective agents causing less depression than propranolol (Wright *et al.* 1979; Wilkinson 1979, 1982). Clonidine, reserpine, minoxidil, and methyldopa (Pohl *et al.* 1974) have little effect on GFR, and the vasodilator prazosin may improve GFR in some cases, despite lowering blood pressure (Curtis and Bateman 1975). The calcium-channel blocker nifedipine probably has minimal clinical effect on renal function; similarly, nicardipine has no measurable effect on GFR or renal plasma flow but has a potent natriuretic effect (Lee *et al.* 1986). The importance of the control of blood pressure by the use of such agents, especially in chronic renal failure, far outweighs any minor fluctuation in GFR due to a functional effect. The study examining the long-term use of ramipril has shown how important blood pressure control is in reducing both proteinuria and rate of decline of GFR in chronic nephropathy (the GISEN Group 1997). The favourable reduction in both of these parameters, however, exceeded that expected from the degree of blood pressure lowering.

A particular caveat, however, regarding the ACE inhibitors applies in their use in patients with generalized atherosclerosis. Hricik (1985) described 11 patients who developed acute renal failure while taking captopril; common to all was renal artery stenosis bilaterally or in a single kidney. The same has been reported in renal transplant recipients with graft artery stenosis (van der Woude *et al.* 1985). Though renal failure is often reversible after discontinuation of the drug, this is not always the case.

The use of ACE inhibitors also carries a risk; those patients with hypertensive nephrosclerosis without renal artery stenosis (Toto *et al.* 1991). Here the perfusion to the glomeruli is already critically reduced by intra-renal small vessel disease. Reversible renal failure associated with ACE inhibitors has also been reported in patients with polycystic kidney disease (Chapman *et al.* 1991). Diabetics with advanced diabetic nephropathy and severe small-vessel disease also may be prone to rapid renal function deterioration on ACE inhibitors (Duclos *et al.* 1992).

Losartan, an angiotensin II-receptor antagonist, is the first of this new antihypertensive class of agent and has been shown to be efficacious and tolerable (Mallion and Goldberg 1996; Ogihara and Yoshinaga 1996). It has also been provisionally shown to induce renal vasodilatation and to reduce proteinuria (de Zeeuw *et al.* 1995). Long-term studies are needed (Burrell 1997), but already there are reports of the occurrence of acute renal failure in renal transplantation (Ostermann *et al.* 1997) and in the presence of bilateral renal artery stenosis (Holm *et al.* 1996) after treatment with losartan.

Acute azotaemia has also been described in patients with chronic heart failure treated with ACE inhibitors (Packer 1989) or with nifedipine (Eicher *et al.* 1988). Care should also be taken in prescribing potent diuretics to patients with congestive cardiac failure who are also taking captopril, as the natriuresis and fall in blood pressure may tip the balance in an already critically compromised renal perfusion (Hogg and Hillis 1986).

A rapid, reversible, acute renal failure, postulated to be due to functional disturbances, has also been described with amphotericin (Sacks and Fellner 1987). Monteiro and colleagues (1993) studied the effects in dogs by directly injecting Amphotericin B into a renal artery. They were able to show a significant decrease in creatinine clearance due to decrease in renal blood flow.

Tubular effects

Proximal tubular damage may lead to a Fanconi syndrome (the features of which include amino-aciduria,

TABLE 14.2
*Drugs associated with impaired
tubular response to ADH*

Amphotericin
Colchicine
Demeclocycline
Glibenclamide
Ifosfamide
Lithium
Methoxyflurane
Rifampicin
Vinblastine

phosphaturia, glycosuria, and renal tubular acidosis). This can be a feature of heavy metal toxicity. In the acute proximal tubular dysfunction that occurs with lead exposure, inclusion bodies consisting of lead–protein complexes are discernible in proximal tubular cells; toxicity can be reversed by treatment with chelating agents (Goyer 1989). Ingestion of outdated tetracyclines can also produce a Fanconi-type syndrome in addition to a concentrating defect (Mavromatis 1965); the effect has been attributed to the tetracycline degradation products anhydrotetracycline and epianhydrotetracycline (Lowe and Tapp 1966). Another report describes a case of lactic acidosis in association with a Fanconi syndrome after ingestion of tetracycline capsules that had been accidentally soaked, dried out, and stored (Montoliu *et al.* 1981).

Another tetracycline, demeclocycline, can produce a reversible, dose-dependent nephrogenic diabetes insipidus, which has nothing to do with the degradation of the drug; patients taking a high dose for prolonged periods, such as acne sufferers, are particularly at risk. The effect can be put to therapeutic use (in adults only) in the treatment of chronic hyponatraemia due to the syndrome of inappropriate ADH secretion. Treatment needs to be monitored closely to avoid dehydration and prerenal uraemia (Oster and Epstein 1977; Perks *et al.* 1979). This and other drugs that are associated with nephrogenic diabetes insipidus are listed in Table 14.2.

The major renal adverse effect of lithium is a nephrogenic diabetes insipidus (Singer *et al.* 1972; Forrest *et al.* 1974; Singer 1981). It is dose dependent (Penney *et al.* 1981) and vasopressin resistant; animal studies have suggested that the resistance may be related to a decrease in vasopressin-receptor density or a downregulation of the vasopressin-regulated water channel Aquaporin-2 (Marples *et al.* 1995; Hensen *et al.* 1996). It is usually reversible after a reduction in dose or discontinuation of the drug (Walker 1993). Bendz and colleagues (1996), however, were unable to demonstrate reversibility up to 9 weeks after discontinuing the drug in a group of 13 patients who had been on lithium for 18 (range 15–24) years. Bucht and Wahlin (1980) had previously found that recovery of the concentrating defect usually takes place slowly over several months and may be incomplete in those that have taken the drug for years. A mild depression of GFR is not uncommon in some patients; this also tends to correlate with duration of treatment (Wallin *et al.* 1982). Gitlin (1993), however, warned of the progressive deterioration in the GFR of some patients (3.7 per cent of his sample of 82 patients) who had been taking lithium for a decade or more.

The elderly are particularly at risk of toxicity. Mild and clinically unimportant polyuria is common; about half of patients taking lithium will demonstrate a concentrating defect (Wallin *et al.* 1982), but serious toxicity is infrequent provided plasma levels are maintained below about 0.6 mmol per litre. Constant levels are promoted by the use of sustained-release preparations (Wallin and Alling 1979). It is recommended by manufacturers that serum concentrations be measured once weekly until stabilization is achieved, then weekly for one month, and monthly thereafter. Massive diuresis may, however, be unpredictable and occur despite therapeutic levels of the drug; it may be further aggravated by hyperglycaemia (Martinez-Maldonado and Terrell 1973).

Salt and water depletion may precipitate toxicity, as lithium is avidly reabsorbed by the proximal tubule 'by mistake' for sodium. Common causes are diarrhoea and vomiting and stringent dieting; patients taking lithium should be warned of these hazards. The concomitant use of diuretics should also be avoided if possible.

Other drugs that may affect blood levels of lithium include NSAID (in particular indomethacin) and tetracyclines. Lithium is more likely to cause diabetes insipidus if combined with tricyclic antidepressants. It appears that with prolonged use or high doses the renal disorder progresses from a purely functional defect to one with structural changes within distal tubular cells and interstitium. Mitochondrial swelling and dilatation of the cisternae of endoplasmic reticulum progress to cell vacuolation, interstitial fibrosis (Aurell *et al.* 1981; Walker *et al.* 1982), tubular fall-out, and occasionally glomerular sclerosis (Bucht *et al.* 1980).

Lithium may also cause a nephrotic syndrome (Bear *et al.* 1985), usually due to a minimal change lesion and usually remitting on withdrawal of the drug (Alexander and Martin 1981; Singer 1981; Tam *et al.* 1996); it may also rarely be responsible for acute renal failure (Lavender *et al.* 1973) due to acute tubular necrosis. Other uncommon adverse effects of lithium that may have an indirect effect on renal function include hypercalcaemia and hypermagnesaemia; a rise in antinuclear antibodies occasionally occurs.

The anaesthetic gas methoxyflurane affects renal tubular function in several ways, but because it has fallen into disuse it will not be discussed here; interested readers should consult the 4th edition of this book. Enflurane anaesthesia can also cause a mild polyuria.

Rifampicin has also been reported to be associated with a nephrogenic diabetes insipidus but with structural tubulo-interstitial damage (Quinn and Wall 1989).

Potassium retention is caused by certain drugs, used singly or in combination. O'Donnell (1988) specifically mentions the grave risk associated with combining ACE inhibitors with potassium-sparing diuretics. The use of high-dose trimethoprim-sulphamethoxazole for *Pneumocystis carinii* pneumonia has unearthed a potentially life-threatening complication, that of hyperkalaemia (Medina *et al.* 1990; Velazquez *et al.* 1993). The hyperkalaemia has now been shown to be due to an amiloride-like effect, with trimethoprim acting directly on the amiloride-sensitive channels (Chou *et al.* 1995). Hyperkalaemia may develop regardless of dose (Perazella and Mahnensmith 1996). Alappan and colleagues (1996) examined the effect of standard doses of trimethoprim-sulphamethoxazole on potassium levels in a group of hospitalized patients. They showed prospectively that over half (62.5 per cent) of patients developed a peak serum potassium concentration of over 5 mmol per litre or greater, and in just under a quarter (21.2 per cent) serum potassium peaked at 5.5 mmol per litre or greater. Renal insufficiency was a risk factor for the development of hyperkalaemia.

Trimethoprim also competitively inhibits the tubular secretion of creatinine (Berglund *et al.* 1975). This effect is only clinically relevant when the GFR is low. Chertow and colleagues (1996) described the development of hypouricaemia with high-dose trimethoprim–sulphamethoxazole used to treat patients with *Pneumocystis carinii* pneumonia. The authors hypothesize that the effect is due to the structural relationship between sulphamethoxazole and probenecid.

Acute renal failure

Acute tubular necrosis

Tubular damage is inevitable with some drugs and develops *pari passu* with their beneficial effect. Examples are amphotericin, cisplatin, and the aminoglycosides; their efficacy in treating specific diseases, however, often precludes the substitution of alternatives and dictates their use. Acute tubular necrosis is characteristically polyuric with some of these drugs (e.g. aminoglycosides), though it can be oliguric. In the single nephron model activation of tubuloglomerular feedback mechanisms best explain the reduction in GFR in nephrotoxic forms of tubular injury (Peterson *et al.* 1989).

Amphotericin increases permeability of tubular cell membranes, and toxicity presents with hypokalaemia, hypomagnesaemia, impaired concentrating ability, and distal renal tubular acidosis. This is followed by a reduction in GFR and non-oliguric acute renal failure. Dehydration should be avoided at all costs; mannitol and sodium bicarbonate infusions may reduce toxicity, and a recent open prospective study evaluating the usefulness of sodium chloride loading to prevent toxicity showed it to be highly successful (Arning and Scharf 1989). The incorporation of amphotericin into liposomes (liposomal amphotericin) significantly reduces renal toxicity (Meunier *et al.* 1991). In addition, reduction in dose and frequency of administration may contain the problem. When toxicity does occur the effects are not always reversible (Butler 1964) and nephrocalcinosis may develop later (Bhathena *et al.* 1978), though it rarely occurs nowadays.

Aminoglycoside antibiotics cause transient renal failure in up to 10–30 per cent of patients and are the cause of the largest proportion of acute drug-induced nephrotoxicity (Tulkens 1989). Typically, non-oliguric renal failure manifests about a week after treatment has started, is seldom severe enough to require dialysis, and is usually reversible, though recovery may be slow. Gentamicin is the most frequent offender, probably because of its regular use and efficacy.

An important caveat in drawing analogies from animal data to man and, indeed, in comparing different animal studies, is illustrated by the aminoglycosides: for example, in the dog, gentamicin is nephrotoxic at two to three times the therapeutic dose, whereas, in the rat, up to 60 times the therapeutic dose may be tolerated (Falco *et al.* 1969); in addition, Fischer Wistar rats appear more susceptible to toxicity than do Sprague-Dawley rats (Soberon *et al.* 1979).

Data from humans and animals indicate that aminoglycoside toxicity is directed predominantly against proximal tubular cells; the drug is concentrated in the renal cortex (Luft *et al.* 1977) and is taken up by proximal tubular cells. In rats and humans there is increased urinary excretion of proximal tubular enzymes before other noticeable changes in renal function; histological damage is initially only seen in proximal tubular cells; and electron microprobe analysis of non-necrotic proximal tubular cells demonstrates abnormalities in electrolyte concentrations not present in the distal tubules (Matsuda *et al.* 1988). Once taken up by the cells, gentamicin remains in a poorly exchangeable pool with tissue half-life of over 100 times that of blood. After binding to the proximal tubular membrane, it is incorporated into the cell in microvesicles and sequenced in lysosomes (an increased number of secondary lysosomes is a characteristic early sign of toxicity); subsequent lysosomal phospholipidosis results in cell death. Therefore their toxicity results from their capacity to interact electrostatically with and disrupt the metabolism of anionic phospholipids (Kaloyanides 1994). There are various other alterations in the structure and function of subcellular components; for example, gentamicin enhances renal cortical mitochondrial generation of reactive oxygen metabolites *in vitro* (Walker and Shah 1988).

Polyaspartic acid, a polyanionic acid, protects against nephrotoxicity of aminoglycosides by complexing with them and preventing their interaction with their intracellular targets (Kaloyanides 1994). A reduction in the risk of developing nephrotoxicity may be possible by an analysis of the patient and drug-related risk factors that have been reported. Excessive dose, or excessive duration of treatment, or both, are clearly the most important factors. The former is probably responsible for the increased frequency of toxicity in the elderly, in whom allowances for a reduced creatinine clearance in the presence of a normal serum creatinine may not be made in calculating dosage. Excessive dose is not the only factor; long-term subtherapeutic doses of gentamicin maintaining the serum aminoglycoside levels below the accepted therapeutic range for 6 months may produce renal failure in rats (Houghton *et al.* 1988). The uptake of aminoglycosides by the kidney is also saturable; thus multiple injections or a continuous infusion may increase the risk of toxicity. Monitoring several trough and peak levels may predict toxicity (Moore *et al.* 1984; Contreras *et al.* 1989). Increasingly aminoglycosides are being given once a day, and in the last 2 years five meta-analyses and one review (Blasel and Konig 1995) have been published indicating that once-daily dosing is as effective as, and no more toxic than, multiple dosing regimens (*Drug and Therapeutics Bulletin* 1997).

Risk factors have been examined by Moore and others (1984), who found nephrotoxicity to be more common, with higher trough and peak levels, in women, and in patients with higher creatinine clearance and those with liver disease. The last observation confirmed data from Cabrera and colleagues (1982), who recognized an increased incidence of aminoglycoside toxicity in patients with advanced cirrhosis, and agrees with experimental evidence that gentamicin toxicity is enhanced after biliary obstruction in rats (Lucena *et al.* 1989).

The concomitant use of other drugs may augment or decrease the risk of toxicity. Animal models have shown that aminoglycoside toxicity may be augmented by protamine (Saito *et al.* 1987), diltiazem (Gomez *et al.* 1989), hydrocortisone (Beauchamp and Pettigrew 1988), potassium depletion, captopril (Klotman *et al.* 1985), and volume depletion (Bennett *et al.* 1976); and it is ameliorated by a higher protein diet (Andrews and Bates 1987), oxygen radical scavengers (Walker and Shah 1988), bicarbonate, and acetazolamide (Aynedjian *et al.* 1988), magnesium supplements (Wong *et al.* 1989), calcium and thyroxine (Ernest 1989), and experimentally induced diabetes mellitus (Teixeria *et al.* 1982). Whether any of these factors are important in humans remains to be established. Drugs that have been associated with increased toxicity in humans include: frusemide, methoxyflurane, cisplatin, amphotericin, clindamycin, cephaloridine, and cephalothin.

The aminoglycoside prescribed is also important; unfortunately, evaluation of comparative nephrotoxicity in humans from the literature is hampered by lack of consistent definition of toxicity, randomization of patients, and satisfactory control groups, and a paucity of double-blind studies. There is little to choose between tobramycin and gentamicin (Kahlmeter and Dahlager 1984; Moore *et al.* 1984), though Smith and colleagues (1980) have found tobramycin to be slightly less nephrotoxic. The toxicity of amikacin may be less still, but again the advantage is probably minimal (Holm *et al.* 1983), and there is little difference between tobramycin and netilmicin (Lerner *et al.* 1983). Netilmicin is associated with less cochlear and vestibular toxicity (Kahlmeter and Dahlager 1984; see also Chapter 22). When it comes to the choice of an aminoglycoside for the treatment of a Gram-negative infection, the evidence for one being less nephrotoxic than another is overshadowed by the results of culture and sensitivity of the organism, when available, and local unit policy in trying to reduce bacterial resistance. Some studies have suggested that newer agents such as the third-generation cephalosporins and aztreonam may be as effective therapeutically as aminoglycosides but with less risk of toxicity (Appel 1990).

Considering the other aminoglycosides, neomycin is far more nephrotoxic than any other aminoglycoside, though as it is only given orally or topically little is absorbed; in chronic renal failure, however, accumulation may occur and renal damage has been described with oral therapy (De Beukelaer *et al.* 1971). Slight proteinuria is common with streptomycin but renal failure is rare (McDermott 1947). Similarly, kanamycin, though frequently producing changes in urine sediment and proteinuria, seldom gives rise to renal failure except when given in doses above the therapeutic range or to patients with impaired renal function (Falco *et al.* 1969).

Other drugs that can cause acute tubular necrosis include some cytotoxic agents, of which cisplatin is the chief offender. Used mainly in the treatment of testicular and ovarian tumours, it was nearly abandoned after Phase 1 trials, because of severe gastrointestinal and renal adverse effects. It was subsequently demonstrated that its nephrotoxicity could be markedly reduced by keeping patients well hydrated before, during, and after its administration (Hayes *et al.* 1977); the risk of nephrotoxicity may also be minimized by administering the drug in three divided doses daily (Donadio *et al.* 1996). Chemotherapy emesis may exacerbate the nephrotoxicity (Cantwell *et al.* 1989), presumably by dehydration, but nausea and vomiting may be effectively controlled by administration of the selective antagonist to serotonin S_3 receptors ondansetron (Cubeddu *et al.* 1990). This is more effective than high-dose metoclopramide (Marty *et al.* 1990).

The principal route of excretion of cisplatin is via the kidney, and accumulation occurs in the cortex. A decrease in renal plasma flow and increase in urinary enzymes is observed very early on in treatment, and hypomagnesaemia, hypocalcaemia, and hypokalaemia commonly occur (Fillastre and Raguenez-Viotte 1989).

The mechanism of toxicity remains unclear but it has been extensively investigated in rats. Certainly, the reduced GFR early on in renal failure due to cisplatin in rats results from reversible changes in renal blood flow and renal vascular resistance (Winston and Safirstein 1985). With 8 mg per kg administered intraperitoneally, damage to proximal, distal, and collecting tubules occurs in association with increased cell proliferation and DNA synthesis, and appearance of fibroblasts in the interstitium (Laurent *et al.* 1988); changes are more severe in the P3 segment of the proximal tubule (Jones *et al.* 1985). With a lower dose (5.5 mg per kg), reversible changes in renal function are accompanied by reversible changes in mitochondrial respiration and calcium accumulation (Gordon and Gattone 1986). In dogs and rats, acute proximal tubular changes precede any alterations in renal haemodynamics (Daugaard 1990).

In rats, protection against toxicity has been demonstrated with the free-radical scavenger o-(β-hydroxyethyl)-rutoside (Dobyan *et al.* 1986) and the calcium-channel blocker nifedipine (Deray *et al.* 1988). In patients given intrapleural or intraperitoneal cisplatin, intravenous thiosulphate has afforded clinically significant protection in some (Markman *et al.* 1985) and a phosphorylated sulphydryl compound, ethiofos, originally developed as a radioprotective agent, may protect the kidneys from toxicity (Mollman 1990). The ACTH (4-9) analogue Org 2766, which significantly prevents or attenuates cisplatin neuropathy, does not appear to affect renal toxicity (Gerritsen van der Hoop *et al.* 1990). Another way to avoid cisplatin toxicity would be to use carboplatin, which appears to have similar antineoplastic effects but fewer adverse effects (Fillastre and Raguenez-Viotte 1989). Acute tubular necrosis has also occurred with the use of the platinum compound TNO-6 (1,1-diaminomethyl cyclohexane sulphato platinum II) (Offerman *et al.* 1985).

Heavy metals may produce acute tubular necrosis or membranous glomerulonephritis (see below). In rats, mercury given intravenously accumulates in the proximal tubular cells of the kidney, preferentially in the S2 and S3 segments within lysosomes (Hultman and Enestrom 1986). The organic mercurial merthiolate has produced fatal acute tubular necrosis on a number of occasions when added in excess as a preservative for drugs given intramuscularly (Axton 1972).

Acute renal failure has also resulted from the absorption of copper sulphate (Holtzman *et al.* 1966) and boric acid (Baliah *et al.* 1969) from skin dressings, and from bismuth thiosulphate given intradermally for warts (Randall *et al.* 1972). Acute renal failure has been reported from Japan in a long-term user of a germanium preparation taken as an elixir. Postmortem examination of the kidney showed acute tubular necrosis, mild proliferation of mesangial matrix, foamy transformation of glomerular epithelial cells, red blood cell casts, and urate crystal deposition (Nagata *et al.* 1985). Chronic renal failure is a more common complication of germanium oxide; a characteristic clinical feature is the absence of proteinuria and haematuria. After discontinuation of the germanium, slow recovery may occur (Sanai *et al.* 1990).

Acute tubular necrosis can occur following paracetamol poisoning. Though usually complicating severe hepatic failure (Wilkinson *et al.* 1974), it may occur without hepatic failure (Pillans and Hall 1985; Davenport and Finn 1988), and perhaps even after therapeutic doses in a few individuals (Gabriel *et al.* 1982); alcoholics are particularly susceptible (Kaysen *et al.* 1985; Keaton 1988). Renal and hepatic damage is prevented by the early administration of *N*-acetylcysteine (Prescott *et al.* 1979). The azotaemia of paracetamol toxicity is typically reversible but may worsen over 7 to 10 days before improving (Blakely and McDonald 1995).

Osmotic nephrosis

Swelling and vacuolation of tubular cells can develop during and after filtration of mannitol and low-molecular-weight dextrans, though these histological changes may not be associated with alterations in tubular function (Engberg 1976). Whether or not the histological changes imply tubular damage has been disputed (Ericsson *et al.* 1967), and the exact mechanism whereby nephrotoxicity occurs is unclear. The patient with acute renal insufficiency associated with dextran-40 reported by Moran and Kapsner (1987), which was rapidly reversed by plasmapheresis argues the case for a hyper-oncotic state where oncotic forces equal or exceed the hydraulic forces that determine GFR.

Mannitol is used predominantly to reduce cerebral oedema, to reduce intraocular pressure in glaucoma, and as a prophylactic agent in the prevention of acute renal failure. Nephrotoxicity is more likely to occur when the cumulative dose is high and there is chronic renal failure; diuretics may also have an additive effect (Horgan *et al.* 1989). The syndrome of mannitol toxicity is clinically manifested by intravascular fluid overload, hyponatraemia with a raised osmolar gap, and confusion as a result of its potent osmotic effect on the brain (Horgan *et al.* 1989; Rello *et al.* 1989).

Though bizarre swelling of proximal tubular cells obliterating the lumen of the nephron has been described in patients developing acute renal failure after receiving dextran-40, many other reasons for developing renal failure were usually present (Morgan *et al.* 1966; Mailloux *et al.* 1967). There are cases reported, however, in which no other cause of acute tubular necrosis was present (Fournier *et al.* 1969). More recently, the gelatin solution Gelofusine has been implicated in the development of renal failure (Hussain and Drew 1989), though other reasons for developing renal failure were present in the patient described. Hyperosmolality related to propylene glycol in an infant treated with enoximone infusion has also been reported (Huggon *et al.* 1990).

Vascular damage

Cyclosporin

Cyclosporin, a drug which has a huge beneficial impact in treating patients with solid organ transplants, unfortunately has a number of adverse effects including nephrotoxicity. The improved pharmacokinetic characteristics of the micro-emulsion formulation of cyclosporin have led to a reduction in inter-individual and intra-individual variation in absorption and bioavailability of cyclosporin and made it easier to use, but no significant differences in adverse events have been reported in liver transplant recipients followed for a year (Grant *et al.* 1996) or in renal transplant recipients

(Pescovitz *et al.* 1997) followed for 2 years. The renal side effects are predominantly non-immunological and dose dependent and may take several different forms: we have divided toxicity initially into two major groups:

1. functional toxicity with minimal or no morphological change;
2. morphological forms of toxicity, which can be further subdivided clinically into acute, subacute, and chronic toxicity; and which morphologically include tubular, vascular, and interstitial change.

Functional toxicity of cyclosporin

Prospective serial renal function tests in patients treated with cyclosporin without renal disease show a sharp reduction in glomerular filtration and effective renal plasma flow, but without a change in filtration fraction, within the first week of treatment (Tegzess *et al.* 1988). This has been demonstrated non-invasively using engymetric radioisotope studies (Nowack *et al.* 1988). This functional disturbance is presumably due to intrarenal haemodynamic changes for which there may be several initiating mechanisms. There are several hypotheses, concerning the renal vasoconstrictive effects of cyclosporin which are probably not mutually exclusive.

First, and most likely, cyclosporin interacts with the kallikrein–prostaglandin humoral system. Arguments for this include the changes that occur in the normal balance of arachidonic acid metabolites. Thromboxane A_2 (a powerful vasoconstrictor) synthesis is augmented by cyclosporin in rats (Coffman *et al.* 1987) and thromboxane A_2 inhibitors attenuate the nephrotoxicity; in addition urinary kallikrein excretion is reduced in humans receiving cyclosporin (Spragg *et al.* 1988). In other animal models, however, treatment with a prostaglandin synthesis inhibitor (indomethacin) did not affect the renal response to cyclosporin, suggesting that prostaglandins may not play an important role in the functional haemodynamics of the renal toxicity (Barros *et al.* 1987).

Secondly, does the renin–angiotensin system play a role in these changes? Activation of the renin–angiotensin system in many disease states stimulates glomerular synthesis of prostacyclin and prostaglandin E_2, their vasodilator properties normally offset the vasoconstrictor effects of angiotensin II; this protective mechanism is lost in cyclosporin-treated animals (Perico *et al.* 1986). There is evidence from *in vivo* and *in vitro* animal experiments that there is activation of this humoral system and elevated plasma renin activity (PRA) but a variable response to captopril when it was used (Baxter *et al.* 1984; Murray *et al.* 1985; Dieperink *et al.* 1986; Barros *et al.* 1987; Kurtz *et al.* 1988). Not all agree, however: Gerkens and Smith (1985) were unable to

detect changes in PRA in rats given cyclosporin and Whitworth and colleagues (1987) showed no rise in sheep given cyclosporin. Others have found that the secretion of, and response to, renin–angiotensin is normal.

Thirdly, cyclosporin has been shown to enhance the release of intracellular free calcium from vascular smooth muscle and mesangial cells (Goldberg *et al.* 1989). A consequence of this may be an exaggerated contractile response by these cells to other stimuli, resulting in a reduction in renal blood flow and glomerular ultrafiltration. Calcium-channel blockers have been shown to exert a protective effect in rats (Barros *et al.* 1987) and may have similar effects in humans (Wagner *et al.* 1987).

Cyclosporin has a direct sympathomimetic effect when infused into conscious rats (Murray *et al.* 1985), but as a renal allograft is denervated this is probably not relevant clinically. Effects mediated through effects on endothelin (Takeda *et al.* 1992) and nitric oxide (NO) have also been implicated (De Nicola *et al.* 1993) and in experimental rats both L-arginine and allopurinol have been shown to protect against cyclosporin nephrotoxicity (Assis *et al.* 1997) adding weight to the probable involvement of NO in this form of haemodynamic toxicity.

Finally, Kahan speculates that there may be a unifying hypothesis linking renal vasoconstriction with the immunosuppressive effects of cyclosporin, through inhibition of gene transcription of proteins concerned with normal vascular tone (Kahan 1989).

In patients with renal transplants, cyclosporin nephrotoxicity may have an additive effect to ischaemic injury in the kidney; this has been demonstrated in the rat (Chow *et al.* 1986; Jablonski *et al.* 1986; Kanazi *et al.* 1986) and may be the reason for the higher incidence of delayed function in human renal allograft recipients treated with cyclosporin (Sheil *et al.* 1983; Hall *et al.* 1985).

In some patients, toxicity is associated with hyperkalaemia that has been attributed to hypoaldosteronism, the additional use of β-blockers to treat hypertension, and a tubular defect of potassium secretion (Adu *et al.* 1983; Petersen *et al.* 1984).

Toxicity of cyclosporin with morphological changes

Acute toxicity may be due to an extension of functional change in that it is commonly seen in renal allografts when the allograft has been harvested under adverse conditions and renal ischaemia is already present. Less commonly, a thrombotic glomerular microangiopathy that clinically and histologically resembles the haemolytic–uraemic syndrome is found (Muirhead *et al.* 1987; Pahl *et al.* 1988). The aetiology of this drug reaction remains speculative; *in vitro* experiments suggest that cyclosporin is directly toxic to endothelial cells (Zoja *et al.* 1986) — a suggestion strengthened by *in vivo* animal (Benigni *et al.* 1988) and patient (Zaal *et al.* 1988) data — and endothelial damage may precipitate the acute angiopathy (Remuzzi and Bertani 1989). This particular complication has been successfully treated by withdrawing cyclosporin and giving intra-arterial streptokinase (Muirhead *et al.* 1987) and FK506 (McCauley *et al.* 1989).

Subacute nephrotoxicity develops between weeks 1–8 of therapy and in the renal transplant patient is suggested by a rising creatinine without signs of graft rejection. Blood levels of cyclosporin are often high but not always so (Holt *et al.* 1986) and the toxicity is usually promptly reversible if the dose of cyclosporin is reduced. Renal biopsy and fine needle aspiration are valuable not so much in the diagnosis of cyclosporin toxicity (no morphological changes are diagnostic, though characteristic features are proximal tubular cell giant mitochondria, vacuolization, and microcalcification [Mihatsch *et al.* 1988*a*]) as in excluding rejection as a cause for deteriorating renal function. The intratubular microcalcification may be related to the reduction in concentration of the calcium-binding protein, calbindin, which has been shown to occur in the kidneys of rats treated with cyclosporin (Aicher *et al.* 1997).

Chronic nephrotoxicity occurs after a longer period of use, usually after one year; it may cause irreversible renal damage in heart transplant recipients (Myers *et al.* 1988). Goldstein and colleagues (1997) recently reviewed their first 9 years' experience with cyclosporin after cardiac transplantation and, disturbingly, report that over a third of 293 patients followed up developed a reduction in creatinine clearance by 6 months and 19 (6.5 per cent) progressed to end-stage renal failure requiring haemodialysis. In patients with autoimmune uveitis treated with cyclosporin, a 50 per cent increase in serum creatinine was observed in 37 per cent of 73 patients (Austin *et al.* 1989). Though the elevation in serum creatinine was rapidly reversed by a reduction in dosage of withdrawal of the drug, after 3 months of treatment renal parenchymal injury did progress in a few patients, despite stable renal function and dose reduction (Austin *et al.* 1989). A vascular basis for this type of toxicity is likely in view of increased renal resistance and hypertension that may precede a serum creatinine rise, illustrated in a patient being treated for chronic inflammatory demyelinating polyradiculopathy (Kolkin *et al.* 1987), and the prominent renal arteriolar changes seen in the biopsies of the patients studied by Austin and colleagues (1989).

Renal histology characteristically shows interstitial striped fibrosis, possibly as a result of tubular loss due to afferent arteriolar vasoconstriction (Palestine *et al.* 1986; Remuzzi and Bertani 1989).

Acute cyclosporin nephrotoxicity has not emerged as a specific risk factor for the development of chronic toxicity in some studies (Greenberg *et al.* 1987) but has in others (Mihatsch *et al.* 1988*b*). Other risk factors for the development of chronic toxicity include high blood trough levels, concomitant use of nephrotoxic drugs, more frequent rejection episodes, and poor primary renal function (Mihatsch *et al.* 1998*b*).

Various drugs can interfere with the metabolism and action of cyclosporin and these are listed in Table 14.3. The nephrotoxicity of endotoxin may also be potentiated by cyclosporin (Cosio *et al.* 1987).

TABLE 14.3
Drugs affecting cyclosporin toxicity

Enhancing toxicity

Aciclovir	additive toxicity	Bennett and Pulliam 1983
Aminoglycosides	additive toxicity	Hows *et al.* 1983
Amphotericin	additive toxicity	Kennedy *et al.* 1983
Ciprofloxacin	additive toxicity	Avent *et al.* 1988
Clarithromycin	additive toxicity	Spicer *et al.* 1997
Clonidine	additive toxicity	Gilbert *et al.* 1995
Colchicine	additive toxicity	Menta *et al.* 1987
Co-trimoxazole	additive toxicity	Thompson *et al.* 1983
Corticosteroids	increase levels	Cockburn 1986
Danazol	increases levels	Passfall *et al.* 1994
Diclofenac	additive toxicity	Deray *et al.* 1987
Diltiazem	increases levels	Wagner *et al.* 1986
Erythromycin	increases levels	Grino *et al.* 1986
Ethanol	increases levels	Paul *et al.* 1987
Frusemide	additive toxicity	Whiting *et al.* 1984
Ketoconazole	increases levels	Dieperink and Moller 1982
Melphalan	additive toxicity	Dale *et al.* 1985
NSAID	additive toxicity	Harris *et al.* 1988

Inhibiting toxicity (and efficacy if reducing blood levels)

Carbamazepine	reduces levels	Lele *et al.* 1985
Dopamine	inhibits toxicity	Kho *et al.* 1987
Enalapril	?inhibits toxicity	McAuley *et al.* 1987
Ethambutol	reduces levels	Leimenstoll *et al.* 1988
Fosfomycin	inhibits toxicity	Sack *et al.* 1987
Imipenem	reduces levels	Mraz *et al.* 1987
Isoniazid	reduces levels	Langhoff and Madsen 1983
Metoprolol	reduces levels	Chan 1986
Nafcillin	reduces levels	Veremis *et al.* 1987
Phenobarbitone	reduces levels	Carstenen *et al.* 1986
Phenytoin	reduces levels	Freeman *et al.* 1984
Prostaglandins	inhibit toxicity	Makowka *et al.* 1986
Rifampicin	reduces levels	Cassidy *et al.* 1985
Spironolactone	?inhibits toxicity	McAuley *et al.* 1987
Warfarin	reduces levels	Snyder 1988

Tacrolimus

Tacrolimus (FK506) has now been used for several years in solid organ transplantation; its effectiveness following liver transplantation is well established and it is also more effective than cyclosporin in preventing acute rejection in cadaveric renal allograft recipients (Pirsch *et al.* 1997). The adverse-effect profile of tacrolimus is also well established; though hyperlipidaemia does not occur as it does with cyclosporin, and hirsutism, gum hypertrophy, and gingivitis are far less frequent, the frequency of nephrotoxicity and hypertension is the same (Woodle *et al.* 1996; Pirsch *et al.* 1997). Neurological adverse effects and post-transplant diabetes mellitus, however, are more frequently associated with the use of tacrolimus. As with cyclosporin, nephrotoxicity is dose dependent (Katari *et al.* 1997). Whole blood levels should be monitored and kept within the therapeutic range (5–15 ng per ml). Nephrotoxicity results in tubular atrophy and fibrosis which is worse if the animals are salt depleted (Stillman *et al.* 1995; Andoh *et al.* 1995). Metabolism is via the cytochrome P-450 3A enzyme system and there a number of clinically significant drug interactions which are similar to those seen with cyclosporin (Mignat 1997).

Other drugs causing vascular damage

Chronic glomerular microangiopathy may complicate metastatic carcinoma particularly when the latter is treated with mitomycin (Hostetter *et al.* 1987; Jain and Seymour 1987; Verweij *et al.* 1987a; Mergenthaler *et al.* 1988). In a carefully monitored study of 44 patients treated with mitomycin, of whom 37 were evaluated, one patient developed a lethal haemolytic–uraemic syndrome after a high dose of mitomycin; the adverse effect was not predictable, but based on this case and a review of the literature the authors concluded that renal toxicity was a dose-dependent adverse effect (Verweij *et al.* 1987b). Plasmapheresis and antiplatelet agents have been used in its treatment (Murgo 1987).

The use of oral contraceptives (Brown *et al.* 1973) and of metronidazole in children (Powell *et al.* 1988) have been implicated as causes of a haemolytic–uraemic syndrome. Postpartum renal failure associated with red cell fragmentation and arteriolar thrombosis may be caused by ergometrine (Robson *et al.* 1968; Williams and Hughes 1974).

Hypersensitivity angiitis due to thiazide diuretics may be associated with renal involvement (Björnberg and Gisslen 1965), though cutaneous vasculitis is much more common. Angiitis has also been attributed to sulphonamides (Berlyne 1972). Other drugs that have induced a granulomatous necrotizing angiitis include allopurinol (Jarzobski *et al.* 1970), carbamazepine (Imai *et al.*

1989), glibenclamide (Clarke *et al.* 1974), phenytoin (Yermakov *et al.* 1983; Gaffey *et al.* 1986), and quinidine (Quin *et al.* 1988). Skin eruption and eosinophilia are consistently found in addition to renal failure. The prognosis is generally poor, but in the case reported by Quin and colleagues (1988) there was a prompt response to prednisone. Fatal renal vasculitis and minimal change glomerulonephritis have also complicated treatment with penicillamine (Falck *et al.* 1979).

Use of streptokinase has been associated with proteinuria and haematuria of glomerular origin (Argent and Adams 1990) and a serum sickness type reaction with vasculitis (Payne *et al.* 1989; Callan *et al.* 1990). Another thrombolytic agent, anistreplase (anisoylated plasminogen–streptokinase complex), has also been reported to cause a vasculitis (Ali *et al.* 1990).

The use of horse sera (De La Pava *et al.* 1962) and vaccines (Bishop *et al.* 1966) has also been described as causing an immune-complex nephritis and vasculitis. The abuse of amphetamines has also been associated with a classical polyarteritis-like syndrome (Citron *et al.* 1970; Bennett *et al.* 1977) and piroxicam has caused a Henoch–Schönlein syndrome with nephritis (Goebel and Mueller-Brodmann 1982).

Glomerular damage

Drug-induced glomerular damage resulting in a rapidly progressive glomerulonephritis is a rare cause of acute renal failure. More common are milder forms of nephritis, such as membranous glomerulonephritis and lupus nephritis, which are discussed later on in the chapter.

Devogelaer and co-workers (1987) provided a review of the literature as well as reporting a case of penicillamine-induced crescentic nephritis, and showed that treatment with withdrawal of the drug and immunosuppression is effective. Circulating antiglomerular basement membrane antibodies (Peces *et al.* 1987) and antimyeloperoxidase antibodies (Gaskin *et al.* 1995) have been demonstrated in similar cases. Glue-sniffing has also been reported to cause Goodpasture's syndrome (Bonzel *et al.* 1987) and mesangiocapillary glomerulonephritis (Venkataraman 1981), as have other solvents (Bernis *et al.* 1985; Lauwerys *et al.* 1985); a proliferative glomerulonephritis with linear IgG deposition along glomerular capillary walls has occurred after exposure to paraquat (Stratta *et al.* 1988).

Rapidly progressive crescentic glomerulonephritis of the non-Goodpasture's type has been described with rifampicin (Murray *et al.* 1987) and hydralazine (Björck *et al.* 1983). We have treated two patients with systemic vasculitis, crescentic nephritis, and perinuclear cytoplasmic antibodies (p-ANCA) in which the antibody is directed against cytoplasmic myeloperoxidase related to penicillamine (Gaskin *et al.* 1995) and hydralazine. The autoantibodies in hydralazine-associated perinuclear ANCA vasculitis are directed against myeloperoxidase and lactoferrin (Short and Lockwood 1995). Crescentic nephritis has also been described in a patient taking enalapril (Bailey and Lynn 1986).

Interstitial damage

Tubulointerstitial disease may occur as a component of nephritis where the primary insult is directed towards the glomerulus, such as in glomerulonephritis or systemic lupus erythematosus; or where the primary insult is vascular, as in vasculitis or the haemolytic–uraemic syndrome. It may also be the primary site of damage either through a direct dose-dependent toxicity (e.g. due to amphotericin) or as a result of a hypersensitivity reaction. The immunoallergic reactions causing interstitial nephritis may be induced by cellular and humoral mechanisms. There are no experimental models at present to substantiate the cellular mechanisms, but the characterization of inflammatory cells in the interstitium of the kidney in cases of drug-induced interstitial nephritis using monoclonal antibodies suggests a cellular basis for the condition (Gimenez and Mampaso 1986). There is also a considerable amount of data to support humoral mechanisms. Serum antitubular basement membrane antibodies have been detected in interstitial nephritis associated with methicillin (Border *et al.* 1974), and Joh and colleagues (1989) have demonstrated that experimental drug-induced acute interstitial nephritis (AIN) in mice is mediated by IgG antihapten antibodies. Other, probably less important, mechanisms include inoculation of Tamm–Horsfall protein into renal substance demonstrated in rabbits (Nagai and Nagai 1987) and tubular crystal deposition as in the case of aciclovir, both of which could spark off an immune reaction. As in drug-induced glomerulonephritis, the different immune reactions leading to AIN may produce a variety of histological and clinical pictures.

The classic type of AIN is best illustrated by the methicillin-induced disease. Methicillin, though not used nowadays, was the first semi-synthetic penicillin used clinically for treating infections caused by penicillinase-producing staphylococci. In one series of 80 children treated with the drug, 15 per cent developed features of AIN (Sanjad *et al.* 1974). Typically, the interstitial infiltrate on microscopy consists of mononuclear cells. Using monoclonal antibody techniques the majority of these cells are identified as T cells with varying numbers of CD4 and CD8 subtypes; these may vary with different drugs and may hint at different pathogeneses (Colvin and Fang 1989). Typically, eosinophils make up 2–10 per cent of the infiltrating cells. In addition, there is usually considerable interstitial oedema and secondary tubular necrosis. The former is in part responsible for the macroscopic swelling of the kidney (which can be picked up by ultrasound or on plain abdominal X-rays) and the loin discomfort frequently felt.

The clinical presentation is usually one of acute renal failure with very little else apart from exposure to the drug. On the other hand, in seriously ill patients multiple-drug regimens are often used, other causes for renal failure are often present, and it is not possible to decide which, if any drug, is responsible. In Pusey's series, the time from exposure to the onset of symptoms ranged from 1–30 days (Pusey *et al.* 1983), but it may be far longer than this. In the case of rifampicin, renal failure is more common with intermittent therapy. A constellation of features suggesting a hypersensitivity reaction may be present, including arthralgia, fever, skin rash, and evidence of abnormal liver function and eosinophilia on blood tests. The urine examination typically reveals mild to moderate proteinuria and haematuria. Eosinophiluria may also be present; Hansel's stain is a simple technique that is superior to Wright's stain for detecting urinary eosinophils (Nolan and Kelleher 1988). The test is sensitive, but it should be remembered that eosinophils may be found in the urine of patients suffering from other renal conditions such as glomerulonephritis. Though other less invasive techniques, such as gallium scanning (Linton *et al.* 1980), have been used in the diagnosis of interstitial nephritis, the diagnosis should be made by renal biopsy whenever possible.

In addition to the classic type of AIN, a histological subtype with a striking granulomatous reaction is well-recognized, acute granulomatous interstitial nephritis. In addition to those mentioned in the classic infiltrate, the cells in this condition include nodular aggregates of histiocytes, eosinophils, and Langhans-type giant cells. Many of the drugs listed can cause this form of AIN, though less commonly than the classic form. Those most often implicated are the penicillins, co-trimoxazole, sulphonamides, allopurinol, and the thiazides. The clinical picture is frequently identical in the acute classical and the acute granulomatous types of interstitial nephritis. The response to withdrawal of the drug and corticosteroids is also similar and it is our policy to treat both these types of AIN with steroids (Pusey *et al.* 1983).

Assuming greater importance as it is becoming a better recognized and frequently diagnosed complication of the NSAID is AIN in association with a

TABLE 14.4
Drugs associated with acute interstitial nephritis

Antibacterials

Amoxycillin	Geller *et al.* 1986
Ampicillin	Maxwell *et al.* 1974; Ruley and Lisi 1974
Aztreonam	Pazmino 1988
Carbenicillin	Appel *et al.* 1978
Cefaclor	Pommer *et al.* 1986
Cefoxitin	Toll *et al.* 1987
Cephalexin	Verma and Kieff 1975
Cephalothin	Drago *et al.* 1976
Cephapirin	Lewis and Rindone 1987
Cephradine	Wiles *et al.* 1979
Ciprofloxacin	Ying and Johnson 1989
Cloxacillin	Grimm *et al.* 1989
Co-trimoxazole	Dry *et al.* 1975; Cryst and Hammer 1988
Gentamicin	Saltissi *et al.* 1979
Methicillin	Galpin *et al.* 1975; Mayaud *et al.* 1975
Mezlocillin	Cushner *et al.* 1985
Minocycline	Walker *et al.* 1979
Nafcillin	Parry *et al.* 1973
Oxacillin	Burton *et al.* 1974
Penicillin	Colvin *et al.* 1974; Orchard and Rooker 1974
Pyrazinamide	Sanwikarja *et al.* 1989
Rifampicin	Nessi *et al.* 1976; Katz and Lor 1986
Sulphonamides	Robson *et al.* 1970
Vancomycin	Bergman *et al.* 1988

Non-steroidal agents

Diclofenac	Cameron 1988
Diflunisal	Wharton *et al.* 1982
Fenoprofen	Finkelstein *et al.* 1982
Glafenine	Andrieu *et al.* 1976
Ibuprofen	Cameron 1988
Indomethacin	Gary *et al.* 1980
Ketoprofen	Cameron 1988
Mefenamate	Cameron 1988
Naproxen	Brezin *et al.* 1979
Nimesulide	Apostolou *et al.* 1997
Phenylbutazone	Russell *et al.* 1978
Piroxicam	Cameron 1988
Pirprofen	Hurault de Ligny *et al.* 1986
Sulindac	Whelton *et al.* 1983
Tolmetin	Bender *et al.* 1984
Zomepirac	Bender *et al.* 1984

Other

Allopurinol	Gelbart *et al.* 1977
Aspirin	McLeish *et al.* 1979
Azathioprine	Saway *et al.* 1988
Captopril	Hooke *et al.* 1982
Carbamazepine	Hogg *et al.* 1981
Cimetidine	Ozawa *et al.* 1987
Clofibrate	Cumming 1980
Contrast agents	Ihle *et al.* 1982
Diazepam	Sadjadi *et al.* 1987
Foscarnet	Nyberg *et al.* 1990
Frusemide	Jennings *et al.* 1986
Methyldopa	Wilson *et al.* 1974
Omeprazole	Assouad 1994
Penicillamine	Feehally *et al.* 1987

(Table 14.4 continued)

(Other)

Phenindione	Galea *et al.* 1963; Lee and Holden 1964
Phenobarbitone	Faarup and Christensen 1974
Phenytoin	Sheth *et al.* 1977; Hyman *et al.* 1978
Recombinant α-interferon	Averbuch *et al.* 1984
Sodium valproate	Lin and Chiang 1988
Sulphinpyrazone	Howard *et al.* 1981
Thiazides	Fuller *et al.* 1976; Goette and Beatrice 1988
Warfarin	Volpi *et al.* 1989

Drugs in bold type are those most commonly associated with AIN.

minimal change type of glomerular lesion (Finkelstein *et al.* 1982; Handa 1986; Marasco *et al.* 1987). As methicillin is the penicillin that has been most studied in classic AIN, so is fenoprofen for this type of renal injury. Usually, the glomerular lesions are non-specific and not severe enough to suggest that they contribute to the renal failure (Bender *et al.* 1984). The interstitial nephritis is often severe and is usually the cause (Ling *et al.* 1990).

Drugs other than the NSAID that have been associated with interstitial nephritis and a minimal change type of glomerular lesion include recombinant α-interferon, ampicillin, lithium, penicillamine, phenytoin (Colvin and Fang 1989), and rifampicin. In the reported cases implicating NSAID, the clinical picture is somewhat different from the classic AIN and granulomatous AIN. Most patients are over 60 years old; only rarely do they manifest the systemic features of an allergic reaction; oliguria is rare; and heavy proteinuria with a nephrotic syndrome is common. As with the other types of AIN, the drug may have been taken only for a short period or for years. Withdrawal of the drug usually results in resolution of both the renal failure and the nephrotic syndrome. Our impression is that steroids may hasten the recovery, though this has not been proved.

There is still much to be learnt; with advancements in immunohistochemistry and molecular biology the pathogenesis of drug-induced AIN should become clearer. A list of drugs that can cause AIN is given in Table 14.4.

Obstruction

Drugs may cause obstruction to urine flow at the level of the nephron by tubular blockage from various proteins or by causing crystalluria and augmenting stone formation; other drugs may cause obstruction lower down in the urinary tract by producing ureteric obstruction from retroperitoneal fibrosis, blood clot and, rarely, tumours; they may also be responsible for bladder-neck obstruction. Drug-induced crystalluria, which may cause acute renal failure due to tubular blockage, is discussed in the section on renal stones and calcium nephropathy later in the chapter.

Tubular blockage

Light-chain casts

Light-chain proteinuria with and without acute renal failure, developing in patients with tuberculosis treated with rifampicin, has been reported by four groups (Graber *et al.* 1975; Kumar *et al.* 1976; Warrington *et al.* 1977; Soffer *et al.* 1987). This unique type of drug reaction was most recently reviewed by Soffer and co-workers in 1987. The cause is unclear but volume depletion may play a role in precipitation (Warrington *et al.* 1977). Renal histology is similar to that seen in the light-chain nephropathy of myeloma, though in the case described by Soffer and colleagues there was no giant-cell reaction to tubular casts. They speculate that this may have been due to the polyclonal origin of the light chains and the short duration of the disease process; light-chain proteinuria usually resolves within 10 days of discontinuing the drug.

Tubular blockage by light chains is also one of many mechanisms whereby myeloma may cause renal failure, and it has been suggested that the risk of precipitation may be aggravated by contrast media (Myers and Witten 1971). Baltzer and colleagues (1978), however, in a review of 89 pyelograms in patients with myeloma, did not find any patient who had suffered a decline in renal function after the procedure. The hazard that attends this investigation is probably dehydration rather than the contrast medium itself. Acute renal failure has also been described in a patient with primary macroglobulinaemia with small-molecule IgM x-chain protein (Matsumoto *et al.* 1985) and in diffuse hypergammaglobulinaemia following intravenous urography (Antman *et al.* 1982).

Tamm–Horsfall protein

The pathophysiology of nephropathy induced by contrast media remains obscure; adverse effects on the kidney include direct tubular toxicity with enzymuria (Goldstein *et al.* 1976) and diuresis; albuminuria (Holtas 1978); changes in renal blood flow, which may in part be due to vasopressin release (Trewhalla *et al.* 1990); and changes in glomerular filtration rate. Contrast media may also promote tubular obstruction. Tamm–Horsfall mucoprotein, predominantly secreted by the tubular cells of the thick ascending limb of Henle's loop (Kumar and Muchmore 1990), is the major constituent of casts and it can be precipitated *in vitro* by adding contrast media to the urine (Schwartz *et al.* 1970). It is possible

that this may occur *in vivo*, although data from Dawnay and others (1985) show no increased rate in excretion of Tamm–Horsfall glycoprotein following routine intravenous urography.

The chances of an otherwise fit person developing acute renal failure after exposure to a contrast medium are minuscule, but higher in the presence of risk factors, including diabetes (Harkonen and Kjellstrand 1979), advanced age (Weinrauch *et al.* 1978), dehydration (Swartz *et al.* 1978), pre-existing renal disease (Byrd and Sherman 1979), and severe cardiac failure (Taliercio *et al.* 1986; Barrett 1994). Weisberg and colleagues (1994) found that there was an increased risk of contrast nephropathy in diabetic patients in association with extreme vascular reactivity (vasoconstriction and vasodilatation). The volume of contrast material used and the type of study performed also played a role in the cases studied retrospectively by Gomes and others (1985), involving 364 patients who were undergoing major arteriography. The incidence of this contrast nephropathy is difficult to assess for various reasons, including variable definitions of nephrotoxicity, differing procedures and doses of contrast used in different studies and the retrospective, uncontrolled nature of many of these reports. There have been three large controlled prospective studies (Cramer *et al.* 1985; Parfrey *et al.* 1989; Schwarb *et al.* 1989). Cramer and colleagues, defining nephrotoxicity as a rise in creatinine of greater than 1.2 mg per dl 2 days after administration of a contrast medium for computed tomography (CT) enhancement, in this study reported an incidence of 2.1 per cent, which was no different from that in controls. Parfrey and colleagues' definition was a rise of 50 per cent or more in baseline creatinine after contrast medium; differing procedures were not randomized, and the incidence of toxicity was 9 per cent in diabetics with pre-existing renal disease compared with 1.6 per cent in controls (who underwent CT scanning or abdominal imaging without contrast medium). Finally, Schwarb and others, defining toxicity as a rise in creatinine of greater than $44\,\mu$mol per litre above baseline within 48 hours, reported toxicity and incidence of toxicity of 10 per cent and 17 per cent in high-risk groups (diabetes, heart failure, and pre-existing renal failure).

The complication may be avoided by critically analysing the potential benefit-to-risk ratio in individual patients and by ensuring good hydration before giving a contrast medium. In addition, it has been shown that intravenous mannitol before or immediately after the medium is given may be beneficial (Anto *et al.* 1981). Cigarroa and colleagues (1989), by adjusting the dose of contrast medium to the severity of azotaemia, found that limiting it reduced the incidence of acute renal dysfunction, particularly in diabetics. The low-osmolality non-ionic agents, in general, exhibit less toxicity, and on theoretical grounds the same should be true for nephrotoxicity (Dawson 1985). The two large clinical studies mentioned above (Parfrey *et al.* 1989; Schwarb *et al.* 1989), however, found no significant difference between groups receiving ionic and non-ionic contrast agents, and acute renal failure has been described following low-osmolality agents (Elliott and Reger 1988). It remains to be seen from the results of future controlled prospective studies if indeed nephrotoxicity is less with these than with conventional contrast agents.

Calcium-channel blockers may exert a protective effect if given before administration of a contrast medium (Neumayer *et al.* 1989), although not all agree (Cacoub *et al.* 1988). The toxic effects of contrast media are discussed in greater detail in Chapter 28.

Myoglobin

A consequence of drug-induced rhabdomyolysis is release of myoglobin into the circulation, and myoglobinuria. Myoglobin has a short half-life in the circulation and is probably not nephrotoxic *per se*, but within the renal tubule it is converted to ferrihaemate, which is a direct tubular cell toxin and causes tubular blockage.

Cocaine and 'crack' (cocaine base) have become the current popular recreational drugs in the affluent society; it has been estimated that three million Americans have tried cocaine and that a further five million use it on a regular basis. Although its life-threatening complications primarily affect the cardiovascular and neurological systems, there are increasingly frequent reports of the association of abuse with hyperpyrexia, rhabdomyolysis, and acute renal failure (Menashe and Roth *et al.* 1988; Gottlieb 1988; Roth *et al.* 1988; Anand *et al.* 1989; Cregler 1989; Jandreski *et al.* 1989; Singhal *et al.* 1989; Ahijado *et al.* 1990). Though in many cases there are other predisposing factors causing rhabdomyolysis, as in the three cases reported by Singal and colleagues, namely, prolonged squatting; lying in an abnormal position, resulting in a compartment syndrome; and violence. Of the 39 cases described by Roth and others (1988), 13 were hyperpyrexial. There are many cases where other predisposing factors are absent. Other recreational drugs that have caused rhabdomyolysis and renal failure include amphetamines (Kendrick *et al.* 1977; Terada *et al.* 1988), heroin (Richter *et al.* 1971; D'Agostino and Arnett 1979; Gibb and Shaw 1985), lysergide (Mercieca and Brown 1984), phencyclidine (Akmal *et al.* 1981), and toluene (Mizutani *et al.* 1989). Ecstasy (3,4-methylenedioxymethamphetamine),

in addition to causing acute renal failure as a consequence of rhabdomyolysis, has been associated with malignant hypertension (Woodrow *et al.* 1995). It should be remembered that drug abuse may expose the user to other toxins that may contaminate the primary drug, for example, arsenic intoxication in cocaine abuse (Lombard *et al.* 1989). Arsenic is also a cause of renal failure (Muehrcke and Pirani 1968; Gerhardt *et al.* 1978). More recently, through the Internet, it has been possible easily to purchase an ingredient of absinthe (wormwood oil) the ingestion of which resulted in acute renal failure secondary to rhabdomyolysis (Weisbord *et al.* 1997). The authors make the point that the Internet provides an easy means of ordering potentially toxic and pharmacologically active substances such as Chinese herbs, discussed later in the chapter as a cause of renal failure.

In many instances, as in cases of alcohol abuse, rhabdomyolysis occurs after a prolonged period of stupor or coma during which limb ischaemia may occur due to compression; alcohol, however, also produces a myopathy that predisposes to this complication in the absence of such precipitants (Haapanen *et al.* 1984). Methanol poisoning has also been described as being complicated by myoglobinuric renal failure (Grufferman *et al.* 1985).

Other drugs that have been associated with renal failure and myoglobinuria include pentamidine (Sensakovic *et al.* 1985), and there is evidence to suggest a particular susceptibility in patients with AIDS (Lachaal and Venuto 1989). Amphotericin (Drutz *et al.* 1970), carbenoxolone (Mitchell 1971), corticosteroids (Heitzman *et al.* 1962), diuretics (Oh *et al.* 1971), and a lotion containing 9-α-fluoroprednisolone (Mijares 1986) share a common pathway — via hypokalaemia — by which they induce rhabdomyolysis and renal failure; this is also the cause of the rhabdomyolysis associated with parenteral nutrition (Nadel *et al.* 1979).

The neuroleptic malignant syndrome (see Chapters 20 and 29), a complication of the use of major tranquillizers, the phenothiazines and haloperidol, may be further complicated by myoglobinuric renal failure (Eiser *et al.* 1982). Rhabdomyolysis and acute renal failure have also been induced by a combination of lovastatin and gemfibrozil (Marais and Larson 1990). The HMG-Co A reductase inhibitors may precipitate rhabdomyolysis, particularly in combination with other lipid-lowering agents (Kogan and Orenstein 1990). Though fibric acid derivatives such as clofibrate, bezafibrate, and fenofibrate have occasionally been associated with rhabdomyolysis, gemfibrozil used alone probably does not have this effect, but it may do so when given with lovastatin, as in 12 cases reported in the literature to date (Pierce *et al.* 1990); so this combination should be discouraged. The concomitant use of cyclosporin with HMG-Co A reductase inhibitors also increases the risk of developing rhabdomyolysis; the predicted odds ratio of developing rhabdomyolysis rises from 0.15 per cent with lovastatin alone to 5 per cent for patients taking lovastatin and gemfibrozil, and to 28 per cent with the combination of lovastatin, gemfibrozil, and cyclosporin (Kogan and Orenstein 1990).

Restoration of blood flow to an ischaemic limb or other tissue by the use of intra-arterial streptokinase can cause massive release of myoglobin into the circulation and cause renal failure (Lang 1985).

Other agents found guilty of causing renal damage by release of myoglobin into the circulation are listed in Table 14.5.

Haemoglobin

An immune-mediated intravascular haemolysis caused by cianidanol has resulted in haemoglobinuria and renal impairment (Rotoli et al. 1985). Drug-induced red cell antibodies of IgG and IgM classes against the antidepressant nomifensine and its metabolites have been found in patients with acute intravascular haemolysis due to this drug, many of whom developed renal impairment (Salama and Mueller-Eckhardt 1985). Acute haemolysis may occur after a second exposure to a single capsule (Fulton et al. 1986), as can chronic haemolysis (Skinner and Ferner 1986).

Retroperitoneal fibrosis

In most cases of retroperitoneal fibrosis no cause can be found, but a careful drug history may uncover one. The first drug to be implicated was methysergide (Graham 1964; Graham et al. 1966). This association was amply confirmed by other reports (Kerbel 1967; Gelford and Cromwell 1968; Bianchine and Freidman 1970; Watts 1973). Fibrosis may also occur around the rectum, sigmoid colon, scrotum, mediastinum, heart valves (Misch 1974), and pleura, causing pleural effusions (Hindle et al. 1970). Whereas methysergide is used in the prophylaxis of migraine, dihydroergotamine and ergotamine tartrate used in the treatment of the acute attack, have also been suspected, though the association is far more tenuous (Verin et al. 1974; Lepage-Savary and Vallières 1982; Malaquin et al. 1989). Other drugs under suspicion include the β-blockers propranolol (Pierce et al. 1981), atenolol (Johnson and McFarland 1980), oxprenolol (McCluskey et al. 1980), timolol (Rimmer et al. 1983), metoprolol (Thompson and Julian 1982), and sotalol (Laakso et al. 1982). Since these reports are few in relation to the use of β-blockers it has been suggested that the association with these drugs may be coincidental

TABLE 14.5
Drugs causing rhabdomyolysis and acute renal failure

Recreational	
Amphetamines	Terada et al. 1988
Cocaine and 'crack'	see text
'Ecstasy'	Fahal et al. 1992
Ethanol	Haapanen et al. 1984
Heroin	Gibb and Shaw 1985
Lysergide	Mercieca and Brown 1984
Methadone	Hojs and Sinkovic 1992
Methanol	Grufferman et al. 1985
Oil of wormwood	Weisbord et al. 1997
Phencyclidine	Akmal et al. 1981
Toluene	Mizutani et al. 1989
Therapeutic	
Amphotericin	Drutz et al. 1970
Bezafibrate	Gorriz et al.1995
Carbenoxolone	Mitchell 1971
Chlorthalidone	Oh et al. 1971
Clofibrate	Langer and Levy 1968
Corticosteroids	Heitzman et al. 1962
Cytarabine	Margolis et al. 1987
Diclofenac	Delrio et al. 1996
Fenofibrate	Giraud et al. 1982
9-α-fluoroprednisolone	Mijares 1986
Gemfibrozil	Gorriz et al. 1996
Haloperidol and phenothiazines	Eiser et al. 1982
Halothane	Rubiano et al. 1987
Lamotrigine	Schaub et al. 1994
Lovastatin	Pierce et al. 1990
Methylene chloride	Miller et al. 1985
Opiates	Blain et al. 1985
Pentamidine	Sensakovic et al. 1985
Streptokinase	Lang 1985
Suxamethonium	Hawker et al. 1985
Suxamethonium and enflurane	Lee et al. 1987
Tacrolimus	Hibi et al. 1995
Overdosage	
Amoxapine	Jennings et al. 1983
Diphenhydramine	Hampel et al. 1983
Doxylamine	Mendoza et al. 1987
Phenazopyridine	Gavish et al. 1986
Sodium valproate	Roodhooft et al. 1990
Terbutaline	Blake and Ryan 1989
Theophylline	Macdonald et al. 1985

(Pryor et al. 1983). Regression usually occurs following withdrawal of the drug, but progression may occur (Schwartz and Dunea 1966), requiring treatment with corticosteroids or by surgical ureterolysis.

Blood-clot obstruction

Urinary tract bleeding may complicate over-anticoagulation, but acute renal failure due to bilateral ureteric clot obstruction is rare (Nade 1972; Rosen 1972). Bilateral ureteric obstruction due to retroperitoneal bleeding has also been described (Kaden and Friedman 1961). In massive haematuria due to other causes, such as haemophilia, the use of the antifibrinolytic agents tranexamic acid and aminocaproic acid has resulted in ureteric obstruction. Haemorrhagic cystitis with severe haemorrhage and clots was observed by Droller and colleagues (1982) in eight of 97 patients receiving cyclophosphamide for malignancy, but this is unlikely to cause clot obstruction. The complication can largely be avoided by ensuring a good diuresis during treatment.

Urinary retention

This rarely causes acute renal failure. The complication is most frequently seen in elderly men with some degree of prostatic hypertrophy; confinement to bed makes things worse. It may also be the cause of confusion in the elderly. The drugs most commonly associated with this form of obstruction are sedatives, drugs with anticholinergic effects, and the opiates.

Glomerulonephritis and the nephrotic syndrome

Drugs may invoke an immune response that may in turn cause glomerulonephritis (Druet 1989) by a variety of mechanisms. Commonly they act as haptens; some may activate complement, possibly within glomeruli, to provoke an inflammatory response (Stark *et al.* 1985); and some (e.g. mercurials) may induce a polyclonal activation of B lymphocytes. Antibodies to glomerular basement membrane antigens can be detected within 8 days after administration of mercury to rats (Michaelson *et al.* 1985). That the T cell repertoire may be involved has been demonstrated by changes in T cell subpopulations before the appearance of such circulating antibodies (Bowman *et al.* 1987). Such drug reactions are largely dose independent.

Less common is damage due to direct glomerular toxicity, which is largely dose dependent. This has been well studied experimentally with the aminonucleoside of puromycin. The hypothesis of 'mesangial overloading' has been invoked as a prelude to glomerular sclerosis found in rats with aminonucleoside nephrosis (Grond *et al.* 1985); disruption of glomerular basement membrane anionic charge sites also occurs early on in this animal model of nephrosis (Mahan *et al.* 1986), and glomerular epithelial cell injury is probably a direct toxic effect of this drug (Diamond and Karnovsky 1986).

Those drugs that cause acute glomerular damage through a serum-sickness type reaction with vasculitis or a Goodpasture's syndrome, with a rapidly progressive glomerulonephritis, are described above in the section

on vascular damage. Drug-induced lupus nephritis is discussed separately later in the chapter.

There are many more drugs that are associated with a more subtle perturbation of the immune system which can none the less produce profound disease in the form of more chronic glomerulonephritis. The most common form of this is a membranous glomerulonephritis, presenting clinically with a nephrotic syndrome. Of the drugs involved, perhaps the best known are gold salts and penicillamine. In common with captopril (also capable of causing a membranous glomerulonephritis [Case *et al.* 1980]), they have sulphydryl groups in their structure, which may be important as patients particularly at risk are poor sulphoxidators. The Class 2 major histocompatibility antigen DR3 confers susceptibility to toxicity from some of these agents (Druet 1989). The HLA major histocompatibility complex is also important in the strong association between Class 1 antigen B35-Cw4 and nephritis developing in patients with rheumatoid arthritis treated with tiopronin, a penicillamine-like compound (Ferraccioli *et al.* 1986). Genetic factors are therefore important in conferring susceptibility. This is further suggested by the fact that patients who develop proteinuria with penicillamine are more likely to do so with gold, and vice versa (Halla *et al.* 1982; Smith *et al.* 1982). Though it has been suggested that when proteinuria is induced by penicillamine given after gold, this may be due to mobilization of gold from tissue deposits by the penicillamine (Dodd *et al.* 1980); it could also be argued that it is more likely to be due to genetic susceptibility.

The incidence of proteinuria in patients being treated with gold for rheumatoid arthritis ranged from one to seven per cent in the series reviewed by Sellars and Wilkinson (1983). It most commonly starts within the first 6 months of treatment but appears to be unrelated to the daily or cumulative dose. Microscopic haematuria and cylinduria may be present and the proteinuria may progress into the nephrotic range. In such cases, renal biopsy usually reveals a membranous glomerulonephritis (Tornroth and Skrivars 1974; Sellars and Wilkinson 1983; Francis *et al.* 1984). Gold is not found in the subepithelial immune deposits but has been detected in mesangial cells (Francis *et al.* 1984). Far less common is a minimal change lesion (Lee *et al.* 1965; Francis *et al.* 1984). Provided that the proteinuria remains less than about 1 g per day, and the gold is controlling the rheumatoid disease, it may be continued with close monitoring. Should the proteinuria be heavier, or if it is felt appropriate to withdraw the gold for other reasons, proteinuria usually diminishes within about 2 months although, rarely, this can take up to 3 years.

Tubular proteinuria and abnormal tubular function have also been described with gold therapy (Iesato *et al.* 1982), and gold deposits have been demonstrated in proximal tubular cells (Yarom *et al.* 1975). Renal tubular dysfunction can be induced in guinea-pigs by injection of sodium aurothiomalate, resulting in excretion of tubular basement membrane antigen and renal tubular epithelial antigen which is followed by an immune complex nephritis and tubulointerstitial change in the majority of animals (Ueda *et al.* 1986).

The nephrotic syndrome has also been described after oral gold (Atero *et al.* 1986), though it is less common than with the parenteral preparation. Three patients described by Tosi and others (1985), who had severe rheumatoid arthritis, were successfully treated with parenteral gold but developed membranous nephropathy; they were switched to oral gold and proteinuria ameliorated within 2–6 months.

As already stated, penicillamine can produce a more aggressive immunological mischief in the susceptible kidney. Not only is its use associated with a rapidly progressive nephritis and vasculitis (see above), but the incidence of membranous glomerulonephritis is approximately four times higher than with gold, averaging 12 per cent in four large series (Day and Golding 1974; Camus *et al.* 1976; Weiss *et al.* 1978; Stein *et al.* 1979). In addition to a membranous lesion, which is by far the most common, IgM nephropathy (Rehan and Johnson 1986) and minimal change nephropathy (Savill *et al.* 1988) have been reported. In contrast with gold, the incidence of most of the major adverse reactions with penicillamine increases with the dose (Day and Golding 1974). An important practical point illustrating this is that concurrent treatment with iron interferes with penicillamine absorption, and the sudden withdrawal of iron therapy has been described as precipitating renal toxicity (Harkness and Blake 1982). Proteinuria usually develops within 3–18 months of treatment and, as with gold, usually settles on withdrawal of the drug, usually over 4 to 24 months but it may be persistent (Camus *et al.* 1976).

It should be remembered that, although the majority of patients with rheumatoid arthritis and concomitant membranous glomerulonephritis are being treated with second-line agents, the nephritis is not always related to one of these drugs (Honkanen *et al.* 1987).

As already mentioned, in the animal model mercury induces a polyclonal activation of B cells that is related to the appearance of autoreactive T cells and causes a nephritis (Pelletier *et al.* 1987). In black Africans living in South Africa, a nephrotic syndrome, which renal biopsy shows to be due to a membranous glomerulo-nephritis, secondary to the use of skin-lightening creams containing mercury, has been well-recognized for many years, although it was not reported in this country until 1987 (Oliveira *et al.* 1987). It has also been described as a hazard in dentistry (Smart 1985).

Other drugs that have caused a membranous glomerulonephritis include tiopronin (thiola, α-mercapto-proprionylglycine) used for the treatment of cystinuria; there may be an association here with the HLA-DR3 antigen (Salvarani *et al.* 1985).

A membranous glomerulonephritis has been described with the use of ketoprofen (Sennesael *et al.* 1986) and flurbiprofen (MacKay 1997), but this is an unusual complication of an NSAID. A nephrotic syndrome on the other hand is a well-recognized complication of NSAID therapy, when it is usually due to minimal change glomerulonephritis in association with an interstitial infiltrate.

Minimal change glomerulonephritis is probably a T cell-mediated disease (Glassock *et al.* 1986); the mechanism whereby NSAID cause this is unknown. Withdrawal of the drug usually results in remission, though the lesion has progressed to focal glomerulosclerosis despite stopping the drug (e.g. fenoprofen [Artinano *et al.* 1986]). The combination of interstitial nephritis and minimal change nephropathy has also been reported with some antibiotics (Baum *et al.* 1986).

Other drugs that have been associated with minimal change glomerulonephritis include captopril (Bailey and Lynn 1987), lithium (Richman *et al.* 1980; Wood *et al.* 1989), practolol (Farr *et al.* 1975), and probenecid (Hertz *et al.* 1972); lithium may also cause a focal segmental glomerulosclerosis (Santella *et al.* 1988) and aggravate proteinuria in diabetics (Pawel *et al.* 1989), but it is far better known for its adverse effect on tubular function discussed earlier in this chapter.

Diffuse and segmental glomerulosclerosis may be caused by intravenous abuse of heroin, pentazocine, or pyribenzamine (May *et al.* 1986). The nephrotic syndrome has also developed after treatment with interferon (Selby *et al.* 1985), mesalazine (5-aminosalicylic acid) (Novis *et al.* 1988), phenytoin (Orlandini and Garini 1989), and quinidine (Chisholm 1985).

Lupus nephritis

The earliest report of what may have been a drug-related lupus (D-RSLE) syndrome appeared in 1945 (Hoffman 1945); subsequently hydralazine was implicated in 1953 (Morrow *et al.* 1953) and procainamide in 1962 (Ladd

1962). A review of the problem is provided by Fritzler and Rubin (1993). The number of drugs that have now been associated with either clinical lupus or serological abnormalities has increased to over 50 (Solinger 1988) and it is estimated that, in the United States, the disease is drug related in about 10 per cent of the 500 000 patients suffering from systemic lupus erythematosus (Hess 1988). We shall confine this discussion to those drugs for which there is definite proof of the association and refer readers to Chapter 18 and to the review on drug-related lupus by Solinger (1988) for details of the more tenuous associations. The drugs most commonly associated with lupus in clinical practice are chlorpromazine, hydralazine, and procainamide. The clinical syndrome may be indistinguishable from idiopathic lupus, although the usual age and sex criteria do not apply and renal involvement is said to be less common, though it most certainly does occur (Alarcón-Segovia et al. 1967). Renal and central nervous system involvement is distinctly uncommon as are the typical malar rash and the other skin manifestations. Fever, arthralgia, pleurisy, and pericarditis commonly occur (Hess 1988). The syndrome usually remits rapidly on withdrawal of the drug.

Genetic factors, which have been most extensively studied with hydralazine, play an important role in susceptibility to drug-related lupus. The syndrome is virtually confined to slow acetylators (Lunde et al. 1977), has a significant association with HLA-DR4 (Batchelor et al. 1980), and, like idiopathic lupus, is commoner in females, and is rare in blacks and carriers of C4 null alleles (Speirs et al. 1989). It has been suggested from studies in a murine model that the drug may interact with T cells in vivo and alter gene expression and induce alloreactivity (Yung et al. 1995).

Immunological abnormalities are common in patients being treated with procainamide; up to 74 per cent of patients on treatment for longer than 2 months will develop antinuclear antibodies though only about one-third will manifest symptoms. More careful analysis of the antinuclear antibodies reveals that they are mainly directed against histone components of the nucleus rather than against non-histone proteins and DNA as in idiopathic lupus (Monestier and Kotzin 1992). Different drugs are associated with different antibody profiles; hydralazine-related antibodies tend to be directed against a broad array of epitopes while procainamide antibodies are mainly directed against the histone complex H2A-H2B and with quinidine H1 and H2B (Hess 1988).

Autoantibodies to double-stranded DNA can, however, occur, as can hypocomplementaemia and anti-cardiolipin antibodies. The latter has been reported in association with multiple pulmonary thromboemboli in a patient treated with procainamide (Asherson et al. 1989).

Though there is no firm evidence to say the drugs that can cause lupus should not be used in idiopathic SLE it would seem prudent to avoid them if there are any alternatives.

Crystalluria, renal calculi, and calcium nephropathy

Nephrocalcinosis, stone formation, and hypercalcaemia are well known complications of pharmacological doses of vitamin D and its analogues. Even in normal doses vitamin D may produce nephrocalcinosis and renal failure in children who are excessively sensitive to the vitamin (Seelig 1969).

In some cases vitamin D is used as treatment for conditions in which its value is doubtful. Schwartzman and Franck in 1987 reported four patients with osteoporosis or osteomalacia who became hypercalcaemic and developed acute renal failure as a result of hypervitaminosis D; although the vitamin is indicated in many forms of osteomalacia, it has yet to be shown conclusively that it is of value in the treatment of osteoporosis. Other situations in which the use of vitamin D can be seriously questioned have resulted in renal failure; for example Todd and others (1987) reported a case of renal failure due to vitamin D used for the treatment of chilblains, and self-medication with preparations containing vitamin D and its analogues may be an important contributory cause of stone formation in the general population (Taylor 1972). Patients with impaired renal function and the elderly appear to be particularly at risk.

Other drugs that may cause hypercalcaemia and thus renal failure when taken in excess include vitamin A (Katz and Tzagournis 1972; Frame et al. 1974) and antacids taken with or without milk (Cameron and Spence 1967; Malone and Horn 1971). Thiazide diuretics, by reducing urinary calcium excretion, may also aggravate the hypercalcaemic effect of antacids (Hakim et al. 1979). Hypercalciuria can also be due to total parenteral nutrition (Adelman et al. 1977) or even the excipient contained in some tablets (Prati et al. 1972).

Nephrocalcinosis and calcium phosphate stone formation may also occur when urinary citrate excretion is reduced, as is the case with acetazolamide, which can cause a renal tubular acidosis (Pepys 1970), and with other carbonic anhydrase inhibitors used to treat glaucoma, such as methazolamide (Shields and Simmons 1976).

Acute hyperphosphataemia from tumour lysis can produce nephrocalcinosis in the face of a normal serum calcium; anuria has occurred in patients with lymphosarcoma (Kanfer *et al.* 1979) and Burkitt's lymphoma (Monballyu *et al.* 1984). There are obvious parallels with hyperuricaemic acute renal failure in the treatment of conditions in which there is lysis of tumour mass and deposition of uric acid crystals in renal tubules, pelvis, and ureters (Mitchell *et al.*. 1965; Maher *et al.* 1969); this should be largely preventable by pretreatment with allopurinol, a high fluid intake to promote diuresis, and alkalinization of the urine. Allopurinol, by inhibiting xanthine oxidase, blocks the transformation of xanthine to uric acid. Xanthine and hypoxanthine, though far more readily soluble than uric acid, may supersaturate the urine and, rarely, result in a xanthine nephropathy (Band *et al.* 1970) and acute renal failure (Ablin *et al.* 1972). When allopurinol has been used in conditions of chronic high production of urate, as in the Lesch–Nyhan syndrome, xanthine stones have occasionally been reported (Landgrebe *et al.* 1975).

Plasma urate levels also rise during weight reduction, and urate nephropathy can be precipitated by sudden reversion to a normal diet or by the inadvertent use of uricosuric agents (Zürcher *et al.* 1977).

Uric acid calculi are common in gout and may be precipitated by the use of uricosuric agents (Gutman and Yu 1968). Suprofen, an NSAID, deserves special mention as a noteworthy example of the value of spontaneous reporting of adverse drug reactions by physicians (Rossi *et al.* 1988). This drug was, within 6 months of marketing, clearly recognized as responsible for a flank-pain syndrome, usually associated with renal failure and haematuria that was reversible and probably due to intratubular precipitation of uric acid crystals with tubular obstruction (Wolfe 1987; Strom *et al.* 1989). Its uricosuric effects appeared no greater than those of other NSAID, yet the syndrome occurred in patients who did not have hyperuricaemia. The drug was similar structurally to ticrynafen, a diuretic that had also been reported to cause acute renal failure due to urate deposition in the kidney, though in those cases ticrynafen had been substituted for a thiazide and thus the patients were 'primed' to a certain extent, as they already had volume contraction and hyperuricaemia (Selby 1979). Phenylbutazone, before it was withdrawn, was also implicated in causing anuria by precipitating uric acid stones or crystals (Weisman and Bloom 1955).

Urinary oxalate excretion is increased by ingestion of large doses of vitamin C, possibly taken as a result of reports in the popular press that in such doses it can cure colds and cancer.

Acute renal failure due to crystallization of drugs in the kidney was a well-recognized complication of use of the sulphonamides in the 1930s, and sulphadiazine was the compound most frequently implicated, probably because it was the one most commonly used to treat infections before the advent of penicillin (Bull *et al.* 1958). In recent years, the use of sulphadiazine has increased, primarily to treat toxoplasmosis in patients with AIDS; two reports have highlighted the fact that it may still cause acute renal failure, though this can largely be prevented by maintaining an alkaline diuresis of at least 2 litres a day during treatment (Sahai *et al.* 1988; Christin *et al.* 1990). The importance of rehydration and an alkaline diuresis was stressed by Fiks and colleagues (1992) following the development of a diffuse calcinosis-induced ARF in a patient on sulphadiazine. The renal failure was reversible.

Aciclovir may cause renal failure from crystalluria and obstructive nephropathy. Four patients with a chronic fatigue syndrome, described by Sawyer and others (1988), developed five episodes of acute renal failure when aciclovir was administered intravenously in high doses, despite precautions to avoid volume contraction. Three patients had birefringent needle-like crystals within leucocytes on urine microscopy; one patient underwent percutaneous renal biopsy revealing foci of interstitial inflammation. On subsequent use of aciclovir in all four patients no adverse effect on renal function was demonstrated. Provided the infusion is given over one hour and the patient is kept well hydrated, serious nephrotoxicity is unlikely to occur (Laskin 1984). Low-dose aciclovir, however, has also been reported as a cause of acute renal failure without recovery of function but, as no biopsy was performed, another cause cannot be ruled out; and if, indeed, the aciclovir was to blame, another pathogenetic mechanism, such as immunological or idiosyncratic, must be invoked (Giustina *et al.* 1988). Two patients (out of 23 given aciclovir) reported by Selby and colleagues (1979) developed a mild rise in blood urea, but renal function improved in both with extra fluid administration, despite completing the course of aciclovir.

Crystals of dihydroxyadenine have been found in the kidneys of patients dying after massive transfusion of stored blood; they were presumably derived from the acid–citrate–dextrose anticoagulant in banked blood (Falk *et al.* 1972). Triamterene can also crystallize out in urine and form stones (Dooley *et al.* 1989). A list of drugs associated with urinary crystals is given in Table 14.6.

TABLE 14.6
Drugs associated with crystalluria

Urate crystals
Cytotoxic drugs
Phenylbutazone
Probenecid
Salicylates
Zoxazolamine

Oxalate crystals
Ascorbic acid
Methoxyflurane
Warfarin

Drug crystals
Aciclovir
Dihydroxyadenine
Mercaptopurine
Sulphonamides
Triamterene

Other crystals
Magnesium trisilicate
Vitamin D

Papillary necrosis and chronic interstitial nephritis (analgesic nephropathy)

History and causes

In 1953 Spuhler and Zollinger described an association between chronic interstitial nephritis and heavy consumption of analgesics; notably Saridone, which contained phenacetin, isopropyl antipyrine, and caffeine. Over the following ten years the incidence of renal papillary necrosis and chronic interstitial nephritis rose, in some countries at an alarming rate. Gloor (1978), from Switzerland, reported an increase in the autopsy rate of papillary necrosis from 2.7 per cent between 1938 and 1942 to 57 per cent between 1958 and 1962. A clinical picture was also forming: papillary necrosis was predominantly occurring in women who had consumed analgesic mixtures, whereas previously it had been an uncommon condition usually found in diabetics or with urinary obstruction. In most cases the mixtures were taken not for their analgesic properties but for their stimulant effects (both caffeine and phenacetin have mood-elevating properties) and occasionally for indications such as rheumatoid arthritis (Moeschlin 1957; Rossi and Muhlethaler 1958; Larsen and Moller 1959; Lindeneg *et al.* 1959; Lindvall 1960; Clausen and Pedersen 1961; Hultengren 1961; Nordenfelt and Ringertz 1961; Bengtsson 1962; Harvald 1968). An exception to the female preponderance was found at Jönköping

(Nordenfelt and Ringertz 1961), where most of the patients were male. This anomaly was traced to the high consumption of Hjorton's powders by male workers at the small-arms factory at Huskvarna, in the belief that they improved work output.

After the diagnosis was accepted as a real entity by nephrologists, the incidence naturally rose and it became well recognized as a cause of chronic renal failure. The global incidence is now falling though it still remains an important cause of end-stage renal failure in some countries; recently, high incidences have been reported from the Czech and Slovak republics (Matousovic *et al.* 1996). There are several reasons for the geographical variation in incidence; they include the availability of the offending analgesic mixtures, local renal-unit interest in the condition, and under-reporting. Underdiagnosis is compounded by patients often concealing or grossly underestimating their intake of analgesics. It has also been suggested that the geographical variation is to some extent due to climate and dehydration. It is interesting to note that the variation can occur within a small geographical area, and this has been blamed on different legislation relating to sales of analgesics (Noels *et al.* 1995). In Belgium, for example, the incidence is 15.6 per cent and in France hardly any cases are reported (Elseviers and De Broe 1993). In other countries the incidence fell after legislative measures were taken: in Sweden the frequency of analgesic nephropathy in the dialysis population fell from 20 per cent in the period 1965–69 to below two per cent in 1982 (Bengtsson 1989); in Australia, which also had one of the highest incidences, the number of new patients with end-stage renal failure due to analgesic nephropathy fell from 16 per cent in 1984 to nine per cent in 1992 (*ANZDATA* 1993).

In their review of the literature of analgesic abuse and renal disease, Buckalew and Schey (1986) demonstrated a highly significant linear relationship between the prevalence of nephropathy, defined as an elevation in serum creatinine, in daily consumers of antipyretic analgesics and the prevalence of habitual consumption in the population from which the habitual consumers were derived (Fig. 14.1). This probably reflects an increase in the number of heavy consumers in those populations with the highest prevalence of regular consumers in a manner analogous to alcohol-induced disease.

The villain of the piece is commonly thought to be phenacetin though it is not the only culprit. The epidemiological data in general strongly implicate phenacetin. Nearly all patients that were reported up to 1975 had consumed mixtures that contained phenacetin, though in the early 1980s it became clear that renal damage also developed with analgesic mixtures that

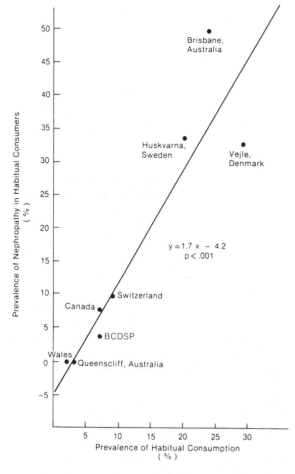

medical patients at autopsy in a teaching hospital peaked at 30 per cent. Following the banning of phenacetin in 1965, both figures fell steadily back to their prewar level. In patients with end-stage renal failure in Michigan who were diagnosed between 1976 and 1984, the risk of end-stage renal failure was significantly related to phenacetin (acetaminophen) consumption (Steenland *et al.* 1990).

FIG. 14.1

The prevalence of analgesic nephropathy in habitual analgesic consumers against the prevalence of analgesic consumption in that population. BCDSP = Boston Cooperative Drug Surveillance Program. (Reproduced with permission from Buckalew, V.M., and Schey, H.M., Renal disease from habitual antipyretic analgesic consumption; an assessment of the epidemiologic evidence. *Medicine* 65, 291–303, © Williams and Wilkins, 1986).

contained no phenacetin (Prescott 1982). There has been a distinct fall in the incidence of analgesic nephropathy in Sweden (Bengtsson 1967; Nordenfelt 1972), Scotland (Murray 1972), Finland (Kasanen 1973), and Denmark (Mabeck and Wichmann 1979), occurring 3–8 years after sales of phenacetin were restricted by legislation or withdrawal from popular proprietaries. In Finland (Silanpaa *et al.* 1982) in the 1950s, the total mortality from renal disease rose from about 500 to 1200 patients per year, and the prevalence of papillary necrosis among

Other substances that have been implicated in the pathogenesis of analgesic nephropathy include *p*-chloracetanilide, a trace contaminant of commercial preparations of phenacetin (Harvald *et al.* 1960; Schnitzer and Smith 1966); the major metabolite of phenacetin, paracetamol (acetaminophen); and aspirin. More recently, however, there has been considerable evidence to suggest that analgesic nephropathy is due to the abuse of analgesic mixtures that contain at least two analgesic compounds and one potentially addictive substance such as caffeine or barbiturates (Elseviers and DeBroe 1994). Though this may be the case in humans (and not all agree, Fox 1996), recent experiments in rats fed a combination of aspirin, paracetamol, and caffeine over 6 months did not result in significant nephrotoxicity or confer additional nephrotoxicity over and above aspirin and paracetamol given as monosubstances (Lehmann *et al.* 1996).

In addition, renal papillary necrosis can develop with the use of the NSAID such as benoxaprofen (Erwin and Boulton-Jones 1982). A high lifetime intake of NSAID other than aspirin (over 5000 pills) is also associated with a higher risk of developing end-stage renal failure (Perneger *et al.* 1994).

Paracetamol is now the commonest ingredient of most compound analgesics and is also commonly used on its own for pain relief. It is concentrated in the renal papilla (Duggin and Mudge 1974) and is clearly a cause of acute tubular necrosis, both in acute poisoning, when it can occur without hepatic failure, as mentioned above. Evidence for its being a cause of analgesic nephropathy is, however, tenuous, though three recent reports indicate that it is nephrotoxic and chronic users may develop renal failure (Sandler *et al.* 1989; Segasothy *et al.* 1988; Perneger *et al.* 1994). The risk of end-stage renal failure is dose dependent and both heavy average use (more than one pill per day) and high cumulative intake (more than 1000 pills in a lifetime) double the odds of its developing (Perneger *et al.* (1994). This relative risk is considerably lower than that previously estimated for phenacetin (Dubach *et al.* 1991).

Very high doses of paracetamol can produce papillary necrosis in rats (Molland 1978); but in a study of 18 patients receiving high doses of paracetamol, Edwards and colleagues (1971) found no significant damage after ingestion of 2–30 kg. Also, in only two cases published prior to 1980 was it considered to be the only culprit (Krikler 1967; Masters 1973). Nevertheless, in a retrospective study of dialysis patients and those who had undergone transplantation, Segasothy and others (1988) described five cases of papillary necrosis that they attributed to the consumption of paracetamol alone; these add to the 10 cases reported earlier by the same group (Segasothy et al. 1984, 1986).

What about aspirin? Papillary necrosis can be caused experimentally in rats and rabbits by doses of aspirin equivalent to or less than the dosage of phenacetin that causes this disease (Clausen 1964; Nanra and Kincaid-Smith 1970), and it does seem to be the major toxin when compared with phenacetin and caffeine in animal experiments; rats, however, have a particularly precarious blood supply to their renal papillae.

In humans, overdosage has been associated with acute renal failure (Campbell and Maclaurin 1958), and in lower dosage there is urinary wastage of proximal tubular cells (Kennedy and Saluga 1970), the excretion of which diminishes with continuation of the drug (Burry et al. 1976); the significance of this is unclear but it is unlikely to be related to the development of papillary necrosis. Aspirin has also been blamed by many for the high incidence of chronic interstitial nephritis in patients with rheumatoid arthritis. Prescott (1982) reported 151 cases of papillary necrosis in patients taking aspirin alone (88 cases) or combined with NSAID (63 cases). Akyol and colleagues (1982), on the other hand, could find no evidence of renal damage (including tests for concentrating defects) in 16 patients who had taken between 5 and 37 kg of aspirin over a long period of time for rheumatoid arthritis. These data are in accord with several other prospective studies that have failed to show any correlation between renal function and aspirin ingestion (Burry 1972; Burry et al. 1976; Wigley 1976; Emkey and Mills 1982). More recently Sandler and others (1989) could find no increased risk in daily users of aspirin whereas there was such a risk with paracetamol, a finding confirmed more recently by Perneger and colleagues (1994).

Many compound analgesics contain caffeine (e.g. Solpadeine tablets in the United Kingdom, Grand Pa powders in South Africa, Bex's and Vincent's in Australia). Apart from adding to the habituation properties of the mixtures, caffeine promotes a diuresis and this could lead to subclinical dehydration and concentration of the other analgesics in the renal medulla. Headache lasting 2–3 days is also caused by caffeine withdrawal from coffee drinkers (mean caffeine intake 435 mg per day) (Dusseldorp and Katan 1990).

In summary: though individual ingredients may be nephrotoxic, the combination of aspirin, phenacetin, and caffeine is particularly dangerous. It should also be stressed that prolonged abuse is required to produce renal failure. Although minor defects in renal function, such as defects in concentrating ability, can be detected after a relatively small cumulative dose (<1 kg), it usually takes 2–3 kg of analgesic before clinically detectable renal disease occurs (Nanra et al. 1978). In six reports from around the world, summarized by Gault and others (1968), the average intake of phenacetin in patients with analgesic nephropathy varied from 6 to over 10 kg taken over 11–12 years. Currently the overall risk of serious adverse renal effects with over-the-counter analgesics appears to be low, but the vast number of people taking these drugs and the ease of access to them mean that adverse effects will continue to the seen (Whelton 1995).

Pathology

This has been reviewed by Gloor (1965, 1974, 1978) and by Nanra and others (1978). The earliest pathological changes are confined to the inner medulla and papillary tips. As the disease advances with continued use of analgesics, the ischaemia extends outwards to involve more of the medulla, and papillae become necrotic and detach. Patchy cortical changes occur initially overlying the necrotic papillae. Microscopically there is atrophy with a patchy interstitial infiltrate, tubular fall-out, and periglomerular fibrosis. Some glomeruli show varying degrees of sclerosis, while others are normal or show compensatory hypertrophy. A heavy deposition of golden-brown granules is a near-constant finding in the cells of the loops of Henle and collecting ducts. Brownish discolouration can also be seen around the ureteric orifices in the bladder at cystoscopy. Of particular interest are characteristic changes in blood vessels: arterial changes are frequently those of benign nephrosclerosis but capillaries, arterioles, and venules are strikingly thickened and stain heavily with periodic acid–Schiff and fat stains. The lumina are often completely obliterated. The microangiopathy in the bladder is virtually pathognomonic of the condition (Mihatsch et al. 1983) but is found in only a minority of patients. Similar vessel changes have also been described in the skin of some patients (Abrahams et al. 1978).

Clinical features

The clinical syndrome is usually characteristic and has been described by many authors, including Hultengren

(1961), Bengtsson (1962), Duggan (1974), and Cove-Smith and Knapp (1978). It is predominantly a disease of females, presenting in their fourth or fifth decade. The patient is frequently asthenic, looks older than her years, and is neurotic and prone to other addictive pastimes, such as smoking and alcohol and purgative abuse. Analgesic use is often denied or minimized, so a history from other family members is often rewarding. Other features include anaemia disproportionate to the degree of renal failure. Factors contributing to this include occult gastro-intestinal blood loss (there is a very high incidence of gastritis and peptic ulceration with mixtures containing aspirin), and haemolysis has been reported with phen-acetin (Moeschlin 1957). The latter may account for the splenomegaly that is occasionally present (Duggan 1974) and the increased incidence of gallstones (Maisel and Priest 1964; Bell et al. 1969). Other features of the clinical syndrome include symptoms of headache, dys-menorrhoea, and dyspepsia; accelerated atherosclerosis with all its attendant complications; often, increased skin pigmentation; and an increased incidence of urinary tract infection and urothelial malignancy.

Diagnosis

The diagnosis is dependent on obtaining a history of prolonged analgesic intake and is suspected from the clinical features mentioned above. In cases where sus-picion is high but consumption is denied, urinalysis for salicylate levels may be helpful. The urine also often contains white cells without infection, protein, or blood. The characteristic radiographic features were reviewed by Lindvall (1978). Diagnostic features of renal papillary necrosis can be seen on intravenous urography, com-puterized tomographic scanning, and ultrasound. As already mentioned, typical features on bladder biopsy are diagnostic.

Prognosis and treatment

Banning over-the-counter sales of analgesic mixtures would go a long way towards preventing analgesic nephropathy. In patients with mild and moderate renal insufficiency, function usually stabilizes or improves if the patient can be persuaded to stop taking analgesics (Kincaid-Smith et al. 1971; Steele and Edwards 1971; Wilson 1972). Even when renal failure is advanced, stopping taking analgesics slows the rate of progression of renal failure, although Cove-Smith and Knapp (1978) suggest that patients with a plasma creatinine of above 400μmol per litre usually progress to end-stage renal failure. Morbidity and mortality from other conditions

related to the analgesic syndrome, such as ischaemic heart disease, are commoner than in other patients with other causes for renal failure; this is also the case in patients who are on dialysis (Schwarz et al. 1984; Balle and Schollmeyer 1990). Following transplantation, the graft may be lost from relapse to the addiction (Furman et al. 1976); there may also be a higher incidence of post-transplant malignant disease in this group (Hauser et al. 1990).

Management of such patients should include regular follow-up to ensure the stopping of taking analgesics and NSAID; good control of hypertension, prompt treat-ment of urinary tract infection or obstruction; regular urinary tract imaging for evidence of progression of disease; and urine cytology in view of the increased incidence of urothelial malignancy in these patients. It is also beneficial to encourage a high fluid intake and to avoid dehydration.

Other urological complications of analgesic abuse

Carcinoma of the renal pelvis in association with anal-gesic nephropathy was initially noted by Hultengren (1961). It subsequently became clear that this was more than a chance association, and the incidence of carci-noma of the pelvis in patients with analgesic nephrop-athy has been reported as 1.5 per cent per annum (Bengtsson et al. 1968). Although carcinoma of the bladder has also been reported (Handa and Tewari 1981; Mihatsch and Knusli 1982), it is far less common than carcinoma of the renal pelvis; this and the close anatom-ical relationship between the tumours and necrotic papillae suggest that the latter may play a role in patho-genesis of the malignancy.

Ureteric strictures, typically in the region of the pelvic brim, also complicate analgesic nephropathy (Lindvall 1960; Hultengren 1961). Other renal complications such as acute interstitial nephritis and functional renal failure were mentioned under the relevant headings earlier in the chapter.

Chinese herb nephropathy

Aristolochic acid (AA), a naturally occurring nephro-toxin and carcinogen, is considered to be the culprit in this condition, causing a relentless and rapidly progress-ive interstitial nephritis (Vanherweghem et al. 1993; Vanherweghem 1994; van Ypersele de Strihou and Van-herweghem 1995; Tanaka et al. 1997). There is also an association with urothelial tumours (van Ypersele de Strihou and Vanherweghem 1995; Reginster et al. 1997).

The disease is spoken of as Chinese herb nephropathy (CHN). Analysis of the Chinese herbs used in the slimming programme for the first patients described with CHN, did not show the presence of aristolochic acid (Vanherweghem *et al.* 1993). It has become recognized over the past several years and was first reported in Belgium, where the unfortunate patients were exposed to it in the form of slimming tablets (Vanherweghem *et al.* 1993; van Ypersele de Strihou and Vanherweghem 1995; Violon 1997). The AA is thought to have been in the herb powder (which was presumed to be *Stephania tetrandra*) in the slimming preparation (van Ypersele de Strihou and Vanherweghem 1995). ^{32}P-post-labelling analysis of DNA adducts formed by AA has demonstrated their presence in the kidneys of five of these patients and in the ureter of one (Bieler *et al.* 1991). Vanherweghem and colleagues (1996) conclude that steroids slow the progressive nature of the disease.

Miscellaneous

Haematuria

Urine dipsticks are very sensitive to blood; occasionally antiseptics used for the cleaning of urine receptacles may contaminate the urine to produce a false result. It is always essential therefore to examine the urine microscopically for red cells; this is also valuable in haemoglobinuria and myoglobinuria (mentioned above under rhabdomyolysis), in which the dipstick may record a large amount of blood with few or no red cells in the urine. Urine microscopy can also help to determine whether the source of the red cells is the glomerulus or the lower urinary tract; this can be done using fresh urine and an ordinary microscope, but is easier with a phase-contrast instrument (Fairley and Birch 1982).

Drugs that interfere with coagulation may cause haematuria. In addition, long-term anticoagulant therapy can cause gross haematuria with clot colic and, rarely, acute renal failure (Nade 1972; Rosen 1972). Bleeding into the retroperitoneal tissues may also obstruct the ureters (Kaden and Friedman 1961). It has also been suggested that warfarin may interfere with the structure of a urinary glycoprotein that normally inhibits crystallization of calcium oxalate, thus leading to an increased propensity for patients being treated with warfarin to form microscopic stones which can irritate the collecting system and cause haematuria (Fowler and Boyarsky 1986).

Cyclophosphamide may cause a haemorrhagic cystitis (Droller *et al.* 1982); characteristic changes are found on bladder biopsy; more sinister is a report of a leiomyosarcoma developing (Rowland and Elbe 1983), as is the review of Ramada *et al.* (1993) reporting on many cases of urothelial carcinomas associated with cyclophosphamide treatment. Haemorrhagic cystitis can be prevented by ensuring a good diuresis and by the use of the drug mesna (sodium 2-mercaptoethanesulphoonate), which is excreted in the urine and binds to acrolein and the toxic metabolite of cyclophosphamide that is responsible for the urotoxic effects in the urine. Hyperbaric oxygenation treatment may have a beneficial effect on cyclophosphamide cystitis (Yazawa *et al.* 1995).

Drugs causing incontinence of urine

Drugs interfering with the normal α-adrenergic stimulation of the proximal urethra may cause incontinence (Kiruluta and Andrews 1983); this may be seen in patients treated with haloperidol, chlorpromazine, or thiohexane. The antihypertensives methyldopa (Raz 1974) and prazosin (Thien *et al.* 1978) have also been implicated.

Drugs affecting tests of renal function

The inhibition of tubular secretion of creatinine may cause a rise in serum creatinine without a change in GFR; this has been described with trimethoprim (Berglund *et al.* 1975) and cimetidine (Larsson *et al.* 1980). As previously mentioned, both drugs can also cause interstitial nephritis.

References

Ablin, A., Stephens, B.G., Hirata, T., *et al.* (1972). Nephropathy, xanthinuria and orotic aciduria complicating Burkitt's lymphoma treated with chemotherapy and allopurinol. *Metabolism* 21, 771.

Abrahams, C., Furman, K.I., and Salant, D. (1978). Dermal micro-angiopathy in patients with analgesic nephropathy. *S. Afr. Med. J.* 54, 393.

Adelman, R.D., Abern, S.B., Merten, D., *et al.* (1977). Hypercalciuria with nephrolithiasis: a complication of total parenteral nutrition. *Pediatrics* 59, 473.

Adu, D., Turney, J., Michael, J., *et al.* (1983). Hyperkalaemia in cyclosporin-treated renal allograft recipients. *Lancet* ii, 370.

Ahijado, F., Garcia de Vinuesa, S., and Luño, J. (1990). Acute renal failure and rhabdomyolysis following cocaine abuse. *Nephron* 54, 268.

Aicher, L., Meier, G., and Norcross, A.J. (1997). Decrease in kidney calbindin-D 28kDa as possible mechanism mediating cyclosporine A- and FK-506-induced calciuria and tubular mineralization. *Biochem. Pharmacol.* 53, 723.

Akmal, M., Valdin, J.R., McCarron, M.M., *et al.* (1981). Rhabdomyolysis with and without acute renal failure in patients with phencyclidine intoxication. *Am. J. Nephrol.* 1, 91.

Akyol, S.M., Thompson, M., and Kerr, D.N.S. (1982). Renal function after prolonged consumption of aspirin. *BMJ* 284, 631.

Alappan, R., Perazella, M.A., and Butter, G.K. (1996). Hyperkalemia in hospitalized patients treated with trimethoprim-sulfamethoxazole. *Ann. Intern. Med.* 124, 316.

Alarcón-Segovia, D., Wakim, K.G., Worthington, J.W., *et al.* (1967). Clinical and experimental studies on the hydralazine syndrome and its relationship to systemic lupus erythematosus. *Medicine* (Baltimore), 46, 1.

Alexander, F. and Martin, J. (1981). Nephrotic syndrome associated with lithium therapy. *Clin. Nephrol.* 15, 267.

Ali, A., Barnes, J.N., Davison, A.J.W., *et al.* (1990). Proteinuria and thrombolytic agents. *Lancet* i, 106.

Allaouchiche, B., Mercatello, A., Tognet, E., *et al.* (1990). Prospective effect of norepinephrine infusion in acute renal insufficiency induced by interleukin 2 therapy. *Nephron* 55, 438.

Anand, V., Siami, G., and Stone, W.J. (1989). Cocaine-associated rhabdomyolysis and acute renal failure. *South. Med. J.* 82, 67.

Andoh, T.F., Burdmann, E.A, Lindsley, I., *et al.* (1995). Functional and structural characteristics of experimental FK 506 nephrotoxicity. *Clin. Exper. Pharm. Physiol.* 22, 646.

Andrews, P.M. and Bates, S.B. (1987). Dietary protein as a risk factor in gentamicin nephrotoxicity. *Renal Failure* 10, 153.

Andrieu, J., Andebrand, C., Chassaigne, M., *et al.* (1976). Anémie hémolytique et insuffisance rénale imputables à la glaférine. *Nouv. Presse Méd.* 5, 2394.

Antman, K.H., Parker, L.M., Goldstein, J.D., *et al.* (1982). Acute renal failure following intravenous pyelography (IVP) in a patient with diffuse hypergammaglobulinemia: a case report. *Med. Pediatr. Oncol.* 10, 289.

Anto, H.R., Chou, S.Y., Porush, J.G., *et al.* (1981). Infusion intravenous pyelography and renal function. Effect of hypertonic mannitol in patients with chronic renal insufficiency. *Arch. Intern. Med.* 141, 1652.

ANZDATA Report (1993). Australia and New Zealand Dialysis and Transplant Registry (ed. A.P.S. Disney). Adelaide, Australia.

Apostolou, T., Sotsiou, F., Yfanti, G., *et al.* (1997). Acute renal failure induced by nimesulide in a patient suffering from temporal arteritis. *Nephrol. Dial. Transplant.* 12, 1493.

Appel, G.B. (1990). Aminoglycoside nephrotoxicity. *Am. J. Med.* 88, 16S.

Appel, G.B., Woda, B.A., Neu, H.C., *et al.* (1978). Acute interstitial nephritis associated with carbenicillin therapy. *Arch. Intern. Med.* 138, 1265.

Argent, N. and Adams, P.C. (1990). Proteinuria and thrombolytic agents. *Lancet* i, 106.

Arning, M. and Scharf, R.E. (1989). Prevention of amphotericin B-induced nephrotoxicity by loading with sodium chloride: a report of 1291 days of treatment with amphotericin B without renal failure. *Klin. Wochenschr.* 67, 1020.

Artinano, M., Etheridge, W.B., Stroehlein, K.B., *et al.* (1986). Progression of minimal-change glomerulopathy to focal glomerulosclerosis in a patient with fenoprofen nephropathy. *Am. J. Nephrol.* 6, 353.

Asherson, R.A., Zulman, J., and Hughes, G.V.R. (1989). Pulmonary thromboembolism associated with procainamide induced lupus syndrome and anticardiolipin antibodies. *Ann. Rheum. Dis.* 48, 232.

Assis, S.M., Monteiro, J.L., and Seguro A.C. (1997). L-Arginine and allopurinol protect against cyclosporine nephrotoxicity. *Transplantation* 63, 1070.

Assouad, M., Vicks, S.L., Pokroy, M.V., *et al.* (1994). Recurrent acute interstitial nephritis on rechallenge with omeprazole. *Lancet* 344, 549.

Atero, F., Rodriguez-Franco, R., Paramo, M.J., *et al.* (1986). Nephrotic syndrome after oral gold. *Br. J. Rheumatol.* 25, 315.

Aurell, M., Svalander, C., Wallin, L., *et al.* (1981). Renal function and biopsy findings in patients on long-term lithium treatment. *Kidney Int.* 20, 663.

Austin, H.A., Palestine, A.G., Sabnis, S.G., *et al.* (1989). Evolution of ciclosporin nephrotoxicity in patients treated for autoimmune uveitis. *Am. J. Nephrol.* 9, 392.

Avent, C.K., Krinsky, D., Kirklin, J.K., *et al.* (1988). Synergistic nephrotoxicity due to ciprofloxacin and cyclosporine. *Am. J. Med.* 85, 452.

Averbuch, S.D., Austin, H.A. 3rd, Sherwin, S.A., *et al.* (1984). Acute interstitial nephritis with the nephrotic syndrome following recombinant leukocyte α-interferon therapy for mycosis fungoides. *N. Engl. J. Med.* 310, 32.

Axton, J.H.M. (1972). Six cases of poisoning after a parenteral organic mercurial compound (Merthiolate). *Postgrad. Med. J.* 48, 417.

Aynedjian, H.S., Nguyen, D., Lee, H.Y., *et al.* (1988). Effects of dietary electrolyte supplementation on gentamicin nephrotoxicity. *Am. J. Med. Sci.* 295, 444.

Bailey, R.R. and Lynn, K.L. (1986). Crescentic glomerulonephritis developing in a patient taking enalapril. *N.Z. Med. J.* 99, 959.

Bailey, R.R. and Lynn, K.L. (1987). Steroid-responsive nephrotic syndrome due to minimal change nephropathy occurring while on captopril. *N.Z. Med. J.* 100, 187.

Baliah, T., MacLeish, H., and Drummond, K.N. (1969). Acute boric acid poisoning: report of an infant successfully treated by peritoneal dialysis. *Can. Med. Assoc. J.* 101, 166.

Balle, C. and Schollmeyer, P. (1990). Morbidity of patients with analgesic-associated nephropathy on regular dialysis treatment and after renal transplantation. *Klin. Wochenschr.* 68, 38.

Baltzer, V.G., Jacob, H., Esselborn, H., *et al.* (1978). Über den Einfluß jodhaltiger Kontrastmittel auf die Nierenfunktion bei Patienten mit multiplem Myelom. Eine retrospektive Studie. *Fortschr. Röontgenstr.* 129, 208.

Band, P.R., Silverberg, D.S., Henderson, J.F., *et al.* (1970). Xanthine nephropathy in a patient with lymphosarcoma treated with allopurinol. *N. Engl. J. Med.* 283, 354.

Barrett, B.J. (1994). Contrast nephrotoxicity. *J. Am. Soc. Nephrol.* 5, 125.

Barros, E.J., Boim, M.A., Ajzen, H., *et al.* (1987). Glomerular hemodynamics and hormonal participation in cyclosporine nephrotoxicity. *Kidney Int.* 32, 19.

Batchelor, J.R., Welsh, K.I., Tinoco, R.M., *et al.* (1980). Hydralazine-induced systemic lupus erythematosus: influence of HLA-DR and sex on susceptibility. *Lancet* i, 1107.

Baum, M., Piel, C.F., and Goodman, J.R. (1986). Antibiotic-associated interstitial nephritis and nephrotic syndrome. *Am. J. Nephrol.* 6, 149.

Baxter, C.R., Duggin, G.G., Hall, B.M., *et al.* (1984). Stimulation of renin release from rat cortical slices by cyclosporin A. *Res. Commun. Chem. Pathol. Pharmacol.* 43, 417.

Bear, R.A., Sugar, L., and Paul, M. (1985). Nephrotic syndrome and renal failure secondary to lithium carbonate therapy. *Can. Med. Assoc. J.* 132, 735.

Beauchamp, D. and Pettigrew, M. (1988). Influence of hydrocortisone on gentamicin-induced nephrotoxicity in rats. *Antimicrob. Agents Chemother.* 32, 992.

Bell, D., Kerr, D.N.S., Swinney, J., *et al.* (1969). Analgesic nephropathy. Clinical course after withdrawal of phenacetin. *BMJ* iii, 378.

Bender, W.L., Whelton, A., Beschorner, W.E., *et al.* (1984). Interstitial nephritis, proteinuria, and renal failure caused by nonsteroidal anti-inflammatory drugs. Immunologic characterization of the inflammatory infiltrate. *Am. J. Med.* 76, 1006.

Bendz, H., Sjodin, I., and Aurell, M. (1996). Renal function on and off lithium in patients treated with lithium for 15 years or more. A controlled, prospective lithium withdrawal study. *Nephrol. Dial. Transplant.* 11, 457.

Bengtsson, U. (1962). A comparative study of chronic non-obstructive pyelonephritis and renal papillary necrosis. *Acta Med. Scand.* (Suppl. 338).

Bengtsson, U. (1967). Analgesic nephropathy — chronic pyelonephritis. In *Proceedings of 3rd International Congress on Nephrology*, Vol. 2 (ed. R.H. Heptinstall), p. 291. Karger, Basel.

Bengtsson, U. (1989). Analgetika-Nephropathie: Langfristige Erfahrungen aus Schweden. *Zeitschr. Urol. Nephrol.* 82, 121.

Bengtsson, U., Angervall, L., Ekman, H., *et al.*(1968). Transitional cell tumors of the renal pelvis in analgesic abusers. *Scand. J. Urol. Nephrol.* 2, 145.

Benigni, A., Chiabrando, C., Piccinelli, A., *et al.* (1988).Increased urinary excretion of thromboxane B2 and 2,3-dinor-TxB2 in cyclosporin A nephrotoxicity. *Kidney Int.* 34, 164.

Bennett, W.M. and Pulliam, J.P. (1983). Cyclosporine nephrotoxicity. *Ann. Intern. Med.* 99, 851.

Bennett, W.M., Hartnett, M.N., Gilbert, D., *et al.* (1976). Effect of sodium intake on gentamicin nephrotoxicity in the rat. *Proc. Soc. Exp. Biol. Med.* 151, 736.

Bennett, W.M., Plamp, C., and Porter, G.A. (1977). Drug-related syndromes in clinical nephrology. *Ann. Intern. Med.* 87, 582.

Berglund, F., Killander, J., and Pompeius, R. (1975). Effect of trimethoprim-sulphamethoxazole on the renal excretion of creatinine in man. *J. Urol.* 114, 802.

Bergman, M.M., Glew, R.H., and Ebert, T.H. (1988). Acute interstitial nephritis associated with vancomycin therapy. *Arch. Intern. Med.* 148, 2139.

Berlyne, G.M. (1972). Renal involvement in the collagen diseases. In *Renal Disease* (3rd edn) (ed. D.A.K. Black), p. 559. Blackwell, Oxford.

Bernis, P., Hamels, J., Quoidbach, A., *et al.* (1985). Remission of Goodpasture's syndrome after withdrawal of an unusual toxic. *Clin. Nephrol.* 23, 312.

Bhathena, D.B., Bullock, W.E., Nuttall, C.E., *et al.*(1978). The effects of amphotericin B therapy on the intrarenal vasculature and renal tubules in man. *Clin. Nephrol.* 9, 103.

Bianchine, J.R. and Freidman, A.P. (1970). Metabolism of methysergide and retroperitoneal fibrosis. *Arch. Intern. Med.* 126, 252.

Bieler, C.A., Stiborova, M., Wiessler, M., *et al.* (1997). ^{32}P-post-labelling analysis of DNA adducts formed by aristolochic acid in tissues from patients with Chinese herbs nephropathy. *Carcinogenesis* 18, 1063.

Bishop, W.B., Carlton, R.F., and Sanders, L.L. (1966). Diffuse vasculitis and death after hyperimmunization with pertussis vaccine. *N. Engl. J. Med.* 274, 616.

Björck, S., Westberg, G., Svalander, C., *et al.* (1983). Rapidly progressive glomerulonephritis after hydralazine. *Lancet* ii, 42.

Björnberg, A. and Gisslen, H. (1965). Thiazides: a cause of necrotising vasculitis? *Lancet* ii, 982.

Blain, P.G., Lane, R.J., Bateman, D.N., *et al.* (1985). Opiate-induced rhabdomyolysis. *Hum. Toxicol.* 4, 71.

Blake, P.G. and Ryan, F. (1989). Rhabdomyolysis and acute renal failure after terbutaline overdose. *Nephron* 53, 76.

Blakely, P. and MacDonald, R. (1995). Acute renal failure due to acetaminophen ingestion: a case report and review of the literature. *J. Am. Soc. Nephrol.* 6, 48.

Blaser, J. and Konig, C. (1995). Once-daily dosing of aminoglycosides, *Eur. J. Clin. Microb. Infect. Dis.* 14, 1029.

Blythe, W.B. (1983). Captopril and renal autoregulation. *N. Engl. J. Med.* 308, 390.

Bonzel, K.E., Muller-Wiefel, D.E., Ruder, H., *et al.* (1987). Anti-glomerular basement membrane antibody-mediated glomerulonephritis due to glue sniffing. *Eur. J. Pediatr.* 146, 296.

Border, W.A., Lehman, D.H., Egan, J.D., *et al.* (1974). Anti-tubular basement-membrane antibodies in methicillin-associated interstitial nephritis. *N. Engl. J. Med.* 291, 381.

Bowman, C., Green, C., Borysiewicz, L., *et al.* (1987). Circulating T-cell populations during mercuric chloride-induced nephritis in the Brown Norway rat. *Immunology* 61, 515.

Brezin, J.H., Katz, S.M., Schwartz, A.B., *et al.* (1979). Reversible renal failure and nephrotic syndrome associated with non-steroidal anti-inflammatory drugs. *N. Engl. J. Med.* 301, 1271.

Brown, C.B., Robson, J.S., Thomson, D., *et al.* (1973). Haemolytic uraemic syndrome in women taking oral contraceptives. *Lancet* i, 1479.

Bucht, G. and Wahlin, A. (1980). Renal concentrating capacity in long-term lithium treatment and after withdrawal of lithium. *Acta Med. Scand.* 207, 309.

Bucht, G., Wahlin, A., Wentzel, T., *et al.* (1980). Renal function and morphology in long-term lithium and combined lithium-neuroleptic treatment. *Acta Med. Scand.* 208, 381.

Buckalew, V.M. and Schey, H.M. (1986). Renal disease from habitual antipyretic analgesic consumption: an assessment of the epidemiologic evidence. *Medicine* (Baltimore) 65, 291.

Bull, G.M., Joekes, A.M., and Lowe, K.G. (1958). Acute renal failure due to poisons and drugs. *Lancet* i, 134.

Burrell, L.M. (1997). A risk-benefit assessment of losartan potassium in the treatment of hypertension. *Drug Saf.* 16, 56.

Burry, H.C. (1972). Reduced glomerular function in rheumatoid arthritis. *Ann. Rheum. Dis.* 31, 65.

Burry, H.C., Dieppe, P.A., Bresnihan, F.B., *et al.* (1976). Salicylates and renal function in rheumatoid arthritis. *BMJ* i, 613.

Burton, J.R., Lichtenstein, N.S., Colvin, R.B., *et al.* (1974). Acute interstitial nephritis from oxacillin. *Johns Hopkins Med. J.* 134, 58.

Butler, W.T. (1964). Amphotericin B toxicity: changes in renal function. *Ann. Intern. Med.* 61, 344.

Byrd, L. and Sherman, R.L. (1979). Radiocontrast-induced acute renal failure: a clinical and physiologic review. *Medicine* (Baltimore) 58, 270.

Cabrera, J., Arroyo, V., Ballesta, A., *et al.* (1982). Aminoglycoside nephrotoxicity in cirrhosis. Value of urinary β_2-microglobulin to discriminate functional renal failure from acute tubular damage. *Gastroenterology* 82, 97.

Cacoub, P., Deray, G., Baumelou, A., *et al.* (1988). No evidence for protective effects of nifedipine against radiocontrast-induced acute renal failure. *Clin. Nephrol.* 29, 215.

Callan, M.F.C., Davies, K.A.A., Merrin, P.K., *et al.* (1990). Proteinuria and thrombolytic agents. *Lancet* i, 106.

Cameron, A.J. and Spence, M.P. (1967). Chronic milk–alkali syndrome after prolonged excessive intake of antacid tablets. *BMJ* iii, 656.

Cameron, J.S. (1988). Allergic interstitial nephritis: Clinical features and pathogenesis. *Q. J. Med.* 66, 97.

Campbell, E.J.M. and Maclaurin, R.E. (1958). Acute renal failure in salicylate poisoning. *BMJ* i, 503.

Camus, J-P., Crouzet, J., Prier, A., *et al.* (1976). Complications du traitement de la polyarthrite rhumatoïde par la D-pénicillamine. *Thérapie* 31, 385.

Cantwell, B.M.J., Carmichael, J., Mannix, K.A., *et al.* (1989). Chemotherapy induced emesis may exacerbate the nephrotoxicity of combined ifosfamide/mesna and cisplatin chemotherapy. *Eur. J. Cancer Clin. Oncol.* 25, 917.

Carstenen, H., Jacobsen, N., and Dieperink, H. (1986). Interaction between cyclosporin A and phenobarbitone. *Br. J. Clin. Pharmacol.* 21, 550.

Case, D.B., Atlas, S.A., Mouradian, J.A., *et al.* (1980). Proteinuria during long-term captopril treatment. *JAMA* 244, 346.

Cassidy, M.J.D., van Zyl-Smit, R., Pascoe, M.D., *et al.* (1985). Effect of rifampicin on cyclosporin A blood levels in a renal transplant recipient. *Nephron* 41, 207.

Chan, M.K. (1986). Cyclosporine pharmacokinetics in end-stage renal failure: the influence of heparin and metoprolol. In: *Proceedings of 2nd Asian Cyclosporine Workshop*, p. 38. Excerpta Medica, Amsterdam.

Chapman, A.B., Gabow, P.A., and Schrier, R.W. (1991). Reversible renal failure associated with angiontensin-converting enzyme inhibitors in polycystic kidney disease. *Ann. Intern. Med.* 115, 769.

Chertow, G.M., Seifter, J.L., Christiansen, C.L., *et al.* (1996). Trimethoprim-sulfamethoxazole and hypouricaemia. *Clin. Nephrol.* 46, 193.

Chisholm, J.C. Jr (1985). Quinidine-induced nephrotic syndrome. *J. Natl Med. Assoc.* 77, 920.

Chou, S.Y., Brown, M., Reiser, I.W., *et al.* (1995). Acute saline loading abrogates the renal potassium retention induced by trimethoprim (TMP). *J. Am. Soc. Nephrol.* 6, 334.

Chow, S.S., Thorner, P., Baumal, R., *et al.* (1986). Cyclosporine and experimental renal ischemic injury. *Transplantation* 41, 152.

Christiansen, N.P., Skubitz, K.M., Nath, K., *et al.* (1988). Nephrotoxicity of continuous intravenous infusion of recombinant interleukin-2. *Am. J. Med.* 84, 1072.

Christin, S., Baumelou, A., Bahri, S., *et al.* (1990). Acute renal failure due to sulfadiazine in patients with AIDS. *Nephron* 55, 233.

Churchill, L., Graham, A., Farina, P., *et al.* (1995). Inhibition of human cyclooxygenase-2 (Cox-2) by meloxicam. *Rheumatol. Eur.* 24 (Suppl. 3), abstract D205.

Ciabattoni, G., Cinotti, G.A., Pierucci, A., *et al.* (1984). Effects of sulindac and ibuprofen in patients with chronic glomerular diseases: evidence for the dependence of renal function on prostacyclin. *N. Engl. J. Med.* 310, 279.

Cigarroa, R.G., Lange, R.A., Williams, R.H., *et al.* (1989). Dosing of contrast material to prevent contrast nephropathy in patients with renal disease. *Am. J. Med.* 86, 649.

Citron, B.P., Halpern, M., McCarron, M., *et al.* (1970). Necrotizing angiitis associated with drug abuse. *N. Engl. J. Med.* 283, 1003.

Clarke, B.F., Campbell, I.W., Ewing, D.J., *et al.* (1974). Generalized hypersensitivity reaction and visceral arteritis with fatal outcome during glibenclamide therapy. *Diabetes* 23, 739.

Clausen, E. (1964). Histological changes in rabbit kidneys induced by phenacetin and acetylsalicylic acid. *Lancet* ii, 123.

Clausen, E. and Pedersen, J. (1961). Necrosis of the renal papillae in rheumatoid arthritis. *Acta Med. Scand.* 170, 631.

Clive, D.M. and Stoff, J.S. (1984). Renal syndromes associated with nonsteroidal antiinflammatory drugs. *N. Engl. J. Med.* 310, 563.

Cockburn, I. (1986). Cyclosporine A: a clinical evaluation of drug interactions. *Transplant. Proc.* 18 (Suppl. 5), 50.

Coffman, T.M., Carr, D.R., Yarger, W.E., et al. (1987). Evidence that renal prostaglandin and thromboxane production is stimulated in chronic cyclosporine nephrotoxicity. Transplantation 43, 282.

Colvin, R.B. and Fang, L.S.T. (1989). Interstitial nephritis. In Renal Pathology, Vol. 1 (ed. C.C. Tisher and B.M. Brenner), p. 728. J.B. Lippincott, Philadelphia.

Colvin, R.B., Burton, J.R., Hyslop, N.E., et al. (1974). Penicillin-associated interstitial nephritis. Ann. Intern. Med. 81, 404.

Contreras, A.M., Gamba, G., Cortes, J., et al. (1989). Serial trough and peak amikacin levels in plasma as predictors of nephrotoxicity. Antimicrob. Agents Chemother. 33, 973.

Cosio, F.G., Innes, J.T., Nahman, N.S. Jr, et al. (1987). Combined nephrotoxic effects of cyclosporine and endotoxin. Transplantation 44, 425.

Cove-Smith, J.R. and Knapp, M.S. (1978). Analgesic nephropathy: an important cause of chronic renal failure. Q. J. Med. 47, 49.

Cramer, B.C., Parfrey, P.S., and Hutchinson, T.A. (1985). Renal function following infusion of radiologic contrast material: a prospective controlled study. Arch. Intern. Med. 145, 87.

Cregler, L.L. (1989). Cocaine-associated myoglobinuric renal failure. Am. J. Med. 86, 632.

Cryst, C. and Hammer, S.P. (1988). Acute granulomatous interstitial nephritis due to co-trimoxazole. Am. J. Nephrol. 8, 483.

Cubeddu, L.X., Hoffman, I.S., Fuenmayor, N.T., et al. (1990). Efficacy of Ondansetron (GR 38032F) and the role of serotonin in cisplatin-induced nausea and vomiting. N. Engl. J. Med. 322, 810.

Cumming, A. (1980). Acute renal failure and interstitial nephritis after clofibrate treatment. BMJ 281, 1529.

Curtis, J.R. and Bateman, F.J.A. (1975). Use of prazosin in management of hypertension in patients with chronic renal failure and in renal transplant recipients. BMJ iv, 432.

Cushner, H.M., Copley, J.B., Bauman, J., et al. (1985). Acute interstitial nephritis associated with mezlocillin, nafcillin, and gentamicin treatment for Pseudomonas infection. Arch. Intern. Med. 145, 1204.

D'Agostino, R.S. and Arnett, E.N. (1979). Acute myoglobinuria and heroin snorting. JAMA 241, 277.

Dale, B.M., Sage, R.E., Norman, J.E., et al. (1985). Bone marrow transplantation following treatment with high-dose melphalan. Transplant. Proc. 17, 1711.

Daugaard, G. (1990). Cisplatin nephrotoxicity: experimental and clinical studies. Dan. Med. Bull. 37, 1.

Davenport, A. and Finn, R. (1988). Paracetamol (acetaminophen) poisoning resulting in acute renal failure without hepatic coma. Nephron 50, 55.

Dawnay, A.B., Thornley, C., Nockler, I., et al. (1985). Tamm-Horsfall glycoprotein excretion and aggregation during intravenous urography. Relevance to acute renal failure. Invest. Radiol. 20, 53.

Dawson, P. (1985). Contrast agent nephrotoxicity: an appraisal. Br. J. Radiol. 58, 121.

Day, A.T. and Golding, J.R. (1974). Hazards of penicillamine therapy in the treatment of rheumatoid arthritis. Postgrad. Med. J. 50 (suppl. 2), 71.

De Beukelaer, M.M., Travis, L.B., Dodge, W.F., et al. (1971). Deafness and acute tubular necrosis following parenteral administration of neomycin. Am. J. Dis. Child. 121, 250.

De la Pava, S., Nigogosyan, G., and Pickren, J.W. (1962). Fatal glomerulonephritis after receiving horse anti-human-cancer serum. Arch. Intern. Med. 109, 67.

Delaney, V.B. and Segel, D.P. (1985). Indomethacin-induced renal insufficiency: recurrence on rechallenge. South. Med. J. 78, 1390.

Delrio, F.M., Park, Y., Herzlich, B., et al. (1996). Case report: diclofenac-induced rhabdomyolysis Am. J. Med. Sci. 312, 95.

De Nicola, L., Thomson, S.C., Wead, L.M., et al. (1993). Arginine feeding modifies cyclosporine nephrotoxicity in rats. J. Clin. Invest. 92, 1859.

Deray, G., Le-Hoang, P., Aupetit, B., et al. (1987). Enhancement of cyclosporine A nephrotoxicity by diclofenac. Clin. Nephrol. 27, 213.

Deray, G., Dubois, M., Beaufils, H., et al. (1988). Effects of nifedipine on cisplatinum-induced nephrotoxicity in rats. Clin. Nephrol. 30, 146.

Devogelaer, J.P., Pirson, Y., Vandenbroucke, J.M., et al. (1987). D-penicillamine induced crescentic glomerulonephritis: report and review of the literature. J. Rheumatol. 14, 1036.

de Zeeuw, D., Gansevoort, R.T., and de Jong, P.E. (1995). Losartan in patients with renal insufficiency. Can. J. Cardiol. 11 (Suppl. F), 41F.

Diamond, J.R. and Karnovsky, M.J. (1986). Focal and segmental glomerulosclerosis following a single intravenous dose of puromycin aminonucleoside. Am. J. Pathol. 122, 481.

Dieperink, H. and Moller, J. (1982). Ketoconazole and cyclosporin. Lancet ii, 1217.

Dieperink, H., Leyssac, P.P., Starklint, H., et al. (1986). Antagonist capacities of nifedipine, captopril, phenoxybenzamine, prostacyclin and indomethacin on cyclosporin A induced impairment of rat renal function. Eur. J. Clin. Invest. 16, 540.

Dobyan, D.C., Bull, J.M., Strebel, F.R., et al. (1986). Protective effects of o-(beta-hydroxyethyl) rutoside on cisplatinum-induced acute renal failure in the rat. Lab. Invest. 55, 557.

Dodd, M.J., Griffiths, I.D., and Thompson, M. (1980). Adverse reactions to D-penicillamine after gold toxicity. BMJ ii, 1498.

Donadio, C., Lucchesi, A., and Gadducci, A. (1996). Minimization of cisplatin nephrotoxicity in high-risk patients. Nephron 73, 325.

Dooley, D.P., Callsen, M.E., and Geiling, J.A. (1989). Triamterene nephrolithiasis. Milit. Med. 154, 126.

Drago, J.R., Rohner, T.J., Sanford, E.J., et al. (1976). Acute interstitial nephritis. J. Urol. 115, 105.

Droller, M.J., Saral, R., and Santos, G. (1982). Prevention of cyclophosphamide-induced haemorrhagic cystitis. Urology 20, 256.

Druet, P. (1989). Contribution of immunological reactions to nephrotoxicity. *Toxicol. Lett.* 46, 55.

Drug and Therapeutics Bulletin (1997). Aminoglycosides once daily? *Drug Ther. Bull.* 35, 36.

Drutz, D.J., Fan, J.H., Tai, T.Y., *et al.* (1970). Hypokalemic rhabdomyolysis and myoglobinuria following amphotericin B therapy. *JAMA* 211, 824.

Dry, J., Leynadier, F., Herman, D., *et al.* (1975). L'association sulfaméthoxazole-triméthoprime (co-trimoxazole). Réaction immunoallergique inhabituelle. *Nouv. Presse Méd.* 4, 36.

Dubach, U.C., Rosner, B., and Stürmer, T. (1991). An epidemiologic study of abuse of analgesic drugs — effects of phenacetin and salicylate on mortality and cardiovascular morbidity (1968 to 1987). *N. Engl. J. Med.* 324, 155.

Duclos, J., Ruiz, I., Sanchez, B., *et al.* (1992). Acute renal insufficiency due to the use of angiotensin converting enzyme inhibitors in 2 patients without renal artery stenosis. *Rev. Med. Chil.* 120, 1282.

Duggan, J.M. (1974). The analgesic syndrome. *Aust. N.Z. J. Med.* 4, 365.

Duggin, G.G. and Mudge, G.H. (1974). Renal distribution of acetaminophen and its conjugates. *Kidney Int.* 6, 38A.

Dusseldorp, M.V. and Katan, M.B. (1990). Headache caused by caffeine withdrawal among moderate coffee drinkers switched from ordinary to decaffeinated coffee: a 12 week double blind trial. *BMJ* 300, 1558.

Edwards, O.M., Edwards, P., Huskisson, E.C., *et al.* (1971). Paracetamol and renal damage. *BMJ* ii, 87.

Eicher, J.C., Morelon, P., Chalopin, J.M., *et al.* (1988). Acute renal failure during nifedipine therapy in a patient with congestive heart failure. *Crit. Care Med.* 16, 1163.

Eiser, A.R., Neff, M.S., and Slifkin, R.F. (1982). Acute myoglobinuric renal failure. A consequence of the neuroleptic malignant syndrome. *Arch. Intern. Med.* 142, 601.

Elliott, C. and Reger, M. (1988). Acute renal failure following low osmolality radiocontrast dye. *Clin. Cardiol.* 11, 420.

Elseviers, M.M. and DeBroe, M.E. (1993). Analgesic nephropathy — still a problem? *Nephron* 64, 505.

Elseviers, M.M. and DeBroe, M.E. (1994). Analgesic nephropathy in Belgium is related to the sales of particular analgesic mixtures. *Nephrol. Dial. Transplant.* 9, 41.

Emkey, R.D. and Mills, J.A. (1982). Aspirin and analgesic nephropathy. *JAMA* 247, 55.

Engberg, A. (1976). Effects of dextran 40 on the proximal renal tubule. *Acta Chir. Scand.* 142, 172.

Ericsson, J.L.E., Andres, G., Bergstrand, A., *et al.* (1967). Further studies on the fine structure of renal tubules in healthy humans. *Acta Pathol. Microbiol. Scand.* 69, 493.

Ernest, S. (1989). Model of gentamicin-induced nephrotoxicity and its amelioration by calcium and thyroxine. *Med. Hypotheses* 30, 195.

Erwin, L. and Boulton Jones, J.M. (1982). Benoxaprofen and papillary necrosis. *BMJ* 285, 694.

Faarup, P. and Christensen, E. (1974). IgE containing plasma cells in acute tubulo-interstitial nephropathy. *Lancet* ii, 718.

Fahal, I.M., Sallo, D.F., Yaqoob, M., *et al.* (1992). Acute renal failure after ecstasy. *BMJ* 305, 29.

Fairley, K.F. and Birch, D.F. (1982). Hematuria: A simple method for identifying glomerular bleeding. *Kidney Int.* 21, 105.

Falck, H.M., Törnroth, T., Kock, B., *et al.* (1979). Fatal renal vasculitis and minimal change glomerulonephritis complicating treatment with penicillamine. *Acta Med. Scand.* 205, 133.

Falco, F.G., Smith, H.M., and Arcieri, G.M. (1969). Nephrotoxicity of aminoglycosides and gentamicin. *J. Infect. Dis.* 119, 406.

Falk, J.S., Lindblad, G.T.O., and Westman, B.J.M. (1972). Histopathological studies on kidneys from patients treated with large amounts of blood preserved with ACD-adenine. *Transfusion* 12, 376.

Farr, M.J., Wingate, J.P., and Shaw, J.N. (1975). Practolol and the nephrotic syndrome. *BMJ* ii, 68.

Feehally, J., Wheeler, D.C., Mackay, E.H., *et al.* (1987). Recurrent acute renal failure with interstitial nephritis due to D-penicillamine. *Renal Failure* 10, 55.

Ferraccioli, G., Peri, F., Nervetti, A., *et al.* (1986). Toxicity due to remission inducing drugs in rheumatoid arthritis. Association with HLA-B35 and Cw4 antigens. *J. Rheumatol.* 13, 65.

Ferrier, C., Beretta-Piccoli, C., Weidmann, P., *et al.* (1989). Hypotension and renal impairment during infusion of atrial natriuretic factor in liver cirrhosis with ascites. *Am. J. Nephrol.* 9, 291.

Fiks, I.N., Folador, C.R., Barbas Filho, J.V., *et al.* (1992). Kidney failure as a complication of the treatment of pulmonary paracoccidioidomycosis. *Rev. Hosp. Fac. Med. Sao Paulo* 47, 103.

Fillastre, J.P. and Raguenez-Viotte, G. (1989). Cisplatin nephrotoxicity. *Toxicol. Lett.* 46, 163.

Finkelstein, A., Fraley, D.S., Stachura, I., *et al.* (1982). Fenoprofen nephropathy: lipoid nephrosis and interstitial nephritis. A possible T-lymphocyte disorder. *Am. J. Med.* 72, 81.

Forrest, J.N., Jr, Cohen, A.D., Torretti, J., *et al.* (1974). On the mechanisms of lithium induced diabetes insipidus in man and the rat. *J. Clin. Invest.* 53, 1115.

Fournier, A., Watchi, J-M., and Reveillaud, R-J. (1969). La néphrose dite osmotique ou vacuolisation hydropique des tubes proximaux. *Presse Méd.* 77, 1987.

Fowler, W.E. and Boyarsky, S. (1986). A possible cause of hematuria in patients taking warfarin. *N. Engl. J. Med.* 315, 65.

Fox, J.M. (1996). No proof for a particular role of combination analgesics causing end-stage renal failure. *Nephrol. Dial. Transplant.* 11, 519.

Frame, B., Jackson, C.E., Reynolds, W.A., *et al.* (1974). Hypercalcemia and skeletal effects in chronic hypervitaminosis A. *Ann. Intern. Med.* 80, 44.

Francis, K.L., Jenis, E.H., Jensen, G.E., *et al.* (1984). Gold-associated nephropathy. *Arch. Pathol. Lab. Med.* 108, 234.

Freeman, D.J., Laupacis, A., Keown, P.A., *et al.* (1984). Evaluation of cyclosporin-phenytoin interaction with observations on cyclosporin metabolites. *Br. J. Clin. Pharmacol.* 18, 887.

Fritzler, M.J. and Rubin, R.L. (1993). Drug-induced lupus. In *Dubois' Lupus Erythematosus* 4th edn (ed. D.J. Wallace and B.H. Hahn), p. 442. Lea and Febiger, Philadelphia.

Fuller, T.J., Barcenas, C.G., and White, M.G. (1976). Diuretic-induced interstitial nephritis. Occurence in a patient with membranous glomerulonephritis. *JAMA* 235, 1998.

Fulton, J.D., Briggs, J.D., Dominiczak, A.F., *et al.* (1986). Intravascular haemolysis and acute renal failure induced by nomifensine. *Scott. Med. J.* 31, 242.

Furman, K.I., Galasko, G.T.F., Meyers, A.M., *et al.* (1976). Post-transplantation analgesic dependence in patients who formerly suffered from analgesic nephropathy. *Clin. Nephrol.* 5, 54.

Gabriel, R., Caldwell, J., and Hartley, R.B. (1982). Acute tubular necrosis, caused by therapeutic doses of paracetamol? *Clin. Nephrol.* 18, 269.

Gaffey, C.M., Chun, B., Harvey, J.C., *et al.* (1986). Phenytoin-induced systemic granulomatous vasculitis. *Arch. Pathol. Lab. Med.* 110, 131.

Galea, E.G., Young, L.N., and Bell, J.R. (1963). Fatal nephropathy due to phenindione sensitivity. *Lancet* i, 920.

Galpin, J.E., Friedman, G.S., Shinaberger, J.H., *et al.* (1975). Acute interstitial nephritis due to methicillin and similar drugs. *Kidney Int.* 8, 411.

Gary, N.E., Dodelson, R., and Eisinger R.P. (1980). Indomethacin-associated renal failure. *Am. J. Med.* 69, 135.

Gaskin, G., Thompson, E.M., and Pusey, C.D. (1995). Goodpasture-like syndrome associated with anti-myeloperoxidase antibodies following penicillamine treatment. *Nephrol. Dial. Transplant.* 10, 1925.

Gault, M.H., Rudwal, T.C., Engles, W.D., *et al.* (1968). Syndrome associated with the abuse of analgesics. *Ann. Intern. Med.* 68, 906.

Gavish, D., Knobler, H., Gottehrer, N., *et al.* (1986). Methemoglobinemia, muscle damage and renal failure complicating phenazopyridine overdose. *Isr. J. Med. Sci.* 22, 45.

Gelbart, D.R., Weinstein, A.B., and Fajardo, L.F. (1977). Allopurinol induced interstitial nephritis. *Ann. Intern. Med.* 86, 196.

Gelford, G.J. and Cromwell, D.K. (1968). Methysergide retroperitoneal fibrosis and retrosigmoid stricture. *AJR* 104, 566.

Geller, R.J., Chevalier, R.L., and Spyker, D.A. (1986). Acute amoxicillin nephrotoxicity following an overdose. *Clin. Toxicol.* 24, 175.

Gerhardt, R.E., Hudson, J.B., Rao, R.N., *et al.* (1978). Chronic renal insufficiency induced by arsenic poisoning. *Arch. Intern. Med.* 138, 1267.

Gerkens, J.F. and Smith, A.J. (1985). Effects of captopril and theophylline on cyclosporine-induced nephrotoxicity in rats. *Transplantation* 40, 213.

Gerritsen van der Hoop, R., Vecht, C.J., van der Burg, M.E.L., *et al.* (1990). Prevention of cisplatin neurotoxicity with an ACTH (4-9) analogue in patients with ovarian cancer. *N. Engl. J. Med.* 322, 89.

Gibb, W.R.G. and Shaw, I.C. (1985). Myoglobinuria due to heroin abuse. *J. R. Coll. Med.* 78, 862.

Gilbert, R, Cassidy, M.J.D., and Kahn D. (1995). Clonidine and cyclosporine. *Nephron* 71, 105.

Gimenez, A. and Mampaso, F. (1986). Characterization of inflammatory cells in drug-induced tubulointerstitial nephritis. *Nephron* 43, 239.

Giraud, P., Casson, M., Paul, R., *et al.* (1982). Toxicité musculaire due au fénofibrate: à propos d'un cas. *Rev. Rheum.* 49, 162.

The Gisen Group (1997). Randomized placebo-controlled trial of effect of ramipril on decline in glomerular filtration rate and risk of terminal renal failure in proteinuric, non-diabetic nephropathy. *Lancet* 349, 1857.

Gitlin, M.J. (1993). Lithium-induced renal insufficiency. *J. Clin. Psychopharmacol.* 13, 276.

Giustina, A., Romanelli, G., Cimino, A., *et al.* (1988). Low-dose acyclovir and acute renal failure. *Ann. Intern. Med.* 108, 312.

Glassock, R.J., Adler, S.G., Ward, H.J., *et al.* (1986). Primary glomerular diseases. In *The Kidney* Vol. 1 (3rd edn) (ed. B.M. Brenner and F.C. Rector), p. 929. W.B. Saunders, Philadelphia.

Gloor, F.J. (1965). Some morphologic features of chronic interstitial nephritis (chronic pyelonephritis) in patients with analgesic abuse. In *Progress in Pyelonephritis* (ed. E.H. Kass), p. 287. Davis, Philadelphia.

Gloor, F.J. (1974). Unsere heutigen Vorstellungen über die Morphologie und Pathogenese der Analgetika-Nephropathie. *Schweiz. Med. Wochenschr.* 104, 785.

Gloor, F.J. (1978). Changing concepts in pathogenesis and morphology of analgesic nephropathy as seen in Europe. *Kidney Int.* 13, 27.

Goebel, K.M. and Mueller-Brodmann, W. (1982). Reversible overt nephropathy with Henoch–Schönlein purpura due to piroxicam. *BMJ* 284, 311.

Goette, D.K. and Beatrice, E. (1988). Erythema annulare centrifugum caused by hydrochlorothiazide-induced interstitial nephritis. *Int. J. Dermatol.* 27, 129.

Goldberg, H.J., Wong, P.Y., Cole, E.H., *et al.* (1989). Dissociation between the immunosuppressive activity of cyclosporine derivatives and their effects on intracellular calcium signaling in mesangial cells. *Transplantation* 47, 731.

Goldstein, D.J., Zuech, N., Sehgal, V., *et al.* (1997). Cyclosporine-associated end-stage nephropathy after cardiac transplantation. Incidence and progression. *Transplantation* 63, 664.

Goldstein, E.J., Feinfeld, D.A., Fleischner, *et al.* (1976). Enzymatic evidence of renal tubular damage following renal angiography. *Radiology* 121, 617.

Gomes, A.S., Baker, J.D., Martin-Paredero, V., *et al.* (1985). Acute renal dysfunction after major arteriography. *AJR* 145, 1249.

Gomez, A., Martos, F., Garcia, R., *et al.* (1989). Diltiazem enhances gentamicin nephrotoxicity in rats. *Pharmacol. Toxicol.* 64, 190.

Gordon, J.A. and Gattone, V.H. (1986). Mitochondrial alterations in cisplatin-induced acute renal failure. *Am. J. Physiol.* 250, F991.

Gorriz, J.L., Sancho, A., Alcoy, E., *et al.* (1995). Rhabdomyolysis and acute renal failure associated with bezafibrate treatment. *Nephrol. Dial. Transplant.* 10, 2371.

Gorriz, J.L., Sancho, A., Lopez-Martin, J.M., *et al.* (1996). Rhabdomyolysis and acute renal failure associated with gemfibrozil therapy. *Nephron* 74, 437.

Gottschall, J.L., Elliot, W., Llanos, E., *et al.* (1991). Thrombocytopenia associated with hemolytic uremic syndrome: a new clinical entity. *Blood* 77, 306.

Goyer, R.A. (1989). Mechanisms of lead and cadmium nephrotoxicity. *Toxicol. Lett.* 46, 153.

Graber, C.D., Patrick, C.C., and Galphin, R.L. (1975). Light chain proteinuria and cellular mediated immunity in rifampin treated patients with tuberculosis. *Chest* 67, 408.

Graham, J.R. (1964). Methysergide for prevention of headache: experience in five hundred patients over three years. *N. Engl. J. Med.* 270, 67.

Graham, J.R., Sury, H.I., LeCompte, P.R., *et al.* (1966). Fibrotic disorders associated with methysergide therapy for headache. *N. Engl. J. Med.* 274, 359.

Grant, D., Rochon, J., and Levy, G. (1996). Comparison of the long-term tolerability, pharmacodynamics, and safety of Sandimmune and Neoral in liver transplant recipients. *Transplant. Proc.* 28, 2232.

Graybill, J.R. (1996). Lipid formulations of amphotericin B. Does the emperor need clothes? *Ann. Intern. Med.* 124, 921.

Greenberg, A., Egel, J.W., Thompson, M.E., *et al.* (1987). Early and late forms of cyclosporine nephrotoxicity: studies in cardiac transplant recipients. *Am. J. Kidney Dis.* 9, 12.

Grimm, P.C., Ogborn, M.R., Larson, A.J., *et al.* (1989). Interstitial nephritis induced by cloxacillin. *Nephron* 51, 285.

Grino, J.M., Sabate, I., Castelao, A.M., *et al.* (1986). Erythromycin and cyclosporine. *Ann. Intern. Med.* 105, 467.

Grond, J., Koudstaal, J., and Elema, J.D. (1985). Mesangial function and glomerular sclerosis in rats with aminonucleoside nephrosis. *Kidney Int.* 27, 405.

Grufferman, S., Morris, D., and Alvarez, J. (1985). Methanol poisoning complicated by myoglobinuric renal failure. *Am. J. Emerg. Med.* 3, 24.

Gutman, A.B. and Yu, T.F. (1968). Uric acid nephrolithiasis. *Am. J. Med.* 45, 756.

Haapanen, E., Pellinen, T.J., and Partanen, J. (1984). Acute renal failure caused by alcohol-induced rhabdomyolysis. *Nephron* 36, 191.

Hakim, R., Tolis, G., Goltzman, D., *et al.* (1979). Severe hypercalcaemia associated with hydrochlorothiazide and calcium carbonate therapy. *Can. Med. Assoc. J.* 121, 591.

Hall, B.M., Tiller, D.J., Duggin, G.G., *et al.* (1985). Post-transplant acute renal failure in cadaver renal recipients treated with cyclosporine. *Kidney Int.* 28, 178.

Halla, J.T., Cassidy, J., and Hardin, J.G. (1982). Sequential gold and penicillamine therapy in rheumatoid arthritis. Comparative study of effectiveness and toxicity and review of the literature. *Am. J. Med.* 72, 423.

Hamblin, T.J. (1990). Interleukin 2. *BMJ* 300, 275.

Hampel, G., Horskotte, H., and Rumpf, K.W. (1983). Myoglobinuric renal failure due to drug-induced rhabdomyolysis. *Hum. Toxicol.* 2, 197.

Handa, S.P. and Tewari, H.D. (1981). Urinary tract carcinoma in patients with analgesic nephropathy. *Nephron* 28, 62.

Harkness, J.A.L. and Blake, D.R. (1982). Penicillamine nephropathy and iron. *Lancet* ii, 1368.

Harkonen, S. and Kjellstrand, C.M. (1979). Intravenous pyelography in nonuremic diabetic patients. *Nephron* 24, 268.

Harris, K.P., Jenkins, D., and Walls, J. (1988). Nonsteroidal antiinflammatory drugs and cyclosporine: a potentially serious adverse interaction. *Transplantation* 46, 598.

Hartman, G.W., Torres, V.E., Leago, G.F., *et al.* (1984). Analgesic-associated nephropathy. *JAMA* 251, 1734.

Harvald, B. (1968). Renal papillary necrosis. A clinical survey of sixty-six cases. *Am. J. Med.* 35, 481.

Harvald, B., Valdorf-Hansen, F., and Nielsen, A. (1960). Effect on the kidney of drugs containing phenacetin. *Lancet* i, 303.

Hauser, A.C., Derfler, K., Stockenhuber, F., *et al.* (1990). Post-transplantation malignant disease in patients with analgesic nephropathy. *Lancet* 335, 58.

Hawker, F., Pearson, I.Y., Soni, N., *et al.* (1985). Rhabdomyolytic renal failure and suxamethonium. *Anaesth. Intens. Care* 13, 208.

Hayes, D.M., Cvitkovic, E., Golbey, R.B., *et al.* (1977). High dose cis-platinum diammine dichloride: amelioration of renal toxicity by mannitol diuresis. *Cancer* 39, 1372.

Heitzman, E.J., Patterson, J.F., and Stanley, M.M. (1962). Myoglobinuria and hypokalemia in regional enteritis. *Arch. Intern. Med.* 110, 117.

Hensen, J., Haenelt, M., and Gross P. (1996). Lithium induced polyuria and renal vasopressin receptor density. *Nephrol. Dial. Transpl.* 11, 622.

Hertz, P., Yager, H., and Richardson, J.A. (1972). Probenecid-induced nephrotic syndrome. *Arch. Pathol.* 94, 241.

Hess, E. (1988). Drug-related lupus. *N. Engl. J. Med.* 318, 1460.

Hibi, S., Misawa, A., Tamai M., *et al.* (1995). Severe rhabdomyolysis associated with tacrolimus. *Lancet* 346, 702.

Hindle, W., Posner, E., Sweetnam, M.T., *et al.* (1970). Pleural effusion and fibrosis during treatment with methysergide. *BMJ* i, 605.

Hoffman, B.J. (1945). Sensitivity to sulfadiazine resembling acute disseminated lupus erythematosus. *Arch. Dermatol. Syph.* 51, 190.

Hogg, K.J. and Hillis, W.S. (1986). Captopril/metolazone induced renal failure. *Lancet* i, 501.

Hogg, R.J., Sawyer, M., Hecox, K., *et al.* (1981). Carbamazepine-induced acute tubulointerstitial nephritis. *J. Pediatr.* 98, 830.

Hojs, R. and Sinkovic, A. (1992). Rhabdomyolysis and acute renal failure following methadone abuse. *Nephron* 62, 362.

Holm, E.A., Randlov, A., and Strandgaard, S. (1996). Brief report: acute renal failure after losartan treatment in a patient with bilateral renal artery stenosis. *Blood Pressure* 5, 360.

Holm, S.E., Hill, B., Lowestad, R., *et al.* (1983). A prospective randomised study of amikacin and gentamicin in serious infections with focus on efficacy, toxicity and duration of serum levels above the MIC. *J. Antimicrob. Chemother.* 12, 393.

Holt, D.W., Marsden, J.T., Johnston, A., *et al.* (1986). Blood cyclosporin concentrations and renal allograft dysfunction. *BMJ* 293, 1057.

Holtas, S. (1978). Proteinuria following nephroangiography. Thesis. Malmo General Hospital, Malmö, Sweden.

Holtzman, N.A., Elliott, D.A., and Heller, R.H. (1966). Copper intoxication. *N. Engl. J. Med.* 275, 347.

Honkanen, E., Tornroth, T., Pettersson, E., *et al.* (1987). Membranous glomerulonephritis in rheumatoid arthritis not related to gold or D-penicillamine therapy: a report of four cases and review of the literature. *Clin. Nephrol.* 27, 87.

Hooke, D., Walker, R.G., Walter, N.M.A., *et al.* (1982). Repeated renal failure with use of captopril in a cystinotic renal allograft recipient. *BMJ* 285, 1538.

Horgan, K.J., Ottaviano, Y.L., and Watson, A.J. (1989). Acute renal failure due to mannitol intoxication. *Am. J. Nephrol.* 9, 106.

Hostetter, A.L., Tubbs, R.R., Ziegler, T., *et al.* (1987). Chronic glomerular microangiopathy complicating metastatic carcinoma. *Hum. Pathol.* 18, 342.

Houghton, D.C., English, J., and Bennett, W.M. (1988). Chronic tubulointerstitial nephritis and renal insufficiency associated with long-term 'subtherapeutic' gentamicin. *J. Lab. Clin. Med.* 112, 694.

Howard, T., Hoy, R.H., Warren, S., *et al.* (1981). Acute renal dysfunction due to sulfinpyrazone therapy in post myocardial infarction cardiomegaly: reversible hypersensitive interstitial nephritis. *Am. Heart J.* 102, 294.

Hows, J.M., Chipping, P.M., Fairhead, S., *et al.* (1983). Nephrotoxicity in bone marrow transplant recipients treated with cyclosporin A. *Br. J. Haematol.* 54, 69.

Hricik, D.E. (1985). Captopril-induced renal insufficiency and the role of sodium balance. *Ann. Intern. Med.* 103, 222.

Huggon, I., James, I., and Macrae, D. (1990). Hyperosmolality related to propylene glycol in an infant treated with enoximone infusion. *BMJ* 301, 19.

Hultengren, N. (1961). Renal papillary necrosis. A clinical study of 103 cases. *Acta Chir. Scand.* (suppl. 277).

Hultman, P. and Enestrom, S. (1986). Localization of mercury in the kidney during experimental acute tubular necrosis studied by the cytochemical silver amplification method. *Br. J. Exp. Pathol.* 67, 493.

Hurault de Ligny, B., Ryckelynck, J.P., Levaltier B., *et al.* (1986). Néphropathie interstitielle avec syndrome néphrotique induite par le pirprofène. *Rev. Méd. Interne* 7, 525.

Hussain, S.P. and Drew, P.J.T. (1989). Acute renal failure after infusion of gelatins. *BMJ* 299, 1137.

Hyman, R.L., Ballow, M., and Knieser, M.R. (1978). Diphenylhydantoin interstitial nephritis. Roles of cellular and humoral immunological injury. *J. Pediatr.* 92, 915.

Iesato, K., Mori, Y., Ueda, S., *et al.* (1982). Renal tubular dysfunction as a complication of gold therapy in patients with rheumatoid arthritis. *Clin. Nephrol.* 17, 46.

Ihle, B.U., Byrnes, C.A., and Simenhoff, M.L. (1982). Acute renal failure due to interstitial nephritis resulting from radio contrast agents. *Aust. N.Z. J. Med.* 12, 630.

Imai, H., Nakamoto, Y., Hirokawa, M., *et al.* (1989). Carbamazepine-induced granulomatous necrotizing angiitis with acute renal failure. *Nephron* 51, 405.

Jain, S. and Seymour, A.E. (1987). Mitomycin C associated hemolytic uremic syndrome. *Pathology* 19, 58.

Jablonski, P., Harrison, C., Howden, B., *et al.* (1986). Cyclosporine and the ischemic rat kidney. *Transplantation* 41, 147.

Jandreski, M.A., Bermes, E.W., Leischner, R., *et al.* (1989). Rhabdomyolysis in a case of free-base cocaine ('crack') overdose. *Clin. Chem.* 35, 1547.

Jarzobski, J., Ferry, J., Wombolt, D., *et al.* (1970). Vasculitis with allopurinol therapy. *Am. Heart J.* 79, 116.

Jennings, A.E., Levy, A.S., and Harrington, J.T. (1983). Amoxapine-associated acute renal failure. *Arch. Intern. Med.* 143, 1525.

Jennings, M., Shortland, J.R., and Maddocks, J.L. (1986). Interstitial nephritis associated with frusemide. *J. R. Soc. Med.* 79, 239.

Joh, K., Shibasaki, T., Azuma, T., *et al.* (1989). Experimental drug-induced allergic nephritis mediated by antihapten antibody. *Int. Arch. Allergy Appl. Immunol.* 88, 337.

Johnson, A.G., Seidemann, P., and Day, R.O. (1994). NSAID-related adverse drug interactions with clinical relevance. An update. *Int. J. Clin. Pharmacol. Ther.* 32, 509.

Johnson, J.N. and McFarland, J.B. (1980). Retroperitoneal fibrosis associated with atenolol. *BMJ* 280, 864.

Jones, T.W., Chorpa, S., Kaufman, J.S., (1985). Cis-diamminedichloroplatinum (II)-induced acute renal failure in the rat: enzyme histochemical studies. *Toxicol. Pathol.* 13, 296.

Kaden, W.S. and Friedman, E.A. (1961). Obstructive uropathy complicating anticoagulant therapy. *N. Engl. J. Med.* 265, 283.

Kahan, B.D. (1989). Drug therapy: Cyclosporine. *N. Engl. J. Med.* 321, 1725.

Kahlmeter, G. and Dahlager, J. (1984). Aminoglycoside toxicity — a review of clinical studies published between 1975 and 1982. *J. Antimicrob. Chemother.* 13, 9A.

Kaloyanides, G.J. (1992). Drug–phosphlipid interactions: role in aminoglycoside nephrotoxicity. *Renal Failure* 14, 251.

Kanazi, G., Stowe, N., Steinmuller, D., *et al.* (1986). Effect of cyclosporine upon the function of ischemically damaged kidneys in the rat. *Transplantation* 41, 782.

Kanfer, A., Richet, G., Roland, J., *et al.* (1979). Extreme hyperphosphataemia causing acute anuric nephrocalcinosis in lymphosarcoma. *Br. Med. J.* i, 1320.

Kasanen, A. (1973). The effect of the restriction of the sale of phenacetin on the incidence of papillary necrosis established at autopsy. *Ann. Clin. Res.* 5, 369.

Katari, S.R., Magnone, M., Shapiro, R., *et al.* (1997). Clinical features of acute reversible tacrolimus (FK 506) nephrotoxicity in kidney transplant recipients. *Clinical Transplantation* 11, 237.

Katz, C.M. and Tzagournis, M. (1972). Chronic adult hypervitaminosis A with hypercalcaemia. *Metabolism* 21, 1171.

Katz, M.D. and Lor, E. (1986). Acute interstitial nephritis associated with intermittent rifampicin use. *Drug Intell. Clin. Pharm.* 20, 789.

Kaysen, G.A., Pond, S.M., Roper, M.H., *et al.* (1985). Combined hepatic and renal injury in alcoholics during therapeutic use of acetaminophen. *Arch. Intern. Med.* 145, 2019.

Keaton, M.R. (1988). Acute renal failure in an alcoholic during therapeutic acetaminophen ingestion. *South. Med. J.* 81, 1163.

Kendrick, W.C., Hull, A.R., and Knochel, J.P. (1977). Rhabdomyolysis and shock after intravenous amphetamine administration. *Ann. Intern. Med.* 86, 381.

Kennedy, A. and Saluga, P.G. (1970). Urinary cytology in experimental toxic renal injury. *Ann. Rheum. Dis.* 29, 546.

Kennedy, M.S., Deeg, H.J., Siegel, M., *et al.* (1983). Acute renal toxicity with combined use of amphotericin B and cyclosporin after marrow transplantation. *Transplantation* 35, 211.

Kerbel, N.C. (1967). Retroperitoneal fibrosis secondary to methysergide bimaleate. *Can. Med. Assoc. J.* 96, 1420.

Kho, T.L., Teule, J., Leunissen, K.M., *et al.* (1987). Nephrotoxic effect of cyclosporine A can be reversed by dopamine. *Transplant. Proc.* 19, 1749.

Kincaid-Smith, P., Nanra, R.S., and Fairley, K.F. (1971). Analgesic nephropathy: a recoverable form of chronic renal failure. In *Renal Infection and Renal Scarring* (ed. P. Kincaid-Smith and K.F. Fairley), p. 385. Mercedes Publishing Services, Melbourne.

Kiruluta, H.G. and Andrews, K. (1983). Urinary incontinence secondary to drugs. *Urology* 22, 88.

Kitahara, T., Hiromura, K., Maezawa, A., *et al.* (1997). Case of propylthiouracil-induced vasculitis associated with anti-neutrophil cytoplasmic antibody (ANCA); review of the literature. *Clin. Nephrol.* 47, 336.

Klotman, P.E., Boatman, J.E., Vlopp, B.D., *et al.* (1985). Captopril enhances aminoglycoside toxicity in potassium-depleted rats. *Kidney Int.* 28, 118.

Kogan, A. and Orenstein, S. (1990). Lovastatin-induced acute rhabdomyolysis. *Postgrad. Med. J.* 66, 294.

Kolkin, S., Nahman, N.S. Jr, and Mendell, J.R. (1987). Chronic nephrotoxicity complicating cyclosporine treatment of chronic inflammatory demyelinating polyradiculoneuropathy. *Neurology* 37, 147.

Krikler, D.M. (1967). Paracetamol and the kidney. *BMJ* ii, 615.

Kumar, S. and Muchmore, A. (1990). Tamm–Horsfall protein — uromodulin (1950–1990). *Kidney Int.* 37, 1395.

Kumar, S., Mehta, J.A., and Trivedi, H.L. (1976). Light chain proteinuria and reversible renal failure in rifampicin-treated patients with tuberculosis. *Chest* 70, 564.

Kurtz, A., Della Bruna, R., and Kühn, K. (1988). Cyclosporine A enhances renin secretion and production in isolated juxtaglomerular cells. *Kidney Int.* 33, 947.

Laakso, M., Arvala, I., Tervonen, S., *et al.* (1982). Retroperitoneal fibrosis associated with sotalol. *BMJ* 285, 1085.

Lachaal, M. and Venuto, R.C. (1989). Nephrotoxicity and hyperkalemia in patients with acquired immunodeficiency syndrome treated with pentamidine. *Am. J. Med.* 87, 260.

Ladd, A.T. (1962). Procainamide-induced lupus erythematosus. *N. Engl. J. Med.* 267, 1357.

Landgrebe, A.R., Nyhan, W.L., and Coleman, M. (1975). Urinary tract stones resulting from the excretion of oxypurinol. *N. Engl. J. Med.* 292, 626.

Lang, E.K. (1985). Streptokinase therapy: complications of intra-arterial use. *Radiology* 154, 75.

Langer, T. and Levy, R.I. (1968). Acute muscular syndrome associated with administration of clofibrate. *N. Engl. J. Med.* 279, 856.

Langhoff, E. and Madsen, S. (1983). Rapid metabolism of cyclosporin and prednisone in kidney transplant patient receiving tuberculostatic treatment. *Lancet* ii, 1031.

Larsen, K. and Møller, C.E. (1959). A renal lesion caused by abuse of phenacetin. *Acta Med. Scand.* 164, 53.

Larsson, R., Bodemar, G., Kagedal, B., *et al.* (1980). The effects of cimetidine on renal function in patients with renal failure. *Acta Med. Scand.* 208, 27.

Laskin, O.L. (1984). Acyclovir. Pharmacology and clinical experience. *Arch. Intern. Med.* 144, 1241.

Laurent, G., Yernaux, V., Nonclercq, D., *et al.* (1988). Tissue injury and proliferative response induced in rat kidney by cis-diamminedichloroplatinum (II). *Virchows Arch. B.* 55, 129.

Lauwerys, R., Bernard, A., Viau, C., *et al.* (1985). Kidney disorders and hematotoxicity from organic solvent exposure. *Scand. J. Work Environ. Health.* 11 (suppl 1), 83.

Lavender, S., Brown, J.N., and Berrill, W.T. (1973). Acute renal failure and lithium intoxication. *Postgrad. Med. J.* 49, 277.

Lee, H.A. and Holden, C.E.A. (1964). Phenindione nephropathy with recovery: studies of morphology and renal function. *Postgrad. Med. J.* 40, 326.

Lee, J.C., Dushkin, M., Eyring, E.J., *et al.* (1965). Renal lesions associated with gold therapy: light and electron microscopic studies. *Arthritis Rheum.* 8, 1.

Lee, S.C., Abe, T., and Sato, T. (1987). Rhabdomyolysis and acute renal failure following use of succinylcholine and enflurane: report of a case. *J. Oral Maxillofac. Surg.* 45, 789.

Lee, S.M., Williams, R., Warnock, D., *et al.* (1986). The effects of nicardipine in hypertensive subjects with impaired renal function. *Br. J. Clin. Pharmacol.* 22, 297S.

Lehmann, H., Hirsch, U., Bauer, E., *et al.* (1996). Studies on the chronic oral toxicity of an analgesic drug combination consisting of acetylsalicylic acid, paracetamol and caffeine in rats including an electron microscopical evaluation of kidneys. *Arzneimittelforschung* 46, 895.

Leimenstoll, G., Schlegelberger, T., and Fulde, R. (1988). Interaction of cyclosporine and ethambutol–isoniazide. *Dtsch. Med. Wochenschr.* 113, 514.

Lele, P., Peterson, P., Yang, S., *et al.* (1985). Cyclosporine and Tegretol — another drug interaction. *Kidney Int.* 27, 344.

Lepage-Savary, D. and Vallières, A. (1982). Ergotamine as a possible cause of retroperitoneal fibrosis. *Clin. Pharm.* 1, 179.

Lerner, A.M., Reyes, M.P., Cone, L.A., *et al.* (1983). Randomised controlled trial of the comparative efficacy, auditory toxicity and nephrotoxicity of tobramycin and netilmicin. *Lancet* i, 1123.

Lewis, J.A. and Rindone, J.P. (1987). Acute interstitial nephritis associated with cephapirin. *Drug. Intell. Clin. Pharm.* 21, 380.

Lin, C.Y. and Chiang, H. (1988). Sodium valproate-induced interstitial nephritis. *Nephron* 48, 43.

Lindeneg, O., Fischer, S., Pedersen, J., *et al.* (1959). Necrosis of the renal papillae and prolonged abuse of phenacetin. *Acta Med. Scand.* 165, 321.

Lindvall, N. (1960). Renal papillary necrosis. A roentgenographic study of 155 cases. *Acta Radiol.* (suppl. 192).

Lindvall, N. (1978). Radiological changes of renal papillary necrosis. *Kidney Int.* 13, 93.

Ling, B.N., Bourke, E., Campbell, W.G. Jr, *et al.*(1990). Naproxen-induced nephropathy in systemic lupus erythematosus. *Nephron* 54, 249.

Linton, A.L., Clark, W.F., Driedger, A.A. (1980). Acute interstitial nephritis due to drugs. Review of the literature with a report of nine cases. *Ann. Intern. Med.* 93, 735.

Lombard, J., Levin, I.H., and Weiner, W.J. (1989). Arsenic intoxication in a cocaine abuser. *N. Engl. J. Med.* 320, 869.

Lowe, M.B. and Tapp, E. (1966). Renal damage caused by anhydro 4-EPI-tetracycline. *Arch. Pathol.* 81, 362.

Lucena, M.I., Gonzalez-Correa, J.A., and Andrade, R.J. (1989). Enhanced gentamicin nephrotoxicity after experimental biliary obstruction in rats. *Pharmacol. Toxicol.* 65, 352.

Luft, F.C., Yum, M.N., Walker, P.D., *et al.* (1977). Gentamicin gradient patterns and morphological changes in human kidneys. *Nephron* 18, 167.

Lunde, P.K.M., Frislid, K., and Hansteen, V. (1977). Disease and acetylation polymorphism. *Clin. Pharmacokinet.* 2, 182.

Lynn, K.L., Bailey, R.R., Swainson, C.P., *et al.* (1985). Renal failure with potassium-sparing diuretics. *N.Z. Med. J.* 98, 629.

Mabeck, C.E. and Wichmann, B. (1979). Mortality from chronic interstitial nephritis and phenacetin consumption in Denmark. *Acta Med. Scand.* 205, 599.

McAuley, F.T., Whiting, P.H., Thomson, A.W., *et al.* (1987). The influence of enalapril or spironolactone on experimental cyclosporin nephrotoxicity. *Biochem. Pharmacol.* 36, 699.

McCauley, J., Bronsther, O., Fung, J., *et al.* (1989). Treatment of cyclosporin-induced haemolytic uraemic syndrome with FK506. *Lancet* ii, 1516.

McCluskey, D., Donaldson, R.A., and McGeown, M.G. (1980). Oxprenolol and retroperitoneal fibrosis. *BMJ* 281, 1459.

McDermott, W. (1947). Toxicity of streptomycin. *Am. J. Med.* 2, 491.

Macdonald, J.B., Jones, H.M., and Cowan, R.A. (1985). Rhabdomyolysis and acute renal failure after theophylline overdose. *Lancet* i, 932.

MacKay (1997). Membranous nephropathy associated with the use of flurbiprofen. *Clin. Nephrol.* 47, 279.

McLeish, K.R., Senitzer, D., and Gohara, A.F. (1979). Acute interstitial nephritis in a patient with aspirin hypersensitivity. *Clin. Immunol. Immunopathol.* 14, 64.

Mahan, J.D., Sisson-Ross, S., and Vernier, R.L. (1986). Glomerular basement membrane anionic charge site changes early in aminonucleoside nephrosis. *Am. J. Pathol.* 125, 393.

Maher, J.F., Raith, C.E., and Schreiner, G.E. (1969). Hyperuricemia complicating leukemia. Treatment with allopurinol and dialysis. *Arch. Intern. Med.* 123, 198.

Mailloux, L., Swartzschwarz, C.D., Capizzi, R., *et al.* (1967). Acute renal failure after administration of low-molecular-weight dextran. *N. Engl. J. Med.* 277, 1113.

Maisel, J.C. and Priest, R.E. (1964). Fatal phenacetin nephritis. *Arch. Pathol.* 77, 646.

Makowka, L., Lopatin, W., Gilas, T., *et al.* (1986). Prevention of cyclosporine (Cya) nephrotoxicity by synthetic prostaglandins. *Clin. Nephrol.* 25 (Suppl. 1), S89.

Malaquin, F., Urban, T., Ostinelli, J., *et al.* (1989). Pleural and retroperitoneal fibrosis from dihydroergotamine. *N. Engl. J. Med.* 321, 1760.

Mallion, J.M. and Goldberg, A.I. (1996). Global efficacy and tolerability of losartan, an angiotensin II subtype 1-receptor antagonist, in the treatment of hypertension. *Blood Press.* (Suppl. 2), 82.

Malone, D.N.S. and Horn, D.B. (1971). Acute hypercalcaemia and renal failure after antacid therapy. *BMJ* i, 709.

Marais, G.E. and Larson, K.K. (1990). Rhabdomyolysis and acute renal failure induced by combination lovastatin and gemfibrozil therapy. *Ann. Intern. Med.* 112, 228.

Marasco, W.A., Gikas, P.W., Azziz-Baumgartner, R., *et al.* (1987). Ibuprofen-associated renal dysfunction. Pathophysiologic mechanisms of acute renal failure, hyperkalemia, tubular necrosis, and proteinuria. *Arch. Intern. Med.* 147, 2107.

Margolis, D., Ross, E., and Miller, K.B. (1987). Rhabdomyolysis associated with high-dose cytarabine. *Cancer Treat. Rep.* 71, 1325.

Markman, M., Cleary, S., and Howell, S.B. (1985). Nephrotoxicity of high-dose intracavitary cisplatin with intravenous thiosulfate protection. *Eur. J. Cancer Clin. Oncol.* 21, 1015.

Marples, D., Christensen, S., Christensen, E.L., *et al.* (1995). Lithium-induced downregulation of aquaporin-2 water channel expression in rat kidney medulla. *J. Clin. Invest.* 95, 1838.

Martinez-Maldonado, M. and Terrell, J. (1973). Lithium carbonate induced nephrogenic diabetes insipidus and glucose intolerance. *Arch. Intern. Med.* 132, 881.

Marty, M., Poullart, P., Scholl, S., *et al.* (1990). Comparison of the 5-hydroxytryptamine$_3$ (serotonin) antagonist ondansetron (GR 38032F) with high-dose metoclopramide in the control of cisplatin-induced emesis. *N. Engl. J. Med.* 322, 816.

Masters, D.R. (1973). Analgesic nephropathy associated with paracetamol. *Proc. R. Soc. Med.* 66, 36.

Matousovic, K., Elseviers, M.M., Devecka, D., *et al.* (1996). Incidence of analgesic nephropathy among patients undergoing renal replacement therapy in Czech republic and Slovak republic. *Nephrol. Dial. Transplant.* 11, 1048.

Matsuda, O., Beck, F.X., Dorge, A., et al. (1988). Electrolyte composition of renal tubular cells in gentamicin nephrotoxicity. Kidney Int. 33, 1107.

Matsumoto, J., Yasaka, T., Ohya, I., et al. (1985). Acute renal failure in primary macroglobulinemia with small-molecule IgM. Arch. Intern. Med. 145, 929.

Matzke, G.R. and Frye, R.F. (1997). Drug administration in patients with renal insufficiency. Minimising renal and extrarenal toxicity. Drug Saf. 16, 205.

Mavromatis, F. (1965). Tetracycline nephropathy. JAMA 193, 191.

Maxwell, D., Szwed, J.J., Wahle, W., et al. (1974). Ampicillin nephropathy. JAMA 230, 585.

May, D.C., Helderman, J.H., Eigenbrodt, E.H., et al. (1986). Chronic sclerosing glomerulopathy (heroin-associated nephropathy) in intravenous T's and Blues abusers. Am. J. Kidney Dis. 8, 404.

Mayaud, C., Kourilsky, D., Kanfer, A., et al. (1975). Interstitial nephritis after methicillin. N. Engl. J. Med. 292, 1132.

Medina, P.I., Mills, J., Leoung, G., et al. (1990). Oral therapy for pneumocystis pneumonia in the acquired immunodeficiency syndrome. N. Engl. J. Med. 323, 776.

Menashe, P.I. and Gottlieb, J.E. (1988). Hyperthermia, rhabdomyolysis, and myoglobinuric renal failure after recreational use of cocaine. South. Med. J. 81, 379.

Mendoza, F., Atiba, J., Kreusky, A., et al. (1987). Rhabdomyolysis complicating doxylamine overdose. Clin. Pediatr. 26, 595.

Menta, R., Rossi, E., Guariglia, A., et al. (1987). Reversible acute cyclosporin nephrotoxicity induced by colchicine administration. Nephrol. Dial. Transplant. 2, 380.

Mercieca, J. and Brown, E.A. (1984). Acute renal failure due to rhabdomyolysis associated with the use of a straitjacket in lysergide intoxication. BMJ 288, 1949.

Mergenthaler, H.G., Binsack, T., and Wilmanns, W. (1988). Carcinoma-associated hemolytic–uremic syndrome in a patient receiving 5-fluorouracil–adriamycin–mitomycin C combination chemotherapy. Oncology 45, 11.

Michaelson, J.H., McCoy, J.P. Jr, Hirszel, P. (1985). Mercury-induced autoimmune glomerulonephritis in inbred rats. I. Kinetics and species specificity of autoimmune responses. Surv. Synth. Pathol. Res. 4, 401.

Mignat, C. (1997). Clinically significant drug interactions with new immunosuppressive agents. Drug Saf. 16, 267.

Mihatsch, M.J. and Knusli, C. (1982). Phenacetin abuse and malignant tumours. An autopsy study covering 25 years (1953–1977). Klin. Wochenschr. 60, 1339.

Mihatsch, M.J., Hoper, H.O., Gudat, F., et al. (1983). Capillary sclerosis of the urinary tract and analgesic nephropathy. Clin. Nephrol. 20, 285.

Mihatsch, M.J., Thiel, G., and Ryffel, B. (1988a). Histopathology of cyclosporine nephrotoxicity. Transplant. Proc. 20, (Suppl. 3), 759.

Mihatsch, M.J., Steiner, K., Abeywickrama, K.H., et al. (1988b). Risk factors for the development of chronic cyclosporine-nephrotoxicity. Clin. Nephrol. 29, 165.

Mijares, R.P. (1986). Hypokalemic rhabdomyolysis secondary to pseudohyperaldosteronism due to the use of a lotion containing 9-α-fluoroprednisolone. Nephron 43, 232.

Miller, L., Pateras, V., Friederici, H., et al. (1985). Acute tubular necrosis after inhalation exposure to methylene chloride. Report of a case. Arch. Intern. Med. 145, 145.

Misch, K.A. (1974). Development of heart valve lesions during methysergide therapy. BMJ ii, 365.

Mitchell, A.B.S. (1971). Duogastrone-induced hypokalaemic nephropathy and myopathy with myoglobinuria. Postgrad. Med. J. 47, 807.

Mitchell, G., Wilken, R.J., and Dixon, P. (1965). Acute renal failure complicating lymphosarcoma. BMJ i, 567.

Mizutani, T., Oohashi, N., and Naito, H. (1989). Myoglobinemia and renal failure in toluene poisoning: a case report. Vet. Hum. Toxicol. 31, 448.

Moeschlin, von S. (1957). Phenacetinsucht und-schaden Innenkörpernamien und interstitielle Nephritis. Schweiz. Med. Wochenschr. 87, 123.

Molland, E.A. (1978). Experimental renal papillary necrosis. Kidney Int. 13, 5.

Mollman, J.E. (1990). Cisplatin neurotoxicity (Editorial). N. Engl. J. Med. 322, 126.

Monballyu, J., Zachee, P., Verberckmoes, R., et al. (1984). Transient acute renal failure due to tumour-lysis-induced severe phosphate load in a patient with Burkitt's lymphoma. Clin. Nephrol. 22, 47.

Monestier, M. and Kotzin, B.L. (1992). Antibodies to histones in systemic lupus erythematosus and drug-induced syndomes. Rheum. Dis. Clin. North Am. 18, 415.

Monteiro, J.L., Seguro, A.C., and Rocha, A. dos S. (1993). Acute nephrotoxicity caused by amphotericin B in the dog. Rev. Hosp. Clin. Fac. Med. Sao Paulo 48, 54.

Montoliu, J., Carrera, M., Darnell, A., et al. (1981). Lactic acidosis and Fanconi's syndrome due to degraded tetracycline. BMJ 283, 1576.

Moore, R.D., Smith, C.R., Lipsky, J.J., et al. (1984). Risk factors for nephrotoxicity in patients treated with aminoglycosides. Ann. Intern. Med. 100, 352.

Moran, M. and Kapsner, C. (1987). Acute renal failure associated with elevated plasma oncotic pressure, N. Engl. J. Med. 317, 150.

Morgan, T.O., Little, J.M., and Evans, W.A. (1966). Renal failure associated with low-molecular-weight dextran infusion. BMJ iii, 737.

Morrow, J.D., Schroeder, H.A., and Perry, H.M. Jr (1953). Studies on the control of hypertension by Hyphex. II. Toxic reactions and side effects. Circulation 8, 829.

Mraz, W., Sido, B., Knedeo, M., et al. (1987). Concomitant immunosuppressive and antibiotic therapy — reduction of cyclosporine A blood levels due to treatment with imipenem/cilastatin. Transplant. Proc. 19, 4017.

Muehrcke, R.C. and Pirani, C.L. (1968). Arsine-induced anuria. Ann. Intern. Med. 68, 853.

Muirhead, N., Hollomby, D.J., and Keown, P.A. (1987). Acute glomerular thrombosis with CsA treatment. Renal Failure 10, 135.

Murgo, A.J. (1987). Plasmapheresis and antiplatelet agents in the treatment of the hemolytic uremic syndrome secondary to mitomycin. *Am. J. Kidney Dis.* 9, 241.

Murray, A.N., Cassidy, M.J.D., and Templecamp, C. (1987). Rapidly progressive glomerulonephritis associated with rifampicin therapy for pulmonary tuberculosis. *Nephron* 46, 373.

Murray, B.M., Paller, M.S., and Ferris, T.F. (1985). Effect of cyclosporine administration on renal hemodynamics in conscious rats. *Kidney Int.* 28, 767.

Murray, R.M. (1972). Analgesic nephropathy: removal of phenacetin from proprietary analgesics. *BMJ* iv, 131.

Myers, B.D., Sibley, R., Newton, L., *et al.* (1988). The long-term course of cyclosporine-associated chronic nephropathy. *Kidney Int.* 33, 590.

Myers, G.H. and Witten, D.N. (1971). Acute renal failure after excretory urography in multiple myeloma. *AJR* 113, 583.

Nade, S. (1972). Acute urinary suppression presumed due to bilateral ureteric obstruction by blood clot. An unusual feature of anticoagulant therapy. *Med. J. Aust.* i, 378.

Nadel, S., Jackson, J., and Ploth, D. (1979). Hypokalemic rhabdomyolysis and acute renal failure. Occurrence following total parenteral nutrition. *JAMA* 241, 2294.

Nagai, T. and Nagai, T. (1987). Tubulointerstitial nephritis by Tamm–Horsfall glycoprotein or egg white component. *Nephron* 47, 134.

Nagata, N., Yoneyama, T., Yanagida, K., *et al.* (1985). Accumulation of germanium in the tissues of a long-term user of germanium preparation died of acute renal failure. *J. Toxicol. Sci.* 10, 333.

Nanra, R.S. and Kincaid-Smith, P. (1970). Papillary necrosis in rats caused by aspirin and aspirin-containing mixtures. *BMJ* iii, 559.

Nanra, R.S., Stuart-Taylor, J., de Leon, A.H., *et al.* (1978). Analgesic nephropathy: etiology, clinical syndrome and clinicopathologic correlations in Australia. *Kidney Int.* 13, 79.

Nessi, R., Bonoldi, G.L., Redaelli, B., *et al.* (1976). Acute renal failure after rifampicin: a case report and survey of the literature. *Nephron* 16, 148.

Neumayer, H.-H., Junge, W., Küfner, A., *et al.* (1989). Prevention of radiocontrast-media-induced nephrotoxicity by the calcium channel blocker nitrendipine: a prospective randomised clinical trial. *Nephrol. Dial. Transplant.* 4, 1030.

New Zealand Rheumatism Association Study. (1974). Aspirin and the kidney. *BMJ* i, 593.

NIH Consensus Conference. (1984). Analgesic associated kidney disease. *JAMA* 251, 3123.

Noels, L.M., Elseviers, M.M., and de Broe, M.E. (1995) Impact of legislative measures on the sales of analgesics and the subsequent prevalence of analgesic nephropathy: a comparative study in France, Sweden and Belgium. *Nephrol. Dial. Transplant.* 10, 167.

Nolan, C.R. and Kelleher, S.P. (1988). Eosinophiluria. *Clin. Lab. Med.* 8, 555.

Nordenfelt, O. (1972). Deaths from renal failure in abusers of phenacetin-containing drugs. *Acta Med. Scand.* 170, 385.

Nordenfelt, O. and Ringertz, N. (1961). Phenacetin takers dead with renal failure, 27 men and 3 women. *Acta Med. Scand.* 170, 385.

Novis, B.H., Korzets, Z., Chen, P., *et al.* (1988). Nephrotic syndrome after treatment with 5-aminosalicylic acid. *BMJ* 296, 1442.

Nowack, C., Garke-Nowack, F., Pretschner, D.P., *et al.* (1988). The engymetric determination of acute functional impairment in kidney graft function caused by cyclosporine A. *Nucl. Med. Commun.* 9, 389.

Nyberg, G., Blohme, I., Persson, H., *et al.* (1990). Foscarnet-induced tubulointerstitial nephritis in renal transplant patients. *Transplant. Proc.* 22, 241.

O'Brien, W.M. (1986). Adverse reactions to nonsteroidal anti-inflammatory drugs. Diclofenac compared with other non-steroidal anti-inflammatory drugs. *Am. J. Med.* 80, 70.

O'Donnell, D. (1988). Renal failure due to enalapril and captopril in bilateral renal artery stenosis: greater awareness needed. *Med. J. Aust.* 148, 525.

Offerman, J.J., Hollema, H., Elema, J.D., *et al.*(1985). TNO-6-induced acute renal failure. A case report. *Cancer* 56, 1511.

Ogihara, T. and Yoshinaga, K. (1996). The clinical efficacy and tolerability of the angiotensin II-receptor antagonist losartan in Japanese patients with hypertension. *Blood Pressure* (Suppl. 2), 78.

Oh, S.J., Douglas, J.E., and Brown, R.A. (1971). Hypokalemic vacuolar myopathy associated with chlorthalidone treatment. *JAMA* 216, 1858.

Oliveira, D.B., Foster, G., Savill, J., *et al.* (1987). Membranous nephropathy caused by mercury-containing skin lightening cream. *Postgrad. Med. J.* 63, 303.

Orchard, R.T. and Rooker, G. (1974). Penicillin hypersensitivity nephritis. *Lancet* i, 689.

Orlandini, G. and Garini, G. (1989). Phenytoin-induced nephrotic syndrome. *Nephron* 52, 109.

Oster, J.R. and Epstein, M. (1977). Demeclocycline-induced renal failure. *Lancet* i, 52.

Ostermann, M., Goldsmith, D.J., Doyle, T., *et al.* (1997). Reversible acute renal failure induced by losartan in a renal transplant recipient. *Postgrad. Med. J.* 73, 105.

Ozawa, T.T., Smith, P., Jr, Vance, D., *et al.* (1987). Acute interstitial nephritis induced by cimetidine. *J. Tenn. Med. Assoc.* 80, 411.

Pacifici, G.M., Viani, A., Franchi, M., *et al.* (1989). Profile of drug-metabolizing enzymes in the cortex and medulla of the human kidney. *Pharmacology* 39, 299.

Packer, M. (1989). Identification of risk factors predisposing to the development of functional renal insufficiency during treatment with converting-enzyme inhibitors in chronic heart failure. *Cardiology* 76 (suppl. 2), 50

Pahl, M.V., Barton, C.H., Ulich, T., *et al.* (1988). Renal dysfunction and microangiopathic changes in a renal transplant patient [clinical conference]. *Am. J. Nephrol.* 8, 72.

Palestine, A.G., Austin, H.A., and Nussenblatt, R.B. (1986). Renal tubular function in cyclosporine-treated patients. *Am. J. Med.* 81, 419.

Parfrey, P.S., Griffiths, S.M., Barrett, B.J., *et al.* (1989). Contrast material-induced renal failure in patients with diabetes mellitus, renal insufficiency, or both. A prospective controlled study. *N. Engl. J. Med.* 320, 143.

Parry, M.F., Ball, W., Conte, J.E., *et al.* (1973). Nafcillin nephritis. *JAMA* 225, 178.

Passfall, J., Schuller, I., and Keller, F. (1994). Pharmacokinetics of cyclosporin during administration of danazol. *Nephrol. Dial. Transpl.* 9, 1807.

Paul, M.D., Parfrey, P.S., Smart, M., *et al.* (1987). The effect of ethanol on serum cyclosporine A levels in renal transplant recipients. *Am. J. Kidney Dis.* 10, 133.

Pawel, B.R., Kaye, W.A., Khan, M.Y., *et al.* (1989). Aggravation of diabetic nephropathy by lithium: a case report and review of the literature. *J. Clin. Psychiatry* 50, 101.

Payne, S.T., Hosker, H.S.R., Allen, M.B., *et al.* (1989). Transient impairment of renal function after streptokinase therapy. *Lancet* ii, 1398.

Pazmino, P. (1988). Acute renal failure, skin rash, and eosinophilia associated with aztreonam. *Am. J. Nephrol.* 8, 68.

Peces, R., Riera, J.R., Arboleya, L.R., *et al.* (1987). Goodpasture's syndrome in a patient receiving penicillamine and carbimazole. *Nephron* 45, 316.

Pelletier, L., Pasquier, R., Vial, M.C., *et al.* (1987). Mercury-induced autoimmune glomerulonephritis: requirement for T-cells. *Nephrol. Dial. Transplant.* 1, 211.

Penney, M.D., Hullin, R.P., Srinivasan, D.P., *et al.* (1981). The relationship between plasma lithium and the renal responsiveness to arginine vasopressin in man. *Clin. Sci.* 61, 793.

Pepys, M.B. (1970). Acetazolamide and renal stone formation. *Lancet* ii, 837.

Perazella, M.A. and Mahnensmith, R.L. (1996). Trimethoprim–sulfamethoxazole hyperkalemia is an important complication regardless of dose. *Clin. Nephrol.* 46, 187.

Perico, N., Zoja, C., Benigni, A., *et al.* (1986). Renin–angiotensin system and glomerular prostaglandins in early nephrotoxicity of ciclosporin. *Contrib. Nephrol.* 51, 120.

Perks, W.H., Walters, E.H., Tams, I.P., *et al.* (1979). Demeclocycline in the treatment of the syndrome of inappropriate secretion of antidiuretic hormone. *Thorax* 34, 324.

Perneger, T.V., Whelton, P.K., and Klag, M.J. (1994). Risk of kidney failure associated with the use of acetominophen, aspirin, and nonsteroidal antiinflammatory drugs. *N. Engl. J. Med.* 331, 1675.

Pescovitz, M.D., Barone G., Choc M.G. Jr, *et al.* (1997). Safety and tolerability of cyclosporine microemulsion versus cyclosporine: two-year data in primary renal allograft recipients. A report of the Neoral Study Group. *Transplantation* 63, 778.

Petersen, K.C., Silberman, H., and Berne, T.V. (1984). Hyperkalaemia after cyclosporin therapy. *Lancet* i, 1470.

Peterson, O.W., Gabbai, F.B., and Myers, R.R. (1989). A single nephron model of acute tubular injury: role of tubuloglomerular feedback. *Kidney Int.* 36, 1037.

Pierce, J.R., Trostle, D.C., and Warner, J.J. (1981). Propranolol and retroperitoneal fibrosis. *Ann. Intern. Med.* 95, 244.

Pierce, L.R., Wysowski, D.K., and Gross, T.P. (1990). Myopathy and rhabdomyolysis associated with lovastatin–gemfibrozil combination therapy. *JAMA* 264, 71.

Pillans, P. and Hall, C. (1985). Paracetamol-induced acute renal failure in the absence of severe liver damage. *S. Afr. Med. J.* 67, 791.

Pohl, J.E.F., Thurston, H., and Swales, J.D. (1974). Hypertension with renal impairment: influence of intensive therapy. *Q. J. Med.* 43, 569.

Pommer, W., Krause, P.H., Berg, P.A., *et al.* (1986). Acute interstitial nephritis and non-oliguric renal failure after cefaclor treatment. *Klin. Wochenschr.* 64, 290.

Pommer, W., Bronder, E., Greiser, E., *et al.* (1989). Regular analgesic intake and the risk of end-stage renal failure. *Am. J. Nephrol.* 9, 403.

Powell, H.R., Davidson, P.M., McCredie, D.A., *et al.* (1988). Haemolytic–uraemic syndrome after treatment with metronidazole. *Med. J. Aust.* 149, 222.

Prati, R.C., Alfrey, A.C., and Hull, A.R. (1972). Spironolactone-induced hypercalciuria. *J. Lab. Clin. Med.* 80, 224.

Prescott, L.F. (1982). Analgesic nephropathy: a reassessment of the role of phenacetin and other analgesics. *Drugs* 23, 75.

Prescott, L.F., Illingworth, R.N., Critchley, J.A.J., *et al.* (1979). Intravenous *N*-acetylcysteine: the treatment of choice for paracetamol poisoning. *BMJ* ii, 1097.

Prisch, J.D., Miller, J., Deierhoi M.H., *et al.* (1997). A comparison of tacrolimus (FK506) and cyclosporine for immunosuppression after cadaveric renal transplantation. FK506 Kidney Transplant Group. *Transplantation* 63, 977.

Pryor, J.P., Castle, W.M., Dukes, D.C., *et al.* (1983). Do beta-adrenoceptor blocking drugs cause retroperitoneal fibrosis? *BMJ* 287, 639.

Pugliese, F. and Cinotti, G.A. (1997). Nonsteroidal anti-inflammatory drugs (NSAIDs) and the kidney. *Nephrol. Dial. Transplant.* 12, 386.

Pusey, C.D., Saltissi, D., Bloodworth, L., *et al.* (1983). Drug associated acute interstitial nephritis: clinical and pathological features and response to high dose steroid therapy. *Q. J. Med.* 52, 194.

Quin, J., Adamski, M., Howlin, K., *et al.* (1988). Quinidine-induced allergic granulomatous angiitis: an unusual cause of acute renal failure. *Med. J. Aust.* 148, 145.

Quinn, B.P. and Wall, B.M. (1989). Nephrogenic diabetes insipidus and tubulointerstitial nephritis during continuous therapy with rifampin. *Am. J. Kidney Dis.* 14, 217.

Ramada Benlloch, F.J., Gonzalvo Perez, V., Blasco Alfonso, E., *et al.* (1993). Urothelial carcinoma after treatment with cyclophosphamide. Review of the literature and presentation of our caseload. *Actas Urol. Esp.* 17, 139.

Randall, R.E., Osheroff, R.J., Bakerman, S., *et al.* (1972). Bismuth nephrotoxicity. *Ann. Intern. Med.* 77, 481.

Raz, S. (1974). Adrenergic influence on the internal sphincter. *Isr. J. Med.* 10, 608.

Reginster, F., Jadoul, M., and Ypersele de Strihou, C. (1997). Chinese herbs nephropathy presentation, natural history and fate after transplantation. *Nephrol. Dial. Transplant.* 12, 81.

Rehan, A. and Johnson, K. (1986). IgM nephropathy associated with penicillamine. *Am. J. Nephrol.* 6, 71.

Reid, G.M. and Muther, R.S. (1987). Nitroprusside-induced acute azotemia. *Am. J. Nephrol.* 7, 313.

Rello, J., Triginer, C., Sànchez, J.M., *et al.* (1989). Acute renal failure following massive mannitol infusion. *Nephron* 53, 377.

Remuzzi, G. and Bertani, T. (1989). Renal vascular and thrombotic effects of cyclosporine. *Am. J. Kidney Dis.* 13, 261.

Richman, A.V., Masco, H.L., Rifkin, S.I., *et al.* (1980). Minimal change disease and the nephrotic syndrome associated with lithium therapy. *Ann. Intern. Med.* 92, 70.

Richter, R.W., Challenor, Y.B., Pearson, J., *et al.* (1971). Acute myoglobinuria associated with heroin addiction. *JAMA* 216, 1172.

Riley, L.J. Jr, Vlasses, P.H., Rotmensch, H.H., *et al.* (1985). Sulindac and Ibuprofen inhibits furosemide-stimulated renin release but not natriuresis in men on a normal sodium diet. *Nephron* 41, 283.

Rimmer, E., Richens, A., Forster, M.E., *et al.* (1983). Retroperitoneal fibrosis associated with timolol. *Lancet* i, 300.

Robson, J.S., Martin, A.M., Ruckley, V.A., *et al.* (1968). Irreversible post-partum renal failure: a new syndrome. *Q. J. Med.* 37, 423.

Robson, M., Levi, J., Dolberg, L., *et al.* (1970). Acute tubulo-interstitial nephritis following sulfadiazine therapy. *Isr. J. Med. Sci.* 6, 561.

Roodhooft, A.M., Van-Dam, K., Haentjens, D., *et al.* (1990). Acute sodium valproate intoxication: occurrence of renal failure and treatment with haemoperfusion-haemodialysis. *Eur. J. Pediatr.* 149, 363.

Rosen, M. (1972). Acute urinary suppression presumed due to bilateral ureteric obstruction by blood clot: an unusual feature of anticoagulant therapy. *Med. J. Aust.* i, 660.

Rossi, A.C., Bosco, L., Faich, G.A., *et al.* (1988). The importance of adverse reaction reporting by physicians. Suprofen and the flank pain syndrome. *JAMA* 259, 1203.

Rossi, von G. and Muhlethaler, J.P. (1958). Phenacetin-abuses und chronische interstitielle Nephritis. *Helv. Med. Acta* 25, 510.

Roth, D., Alarcon, F.J., Fernandez, J.A., *et al.* (1988). Acute rhabdomyolysis associated with cocaine intoxication. *N. Engl. J. Med.* 319, 673.

Rotoli, B., Giglio, F., Bile, M., *et al.* (1985). Immune-mediated acute intravascular hemolysis caused by cianidanol (catergen). *Haematologica Pavia* 70, 495.

Rowland, R.G. and Elbe, J.N. (1983). Bladder leiomyosarcoma and pelvic fibroblastic tumour following cyclophosphamide therapy. *J. Urol.* 130, 344.

Rubiano, R., Chang, J.L., and Carroll, J. (1987). Acute rhabdomyolysis following halothane anesthesia without succinylcholine. *Anesthesiology* 67, 856.

Ruley, E.J. and Lisi, L.M. (1974). Interstitial nephritis and renal failure due to ampicillin. *J. Pediatr.* 84, 878.

Russell, G.I., Bing, R.F., Walls, J., *et al.* (1978). Interstitial nephritis in a case of phenylbutazone hypersensitivity. *BMJ* i, 1322.

Sack, K., Schulz, E., Marre, R., *et al.* (1987). Fosfomycin protects against tubulotoxicity induced by cis-diamine-dichloroplatin and cyclosporin A in the rat. *Klin. Wochenschr.* 65, 525.

Sacks, P. and Fellner, S.K. (1987). Recurrent reversible acute renal failure from amphotericin. *Arch. Intern. Med.* 147, 593.

Sadjadi, S.A., McLaughlin, K., and Shah, R.M. (1987). Allergic interstitial nephritis due to diazepam. *Arch. Intern. Med.* 147, 579.

Sahai, J., Heimberger, T., Collins, K., *et al.* (1988). Sulfadiazine-induced crystalluria in a patient with the aquired immunodeficiency syndrome: a reminder. *Am. J. Med.* 84, 791.

Saito, T., Sumithran, E., Glasgow, E.F., *et al.* (1987). The enhancement of aminonucleoside nephrosis by the co-administration of protamine. *Kidney Int.* 32, 691.

Salama, A. and Mueller-Eckhardt, C. (1985). The role of metabolite-specific antibodies in nomifensine-dependent immune hemolytic anemia. *N. Engl. J. Med.* 313, 469.

Saltissi, D., Pusey, C.D., and Rainford, D. (1979). Recurrent acute renal failure due to antibiotic-induced interstitial nephritis. *Br. Med. J.* i, 1182.

Salvarani, C., Macchioni, P., Rossi, F., *et al.* (1985). Nephrotic syndrome induced by tiopronin: association with the HLA-DR3 antigen. *Arthritis Rheum.* 28, 595.

Sanai, T., Okuda, S., Onoyama, K., *et al.* (1990). Germanium dioxide-induced nephropathy: a new type of renal disease. *Nephron* 54, 53.

Sandler, D.P., Smith, J.C., Weinberg, C.R., *et al.* (1989). Analgesic use and chronic renal disease. *N. Engl. J. Med.* 320, 1238.

Sanjad, S.A., Haddad, G.G., and Nassar, V.H. (1974). Nephropathy, an underestimated complication of methicillin therapy. *J. Pediatr.* 84, 873.

Santella, R.N., Rimmer, J.M., and MacPherson, B.R. (1988). Focal segmental glomerulosclerosis in patients receiving lithium carbonate. *Am. J. Med.* 84, 951.

Sanwikarja, S., Kauffmann, R.H., te Velde, J., *et al.* (1989). Tubulointerstitial nephritis associated with pyrazinamide. *Neth. J. Med.* 34, 40.

Savill, J.S., Chia, Y., and Pusey, C.D. (1988). Minimal change nephropathy and pemphigus vulgaris associated with penicillamine treatment of rheumatoid arthritis. *Clin. Nephrol.* 29, 267.

Saway, P.A., Heck, L.W., Bonner, J.R., *et al.* (1988). Azathioprine hypersensitivity. *Am. J. Med.* 84, 960.

Sawyer, M.H., Webb, D.E., Balow, J.E., *et al.* (1988). Acyclovir-induced renal failure. Clinical course and histology. *Am. J. Med.* 84, 1067.

Schaub, J.E., Williamson, P.J., Barnes, W. *et al.* (1994). Multisystem adverse reaction to lamotrigine. *Lancet* 344, 481.

Schnitzer, B. and Smith, E.B. (1966). Effects of the metabolites of phenacetin on the rat. *Arch. Pathol.* 81, 264.

Schwarb, S.J., Hlatky, M.A., Pieper, K.S., *et al.* (1989). Contrast nephrotoxicity: a randomised control trial of a nonionic and an ionic radiographic contrast agent. *N. Engl. J. Med.* 320, 149.

Schwartz, F.D. and Dunea, G. (1966). Progression of retroperitoneal fibrosis despite cessation of treatment with methysergide. *Lancet* i, 955.

Schwartz, R.H., Berdon, W.E., Wagner, J., *et al.* (1970). Tamm–Horsfall urinary mucoprotein precipitation by urographic contrast agents: *in vitro* studies. *AJR* 108, 698.

Schwartzman, M.S. and Franck, W.A. (1987). Vitamin D toxicity complicating the treatment of senile, postmenopausal, and glucocorticoid-induced osteoporosis. *Am. J. Med.* 82, 224.

Schwarz, A., Pommer, W., Keller, F., *et al.* (1984). Morbidity of patients with analgesic-associated nephropathy and endstage renal failure. *Proc. Eur. Dial. Transplant Assoc. Eur. Ren. Assoc.* 21, 311.

Seelig, C.B., Maloley, P.A, and Campbell, J.R. (1990). Nephrotoxicity associated with concomitant ACE inhibitor and NSAID therapy. *South. Med. J.* 83, 1144.

Seelig, M.S. (1969). Vitamin D and cardiovascular, renal, and brain damage in infancy and childhood. *Ann. N.Y. Acad. Sci.* 147, 537.

Segasothy, M., Kong, B.C.T., Kamal, A., *et al.* (1984). Analgesic nephropathy associated with paracetamol. *Aust. N.Z. J. Med.* 14, 23.

Segasothy, M., Cheong, I., Kong, B.C.T., *et al.* (1986). Further evidence of analgesic nephropathy in Malaysia. *Med. J. Malaysia* 41, 377.

Segasothy, M., Suleiman, A.B., Puvaneswary, M., *et al.* (1988). Paracetamol: a cause for analgesic nephropathy and endstage renal disease. *Nephron* 50, 50.

Selby, P., Kohn, J., Raymond, J., *et al.* (1985). Nephrotic syndrome during treatment with interferon. *BMJ* 290, 1180.

Selby, P.J., Powles, R.L., Jameson, B., *et al.* (1979). Parenteral acyclovir therapy for herpes virus infections in men. *Lancet* ii, 1267.

Selby, T. (1979). Acute renal failure from ticrynafen. *N. Engl. J. Med.* 301, 1180.

Sellars, L. and Wilkinson, R. (1983). Adverse effects of antirheumatic drugs on the kidney. *Adverse Drug React. Acute Poisoning Rev.* 2, 51.

Sennesael, J., van den Houte, K., and Verbeelen, D. (1986). Reversible membranous glomerulonephritis associated with ketoprofen. *Clin. Nephrol.* 26, 213.

Sensakovic, J.W., Suarez, M., Perez, G., *et al.* (1985). Pentamidine treatment of *Pneumocystis carinii* pneumonia in the acquired immunodeficiency syndrome. Association with acute renal failure and myoglobinuria. *Arch. Intern. Med.* 145, 224.

Sheil, A.G.R., Hall, B.M., Tiller, D.J., *et al.* (1983). Australian trial of cyclosporine (CsA) in cadaveric donor renal transplantation. *Transplant. Proc.* 15 (Suppl. 1), 2485.

Sheilds, M.B. and Simmons, R.J. (1976). Urinary calculus during methazolamide therapy. *Am. J. Ophthalmol.* 81, 622.

Sheth, K.J., Casper, J.T., and Good, T.A. (1977). Interstitial nephritis due to phenytoin hypersensitivity. *J. Pediatr.* 91, 438.

Short, A.K. and Lockwood, C.M. (1995). Antigen specificity in hydralazine associated ANCA positive vasculitis. *Q. J. Med.* 88, 775.

Silanpaa, M., Kasanen, A., and Elonen, A. (1982). Changes of panorama in renal disease mortality in Finland after phenacetin restriction. *Acta Med. Scand.* 212, 313.

Singer, I. (1981). Lithium and the kidney. *Kidney Int.* 19, 374.

Singer, I., Rotenberg, D., and Puschett, J. B. (1972). Lithium induced nephrogenic diabetes insipidus: *In vivo* and *in vitro* studies. *J. Clin. Invest.* 51, 1081.

Singhal, P., Horowitz, B., Quinones, M.C., *et al.* (1989). Acute renal failure following cocaine abuse. *Nephron* 52, 76.

Skinner, R. and Ferner, R.E. (1986). Acute renal failure without acute intravascular haemolysis after nomifensine overdosage. *Hum. Toxicol.* 5, 279.

Smart, E.R. (1985). The hazards of mercury in dentistry. *Rev. Environ. Health.* 5, 59.

Smith, C.R., Lipsky, J.J., Laskin, O.L., *et al.* (1980). Doubleblind comparison of the nephrotoxicity and auditory toxicity of gentamicin and tobramycin. *N. Engl. J. Med.* 302, 1106.

Smith, P.J., Swinburn, W.R., Swinson, D.R., *et al.* (1982). Influence of previous gold toxicity on subsequent development of penicillamine toxicity. *Br. Med. J.* 285, 595.

Snyder, D.S. (1988). Interaction between cyclosporine and warfarin. *Ann. Intern. Med.* 108, 311.

Soberon, L., Bowman, R.L., Pasoriza-Munoz, E., *et al.* (1979). Comparative nephrotoxicities of gentamicin, netilmicin and tobramycin in the rat. *J. Pharmacol. Exp. Ther.* 210, 334.

Soffer, O., Nassar, V.H., Campbell, W.G. Jr, *et al.* (1987). Light chain cast nephropathy and acute renal failure associated with rifampin therapy. Renal disease akin to myeloma kidney. *Am. J. Med.* 82, 1052.

Solinger, A.M. (1988). Drug-related lupus. Clinical and etiologic considerations. *Rheum. Dis. Clin. North Am.* 14, 187.

Speirs, C., Fielder, A.H.L., Chapel, H., *et al.* (1989). Complement system protein C4 and susceptibility to hydralazineinduced systemic lupus erythematosus. *Lancet* i, 922.

Spicer, S.T., Liddle, C., Chapman, J.R., *et al.* (1997). The mechanism of cyclosporin toxicity induced by clarithromycin. *Br. J. Clin. Pharmacol.* 43, 194.

Spragg, J., Weinblatt, M.E., Coblyn, J., *et al.* (1988). Effect of cyclosporine on urinary kallikrein excretion in patients with rheumatoid arthritis. *J. Lab. Clin. Med.* 112, 324.

Spuhler, O. and Zollinger, H.U. (1953). Die chronische interstitielle Nephritis. *Z. Klin. Med.* 151, 1.

Stark, H., Alkalay, A., Ben-Bassat, M., *et al.* (1985). Levaninduced glomerulitis in rabbits: a possible role for direct complement activation in situ. *Br. J. Exp. Pathol.* 66, 165.

Steele, T.W. and Edwards, K.D.G. (1971). Analgesic nephropathy. Changes in various parameters of renal function following cessation of analgesic abuse. *Med. J. Aust.* i, 181.

Steenland, N.K., Thun M.J., Ferguson C.W., *et al.* (1990). Occupational and other exposures associated with male end-stage renal disease: a case control study. *Am. J. Public Health* 80, 153.

Stein, H.B., Patterson, A.C., Offer, R.C., *et al.* (1979). Adverse effects of D-penicillamine in rheumatoid arthritis. *Ann. Intern. Med.* 91, 24.

Stillman, I.E., Andoh, T.F., Burdmann, E.A., *et al.* (1995). FK506 nephrotoxicity: morphologic characterization of a rat model. *Lab. Invest.* 73, 794.

Stratta, P., Mazzucco, G., Griva, S., *et al.* (1988). Immunemediated glomerulonephritis after exposure to paraquat. *Nephron* 48, 138.

Strom, B.L., West, S.L., Sim, E., *et al.* (1989). The epidemiology of the acute flank pain syndrome from suprofen. *Clin. Pharmacol. Ther.* 46, 693.

Swartz, R.D., Rubin, J.E., Leeming, B.W., *et al.* (1978). Renal failure following major angiography. *Am. J. Med.* 65, 31.

Tahan, S.R., Diamond, J.R., Blank, J.M., *et al.* (1985). Acute hemolysis and renal failure with rifampicin-dependent antibodies after discontinuous administration. *Transfusion* 25, 124.

Takeda, M., Breyer, M.D., Noland, T.D., *et al.* (1992). Endothelin-1 receptor antagonist: effects on endothelin- and cyclosporine-treated mesangial cells. *Kidney Int.* 42, 17.

Taliercio, C.P., Vlietstra, R.E., Fisher, L.D., *et al.* (1986). Risks for renal dysfunction with cardiac angiography. *Ann. Intern. Med.* 104, 501.

Tam, V.K., Green, J., Schwieger, J., *et al.* (1991). Nephrotic syndrome and renal insufficiency associated with lithium therapy. *Am. J. Kidney Dis.* 27, 715.

Tanaka, A., Shinai, S., Kasuno, K., *et al.* (1997). Chinese herbs nephropathy in Kansai area: a warning report. *Nippon. Jinzo Gakkai. Shi.* 39, 438.

Taylor, W.H. (1972). Renal calculi and self-medication with multi-vitamin preparations containing vitamin D. *Clin. Sci.* 42, 515.

Tegzess, A.M., Doorenbos, B.M., Minderhound, J.M., *et al.* (1988). Prospective serial renal function studies in patients with non-renal disease treated with cyclosporine A. *Transplant. Proc.* 20 (Suppl. 2), 390.

Teixeria, R.B., Kelly, J., Alpert, H., *et al.* (1982). Complete protection from gentamicin-induced acute renal failure in the diabetes mellitus rat. *Kidney Int.* 21, 600.

Terada, Y., Shinohara, S., Matui, N., *et al.* (1988). Amphetamine-induced myoglobinuric acute renal failure. *Jpn J. Med.* 27, 305.

Thien, T.H., Delaere, K.P.J., Debruyne, F.M.T., *et al.* (1978). Urinary incontinence caused by prazosin. *BMJ* i, 622.

Thompson, J. and Julian, D.G. (1982). Retroperitoneal fibrosis associated with metoprolol. *BMJ* 284, 83.

Thompson, J.F., Chalmers, D.H., Hunnisett, A.G., *et al.* (1983). Nephrotoxicity of trimethoprim and cotrimoxazole in renal allograft recipients treated with cyclosporine. *Transplantation* 36, 204.

Todd, M.A., Bailey, R.R., Espiner, E.A., *et al.* (1987). Vitamin D2 for the treatment of chilblains — a cautionary tale. *N.Z. Med. J.* 100, 465.

Toll, L.L., Lee, M., and Sharifi, R. (1987). Cefoxitin-induced interstitial nephritis. *South. Med. J.* 80, 274.

Tornroth, T. and Skrivars, B. (1974). Gold nephropathy prototype of membranous glomerulonephritis. *Am. J. Pathol.* 75, 573.

Tosi, S., Cagnoli, M., Guidi, G., *et al.* (1985). Injectable gold dermatitis and proteinuria: retreatment with auranofin. *Int. J. Clin. Pharmacol. Res.* 5, 265.

Toto, R,D., Mitchell, H.C., Lee, H.C., *et al.* (1991). Reversible renal insufficiency due to angiotensin converting enzyme inhibitors in hypertensive nephrosclerosis. *Ann. Intern. Med.* 115, 513.

Trewhalla, M., Dawson, P., Forsling, M., *et al.* (1990). Vasopressin release in response to intravenously injected contrast media. *Br. J. Radiol.* 63, 97.

Tulkens, P.M. (1989). Nephrotoxicity of aminoglycoside antibiotics. *Toxicol. Lett.* 46, 107.

Ueda, S., Wakashin, M., Wakashin, Y., *et al.* (1986). Experimental gold nephropathy in guinea pigs: detection of autoantibodies to renal tubular antigens. *Kidney Int.* 29, 539.

van der Woude, F.J., van Son, W.J., Tegzess, A.M., *et al.* (1985). Effect of captopril on blood pressure and renal function in patients with transplant renal artery stenosis. *Nephron* 39, 184.

Vanherweghem, J.L. (1994). A new form of nephropathy secondary to the absorption of Chinese herbs. *Bull. Med. Acad. R. Med. Belg.* 149, 128.

Vanherweghem, J.L, Depierreux, M., Tielemans, C., *et al.* (1993). Rapidly progressive interstitial renal fibrosis in young women: association with slimming regimen including Chinese herbs. *Lancet* 41, 387.

Vanherweghem, J.L., Abromowicz, D., Tielemans, C., *et al.* (1996). Effects of steroids on the progression of renal failure in chronic interstitial renal fibrosis: a pilot study in Chinese herbs nephropathy. *Am. J. Kidney Dis.* 27, 209.

van Ypersele de Strihou, C. and Vanherweghem J.L. (1995). The tragic paradigm of Chinese herbs nephropathy. *Nephrol. Dial. Transplant.* 10, 157.

Vanucci, L. and Mosca, F. (1989). Profile of drug-metabolizing enzymes in the cortex and medulla of the human kidney. *Pharmacology* 39, 299.

Velazquez, H., Perazella, M.A., Wright, F S., *et al.* (1993). Renal mechanisms of trimethoprim-induced hyperkalemia. *Ann. Intern. Med.* 119, 296.

Venkataraman, G. (1981). Renal damage and glue sniffing. *Br. Med. J.* 283, 1467.

Veremis, S.A., Maddux, M.S., Pollak, R., *et al.* (1987). Subtherapeutic cyclosporine concentrations during nafcillin therapy. *Transplantation* 43, 913.

Verin, P., Bresque, E., Vizdy, A., *et al.* (1974). Fibrose rétropéritonéale et dérivés de l'ergot. *Bull. Soc. Ophtalmol. Fr.* 31, 281.

Verma, S. and Kieff, E. (1975). Cephalexin-related nephropathy. *JAMA* 234, 618.

Verweij, J., van der Burg, M.E., and Pinedo, H.M. (1987a). Mitomycin C-induced hemolytic uremic syndrome. Six case reports and review of the literature on renal, pulmonary and cardiac side effects of the drug. *Radiother. Oncol.* 8, 33.

Verweij, J., de Vries, J., and Pinedo, H.M. (1987b). Mitomycin C-induced renal toxicity, a dose-dependent side effect? *Eur. J. Cancer Clin. Oncol.* 23, 195.

Violon, C. (1997). Belgian (Chinese herb) nephropathy: why? *J. Pharm. Belg.* 52, 7.

Volpi, A., Ferrario, G.M., Giordano, F., *et al.* (1989). Acute renal failure due to hypersensitivity interstitial nephritis induced by warfarin sodium. *Nephron* 52, 196.

Wagner, K., Albrecht, S., and Neumayer, H.H. (1986). Prevention of delayed graft function in cadaveric kidney transplantation by a calcium antagonist. *Transplant. Proc.* 18, 510.

Wagner, K., Albrecht, S., and Neumayer, H.H. (1987). Prevention of posttransplant acute tubular necrosis by the calcium antagonist diltiazem: a prospective randomized study. *Am. J. Nephrol.* 7, 287.

Walker, P.D. and Shah, S.V. (1988). Evidence suggesting a role for hydroxyl radical in gentamicin-induced acute renal failure in rats. *J. Clin. Invest.* 81, 334.

Walker, R.G. (1993). Lithium nephrotoxicity. *Kidney Int.* (Suppl. 42), S93.

Walker, R.G., Thomson, N.M., Dowling, J.P., *et al.* (1979). Minocycline-induced acute interstitial nephritis. *BMJ* i, 524.

Walker, R.G., Bennet, W.M., Davies, B.M., *et al.* (1982). Structural and functional effects of long-term lithium therapy. *Kidney Int.* 21 (Suppl. 11), S13.

Walker, R.J., Fawcett, J.P., Flannery, E.M., *et al.* (1994). Indomethacin potentiates exercise-induced reduction in renal haemodynamics in athletes. *Med. Sci. Sports Exerc.* 26, 1302.

Wallin, L. and Alling, C. (1979). Effect of sustained-release lithium tablets on renal function. *BMJ* ii, 1332.

Wallin, L., Alling, C., and Aurell, M. (1982). Impairment of renal function in patients on long-term lithium treatment. *Clin. Nephrol.* 18, 23.

Warren, D.J. (1976). Beta-adrenergic receptor blockade and renal function. *Am. Heart J.* 91, 265.

Warrington, R.J., Hogg, G.R., Paraskevas, F., *et al.* (1977). Insidious rifampin-associated renal failure with light-chain proteinuria. *Arch. Intern. Med.* 137, 927.

Watts, H.G. (1973). Retroperitoneal fibrosis. *N.Z. Med. J.* 78, 247.

Weinberg, M.S., Quigg, R.J., Salant, D.J., *et al.* (1985). Anuric renal failure precipitated by indomethacin and triamterene. *Nephron* 40, 216.

Weinrauch, L.A., Robertson, W.S., and D'Elia, J.A. (1978). Contrast media-induced acute renal failure. Use of creatinine clearance to determine risk in elderly diabetic patients. *JAMA* 239, 2018.

Weisberg, L.S., Kurnik, P.B., and Kurnik, B.R. (1994). Risk of radiocontrast nephropathy in patients with and without diabetes mellitus. *Kidney Int.* 45, 259.

Weisbord, S.D., Soule, J.B., and Kimmel, P.L. (1997). Poison on line — acute renal failure caused by oil of wormwood purchased through the Internet. *N. Engl. J. Med.* 337, 825.

Weisman, J.I. and Bloom, B. (1955). Anuria following phenylbutazone therapy. *N. Engl. J. Med.* 252, 1086.

Weisman, S.M., Felsen, D., and Vaughan, E.D. Jr (1985). Indications and contraindications for the use of nonsteroidal antiinflammatory drugs in urology. *Semin. Urol.* 3, 301.

Weiss, A.S., Markenson, J.A., Weiss, M.S., *et al.* (1978). Toxicity of D-penicillamine in rheumatoid arthritis. *Am. J. Med.* 64, 114.

Wharton, J.G., Oliver, D.O., and Dunnill, M.S. (1982). Acute renal failure associated with diflunisal. *Postgrad. Med. J.* 58, 104.

Whelton, A. (1995). Renal effects of over-the-counter analgesics. *J. Clin. Pharm.* 35, 454.

Whelton, A., Bender, W., Vaghaiwalla, F., *et al.* (1983). Sulindac and renal impairment. *JAMA* 249, 2892.

Whiting, P.H., Cunningham, C., Thomson, A.W., *et al.* (1984). Enhancement of high dose cyclosporin A toxicity by frusemide. *Biochem. Pharmacol.* 33, 1075.

Whitworth, J.A., Mills, E.H., Coghlan, J.P., *et al.* (1987). The haemodynamic effects of cyclosporine A in sheep. *Clin. Exp. Pharmacol. Physiol.* 14, 573.

Wiesberg, L.S., Kurnik, P.B., and Kurnik, B.R. (1994). Risk of radiocontrast nephropathy in patients with and without diabetes mellitus. *Kidney Int.* 45, 259.

Wigley, R.A.D. (1976). The New Zealand experience. *Aust. N.Z. J. Med.* 6 (suppl. 1), 37.

Wiles, C.M., Assem, E.S.K., and Cohen, S.L. (1979). Cephradine-induced interstitial nephritis. *Clin. Exp. Immunol.* 36, 342.

Wilkinson, R. (1979). Beta-blockers, blood sugar control, and renal function. *BMJ* i, 617.

Wilkinson, R. (1982). Beta-blockers and renal function. *Drugs* 23, 195.

Wilkinson, S.P., Blendis, L.M., and Williams, R. (1974). Frequency and type of renal and electrolyte disorders in fulminant hepatic failure. *BMJ* i, 186.

Wilkinson, S.P., Stewart, W.K., Spiers, E.M., *et al.* (1989). Protracted systemic illness and interstitial nephritis due to minocycline. *Postgrad. Med. J.* 65, 53.

Williams, G. and Hughes, M. (1974). Post-partum renal failure. *J. Pathol.* 114, 149.

Wilson, D.R. (1972). Analgesic nephropathy in Canada: a retrospective study of 351 cases. *Can. Med. Assoc. J.* 107, 752.

Wilson, M., Brown, D.J., Brown, R.W., *et al.* (1974). Renal failure from alpha-methyldopa therapy. *Aust. N.Z. J. Med.* 4, 415.

Winearls, C.G. and Kerr, D.N.S. (1985). In *Textbook of Adverse Drug Reactions* (3rd edn) (ed. D.M. Davies), p. 291. Oxford University Press.

Winston, J.A. and Safirstein, R. (1985). Reduced renal blood flow in early cisplatin-induced acute renal failure in the rat. *Am. J. Physiol.* 249, F490.

Wolfe, S.M. (1987). Suprofen-induced transient flank pain and renal failure. *N. Engl. J. Med.* 316, 1025.

Wong, E.G.C., Rowe, P.H., Blumenkrantz, M.J., *et al.* (1974). Nephrotoxicity associated with use of methoxyflurane. *Nephron* 13, 174.

Wong, N.L., Magil, A.B., and Dirks, J.H. (1989). Effect of magnesium diet in gentamicin-induced acute renal failure in rats. *Nephron* 51, 84.

Wood, I.K., Parmelee, D.X., and Foreman, J.W. (1989). Lithium-induced nephrotic syndrome. *Am. J. Psychiatry* 146, 84.

Woodle, E.S., Thistlethwaite, J.R., Gordon, J.H., *et al.* (1996). A multicenter trial of FK506 (tacrolimus) therapy in refractory acute renal allograft rejection: A report of the Tacrolimus Kidney Transplantation Rescue Study Group. *Transplantation* 62, 594.

Woodrow, G., Harnden, P., and Turney, J.H. (1995). Acute

renal failure due to accelerated hypertension following ingestion of 3,4-methylenedioxymethamphetamine ('Ecstasy'). *Nephrol. Dial. Transplant.* 10, 399.

Wright, A.D., Barber, S.G., Kendall, M.J., *et al.* (1979). Beta-adrenoceptor-blocking drugs and blood sugar control in diabetes mellitus. *Br. Med. J.* i, 159.

Yarom, R., Stein, H., Peters, P.D., *et al.* (1975). Nephrotoxic effect of parenteral and intraarticular gold. *Arch. Pathol.* 99, 36.

Yazawa, H., Nakada, T., Sasagawa I. *et al.* (1995). Hyberbaric oxygenation therapy for cyclophosphamide-induced haemorrhagic cystitis. *Int. Urol. Nephrol.* 27, 381.

Yermakov, V.M., Hitti, I.F., and Sutton, A.L. (1983). Necrotizing vasculitis associated with diphenylhydantoin: two fatal cases. *Hum. Pathol.* 14, 182.

Ying, L.S. and Johnson, C.A. (1989). Ciprofloxacin-induced interstitial nephritis. *Clin. Pharm.* 8, 518.

Yung, R.L., Quddus, J., and Chrisp, C.E. (1995). Mechanisms of drug-induced lupus 1. Cloned Th cells modified with DNA methylation inhibitors *in vitro* cause autoimmunity *in vivo*. *J. Immunol.* 154, 3025.

Zaal, M.J., de Vries, J., and Boen-Tan, Y.T. (1988). Is cyclosporin toxic to endothelial cells? *Lancet* ii, 956.

Zipser, R.D. and Henrich, W.L. (1986). Implications of nonsteroidal anti-inflammatory drug therapy. *Am. J. Med.* 80, 78.

Zoja, C., Furci, L., Ghilardi, F., *et al.* (1986). Cyclosporin-induced endothelial cell injury. *Lab. Invest.* 55, 455.

Zürcher, H.U., Meier, H.R., Huber, M., *et al.* (1977). Akutes Nierenversagen als Komplikation von Fastenkuren. *Schweiz. Med. Wochenschr.* 107, 1025.

15. Endocrine disorders

V. T. F. YEUNG, W. B. CHAN, and C. S. COCKRAM

Introduction

Drugs having actions on endocrine systems can be classified into two major categories: (1) those used primarily in the management of endocrine problems; and (2) those used primarily for other disorders but fortuitously affecting endocrine function.

The mechanisms of their actions are best understood in the light of their effects on control of hormone secretion and hormone action. Carbimazole and thyroxine, when given in excess, produce hypothyroidism and hyperthyroidism respectively. Amiodarone and lithium, however, may produce hypothyroidism or (less commonly) hyperthyroidism. Even these apparently contradictory effects can be explained by alterations in iodine metabolism and possibly also in immunomodulation. Excessive doses of glucocorticoids for a prolonged period will produce both Cushing's syndrome and suppression of the hypothalamic–pituitary–adrenal axis with a concomitant fall in endogenous glucocorticoid production. Ketoconazole, an antifungal agent acting on the fungal cytochrome P-450-dependent enzyme, induces adrenal crisis because of the concomitant and dose-dependent effect on the mammalian steroidogenic enzymes. Some psychotherapeutic agents, owing to their pharmacological effects on central dopaminergic or serotoninergic pathways, lead incidentally to hyperprolactinaemia and galactorrhoea. Even gynaecomastia, a superficially bizarre adverse effect of spironolactone, is in fact a dose-dependent oestrogen-like action of the drug. Thus, the adverse effects of drugs on endocrine function, although diverse, can mainly be explained as dose-related pharmacological reactions (augmented or Type A) rather than idiosyncratic (bizarre or Type B) reactions.

Drugs can also interfere with the investigation and diagnosis of endocrine disease by interfering with assay and measurement procedures. For example, certain medications can affect binding of hormone to binding proteins in blood, such as thyroxine-binding globulin. This can result in misdiagnosis of hyperthyroidism or hypothyroidism unless appropriate assay procedures are carried out. Other drugs can interfere with such hormonal assays as those for vanillylmandelic acid (VMA) or 5-hydroxyindole acetic acid (5-HIAA), either directly or by effects on the assayed metabolites, again potentially leading to erroneous diagnoses.

Knowledge of adverse effects of drugs is therefore essential to the diagnosis of drug-induced endocrine disorders and avoidance of misinterpretation of the results of endocrine investigations.

The hypothalamic–pituitary–thyroid axis

The thyroid gland synthesizes, stores, and secretes the thyroid hormones thyroxine and tri-iodothyronine. This function is controlled by pituitary thyroid-stimulating hormone (TSH), although there may be partial autoregulation by the thyroid itself. TSH is a glycoprotein hormone secreted under the control of hypothalamic neurohormones: stimulation by thyrotrophin-releasing hormone (TRH) and inhibition by dopamine and somatostatin. There is also evidence that noradrenaline, serotonin, and possibly other central neurotransmitters interact with the hypothalamic regulatory hormones in the control of thyrotrophin function. The thyroid hormones exert feedback control on the secretion of TSH at both the hypothalamic and pituitary levels. A reduced circulating thyroid hormone level stimulates the secretion of TSH. Conversely, an excess of the circulating thyroid hormones inhibits the release of TSH and probably TRH production. Other hormones, including sex hormones and corticosteroids, can also modulate TSH secretion.

More than 99 per cent of thyroxine (T_4) and tri-iodothyronine (T_3) in the blood are bound to proteins (mainly thyroxine-binding globulin, TBG), and only one to two per cent of circulating thyroid hormone is in the form of T_3. T_4 is converted peripherally, however, into T_3, which is three to four times as potent, and the inactive metabolite reverse T_3 (rT_3). It is believed that the small amounts of free T_4 (FT_4) and free T_3 (FT_3) mediate the biological actions, whereas the protein-bound fractions are inactive and serve as a storage pool of hormones.

Drugs affecting TRH and TSH production

Impaired TSH secretion

Therapeutic doses of thyroid hormones, particularly with T_4 greater than 200 μg per day, can suppress TSH secretion (Evered et al. 1973; Erfurth and Hedner 1982). Pharmacological doses of glucocorticoids can impair basal and TRH-stimulated TSH concentrations (Wilber and Utiger 1969; Nicoloff et al. 1970; Otsuki et al. 1973). Dopamine and dopaminergic agents such as levodopa and bromocriptine inhibit basal TSH secretion and reduce the TSH response to TRH stimulation (Miyai et al. 1974; Refetoff et al. 1974; Kaptein et al. 1980), and some authors have questioned the safety of prolonged use of dopamine in critically ill patients because of the possibility of inducing secondary hypothyroidism and thus worsening the prognosis (Varl et al. 1988). Serotonin antagonists (metergoline, cyproheptadine), used for treatment of hyperprolactinaemia and for appetite stimulation, have been found to decrease TSH secretion (Ferrari et al. 1976; Delitala et al. 1978). Reserpine, a classic depletor of biogenic monoamines, and phentolamine, an α-blocking agent, reduce basal TSH and block the TSH response to cold stimulation (Tuomisto et al. 1973). Lowering of basal serum TSH concentration also occurs in patients with chronic renal failure treated with heparin. This was once attributed to increased FT_4 and FT_3 concentrations induced by heparin but is now regarded as an artefact (see section on Free thyroid hormone assays) (Mendel et al. 1987; Vagenakis 1988).

Enhanced TSH secretion

The neuroleptics chlorpromazine and haloperidol and other dopamine-receptor blocker drugs such as metoclopramide and sulpiride can raise basal TSH and enhance the TSH response to TRH (Kirkegaard et al. 1977, 1978; Massara et al. 1978; Scanlon et al. 1979). Theophylline increases TSH and T_4, possibly through β-adrenergic stimulation of the hypothalamus (Faglia et al. 1972; Hikita et al. 1989). Since TSH release is under feedback control by thyroid hormones, any goitrogenic medications that produce hypothyroidism can lead to compensatory increases in TSH concentrations.

Drugs affecting the thyroid

Iodine

Iodine preparations have diverse effects upon the thyroid. Acute administration of high doses of iodine inhibits the release of hormone from the thyroid. This effect is transient but has been used in the preparation of patients for thyroid surgery and in the management of thyroid crisis. Further, the iodine can suppress thyroid hormone formation, which is known as the Wolff–Chaikoff effect (Wolff and Chaikoff 1948). Prolonged exposure to iodide is accompanied by reduction in iodide trapping and inhibition of synthesis of thyroid hormones, leading to hypothyroidism and goitre formation in susceptible subjects (Wolff 1969; Vagenakis and Braverman 1975).

Iodide may exacerbate or cause relapse in patients with previous hyperthyroidism (Jod–Basedow phenomenon). In addition, iodide-induced thyrotoxicosis can occasionally occur in patients with no previous thyroid disease (Fradkin and Wolff 1983; Clark and Hutton 1985).

Hyperthyroidism

Inorganic iodide in the form of potassium iodide used as a cough expectorant can induce thyrotoxicosis, albeit uncommonly (Fradkin and Wolff 1983).

Organic iodine is more often incriminated in causing thyrotoxicosis. Drugs containing organic iodine include amiodarone, iodochlorhydroxyquinoline, the uricosuric benziodarone, and radiographic contrast media. Features of iodine-induced thyrotoxicosis include an absence of exophthalmos, a low incidence of antithyroid antibodies, and a low uptake of radioiodine, and a tendency for the hyperthyroidism to be self-limiting (1–6 months) on cessation of the medication. Radioiodine contrast agents, including ipodate, iopanic acid, and tyropanoate have been employed to treat thyrotoxicosis with variable success. Amongst these agents, iopanate seems to be most effective. The mechanism is not fully understood, but appears to include inhibition of conversion of T_4 to T_3. Only those iodine-containing contrast media taken up by the liver and excreted in the bile appear to have this property (Laurberg 1985; Roti et al. 1985; Arem and Munipalli 1996). Their long-term effect awaits further evaluation.

Amiodarone is a widely used antiarrhythmic agent containing 37% iodine by weight. As much as 18 mg of iodine per day may be released from the usual maintenance dose (200–600 mg) of the drug, which is considerably in excess of the usual daily dietary intake of less than 200 μg (Kennedy et al. 1989). The heavy iodine load is largely responsible for its profound effect on thyroid function, although the drug might also initiate an auto-immune process (Wiersinga and Trip 1986; Kennedy *et al.* 1988). Amiodarone causes increases in T_4 and rT_3 and a reduction of T_3 (Gammage and Franklyn 1987). The effect becomes evident a week after initiating therapy and is due to suppression of peripheral deiodination of T_4 to T_3 by inhibition of the enzyme 5'-monodeiodinase (Melmed *et al.* 1981; Aanderud *et al.* 1984). These changes are accompanied by an increase in the basal and TRH-stimulated TSH levels, mostly within the normal range and in the first few weeks (Burger *et al.* 1976). Continuation of amiodarone is associated with a further rise in plasma T_4, free T_4, rT_3 and a fall in plasma T_3. TSH levels return gradually to pretreatment values and a steady state of thyroid hormone concentrations is reached by 3–4 months (Melmed *et al.* 1981). Clinically significant hyperthyroidism ranges from 1–23 per cent in different reports from different geographical areas. It tends to be higher in areas of iodine deficiency (Martino *et al.* 1984), and thyroid dysfunction is more common in subjects with a past history or family history of thyroid disease and in people with goitre (Amico *et al.* 1984). Autoimmunity does not, however, seem to play a significant role in the development of amiodarone-induced thyrotoxicosis (Martino *et al.* 1986*a*). Because of its non-specific adrenoceptor-blocking properties, amiodarone can mask many of the clinical features of hyperthyroidism. Weight loss and tiredness are often the presenting symptoms. Thyrotoxicosis should also be suspected if the heart rate exceeds the pretreatment value or when arrhythmia recurs or worsens during amiodarone therapy (Gammage and Franklyn 1987; Nademanee *et al.* 1989). No single hormonal test reliably predicts thyroid dysfunction associated with amiodarone therapy. If hyperthyroidism is suspected on clinical grounds, an increase in serum T_3, in addition to an increase in T_4, confirms the diagnosis, which is supported further by a suppressed TSH concentration or an absent TSH response to TRH. A normal T_3 does not, however, rule out hyperthyroidism since the value observed might be lowered by concomitant non-thyroidal illness. Further, many euthyroid patients on treatment with amiodarone can exhibit a blunted TSH response to TRH. Treatment of amiodarone-induced thyrotoxicosis may be difficult. Patients without goitre tend to remit spontaneously with discontinuation of medication (Martino *et al.* 1986*b*; Mechlis *et al.* 1987). Hyperthyroidism can be severe, however, and in some patients amiodarone may be the only effective drug for the underlying arrhythmia and therefore not able to be stopped. Treatment with radioactive iodine will not be effective, since its uptake is blocked; and thyroidectomy is contraindicated in patients with uncontrolled hyperthyroidism and underlying cardiac disease. In these cases, a combination of potassium perchlorate and thionamide, which prevents further iodine uptake and inhibits hormone synthesis, has been used with success (Martino *et al.* 1987*a*; Reichert and de Rooy 1989).

Lithium has been associated with thyrotoxicosis (Cubitt 1976; Reus *et al.* 1979) and there has been a report of hypothyroidism followed by hyperthyroidism during lithium treatment (McDermott *et al.* 1986). It is postulated that the underlying event is an iodide-induced thyrotoxicosis in susceptible patients due to blockade by lithium of thyroid iodine release and hence expansion of the intrathyroidal iodide pool.

Reversible hyperthyroxinaemia can be induced by heavy amphetamine abuse, which also produces clinical features resembling those of thyrotoxicosis (Morley *et al.* 1980). The elevation of T_4 concentration is apparently secondary to increased TSH secretion as a result of amphetamine effects on the hypothalamus or pituitary. One biochemical feature that may help to distinguish this from Graves' disease is that T_4 is inappropriately raised compared with T_3. Thyrotoxicosis with a similar thyroid hormone profile can also result from deliberate or accidental intake of exogenous thyroid hormones, as demonstrated by thyrotoxicosis due to consumption of hamburgers in the USA (Cohen III *et al.* 1989).

Other drugs reported to cause hyperthyroidism include α-interferon and antihaemophilic factor (Winter and Smail 1980; Burman *et al.* 1985; Fentiman *et al.* 1985), probably due to cross reactivity with the TSH receptor.

Hypothyroidism

Hypothyroidism can occur with prolonged administration of iodide. Locally applied iodine, such as povidone–iodine, when used in the neonate has been shown to cause transient hypothyroidism (Smerdely *et al.* 1989; Parravicini *et al.* 1996). It can also be caused by over-treatment with antithyroid medications such as carbimazole and propylthiouracil. Many drugs not primarily employed for treatment of thyroid disorders can induce hypothyroidism and goitre by affecting the trapping of iodine or interfering with the synthesis or release of thyroid hormones. These are listed in Table 15.1.

Monovalent anions, such as perchlorate, block the uptake of iodine (Morgans and Trotter 1954). Amiodarone directly affects the trapping of iodine, but its dominant effect is inhibition of the synthesis and release of thyroid hormones (Wolff 1969). The incidence of hypothyroidism varies from 0.75–10 per cent (Borowski

TABLE 15.1
*Drugs inhibiting the synthesis and release
of thyroid hormones*

Inhibition of iodine trapping

Lithium (acute effect)
Potassium perchlorate

Inhibition of organification and iodotyrosine coupling

Adrenal suppressants	aminoglutethimide high-dose ketoconazole
Antiarrhythmic	amiodarone
Antirheumatic drugs	oxyphenbutazone phenylbutazone
Antithyroid drugs	carbimazole methimazole propylthiouracil
Antituberculous drugs	ethionamide rifampicin sodium aminosalicylate (PAS)
Sulphonamides	co-trimoxazole sulphadiazine
Miscellaneous	chlorpromazine pentazocine sulphonylureas

Inhibition of release

Amiodarone
Iodide (large doses)
Lithium (chronic effect)

et al. 1985). In areas of iodine repletion, hypothyroidism is a more common complication than thyrotoxicosis (Martino *et al.* 1984). The presence of serum thyroid antibodies indicates a greater risk of development of amiodarone-induced hypothyroidism. About 50 per cent have circulating antithyroid antibodies at diagnosis. In patients without underlying thyroid disorders, the hypothyroidism remits spontaneously whereas it may persist in patients with underlying thyroid problems, particularly in those with positive thyroid antibodies (Martino *et al.* 1987b). On the other hand, amiodarone treatment does not seem to increase the incidence of antithyroid antibodies (Safran *et al.* 1988). Therefore, in some cases, hypothyroidism may represent unmasking of autoimmune thyroiditis in susceptible subjects, whereas in others the inhibitory effect of iodine on the thyroid may be the only factor. Classical hypothyroid symptoms may occur, but the hypothyroidism is often relatively asymptomatic (subclinical) and detected by thyroid function tests in patients with minimal symptoms (Hawthorne *et al.* 1985). The diagnosis of amiodarone-induced hypothyroidism is confirmed by the demon-

stration of raised TSH levels and decreased thyroid hormones, although T_4 may remain within the normal range (Kennedy *et al.* 1989; Nademanee *et al.* 1989). Treatment is with T_4 replacement as guided by the clinical state, if amiodarone cannot be discontinued. Complete normalization of TSH levels may be unfavourable in some patients, because a dose sufficient to achieve this may lead to exacerbation of underlying cardiac problems.

Lithium is another goitrogenic agent commonly used in manic-depressive disorders. The reported prevalence of goitre in patients treated with this drug varies from 0–61.5 per cent (Lazarus 1982). Acutely, lithium blocks the uptake of iodine and release of thyroid hormones, possibly by inhibiting TSH-stimulated adenylate cyclase and blocking the effect of cyclic AMP on the biosynthetic pathway (Singer and Rotenberg 1973). During long-term administration, the uptake of iodine is enhanced but the release of thyroid hormones remains impaired. In the past, hypothyroidism was considered to be a common complication of lithium treatment, the incidence ranging from 10–34 per cent in various lithium clinics (Hullin 1978). More recent long-term studies by Smigan and others (1984) and Maarbjerg and colleagues (1987) show, however, that although T_3 and T_4 tend to fall in the first few months of treatment, they return to pretreatment levels after 12 months and can exceed the pre-lithium values afterwards. Conversely, TSH tends to rise in the first few months but gradually returns to pretreatment levels after more than 12 months. Only about two per cent of patients develop clinical features of hypothyroidism and require thyroxine replacement. Single deviant thyroid hormone results during lithium treatment can, therefore, be transient and it now seems wise to subject the patient to re-examination at intervals before starting thyroxine, unless clinical features of hypothyroidism become overt.

Other agents that have antithyroid potential include the adrenal suppressants aminoglutethimide (Hughes and Burley 1970) and ketoconazole (Namer *et al.* 1986); the antituberculous drugs *p*-aminosalicylic acid (Mac-Gregor and Somner 1954), ethionamide (Moulding and Fraser 1970), and possibly rifampicin (Isley 1987); sulphonamides (Milne and Greer 1962; Cohen *et al.* 1980); and the NSAID phenylbutazone (Morgans and Trotter 1955; Aboidun *et al.* 1973) and oxyphenbutazone (Lane *et al.* 1977). These agents apparently act through inhibition of synthesis of thyroid hormone by blocking organic binding of iodine. Hypothyroidism can also be caused by sodium nitroprusside, because of blockade of iodine uptake by the thiocyanate ion (Nourok *et al.* 1964).

Immunomodulatory agents used to treat malignancy, including combinations of interleukin-2 with α-interferon or lymphokine-activated killer cells, filgrastim (a haemopoietic growth factor), and molgramostim (human recombinant granulocyte–macrophage colony-stimulating factor), have been reported to cause hypothyroidism, possibly either by cross reactivity of thyroid-stimulating hormone with membrane receptors for interferon or autoimmune mechanisms. Thyroid antibodies are frequently reported in these cases (Atkins *et al.* 1988; Pichert *et al.* 1990; Hansen *et al.* 1993; de Luis and Romero 1996).

There have been isolated case reports of hypothyroidism following treatment with cyclophosphamide (Coffey 1971) and possible aggravation of hypothyroidism after pentazocine (Evans *et al.* 1972) and chlorpromazine (Mitchell *et al.* 1959).

Although sulphonylureas are known to lower circulating thyroid hormone concentrations, possibly by suppressing organification of iodine, no increased incidence of hypothyroidism with the use of these drugs has been demonstrated.

Drugs interfering with thyroid function tests

Interference with total hormone measurements due to effects on thyroid-hormone-binding proteins

Since more than 99 per cent of thyroid hormones are protein-bound (mainly as TBG), drug-induced changes in the concentration of transport proteins or inhibition of binding to these proteins can give rise to falsely high or low values, leading to misdiagnosis of hypothyroidism or hyperthyroidism. Table 15.2 provides a list of drugs with these effects.

The use of oestrogens and oral contraceptives is associated with an increase in serum T_4 and thyroxine-binding globulin concentration due to increased hepatic synthesis of TBG (Engbring and Engstrom 1959; Bockner and Roman 1967; Doe *et al.* 1967; Laurell *et al.* 1967; Walden *et al.* 1986). In heroin and methadone addicts, increases in TBG concentration and hence serum T_4 and T_3 levels may occur (Azizi *et al.* 1974). Similar phenomena have also been observed following therapy with the lipid-lowering agent clofibrate and the cytotoxic agent fluorouracil (McKerron *et al.* 1969; Beex *et al.* 1976).

Androgens (including danazol) and anabolic steroids reduce the TBG and serum T_4 concentrations despite an increase in TBPA capacity (Engbring and Engstrom 1959; Braverman and Ingbar 1967; Dickinson *et al.* 1969; Barbosa *et al.* 1971; Pannall and Maas 1977). Growth hormone (GH) may induce a fall in serum T_4 by enhancing peripheral deiodination of T_4 to T_3, thus unmasking

TABLE 15.2
Drugs affecting thyroid-hormone-binding protein

Increase in TBG levels

    Clofibrate
    Fluorouracil
    Oestrogens (including oral contraceptives)
    Opiates (heroin, methadone)

Decrease in TBG levels

    Androgens
    Colaspase (asparaginase)
    Colestipol/niacin (nicotinic acid)
    Danazol
    Glucocorticoids

Interference with hormone binding to transport proteins

    o,p'-DDD (mitotane)
    Diazepam
    Fenclofenac
    Frusemide
    Phenylbutazone
    Phenytoin
    Salicylates
    Sulphonylureas

the co-existing secondary hypothyroidism during treatment for GH deficiency (Jorgensen *et al.* 1989; Laurberg 1994). Acute transient reduction in TBG and T_4 values occurs during treatment with colaspase (asparaginase) for acute leukaemia (Garnick and Larsen 1979; Heidemann *et al.* 1980). Combined colestipol (a bile acid sequestrant) and nicotinic acid therapy for hypercholesterolaemia has been reported to lower T_4 significantly, 19 per cent of patients having values in the hypothyroid range (Cashin-Hemphill *et al.* 1987). Large doses of glucocorticoids suppress TBG binding capacity but enhance that of the thyroxine-binding prealbumin. These effects tend to offset each other, and therefore the decrease in thyroid hormones (Werner and Platman 1965; Oppenheimer and Werner 1966) could be due to other mechanisms, such as reduction in thyroid secretion (Chopra *et al.* 1975).

A number of drugs compete with thyroid hormones for TBG, and reduce total thyroid hormone levels. Such displacement often leads to increased metabolism and turnover of the free hormones. Salicylates compete with thyroid-hormone binding to transport proteins, resulting in a reduction of total T_4 and T_3 concentrations but elevation of the free hormones (Larsen 1972) that could account for the reduced basal and TRH-stimulated TSH concentrations as well as the hypermetabolic effects (Dussault *et al.* 1976; Langer *et al.* 1978). Both phenytoin and fenclofenac inhibit thyroid-hormone binding to TBG (Wolff *et al*. 1961; Chin and Schussler 1968; Taylor *et al*. 1980) and lead to alteration of hormone metabolism, although the displacement itself plays only a minor role in the reduction of serum concentrations of thyroid hormones (see below). *o,p'*-DDD, a compound that is chemically similar to phenytoin, also lowers the T_4 concentration by competitive binding to TBG (Marshall and Tompkins 1968). High concentrations of frusemide cause a dose-dependent inhibition of T_4 binding and may contribute to the low T_4 state in critically ill patients (Stockigt *et al*. 1984). Diazepam (Schussler 1971) and sulphonylureas (Hershman *et al*. 1968) also compete for thyroid-hormone binding proteins but the effects are not of clinical significance.

With the increasing availability of reliable assays for free T_4 and free T_3, and sensitive TSH assays, problems of interpretation of binding protein effects on thyroid function assessment have been lessened.

Interference due to alteration of thyroid hormone metabolism

Phenytoin increases the metabolism and clearance of thyroid hormones, presumably due to hepatic enzyme induction. This leads to reduction of both total and free thyroid hormone concentrations. The patients are clinically euthyroid, however, and TSH levels remain normal (Larsen *et al*. 1970; Liewendahl *et al*. 1978; Yeo *et al*. 1978; Cavalieri *et al*. 1979). This may be explained by achievement of a new steady state in which the increased rate of thyroid hormone clearance is balanced by a reduction in the free thyroid hormone pool or increased generation of T_3 from T_4 (Faber *et al*. 1985) or both.

Fenclofenac, an NSAID with structural similarity to thyroxine, is the most potent drug known to interfere with the binding of thyroid hormones to serum protein. It displaces T_4 and T_3 from TBG (Taylor *et al*. 1980), leading to transient reduction in TSH and a reduced TSH response to TRH (Kurtz *et al*. 1981). This gradually returns to normal after 2–4 weeks of treatment, as a new steady state is achieved between bound and free hormone pools. Free T_4 and T_3 concentrations tend to remain at low normal levels, however, presumably due to increased clearance with formation of a new steady state. Despite these biochemical changes there is no observable clinical disturbance.

β-Blockers such as propranolol and nadolol reduce the concentrations of T_3 relative to T_4 (Lotti *et al*. 1977; Peden *et al*. 1982). They appear to block 5'-deiodination and diminish the peripheral conversion of T_4 to T_3 (Heyma *et al*. 1980). Hyperthyroxinaemia has been reported in euthyroid patients taking high doses of

propranolol (Cooper *et al*. 1982). Studies with other β-blockers (Nilsson *et al*. 1979; How *et al*. 1980) suggest that the benefits on control of thyrotoxic symptoms are more related to sympathetic inhibitory activity than to their action on peripheral T_4/T_3 metabolism.

As with amiodarone, the radiographic contrast agents ipodate and iopanoic acid block the T_4 conversion to T_3 in peripheral tissues and in the anterior pituitary (Kaplan and Utiger 1978; Larsen *et al*. 1979). Administration of these agents leads to decreased serum T_3 and increased rT_3. There is also enhancement of basal and TRH-stimulated TSH concentrations, possibly in response to the reduction in circulating and intrapituitary T_3 (Burgi *et al*. 1976; Suzuki *et al*. 1979). These hormonal changes return to normal after 2 weeks of exposure (Suzuki *et al*. 1981).

Propylthiouracil, though predominantly an inhibitor of synthesis of thyroid hormone, also suppresses the conversion of T_4 to T_3 and leads to preferential formation of the inactive metabolite reverse T_3 (rT_3) shortly after administration in high dosage. This may be an advantage, at least theoretically, in the treatment of thyrotoxicosis, particularly in severe cases (Westgren *et al*. 1977; Laurberg and Weeke 1978). High doses of glucocorticoids have a similar effect on T_4/T_3 metabolism (Chopra *et al*. 1975; Burr *et al*. 1976). This provides a rational basis for the use of propylthiouracil and steroids in the emergency management of thyroid storm.

Serum total T_4 and free T_4 may be decreased by rifampicin, presumably due to enhanced hepatic metabolism and biliary excretion. In contrast, the level of T_3 increases but the mechanism of this still awaits elucidation (Ohnhaus *et al*. 1981).

Interference of indirect methods of thyroid hormone measurement (*in vitro* uptake tests)

The *in vitro* uptake tests measure the unoccupied thyroid hormone binding sites on TBG. The tests involve the use of T_3 or T_4 labelled with [125]Iodine and some form of synthetic absorbent (usually an ion-exchange resin) to measure the proportion of radioactive hormone that is not tightly bound to serum proteins, and are accordingly named the resin T_3 or T_4 uptake tests. The uptake of the tracer is inversely proportional to the number of unsaturated binding sites. Thus, the uptake is increased when the amount of TBG decreases owing to excess thyroid hormone or reduction of TBG level. Conversely, an increase in the amount of unsaturated TBG due to a low serum thyroid hormone concentration or an increase of TBG results in a reduced uptake value. The techniques provide an indirect measure of total serum thyroxine, and the free thyroxine index thus derived corrects for changes in TBG levels induced by drugs. The uptake test results are still invalidated, however, by compounds that compete with thyroid hormone binding to TBG. The need for these tests in clinical practice has been reduced by the increased availability of assays that directly measure free T_4 and free T_3 concentrations.

Interference with free thyroid hormone assays

In the past, the direct measurement of free thyroid hormones in serum using equilibrium dialysis was limited to a few research laboratories. The advent of the simple free thyroid hormone assay employing labelled hormone tracers or, more commonly, labelled hormone analogues, has made the technique widely available and greatly obviated the problem of interference by drugs affecting the binding capacity of serum proteins (e.g. oral contraceptives, phenytoin). The labelled T_4 analogue binds to the hormone antibody and, theoretically, not to carrying proteins, thus competing only with the free hormones in the serum. It does bind to albumin (Pearce and Byfield 1986), however, and in one labelled-analogue radioimmunoassay heparin can produce low free T_4 results as an artefact (Mardell and Gamlen 1982). This is due to activation of lipoprotein lipase and production of free fatty acids that compete with the analogue for the binding sites on albumin. Interference by heparin also occurs with free T_4 measurement by equilibrium dialysis. Contrary to the analogue assay, however, the free fatty acids generated lead to falsely elevated free T_4 values (Mendel et al. 1987).

Effects on *in vivo* tests of thyroid gland activity

Thyroid radioiodine uptake, previously used for diagnosis of hypothyroidism and hyperthyroidism, has now been largely superseded by measurement of serum free hormones. It is still used in some centres, however, for estimating the dose of radioiodide to be delivered in the therapy of thyrotoxicosis and thyroid carcinoma and remains a valuable investigation in the diagnosis of thyrotoxicosis secondary to transient thyroiditis, iodine excess, exogenous thyroxine, or drugs such as lithium and amiodarone when radioiodine uptake is suppressed despite the presence of thyrotoxicosis. Uptake studies and thyroid scanning can be significantly affected by changes in the body iodine pool caused by intake of iodine-containing drugs and radiographic contrast media. The antithyroid or goitrogenic medications can also interfere with trapping and retention of iodide and thus the results of these investigations.

Hypothalamic–pituitary–adrenal axis

Synthesis and secretion of cortisol are controlled by

ACTH (corticotrophin), a 39-aminoacid polypeptide derived from the precursor molecule pro-opiomelanocortin. Hypothalamic corticotrophin-releasing hormone (CRH) is the predominant regulator of ACTH formation and release by the pituitary. A parallel effect is seen with β-endorphin and with other pro-opiomelanocortin-related gene products. In man CRH is a 41-amino acid straight chain peptide (Vale et al. 1983). Among hormones of hypothalamic origin that can influence ACTH secretion (oxytocin, adrenaline, somatostatin, and vasoactive intestinal peptide), arginine vasopressin is most important in modulating pituitary ACTH release and it potentiates the action of CRH significantly (Gillies et al. 1982; De Bold et al. 1984). The cytokines interleukins 1 and 6 have been shown to enhance ACTH release, principally through stimulation of CRH (Sapolsky et al. 1987; Uehara et al. 1987; Naitoh et al. 1988). In this way they may act as an interface for communication between the endocrine and immune system.

Drugs affecting CRH and ACTH

Impaired CRH and ACTH secretion

CRH and ACTH secretion is impaired by negative feedback effects of glucocorticoids exerted at the hypothalamus and pituitary. Acute inhibition by corticosteroids occurs rapidly (within minutes) and is mediated via a membrane-dependent effect on the secretion of the hormones. Continued slow-onset feedback, however, involves suppression of hormone formation via an inhibitory effect on gene transcription (Taylor and Fishman 1988).

Physiological replacement doses of glucocorticoid hormones (hydrocortisone 20–30 mg, prednisone 7.5 mg or dexamethasone 0.5 mg daily) given for up to 18 months do not seem to cause suppression of ACTH secretion and cortisol levels (Livanou et al. 1967). High-dose glucocorticoid administration of short duration, such as in the treatment of acute severe asthma, also produces only transient (<10 days) hypothalamic–pituitary–adrenal axis (HPA) suppression (Zora et al. 1986).

Marked suppression of the HPA axis can, however, occur with the prolonged use of supraphysiological doses of glucocorticoids. It may also follow chronic topical application of steroids, especially fluorinated preparations, because of systemic absorption (Sneddon 1976). Adrenal hypofunction can also develop with high doses of inhaled steroid (e.g. >1500 μg beclomethasone dipropionate) for treatment of asthma (Smith and Hodson 1983). The recovery of suppressed pituitary–adrenal function after cessation of therapy has been reported to take as long as 9 months (Graber *et al.* 1965), and our own experience suggests that much longer intervals are occasionally required. During this recovery period and for an additional 1–2 years, the patient will need steroid cover during periods of stress (Bayliss 1975).

Cyproterone acetate, an antiandrogen, may also reduce basal and stress-induced rises in ACTH if given for more than 3 months (Jeffcoate *et al.* 1976; Smals *et al.* 1978).

Increased ACTH production

The administration of amphetamines stimulates production of ACTH (Besser *et al.* 1969). Metoclopramide can cause increases in ACTH and cortisol secretion, possibly through an antidopaminergic action on the central pituitary dopamine receptors (Nishida *et al.* 1983a, 1987). Metyrapone and aminoglutethimide, by blocking the synthesis of cortisol, can stimulate secretion of ACTH by secondary reduction in negative feedback (Dexter *et al.* 1967). ACTH secretion also increases in response to mifepristone (RU 486), a glucocorticoid receptor blocker with potential use for treatment of Cushing's syndrome, and can in turn stimulate further cortisol production, thus overcoming the effect of the drug in patients with pituitary-dependent Cushing's syndrome (Schteingart 1989; Bamberger and Chrousos 1995). A feedback rise of ACTH secretion in this condition also occurs in response to metyrapone and may serve both to attenuate the effectiveness of the drug in treating Cushing's disease and to increase the likelihood of potentially troublesome adverse effects such as hirsutism.

Drugs affecting the adrenal cortex

Cushing's syndrome

Iatrogenic Cushing's syndrome can occur with the administration of pharmacological doses of glucocorticoids or ACTH. Prolonged and excessive alcohol ingestion can also lead to alcoholic pseudo-Cushing's syndrome (Lamberts *et al.* 1979) which improves rapidly following withdrawal of alcohol. The disorder is most likely to be due to a centrally mediated mechanism with hypersecretion of pituitary ACTH and secondary stimulation of the adrenals (Kapcala 1987; Kirkman and Nelson 1988).

Hypoadrenalism

Adrenocortical failure can develop in patients who have been previously treated with suppressive doses of glucocorticoids if appropriate steroid cover is not given follow-

ing withdrawal. Hypoadrenalism can also occur in patients with Cushing's syndrome treated with aminoglutethimide, metyrapone, trilostane, or *o,p'*-DDD, which block the steroid biosynthetic pathway. Both aminoglutethimide and *o,p'*-DDD inhibit the cholesterol side-chain-cleavage enzymes and 11-β-hydroxylase (Hughes and Burley 1970). Trilostane acts by blocking 3-β-hydroxysteroid dehydrogenase (Engelhardt and Weber 1994). In addition, *o,p'*-DDD, or more probably its metabolites, destroys cell mitochondria, leading to adrenocortical cell death (Sparagana 1987). Metyrapone inhibits 11-β-hydroxylase and blocks the final step of cortisol synthesis.

Ketoconazole is an imidazole derivative with a potent inhibitory effect on adrenal steroidogenesis. It interferes with the P-450 cytochrome enzymes, which include 17-20 desmolase (side-chain cleavage), 11- and 21-hydroxylase, 17-20 lyase, and 17- and 18-hydroxylase (Sonino 1987; Trachtenberg and Zadra 1988). Acute hypoadrenalism has been reported with both high-dose ketoconazole treatment in Cushing's syndrome and low-dose ketoconazole treatment of fungal infections (Best *et al.* 1987; McCance *et al.* 1987). Itraconazole and fluconazole have been shown to have similar effects but with a lower incidence (Gradon and Sepkowitz 1991; Sharkey *et al.* 1991). Etomidate, a short-acting general anaesthetic, is another example of an imidazole derivative with significant inhibitory effects on 11-β-hydroxylase (Preziosi and Vacca 1988). Its use has also been associated with the development of adrenal insufficiency (Ledingham and Watt 1983).

Rifampicin, used in the treatment of mycobacterial infections, has been reported to precipitate acute adrenal insufficiency in patients with compromised adrenal reserve. This action is probably due to enhanced glucocorticoid metabolism, which presumably occurs through induction of microsomal enzymes (Kyriazopoulou *et al.* 1984). It is recommended that treatment with rifampicin in these patients be accompanied by doubling or tripling the dose of replacement steroids. Aminoglutethimide has also been reported to accelerate the degradation of some glucocorticoids, such as dexamethasone (but not hydrocortisone), and this may influence the decision regarding choice of replacement therapy in such patients (Santen *et al.* 1977).

Suramin, used to treat human trypanosomiasis and also tested as an agent for AIDS and certain malignancies, can induce hypoadrenalism by blocking the P-450 cytochrome enzymes (Stein *et al.* 1986; Cheson *et al.* 1987; Ashby *et al.* 1989). Both dicoumarol and warfarin can cause hypoadrenalism by causing adrenal haemorrhage (Dreher *et al.* 1971).

Interference with biochemical tests

Spironolactone, monamine oxidase inhibitors, and minor tranquillizers such as hydroxyzine and chlordiazepoxide can interfere with the colour reaction of the Porter–Silber reactions for measurement of urinary 17-hydroxycorticosteroids (17-OHCS), giving rise to spuriously increased values (Borushek and Gold 1964). Interference with the β-glucuronidase employed in the assay (e.g. by high urinary acetylsalicylic acid concentrations) will lead to falsely low values. Likewise, the Zimmerman reaction for measurement of urinary 17-ketogenic steroids and 17-ketosteroids can be affected by acebutolol (Ooiwa *et al.* 1988), penicillin, and minor tranquillizers (Borsushek and Gold 1964).

Oestrogen, in the form of an oral contraceptive, is the most common drug to cause elevation of plasma cortisol concentrations secondary to change in the concentration of cortisol-binding globulin (CBG). Drugs that are inducers of hepatic mixed function oxidases (phenytoin, phenobarbitone, and *o,p'*-DDD) modify the metabolism of cortisol and related steroids, resulting in increased urinary excretion of 6-hydroxylated steroids and other multihydroxylated derivatives (Bledsoe *et al.* 1964; Werk *et al.* 1964; Burstein and Klaiber 1965). As a consequence, urinary 17-OHCS and 17-ketogenic steroid determinations may be falsely low. These agents also interfere with dexamethasone suppression and metyrapone stimulation tests by inducing enzymes that inactivate these compounds, thus rendering the tests ineffective and potentially leading to erroneous diagnoses of Cushing's syndrome (Meikle *et al.* 1969; Jubiz *et al.* 1970).

In general, radioimmunoassay and related tests on blood and urine show little clinically important cross-reactivity at usual doses with drugs such as dexamethasone and other steroid-based preparations. One important result is that drug-induced Cushing's syndrome secondary to administration of dexamethasone or prednisolone will usually be associated with lowered plasma and urine cortisol concentrations, which will not be the case if the exogenous steroid is hydrocortisone.

Aldosterone synthesis

Aldosterone production is regulated mainly by changes in blood volume, mediated through the renin–angiotensin system (RAS), which interacts with the sympathetic nervous system and prostaglandins. Other factors controlling its secretion include changes in potassium and ACTH. The RAS is now known to play important pathophysiological roles in left ventricular hypertrophy and heart failure (Dahlöf 1993; Johnston *et al.* 1993).

Secondary hyperaldosteronism occurs with the use of thiazide or loop diuretics (Vaughan *et al.* 1978; Griffing and Melby 1989). Lithium therapy has been associated with elevated aldosterone concentration and sodium retention (Murphy *et al.* 1969). Females taking oral contraceptives have raised plasma renin activity and aldosterone concentrations, which may account for the development of hypertension in some susceptible subjects (Beckerhoff *et al.* 1973). Metoclopramide stimulates the secretion of aldosterone through both an ACTH-dependent effect and an antidopaminergic adrenal action (Nishida *et al.* 1983*b*). Hyperaldosteronism with hypertension, relative hypernatraemia and hypokalaemia may be mimicked by the ingestion of large quantities of licorice (Conn *et al.* 1968) or injudicious use of mineralocorticoid agents such as 9-fludrocortisone (Armbruster *et al.* 1975; Whitworth *et al.* 1986) and it is a possible risk of carbenoxolone therapy (Pinder *et al.* 1976; Nicholls and Espiner 1983). Recent evidence suggests that the mineralocorticoid effect of licorice and carbenoxolone is primarily mediated through inhibition of the enzyme 11β-hydroxysteroid dehydrogenase, which catalyzes conversion of cortisol to cortisone, so leading to significant enhancement of the mineralocorticoid effect of cortisol (Stewart *et al.* 1987, 1990; MacKenzie *et al.* 1990).

Angiotensin-converting-enzyme (ACE) inhibitors such as captopril and enalapril can produce hyperreninaemic hypoaldosteronism which manifests as hyperkalaemia with a hyperchloraemic metabolic acidosis (Sakemi *et al.* 1988). The newer classes of drugs acting on the RAS and used for the treatment of hypertension and congestive heart failure include renin-receptor inhibitor and angiotensin II-receptor antagonists. Remikiren, a renin receptor blocker, induces rise in plasma renin activity and reduction in angiotensin II level (Himmelmann *et al.* 1996). Losartan, a non-peptide specific angiotensin II receptor antagonist, leads to increase in plasma renin activity and angiotensin II concentration, with concomitant reduction in aldosterone level (Bauer *et al.* 1995; Goldberg *et al.* 1995). These changes in hormone levels are to be expected when the mechanism of actions of these drugs and feed-back hormonal control are considered.

Adrenaline has been shown to increase renin concentrations, while aldosterone concentrations remain unaffected (Kruse *et al.* 1994). β_2-Agonists, such as nebulized albuterol, have been shown to increase renin and aldosterone in a dose-dependent manner (Millar *et al.* 1997). Piribedil, a dopamine (D_1) agonist with potential use as an antihypertensive agent, causes lowering of blood pressure and increase in renin and aldosterone, probably through vasodilatation. Bromocriptine, a D_2 agonist, causes a fall in blood pressure and aldosterone concentration, probably through reduction in sympathetic tone (Luchsinger *et al.* 1992). α-Adrenoceptor blockers induce an acute rise in renin and aldosterone, but no long-term clinical effects have been demonstrated (Tomiyama *et al.* 1992).

Non-steroidal anti-inflammatory agents (such as indomethacin, ibuprofen, piroxicam, and naproxen) can lead to hyporeninaemic hypoaldosteronism and thus hyperkalaemia through inhibition of prostaglandin synthesis (Tan *et al.* 1979; Miller *et al.* 1984; Mactier and Khanna 1988).

Even at low doses, standard or low-molecular-weight heparins given for thromboembolic disorders can produce hypoaldosteronism, usually with a compensatory increase in renin concentration (Sherman and Ruddy 1986; Levesque *et al.* 1990). The effect is thought to occur by inhibition of the conversion of corticosterone to 18-hydroxycorticosterone (Conn *et al.* 1966). Thus, patients with a compromised renin–angiotensin–aldosterone system, as in diabetes mellitus or chronic renal insufficiency, are more prone to the development of hyperkalaemia with heparin administration (Edes and Sunderrajan 1985; Kutyrina *et al.* 1987).

Growth hormone has been shown to increase plasma renin and aldosterone concentrations (Hoffman *et al.* 1996). This can, at least partly, account for the hypertension induced by GH. Magnesium sulphate, used in pre-eclampsia and tested for treatment of myocardial infarction, also suppresses aldosterone and increases renin concentrations (Ichihara *et al.* 1993).

Adrenal medulla

Adverse drug reactions in phaeochromocytoma

These are discussed fully in Chapter 9.

Drug interference with biochemical tests

Drug-induced alterations are perhaps the most common cause of erroneous interpretation of measurement of plasma or urinary catecholamines and their metabolites. Samples should preferably be collected under drug-free conditions. If this is not possible, a knowledge and avoidance of the principal offending medications is important. Drugs that alter sympathochromaffin physiology can affect the secretion of catecholamines or their metabolites, and certain other drugs can interfere with fluorimetric or non-specific chromatographic assays (Rayfield *et al.* 1972; Cryer 1985; Feldman 1987; Sheps *et al.* 1988). These are summarized in Table 15.3.

TABLE 15.3
Drugs interfering with tests of adrenal medullary function

Catecholamines and metanephrines

Elevation	α-Adrenergic antagonists
	phenoxybenzamine, phentolamine, prazosin
	β-Adrenergic agonists
	isoprenaline, terbutaline
	β-Adrenoceptor blockers
	propranolol and related drugs
	Diuretics (if Na⁺ depletion occurs)
	Indirectly acting sympathomimetics
	amphetamines, ephedrine
	Tricyclic antidepressants
	Vasodilators
	calcium-channel blockers (acutely)
	minoxidil, nitrates, phenothiazines, theophylline,
	Miscellaneous
	erythromycin
	labetalol, methyldopa, tetracycline
Reduction	ACE inhibitors
	α_2-Adrenergic agonist
	clonidine
	Monoamine oxidase inhibitors
	Miscellaneous
	bromocriptine, dexamethasone, α-methyl-paratyrosine

Urinary vanillylmandelic acid (VMA)

Elevation (due to assay interference)	Aspirin
	Nalidixic acid
	Penicillin
	Sulphonamides
Reduction	Clofibrate
	Methyldopa
	Monoamine oxidase inhibitors

N.B. Methyldopa characteristically produces elevated catecholamines, but not VMA, in some conventional chromatographic systems, owing to the production of *o*-methyl metabolites; the interference can be overcome with high-pressure liquid chromatography (HPLC).

Hypothalamic–pituitary–gonadal axis

In both sexes, the hypothalamus is the integrative centre of the reproductive axis. It receives messages from the central nervous system and from the gonads, which regulate the synthesis and release of gonadotrophin-releasing hormones (GnRH or LHRH). In addition, certain neurotransmitters (catecholamines, serotonin, acetylcholine) and endogenous opioid peptides have modulatory effects on GnRH release.

Episodic, pulsatile release of GnRH is essential for the synthesis and release of the gonadotrophins, namely luteinizing hormone (LH) and follicle-stimulating hormone (FSH), which are glycoproteins synthesized in the anterior pituitary. LH and FSH then bind to receptors at the target cells. In the male, LH stimulates synthesis of testosterone from Leydig cells and FSH promotes spermatogenesis in the germinal epithelium. In the female, FSH action leads to formation of the Graaffian follicle which contains the ovum, and LH stimulates production of oestrogen from the follicle and subsequently progesterone from the corpus luteum following ovulation.

The secretion of GnRH and FSH/LH are under negative feedback control from testosterone and oestradiol. In addition, FSH secretion is inhibited by inhibin, a glycoprotein composed of interlinked α- and β-subunits, which is produced in the Sertoli cells of the testis and the granulosa cells of the ovary. In the female, there is also a positive feedback mechanism whereby LH and FSH surge in midcycle in response to increasing oestrogen secretion, and induce ovulation.

Drugs affecting gonadotrophin and gonadal sex hormone secretion

Gonadotrophin and sex hormone dysfunction

Pituitary gonadotrophin secretion can be inhibited by glucocorticoid excess, resulting in testicular or ovarian dysfunction with suppressed spermatogenesis and lowering of gonadal sex hormone levels (Sakakura *et al.* 1973; MacAdams *et al.* 1986; McClure 1987). Opiates such as heroin and methadone lower testosterone levels without concomitant elevation of gonadotrophin levels. The phenomenon could be due to direct central actions of the drugs and their effects on peripheral androgen metabolism (Mendelson *et al.* 1975). Ketoconazole decreases testicular production of testosterone by blocking 17,20-desmolase and 17-α-hydroxylase (Rajfer *et al.* 1986). Danazol, used in the treatment of endometriosis and angioedema, decreases the binding capacity of sex-hormone-binding globulin and increases free testosterone levels, which partially accounts for its adverse effects of hirsutism and virilization (Pugeat *et al.* 1987). A metabolite of danazol may also interfere with certain testosterone assays leading to falsely high results.

Drugs used in treatment of metastatic prostatic carcinoma tend to have significant effects on reproductive hormones. Prolonged oestrogen therapy may cause irreversible testicular damage and loss of the feedback response of the hypothalamic–pituitary–gonadal axis (Wortsman *et al.* 1989). The steroid antiandrogen cyproterone acetate, in addition to competitive antagonism at the target organ receptors, lowers LH, FSH and, consequently, testosterone levels and sperm count because of its strong progestational activity (Namer 1988). On the other hand, the non-steroid antiandrogens flutamide and anandron are specific androgen-receptor blockers without intrinsic activity. They can establish an effective peripheral androgen resistance despite increases in gonadotrophin and testosterone levels (Migliari *et al.* 1988).

Long-acting LHRH analogues used for treatment of such disorders as central precocious puberty, endometriosis, and prostatic and breast carcinoma act by abolishing the pulsatile nature of LHRH stimulation, thereby desensitizing the pituitary with reduction in gonadotrophin and hence gonadal sex hormone production, and producing 'medical castration'. The majority of women experience some degree of hot flushes, vaginal dryness, and loss of libido, with the potential long-term complication of osteoporosis; whereas in men decreased libido and impotence may be produced (Santen and Bourguignon 1987; Fraser and Baird 1987).

Oral contraceptives were once thought to increase the incidence of amenorrhoea. More recent studies have shown, however, that the incidence of post-pill amenorrhoea is similar to that of the development of spontaneous secondary amenorrhoea in the general population and that subsequent fertility is probably not impaired by previous use of oral contraceptives (Archer and Thomas 1981; Hull *et al.* 1981).

Drugs that induce hyperprolactinaemia, by various mechanisms (see section on Hyperprolactinaemia), can interfere with reproductive function at the level of hypothalamus, pituitary, or gonads.

Gonadal dysfunction after chemotherapy

In man, progressive dose-related depletion of germinal epithelium resulting in azoöspermia and infertility can occur with cytotoxic agents, particularly alkylating agents such as mustine hydrochloride, cyclophosphamide, chlorambucil, procarbazine, and busulphan (Miller 1971; Bajorunas 1980; Waxman *et al.* 1982). The Leydig cells remain morphologically intact, although they may be functionally abnormal. Other drugs that have been found to be toxic to the germinal epithelium include vinblastine, doxorubicin, cytarabine, and *o,p'*-DDD. The effects of newer agents such as ifosfamide, cisplatin and high-dose methotrexate are less clear and await further elucidation (Sparagana 1987; Aubier *et al.* 1989;

Sherins and Mulvihill 1989). Ovarian failure also occurs in at least 50 per cent of female patients treated with single alkylating agents (Sherins and Mulvihill 1989). High-dose methotrexate is the only antimetabolite that has been assessed; it does not appear to have immediate ovarian toxicity (Shamberger *et al.* 1981).

Combination chemotherapy has a profound impact on spermatogenesis: 80 per cent of men who have received MOPP (mustine hydrochloride, vincristine, procarbazine, and prednisone) or a similar regimen for treatment of Hodgkin's lymphoma develop azoöspermia (Chapman *et al.* 1979*a*). This regimen also produces ovarian dysfunction in over 50 per cent of women (Chapman *et al.* 1979*b*; Horning *et al.* 1981; Waxman *et al.* 1982). In general, young patients (under age 30) tolerate the drug better and have higher chances of recovery from azoöspermia or amenorrhoea. A combination of doxorubicin, bleomycin, vinblastine, and DTIC (ABVD) is cited as equally efficacious and less toxic to the gonads than the classical MOPP regimen, oligospermia being induced in only 54 per cent of patients and full recovery of spermatogenesis occurring in all patients within 18 months (Viviani *et al.* 1985).

Basal FSH rises as a result of germinal aplasia. Basal LH may either increase or, more commonly, remain normal (Waxman *et al.* 1982; Sherins and Mulvihill 1989). Booth and others (1987) have shown that, although still within the normal range, both levels and production of testosterone are in fact significantly reduced, signifying altered Leydig cell function and in line with the fact that challenge with LHRH usually results in excessive responses of both gonadotrophins.

Virilization

Anabolic steroids used in the treatment of aplastic anaemia, hereditary angioedema, and breast cancer have variable degrees of androgenic effect (Wynn and Path 1968). They can therefore cause virilization ranging from mild hirsutism to clitoromegaly, deepening of voice, and muscle development when given to women, and may produce precocious puberty or acceleration of bone age in young children. Furthermore, by suppressing endogenous gonadotrophin secretion, they can inhibit spermatogenesis, which provides a theoretical basis for clinical trials of androgens as male contraceptives (Swerdloff *et al.* 1978).

Most progestogens are weakly androgenic. They have been used for prevention of abortion, although this effect is controversial. Because of the enormous capacity of the placenta to aromatize the naturally occurring androgens to oestrogens, however, even high doses of progesterone and 17-α-hydroxyprogesterone have not

been shown to be teratogenic (Chez 1978; Check *et al.* 1986). On the other hand, synthetic androgens and progestogens often cannot be aromatized, and norethisterone in doses of 10–20 mg daily can cause masculinization of the female fetus (Schardein 1980).

Cyproterone acetate, used in humans for the treatment of hirsutism, causes feminization in male fetal rats (Neumann 1978). Although feminization has not been reported in humans (Laudahn 1984), the drug should be avoided during pregnancy. Addition of oestrogen in a reversed sequential regimen can provide effective contraception and decrease the menstrual irregularity resulting from the strong progestational property and long elimination half-life of cyproterone acetate (Biffignandi and Molinatti 1987).

Gynaecomastia

Gynaecomastia is enlargement of the male breast due to an increase in the glandular and stromal tissue. A wide variety of drugs can produce it (Table 15.4), mainly as a result of alteration of the balance between testosterone and oestradiol effects (Carlson 1980).

The use of oestrogens or compounds with oestrogen-like activity can induce severe gynaecomastia in men. Breast enlargement is common among men treated with the synthetic oestrogen diethylstilboestrol (DES) for prostatic carcinoma (Wolf *et al.* 1969; Hendrickson and Anderson 1970). Oral contraceptives, used in haemophilia, can induce gynaecomastia (Brandt 1973). Human chorionic gonadotropin (hCG), LHRH, and menotropins (mixture of FSH and LH), used for induction of puberty and fertility in patients with hypogonadotrophic hypogonadism, result in gynaecomastia by preferential stimulation of oestrogen production (Morse *et al.* 1962; Okada *et al.* 1992).

Anabolic steroids, such as nandrolone and testosterone cypionate taken by body-builders and athletes, can lead to gynaecomastia as a result of peripheral aromatization into oestrogens (Spano and Ryan 1984; Goldberg 1996).

The major mechanism of production of gynaecomastia with cimetidine and spironolactone seems to be inhibition of dihydrotestosterone binding to its cellular receptor protein (Loriaux *et al.* 1976; Funder and Mercer 1979). In addition, cimetidine causes an increase in serum oestradiol concentration by inhibiting its 2-hydroxylation (Galbraith and Michnovicz 1989), and spironolactone has a partial suppressive effect on the 17-hydroxylation, which could explain its adverse effect of menstrual irregularity in females (Loriaux *et al.* 1976). Ketoconazole and itraconazole, through their suppressive effect on androgen and glucocorticoid synthesis, depress serum testosterone concentrations more than serum oestradiol and produce an elevated oestradiol–testosterone ratio (Pont *et al.* 1985; Tucker *et al.* 1990). Reduction in free testosterone concentration due to increased amount of sex-hormone-binding globulin and enhanced conversion of testosterone to oestradiol could explain the gynaecomastia due to phenytoin (Monson and Scott 1987) and diazepam (Moerck and Magelund 1979; Bergman *et al.* 1981).

Cytotoxic agents (Trump *et al.* 1982), antiandrogens such as cyproterone acetate (Geller *et al.* 1968), flutamide (Caine *et al.* 1975), nilutamide (Decensi *et al.* 1991) and finasteride, a 5-α-reductase inhibitor (Steiner 1996), and the adrenal toxic agent *o,p'*-DDD (Luton *et al.* 1979; Slooten *et al.* 1984) can all cause gynaecomastia either by direct testicular damage or reduction of the effect of testosterone.

TABLE 15.4
Drugs producing gynaecomastia

With oestrogenic activity
Conjugated or synthetic oestrogens
Digitoxin
Oral contraceptives

Stimulating oestrogen secretion
Anabolic steroids
Human chorionic gonadotrophin (hCG)
Luteinizing-hormone-releasing hormone (LHRH)
Menotropins

Reducing testosterone synthesis/effect
Antiandrogens (cyproterone acetate, flutamide)
Cimetidine
Cytotoxic agents (busulfan, nitrosoureas, *o,p'*-DDD, vincristine)
Diazepam
Ketoconazole
Phenytoin
Spironolactone

Unknown mechanisms
Auranofin
Calcium-channel blockers
Captopril
Digoxin
Ethionamide
Etretinate
Isoniazid
Major tranquillizers (? prolactin effect)
Marihuana
Methadone
Methyldopa
Metronidazole
Penicillamine
Reserpine
Thiacetazone

Although hyperprolactinaemia is not considered a direct cause of gynaecomastia, prolactin may contribute to breast enlargement through indirect effects on gonadal and possibly adrenal function. This may explain the effect of centrally acting antihypertensive agents such as methyldopa (*Journal of the American Medical Association* 1963), reserpine (Robinson 1957), and clonidine (Weiss 1991); the psychotherapeutic drugs, including phenothiazines (Margolis and Gross 1967) and tricyclic antidepressants; and the antiemetic domperidone (Keating and Rees 1991). Gynaecomastia has also been reported following treatment with the calcium-channel blockers verapamil and nifedipine, elevated prolactin values having been demonstrated with verapamil (Clyne 1986; Tanner and Bosco 1988).

Digitoxin has inherent oestrogen-like properties (Le Winn 1953), but digoxin probably produces gynaecomastia through a 'refeeding' mechanism in debilitated men. Isoniazid (Koang *et al.* 1955), ethionamide, and thiacetazone (Chunhaswasdikul 1974) may similarly act through a refeeding mechanism in men suffering from tuberculosis.

The mechanism of gynaecomastia remains unclear, a number of medications occasionally being reported to be associated with it. These include methadone (Thomas 1976), marihuana (Harmon and Aliapoulios 1972), angiotensin-converting-enzyme inhibitors (Markusse and Meyboom 1988; Nakamura *et al.* 1990; Llop 1994), omeprazole (Convens *et al.* 1991; Santucci *et al.* 1991); minoxidil (Smith 1980), amiloride (Vidt 1981), bumetanide (Dixon 1981), cyclosporin (Rahman and Ing 1989), penicillamine (Reid *et al.* 1982; Kahl *et al.* 1985), auranofin (Williams 1988), etretinate (Carmichael and Paul 1989), and metronidazole (Fagan *et al.* 1985).

Hypothalamic–pituitary–prolactin secretion

Prolactin is a polypeptide trophic hormone secreted from the anterior pituitary. Its secretion is primarily under the inhibitory control of hypothalamic dopamine, whereas the hypothalamic serotonergic system is stimulatory. A prolactin-releasing factor, probably regulated by serotonin, has been identified in hypothalamic extracts but not yet characterized. Thyrotrophin-releasing hormone is also a potent stimulator of prolactin release but is of uncertain physiological significance. Excessive secretion of prolactin may result in galactorrhoea, amenorrhoea, impotence, and infertility. Several possible mechanisms may be responsible for its effect on the menstrual cycle and fertility (Frantz 1978). First, prolactin could act at the hypothalamic level to interfere with either the tonic or the cyclic release of luteinizing-hormone-releasing hormone (LHRH). Secondly, high prolactin concentrations could desensitize the pituitary gland to the action of LHRH, leading to impaired gonadotrophin secretion. Thirdly, excessive prolactin could interfere with the steroidogenic action of gonadotrophin at the ovarian level. In addition, hyperprolactinaemia inhibits 5-α-reductase and hence peripheral conversion of testosterone to dihydrotestosterone, so interfering with spermatogenesis and other peripheral actions of testosterone (Carter *et al.* 1978).

Galactorrhoea has been associated with a wide variety of drugs that induce prolactin secretion (Table 15.5). Many of these substances act on the hypothalamus by either inhibiting the action of dopamine or enhancing the effect of serotonin. For instance, reserpine and methyldopa deplete catecholamine stores. The major tranquillizers, the phenothiazines and butyrophenones, block the dopamine receptors (Turkington 1972; Tolis *et al.* 1974). Metoclopramide and sulpiride are orthopramides that produce hyperprolactinaemia, presumably through their inhibitory effect on dopamine (McCallum et al. 1976; Aono *et al.* 1978). The tricyclics probably stimulate prolactin release by blocking the reuptake

TABLE 15.5
Drugs causing galactorrhoea

Benzodiazepines	chlordiazepoxide
Butyrophenones	haloperidol
Cimetidine	
Dexamphetamine, fenfluramine	
Methyldopa	
Monoamine oxidase inhibitors	
Oestrogens and oral contraceptives	
Orthopramides	bromopride
	metoclopramide
	sulpiride
Phenothiazines	chloropromazine
	perphenazine
	prochlorperazine
	promazine
	trifluoperazine
Rauwolfia alkaloids	reserpine
Tricyclic compounds	amitriptyline
	clomipramine
	imipramine
Verapamil	

of serotonin or enhancing the sensitivity of the postsynaptic serotonin receptors (Charney *et al.* 1984; Gadd *et al.* 1987). Monoamine oxidase inhibitors may shift the balance between dopaminergic inhibition and serotonergic stimulation of prolactin release (Slater *et al.* 1977). Fluoxetine, a second-generation antidepressant widely prescribed for depression and obsessive compulsive disorders, is a selective inhibitor of serotonin reuptake which can lead to hyperprolactinameia and rarely, galactorrhoea (Urban and Velduis 1991; Iancu *et al.* 1992). Prolactin concentrations also increase with fenfluramine, an anorexiant drug used in the treatment of obesity and capable of serotonergic stimulation (Barbieri *et al.* 1983).

Other drugs produce hyperprolactinaemia through less well-defined mechanisms. Oestrogens increase mean serum prolactin levels and also enhance responsiveness to prolactin-releasing stimuli (Frantz 1978). Administration of cimetidine has been reported rarely to increase prolactin secretion and produce galactorrhoea, suggesting that brain histamine could play a role in prolactin release (Bohnet *et al.* 1978; Ehrinpreis *et al.* 1989). Ranitidine produces similar effects when administered at high intravenous doses, but it does not lead to hyperprolactinaemia when given orally at the maintenance dosage. This is likely to be due to its poor penetration of the blood–brain barrier (Knigge *et al.* 1981; Delitala *et al.* 1981). Likewise, the possibility of opioid regulation is reflected by hyperprolactinaemia due to morphine and methadone (Frantz 1978). Verapamil has been found to elevate basal and TRH-stimulated prolactin concentrations, possibly via an inhibitory effect on dopaminergic tone (Gluskin *et al.* 1981; Nielsen-Kudsk *et al.* 1990). Other drugs which can induce prolactin release include cyproterone acetate (Goldenberg and Bruchovsky 1991) and bezafibrate (Monk and Todd 1987). Galactorrhoea has also been associated with benzodiazepines, though without hyperprolactinaemia (Kleinberg *et al.* 1977).

Treatment of troublesome drug-induced hyperprolactinaemia requires withdrawal of the offending medication if the clinical setting allows. The prolactin level and disturbed menstrual cycle should then return to normal within a few weeks, with restoration of fertility.

Drugs that inhibit prolactin release include levodopa; the ergot alkaloids (bromocriptine, pergolide), which act as dopamine agonists; and the serotonin-antagonist metergoline. These drugs are effective in reversing galactorrhoea and restoring ovulatory menses in patients with hyperprolactinaemia, whether due to a tumour or other causes (Vance *et al.* 1984; Bohnet *et al.* 1986). Further, the ergot derivatives can shrink prolactin-secreting pituitary tumours (Kleinberg *et al.* 1983; Vance *et al.* 1984) and are now a well-established means of treating such disorders.

Growth hormone

Growth hormone (GH) is synthesized in the somatotrophs of the pituitary. Its release is regulated by a balance between the actions of hypothalamic-growth-hormone-releasing hormone (GHRH) and somatostatin. These, in turn, are influenced by interactions between various neurotransmitters and neuropeptides at the hypothalamic or suprahypothalamic levels. Most of the growth-promoting effects of GH are mediated by somatomedins, principally insulin-like growth factor-1 (IGF 1) or somatomedin-C. Drugs may influence growth through their effects on GH secretion at the hypothalamic or pituitary level or through antagonism of its peripheral actions through effects on IGF 1. In addition, they may indirectly inhibit growth through interference with the metabolism of thyroid hormones or cortisol, which are also required for normal growth.

In children, prolonged treatment with corticosteroids, for example in asthma, has been associated with poor growth (Preece 1976; Chang *et al.* 1982). Although, however, large doses of glucocorticoids and Cushing's syndrome inhibit growth hormone secretion in adults, the suppression seems to be less significant in children (Strickland *et al.* 1972). Also, the administration of GH together with glucocorticoid does not reverse steroid-induced growth retardation in children (Solomon and Schoen 1976) and serum IGF 1 concentrations are not necessarily low in patients with glucocorticoid excess. These, together with other observations (Loeb 1976), suggest that the inhibitory effects of glucocorticoids on growth are due to direct actions on target tissue rather than alteration of GH secretion. The mechanisms are undoubtedly more complex than previously suspected.

Testosterone and its metabolite dihydrotestosterone are potent anabolic agents that enhance linear growth and weight gain. Androgen administration to prepubertal human children increases peak plasma GH levels after provocative stimuli but does not have consistent direct effects on plasma levels of IGF 1 (Craft and Underwood 1984). Therefore, the elevated plasma IGF 1 concentrations observed during puberty are probably secondary to sex-hormone-stimulated increases in GH secretion. Caution has to be exercised, however, in using androgens to stimulate growth, since they can lead to premature closure of epiphysial plates and a reduction in final adult height. Androgen replacement should not be commenced in young patients with hypopituitarism until other pituitary hormones have exerted their stimulatory effects on growth.

Although oestrogens increase basal plasma GH levels and enhance GH response to provocative stimuli, pharmacological doses of oestrogens reduce the concentrations of somatomedins (von Puttkamer *et al.* 1977) and enhance epiphysial maturation (Strickland and Sprinz 1973). This is the rationale for treating excessively tall girls with high-dose oestrogens (Wettenhall *et al.* 1975; Crawford 1978).

Thyroid hormones can influence growth by effects on the synthesis and secretion of GH by the pituitary gland, enhancement of the GH response to GHRH *in vitro* and *in vivo* (Wehrenberg *et al.* 1986) and possibly by an additional direct action on cartilage growth plates. Hypothyroid patients frequently have severely blunted GH responses to provocative stimuli, and they tend to have low serum Sm-C/IGF 1 levels (Chernausek *et al.* 1983). Hypothyroidism can be iatrogenic, and withdrawal of the offending medication, by correcting hypothyroidism, will lead to recovery of growth (Wilkinson *et al.* 1972).

A number of drugs that affect neurotransmitter (biogenic amines, GABA, and opioids) activity can influence growth hormone secretion. Drugs that stimulate GH secretion include levodopa (Huseman and Hassing 1984); apomorphine (Massara *et al.* 1985); bromocriptine and clonidine, which act via the dopaminergic or α-adrenergic pathways (Martin and Reichlin 1987); the serotonin precursors tryptophan and 5-OH-tryptophan, which increase central serotonin level (Martin *et al.* 1978); the GABA-ergic drugs muscimol, baclofen, and diazepam; some opiates such as methadone and nalorphine (Bercu and Diamond 1986); and β-blockers such as propranolol. The dopamine antagonist metoclopramide paradoxically stimulates GH secretion (Cohen *et al.* 1979), which may be due to blockade of the presynaptic receptors leading to increased secretion of dopamine, or to its actions on other monoaminergic pathways. On the other hand, GH secretion, mostly that associated with sleep and insulin-induced hypoglycaemia, is inhibited by the α-blockers phenoxybenzamine and phentolamine; the dopamine-receptor blockers chlorpromazine and haloperidol; the amine depletor reserpine; the serotonin-receptor blocker cyproheptadine; and the β-agonists such as isoprenaline. The anticholinergic agents atropine and pirenzepine also block exercise-associated and drug-induced GH secretion (Casanueva *et al.* 1984; Chiodera *et al.* 1984). Conversely, pyridostigmine augments GH secretion and release through its anticholinesterase activity (Ross *et al.* 1987). These drugs have been widely used for study of neuroendocrine control of GH secretion and sometimes applied clinically for screening tests of GH reserve (Cohen *et al.* 1979; Lanes and Hurtado 1982). Their long-term effects on GH secretion and growth, however, still remain unclear.

Posterior pituitary

Vasopressin (ADH)

The posterior pituitary is principally made up of the axon terminals of the supraoptic and paraventricular nuclei in the hypothalamus. Vasopressin (antidiuretic hormone or ADH) and oxytocin are synthesized in both nuclei as parts of large precursor molecules and packaged with their respective neurophysins in neurosecretory granules that migrate along the axons to the posterior pituitary. A large number of stimuli, for example, emesis and hypoglycaemia, can cause release of vasopressin. Under physiological conditions, however, the major regulator is the plasma osmotic pressure, which is believed to exert its influence through specific osmoreceptor neurons situated at the anterior hypothalamus. Drugs affecting vasopressin release and producing the conditions discussed in the two following sections are listed in Table 15.6.

The syndrome of inappropriate secretion of ADH (SIADH)

The syndrome of inappropriate secretion of ADH has been associated with the use of a variety of antipsychotic medications, namely, phenothiazines (De Rivera 1975; Rao *et al.* 1975; Matuk and Kalyanaraman 1977; Hwang and Magraw 1989), tricyclic antidepressants (Ajlouni *et al.* 1974; Luzecky 1974; Dhar and Ramos 1978; Liskin *et al.* 1984; Mitsch and Lee 1986), and monoamine oxidase inhibitors (Peterson *et al.* 1978; Giese *et al.* 1989), presumably through increased secretion or potentiation of actions of vasopressin. Selective serotonin-reuptake inhibitors, for example, fluoxetine and sertraline, can also cause SIADH, particularly in the elderly (Kazal *et al.* 1993; Bradley *et al.* 1996; Burke and Fanker 1996). Chlorpropamide causes antidiuresis, probably through enhancement of both the release and peripheral actions of ADH (Miller and Moses 1970; Moses *et al.* 1973*a*; Singer and Forrest 1976). Carbamazepine, structurally related to tricyclic antidepressants, also induces water

TABLE 15.6
Drugs affecting vasopressin release or function

I. Leading to SIADH

Chemotherapeutic agents	cisplatin cyclophosphamide melphalan vinblastine vincristine
Monoamine oxidase inhibitors	phenelzine tranylcypromine
Phenothiazines	fluphenazine thioridazine
Tricyclic antidepressants	amitriptyline desipramine imipramine
Serotonin-reuptake inhibitors	fluoxetine sertraline
Miscellaneous	carbamazepine chlorpropamide haloperidol thiothixene vasopressin and its long-acting derivatives

II. Leading to diabetes insipidus (DI) (nephrogenic)

Democycline
Ifosfamide
Lithium carbonate
  (short-term
  administration
  causes central DI)
Methoxyflurane

intoxication through stimulation of ADH release (Rado 1973; Kimura *et al.* 1974). Sodium valproate, another antiepileptic drug, has also been reported to cause SIADH (Ikeda *et al.* 1995). Certain cytotoxic drugs also predispose to development of SIADH. They include cyclophosphamide (DeFronzo *et al.* 1973), high-dose melphalan (Greenbaum-Lefkoe *et al.* 1985), vincristine (Robertson *et al.* 1973; Stuart *et al.* 1975), vinblastine (Antony *et al.* 1980), and cisplatin (Littlewood and Smith 1984; Ritch 1988). The water-retaining properties of these drugs are particularly noteworthy, since patients on cyclophosphamide or cisplatin require vigorous hydration to prevent the occurrence of cystitis or nephrotoxicity, and electrolyte disturbance can easily develop if the electrolytes are not monitored closely. Clofibrate enhances the release of ADH, although clinically significant hyponatraemia has not been reported (Moses *et al.* 1973*b*).

Diabetes insipidus

Short-term lithium administration inhibits ADH secretion from the posterior pituitary, while prolonged use can lead to symptomatic nephrogenous diabetes insipidus in 10–30 per cent of patients (Forrest *et al.* 1974; Baylis and Heath 1978; Mannisto 1980). The disorder tends, however, to be mild and reversible in most patients on stopping the medication. Demeclocycline produces dose-dependent nephrogenic diabetes insipidus (Castell and Sparks 1965; Feldman and Singer 1974) and has been used for the treatment of SIADH. Nephrotoxicity with polyuria has also been associated with the general anaesthetic agent methoxyflurane, owing to the formation of inorganic fluoride from its metabolism (Mazze *et al.* 1971; Cousins *et al.* 1974). There has also been a case report of ifosfamide, a derivative of cyclophosphamide, causing diabetes insipidus in a patient treated for breast cancer. The underlying mechanism is, however, unclear (DeFronzo *et al.* 1974). Certain other drugs have been reported to cause nephrogenic diabetes insipidus due to tubular damage. These include rifampicin (Quinn and Wall 1989), foscarnet (Farese *et al.* 1990; Navarro *et al.* 1996), and mesalazine (Masson 1992).

Oxytocin

The regulation of oxytocin secretion and its physiological role are still largely unknown, although breast-feeding is a recognized stimulus for oxytocin release in post-partum lactating women.

No clinical disorder due to deranged secretion of the hormone is known. Occasionally, however, high-dose oxytocin infusion has been associated with water intoxication, probably as a result of the antidiuretic potential of oxytocin together with simultaneous infusion of dextrose solution (Ahmad *et al.* 1975). Syntocinon infusion can occasionally lead to severe hyponatraemia during labour, particularly if labour is prolonged and dextrose is infused at the same time (personal observations).

Parathyroids and vitamin D

Several drugs have been reported to affect parathyroid function and vitamin D metabolism. Since drugs affecting vitamin D metabolism will be discussed in detail in Chapter 17, they are only briefly mentioned here.

Lithium treatment for manic-depressive illness is associated with mild hyperparathyroidism, apparently by interference with the normal negative feedback process whereby parathyroid hormone (PTH) secretion is suppressed in response to elevation of the calcium level (Christiansen *et al.* 1980; McIntosh *et al.* 1987). The resulting chronic stimulation of the parathyroids has been found to cause an increase in gland size and may lead to hyperplasia or adenoma (Garfinkel *et al.* 1973; Mallette *et al.* 1989; Stancer and Forbath 1989).

Although thiazide diuretics (Christensson *et al.* 1977; Kohri *et al.* 1987) and diltiazem (Seely *et al.* 1989) have been reported to cause an increase of PTH concentrations, the clinical significance of this remains doubtful.

Ketoconazole lowers serum 1,25-dihydroxyvitamin D (1,25[OH]$_2$D) concentration by inhibition of renal 1-α-hydroxylase, a cytochrome-P-450-dependent enzyme (Glass and Eil 1986, 1988). It has recently been employed to treat a patient with sarcoidosis-associated hypercalcaemia (Adams *et al.* 1990). In theory, chronic administration of ketoconazole in high dosage may induce osteomalacia, but this remains unsubstantiated. Anticonvulsants such as phenytoin and phenobarbitone occasionally induce osteomalacia (Winnacker *et al.* 1977) by increasing hepatic conversion of vitamin D and 25-hydroxyvitamin D (25[OH]D) to more polar biologically inactive metabolites. Consequently the serum 25[OH]D is lowered. Serum 1,25[OH]$_2$D is usually normal (Hahn 1980), however. This, together with the fact that, in animals, phenytoin inhibits intestinal absorption of calcium and that phenytoin and phenobarbitone inhibit mobilization of calcium from bone *in vitro*, suggests that the drugs may cause bone disease by blocking the actions of 1,25[OH]$_2$D in target organs, rather than by a direct effect on 1,25[OH]$_2$D synthesis.

Although biphosphonates, now important as therapeutic agents for the treatment of disorders associated with excessive osteoclastic activities such as Paget's disease and malignant hypercalcaemia, can lead to a transient decrease in plasma calcium and elevation of PTH (Papapoulos *et al.* 1986; Fraser *et al.* 1991), they do not tend to induce chronic stimulation of PTH secretion (Landman and Papapoulos 1995). Vitamin D analogues, used for treatment of renal osteodystrophy and osteoporosis, also cause a reduction of PTH concentration (Dunlay *et al.* 1989; Quesada *et al.* 1992).

Gut hormones

Endocrine cells situated along the gastro-enteropancreatic axis secrete hormones which not only regulate gastrointestinal functions (e.g. gastrin in stimulating gastric acid release, cholecystokinin in gall-bladder function) but also affect glucose control (insulin and glucagon). Many hormones originally isolated from the gut have also been identified as important neuropeptides in the nervous system, and vice versa (e.g. vasoactive intestinal polypeptide, cholecystokinin, and somatostatin). A major stimulus to exploration of this complex area of endocrinology is the existence of the relatively rare but intriguing gut-hormone-secreting tumours. Thus far there are relatively few reports on the effects of drugs on the secretion and measurement of these hormones.

Raised urinary 5-hydroxyindoleacetic acid (5-HIAA) derived from metabolism of serotonin is the classical finding for diagnosis of carcinoid tumours. The assay can, however, be influenced by a number of medications. The more commonly used drugs that may produce false positive results include paracetamol, fluorouracil, Lugol's iodine, melphalan, mephenesin, methocarbamol, reserpine, and glyceryl guaiacolate (in some cough syrups), whereas false negatives occur with heparin, imipramine, isoniazid, methyldopa, monoamine oxidase inhibitors, phenothiazines, and *p*-chlorophenylalanine, the latter two drugs often being employed for symptomatic treatment of carcinoid symptoms (Cryer 1988; Roberts 1988).

Radioimmunoassay of gastrin is essential for the diagnosis of the Zollinger–Ellison syndrome. Acid-reducing drugs such as H_2-receptor antagonists, anticholinergics, and proton-pump inhibitors such as omeprazole can, however, lead to elevation of gastrin levels owing to loss of acid inhibition (Debas 1987; Sharma *et al.* 1987; Gaginella *et al.* 1989). These medications should therefore be excluded when gastrin measurements are to be made. Tolbutamide has been found to suppress gastrin release in man, but the physiological significance of this is not clear (Chiba *et al.* 1988).

The long-acting somatostatin analogue Sandostatin has been used to treat a variety of gut-hormone-secreting tumours as well as acromegaly. Steatorrhoea is a recognized adverse effect, and inhibition of endocrine secretions could contribute to the pathogenesis (Lembcke *et al.* 1987). Gallstone formation due to suppression of cholecystokinin and hence of gall-bladder contractility is another potential problem (Comi 1989). Since Sandostatin inhibits the secretion of insulin, one would expect an impairment of glucose tolerance. This does not appear, however, to be a major problem (Ch'ng *et al.* 1986; Halse *et al.* 1990), probably because of its concomitant inhibitory effect on other counter-regulatory hormones, which oppose the action of insulin.

References

Aanderud, S., Sundsfjord, J., and Aarbakke, J. (1984). Amiodarone inhibits the conversion of thyroxine to triiodothyronine in isolated rat hepatocytes. *Endocrinology* 115, 1605.

Abiodun, M.O., Bird, R., Havard, C.W., *et al.* (1973). The effects of phenylbutazone on thyroid function. *Acta Endocrinol.* 72, 257.

Adams, J.S., Sharma, O.P., Diz, M.M., *et al.* (1990). Ketoconazole decreases the serum 1,25-dihydroxyvitamin D and calcium concentration in sarcoidosis-associated hypercalcemia. *J. Clin. Endocrinol. Metab.* 70, 1090.

Ahmad, A.J., Clark, E.H., and Jacobs, H.S. (1975). Water intoxication associated with oxytocin infusion. *Postgrad. Med. J.* 51, 249.

Ajlouni, K., Kern, M.W., Tures, J.F., *et al.* (1974). Thiothixene-induced hyponatremia. *Arch. Intern. Med.* 134, 1103.

Amico, J.A., Richardson, V., Alpert, V., *et al.* (1984). Clinical and chemical assessment of thyroid function during therapy with amiodarone. *Arch. Intern. Med.* 144, 487.

Antony, A., Robinson, W.A., Roy, C., *et al.* (1980). Inappropriate antidiuretic hormone secretion after high dose vinblastine. *J. Urol.* 123, 783.

Aono, T., Shioji, T., Kinugasa, T., *et al.* (1978). Clinical and endocrinological analyses of patients with galactorrhea and menstrual disorders due to sulpiride or metoclopramide. *J. Clin. Endocrinol. Metab.* 47, 675.

Archer, D.F. and Thomas, R.L. (1981). The fallacy of the postpill amenorrhea syndrome. *Clin. Obstet. Gynecol.* 24, 943.

Arem, R. and Munipalli, B. (1996). Ipodate therapy in patients with severe destruction-induced thyrotoxicosis. *Arch. Intern. Med.* 156, 1752.

Armbruster, H., Vetter, W., Reck, G., *et al.* (1975). Severe arterial hypertension caused by chronic abuse of a topical mineralocorticoid. *Int. J. Clin. Pharmacol.* 12, 170.

Ashby, H., DiMattina, M., Linehan, W.M., *et al.* (1989). The inhibition of human adrenal steroidogenic enzyme activities by suramin. *J. Clin. Endocrinol. Metab.* 2, 505.

Atkins, M.B., Mier, J.W., Parkinson, D.R., *et al.* (1988). Hypothyroidism after treatment with interleukin-2 and lymphokine-activated killer cells. *N. Engl. J. Med.* 318, 1557.

Aubier, F., Flamant, F., Brauner, R., *et al.* (1989). Male gonadal function after chemotherapy for solid tumors in childhood. *J. Clin. Oncol.* 7, 304.

Azizi, F., Vagenakis, A.G., Portnay, G.I., *et al.* (1974). Thyroxine transport and metabolism in methadone and heroin addicts. *Ann. Intern. Med.* 80, 194.

Bajorunas, D.R. (1980). Disorders of endocrine function following cancer therapies. *Clin. Endocrinol. Metab.* 9, 405.

Bamberger, C.M. and Chrousos, G.P. (1995). The glucocorticoid receptor and RU 486 in man. *Ann. N.Y. Acad. Sci.* 761, 296.

Barbieri, C., Magnoni, V., Rauhe, W.G., *et al.* (1983). Effect of fenfluramine on prolactin secretion in obese patients: evidence for serotoninergic regulation of prolactin in man. *Clin. Endocrinol.* 19, 705.

Barbosa, J., Seal, U.S., and Doe, R.P. (1971). Effects of anabolic steroids on hormone-binding proteins, serum cortisol and serum nonprotein-bound cortisol. *J. Clin. Endocrinol. Metab.* 32, 232.

Bauer, I.H., Reams, G.P., Wu, Z., *et al.* (1995). Effect of losartan on the renin-angiotensin-aldosterone axis in essential hypertension. *J. Hum. Hypertens.* 9, 237.

Baylis, P.H. and Heath, D.A. (1978). Water disturbances in patients treated with oral lithium carbonate. *Ann. Intern. Med.* 88, 607.

Bayliss, R.I.S. (1975). The use of corticosteroids and corticotrophins in non-endocrine diseases. *Prescribers' J.* 15, 46.

Beckerhoff, R., Vetter, W., Armbruster, H., *et al.* (1973). Plasma aldosterone during oral-contraceptive therapy. *Lancet* i, 1218.

Beex, L.V.A., Ross, A., Smals, A.G.H., *et al.* (1976). 5-Fluorouracil and the thyroid. *Lancet* i, 866.

Bercu, B.B. and Diamond, F.B. Jr (1986). Growth hormone neurosecretory dysfunction. *Clin. Endocrinol. Metab.* 15, 537.

Bergman, D., Futterweit, W., Segal, R., *et al.* (1981). Increased oestradiol in diazepam-related gynaecomastia. *Lancet* ii, 1225.

Besser, G.M., Butler, P.W.P., Landon, J., *et al.* (1969). Influence of amphetamines on plasma corticosteroid and growth hormone levels in man. *Br. Med. J.* iv, 528.

Best, T.R., Jenkins, J.K., Murphy, F.Y., *et al.* (1987). Persistent adrenal insufficiency secondary to low-dose ketoconazole therapy. *Am. J. Med.* 82, 676.

Biffignandi, P. and Molinatti, G.M. (1987). Antiandrogens and hirsutism. *Horm. Res.* 28, 242.

Bledsoe, T., Island, D.P., Ney, R.L., *et al.* (1964). An effect of *o,p'*-DDD on the extra-adrenal metabolism of cortisol in man. *J. Clin. Endocrinol.* 24, 1303.

Bockner, V. and Roman, W. (1967). The influence of oral contraceptives on the binding capacity of serum proteins. *Med. J. Aust.* ii, 1187.

Bohnet, H.G., Greiwe, M., Hanker, J.P., *et al.* (1978). Effects of cimetidine on prolactin, LH, and sex steroid secretion in male and female volunteers. *Acta Endocrinol.* 88, 428.

Bohnet, H.G., Kato, K., and Wolf, A.S. (1986). Treatment of hyperprolactinemic amenorrhea with metergoline. *Obstet. Gynecol.* 67, 249.

Booth, J.D., Merriam, G.R., Clark, R.V., *et al.* (1987). Evidence for Leydig cell dysfunction in infertile men with a selective increase in plasma follicle-stimulating hormone. *J. Clin. Endocrinol. Metab.* 64, 1194.

Borowski, G.D., Garofano, C.D., Rose, L.I., *et al.* (1985). Effect of long-term amiodarone therapy on thyroid hormone levels and thyroid function. *Am. J. Med.* 78, 443.

Borushek, S. and Gold, J.J. (1964). Commonly used medications that interfere with routine endocrine laboratory procedures. *Clin. Chem.* 10, 41.

Bradley, M.E., Foote, Lee En, Merkle, L. (1996). Sertraline-associated syndrome of inappropriate antidiuretic hormone: case report and review of the literature. *Pharmacotherapy* 16, 680.

Brandt, N.J., Cohn, J., and Hilder, M. (1973). Controlled trial of oral contraceptives in haemophilia. *Scand. J. Haematol.* 11, 225.

Braverman, L.E. and Ingbar, S.H. (1967). Effects of norethandrolone on the transport in serum and peripheral turnover of thyroxine. *J. Clin. Endocrinol. Metab.* 27, 389.

Burger, A., Dinichert, D., Nicod, P., *et al.* (1976). Effect of amiodarone on serum triiodothyronine, reverse triiodothyronine, thyroxin, and thyrotropin: a drug influencing peripheral metabolism of thyroid hormones. *J. Clin. Invest.* 58, 255.

Burgi, H.W., Wimpfheimer, C., Burger, A., *et al.* (1976). Changes of circulating thyroxine, triiodothyronine and reverse triiodothyronine after radiographic contrast agents. *J. Clin. Endocrinol. Metab.* 43, 1203.

Burke, D. and Fanker, S. (1996). Fluoxetine and the syndrome of inappropriate secretion of antidiuretic hormone (SIADH). *Aust. N.Z. J. Psychiatry* 30, 295.

Burman, P., Karlsson, F.A., Oberg, K., *et al.* (1985). Autoimmune thyroid disease in interferon-treated patients. *Lancet* i, 100.

Burr, W.A., Ramsden, D.B., Griffiths, R.S., *et al.* (1976). Effect of a single dose of dexamethasone on serum concentrations of thyroid hormones. *Lancet* ii, 58.

Burstein, S. and Klaiber, E.L. (1965). Phenobarbital-induced increase in 6 β-hydroxycortisol excretion: clue to its significance in human urine. *J. Clin. Endocrinol. Metab.* 25, 293.

Caine, M., Perlberg, S., and Gordon, R. (1975). The treatment of benign prostatic hypertrophy with flutamide (SCH 13521): a placebo-controlled study. *J. Urol.* 114, 564.

Carlson, H.E. (1980). Current concepts: gynecomastia. *N. Engl. J. Med.* 303, 795.

Carmichael, A.J. and Paul, C.J. (1989). Reversible gynaecomastia associated with etretinate. *Br. J. Dermatol.* 120, 317.

Carter, J.N., Tyson, J.E., Tolis, G., *et al..* (1978). Prolactin-secreting tumors and hypogonadism in 22 men. *N. Engl. J. Med.* 299, 847.

Casanueva, F.F., Villanueva, L., Cabraves, J.A., *et al.* (1984). Cholinergic mediation of growth hormone secretion elicited by arginine, clonidine, and physical exercise in man. *J. Clin. Endocrinol. Metab.* 59, 526.

Cashin-Hemphill, L., Spencer, C.A., Nicoloff, J.T., *et al.* (1987). Alterations in serum thyroid hormonal indices with colestipol-niacin therapy. *Ann. Intern. Med.* 107, 324.

Castell, L.D.O. and Sparks, C.H.A. (1965). Nephrogenic diabetes insipidus due to demethylchlortetracycline hydrochloride. *JAMA* 193, 137.

Cavalieri, R.R., Gavin, L.A., Wallace, A., *et al.* (1979). Serum thyroxine, free T_4, triiodothyronine, and reverse-T_3 in diphenylhydantoin treated patients. *Metabolism* 28, 1161.

Chang, K.C., Miklich, D.R., Barwise, G., *et al.* (1982). Linear growth of chronic asthmatic children: the effects of the disease and various forms of steroid therapy. *Clin. Allergy* 12, 369.

Chapman, R.M., Sutcliffe, S.B., Rees, L.H., *et al.* (1979*a*). Cyclical combination chemotherapy and gonadal function. *Lancet* i, 285.

Chapman, R.M., Sutcliffe, S.B., and Malpas, J.S. (1979*b*). Cytotoxic-induced ovarian failure in women with Hodgkin's disease. *JAMA* 242, 1877.

Charney, D.S., Heninger, G.R., and Sternberg, D.E. (1984). Serotonin function and mechanism of action of antidepressant treatment. *Arch. Gen. Psychiatry* 41, 359.

Check, J.H., Rankin, A., and Teichman, M. (1986). The risk of fetal anomalies as a result of progesterone therapy during pregnancy. *Fertil. Steril.* 45, 575.

Chernausek, S.D., Underwood, L.E., Utiger, R.D., *et al.* (1983). Growth hormone secretion and plasma somatomedin-C in primary hypothyroidism. *Clin. Endocrinol.* 19, 337.

Cheson, B.D., Levine, A.M., Mildvan, D., *et al.* (1987). Suramin therapy in AIDS and related disorders: report of the US Suramin Working Group. *JAMA* 258, 1347.

Chez, R.A. (1978). Proceedings of the Symposium: Progesterone, progestins, and fetal development. *Fertil. Steril.* 30, 16.

Chiba, T., Okimura, Y., Kodama, H., *et al.* (1988). Tolbutamide inhibits gastrin release in man. *Horm. Metabol. Res.* 20, 641.

Chin, W. and Schussler, G.C. (1968). Decreased serum free thyroxine concentration in patients treated with diphenylhydantoin. *J. Clin. Endocrinol.* 28, 181.

Chiodera, P., Coiro, V., Speroni, G., *et al.* (1984). The growth hormone response to thyrotropin-releasing hormone in insulin-dependent diabetes involves a cholinergic mechanism. *J. Clin. Endocrinol. Metab.* 59, 794.

Ch'ng, J.L.C., Anderson, J.V., Williams, S.J., *et al.* (1986). Remission of symptoms during long term treatment of metastatic pancreatic endocrine tumours with long acting somatostatin analogue. *Br. Med. J.* 292, 981.

Chopra, I.J., Williams, D.E., Orgiazzi, J., *et al.* (1975). Opposite effects of dexamethasone on serum concentrations of 3,3′,5′-triiodothyronine (reverse T_3) and 3,3′,5-triiodothyronine (T_3). *J. Clin. Endocrinol. Metab.* 41, 911.

Christensson, T., Hellstrom, K., and Wengle, B. (1977). Hypercalcemia and primary hyperparathyroidism. Prevalence in patients receiving thiazides as detected in a health screen. *Arch. Intern. Med.* 137, 1138.

Christiansen, C., Baastrup, P.C., and Transbol, I. (1980). Development of 'primary' hyperparathyroidism during lithium therapy: longitudinal study. *Neuropsychobiology* 6, 280.

Chunhaswasdikul, B. (1974). Gynecomastia in association with administration of thiacetazone in the treatment of tuberculosis. *J. Med. Assoc. Thailand* 57, 323.

Clark, F. and Hutton, C.W. (1985). The effect of drugs upon the assessment of thyroid function. *Adverse Drug React. Acute Poisoning Rev.* 4, 59.

Clyne, C.A.C. (1986). Unilateral gynaecomastia and nifedipine. *BMJ* 292, 380.

Coffey, V.J. (1971). Myxoedema during cyclophosphamide therapy. *Br. Med. J.* iv, 682.

Cohen, H.N., Hay, I.O., Thomson, J.A., *et al.* (1979). Metoclopramide stimulation: a test of growth hormone reserve in adolescent males. *Clin. Endocrinol.* 11, 89.

Cohen, H.N., Beastall, G.H., Ratcliffe, W.A., *et al.* (1980). Effect on human thyroid function of sulphonamide and trimethoprim combination drugs. *BMJ* 281, 646.

Cohen III, J.H., Ingbar, S.H., and Braverman, L.E. (1989). Thyrotoxicosis due to ingestion of excess thyroid hormone. *Endocrinol. Rev.* 10, 113.

Comi, R.J. (1989). Pharmacology and use in pituitary tumors. In: P. Gorden (moderator). Somatostatin and somatostatin analogue (SMS 201-995) in treatment of hormone-secreting tumors of the pituitary and gastrointestinal tract and non-neoplastic diseases of the gut. *Ann. Intern. Med.* 110, 35.

Conn, J.W., Rovner, D.R., Cohen, E.L., *et al.* (1966). Inhibition by heparinoid of aldosterone biosynthesis in man. *J. Clin. Endocrinol.* 26, 527.

Conn, J.W., Rovner, D.R., and Cohen, E.L. (1968). Licorice-induced pseudoaldosteronism: hypertension, hypokalemia, aldosteronopenia, and suppressed plasma renin activity. *JAMA* 205, 80.

Convens, C., Verhelst, J., Mahler, C. (1991). Painful gynaecomastia during omeprazole therapy. *Lancet* 338, 1153.

Cooper, D.S., Daniels, G.H., Ladenson, P.W., *et al.* (1982). Hyperthyroxinemia in patients treated with high-dose propranolol. *Am. J. Med.* 73, 867.

Cousins, M.J., Mazze, R.I., Kosek, J.C., *et al.* (1974). The etiology of methoxyflurane nephrotoxicity. *J. Pharmacol. Exp. Ther.* 190, 530.

Craft, W.H. and Underwood, L.E. (1984). Effect of androgens on plasma somatomedin-C/insulin-like growth factor I responses to growth hormone. *Clin. Endocrinol.* 20, 549.

Crawford, J.D. (1978). Treatment of tall girls with estrogen. *J. Pediatr.* 62 (Suppl.), 1189.

Cryer, P.E. (1985). Pheochromocytoma. *Clin. Endocrinol. Metab.* 14, 203.

Cryer, P.E. (1988). The carcinoid syndrome. In *Cecil Textbook of Medicine*, Vol. 2 (18th edn) (ed. J.B. Wyngaarden and L.H. Smith), p. 1467. W.B. Saunders, Philadelphia.

Cubitt T. (1976). Lithium and thyrotoxicosis. *Lancet* i, 1247.

Debas, H.T. (1987). Gastrin. *Clin. Invest. Med.* 10, 222.

DeBold, C.R., Sheldon, W.R., DeCherney, G.S., *et al.* (1984). Arginine vasopressin potentiates adrenocorticotropin release induced by ovine corticotropin-releasing factor. *J. Clin. Invest.* 73, 533.

Decensi, A., Guarneri, D., Paoletti, M.C., *et al.* (1991). Phase II study of the pure non-steroidal antiandrogen nilutamide in prostatic cancer. *Eur. J. Cancer* 27, 1100.

DeFronzo, R.A., Braine, H., Colvin, O.M., *et al.* (1973). Water intoxication in man after cyclophosphamide therapy. *Ann. Intern. Med.* 78, 861.

DeFronzo, R.A., Abeloff, M., Braine, H., *et al.* (1974). Renal dysfunction after treatment with isophosphamide (NSC-109724). *Cancer Chemother. Rep.* 58, 375.

Delitala, G., Rovasio, P.P., Masala, A., *et al.* (1978). Metergoline inhibition of thyrotropin and prolactin secretion in primary hypothyroidism. *Clin. Endocrinol.* 8, 69.

Delitala, G., Stubbs, W.A., Wass, J.A., *et al.* (1979). Effects of the H2-receptor antagonist cimetidine on pituitary hormones in man. *Clin Endocrinol* 11, 161.

de Luis, D.A. and Romero, E. (1996). Reversible thyroid dysfunction with filgrastim. *Lancet* 348, 1595.

De Rivera, J.L.G. (1975). Inappropriate secretion of antidiuretic hormone from fluphenazine therapy. *Ann. Intern. Med.* 82, 811.

Dexter, R.N., Fishman, L.M., Ney, R.L., *et al.* (1967). Inhibition of adrenal corticosteroid synthesis by aminoglutethimide: studies of the mechanism of action. *J. Clin. Endocrinol.* 27, 473.

Dhar, S.K. and Ramos, R.R. (1978). Inappropriate antidiuresis during desipramine therapy. *Arch. Intern. Med.* 138, 1750.

Dickinson, P., Zinneman, H.N., Swaim, W.R., *et al.* (1969). Effects of testosterone treatment on plasma proteins and aminoacids in man. *J. Clin. Endocrinol. Metab.* 29, 837.

Dixon, D.W., Barwolf-Gohlke, C., and Gunnar R.M. (1981). Comparative efficacy and safety of bumetanide and furosemide in long-term treatment of edema due to congestive heart failure. *J. Clin. Pharmacol.* 21, 680.

Doe, R.P., Mellinger, G.T., Swaim, W.R., *et al.* (1967). Estrogen dosage effects on serum proteins: a longitudinal study. *J. Clin. Endocrinol.* 27, 1081.

Dreher, W.H., MacIndoe, J.H., Magnin, G.E., *et al.* (1971). Acute adrenal insufficiency secondary to anticoagulant therapy. *Wis. Med. J.* 70, 144.

Dunlay, R., Rodriguez, M., Felsenfeld, A.J., *et al.* (1989). Direct inhibitory effect of calcitriol on parathyroid function (sigmoid curve) in dialysis. *Kidney Int.* 36, 1093.

Dussault, H.H., Turcotte, R., and Guyda H. (1976). The effect of acetylsalicylic acid on TSH and PRL secretion after TRH stimulation in the human. *J. Clin. Endocrinol. Metab.* 43, 232.

Edes, T.E. and Sunderrajan, E.V. (1985). Heparin-induced hyperkalemia. *Arch. Intern. Med.* 145, 1070.

Ehrinpreis, M.N., Dhar, R., and Narula, A. (1989). Cimetidine-induced galactorrhea. *Am. J. Gastroenterol.* 84, 563.

Engbring, N.H. and Engstrom, W.W. (1959). Effects of estrogen and testosterone on circulating thyroid hormone. *J. Clin. Endocrinol. Metab.* 19, 783.

Engelhardt, D., and Weber, M.M. (1994). Therapy of Cushing's syndrome with steroid biosynthesis inhibitors. *J. Steroid Biochem. Mol. Biol.* 49, 261.

Erfurth, E.M. and Hedner, P. (1982). Importance of thyroxine in suppressing secretion of thyroid-stimulating hormone after thyroidectomy. *Br. Med. J.* 284, 941.

Evans, B.M., Dunne, J., and Surveyor, I. (1972). Pentazocine in thyroid failure. *BMJ* ii, 716.

Evered, D., Young, E.T., Ormston, B.J., *et al.* (1973). Treatment of hypothyroidism: a reappraisal of thyroxine therapy. *BMJ* iii, 131.

Faber, J., Lumholtz, I.B., and Kirkegaard, C. (1985). The effects of phenytoin (diphenylhydantoin) on the extrathyroidal turnover of thyroxine, 3,5,3'-triiodothyronine, 3,3',5'-triiodothyronine and 3',5'-triiodothyronine in man. *J. Clin. Endocrinol. Metab.* 61, 1093.

Fagan, T.C., Johnson, D.G., and Grosso, D.S. (1985). Metronidazole-induced gynecomastia. *JAMA* 254, 3217.

Faglia, G., Ambrosi, B., Beck-Peccoz P., *et al.* (1972). The effect of theophylline on plasma thyrotropin (HTSH) response to thyrotropin releasing factor (TRF) in man. *J. Clin. Endocrinol. Metab.* 34, 906.

Farese, R.V. Jr, Schambelan, M., Hollander, H., *et al.* (1990). Nephrogenic diabetes insipidus associated with foscarnet treatment of cytomegalovirus retinitis. *Ann. Intern. Med.* 112, 955.

Feldman, H.A. and Singer, I. (1974). Comparative effects of tetracyclines on water flow across toad urinary bladders. *J. Pharmacol. Exp. Ther.* 190, 358.

Feldman, J.M. (1987). Falsely elevated urinary excretion of catecholamines and metanephrines in patients receiving labetalol therapy. *J. Clin. Pharmacol.* 27, 288.

Fentiman, I.S., Thomas B.S., Balkwill, F.R., *et al.* (1985). Primary hypothyroidism associated with interferon therapy of breast cancer. *Lancet* i, 1166.

Ferrari, C., Paracchi, A., Rondena, M., *et al.* (1976). Effect of two serotonin antagonists on prolactin and thyrotropin secretion in man. *Clin. Endocrinol.* 5, 575.

Forrest, J.N. Jr, Cohen, A.D., Torretti, J., *et al.* (1974). On the mechanism of lithium-induced diabetes insipidus in man and the rat. *J. Clin. Invest.* 53, 1115.

Fradkin, J.E. and Wolff, J. (1983). Iodide-induced thyrotoxicosis. *Medicine* 62, 1.

Frantz, A.G. (1978). Prolactin. *N. Engl. J. Med.* 298, 201.

Fraser, H.M. and Baird, D.T. (1987). Clinical applications of LHRH analogues. *Baillière's Clin. Endocrinol. Metab.* 1, 43.

Fraser, W.D., Logue, F.C., Gallacher, S.J., *et al.* (1991). Direct and indirect assessment of the parathyroid hormone response to pamidronate therapy in Paget's disease of bone and hypercalcemia of malignancy. *Bone Miner.* 12, 113.

Funder, J.W. and Mercer, J.E. (1979). Cimetidine, a histamine H_2 receptor antagonist, occupies androgen receptors. *J. Clin. Endocrinol. Metab.* 48, 189.

Gadd, E.M., Norris, C.M., and Beeley, L. (1987). Antidepressants and galactorrhoea. *Int. Clin. Psychopharmacol.* 2, 361.

Gaginella, T.S., O'Dorisio, T.M., Mekhjian, H.S., *et al.* (1989). Tumors of the gastroenteropancreatic axis. In *Sandostatin in the Treatment of GEP Endocrine Tumors* (ed. T.M. O'Dorisio), p. 23. Springer-Verlag, Berlin.

Galbraith, R.A. and Michnovicz, J.J. (1989). The effect of cimetidine on the oxidative metabolism of estradiol. *N. Engl. J. Med.* 321, 269.

Gammage, M.D. and Franklyn, J.A. (1987). Amiodarone and the thyroid. *Q. J. Med.* 62, 83.

Garfinkel, P.E., Calvin, E., and Harvey, C.S. (1973). Hypothyroidism and hyperparathyroidism associated with lithium. *Lancet* ii, 331.

Garnick, M.B. and Larsen, P.R. (1979). Acute deficiency of thyroxine-binding globulin during L-asparaginase therapy. *N. Engl. J. Med.* 301, 252.

Geller, J., Vazakas, G., Fruchtman, B., *et al.* (1968). The effect of cyproterone acetate on advanced carcinoma of the prostate. *Surg. Gynecol. Obstet.* 127, 748.

Giese, A.A., Leibenluft, E., Green, S., *et al.* (1989). Phenelzine-associated inappropriate ADH secretion. *J. Clin. Psychopharmacol.* 9, 309.

Gillies, G.E., Linton, E.A., and Lowry, P.J. (1982). Corticotropin releasing activity of the new CRF is potentiated several times by vasopressin. *Nature* 299, 355.

Glass, A.R. and Eil, C. (1986). Ketoconazole-induced reduction in serum 1,25-dihydroxyvitamin D. *J. Clin. Endocrinol. Metab.* 63, 766.

Glass, A.R. and Eil, C. (1988). Ketoconazole-induced reduction in serum 1,25-dihydroxyvitamin D and total serum calcium in hypercalcemic patients. *J. Clin. Endocrinol. Metab.* 66, 934.

Gluskin, L.E., Strasberg, B., and Shah, J.H. (1981). Verapamil-induced hyperprolactinemia and galactorrhea. *Ann. Intern. Med.* 95, 66.

Goldberg, L. (1996). Adverse effects of anabolic steroids. *JAMA* 276, 257.

Goldberg, M.R., Bradstreet, T.E., McWilliam, E.J., *et al.* (1995). Biochemical effects of losartan, a nonpeptide angiotensin II receptor antagonist, on the renin–angiotensin–aldosterone system in hypertensive patients. *Hypertension* 25, 37.

Goldenberg, S.L. and Bruchovsky, N. (1991). Use of cyproterone acetate in prostate cancer. *Urol. Clin. North Am.* 18, 111.

Graber, A.L., Ney, R.L., Nicholson, W.E., *et al.* (1965). Natural history of pituitary–adrenal recovery following long-term suppression with corticosteroids. *J. Clin. Endocrinol.* 25, 11.

Gradon, J.D. and Sepkowitz, D.V. (1991). Fluconazole-associated acute adrenal insufficiency. *Postgrad. Med. J.* 67, 1084.

Greenbaum-Lefkoe, B., Rosenstock, J.G., Belasco, J.B., *et al.* (1985). Syndrome of inappropriate antidiuretic hormone secretion: a complication of high-dose intravenous melphalan. *Cancer* 55, 44.

Griffing, G.T. and Melby, J.C. (1989). Reversal of diuretic-induced secondary hyperaldosteronism and hypokalemia by trilostane, an inhibitor of adrenal steroidogenesis. *Metabolism* 38, 353.

Hahn, T.J. (1980). Drug-induced disorders of vitamin D and mineral metabolism. *Clin. Endocrinol. Metab.* 9, 107.

Halse, J., Harris, A.G., Kvistborg, A., *et al.* (1990). A randomized study of SMS 201-995 versus bromocriptine treatment in acromegaly: clinical and biochemical effects. *J. Clin. Endocrinol. Metab.* 70, 1254.

Hansen, P.B., Johnsen, H.E., and Hippe, E. (1993). Autoimmune hypothyroidism and granulocyte-macrophage colony-stimulating factor. *Eur. J. Haematol.* 50, 183.

Harmon, J. and Aliapoulios, M.A. (1972). Gynecomastia in marihuana users. *N. Engl. J. Med.* 287, 936.

Hawthorne, G.C., Campbell, N.P.S., Geddes, J.S., *et al.* (1985). Amiodarone-induced hypothyroidism. A common complication of prolonged therapy: a report of eight cases. *Arch. Intern. Med.* 145, 1016.

Heidemann, P., Peters, H.H., and Stubbe, P. (1980). Influence of L-asparaginase and oxandrolone on serum thyroxine-binding globulin. *Acta Endocrinol.* 94 (Suppl. 234) (Abstract 20), 19.

Hendrickson, D.A., Anderson, W.R. (1970). Diethylstilbestrol therapy gynecomastia. *JAMA* 213, 468.

Hershman, J.M., Craane, T.J., and Colwell, J.A. (1968). Effect of sulfonylurea drugs on the binding of triiodothyronine and thyroxine to thyroxine-binding globulin. *J. Clin. Endocrinol. Metab.* 28, 1605.

Heyma, P., Larkins, R.G., and Campbell, D.G. (1980). Inhibition of propranolol of 3,5,3'-triiodothyronine formation from thyroxine in isolated rat renal tubules: an effect independent of β-adrenergic blockade. *Endocrinology* 106, 1437.

Hikita, T., Fukutani, K., Yamamoto, Y., *et al.* (1989). Effect of aminophylline injection on the pituitary–thyroid axis in asthmatics. *Jpn J. Med.* 28, 303.

Himmelmann, A., Bergbrant, A., Hansson, L., *et al.* (1996). Remikiren (Ro 42-5892)—an orally active renin inhibitor in essential hypertension. Effects on blood pressure and the renin-angiotensin-aldosterone system. *Am. J. Hypertens.* 9, 517.

Hoffman, D.M., Crampton, L., Sernia, C., *et al.* (1996). Short-term growth hormone (GH) treatment of GH-deficient adults increases body sodium and extracellular water, but not blood pressure. *J. Clin. Endocrinol. Metab.* 81, 1123.

Horning, S.J., Hoppe, R.T., Kaplan, H.S., *et al.* (1981). Female reproductive potential after treatment for Hodgkin's disease. *N. Engl. J. Med.* 304, 1377.

How, J., Khir, A.S.M., and Bewsher, P.D. (1980). The effect of atenolol on serum thyroid hormones in hyperthyroid patients. *Clin. Endocrinol.* 13, 299.

Hughes, S.W.M. and Burley, D.M. (1970). Aminoglutethimide: a 'side-effect' turned to therapeutic advantage. *Postgrad. Med. J.* 46, 409.

Hull, M.G.R., Bromham, D.R., Savage, P.E., *et al.* (1981). Normal fertility in women with post-pill amenorrhoea. *Lancet* i, 1329.

Hullin, R.P. (1978). The place of lithium in biological psychiatry. In *Lithium in Medical Practice* (ed. F.N. Johnson and S. Johnson), p. 433. MTP Press, Lancaster.

Huseman, G.A. and Hassing, J.M. (1984). Evidence for dopaminergic stimulation of growth velocity in some hypopituitary children. *J. Clin. Endocrinol. Metab.* 58, 419.

Hwang, A.S. and Magraw, R.M. (1989). Syndrome of inappropriate secretion of antidiuretic hormone due to fluoxetine. *Am. J. Psychiatry* 146, 399.

Iancu, K., Ratzoni, G., Weitzman, A., *et al.* (1992). More fluoxetine experience. *J. Am. Acad. Child. Adolesc. Psychiatry* 31, 755.

Ichihara, A., Suzuki, H., and Saruta, T. (1993). Effects of magnesium on the renin-angiotensin-aldosterone system in human subjects. *J. Lab. Clin. Med.* 122, 432.

Ikeda, K., Moriyasu, H., Yasaka, M., *et al.* (1994). Valproate related syndrome of inappropriate secretion of antidiuretic hormone (SIADH) — a case report. *Rinsho Shinkeigaku* 34, 911.

Isley, W.L. (1987). Effect of rifampin therapy on thyroid function tests in a hypothyroid patient on replacement L-thyroxine. *Ann. Intern. Med.* 107, 517.

Jeffcoate, W.J., Edwards, C.R.W., Rees, L.H., *et al.* (1976). Cyproterone acetate. *Lancet* ii, 1140.

Journal of the American Medical Association. (1963). AMA Council on drugs: A new antihypertensive — methyldopa (Aldomet). *JAMA* 186, 504.

Jorgensen, J.O., Pedersen, S.A., Laurberg, P., *et al.* (1989). Effects of growth hormone therapy on thyroid function of growth hormone-deficient adults with and without concomitant thyroxine-substituted central hypothyroidism. *J. Clin. Endocrinol. Metab.* 69, 1127.

Jubiz, W., Meikle, A.W., Levinson, R.A., *et al.* (1970). Effect of diphenylhydantoin on the metabolism of dexamethasone: mechanism of the abnormal dexamethasone suppression in humans. *N. Engl. J. Med.* 283, 11.

Kahl, L.E., Medsger, T.A., and Klein, I. (1985). Massive breast enlargement in a patient receiving D-penicillamine for systemic sclerosis. *J. Rheumatol.* 12, 990.

Kapcala, L.P. (1987). Alcohol-induced pseudo-Cushing's syndrome mimicking Cushing's disease in a patient with an adrenal mass. *Am. J. Med.* 82, 849.

Kaplan, M.M. and Utiger, R.D. (1978). Iodothyronine metabolism in rat liver homogenates. *J. Clin. Invest.* 61, 459.

Kaptein, E.M., Spencer, C.A., Kamiel, M.B., *et al.* (1980). Prolonged dopamine administration and thyroid hormone economy in normal and critically ill subjects. *J. Clin. Endocrinol. Metab.* 51, 387.

Kazal, L.A. Jr, Hall, D.L., Miller, L.G., *et al.* (1993). Fluoxetin-induced SIADH: a geriatric occurrence? *J. Fam. Pract.* 36, 341.

Keating, J.P. and Rees, M. (1991). Gynaecomastia after long-term administration of domperidone. *Postgrad. Med. J.* 67 401.

Kennedy, R.L., Jones, T.H., and Shaukat, H.N. (1988). Amiodarone and thyroid immunity. *BMJ* 297, 621.

Kennedy, R.L., Griffiths, H., and Gray, T.A. (1989). Amiodarone and the thyroid. *Clin. Chem.* 35, 1882.

Kimura, T., Matsui, K., Sato, T., *et al.* (1974). Mechanism of carbamazepine (Tegretol)-induced antidiuresis: evidence for release of antidiuretic hormone and impaired excretion of a water load. *J. Clin. Endocrinol. Metab.* 38, 356.

Kirkegaard, C., Bjoerum, C.N., Cohn, D., *et al.* (1977). Studies of the influence of biogenic amines and psychoactive drugs on the prognostic value of the TRH stimulation test in endogenous depression. *Psychoneuroendocrinology* 2, 131.

Kirkegaard, C., Bjoerum, N., Cohn, D., *et al.* (1978). Thyrotrophin-releasing hormone (TRH) stimulation test in manic-depressive illness. *Arch. Gen. Psychiatry* 35, 1017.

Kirkman, S. and Nelson, D.H. (1988). Alcohol-induced pseudo-Cushing's disease: a study of prevalence with review of the literature. *Metabolism* 37, 390.

Kleinberg, D.L., Noel, G.L., and Frantz, A.G. (1977). Galactorrhea: a study of 235 cases, including 48 with pituitary tumors. *N. Engl. J. Med.* 296, 589.

Kleinberg, D.L., Boyd III, A.E., Wardlaw, S., *et al.* (1983). Pergolide for the treatment of pituitary tumors secreting prolactin or growth hormone. *N. Engl. J. Med.* 309, 704.

Knigge, U., Wollesen, F., Dejgarrd, A., *et al.* (1981). Comparison between dose-responses of prolactin, thyroid stimulating hormone and growth hormone to two different histamine H2-receptor antagonists in normal men. *Clin. Endocrinol.* 15, 585.

Koang, N.K., Hu, T.C., Tch'en, K.L., *et al.* (1955). Gynecomastia during administration of INH (isonicotinic hydrazide) for pulmonary tuberculosis. *Chin. Med. J.* 73, 214.

Kohri, K., Takada, M., Katoh, Y., *et al.* (1987). Parathyroid hormone and electrolytes during long term treatment with allopurinol and thiazide. *Br. J. Urol.* 59, 503.

Kruse, H.J., Kreutz, R., Staib, S., *et al.* (1994). Dissociation of renin and aldosterone during low dose epinephrine infusion. *Am. J. Hypertens.* 7, 913.

Kurtz, A.B., Capper, S.J., Clifford, J., *et al.* (1981). The effect of fenclofenac on thyroid function. *Clin. Endocrinol.* 15, 117.

Kutyrina, I.M., Nikishova, T.A., and Tareyeva, I.E. (1987). Effects of heparin-induced aldosterone deficiency on renal function in patients with chronic glomerulonephritis. *Nephrol. Dial. Transplant.* 2, 219.

Kyriazopoulou, V., Parparousi, O., and Vagenakis, A.G. (1984). Rifampicin-induced adrenal crisis in Addisonian patients receiving corticosteroid replacement therapy. *J. Clin. Endocrinol. Metab.* 59, 1204.

Lamberts, S.W.J., Klijn, J.G.M., de Jong, F.H., *et al.* (1979). Hormone secretion in alcohol-induced pseudo-Cushing's syndrome. *JAMA* 242, 1640.

Landman, J.O., Papapoulos, S.E. (1995). Uninterrupted oral bisphosphonate (pamidronate) therapy is not associated with chronic stimulation of parathyroid hormone secretion. *Osteoporosis International* 5, 93.

Lane, R.J.M., Clark, F., and McCollum, J.K. (1977). Oxyphenbutazone-induced goitre. *Postgrad. Med. J.* 53, 93.

Lanes, R. and Hurtado, E.J. (1982). Oral clonidine — an effective growth hormone releasing agent in prepubertal subjects. *J. Pediatr.* 100, 710.

Langer, P., Foldes, O., Michajlovskij, N., *et al.* (1978). Short-term effect of acetylsalicylic acid analogue on pituitary–thyroid axis and plasma cortisol level in healthy human volunteers. *Acta Endocrinol.* 88, 698.

Larsen, P.R. (1972). Salicylate-induced increases in free triiodothyronine in human serum: evidence of inhibition of triiodothyronine binding to thyroxine-binding globulin and thyroxine-binding prealbumin. *J. Clin. Invest.* 51, 1125.

Larsen, P.R., Atkinson, A.J. Jr, Wellman, H.N., *et al.* (1970). The effect of diphenylhydantoin on thyroxine metabolism in man. *J. Clin. Invest.* 49, 1266.

Larsen, P.R., Dick, T.E., Markovitz, B.P., *et al.*(1979). Inhibition of intrapituitary thyroxine to 3,5,3'-triiodothyronine conversion prevents the acute suppression of thyrotropin release by thyroxine in hypothyroid rats. *J. Clin. Invest.* 64, 117.

Laudahn, G. (1984). Sex hormones. In *Clinical Pharmacology in Pregnancy* (ed. H.P. Kuemmerle and K. Brendel), p. 294. Thieme-Stratton, New York.

Laurberg P. (1985). Multisite inhibition by ipodate of iodothyronine secretion from perfused dog thyroid. *Endocrinology* 117, 1639.

Laurberg, P. and Weeke, J. (1978). Opposite variations in serum T_3 and reverse T_3 during propylthiouracil treatment of thyrotoxicosis. *Acta Endocrinol.* 87, 88.

Laurberg, P., Jakobsen, P.E., Hoeck, H.C. *et al.* (1994). Growth hormone and thyroid function: is secondary thyroid failure underdiagnosed in growth hormone deficient patients? *Thyroidology* 6, 73.

Laurell, C.-B., Kullander, S., and Thorell, J. (1967). Effect of administration of a combined estrogen-progestin contraceptive on the level of individual plasma proteins. *Scand. J. Clin. Lab. Invest.* 22, 337.

Lazarus, J.H. (1982). Endocrine and metabolic effects of lithium. *Adverse Drug React. Acute Poisoning Rev.* 1, 181.

Ledingham, I.M. and Watt, I. (1983). Influence of sedation on mortality in critically ill multiple trauma patients. *Lancet* i, 1270.

Lembcke, B., Schleser, C.S., Schleser, S., *et al.* (1987). Effect of the somatostatin analogue sandostatin (SMS 201-995) on gastrointestinal, pancreatic and biliary function and hormone release in normal men. *Digestion* 36, 108.

Levesque, H., Verdier, S., Cailleux, N., *et al.* (1990). Low molecular weight heparins and hypoaldosteronism. *BMJ* 300, 1437.

LeWinn, E.B. (1953). Gynecomastia during digitalis therapy: Report of eight additional cases with liver-function studies. *N. Engl. J. Med.* 248, 316.

Liewendahl, K., Majuri, H., and Helenius, T. (1978). Thyroid function tests in patients on long-term treatment with various anticonvulsant drugs. *Clin. Endocrinol.* 8, 185.

Liskin, B., Walsh, B.T., Roose, S.P., *et al.* (1984). Imipramine-induced inappropriate ADH secretion. *J. Clin. Psychopharmacol.* 4, 146.

Littlewood, T.J. and Smith, A.P. (1984). Syndrome of inappropriate antidiuretic hormone secretion due to treatment of lung cancer with cisplatin. *Thorax* 39, 636.

Livanou, T., Ferriman, D., and James, V.H.T. (1967). Recovery of hypothalamo–pituitary–adrenal function after corticosteroid therapy. *Lancet* ii, 856.

Llop, R. (1994). Gynecomastia associated with enalapril and diazepam. *Annals of Pharmacotherapy* 28, 671.

Loeb, J.N. (1976). Corticosteroids and growth. *N. Engl. J. Med.* 295, 547.

Loriaux, D.L., Menard, R., Taylor, A., *et al.* (1976). Spironolactone and endocrine dysfunction. *Ann. Intern. Med.* 85, 630.

Lotti, G., Delitala, G., Devilla, L., *et al.* (1977). Reduction of plasma triiodothyronine (T_3) induced by propranolol. *Clin. Endocrinol.* 6, 405.

Luchsinger, A., Velsasco, M., Urbina, A., *et al.* (1992). Comparative effects of dopaminergic agonists on cardiovascular, renal and renin-angiotensin system in hypertensive patients. *J. Clin. Pharmacol.* 32, 55.

Luton, J.P., Mahoudeau, J.A., Bouchord, P., *et al.* (1979). Treatment of Cushing's syndrome by *o,p'*-DDD. Survey of 62 cases. *N. Engl. J. Med.* 300, 459.

Luzecky, M.H. (1974). The syndrome of inappropriate secretion of antidiuretic hormone associated with amitriptyline administration. *South. Med. J.* 67, 495.

Maarbjerg, K., Vestergaard, P., and Schou, M. (1987). Changes in serum thyroxine (T_4) and serum thyroid stimulating hormone (TSH) during prolonged lithium treatment. *Acta Psychiatr. Scand.* 75, 217.

MacAdams, M.R., White, R.H., and Chipps, B.E. (1986). Reduction of serum testosterone levels during chronic glucocorticoid therapy. *Ann. Intern. Med.* 104, 648.

McCallum, R.W., Sowers, J.R., Hershman, J.M., *et al.* (1976). Metoclopramide stimulates prolactin secretion in man. *J. Clin. Endocrinol. Metab.* 42, 1148.

McCance, D.R., Hadden, D.R., Kennedy, L., *et al.* (1987). Clinical experience with ketoconazole as a therapy for patients with Cushing's syndrome. *Clin. Endocrinol.* 27, 593.

McClure, R.D. (1987). Endocrine investigation and therapy. *Urol. Clin. North Am.* 14, 471.

McDermott, M.T., Burman, K.D., Hofeldt, F.D., *et al.* (1986). Lithium-associated thyrotoxicosis. *Am. J. Med.* 80, 1245.

MacGregor, A.G. and Somner, A.R. (1954). The anti-thyroid action of para-aminosalicylic acid. *Lancet* ii, 931.

McIntosh, W.B., Horn, E.H., Mathieson, L.M., *et al.* (1987). The prevalence, mechanism and clinical significance of lithium-induced hypercalcaemia. *Med. Lab. Sci.* 44, 115.

MacKenzie, M.A., Hoefnagels, W.H.L., Jansen, R.W.M., *et al.* (1990). The influence of glycyrrhetinic acid on plasma cortisol and cortisone in healthy young volunteers. *J. Clin. Endocrinol. Metab.* 70, 1637.

McKerron, C.G., Scott, R.L., Asper, S.P., *et al.* (1969). Effects of clofibrate (atromid S) on the thyroxine-binding capacity of thyroxine-binding globulin and free thyroxine. *J. Clin. Endocrinol.* 29, 957.

Mactier, R.A. and Khanna, R. (1988). Hyperkalemia induced by indomethacin and naproxen and reversed by fludrocortisone. *South. Med. J.* 81, 800.

Mallette, L.E., Khouri, K., Zengotita, H., *et al.* (1989). Lithium treatment increases intact and midregion parathyroid hormone and parathyroid volume. *J. Clin. Endocrinol. Metab.* 68, 654.

Mannisto, P.T. (1980). Endocrine side-effects of lithium. In *Handbook of Lithium Therapy* (ed. F.N. Johnson), p. 310. MTP Press, Lancaster.

Mardell, R. and Gamlen, T.R. (1982). Artifactual reduction in circulating free thyroxine concentration by radioimmunoassay. *Lancet* i, 973.

Margolis, I.B. and Gross, C.G. (1967). Gynecomastia during phenothiazine therapy. *JAMA* 199, 942.

Markusse, H.M. and Meyboom, R.H.B. (1988). Gynaecomastia associated with captopril. *BMJ* 296, 1262.

Marshall, J.S. and Tompkins, L.S. (1968). Effect of *o,p''*-DDD and similar compounds on thyroxine binding globulin. *J. Clin. Endocrinol.* 28, 386.

Martin, J.B. and Reichlin, S. (1987). Neuropharmacology of anterior pituitary regulation. In *Clinical Neuroendocrinology* (2nd edn), p. 45. F.A. Davis, Philadelphia.

Martin, J.B., Durand, D., Gurd, W., *et al.* (1978). Neuropharmacological regulation of episodic growth hormone and prolactin secretion in the rat. *Endocrinology* 102, 106.

Martino, E., Safran, M., Aghini-Lombardi, F., *et al.* (1984). Environmental iodine intake and thyroid dysfunction during chronic amiodarone therapy. *Ann. Intern. Med.* 101, 28.

Martino, E., Macchia, E., Aghini-Lombardi, F., *et al.* (1986*a*). Is humoral thyroid autoimmunity relevant in amiodarone iodine-induced thyrotoxicosis (AIIT)? *Clin. Endocrinol.* 24, 627.

Martino, E., Aghini-Lombardi, F., Mariotti, S., *et al.* (1986*b*). Treatment of amiodarone associated thyrotoxicosis by simultaneous administration of potassium perchlorate and methimazole. *J. Endocrinol. Invest.* 9, 201.

Martino, E., Aghini-Lombardi, F., Mariotti, S., *et al.* (1987*a*). Amiodarone: a common source of iodine-induced thyrotoxicosis. *Horm. Res.* 26, 158.

Martino, E., Aghini-Lombardi, F., Mariotti, S., *et al.* (1987*b*). Amiodarone iodine-induced hypothyroidism: risk factors and follow-up in 28 cases. *Clin. Endocrinol.* 26, 227.

Massara, F., Camanni, F., Belforte, L., *et al.* (1978). Increased thyrotrophin secretion induced by sulpiride in man. *Clin. Endocrinol.* 9, 419.

Massara, F., Tangolo, D., and Godano, A. (1985). The effect of metaclopramide, domperidone and apomorphine on GH secretion in children and adolescents. *Acta Endocrinol.* 108, 451.

Masson, E.A. and Phodes, J.M. (1992). Mesalazine associated nephrogenic diabetes insipidus presenting as weight loss. *Gut* 33, 563.

Matuk, F. and Kalyanaraman, K. (1977). Syndrome of inappropriate secretion of antidiuretic hormone in patients treated with psychotherapeutic drugs. *Arch. Neurol.* 34, 374.

Mazze, R.I., Shue, G.L., and Jackson, S.H. (1971). Renal dysfunction associated with methoxyflurane anesthesia: a randomized, prospective clinical evaluation. *JAMA* 216, 278.

Mechlis, S., Lubin, E., Laor, J., *et al.* (1987). Amiodarone-induced thyroid gland dysfunction. *Am. J. Cardiol.* 59, 833.

Meikle, A.W., Jubiz, W., Matsukura, S., *et al.* (1969). Effect of diphenylhydantoin on the metabolism of metyrapone and release of ACTH in man. *J. Clin. Endocrinol.* 29, 1553.

Melmed, S., Nademanee, K., Reed, A.W., *et al.* (1981). Hyperthyroxinemia with bradycardia and normal thyrotropin secretion after chronic amiodarone administration. *J. Clin. Endocrinol. Metab.* 53, 997.

Mendel, C.M., Frost, P.H., Kunitakis, P.H., *et al.* (1987). Mechanisms of heparin-induced increase in the concentration of free thyroxine in plasma. *J. Clin. Endocrinol. Metab.* 65, 1259.

Mendelson, J.H., Mendelson, J.E., and Patch, V.D. (1975). Plasma testosterone levels in heroin addiction and during methadone maintenance. *J. Pharmacol. Exp. Ther.* 192, 211.

Migliari, R., Balzano, S., Scarpa, R.M., *et al.* (1988). Short term effects of flutamide administration on hypothalamic–pituitary–testicular axis in man. *J. Urol.* 139, 637.

Millar, E.A., Connell, J.M., and Miller, D.G. (1971) Alkylating agents and human spermatogenesis. *JAMA* 217, 1662.

Millar, E.A., Connell, J.M., and Thomson, N.C. (1997). The effect of nebulized albuterol on the activity of the renin-angiotensin system in asthma. *Chest* 111, 71.

Miller, K.P., Lazar, E.J., Fotino, S. (1984). Severe hyperkalemia during piroxicam therapy. *Arch. Intern. Med.* 144, 2414.

Miller M. and Moses, A.M. (1970). Mechanism of chlorpropamide action in diabetes insipidus. *J. Clin. Endocrinol.* 30, 488.

Milne, K. and Greer, M.A. (1962). Comparison of the effects of propylthiouracil and sulfadiazine on thyroidal biosynthesis and the manner in which they are influenced by supplemental iodide. *Endocrinology* 71, 580.

Mitchell, J.R.A., Surridge, D.H.C., and Wilson, R.G. (1959). Hypothermia after chlorpromazine in myxedematous psychosis. *BMJ* ii, 932.

Mitsch, R.A. and Lee, A.K. (1986). Syndrome of inappropriate antidiuretic hormone with imipramine. *Drug Intell. Clin. Pharm.* 20, 787.

Miyai, K., Onishi, T., Hosokawa, M., *et al.* (1974). Inhibition of thyrotropin and prolactin secretions in primary hypothyroidism by 2-Br-α-ergocryptine. *J. Clin. Endocrinol. Metab.* 39, 391.

Moerck, H.J. and Magelund G. (1979). Gynaecomastia and diazepam abuse. *Lancet* i, 1344.

Monk, J.P. and Todd, P.A. (1987). Bezafibrate: a review of its pharmacodynamic and pharmacokinetic properties, and therapeutic use in hyperlipidaemia. *Drugs* 33, 539.

Monson, J.P. and Scott, D.F. (1987). Gynaecomastia induced by phenytoin in men with epilepsy. *BMJ* 294, 612.

Morgans, M.E. and Trotter, W.R. (1954). Treatment of thyrotoxicosis with potassium perchlorate. *Lancet* i, 10, 749.

Morgans, M.E. and Trotter, W.R. (1955). The anti-thyroid effect of phenylbutazone. *Lancet* ii, 164.

Morley, J.E., Shafer, R.B., Elson, M.K., *et al.* (1980). Amphetamine-induced hyperthyroxinemia. *Ann. Intern. Med.* 93, 707.

Morse, W.I., Clark A.F., Macleod, S.C., *et al.* (1962). Urine estrogen responses to human chorionic gonadotropin in young, old and hypogonadal men. *J. Clin. Endocrinol.* 22, 678.

Moses, A.M., Numann, P., and Miller, M. (1973*a*). Mechanism of chlorpropamide-induced antidiuresis in man: evidence for release of ADH and enhancement of peripheral action. *Metabolism* 22, 59.

Moses, A.M., Howanitz, J., van Gemert, M., *et al.* (1973*b*). Clofibrate-induced antidiuresis. *J. Clin. Invest.* 52, 535.

Moulding, T. and Fraser, R. (1970). Hypothyroidism related to ethionamide. *Am. Rev. Respir. Dis.* 101, 90.

Murphy, D.L., Goodwin, F.K., and Bunney, W.E. Jr (1969). Aldosterone and sodium response to lithium administration in man. *Lancet* ii, 458.

Nademanee, K., Piwonka, R.W., Singh, B.N., *et al.* (1989). Amiodarone and thyroid function. *Prog. Cardiovasc. Dis.* 31, 427.

Naitoh, Y., Fukato, J., Tominaga, T., *et al.* (1988). Interleukin-6 stimulates the secretion of adrenocorticotropic hormone in conscious freely-moving rats. *Biochem. Biophys. Res. Commun.* 155, 1459.

Nakamura, Y., Yoshimoto, K., and Saima, S. (1990). Gynaecomastia induced by angiotensin converting enzyme inhibitor. *BMJ* 300, 41.

Namer, M. (1988). Clinical applications of antiandrogens. *J. Steroid. Biochem.* 31, 719.

Namer, M., Khater, R., Frenay, M., *et al.* (1986). High dose of ketoconazole in the treatment of advanced breast cancers. *Bull. Cancer* 73, 89.

Navarro, J.F., Quereda, C., Gakkego, N., *et al.* (1996). Nephrogenic diabetes insipidus and renal tubular acidosis secondary to foscarnet therapy. *Am. J. Kidney Dis.* 27, 413.

Neumann, F. (1978). Antiandrogens. In *Advances in Gynaecological Endocrinology* (ed. H.S. Jacobs). Proceedings of the 6th Study Group of the Royal College of Obstetricians and Gynaecologists, p. 335.

Nicholls, M.G. and Espiner, E.A. (1983). Liquorice, carbenoxolone and hypertension. In *Handbook of Hypertension, Vol. 2: Clinical Aspects of Secondary Hypertension* (ed. J.I.S. Robertson), p. 189. Elsevier, Amsterdam.

Nicoloff, J.T., Fisher, D.A., and Appleman, M.D. Jr. (1970). The role of glucocorticoids in the regulation of thyroid function in man. *J. Clin. Invest.* 49, 1922.

Nielsen-Kudsk, J.E., Bartels, P.D., and Dalby, J. (1990). Effects of verapamil on diurnal and thyrotropin-releasing hormone-stimulated prolactin levels in man. *J. Clin. Endocrinol. Metab.* 70, 1269.

Nilsson, O.R., Karlberg, B.E., Kagedal, B., *et al.* (1979). Non-selective and selective β_1-adrenoceptor blocking agents in the treatment of hyperthyroidism. *Acta Med. Scand.* 206, 21.

Nishida, S., Matsuki, M., Nagase, Y., *et al.* (1983a). Stress-mediated effect of metoclopramide on cortisol secretion in man. *J. Clin. Endocrinol. Metab.* 56, 839.

Nishida, S., Matsuki, M., Nagase, Y., *et al.* (1983b). Adrenocorticotropin-mediated effect of metoclopramide on plasma aldosterone in man. *J. Clin. Endocrinol. Metab.* 57, 981.

Nishida, S., Matsuki, M., Adachi, N., *et al.* (1987). Pituitary–adrenocortical response to metoclopramide in patients with acromegaly and prolactinoma: a clinical evaluation of catecholamine-mediated adrenocorticotropin secretion. *J. Clin. Endocrinol. Metab.* 64, 995.

Nourok, D.S., Glassock, R.J., Solomon, D.H., *et al.* (1964). Hypothyroidism following prolonged sodium nitroprusside therapy. *Am. J. Med. Sci.* 248, 129.

Ohnhaus, E.E., Burgi, H., Burger, A., *et al.* (1981). The effect of antipyrine, phenobarbital and rifampicin on thyroid hormone metabolism in man. *Eur. J. Clin. Invest.* 11, 381.

Okada, Y., Kondo, T., Okamoto, S., *et al.* (1992). Induction of ovulation and spermatogenesis in hypogonadotropic GH-deficient patients. *Endocrinol. Jpn* 39, 31.

Ooiwa, H., Shimamoto, K., Nakagawa, M. *et al.* (1988). The interference of acebutolol administration in the measurement of urinary 17-ketosteroid by Zimmermann's method. *Endocrinol. Jpn* 35, 485.

Oppenheimer, J.H. and Werner, S.C. (1966). Effect of prednisone on thyroxine-binding proteins. *J. Clin. Endocrinol.* 26, 715.

Otsuki, M., Dakoda, M., and Baba, S. (1973). Influence of glucocorticoids on TRF-induced TSH response in man. *J. Clin. Endocrinol. Metab.* 36, 95.

Pannall, P.R. and Maas, D.A. (1977). Danazol and thyroid-function tests. *Lancet* i, 102.

Papapoulos, S.E., Harinck, H.I., Bijvoet, O.L., *et al.* (1986). Effects of decreasing serum calcium on circulating para-thyroid hormone and vitamin D metabolites in normocalcaemic and hypercalcaemic patients treated with APD. *Bone Miner.* 1, 69.

Parravicini, E., Fontana, C., Paterlini G.L., *et al.* (1996). Iodine, thyroid function, and very low birth weight infants. *Pediatrics* 98, 730.

Pearce, C.J. and Byfield, P.G.H. (1986). Free thyroid hormone assays and thyroid function. *Ann. Clin. Biochem.* 23, 230.

Peden, N.R., Isles, T.E., Stevenson, I.H., *et al.* (1982). Nadolol in thyrotoxicosis. *Br. J. Clin. Pharmacol.* 13, 835.

Peterson, J.C., Pollack, W.R., and Mahoney, J.J. (1978). Inappropriate antidiuretic hormone secondary to a monoamine oxidase inhibitor. *JAMA* 239, 1422.

Pichert, G., Jost, L.M., Zobeli, L., *et al.* (1990). Thyroiditis after treatment with interleukin-2 and interferon alpha-2a. *Br. J. Cancer* 62, 100.

Pinder, R.M., Brogden, R.N., Sawyer, P.R., *et al.* (1976). Carbenoxolone: a review of its pharmacological properties and therapeutic efficacy in peptic ulcer disease. *Drugs* 11, 245.

Pont, A., Goldman, E.S., Sugar, A.M., *et al.* (1985). Ketoconazole-induced increase in estradiol-testosterone ratio. *Arch. Intern. Med.* 145, 1429.

Preece, M.A. (1976). The effect of administered corticosteroids on the growth of children. *Postgrad. Med. J.* 52, 625.

Preziosi, P. and Vacca, M. (1988). Adrenocortical suppression and other endocrine effects of etomidate. *Life Sci.* 42, 477.

Pugeat, M., Lejeune, H., Dechaud, H., *et al.* (1987). Effects of drug administration on gonadotropins, sex steroid hormones and binding proteins in humans. *Horm. Res.* 28, 261.

Quesada, J.M., Coopmans, W., Ruiz, B., *et al.* (1992). Influence of vitamin D on parathyroid function in the elderly. *J. Clin. Endocrinol. Metab.* 75, 494.

Quinn, B.P. and Wall, B.M. (1989). Nephrogenic diabetes insipidus and tubulointerstitial nephritis during continuous therapy with rifampin. *Am. J. Kidney Dis.* 14, 217.

Rado, J.P. (1973). Water intoxication during carbamazepine treatment. *BMJ* iii, 479.

Rahman, M.A. and Ing, T.S. (1989). Cyclosporine and magnesium and metabolism. *J. Lab. Clin. Med.* 114, 213.

Rajfer, J., Sikka, S.C., Rivera, F., *et al.* (1986). Mechanism of inhibition of human testicular steroidogenesis by oral ketoconazole. *J. Clin. Endocrinol. Metab.* 63, 1193.

Rao, K.J., Miller, M., and Moses, A. (1975). Water intoxication and thioridazine (Mellaril). *Ann. Intern. Med.* 82, 61.

Rayfield, E.J., Cain, J.P., Casey, M.P., *et al.* (1972). Influence of diet on urinary VMA excretion. *JAMA* 221, 704.

Refetoff, S., Fang, V.S., Rapoport, B., *et al.* (1974). Inter-relationships in the regulation of TSH and prolactin secretion in man: effects of L-dopa, TRH and thyroid hormone in various combinations. *J. Clin. Endocrinol. Metab.* 38, 450.

Reichert, L.J.M. and de Rooy, H.A.M. (1989). Treatment of amiodarone induced hyperthyroidism with potassium perchlorate and methimazole during amiodarone treatment. *BMJ* 298, 1547.

Reid, D.M., Martynoga, A.G., and Nuki, G. (1982). Reversible gynaecomastia associated with D-penicillamine in a man with rheumatoid arthritis. *BMJ* 285, 1083.

Reus, V.I., Gold, P., and Post, R. (1979). Lithium-induced thyrotoxicosis. *Am. J. Psychiatry* 136, 724.

Ritch, P.S. (1988). Cis-dichlorodiammineplatinum II-induced syndrome of inappropriate secretion of antidiuretic hormone. *Cancer* 61, 448.

Roberts II, L.J. (1988). Carcinoid syndrome and disorders of systemic mast-cell activation including systemic mastocytosis. *Endocrinol. Metab. Clin. North Am.* 17, 415.

Robertson, G.L., Bhoopalam, N., and Zelkowitz, L.J. (1973). Vincristine neurotoxicity and abnormal secretion of antidiuretic hormone. *Arch. Intern. Med.* 132, 717.

Robinson, B. (1957). Breast changes in the male and female with chlorpromazine or reserpine therapy. *Med. J. Aust.* ii, 239.

Ross, R.J.M., Tsagarakis, S., Grossman, A., *et al.* (1987). GH feedback occurs through modulation of hypothalamic somatostatin under cholinergic control: studies with pyridostigmine and GHRH. *Clin. Endocrinol.* 27, 727.

Roti, E., Robuschi, G., Manfredi, A., *et al.* (1985). Comparative effects of sodium ipodate and iodide on serum thyroid hormone concentrations in patients with Graves' disease. *Clin. Endocrinol.* 22, 489.

Safran, M., Martino, E., Aghini-Lombardi, F., *et al.* (1988). Effect of amiodarone on circulating antithyroid antibodies. *BMJ* 297, 456.

Sakakura, M., Takebe, K., and Nakagawa, S. (1973). Inhibition of luteinizing hormone secretion induced by synthetic LRH by long-term treatment with glucocorticoids in human subjects. *J. Clin. Endocrinol. Metab.* 40, 774.

Sakemi, T., Ohchi, N., Sanai, T., *et al.* (1988). Captopril-induced metabolic acidosis with hyperkalemia. *Am. J. Nephrol.* 8, 245.

Santen, R.J. and Bourguignon, J-P. (1987). Gonadotropin-releasing hormone: physiological and therapeutic aspects, agonists and antagonists. *Horm. Res.* 28, 88.

Santen, R.J., Wells, S.A., Runic, S., *et al.* (1977). Adrenal suppression with aminoglutethimide. I: Differential effects of aminoglutethimide on glucocorticoid metabolism as a rationale for use of hydrocortisone. *J. Clin. Endocrinol. Metab.* 45, 469.

Santucci, ? Farroni, F., Fiorucci, S., *et al.* (1991). Gynecomastia during omeprazole therapy. *N. Engl. J. Med.* 324, 635.

Sapolsky, R., Rivier, C., Yamamoto, G., *et al.* (1987). Interleukin-1 stimulates the secretion of hypothalamic corticotropin-releasing factor. *Science* 238, 522.

Scanlon, M.F., Weightman, D.R., Shale, D.J., *et al.* (1979). Dopamine is a physiological regulator of thyrotrophin (TSH) secretion in normal man. *Clin. Endocrinol.* 10, 7.

Schardein, J.L. (1980). Congenital abnormalities and hormones during pregnancy: a clinical review. *Teratology* 22, 251.

Schteingart, D.E. (1989). Cushing's syndrome. *Endocrinol. Metab. Clin. North Am.* 18, 311.

Schussler, G.C. (1971). Diazepam competes for thyroxine binding. *J. Pharmacol. Exp. Ther.* 178, 204.

Seely, E.W., LeBoff, M.S., Brown, E.M., *et al.* (1989). The calcium channel blocker diltiazem lowers serum parathyroid hormone levels in vivo and in vitro. *J. Clin. Endocrinol. Metab.* 68, 1007.

Shamberger, R.C., Rosenberg, S.A., Seipp, C.A., *et al.* (1981). Effects of high-dose methotrexate and vincristine on ovarian and testicular functions in patients undergoing postoperative adjuvant treatment of osteosarcoma. *Cancer Treat. Rep.* 65, 739.

Sharkey, P.K., Rinaldi, M.G., Dunn, J.F., *et al.* (1991). High-dose itraconazole in the treatment of severe mycoses. *Antimicrob. Agents Chemother.* 35, 707.

Sharma, B., Axelson, M., Pounder, R.P., *et al.* (1987). Acid secretory capacity and plasma gastrin concentration after administration of omeprazole to normal subjects. *Aliment. Pharmacol. Ther.* 1, 67.

Sheps, S.G., Jiang, N.S., and Klee, G.G. (1988). Diagnostic evaluation of pheochromocytoma. *Endocrinol. Metab. Clin. North Am.* 17, 397.

Sherins, R.J. and Mulvihill, J.J. (1989). Gonadal dysfunction. In *Cancer: Principles and Practice of Oncology* (3rd edn) (ed. V.T. DeVita Jr, S. Hellman, and S.A. Rosenberg), p. 2170. J.B. Lippincott, Philadelphia.

Sherman, R.A. and Ruddy, M.C. (1986). Suppression of aldosterone production by low-dose heparin. *Am. J. Nephrol.* 6, 165.

Singer, I. and Forrest, J.N. Jr (1976). Drug-induced states of nephrogenic diabetes insipidus. *Kidney Int.* 10, 82.

Singer, I. and Rotenberg, D. (1973). Mechanisms of lithium action. *N. Engl. J. Med.* 289, 254.

Slater, S.L., Lipper, S., Shiling, D.J., *et al.* (1977). Elevation of plasma-prolactin by monoamine-oxidase inhibitors. *Lancet* ii, 275.

Slooten, H.V., Moolenaar, A.J., van Seters, A.P., *et al.* (1984). The treatment of adrenocortical carcinoma with *o,p'*-DDD: prognostic simplifications of serum level monitoring. *Eur. J. Cancer Clin. Oncol.* 20, 47.

Smals, A.G.H., Kloppenborg, P.W.C., Goverde, H.J.M., *et al.* (1978). The effect of cyproterone acetate on the pituitary–adrenal axis in hirsute women. *Acta Endocrinol.* 87, 352.

Smerdely, P., Lim, A., Boyages, S.C., *et al.* (1989). Topical iodine-containing antiseptics and neonatal hypothyroidism in very-low-birth weight infants. *Lancet* ii, 661.

Smigan, L., Wahlin, A., Jacobsson, L., *et al.* (1984). Lithium therapy and thyroid function tests: a prospective study. *Neuropsychobiology* 11, 39.

Smith, G.H. (1980). Minoxidil. *Drug Intell. Clin. Pharm.* 14, 477.

Smith, M.J. and Hodson, M.E. (1983). Effects of long term inhaled high dose beclomethasone dipropionate on adrenal function. *Thorax* 38, 676.

Sneddon, I.B. (1976). Clinical use of topical corticosteroids. *Drugs* 11, 193.

Solomon, I.L. and Schoen, E.J. (1976). Juvenile Cushing syndrome manifested primarily by growth failure. *Am. J. Dis. Child.* 130, 200.

Sonino, N. (1987). The use of ketoconazole as an inhibitor of steroid production. *N. Engl. J. Med.* 317, 812.

Spano, F. and Ryan, W.G. (1984). Tamoxifen for gynecomastia induced by anabolic steroids? *N. Engl. J. Med.* 311, 861.

Sparagana, M. (1987). Primary hypogonadism associated with *o,p'*-DDD (mitotane) therapy. *Clin. Toxicol.* 25, 463.

Stancer, H.C. and Forbath, N. (1989). Hyperparathyroidism, hypothyroidism, and impaired renal function after 10 to 20 years of lithium treatment. *Arch. Intern. Med.* 149, 1042.

Stein, C.A., Saville, W., Yarchoan, R., *et al.* (1986). Suramin and function of the adrenal cortex. *Ann. Intern. Med.* 104, 286.

Steiner, J.F. (1996). Clinical pharmacokinetics and pharmacodynamics of finasteride. *Clin. Pharmacokinet.* 30, 16.

Stewart, P.M., Wallace, A.M., Valentino, R., *et al.* (1987). Mineralocorticoid activity of liquorice: 11-β-hydroxysteroid dehydrogenase deficiency comes of age. *Lancet* ii, 821.

Stewart, P.M., Wallace, A.M., Atherden, S.M., *et al.* (1990). Mineralocorticoid activity of carbenoxolone: contrasting effects of carbenoxolone and liquorice on 11-β-hydroxysteroid dehydrogenase activity in man. *Clin. Sci.* 78, 49.

Stockigt, J.R., Lim, C.F., Barlow, J.W., *et al.* (1984). High concentrations of furosemide inhibit serum binding of thyroxine. *J. Clin. Endocrinol. Metab.* 59, 62.

Strickland, A.L. and Sprinz, H. (1973). Studies of the influence of estradiol and growth hormone on the hypophysectomized immature rat epiphyseal cartilage growth plate. *Am. J. Obstet. Gynecol.* 115, 471.

Strickland, A.L., Underwood, L.E., Voina, S.J., *et al.* (1972). Growth retardation in Cushing's syndrome. *Am. J. Dis. Child.* 123, 207.

Stuart, M.J., Cuaso, C., Miller, M., *et al.* (1975). Syndrome of recurrent increased secretion of antidiuretic hormone following multiple doses of vincristine. *Blood* 45, 315.

Suzuki, H., Kadena, N., Takeuchi, K., *et al.* (1979). Effects of three-day oral cholecystography on serum iodothyronines and TSH concentrations: comparison of the effects among some cholecystographic agents and the effects of iopanoic acid on the pituitary–thyroid axis. *Acta Endocrinol.* 92, 477.

Suzuki, H., Noguchi, K., Nakahata, M., *et al.* (1981). Effect of iopanoic acid on the pituitary–thyroid axis: time sequence of changes in serum iodothyronines, thyrotropin, and prolactin concentrations and responses to thyroid hormones. *J. Clin. Endocrinol. Metab.* 53, 779.

Swerdloff, R.S., Palacios, A., McClure, R.D., *et al.* (1978). Male contraception: clinical assessment of chronic administration of testosterone enanthate. *Int. J. Androl.* 2, 731.

Tan, S.Y., Shapiro, R., Franco, R., *et al.* (1979). Indomethacin-induced prostaglandin inhibition with hyperkalemia. *Ann. Int. Med.* 90, 783.

Tanner, L.A. and Bosco, L.A. (1988). Gynecomastia associated with calcium channel blocker therapy. *Arch. Intern. Med.* 148, 379.

Taylor, A.L. and Fishman, L.M. (1988). Corticotropin-releasing hormone. *N. Engl. J. Med.* 319, 213.

Taylor, R., Clark, F., and Griffiths, I.D. (1980). Prospective study of effect of fenclofenac on thyroid function tests. *BMJ* 281, 911.

Thomas, B.L. (1976). Methadone-associated gynecomastia. *N. Engl. J. Med.* 294, 169.

Tolis, G., Somma, M., Campenhout, J.V., *et al.* (1974). Prolactin secretion in sixty-five patients with galactorrhea. *Am. J. Obstet. Gynecol.* 118, 91.

Tomiyama, T., Baba, T., Murabayashi, S., *et al.* (1992). Acute effect of an alpha 1-adrenoreceptor antagonist on urinary sodium excretion, plasma atrial natriuretic peptide, arginine vasopressin, and the renin-aldosterone system in healthy subjects. *Eur. J. Clin. Pharmacol.* 43, 17.

Trachtenberg, J. and Zadra, J. (1988). Steroid synthesis inhibition by ketoconazole: sites of action. *Clin. Invest. Med.* 11, 1.

Trump, D.L., Pavy, M.D., and Staal, S. (1982). Gynaecomastia in men following antineoplastic therapy. *Arch. Intern. Med.* 142, 511.

Tucker, R.M., Haq, Y., Denning, D.W., *et al.* (1990). Adverse events associated with itraconazole in 189 patients on chronic therapy. *J. Antimicrob. Chemother.* 26, 561.

Tuomisto, J., Ranta, T., Saarinen, A., *et al.* (1973). Neurotransmission and secretion of thyroid stimulating hormones. *Lancet* ii, 510.

Turkington, R.W. (1972). Prolactin secretion in patients treated with various drugs. *Arch. Intern. Med.* 130, 349.

Uehara, A., Gottschall, P.E., Dahl, R.R., *et al.* (1987). Interleukin-1 stimulates ACTH release by an indirect action which requires endogenous corticotropin releasing factor. *Endocrinology* 121, 1580.

Urban, R.J. and Veldhuis, J.D. (1991). A selective serotonin reuptake inhibitor, fluoxetine hydrochloride, modulates the pulsatile release of prolactin in post-menopausal women. *Am. J. Obstet. Gynecol.* 164, 147.

Vagenakis, A.G. (1988). Pituitary–thyroid interaction: effects of thyroid hormone, non thyroidal illness and various agents on TSH secretion. *Acta Med. Austriaca* 15, 52.

Vagenakis, A. and Braverman, L. (1975). Adverse effects of iodides on thyroid function. *Med. Clin. North Am.* 59, 1075.

Vale, W., Rivier, C., Brown, M.R., *et al.* (1983). Chemical and biological characterization of corticotropin releasing factor. *Recent Prog. Horm. Res.* 39, 245.

Vance, M.L., Evans, W.S., and Thorner, M.O. (1984). Diagnosis and treatment: drugs five years later — bromocriptine. *Ann. Intern. Med.* 100, 78.

Varl, B., Tos, L., and Cokic, M. (1988). Influence of dopamine on the thyroid hormones and thyrotropin in acute respiratory distress syndrome. *Acta Med. Austriaca* 15, 59.

Vaughan, E.D. Jr, Carey, R.M., Peach, M.J., *et al.* (1978). The renin response to diuretic therapy : a limitation of antihypertensive potential. *Circ. Res.* 42, 376.

Vidt, D.G. (1981). Mechanism of action, pharmacokinetics, adverse effects, and therapeutic uses of amiloride hydrochloride, a new potassium-sparing diuretic. *Pharmacotherapy* 1, 179.

Viviani, S., Santoro, A., Ragni, G., *et al.* (1985). Gonadal toxicity after combination chemotherapy for Hodgkin's disease: comparative results of MOPP vs ABVD. *Eur. J. Cancer Clin. Oncol.* 21, 601.

von Puttkamer, K., Bierich, J.R., Brugger, F., *et al.* (1977). Oestrogen treatment of girls with increased growth. *Dtsch. Med. Wochenschr.* 102, 983.

Walden, C.E., Knopp, R.H., and Johnson, J.L. (1986). Effect of estrogen/progestin potency on clinical chemistry measures. *Am. J. Epidemiol.* 123, 517.

Waxman, J.H.X., Terry, Y.A., Wrigley, P.F.M., *et al.* (1982). Gonadal function in Hodgkin's disease: long-term follow-up of chemotherapy. *BMJ* 285, 1612.

Wehrenberg, W.B., Esch, F., Baird, A., *et al.* (1986). Growth hormone-releasing factor: a new chapter in neuroendocrinology. *Horm. Res.* 24, 82.

Weiss, R.J. (1991). Effects of antihypertensive agents on sexual function. *Am. Fam. Physician* 44, 2075.

Werk, E.E., MacGee, J., and Sholiton, L.J. (1964). Effect of diphenylhydantoin on cortisol metabolism in man. *J. Clin. Invest.* 43, 1824.

Werner, S.C. and Platman, S.R. (1965). Remission of hyperthyroidism (Graves' disease) and altered pattern of serum-thyroxine binding induced by prednisone. *Lancet* ii, 751.

Westgren, U., Melander, A., Wahlin, E., *et al.* (1977). Divergent effects of 6-propylthiouracil on 3,5,3'-triiodothyronine (T_3) and 3,3',5'-triiodothyronine (rT_3) serum levels in man. *Acta Endocrinol.* 85, 345.

Wettenhall, H.N.B., Cahill, C., and Roche, A.F. (1975). Tall girls: a survey of 15 years of management and treatment. *J. Pediatr.* 86, 602.

Whitworth, J.A., Butkus, A., Coghlan, J.P., *et al.* (1986). 9-alpha-fluorocortisol-induced hypertension: a review. *J. Hypertens.* 4, 133.

Wiersinga, W.M. and Trip, M.D. (1986). Amiodarone and thyroid hormone metabolism. *Postgrad. Med. J.* 62, 909.

Wilber, J.F. and Utiger, R.D. (1969). The effect of glucocorticoids on thyrotropin secretion. *J. Clin. Invest.* 48, 2096.

Wilkinson, R., Anderson, M., and Smart, G.A. (1972). Growth-hormone deficiency in iatrogenic hypothyroidism. *BMJ* ii, 87.

Williams, H.J. (1988). Gynecomastia as a complication of auranofin therapy. *J. Rheumatol.* 15, 1863.

Winnacker, J.L., Yeager, H., Saunders, J.A., *et al.* (1977). Rickets in children receiving anticonvulsant drugs. *Am. J. Dis. Child.* 131, 286.

Winter, J.S.D. and Smail, P.J. (1980). Raised serum thyroxine in patient on haemophilia therapy. *Lancet* ii, 652.

Wolf, H., Madsen, P.O., and Vermund, H. (1969). Prevention of estrogen-induced gynecomastia by external irradiation. *J. Urol.* 102, 607.

Wolff, J. (1969). Iodide goiter and the pharmacologic effects of excess iodide. *Am. J. Med.* 47, 101.

Wolff, J. and Chaikoff, I.L. (1948). Plasma inorganic iodide as a homeostatic regulator of thyroid function. *J. Biol. Chem.* 174, 555.

Wolff, J., Standaert, M.E., and Rall, J.E. (1961). Thyroxine displacement from serum proteins and depression of serum protein-bound iodine by certain drugs. *J. Clin. Invest.* 40, 1373.

Wortsman, J., Hamidinia, A., and Winters, S.J. (1989). Hypogonadism following long-term treatment with diethylstilbestrol. *Am. J. Med. Sci.* 297, 365.

Wynn, V. and Path, F.C. (1968). The anabolic steroids. *Practitioner* 200, 509.

Yeo, P.P.B., Bates, D., Howe, J.G., *et al.* (1978). Anticonvulsants and thyroid function. *BMJ* i, 1581.

Zora, J.A., Zimmerman, D., Carey, T.L., *et al.* (1986). Hypothalamic–pituitary–adrenal axis suppression after long-term, high-dose glucocorticoid therapy in children with asthma. *J. Allergy Clin. Immunol.* 77, 9.

16. Disorders of metabolism 1

W. Y. SO, J. C. N. CHAN, and C. S. COCKRAM

Carbohydrate metabolism

Diabetes mellitus

Diabetes mellitus is a clinical state characterized by hyperglycaemia and usually accompanied by glycosuria. This results from either an absolute or relative deficiency of insulin commonly combined with resistance to it. Presentation may either be acute, with diabetic keto-acidosis or hyperosmolar non-ketotic coma; or insidious, with polyuria, polydipsia, and weight loss. It may also be detected incidentally by screening or in the presence of concurrent illness. Elderly patients with less severe biochemical disturbance may present with one of the complications of diabetes mellitus. Not uncommonly, patients with Type 2 diabetes present with diabetic complications after a lengthy period of undiagnosed disease.

Diagnostic criteria

In most clinical situations, oral glucose tolerance testing (OGTT) is not required to establish the diagnosis of diabetes mellitus. The current recommendations of the World Health Organization (WHO 1985) are at present under review (McCance *et al.* 1997). According to recent recommendations (of the Expert Committee on the Diagnosis and Classification of Diabetes Mellitus), there are three ways of diagnosing diabetes. In the presence of symptoms of diabetes mellitus, either a random venous plasma glucose concentration equal to or exceeding 11.1 mmol per litre, or a fasting glucose concentration equal to or exceeding 7.0 mmol per litre confirms the diagnosis. In the absence of symptoms or when the metabolic abnormality is less overt, the values of fasting plasma glucose concentration equal to or exceeding 7.0 mmol per litre or 2-hour plasma glucose concentration equal to or exceeding 11.1 mmol per litre should be confirmed on two occasions. These modified criteria employ a lower, fasting plasma glucose cut-off of 7.0 mmol per litre compared with the previously recommended diagnostic value of 7.8 mmol per litre. A fasting plasma glucose concentration equal to or less than 6.1 mmol per litre or a random plasma glucose concentration equal to or less than 7.8 mmol per litre excludes the diagnosis of diabetes mellitus. The recent recommendations also recognize a group of subjects with impaired fasting glucose (IFG), in whom the fasting plasma glucose concentration is between 6.1 and 7.0 mmol per litre. Impaired glucose tolerance (IGT) is defined as the presence of a fasting plasma glucose concentration less than 7.0 mmol per litre and a 2-hour plasma glucose concentration equal to or greater than 7.8 mmol per litre but less than 11.1 mmol per litre following a 75 g oral glucose load. The new proposed classification (as described below) emphasizes the fact that all types of diabetes can range between normoglycaemia, on the one hand, to a requirement for insulin treatment for glycaemic control at the other end of the spectrum. Thus IGT and IFG become intermediate states for all types of diabetes. Type 1 diabetes requires insulin treatment for survival as well as for glycaemic control.

Classification of diabetes mellitus

Diabetes mellitus is classically divided into Type 1 (insulin-dependent, IDDM) and Type 2 (non-insulin-dependent (NIDDM). The existing WHO (1985) classification into IDDM and NIDDM is largely treatment based, while that into Type 1 and 2 was based on the demonstration of β-cell destruction and immunological phenomena in Type 1 patients. However, with increasing recognition of heterogeneity, the Expert Committee is proposing changes to this classification. These changes include removing the terms IDDM and NIDDM. Type 1 diabetes is subdivided into immune-mediated and idiopathic subgroups. Type 2 diabetes is recognized to encompass a range from predominantly insulin resistance with relative insulin deficiency to a predominant insulin secretory defect with insulin resistance. Other distinct clinical types of diabetes with a recognizable underlying cause will be listed separately. The latter include diabetes due to genetic defects of β-cell function or insulin action, diseases of the exocrine pancreas, endocrinopathies, drugs or chemicals, or infections, as well as uncommon forms of immune-mediated diabetes and other genetic syndromes sometimes associated with diabetes. Gestational diabetes mellitus is also listed separately (Expert Committee on the Diagnosis and Classification of Diabetes Mellitus 1997).

Insulin deficiency and insulin resistance

An understanding of the mechanisms regulating glucose homoeostasis is essential to understand the hyperglycaemic and hypoglycaemic actions of drugs. Blood glucose concentration is closely regulated in man and is maintained by a balance between insulin release and action and counter-regulatory responses.

Insulin lowers blood glucose by suppressing hepatic glucose production and adipose tissue lipolysis. It enhances the uptake of glucose for utilization in energy production or storage as glycogen or triglyceride in liver, muscle, and adipose tissue. The main stimulus to insulin secretion is an increase in glucose concentration. Other physiological insulin secretagogues include free fatty acids (FFA), ketone bodies, and amino acids. These stimuli alter cation flux across calcium and potassium channels of the pancreatic β-cell membrane and result in a rise in intracellular free calcium concentration which is followed by a pulsatile release of insulin (Howell 1988).

Diminished sensitivity to insulin action (insulin resistance) may result from diminished tissue blood flow, insulin receptor changes, or intracellular changes in post-receptor or insulin-signalling pathways in various tissues (DeFronzo 1988; Taylor *et al.* 1994). Hyperglycaemia *per se* may impair insulin secretion and induce insulin resistance (Rossetti *et al.* 1990). Once hyperglycaemia is established, the relative roles of insulin resistance and insulin deficiency may be difficult to distinguish.

Counter-regulatory hormones

Decrements in plasma glucose within the physiological range ($\sim$4.6 mmol per litre) decrease insulin secretion. Further falls in glucose concentrations to just outside the physiological range ($\sim$3.8 mmol per litre) increase the secretion of glucose counter-regulatory hormones. Further glucose decrements elicit the symptoms of hypoglycaemia ($\sim$3.0 mmol per litre) while even greater falls cause cognitive dysfunction ($\sim$2.7 mmol per litre). Counter-regulatory hormones include glucagon, adrenaline, cortisol, and growth hormone (GH). These hormones have insulin-antagonistic effects both in the liver and in the peripheral tissues. The insulin-antagonistic effects of glucagon and adrenaline are of rapid onset whereas those of cortisol and GH are observed after a lag period. Glucagon is the most important hormone for acute glucose counter-regulation. When the release of glucagon is deficient, as in patients with Type 1 diabetes, adrenaline becomes the most important hormone for glucose recovery during hypoglycaemia. Cortisol and GH contribute to counter-regulation during prolonged hypoglycaemia but adrenaline is also of utmost importance in this condition (Cryer 1994; Lager 1991).

Glucagon has potent stimulatory effects on hepatic gluconeogenesis and glycogenolysis. The catecholamines (noradrenaline and, especially, adrenaline) enhance glucagon secretion, inhibit the activity of glycogen synthase, and stimulate lipolysis, glycogenolysis, and gluconeogenesis. Catecholamines also have a dual action on pancreatic β-cells. Physiologically, the β-adrenergic effect of catecholamines, mainly mediated by noradrenaline, limits insulin secretion and predominates over the β-adrenergic (insulin-releasing) effect, mediated mainly by adrenaline. Together, catecholamines and glucagon mobilize fuel stores in the liver, fat, and skeletal muscle to produce simple energy substrates, such as glucose and FFA, for cellular metabolism during hypoglycaemia or stress.

Cortisol promotes lipogenesis, increases protein breakdown, and promotes gluconeogenesis. It induces insulin resistance by diminishing the rate of glycogen synthesis, reducing capillary density and altering muscle fibre composition in muscle (Holmäng and Björntorp 1992). Cortisol also increases the synthesis and release of adrenaline from the adrenal medulla. (Critchley *et al.* 1982; Axelrod and Reisine 1984; Critchley *et al.* 1988).

The effects of GH on intermediary metabolism are more complex. Growth hormone exerts both insulin-like and insulin-antagonistic effects. The growth effects of GH are mainly mediated by insulin-like growth factor 1 (IGF-1), which shares some of the pathways of action of insulin. However, growth hormone inhibits glucose transport and utilization in peripheral tissues and increases lipolysis with elevation of FFA levels. These metabolic effects of GH and cortisol contribute to the dawn phenomenon (decreased insulin effects in the early morning) and insulin resistance seen after hypogly-caemic episodes (Lager 1991; Froesch et al. 1994).

Drug-induced hyperglycaemia

Although many drugs have potential adverse effects on glucoregulation, euglycaemia is usually maintained by a compensatory increase in endogenous insulin. However, in diabetic subjects or predisposed individuals who may have relative insulinopenia, glucose intolerance may be unmasked or may deteriorate in the presence of these drugs.

Hormones

Corticosteroids

In a case–control study involving 11 855 patients newly started on an oral antidiabetic agent or insulin, in the subgroup of patients using oral glucocorticoids, the esti-mated relative risk for the development of hypergly-caemia requiring treatment was 2.2 when compared with non-users. The risk increased proportionally with dos-age. When dosage is expressed in hydrocortisone equiv-alents (milligrams), the odds ratio was 1.77 for 1–39 mg per day, 3.0 for 40–79 mg per day, 5.82 for 80–119 mg per day and 10.34 for 120 mg per day or more (Gurwitz et al. 1994). Severe hyperglycaemia requiring insulin treat-ment frequently develops during steroid treatment for malignant conditions or immunosuppression for organ transplantation (Weissman et al. 1987; Walker 1988; D. Roth et al. 1989), as well as for bronchopulmonary dysplasia in neonates (Kazzi et al. 1990; Spear et al. 1993). These adverse metabolic effects have also been reported in diabetic patients receiving tetracosactrin as an intra-articular steroid injection (Feuerstein et al. 1992). For equivalent anti-inflammatory dosages, ad-ministration of methylprednisolone is associated with a greater hyperinsulinaemic response than hydrocortisone (Bruno et al. 1994). Although a third-generation cortico-steroid known as deflazacort has recently been shown to have fewer adverse metabolic effects, more data are necessary to confirm its relative lack of significant hyper-glycaemic action (A. Ferrari et al. 1991; Cerqueti et al. 1993).

Sex steroids

Earlier prospective data have shown that oral contracep-tive pill users have a higher incidence of impaired glucose tolerance (16 per cent) than non-users (eight per cent) (Duffy and Ray 1984; Perlman et al. 1985). Users also had higher fasting serum insulin, triglycerides and 2-hour post-glucose-loading plasma glucose concen-trations than non-users (Eschwège et al. 1991). However,

in a 12-year prospective study (Rimm et al. 1992), the risk of developing Type 2 diabetes was not significantly increased among women using oral contraceptives. These differences may be related to dosages and types of sex steroid used. The adverse effects of oral contracep-tive pills on carbohydrate metabolism are mainly due to the progestogens (Skouby 1988), with norethidrone hav-ing the least, and norgestrel the greatest, hypergly-caemic effect (Spellacy et al. 1981; Spellacy 1982). Severe hyperglycaemia has also been reported following med-roxyprogesterone therapy (Bottino and Tashima 1976; Panwalker 1992). The exact mechanism for this effect of progestogens remains to be clarified. Decreased insulin sensitivity at a cellular level in peripheral tissues has been observed during the luteal phase of the menstrual cycle and in women using oral contraceptive pills (De Pirro et al. 1981). Diminution of glycogen synthase activity and increased plasma cortisol levels have also been observed in contraceptive pill users (Munck 1971).

Most studies support a neutral metabolic effect of low dose oral contraceptive pills in women with Type 1 diabetes. However, results remain inconclusive in women with Type 2 or gestational diabetes (Skouby et al. 1991). In Caucasian women, the short-term use (e.g. 6 months) of low-dose combined oral contraceptive preparations was not associated with a significant deterioration in glycaemic control. However, an increased insulin re-sponse to oral glucose loading in these women suggests a degree of insulin resistance (van der Vange et al. 1987; Miccoli et al. 1989; Molsted-Pederson et al. 1991; Skouby et al. 1991). Similar treatment regimens have resulted in deterioration in glycaemic control and development of diabetes in Chinese women with a history of gestational diabetes mellitus. The risk factors for glucose intoler-ance in these women included a positive family history of diabetes, increasing age, obesity, a past history of large babies or stillbirths, and a prior history of abnormal glucose tolerance (Kung et al. 1987). Similar findings have also been reported in Kenyan women, some of whom developed glucose intolerance as early as one month after starting treatment with low-dose oral con-traceptive pills (Kamau et al. 1990). These findings there-fore emphasise the importance of ethnic or host factors, disease states, and other determinants in the manifes-tation of adverse effects of oral contraceptive pills.

While oestrogens and progestogens prescribed in pharmacological dosages may cause insulin resistance and hyperinsulinaemia in women of reproductive age, postmenopausal women are known to have both increased atherogenic risk and hyperinsulinaemia (Mathews et al. 1989; Eschwège et al. 1991; Ko et al. 1997). These metabolic changes can be improved by postmenopausal hormone replacement therapy, although long-term data are required to confirm a protective effect on glucose intolerance and related clinical events (Jacobs and Loeffler 1992). These findings also emphasize the differential effects of sex hormones, given in replacement as opposed to pharmacological dosages, on intermediary metabolism.

Growth hormone

There is now convincing evidence showing that adults deficient in growth hormone (GH) have increased body fat, insulin resistance, and abnormal metabolic indices, all of which can be reversed by GH replacement therapy (Rosenbaum et al. 1989; Bengtsson et al. 1993; De Boer et al. 1995). Beneficial effects of GH therapy on body fat composition have also been demonstrated in normal elderly subjects with reduced GH levels. However, GH therapy was associated with a high incidence of adverse effects (including arthralgia, carpal tunnel syndrome, and increased plasma glucose concentrations) in these elderly subjects (Ho and Hoffman 1993). In catabolic patients, GH therapy has been rarely associated with severe hyperglycaemia during nutritional support (Lehmann and Cerra 1992; Garg 1996). Hence, while GH replacement therapy in GH-deficient patients is now accepted, such therapy remains highly controversial in elderly subjects (De Boer et al. 1995).

Sympathomimetics

β-Adrenoceptor agonists

Sympathomimetic drugs, often given as a tocolytic therapy to halt premature labour, can be associated with the development of hyperglycaemia (Ingemarsson et al. 1985), especially when given together with betamethasone (Adam et al. 1993). Compared with non-diabetic individuals, diabetic subjects have higher plasma glucose, FFA, ketones, and glycerol concentrations in response to intravenous salbutamol infusion (Gündogdu et al. 1979). These adverse effects may be ameliorated by a reduction in dosage and are usually reversible upon discontinuation (Leslie and Coats 1977; Spellacy et al. 1978; Kirkpatrick et al. 1980). When low-dose intravenous salbutamol is administered to normal volunteers, there is no significant increase in plasma glucose concentration. However, with higher dosages, the hyperglycaemic actions of salbutamol predominate, resulting in relative insulinopenia and glucose intolerance (Huupponen and Pihlajamäki 1986). These findings emphasize the importance of host factors (such as pancreatic β-cell function) in determining individual responses to agents which, potentially, can cause hyperglycaemia. The hyperglycaemic effects of β-sympathomimetics

have also been reported in asthmatic children given high dosages of nebulized salbutamol (Dawson et al. 1995), and in association with the use of cough linctus (MacRury et al. 1987) and local anaesthetic solutions (Karch 1993; Meechan and Welbury 1993).

Theophylline

The β-sympathomimetic activity of theophylline is related to its inhibitory effect on the enzyme, phosphodiesterase, and resulting increases in cyclic AMP. Cardiac arrhythmias, hyperglycaemia, hypokalaemia, and metabolic acidosis have all been observed following theophylline overdosage, and these may be due to enhanced adrenergic activity and tissue responsiveness (Sessler 1990; Hagley et al. 1994). The glucose and potassium disturbances often parallel changes in plasma adrenaline concentrations (Shannon 1994). The clinical features of acute toxicity correlate well with serum theophylline concentration, but these relationships are weak in patients with chronic toxicity in whom extremes of age and pre-existing medical conditions are important predictors for life-threatening events (Shannon and Lovejoy 1990, 1992).

Cardiovascular drugs

Several large-scale studies have now demonstrated that treatment with antihypertensive agents is associated with an increased risk of glucose intolerance. This may be in part due to the close associations between glucose intolerance and hypertension (DeFronzo and Ferrannini 1991). Thus, the use of antihypertensive agents, notably diuretics and β-blockers, which have adverse effects on intermediary metabolism, may unmask diabetes in predisposed subjects or worsen glycaemic control in diabetic subjects (Yudkin 1991). The risk may be as high as fivefold for thiazide diuretics and sixfold for β-blocking agents (Lewis et al. 1976; Skarfors et al. 1989; Bengtsson et al. 1992). The relative risk for the initiation of antidiabetic drug therapy has been reported to be 1.4 for patients receiving thiazide diuretics and ranged from 1.56 to 1.77 for patients receiving other antihypertensive medications. With the exception of thiazides, the risk is more related to the number of antihypertensive agents used and to drug dosages rather than to individual agents (Gurwitz et al. 1993).

Diuretics

The adverse effect of diuretics on glucose metabolism has been linked to a reduction in total body potassium which correlates with a reduction in insulin secretion (Helderman et al. 1983). Hypokalaemia occurs in up to 30 per cent and glucose intolerance develops in three per

ients treated with diuretics. The adverse effect
se metabolism is dose dependent and can be
by giving a lower dosage or concurrent treat-
with antikaliuretics or adequate potassium supplements. It is usually reversible (Knauf 1993). Insulin
resistance has also been reported in association with
diuretic treatment (Pollare *et al.* 1989; P. Ferrari *et al.*
1991). Short-term study has suggested that indapamide,
an indoline diuretic structurally related to thiazides,
does not adversely affect glucose homoeostasis (Roux
and Courtois 1981). However, treatment for longer than
24 weeks has been associated with significant deterioration in glycaemic control in diabetic patients (Osei *et
al.* 1986).

Hyperglycaemic hyperosmolar non-ketotic coma
(particularly in the elderly) may also be precipitated by
thiazides, including indapamide (Fonseca and Phear
1982), chlorthalidone (Curtis *et al.* 1972), metolazone
(Rowe and Mather 1985), bumetanide (Hall 1982), and
frusemide (Tasker and Mitchell-Heggs 1976).

β-Adrenoreceptor blocking agents

Although there is *in vitro* evidence to show that both
secretion and action of insulin may be impaired by
β-blocking agents, *in vivo* data are not conclusive
(Wicklmayr *et al.* 1990). Glucose tolerance is usually
unaffected by β-adrenoceptor blockers in normal subjects although deterioration in glycaemic control has
been observed in patients with Type 2 diabetes due
to inhibition of insulin release (Wright *et al.* 1979).
Epidemiological data also give support to potential adverse effects of β-blocking agents on glucose metabolism, especially when combined with other agents such
as diuretics and this can occasionally be severe (Podolsky
and Pattavina 1973; Lewis *et al.* 1976; Dornhorst *et al.*
1985; Josselson and Sadler 1986; Skarfors *et al.* 1989;
Bengtsson *et al.* 1992). In view of their proven benefit
upon clinical end-points, β-blocking agents remain important in the treatment of hypertension. They should
be used with due awareness in diabetic patients or subjects at risk of developing glucose intolerance, such as
obese subjects (Tse and Kendall 1994).

Calcium-channel-blocking agents

Intracellular calcium metabolism is involved in the regulation of insulin secretion. However, the effects of
calcium-channel-blocking agents on glucoregulation remain controversial and may vary between different
drugs. Based on over 1000 clinical trials, the current
consensus is that the use of these drugs in standard
dosages is associated with neutral effects on glucose
metabolism in both normal and diabetic subjects (Trost
1990; Lithell 1991; J. Chan *et al.* 1994). However, it is

noteworthy that severe hyperglycaemia has been reported following both therapeutic and overdoses of nicardipine (Ahmad 1992), nifedipine (Greenwood 1982;
Sharma *et al.* 1990), and verapamil (Enyeart *et al.* 1983;
Heyman 1989; A. Roth *et al.* 1989).

Other antihypertensive agents

The known hyperglycaemic effect of diazoxide is due to
a combination of reduced insulin secretion and increased
counter-regulatory responses as reviewed previously by
Chan and Cockram (1991). Limited data on centrally
acting drugs and other vasodilators suggest neutral
effects on glucose tolerance (Holland and Pool 1988).
There have been anecdotal reports of severe hyperglycaemia following the use of clonidine either alone
(Mimouni and Mimouni 1993) or in combination with
metoprolol (Josselson and Sadler 1986).

Antiarrhythmic agents

Although there has been a report of hyperglycaemia and
hypertriglyceridaemia following the use of amiodarone
(Politi *et al.* 1984), no adverse effect on carbohydrate
metabolism was observed in 10 non-diabetic subjects
treated with amiodarone for 10 months (Lakhdar *et al.*
1988). The use of encainide, a new Class IC antiarrhythmic drug, has been associated with hyperglycaemia and increased plasma glucagon concentrations
(Salerno *et al.* 1988; Winter *et al.* 1992).

Psychotropic drugs

Although a number of psychotropic drugs have been
reported to cause hyperglycaemia, including chlordiazepoxide (Zumoff and Hellman 1977), loxapine,
amoxapine (Tollefson and Lesar 1983), phenothiazines
(Arneson 1964), clozapine (Kamran *et al.* 1994), and
mianserin (Marley and Rohan 1993), these effects are
probably of minor importance. Intraventricular morphine causes hyperglycaemia and increases plasma prolactin and GH in patients with cancer pain (Kamran *et al.*
1994). The opiate antagonists naloxone and nalmefene,
enhance the release of adrenaline in dog models (Critchley
et al. 1988) and naloxone increases insulin secretion in
man (Giugliano *et al.* 1982). Cocaine enhances the release of adrenaline with subsequent hyperglycaemia
(Olsen 1995). Caffeine overdosage may result in hypokalaemia, hyperglycaemia, and high blood pressure
(Leson *et al.* 1988). These findings point to possible
interactions between endogenous opiates, catecholamines, and brain amines in the regulation of glucose
and insulin metabolism.

Both hypo- and hyperglycaemia have been reported to
develop during lithium treatment (Craig *et al.* 1977;

Waziri and Nelson 1978). Hyperglycaemia occurs especially in the presence of lithium-induced nephrogenic diabetes insipidus (Lee *et al.* 1971; Martinez-Maldonaldo and Terrell 1973; Vendesborg 1979). Extracellular volume depletion with excessive reabsorption of glucose from the renal tubules has been proposed as a possible mechanism (Singer and Rotenberg 1973).

Immunosuppressive and immunomodulating agents

Glucose intolerance develops in approximately 11 per cent of patients treated with cyclosporin (Gunnarsson *et al.* 1983; D. Roth *et al.* 1989). However, identification of this effect is often difficult because of concurrent use of corticosteroids. Cyclosporin deposits have been observed in the pancreas of patients who have received the drug. Both defective insulin secretion (D. Roth *et al.* 1989) and increased insulin resistance (Gunnarsson *et al.* 1983) have been proposed as possible mechanisms for cyclosporin-associated hyperglycaemia. Risk factors include a positive family history of diabetes, age greater than 45 years, obesity, male sex, and certain HLA types (Sumrani *et al.* 1991).

Significant deterioration in glucose tolerance may also develop with agents such as colaspase (Iyer *et al.* 1993; Wang *et al.* 1993; Cetin *et al.* 1994), homoharringtonine (Sylvester *et al.* 1989), interleukin-6 (Weber *et al.* 1994), FK-506 (Tabasco *et al.* 1993; Krentz *et al.* 1994c; Takahara *et al.* 1994), pibenzimol (Patel *et al.* 1991), α-interferon (Jones and Itri 1986), and isotretinoin (Timperley 1996).

Antimicrobial agents and other drugs

Pentamidine, an antiprotozoal agent, has a multiphasic effect on glucose metabolism (similar to streptozotocin) with acute hypoglycaemia due to a cytolytic effect on the pancreas followed by insulinopenia with hyperglycaemia (Bouchard *et al.* 1982). Diabetes mellitus has been reported in patients treated with pentamidine for kala azar (Jha and Sharma 1984), leishmaniasis (Belehu and Naafs 1982), or *Pneumocystis carinii* infection (Coyle *et al.* 1996). Diabetes mellitus can persist despite discontinuation, and insulin therapy may be necessary (Bouchard *et al.* 1982; Jha and Sharma 1984; Shen *et al.* 1989; Coyle *et al.* 1996). Pentamidine isethionate appears less toxic to the pancreas than pentamidine mesylate (Belehu and Naafs 1982).

Didanosine, a purine nucleoside analogue used as an antiviral agent, has been reported to cause both hyper- and hypoglycaemia (Bouvet *et al.* 1990; Munshi *et al.* 1994). The hyperglycaemic effect may be an indication of pancreatitis (Albrecht *et al.* 1993).

Other drugs reported to cause hyperglycaemia include thiopentone (Amar *et al.* 1993), phenytoin (Fariss and Lutcher 1971; al-Rubeaan and Ryan 1991), niacin (Schwartz 1993), endosulfan (Blanco-Coronado *et al.* 1992), glycerol (Oakley and Ellis 1976; Sears 1976), isoniazid (Dickson 1962; Whitefield 1971), nalidixic acid (Fraser and Harrower 1977), rifampicin (Takasu *et al.* 1982), clofazimine, and the antischistosomal and taenicidal drug praziquantel (Webbe 1994).

Despite the large number of single case reports of drug-related glucose intolerance, in the majority of cases the underlying mechanisms remain uncertain. Clinicians should use these drugs with due caution, especially in diabetic patients. In subjects who develop hyperglycaemia, glucose tolerance should be formally tested following discontinuation of the culprit agent.

Hyperosmolar non-ketotic diabetic coma (HNC)

This condition is characterized by severe dehydration, hyperosmolality, and hyperglycaemia in the absence of ketosis. It occurs typically in elderly patients with or without known Type 2 diabetes and is frequently precipitated by concurrent illness. It carries a high mortality and morbidity and is not infrequently complicated by thromboembolic disease, such as myocardial infarction or cerebrovascular accident.

HNC is believed to be secondary to relative insulin deficiency which fails to control hyperglycaemia but suppresses lipolysis and ketogenesis. Drugs implicated in precipitating it include diuretics (Fonseca and Phear 1982), dexamethasone (Spenny *et al.* 1969), phenytoin (Goldberg and Sandbar 1969), and glycerol (Sears 1976). Diuretics are particularly important in view of their common use. Treatment with thiazide (Curtis *et al.* 1972), and thiazide-related compounds including indapamide (Fonseca and Phear 1982), metolazone (Rowe and Mather 1985), and diazoxide (Lancaster-Smith *et al.* 1974) has been associated with the development of HNC. Loop diuretics such as frusemide (Tasker and Mitchell-Heggs 1976) and bumetanide (Hall 1982) have also been implicated. Although deterioration in glucose tolerance is well recognized with diuretic therapy, the severity of HNC does not correlate with the magnitude of dehydration or potassium loss. A few cases appear to be precipitated by concomitant therapy with β-adrenoceptor-blockers (Podolsky and Pattavina 1973; Fonseca and Phear 1982; Rowe and Mather 1985; Josselson and Sadler 1986). The latter may worsen hyperglycaemia due to unopposed α-stimulation of gluconeogenesis and inhibition of insulin secretion. When

β-adrenoceptor-blocking agents and diuretics are used in combination in predisposed subjects under stressful situations, severe hyperglycaemia can occur and may progress to HNC.

Drug-induced hypoglycaemia

Hypoglycaemia is arbitrarily defined as a plasma glucose below 2.2 mmol per litre. However, the glucose level at which symptoms appear is variable. The neurohormonal response to hypoglycaemia results in a symptom complex which can be autonomic or neuroglycopenic in nature. Autonomic stimulation results in typical symptoms of sweating, tremor, tachycardia, and pallor. Neuroglycopenia may lead to diverse symptoms such as blurred vision, circumoral paraesthesia, poor concentration, ataxia, and hemiplegia. These symptoms can progress to irrational behaviour, automatism, confusion, and coma. Autonomic symptoms usually precede neuroglycopenic symptoms although diabetic patients with long duration of disease or tight control may have 'hypoglycaemic unawareness'.

In response to hypoglycaemia, counter-regulatory hormones (glucagon and catecholamines) are rapidly released to increase hepatic glucose production. Increased cortisol and GH secretion than assists in restoring plasma glucose concentration.

Drug-induced hypoglycaemia may result from therapeutic drug use in diabetic patients, deliberate or accidental overdosage, drug interactions, inadvertent use or incorrect drug dispensing, and drug-induced hepatotoxicity and nephrotoxicity (Seltzer 1989). The liver and kidneys are important organs for both glucose metabolism and drug elimination. The liver is the major site for glycogenesis, glycogenolysis, and gluconeogenesis and is vital for glucose homoeostasis. It is also an important site of drug metabolism. Hepatotoxic drugs can lead to hypoglycaemia through direct toxicity, though there is poor correlation between the degree of liver damage and susceptibility to hypoglycaemia (Arky 1989). Patients with renal failure are predisposed to hypoglycaemia by several mechanisms. These include poor nutrition and calorie deprivation, impaired glycolysis and gluconeogenesis, reduced production of precursor of gluconeogenic substrate (e.g. alanine), defective counter-regulatory hormone secretion, and reduced insulin clearance. Such patients are also at increased risk of drug-induced hypoglycaemia due to impaired drug clearance, altered pharmacokinetics, and alterations in protein binding (Arem 1989).

Insulin, sulphonylureas, and alcohol account for the majority of cases of drug-induced hypoglycaemia. The combination of an oral antidiabetic agent, or insulin, and alcohol explains most hypoglycaemic deaths. Salicylate poisoning remains the most important cause of hypoglycaemia in the first 2 years of life, while alcohol alone predominates during the next 8 years. Between the ages of 11 and 50 years, insulin and oral antidiabetic agents alone, or in combination with alcohol, account for the majority of cases of hypoglycaemia, some of which result from intentional overdosage. Over the age of 60 years, sulphonylurea therapy is by far the most important cause of hypoglycaemia (Seltzer 1989).

Hypoglycaemic agents

There is now clear evidence showing that optimal glycaemic control can delay the onset and progression of microangiopathic complications in both Type 1 (Reichard *et al.* 1991; DCCTRG 1993) and Type 2 diabetic patients (Ohkubo *et al.* 1995). Nevertheless, this is associated with a three-to-six-times increased risk of significant hypoglycaemia (The DCCTRG 1991). A good understanding of the mechanisms underlying these iatrogenic hypoglycaemic episodes should help clinicians to achieve euglycaemia while minimizing risk.

Insulin

Episodes of hypoglycaemia are almost inevitable in Type 1 diabetic patients and can be associated with significant physical and psychosocial morbidity. Ten per cent or more of patients with diabetes have at least one severe episode of hypoglycaemia yearly and three per cent experience recurrent episodes (Patrick *et al.* 1991; Everett and Kerr 1994). The frequency of mild to moderate symptomatic hypoglycaemia has been reported to be 1.8 episodes per week in insulin-treated patients (Cryer *et al.* 1994). In the Diabetes Control and Complications Trial (DCCT), the average incidence of severe hypoglycaemic episodes requiring assistance was reported to be 19 and 62 episodes per 100 patient-years in the conventionally and intensively treated groups respectively. Thus, an incidence of severe, temporarily disabling hypoglycaemia, often with coma or seizure, can be estimated to occur once every 1.6 years in intensively treated patients as compared with once every 5 years in conventionally treated patients (DCCTRG 1993, 1995). Although the incidence of sulphonlyurea-induced hypoglycaemia in Type 2 diabetic patients is lower than that of insulin-induced hypoglycaemia in Type 1 patients, the frequency of severe hypoglycaemia appeared to be similar between insulin-treated Type 1 and Type 2 patients, matched for duration of insulin therapy (Hepburn *et al.* 1993).

Asymptomatic hypoglycaemia is particularly common at night, reportedly occurring in 56 per cent of Type 1 diabetic patients. In the DCCT, over 50 per cent of severe hypoglycaemic episodes occurred during sleep. Warning symptoms were absent in 36 per cent of episodes that occurred while the patients were awake. Mismatch of food intake, exercise, and insulin injection, increased insulin sensitivity (as in hypopituitarism and hypoadrenalism), alcohol intake, and reduced insulin clearance with progressive renal insufficiency explain some of the hypoglycaemic episodes in Type 1 diabetic patients. A history of severe hypoglycaemia, long duration of disease, higher baseline glycosylated haemoglobin (HBA$_{1c}$), a lower recent HBA$_{1c}$ and higher baseline insulin dosages were all predictors of severe hypoglycaemia in the DCCT (DCCTRG 1991).

Insulin overdosage may result in refractory hypoglycaemia and fatality, particularly if combined with alcohol ingestion. The diagnosis can be made by the concurrent measurement of plasma insulin and C-peptide concentrations, the latter being inappropriately low compared with the former. The effects of massive insulin overdosage are something of a paradox. On the one hand, huge overdoses with exceptionally high plasma insulin levels have been tolerated with minimal symptomatology and have responded favourably to modest dextrose infusions. On the other hand, deaths do occur following such insulin overdosage but are usually in association with alcohol, often compounded by poor calorie intake. The counter-regulatory responses which normally prevent severe hypoglycaemia are impaired by the inhibitory effects of alcohol on hepatic gluconeogenesis. The resulting refractory hypoglycaemia results in potentially fatal brain damage (Critchley et al. 1984).

Hypoglycaemic unawareness and defective counter-regulation

Iatrogenic hypoglycaemia in Type 1 diabetes results from an interplay between absolute or relative therapeutic insulin excess and compromised glucose counter-regulation. The hypoglycaemic symptoms due to the activation of the counter-regulatory systems serve as important warning symptoms for corrective action. On the other hand, neuroglycopenic symptoms may be easily missed by patients, especially in the absence of autonomic symptoms, resulting in rapid loss of consciousness (Cryer et al. 1994).

With increasing disease duration, Type 1 diabetic patients experience increasing frequencies of hypoglycaemia. This is mainly due to impaired counter-regulation and reduced symptomatic awareness. The latter is manifested in a reduction in the blood glucose concentration at which activation of the autonomic/

sympathoadrenal responses to hypoglycaemia occur (Hepburn et al. 1990; Cryer et al. 1994).

Apart from the loss of glucagon response with increasing duration of disease, Type 1 diabetic patients also have reduced catecholamine responses during exercise-induced hypoglycaemia (Schneider et al. 1991). During hypoglycaemia, there is a linear correlation between glucagon and glucose responses in Type 1 diabetic patients, but the slope of the regression line is less steep than in control subjects. The increment in glucagon is directly related to that in adrenaline but inversely to that in insulin (Liu et al. 1993). In patients with hypoglycaemic unawareness, counter-regulatory responses occur at a significantly lower plasma glucose concentration than 'aware' patients and with a predominance of neuroglycopenic symptoms (Hepburn et al. 1991). Improvement of hypoglycaemic awareness is not always accompanied by recovery of counter-regulatory responses (or vice versa) suggesting a dissociation between these two processes (Kern et al. 1990; Egger et al. 1991b; Lingenfelser et al. 1991; Dagogo et al. 1994; Meneilly et al. 1995).

Hypoglycaemic unawareness and intensive insulin treatment

Apart from defective counter-regulation, iatrogenic hypoglycaemia and intensive insulin therapy are the other main factors contributing to hypoglycaemic unawareness. In intensively treated patients, counter-regulatory mechanisms may occur only when plasma glucose concentrations fall below 2.5 mmol per litre. Recovery from hypoglycaemia is adversely affected by a blunted glucagon response, delayed adrenaline release, and suppressed gluconeogenesis (Hoffman et al. 1991; Caprio et al. 1992; Davis et al. 1994; Fanelli et al. 1994). The glucagon response is also suppressed by high insulin levels (Liu et al. 1991, 1992). Responsiveness may be improved by meticulous avoidance of hypoglycaemia without significant compromise to glycaemic control (Hoffman et al. 1991; Cranston et al. 1994; Dagogo et al. 1994; Fanelli et al. 1994).

Hypoglycaemic unawareness and human insulin

Following the introduction of human insulin, concern arose over reports of reduced awareness of hypoglycaemia and increased frequency of hypoglycaemic episodes when patients were changed from animal to human insulin (Hepburn et al. 1988; Egger et al. 1991a,b). There is now a wealth of literature showing that the numbers of hypoglycaemic episodes and counter-regulatory responses are similar during hypoglycaemic episodes induced by either human or animal insulin.

There is also no difference in the plasma glucose threshold at which these responses are triggered, which on average is between 2 and 3 mmol per litre (Cryer 1994; Jorgensen *et al.* 1994). The evidence for this comes from both Type 1 (Bendtson and Binder 1991; Muhlhauser *et al.* 1991; Patrick *et al.* 1991; Colagiuri *et al.* 1992; Ferrer *et al.* 1992; Lingenfelser *et al.* 1992, 1993; MacLeod *et al.* 1995) and Type 2 diabetic patients (Meneilly *et al.* 1995) as well as normal subjects (Heine *et al.* 1989). Compared with regular human insulin, the new insulin analogue, Lispro, is associated with a lower rate of hypoglycaemia, possibly due to its more rapid onset and shorter duration of action (Wilde and McTavish 1997). However the very rapid onset of action needs to be carefully explained to patients receiving Lispro to ensure that food intake is not delayed following injection.

Sulphonylureas

Sulphonylureas are potent hypoglycaemic agents and inhibit hepatic glucose production, even in the fasting state due to unrestrained insulin secretion at low glucose concentrations. Sulphonylureas stimulate closure of potassium channels of the pancreatic β-cells leading to acute insulin release. The long-term use of these drugs is also associated with improved insulin sensitivity (Gerich 1989), but this may be secondary to improved glycaemic control (Rossetti *et al.* 1990).

The incidence of severe hypoglycaemia in patients taking a sulphonylurea has been estimated at 1.9 to 2.5 episodes per 100 patient-years compared with nine to 62 per 100 patient-years in insulin-treated patients (Krentz *et al.* 1994*a*). However, in view of the large number of Type 2 diabetic patients worldwide, the impact of sulphonylurea-induced hypoglycaemia is enormous (Cryer *et al.* 1994). The mortality rate associated with sulphonylurea-induced hypoglycaemia has been reported to be four to seven per cent (Koda-Kimble 1992). In the elderly, after adjusting for confounding factors, glibenclamide and chlorpropamide carry twice as great a risk of severe hypoglycaemia as does glipizide (Shorr *et al.* 1996). In one study, 20 per cent of patients taking a sulphonylurea reported at least one episode of symptomatic hypoglycaemia in the preceding 6 months and six per cent reported monthly episodes (Jennings *et al.* 1989). These patients were generally older and often had altered awareness (Hepburn *et al.* 1993) and little knowledge of hypoglycaemia (Thomson *et al.* 1991). Sulphonylurea-induced hypoglycaemia is associated with significant morbidity, permanent neurological deficits occurring in five per cent of survivors. Compared with Type 1 diabetes, counter-regulatory responses and effects of hypoglycaemia on cognitive function in Type 2

diabetes have been less well studied. De Mattia and colleagues (1996) demonstrated reduced serum levels of circulating catecholamines and insulin in a group of Type 2 diabetic patients taking captopril. Other workers have shown that at a plasma glucose concentration of 2.8 mmol per litre, elderly Type 2 diabetic patients have lower GH and glucagon responses but higher adrenaline and cortisol responses compared with normal subjects of similar age (Meneilly *et al.* 1994).

Although hypoglycaemia can occur with any sulphonylurea, chlorpropamide and glibenclamide remain the most important agents causing severe hypoglycaemia. It has been estimated that if the standardized incidence ratio for hypoglycaemia was 100 for chlorpropamide, that for glibenclamide would be 111, while for glipizide and tolbutamide it would be 46 and 21 respectively (Ferner and Neil 1988). Prospective studies have shown a lower risk of hypoglycaemia with short-acting sulphonylureas such as gliclazide and glipizide in comparison with glibenclamide (Harrower 1994; Krentz *et al.* 1994*c*; Tessier *et al.* 1994), but fatal cases of hypoglycaemia have still been reported with glipizide (Asplund *et al.* 1991). Hospitalization rates following hypoglycaemia have been reported to be 5.8 per 1000 person-years for chlorpropamide, 16 per 1000 patient-years for glibenclamide, and 9.1 per 1000 patient-years for insulin (Sugarman 1991). The prolonged hypoglycaemic effect of glibenclamide, even at low dosage, may result from an active metabolite or accumulation of the drug within the islets (Gerich 1989).

Table 16.1 summarizes the risk factors for iatrogenic hypoglycaemia. In Type 2 diabetes, increased age, poor nutrition, drug interactions, and hepatic or renal disease leading to altered drug metabolism and excretion are particularly important causes (Chan *et al.* 1992*a*,*b*; Cryer *et al.* 1994).

Mistaken dispensing of sulphonylureas remains an important cause of unexplained hypoglycaemia in non-diabetic subjects. This is often due to a similarity in the in the shape and colour of the tablets or to unclear prescriptions. This can be prevented by instructing patients to carefully identify their drugs, introducing typed prescription forms using generic names, and avoiding tablets with similar names or appearance (Huminer *et al.* 1989; Sledge and Broadstone 1993; T. Chan *et al.* 1994).

Drug interactions with hypoglycaemic agents

Interacting drugs may alter the pharmacokinetics of hypoglycaemic agents by enhancing or reducing drug absorption, by accelerating or inhibiting drug

Table 16.1
*Some common risk factors for hypoglycaemia
in diabetic patients*

Past history of hypoglycaemia
Defective counter-regulation especially in Type 1 diabetic
  patients with long duration of disease
Hypoglycaemic unawareness
Intensive insulin therapy
Overzealous glycaemic control
Errors of dosage and timing
Old age
Missed meals
Exercise
Co-existing diseases — e.g. renal or liver disease
Reduced calorie intake
Recent weight loss
Drug interactions — e.g. alcohol, β-blocking agents, other
  antihyperglycaemic agents
Increased insulin sensitivity — e.g. hypoadrenalism and
  hypopituitarism, post-partum state
Change of insulin preparation
Psychological problems — deliberate overdosage,
  manipulative behaviour

metabolism and elimination, or (rarely) by affecting the equilibrium between free and bound drug in the circulation. Pharmacodynamic interactions can also occur. These include direct effects on glucose homoeostasis including pancreatic β-cell function, insulin resistance, and secretion of counter-regulatory hormones. Apart from ethanol, which inhibits gluconeogenesis, β-blocking agents, salicylates, phenylbutazone, monoamine oxidase inhibitors, sulphonamides, co-trimoxazole (Jackson and Bressler 1981), H_2-receptor-blocking agents (Feely and Peden 1983; Lee et al. 1987; MacWalter et al. 1985), and tricyclic antidepressants (Shrivastava and Edwards 1983; True et al. 1987) have also been reported to potentiate the effects of hypoglycaemic agents. The suggested mechanisms underlying some of these interactions often remain unproved.

Other antihyperglycaemic drugs
Other antidiabetic drugs in common therapeutic usage lower blood glucose concentrations in subjects with hyperglycaemia but do not reduce blood glucose concentrations during euglycaemia. These agents do not cause an excessive fall in blood glucose because they do not inhibit hepatic glucose production and have little effect, if any, on counter-regulation. Thus, when given alone, they do not cause hypoglycaemia, but they may potentiate the hypoglycaemic actions of insulin or sulphonylureas. The biguanide metformin has a mild inhibitory effect on gluconeogenesis but sustains hepatic glucose

output through an increased supply of gluconeogenic substrates in the form of lactate from the intestine (Bailey 1992). α-Glucosidase inhibitors (e.g. acarbose) reduce the rate of glucose entry into the circulation from the intestine (Lebovitz 1993).

Ethanol

The inhibitory effects of alcohol on gluconeogenesis are particularly important in subjects with insufficient glycogen reserve, such as during the fasting state or in malnourished individuals. Thus, there have been reports of young men presenting with hypoglycaemic coma after drinking low-calorie alcoholic beverages without food and playing energetic sports. Alcohol may also enhance the plasma insulin response to a glucose load in both normal and mildly diabetic subjects, resulting in symptomatic reactive hypoglycaemia (McDonald 1980; Arky 1989). In alcoholism, despite higher resting plasma cortisol concentrations, the adrenocorticotrophin (ACTH) response to insulin-induced hypoglycaemia is attenuated suggesting alterations in the control of the hypothalamic–pituitary–adrenal axis (Berman et al. 1990). In both Type 1 diabetic patients and normal subjects, during insulin-induced hypoglycaemia, alcohol intake is associated with suppression of lipolysis and reduced plasma FFA which may contribute to delayed recovery from hypoglycaemia (Avogaro et al. 1993). By contrast, in Type 2 diabetes, ingestion of a moderate amount of alcohol with a light meal is not associated with significant changes in glucose, insulin, FFA, or triacylglycerol (Christiansen et al. 1993). Insulin overdosage combined with alcohol ingestion may result in refractory hypoglycaemia due to the inhibitory effects of alcohol on counter-regulation (Critchley et al. 1984).

In patients with acute alcohol intoxication and altered consciousness, hypoglycaemia should always be excluded. However, in a study involving 474 non-diabetic patients, the investigators were unable to identify any difference in the frequency of hypoglycaemia between intoxicated and non-intoxicated patients (Sporer et al. 1995). Ethanol is often present in pharmaceuticals, cosmetics, detergents, beverages, and household products. Ingestion of these products by children may occasionally result in serious poisoning. Asymptomatic hypoglycaemic children may be observed at home but all symptomatic children should be admitted for medical evaluation (Vogel et al. 1995). Severe intoxication resulting in hypoglycaemia, metabolic acidosis, coma, seizure, and death has been reported following ingestion of rice wine (Yang et al. 1995) and mouthwash (Hornfeldt 1992) by children.

Aspirin and paracetamol

Aspirin rarely produces hypoglycaemia in normal subjects at therapeutic dosage but may potentiate the effect of hypoglycaemic treatments in diabetic subjects, especially in the presence of liver or renal impairment (Jackson and Bressler 1981). Similar effects have been reported with other non-steroidal anti-inflammatory drugs such as indomethacin (Jackson and Bressler 1981) and piroxicam (Diwan et al. 1992). Aspirin-induced hyperinsulinaemia with reduced gluconeogenesis can be ameliorated by an infusion of prostaglandin E_2 (Giugliano et al. 1985). Other workers suggest that aspirin-induced hyperinsulinaemia may result from insulin resistance and reduced clearance of insulin, since there is a lack of change in plasma C peptide concentration (Bratusch-Marrain et al. 1985).

Profound hypoglycaemia may develop when large amounts of salicylate-containing compounds are ingested, particularly in children with accidental poisoning (Seltzer 1989). An elderly man with psoriasis and renal impairment developed severe intoxication with a serum salicylate concentration of 3.2 mmol per litre due to systemic absorption of topical salicylate from the abnormal skin. The patient was successfully treated by haemodialysis (Raschke et al. 1991).

Following ingestion of toxic doses of paracetamol (7–35 g), both hypoglycaemia and transient hyperglycaemia have been reported (Thomson and Prescott 1966). These effects may be due to paracetamol-induced hepatic injury (Davidson et al. 1966; Prescott et al. 1971).

Cardiovascular drugs

Numerous cardiovascular drugs alter intermediary metabolism and the use of such agents may sometimes precipitate diabetes or induce hypoglycaemia in susceptible individuals (Lithell 1991; Yudkin 1991).

β-Adrenoreceptor blocking agents

Owing to the diverse effects of catecholamines on intermediary metabolism and insulin secretion, β-adrenoceptor-blocking agents, alone or in combination with other drugs, can predispose to either hyperglycaemia or hypoglycaemia depending on the circumstances.

Although there have been reports of hypoglycaemia during exercise in normal subjects receiving β-blocking agents (Holm et al. 1981), the effects of these drugs on counter-regulation have not been critically compared. In a cross-over study involving treatment (for one week) with non-selective (propranolol) and selective (atenolol and metoprolol) β-blocking agents in normal volunteers, the expected increase in heart rate during insulin-induced hypoglycaemia was inhibited by atenolol but not by metoprolol. Pretreatment with propranolol was associated with a significant pressor effect, bradycardia, and diminished hand tremor. All three β-blocking agents augmented sweating. However, awareness of hypoglycaemic symptoms and slowing of reaction times were similar in both treated and placebo groups (Kerr et al. 1990).

Under experimental conditions, administration of β-blocking agents is associated with delayed glucose recovery and elevation of glycaemic threshold (lower plasma glucose levels required) for symptoms in Type 1 diabetic patients (Seltzer 1989). The use of local ocular application of timolol for glaucoma was reported to have caused hypoglycaemia in a Type 1 diabetic patient (Angelo-Nielson 1980). Thus, despite lack of conclusive evidence regarding their effects on glucoregulation, β-blocking agents should be used with caution in diabetic patients. The use of a single 30 mg intravenous dose of labetalol, given 20 minutes prior to caesarean delivery at 35 weeks of gestation for severe pregnancy hypertension, was associated with hypotension, hypoglycaemia, and bradycardia in preterm twins (Klarr et al. 1994).

Angiotensin-converting-enzyme inhibitors and α-blocking agents

Several studies have demonstrated the hypoglycaemic effects of captopril in diabetic, hypertensive subjects (Winocour et al. 1986; Shionoiri et al. 1987; Zanella et al. 1988; Pollare et al. 1989). Ferriere and colleagues (1985) reported cases of hypoglycaemia in both Type 1 and 2 diabetic patients after introduction of captopril therapy and demonstrated enhanced insulin sensitivity with increased glucose disposal. Hypoglycaemia has occurred in diabetic patients with previously stable glycaemic control within 7 hours to up to one week after initiating treatment with captopril or enalapril. Most of the data now support the notion that ACE inhibitors improve insulin resistance and glycaemic control in both diabetic and non-diabetic patients and may lead to hypoglycaemic episodes, requiring a reduction in the dosage of hypoglycaemic agents (Pollare et al. 1989; Lithell 1991). The use of ACE inhibitors has also been reported to be associated with an increased risk of hospital admission for hypoglycaemia with an odds ratio of 2.8 amongst users of insulin and 4.1 amongst users of oral hypoglycaemic agents (Herings et al. 1995). However, in this study, 74 per cent of the cases but only 42 per cent of the controls were using insulin, and the groups were not fully matched for frequency of past hypoglycaemia, duration of therapy, and degree of glycaemic control.

The mechanism for the effects of ACE inhibitors on glucose metabolism remains uncertain. It has often been assumed that angiotensin II has diabetogenic effects. However, more recent studies have shown that both pressor and subpressor doses of angiotensin II increase insulin-mediated glucose uptake in healthy subjects and Type 2 diabetic patients. Postulated mechanisms include redistribution of blood flow by angiotensin II with increased perfusion of skeletal muscle, as well as a direct effect of angiotensin II on insulin-mediated glucose disposal (Morris and Donnelly 1996). On the other hand, the beneficial metabolic effects of ACE inhibitors may result from accumulation of bradykinin. In experimental studies, local accumulation of bradykinin, which has an insulin-like activity due to kininase II inhibition, was associated with increased peripheral insulin sensitivity, enhanced forearm glucose uptake, and reduced hepatic glucose production (Jauch et al. 1987). In a comparative study between captopril and hydrochlorothiazide, patients receiving captopril showed no change in basal insulin, but an increase in the early, and decrease in the late, insulin peak suggestive of enhanced insulin sensitivity. This is in contrast to the increase of levels, both basal insulin and in the late peak in the patients taking hydrochlorothiazide (Pollare et al. 1989).

Given the known interactions between the renin–angiotensin system and the sympathoadrenal system (Axelrod and Reisine 1984; Zimmerman et al. 1984), it is plausible that the effects of ACE inhibition on glucose metabolism may be mediated by changes in other hormones. For example, angiotensin II enhances the release of adrenaline from the adrenal medulla (Critchley et al. 1982, 1988), and augments the release of catecholamines presynaptically and their effects postsynaptically (Zimmerman et al. 1984). De Mattia and colleagues (1996) demonstrated reduced serum levels of circulating catecholamines and insulin in a group of Type 2 diabetic patients treated with captopril. In both animal and human studies, the release of adrenaline can be attenuated by pretreatment with ACE inhibitors (Critchley et al. 1988; Madsen et al. 1992). The potential metabolic effects of catecholamines are also implied by the beneficial effects of α-blocking agents on insulin sensitivity, glycaemic control, and lipid metabolism (Lund-Johnson et al. 1993; Shionoiri et al. 1994).

Antiarrhythmic drugs

Disopyramide, a quinidine-like Class Ia antiarrhythmic drug, is known to be associated with hypoglycaemia. Croxson et al. (1987) detected failure of suppression of insulin during hypoglycaemia in a patient treated with disopyramide and proposed that the drug might stimulate insulin release, in the same way as quinidine and quinine. In a review of 14 cases of disopyramide-induced hypoglycaemia, nine had significantly impaired renal function. Elderly, and malnourished patients were also at particular risk and toxicity could occur with normal therapeutic dosages (Cacoub et al. 1989). Hypoglycaemia, with non-suppression of insulin secretion, and inadequate counter-regulatory responses, has also been reported during treatment with disopyramide, alone or in combination with other hypoglycaemic agents (Smith et al. 1992). The action of other hypoglycaemic agents can be potentiated in the presence of disopyramide (Stapleton and Gillman 1983). Cibenzoline, a type of Class I drug has recently been reported to cause hypoglycaemia (Hilleman et al. 1987; Gachot et al. 1988; Jeandel et al. 1988).

Lipid-lowering agents

Aberrant fat metabolism may be causally linked to the development of insulin resistance. Increased lipolysis and oxidation of FFA enhance gluconeogenesis and induce insulin resistance by inhibiting the peripheral uptake of glucose (Randle et al. 1963; Björntorp 1994). Accumulation of triglyceride and long-chain FFA inhibit the expression of glycogen synthase and insulin receptors in muscle and liver (Saha et al. 1994). Experimentally, lipid-lowering agents and drugs, such as acipimox, that inhibit the formation of FFA have been shown to improve insulin sensitivity (Donnelly and Morris 1994). The relevance of these findings to clinical practice remains uncertain, although a case of hypoglycaemia in association with gemfibrozil combined with glibenclamide has been reported (Ahmad 1991).

Sympathomimetic drugs

The use of sympathomimetics such as ritodrine to halt premature labour is associated with increased incidence of neonatal hyperinsulinaemic hypoglycaemia due to β-adrenergic stimulatory effects on insulin secretion (Brazy and Pupkin 1979). Babies exposed to ritodrine up to the date of delivery were at greater risk than babies whose exposure was stopped at least one week before delivery (Musci et al. 1988). Hyperinsulinaemic hypoglycaemia occurred in a mother with a triple pregnancy treated with ritodrine for premature labour. It was proposed that the insulinotropic effect of ritodrine augmented the hyperinsulinaemic state of the triplet pregnancy (Caldwell et al. 1987). Symptomatic hypoglycaemia has also been reported in a child 16 hours after acute albuterol overdose (Wasserman and Amitai 1992).

Hormones

Octreotide, a long-acting analogue of somatostatin, suppresses the release of insulin and C-peptide in both basal and stimulated states. During insulin-induced hypoglycaemia, octreotide also suppresses the secretion of glucagon and GH (Krentz *et al.* 1994*a*). In the treatment of acromegaly with octreotide, suppression of insulin secretion can lead to initial hyperglycaemia. As the high circulating GH concentrations fall with octreotide therapy, the adverse effects of GH on lipid and glucose metabolism are expected to improve (Lamberts *et al.* 1985). Hypoglycaemic reactions have also been reported during treatment of insulinoma (Stehouwer *et al.* 1989), acromegaly (Popvic *et al.* 1989) and metastatic carcinoid tumours (Brunner *et al.* 1989) with octreotide. This may be due to the inhibitory effect of somatostatin on release of counter-regulatory hormones and on gut polypeptides. The latter may lead to reduced glucose absorption. Octreotide has also been successfully used to treat refractory hyperinsulinaemic hypoglycaemia following massive sulphonylurea overdosage (Boyle *et al.* 1993; Krentz *et al.* 1993) and during quinidine therapy for falciparum malaria (Phillips *et al.* 1986*a*, 1993).

Many of the growth-promoting effects of GH are mediated by IGF-I which also has affinity for insulin receptors (Jérôme *et al.* 1995). Recombinant human IGF-1 (rhIGF-1) has been shown to reduce plasma glucose and insulin concentrations in normal individuals without causing clinically significant hypoglycaemia (Morgan *et al.* 1993). Preliminary studies in a small number of hyperinsulinaemic patients, including those with Type 2 diabetes, show that short-term treatment with IGF-I in appropriate dosage improves glycaemic profiles, enhances insulin sensitivity, and decreases insulin and GH concentrations (Zenobi *et al.* 1992, 1993; Froesch *et al.* 1994). However, in view of the growth-promoting effects of IGF-I, studies are required to confirm its long-term safety and efficacy.

Antimalarial drugs

Spontaneous hypoglycaemia can occur in patients with severe *Plasmodium falciparum* infection through depletion of hepatic glycogen reserves in the host and the parasites' metabolic demand for glucose. However, hyperinsulinaemic hypoglycaemia occurs not uncommonly in patients treated with quinine, quinidine, or mefloquine for this infection (White *et al.* 1983), particularly children (Okitolonda *et al.* 1987) and pregnant women (Looareesuwan *et al.* 1985). A stimulatory effect of quinine on insulin release from pancreatic β-cells has been postulated, but direct inhibition of hepatic gluco-

neogenesis and increased glucose utilization by the parasites may also play contributory roles (White *et al.* 1983; Looareesuwan *et al.* 1985; Okitolonda *et al.* 1987; Krishna *et al.* 1994; Assan *et al.* 1995*a*). In patients receiving quinine who had severe life-threatening hypoglycaemia, plasma insulin concentrations remained inappropriately high at a plasma glucose as low as 1.2 mmol per litre, but the glucose counter-regulatory responses, indicated by plasma cortisol, GH, catecholamines, and glucagon concentrations remained intact (Phillips *et al.* 1993). Refractory hypoglycaemia with quinine-induced hyperinsulinaemia can be successfully treated by long-acting somatostatin analogues such as octreotide, which inhibits insulin release and reduces the need for large volumes of intravenous dextrose (Phillips *et al.* 1986*b*, 1993).

Although hypoglycaemia has been reported mainly with quinine therapy (White *et al.* 1983; Phillips *et al.* 1986*a*), chloroquine-induced hypoglycaemia has been reported (Abu-Shakra and Lee 1994) and may lead to death in overdosage (Bamber and Redpath 1987). Quinine sulphate prescribed in a standard dose of 600 mg twice daily for cramps produced a reduction in plasma glucose of 1.0 mmol per litre 3–5 hours later in both normal subjects and Type 2 diabetic patients. However, the decrement is unlikely to cause clinically significant hypoglycaemia (Dyer *et al.* 1994).

Pentamidine

This is an antiprotozoal agent used in the treatment of leishmaniasis, trypanosomiasis, and *Pneumocystis carinii* pneumonia. Like streptozotocin and alloxan, pentamidine is toxic to pancreatic β-cells. It may cause haemorrhagic pancreatitis and produce a multiphasic effect on blood glucose concentrations. Severe hypoglycaemia due to acute release of insulin and consequent hyperinsulinaemia can be followed by persistent hyperglycaemia from destruction of islet cells (Sharpe 1983; Salmeron *et al.* 1986; Herchline *et al.* 1991). This hypoglycaemia occurs suddenly, early during therapy, and may be recurrent as well as life-threatening. Islet cell antibodies, insulin antibodies, and insulitis are not detected. Pentamidine-induced dysglycaemia can occur in up to 50 per cent of patients with the acquired immune deficiency syndrome (AIDS) (Stahl-Bayliss *et al.* 1986; Perronne *et al.* 1990). Drug accumulation due to excessive dosage and renal impairment, as well as a severe clinical course with shock and hypoxia, are risk factors for pentamidine-induced dysglycaemia (Waskin *et al.* 1988; Assan *et al.* 1995*b*). Hypoglycaemia has also been reported following the use of pentamidine by inhalation

(Karboski and Godley 1988). In the light of its pancreatic β-cell toxicity, pentamidine is now infrequently used.

Trimethoprim/sulphamethoxazole (co-trimoxazole)

Apart from potentiating the effects of sulphonylureas (Jackson and Bressler 1981), high-dose co-trimoxazole given alone for the treatment of *Pneumocystis carinii* pneumonia has also been reported to induce hypoglycaemia with unsuppressed plasma C-peptide levels in patients with AIDS (Poretsky and Moses 1984; Schattner *et al.* 1988) and in renal transplant recipients (Johnson *et al.* 1993). These findings suggest that co-trimoxazole may mimic sulphonylurea agents and stimulate pancreatic β-cells to secrete insulin (Schattner *et al.* 1988). However, this antimicrobial is very widely used and does not appear to have a significant effect on glucose homoeostasis when given in standard therapeutic dosage.

Lithium and other psychotropic drugs

Huntsinger (1987) previously reported a case of lithium-induced hypoglycaemia in a Type 2 diabetic patient. Lithium mimics the action of insulin by inhibiting adenyl cyclase activity and production of cyclic AMP which mediates the actions of many counter-regulatory hormones (including adrenaline, adrenocorticotrophic hormone [ACTH], and glucagon). Hence, hypoglycaemia may ensue due to increased glucose uptake by peripheral tissues as well as decreased lipolysis and hepatic glucose production.

Phenothiazine and some other thioxanthene derivatives have caused hypoglycaemia when used in combination with orphenadrine (Buckle and Guillebaud 1967; Korenyi and Lowenstein 1968). Bromperidol, a butyrophenone neuroleptic, has also had this effect, as have some of the tricyclic antidepressants (e.g. imipramine) by increasing sensitivity to insulin (Kathol *et al.* 1991). Monoamine oxidase inhibitors, selective serotonin reuptake inhibitors, and phenylpiperazine-class drugs may also lower blood glucose (Rowland *et al.* 1994; Warnock and Biggs 1997).

Other drugs

Treatment with selegiline produced profound hypoglycaemia accompanied by hyperinsulinaemia in an elderly woman with Parkinson's disease. Molecular modeling techniques show that both selegiline and glucose show similar stereochemical complementarity to a specific site in partially unwound DNA. However, the clinical relevance of these findings remains uncertain (Rowland *et al.* 1994).

Chloroquinoxaline sulphonamide (CQS) is a halogenated heterocyclic sulphanilamide active against solid tumours. In phase I and II studies, cases of hyperinsulinaemic hypoglycaemia have been reported following its use (Rigas *et al.* 1992, 1995).

A woman suffering from rheumatoid arthritis developed recurrent hypoglycaemia due to insulin antibodies related to a granuloma induced by gold thioglucose. After resection of the granuloma, the frequency of hypoglycaemic attacks decreased, as did the levels of insulin antibody (Yao *et al.* 1992).

Hypoglycaemia in association with liver damage has occurred following exposure to anaesthetic agents, including halothane (Bichel *et al.* 1994) and enflurane (Schneider 1995). Other agents which have caused hypoglycaemia include aluminium phosphide (Patial *et al.* 1990; Singh *et al.* 1994), maprotiline (Zogno *et al.* 1994), calcium hopantenate (Otsuka *et al.* 1990), propoxyphene (Almirall *et al.* 1989), valproate (Almirall *et al.* 1989), and acadesine (a purine nucleoside analogue under investigation as a cardioprotective agent in heart surgery) (Dixon *et al.* 1991).

In many reported cases of hypoglycaemia, underlying mechanisms remain unclear. The adverse events often occur in patients receiving several drugs and suffering from such conditions as renal or hepatic failure. Hence, it can be difficult to determine if the hypoglycaemia was a direct effect of the drug, the result of interaction with another drug, or due to otherwise unrelated underlying disease.

Prevention and treatment of hypoglycaemia in diabetes

Iatrogenic hypoglycaemia and intensive insulin treatment may result in hypoglycaemic unawareness which is associated with an increased risk of severe hypoglycaemia. Rational and individualized treatment with meticulous avoidance of hypoglycaemia may restore normal awareness of hypoglycaemic symptoms without adversely affecting glycaemic control (Cryer *et al.* 1994). Great care is required to achieve a balance between optimal glycaemic control and risk of hypoglycaemia, particularly in older patients, those with multiple diseases, and those exposed to polypharmacy. Identification of the precipitating causes of hypoglycaemia (Table 16.1), patient education with particular emphasis on self-care and self-monitoring, and avoidance of overzealous glycaemic control are probably the most effective means to prevent iatrogenic hypoglycaemia.

TABLE 16.2
Possible hypoglycaemic mechanisms of some commonly used drugs

Counter-regulatory responses decreased	Increased insulin secretion	Increased insulin sensitivity
ACE inhibitors	Aspirin	ACE inhibitors
β-Blocking agents	Cibenzoline	α-Blocking
Ethanol	Co-trimoxazole	agents
Octreotide	Disopyramide	Recombinant
	Ethanol	human
	Insulin	insulin-like
	Pentamidine	growth factor
	Quinine	(rhIGF-I)
	Sulphonylureas	
	β-Sympatho-	
	mimetics	

TABLE 16.3
Possible hyperglycaemic mechanisms of some commonly used drugs

Counter-regulatory responses increased	Reduced insulin secretion	Decreased insulin sensitivity
β-sympathomimetics	β-blocking agents	β-blocking agents
Corticosteroids	Diazoxide	Corticosteroids
Diazoxide	Diuretics	Diuretics
Growth hormone	Octreotide	

Treatment of mild episodes of hypoglycaemia is by the intake of 20 g of rapidly absorbed glucose followed by more complex forms of carbohydrates to prevent recurrence (Binder and Bendtson 1992). Glucose given orally appears to act faster than saccharose (Georgakopoulos *et al.* 1990). Severe hypoglycaemic episodes with an impaired level of consciousness should be treated with either intravenous dextrose (0.2–5 g per kg) or glucagon (0.5–1 mg) injected intramuscularly or intravenously. The glycaemic response and recovery of a normal level of consciousness is 1–2 minutes slower after glucagon than after glucose and thus the latter is the treatment of choice, if available. However, non-medical personnel and relatives find administration of glucagon easier and more practical (Soltesz 1993). An intranasal spray of 7.5 mg glucagon with deoxycholic acid as surfactant has been shown to be effective in correcting insulin-induced hypoglycaemia, although its routine clinical use remains to be evaluated (Slama *et al.* 1990; Rosenfalck *et al.* 1992).

Theophylline (a phosphodiesterase inhibitor) mimics the actions of counter-regulatory hormones by inhibiting the breakdown of cyclic AMP. Administration of theophylline in bronchodilator dosage enhances glucose recovery after hypoglycaemia in healthy subjects and Type 1 diabetic patients (Hvidberg *et al.* 1994). Prolonged and recurrent hypoglycaemia may occur with sulphonylureas, requiring prolonged administration of intravenous dextrose. In refractory hypoglycaemia due to hyperinsulinaemia (as in sulphonylurea overdosage) unresponsive to large doses of intravenous glucose, octreotide may inhibit the release of insulin and restore euglycaemia (Boyle *et al.* 1993; Krentz *et al.* 1993).

Conclusions

The effects of a drug on glucose metabolism may be due to a combination of factors involving the secretion and action of insulin, counter-regulatory hormones and responses (Tables 16.2 and 16.3). Host factors, such as inherent glucoregulation, concurrent disease, organ function and concomitant medications are also important. Insulin and sulphonylureas are by far the most important agents causing hypoglycaemia. Alcohol, overzealous glycaemic control, hypoglycaemic unawareness, defective counter-regulation especially in Type 1 diabetes, renal impairment, and ageing are all important predisposing factors. Antihyperglycaemic agents such as metformin and α-glucosidase inhibitors do not on their own cause hypoglycaemia, but may enhance the hypoglycaemic potential of insulin and sulphonylureas.

Diuretics, β-blocking agents, sympathomimetics, corticosteroids, and sex hormones are drugs in common usage which may have deleterious effects on carbohydrate metabolism. These effects are of particular relevance to diabetic patients or subjects at risk of glucose intolerance. An understanding of the mechanisms of glucoregulation allows the prediction of drug-induced adverse effects on carbohydrate metabolism and the implementation of more rational therapy.

Finally, the adverse metabolic effects of a drug, and the underlying mechanisms, may provide insights into the control of glucoregulation and its potential for modulation. Effects which are disadvantageous in one situation may be advantageous in another. Hence, the hypoglycaemic potential of a drug may be turned to therapeutic advantage in patients with glucose intolerance. Similarly, the hyperglycaemic potential of a drug may be used to advantage in refractory hypoglycaemia.

Lactic acidosis

Lactate homoeostasis is dependent upon a balance between production and utilization. Complete oxidation of carbohydrate to carbon dioxide and water during gly-colysis occurs in the cellular mitochondria. Lactate, an end product of incomplete oxidation, is normally util-ized by the liver and kidney for gluconeogenesis, and these organs play an important role in the homoeostasis of lactate metabolism. When there is inadequate tissue perfusion or mitochondrial dysfunction, increased an-aerobic glycolysis results in overproduction of lactate from pyruvate. Lactate is a strong organic acid which rapidly dissociates forming hydrogen ions which can accumulate, leading to acidosis. Significant lactic aci-dosis is considered to be present when there is a systemic $pH \leqslant 7.25$ occurring in association with a lactate concen-tration $\geqslant 5$ mEq per litre and this is characterized by an increase in the anion gap $([Na^+]+[K^+])-([Cl^-]+[HCO_3^-])$ (Kreisberg 1984). Lactic acidosis typically occurs in the presence of poor tissue perfusion or oxygenation, such as during shock, sepsis, and cardiac failure (Type A lactic acidosis). Type B lactic acidosis occurs in association with certain drugs or toxins and disease states in which poor tissue oxygenation is not a typical feature except as a terminal event.

Many drugs or chemicals are known to be associated with lactic acidosis. Biguanides act on the mitochondrial membranes causing inhibition of gluconeogenesis with the resultant increase in gluconeogenic precursors of lactate, pyruvate, and alanine. This predisposes the patient to lactic acidosis, especially in the presence of impaired renal or hepatic function. Metformin, which is excreted by the kidney, has been reported to lead to lactic acidosis in 0.4 cases per 10 000 treatment years, with a mortality of 30 per cent. Mortality from phen-formin-related lactic acidosis is higher at 70 per cent (Berger et al. 1986). In another review, by Campbell (1985), there were 18 deaths in 43 cases of metformin-associated lactic acidosis, and 40 had documented con-traindications. Phenformin has now been withdrawn from the market in most countries. Metformin should be used with caution in the elderly, and in patients known to have renal, cardiac, or hepatic impairment.

Poisoning with methanol or ethylene glycol can lead to severe formate and lactic acidosis due to depression of the $NAD/NADH^+$ ratio, which enhances the conversion of pyruvate to lactate (*The Lancet* 1983). Ethanol is known to increase the lactate concentration in the blood, and both oral alcohol poisoning and intravenous therapy with alcohol for premature labour have resulted in severe lactic acidosis (Ott et al. 1976).

Lactic acidosis has been reported to occur in patients treated with nalidixic acid, and Phillips and colleagues (1979) suggested that nalidixic acid may cause both an increase in lactate production and reduction in hepatic uptake. Outdated tetracycline tablets (of now outmoded formulations) degrade to form toxic chemicals of 4-epi-anhydrotetracycline and anhydrotetracycline that are known to cause Fanconi's syndrome. Montoliu and others (1981) reported a case of lactic acidosis associated with Fanconi's syndrome following the ingestion of de-graded tetracycline tablets and both toxic chemicals were detectable on biochemical analysis of the tablets. Sodium nitroprusside therapy for severe hypertension can lead to accumulation of cyanmethaemoglobin and free cyanide ions, which are known to cause lactic aci-dosis (Humphrey and Nash 1978). Mann and others (1985) reported a case of lactic acidosis in a patient treated with lactulose for hepatic encephalopathy. Sig-nificant reabsorption of the lactic acid from the break-down of lactulose in the presence of poor gut motility was proposed as a possible mechanism. Papaverine, which inhibits cellular oxidative pathways, was reported to cause severe lactic acidosis in a patient who took an overdose (Vaziri et al. 1981). Other agents known to be associated with lactic acidosis include salicylates, fructose, sorbitol, adrenaline, and isoniazid (Kreisberg 1984).

Fat metabolism

Cholesterol and triglycerides are hydrophobic com-pounds and their transport in plasma is facilitated by combination with phospholipids and a class of hydro-philic polypeptides, known as apoproteins, to form com-plexes called lipoproteins. Fatty acids on the other hand are transported in plasma bound to albumin.

Compositions of lipoproteins

There are several classes of apoproteins (apo A, consist-ing of apo A-I and apo A-II; apo B; apo C consisting of apo C-I, apo C-II, apo C-III; and apo E) which are mainly synthesized in the liver or intestinal mucosa. The various combinations of apolipoproteins with choles-terol and triglycerides result in the formation of five classes of lipoproteins which vary in their composition, functions, and other properties.

Chylomicrons consist mainly of dietary triglyceride with only a small amount of apoprotein. The very-low-density lipoproteins (VLDL) consist of endogenously synthesized triglycerides and are substantially smaller and denser than the chylomicrons, because of the incor-poration of apoproteins, mainly of the apo B type. The VLDL is converted via intermediate-density lipoprotein (IDL) to low-density lipoprotein (LDL), which consists mainly of cholesterol and apo B. High-density lipo-protein (HDL) is the most dense form, with apo A as its major apoprotein and equal amounts of cholesterol and phospholipid. HDL has a major role in reverse transport of cholesterol from peripheral tissues to liver for the excretion of cholesterol. Apo E is mainly associated with VLDL and chylomicron remnants.

There are four enzymes involved in plasma lipid trans-port. Activity of lecithin cholesterol acyltransferase (LCAT) is stimulated by apo A-I and is involved in the synthesis of cholesterol ester. Lipoprotein lipase, found mainly in the liver and adipose tissue, splits triglycerides in chylomicrons and VLDL to glycerol and free fatty acids and its activity is stimulated by apo C-II. Hepatic lipase mainly hydrolyses triglycerides in the VLDL rem-nants. Mobilizing lipase releases free fatty acids from adipose tissue and is activated through the adenyl cyclase system by catecholamines, growth hormone, and gluco-corticoids, and is inhibited by glucose and insulin.

Transport and metabolism of lipoproteins

Exogenous (dietary) lipid is transported by chylo-microns, which are resynthesized in the intestinal mucosa from the breakdown products of dietary tri-glycerides and cholesterol in the gastrointestinal tract. They consist principally of triglycerides and contain apo A and apo B. In the circulation, apo A is transferred to HDL, where the chylomicrons acquire apo C and apo E from HDL. Apo C-II then activates lipoprotein lipase in the peripheral tissues, mainly adipose tissue, muscle, and liver, where triglycerides are released from the chylomicrons. The fatty acids liberated from hydrolysis of triglycerides are then stored or used as a source of energy. The chylomicron remnants consisting of apo B, apo E, and cholesterol esters are taken up by the liver and catabolised. The sterol is then excreted in the bile.

In the fasting state, VLDL is synthesized in the liver and, to a lesser extent, the intestinal mucosa, and con-tains mainly triglycerides and some unesterified choles-terol with apo B and lesser amounts of apo E. Apo C is acquired from HDL and VLDL remnants in the plasma. Lipoprotein lipase, activated by apo C-II, removes tri-glycerides from VLDL in the adipose and other tissue. The apo C, unesterified cholesterol, and phospholipid are progressively transferred to HDL. The catabolism of VLDL results in the formation of IDL which is further hydrolysed to form LDL, consisting mainly of choles-terol and apo B. LDL either binds to apo B receptors in the liver, and is taken up when cholesterol esters are hydrolysed and apo B destroyed, or to receptors on peripheral tissues such as the adrenals where cholesterol

is used for synthesis of steroids. A small proportion of LDL is taken up by the scavenger cells of the monocyte–macrophage system.

HDL is formed in the liver and intestinal mucosa and contains mainly apo C, apo E, equal amounts of choles-terol and phospholipid, and very little triglyceride. In the circulation, HDL acquires apo A-I mainly from chylomicrons, to which it transfers apo C and apo E. Apo A-I is a co-factor for LCAT, which esterifies free cholesterol on HDL. The more hydrophobic esterified cholesterol passes into the core of the HDL particle while the surface accepts more cholesterol and lipo-proteins from other tissues for further esterification. The cholesterol ester is transferred from the HDL core to VLDL and LDL by a transfer protein (cholesteryl ester transfer protein) and is then taken up again by the liver and peripheral tissues through the recognition of apo B on LDL by apo B receptors.

Significance of dyslipoproteinaemia

The association of hypercholesterolaemia with coronary arterial disease has long been recognized. Most studies have now shown a positive association between elevated plasma LDL-C and remnant VLDL-C concentrations and ischaemic heart disease. On the other hand, HDL-C appears to confer a protective effect, and a high HDL-C: total cholesterol ratio indicates low risk. An inverse relationship between HDL-C and LDL-C is frequently observed. In addition, the subfraction HDL_2-C of HDL-C has recently been shown to be the specific component responsible for this protective role, while HDL_3-C is associated with atherogenesis. Although hypertriglycer-idaemia itself is less clearly associated with increased risk of coronary arterial disease, very high levels of chylo-microns and VLDL-C are associated with recurrent pancreatitis.

Classification of dyslipoproteinaemia

Hyperlipidaemia may be defined as an elevation of cholesterol or triglyceride or both. The elucidation of the complex mechanism of lipid transport and metab-olism, however, has allowed the recognition of the im-portant roles played by apoproteins in the pathogenesis of disorders of lipid metabolism. Hyperlipoprotein-aemia (dyslipoproteinaemia) is defined as an abnor-mality involving either the lipids or lipoproteins or both.

There are five types of hyperlipoproteinaemia accord-ing to the World Health Organization classification. Type I is characterized by gross hypertriglyceridaemia and hyperchylomicronaemia due to a deficiency of lipo-protein lipase or apo C-II, which activates lipoprotein lipase; pancreatitis is a well-recognized complication. Types IIa and IIb (familial hypercholesterolaemia) are characterized by elevation of LDL-C, and represent a result of defective cholesterol metabolism. In about five per cent of patients, defective expression or reduced activity of tissue apo B receptor for LDL, due to a genetic defect, has been identified. Patients with Type II hyperlipoproteinaemia are at increased risk of ischaemic heart disease. Type III is an uncommon disorder due to a defective catabolism of remnants of chylomicrons and VLDL resulting from an abnormality of apo E. LDL is characteristically depressed with abnormally high concentrations of VLDL remnants (IDL). These subjects are also at increased risk of arteriosclerosis. Types IV and V are due to defects in either the production or catabolism of VLDL, resulting in hypertriglyceridaemia with marked increase in VLDL and decrease in LDL and HDL. Some of these patients may have familial lipoprotein lipase deficiency, as with Type I; recurrent attacks of acute pancreatitis are a known complication of this form of dyslipoproteinaemia.

Although dyslipoproteinaemia can be genetically acquired, a large proportion is related to dietary intake. In addition, it may accompany disease states such as the nephrotic syndrome, diabetes mellitus, and hypothyroidism. Drugs that alter the synthesis or clearance of apolipoproteins by actions on different enzymes may result in abnormal lipid metabolism. Such adverse effects can be particularly important in the presence of a pre-existing dyslipoproteinaemic state.

Drugs affecting lipid metabolism

Diuretics

Thiazides and related diuretics have been known to increase serum lipids significantly. Although most studies have demonstrated significant increases in total cholesterol (range 4–13 per cent), total triglyceride (range 14–37 per cent), LDL-C (range 7–29 per cent), and VLDL-C (7–56 per cent) in response to thiazides, the response is variable both between individuals and within individuals over time (Ames 1986a). Two large multicentre studies have examined lipids in patients treated with antihypertensive drugs for 1 to 4 years. Materson and others (1993) showed similar initial rises in total cholesterol between patients treated with thiazides and patients treated with other drugs. Neaton and others (1993) showed that after 4 years of treatment, there was an increase in HDL-C and decrease in triglycerides. These results suggest that initial unfavourable lipid changes may be transient. Later beneficial changes were quantitatively similar to those seen with ACE inhibitors

and calcium-channel-blocking agents. Treatment with indapamide has also been reported recently to result in favourable elevations in HDL-C and an increase in apoprotein A-I and A-II lipoprotein fractions (Ames 1996).

The pathogenesis of diuretic-induced dyslipoproteinaemia is largely unknown. Again, Ames discussed the possible mechanisms in his review (1986a). Potassium-sparing diuretics have been reported to have no effect on lipid metabolism (Ames and Hill 1978; Amery et al. 1982), although a change of diuretic therapy to potassium-sparing agents failed to improve existing lipid abnormalities (Ames and Peacock 1984). Dyslipoproteinaemia does not seem to occur in premenopausal women taking thiazides, which suggests a protective hormonal effect on lipid metabolism changes associated with thiazide therapy (Boehringer et al. 1982). Glycosylation of lipoproteins may provide a link between disturbances of lipid metabolism secondary to thiazide therapy, and possibly other drugs such as β-adrenoceptor-blocking agents, which may worsen glucose tolerance.

β-Adrenoceptor-blocking agents

There is evidence that non-cardioselective β-adrenoceptor blocking agents (e.g. propranolol) have adverse effects on lipid metabolism, resulting in increased serum triglyceride and decreased HDL-C levels (Gemma et al. 1982; Otero et al. 1983; Lehren 1987). However, cardioselective β-adrenoceptor-blocking agents, especially those with intrinsic sympathomimetic activity (ISA) (e.g. pindolol and acebutolol) and those with combined α and β activity (e.g. labetalol) appear to have no adverse effect on lipid metabolism (Fogari et al. 1989). Newer agents such as celiprolol, with cardioselectivity and ISA, appear to have favourable effects with decreases in total cholesterol and triglyceride. Durrington and colleagues (1985) reported a reduction in the cardioprotective HDL_2 subfraction of cholesterol, which is most apparent in patients treated with propranolol and atenolol. In patients with pre-existing hypertriglyceridaemia, there was reduced clearance of triglycerides. This was not found in normolipidaemic patients, or in patients treated with β-adrenoceptor-blocking agents with ISA. Increased hepatic synthesis of VLDL is the major determinant of the concentration of triglycerides. Hence, reduced hepatic production secondary to β-blockade may minimize the adverse effect on triglyceride clearance, which becomes apparent only with pre-existing hypertriglyceridaemia.

Durrington and Cairns (1982) first reported cases of acute pancreatitis and massive hypertriglyceridaemia associated with the use of metoprolol and atenolol therapy. They suggested that this was a result of reduced clearance of triglycerides due to unopposed α-adrenergic stimulation which reduced lipoprotein lipase activity. Since then, there have been further reports of acute pancreatitis and hypertriglyceridaemia in patients treated with atenolol (Haitas *et al.* 1988) or nadolol (O'Donoghue 1989). In some cases, genetic predisposition and alcoholism are probable contributory factors.

Other antihypertensive agents

Lehren (1987) and Ames (1986*b*) reviewed the effects of α-adrenergic-blocking agents and concluded that most studies have shown prazosin to have a favourable effect on lipid metabolism, with a reduction in triglyceride, cholesterol, and LDL-C, and elevation of HDL-C. In his extensive review, Ames (1986*b*) examined the effects of other antihypertensive agents on lipid metabolism. The few studies on calcium-channel-blocking agents suggested either a neutral or favourable effect, while only limited information was available on centrally acting drugs. Methyldopa has been associated with an unfavourable reduction in the ratio of HDL-C to total cholesterol, although this is not conclusive. Clonidine appears to have neutral effects on lipid profile. Angiotensin-converting-enzyme inhibitors do not appear to be associated with adverse effects on lipid metabolism, and some drugs, such as cilazapril, may even show beneficial effects (Pollare *et al.* 1989; De Cesaris 1993; Shionoiri *et al.* 1994) although more (and longer) studies are required.

Corticosteroids and immunosuppressive drugs

Ibels and others (1975) reported that Type IV dyslipoproteinaemia with hypertriglyceridaemia was common among uraemic and dialysis patients. Their serum cholesterol levels were often normal although very variable. Following transplantation, however, hypercholesterolaemia was found more commonly in these patients than in uraemic or dialysis patients, and the pattern of dyslipoproteinaemia was more variable, with Types IIa, IIb, and IV occurring equally frequently, suggesting a multifactorial aetiology attributable to obesity, prednisone therapy, and degree of residual uraemia. Transplant patients who were receiving prednisone and azathioprine had a significantly higher incidence of coronary arterial disease than uraemic patients and patients on haemodialysis. This was thought to be related to the hyperlipidaemic properties of the corticosteroids used for immunosuppression (Ibels *et al.* 1977).

The dyslipoproteinaemia associated with corticosteroid therapy includes elevations of triglycerides, cholesterol, VLDL-C, and LDL-C. This is often, though not always, accompanied by a low level of HDL-C. Although Jefferys and colleagues (1980) observed a lower level of HDL-C in females treated with corticosteroids, this sex difference was not found in corticosteroid-treated patients after renal transplantation (Ettinger *et al.* 1987*a*).

The pathogenesis of dyslipoproteinaemia associated with corticosteroid therapy is currently being investigated and appears multifactorial. Taskinen (1987) reported a correlation between plasma concentration of VLDL-C and HDL-C and enzymatic activities of lipoprotein lipase in both healthy subjects and patients with abnormal lipoprotein metabolism. Reduction of activity of lipoprotein lipase with impaired catabolism of VLDL-C following corticosteroid therapy has been demonstrated in *in vitro* studies (Krause *et al.* 1981). This abnormality was not found, however, in patients with systemic lupus erythematosus treated with corticosteroids (Ettinger and Hazzard 1988). The hyperinsulinaemic state associated with corticosteroid therapy can increase hepatic production of VLDL and HDL and impair receptor uptake of LDL particles (Henze *et al.* 1983; Hirsch and Mazzone 1986). Ettinger and Hazzard (1988) reported an elevation of plasma apo B in patients with systemic lupus erythematosus treated with corticosteroids, which might explain the increased synthesis of VLDL apo B. Patients with coronary arterial disease have been reported to have significantly lower Apo A-I and Apo-II and elevated Apo B with hypertriglyceridaemia, which are considered to be independent risk factors for arteriosclerosis (Kukita *et al.* 1985).

The effect of corticosteroids on HDL-C is less well known. Ettinger and co-workers (1987*b*) reported a lack of correlation between the change in cholesterol level and that of HDL-C. Irrespective of the absolute HDL-C level, abnormalities of the subfractions of HDL-C are probably of more importance. Jung and others (1982) reported an abnormal composition of HDL-C with increased apo A:HDL-C ratio and decreased apo A:HDL-triglyceride ratio that may impair the transport of cholesterol. Ettinger and colleagues (1987*a,b*) reported an increase in HDL$_3$-C and decrease in the cardioprotective HDL$_2$-C subfraction in patients treated with corticosteroids following renal transplantation and for systemic lupus erythematosus. The adverse effects of corticosteroids on lipid metabolism appear to be dose related. Significantly higher levels of triglyceride and cholesterol were found in post-renal-transplant patients who required methylprednisolone (Ibels *et al.* 1975). A positive correlation between the prednisone dosage and severity of hyperlipidaemia has been observed (Ibels *et al.* 1978; Ponticelli *et al.* 1978; Cattran *et al.* 1979; Ettinger *et al.* 1987*b,c*) but this was ameliorated by the administration of an alternate day regimen (Cattran *et al.* 1979; Curtis 1982; Ettinger *et al.* 1987a).

Transient hyperlipidaemia has also been reported during cyclosporin therapy (Steinherz 1994). In contrast, patients treated with aldesleukin, a human recombinant interleukin-2 product, showed reversible hypocholesterolaemia and increased remnant proteins. The clinical significance of these effects remain unclear (Wilson *et al.* 1989). Severe hypertriglyceridaemia and decreased HDL-C have been reported following the use of α-interferon (Olsen *et al.* 1988). Didanosine, an antiviral agent, has been reported to increase circulating triglyceride in one-third of patients (Yarchoan *et al.* 1990).

Oral contraceptives and other sex hormones

The Framingham Study (Castelli 1984) has shown that women under the age of 40 have a lower risk of arteriosclerosis. This was thought due to a protective effect of higher levels of HDL-C in females. With increasing age, the risk parallels that of males, with increasing levels of total and LDL-C. The Lipid Research Clinics Program Prevalence Study (LaRosa *et al.* 1986) showed a 30 per cent prevalence of dyslipoproteinaemia in women using gonadal hormones, compared with women who were non-users, although the HDL-C:LDL-C ratio was more favourable in the users. With increasing identification and understanding of the nature of various subfractions of HDL-C, interpretation of HDL-C becomes incomplete without analysis of these subfractions. It has been suggested that the HDL_2-C subfraction confers protection against arteriosclerosis, while HDL_3-C is associated with increased risk of coronary arterial disease (Ballantyne *et al.* 1982; Brensike *et al.* 1984; Levy *et al.* 1984).

Oestrogen and progestogen components of oral contraceptive steroids and postmenopausal replacement therapy have opposing effects on lipid metabolism. Oestrogens increase hepatic production of VLDL-C and HDL-C, reduce activity of lipoprotein lipase, and increase HDL-C and HDL_2 subfractions, while progestogens have opposite effects (Wahl *et al.* 1983; Knopp 1986). Hence, adverse effects on lipid metabolism are dependent on the relative potency and composition of the progestogen in the formulation. Miccoli and others (1989) compared the effects of three conventional formulations of low-dose oral contraceptives (two monophasic and one triphasic) on lipid and glucose metabolism. Plasma glucose remained unchanged, while triglycerides increased in all three groups of patients; total and LDL-C were unaffected. HDL-C was increased in the women taking the two monophasic formulations. The overall effect, however, was negligible. In another

study, by Notelovitz and colleagues (1989), the effects of triphasic and monophasic pills on plasma lipid and lipoproteins were studied. Similar effects were seen in both groups: total, LDL-C, and HDL_3-C, apolipoproteins A-I and B, and triglyceride increased while HDL-C and HDL_2-C decreased. The changes were mild, however, and the authors concluded that they were unlikely to be of clinical significance.

Knopp (1986), in his review of the subject, concluded that the risk of arteriosclerosis and myocardial infarction in young women using oral contraceptive steroids is associated with increasing progestogen dose. Oestrogen therapy elevates HDL-C and HDL_2-C and confers a protective effect against myocardial infarction in postmenopausal women. The addition of a progestogen, however, may have a deleterious effect on lipoprotein metabolism, cancelling any benefit associated with oestrogen. Further long-term, detailed, prospective studies are required to characterize the effects of oral contraceptives on lipid metabolism and arteriosclerosis fully. Until such time, lipid profiles should be taken regularly in women who are contemplating the use of oral contraceptives, particularly in the presence of other risk factors, and their use is perhaps best avoided in patients with known dyslipoproteinaemic disorders.

Although oestrogen therapy selectively inhibits hepatic triglyceride lipase activity, the effect is only mild and rarely leads to clinically significant hypertriglyceridaemia (Applebaum *et al.* 1977). In patients with familial hyperlipidaemia, however, reduced clearance of plasma triglyceride secondary to oestrogen therapy has been reported to cause acute pancreatitis due to massive hypertriglyceridaemia (Glueck *et al.* 1972; Davidoff *et al.* 1973; Stuyt *et al.* 1986).

Androgenic steroids, in particular anabolic steroids, can lower HDL-C. Mechanisms probably include impaired triglyceride clearance by lipoprotein lipase and accelerated HDL metabolism. Danazol and buserelin (a synthetic gonadotropin-releasing-hormone agonist), can increase LDL-C and danazol may also decrease HDL-C (Dlugi 1988; Brogden 1990).

Tamoxifen

Tamoxifen, a non-steroidal oestrogen antagonist, is frequently used as adjuvant therapy for breast carcinoma. Rossner and Wallgren (1984) observed small changes in both lipid and lipoprotein concentrations following tamoxifen therapy. Concentrations of triglycerides and VLDL triglyceride both increased, while total cholesterol and LDL-C fell. This was accompanied by a reduction of orosomucoid and haptoglobin concentrations, and implied an oestrogen-like effect of tamoxifen on protein and lipoprotein metabolism. Brun and others (1986) reported a case of severe lipidaemia induced by tamoxifen with high plasma triglyceride, VLDL-C, and VLDL-apo B concentrations, and low levels of LDL-C and LDL-apo B. They demonstrated a reduction in the activities of lipoprotein ipase and hepatic triglyceride lipase, which impeded the conversion of VLDL-C to LDL-C. A fatal case of acute pancreatitis following tamoxifen has also been reported (Noguchi *et al.* 1987).

Ethanol

Chait and Brunzell (1990) reviewed the effects of alcohol intake on lipid metabolism. Alcohol increases HDL-C but appears to have little effect on LDL-C. Elevations of both HDL_3-C and HDL_2-C have been demonstrated. Dyslipoproteinaemia can also result from alcoholic liver disease. Ethanol competes with fatty acids in the liver for oxidation. The fatty acids are otherwise incorporated into triglycerides leading to an increased hepatic synthesis of VLDL. The increased production of VLDL particles is usually compensated for by increased clearance via the lipoprotein lipase system. If the secretion of VLDL is impaired, however, as in the case of liver disease or in the presence of pre-existing dyslipoproteinaemia, small increases in VLDL production may saturate the removal system, resulting in significant hypertriglyceridaemia and hyperchylomicronaemia.

Anticonvulsants

HDL-C and apolipoproteins have been reported to be elevated in epileptic children receiving carbamazepine, phenobarbitone, and valproic acid. These changes were independent of dosage and duration of treatment (Calandre *et al.* 1991). Phenytoin has been shown to increase triglycerides and HDL-C level, probably by increasing apo A, although the exact mechanism remains uncertain.

Other drugs

Dose-related increases in total cholesterol, triglycerides, and LDL-C, and decreases in HDL-C, are associated with the use of retinoids (isotretinoin and etretinate). These adverse effects are seen particularly in predisposed subjects such as diabetic patients, alcoholics, obese subjects, or those with a positive family history of hyperlipidaemia. These abnormalities usually resolve upon discontinuation of therapy (Chait and Brunzell 1990; Kurie *et al.* 1996). Ritonavir, a protease inhibitor used in the treatment of HIV infection, is reported to cause significant increases in circulating total cholesterol

and triglyceride (Markowitz 1995). Amiodarone has been reported to cause hypertriglyceridaemia but the pattern of the lipoproteins was not examined in detail (Lakhadar *et al.* 1988). Itraconazole treatment is associated with hypertriglyceridaemia (Tucker 1991) while ketoconazole causes transient hypercholesterolaemia (Rosenblatt 1980) and hypertriglyceridaemia (Rollman 1985).

References

Abu-Shakra, M. and Lee, P. (1994). Hypoglycemia: an unusual adverse reaction to chloroquine. *Clin. Exp. Rheumatol.* 12, 95.

Adam, K., Ou, C.N., and Cotton, D.B. (1993). Combined effect of terbutaline and betamethasone on glucose homeostasis in preterm labor. *Fetal Diagn. Ther.* 8, 187.

Ahmad, S. (1991). Gemfibrozil: interaction with glyburide. *South. Med. J.* 84, 102.

Ahmad, S. (1992). Nicardipine-induced hyperglycemia. *Am. Fam. Physician* 45, 449.

Albrecht H., Stellbrink H.J., and Arastec K. (1993). Didanosine-induced disorders of glucose tolerance. *Ann. Intern. Med.* 119, 1050.

Almirall, J., Montoliu, J., Torras, A., *et al.* (1989). Propoxyphene induced hypoglycaemia in a patient with chronic renal failure. *Nephron* 53, 273.

al-Rubeaan, K. and Ryan, E.A. (1991). Phenytoin-induced insulin insensitivity. *Diabetic Med.* 8, 968.

Amar, D., Shamoon, H., Lazar, E.J., *et al.* (1993). Acute hyperglycaemic effect of anaesthetic induction with thiopentone. *Acta Anaesthesiol. Scand.* 37, 571.

Amery, A., Birkenhager, W., Bulpitt, C.P., *et al.* (1982). Influence of antihypertensive therapy on serum cholesterol in elderly hypertensive patients. *Acta Cardiologica* 37, 235.

Ames, R.P. (1986a). The effects of antihypertensive drugs on serum lipids and lipoproteins. I. Diuretics. *Drugs* 32, 260.

Ames, R.P. (1986b). The effects of antihypertensive drugs on serum lipids and lipoproteins. II. Non diuretic drugs. *Drugs* 32, 335.

Ames R.P. (1996). A comparison of blood lipid and blood pressure responses during the treatment of systemic hypertension with indapamide and with thiazides. *Am. J. Cardiol.* 77, 12B.

Ames, R.P. and Hill, P. (1978). Raised serum lipid concentrations during diuretic treatment of hypertension: a study of predictive indexes. *Clin. Sci. Mol. Med.* 55 (Suppl. 4), 311S.

Ames, R.P. and Peacock, P. (1984). Serum cholesterol during treatment of hypertension with diuretic drugs. *Arch. Intern. Med.* 144, 710.

Angelo-Nielson K. (1980). Timolol topically and diabetes mellitus. *JAMA* 244, 2263.

Applebaum, D.M., Goldberg, A.P., Pykalisto, O.J., *et al.* (1977). Effect of estrogen on post-heparin lipolytic activity:

Selective decline in hepatic triglyceride lipase. *J. Clin. Invest.* 59, 601.

Arem R. (1989). Hypoglycemia associated with renal failure. *Endocrinol. Metab. Clin. North Am.* 18, 103.

Arky, R.A. (1989). Hypoglycaemia associated with liver disease and ethanol. *Endocrinol. Metab. Clin. North Am.* 18, 75.

Arneson, G.A. (1964). Phenothiazine derivatives and glucose metabolism. *J. Neuropsychiatry* 5, 181.

Asplund, K., Wiholm, B.E., and Lundman, B. (1991). Severe hypoglycaemia during treatment with glipizide. *Diabetic Med.* 8, 726.

Assan, R., Perronne, C., Chotard, L., *et al.* (1995a). Mefloquine-associated hypoglycaemia in a cachectic AIDS patient. *Diabète Métab.* 21, 54.

Assan, R., Perronne, C., Assan, D., *et al.* (1995b). Pentamidine-induced derangements of glucose homeostasis. Determinant roles of renal failure and drug accumulation. A study of 128 patients. *Diabetes Care* 18, 47.

Avogaro, A., Beltramello, P., Gnudi, L., *et al.* (1993). Alcohol intake impairs glucose counterregulation during acute insulin-induced hypoglycemia in IDDM patients. Evidence for a critical role of free fatty acids. *Diabetes* 42, 1626.

Axelrod, J. and Reisine, T.D. (1984). Stress hormones: Their interaction and regulation. *Science* 224, 452.

Bailey, C.J. (1992). Hypoglycaemic, antihyperglycaemic and antidiabetic drugs. *Diabetic Med.* 9, 482.

Ballantyne, F.C., Clark, F.S., Simpson, H.S., *et al.* (1982). High density and low density lipoprotein subfractions in survivors of myocardial infarction and in control subjects. *Metabolism* 31, 433.

Bamber, M.G. and Redpath, A. (1987). Chloroquine and hypoglycaemia. *Lancet* i, 1211.

Belehu, A. and Naafs, B. (1982). Diabetes mellitus associated with pentamidine mesylate. *Lancet* i, 1463.

Bendtson, I. and Binder, C. (1991). Counterregulatory hormonal response to insulin-induced hypoglycaemia in insulin-dependent diabetic patients: a comparison of equimolar amounts of porcine and semisynthetic human insulin. *J. Intern. Med.* 229, 293.

Bengtsson, C., Blohme, G., Lapidus, L., *et al.* (1992). Diabetes incidence in users and non-users of antihypertensive drugs in relation to serum insulin, glucose tolerance and degree of adiposity: a 12-year prospective population study of women in Gothenburg, Sweden. *J. Intern. Med.* 231, 583.

Bengtsson, B.A., Eden, S., Lonn, L., *et al.* (1993). Treatment of adults with growth hormone (GH) deficiency with recombinant human GH. *J. Clin. Endocrinol. Metab.* 76, 309.

Berger, W., Caduff, F., Pasquel, M., *et al.* (1986). The relatively frequent incidence of severe sulfonylurea-induced hypoglycaemia in the last 25 years in Switzerland. Results of 2 surveys in Switzerland in 1969 and 1984. *Schweiz. Med. Wochenschr.* 116, 45.

Berman, J.D., Cook, D.M., Buchman, M., *et al.* (1990). Diminished adrenocorticotropin response to insulin-induced hypoglycemia in nondepressed, actively drinking male alcoholics. *J. Clin. Endocrinol. Metab.* 71, 712.

Bichel, T., Canivet, J.L., Damas, P., *et al.* (1994). Malignant hyperthermia and severe hypoglycemia after reexposure to halothane. *Acta Anaesthesiol. Belg.* 45, 23.

Binder, C. and Bendtson, I. (1992). Endocrine emergencies. Hypoglycaemia. *Baillière's Clin. Endocrinol. Metab.* 6, 23.

Björntorp, P. (1994). Fatty acids, hyperinsulinemia, and insulin resistance: which comes first? *Curr. Opin. Lipidol.* 5, 166.

Blanco-Coronado, J.L., Repetto, M., Ginestal, R., *et al.* (1992). Acute intoxication by endosulfan. *J. Toxicol. Clin. Toxicol.* 30, 575.

Boehringer, K., Weidmann, P., Mordasini, R., *et al.* (1982). Menopause-dependent plasma lipoprotein alterations in diuretic treated women. *Ann. Intern. Med.* 91, 206.

Bottino, J.C. and Tashima, C.K. (1976). Medroxyprogesterone acetate and diabetes mellitus *Ann. Intern. Med.* 84, 341.

Bouchard, P., Sai, P., Reach, G., *et al.* (1982). Diabetes mellitus following pentamidine-induced hypoglycaemia in humans. *Diabetes* 31, 40.

Bouvet, E., Casalino, E., Prevost, M.H., *et al.* (1990). Fatal case of 2,3-dideoxyinosine-associated pancreatitis. *Lancet*, 336, 1515.

Boyle, P.J., Justice, K., Krentz, A., *et al.* (1993). Octreotide reverses hyperinsulinemia and prevents hypoglycemia induced by sulfonylurea overdoses. *J. Clin. Endocrinol. Metab.* 76, 752.

Bratusch-Marrain, P.R., Vierhapper, H., Komjati, M., *et al.* (1985). Acetyl-salicylic acid impairs insulin-mediated glucose utilization and reduces insulin clearance in healthy and non-insulin-dependent diabetic man. *Diabetologia* 28, 671.

Brazy, J.E. and Pupkin, M.J. (1979). Effects of maternal isoxsuprine administration on preterm infants. *J. Pediatr.* 94, 444.

Brensike, J.F., Levy, R.I., Kelsey, S.F., *et al.* (1984). Effects of therapy with cholestyramine on progression of coronary arteriosclerosis: Results of the NHLBI Type II Coronary Intervention Study. *Circulation* 69, 313.

Brogden, R.N., Buckley, M.M.T., Ward, A. (1990). Buserelin. A review of its pharmacodynamic and pharmacokinetic properties and clinical profile. *Drugs* 39, 399.

Brun, L.D., Gage, C., Rousseau, C., *et al.* (1986). Severe lipemia induced by tamoxifen. *Cancer* 57, 2123.

Brunner, J.E., Kruger, D.F., Basha, M.A., *et al.* (1989). Hypoglycemia after administration of somatostatin analog (SMS 201-995) in metastatic carcinoid. *Henry Ford Hosp. Med. J.* 37, 60.

Bruno, A., Carucci, P., Cassader, M., *et al.* (1994). Serum glucose, insulin and C-peptide response to oral glucose after intravenous administration of hydrocortisone and methylprednisolone in man. *Eur. J. Clin. Pharmacol.*, 46, 411.

Buckle, R.M. and Guillebaud, J. (1967). Hypoglycaemic coma occurring during treatment with chlorpromazine and orphenadrine. *BMJ* iv, 599.

Cacoub, P., Deray, G., Baumelou, A., *et al.* (1989). Disopyramide-induced hypoglycaemia: case report and review of the literature. *Fundam. Clin. Pharmacol.* 3, 527.

Calandre, E.P., Rodriquez-Lopez C., Blazquez A., *et al.* (1991). Serum lipids, lipoproteins and apolipoproteins A and B in epileptic patients treated with valproic acid, carbamazepine or phenobarbital. *Acta Neurol. Scand.* 83, 250.

Caldwell, G., Scougall, I., Boddy, K., *et al.* (1987). Fasting hyperinsulinemic hypoglycaemia after ritodrine therapy for premature labor. *Obstet. Gynaecol.* 70, 478.

Campbell, I.W. (1985). Metformin and the sulphonylureas: the comparative risk. *Horm. Metab. Res. Suppl.* 15, 105.

Caprio, S., Napoli, R., Sacca, L., *et al.* (1992). Impaired stimulation of gluconeogenesis during prolonged hypoglycemia in intensively treated insulin-dependent diabetic subjects. *J. Clin. Endocrinol. Metab.* 75, 1076.

Castelli, W.P. (1984). Epidemiology of coronary heart disease: The Framingham study. *Am. J. Med.* 76 (Suppl. 2A), 4.

Cattran, D.C., Steiner, G., Wilson, D.R., *et al.* (1979). Hyperlipidemia after renal transplantation: natural history and pathophysiology. *Ann. Intern. Med.* 91, 554.

Cerqueti, P.M., Sacca, S.C., Allegri, P., *et al.* . (1993). Deflazacort in the treatment of uveitis: a comparative study versus prednisone. *Allergol. Immunopathol.* (Madrid), 21, 107.

Cetin, M., Yetgin, S., Kara, A., *et al.* (1994). Hyperglycemia, ketoacidosis and other complications of L-asparaginase in children with acute lymphoblastic leukemia. *J. Med.* 25, 219.

Chait, A. and Brunzell, J.D. (1990). Acquired hyperlipidemia (secondary dyslipoproteinemias). *Endocrinol. Metab. Clin. North Am.* 2, 259.

Chan, J.C.N. and Cockram, C.S. (1991). Drug-induced disturbances of carbohydrate metabolism. *Adverse Drug React. Toxicol. Rev.* 10, 1.

Chan, J.C.N., Yeung, V.T.F., Leung, D.H.Y., *et al.* (1994). The effects of enalapril and nifedipine on carbohydrate and lipid metabolism, in NIDDM. *Diabetes Care* 17, 859.

Chan, J.C.N., Cockram, C.S., and Critchley, J.A.J. (1996). Drug-induced disorders of glucose metabolism: mechanisms and management. *Drug Saf.* 15, 135.

Chan, T.Y.K., Chan, J.C.N., and Critchley, J.A.J. (1992a). Severe hypoglycaemia in Chinese patients with non-insulin-dependent diabetes treated with insulin or sulphonylureas. *Pharmacoepidemiol. Drug Saf.* 1, 207.

Chan, T.Y.K., Chan, J.C.N., Tomlinson, B., *et al.* (1992b). Adverse reactions to drugs as a cause of admission to a general teaching hospital in Hong Kong. *Drug Saf.* 7, 235.

Chan, T.Y.K., Chan, J.C.N., Choi, S.S., *et al.* (1994). Recurrent glibenclamide-induced hypoglycemia: the importance of obtaining a comprehensive medication history. *Ann. Pharmacother.* 28, 119.

Christiansen, C., Thomsen, C., Rasmussen, O., *et al.* (1993). Acute effects of graded alcohol intake on glucose, insulin and free fatty acid levels in non-insulin-dependent diabetic subjects. *Eur. J. Clin. Nutr.* 47, 648.

Colagiuri, S., Miller, J.J., and Petocz, P. (1992). Double-blind crossover comparison of human and porcine insulins in patients reporting lack of hypoglycaemia awareness. *Lancet* 339, 1432.

Coyle, P., Carr, A.D., Depczynski, B.B., *et al.* (1996). Diabetes mellitus associated with pentamidine use in HIV-infected patients. *Med. J. Aust.*, 165, 587.

Craig, J., Abu-Saleh, M., Smith, B., *et al.* (1977). Diabetes mellitus in patients on lithium. *Lancet* ii, 1028.

Cranston, I., Lomas, J., Maran, A., *et al.* (1994). Restoration of hypoglycaemia awareness in patients with long duration insulin-dependent diabetes. *Lancet* 344, 283.

Critchley, J.A.J., Ellis, P., Henderson, C.G., *et al.* (1982). The role of the pituitary adrenocortical axis in reflex responses of the adrenal medulla. *J. Physiol.* 323, 533.

Critchley, J.A.J., Proudfoot, A.T., Boyd, S.G., *et al.* (1984). Deaths and paradoxes after intentional insulin overdosage. *BMJ* 289, 225.

Critchley, J.A.J., MacLean, M.R., and Ungar, A. (1988). Inhibitory regulation by co-released peptides of catecholamine secretion by the canine adrenal medulla. *Br. J. Pharmacol.* 93, 383.

Croxson, M.S., Shaw, D.W., Henley, P.G., *et al.* (1987). Disopyramide-induced hypoglycaemia and increased serum insulin. *N.Z. Med. J.* 100, 407.

Cryer, P.E. (1994). Banting Lecture. Hypoglycemia: the limiting factor in the management of IDDM. *Diabetes* 43, 1378.

Cryer, P.E., Fisher, J.N., and Shamoon, H. (1994). Hypoglycaemia. *Diabetes Care* 17, 734.

Curtis, J., Horrigan, F., and Ahearn, D. (1972). Chlorthalidone-induced hyperosmolar hyperglycaemic non-ketotic coma. *JAMA* 220, 1592.

Curtis, J.J., Galla, J.H., Woodward, S.Y., *et al.* (1982). Effect of alternate day prednisone on plasma lipids in renal transplant recipients. *Kidney Int.* 22, 42.

Dagogo, J.S., Rattarasam, C., and Cryer, P.E. (1994). Reversal of hypoglycemia unawareness, but not defective glucose counterregulation, in IDDM. *Diabetes* 43, 1426.

Davidoff, F., Tishler, S., and Rosoff, C. (1973). Marked hyperlipidemia and pancreatitis associated with contraceptive therapy. *N. Engl. J. Med.* 289, 552.

Davidson, D.G.D. and Eastham, W.N. (1966). Acute liver necrosis following overdose of paracetamol. *BMJ* ii, 497.

Davis, M., Mellman M., Friedman S., *et al.* (1994). Recovery of epinephrine response but not hypoglycemic symptom threshold after intensive therapy in type 1 diabetes. *Am. J. Med.* 97, 535.

Dawson, K.P., Penna, A.C., and Manglick, P. (1995). Acute asthma, salbutamol and hyperglycaemia. *Acta Paediatr.* 84, 305.

DCCTRG (Diabetes Control and Complications Trial Research Group). (1991). Epidemiology of severe hypoglycemia in the diabetes control and complications trial. *Am. J. Med.* 90, 450.

DCCTRG (Diabetes Control and Complications Trial Research Group) (1993). The effect of intensive treatment of diabetes on the development and progression of long-term complications in insulin-dependent diabetes mellitus. *N. Engl. J. Med.* 329, 977.

DCCTRG (Diabetes Control and Complications Trial Research Group) (1995). Adverse events and their association with treatment regimens in the diabetes control and complications trial. *Diabetes Care* 18, 1415.

De Boer, H., Blok, G-J., and Van der Veen, E.A. (1995). Clinical aspects of growth hormone deficiency in adults. *Endocr. Rev.* 16, 63.

De Cesaris, R., Ranieri, G., Filitte, V., *et al.* (1993). Glucose and lipid metabolism in essential hypertension: Effects of diuretics and ACE-inhibitors. *Cardiology* 83, 165.

DeFronzo, R. (1988). Lilly Lecture 1987. The triumvirate: B-cell, muscle, liver: a collusion responsible for NIDDM. *Diabetes* 37, 667.

DeFronzo, R.A. and Ferrannini, E. (1991). Insulin resistance. A multifaceted syndrome responsible for NIDDM, obesity, hypertension, dyslipidemia, and atherosclerotic cardiovascular disease. *Diabetes Care* 14, 173.

De Mattia, G., Ferri, C., Cassone-Faldetta, M., *et al.* (1996). Circulating catecholamines and metabolic effects of captopril in NIDDM patients. *Diabetes Care* 19, 226.

De Pirro, R., Forte, F., Bertoli, A., *et al.* (1981). Changes in insulin receptors during oral contraception. *J. Clin. Endocrinol. Metab.* 52, 29.

Dickson, I. (1962). Glycosuria and diabetes following INAH therapy. *Med. J. Aust.* i, 325.

Diwan, P.V., Sastry, M.S., and Satyanarayana, N.V. (1992). Potentiation of hypoglycemic response of glibenclamide by piroxicam in rats and humans. *Indian J. Exp. Biol.* 30, 317.

Dixon, R., Gourzis, J., McDermott, D., *et al.* (1991). AICA-riboside: safety, tolerance, and pharmacokinetics of a novel adenosine-regulating agent. *J. Clin. Pharmacol.* 31, 342.

Dlugi, A.M., Rafo S., D'Amico, J.F., *et al.* (1988). A comparison of the effects of buserelin versus danazol on plasma lipoproteins during treatment of pelvic endometriosis. *Fertil. Steril.* 49, 913.

Donnelly, R. and Morris, A.D. (1994). Drugs and insulin resistance: clinical methods of evaluation and new pharmacological approaches to metabolism. *Br. J. Clin. Pharmacol.* 37, 311.

Dornhorst, A., Powell, S.H., and Pensky, J. (1985). Aggravation by propranolol of hyperglycaemic effect of hydrochlorothiazide in type II diabetics without alteration of insulin secretion. *Lancet* i, 123.

Duffy, T.J. and Ray, R. (1984). Oral contraceptive use: Prospective follow-up of women with suspected glucose intolerance. *Contraception* 30, 197.

Durrington, P.N. and Cairns, S.A. (1982). Acute pancreatitis, a complication of beta-blockade. *BMJ* 284, 1016.

Durrington, P.N., Brownlee, W.C., and Large, D.M. (1985). Short term effects of beta-adrenoceptor blocking drugs with and without cardioselectivity and intrinsic sympathomimetic activity on lipoprotein metabolism in hypertriglyceridaemic patients and in normal men. *Clin. Sci.* 69, 713.

Dyer, J.R., Davis, T.M., Oiele, C., *et al.* (1994). The pharmacokinetics and pharmacodynamics of quinine in the diabetic and non-diabetic elderly. *Br. J. Clin. Pharmacol.*, 38, 205.

Egger, M., Smith, G.D., Imhoof, H., *et al.* (1991a). Risk of severe hypoglycaemia in insulin treated diabetic patients transferred to human insulin: a case control study. *BMJ* 303, 617.

Egger, M., Smith, G.D., Teuscher, A.U., *et al.* (1991 b). Influence of human insulin on symptoms and awareness of hypoglycaemia: a randomised double blind crossover trial. *BMJ* 303, 622.

Enyeart, J.L., Price, W.A., Hoffman, D.A., *et al.* (1983). Profound hyperglycemia and metabolic acidosis after verapamil overdose. *J. Am. Coll. Cardiol.* 2, 1228.

Eschwège, E., Fontbonne, A., Simon, D., *et al.* (1991). Oral contraceptives, insulin resistance and ischaemic vascular disease. *Int. J. Gynaecol. Obstet.* 31, 263.

Ettinger, W.H. Jr and Hazzard, W.R. (1988). Elevated apolipoprotein-B levels in corticosteroid-treated patients with systemic lupus erythematosus. *J. Clin. Endocrinol. Metab.* 67, 425.

Ettinger, W.H., Bender, W.L., Goldberg, A.P., *et al.* (1987a). Lipoprotein lipid abnormalities in healthy renal transplant recipients: persistence of low HDL$_2$ cholesterol. *Nephron* 47, 17.

Ettinger, W.H., Goldberg, A.P., Applebaum-Bowden, D., *et al.*. (1987b). Dyslipoproteinemia in systemic lupus erythematosus: effect of corticosteroids. *Am. J. Med.* 83, 503.

Ettinger, W.H., Klinefelter, H.K., and Kwiterovich, P.O. (1987c). Effect of short term, low dose prednisone on plasma lipids. *Atherosclerosis* 63, 167.

Everett, J. and Kerr D. (1994). Changing from porcine to human insulin. *Drugs* 47, 286.

Expert Committee on the Diagnosis and Classification of Diabetes Mellitus. (1997). Report. *Diabetes Care* 20, 1183.

Fanelli, C., Pampanelli, S., Epifano, L., *et al.* (1994). Long-term recovery from unawareness, deficient counterregulation and lack of cognitive dysfunction during hypoglycaemia, following institution of rational, intensive insulin therapy in IDDM. *Diabetologia* 37, 1265.

Fariss, B.L. and Lutcher, C.L. (1971). Diphenylhydantoin-induced hyperglycaemia and impaired insulin release: effect of dosage. *Diabetes* 20, 177.

Feely, J. and Peden, N. (1983). Enhanced sulfonlyurea-induced hypoglycaemia with cimetidine. *Br. J. Clin. Pharmacol.* 16, 607P.

Ferner, R.E. and Neil, H.A.W. (1988). Sulphonylureas and hypoglycaemia. *BMJ* 296, 949.

Ferrari, A., Pasqualetti, D., Del, B.P., *et al.* (1991). Prednisone versus deflazacort in the treatment of autoimmune thrombocytopenic purpura: evaluation of clinical response and immunological modifications. *Haematologica* 76, 342.

Ferrari, P., Rosman, J., and Weidmann, P. (1991). Antihypertensive agents, serum lipoproteins and glucose metabolism. *Am. J. Cardiol.* 67 , 26B.

Ferrer, J.P., Esmatjes, E., Gonzalez, C.J., *et al.* (1992). Symptomatic and hormonal hypoglycaemic responses to human and porcine insulin in patients with type I diabetes mellitus. *Diabetic Med.* 9, 522.

Ferriere, M., Lachkar, H., Richard, J., *et al.* (1985). Captopril and insulin sensitivity. *Ann. Intern. Med.* 102, 134.

Feuerstein, B.L., Lebowitz M.R., Blumenthal S.A., *et al.* (1992). Severe hyperkalemia in two patients with diabetes after cosyntropin administration. *J. Diabet. Complications* 6, 203.

Fogari, R., Zoppi A., Pasotti C., *et al.* (1989). Plasma lipids during chronic antihypertensive therapy with different beta-blockers. *J. Cardiovasc. Pharmacol.* 14 (Suppl. 7), S28.

Fonseca, V. and Phear, D.N. (1982). Hyperosmolar non-ketotic diabetic syndrome precipitated by treatment with diuretics. *BMJ* 284, 36.

Fraser, A.G. and Harrower, A.D.B. (1977). Convulsions and hyperglycaemia associated with nalidixic acid. *BMJ* ii, 1518.

Froesch, E.R., Zenobi, P.D., and Hussain, M. (1994). Metabolic and therapeutic effects of insulin-like growth factor 1. *Horm. Res.* 42, 66.

Gachot, B.A., Bezier, M., Cherrier, J.F., *et al.* (1988). Cibenzoline and hypoglycaemia. *Lancet* 2, 280.

Garg, S.K., Carmain, I.A., Brady K.C., *et al.* (1996). Pre-meal insulin analogue insulin lispro vs Humulin® insulin treatment in young subjects with Type I diabetes. *Diabetic Med.* 13, 47.

Gemma, G., Montanari, G., Suppa, G., *et al.* (1982). Plasma lipid and lipoprotein changes in hypertensive patients treated with propranolol and prazosin. *J. Cardiovasc. Pharmacol.* 4 (Suppl. 2), S233.

Georgakopoulos, K., Katsilambros, N., Fragaki, M., *et al.* (1990). Recovery from insulin-induced hypoglycemia after saccharose or glucose administration. *Clin. Physiol. Biochem.* 8, 267.

Gerich, J.E. (1989). Oral hypoglycemic agents. *N. Engl. J. Med.* 321, 1231.

Giugliano, D., Ceriello, A., di Pinto, P., *et al.* (1982). Impaired insulin secretion in human diabetes mellitus. The effect of naloxone-induced opiate receptor blockade. *Diabetes* 31, 367.

Giugliano, D., Ceriello, A., Saccomanno, F., *et al.* (1985). Effects of salicylate, tolbutamide, and prostaglandin E$_2$ on insulin responses to glucose in non-insulin-dependent diabetes mellitus. *J. Clin. Endocrinol. Metab.* 61, 160.

Gleuck, C.J., Scheel, D., Fishback, J., *et al.* (1972). Estrogen induced pancreatitis in patients with previous covert type V hyperlipoproteinemia. *Metabolism* 21, 657.

Goldberg, E.M. and Sanbar, S.S. (1969). Hyperglycaemic, nonketotic coma following administration of Dilantin (diphenylhydantoin). *Diabetes* 18, 101.

Greenwood, R.H. (1982). Hyperglycaemic effect of nifedipine. *BMJ* 284, 50.

Gündogdu, A.S., Brown, P.M., Juul, S., *et al.* (1979). Comparison of hormonal and metabolic effects of salbutamol infusion in normal subjects and insulin-requiring diabetics. *Lancet* ii, 1317.

Gunnarsson, R., Klintmalm, G., Lundgren, G., *et al.* (1983). Deterioration in glucose metabolism in pancreatic transplant recipients given cyclosporin. *Lancet* ii, 571.

Gurwitz, J.H., Bohn, R.L., Glynn, R.J., *et al.* (1993). Antihypertensive drug therapy and the initiation of treatment for diabetes mellitus. *Ann. Intern. Med.* 118, 273.

Gurwitz, J.H., Bohn, R.L., Glynn, R.J., *et al.* (1994). Glucocorticoids and the risk for initiation of hypoglycemic therapy. *Arch. Intern. Med.* 154, 97.

Hagley, M.T., Traeger, S.M., and Schuckman, H. (1994). Pronounced metabolic response to modest theophylline overdose. *Ann. Pharmacother.* 28, 195.

Haitas, B., Disler, L.J., Joffe, B.I., *et al.* (1988). Massive hypertriglyceridemia associated with atenolol. *Am. J. Med.* 85, 586.

Hall, S. (1982). Hyperosmolar non-ketotic diabetic syndrome precipitated by treatment with diuretics. *BMJ* 284, 665.

Harrower, A.D. (1994). Comparison of efficacy, secondary failure rate and complications of sulfonylureas. *J. Diabet. Complications* 8, 201.

Heine, R.J., van der Heyden, E.A., and van der Veen, E.A. (1989). Responses to human and porcine insulin in healthy subjects. *Lancet* 2, 946.

Helderman, J.H., Elahi, D., Andersen, D.K., *et al.* (1983). Prevention of the glucose tolerance of thiazide diuretics by maintenance of body potassium. *Diabetes* 32, 106.

Henze, K., Chait, A., Albers, J.J., *et al.* (1983). Hydrocortisone decreases the internalization of low density lipoprotein in cultured human fibroblasts and arterial smooth muscle cells. *Eur. J. Clin. Invest.* 13, 171.

Hepburn, D.A., Patrick, A.W., Eadington, D.W., *et al.* (1988). How common are changes in hypoglycaemic awareness after conversion from animal to human insulins? *Diabetic Med.* 5 (Suppl. 2), 7.

Hepburn, D.A., Patrick, A.W., Eadington, D.W., *et al.* (1990). Unawareness of hypoglycaemia in insulin-treated diabetic patients: prevalence and relationship to autonomic neuropathy. *Diabetic Med.* 7, 711.

Hepburn, D.A., Patrick, A.W., Brash, H.M., *et al.* (1991). Hypoglycaemia unawareness in type 1 diabetes: a lower plasma glucose is required to stimulate sympatho-adrenal activation. *Diabetic Med.* 8, 934.

Hepburn, D.A., MacLeod, K.M., Pelt, A.C., *et al.* (1993). Frequency and symptoms of hypoglycaemia experienced by patients with type 2 diabetes treated with insulin. *Diabetic Med.* 10, 231.

Herchline, T.E., Plouffe, J.F., and Para, M.F. (1991). Diabetes mellitus presenting with ketoacidosis following pentamidine therapy in patients with acquired immunodeficiency syndrome. *J. Infect.* 22, 41.

Herings, R.M.C., de Boer, A., Stricker, B.H.C., *et al.* (1995). Hypoglycaemia associated with use of inhibitors of angiotensin converting enzyme. *Lancet* 345, 1195.

Heyman, S.N. (1989). Verapamil intoxication and hyperglycaemia. *J. Emerg. Med.* 7, 407.

Hilleman, D.E., Mohiuddin, S.M., Ahmed, T.S., *et al.* (1987). Cibenzoline-induced hypoglycaemia. *Drug Intell. Clin. Pharm.* 21, 38.

Hirsch, L.J. and Mazzone, T. (1986). Dexamethasone-modulated lipoprotein metabolism in cultured human monocyte-derived macrophages: stimulation of scavenger receptor activity. *J. Clin. Invest.* 77, 485.

Ho, K.K. and Hoffman, D.M. (1993). Aging and growth hormone. *Horm. Res.* 40, 80.

Hoffman, R.P., Singer, G.C., Drash, A.L., *et al.* (1991). Plasma catecholamine responses to hypoglycemia in children and adolescents with IDDM. *Diabetes Care* 14, 81.

Holland, O.B. and Pool, P.E. (1988). Metabolic changes with antihypertensive therapy of the salt-sensitive patient. *Am. J. Cardiol.* 61, 53H.

Holm, G. (1983). Adrenergic regulation of insulin release. *Acta Med. Scand.* (Suppl. 627), 21.

Holm, G., Herlitz, J., and Smith, U. (1981). Severe hypoglycaemia during physical exercise and treatment with beta-blockers. *BMJ* 282, 1360.

Holmäng, P. and Björntorp, P. (1992). The effects of cortisol on insulin sensitivity in muscle. *Acta Physiol. Scand.* 144, 425.

Hornfeldt, C.S. (1992). A report of acute ethanol poisoning in a child: mouthwash versus cologne, perfume and after-shave. *J. Toxicol. Clin. Toxicol.* 30, 115.

Howell, S.L. (1988). Regulation and mechanism of insulin secretion. In *Clinical Diabetes — An Illustrated Text* (ed. M.G. Besser, H.J. Bodansky, and A.G. Cudworth), p. 2.1. J.B. Lippincott, Philadelphia.

Huminer, D., Shlomo, D., Rosenfeld, J.B., *et al.* (1989). Inadvertent sulfonylurea-induced hypoglycaemia. *Arch. Intern. Med.* 149, 1890.

Humphrey, S.H. and Nash, D.A. (1978). Lactic acidosis complicating sodium nitroprusside therapy. *Ann. Intern. Med.* 88, 58.

Huntsinger, N.J. (1987). Hypoglycaemic effect of lithium. *Biol. Psychiatry* 22, 798.

Huupponen, R. and Pihlajamäki, K. (1986). Effect of blood glucose level on the metabolic response of intravenous salbutamol. *Int. J. Clin. Pharmacol. Ther. Toxicol.* 24, 374.

Hvidberg, A., Rasmussen, M.H., Christensen, N.U., *et al.* (1994). Theophylline enhances glucose recovery after hypoglycemia in healthy men and in type I diabetic patients. *Metabolism* 43, 776.

Ibels, L.S., Simons, L.A., King, J.O., *et al.* (1975). Studies on the nature and cause of hyperlipidemia in uraemia, maintanence dialysis and renal transplantation. *Q. J. Med.* 44, 601.

Ibels, L.S., Stewart, J.H., Mahoney, J.F., *et al.* (1977). Occlusive arterial disease in uremic and hemodialysis patients and renal transplant recipients. A study of the incidence of arterial disease and of the prevalence of risk factors\implicated in the pathogenesis of arteriosclerosis. *Q. J. Med.* 46, 197.

Ibels, L.S., Alfrey, A.C., and Weil, R. (1978). Hyperlipidemia in adult, pediatric and diabetic renal transplant recipients. *Am. J. Med.* 64, 634.

Ingemarsson, I., Amlkumaran, S., and Kottegoda, S.R. (1985). Complication of beta-mimetic therapy in preterm labour. *Aust. N.Z. J. Obstet. Gynaecol.* 25, 182.

Iyer, R.S., Rao, S.R., Pal, S., *et al.* (1993). L-asparaginase related hyperglycemia. *Indian J. Cancer* 30, 72.

Jackson, J.E. and Bressler, R. (1981). Clinical pharmacology of sulphonylurea hypoglycaemic agents. 2. *Drugs* 22, 295.

Jacobs, H.S. and Loeffler, F.E. (1992). Postmenopausal hormone replacement therapy. *BMJ* 305, 1403.

Jauch, K-W., Hartl, W., Guenther, B., *et al.* (1987). Captopril enhances insulin responsiveness of forearm muscle tissue in non-insulin-dependent diabetes mellitus. *Eur. J. Clin. Invest.* 17, 448.

Jeandel, C., Preiss, M.A., Pierson, H., *et al.* (1988). Hypoglycaemia induced by cibenzoline. *Lancet* i, 1232.

Jefferys, D.B., Lessof, M.H., and Mattock, M.B. (1980). Corticosteroid treatment, serum lipids and coronary artery disease. *Postgrad. Med. J.* 56, 491.

Jennings, A.M., Wilson, R.M., and Ward, J.D. (1989). Symptomatic hypoglycaemia in NIDDM patients treated with oral hypoglycaemic agents. *Diabetes Care* 12, 203.

Jérôme, B., Bluet-Pajot, M.T., and Epelbaum, J. (1995). Neuroendocrine regulation of growth hormone. *Eur. J. Endocrinol.* 132, 12.

Jha, T.K. and Sharma, V.K. (1984). Pentamidine-induced diabetes mellitus. *Trans. R. Soc. Trop. Med. Hyg.* 78, 252.

Johnson, J.A., Kappel, J.E., and Sharif, M.N. (1993). Hypoglycemia secondary to trimethoprim/sulfamethoxazole administration in a renal transplant patient. *Ann. Pharmacother.* 27, 304.

Jones, G.J. and Itri, L.M. (1986). Safety and tolerance of recombinant interferon alfa-2a (Roferon®-A) in cancer patients. *Cancer* 57 (Suppl.), 1709.

Jorgensen, L.N., Dejgaard, A., and Pramming, S.K. (1994). Human insulin and hypoglycaemia; a literature survey. *Diabetic Med.* 11, 925.

Josselson, J. and Sadler, J.H. (1986). Nephrotic-range proteinuria and hyperglycaemia associated with clonidine therapy. *Am. J. Med.* 80, 545.

Jung, K., Neumann, R., Scholz, D., *et al.* (1982). Abnormalities in the composition of serum high density lipoprotein in renal transplant recipients. *Clin. Nephrol.* 17, 191.

Kamau, R.K., Maina, F.W., Kigondu, C., *et al.* (1990). The effect of low-oestrogen combined pill, progestogen-only pill and medroxyprogesterone acetate on oral glucose tolerance test. *East Afr. Med. J.* 67, 550.

Kamran, A., Doraiswamy, P.M., Jane, J.L., *et al.* (1994). Severe hyperglycemia associated with high doses of clozapine. *Am. J. Psychiatry* 151, 1395.

Karboski, J.A. and Godley, P.J. (1988). Inhaled pentamidine and hypoglycemia. *Ann. Intern. Med.* 108, 490.

Karch, S.B. (1993). High-dose epinephrine. *Am. J. Emerg. Med.* 11, 423.

Kathol, R.G., Jaeckle, R., Wysham, C., *et al.* (1991). Imipramine effect on hypothalamic–pituitary–adrenal axis response to hypoglycaemia. *Psychiatry Res.* 41, 45.

Kazzi, N.J., Brans, Y.W., and Poland, R.L. (1990). Dexamethasone effects on the hospital course of infants with bronchopulmonary dysplasia who are dependent on artificial ventilation. *Pediatrics* 86, 722.

Kern, W., Lieb, K., Kerner, W., *et al.* (1990). Differential effects of human and pork insulin-induced hypoglycemia on neuronal functions in humans. *Diabetes* 39, 1091.

Kerr, D., MacDonald, I.A., Heller, S.R., *et al.* (1990). Beta-adrenoceptor blockade and hypoglycaemia. A randomised, double-blind, placebo controlled comparison of metoprolol CR, atenolol and propranolol LA in normal subjects. *Br. J. Clin. Pharmacol.* 29, 685.

Kirkpatrick, C., Quenon, M., and Desir, D. (1980). Blood anions and electrolytes during ritodrine infusion in preterm labor. *Am. J. Obstet. Gynecol.* 138, 523.

Klarr, J.M., Bhatt, M.V., and Donn, S.M. (1994). Neonatal adrenergic blockade following single dose maternal labetalol administration. *Am. J. Perinatol.* 11, 91.

Knauf, H. (1993). The role of low-dose diuretics in essential hypertension. *J. Cardiovasc. Pharmacol.* 22 (Suppl. 6), S1.

Knopp, R.H. (1986). Arteriosclerosis risk. The roles of oral contraceptives and postmenopausal estrogens. *J. Reprod. Med.* 31 (Suppl.), 913.

Ko, G.T.C., Chan, J.C.N., Woo, J., *et al.* (1997). The effect of age on cardiovascular risk factors in Chinese women. *Int. J. Cardiol.* 61, 221.

Koda-Kimble, M.A. (1992). Diabetes Mellitus. In *Applied Therapeutics — The Clinical Use of Drugs* (5th edn) (ed. M.A. Koda-Kimble and L.Y. Young). Applied Therapeutics, Vancouver.

Korenyi, C. and Lowenstein, B. (1968). Chlorpromazine induced diabetes. *Dis. Nerv. Syst.* 29, 887.

Krause, I., Bar-on, H., and Shaffir, E. (1981). Origin and pattern of glucocorticoid-induced hyperlipidemia in rats. *Biochim. Biophys. Acta* 663, 69.

Kreisberg, R.A. (1984). Pathogenesis and management of lactic acidosis. *Annu. Rev. Med.* 35, 181.

Krentz, A.J., Boyle, P.J., Justice, K., *et al.* (1993). Successful treatment of severe refractory sulfonylurea-induced hypoglycemia with octreotide. *Diabetes Care* 16, 184.

Krentz A.J., Ferner R.E., Bailey, C.J. (1994a). Comparative tolerability profiles of oral antidiabetic agents. *Drug Saf.* 11, 223.

Krentz, A.J., Boyle, P.J., MacDonald, L.M., *et al.* (1994b). Octreotide: a long-acting inhibitor of endogenous hormone secretion for human metabolic investigations. *Metabolism* 43, 24.

Krentz, A.J., Dmitrewski, J., Mayer, D., *et al.* (1994c). Tacrolimus (FK506) versus cyclosporin in prevention of liver allograft rejection. *Lancet* 344, 948.

Krishna, S., Waller, D.W., ter Kuile, F., *et al.* (1994). Lactic acidosis and hypoglycaemia in children with severe malaria: pathophysiological and prognostic significance. *Trans. R. Soc. Trop. Med. Hyg.* 88, 67.

Kukita, H., Hamada, H.M., Hiwada, K., *et al.* (1985). Clinical significance of measurements of serum apolipoprotein A-I, A-II and B in hypertriglyceridemic male patients with and without coronary heart disease. *Atherosclerosis* 55, 143.

Kung, A.W.C., Ma, J.T.C., Wong, V.C.W., *et al.* (1987). Glucose and lipid metabolism with triphasic oral contraceptives in women with history of gestational diabetes. *Contraception* 35, 257.

Kurie, J.M., Lee, J.S., Griffin, T., *et al.* (1996). Phase I trial of 9-cis retinoic acid in adults with solid tumors. *Clin. Cancer Res.* 2, 287.

Lager, I. (1991). The insulin-antagonistic effect of the counter-regulatory hormones. *J. Intern. Med.* 229 (Suppl. 2), 41.

Lakhdar, A.A., Farish, E., Dunn, F.G., *et al.* (1988). Amiodarone therapy and glucose tolerance — a prospective trial. *Eur. J. Clin. Pharmacol.* 34, 651.

Lamberts, S.W.J., Uitterlinden, P., Verschoor, L., *et al.* (1985). Long-term treatment of acromegaly with the somatostatin analogue SMS 201-995. *N. Engl. J. Med.* 313, 1576.

Lancaster-Smith, M., Leigh, N.I., and Thompson, H.H. (1974). Death following non-ketotic hyperglycaemic coma during diazoxide therapy and peritoneal dialysis. *Postgrad. Med. J.* 50, 175.

The Lancet (1983). Methanol poisoning. *Lancet* i, 910.

LaRosa, J.C., Chambless, L.E., Criqui, M.H., *et al.* (1986). Patterns of dyslipoproteinemia in selected North American populations. The Lipid Research Clinics Program Prevalence Study. *Circulation* 73 (Suppl. I) I 12.

Lebovitz, HE. (1993). Oral antidiabetic agents: the emergence of alpha glucosidase inhibitors. *Drugs* 44 (Suppl. 3), 21.

Lee, K., Mize, R., and Lowenstein, S.R. (1987). Glyburide-induced hypoglycemia and ranitidine. *Ann. Intern. Med.* 107, 261.

Lee, R.V., Jampol, L.M., and Brown, W.V. (1971). Nephrogenic diabetes insipidus and lithium intoxication — complications of lithium carbonate therapy. *N. Engl. J. Med.* 284, 93.

Lehmann, S. and Cerra, F.B. (1992). Growth hormone and nutritional support: adverse metabolic effects. *Nutr. Clin. Pract.* 7, 27.

Lehren, P. (1987). Comparison of effects on lipid metabolism of antihypertensive drugs with alpha- and beta-adrenergic antagonist properties. *Am. J. Med.* 82 (Suppl. 1A), 31.

Leslie, D. and Coats, P.M. (1977). Salbutamol-induced diabetic ketoacidosis. *BMJ* ii, 768.

Leson, C.K., McGuigan, M.A., and Bryson, S.M. (1988). Caffeine overdose in an adolescent male. *J. Toxicol. Clin. Toxicol.* 26, 407.

Levy, R.I., Brensike, J.F., Epstein, S.E., *et al.* (1984). The influence of changes in lipid values induced by cholestyramine and diet on progression of coronary artery disease: Results of the NHLBI Type II Coronary Intervention Study. *Circulation* 69, 325.

Lewis, P.J., Kohner, E.M., Petrie, A., *et al.* (1976). Deterioration of glucose tolerance in hypertensive patients on prolonged diuretic treatment. *Lancet* i, 564.

Lingenfelser, T., Overkamp, D., Renn, W., *et al.* (1991). Different awareness of hypoglycaemia induced by human or purified pork insulin in type 1 diabetic patients. *Diabetes Res. Clin. Pract.* 13, 29.

Lingenfelser, T., Renn, W., Plonz, C., *et al.* (1992). Catecholamine response during human and pork insulin-induced hypoglycemia in IDDM patients. *Diabetes Care* 15, 261.

Lingenfelser, T., Pickert, A., Pfohl, M., *et al.* (1993). Hypothalamic–pituitary activation does not differ during human and porcine insulin-induced hypoglycemia in insulin-dependent diabetes mellitus. *Clin. Invest.* 72, 56.

Lithell, H.O.L. (1991). Effect of antihypertensive drugs on insulin, glucose, and lipid metabolism. *Diabetes Care* 40, 203.

Liu, D., Moberg, E., Kollind, M., *et al.* (1991). A high concentration of circulating insulin suppresses the glucagon response to hypoglycemia in normal man. *J. Clin. Endocrinol. Metab.* 73, 1123.

Liu, D.T., Adamson, U.C., Lins, P.E., *et al.* (1992). Inhibitory effect of circulating insulin on glucagon secretion during hypoglycemia in type I diabetic patients. *Diabetes Care* 15, 59.

Liu, D., Adamson, U., Lins, P.E., *et al.* (1993). An analysis of the glucagon response to hypoglycaemia in patients with type 1 diabetes and in healthy subjects. *Diabetic Med.* 10, 246.

Looareesuwan, S., Phillips, R.E., White, N.J., *et al.* (1985). Quinine and severe falciparum malaria in late pregnancy. *Lancet* ii, 4.

Lund-Johnson, P., Hjermann, I., Iversen, B.M., *et al.* (1993). Selective alpha-1 inhibitors: first or second-line antihypertensive agents? *Cardiology* 83, 150.

McCance, D.R., Hanson, R.L., Pettitt, D.J., *et al.* (1997). Diagnosing diabetes mellitus — do we need new criteria? *Diabetologia* 40, 247.

McDonald, J. (1980). Alcohol and diabetes. *Diabetes Care* 3, 629.

MacLeod, K.M., Gold, A.E., and Frier, B.M. (1995). A trial of human and porcine insulins in Type I diabetic patients. *Diabetic Med.* 12, 134.

MacRury, S., Neilson, R., and Goodwin, K. (1987). Benylin dependence, metabolic acidosis and hyperglycemia. *Postgrad. Med. J.* 63, 587.

MacWalter, R.S., El Debani, A.H., Feely, J., *et al.* (1985). Potentiation by ranitidine of the·hypoglycaemic response to glypizide in diabetic patients. *Br. J. Clin. Pharmacol.* 19, 121P.

Madsen, B.K., Holmer, P., Ibsen, H., *et al.* (1992). The influence of captopril on the epinephrine response to insulin-induced hypoglycemia in humans. The interaction between the renin-angiotensin system and the sympathetic nervous system. *Am. J. Hypertens.* 5, 361.

Mann, N.S., Russman, H.B., Mann, S.K., *et al.* (1985). Lactulose and severe lactic acidosis. *Ann. Intern. Med.* 103, 637.

Markowitz M., Saag M., Powderly W.O., *et al.* (1995). A preliminary study of ritonavir, an inhibitor of HIV-I protease, to treat HIV-I infection. *N. Engl. J.Med.* 333, 1534.

Marley, J. and Rohan, A. (1993). Mianserin-induced hyperglycaemia. *Lancet* 342, 1430.

Martinez-Maldonaldo, M. and Terrell, J. (1973). Lithium carbonate-induced nephrogenic diabetes insipidus and glucose-intolerance. *Arch. Intern. Med.* 132, 881.

Materson, B.J., Reda, D.J., Cushman M.S., *et al.* (1993). Single-drug therapy for hypertension in men. A comparison of six antihypertensive agents with placebo. *N. Engl. J. Med.* 328, 914.

Mathews, K.A., Meilahn, E., and Lewis, M.P.M. (1989). Menopause and risk factors for CHD. *N. Engl. J. Med.* 321, 641.

Meechan, J.G. and Welbury, R.R. (1993). Metabolic responses to oral surgery under local anaesthesia and sedation with intravenous midazolam: the effects of two different local anaesthetics. *Anesth. Prog.* 39, 9.

Meneilly, G.S., Cheung, E., and Tuokko, H. (1994). Counterregulatory hormone responses to hypoglycemia in the elderly patient with diabetes. *Diabetes* 43, 403.

Meneilly, G.S., Cheung, E., and Tuokko, H. (1995). Differential effects of human and animal insulin on the responses

to hypoglycemia in elderly patients with NIDDM. *Diabetes* 44, 272.

Miccoli, R., Orlandi, M.C., Fruzzetti, F., *et al.* (1989). Metabolic effects of three new low dose pills: a six month experience. *Contraception* 39, 643.

Mimouni, B.A. and Mimouni, M. (1993). Clonidine-induced hyperglycemia in a young diabetic girl. *Ann. Pharmacother.* 27, 980.

Molsted-Pederson, L., Skouby, S.O., and Skouby, P.D. (1991). Preconception counselling and contraception after gestational diabetes. *Diabetes Care* 40 (Suppl. 2), 147.

Montoliu, J., Carrera, M., Darnell, A., *et al.* (1981). Lactic acidosis and Fanconi's syndrome due to degraded tetracycline. *BMJ* 283, 1576.

Morgan, J.M., Saris, S.D., Capuzzi, D.M., *et al.* (1993). Hypoglycemic and insulin response to a continuous intravenous infusion of CGP-35126 recombinant human insulin-like growth factor-I (rhIGF-I) in healthy males. *J. Clin. Pharmacol.* 33, 366.

Morris, A.D. and Donnelly, R. (1996). Angiotensin II: an insulin-sensitizing vasoactive hormone? *J. Clin. Endocrinol. Metab.* 81, 1303.

Muhlhauser, I., Heinemann, L., Fritsche, E., *et al.* (1991). Hypoglycemic symptoms and frequency of severe hypoglycemia in patients treated with human and animal insulin preparations. *Diabetes Care* 14, 745.

Munck, A. (1971). Glucocorticoid inhibition of glucose uptake by peripheral tissues: old and new evidence, molecular mechanisms, and physiological significance. *Perspect. Biol. Med.* 14, 265.

Munshi, M.N., Martin, R.E., and Fonseca, V.A. (1994). Hyperosmolar nonketotic diabetic syndrome following treatment of human immunodeficiency virus infection with didanosine. *Diabetes Care* 17, 316.

Musci, M.N. Jr, Abbasi, S., Otis, C., *et al.* (1988). Prolonged fetal ritodrine exposure and immediate neonatal outcome. *J. Perinatol.* 8, 27.

Neaton J.D., Grimm R.H. Jr, Prineas, R.J., *et al.* (1993). Treatment of mild hypertension study. Final results. *JAMA* 270, 713.

Noguchi, M., Taniya, T., Tajiri, K., *et al.* (1987). Fatal hyperlipaemia in a case of metastatic breast cancer treated by tamoxifen. *Br. J. Surg.* 74, 586.

Notelovitz, M., Feldman, E.B., and Gillespy, M. (1989). Lipid and lipoprotein changes in women taking low dose triphasic oral contraceptives: a controlled comparative 12-month clinical trial. *Am. J. Obstet. Gynecol.* 160, 1269.

Oakley, D.E. and Ellis, P.P. (1976). Glycerol and hyperosmolar nonketotic coma. *Am. J. Ophthalmol.* 81, 469.

O'Donoghue, D.J. (1989). Acute pancreatitis due to nadolol-induced hypertriglyceridaemia. *Br. J. Clin. Pract.* 43, 74.

Ohkubo, Y., Kishikawa, H., Araki, E., *et al.* (1995). Intensive insulin therapy prevents the progression of diabetic microvascular complications in Japanese patients with NIDDM: a randomised prospective 6-year study. *Diab. Res. Clin. Pract.* 28, 103.

Okitolonda, W., Delacollette, C., Malengreau, M., *et al.* (1987). High incidence of hypoglycaemia in African patients treated with intravenous quinine for severe malaria. *BMJ* 295, 716.

Olsen, E.A., Lichtenstein, G.R, and Wilkinson, W.E. (1988). Changes in serum lipids in patients with condylomata acuminata treated with interferon alfa-n1 (Wellferon). *J. Am. Acad. Dermatol.* 19, 286.

Olsen, G.D. (1995). Potential mechanisms of cocaine-induced developmental neurotoxicity: a mini-review. *Neurotoxicology* 16, 159.

Osei, K., Holland, G., and Falko, J.M. (1986). Indapamide. Effects on apoproteins, lipoproteins and glucoregulation in ambulatory diabetic patients. *Arch. Intern. Med.* 146, 1973.

Otero, M.L., Pinilla, C.F., and Claros, N.M. (1983). The effect of long-term therapy of essential hypertension with atenolol and chlorthalidone on carbohydrate tolerance. *Primary Cardiology* 6 (Suppl. 1), 193.

Otsuka, M., Akiba, T., Okita, Y., *et al.* (1990). Lactic acidosis with hypoglycemia and hyperammonemia observed in two uremic patients during calcium hopantenate treatment. *Jpn J. Med.* 29, 324.

Ott, A., Hayes, J., and Polin, J. (1976). Severe lactic acidosis associated with intravenous alcohol for premature labor. *Obstet. Gynecol.* 48, 362.

Panwalker, A. (1992). Hyperglycemia induced by megestrol acetate. *Ann. Intern. Med.* 116, 878.

Patel, S.R., Kvols, L.K., Rubin, J., *et al.* (1991). Phase I-II study of pibenzimol hydrochloride (NSC 322921) in advanced pancreatic carcinoma. *Invest. New Drugs* 9, 53.

Patial, R.K., Bansal, S.K., Kashyap, S., *et al.* (1990). Hypoglycaemia following zinc phosphide poisoning. *J. Assoc. Physicians India* 38, 306.

Patrick, A.W., Bodmer, C.W., Tieszen, K.L., *et al.* (1991). Human insulin and awareness of acute hypoglycemic symptoms in insulin dependent diabetes. *Lancet* 338, 528.

Perlman, J.A., Russell-Briefel, R., Ezzati, T., *et al.* (1985). Oral glucose tolerance and the potency of contraceptive progestins. *J. Chronic Dis.* 38, 857.

Perronne, C., Bricaire, F., Leport, C., *et al.* (1990). Hypoglycaemia and diabetes mellitus following parenteral pentamidine mesylate treatment in AIDS patients. *Diabetic Med.* 7, 585.

Phillips, P.J., Need, A.G., Thomas, D.W., *et al.* (1979). Nalidixic acid and lactic acidosis. *Aust. N.Z. J. Med.* 9, 694.

Phillips, R.E., Looareesuwan, S., and White, N.J., *et al.* (1986a). Hypoglycaemia and antimalarial drugs: quinidine and release of insulin. *BMJ* 292, 1319.

Phillips, R.E., Warrell, D.A., Looareesuwan, S., *et al.* (1986b). Effectiveness of SMS 201-995, a synthetic long-acting somatostatin analogue in treatment of quinine-induced hyperinsulinaemia. *Lancet* i, 713.

Phillips, R.E., Looareesuwan, S., Molyneux, M.E., *et al.* (1993). Hypoglycaemia and counterregulatory hormone responses in severe falciparum malaria: treatment with Sandostatin. *Q. J. Med.* 86, 233.

Podolsky, S. and Pattavina, C.G. (1973). Hyperosmolar nonketotic diabetic coma: a complication of propranolol therapy. *Metabolism* 22, 685.

Politi, A., Poggio, G., and Margiotta, A. (1984). Can amiodarone induce hyperglycaemia and hypertriglyceridaemia? *BMJ* 288, 285.

Pollare, T., Lithell, H., and Berne, C. (1989). A comparison of the effects of hydrochlorothiazide and captopril on glucose and lipid metabolism in patients with hypertension. *N. Engl. J. Med.* 28, 868.

Ponticelli, C., Barbi, G.L., Cantaluppi, A., *et al.* (1978). Lipid disorders in renal transplant recipients. *Nephron* 20, 189.

Popovic, V., Nesovic, M., Micic, D., *et al.* (1989). Hypoglycaemia in acromegalic patients with long acting somatostatin analogue (SMS 201-995). *Horm. Metab. Res.* 21, 282.

Poretsky, L. and Moses, A.C. (1984). Hypoglycaemia associated with trimethoprim/sulphamethoxazole therapy. *Diabetes Care* 7, 508.

Prescott, L.F., Roscoe, P., Wright, N., *et al.* (1971). Plasma paracetamol half-life and hepatic necrosis in patients with paracetamol overdose. *Lancet* 1, 519.

Randle, P.J., Hales, C.N., Garland, P.B., *et al.* 1963). The glucose fatty-acid cycle: its role in insulin sensitivity and the metabolic disturbances of diabetes mellitus. *Lancet* ii, 785.

Raschke, R., Arnold, C.P., Richeson, R., *et al.* (1991). Refractory hypoglycemia secondary to topical salicylate intoxication. *Arch. Intern. Med.*, 151, 591.

Reichard, P., Britz, A., and Rosenqvist, U. (1991). Intensified conventional insulin treatment and neuropsychological impairment. *BMJ* 303, 1439.

Rigas, J.R., Tong, W.P., Kris, M.G., *et al.* (1992). Phase I clinical and pharmacological study of chloroquinoxaline sulfonamide. *Cancer Res.* 52, 6619.

Rigas, J.R, Francis, P.A., Miller, V.A., *et al.* (1995). Clinical and pharmacology study of chloroquinoxaline sulfonamide given on a weekly schedule. *Cancer Chemother. Pharmacol.* 35, 483.

Rimm E.B., Manson J.E., Stampfer M.J., *et al.* (1992). Oral contraceptive use and the risk of type 2 (non-insulin-dependent) diabetes mellitus in a large prospective study of women. *Diabetologia* 35, 967.

Rollman, O., Jameson, S., and Lithell, H. (1985). Effects of long-term ketoconazole therapy and serum lipid levels. *Eur. J. Clin. Pharmacol.* 29, 241.

Rosenbaum, M., Gertner, J.M., and Leibel, R.L. (1989). Effects of systemic growth hormone (GH) administration on regional adipose tissue distribution and metabolism in GH deficient children. *J. Clin. Endocrinol. Metab.* 69, 1274.

Rosenblatt, H.M., Byrne, W., Ament, M.E., *et al.* (1980). Successful treatment of chronic mucocutaneous candidiasis with ketoconazole. *J. Pediatr.* 97, 657.

Rosenfalck, A.M., Bendtson, I., Jorgensen, S., *et al.* (1992). Nasal glucagon in the treatment of hypoglycaemia in type 1 (insulin-dependent) diabetic patients. *Diabetes Res. Clin. Pract.* 17, 43.

Rossetti, L., Giaccari, A., and DeFronzo, R.A. (1990). Glucose toxicity. *Diabetes Care* 13, 610.

Rossner, S. and Wallgren, A. (1984). Serum lipoproteins and proteins after breast cancer surgery and effects of tamoxifen. *Atherosclerosis* 52, 339.

Roth, A., Miller, H.I., Belhassen, B., *et al.* (1989). Slow-release verapamil and hyperglycemic metabolic acidosis. *Ann. Intern. Med.* 110, 171.

Roth, D., Milgrom, M., Esquenazi, V., *et al.* (1989). Post-transplant hyperglycaemia. Increased incidence in cyclosporine-treated renal allograft recipients. *Transplantation* 47 278.

Roux, P. and Courtois, H. (1981). Blood sugar regulation during treatment with indapamide in hypertensive diabetics. *Postgrad. Med. J.* 57 (Suppl. 2), 70.

Rowe, P. and Mather, H.G. (1985). Hyperosmolar non-ketotic diabetes mellitus associated with metolazone. *BMJ* 291, 25.

Rowland, M.J., Bransome, E.J., and Hendry, L.B. (1994). Hypoglycemia caused by selegiline, an antiparkinsonian drug: can such side effects be predicted? *J. Clin. Pharmacol.* 34, 80.

Saha, A.K., Kurowski, T.G., Colca, J.R., *et al.* (1994). Lipid abnormalities in tissues of the KKA^y mouse: effects of pioglitazone on malonyl-CoA and diacylglycerol. *Am. J. Physiol.* 267, E95.

Salerno, D.M., Fifield, J., Krejci, J., *et al.* (1988). Encainide-induced hyperglycaemia. *Am. J. Med.* 84, 39.

Salmeron, S., Petitpretz, P., Katalama, C., *et al.* (1986). Pentamidine and pancreatitis. *Ann. Intern. Med.* 105, 140.

Schattner, A., Rimon, E., Green, L., *et al.* (1988). Hypoglycaemia induced by co- trimoxazole in AIDS. *BMJ* 297, 742.

Schneider, M. (1995). Fatal hepatic necrosis following cardiac surgery and enflurane anaesthesia. *Anaesth. Intensive Care* 23, 225.

Schneider, S.H., Vitug, A., Ananthakrishnan, R., *et al.* (1991). Impaired adrenergic response to prolonged exercise in type I diabetes. *Metabolism* 40, 1219.

Schwartz, M.L. (1993). Severe reversible hyperglycemia as a consequence of niacin therapy. *Arch. Intern. Med.* 153, 2050.

Sears, E.S. (1976). Nonketotic hyperosmolar hyperglycemia during glycerol therapy for cerebral edema. *Neurology* 26, 89.

Seltzer, H.S. (1989). Drug-induced hypoglycaemia. A review of 1418 cases. *Endocrinol. Metab. Clin. North Am.* 18, 163.

Sessler, C.N. (1990). Theophylline toxicity: clinical features of 116 consecutive cases. *Am. J. Med.* 86, 567.

Shannon, M. (1994). Hypokalemia, hyperglycemia and plasma catecholamine activity after severe theophylline intoxication. *J. Toxicol. Clin. Toxicol.* 32, 41.

Shannon, M. and Lovejoy, F.H.J. (1990). The influence of age vs peak serum concentration on life-threatening events after chronic theophylline intoxication. *Arch. Intern. Med.* 150, 2045.

Shannon, M. and Lovejoy, F.H.J. (1992). Effect of acute versus chronic intoxication on clinical features of theophylline poisoning in children. *J. Pediatr.* 121, 125.

Sharma, S.N., Iyengar, S.S., and Hegde, K.P. (1990). Nifedipine induced hyperglycaemia. *J. Assoc. Physicians India* 38, 673.

Sharpe, S.M. (1983). Pentamidine and hypoglycemia. *Ann. Intern. Med.* 99, 128.

Shen, M., Orwoll, E.S., Conte, J.E. Jr, *et al.* (1989). Pentamidine-induced pancreatic beta cell dysfunction. *Am. J. Med.* 86, 726.

Shionoiri, H., Miyakawa, T., Takasaki, I., *et al.* (1987). Glucose tolerance during chronic captopril therapy in patients with essential hypertension. *J. Cardiovasc. Pharmacol.* 9, 160.

Shionoiri, H., Gotoh, E., Ito, T., *et al.* (1994). Long-term therapy with terazosin may improve glucose and lipid metabolism in hypertensives: a multicenter prospective study. *Am. J. Med. Sci.* 307 (Suppl. 1), S91.

Shorr, R.I., Ray, W.A., Daugherty, J.R., *et al.* (1996). Individual sulphonylureas and serious hypoglycaemia in older people. *J. Am. Geriatr. Soc.* 44, 751.

Shrivastava, R.K. and Edwards, D. (1983). Hypoglycemia associated with imipramine. *Biol. Psychiatry* 18, 1509.

Singer, I. and Rotenberg, D. (1973). Mechanisms of lithium action. *N. Engl. J. Med.* 289, 254.

Singh, B., Gupta, S., Minocha, S.K., *et al.* (1994). Hypoglycaemia in aluminium phosphide poisoning. *J. Assoc. Physicians India* 42, 663.

Skarfors, E.T., Lithell, H.O., Selinus, I., *et al.* (1989). Do antihypertensive drugs precipitate diabetes in predisposed men? *BMJ* 298, 1147.

Skouby S.O. (1988). Oral contraceptives: hormonal dose and effects on carbohydrate metabolism. *Matruitas* 1 (Suppl.), 111.

Skouby, S.O., Mølsted-Pedersen, L., and Petersen, K.R. (1991). Contraception for women with diabetes: an update. *Baillière's Clin. Obstet. Gynaecol.* 5, 493.

Slama, G., Alamowitch, C., Desplanque, N., *et al.* (1990). A new non-invasive method for treating insulin-reaction: intranasal lyophilized glucagon. *Diabetologia* 33, 671.

Sledge, E.D. and Broadstone, V.L. (1993). Hypoglycemia due to a pharmacy dispensing error. *South. Med. J.* 86, 1272.

Smith, R.C., Sullivan, M., and Getter, J. (1992). Inadequate adrenergic response to disopyramide-induced hypoglycemia. *Ann. Pharmacother.* 26, 490.

Soltesz, G. (1993). Hypoglycaemia in the diabetic child. *Baillière's Clin. Endocrinol. Metab.* 7, 741.

Spear, M.L., Reeves, G., and Pearlman, S.A. (1993). Diabetic ketoacidosis after steroid administration for bronchopulmonary dysplasia: a case report. *J. Perinatol.* 13, 232.

Spellacy, W.N. (1982). Carbohydrate metabolism during treatment with estrogen, progestogen and low-dose oral contraceptives. *Am. J. Obstet. Gynecol.* 142, 732.

Spellacy, W.N., Cruz, A.C., Buhi, W.C., *et al.* (1978). The acute effects of ritodrine infusion on maternal metabolism: measurements of levels of glucose, insulin, glucagon, triglycerides, cholesterol, placental lactogen, and chorionic gonadotrophin. *Am. J. Obstet. Gynecol.* 131, 637.

Spellacy, W.N., Buhi, W.C., and Birk, S.A. (1981). Prospective studies of carbohydrate metabolism in 'normal' women using norgestrel for eighteen months. *Fertil. Steril.* 35, 167.

Spenney, J.G., Eure, C.A., and Kreisberg, R.A. (1969). Hyperglycemic, hyperosmolar, non-ketoacidotic diabetes: a complication of steroid and immunosuppressive therapy. *Diabetes* 18, 107.

Sporer, K.A., Ernst, A.A., Conte, R., *et al.* (1995). The incidence of ethanol-induced hypoglycaemia. *Am. J. Emerg. Med.* 10, 403.

Stahl-Bayliss, C.M., Kalman, C.M., and Laskin, O.L. (1986). Pentamidine-induced hypoglycaemia in patients with the acquired immune deficiency syndrome. *Clin. Pharmacol. Ther.* 39, 271.

Stapleton, J.T. and Gillman, M.W. (1983). Hypoglycemic coma due to disopyramide toxicity. *South. Med. J.* 76, 1453.

Stehouwer, C.D., Lems, W.F., Fischer, H.R., *et al.* (1989). Aggravation of hypoglycaemia in insulinoma patients by the long-acting somatostatin analogue octreotide (Sandostatin). *Acta Endocrinol.* 21, 34.

Steinherz, P.G.(1994). Transient, severe hyperlipidemia in patients with acute lymphoblastic leukemia treated with prednisone and asparaginase. *Cancer* 74, 3234.

Stuyt, P.M.J., Demacker, P.N.M., and Stalenhoef, A.F.H. (1986). Pancreatitis induced by oestrogen in a patient with type I hyperlipoproteinaemia. *BMJ* 293, 734.

Sugarman, J.R. (1991). Hypoglycemia associated hospitalizations in a population with a high prevalence of non-insulin-dependent diabetes mellitus. *Diabetes Res. Clin. Pract.* 14, 139.

Sumrani, N., Delaney, V., Ding, Z., *et al.* (1991). Post-transplant diabetes mellitus in cyclosporine-treated renal transplant recipients. *Transplant. Proc.* 23, 1249.

Sylvester, R.K., Lobell, M., Ogden, W., *et al.* (1989). Homoharringtonine-induced hyperglycaemia. *J. Clin. Oncol.* 7, 392.

Tabasco, M.J., Mieles, L., Carroll, P., *et al.* (1993). Insulin requirements after liver transplantation and FK-506 immunosuppression. *Transplantation* 56, 862.

Takahara, S., Kokaclo, Y., Kameoka, H., *et al.* (1994). Monitoring of FK506 blood levels in kidney transplant recipients. *Transplant. Proc.* 26, 2106.

Takasu, N., Yamada, T., Miura, H., *et al.* (1982). Rifampicin-induced early phase hyperglycemia in humans. *Am. Rev. Respir. Dis.* 125, 23.

Tasker, P.R.W. and Mitchell-Heggs, P.F. (1976). Non-ketotic diabetic precoma associated with high dose frusemide therapy. *BMJ* i, 626.

Taskinen, M.R. (1987). Lipoprotein lipase in hypertriglyceridemias. In *Lipoprotein Lipase* (ed. J. Borensztajn), p. 201. Evener, Chicago.

Taylor, S.I., Accili, D., and Imai, Y. (1994). Insulin resistance or insulin deficiency. Which is the primary cause of NIDDM? *Diabetes* 43, 736.

Tessier, D., Dawson, K., Tetrault, J.P., *et al.* (1994). Glibenclamide vs gliclazide in type 2 diabetes of the elderly. *Diabetic Med.* 11, 974.

Thomson, J.S. and Prescott, L.F. (1966). Liver damage and impaired glucose tolerance after paracetamol overdosage. *BMJ* 2, 506.

Thomson, F.J., Masson, E.A., Leeming, J.T., *et al.* (1991). Lack of knowledge of symptoms of hypoglycaemia by elderly diabetic patients. *Age Ageing* 20, 404.

Timperley, A.C., Withnall, R.D.J., and Rainford D.J. (1996). The development of insulin-dependent diabetes mellitus in a renal transplant patient receiving oral isotretinoin. *Nephrol. Dialysis Transplant.* 11, 753.

Tollefson, G. and Lesar, T. (1983). Non-ketotic hyperglycemia associated with loxapine and amoxapine: case report. *J. Clin. Psychiatry* 44, 347.

Trost, B.N. (1990). Glucose metabolism and calcium antagonists. *Horm. Metab. Res. Suppl.* 22, 48.

True, B.L., Perry, P.J., and Burns, E.A. (1987). Profound hypoglycaemia with the addition of a tricyclic antidepressant to maintenance sulfonylurea therapy. *Am. J. Psychiatry* 144, 1220.

Tse, W.Y. and Kendall, M. (1994). Is there a role for beta-blockers in hypertensive diabetic patients? *Diabetic Med.* 11, 137.

Tucker, R.M., Haq, Y., Denning, D.W., *et al.* (1991). Adverse events associated with itraconazole in 189 patients on chronic therapy. *J. Antimicrob. Chemother.* 26, 561.

van der Vange, N., Kloosterboer, H.J., and Haspels, A.A. (1987). Effect of seven low-dose combined oral contraceptive preparations on carbohydrate metabolism. *Am. J. Obstet. Gynecol.* 156, 918.

Vaziri, N.D., Stokes, J., and Treadwell, T.R. (1981). Lactic acidosis, a complication of papaverine overdose. *Clin. Toxicol.* 18, 417.

Vendesborg, P.B. (1979). Lithium treatment and glucose tolerance in manic melancholic patients. *Acta Psychiatr. Scand.* 59, 306.

Vogel, C., Caraccio, T., Mofenson, H., *et al.* (1995). Alcohol intoxication in young children. *J. Toxicol. Clin. Toxicol.* 33, 25.

Wahl, P., Walden, C., Knopp, R., *et al.* (1983). Effect of estrogen/progestin potency on lipid/lipoprotein cholesterol. *N. Engl. J. Med.* 308, 862.

Walker, E.D. (1988). Hyperglycemia. A complication of chemotherapy in children. *Cancer Nurs.* 11, 18.

Wang, Y.J., Chu, H.Y., Shu, S.G., *et al.* (1993). Hyperglycemia induced by chemotherapeutic agents used in acute lymphoblastic leukemia: report of three cases. *Chung Hua i Hsueh Tsa Chih (Chinese Medical Journal)* 1, 457.

Warnock, J.K. and Biggs, F. (1997). Nefazodone-induced hypoglycemia in a diabetic patient with major depression. *Am. J. Psychiatry* 154, 288.

Waskin, H., Stehr-Green, J.K., Helmick, C.G., *et al.* (1988). Risk factors for hypoglycaemia associated with pentamidine therapy for pneumocystis pneumonia. *JAMA* 260, 345.

Wasserman, D. and Amitai, Y. (1992). Hypoglycemia following albuterol overdose in a child. *Am. J. Emerg. Med.* 10, 556.

Waziri, R. and Nelson, J. (1978). Lithium in diabetes mellitus: A paradoxical response. *J. Clin. Psychiatry* 39, 623.

Webbe, G. (1994). Human cysticercosis: parasitology, pathology, clinical manifestations and available treatment. *Pharmacol. Ther.* 64, 175.

Weber, J., Gunn, H., Yang, J., *et al.* (1994). A phase I trial of intravenous interleukin-6 in patients with advanced cancer. *Journal of Immunotherapy with Emphasis on Tumor Immunology* 15, 292.

Weissman, D.E., Dufer, D., Vogel, V., *et al.* (1987). Corticosteroid toxicity in neuro-oncology patients. *J. Neuro-oncol.* 5, 125.

White, N.J., Warrell, D.A., Chanthavanich, P., *et al.* (1983). Severe hypoglycaemia and hyperinsulinemia in falciparum malaria. *N. Engl. J. Med.* 309, 61.

Whitefield, C.L. (1971). Isoniazid overdose: report of 40 patients, with a critical analysis of treatment and suggestions for prevention. *Am. Rev. Resp. Dis.* 103, 887.

Wicklmayr, M., Rett, K., Deitze, G., *et al.* (1990). Effects of beta-blocking agents on insulin secretion and glucose disposal. *Horm. Metab. Res. Suppl.* 22, 29.

Wilde, M.I. and McTavish, D. (1997). Insulin Lispro. A review of its pharmacological properties and therapeutic use in the management of diabetes mellitus. *Drugs* 54, 597.

Wilson, D.E., Birchfield, G.R., Hejazi, J.S., *et al.* (1989). Hypocholesterolemia in patients treated with recombinant interleukin-2: appearance of remnant-like lipoproteins. *J. Clin. Oncol.* 7, 1573.

Winocour, P., Waldek, S., and Anderson, D.C. (1986). Captopril and blood glucose. *Lancet* ii, 461.

Winter, W.E., Funahashi, M., and Koons, J. (1992). Encainide-induced diabetes: analysis of islet cell function. *Res. Commun. Chem. Pathol. Pharmacol.* 76, 259.

World Health Organisation (WHO) (1985). Technical report series No. 727, p. 10. WHO, Geneva.

Wright, A.D., Barber, S.G., Kendall, M.J., *et al.* (1979). Beta-adrenoreceptor-blocking drugs and blood sugar control in diabetes mellitus. *BMJ* i, 159.

Wright, J., Abolfathi, A., Penman, E., *et al.* (1980). Pancreatic somatostatinoma presenting with hypoglycemia. *Clin. Endocrinol.* 12, 603.

Yang, C.C., Yang, L.Y., and Deng, J.F. (1995). Hypoglycemia following ethanol ingestion in children: report of a case. *Journal of the Formosan Medical Association* 94, 267.

Yao, K., Uchigata, Y., Kyono, H., *et al.* (1992). Human insulin-specific immunoglobulin G antibody and hypoglycemic attacks after the injection of gold thioglucose. *J. Endocrinol. Invest.* 15, 43.

Yarchoan, R., Pluda, J.M., Thomas, R.V., *et al.* (1990). Long-term toxicity/activity profile of 2′,3′-dideoxyinosine in AIDS or AIDS-related complex. *Lancet* 336, 526.

Yudkin, J.S. (1991). Hypertension and non-insulin dependent diabetes. *BMJ* 303, 730.

Zanella, M.T., Santiago, R.C.M., de Sa, J.R., *et al.* (1988). Hypertension and diabetes: clinical problems. *Drugs* 35 (Suppl. 6), 135.

Zenobi, P.D., Holzmann, P., Glatz, Y., *et al.* (1992). Insulin-like growth factor I improves glucose and lipid metabolism in type 2 diabetes mellitus. *J. Clin. Invest.* 90, 2234.

Zenobi, P.D., Holzmann, P., Glatz, Y., *et al.* (1993). Improvement of lipid profile in type 2 (non-insulin-dependent) diabetes mellitus by insulin-like growth factor I. *Diabetologia* 36, 465.

Zimmerman, B.G., Sybertz, E.J., and Wong, P.C. (1984). Interaction between sympathetic and renin–angiotensin systems. *J. Hypertens.* 2, 581.

Zogno, M.G., Tolfo, L., and Draghi, E. (1994). Hypoglycemia caused by maprotiline in a patient taking oral antidiabetics. *Ann. Pharmacother.* 28, 406.

Zumoff, B. and Hellman, L. (1977). Aggravation of diabetic hyperglycemia by chlordiazepoxide. *JAMA* 237, 1960.

17. Disorders of metabolism 2

R. SWAMINATHAN

Acid–base balance

Acidosis

Respiratory acidosis

In respiratory acidosis, the blood hydogen ion concentration is increased, pH is reduced, and pCO_2 is elevated. The bicarbonate concentration is normal in acute respiratory acidosis and becomes elevated in chronic respiratory acidosis. Drugs may cause respiratory acidosis by reducing ventilation either by depressing the respiratory centre or by interfering with the neuromuscular transmission.

Any drug that causes coma or reduces consciousness may depress the respiratory centre and lead to respiratory acidosis. This is most commonly seen with overdosage (Rose 1994) but some drugs can cause respiratory depression in therapeutic doses. Such drugs include narcotics, barbiturates, benzodiazepines, non-barbiturate hypnotics, and alcohols (Rose 1994). Morphine and heroin reduce the hypoxic and hypercapnic ventilatory drives in normal subjects when given in therapeutic doses, and in overdose there is respiratory depression. The respiratory acidosis in heroin overdose is often complicated by pulmonary oedema, which further reduces gas exchange. Narcotic analgesics given to the mother during labour can cause respiratory depression and acidosis in the neonate. Buprenorphine and pethidine used in the postoperative period have been reported to cause respiratory acidosis severe enough to require mechanical ventilation (Carl et al. 1987). The degree of depression by barbiturates is directly related to the level of drug within the nervous system. In patients with underlying lung disease, barbiturates may cause acute respiratory acidosis. Acute respiratory failure and respiratory acidosis are universally seen with severe overdoses of barbiturates. Benzodiazepines, in therapeutic doses, will depress respiration in patients with chronic obstructive airways disease and produce CO_2 retention; in higher doses, respiratory depression is seen even in normal subjects, but it is not as severe as that with barbiturates unless other depressants such as alcohol are taken. The muscle-relaxant property of benzodiazepines further aggravates the respiratory depression in patients with chronic obstructive airways disease, in whom the work of respiration is increased (Sybrecht 1983). Other non-barbiturate hypnotic sedatives, especially when taken in combination with alcohol or other depressants, can cause severe depression of respiration in cases of overdose. Alcohol, both ethanol and methanol, can cause significant respiratory depression in acute intoxication. Isopropanol, which is used as a sterilizing agent, rubbing alcohol, and in aftershave lotions, causes respiratory depression when ingested or absorbed via skin by its direct toxic effect on the respiratory centre (Pappas et al. 1991; Vale et al. 1996). Anaesthetic agents such as fentanyl may cause delayed respiratory depression (Lehot 1989). Very high concentrations of salicylate depress the respiratory centre and can lead to respiratory depression (Meredith et al. 1996). Non-steroidal anti-inflammatory agents (NSAID) which are propionic acid derivatives (such as ibuprofen) can cause hypoventilation (Smolinske et al. 1990).

Respiratory acidosis can also be caused by an effect on the respiratory muscles. Such events are seen with muscle relaxants, drug-induced hypokalaemia, and hypophosphataemia (Newmann et al. 1977; Crook and Swaminathan 1996). A similar effect is seen with some antibiotics which block the neuromuscular junction and cause a peripheral myopathy. This effect is seen at high dosage and the antibiotics that have been implicated include the aminoglycosides, polymyxins A, B, and E, bacitracin, clindamycin, lincomycin, colistin, and the tetracyclines (Rutten et al. 1980). Large amounts of carbohydrate administered intravenously (Jih et al. 1996) or via dialysis (Cohn et al. 1990) can cause respiratory acidosis, especially in the presence of pre-existing respiratory disease.

Sodium valproate in normal therapeutic dose caused respiratory failure and the association was confirmed by withdrawal and rechallenge with the drug. This effect could be due to muscle weakness related to carnitine deficiency or mitochondrial dysfunction (Trehan and Clark 1993).

Treatment

Respiratory acidosis can be treated by discontinuing the drug concerned and increasing the removal of the drug from the body in cases of overdose. Specific antidotes if available, such as in the case of morphine poisoning, should also be given. Artificial ventilation may be required in severe cases.

Metabolic acidosis

Metabolic acidosis is characterized by a low arterial pH, a reduced plasma bicarbonate, and a compensatory decrease in pCO_2. Drugs can cause metabolic acidosis by increasing the acid load, by increasing the loss of bicarbonate, or by interfering with hydrogen ion excretion. It can be classified according to whether there is an increased anion gap or normal anion gap (hyperchloraemic acidosis) (Table 17.1).

Metabolic acidosis with an increased anion gap

The biguanides metformin and phenformin are well recognized as a cause of lactic acidosis (Campbell 1985; Bailey and Turner 1996). The reported incidence of lactic acidosis with phenformin ranged from 0.25 to 1 case per 1000 patient-years (Hermann and Melander 1992) and it is estimated to be 10 to 20 times greater than that for metformin (Krentz *et al.* 1994). In many countries, phenformin was withdrawn from clinical use in the 1970s due to this high incidence of lactic acidosis (Bailey and Turner 1996). The incidence of lactic acidosis induced by metformin has been estimated to be 0.01 to 0.08 (average 0.03) case per 1000 patient-years (Bailey 1992; Hermann and Melander 1992) and the mortality associated with lactic acidosis is about 50 per cent (Bailey 1992). Metformin is not metabolised and is excreted unchanged in urine (Hermann and Melander 1992) and, therefore, in patients with renal impairment, blood concentrations are likely to be high; this increases the risk of lactic acidosis (Harrower 1996). Other factors that increase the risk of lactic acidosis are the presence of hepatic disease (Bailey 1992) or other factors which increase lactate concentration, for example, alcohol abuse, and shock. Some authors suggest that in most cases lactic acidosis occurs as a result of overlooking one or more of the contraindications to its use (Campbell 1985; Bailey and Turner 1996; Campbell *et al.* 1996).

TABLE 17.1
Causes of drug-induced metabolic acidosis

With increased ion gap

  Biguanides

  Alcohols — ethanol, methanol, ethylene glycol, propylene glycol, benzyl alcohol, diethylene glycol

  Polyhydric sugars — fructose, sorbitol, xylitol

  Salicylate

  Paracetamol

  Others — β-agonists and catecholamines, folk remedies (sulphur), germanium, isoniazid, Lugol's iodine, nalidixic acid, niacin, nitroprusside, nucleoside analogues (fialuridine, fludarabine, zidovudine), paraldehyde, pentamidine, povidone–iodine, propionic acid derivatives (ibuprofen and fenoprofen), streptozotocin, verapamil

With normal anion gap

1. Gastrointestinal loss of bicarbonate
   cholestyramine, laxatives, purgatives

2. Renal loss of bicarbonate (Type 2 renal tubular acidosis)
   arginine hydrochloride, carbonic anhydrase inhibitors, gentamicin, heavy metals (lead, cadmium, mercury), mercaptopurine, methyl-3-chromone, outdated tetracyclines, streptozotocin, sulphanilamide, tacrolimus (FK506), valproic acid

3. Decreased hydrogen ion secretion (Type 1 renal tubular acidosis)
   amiloride, amphotericin, analgesic abuse, cyclamate, cyclosporin, lithium, non-steroidal anti-inflammatory drugs, toluene

4. Ingestion of acids
   ammonium chloride, hydrochloric acid, L-arginine and L-lysine

Furthermore, a significant number of cases are associated with overdosage (Innerfield 1996). Metformin does not increase fasting plasma lactate concentrations (De Fronzo *et al.* 1995; Stamvoll *et al.* 1995). Although conversion of lactate to glucose was decreased by metformin, lactate oxidation was increased and lactate turnover and lactate metabolism by muscle were unaltered (Stamvoll *et al.* 1995). This action of metformin is unlike that of phenformin, which inhibits mitochondrial oxidation of lactate, thereby increasing the risk of lactic acidosis (Crofford 1995). Furthermore, phenformin lactic acidosis has been associated with an inborn error of hepatic hydroxylation enzymes (Kreisberg and Wood 1983; Oates *et al.* 1983). The decreased conversion of lactate to glucose due to metformin may become significant if there are associated conditions such as hepatic disease which impair the removal of lactate and hence increase the risk of lactic acidosis.

Treatment of biguanide-induced lactic acidosis is unsatisfactory, and mortality is relatively high. Treatment with insulin and glucose has been recommended (Kreisberg and Wood 1983) together with bicarbonate (Ryder 1987). However, intravenous bicarbonate may paradoxically aggravate the intracellular acidosis. An equimolar mixture of sodium bicarbonate and sodium carbonate (carbicarb) has been suggested as an alternative (Stacpoole 1993). Dichloroacetate, which has also been proposed as an alternative in the treatment of the lactic acidosis, was found to be ineffective in a recent placebo-controlled study (Stacpoole *et al.* 1992). Haemodialysis is now recommended as the treatment of choice to remove the drug as well as the lactate (Gan *et al.* 1992; Bailey and Turner 1996).

Ethanol may cause a metabolic acidosis that is mainly due to ketoacids (Rose 1994); this may be seen in nearly a quarter of alcoholic patients admitted to hospital (Elisaf *et al.* 1994). Factors contributing to the acidosis include increased mobilization of free fatty acids, relative or absolute deficiency of insulin, and changes in the ketogenic capacity of the liver. Ethanol intoxication may also give rise to lactic acidosis by increasing lactate production and inhibiting alternate pathways for pyruvate removal (Stacpoole 1993).

Methanol is metabolised to formaldehyde and then to formic acid, and severe metabolic acidosis with a high anion gap follows its ingestion, usually after a delay, reaching a peak at 12 hours. The acidosis is mainly due to formic acid, although other metabolites may contribute (Bennett *et al.* 1953; Rose 1994). Treatment involves the use of ethanol to inhibit metabolism of methanol, and dialysis.

Ethylene glycol has many metabolites and of these glycolic and oxalic acids are the most toxic and responsible for the high anion-gap metabolic acidosis which follows ingestion (Rose 1994). The acidosis is further complicated by renal failure. The concentration of lactate levels is only slightly elevated, except when there is circulatory failure. An unusual case of ethylene glycol poisoning with normal anion gap, due to occult bromide intoxication, has been reported (Heckerling 1987). The treatment of ethylene glycol poisoning consists of ethanol infusion to reduce the metabolism of ethylene glycol to toxic metabolites, together with dialysis to eliminate toxic metabolites.

Diethylene glycol, which is used as a solvent and as an additive to wines, is metabolised to 2-hydroxyethoxy acetic acid (Vale *et al.* 1996) and causes metabolic acidosis, hepatotoxicity, and renal failure. Deaths from diethylene glycol poisoning as a result of application of a burn cream containing this glycol have been reported (Canterall *et al.* 1987). As with other glycols, treatment consists of ethanol administration to block the metabolism of diethylene glycol and dialysis or haemofiltration (Vale *et al.* 1996).

Propylene glycol (1,2-propanediol) is a clear, colourless, odourless, and viscous liquid with a sweet taste that is used as a vehicle for a large number of drugs that are insufficiently soluble or are unstable in water (Reynolds 1989). Although a large proportion (up to 45 per cent) of propylene glycol is excreted unchanged in the urine, a significant amount is metabolised to lactate and pyruvate in the liver, and when large amounts are administered as a vehicle, lactic acidosis may result, especially in the presence of renal impairment (Kelner and Bailey 1985). In a study of 28 patients receiving nitroglycerin (containing propylene glycol) intravenously, six patients (21 per cent) had high lactate concentrations (Demey *et al.* 1988); the authors, however, dismissed the elevation as being of minor clinical significance. Kelner and Bailey (1985), on the other hand, found elevated lactate concentrations (up to 24 mmol per litre) in patients receiving intravenous solutions containing propylene glycol and suggested that it may be an important cause of lactic acidosis in hospitalized patients. More recently, van de Wiele and colleagues (1995) described a case of lactic acidosis induced by propylene glycol toxicity due to intravenous administration of etomidate, which has 35% propylene glycol as vehicle.

Benzyl alcohol is used in subcutaneous or intramuscular injections for its disinfectant and anaesthetic action (Reynolds 1989), and can cause metabolic acidosis. Menon and co-workers (1984) reported that the use of benzyl alcohol in neonatal intensive care units was associated with metabolic acidosis and they observed an improvement in survival after its use was discontinued.

In the above situations the presence of an osmolar gap (difference between measured and calculated osmolality) usually gives a clue to the presence of unidentified osmoles such as alcohols (M. Demedts *et al.* 1994).

Polyhydric sugars, fructose, xylitol, and sorbitol, have been used as substitutes for glucose in parenteral nutrition and have been associated with lactic acidosis (Kashner 1986). Metabolism of fructose causes depletion of hepatic adenosine triphosphate, which leads to an increase in glycolysis and lactate concentration (Stacpoole 1993). Sorbitol and xylitol act in the same way in that they cause depletion of adenine nucleotides (Krebs *et al.* 1975). Fructose can cause a striking, dose-related, renal tubular acidosis in the very occasional patient with the rare disease hereditary fructose intolerance (DuBose *et al.* 1996).

In three patients with the hyperosmolar syndrome, infusion of 5% fructose caused severe lactic acidosis (Druml *et al.* 1989) and in such patients infusion of fructose and xylitol is a life-threatening risk (DuBose *et al.* 1996).

Salicylate intoxication, in addition to causing respiratory alkalosis by direct stimulation of the respiratory centre, can also cause metabolic acidosis (Rose 1994). The toxicity of salicylate is in part due to uncoupling of oxidative phosphorylation in mitochondria, resulting in disturbances of carbohydrate, lipid, and protein metabolism leading to increased lactate as well as ketoacids (Meredith *et al.* 1996). The increased anion gap seen in salicylate overdose is therefore due to accumulation of lactate, ketoacids, salicylate, and other organic acids (Rose 1994). Salicylate intoxication in adults usually causes respiratory alkalosis or mixed metabolic acidosis and respiratory alkalosis, whereas in children and infants metabolic acidosis is more prominent. Salicylate intoxication can result not only from taking aspirin but also methyl salicylate ('oil of wintergreen') by mouth (Chan *et al.* 1995) and from percutaneous absorption of keratolytic agents (Germann *et al.* 1996; Meredith *et al.* 1996). Fatal salicylate overdosage of bismuth subsalicylate, available in some countries, has been described (Sainsbury 1991). If aspirin is taken in enteric-coated tablets, absorption and development of symptoms may be delayed (Pierce *et al.* 1991). Treatment of salicylate intoxication involves increasing the elimination of the drug by forced alkaline diuresis or haemodialysis.

Although the major manifestation of paracetamol toxicity is liver failure, metabolic acidosis with high lactate concentrations has been described in paracetamol overdose (Meredith et al. 1996). In these cases the anion gap is increased. High lactate concentrations are frequently found during the first 15 hours after taking paracetamol and these are not significant clinically except in severe paracetamol poisoning. The high lactate is due to increased lactate production as a result of inhibition of mitochondrial respiration (Meredith *et al.* 1996). Metabolic acidosis is more common in those presenting too late (more than 15 hours after taking an overdose) for treatment with *N*-acetylcysteine, in whom it is due to decreased lactate clearance as a result of liver damage and increased lactate production resulting from poor tissue perfusion.   Paraldehyde has been reported to cause high anion-gap metabolic acidosis (Linter and Linter 1986). It is usually seen in chronic alcoholics who drink large amounts of paraldehyde. Although paraldehyde is metabolised to acetic acid, the metabolic acidosis is due to accumulation of multiple organic acids. Severe lactic acidosis following paraldehyde administration has also been reported (Linter and Linter 1986).

Isoniazid poisoning has been associated with lactic acidosis when it is usually secondary to the grand mal fits that result from the decreased tissue concentrations of pyridoxal 5-phosphate and γ-aminobutyric acid (GABA) (Proudfoot *et al.* 1996). The acidosis can be very severe (Hankins *et al.* 1987) but usually disappears within several hours of control of the fits (Chin *et al.* 1979). Acute metabolic acidosis due to β-hydroxybutyrate, however, has been reported in isoniazid toxicity (Pahl *et al.* 1984). The incidence of isoniazid toxicity is high in certain groups (Proudfoot *et al.* 1996; Tai *et al.* 1996) but this is most likely due to the ready availability of antituberculous drugs rather than to racial differences. Patients with isoniazid poisoning have been successfully treated with large doses of intravenous pyridoxine hydrochloride (Watkins *et al.* 1990; Tai *et al.* 1996).

Nicotinic acid used in the treatment of hyperlipidaemia, can cause lactic acidosis in high doses (Earthman *et al.* 1991). Toxicity is more likely with sustained-release preparations (Dalton and Berry 1992), and when alcohol is taken at the same time (Schwab and Bachhuber 1991).

Nitroprusside, used in hypertensive crises or to produce controlled hypotension during surgery, is converted to cyanide (Przybylo *et al.* 1995) through a chemical reaction with haemoglobin, and cyanide poisoning can occur, usually after the use of large doses of nitroprusside over a prolonged period. Lactic acidosis is a feature of cyanide poisoning (Borron and Baud 1996) due to inhibition of oxidative phosphorylation, electron transport, and cellular respiration by the cyanide. Sodium azide may be converted endogenously to cyanide and severe metabolic acidosis may result from sodium azide ingestion (DuBose *et al.* 1996).

Catecholamines and other sympathomimetics may rarely produce lactic acidosis as a result of increased glycogenolysis, glycolysis, reduced tissue blood flow, and reduced oxygenation (Rose 1994). In patients with vascular collapse, catecholamines may exaggerate an already present lactic acidosis (Day *et al.* 1996). β-Adrenergic drugs such as ritodrine (Braden *et al.* 1985*a*) and theophylline in therapeutic doses (Braden *et al.* 1985*b*) or in toxic doses (Bernard 1991) can cause metabolic acidosis. In most cases, lactic acidosis was found, although ketoacidosis has also been reported (Ryan *et al.* 1989). Acidosis is more likely to occur in alcoholic patients treated with β-adrenergic drugs such as salbutamol, as alcohol metabolism reduces lactate clearance (Taboulet *et al.* 1995). Sympathomimetics such as terbutaline, used as a tocolytic agent, cross the placenta and can cause toxicity including metabolic acidosis in infants (Thorkelsson and Loughead 1991).

Lactic acidosis has been reported with the use of streptozotocin, Lugol's iodine, nalidixic acid, with papaverine, which inhibits cellular respiration, and with povidone–iodine used in ointment for burns (Rose 1994; DuBose et al. 1996). However, some of the cases of metabolic acidosis ascribed to povidone–iodine reported in the literature have been in patients with sepsis or other form of morbidity, so the metabolic disturbances may have been caused by other factors (Steen 1993).

Pentamidine, used in treatment of patients with AIDS complicated by *Pneumocystis carinii*, has been reported to cause ketoacidosis (Lambertus et al. 1988).

Verapamil, a calcium-channel blocker, has been reported to cause metabolic acidosis (Roth et al. 1989) together with other toxic effects, including renal failure (Pritza et al. 1991). Most of the cases of verapamil toxicity were with the sustained-release form (Ashraf et al. 1995) and this form of verapamil should be used with caution in patients with renal impairment (Pritza et al. 1991).

Propionic acid derivatives, such as ibuprofen, fenoprofen, and naproxen taken in large doses as in self-poisoning, can cause metabolic acidosis (Kolodzik et al. 1990; Smolinske et al. 1990; Le et al. 1994; Mattana et al. 1997). The acidosis is likely to be due to renal failure with a contribution from lactate as a result of hypoxia following respiratory failure (Mattana et al. 1997).

Valproate toxicity mainly affects the liver but fatal cases are associated with severe lactic acidosis (Siemes et al. 1993). Overdosage with misoprostol, a prostaglandin E_1 analogue, has been reported to cause metabolic acidosis in a pregnant woman (Bond and Van Zee 1994).

The nucleoside analogue fialuridine, used in the treatment of chronic hepatitis B, caused lactic acidosis in seven out of 15 patients (McKenzie et al. 1995). Zidovudine, another analogue, used in patients with AIDS, caused severe lactic acidosis (Olano et al. 1995). Fludarabine, an analogue used in the treatment of malignancy, also caused metabolic acidosis (Hood and Finley 1991). In these cases the toxicity is thought to be due to the effect of the drugs on mitochondria.

Germanium, available without a prescription in many countries, is used as treatment of many conditions, including AIDS and cancer. Severe lactic acidosis and renal and liver failure associated with germanium have been reported (Krapf et al. 1992).

Ingestion of folk remedies containing sulphur is associated with generation of sulphuric acid that is normally excreted rapidly in the urine. In the presence of renal failure, ingestion of sulphur may result in severe metabolic acidosis (Rose 1994). Administration of prednisolone to patients with the Kearns–Sayre syndrome (progressive external ophthalmoplegia, heart block, elevated CSF protein, and ragged muscle fibres) was associated with fatal acidosis — lactic acidosis as well as ketoacidosis (Bachynski et al. 1986). The use of cetrimonium bromide ('Cetavlon') to sterilize a hydatid cyst during surgery was reported to cause high anion-gap metabolic acidosis (Momblano et al. 1984), probably from absorption of the cetrimonium bromide. Use of pethidine in labour was associated with metabolic acidosis in the newborn (Kariniemi and Rosti 1986). Intravesical irrigation with alum in the treatment of intractable haematuria caused a fatal metabolic acidosis in an elderly patient with poor renal function (Shoskes et al. 1992).

Metabolic acidosis with normal anion gap

Gastrointestinal loss of bicarbonate can give rise to metabolic acidosis with normal anion gap and high plasma chloride; this is seen in laxative abuse (Rose 1994). Cholestyramine, used in the treatment of hypercholesterolaemia, acts as an anion exchange resin and exchanges chloride for endogenous bicarbonate, leading to metabolic acidosis (Blom and Monasch 1983). Ingestion of calcium chloride and magnesium sulphate can also lead to a hypochloraemic acidosis (DuBose et al. 1996).

Bicarbonate reabsorption in the tubules is mediated by carbonic anhydrase, and carbonic anhydrase inhibitors such as acetazolamide will cause normal anion-gap metabolic acidosis (Sporn et al. 1991). As acetazolamide is cleared by the kidney, the blood concentration is related to creatinine clearance and the risk of acidosis is greater in patients with renal impairment (Chapron et al. 1989). The incidence of severe acidosis in elderly patients has been reported to be 3.7 per cent, moderate acidosis 37 per cent, and mild acidosis 14.8 per cent (Heller et al. 1985). Concomitant treatment with salicylates increased the risk of acidosis (Cowan et al. 1984). Streptozotocin and sulphanilamide produce acidosis in a similar way to acetazolamide (Kreisberg and Wood 1983). Mafenide acetate, used topically in treating burns, is absorbed and inhibits carbonic anhydrase, causing metabolic acidosis (Asch et al. 1970).

Drugs can also cause acidosis by inducing a Fanconi syndrome. Drugs thus implicated are: tetracyclines degraded by prolonged storage, methyl-3-chromone, mercaptopurine, gentamicin, sodium valproate, and heavy metals such as lead, mercury, and cadmium (Rose 1994). The offending agents in the case of tetracycline are the degradation products rather than the parent drug; this syndrome is now rarely seen as the formulation of tetracycline has been changed. Ifosfamide, an isomer of cyclophosphamide, causes proximal tubular acidosis (Antman *et al.* 1990) in up to 25 per cent of children treated (Skinner *et al.* 1996). Renal tubular acidosis has also followed the use of methoxyflurane, foscarnet (Navarro *et al.* 1995), and co-trimoxazole during treatment of AIDS (Domingo *et al.* 1995).

Distal acidification defects will give rise to metabolic acidosis and are seen with amphotericin, lithium, toluene, and cyclamate, and in analgesic nephropathy (Rose 1994; DuBose *et al.* 1996). Amphotericin interacts with the tubular membrane and causes increased permeability, allowing back-diffusion of hydrogen ions (Rose 1994). Toluene and lithium have been thought to act in a similar fashion, though in the case of lithium some studies do not support this (Rose 1994). Although a renal acidification defect is seen in patients treated with lithium, metabolic acidosis is not often seen (Boton *et al.* 1987). An unusual case of toluene-induced metabolic acidosis in which ketoacids were found has been described (Jone and Wu 1988). Toluene sniffing by their mothers has been associated with tubular acidosis in the newborn (Erramouspe *et al.* 1996).

Recent studies suggest that the acidosis due to toluene is caused by accumulation of hippuric acid rather than distal renal tubular acidosis (Carlisle *et al.* 1991). Edetic acid (ethylenediamine tetra-acetic acid, EDTA) used as a chelating agent has caused renal tubular acidosis (Magee 1985).

Impairment in hydrogen ion secretion is also seen in Type 4 renal tubular acidosis, which is due to aldosterone deficiency or aldosterone resistance. This is associated with hyperkalaemia (DuBose 1997). Type 4 renal tubular acidosis has been reported with indomethacin, amiloride, triamterene, captopril, and spironolactone (Rose 1994). Patients with intrinsic renal disease are more susceptible (O'Connell and Colledge 1993). Analgesics, particularly phenacetin, may also cause Type 4 renal tubular acidosis. Phenacetin metabolites damage the renal medulla to cause a chronic tubulointerstitial nephritis, generalized dysfunction of distal tubules, and insensitivity to aldosterone (Kreisberg and Wood 1983).

Ingestion of acids can also cause normal anion-gap acidosis. This is seen following administration of ammonium chloride, which may be present in cough mixtures (Rose 1994), hydrochloric acid, and the cationic amino acids arginine, lysine, and histidine, the chloride forms of which are used in parenteral nutrition (DuBose *et al.* 1996). The acid load of total parenteral nutrition can be reduced by supplementation with acetate (Berkel-

hammer *et al.* 1988). Concurrent administration of potassium-sparing diuretics to patients receiving total parenteral nutrition caused metabolic acidosis which disappeared on discontinuing the diuretic (Kushner and Sitrin 1986). Severe metabolic acidosis may follow the ingestion of household bleach (NaOCl) owing to the formation of hypochlorous acid in the stomach (Ward and Routledge 1988).

The immunosuppressive agents cyclosporin and tacrolimus, can both cause hyperchloraemic metabolic acidosis (Aguilera *et al.* 1992; O'Gorman *et al.* 1995; McDiarmid 1996). Cyclosporin A caused hyperchloraemic metabolic acidosis in about 17 per cent of renal transplant recipients (Stahl *et al.* 1986). The effect of cyclosporin is predominantly due to a defect in the distal acidification (distal renal tubular acidosis) (Aguilera *et al.* 1992), whereas tacrolimus (FK506) is thought to cause a proximal tubular acidosis (O'Gorman *et al.* 1995). Metabolic acidosis developed in seriously ill children who received chloramphenicol intravenously (Evans and Kleiman 1986), but the cause of the acidosis was not clear. Cisplatin treatment was reported to cause a renal acidification defect in four of 12 patients, but there was no clinical metabolic acidosis (Swainson *et al.* 1985). Cocaine poisoning has been associated with respiratory and metabolic acidosis (Jonsson *et al.* 1983).

Dextran, which is used as a plasma substitute, can cause metabolic acidosis as result of anaphylactic reactions (Ljungstrom and Renck 1987) or of development of acute renal failure (Kurnik *et al.* 1991).

Some stored blood has relatively low pH and if large amounts are given metabolic acidosis may occur (Koch 1996).

Treatment

In the treatment of metabolic acidosis the offending drug should be withdrawn and in severe cases bicarbonate may be infused to correct the acidosis; enough bicarbonate should be infused to raise the pH to about 7.2. Correction of pH to 7.4 with bicarbonate is not recommended (Adrogue and Madias 1998*a*).

Alkalosis

Respiratory alkalosis

In respiratory alkalosis there is a primary decrease in pCO_2 owing to an increase in ventilation, and the pH is increased. Bicarbonate concentration will be low in chronic respiratory alkalosis. Any drug that stimulates respiration may cause respiratory alkalosis.

Salicylate in high doses causes hyperventilation, and respiratory alkalosis is a common feature of salicylate intoxication, the hyperventilation being characterized by an increase in rate and depth (Meredith *et al.* 1996). The respiratory stimulation is due to a direct effect on the respiratory centre; the mechanism is not known, but possibly involves uncoupling of oxidative phosphorylation and local changes in pH within the central nervous system (Meredith *et al.* 1996). Salicylate also causes a metabolic acidosis due to its effect on metabolism, and the acid–base picture can therefore be variable. Gabow and colleagues (1978) have reported that 78 per cent of patients with salicylate intoxication show respiratory alkalosis. Other pharmacological agents, such as nikethamide and xanthines in high doses, can cause respiratory alkalosis. Leson and co-workers (1988) described the disorder in a case of caffeine overdose in a 16-year-old male who ingested 6–8 g of caffeine. Nortriptyline has been reported to cause severe respiratory alkalosis that required mechanical ventilation to correct (Sunderrajan *et al.* 1985).

Treatment

Withdrawal of the offending drug may be the only treatment required. In cases of overdose, efforts to accelerate the elimination of the drug may be necessary. Very rarely, mechanical ventilation may be required.

Metabolic alkalosis

Metabolic alkalosis is characterized by an elevation of pH and plasma bicarbonate with a compensatory decrease in pCO_2. It can be induced by increased retention of bicarbonate or increased loss of acid. The causes of drug-induced metabolic alkalosis are listed in Table 17.2.

It is important to note that in most situations of metabolic alkalosis the mechanism responsible for alkalosis not only generates the alkalosis but also maintains it (Rose 1994).

Loss of hydrogen ions

Drugs that cause protracted vomiting can cause sufficient loss of acid to cause metabolic alkalosis. Occasionally, anticancer agents such as cisplatin can cause severe vomiting that cannot be controlled by antiemetics. Severe hypochloraemic metabolic alkalosis has been described in an infant as a result of increased gastric acid secretion induced by tolazoline (Adams *et al.* 1980). Chronic intake of antacids such as magnesium hydroxide has been reported to cause metabolic alkalosis, especially in combination with cation-exchange resins (sodium polystyrene sulphonate), which are used in the treatment of hyperkalaemia. When magnesium hydroxide is ingested alone, the hydrogen ions of the gastric juice are buffered by the hydroxyl component of the

TABLE 17.2
Causes of drug-induced metabolic alkalosis

Loss of hydrogen ions

Gastrointestinal loss
drug-induced vomiting (e.g. cytotoxic drugs)
antacid therapy — especially in combination with cation-exchange resins

Renal loss
diuretics
carbenicillin and other penicillin derivatives
mineralocorticoid-like activity (e.g. carbenoxolone)

Retention of bicarbonate
administration of bicarbonate or its precursors
massive blood transfusion and plasma protein infusion
milk–alkali syndrome

Shift of hydrogen ions into cells
hypokalaemia
refeeding

compound leaving the magnesium to form insoluble complexes with bicarbonate, fats, and phosphates. This leaves only a small amount of bicarbonate to be absorbed and this does not cause alkalosis as long as renal function is normal. In the presence of the cation-exchange resin some of the magnesium binds to the resin leaving free bicarbonate to be absorbed. The net result is a gain of alkali and metabolic alkalosis. This is further aggravated by the presence of renal impairment, which reduces the ability to excrete the excess bicarbonate (Rose 1994). Inadvertent administration of antacids included as 'fillers' or buffers in tablets as, for example, in 'Panadol soluble', may cause alkalosis (Acomb *et al.* 1985).

Diuretics — both loop and thiazide types — are common causes of metabolic alkalosis, the severity of which varies with the degree of diuresis and the extent of depletion of extracellular fluid. The factors contributing to the alkalosis are volume contraction and increased urinary loss of hydrogen ions. The latter is due to increased secretion as a result of three factors: secondary hyperaldosteronism, increased distal flow, and the associated hypokalaemia (Rose 1994; DuBose *et al.* 1996). Metabolic alkalosis is a significant problem in neonates and infants treated with diuretics (Laudignon *et al.* 1989), and in adults from surreptitious ingestion of diuretics (DuBose *et al.* 1996). Diuretic-induced alkalosis can be severe enough to mask co-existing metabolic acidosis as, for example, in a diabetic patient with ketosis who presented initially with alkalosis (Cronin *et al.* 1984).

Excess mineralocorticoids or mineralocorticoid-like activity will cause metabolic alkalosis and hypokalaemia.

The alkalosis is due to a direct effect of these agents on hydrogen ion secretion in the distal tubules concurrently with increasing sodium reabsorption. The hypokalaemia caused by these agents maintains the alkalosis (Rose 1994). The causes are further discussed under Hypokalaemia.

Carbenicillin and other penicillins, when given in high doses, can cause metabolic alkalosis and hypokalaemia owing to the presence of carbenicillin in the renal tubular fluid as a non-reabsorbable anion (see Hypokalaemia).

Retention of bicarbonate

Sodium bicarbonate administered in the treatment of metabolic acidosis may result in metabolic alkalosis if large amounts are given. This is typically seen in situations where the underlying cause of the acidosis, for example, diabetic ketoacidosis or the lactic acidosis of cardiac arrest (Adrogue and Madias 1998*a*), is treated. Therapeutic ingestion of large quantities of sodium bicarbonate is associated with severe metabolic alkalosis (Mennen and Slovis 1988; Thomas and Stone 1994). Topical application of baking soda for the treatment of a napkin rash has caused the disorder (Gonzalez and Hogg 1981).

Administration of precursors such as lactate, acetate, citrate, or gluconate, which are rapidly metabolised to bicarbonate in the body, may lead to metabolic alkalosis. Preserved blood contains about 17 mmoles of citrate per unit and transfusion of large quantities of blood may lead to alkalosis (DuBose *et al.* 1996). Administration of human plasma protein fraction, which contains 40–50 mmol per litre of acetate, may have a similar result (Rahilley and Berl 1979). Citrate is used as an anticoagulant in haemodialysis and alkalosis may follow its use, especially in the long term (van der Meulen *et al.* 1992). Alkalosis can be avoided by reducing the buffer content of the dialysate (van der Meulen *et al.* 1992). Use of acetate and bicarbonate in regular haemodialysis will cause elevation of the bicarbonate concentration of plasma, although the rise in plasma bicarbonate is lower in the case of acetate (Scheppach *et al.* 1988). The milk–alkali syndrome, in which the alkalosis is due to ingestion of large amounts of alkali, is discussed under Calcium.

Shift of hydrogen ions into cells

Alkalosis may also result from a shift of hydrogen ions into cells. This, in addition to other mechanisms, occurs in hypokalaemia, raising the pH of extracellular fluid (Rose 1994). Refeeding after a prolonged fast can also raise the pH acutely, probably from intracellular shift of hydrogen ions as there is no volume depletion nor any abnormal increase in hydrogen ion excretion (DuBose *et al.* 1996).

Treatment

Withdrawal of the drug concerned and correction of any volume depletion and potassium depletion (if present) are enough to correct the metabolic alkalosis. Rarely, treatment with hydrochloric acid or ammonium chloride may be necessary (Brimioulle *et al.* 1989). In situations such as diuretic-induced alkalosis it is important to correct the chloride depletion as well (Adrogue and Madias 1998*b*).

Sodium and water balance

In an adult weighing 70 kg there are approximately 4000 millimoles of sodium and 42 litres of water. Sodium is mainly present in the extracellular fluid (ECF) and 60 per cent of the body water is intracellular. Sodium ion and its accompanying anions are the major determinants of ECF osmolality, which in turn is responsible for movement of water between ECF and intracellular fluid (ICF). Changes in body sodium are therefore usually accompanied by changes in water, and thus loss of body sodium will cause depletion of ECF volume and increase in body sodium will lead to expansion of ECF, and oedema. Volume depletion may be present without any change in plasma sodium concentration, or it may give rise to a low plasma osmolality and hyponatraemia (see below). Changes in water content lead to changes in plasma osmolality and plasma sodium concentration.

Hypernatraemia

An increase in plasma sodium concentration can arise either due to administration of sodium (without water) or due to loss of water. The latter, water depletion, is the commonest cause of hypernatraemia in clinical practice.

Rapid infusion of hypertonic saline or sodium bicarbonate can lead to sodium overload and hypernatraemia. In infants, hypernatraemia may result from incorrect use of oral rehydration (glucose–electrolyte) solutions (Kahn and Blum 1980), from high-salt feeds (Meadow 1993) or from administration of sodium bicarbonate (Simmons *et al.* 1974). In adults, sodium bicarbonate infusion during cardiopulmonary resuscitation (Mattar *et al.* 1974), accidental administration of hypertonic saline (Walter and Maresch 1987), or massive salt ingestion (Moder and Hurley 1990) may cause hypernatraemia. Severe hypernatraemia may also follow the absorption of sodium from wound packs soaked in antiseptic containing buffered sodium hypochlorite solution in hypertonic saline (Thorp *et al.* 1987). Hypernatraemia can also result from infusion of sodium sulphate (Heckman and Walsh 1967), sodium phosphate enemas (Fass *et al.* 1993), sodium citrate tablets, sodium emetics (Robertson 1977) and intra-amniotic administration of saline (Rose 1994; DuBose *et al.* 1996). The use of cation-exchange resins in the sodium phase may lead to excessive intake of sodium and hypernatraemia (Reynolds 1989). Overdosage or excessive use of baking soda as an antacid can lead to hypernatraemia (Thomas and Stone 1994), especially in children (Schindler and Hiner 1988). Some antacids can contribute substantial amounts of sodium, and can lead to hypernatraemia when given in large doses. Severe hypernatraemia (plasma sodium concentration 171 mmol per litre), hyperosmolality (400 mosmol per kg), cerebral dehydration and coma as a result of administration of large doses of the antacid magnesium trisilicate, which contains 600 mmol of sodium, have been reported (Faraj 1989). A moderate rise in plasma sodium concentration follows the administration of mineralocorticoids, or other steroids, or drugs like carbenoxolone that have mineralocorticoid-like activity (see Hypokalaemia). Hypernatraemia and acidosis can result from topical treatment of burns with povidone–iodine (Scoggin *et al.* 1977) and after sodium valproate intoxication (Schnabel *et al.* 1984). Hypernatraemia has also been reported with the use of large doses of sodium penicillin (Wright and Wilkowske 1987).

Hypernatraemia as a result of excessive loss of water may arise from loss of water either from the gastrointestinal tract or by the kidney. Therapeutic administration of lactulose (Nanji and Lauener 1984) or sorbitol (in the form of activated charcoal–sorbitol suspension) has caused severe hypernatraemic dehydration (Farley 1986; Moore 1988). The mechanism of hypernatraemia is a shift of water into the gut lumen as a result of the osmotic load (Farley 1986). Cathartics can cause hypernatraemia when used in the management of overdose (Caldwell *et al.* 1987) or when abused.

Loss of water in the urine results from inability to concentrate urine and conserve water. This may arise either as a result of inhibition of antidiuretic hormone (ADH) secretion or from inhibition of action of ADH on the renal tubules (nephrogenic diabetic insipidus). Ethanol and phenytoin inhibit ADH secretion (Robertson and Berl 1996). Hypernatraemia as been found in 2 per cent of alcoholic patients (Elisaf *et al.* 1994), and severe hypernatraemic coma is seen in phenytoin intoxication (Luscher *et al.* 1983). Lithium, demeclocycline, and methoxyflurane can cause nephrogenic diabetes insipidus (Robertson and Berl 1996): 20–25 per cent of

patients on lithium therapy are reported to have polyuria and polydipsia, and impaired concentrating ability has been found in 54 per cent of patients on lithium therapy (Boton *et al.* 1987). Lithium reduces the effectiveness of ADH by decreasing the generation of cyclic AMP and by inducing a postcyclic AMP defect (Yamaki *et al.* 1991). Hypernatraemia arises in patients treated with lithium, because of intoxication with the drug (Robertson 1995) or as a result of failure to maintain water intake. Demeclocyline can also cause reversible nephrogenic diabetes insipidus (Robertson and Berl 1996). The chemotherapeutic agent ifosfamide has been reported to cause nephrogenic diabetes insipidus in addition to other nephrotoxic effects (Skinner *et al.* 1990). Other drugs reported to cause nephrogenic diabetic insipidus are rifampicin and foscarnet (Robertson 1995).

Hypernatraemia may be seen in osmotic diuresis induced by high-protein infant feeding, intravenous hyperalimentation, and mannitol administration (Robertson and Berl 1996). Impairment in concentrating ability, and consequently hypernatraemia, occurs in hypokalaemia and hypercalcaemia (Rose 1994). For causes of drug-induced hypokalaemia and hypercalcaemia see the relevant sections.

It is important to note that hypernatraemia develops in all the above instances as a result of failure to maintain adequate water intake.

Treatment

Therapy for hypernatraemia depends on whether there is excess sodium or a true water depletion (Rose 1994). In absolute water depletion the deficit should be corrected slowly over a 48-hour period with water by mouth or with intravenous dextrose solution, as rapid correction may lead to cerebral oedema (Rose 1994). In cases of hypernatraemia due to sodium excess, in addition to giving sodium-free solutions, attempts should be made to encourage the excretion of sodium (e.g. by administration of a loop diuretic) in order to prevent volume overload. In patients with poor renal function, dialysis may be necessary.

Hyponatraemia

Hyponatraemia can arise either from volume depletion or from impaired ability to excrete (Table 17.3). Volume depletion can occur without hyponatraemia.

Volume depletion

Volume depletion without hyponatraemia may arise as a result of loss of sodium and water — either from the gastrointestinal tract or the kidney. Drugs that cause persistent vomiting or diarrhoea (cathartic agents) will lead to volume depletion. Volume depletion due to renal loss of sodium and water may arise due to agents which cause negative sodium balance, such as diuretics.

TABLE 17.3
Drugs causing hyponatraemia classified according to their mechanism of action

A. Volume depletion
  1. Gastrointestinal loss (e.g. cathartic agents)
  2. Renal salt loss
    carboplatin, cisplatin, diuretics, ketoconazole

B. Decreased ability to excrete water
  1. Diuretics
  2. Increased production of ADH
    anticancer drugs
      cyclophosphamide, vincristine, vinblastine
    antidepressants
      selective serotonin reuptake inhibitors
        fluoxetine, fluvoxamine, paroxetine, sertraline
      tricyclic antidepressants
        amitriptyline, imipramine
      monoamine-oxidase inhibitors
    antipsychotic drugs
      phenothiazines, trifluoperazine, thioridazine, thiothixene, haloperidol
    others
      carbamazepine, oxcarbazepine, lorcainide
  3. Drugs potentiating action of antidiuretic hormone
    carbamazepine, oxcarbazepine
    cyclophosphamide
    sulphonylureas
      chlorpropamide, tolbutamide
    somatostatin
    NSAID
      naproxen, ibuprofen, indomethacin
  4. Exogenous antidiuretic activity
    vasopressin, desmopressin
    oxytocin

C. Shift of water out of the cell
  mannitol
  glycerol

D. Miscellaneous
  ACE inhibitors
    captopril, enalapril, lisinopril
  bladder irrigation fluids
    1.5% glycine

Drugs may induce volume depletion with hyponatraemia. Some drugs produce volume depletion by causing salt wasting by their toxic effects on the kidney. Cisplatin (*cis*-diamminedichloroplatinum) (Hutchison *et al.* 1988) and carboplatin (Welborn *et al.* 1988) cause renal salt loss and hyponatraemia by their effect on the proximal tubule (Daugaard 1990). Hyponatraemia is particularly common with high-dose therapy — the incidence varying from 4 per cent (Giaccone *et al.* 1985) to 33 or 43 per cent (Lee and Shin 1992; Santana *et al.* 1992). Standard doses of cisplatin do not affect renal handling of sodium (Daugaard *et al.* 1987). Cisplatin has also been shown to cause inappropriate antidiuretic hormone secretion (Otsuka *et al.* 1996).

Ketoconazole, a drug which blocks adrenal steroidogenesis, has been reported to cause hyponatraemia (Pillans *et al.* 1985) probably by a mechanism similar to that in Addison's disease.

Decreased ability to excrete water

Hyponatraemia is a well-recognized complication of diuretic therapy (Ashraf *et al.* 1981; Ayus 1986; McInnes 1996). In over 90 per cent of cases the cause is a thiazide-like diuretic either alone or in combination with other drugs (Sonnenblick *et al.* 1993). In recent times the problem has lessened as lower dosages of thiazides are used in treating hypertension (McInnes 1996). Hyponatraemia is more likely to occur in elderly females (Baglin *et al.* 1995) and those with congestive heart failure — it has been reported to develop in up to 12 per cent of elderly people taking diuretics (Baglin *et al.* 1992). The high incidence in elderly females may merely be a reflection of the widespread use of diuretics in this group (McInnes 1996). Hyponatraemia is usually mild and asymptomatic, but severe hyponatraemia may occasionally occur, especially in patients who also drink large volumes of water (Friedman *et al.* 1989). It usually develops within a few weeks of starting therapy in the case of thiazides, and in the case of loop diuretics after several months of treatment (McInnes 1996). With thiazides, a new steady state is reached after a few weeks of therapy and fluid intake and output again become equal (Rose 1994). If plasma sodium concentration decreases further in a patient who is receiving long-term diuretics, it is usually because of an additional problem such as vomiting, diarrhoea, or increased water intake (Kone *et al.* 1986), or an increase in drug dosage.

The combination of hydrochlorothiazide and amiloride (co-amilozide, 'Moduretic') has been consistently reported to cause hyponatraemia; Byatt and colleagues (1990) reported the incidence due to co-amilozide to be twice that of other diuretics.

The factors contributing to the hyponatraemia are increased ADH release due to volume depletion (Ghose 1985; Burnier and Brunner 1992), potassium depletion, and direct inhibition of urinary dilution (Rose 1994). The last mechanism particularly applies to thiazides, which act on the distal tubule in the renal cortex and do not interfere with the ability of ADH to increase water retention. Loop diuretics, by virtue of their action on the medullary thick ascending limb, diminish the interstitial osmolality and thus the ADH released in response to volume depletion is not effective in increasing water reabsorption (Rose 1994). The effect of diuretics is potentiated by some drugs, such as aminoglutethimide, which blocks the synthesis of aldosterone (Bork and Hansen 1986) and NSAID, such as ibuprofen, which block prostaglandin synthesis (Goodenough and Lutz 1988).

Carbamazepine and oxcarbazepine are now well recognized as drugs which cause a decrease in plasma sodium concentration in a dose-related fashion (Ashton et al. 1977; Dam 1994). Usually mild, in some cases it can give rise to symptomatic or severe hyponatraemia (van Amelsvoort et al. 1994; Gandelman 1994). The incidence of hyponatraemia has been reported to vary from 4.8 to 40 per cent (van Amelsvoort et al. 1994) and the risk is higher in the elderly (Leppik 1992) and in those with a higher serum carbamazepine concentration (>6 mg per litre). Occasionally, hyponatraemia has occurred with low-dose carbamazepine therapy (Appleby 1984). Friis and co-workers (1993) found hyponatraemia in 25 per cent of patients taking oxcarbazepine.

The mechanism by which carbamazepine induces hyponatraemia is uncertain (van Amelsvoort et al. 1994). Although carbamazepine inhibits the excretion of a water load, it has no intrinsic antidiuretic action. Several studies have shown that it increases the plasma ADH concentration (Smith and Espir 1977), but other studies have not confirmed this (Thomas et al. 1978), and this has led to the suggestion that carbamazepine potentiates the effect of ADH. A study in normal subjects, however, failed to show either an increase in ADH secretion or increased sensitivity to ADH as assessed by the slope of the relationship between ADH and urine osmolality (Thomas et al. 1978) and it has been suggested that the effect of carbamazepine is to modify the threshold of the hypothalamic osmoreceptors (van Amelsvoort et al. 1994). Simultaneous administration of a thiazide increases the risk of hyponatraemia (Yassa et al. 1988), and on the other hand hyponatraemia can be prevented by simultaneous administration of lithium (Vieweg et al. 1987).

Cyclophosphamide, especially when administered intravenously in high doses, can cause hyponatraemia (Bressler and Huston 1985). To avoid renal toxicity during such therapy, a high fluid intake is recommended and this, together with the increased ADH secretion, can lead to severe and occasionally fatal hyponatraemia (Harlow et al. 1979). It has also been suggested that cyclophosphamide potentiates the action of ADH (Rose 1994). Recently a case of water intoxication following low-dose cyclophosphamide has been reported (McCarron et al. 1995).

Vincristine and vinblastine have been reported to cause hyponatraemia by an inappropriate elevation of ADH (Zavagli et al. 1988; Robertson and Berl 1996). Renal loss of sodium as a result of tubular damage has been suggested as a contributing factor (Zavagli et al. 1988).

Many psychotropic drugs are known to cause hyponatraemia (Table 17.3) (Koide 1991; Siegler et al. 1995; Spigset and Hedenmalm 1995; Thomas and Verbalis 1995). Antidepressants cause hyponatraemia (Spigset and Hedenmalm 1997) in a significant number of cases, especially in the elderly. Patients receiving phenothiazines were noted to have a significantly lower plasma sodium concentration (Kimelman and Albert 1984) and severe hyponatraemia developed when there was an added stimulus to ADH secretion such as volume depletion (Kimelman and Albert 1984). Trifluoperazine therapy worsened the hyponatraemia in a patient with the syndrome of inappropriate secretion of antidiuretic hormone (SIADH) due to carcinoma of the lung (Kennedy et al. 1987), suggesting that these drugs may potentiate the release of ADH even from the tumour. Selective serotonin reuptake inhibitors (SSRI), such as fluoxetine (ten Holt et al. 1994), fluvoxamine, paroxetine, and sertraline have been reported to cause hyponatraemia, especially in the elderly (Liu et al. 1996), and in their review of the literature on hyponatraemia and SSRI these workers identified 736 cases of hyponatraemia and SIADH. Of these, fluoxetine was involved in 75 per cent of cases, paroxetine and sertraline in 12 per cent each, and fluvoxamine in 1.5 per cent. The median time to development of hyponatraemia after treatment began was 13 (range 3–120) days; most cases occurred in the elderly.

Although hyponatraemia has been described with large numbers of psychotropic drugs, the mechanism is not clear (Robertson and Berl 1996). In most cases it has not been established that these drugs impair water excretion; rechallenge has rarely caused hyponatraemia under controlled conditions; and measurement of serum ADH has failed to show any effect from them. Thus it has been suggested that the hyponatraemia may not be due to the drugs themselves (Robertson and Berl 1996). Compulsive water-drinking may be an important contributory factor to the development of hyponatraemia with psychotropic drugs (Assal and Chauchot 1994).

Clofibrate (chlorphenoxyisobutyrate) has a well-documented antidiuretic effect (Rose 1994) due to stimulation of ADH secretion; it does not affect the renal response to ADH. It seldom causes significant hyponatraemia when used in therapeutic doses, three to four times the therapeutic dose being required to produce hyponatraemia (Rado et al. 1975).

Lorcainide, an antiarrhythmic drug, has been reported to cause a plasma sodium concentration decrease which in the majority of patients returned to normal within 3–12 months of treatment (Somani *et al.* 1984). In one patient, severe hyponatraemia developed when hydrochlorothiazide was given in addition. The mechanism was suggested to be inappropriate ADH secretion. Hyponatraemia has been reported in association with methyldopa (Varkel *et al.* 1988), propafenone (Dirix *et al.* 1988), and amantadine (Lammers and Roos 1993).

Chlorpropamide, a sulphonylurea used in the treatment of diabetes mellitus, is the most common cause of drug-induced SIADH-like syndrome. The incidence of hyponatraemia in patients taking chlorpropamide was found to be 7 per cent by Hirokawa and Gray (1992). A decrease in plasma sodium concentration was observed with all sulphonylureas but hyponatraemia is less frequent with tolbutamide or glibenclamide (Krans 1996). Significant risk factors for the development of hyponatraemia following chlorpropamide are increasing age and concurrent administration of diuretics (Kadowaki *et al.* 1983; Zalin *et al.* 1984) and the use of ACE inhibitors (Hirokawa and Gray 1992). Chlorpropamide is thought to act directly on the ADH receptor and potentiate the effect of ADH on the renal tubules. Medullary hypertonicity is increased and there is increased cyclic AMP production as well as inhibition of prostaglandin synthesis (Rose 1994; Robertson and Berl 1996). In addition to the direct action on the tubules there is some evidence to suggest that chlorpropamide may also increase ADH release (Kimura *et al.* 1995).

NSAID potentiate the action of ADH by inhibiting the synthesis of prostaglandins, which normally antagonize the action of ADH (Patrono and Dunn 1987). In spite of their widespread use, however, hyponatraemia rarely develops, as ADH secretion is inhibited following initial retention of water. These drugs may nevertheless increase the risk of the disorder in patients who have other risk factors for development of hyponatraemia, such as volume depletion or causes of impaired urinary dilution (Goodenough and Lutz 1988; Rault 1993; Rose 1994; Wen 1997). Symptomatic hyponatraemia has been occasionally reported with the use of indomethacin and diclofenac (Petersson *et al.* 1987), piroxicam (Biscarini 1996), ibuprofen (Dunn and Buckley 1986), and naproxen (Alun-Jones and Williams 1986). Hyponatraemia has been described in infants whose mothers were given NSAID before delivery (Bavoux 1992). NSAID have also been reported to potentiate the hyponatraemic effect of low-dose cyclophosphamide (Webberley and Murray 1989).

Somatostatin and its analogues cause a reduction in free-water clearance and severe hyponatraemia developed in two patients after 2–3 weeks of continuous intravenous infusion (Halma *et al.* 1987). The authors suggested that somatostatin increases the sensitivity of the collecting tubules to ADH.

Bromocriptine, a dopaminergic agonist, was reported to cause hyponatraemia which reappeared when the patient was rechallenged with bromocriptine (Marshall *et al.* 1982). The mechanism of action is not understood.

Newer antineoplastic agents such as interleukin-2 (Shulman *et al.* 1996), levamisole, interleukin-4, and α-interferon have been reported to cause hyponatraemia (Bennett *et al.* 1986; Lei *et al.* 1995; Whitehead *et al.* 1995), the mechanism of which is not clear.

Hyponatraemia during treatment with co-trimoxazole has been reported (Ahn and Goldman 1985), especially in association with diuretics. It was suggested that co-trimoxazole may have an effect similar to that of chlorpropamide, and hyponatraemia seems to occur when there is an added factor, such as the use of a diuretic or increased fluid load, as in the case reported by Ahn and Goldman (1985).

Antidiuretic hormone (ADH, vasopressin), or its synthetic analogues desmopressin (DDAVP) and terlipressin, and oxytocin, which has significant antidiuretic effect, will cause hyponatraemia, especially when accompanied by administration of large amounts of fluid (without sodium). Hyponatraemia and convulsions have been reported with the use of DDAVP in the treatment of enuresis (Hamed *et al.* 1993; Eckford *et al.* 1994; Robson and Leung 1994), nocturnal polyuria (Valiquette *et al.* 1996) and haemorrhage (Smith *et al.* 1989; Weinstein *et al.* 1989). Infusion of oxytocin with 5% dextrose to induce labour has caused severe hyponatraemia and seizures in both mothers and the newborn (Schwartz and Jones 1978). Hyponatraemia that followed the infusion of ACTH (in 5% dextrose) over 12–45 hours (Baumann 1979) was probably due to contamination of the ACTH with ADH.

The use of 1.5% glycine solution for irrigation before or during surgery such as transurethral prostatectomy (Sunderrajan *et al.* 1984), percutaneous lithotripsy (Schultz *et al.* 1983), or transcervical resection of endometrium (Baumann *et al.* 1990) has been shown to lower the plasma sodium concentration. In a few patients, severe symptomatic and sometimes fatal hyponatraemia develops (Rao 1987).

Angiotensin-converting-enzyme (ACE) inhibitors used in the treatment of hypertension and heart failure have variable effects on plasma sodium concentration. They increase the plasma sodium concentration when the pretreatment concentration is low (Nicholls 1987), but when the initial plasma sodium concentration is normal it may fall (Nicholls 1987). Although the plasma sodium concentration decreases in these patients, symptomatic or severe hyponatraemia is not common. Several case reports of hyponatraemia in association with captopril (Al-Mufti and Arieff 1985), enalapril (Castrillon *et al.* 1993), and lisinopril (Hume *et al.* 1990; Subramanian and Ayus 1992) have appeared in the literature. In some instances the hyponatraemia was severe (Hume *et al.* 1990; Subramanian and Ayus 1992) especially with lisinopril in combination with thiazides. These patients had features similar to SIADH, that is, a decreased ability to excrete water.

Silver nitrate solutions used in the topical therapy of burns can cause hyponatraemia, as the solution is hypotonic and large amounts can be absorbed from the skin (Connelly 1970).

Hyponatraemia is a common finding in patients with HIV infection and in some of these it is associated with drugs like trimethoprim, vidarabine, miconazole, and pentamidine (Bevilacqua 1994).

Infusion of hypertonic solutions of mannitol, glycerol, or glucose can cause hyponatraemia by shifting water from the intracellular space (Borges *et al.* 1982; Rose 1994). The decrease in plasma sodium concentration is profound and prolonged if the agent is not eliminated or metabolised. Mannitol, often used in patients with reduced renal function, can cause severe hyponatraemia (Borges *et al.* 1982).

Treatment

Treatment of hyponatraemia involves treatment of the underlying cause, discontinuing the offending drug, and correcting any abnormality in ECF volume. Once the offending drug is removed and the volume abnormality is corrected (i.e. by volume replacement in the case of depletion or water restriction in the case of water overload) plasma sodium will eventually return to normal. There is controversy as to whether the low plasma sodium itself should be reversed (Robertson and Berl 1996). In general, it is agreed that the plasma sodium should be corrected actively when the hyponatraemia is acute and symptomatic or if the hyponatraemia is severe (i.e. plasma Na<110 mmol per litre) (Arieff 1986). The correction of low plasma sodium concentration involves the use of normal or hypertonic saline. A loop diuretic is added in cases in which there is water overload (Rose 1994); the latter is required to prevent fluid overload, especially in the elderly.

Despite the dangers of hyponatraemia, rapid correction has been shown to cause a central demyelinating lesion of the pons (Robertson and Berl 1996; Laureno and Karp 1997). There is now general agreement that serum sodium concentration should be corrected slowly, probably by no more than 0.5 mmol per litre per hour until the plasma sodium concentration reaches 120 mmol per litre, when the patient is likely to be out of danger. Further correction of hyponatraemia is carried out slowly over several days. It may, however, be necessary to raise plasma sodium more quickly (i.e. 1–2 mmol per litre per hour) if the patient has seizures. The importance of correction of hyponatraemia is highlighted in a study of 11 patients with severe hyponatraemia for which no specific treatment was given. All these patients died and at postmortem there was evidence of tentorial herniation (Fraser and Arieff 1990).

Other methods of treatment include agents which inhibit the action of ADH such as demeclocycline and newer agents such as AVP V2 receptor antagonists (Shimizu 1995) and α-opioid antagonists (Gines and Jimenez 1996).

Potassium

Total potassium content in an adult is 3000–4000 millimoles (50–55 mmol per kg body-weight) and 98 per cent of this is found in the cells, in contrast to sodium, which is mainly an extracellular cation. The distribution of potassium is reflected in the concentration difference between the two compartments, 4–5 mmol per litre in extracellular fluid and 140 mmol per litre in intracellular fluid. This concentration gradient is maintained by the active sodium–potassium pump (the Na^+, K^+ pump) in the cell membrane, which pumps sodium ions out of and potassium ions into the cell in a ratio of 3:2. Drugs may cause disturbances in plasma potassium concentration either by altering the distribution between intracellular and extracellular compartments or by altering external potassium balance.

Hyperkalaemia

Drugs may cause hyperkalaemia by one of three mechanisms: a shift from the intracellular compartments, increased intake, or reduced renal excretion (Table 17.4). Chronic hyperkalaemia is always associated with impaired renal excretion.

Transcellular shift

Shift of potassium out of cells is a relatively common cause of acute hyperkalaemia in clinical practice. The

Causes of drug-induced hyperkalaemia

1. Transcellular shift
   cardiac glycosides, β-blockers, suxamethonium,
   arginine, chemotherapeutic agents, drug-induced
   acidosis (e.g. lactic acidosis from biguanides)

2. Increased potassium intake
   potassium supplements, salt substitutes,
   potassium penicillin

3. Decreased renal excretion
   drug-induced renal failure
   decreased delivery of sodium to distal tubules
     any drug that causes volume depletion
     (e.g. cytotoxic drugs)
   hypoaldosteronism
     angiotensin-converting-enzyme inhibitors,
     NSAID, heparin, cyclosporin, tacrolimus
   decreased tubular secretion of potassium
     amiloride, spironolactone, triamterene
     trimethoprim

transcellular gradient is maintained by the active sodium pump, which is specifically modified by cardiac glycosides (Smith 1988), administration of which can lead to an increase in plasma potassium concentration. In therapeutic concentrations digitalis causes only a small increase. However, the increase in potassium seen during exercise may be exacerbated by cardiac glycosides (Norgaard *et al.* 1991) and a case of exercise-associated cardiac arrhythmia attributed to digitalis has been reported (Gosselink *et al.* 1993). Severe hyperkalaemia has been reported with accidental or suicidal overdose of digitalis (Reza *et al.* 1974; Taboulet *et al.* 1993).

Catecholamines promote potassium entry into cells by activation of the sodium pump (Moratinos and Reverte 1993) mediated by the β_2-adrenergic receptors, and β-adrenergic blockers interfere with this β_2-adrenergic-stimulated potassium entry into cells. Hyperkalaemia due to the use of β-adrenergic blockers is rare and in most instances the rise in plasma potassium concentration is less than 0.5 mmol per litre (Sterns *et al.* 1981), as the potassium entering the extracellular compartment is rapidly excreted by the kidney. Hyperkalaemia can occur, however, if there is increased potassium to dispose of, as in severe exercise (Carlsson *et al.* 1978; Lindinger 1995), increased potassium load, hypoaldosteronism, or cardiac surgery (Kamel *et al.* 1996). Occasionally severe hyperkalaemia develops with β-blockers (Bory *et al.* 1993), and hyperkalaemia has also been reported with the use of timolol eye-drops (Diggory *et al.* 1995).

Suxamethonium, a muscle relaxant, causes an immediate increase in serum potassium as a result of opening of the receptor-linked ion channels causing movement of potassium out of cells. In patients taking β-blockers this rise may be exaggerated and prolonged (Kamel *et al.* 1996). Dangerous hyperkalaemia may occur in renal failure patients with pre-existing high serum potassium (Koide and Waud 1972). Severe hyperkalaemia associated with ventricular fibrillation and cardiac arrest due to suxamethonium has been reported in the following conditions: burns, severe trauma, spinal cord injury, hemiplegia, multiple sclerosis, tetanus, encephalitis, and metastatic rhabdomyosarcoma (Yentis 1990; Schwartz *et al.* 1992; Leuwer and Motsch 1996).

Infusion of arginine hydrochloride can cause hyperkalaemia (Bushinsky and Gennari 1978), probably due to the movement of potassium out of cells associated with the entry of cationic arginine. Risk of hyperkalaemia is higher in those with impaired ability to metabolise or eliminate arginine (patients with liver and renal disease) and in those with impaired ability to excrete potassium. Several patients with hepatic or renal disease who developed life-threatening hyperkalaemia after infusion of arginine have been described (Bushinsky and Gennari 1978).

Increased catabolism or necrosis of tissues, as in the tumour-lysis syndrome or rhabdomyolysis, will cause rapid release of potassium from cells and may cause hyperkalaemia even when renal failure is absent (Arrambide and Toto 1993). Treatment of malignant lymphomas, leukaemia, and Hodgkin's disease with cytotoxic drugs, and massive haemolysis have all been reported to cause hyperkalaemia (Kamel *et al.* 1996).

Drug-induced metabolic acidosis can lead to hyperkalaemia due to the shift of potassium out of cells in exchange for movement of hydrogen ions into the cells (Bushinsky and Cox 1985 — see Metabolic acidosis). The degree of hyperkalaemia depends on the severity and nature of the metabolic acidosis (Kamel *et al.* 1996).

Increased intake

When renal function is normal, increased potassium intake is not a frequent cause of hyperkalaemia. With increased oral intake its excretion will increase with only a small increase in plasma potassium concentration. Severe hyperkalaemia may occur if the daily intake is greater than 160 millimoles (Rose 1994) or if potassium is infused rapidly. Severe hyperkalaemia and cardiac arrest were reported after bolus injection of potassium penicillin (Mercer and Logic 1973), following high-dose glucose–insulin–potassium for inotropic support (Böhrer *et al.* 1988), and during rapid correction of hypokalaemia (Kruse and Carlson 1990). The most frequent sources of exogenous potassium are the various potassium supplements (Kamel *et al.* 1996). Hyperkalaemia can follow the ingestion of large amounts of 'salt substitutes' (McCaughan 1984; Swales 1991) or over-the-counter potassium supplements (Browning and Channer 1981), and a case of fatal hyperkalaemia from a salt substitute has been described (Restuccio 1992). The use of potassium supplements or salt substitutes is more likely to cause hyperkalaemia when there is increased proximal tubular reabsorption of sodium, as with salt restriction. Salt restriction will limit sodium delivery to distal tubules and therefore limit potassium secretion. Hyperkalaemia as a result of accidental poisoning with a sustained-release potassium preparation has been reported (Steedman 1988). The risk of hyperkalaemia is also higher in those taking NSAID, ACE inhibitors and potassium-sparing diuretics (Swales 1991). Hyperkalaemia is also likely to occur with the use of stored blood for exchange transfusion (Kamel et al. 1996), owing to the leakage of potassium from red cells during storage, and it may be life-threatening in patients with pre-existing hyperkalaemia (Koch 1996), or in infants (Sato et al. 1991). In any of the above situations of increased potassium intake, hyperkalaemia is more common if there is impairment of potassium excretion. Several cases of hyperkalaemia during dialysis due to inadvertent use of a high-potassium dialysate have been described (Brady et al. 1988).

Decreased renal excretion

Renal handling of potassium involves filtration, reabsorption, and distal tubular secretion; the amount of potassium excreted depends on the amount of potassium secreted. A drug may cause hyperkalaemia by decreasing the functional renal mass, by reducing sodium delivery to distal tubules, by causing hypoaldosteronism, or by interfering with tubular secretion of potassium.

In states of volume depletion, the proximal tubular reabsorption of sodium is increased, leading to decreased delivery of sodium to the distal tubules, and this limits the capacity to secrete potassium in exchange for sodium. Drugs that cause volume depletion (see section on Sodium) may lead to hyperkalaemia, especially if potassium supplements are being given at the same time (Rose 1994).

Drugs that interfere with the renin–angiotensin–aldosterone axis or that block the action of aldosterone cause hyperkalaemia. The best examples are ACE inhibitors, which block the conversion of angiotensin I to II and thereby decrease the synthesis of aldosterone. Decrease in potassium secretion follows and plasma potassium concentration rises. If renal function is normal the rise is usually less than 0.5 mmol per litre (Veterans Administration Co-operative Study 1984).

However, it is greater after exercise (Sullivan et al. 1992), in patients who have renal insufficiency (Doman et al. 1993; Antonios and MacGregor 1995; Alderman et al. 1996), in those who are also taking potassium-sparing diuretics or potassium supplements (Good et al. 1995; Keilani et al. 1995), and in diabetic patients with mild renal impairment (Shionoiri 1993). The risk of hyperkalaemia is particularly high when ACE inhibitors are the cause of renal failure (Speires et al. 1988), and with long-acting preparations (DiBianco 1986). Hyperkalaemia was the cause of withdrawal of enalapril therapy in 0.3 per cent of patients. The rapid rise in serum potassium concentration seen in patients with chronic renal failure treated with ACE inhibitors was shown to be due to their inability to increase aldosterone secretion in response to the hyperkalaemia (Zanella et al. 1985).

Prostaglandins promote renin secretion and facilitate aldosterone release. Hence, NSAID that inhibit prostaglandin synthesis cause hyporeninaemic hypoaldosteronism and may cause hyperkalaemia (Rotenberg and Giannini 1992; Murray and Brater 1993; Howes 1995; Wen 1997). Inhibition of vasodilatory prostaglandins also decreases the delivery of sodium and potassium secretion (Whelton and Hamilton 1991). The increase in plasma potassium concentration seen with NSAID is usually small or negligible in patients with normal renal function, even in the elderly (Allred et al. 1989). Significant hyperkalaemia has been reported with indomethacin (Mactier and Khanna 1988), ibuprofen (Marasco et al. 1987), and sulindac (Horowitz et al. 1988). The incidence of hyperkalaemia with NSAID can be as high as 26 per cent in the presence of pre-existing mild to moderate renal failure (Zimran et al. 1985). It is less with sulindac (Nesher et al. 1988), which does not interfere with renal prostaglandin synthesis, than with other NSAID. The risk of hyperkalaemia is also high when NSAID is given together with ACE inhibitors (Howes 1995). Overdose with ibuprofen in a young healthy adult caused fulminant hyperkalaemia (8.3 mmol per litre) and cardiac arrhythmias (Menzies et al. 1989). Hyperkalaemia has also been reported in the newborn as a result of mothers' use of NSAID.

Calcium-channel blockers have been reported to inhibit aldosterone secretion in response to angiotensin II, ACTH, and potassium (Freed et al. 1991). Diltiazem and nifedipine decreased serum aldosterone concentration by 30–40 per cent (Krishna et al. 1991). However, hyperkalaemia is uncommon (Freed et al. 1991).

Heparin can cause hyperkalaemia (Brown et al. 1996), and this is seen in about 7–8 per cent of patients (Gonzalez-Martin et al. 1991). Hyperkalaemia is more frequent in patients with diabetes mellitus or metabolic acidosis and those on long-term therapy (Gonzalez-Martin *et al.* 1991). The effect is due to the inhibition of aldosterone synthesis in the zona glomerulosa. This inhibitory effect is seen with both unfractionated heparin (UFH) and low molecular weight heparin (LMWH) (Siebels *et al.* 1992). Inhibition of aldosterone synthesis is seen in daily doses above 10 000 IU of UFH or 2500 IU of LMWH. Above this dose the inhibition was dose related (Siebels *et al.* 1992; Oster *et al.* 1995). The mechanism of inhibition appears to involve reduction in number and affinity of the angiotensin II receptors (Oster *et al.* 1995). Hyperkalaemia is more pronounced in patients with reduced renal function and in diabetic patients (Uribarri *et al.* 1990), who are unable to compensate for the reduction in aldosterone by increasing renin production by juxtaglomerular cells (Aull *et al.* 1990).

Benzalkonium chloride is used in the bonding process of heparin-bonded umbilical catheters, and elevated serum potassium concentrations have been seen with the use of such catheters (Gaylord *et al.* 1991). This effect was shown, however, to be an artefact due to an effect of the benzalkonium chloride on the ion-selective electrodes (Gaylord *et al.* 1991).

Cyclosporin used as an immunosuppressive agent in renal transplantation causes hyperkalaemia (Min and Monaco 1991; Williams 1991). In a multicentre trial the mean plasma potassium concentration in patients treated with cyclosporin was found to be significantly raised (European Multicentre Trial 1982). Adu and co-workers (1983) reported sustained hyperkalaemia inappropriate for the degree of impairment of renal function in 16 per cent of patients, all of whom had hyperchloraemic acidosis with defective renal tubular secretion of potassium. Factors contributing to the hyperkalaemia are hypoaldosteronism, renal tubular damage (Bantle *et al.* 1985), and reduced prostaglandin secretion (Bennett *et al.* 1988). An inappropriate renal response to hyperkalaemia as measured by the transtubular potassium gradient was demonstrated (Kamel *et al.* 1992). Furthermore cyclosporin-induced reduction in distal tubular flow rate decreased potassium excretion (Laine and Holmberg 1995). The use of β-blockers, which blunt the aldosterone response to hyperkalaemia, further worsens it. Tacrolimus, a macrolide immunosuppressive agent more potent than cyclosporin, also causes hyperkalaemia (McDiarmid 1996).

The potassium-sparing diuretics amiloride, triamterene, and spironolactone reduce the secretion of potassium and hydrogen ions in the collecting tubules; as a result, hyperkalaemia and metabolic acidosis may follow (Hollenberg and Mickiewicz 1989; Kamel *et al.* 1996). This is more likely in the presence of a potassium load, such as potassium supplements or 'salt substitutes' (McCaughan 1984), or if there is reduced renal function or simultaneous administration of ACE inhibitors or NSAID (Burnakis and Mioduch 1984; Kamel *et al.* 1996), and life-threatening hyperkalaemia has been reported in patients taking these diuretics (Lawson *et al.* 1982).

Trimethoprim, which is an antimicrobial agent, has actions similar to the potassium-sparing diuretic triamterene, and can cause hyperkalaemia (Greenberg *et al.* 1993). It blocks apical-membrane sodium channels in the distal nephron and causes a reduction in transepithelial voltage and hence in potassium secretion (Velazquez *et al.* 1993). Serum potassium increased by 0.6 mmol per litre and about 50 per cent of subjects developed hyperkalaemia in one study (Velazquez *et al.* 1993). The effect is greater in the elderly (Perazella 1996; Witt *et al.* 1996). In combination with other drugs such as ACE inhibitors severe hyperkalaemia may result (Bugge 1996). In doses used in the treatment of *Pneumocystis carinii* pneumonia in AIDS patients, hyperkalaemia is much more frequent (Medina *et al.* 1990; Choi *et al.* 1993). Pentamidine, another drug used for AIDS, causes hyperkalaemia in a large percentage of patients (Briceland and Bailie 1991; O'Brien *et al.* 1997), as high as 100 per cent in patients treated for more than 6 days (Kleyman *et al.* 1995). This 'cationic' drug is excreted in the urine and, like triamterene, blocks sodium channels and causes a reduction in potassium secretion (Kleyman *et al.* 1995).

Increase in plasma potassium concentration follows treatment with erythropoietin (Eschbach *et al.* 1989), though frank hyperkalaemia has not been reported. Aminoglutethimide, a drug that inhibits adrenal hormone synthesis, has been reported to cause severe hyperkalaemia (Davies *et al.* 1989), but this complication is very rare. Lovastatin, an inhibitor of HMG-CoA reductase, caused hyperkalaemia in diabetic patients with renal impairment taking ACE inhibitors (Edelman and Witztum 1989). The authors suggested that the myopathy induced by lovastatin and the resulting release of potassium, combined with renal insufficiency and the use of ACE inhibitors, caused the hyperkalaemia.

Prolonged infusion of ACTH for infantile spasm has been associated with hyperkalaemia (Zeharia *et al.* 1987) shortly after cessation of the infusion. The exact mechanism of this hyperkalaemia is not well understood.

Hyperkalaemia is seen in acute fluoride toxicity (Cummings and McIvor 1988) and in malignant hyperthermia induced by anaesthetic agents, such as isoflurane, in susceptible subjects (Simons and Goldman 1988). Hetastarch, a colloidal plasma-volume expander,

TABLE 17.5
Drug-induced hypokalaemia

1. Increased entry into cells (redistribution)
   β-adrenergic agonists, drug-induced metabolic
   alkalosis, insulin

2. Increased gastrointestinal losses
   laxative or purgative abuse, vomiting

3. Increased renal loss
   diuretics, increased mineralocorticoid activity,
   corticosteroids, carbenoxolone, penicillins,
   amphotericin, hypomagnesaemia, drug-induced
   renal tubular acidosis, gossypol, levodopa

4. Miscellaneous
   fluconazole, haloperidol, ifosfamide/mesna,
   mithramycin, zimeldine

has caused hyperkalaemia when used as a pump-priming
fluid during cardiopulmonary bypass (Schmidt and Sesin
1987).

Severe hyperkalaemia has been reported in pregnant
intravenous drug abusers who were treated with prolonged parenteral magnesium sulphate for toxaemia
(Spital and Greenwell 1991).

Hypokalaemia

Drugs may cause hypokalaemia without potassium depletion as a result of transcellular shift or they may cause
hypokalaemia and potassium depletion by increasing the
loss of potassium (Table 17.5).

Transcellular shift

In alkalosis, hydrogen ions move from the ICF to ECF
and minimize the elevation of ECF pH. Electro-
neutrality is preserved by potassium ions entering the
cells. Hypokalaemia is more likely with metabolic alkalosis than respiratory alkalosis (Halperin and Scheich
1994). It is usually mild, and the fall in plasma potassium
concentration usually less than 0.4 mmol per litre for
each 0.1 unit of pH increase. Administration of sodium
bicarbonate to correct metabolic acidosis can cause
hypokalaemia, due to a rapid shift of potassium into the
cells (Kamel *et al.* 1996). It is important to note that
hypokalaemia and metabolic alkalosis are commonly
found together, either because the causative agent, such
as a diuretic, induces both low potassium and high pH, or
because the alkalosis may be the result of hypokalaemia
and a consequent increase in the tubular secretion of
hydrogen ions (Kamel *et al.* 1996).

Insulin increases potassium uptake into cells by
stimulating the Na^+, K^+ pump. The effect is maximal 60–
90 min after an injection of insulin and persists for more

than 3 hours. Hypokalaemia can occur during the treatment of diabetic ketoacidosis when there is potassium
depletion. A decrease in plasma potassium is also seen
after a glucose load or administration of insulin as, for
example, in the performance of an insulin tolerance test.
Spuriously low potassium concentrations may also be
found in specimens from patients given insulin, if blood
samples are left standing for several hours before separation of plasma from red cells (Kalsheker and Hales
1985). The mechanism of this effect is not fully understood but it is thought to be due to a shift of potassium into red cells *in vitro* during storage, somehow
triggered by insulin administration *in vivo* (Kalsheker
and Hales 1985).

Sympathomimetic agents, including β₂-agonists, theophylline, dopamine, and dobutamine, promote potassium uptake into liver as well as peripheral tissues —
muscle being the major site (Brown *et al.* 1983;
Moratinos and Reverte 1993). The increased cellular
uptake is due to a direct effect of β-agonists, as well as to
an indirect effect through stimulation of insulin secretion
(Kamel *et al.* 1996). Hypokalaemia has been reported
after administration of β-adrenergic agonists, including
adrenaline, fenoterol (Burgess *et al.* 1989), ritodrine
(Shin and Kim 1988; Braden *et al.* 1997), salbutamol
(Udezue *et al.* 1995), and terbutaline (Rahman *et al.*
1992*a*). Infusion of terbutaline in therapeutic doses decreases plasma potassium below the reference range in
all patients, the decrease in potassium being largely
reversed within 30 minutes after the drug is discontinued. Both intravenous administration (Rey *et al.*
1989) and inhalation of β₂-agonists, decrease the plasma
potassium concentration (Burgess *et al.* 1989; Wong *et
al.* 1990). The effect is more pronounced in women than
in men (Rahman *et al.* 1992*b*; Taylor *et al.* 1993). The
effect of fenoterol and terbutaline lasts longer than that
of salbutamol (4 hours vs 2 hours) (Burgess *et al.* 1989).
The most potent hypokalaemic β₂-agonist is fenoterol,
followed by terbutaline and salbutamol (Burgess *et al.*
1989; Wong *et al.* 1990). Fenoterol, as a tocolytic agent,
causes significant hypokalaemia (Bouillon *et al.* 1996)
but this does not produce any clinically significant effects
(Hildebrant *et al.* 1997). Prior administration of thiazide
diuretics aggravated the hypokalaemia and ECG effects
of the β₂-agonist salbutamol (Lipworth *et al.* 1989).
Frusemide also exaggerated the hypokalaemic effect of
inhaled terbutaline (Newnham *et al.* 1991). These interactions may increase the risk of arrhythmias, especially if
there is concomitant hypoxaemia, ischaemic heart disease, or acidosis (Lipworth *et al.* 1989). Concurrent
administration of corticosteroids and inhaled β₂-agonists
exaggerated the fall in plasma potassium (Taylor *et al.*

1992). In children treated with nebulized salbutamol for acute asthmatic attacks, hypokalaemia was seen in 39 per cent of patients (Singhi *et al.* 1996) and therefore monitoring of serum potassium was recommended. The hypokalaemic effect of intravenous salbutamol is potentiated by theophylline (Whyte *et al.* 1988), and theophylline in therapeutic doses significantly decreases plasma potassium (Zantvoort *et al.* 1986). Hypokalaemia is more frequent and severe in poisoning or overdose (Anderson *et al.* 1991) and is related to serum theophylline concentration (Flack *et al.* 1994). In one study, 85 per cent of patients admitted with acute theophylline poisoning had plasma potassium concentrations below 3.5 mmol per litre and 45 per cent below 3.0 mmol per litre. The degree of hypokalaemia correlated with the peak serum theophylline concentration (Amitai and Lovejoy 1988). The frequency of hypokalaemia in chronic theophylline poisoning is 32 per cent (Shannon and Lovejoy 1989). The reason why the frequency of hypokalaemia in chronic theophylline intoxication is lower has not been fully explained. Theophylline-induced hypokalaemia may contribute to the sudden respiratory arrest seen in asthmatic subjects (Kolski *et al.* 1988). Hypokalaemia has also been reported in an individual who took an overdose (6–8g) of caffeine (Leson *et al.* 1988), and after overdose with salbutamol (King *et al.* 1992; Leikin *et al.* 1994). The hypokalaemia induced by β_2-agonists could be prevented by the administration of β-blockers (J. Reid *et al.* 1986.

Ingestion of large doses of chloroquine has been reported to cause severe hypokalaemia (Jaeger *et al.* 1987; Lofaso *et al.* 1987; Clemessy *et al.* 1995). In an analysis of 191 cases of chloroquine poisoning, plasma potassium concentrations were found to correlate inversely with blood chloroquine concentrations (Clemessy *et al.* 1995). This study also showed that the hypokalaemia was unlikely to be due to potassium depletion and the most likely explanation of the hypokalaemia is transcellular shift.

Treatment with granulocyte–macrophage colony-stimulating factor (GM-CSF) causes hypokalaemia due to increased intracellular uptake as a result of massive leucocytosis (Viens *et al.* 1989; Kamel *et al.* 1996).

Gastrointestinal losses

Drugs that cause vomiting may lead to hypokalaemia through a combination of factors: loss of potassium in gastric juice, metabolic alkalosis due to loss of acid, and increased renal losses.

Loss of potassium in stools due to chronic laxative abuse will lead to hypokalaemia (Sladen 1972) and a

pseudo-Bartter's syndrome has been described (Meyers *et al.* 1990). Potassium loss can amount to 50–60 mmol per litre of stool, and together with this there may be renal loss of potassium due to secondary hyperaldosteronism.

Renal losses

Both loop and thiazide diuretics cause hypokalaemia and this accounted for 3.4 per cent of all admissions to an acute medical unit (Fitzgerald *et al.* 1989). The loss of potassium induced by diuretics is due to increased flow to the distal tubules as a result of inhibition of sodium chloride reabsorption in the proximal segments. The relative dilution of potassium in the tubular fluid allows more potassium to be secreted, as the secretion of potassium is normally limited by the concentration gradient between distal tubular fluid and cells. In addition to the increased flow rate there may be secondary hyperaldosteronism due to the induction of volume depletion (Rose 1994) and any underlying disease such as heart failure. Hypomagnesaemia induced by diuretics may further aggravate the renal loss of potassium. When the diuretic dose is not altered the loss of potassium stops after 2 weeks and a new steady state is reached when intake and output are again equal (Rose 1994).

The magnitude, frequency, and extent of hypokalaemia have been studied extensively. The incidence of hypokalaemia (plasma K$^+$<3.5 mmol per litre) is dose related (Siegel *et al.* 1992), and increases from 25 per cent with 50 mg hydrochlorothiazide per day to 40–50 per cent with 100 mg per day (Morgan and Davidson 1980; Knochel 1984) and is higher with longer-acting diuretics such as chlorthalidone (Morgan and Davidson 1980; Siegel *et al.* 1992). In a recent survey, hypokalaemia was found in nearly 25 per cent of patients on diuretics (Widmer *et al.* 1995). The incidence of hypokalaemia with frusemide was 5 per cent (Morgan and Davidson 1980). The question whether potassium depletion accompanies this hypokalaemia has been debated, as plasma potassium concentration does not reflect total body potassium status. Measurement of total body potassium in patients treated with diuretics for prolonged periods showed a deficit of about 200 millimoles or 5 per cent of total body potassium (Morgan and Davidson 1980), and muscle potassium was also found to be low (Dorup 1994). However, these changes may be due to the cardiac failure itself (McInnes 1996).

There has been intense debate as to whether diuretic-induced hypokalaemia may cause ill effects. It is well known that hypokalaemia will increase the risk of digoxin toxicity (Prichard *et al.* 1992). Diuretic-induced hypokalaemia has been implicated in ventricular arrhythmias and possibly sudden death (Poole-Wilson 1987; Dyckner 1990; Frohlich 1992). However, recent large studies have failed to confirm a relationship between diuretic-induced hypokalaemia and ventricular arrhythmias (Neaton et al. 1993; Kostis et al. 1994), and recent reviews suggest that the risk of hypokalaemia from diuretics is exaggerated (McInnes 1996; Papademetriou 1994).

Increased mineralocorticoid activity will lead to hypokalaemia and potassium depletion. Ingestion of licorice or licorice-containing tobacco can cause hypokalaemia (Blachley and Knochel 1980; Sunderam and Swaminathan 1981). Glycyrrhizic acid present in licorice inhibits the enzyme 11β-hydroxysteroid dehydrogenase and thereby inhibits the conversion of cortisol to cortisone in the kidney (Whorwood et al. 1993). The resulting high concentration of cortisol binds to the mineralocorticoid receptor and causes hypokalaemia (Farese et al. 1991). The administration of a thiazide diuretic (Sunderam and Swaminathan 1981) or sodium bicarbonate aggravates the hypokalaemia and can precipitate symptoms. Carbenoxolone, which is synthesized from glycyrrhetinic acid, can cause hypokalaemia by a similar mechanism (Dickinson and Swaminathan 1978) in 43 per cent of patients (Ganguli and Mohamed 1980). The effect is dose dependent and the elderly are more susceptible to it. The use of 9α-fluoroprednisolone in nasal sprays, in antihaemorrhoid ointments (Marin et al. 1989), and other topical preparations (Lauzurica et al. 1988) has been reported to be able to cause severe hypokalaemia. Gossypol, which is used as a male contraceptive, inhibits 11β-hydroxysteroid dehydrogenase and causes hypokalaemia (Sang et al. 1991).

Penicillins are frequently used as sodium salts and, especially when given in large doses, may give rise to increased potassium secretion in the distal tubules. The presence of the penicillin anion, which cannot be reabsorbed, leads to increased secretion of potassium and hydrogen ions, giving rise to hypokalaemia and metabolic alkalosis (Lipner et al. 1975). Hypokalaemia has been reported with the use of amoxycillin, ampicillin, carbenicillin, cephalexin, nafcillin, oxacillin, penicillin, and ticarcillin (Kamel et al. 1996). It is more common with carbenicillin because of the large doses used and high sodium content.

Amphotericin causes hypokalaemia (DuBose et al. 1996) by increasing urinary losses as a result of renal tubular acidosis (discussed under Acidosis). Increased urinary loss of potassium is due to an interaction of the drug with the membrane, causing increased potassium permeability for sodium and potassium which leads to a high luminal potassium concentration and potassium wasting (Kamel et al. 1994). Hypokalaemia is seen in up to 50 per cent of patients; it can be prevented by administration of amiloride (Smith et al. 1988). Polymyxin B has also been reported to cause renal damage and hypokalaemia (Ruef et al. 1996).

Hypomagnesaemia and hypokalaemia are seen together in up to 40 per cent of cases (Swaminathan 1998). In some instances this is due to impairment of reabsorption of potassium and magnesium by a common causative factor (Sutton and Dirks 1996) as, for example, in cisplatin toxicity (Rodriguez et al. 1989). In addition, hypomagnesaemia can lead to hypokalaemia by a poorly understood mechanism (Whang et al. 1985). Increased aldosterone secretion and impaired distal tubular transport of chloride (Kamel et al. 1994) may play important roles. In the presence of hypomagnesaemia, the hypokalaemia is refractory to potassium replacement (Rodriguez et al. 1989).

Increased loss of potassium in the urine occurs in renal tubular acidosis. The reduction in bicarbonate reabsorption in proximal renal tubular acidosis induced by drugs leads to increased delivery of sodium and bicarbonate to the distal tubules, causing potassium loss. In distal renal tubular acidosis, the reduction in hydrogen ion secretion enhances the exchange of potassium for sodium and results in loss of potassium (Kamel et al. 1994).

Levodopa increases potassium loss in the urine by an unknown mechanism and can cause hypokalaemia in up to 10 per cent of patients treated by this drug alone (Granerus et al. 1977). This is now less common, however, since the combination with peripheral dopadecarboxylase inhibitors has come into use.

Miscellaneous

Zimeldine, a selective blocker of serotonin uptake, was associated with hypokalaemia in a case of overdose (Lilijeqvist and Edvardsson 1989). Chemotherapy with ifosfamide and mesna leads to hypokalaemia which is occasionally fatal (Husband and Watkin 1988).

Hypokalaemia has been described in haloperidol overdosage (Aunsholt 1989) and in a patient receiving mithramycin for Paget's disease (Bashir and Tomson 1988).

Non-ionic radiographic contrast media were reported to cause a small (5.1 per cent) decrease in plasma potassium concentration, probably due to the high osmolality of the contrast medium and consequent haemodilution (Brunet et al. 1989).

ACE inhibitors are recognized to cause hyperkalaemia, but D'costa et al. (1990) reported that some patients taking diuretics and ACE inhibitors developed hypokalaemia; the mechanism and the significance of this observation are not clear.

Treatment with nisoldipine has been reported to cause a significant decrease in plasma potassium concentration — although within the reference range (Takahashi *et al.* 1989). This effect is presumably due to the increase in plasma catecholamines.

Hypokalaemia has been described in a man after 2 weeks of treatment with nifedipine (Tishler and Armon 1986); the serum potassium concentration returned to normal on withdrawal of the drug and fell again on rechallenge. Nifedipine may enhance the potassium loss induced by thiazides (Murphy *et al.* 1982). In a 4-year study with amlodipine, however, serum potassium did not show any significant change (Neaton *et al.* 1993). Hypokalaemia in association with torsade de pointes has been reported with the use of bepridil (Prystowsky 1992) especially in combination with diuretics (Singh 1992).

The antifungal agent itraconazole has been reported to cause hypokalaemia especially with high doses (Lyman and Walsh 1992; Wheat *et al.* 1993), but only a few instances have been reported wih fluconazole (Tester-Dalderup 1996).

Calcium

Most of the calcium in the body is in the skeleton, and the extracellular fluid calcium accounts for only a small percentage of the total body calcium. The concentration of calcium in plasma (2.25–2.60 mmol per litre), however, is kept within narrow limits by homoeostatic mechanisms. In plasma the calcium is present in three forms: ionized (about 45 per cent); protein-bound, mainly to albumin (about 40 per cent); and complexed (about 15 per cent). It is the ionized calcium concentration that is physiologically important. Clinical laboratories, however, measure the total plasma calcium concentration, and therefore an awareness of the changes in total calcium concentration caused by changes in protein concentration is important.

The plasma ionized calcium concentration is regulated by parathyroid hormone (PTH) and vitamin D. Calcitonin, the third calcium-regulating hormone, does not play an important role. In addition to PTH and vitamin D, several other factors, such as thyroid hormones, growth hormone (GH), and glucocorticoids, influence the plasma calcium concentration. The effects of all these factors are mediated by their action on one or more of three organs: kidney, bone, and intestine. Of these three, the kidney plays an important role because of the large amount of calcium it handles (240 mmol per day compared with intestinal absorption of about 1–2 mmol

TABLE 17.6
Causes of drug-induced hypercalcaemia

Increased absorption from the intestine
  milk–alkali syndrome
  vitamin D and its metabolites

Increased mobilization from bone
  vitamin A and its derivatives (etretinate, acitretin, isotretinoin)
  vitamin D and its metabolites
  calcipotriol, tacalcitol

Decreased renal excretion
  calcium-channel blockers
  lithium
  thiazides
  tamoxifen
  theophylline

TABLE 17.7
Causes of drug-induced hypocalcaemia

Decreased absorption from the intestine
  alteration in vitamin D metabolism — alcohol, anticonvulsants, glutethimide

Decreased bone mobilization
  calcitonin, diphosphonates, drug-induced hypomagnesaemia, gallium nitrate, mithramycin

Increased renal excretion
  loop diuretics, magnesium sulphate

Complexing of calcium
  EDTA, desferrioxamine, foscarnet, neomycin, phosphate

per day) (Nordin 1990). Drugs may affect one or more of the organs involved in calcium regulation. The causes of drug-induced abnormalities of serum calcium concentration are listed in Tables 17.6 and 17.7.

Hypercalcaemia

Increased intestinal absorption

The milk–alkali syndrome, caused by ingestion of large quantities of milk and antacids for prolonged periods of time by patients with peptic ulcer used to be a relatively common cause of hypercalcaemia. It then became relatively uncommon (Shek *et al.* 1990), but it is becoming more common again with the promotion of calcium carbonate as treatment for osteoporosis and dyspepsia, and in one study accounted for 12 per cent of hypercalcaemias (Beall and Scofield 1995). A case of severe hypercalcaemic crisis in pregnancy requiring dialysis has been described (Kleinman *et al.* 1991). The mechanism of the hypercalcaemia is thought to involve the production of alkalosis from the absorption of large amounts of alkali, promoting renal tubular reabsorption of calcium

(Orwell 1982; Sutton and Dirks 1996). This is accompanied by increased calcium absorption leading to hypercalcaemia. In some patients, renal failure further limits calcium excretion. Serum PTH concentrations are suppressed (Beall and Scofield 1995). The importance of increased renal tubular absorption in the pathogenesis of hypercalcaemia in the milk–alkali syndrome is illustrated by the absence of hypercalcaemia in absorptive hypercalciuria.

Calcium carbonate has also been used as a substitute for aluminium hydroxide in the control of plasma phosphate in patients on haemodialysis. Plasma calcium concentration has been shown to increase with the use of calcium carbonate (Anelli *et al.* 1989) and hypercalcaemia has been reported. A case of severe hypercalcaemia, nephrocalcinosis, and renal failure secondary to ingestion of calcium carbonate, has been reported (Blau and Hoyman 1997). Mild hypercalcaemia has been observed with the use of calcium acetate in patients on haemodialysis (Emmett *et al.* 1991). Calcium ion-exchange resins used in the management of hyperkalaemia in patients who are in renal failure may precipitate hypercalcaemia (Sevitt and Wrong 1968). Hypercalcaemia has also been reported following the use of haemostatic compresses (Sorbacal) containing 4.6–6.8% calcium acetate by weight (Texier *et al.* 1982).

Vitamin D and its metabolites, 25-hydroxycholecalciferol (25-OHD$_3$) and 1,25-dihydroxycholecalciferol (1,25-DHCC), and alphacalcidol (1α-hydroxycholecalciferol [1α-OHD$_3$]), when taken in large doses can cause hypercalcaemia from increased intestinal absorption of calcium and increased bone resorption. Hypercalcaemia may also arise as a result of overdosage with these preparations following self-medication or in the treatment of hypocalcaemic states (Chapuy and Meunier 1990) or during use of supplementary calcium by the elderly to prevent osteoporosis (Byrne *et al.* 1995). The duration of hypercalcaemia after withdrawal of the drug depends on the preparation used, with vitamin D > dihydrotachysterol > 25-OHD$_3$ > 1α-OHD$_3$ > 1,25-DHCC (Kanis and Russell 1977). The duration of hypercalcaemia is usually much longer than the serum half-lives of the metabolites, because of the persistence of its physiological action. For example, the serum half-life of 1,25-DHCC is a few hours but the hypercalcaemia following 1,25-DHCC may persist for 1–2 days. Danazol may potentiate the effect of 1α-OHD$_3$ (Hepburn *et al.* 1989).

Increased mobilization from bone

Calcipotriol is a vitamin D analogue used in the treatment of psoriasis (Berth Jones and Hutchinson 1992).

This is 100–200 times less potent than the natural hormone 1,25 DHCC in its effects on calcium metabolism (Kragballe and Iverson 1993) and several studies showed no significant effect on serum calcium concentration (Langner *et al.* 1993). However, hypercalcaemia as a result of percutaneous absorption has been reported in patients using large doses of calcipotriol (Dwyer and Chapman 1991; Berth Jones and Hutchinson 1992; Cunliffe *et al.* 1992; Bourke *et al.* 1993) and even with the recommended dose (Hardman *et al.* 1993; Russell and Young 1994). A case of severe hypercalcaemic crisis after excessive use of calcipotriol (Hoeck *et al.* 1994) highlights the danger of exceeding the recommended dose (Berth Jones and Hutchinson 1992).

Vitamin A in toxic doses causes hypercalcaemia due to increased bone resorption. Hypercalcaemia following vitamin A intoxication has been reported in haemodialysed patients (Fishbane *et al.* 1995) and in those taking 50–100 000 units of vitamin A per day (Sutton and Dirks 1996).

The vitamin A derivatives etretinate, acitretin, and isotretinoin are used in dermatological practice and in the treatment of some malignancies. When used in the treatment of neuroblastoma, isotretinoin (13 *cis*-retinoic acid) caused hypercalcaemia in 23 per cent of patients (Villablanca *et al.* 1993). Initial trial of a retinoid receptor agonist in patients with advanced cancer showed hypercalcaemia as a minor adverse effect (Miller *et al.* 1997).

Decreased renal excretion

Thiazides reduce the excretion of calcium by increasing the reabsorption of calcium in the proximal tubules, as a result of extracellular volume contraction, as well as by an increase in reabsorption at the distal tubules (Sutton and Dirks 1996). The use of thiazide diuretics is associated with an increase in serum calcium concentration. The degree of hypercalcaemia is mild (total serum calcium usually <2.75 mmol per litre) and is mostly due to haemoconcentration. The plasma calcium returns to normal within 2 weeks of withdrawing the thiazides. True hypercalcaemia, however, may develop during thiazide therapy under conditions of high bone turnover such as primary hyperparathyroidism (Strong *et al.* 1991) and in elderly subjects taking supplementary vitamin D or calcium (Boulard *et al.* 1994; Sutton and Dirks 1996).

Lithium therapy has been reported to increase plasma calcium concentration, decrease serum phosphate concentration, and decrease urinary calcium excretion (Mallette and Eichhorn 1986). Various figures for the incidence of hypercalcaemia have been reported. In patients treated for a mean of 7.4 years the incidence was

20.9 per cent (Linder *et al.* 1993); in those treated over 10 years (Nordenstrom *et al.* 1994), 42 per cent; and in those treated for 1–30 years, 25 per cent (Kallner and Petterson 1995). In a recent survey of 142 patients treated for at least 15 years, however, the prevalence of persistent hypercalcaemia was only 3.6 per cent (Bendz *et al.* 1996). These differences in prevalence of hypercalcaemia could be due to differences in the dosage of lithium used. The serum concentration of parathyroid hormone measured by specific assays was inappropriately high for the prevailing plasma calcium concentration (Kallner and Petterson 1995; Nordenstrom *et al.* 1994). At least 45 case reports of hyperparathyroidism associated with lithium therapy have appeared in the world literature (Taylor and Bell 1993; Bachmeyer *et al.* 1995). Study of parathyroid glands removed at surgery showed predominantly hyperplasia without adenomatous change (Nordenstrom *et al.* 1992). Lithium reduces renal calcium excretion and increases its intestinal absorption (Mallette and Eichhorn 1986) and serum calcium concentration increases. At the same time lithium reduces the sensitivity of the parathyroid cells, possibly by decreasing the binding of calcium to the calcium-binding sites on the parathyroid cell membrane (Mallette 1991). The calcium concentration required to inhibit PTH secretion is therefore higher in patients taking lithium (McHenry and Racke 1993). The effects on the kidney and intestine are transient, however, so that positive calcium balance is only seen for a short period, after which a steady state is reached (Mallette 1991). Most patients with lithium-induced hypercalcaemia are asymptomatic.

Tamoxifen treatment of patients with metastatic breast cancer has been reported to cause severe hypercalcaemia in a small proportion of patients (Larsen *et al.* 1990; Daugaard 1993; Ellis and Tattersall 1995); those with osteolytic bone metastases appear to be at greater risk and the incidence varies greatly (Dukes 1996*a*). Parathyroid hormone-related peptide (PTHrP) concentrations in a patient with hypercalcaemia due to tamoxifen were three times normal at the onset of the hypercalcaemia, which suggests that PTHrP may be involved in its development (Berruti *et al.* 1996).

Hypercalcaemia following exposure to manganese has been reported (Roels *et al.* 1987). The high ionized calcium concentration found in infants born to mothers receiving magnesium sulphate therapy has been suggested to be due to displacement of calcium from albumin by the magnesium (Liu *et al.* 1988*b*).

In theophylline poisoning up to 20 per cent of patients have hypercalcaemia, probably related to β-adrenergic stimulation (McPherson *et al.* 1986).

Calcium-channel blockers have been reported to cause abnormalities in plasma calcium and PTH concentrations. Studies reported up to now, however, have produced conflicting results and, so far, frank hypercalcaemia with the use of calcium-channel blockers has not been reported. Verapamil (Resnick *et al.* 1989), nifedipine (Resnick *et al.* 1987), felodipine (Hespel *et al.* 1987), and nisoldipine (Odigwe *et al.* 1986) have been reported to increase ionized calcium concentration. Other studies, however, have not been able to show any increase (Benjamin *et al.* 1988; Graves *et al.* 1988). Diltiazem lowered serum PTH, increased urinary calcium, and decreased phosphate excretion (Seely *et al.* 1989), whereas felodipine had no effect (Villiger *et al.* 1993). Calcium-channel blockers were reported to have worsened hypercalcaemia in patients with hyperparathyroidism (Samani 1991) and in patients with breast cancer (Sinzinger *et al.* 1991). It was suggested that in these cases the effect was mediated by stimulation of prostaglandin synthesis by the calcium antagonists (Sinzinger *et al.* 1991).

Danazol, a weak androgen, and progestogens have been reported to cause hypercalcaemia (Dukes 1996*b*). Administration of GH to critically ill surgical patients is associated with hypercalcaemia in 43 per cent of cases (Knox *et al.* 1995) probably due to reduced renal excretion.

Treatment

Plasma calcium concentrations raised by drugs usually return to normal once the drug is withdrawn. If the plasma calcium is very high or is associated with ill effects, then active treatment may be required. The first step is rehydration and treatment with frusemide. Other measures are administration of a glucocorticoid, calcitonin, or sodium phosphate or diphosphonates (Thiebaud et al. 1986; Sutton and Dirks 1996). Very rarely, haemodialysis may be required to lower serum calcium when other methods fail.

Hypocalcaemia

As 40 per cent of plasma calcium is bound to plasma proteins, mainly albumin, hypoalbuminaemia is the commonest cause of apparent hypocalcaemia in clinical practice. Correcting the plasma total calcium concentration for low albumin using one of the many available formulae will help in detecting true hypocalcaemia.

Decreased intestinal absorption

Hypocalcaemia has been reported to occur in up to 48 per cent of epileptic patients on anticonvulsant therapy (Weinstein *et al.* 1984). This is thought to be due to altered metabolism of vitamin D (see below under Vitamin D for further details).

Corticosteroids are used in the treatment of some forms of hypercalcaemia. The decrease in plasma calcium is at least partly due to reduction in intestinal calcium absorption (Lukert and Raisz 1990). Frank hypocalcaemia, however, is not likely to be seen with the use of corticosteroids.

Decreased mobilization from bone

Hypomagnesaemia of any aetiology causes hypocalcaemia, due to a combination of decreased release of PTH, resistance to the action of PTH, decreased concentration of 1,25 DHCC, and resistance to the action of 1,25 DHCC (Swaminathan 1998; Rude and Oldham 1990). Administration of calcium alone does not correct the hypocalcaemia. Hypomagnesaemia due to cisplatin or gentamicin treatment (Nanji and Denegri 1984) can, for example, cause severe hypocalcaemia. Blom and colleagues (1985), however, have reported that, in cisplatin treatment, serum calcium concentration decreased in spite of magnesium supplementation and the serum calcium returned spontaneously to normal some months after the last course of cisplatin. This effect may be due to a direct effect of cisplatin on the release of PTH (Aggarwal and Fadool 1993).

Drugs used in the treatment of severe hypercalcaemia such as mithramycin, calcitonin, clodronate, gallium nitrate (Baselga et al. 1993) and pamidronate (Purohit et al. 1994) may cause hypocalcaemia by reducing bone resorption. Colchicine may also cause hypocalcaemia by inhibiting bone resorption (Heath et al. 1972).

Increased renal excretion

Loop diuretics can exacerbate hypocalcaemia in hypoparathyroidism by increasing the urinary excretion of calcium (Gabow et al. 1977).

Magnesium sulphate used in the treatment of preeclampsia has been found to lower the plasma calcium concentration (Lamm et al. 1988) and this is accompanied by an increase in urinary calcium excretion, and a decrease in renal cyclic-AMP excretion (Suzuki et al. 1986). The increased renal loss of calcium induced by magnesium is the main factor in lowering the plasma calcium (Sutton and Dirks 1996).

Radioactive iodine (^{131}I), used in the management of thyroid cancer, has been reported to cause a significant decrease in plasma calcium concentration. In one study, 58 per cent of patients who received ^{131}I had hypocalcaemia and this was not related to age, sex, or the amount of ^{131}I uptake by the thyroid (Glazebrook 1987). The hypocalcaemia is due to PTH deficiency and is related to pretreatment plasma calcium concentration, which was lower in those who subsequently developed hypocalcaemia.

Sodium phosphate, administered intravenously, orally, or rectally (Craig et al. 1994) may cause hypocalcaemia (Crook and Swaminathan 1996; Sutton and Dirks 1996).

EDTA chelates divalent cations and can be used to lower the plasma calcium concentration in hypercalcaemic states. The EDTA–calcium complex is excreted by the kidney. The rate and amount of administration of EDTA determine the fall in plasma calcium. Hypocalcaemia may be caused by too rapid infusion of EDTA (Sutton and Dirks 1996), but the hypocalcaemia is short-lived. By complexing calcium, neomycin may cause hypocalcaemia (Yao et al. 1980). Desferrioxamine used to treat aluminium overload caused hypocalcaemia in an infant (Klein et al. 1989) and in dialysis patients (McCarthy et al. 1990).

Polymyxin B, by its nephrotoxic effect, can cause hypocalcaemia (Ruef et al. 1996).

Infusion of adrenaline or administration of the sympathomimetic agent ritodrine lowers plasma ionized calcium concentration (Kawarabayashi et al. 1989). The mechanism and significance of these findings are not clear.

Neuroleptics used in psychiatric patients are associated with low serum ionized calcium concentrations, together with neuroleptic-induced extrapyramidal symptoms (Kuny and Binswanger 1989).

When large amounts of blood containing preservative acid citrate dextrose are transfused, hypocalcaemia may follow (Sutton and Dirks 1996). In one study of patients receiving 20 or more units of blood within 24 hours, the ionized calcium concentration was less than 0.70 mmol per litre in 53 per cent (Wilson et al. 1987). The hypocalcaemia is caused by complexing of calcium by citrate. Significant hypocalcaemia may also occur during therapeutic plasma exchange (Choudhary and Hughes 1995). Infusion of citrate-containing radiocontrast media may also cause hypocalcaemia (Mallette and Gomez 1983).

Oestrogen replacement therapy in the menopause will cause a significant decrease in plasma calcium concentration (Sutton and Dirks 1996) and a case of severe hypocalcaemia following oestrogen treatment of a patient with metastatic carcinoma of the prostate has been described (Dukes 1996a). The mechanism of action of oestrogens in lowering the plasma calcium concentration is thought to be resetting of the threshold for secretion of PTH.

The antiviral drugs foscarnet and ganciclovir, used in the treatment of cytomegalovirus infections, can cause hypocalcaemia (Jacobson 1997). The hypocalcaemia seen during the infusion of the drug can be severe and symptomatic, is due to its chelation of calcium (Jacobson *et al.* 1991; Jacobson 1992); it may limit the dose that can be used in about 20 per cent of patients, and may limit the dosage. Foscarnet, by its effects on the kidney, causes renal tubular acidosis, hypomagnesuria and chronic hypocalcaemia (Gearhart and Sorg 1993; Navarro *et al.* 1995).

Fluorescein used in angiography was found to cause a significant decrease in ionized calcium concentration, probably due to complexing of calcium by the fluorescein (Turetta *et al.* 1985). Cysteamine, used in the treatment of paracetamol intoxication, reduced serum calcium concentration when administered to normal subjects (Copeland *et al.* 1986).

Heparin caused apparent hypocalcaemia in haemodialysis patients by the formation of calcium soaps with fatty acids released *in vitro* (Godolphin *et al.* 1979).

Indomethacin administration has been associated with increased urinary calcium excretion (Ambanelli *et al.* 1982).

Treatment

Treatment of hypocalcaemia consists of withdrawal of the offending drug and the administration of calcium supplements (Sutton and Dirks 1996).

Bone disease

Drugs may interfere with metabolism of calcium, phosphate, vitamin D, or bone to cause metabolic bone disease ranging from osteoporosis, in which there is a reduction in volume of bone tissue, to osteomalacia or rickets, characterized by increased osteoid tissue. In some instances of drug-induced metabolic bone disease the bone morphology is more complicated.

Corticosteroid-induced osteoporosis

The effect of glucocorticoids on bone is well recognized, and with their widespread use as anti-inflammatory and immunosuppressive agents, glucocorticoid-induced osteoporosis has become a significant problem (Reid *et al.* 1994). Recent studies show that nearly 0.5 per cent of the community uses corticosteroids (Walsh *et al.* 1996), and their use is increasing (Eastell 1995). Corticosteroids appear to cause a preferential loss of trabecular bone (Reid and Grey 1993), most severe in vertebrae and ribs (Wolinsky-Friedland 1995), resulting in compression fractures of vertebrae and fractures of the ribs and pubic rami (Adinoff and Hollister 1983). However, bone mass studies show that bone loss at cortical bone such as in the femoral neck can be similar to that in trabecular bone (Sambrook *et al.* 1990).

The prevalence of vertebral fractures in patients with rheumatoid arthritis may be as high as 34 per cent (Michel *et al.* 1991). In some studies using a morphometric method, however, the prevalence of vertebral fracture was found to be only 12 per cent in patients with rheumatoid arthritis and there was no increased prevalence in those treated with low-dose corticosteroids (Spector *et al.* 1993). In asthmatic patients, where the dose of corticosteroids is likely to be higher, the prevalence of fracture as high as 42 per cent has been found (Adinoff and Hollister 1983). The risk of hip fracture is doubled with corticosteroid treatment (Cooper *et al.* 1995).

Bone loss occurs rapidly during the early part of treatment (Olbricht and Benker 1993; Sambrook *et al.* 1990) but with prolonged treatment it slows (Lo Cascio *et al.* 1990). Quantitative computerized tomographic (CT) studies show a 40 per cent reduction in vertebral bone density in patients treated with moderate doses of corticosteroids (Laan *et al.* 1993). Factors contributing to the amount of bone loss are total cumulative dose, daily dose, duration of treatment, sex, age and menopausal status (Reid and Heap 1990; Reid *et al.* 1994; Wolinksy-Friedland 1995). Several studies have shown that the degree and prevalence of bone loss is related to cumulative dosage (Ruegsegger *et al.* 1983). The incidence of osteopenia varies from about 23 per cent in those taking a cumulative dose of less than 10 g (prednisolone equivalent) to 78 per cent in those who received more than 30 g (Dykman *et al.* 1985). Alternate-day treatment is not protective, showing that cumulative dose is the more important risk factor (Gluck *et al.* 1981; Reid 1989). When used in high doses, inhaled corticosteroids cause reduction in bone mass (Packe *et al.* 1996). Topical (dermal, ocular) corticosteroids have not been reported to affect bone turnover (Reid and Harvie 1997). In addition to these factors there seems to be large individual variation in the response to corticosteroids (Olbricht and Benker 1993; Reid and Grey 1993; Reid *et al.* 1994).

Glucocorticoids decrease bone formation and increase bone resorption (Adachi 1997; Reid and Harvie 1997). Most probably they suppress osteoblast formation by a direct effect on osteoblasts, and this is supported by the demonstration of glucocorticoid receptors in osteoclasts. Reduced osteoblast function is shown by reduced serum osteocalcin (Reid *et al.* 1986; Caporali *et al.* 1991; Lane *et al.* 1996) and by histomorphometric studies (Aaron *et al.* 1989). Glucocorticoids not only inhibit the synthesis of bone collagen by pre-existing osteoblasts but also reduce the conversion of precursor cells to functioning osteoblasts (Adachi 1997). They may also affect the production and action of many cytokines and growth factors produced in bone cells (Reid and Harvie 1997; Reid and Grey 1993; Delany et al. 1994), and may also influence osteoblast function by modulating the effect of PTH and 1,25 vitamin D on these cells (Adachi 1997). They may also influence bone indirectly by reducing sex hormones in men (Morrison et al. 1994) and in postmenopausal women (Crilly et al. 1978).

Serum PTH concentrations have been reported to be increased during corticosteroid treatment (Lukert and Raisz 1990) but some of the newer assays for PTH have not confirmed this (Bikle et al. 1993). However, the increased bone resorption can be abolished by parathyroidectomy (Kukreja et al. 1976). The hyperparathyroidism induced by glucocorticoids is thought to be secondary to negative calcium balance as a result of glucocorticoid-induced decrease in calcium absorption (Lukert and Raisz 1990) and hypercalciuria (Suzuki et al. 1983) by a direct effect on the kidney (Reid and Ibbertson 1987).

A number of potential methods are now available to prevent glucocorticoid-induced bone loss (Reid 1997). In addition to using the lowest possible dose, it has been suggested that a newer steroid such as deflazacort would cause less effect on bone (LoCascio et al. 1984; Olgaard et al. 1992), though it still causes some bone loss (Krogsgaard et al. 1996; Messina et al. 1992).

Calcium supplements with vitamin D (Warady et al. 1994) and hormone replacement therapy (Lukert et al. 1992), bisphosphonates (Diamond et al. 1995), or calcitonin (Montemurro et al. 1991) administered concurrently with glucocorticoids may be beneficial in inhibiting bone loss. Intermittent etidronate therapy has recently been shown to reduce the loss of vertebral and trochanteric bone in patients treated with corticosteroids (Adachi et al. 1997).

Treatment

Treatment of established glucocorticoid-induced bone loss includes attempts to increase bone formation by agents such as fluoride or sex hormone and the use of antiresorptive agents such as bisphosphonates (Struys et al. 1995; Reid et al. 1996) in addition to calcium supplements and vitamin D metabolites (Dechant and Goa 1994). Calcium supplementation decreases bone loss (Sambrook et al. 1993). Combination of calcium and calcitriol prevents bone loss in the lumbar spine but not in proximal femur (Sambrook et al. 1993) or forearm (Adachi et al. 1996).

Anticonvulsant-induced bone disease

Metabolic bone disease has been reported to occur in 10–60 per cent of patients treated long-term with anticonvulsants (Hoikka et al. 1982; Wolinksky-Friedland 1995), and the incidence of pathological fracture is 10 per cent (Nilsson et al. 1986). Bone mass measurements show a 10–30 per cent decrease in total body mineral content (Tjellsen et al. 1985; Takeshita et al. 1989). Sodium valproate monotherapy was shown to cause a 14 per cent reduction in bone density in children while carbamazepine had no effect. The fall in bone density increased with duration of therapy (Sheth et al. 1995). Quantitative ultrasound studies of the calcaneus in young patients (mean age 19 years) on anticonvulsant therapy showed significant bone loss (Pluskiewicz and Nowakowska 1997). The type of abnormality described varies from osteomalacia to osteopenia and mineralization disorders (Wolinksky-Friedland 1995). Earlier reports showed that the predominant feature was osteomalacia or rickets, but more recent studies show that anticonvulsant-induced bone disease is a high bone turnover state (Shane 1996), the pathogenesis of which is not entirely clear. The osteomalacia picture seen is probably due to alteration in vitamin D metabolism (see section on vitamin D). In addition, anticonvulsants may have a direct effect on intestinal absorption of calcium and a direct effect on bone resorption and formation (Shane 1996).

Anticoagulant-induced osteoporosis

Long-term treatment with heparin is associated with osteoporosis (Levine 1986; Bardin and Lequesne 1989; Dahlman et al. 1990; Monreal et al. 1991) and fractures of the lumbar spine and ribs have been reported (Wolinsky-Friedland 1995). A study of pregnant women after heparin therapy found low bone density in up to 30 per cent (Barbour et al. 1994; Dahlman et al. 1994). In a larger study, osteoporotic vertebral fractures were seen in 2.2 per cent of patients (Dahlman 1993). The development of osteopenia is thought to be related to the dose and duration of therapy (Wolinsky-Friedland 1995; Douketis et al. 1996), though Barbour and colleagues (1994) were unable to demonstrate this relationship in their study. The osteopenic effect is predominantly seen with high-molecular-weight unfractionated heparin, although recently a case of vertebral fracture in a young woman receiving low-dose LMWH heparin has been reported (Sivakumaran et al. 1996). The mechanism of heparin-induced osteoporosis is not clear. Histomorphometric studies show increased bone resorption and decreased bone formation (Wolinksky-Friedland 1995; Muir et al. 1997). In a short-term (10-day) study of low-dose heparin, however, no biochemical evidence of increased bone resorption was found, although there was a significant decrease in alkaline phosphatase (van der Wiel *et al.* 1993) and osteocalcin (Cantini *et al.* 1995), suggesting decreased bone formation. *In vitro* studies show that heparin increases the bone resorption-stimulating activity of serum (Fuller *et al.* 1991) and animal studies show that unfractionated and high-molecular-weight heparin, but not LMWH, reduce bone density (Murray *et al.* 1995). LMWH only reduces bone formation (Muir *et al.* 1997) and this effect is less than that of unfractionated heparin (Nishiyama *et al.* 1997). *In vitro* studies also demonstrate that the bone-resorbing effect of heparin is dependent on molecular size and sulphation (Shaughnessy *et al.* 1995). Heparin does not, however, affect the bone-resorbing effect of IL-1β (Panagakos *et al.* 1995).

Osteocalcin is an α-carboxyl-glutamyl protein that may have a regulatory role in bone metabolism (Booth 1997). Serum concentrations of osteocalcin reflect osteoblastic activity (Swaminathan 1997). It is a vitamin K-dependent protein and therefore administration of vitamin K antagonists may reduce the carboxylation or inhibit the synthesis of this protein, or both (Furie and Furie 1990), and this in turn may affect bone (Vermeer *et al.* 1995). Vitamin K administration will reverse the carboxylation defect of osteocalcin (Pineo and Hull 1993; Douglas *et al.* 1995). Serum osteocalcin concentrations were found to be decreased in patients treated with vitamin K antagonists (Lafforgue *et al.* 1997) and greater proportion of circulating osteocalcin was under-carboxylated (Menon *et al.* 1987). Animal studies demonstrate that warfarin reduces osteocalcin in bone and causes significant osteopenia (Pastoureau *et al.* 1993). Bone density studies in patients taking warfarin have produced conflicting results — some showing no effect (Rosen *et al.* 1993; Lafforgue *et al.* 1997), others showing significant reduction (Philip *et al.* 1995).

Aluminium and bone disease

Aluminium is an aetiological factor in the pathogenesis of one form of bone disease seen in dialysis patients (Gonzalez and Martin 1992; Alfrey 1993; Hruska 1997). It is less common since the introduction of water purification and the use of phosphate binders that contain no aluminium (Gonzalez and Martin 1992). The bone disease associated with aluminium is resistant to vitamin D and its biologically active metabolites. Its mechanism is not fully understood (Jeffery *et al.* 1996). Aluminium impairs the mineralization of bone and it also directly affects the numbers or function of osteoblasts. In ad-

dition, aluminium has complex effects on PTH secretion and vitamin D metabolites (for a review see Jeffery *et al.* 1996).

Bone disease of total parenteral nutrition

Metabolic bone disease is a relatively common complication of long-term parenteral nutrition (Nomura *et al.* 1993; von Wowern *et al.* 1996). In patients receiving this treatment at home, incidences ranging from 42–100 per cent have been reported. The metabolic basis of the bone disease seen in home parenteral nutrition is complex (for a review, see Klein and Coburn 1994). There is altered bone remodelling following total parenteral nutrition (Lawson *et al.* 1995). Many factors contribute to the development of the bone disease, including inadequate calcium, inadequate phosphate, hypercalciuria (due to such factors as high protein intake, acidosis, high sodium content, hypertonic dextrose, and insulin), and aluminium toxicity (see section on Aluminium), continuous instead of intermittent supply of nutrients, effects on cytochrome P450 isoenzymes (Klein and Coburn 1994) and sensitivity to vitamin D (Klein and Coburn 1994). As patients on long-term parenteral nutrition are at high risk of developing metabolic bone disease, they should be carefully monitored. With current parenteral nutrition regimens there was no significant reduction in bone density suggesting that aluminium and vitamin D_2 may have played an important role in the past (Saitta *et al.* 1993). In selected patients (with suppressed PTH) withdrawal of vitamin D supplement increased bone density (Verhage *et al.* 1995).

Bone disease associated with other drugs

Loss of oestrogens is associated with accelerated loss of bone (Nordin *et al.* 1984), and low oestrogen concentrations may result from treatment with long-acting gonadotrophin-releasing hormone (GnRH) agonists (Polan and Barbieri 1990; Judd 1992; Stevenson 1995) or neuroleptics. Treatment with leuprolide, a GnRH antagonist, caused a significant reduction in bone density which returned to normal after treatment (Wheeler *et al.* 1993). Long-term treatment with GnRH analogues caused osteoporosis in both sexes (Fogelman 1992; Goldray *et al.* 1993). Hyperprolactinaemia induced by neuroleptics suppresses oestrogen concentration (Ataya *et al.* 1988). Patients taking antipsychotic drugs have increased urinary calcium and hydroxyproline excretion and this may contribute to osteopenia and the increased risk of hip fracture associated with antipsychotic treatment (Higuchi *et al.* 1987). The antioestrogenic drug tamoxifen did not cause significant reduction in bone density in a patient with mastalgia treated for 3–6 months (Fentiman *et al.* 1989) and it may protect the skeleton against corticosteroid-induced bone loss (Fentimen and Fogelman 1993).

Ketoconazole caused an increase in bone fragility in animals. Danazol treatment has been reported to cause either no change in bone density (Stevenson *et al.* 1989) or an increase (Dawood *et al.* 1995).

Long-term infusion (up to 13 weeks) of magnesium sulphate for prevention of premature labour can cause congenital rickets (Lamm *et al.* 1988), probably as a result of suppression of the fetal parathyroid glands.

Chemotherapy for malignant conditions may cause abnormalities in calcium, magnesium, and vitamin D metabolism. In children treated for acute lymphoblastic leukaemia, bone mineral content was found to be low 6 months after the end of treatment (Atkinson *et al.* 1989).

Earlier studies indicated that lithium treatment was associated with reduced bone density. However, more recent studies showed no significant differences in bone density between patients taking lithium for 10 years or longer and control subjects (Nordenstrom *et al.* 1994).

Miscellaneous drugs that may affect bone include cyclosporin (Buchinsky *et al.* 1996; Rich *et al.* 1992), methotrexate (May *et al.* 1996), prostaglandin in neonates (Kaufman and El Chaar 1996), and tacrolimus. Animal studies have shown that all these drugs produce changes in bone metabolism (Epstein and Shane 1996). Transplantation is associated with osteoporosis (Epstein *et al.* 1995), perhaps related to cyclosporin treatment (Wolpaw *et al.* 1994; Callegari 1997), although some studies have shown cyclosporin to increase bone density (Arolidi *et al.* 1997) in renal transplant patients. Theophylline increases urinary excretion of calcium and phosphate and may have an effect on bone (Prince *et al.* 1988). Caffeine increases urinary calcium excretion (Heaney and Recker 1982) and in epidemiological studies high caffeine consumption is associated with lowered bone density (Barrett-Connor *et al.* 1994).

Excessive alcohol intake is an established risk factor for osteoporosis (Spector *et al.* 1992; Reid and Harvie 1997). The possible causes of alcohol-related bone disease include poor nutrition, a toxic effect of alcohol on bone metabolism and osteoblast function, liver dysfunction, vitamin D deficiency, abnormalities in vitamin D metabolism, and alcohol-induced gonadal dysfunction (Wolinsky-Friedland 1995; Reid and Harvie 1997).

Treatment of a patient with severe congenital neutropenia with G-M CSF was associated with severe osteoporosis (Bishop *et al.* 1995) and exacerbation of osteoporosis has been observed in other patients (Bonilla et al. 1994). Bone density was found to be lowered in

women using depot medroxyprogesterone acetate as contraceptive. When they stopped, bone density returned to normal (Cundy *et al.* 1994).

Bismuth used as an antacid can cause osteolytic lesions and fractures (Dukes 1996a). Oral zinc therapy can cause copper deficiency as well as osteopenia (Patterson *et al.* 1985). High doses of ascorbic acid have been shown to increase bone resorption in animal studies (Helsing 1996). Repeated intravenous injection of polyvinylpyrrolidone (Povidone) as a plasma expander over a 10-year period was associated with pathological fractures due to deposition of this compound in bone cells (Kepes *et al.* 1993).

Phosphate

Most of the phosphorus in the body, like potassium, is intracellular and only a small fraction is present in plasma. In plasma, phosphate exists in two main forms: organic (ester and lipid phosphates) and inorganic (orthophosphate). Fifteen per cent of plasma inorganic phosphate is bound to protein, and the rest is dialysable. The concentration of plasma inorganic phosphate in health varies with age, sex, and time of day (Crook and Swaminathan 1996). Drugs may cause changes in plasma phosphate concentration by affecting the distribution between the intracellular and extracellular compartments, or by altering the intestinal absorption or renal excretion (Knochel and Agarwal 1996) (Table 17.8).

Hypophosphataemia

Intracellular shift

An acute shift of phosphate from the extracellular to the intracellular compartment is frequently responsible for hypophosphataemia. The most frequent cause of this redistribution is the intravenous administration of carbohydrates with or without insulin (Crook and Swaminathan 1996). When glucose or other carbohydrates enter cells, they are accompanied by phosphate, because of phosphorylation of hexose intermediates within the cell. One mole of glucose uses four moles of phosphate in the glycolytic process. In hospital patients, infusion of carbohydrates accounted for 43–73 per cent of all the cases of hypophosphataemia (Swaminathan *et al.* 1979). Even smaller amounts of glucose in the form of 5% dextrose solution or dextrose saline (4% dextrose) cause a moderate decrease in plasma phosphate (0.25–0.35 mmol per litre). In starving and cirrhotic patients this effect is aggravated by the exaggerated insulin response, whereas in diabetic patients and those with

TABLE 17.8
Causes of drug-induced hypophosphataemia

A. Distribution into cells
β-adrenoceptor agonists — adrenaline,
bronchodilators, carbohydrate administration
(e.g. total parenteral nutrition), insulin-like
growth factors, parenteral iron (saccharated iron
oxide) respiratory alkalosis induced by drugs

B. Reduced intestinal absorption
antacids, sucralfate, laxatives

C. Increased excretion
diuretics, glucocorticoids, ifosfamide, metabolic
alkalosis, paracetamol

D. Miscellaneous mechanisms
anticonvulsants, foscarnet, oestrogens,
pamidronate and gallium nitrate, tumour
necrosis factor-α, interleukin-2

muscular dystrophy the effect is the opposite (Crook and Swaminathan 1996). In severely malnourished subjects life-threatening hypophosphataemia may occur during refeeding (Bufano *et al.* 1990; van Dissel *et al.* 1992; Brooks and Melnik 1995). Severe, sometimes symptomatic, hypophosphataemia is caused by glucose–insulin–potassium therapy (Swaminathan *et al.* 1978) and by intravenous feeding regimens containing high concentrations of glucose without phosphate supplements (Travis *et al.* 1971). The degree of hypophosphataemia is related to the number of calories infused and the nutritional state, being severe in starving, malnourished individuals and alcoholics. Severe hypophosphataemia (0.16–0.39 mmol per litre) has also been reported following enteral feeding of carbohydrates (Crook *et al.* 1996). Insulin administration without glucose has similar hypophosphataemic effects, and profound hypophosphataemia is not uncommon during treatment of diabetic ketoacidosis and hyperosmolar coma with insulin (Knochel and Agarwal 1996).

Administration of carbohydrates other than glucose, such as fructose, xylitol, or sorbitol, causes hypophosphataemia that is more severe than that seen after glucose. This is due to unregulated uptake of fructose by the liver and subsequent formation of fructose-1-phosphate (Knochel and Agarwal 1996).

Respiratory alkalosis caused by drugs such as salicylates can lower plasma phosphate. This is largely due to transcellular shift of phosphates with a contribution from increased phosphate excretion (Crook and Swaminathan 1996). Respiratory alkalosis increases intracellular pH which stimulates phosphofructokinase activity resulting in increased glycolysis (Knochel and Agarwal 1996). Plasma phosphate concentration can be

as low as 0.3 mmol per litre in respiratory alkalosis (Crook and Swaminathan 1996).

Administration of adrenaline causes hypophosphataemia and this effect of adrenaline is β-adrenoceptor-mediated and believed to be caused by a shift of phosphate into cells due to increased glycogenolytic activity. Administration of catecholamines and β-adrenergic agonists, among other drugs, contribute to the hypophosphataemia in the critically ill (Brown and Greenwood 1994). Phosphate depletion is common in patients with chronic obstructive airways disease and is probably the result of bronchodilator therapy (Fiaccadori *et al.* 1994). Hypophosphataemia developed in 54 per cent of patients with acute severe asthma admitted for emergency bronchodilator therapy, and serum phosphate and serum theophylline concentrations were negatively correlated (Brady *et al.* 1989). Similar effects were found in a larger study of 569 patients with serum theophylline concentrations <5.5 mmol per litre (Flack *et al.* 1994). The risk of developing hypophosphataemia was calculated to be increased 2.7 times in this group. Hypophosphataemia is a feature of theophylline overdose (Filejski *et al.* 1993) even when the plasma concentration of theophylline was only moderately high (Hagley *et al.* 1994).

Acetate in concentrations ranging from 2–140 mmol per litre is used in dialysis fluids and lavage fluids used in surgery. The use of acetate may lower plasma phosphate concentration, probably because of a transcellular shift (Veech and Gitomer 1988).

Insulin-like growth factor (IGF1) when used in Type 1 diabetic patients with insulin resistance caused acute symptomatic hypophosphataemia (Usala *et al.* 1994).

Reduced intestinal absorption

Decreased absorption of phosphate from the intestine accounts for the hypophosphataemia induced by chronic use of phosphate binders. These agents not only reduce the absorption of dietary phosphate, but also that of secreted phosphate and cause a net negative balance (Knochel and Agarwal 1996). Prolonged use of antacids may lead to osteomalacia (Chines and Pacifici 1990; Boutsen *et al.* 1996) or rickets (Foldes *et al.* 1991). The use of antacids accounted for about 2 per cent of the hypophosphataemia in one survey (Juan and Elrazak 1979). Prolonged use of laxatives can also lead to hypophosphataemia (Meyers *et al.* 1990).

Increased excretion

Metabolic alkalosis causes an increased loss of phosphate in the urine and thereby causes hypophosphataemia (Knochel and Agarwal 1996).

Diuretics, especially those that inhibit sodium reabsorption in segments of the nephron that also transport phosphate, may cause hypophosphataemia. Thus, diuretics such as acetazolamide frequently cause phosphaturia and hypophosphataemia, whereas those that act on the loop of Henle, such as frusemide, bumetanide, and ethacrynic acid, do not produce phosphaturia. Distally acting diuretics such as thiazides and chlorthalidone rarely produce significant hypophosphataemia, despite the fact that 10–15 per cent of phosphate is reabsorbed in the distal segments, because there is a compensatory increase in phosphate transport in the proximal segment in response to a mild depletion (Knochel and Agarwal 1996). Other diuretics, such as metolazone and osmotic diuretics, also reduce proximal tubular reabsorption and can cause increased phosphate excretion and thus lower plasma phosphate.

Glucocorticoids in pharmacological doses have been shown to cause increased phosphate excretion (Knochel and Agarwal 1996), and this may account for the low phosphate concentrations seen during corticosteroid therapy (Nuti et al. 1984) and ACTH infusions for infantile spasm (Riikonen et al. 1986).

Hypophosphataemia is a feature of paracetamol poisoning. This was demonstrated to be due to phosphaturia (Meredith et al. 1996) and the severity of hypophosphataemia correlated with severity of hepatotoxicity (Jones et al. 1989). It has been suggested that paracetamol may have a direct effect on the renal tubules, although the role of other factors such as respiratory alkalosis, glucose infusion, and volume expansion cannot be excluded (Knochel and Agarwal 1996). Estramustine has been reported to cause significant hypophosphataemia during the first 6 weeks of treatment of metastatic prostatic cancer. The cause of hypophosphataemia is increased phosphate excretion, as shown by a reduced renal tubular threshold for phosphate reabsorption ($TmPO_4$/GFR) (Citrin et al. 1986). It was also suggested that this is probably an oestrogenic effect of estramustine.

Miscellaneous

Oestrogen administration lowers plasma phosphate concentration (Selby and Peacock 1986). The exact mechanism of this oestrogen effect is not clear; it has been suggested to be due to increased bone formation. Ifosfamide, a drug used for the treatment of solid tumours, produces hypophosphataemia and phosphaturia because of its renal toxicity and the decrease in plasma phosphate concentration was related to total dose (Skinner et al. 1996). In children this results in hypophosphataemic rickets (Skinner et al. 1989). Anticonvulsant therapy has been reported to cause a lower plasma phosphate concentration (Patweri et al. 1996), and this effect of anticonvulsants is probably through their effect on vitamin D metabolism (see sections on Calcium, Bone, and Vitamin D).

Patients treated for malignant hypercalcaemia with pamidronate, a potent inhibitor of osteoclast-mediated bone resorption, were reported to show a significant decrease in plasma phosphate concentration (Nussbaum et al. 1993). Gallium nitrate, another hypocalcaemic drug, was found to reduce plasma phosphate concentration by 27 per cent (Warrell et al. 1991). Foscarnet, used in the treatment of cytomegalovirus infections, caused significant hypophosphataemia (Gearhart and Sorg 1993) among other electrolyte disturbances. Tumour necrosis factor-α and interleukin-2 have been reported to cause hypophosphataemia (Kozeny et al. 1988; Webb et al. 1988; Vial and Descotes 1996) and intrahepatic administration of tumour necrosis factor produced a transient hypophosphataemia (del Giglio et al. 1991).

Hypophosphataemia was reported in cirrhotic patients given erythropoietin (Kajikawa et al. 1993).

Treatment

Hypophosphataemia, especially when it is severe and prolonged, requires treatment with phosphate supplements either orally or parenterally, as it has been shown that the disorder can have adverse effects (Crook and Swaminathan 1996).

Hyperphosphataemia

Increased plasma phosphate concentration can arise from increased absorption or reduced excretion of phosphate. Increase in phosphate intake only produces mild elevation of serum phosphate, as the renal excretion is efficient. If the amount administered is large, plasma phosphate will increase. Hyperphosphataemia may occur in infants fed unadapted cows' milk (Venkataraman et al. 1985). Hyperphosphataemia, hypocalcaemia, and tetany due to absorption of phosphate from the colon following enemas with a high phosphate content have been reported in children (Fass et al. 1993; Hunter et al. 1993) and in adults (Rao et al. 1976), occasionally resulting in death (Korzets et al. 1992), especially patients with ileus (Fass et al. 1993). Oral sodium phosphate, which is used as a colonic cleansing agent, causes significant hyperphosphataemia (Cohen et al. 1994; Huynh et al. 1995). Hyperphosphataemia is also seen after the use of laxatives containing phosphate (McConnel 1971; Ilberg et al. 1978). Over-treatment of hypophosphataemia or hypercalcaemia by oral or intravenous phosphate can lead to hyperphosphataemia, especially if the renal function is poor. A patient with renal failure treated with oral phosphate developed hyperphosphataemia, hypocalcaemia, laryngeal spasm and vocal cord paralysis (Lye and Leong 1994).

Drugs that cause renal failure (see Chapter 14) will cause hyperphosphataemia. Rhabdomyolysis causes release of intracellular phosphate and hence hyperphosphataemia, particularly if renal function is impaired. For instance, opiate overdosage has been reported to cause rhabdomyolysis and hyperphosphataemia which lasted for 7–10 days (Blain et al. 1985).

Hyperphosphataemia may also result from hypervitaminosis D and hypervitaminosis A. In hypervitaminosis D there is increased intestinal absorption and, in addition, reduced renal excretion due to suppression of PTH (Chapuy and Meunier 1990). Calcitriol treatment of the hyperparathyroidism of end-stage renal failure has caused significant hyperphosphataemia (Bechtel et al. 1995). A neonate who ingested 60 times the recommended daily dose of vitamin A for 11 days developed hyperphosphataemia; this was probably due to accelerated bone resorption (Bush and Dahms 1984).

Administration of recombinant human erythropoietin to patients with renal failure on regular haemodialysis caused a small but significant increase in plasma phosphate (Eschbach et al. 1989). Treatment with GnRH analogues for 6 months caused a pronounced increase in serum phosphate concentration probably by increasing bone resorption (Gudmundsson et al. 1987). Diphosphonate administration has been associated with hyperphosphataemia (Russell et al. 1974); this effect is not seen until 2 weeks after starting treatment and is due partly to reduced renal clearance of phosphate and partly to a shift of intracellular phosphate (Walton et al. 1975).

Transfusion of stored blood can lead to significant hyperphosphataemia (Crook and Swaminathan 1996).

Severe hyperphosphataemia and hypocalcaemia may also occur following chemotherapy of certain malignant diseases, especially lymphomas, because of rapid release of phosphate from lysing cells (Knochel and Agarwal 1996). Administration of growth hormone and IGF1 is known to cause increased tubular reabsorption of phosphate and an increase in plasma phosphate, although severe hyperphosphataemia is rare (Knochel and Agarwal 1996).

Propranolol and metoprolol caused an increase in plasma phosphate concentrations in hyperthyroid subjects, probably because of a shift of phosphate from cells as a result of β-blockade (Feely 1981).

Treatment

Treatment of hyperphosphataemia is the treatment of the underlying cause and the renal failure (if present). Occasionally, additional measures may be required and administration of phosphate binders is suggested. Intravenous sodium bicarbonate or acetazolamide, or both, will increase phosphate excretion, but in severe cases dialysis may be required (Crook and Swaminathan 1996).

Magnesium

Magnesium is the most abundant intracellular cation after potassium. Less than 1 per cent of the body magnesium is in the ECF and, consequently, plasma magnesium is not a good indicator of whole-body magnesium status (Swaminathan 1998). The plasma magnesium concentration ranges from 0.68–1.0 mmol per litre in healthy subjects and of this 60 per cent is ionized, 25 per cent bound to protein, and 15 per cent complexed. Intracellular magnesium plays a critical role in many metabolic processes, and intracellular magnesium concentration is maintained at the expense of ECF and bone magnesium. Approximately 30–40 per cent of ingested magnesium is absorbed; factors controlling its absorption are not well understood, but vitamin D metabolites and PTH are known to be involved. Magnesium absorption can be reduced by intraluminal complexing agents such as phytate. The major organ regulating magnesium homoeostasis is the kidney, in which magnesium is filtered and reabsorbed. Factors that influence reabsorption by the tubules include PTH, changes in plasma magnesium concentration, and ECF volume (Sutton and Dirks 1996; Swaminathan 1998).

Hypermagnesaemia

Hypermagnesaemia is a relatively unusual finding, as the normal kidney can excrete excess magnesium by rapidly reducing tubular reabsorption to almost negligible amounts. Hypermagnesaemia, when it occurs, is usually due to excessive administration of magnesium salts or magnesium-containing drugs in the presence of renal impairment (Sutton and Dirks 1996). However, even in the absence of renal impairment, hypermagnesaemia may occur if the intake of magnesium is very high. The use of antacids containing magnesium caused hypermagnesaemia, hypotension, respiratory depression, and coma in an adult (Ferdinandus et al. 1981), and hypermagnesaemia and intestinal perforation were described in a premature infant following antacid administration

(Brand and Greer 1990). The magnesium content of antacid preparations can be as high as 7.0 millimoles in 5 ml. Hypermagnesaemia has been described with the administration of magnesium-containing cathartics for drug overdose (Smilkstein *et al.* 1988; Woodard *et al.* 1990) or for non-emergency therapeutic purposes, and this effect can occur in patients with normal renal function (Gren and Woolf 1989; Clark and Brown 1992; Golzarian *et al.* 1994; Fung *et al.* 1995; Nordt *et al.* 1996; Qureshi and Melonakos 1996). Abuse of laxatives containing magnesium can lead to severe hypermagnesaemia (serum concentration > 8.0 mmol per litre), quadriparesis, and neuromuscular dysfunction (Castelbaum *et al.* 1989). Intravenous or intramuscular administration of magnesium sulphate may cause hypermagnesaemia (Rogiers *et al.* 1989; Vissers and Purssell 1996).The use of magnesium salts in the treatment of pre-eclampsia can cause hypermagnesaemia in both mother and infant (Brady and Williams 1967; Hill *et al.* 1985). Magnesium intoxication may follow the use of magnesium sulphate in rectal enemas (Swaminathan 1998), of urological irrigation solutions containing magnesium salts (Fassler *et al.* 1985), of Renacidin (a proprietary urinary stone-dissolving agent containing magnesium salts and citric acid [Wilson *et al.* 1986]), and of Epsom salts for bowel preparation (Aucamp *et al.* 1981). Potassium-sparing diuretics tend to increase serum magnesium concentration, but rarely cause significant hypermagnesaemia (Davies and Fraser 1993).

Treatment

Treatment of magnesium intoxication involves removal or withdrawal of the drug concerned and, if the patient is symptomatic, supportive therapy such as ventilation, rehydration, and intravenous calcium. Occasionally, dialysis may be required to remove the magnesium, especially in those with renal insufficiency (Sutton and Dirks 1996).

Hypomagnesaemia

Drugs that cause hypomagnesaemia are classified according to their possible mechanisms of action, which are listed in Table 17.9.

Redistribution

Redistribution of magnesium into ICF can cause hypomagnesaemia; it is seen in situations which are similar to those for redistribution of potassium. It occurs in

TABLE 17.9
Causes of drug-induced hypomagnesaemia

1. Redistribution between extracellular and intracellular fluids
   acute metabolic alkalosis, catecholamines and β-agonists, insulin, oral or intravenous nutrition

2. Decreased gastrointestinal absorption
   drug-induced malabsorption (e.g. from neomycin), laxative abuse

3. Increased renal loss
   aminoglycosides, amphotericin, diuretics, cisplatin, cyclosporin

4. Others
   anticonvulsants, cytotoxic drugs, lithium, pentamidine

malnourished or starving children during refeeding (Caddell and Olson 1973), and in patients fed intravenously with glucose and aminoacids without an adequate amount of magnesium (Swaminathan 1998) and during treatment of diabetic ketoacidosis (McMullen 1977). Insulin administration decreases plasma magnesium concentration by 15–20 per cent, and hypomagnesaemia has been reported in 47 per cent of children undergoing an insulin hypoglycaemia test (Ratzmann and Zollner 1985).

Adrenaline infusion has been shown to cause a decrease in plasma magnesium concentration (Whyte *et al.* 1987), as has also been reported following the administration of ritodrine (Kawarabayashi *et al.* 1989), rimiterol (Haffner and Kendall 1992), salbutamol, terbutaline (Bremme *et al.* 1986), and other β-agonists (Whyte *et al.* 1987; Rolla and Bucca 1988; Lipworth *et al.* 1989). This effect is due to β-adrenoreceptor-stimulated magnesium transport (Sutton and Dirks 1996). Theophylline, especially in toxic doses, is reported to cause hypomagnesaemia (Robertson 1985; Parr *et al.* 1990; Hagley *et al.* 1994). In addition to transcellular shift, intravenous administration of theophylline can cause increased magnesium excretion (Knutsen *et al.* 1994). Patients taking theophylline have an increased risk of developing hypomagnesaemia (Flack *et al.* 1994) accompanied by other metabolic abnormalities, including hypokalaemia, hyponatraemia, hypophosphataemia, and hyperglycaemia. Shift of magnesium into the cells is also responsible for the decrease in plasma magnesium concentration during acute metabolic alkalosis (Sutton and Dirks 1996). Massive blood transfusion may cause hypomagnesaemia (Kulkarin *et al.* 1992) due to chelation of magnesium by citrate. In this situation the total magnesium concentration may not decrease but ionized magnesium is reduced.

Decreased gastrointestinal absorption

Hypomagnesaemia, with reduced urinary magnesium, may be seen in any drug-induced malabsorption syndrome, such as those due to cholestyramine, neomycin, or chronic abuse of laxatives (Sutton and Dirks 1996).

Increased renal excretion

Both thiazide and loop diuretics have been reported to cause hypomagnesaemia (Ryan 1987; Preuss and Burris 1996), and some studies show that with long-term diuretic therapy muscle magnesium content, as well as the number of sodium pumps, decreases (Dorup 1994). This in turn is thought to increase the risk of ventricular arrhythmias, sudden death (Ryan 1987), and digoxin toxicity (Martin et al. 1988). This view, however, has been questioned recently (Ramsay et al. 1994; McInnes 1996). Many of the reports on the role of diuretics causing hypomagnesaemia are not based on properly controlled trials (McInnes 1996). In a review of this topic, Davies and Fraser (1993) conclude that well-controlled trials, of which there are few, do not substantiate claims that diuretics play a role in causing magnesium deficiency. The vast majority of patients taking conventional doses of thiazide diuretics (e.g. bendrofluazide 2.5 mg per day) do not need magnesium supplements. Some of the confusion in the literature comes from the lack of a suitable method of assessing magnesium status (Swaminathan 1998). However, patients who are taking large doses of diuretics or those who are on a poor diet or in soft water areas, or with malabsorption may be at greater risk of magnesium deficiency and may need regular monitoring. Hypomagnesaemia and tetany have been described in cases of surreptitious use of frusemide (Brucato et al. 1993; Olveira Fuster et al. 1996).

The chemotherapeutic agent cisplatin can cause nephrotoxicity and hypomagnesaemia, secondary to renal magnesium wasting (Jones and Chesney 1995; Folb 1996). The incidence of hypomagnesaemia has been reported to be as high as 50–100 per cent (Lam and Adelstein 1986), though symptomatic hypomagnesaemia is less common (Ashraf et al. 1983), up to 10 per cent in one study (Salem et al. 1984). The hypomagnesaemia is dose related (Lam and Adelstein 1986), cumulative in sequential therapy with repeated courses (Swainson et al. 1985), and more common with continuous infusion than with intermittent bolus injections (Forastiere et al. 1988), suggesting that the total exposure to free platinum contributes to the toxicity. Hypomagnesaemia and magnesium wasting induced by cisplatin can become chronic in some patients and may be present several years after treatment (Ariceta et al. 1991; Brock

et al. 1991; Markmann et al. 1991). In chronic magnesium wasting there is accompanying hypocalciuria and hypokalaemic metabolic acidosis. The exact mechanism and site of this effect is not known, but a lesion in the distal tubules has been suggested (Mavichak et al. 1988). Carboplatin, a newer analogue, is associated with a lower incidence (< 10 per cent) of hypomagnesaemia (Ettinger et al. 1994). Intravenous thiosulphate administered with cisplatin lowered the incidence of hypomagnesaemia (Markman et al. 1986). This was probably due to inactivation of cisplatin by thiosulphate before it reached the kidney. Giving magnesium with cisplatin also reduced the renal toxicity of the latter (Wilcox et al. 1986).

Hypomagnesaemia has been reported in 4.5 per cent of patients receiving aminoglycoside treatment, although there have been reports of up to 30 per cent (Zaloga et al. 1984). It is usually seen in patients on prolonged treatment or high doses, or both (Bar et al. 1975) and has been seen with gentamicin (Beatty et al. 1989), tobramycin (Watson et al. 1984; Slayton et al. 1996), amikacin (Wu et al. 1996) as well as with the antituberculous agents viomycin and capreomycin (Bar et al. 1975; Green et al. 1985). Symptomatic hypomagnesaemia with tetany has been reported (Wilkinson et al. 1986), especially in the elderly (Kes and Reiner 1990) or if there are other associated conditions causing magnesium loss (Shiah et al. 1994) or poor intake. Aminoglycosides accumulate preferentially in the proximal tubule, leading to cell damage (Ali et al. 1992). Juxtaglomerular hyperplasia with hyperreninaemia and secondary hyperaldosteronism has also been reported (Ali et al. 1992). Infusion of gentamicin into rats causes a rapid decrease in magnesium before development of nephrotoxicity (Foster et al. 1992) and excretion of proximal tubular enzymes such as alanine aminopeptidase is increased during aminoglycoside treatment (Davey et al. 1983).

Cyclosporin and cyclophosphamide, used for immunosuppression, are associated with renal toxicity and hypomagnesaemia. Cyclosporin has been shown to increase magnesium excretion (Barton et al. 1987, 1989). The hypomagnesaemia is usually mild and asymptomatic although severe symptomatic magnesium deficiency is occasionally seen in bone marrow transplant patients (Thompson et al. 1984; June et al. 1986). Hypomagnesaemia developed in 88 per cent of bone marrow transplant recipients given cyclosporin or cyclophosphamide (Kone et al. 1988). In another study of renal transplant recipients, in which cyclosporin was associated with reduction in serum magnesium concentration and inappropriately increased urinary excretion of magnesium, nearly all patients required magnesium supplements (Barton *et al.* 1987). Severe hypomagnesaemia and neurotoxicity following cyclosporin therapy resolved or did not recur with adequate magnesium replacement (Thompson *et al.* 1984; June *et al.* 1986).

Total serum magnesium concentration during cyclosporin treatment was low (Barton *et al.* 1987; Scoble *et al.* 1990) or normal (Haag-Weber *et al.* 1990); ionized magnesium concentration was reduced in renal transplant patients, the reduction correlating with blood cyclosporin concentration (Markell *et al.* 1993). Myocardial magnesium was diminished in cardiac patients treated with cyclosporin (Millane *et al.* 1992); muscle magnesium (Qureshi *et al.* 1994) and red cell and leucocyte magnesium content were reduced (al-Khursany *et al.* 1992) in renal transplant patients. On the other hand, tissue magnesium content was increased in rats given cyclosporin (Barton *et al.* 1989; Nozue *et al.* 1993) and mononuclear cell magnesium content was also increased in patients with nephrosis treated with cyclosporin for short periods (Nozue *et al.* 1992). Muscle magnesium content in transplant patients was not decreased (Frost *et al.* 1993). These conflicting results could be explained on the basis that short-term treatment with cyclosporin causes hypomagnesaemia due to an intracellular shift of magnesium, whereas in long-term treatment magnesium deficiency is a result of renal magnesium wasting. The immunosuppressive agent tacrolimus (FK 506) also produced hypomagnesaemia in rats (Ryffel *et al.* 1994).

Amphotericin, a highly nephrotoxic agent, has been reported to cause mild but reversible hypomagnesaemia (Barton *et al.* 1984). Pentamidine may cause renal magnesium wasting (Wharton *et al.* 1987; Burnett and Reents 1990; Shah *et al.* 1990; Gradon *et al.* 1991). This drug accumulates in the kidney and can be detected up to a year after treatment (Shah *et al.* 1990). Up to 70 per cent of AIDS patients treated with foscarnet for cytomegalovirus retinitis were hypomagnesaemic (Palestein *et al.* 1991). The exact mechanism for this is not clear (Palestein *et al.* 1991; Gearhart and Sorg 1993).

Mild hypomagnesaemia has been reported in a case of accidental overdose with lithium (Corbett *et al.* 1989); hypomagnesaemia and hypocalcaemia were reported after treatment with mitoxantrone, an antineoplastic drug (Griffiths and Parry 1988), and other cytotoxic drugs (Wandrup and Kancir 1986). Chronic anticonvulsant treatment is associated with deficiency of magnesium, the incidence of which increases with duration of treatment (Steidl *et al.* 1987). This effect may be related to the effect of anticonvulsants on vitamin D metabolism. Oral contraceptives caused a decrease in plasma magnesium concentration (Stanton and Lowenstein 1987; Newhouse *et al.* 1993).

Trace elements

Copper

Copper is an essential trace element, contained in several important enzymes such as cytochrome C oxidase (Linder and Hazegh-Azam 1996). Adult man has about 80–150 mg of copper, of which about 50 per cent is in muscle and bone, but the highest concentration is in liver (Milne 1994). The dietary intake of copper is approximately 2 mg per day and about 50 per cent of this is absorbed (Linder and Hazegh-Azam 1996; Olivares and Uauy 1996). In plasma, 90–95 per cent of copper is bound to the α_2-globulin caeruloplasmin; 10 per cent is associated with or loosely bound to albumin; and a small fraction is complexed with low-molecular-weight compounds such as amino acids (Taylor 1996).

A copper-deficiency syndrome, with low red cell and plasma copper concentrations, is seen in patients receiving total parenteral nutrition containing no copper (Fujita *et al.* 1989). In some infants receiving total parenteral nutrition, an unusual skeletal disorder resembling that seen in scurvy has been described (Sivasubramanian *et al.* 1978). Copper deficiency has also been associated with oral zinc therapy (Porter *et al.* 1977; Prasad *et al.* 1978; Abdulla 1979; Fiske *et al.* 1994) due to the effect of zinc on copper absorption. Penicillamine, a potent chelator of metals used in the treatment of Wilson's disease, lead poisoning, and rheumatoid arthritis, increases urinary copper excretion (Milanino *et al.* 1993), and may lead to copper deficiency, which may play a role in the alopecia, loss of taste (Knudsen and Weisman 1978), and anaemia (Cutolo *et al.* 1982) reported in these patients. Of the other chelating agents used in lead poisoning, calcium EDTA increases copper excretion whereas succimer (DMSA) does not (Chisolm 1990). Thiamazole, which forms complexes with copper, may also lead to loss of taste (Hanlon 1975).

Severe copper deficiency as a result of taking a gel containing bismuth, aluminium, magnesium, and sodium has been reported in a patient with pyloric stenosis (van Kalmthout *et al.* 1982). Anticonvulsants have been reported to cause variable effects on serum copper (Kaji *et al.* 1992; Kuzuya *et al.* 1993; Sozuer *et al.* 1995).

Levonorgestrel implants (Norplant) caused a significant decrease in copper and zinc concentrations after use for 3 months but not after a year or more (Ismail *et al.* 1992). Copper concentration was reduced by iron folate supplementation during pregnancy (Burns and Paterson 1993) and by zidovudine treatment (Baum *et al.* 1991).

Copper toxicity has been reported as a complication of long-term haemodialysis (Blomfield et al. 1971), and with the use of copper-containing intrauterine contraceptive devices (Milne 1994). Plasma copper concentrations increase after treatment with oral contraceptives (Newhouse et al. 1993), and after oral ethinyloestradiol treatment in postmenopausal women (Chilvers et al. 1985). Serum caeruloplasmin concentration was also increased (Milne and Johnson 1993), owing to increased synthesis by the liver. Chilvers and associates (1985) showed that 80 per cent of the increase in plasma copper is due to a rise in caeruloplasmin-bound copper and 20 per cent to an increase in copper bound to albumin.

Excretion of copper is low in drug addicts compared with healthy subjects, suggesting that drugs of abuse may affect copper metabolism (Iyengar et al. 1994).

Zinc

Zinc is an essential element, and is a co-factor in many metalloenzymes. Over 200 zinc-dependent enzymes have been described (Milne 1994). Total body zinc content in adult man is 1.4–2.3 g, of which 70–80 per cent is in bone, skin, and muscle. The zinc concentration of red cells is about 10 times that of plasma, because of their high content of carbonic anhydrase. The average intake of zinc is about 15 mg per day, of which approximately 20–30 per cent is absorbed (Milne 1994). About 98 per cent of the zinc in plasma is bound to protein, 60–70 per cent to albumin, 30–40 per cent to α_2-macroglobulin, and less than 2 per cent to transferrin and free amino acids (Milne 1994). Although it is plasma zinc that is usually measured, this is not a good measure of zinc status (Taylor 1996).

When zinc is not included during parenteral nutrition, plasma and red cell zinc fall progressively (Kay et al. 1976). The risk of zinc deficiency is greater in those with hypercatabolic states (Jeejeebhoy 1984; Taylor 1996) and it is recommended that adults require at least 2.5 mg of zinc a day.

The chelating agent EDTA increases zinc excretion and can lead to zinc deficiency whereas succimer does not cause significant increase in zinc excretion (Chisolm 1990). Zinc deficiency has been reported in patients receiving penicillamine therapy (Milanino et al. 1993). Plasma zinc concentration was found to be lower in rheumatoid arthritic patients treated with NSAID or corticosteroids, or both (Milanino et al. 1993). Thiazide diuretics increase urinary excretion of zinc (Wester 1975) and may lead to zinc deficiency as shown by reduced hair zinc content although plasma zinc may be normal (Mountokalakis et al. 1984). Cisplatin causes increased urinary loss of zinc and decreases plasma zinc concentration (Sweeney et al. 1989). Low plasma zinc concentrations seen after treatment with oestrogens (Chilvers et al. 1985) are a result of decreased albumin concentration leading to a decrease in the amount of albumin-bound zinc. Captopril increases zinc excretion (Golik et al. 1990a; Peczkowska et al. 1997). The increase in zinc excretion after enalapril is not as great as that after captopril (Golik et al. 1990b). The reduced taste acuity seen after captopril treatment resembles that accompanying zinc deficiency (Ackerman and Kasbekar 1997) and increased urinary zinc excretion and low plasma zinc concentration were associated with hypogeusia in patients taking captopril (Abu-Hamdan et al. 1988). In patients on long-term treatment serum zinc (Rubio Luengo et al. 1995) and red cell zinc (Golik et al. 1990b) concentrations fell, but in the short term there were no changes (O'Connor et al. 1987; Neil-Dwyer and Marus 1989). Animal studies suggest that captopril may cause a tissue redistribution of zinc and copper as well as increasing excretion, as zinc and copper content falls in liver, for example, while rising in the testis (Kotsaki-Kovatsi et al. 1997).

Reduced zinc absorption is observed with the use of high-fibre diets (e.g. containing bran) which contain phytate, with the use of ferrous sulphate or substances with a high inorganic iron content (Taylor 1996), and the use of aluminium hydroxide (Abu-Hamdan et al. 1986). Folic acid supplements, commonly used in pregnancy, are thought to reduce intestinal absorption of zinc. This is especially important, as zinc deficiency has been associated with low-birth-weight babies. Milne and co-workers (1984) found that faecal excretion of zinc was increased significantly, and urinary zinc was reduced, by folate supplementation in normal men, especially when dietary zinc was low, and they suggested that folate may form insoluble complexes and thereby reduce absorption. Simmer and colleagues (1987) also found reduced zinc absorption during folate supplementation. On the other hand, folate had no effect on zinc absorption (Keating et al. 1987) and plasma and red cell zinc concentrations were not altered by folate supplementation for 4 months (Butterworth et al. 1988) in normal men (Milne et al. 1990) or in haemodialysis patients (Reid et al. 1992). A detailed study of zinc metabolism using plasma, red cell, and urinary zinc, and red cell metallothionine did not show any effect of folate supplementation (Kauwell et al. 1995). In premature infants there was a negative correlation between serum folate and serum zinc concentration (Fuller et al. 1992) and zinc concentration in breast milk was reduced by folate supplementation during the postpartum period (Keizer et al. 1995).

These conflicting results could be explained by the observation that zinc absorption and serum zinc concentration are reduced when the initial fractional absorption is high, that is, during increased demand or reduced dietary intake (Milne 1994).

The use of oral contraceptives is associated with a decrease in plasma zinc and an increase in red cell zinc (Milne 1994). Corticosteroid therapy causes a rapid decrease in plasma zinc and a marked increase in urinary zinc (Peretz *et al.* 1989*b*). Zinc deficiency, or increased excretion of zinc, has been associated with cisplatin (Sweeney *et al.* 1989), anabolic steroids (Milne 1994), anticonvulsants (Kuzuya *et al.* 1993; Sozuer *et al.* 1995), the magnetic-resonance contrast agents gadolinium HP-D03A and gadolinium DTPA-BMA (Puttagunta *et al.* 1996), drugs of abuse (Iyengar *et al.* 1994), exposure to cadmium (Thijs *et al.* 1992), indomethacin (Ambanelli *et al.* 1982), and treatment with zidovudine (Baum *et al.* 1991). Anticonvulsants have also been reported to have no effect (Yuen *et al.* 1988; Kaji *et al.* 1992).

Marked increases in serum zinc concentration due to inadvertent administration of excessive doses of zinc (Brocks *et al.* 1977) have been reported in patients receiving total parenteral nutrition. The diuretic chlorthalidone was associated with raised plasma and hair zinc concentrations (Geissler *et al.* 1986). The significance of this effect is not clear. Glucose polymers used as energy source were found to increase the absorption of zinc (Bei *et al.* 1986). Acute zinc toxicity has been reported in haemodialysis patients (Gallery *et al.* 1972), and toxicity may be seen when zinc is used to treatment of subfertile men, to improve cellular immunity, or for tropical ulcers (Taylor 1996).

Aluminium

Aluminium toxicity is well recognized in patients undergoing dialysis for chronic renal failure (Salusky *et al.* 1991; Alfrey 1993; Golub and Domingo 1996), in uraemic and non-uraemic subjects receiving aluminium-containing antacids (Golub and Domingo 1996), and in patients receiving total parenteral nutrition (Klein 1995). The manifestations of toxicity include encephalopathy, osteomalacic dialysis osteodystrophy, and microcytic anaemia (Jeffrey *et al.* 1996). Possible sources of aluminium are the tap water used in the preparation of the dialysate (Golub and Domingo 1996), phosphate binding agents containing aluminium (Golub and Domingo 1996), parenteral solutions (Klein 1995; Leung 1995), aluminium in infant formulae (Simmer *et al.* 1990; Sahin *et al.* 1995), and aluminium cookware (Mendis 1988). The tissue accumulation of aluminium occurs mainly as a result of the inability of patients with chronic renal failure receiving haemodialysis or peritoneal dialysis to excrete the aluminium. However, aluminium toxicity is now recognized in patients with renal failure who are not being dialysed and in patients with normal renal function (Sedman 1992; Golub and Domingo 1996). Evidence of aluminium loading, as shown by increased concentrations of aluminium in plasma, urine, and bone, has been found in infants receiving intravenous therapy contaminated with aluminium (Klein 1995). Concomitant administration of citrate and aluminium has been shown to increase the absorption of aluminium in patients in renal failure (Lindberg *et al.* 1993; Sakhaee *et al.* 1993). Contamination of calcium supplements with aluminium is another possible source of aluminium toxicity (Whiting 1994). Elevated aluminium concentrations have been described in patients receiving large amounts of albumin intravenously (Kelly *et al.* 1989; Klein *et al.* 1990). Intravesical irrigation with alum has been reported to cause aluminium toxicity (Perazella and Brown 1993), especially when there is renal impairment (Murphy *et al.* 1992; Shoskes *et al.* 1992). Serum aluminium was also reported to be high in critically ill patients as a result of antacid treatment (Ittel *et al.* 1991).

Treatment involves the use of aluminium-free antacids and water, and desferrioxamine to remove the aluminium (Sprague *et al.* 1986).

Lead

Lead poisoning from ingestion of traditional remedies (*kushtas*) (Haq and Asghar 1989) or use of oriental cosmetics (*surma*) is seen in Asian communities (Sprinkle 1995), in Britain (Healy and Aslam 1986), North America (*MMWR* 1984), in Middle Eastern countries (Abu Melha *et al.* 1987), and in the Mexican community in the USA (*MMWR* 1983). The lead content of these preparations can be as high as 82.5%. A case of lead poisoning due to the use of an Indian herbal remedy for diabetes has been described (Keen *et al.* 1994).

Lead poisoning has been reported in association with the use of contaminated water to reconstitute infant feeds (Shannon and Graef 1989), illicit methamphetamine (*MMWR* 1989), contaminated heroin (Antonini *et al.* 1989), and with illegally distilled alcohol (Alkhawajah 1992; Pegues *et al.* 1993). Lead intoxication possibly from contamination of calcium supplements has been reported (Whiting 1994).

Mercury

Mercury poisoning or increased blood mercury concentrations may be found in patients given normal human immunoglobulin, which contains the organic mercurial thiomersal as preservative. Over 70 per cent of hypo-gammaglobulinaemic patients given immunoglobulin have increased urinary excretion of mercury (Heaney *et al.* 1979). Increased concentrations of mercury in blood, brain, and kidney are found in subjects with mercury-amalgam dental fillings and this risk has recently been reviewed (Levy 1995). Mercury concentrations may reach toxic levels following postoperative wound treatment with the antiseptic merbromine (mercurochrome), because of absorption from the wound surface (Kloppel and Weiler 1985). Mercury poisoning may also occur after the use of 'traditional' medicines with a high mercury content (Kang-Yum and Oransky 1992; Hardy *et al.* 1995).

Silver

Increased intake of silver, and possibly poisoning, may occur after ingestion of traditional *kushtas* used by the Indo-Pakistan community. These remedies have been reported to contain mercury and silver in addition to lead (Haq and Asghar 1989). The use of anti-smoking lozenges containing silver acetate may cause silver poisoning (Shelton and Goulding 1979) and the use of anti-smoking chewing gum containing silver acetate increases the concentrations of silver in serum and skin biopsies (Jensen *et al.* 1988). The use of silver sulpha-diazine as a topical antimicrobial agent in burns patients is associated with absorption of silver from the raw skin surface and silver toxicity (Payne *et al.* 1992). Serum silver concentrations were found to be high and urinary silver excretion 1000-fold greater in patients with more than 60 per cent burns treated with silver sulphadiazine (Boosalis *et al.* 1987). Recent evidence shows that absorption of silver from burns is enhanced due to the solubilizing effect of human serum on silver (Tsipouras *et al.* 1995). Another potential source of silver toxicity is from the use of iontophoretic devices (Hollinger 1996).

Fluoride

Fluoride has been used in the treatment of osteoporosis, as it stimulates bone formation and increases cancellous bone mass. Accidental fluoride overdosage may occur due to the use of excess hydrofluorosilicic acid in the water supply (Petersen *et al.* 1988).

When fluorinated anaesthetics such as halothane, methoxyflurane, enflurane, and isoflurane are metab-olised, fluoride is released into the circulation, resulting in an increase in plasma fluoride concentration (Oikkonen and Meretoja 1989). Peak concentrations of serum fluor-ide are seen 3 days after anaesthesia with methoxyflur-ane, 24 hours after halothane, and soon after the end of anaesthesia with enflurane or isoflurane (Cousins *et al.* 1987). This difference is accounted for by the high lipid solubility of methoxyflurane. After sevoflurane anaes-thesia plasma fluoride concentration rises to a peak within 1 hour but only reaches a high value ($750\,\mu$mol per litre) in seven per cent of patients; it then declines rapidly, reaching preoperative values within a day (Kharasch 1995). Plasma fluoride does not rise after desflurane anaesthesia unless the exposure is prolonged (Kharasch 1996); a different metabolite, trifluoroacetate, is increased after desflurane but to only a tenth of the extent that occurs with isoflurane.

Prolonged use of isoflurane in the management of tetanus has caused potentially toxic concentrations of fluoride (J.J. Stevens *et al.* 1993). The peak fluoride concentration was higher with methoxyflurane than with enflurane or isoflurane and the high fluoride concen-trations may account for the nephrotoxicity of methoxy-flurane (Mazze 1984). When isoflurane was compared with enflurane, serum fluoride was higher with enflurane (Oikkonen 1984). The urinary excretion of fluoride is increased after isoflurane and enflurane but not after halothane (Cousins *et al.* 1987; Davidkova *et al.* 1988; Kofke *et al.* 1989). Ethanol affects defluorination of enflurane (Pantuck *et al.* 1985). The fluoride concen-tration in silver fluoride used in dental practice can be very high and may cause fluoride toxicity, especially in children (Gotjamanos and Afonso 1997).

Administration of aluminium hydroxide decreases plasma fluoride concentrations by 50 per cent, by reduc-ing net absorption (Spencer *et al.* 1985).

Porphyrins

Porphyrins are a group of cyclic tetrapyrrole compounds that are red in colour. They are intermediates in the synthesis of haem and cytochromes. Porphyrias are a group of metabolic disorders of haem biosynthesis in which there is increased formation of porphyrins and their precursors (Moore 1993; McColl *et al.* 1996; Elder *et al.* 1997). Porphyrias are classified as either hepatic or erythroid, depending on the principal site of expression of the specific enzyme defect (Table 17.10). In addition to these inherited disorders, several different diseases, particularly anaemias, hepatobiliary diseases, or toxins may cause secondary porphyrinuria.

The erythropoietic porphyrias do not appear to be affected or aggravated by drugs or toxins. On the other hand, a wide variety of drugs can affect the hepatic

TABLE 17.10
Classification of porphyrias

Erythropoietic

Congenital erythropoietic porphyria	++	Uroporphyrin and coproporphyrin in urine
Erythropoietic protoporphyria	++	Protoporphyrin in stool

Hepatic

ALA dehydratase deficiency porphyria (plumboporphyria)	−	ALA in urine
Acute intermittent porphyria	−	ALA and PBG in urine
Hereditary coproporphyria	+	ALA, PBG and coproporphyrin
Variegate porphyria	+	ALA, PBG, and coproporphyrin
Porphyria cutanea tarda	++	Uroporphyrin
Hepatoerythropoietic porphyria	+	Uroporphyrin

−	no photosensitivity	ALA: δ-amino laevulinic acid
+	photosensitivity ±	PBG: Porphobilinogen
++	marked photosensitivity	

porphyrias. The porphyrias can also be divided into acute and non-acute, both of which can be affected by drugs. The acute porphyrias are disorders in which patients may present with acute attacks. They include acute intermittent porphyria, variegate porphyria, hereditary coproporphyria, and plumboporphyria (amino laevulinic acid [ALA] dehydratase deficiency porphyria).

Acute porphyrias

Patients with acute porphyria may present with acute abdominal pain, mental dysfunction, and peripheral neuropathy (Moore 1993; Elder *et al.* 1997). During an attack the urine develops a dark red-brown colour, deepening with exposure to light. Acute attacks are precipitated by various factors, including alcohol, infection, hormones, reduced calorie intake (as in fasting or dieting), and drugs (Kauppinen and Mustajoki 1992). A comprehensive list of drugs that have been reported to precipitate acute attacks, and drugs that have been shown to be porphyrinogenic in experimental animals or in cell culture systems has been published (Bonkovsky 1993; Kappas *et al.* 1995). A fuller list of drugs, including those which are thought to be safe in porphyrias is given by McColl and colleagues (1996). A selected list of drugs reported to have caused acute attacks of porphyria is given in Table 17.11; it includes drugs such as barbiturates and phenytoin that induce hepatic microsomal

TABLE 17.11
Drugs that have been reported to be associated with acute attacks of porphyria

Hypnotics, sedatives, and tranquillizers
  barbiturates, carbromal, carisoprodol, chlordiazepoxide, dichloralphenazone, ethchlorvynol, glutethimide, meprobamate, methylpyrrolone
Anticonvulsants
  barbiturates (phenobarbitone, primidone) carbamazepine, hydantoins (phenytoin)
Antibacterial, antifungal, and antimalarial agents
  chloramphenicol, erythromycin, flucloxacillin, griseofulvin, pivampicillin, pyrazinamide, sulphonamides
Hormones and antidiabetic drugs
  chlorpropamide, oral contraceptives, progesterone methandrostenolone
Miscellaneous
  alphaxalone:alphadolone (Althesin), bemegride, carbromal, dimenhydrinate, enalapril, enflurane, ergot compounds (dihydroergotamine), ethanol, flufenamic acid, frusemide, halothane, hydrochlorothiazide, hydroxyzine, hyoscine butylbromide, imipramine, lisinopril, metoclopramide, methyldopa, methylsulphonal, nifedipine, nikethamide, orphenadrine, oxymetazoline, pentazocine, pentylenetetrazol, piroxicam, prilocaine, terfenadine, theophylline, thiopentone sodium, verapamil

(Adapted from McColl *et al.* 1996)

enzymes. However, there are no common factors or features among these drugs, and it is difficult to predict whether or not a drug will precipitate an acute attack.

Treatment

Treatment of acute porphyrias consists of symptomatic and specific therapy (Kappas *et al.* 1995). Specific therapies are few and include high carbohydrate intake which suppresses the synthesis of aminolaevulinate, and haem arginate (haematin) which reduces aminolaevulinate and porphobilinogen. Early treatment with haem arginate is thought to be highly effective (Mustajoki and Nordmann 1993). Recently, cimetidine has been used as a cheaper alternative to haem arginate (Rogers 1997). In women with acute intermittent porphyria who develop frequent exacerbations related to the menstrual cycle, LHRH analogues have been used to prevent the cyclical attacks by hormonal manipulation (Anderson 1989; Anderson *et al.* 1990). Although LHRH analogues prevent the cyclical attacks they do not normalise abnormal porphyrin precursor excretion nor prevent acute attacks precipitated by other factors (Elder *et al.* 1997).

Non-acute porphyria (cutaneous porphyrias)

Porphyria cutanea tarda (PCT), the most common form of porphyria, is characterized by a deficiency of hepatic uroporphyrinogen decarboxylase activity. PCT can be inherited or acquired (sporadic). In the acquired form, the enzyme defect is confined to the liver and is often triggered by environmental agents, amongst which alcohol is the best-recognized, though its mechanism of action is not well understood (Kappas *et al.* 1995). Oestrogen administration for prostatic carcinoma (Weimar *et al.* 1978; Coulson and Misch 1989), or to postmenopausal women, or in the form of the contraceptive pill (Behm and Unger 1974; Kappas *et al.* 1995) has been associated with the aggravation or precipitation of PCT. That exogenous, but not endogenous, oestrogen can precipitate PCT suggests that the first-pass effect of oestrogen is important (Urbanek and Cohen 1994). Iron has been shown to be another important factor in the pathogenesis (Kappas *et al.* 1995). Other compounds that have been implicated in this way include polychlorinated hydrocarbons (Calvert *et al.* 1994; Kappas *et al.* 1995; McColl *et al.* 1996), diazinon (an organophosphorus insecticide) (Bleakley *et al.* 1979), rifampicin (Millar 1980), cyclophosphamide (Manzione *et al.* 1988), and zidovudine (Ong *et al.* 1988), HMG-CoA reductase inhibitors ('statins') (Perrot *et al.* 1994), and khellin and UV radiation (KUVA) therapy (Jansen *et al.* 1995).

Several drugs have been reported to cause skin lesions similar to PCT but without disturbances in porphyrin metabolism. This is called 'pseudoporphyria' and it has been described in association with amiodarone (Parodi *et al.* 1988), bumetanide (McInnes 1996), carisoprodol/aspirin (Hazen 1994), chlorthalidone (Baker *et al.* 1989), cyclophosphamide (Sola *et al.* 1987), cyclosporin, etretinate (McDonagh and Harrington 1989), frusemide, hydrochlorothiazide/triamterene (Dyazide) (Motley 1990), isotretinoin (Riordan *et al.* 1993), naproxen (Shelley *et al.* 1987; Creemers *et al.* 1995) and other NSAID, nalidixic acid, nifedipine, oxaprozin (Ingrish and Rietschel 1996), pyridoxine, rifampicin, and tetracycline.

Treatment

Apart from removing the offending agent, phlebotomy and chloroquine are the main forms of treatment (Ashton *et al.* 1984; Kappas *et al.* 1995). Cimetidine has also been used successfully (Horie *et al.* 1996), and desferrioxamine in haemodialysis-related PCT (Praga *et al.* 1987).

Erythropoietic protoporphyria

Erythropoietic protoporphyria is an inherited porphyria associated with decreased activity of ferrochelatase and characterized by cutaneous photosensitivity (Kappas *et al.* 1995; Fritsch *et al.* 1997). No precipitating agents are known (Kappas *et al.* 1995). It is characterized by high concentration of protophyrin in erythrocytes, plasma, bile, and faeces, but not in urine.

Secondary porphyrinuria

Moderate elevation of porphyrin excretion is associated with several diseases (such as anaemias and hepatobiliary diseases), drugs, and toxins (McColl *et al.* 1996). Lead poisoning is a well-recognized cause of secondary porphyrinuria: the lead inhibits PBG synthase and causes increased excretion of ALA and coproporphyrin (Nuttall 1994). Other heavy metals, such as mercury, bismuth, copper, silver, gold, and arsenic, cause coproporphyrinuria, but without elevation of urinary ALA (Nuttall 1994). Alcohol (especially in large amounts), hexachlorobenzene, sedatives, hypnotics (such as chloral hydrate), morphine, ether, and nitrous oxide can all cause coproporphyrinuria (Nuttall 1994).

Uric acid

Uric acid is the end-product of metabolism of purines of endogenous and dietary origin. Dietary purines may contribute up to 50 per cent of uric acid production. About 25 per cent of the uric acid produced is excreted through the intestines and this proportion increases in chronic renal failure (Becker and Roessler 1995). Uric acid is present in plasma almost entirely as a monovalent anion; there is very little protein-binding, and more than 95 per cent of plasma urate is freely filtered by the glomeruli (Fuiano *et al.* 1989). The amount of urate excreted is about 10 per cent of the filtered load. During the passage through the tubules, filtered urate is almost entirely reabsorbed in the proximal tubules. An amount equivalent to about 50 per cent of the filtered load is secreted in the mid-proximal tubule and most of this is reabsorbed in the late proximal tubule (Becker and Roessler 1995), leaving an amount equivalent to about 10 per cent of the filtered load to be excreted. Drugs may influence the production and/or excretion of uric acid (German and Holmes 1986) (Table 17.12).

Hyperuricaemia and gout

Increased production of urate

Apart from genetic causes of overproduction of urate, several acquired factors can increase the production of uric acid. Hyperuricaemia and gout are well-recognized complications of conditions in which there is increased

TABLE 17.12
Drugs causing hyperuricaemia and hypouricaemia

Hyperuricaemia
  Over-production
    alcohol, cytotoxic drugs, fructose, nitroglycerin,
    theophylline

  Decreased excretion
    cyclosporin, drug-induced acidosis — lactic or
    ketoacidosis, drug-induced ECF volume
    contraction, low-dose aspirin, nicotinic acid,
    pyrazinamide, thiazide diuretics, vasopressin

Hypouricaemia
  Reduced production
    allopurinol, azathioprine

  Increased excretion
    anticonvulsants, aspirin, oral anticoagulants,
    radiographic contrast media, uricosuric agents

turnover of uric acid, such as myeloproliferative and haemolytic disorders (Becker and Roessler 1995). It is further aggravated by treatment with cytotoxic agents. Hyperuricaemia is also seen during treatment of other malignant disorders with cytotoxic drugs.

Hyperuricaemia and gout are more common in alcoholics (German and Holmes 1986). Beer contains sufficient purines to increase the purine load in beer drinkers, and alcohol itself increases uric acid production (Faller and Fox 1982; Yamamoto *et al.* 1997). The increased lactate concentration found in alcoholics may further reduce uric acid excretion (Becker and Roessler 1995).

Rapid intravenous administration of fructose increases uric acid concentration: the rapid phosphorylation of fructose leads to dephosphorylation of adenine nucleotides, which are subsequently degraded to uric acid (Becker and Roessler 1995; Yamamoto *et al.* 1997). The rate of administration of fructose is important in determining hyperuricaemia. Lactic acidosis caused by fructose further increases serum uric acid concentration by reducing renal excretion (Woods and Alberti 1972). Xylitol administration also increases serum uric acid concentration by increasing production (Yamamoto *et al.* 1995).

Serum uric acid concentrations are about 50 per cent higher than normal in asthmatics treated with theophylline and there is a significant correlation between serum theophylline and uric acid concentrations. As intravenous theophylline failed to affect the renal clearance of urate and *in vitro* studies showed that theophylline inhibited the enzyme hypoxanthine guanine phosphoribosyl transferase, it has been suggested that the effect of theophylline is on production of urate (Morita *et al.* 1984).

In patients receiving intravenous nitroglycerin for unstable angina, acute gout developed and serum uric acid increased. This was attributed to the alcohol content of the intravenous nitroglycerin preparation (Shergy *et al.* 1988).

Decreased excretion

In volume depletion there is increased reabsorption of urate, leading to an increased plasma uric acid concentration (Feinstein *et al.* 1984). Thus, any drug causing volume depletion may lead to hyperuricaemia. Hyperuricaemia is also a feature of renal failure induced by drugs (see Chapter 14).

Although tacrolimus (FK 506) causes minimal change in uric acid (Starzl *et al.* 1990), a case of severe hyperuricaemia and renal failure has been reported to have been precipitated in a patient with gout (Williams and Lewis 1992).

Salicylate at all doses inhibits uric acid secretion, but at high doses it reduces tubular reabsorption. Thus, low-dose salicylate causes hyperuricaemia and high doses lead to hypouricaemia (Becker and Roessler 1995; Emmerson 1996).

Hyperuricaemia is frequently found in patients on diuretic treatment (Kahn 1988). In most patients the increase in serum urate is small and has no clinically significant effect (Baglin *et al.* 1995; Schmitz and Trimble 1995). Increased proximal tubular reabsorption as a result of diuretic-induced volume depletion is the important mechanism leading to hyperuricaemia (Scott and Higgens 1992). Urate reabsorption varies directly with sodium reabsorption in the proximal tubule, which is increased as a consequence of diuretic-induced volume depletion. Angiotensin II may play a part in mediating this by enhancing the activity of Na^+–H^+ exchange, which leads to a parallel increase in urate–OH^- exchange (Rose 1994). The majority of patients with hyperuricaemia induced by diuretics are asymptomatic and gout develops in only 3–5 per cent (Moser 1990), mainly in those with a predisposition to gout (such as a family history of gout, obesity, and high alcohol intake) (Moser 1992). Frusemide, in addition to volume depletion, increases lactic acid concentrations and the risk of gout is higher with loop diuretics than thiazides (Waller and Ramsay 1989). All diuretics, apart from amiloride (Fogari *et al.* 1995), triamterene, spironolactone (Jeunemaitre *et al.* 1987), and the uricosuric group of diuretics, will cause an increase in serum uric acid concentration. Myers (1987), however, found that the increase in uric acid after a combination of amiloride and thiazide was greater than after thiazide alone, suggesting that amiloride may have an effect on renal handling of uric acid. Elderly women are particularly prone to diuretic-induced tophaceous gout (Macfarlane and Dieppe 1985). The effect of diuretics on serum uric acid is dose related (Carlsen et al. 1990) and hyperuricaemia could be avoided by low-dose therapy (Weir et al. 1996).

The antituberculous drug pyrazinamide has a dose-related effect on uric acid concentration (Sanwikarja et al. 1989) and it increases the risk of gout through inhibition of urate secretion by pyrazionic acid, its main metabolite. Hyperuricaemia occurs in 74–81 per cent of patients treated with pyrazinamide, and arthralgia, but no significant arthritis, was reported in 16 per cent (Khanna and Kumar 1991; Al Majed et al. 1995). Allopurinol, a hypouricaemic agent that reduces uric acid synthesis, has no effect on the hyperuricaemia induced by pyrazionic acid (Lacroix et al. 1988). Ethambutol, another antituberculous drug, also causes hyperuricaemia (German and Holmes 1986; Emmerson 1996) in about 52 per cent of patients and the combination of ethambutol and pyrazinamide caused hyperuricaemia in 91 per cent (Khanna and Kumar 1991).

Cyclosporin treatment is associated with hyperuricaemia in both renal transplant (Palestine et al. 1986) and heart transplant (Burack et al. 1992) recipients, and also in patients receiving it for diseases unrelated to transplantation (Ellis et al. 1991; Deray et al. 1992). Hyperuricaemia occurs in about 30–55 per cent of renal transplant recipients during the first 2 years (Kahan et al. 1987) and in 77 per cent of heart transplant recipients (Burack et al. 1992). This is associated with gout in 12–24 per cent of patients (West et al. 1987; Noordzij et al. 1991; Burack et al. 1992; Ben Hmida et al. 1995). Gout develops in patients receiving diuretics, especially in males (Rossi et al. 1993); the incidence in renal transplant patients varies from 5 to 24 per cent (Ben Hmida et al. 1995) and tophi develop rapidly (Baethge et al. 1993). Studies of urate metabolism showed that the hyperuricaemia is due to decreased urate clearance (Lin et al. 1989). A recent study in which children treated with cyclosporin after receiving renal transplants were investigated with detailed analysis of renal handling showed that increased proximal reabsorption rather than decreased secretion was the mechanism (Laine and Holmberg 1996). Impaired fractional clearance of urate did not improve up to 18 months after changing cyclosporin to azathioprine in seven patients (Noordzij et al. 1991), but in a more recent study serum uric acid concentration decreased after stopping cyclosporin, showing that its effect is reversible (Hilbrands et al. 1996).

Nicotinic acid in pharmacological doses reduces uric acid excretion and causes hyperuricaemia (Emmerson 1996).

Lead poisoning is also associated with hyperuricaemia and gout (Goyer 1989), probably due to the effects of lead on the kidney.

Ramipril, an ACE inhibitor, increased serum uric acid in hypertensive subjects (Walter et al. 1987). Renal impairment may be responsible for the hyperuricaemia seen in some patients receiving azapropazone and that seen in amoxapine overdose (Sipila et al. 1986). The anticoagulant warfarin was reported to increase uric acid concentration, probably as a result of increased production (Menon et al. 1986), but this was not confirmed by others (Walker et al. 1988). In those treated with the β-blockers propranolol and timolol, there was a tendency for serum uric acid concentration to increase (Pedersen and Mikkelsen 1979; Helgeland 1983). Treatment with the H_2-receptor antagonists cimetidine and ranitidine (Einarson et al. 1985), and with levodopa (Honda and Gindin 1972), was reported to cause gouty arthritis. The use of the anaesthetic agent methoxyflurane was associated with increased serum uric acid concentrations, probably due to the nephrotoxic effect of fluoride on distal tubular function (Hamilton and Robertson 1974).

Ibuprofen causes an increase in serum uric acid concentration (Chalmers 1971). Amrinone, a selective phosphodiesterase inhibitor, causes hyperuricaemia (Johnston et al. 1984). Treatment with granulocyte-macrophage colony-stimulating factor has been reported to increase serum urate (Grant et al. 1992).

Omeprazole, which acts on the gastric H^+/K^+ ATPase has been reported to have caused gout in two patients who had no previous history of gout, hyperuricaemia, or other predisposing factors; in one, rechallenge caused gout again (Kraus and Flores Suarez 1995).

Hypouricaemia

Hypouricaemia due to decreased production is seen with the use of xanthine oxidase inhibitors such as allopurinol and azathioprine (Emmerson 1996).

Increased urate excretion is seen in volume expansion and this has been suggested as the mechanism of the hypouricaemia and hyponatraemia in the syndrome of inappropriate secretion of antidiuretic hormone (SIADH) (Prospert et al. 1993). Uricosuric drugs such as probenecid, sulphinpyrazone, benzbromarone, and benziodarone all reduce serum urate by increasing urate clearance (Scott 1991). High doses of aspirin and phenylbutazone have a similar effect (Becker and Roessler 1995).

Many radiographic contrast media (such as iopanoic acid, sodium diatrizoate, and meglumine iodipamide) are uricosuric and cause a decrease in the serum urate concentration (Postlethwaite and Kelley 1971). Serum uric acid concentrations were found to be lowered in epileptic patients on long-term antiepileptic drugs, especially phenytoin (Krause *et al.* 1987). A number of anticoagulants, such as ethylbiscoumacetate, phenindione, and dicoumarol, cause hypouricaemia (Becker and Roessler 1995; Caron *et al.* 1996). Other drugs that have been shown to lower serum urate are etofibrate (a complex of clofibrate and nicotinic acid) retard (Degenring *et al.* 1983), the anticholinergic agents glycopyrrolate, glyceryl guaiacolate (a common component of cough mixtures), the antipsychotic drug chlorprothixene (Shalev *et al.* 1987a), and prednisone and other adrenal steroids.

Urinastatin, a proteinase inhibitor, reduces serum uric acid concentration in patients treated with cisplatin (Umeki *et al.* 1989). Traxanox and tienilic acid reduce serum uric acid and increase uric acid excretion in hypertensive patients (Fujimura *et al.* 1989). Oxaprozin, a propionic acid analogue, was reported to cause a fall in serum uric acid and increased excretion of uric acid in healthy volunteers (Goldfarb *et al.* 1985). Indacrinone, a loop diuretic, has a uricosuric effect and causes hypouricaemia (Vlasses *et al.* 1984). Any drug or agent that causes a Fanconi-type syndrome will cause hypouricaemia (see section on Acidosis and Chapter 14).

Cilazapril, when administered with hydrochlorothiazide, reduces the incidence of hyperuricaemia as compared with hydrochlorothiazide alone (Pordy 1994). Losartan, a selective angiotensin II receptor antagonist, decreases serum uric acid concentration (Burnier *et al.* 1995; Soffer *et al.* 1995; Burrell 1997) by increasing uric acid excretion. Administration of co-trimoxazole decreases uric acid by 37 per cent in patients with AIDS (Chertow *et al.* 1996).

Oxalate

Healthy subjects excrete less than 0.45 millimoles of oxalate a day (Williams and Wandzilak 1989; Watts 1996). Approximately 10–20 per cent of urinary oxalate comes from dietary sources such as cocoa, tea, beans, celery, beetroot, chocolate, nuts, rhubarb, and spinach, while the rest comes from endogenous metabolism of precursors, mainly glyoxylate and ascorbic acid. About 35–50 per cent of the total oxalate comes from ascorbic acid (Williams and Wandzilak 1989); the major sources of glyoxylate include glycine, glycolic acid, and serine (Williams and Wandzilak 1989). Oxalate is excreted almost exclusively in the urine, and renal tubular se-

cretion plays an important role (Watts 1996). There are three types of primary hyperoxaluria. Type I is due to a defect in the (peroxisomal) enzyme alanine glyoxylate aminotransferase; type II, which is rare, is due to a defect in the enzyme glyoxylate reductase (Watts 1996); and type III is primary absorptive hyperoxaluria. Secondary hyperoxaluria can result from excessive production of oxalate, due either to an increase in endogenous synthesis or increased intake of oxalate precursors.

Increased excretion of oxalate

Ingestion of ethylene glycol leads to hyperoxaluria (Rose 1994) due to conversion of ethylene glycol to glycoaldehyde and glycolate in the liver. Hyperoxaluria and renal failure may follow administration of the anaesthetic agent methoxyflurane, which is metabolised to oxalate (McIntyre *et al.* 1973). Abuse of methoxyflurane was reported to cause hyperoxaluria and widespread retinal crystalline deposits (Frascino *et al.* 1970; Novak *et al.* 1988). Xylitol, which has been used in parenteral nutrition as a source of calories, may also lead to hyperoxaluria (Rofe *et al.* 1979). This may also follow the use of glycine-rich fluid during prostatectomy (Fitzpatrick *et al.* 1981). Increased intake of ascorbic acid can lead to hyperoxaluria (Schmidt *et al.* 1981), which is a potential adverse effect of high pharmacological doses ('megadoses') of the vitamin. Total parenteral nutrition is associated with increased oxalate excretion in low-birth-weight infants. This is due to the presence of the oxalate precursors glycine and ascorbic acid (Campfield and Braden 1989).

Naftidrofuryl oxalate infusion used for arteriosclerosis obliterans increases serum and urinary oxalate and in two patients renal failure developed (Le Meur *et al.* 1995).

Hyperoxaluria due to increased intestinal absorption follows oral phosphate administration in the treatment of hypophosphataemic rickets (Reusz *et al.* 1990). Long-term administration (for 6 months) of the somatostatin analogue octreotide to a patient with carcinoid tumour caused hyperoxaluria and renal stones, probably due to increased intestinal absorption of oxalate (Ranft and Eibl-Eibesfeldt 1990). Pyridoxilate, used in the treatment of angina pectoris or arteritis, contains an equimolar combination of glyoxylate and pyridoxine and causes increased excretion of oxalate and formation of renal stones (Daudon *et al.* 1987). Ingestion of 250 g of sucrose daily for 7 days increased oxalate excretion (Li *et al.* 1986). When bumetanide was infused, excretion increased, either from increased renal tubular secretion or decreased reabsorption (Young 1995).

Decreased excretion of oxalate

Administration of magnesium (Berg *et al.* 1986) or calcium (Barilla *et al.* 1978) reduces the excretion of oxalate, presumably by precipitating oxalate in the intestinal lumen. Cholestyramine binds to oxalate in the intestine and reduces its excretion. Aluminium hydroxide has similar actions (Nordenvall *et al.* 1983). Allopurinol, in addition to reducing uric acid excretion, also reduces oxalate excretion (Ettinger *et al.* 1986). Treatment of recurrent stone-formers with pyridoxine (Harrison *et al.* 1981), and severe hyperoxalaemia associated with chronic disease (Le Meur *et al.* 1995) have been reported to lower the excretion of oxalate. Oral citrate and an extract from banana stem (Family Musaceae) reduced oxalate excretion in an animal model (Poonguzhali and Chegu 1994). Verapamil given to hyperoxalaemic subjects caused reduction in oxalate excretion (Umekawa *et al.* 1996). In a phase 1 trial, (1)-2-oxothiazolidine-4-carboxylate decreased oxalate excretion in healthy subjects (Holmes *et al.* 1997).

Proteins

Protein metabolism can be affected by many drugs and hormones. Of the hormones, glucocorticoids and thyroxine are catabolic and cause a net negative balance. Oestrogens stimulate androgens and tend to decrease the synthesis of several plasma proteins by the liver (see below). Androgens are anabolic at the tissue level and increase the tissue protein content, and this is accompanied by a positive nitrogen balance.

Total plasma protein

Increase in total plasma protein

Agents or drugs that produce volume depletion will cause an increase in plasma total protein concentration (see section on Sodium and water). Vasopressor drugs like adrenaline, noradrenaline, and angiotensin will raise the plasma protein concentration owing to vasoconstriction and loss of protein-free fluid to the extravascular space (Young 1995). Drugs and agents that increase hepatic protein synthesis, like growth hormone or insulin, will cause an increase in plasma total protein concentration. Plasma protein concentrations are reported to be raised in heroin and cocaine addicts (Marks and Chapple 1967). Felodipine infusion and isotretinoin treatment are reported to cause a small but significant increase in total protein concentration (Young 1995).

Decreased plasma protein concentration

The concentration of total protein will decrease in all situations in which there is an increase in ECF volume or total body water (see section on Sodium and water). Oestrogens and oestrogen-containing contraceptives can decrease total protein concentration (Sadik *et al.* 1985). A significant (13.7 per cent) decrease in total protein was produced by a non-ionic radiographic contrast medium (Brunet *et al.* 1989) and this could not be explained by dilution. Exposure to lead, and toxicity from vitamin A (Helsing 1996), cause hypoproteinaemia.

Artefacts

Many drugs or agents can interfere with total protein determination and cause spuriously low or high results. Drugs that have been reported as causing an apparent increase in total protein concentration are aspirin, carbenicillin and other penicillins, cephalothin, chloramphenicol, rifampicin, and sulphasalazine, dextrans, and radiographic contrast media. Drugs that cause an apparent decrease are aspirin, caproxamine, cefotaxime, dextran 40, fluosol-DA, and sodium valproate (Young 1995). The effect depends on the method of determination of total protein. For example, aspirin decreases the total protein concentration measured by the biuret method, but increases it when measured by spectrophotometry (Young 1995).

Albumin

Albumin, which has a molecular weight of about 68 000, is synthesized in the liver and accounts for 40–60 per cent of the total protein concentration in plasma.

Increase in plasma albumin

Plasma albumin concentrations will be high in situations similar to those that increase total plasma protein.

Decrease in plasma albumin

The plasma albumin concentration will decrease in hepatocellular disease caused by drugs (see Chapter 13) and in drug-induced malabsorption syndromes (see Chapter 12). Decreased albumin synthesis is probably responsible for the decrease in albumin concentration seen after administration of oestrogen and the contraceptive pill (Sadik *et al.* 1985). Contraceptive pills with low oestrogen content or steroids with an oestrogenic effect do not affect plasma albumin concentration (Hawkins and Benster 1977). Phenytoin has been reported by some to cause a decrease in plasma albumin concentration (Andreasen *et al.* 1973), whereas others failed to find any effect (Parker and Shearer 1979). Sodium valproate decreased plasma albumin levels (Itoh *et al.* 1982), but other anticonvulsants had no effect (Salway 1989). Other drugs that have been reported to cause a decrease in plasma albumin concentration include amiodarone, colaspase (asparaginase), flurbiprofen, ibuprofen, indomethacin, oxyphenisatin (Reynolds *et al.* 1989), and nitrofurantoin (Holmes *et al.* 1980; Young 1995). The clinical significance of these findings remains to be established. Marked hypoalbuminaemia developed in four of nine patients treated with granulocyte-macrophage colony-stimulating factor (Kaczmarski and Mufti 1990). Dapsone, the antileprosy drug, caused severe hypoalbuminuria and oedema when used in the treatment of dermatitis herpetiformis (Cowan and Wright 1981).

Artefacts

Penicillins, caproxamine, clofibrate, heparin, and salicylate interfere with some methods of albumin measurement and cause an apparent decrease in albumin concentration (Young 1995).

Prealbumin

Prealbumin, which has a molecular weight of 54 000, is synthesized in the liver, and because of its short half-life serves as a sensitive marker of protein malnutrition. It acts as a carrier protein for thyroid hormone and for vitamin A in association with retinol-binding protein.

Increase in plasma prealbumin

The prealbumin concentration is increased by androgens and anabolic steroids (Culberg 1984), carbamazepine, danazol, dronabinol (Struwe *et al.* 1993), medroxyprogesterone (Downer *et al.* 1993), betamethasone (Gamstedt *et al.* 1981), prednisolone, and propranolol (Franklyn *et al.* 1985*a*). Ornithine α-ketoglutarate given in addition to intravenous nutrition further improved nitrogen balance and prealbumin concentration (Erstad *et al.* 1994). Infusion of human tumour necrosis factor-α (TNFα) did not significantly change the serum concentration of prealbumin (Hardin *et al.* 1993). Treatment of patients with multiple injuries with human growth hormone (GH) also failed to change prealbumin concentration (Roth *et al.* 1995).

Decrease in plasma prealbumin

Plasma concentrations of prealbumin decrease during pregnancy and after administration of oestrogens or oral contraceptives (Barbosa *et al.* 1971). Amiodarone decreases prealbumin concentration by about 20 per cent (Franklyn *et al.* 1985*b*). Human recombinant inter-leukin-6 used as a chemotherapeutic agent decreases prealbumin concentration (Nieken *et al.* 1995).

Retinol-binding protein

Retinol-binding protein (RBP) is a small protein of 21 000 molecular weight that is synthesized in the liver. In association with prealbumin it transports vitamin A. Plasma RBP concentration is a useful indicator of protein nutritional status.

Increase in plasma RBP

Like other plasma proteins — for example, sex-hormone-binding globulin (SHBG), thyroxine-binding globulin (TBG) — RBP concentrations are increased by oestrogens and oral contraceptives (Amatayakul *et al.* 1994), and by the anticonvulsants phenobarbitone, phenytoin, and carbamazepine (Kozlowski *et al.* 1987). Cord blood RBP concentrations are increased in babies born to mothers who have been given betamethasone before delivery (Georgieff *et al.* 1988). Medroxyprogesterone administration to cancer patients with cachexia increases RBP concentration significantly (Downer *et al.* 1993).

Decrease in plasma RBP

Administration of GH to GH-deficient children caused a significant reduction in RBP (Kemp and Canfield 1983).

Cortisol-binding globulin

Cortisol-binding globulin (CBG) is an α-globulin which carries about 90 per cent of circulating cortisol. It is increased by oestrogens (Barbosa *et al.* 1971) and oestrogen-containing contraceptive pills, and anabolic steroids, and decreased by androgens (Barbosa *et al.* 1971). Premature neonates treated with dexamethasone showed a 42 per cent decrease in CBG (Kari *et al.* 1996). Mitotane increased CBG two to threefold within one month of starting treatment (Van Seters and Moolenaar 1991).

Thyroxine-binding globulin

TBG binds and transports the thyroid hormones T_4 and T_3.

Increase in plasma TBG

Oestrogens and oral contraceptives increase TBG concentration (Carey 1971), an effect similar to that in pregnancy (Swaminathan *et al.* 1989). The increase in

TBG is dose dependent. Tamoxifen, with its weak oestrogen effect, has been reported by some to increase TBG (Gordon *et al.* 1986), whereas others did not find any effect (Jensen 1985). Carbamazepine increased TBG in hypothyroid patients (Aanderud *et al.* 1981) but had no effect in euthyroid volunteers (Connell *et al.* 1984*a*) or epileptics (De Luca *et al.* 1986) during short-term treatment, but a decrease in TBG concentration was reported with longer-term treatment with carbamazepine (Strandjord *et al.* 1981). Clofibrate, long-term methadone treatment, clomipramine, perphenazine, and other phenothiazines, are some of the other drugs reported to increase plasma TBG concentration (Young 1995). Mitotane increased TBG together with SHBG and CBG (Van Seters and Moolenaar 1991). Chronic GH treatment increased TBG concentration (Schmitt *et al.* 1997).

Decrease in plasma TBG

Androgens and steroids, such as danazol and stanozolol, with androgenic properties decrease TBG concentration (Deyssig and Weissel 1993; Arafah 1994). Other drugs reported to decrease plasma TBG concentration are amiodarone (Davies and Franklyn 1991), colaspase, colestipol, co-trimoxazole, fenclofenac (Ratcliffe *et al.* 1980), fluoxymesterone, glucocorticoids (Gamstedt *et al.* 1981), nadolol, oxandrolone, phenytoin (Young 1995), and propranolol (Franklyn *et al.* 1985*a*). Phenytoin has also been reported to have no effect on TBG (Larsen *et al.* 1970), but this apparent lack of effect may have been from short duration of treatment; TBG concentrations were within the reference range in subjects treated with fenclofenac (Salway 1989).

Sex-hormone-binding globulin

SHBG is a glycoprotein with a high affinity for sex steroid hormones, in particular 5α-dihydrotestosterone and testosterone, but less for oestradiol (Lindstedt *et al.* 1985).

Increase in serum SHBG

SHBG concentrations are increased by oestrogens and oral contraceptives (Lindstedt *et al.* 1985; Sobbrio *et al.* 1991). Of the oestrogens, ethinyloestradiol was more potent than oestradiol valerate (Mall-Haefeli *et al.* 1983). Furthermore, oestrogen was less effective when administered percutaneously than when given orally (Stomati *et al.* 1996). The increase in SHBG induced by oestrogens is sometimes used as a sensitive indicator of oestrogen effect. Oestrogen-containing oral contraceptive pills increase the SHBG concentration by 46–213 per

cent (Murphy *et al.* 1990). Dexamethasone increased SHBG concentrations by 35.5 per cent in hirsute women (Cunningham *et al.* 1985), whereas large doses of glucocorticoids decrease SHBG concentration (Lindstedt *et al.* 1985). Excessive administration of thyroid hormone (Ruder *et al.* 1971), or of anticonvulsants like carbamazepine, phenobarbitone, phenytoin, primidone, or sodium valproate, increases SHBG concentrations (Beastall *et al.* 1985; Isojarvi *et al.* 1991, 1995). The increase induced by carbamazepine was seen within 7 days of starting the drug (Connell *et al.* 1984*b*); in epileptics treated with phenytoin the concentrations increased by 110 per cent (Toone *et al.* 1980). Of the anticonvulsants, phenytoin caused the highest rise in SHBG (Murialdo *et al.* 1994). Rifampicin, the antituberculous drug, caused 47–75 per cent increase in SHBG concentrations (Lonning *et al.* 1989). The synthetic antioestrogen clomiphene citrate produces a moderate rise (Marshall *et al.* 1972). Tamoxifen, like clomiphene, increases serum SHBG (Kedar *et al.* 1994; Lonning *et al.* 1995). Droloxifene, a new antioestrogen, increased SHBG, and this effect was dose dependent (Rauschning and Pritchard 1994). The antifungal agent ketoconazole, which affects steroidogenesis, increases the serum SHBG concentration (Heyns *et al.* 1985), whereas fluconazole produced no significant rise in SHBG (Devenport *et al.* 1989). Cimetidine had no effect on serum SHBG (Michnovicz and Galbraith 1991). Exogenous administration of IGF1 increased SHBG concentration in patients with Laron syndrome (somatomedin-deficient dwarfism) or GH deficiency (Gafny *et al.* 1994). Mitotane increased SHBG to two to three times pretreatment values (Van Seters and Moolenaar 1991).

Decrease in serum SHBG

A fall in serum SHBG concentration occurs during treatment with androgens (Lindstedt *et al.* 1985) or androgenic steroids such as danazol and stanozolol (Bagatell and Bremner 1996). Progestogens such as medroxyprogesterone acetate, levonorgestrel, lynoestrenol, megestrol, and desogestrel, cause a decrease in SHBG concentrations (Amatayakut 1994; Amatayakut *et al.* 1994). Cyproterone acetate, which has some progestogenic activity, decreases SHBG concentrations in hirsute women (Vincens *et al.* 1989). Simvastatin treatment decreased serum SHBG concentration by 19 per cent in insulin-dependent diabetic subjects (Kjaer *et al.* 1992). Administration of GH decreases SHBG concentration (Gafny *et al.* 1994). Gemfibrozil treatment of dysplipidaemic patients causes a significant (10 per cent) decrease in SHBG concentration (Hautanen *et al.* 1994). Finasteride, a 5α-reductase inhibitor, and nomegestrol implants, did not cause any significant effect on serum SHBG (Fruzzetti *et al.* 1994; Barbosa *et al.* 1996). Cimetidine has been reported to decrease SHBG concentration (Young 1995).

Haptoglobin

Haptoglobin, which binds free haemoglobin in plasma, is an acute-phase reactant and is a glycoprotein which moves in the α_2 region.

Increase in plasma haptoglobin

Androgens and steroids with androgenic activity increase plasma haptoglobin concentration (Barbosa *et al.* 1971). High doses of medroxyprogesterone acetate used in the treatment of prostatic and renal carcinoma caused a significant increase in haptoglobin concentration (Nilsson *et al.* 1989). Treating cancer patients with recombinant interleukin-6 increased haptoglobin concentrations (Nieken *et al.* 1995).

Decrease in plasma haptoglobin

Haptoglobin concentrations decrease whenever there is free haemoglobin in the circulation, and drugs like dapsone that cause haemolytic anaemia (see Chapter 24) will cause a decrease in plasma haptoglobin (Young 1995). Oestrogens and oestrogen-containing contraceptives and colaspase decrease the plasma haptoglobin concentration, probably by reducing hepatic synthesis (Young 1995). Dextran, a plasma expander, decreases haptoglobin, possibly by forming a complex (Skrede *et al.* 1973). Treatment of rheumatoid arthritis patients with adrenal corticosteroids decreased plasma haptoglobin (McConkey *et al.* 1973), possibly due to a decrease in acute-phase response.

Spuriously low haptoglobin concentrations due to chlorpromazine interference with the assay have been reported (Sher 1982).

Caeruloplasmin

Caeruloplasmin, the principal copper-containing protein of plasma, is an antioxidant, and is a late acute-phase reactant.

Increase in plasma caeruloplasmin

Oestrogens increase the synthesis of caeruloplasmin, and elevated concentrations are seen in patients taking oestrogens and oestrogen-containing contraceptive pills (Song *et al.* 1989; Amatayakul *et al.* 1994). Norethindrone (Taietal and Kafrissen 1995) and tamoxifen,

because of their oestrogenic effects, increase caeruloplasmin concentrations (Song *et al.* 1989). The anticonvulsants phenobarbitone, phenytoin, and carbamazepine, either alone or in combination, increase caeruloplasmin concentrations (Werther *et al.* 1986). Elevated concentrations of serum caeruloplasmin are found in copper poisoning (Young 1995). As caeruloplasmin is an acute-phase protein, it is increased in many conditions, such as rheumatoid arthritis. Exposure to vinyl chloride monomer (Wagnerova *et al.* 1988) and lead (Wagnerova *et al.* 1986) caused an increase in caeruloplasmin concentrations. D-Penicillamine interferes with the function of caeruloplasmin (Meyboom and Brodie-Meijer 1996).

Decrease in plasma caeruloplasmin

Colaspase decreases the synthesis and plasma concentration of caeruloplasmin (Oettgen *et al.* 1970), and levonorgestrel causes a significant fall (Shaaban *et al.* 1984). Plasma caeruloplasmin concentrations are also low in malnutrition, malabsorption, the nephrotic syndrome, and severe liver disease.

Transferrin

Transferrin is the principal transporter of iron in plasma. It is a β-globulin with a molecular weight of 77 000, and its concentration falls during acute-phase reactions.

Increase in serum transferrin

A progressive increase in transferrin is seen in pregnancy (Rosenmund *et al.* 1986). Oestrogens and oral contraceptives have a similar effect but not to the same degree (Horne *et al.* 1970). Low-oestrogen oral contraceptives have no effect on transferrin concentrations (Rosenmund *et al.* 1986). Increased plasma concentrations were found in the cord blood of infants whose mothers had had betamethasone treatment prior to delivery (Georgieff *et al.* 1988). Transferrin exists in plasma in different isoforms differing in their carbohydrate content. Alcohol abuse increases one of these (carbohydrate-deficient transferrin [Crabb 1990]), as does exposure to organic solvents (Petren and Vesterberg 1987). Serum transferrin is increased by GH administration to GH-deficient children (Kemp and Canfield 1983) and by danazol during treatment of endometriosis (Young 1995).

Decrease in plasma transferrin

Testosterone (Barbosa *et al.* 1971), colaspase (Oettgen *et al.* 1970), and cortisone cause a reduction in plasma transferrin by decreasing synthesis. High-molecular-weight dextrans (e.g. dextran 70) decrease plasma transferrin, but low-molecular-weight dextrans (e.g. dextran 40) do not (Skrede *et al.* 1973). Interleukin-6 therapy significantly reduces serum transferrin (Nieken *et al.* 1995).

Fibrinogen

Fibrinogen, a large dimeric protein, is converted by thrombin to fibrin, which polymerizes to form an insoluble gel.

Increase in plasma fibrinogen concentration

Plasma fibrinogen concentration is increased, owing to increased synthesis in the liver, by oestrogens and oestrogen-containing oral contraceptives. With the latter, the increase occurs within 1–3 months of starting their use (Ernst 1992), and this may contribute to an increase in cardiovascular risk. Plasma fibrinogen is also increased in drug addiction, particularly in opiate users (Galante *et al.* 1994). Aspirin, gemfibrozil, pyrazinamide, and xanthine raise fibrinogen concentrations in some patients (Young 1995). Transdermal nicotine had no effect on plasma fibrinogen, whereas smoking increased it (Benowitz *et al.* 1993).

Decrease in plasma fibrinogen concentration

Androgens and anabolic steroids (Barbosa *et al.* 1971), niceritrol (Matsunaga *et al.* 1992), celiprolol (Hermann and Mayler 1988), bezafibrate (Pazzucconi *et al.* 1992; Specht Leible 1993), clofibrate (Chakrabarti *et al.* 1968), dextrans (Skrede *et al.* 1973), fluroxene (Johnston *et al.* 1973), kanamycin, sodium valproate (Sussman and McLain 1979), mesoglycan (Orefice *et al.* 1992), ticlopidine (De Maat *et al.* 1996), and urapidil (Haenni and Lithell 1996) all decrease plasma fibrinogen, and ticlopidine prevents the rise in plasma fibrinogen usually seen after surgery (Kroft *et al.* 1993). The decrease in fibrinogen with sodium valproate was greater when given with other anticonvulsants (Dukes 1996*c*). Pravastatin, but not simvastatin, decreases plasma fibrinogen in hyperlipoproteinaemic subjects (Tsuda *et al.* 1996). Simvastatin in combination with ciprofibrate reduces plasma fibrinogen (Kontopoulos *et al.* 1996) and ciprofibrate has significantly more effect than gemfibrozil (De Maat *et al.* 1997).

Octreotide decreased plasma fibrinogen concentration in type I diabetic patients (Norgaard *et al.* 1990). The antiplatelet drug ticlopidine decreased plasma fibrinogen in patients with peripheral vascular disease (Randi *et al.* 1991).

Immunoglobulins (γ-globulin)

Increase in plasma immunoglobulin concentration

An increase in γ-globulin concentration followed treatment with aminopyrine, cimetidine, colaspase, interferon-α, methimazole, nitrofurantoin, phenytoin, propylthiouracil, and tubocurarine (Young 1995). Serum concentrations of immunoglobulins A, G, and M are increased by administration of colaspase (Oettgen *et al.* 1970), methyldopa, and nitrofurantoin (Young 1995). Oxyphenisatin increased IgG and IgM by causing chronic active hepatitis (Dietrichson 1975). Chlorpromazine treatment in schizophrenic patients increases IgM concentration in a dose-dependent manner (Zarrabi *et al.* 1979).

Decrease in plasma immunoglobulins

A fall in plasma immunoglobulins follows the administration of gold (Dukes 1996*b*), glucocorticoids, methotrexate, and phenytoin; dextrans decreased plasma IgA and IgM (Young 1995). In one study, phenytoin decreased IgA concentration in 9 per cent of treated children (Ruff *et al.* 1987). Administration of thyroxine to infants with hypothyroidism decreased serum IgA concentrations (Seager 1984).

Serum enzymes

Enzymes found in the blood can be classified according to their site of function: (a) enzymes that act or function in plasma (plasma-specific enzymes) — enzymes involved in the blood-clotting mechanism and those involved with fibrinolysis are examples; (b) enzymes that are secreted — enzymes of the gastrointestinal tract exemplify this group; (c) cellular enzymes that function intracellularly — most clinically relevant enzymes fall into this third category, and this section is mainly concerned with cellular enzymes. These intracellular enzymes are present in various compartments of the cell such as cytoplasm, mitochondria, and lysosomes. They are present in small amounts in the serum of normal subjects, and the amount increases in various disease processes. This increase is used diagnostically. The pathophysiological mechanisms involved in changes in serum enzymes are, however, not fully understood (Pappas 1989). Some of the factors thought to influence the concentration of serum enzymes in health and disease are: the rate of release of the enzyme (due to cell death or injury and increased synthesis); rate of clearance of the enzyme; and leakage of the enzyme from the cells (for a review see Pappas 1989).

Drugs may cause changes in serum enzymes due to injury or damage to an organ (e.g. large doses of paracetamol cause elevation of aspartase aminotransferase [AST]) or due to increased synthesis (e.g. increased synthesis of γ-glutamyl transferase [GGT] by alcohol or barbiturates).

Creatine kinase

Creatine kinase (ATP; creatine *N*-phosphotransferase; EC2.7.3.2, CK) is widely distributed throughout the human body but is particularly concentrated in muscle tissues. Three cytosolic isoenzymes (CK-MM, CK-MB, CK-BB) and one mitochondrial isoenzyme of CK have been identified (Apple 1989). The tissue sources are primarily skeletal muscle for CK-MM, heart for CK-MB, and brain for CK-BB (Lott and Stang 1989). In the circulation, the tissue forms of the enzyme are converted to serum forms by loss of the C-terminal residue. The resulting serum isoforms are termed MM_1, MM_2, MM_3, MB_1, and MB_2 (Jones and Swaminathan 1990).

Increase in serum CK activity

Increase in serum CK activity may follow strenuous exercise (Robertshaw and Swaminathan 1993) or intramuscular injections (Jones and Swaminathan 1990). Several drugs can cause elevation of CK activity, some by causing rhabdomyolysis. The mechanism by which other drugs cause an elevation in CK activity may be a disturbance in membrane function or an actual toxic effect on the cells.

Aminocaproic acid therapy causes acute muscle cell injury and elevation of CK activity in a few patients (Argov and Mastaglia 1988). Clofibrate treatment causes a mild increase in serum CK activity in some patients (Dujovne *et al.* 1976), but a more pronounced rise is seen in obese patients (Belaiche *et al.* 1977) and those with renal failure (Pierides and Alvasez-Ude 1975). Some of these patients had acute muscle cramp, weakness, and aching, which disappeared on stopping clofibrate treatment (Argov and Mastaglia 1988). Nicotinic acid has also been associated with myopathy and elevated CK activity and this occurred with both crystalline and sustained-release preparations (Gharavi *et al.* 1994). Fenofibrate (Rigal *et al.* 1989) and beclofibrate (Capurso 1991) increased CK values in 0.8 per cent and 0.4 per cent of patients respectively. Myopathy has been reported with gemfibrozil (Magarian *et al.* 1991) and ciprofibrate (Delangre *et al.* 1990), and rhabdomyolysis has been reported in bezafibrate overdose (Bedani *et al.* 1994). A small increase in CK activity has been found after long-term administration of halofenate (Dujovne *et al.* 1976).

In alcoholics, elevated CK activity due to alcoholic rhabdomyolysis may be seen (DiSilvio 1978). Drugs such as thiazide diuretics, carbenoxolone, licorice, purgatives, and amphotericin cause skeletal muscle damage and a moderate rise in CK activity due to hypokalaemia (Sunderam and Swaminathan 1981; Argov and Mastaglia 1988). Diclofenac treatment for arthritis caused rhabdomyolysis mild renal failure in one patient (Delrio *et al.* 1996). Pentazocine taken together with alcohol caused rhabdomyolysis (Tsai *et al.* 1987).

Other drugs or agents that cause rhabdomyolysis are drugs of abuse such as opiates and heroin (Argov and Mastaglia 1988), methylenedioxymethamphetamine (MDMA, 'Ecstasy') (Screaton *et al.* 1992; Williams and Unwin 1997), amphetamines and phenylpropanolamine, phencyclidine, and drugs which cause hypophosphataemia (see section on Phosphate).

Elevated serum CK activity as a result of rhabdomyolysis has been found with colchicine, cyclosporin, famotidine, labetalol (Willis *et al.* 1990), and suxamethonium (Arellano and Krupp 1991).

The phenothiazines prochloperazine, perphenazine, and thioridazine, and the butyrophenone haloperidol have been shown to increase CK activity in some patients (Pearlman *et al.* 1988), and in others withdrawal of the drugs caused elevation of CK (Malas and van Kammen 1982) and sometimes a neuroleptic malignant syndrome (Goldwasser *et al.* 1989). Clozapine causes marked elevation of CK (Kirson *et al.* 1995) and has been reported to produce the neuroleptic malignant syndrome (Reddig *et al.* 1993). In 10 per cent of patients taking antipsychotic drugs, such as clozapine, haloperidol, loxapine, melperone, olanzipine, and risperidone, marked elevation of activity of the serum CK MM isoenzyme was found (Meltzer *et al.* 1996). Elevated CK values were observed in overdose with the tricyclic antidepressants imipramine (Sueblinvong and Wilson 1969) and amitriptyline (Guthrie and Lott 1986).

The β-blockers carteolol, labetalol, bucindolol, pindolol, and propranolol caused elevation of serum CK activity, more markedly and commonly in the case of pindolol; isoenzyme studies showed the elevation to be due mainly to the MM isoenzyme (Saruta *et al.* 1985). Peaks of CK were seen 1–5 days after stopping pindolol. Xamoterol, a $β_1$-selective partial agonist did not show this effect, suggesting that the rise in CK activity is due to $β_2$-selective agonist activity (Tomlinson *et al.* 1990).

The β-adrenoreceptor agonist salbutamol has been associated with muscle cramps and elevated CK activity (Lisi 1989). This increase was seen to be due to the CK-MB isoenzyme (Chazan *et al.* 1992, 1994). Elevated

CK-MB activity has also been seen in children with status asthmaticus treated with isoprenaline (Maguire *et al.* 1986) and theophylline (Ng *et al.* 1985). Increases in skeletal muscle CK activity were seen in patients treated with terbutaline (Sykes *et al.* 1991). Theophylline overdosage is associated with gross elevation of total CK and the MM isoenzyme (Modi *et al.* 1985). The elevation is partly due to hypokalaemia-induced muscle damage and partly to CK release from muscle as a result of generalized seizures.

Quinidine therapy was reported to cause gross elevation in CK and CK-MM isoenzyme activity in one patient (Weiss *et al.* 1979); the CK values returned to normal once the drug was stopped and increased again when it was restarted.

Elevation of CK activity and mild myopathy have been found in patients treated with bumetanide, danazol, emetine, lithium, metolazone, stanozolol, and vincristine (Swash and Schwarz 1997). In overdosage with such drugs as barbiturates, glutethimide, and amoxapine (Abero *et al.* 1982), CK levels are elevated, probably as a result of crush injury (Lott and Wolf 1986). Elevated total CK, CK-MB, and BB values were found in a case of salicylate overdose (Vladutiu and Reitz 1980). Isotretinoin, a retinoid used in the treatment of acne, caused a marked increase in serum CK activity (McBurney and Rosen 1984). The chemotherapeutic agents 5-fluorouracil and levamisole were associated with marked elevations of CK (Cersosimo and Lee 1996).

Radiographic contrast agents caused an elevation of serum CK activity after 24 hours (Carlsson *et al.* 1985) and isoenzyme studies showed that there is elevation of BB isoenzyme, probably due to breakdown of the blood--brain barrier (Pfeiffer *et al.* 1987).

HMG-CoA reductase inhibitors cause elevation of CK activity and in some cause rhabdomyolysis and even renal failure. The increase is seen in a small proportion of patients (up to 3 per cent) and the elevation of CK activity is usually less than three times the upper limit of normal (Glueck *et al.* 1990; Thompson *et al.* 1991; Knopp *et al.* 1996). It is also seen with simvastatin, lovastatin (Glueck *et al.* 1990; Mantell *et al.* 1990; Thompson *et al.* 1991), and pravastatin (Knopp *et al.* 1996), but not with fluvastatin (Jokubaitis *et al.* 1994). Rhabdomyolysis has been reported with simvastatin (Deslypere and Vermeuten 1991; Berland *et al.* 1991). These drugs decrease serum concentrations of co-enzyme Q (ubiquinone) (Laaksonen *et al.* 1994, 1995), which is part of the oxidative respiratory pathway, and a decrease in this could lead to myocyte dysfunction and a rise in CK. Twenty-four cases of rhabdomyolysis have

been reported following lovastatin treatment (Mantell *et al.* 1990) and in many of these there were other medications which increased the risk. Concurrent administration of cyclosporin, erythromycin, nicotinic acid, or gemfibrozil increases the risk of myopathy (Marais *et al.* 1990; Pierce *et al.* 1990).

Intramuscular injections of ampicillin, carbenicillin, chlordiazepoxide, digoxin, fluphenazine, lignocaine, pentazocine, and pethidine have been reported to cause elevation of CK activity (Salway 1989). In many cases the degree of elevation was greater than expected from the injection, suggesting that the drugs caused muscle damage in some manner. Myalgia and elevated CK activity were noted during treatment with recombinant growth hormone (Bach *et al.* 1992; Momoi *et al.* 1995) and in one case this was traced to the presence of glycerol and *m*-cresol in the diluent (Bach *et al.* 1992).

A small increase in CK activity has followed long-term administration of captopril (Katayama *et al.* 1987) and miconazole (Young 1995).

Corticosteroids cause a myopathy and elevate CK activity in some patients and decrease it in others. In subjects who are susceptible to malignant hyperthermia, halothane, lignocaine, and suxamethonium can cause gross elevation of CK activity (Argov and Mastaglia 1988), and even in insusceptible subjects, suxamethonium can cause some elevation (Umino *et al.* 1985); the increase is smaller if patients are first treated with dantrolene (Laurence and McKean 1990). Sevoflurane, but not isoflurane, caused a marked elevation of CK when given to a child in addition to suxamethonium (Kudoh *et al.* 1994).

Decrease in serum CK activity

A decrease from initially high values is seen in schizophrenic patients treated with a phenothiazine (Young 1995). Decreased CK values are also seen in women during the luteal phase of menstruation, in women taking alcohol, in pregnancy, and in some patients given prednisolone (Young 1995).

Artefacts

Decrease in serum CK activity may result from the *in vitro* effects of aspirin, clothiapine, EDTA, heparin, pindolol (Young 1995), and dipyrone (Gascon *et al.* 1993). Freezing and thawing of samples decreases the activity by 50 per cent. Thiols such as cysteine and cystine increase the measured CK activity (Young 1995).

Lactate dehydrogenase

Lactate dehydrogenase (LD, EC 1.1.1.27), a zinc-containing enzyme, catalyses the oxidation of lactate to pyruvate and is present in the cytoplasm of all cells. Highest activity is found in skeletal muscle, liver, heart, kidney, and red blood cells. LD is a tetramer composed of two subunits, H and M, and five isoenzymes can be demonstrated.

Increase in serum LD activity

Since LD is present in high concentrations in muscle, heart, liver, and red blood cells, drugs that cause damage to these organs or cells can be expected to cause elevation of serum LD activity.

Heparin causes increase in serum LD activity and isoenzyme studies show that this is of hepatic origin (Dukes *et al.* 1984).

Hepatic necrosis or injury caused by drugs such as paracetamol, halothane (Sherlock 1971), and xylitol, and drugs that cause cholestasis, such as imipramine, will lead to an elevation of LD activity. Drugs that cause muscle damage and release CK will also cause an elevation of LD activity (e.g. in rhabdomyolysis induced by alcohol). A transient rise in LD activity was seen after treatment with GM-CSF (Schriber and Negrin 1993; Grant and Heel 1992).

Decrease in serum LD activity

Serum LD tends to decrease with age. Fluoride and clofibrate cause a decrease (Young 1995), probably by decreasing release of the enzyme.

Artefacts

Drugs or chemicals that have been shown to decrease serum LD by analytical interference are oxalate, acetylsalicylic acid, ascorbic acid, cefotaxime, dipyrone, ketoprofen, methotrexate, and theophylline. Paracetamol, fluosol-DA, caffeine, phenobarbitone, rifampicin, and triamterene have been reported to increase the activity of LD (Young 1995).

Aminotransferases (transaminases)

This a group of enzymes that catalyse the reversible transfer of the amino group from an α-amino compound to an oxo acid. Although there are over 50 such enzymes, only two, aspartate aminotransferase (AST, EC 2.6.1.1) and alanine aminotransferase (ALT, EC 2.6.1.2) are commonly measured in clinical practice. Both are widely distributed in tissues and high concentrations of AST are found in liver, heart, skeletal muscle, and kidney, whereas high concentrations of ALT are found mainly in the liver. Isoenzymes of AST and ALT exist in both mitochondria and cytoplasm.

Aspartate aminotransferase

AST is a dimer of two identical subunits, and two isoenzymes have been identified: a mitochondrial form and a cytoplasmic form.

Increase in AST

Increased serum AST activity may originate from liver, heart, or skeletal muscle. It is elevated in any type of hepatocellular injury, and over 300 drugs that are hepatotoxic have been incriminated (Young 1995) (see also Chapter 13).

Anticonvulsant treatment with phenytoin, carbamazepine, or sodium valproate causes a significant increase in AST activity in about 40 per cent of patients (Aldenhovel 1988). It is not clear, however, whether this is entirely due to the anticonvulsants (Rao *et al.* 1993). Sulphasalazine (salazosulphapyridine) (Dougados *et al.* 1987) increased serum AST concentrations. Increases have also been reported with ritodrine and fenoterol (Rej 1989), in the latter case in cord blood of neonates born to mothers being treated with fenoterol (Kovacs *et al.* 1985). Heparin therapy causes elevation of AST activity (Dukes *et al.* 1984; Monreal *et al.* 1989). This is more common with conventional heparin than with the low-molecular-weight form (Monreal *et al.* 1989) and it occurs 5–10 days after starting treatment (Guevara *et al.* 1993). The exact mechanism of this increase is not known but may involve induction of enzymes. In patients treated with HMG-CoA reductase inhibitors such as lovastatin and simvastatin, increases in AST activity are due to muscle damage (Bradford *et al.* 1994). Another hypocholesterolaemic agent, pyridylcarbinol (Ronicol retard), has also been reported to increase AST activity (Keller *et al.* 1988). The antimicrobial agents teicoplanin (Bibler *et al.* 1987) and aztreonam (Miller *et al.* 1983), and the antifungal agents ketoconazole, fluconazole, itraconazole, and clotrimazole (Tester-Dalderup 1996), are known to cause elevation of AST activity. The NSAID fenbufen and suprofen also do so, owing to their hepatotoxic effects. Diethylcarbamazine and the antimetabolite 5-fluoro-2-deoxyceridine cause significant but reversible elevation of AST activity (Young 1995). Isoflurane, like halothane, has been reported to cause postoperative elevation of transaminase activity (Gunza 1992). Theophylline administration was reported to increase aminotransferase in an animal study and the increase was dose related (Dodig *et al.* 1994). Losartan, an angiotensin I receptor antagonist, caused elevation of transaminase activity (Elliott 1996), and the same occurs in 2.5 per cent of patients taking gemfibrozil and lovastatin together (Glueck *et al.* 1990).

The anabolic steroid nandrolone caused elevation of AST activity in one out of 29 elderly females with hip fracture (Sloan *et al.* 1992). Mexiletine raises it in a few patients (Campbell 1987). Unexplained increases in transaminase activity have been reported in about 28 per cent of patients treated with streptokinase (Maclennan *et al.* 1990; Freimark *et al.* 1991).

Serum AST activity is increased in drug-induced disorders of muscle. All the drugs that increase serum CK activity (see above) will therefore also elevate AST activity.

Decrease in serum AST activity

Drugs affecting vitamin B_6 status or which react with pyridoxal phosphate reduce serum AST activity (Rej 1989). The effect of cefazolin in decreasing AST concentrations in experimental animals may be due to the reaction of the drug with pyridoxal phosphate (Dhami *et al.* 1979). Haemodialysis may decrease AST concentrations, owing to loss of pyridoxal phosphate (Wolf *et al.* 1972). In haemophiliac patients, treatment with stanozolol caused a decrease in AST activity that was abnormal at the start of the treatment (Greer *et al.* 1985). A significant decrease in AST activity was reported in users of high-oestrogen oral contraceptives (Walden *et al.* 1986).

Artefacts

Drugs that have been reported to interfere with the measurement of AST activity and give spurious results include ascorbic acid in large doses (Barnes 1975), chlordiazepoxide, fluorescein, ibuprofen, isoniazid (Young 1995) metronidazole, pindolol, and rifampicin. Low aminotransferase values are seen in dialysis patients and these are thought to be the result of inhibition of the enzyme activity by a 'uraemic toxin' (Chimata *et al.* 1994).

Alanine aminotransferase

Serum ALT activity is increased by drugs that affect the liver (see section on AST above). It is low in patients taking vigabatrin and this is thought to be due to the drug binding to the enzyme and reducing its activity (Ryan *et al.* 1996; Richens *et al.* 1997). Unfiltered coffee beans elevate serum ALT and this is due to the effect of the coffee diterpenes cafestol and kahweol (Urgert *et al.* 1997).

Alkaline phosphatase

Alkaline phosphatase (ALP, E.C. 3.1.3.1) refers to a group of non-specific phosphomonoesterases that hydrolyse phosphate monoesters and are ubiquitous and found attached to plasma membranes. The natural substrate and the specific function of ALP are not known. The ALP are glycoproteins and there are at least four genes that code for the main groups of ALP isoenzymes: the intestinal, placental, placental-like, and hepatic/renal/bone (or tissue-non-specific) isoenzyme groups. Of the four groups, the hepatic/renal/bone isoenzyme has received most attention in clinical practice. Changes in plasma ALP activity occur most frequently from hepatic or skeletal causes. A variety of methods, including immunoassays, are available for the identification and quantitation of the different isoenzymes (Swaminathan 1997).

Increase in serum ALP activity

In clinical practice, increases in serum ALP are most often seen in liver or bone disease.

Hepatic origin

The liver isoenzyme is located in the exterior surface of the bile canalicular membrane and serum ALP activity rises when the bile duct is obstructed. This forms the basis of its clinical usefulness. An increase in serum ALP activity is seen in many types of liver disease, including hepatitis, cholestasis, and space-occupying lesions. ALP values are usually higher in biliary tract obstruction than in hepatocellular lesions. A large number of drugs can cause elevation of serum ALP activity of hepatic origin (Young 1995). The mechanism of the increase is either a hepatocellular effect as with paracetamol, or cholestasis as with anabolic steroids (see Chapter 13).

Skeletal origin

Increase in osteoblastic activity will elevate serum ALP activity, as will drugs that cause metabolic bone disease, such as anticonvulsants (see section on Bone disease and Chapter 18). An increase in ALP activiy was seen in patients treated with verapamil and this was associated with a slight rise in PTH concentration (Lim and MacDonald 1996).

An ALP isoenzyme with unusual mobility found in a patient who had taken an overdose of colchicine was identified as being of renal origin (Rosalki *et al.* 1989).

Decrease in serum ALP activity

A decrease in serum ALP activity has been reported with the use of bezafibrate, clofibrate, contraceptives and oestrogens (Young 1995), danazol, fluoride, stanozolol, and sulphonamides. The decrease in ALP activity seen after bezafibrate was 25 per cent and this was mainly the result of a reduction in the liver isoenzyme (Day *et al.* 1993).

Artefacts

Several drugs and compounds cause an apparent decrease in serum ALP activity by interference with analytical methods. These include cefotaxime, cystine, cysteine, detergents, EDTA, fluorides, ibuprofen, methotrexate, nitrofurantoin (Young 1995), oxalate, pindolol, theophylline, and zinc. It is important to note that not all methods of ALP determination are affected to the same extent by any particular interfering agent.

γ-Glutamyltransferase

γ-Glutamyltransferase (GGT, EC 2.3.2.2) is a membrane-bound enzyme found in cells that show high secretory or absorptive capacity, such as the epithelial cells lining the biliary tract, hepatic canaliculi, renal tubules, and intestinal brush borders. High activity is found in kidney, liver, pancreas, and intestine. Most of the GGT found in serum comes from liver.

Increase in serum GGT activity

Serum GGT is elevated in all types of hepatobiliary disease, including hepatocellular damage, cholestasis, and space-occupying lesions. Examples of drugs that elevate GGT by causing hepatocellular damage include paracetamol, captopril, halothane, enflurane, methyldopa, streptokinase, and G-M CSF (Gunther et al. 1992). Haloperidol, warfarin, sulindac, and phenothiazines are examples of drugs that elevate GGT by causing cholestasis (Young 1995).

Serum GGT activity is also elevated by drugs that cause induction of microsomal enzymes as a result of enhanced synthesis of GGT and release of membrane-bound GGT. Alcohol and anticonvulsant drugs are well known to cause elevation of serum GGT activity by this mechanism. Anticonvulsants elevate GGT in a variable proportion of patients (Braide and Davies 1987; Aldenhovel 1988) depending on the age and sex of the patient, the choice of drug, and the duration of treatment (Braide and Davies 1987). The serum GGT activity was higher in patients treated with phenytoin than in those given phenobarbitone; elevation occurred 6 months after starting treatment.

Bone cement used in joint replacement has been shown to cause elevation in serum GGT activity (Pople and Phillips 1988). Anabolic steroids cause a small but significant increase in GGT activity in healthy subjects (Alen 1985); oral contraceptives have a similar significant effect to an extent varying with the composition of the preparation (Calic et al. 1989). Heparin treatment caused an increase in GGT activity in some patients (Lambert et al. 1986).

Decrease in serum GGT activity

A decrease in GGT activity is reported with clofibrate (Ferrari et al. 1976) and bezafibrate (Day et al. 1993).

Artefacts

Cefotaxime and heparin cause an apparent reduction in GGT measured by some methods (Young 1995).

Amylase

Amylases (EC 3.2.1.1) are calcium-containing metalloenzymes that hydrolyse α-1,4-glycosidic bonds in glucose polymers such as starch, glycogen, and dextrin. The amylase molecule consists of a single peptide chain. Although pancreatic and salivary amylases are secretory enzymes, some amylase is found in the serum.

Increase in serum amylase

Drugs that cause spasm of the sphincter of Oddi, such as cholinergics and narcotics, may cause elevation of serum amylase (Young 1995), but the commonest cause of an elevated amylase is pancreatitis; the drugs most often associated with this disease are discussed in Chapter 12.

In smokers, basal serum amylase activity is double that in non-smokers (Dubick et al. 1987), and this is further increased after injection of secretin (but there is no increase in non-smokers). The plasma volume expander hydroxyethyl starch solution significantly increased serum amylase activity (Korttila et al. 1984). Hyperamylasaemia is frequently found in patients with AIDS. The increase in amylase is primarily salivary in type but pancreatitis may also occur. Hyperamylasaemia is associated with the use of pentamidine (Murthy et al. 1992), didanosine, and dideoxyinosine (Rathbun and Martin 1992; Brivet et al. 1994; Foo and Konecny 1997). Ritodrine or ephedrine treatment in pregnant women causes elevation of serum amylase in nearly 50 per cent of subjects and isoenzyme studies showed that the elevation is due to salivary amylase (Takahashi et al. 1997).

Decrease in serum amylase activity

During administration of 20% glucose and 8% amino acid solution, serum pancreatic isoamylase decreased and the decrease was proportional to the plasma glucose concentration (Skrha et al. 1986). Decreased serum amylase activity was also found with propylthiouracil and anabolic steroids (Tuzhilin et al. 1982). Chloroquine treatment caused a decrease in amylase activity (Ogonor 1993).

Cholinesterase

Serum cholinesterase (EC 3.1.1.7), or pseudocholinesterase, is synthesized by the liver and hydrolyses acetylcholine esters. It is a large mucoprotein and there are several variants (Evans 1986). Its function is still not fully understood.

Low cholinesterase activity may be genetically determined, or be secondary to liver disease, malnutrition, or recent infection (Sawhney and Lott 1986). Drugs can lower the activity of serum cholinesterase either by inhibiting the enzyme directly or by reducing the hepatic synthesis of the enzyme. Serum cholinesterase can be inhibited by a variety of chemicals, including many organophosphorus compounds, and carbamates, such as physostigmine and neostigmine (Sawhney and Lott 1986). Very low or undetectable serum cholinesterase activity is seen in severe poisoning with organophosphorus insecticides such as parathion (Sawhney and Lott 1986). Metriphonate, an organophosphorus compound used in the treatment and control of urinary schistosomiasis, causes a marked fall in serum cholinesterase activity. Workers in the insecticide industry also have low serum cholinesterase activity from chronic exposure to insecticides (Sawhney and Lott 1986).

Low concentrations of serum cholinesterase are seen after paracetamol poisoning and after treatment with streptokinase, colaspase, and oestrogens, (Calic et al. 1989), anabolic steroids (Barbosa et al. 1971) and danazol. Other drugs that have been reported to cause reversible inhibition of serum cholinesterase include antimalarial drugs, barbiturates, caffeine, chlorpromazine and other phenothiazines, cyclophosphamide (Zsigmund and Robins 1972), ether, folic acid, iodipamide, quinine, quinidine, metriphonate, theophylline, sulphonamides, and vitamin K (Sawhney and Lott 1986; Young 1995). Irreversible inhibition of the enzyme is seen with alkyl fluorophosphates.

Acid phosphatase

Acid phosphatase (ACP, EC 3.1.3.2) refers to a group of non-specific phosphatases that show maximal activity near pH 5.0. It exists in multimolecular form and is distributed widely in the body. Highest ACP activity is found in the prostate.

Increase in serum ACP activity

Administration of androgens to females increases serum ACP activity. In patients with prostatic carcinoma treated with the GnRH analogue buserelin there was an initial increase in ACP activity associated with an increase in testosterone, followed by a fall of both ACP activity and testosterone concentration (Huhtaniemi et al. 1985). Clofibrate has been reported to increase ACP activity (Young 1995). Digital examination of the prostate leads to an elevation of serum ACP activity during the ensuing 24 hours (Pearson et al. 1983).

Decrease in serum ACP activity

Fluoride is said to decrease serum ACP activity (Young 1995). Treatment of prostatic carcinoma with oestrogen will reduce the raised ACP concentrations (Grayhack 1984; Maatman et al. 1984). Treatment with a GnRH analogue for 2–3 weeks reduced the raised ACP concentrations seen in patients with prostatic carcinoma (Huhtaniemi et al. 1985). Ketoconazole, an oral antimycotic agent with potent inhibitory effects on adrenal and gonadal steroid synthesis, has been used successfully in the treatment of prostatic carcinoma, with reduction in serum ACP activity (Sonino 1987).

Artefacts

Haemolysis can increase, and inappropriate storage of samples can decrease, the serum ACP activity. Fluoride, oxalate, copper, alcohol, and detergent decrease, and in certain immunoassay procedures sodium azide falsely elevates, ACP activity (Young 1995).

Angiotensin-converting enzyme

Angiotensin-converting enzyme (ACE, EC 3.4.15.1) converts angiotensin I to angiotensin II by cleavage of a dipeptide. It also inactivates bradykinins.

Increase in serum ACE activity

Administration of tri-iodothyronine has been observed to increase serum ACE activity (Graninger et al. 1986).

Decrease in serum ACE activity

Decrease in serum ACE activity is seen with the use of ACE inhibitors such as captopril (Kamoun et al. 1982), enalapril (Jackson and Johnston 1984), ramipril (Crozier et al. 1987), and perindopril (Bussien et al. 1986). Captopril acts more rapidly (within 30 minutes) than does enalapril (1–4 hours). The inhibitory effect of captopril is markedly reduced with storage of the serum and, furthermore, it is reversed by dilution of the sample or following dialysis. Enalapril, on the other hand, does not lose its inhibitory effect during storage or dilution (Lieberman 1989). Administration of magnesium sulphate in the treatment of hypertension of pregnancy decreased serum ACE (Fuentes and Goldkrand 1987). Prednisone reduced serum ACE activity in those who had an elevated value initially (Romer and Jacobsen 1982).

Artefacts

Freezing and thawing of serum increases ACE activity by

15 per cent. Uric acid at high concentrations can increase activity; EDTA, hydroxyquinoline, methylprednisolone, and phenanthroline can decrease activity of ACE measured by some methods (Young 1995).

Vitamins

Water-soluble vitamins

The vitamin B complex

Vitamin B₁ (thiamine)

Thiamine, in its co-enzyme form thiamine pyrophosphate (TPP), is essential for decarboxylation and transketolase reactions. Thiamine deficiency leads to neurological effects — peripheral neuropathy (dry beriberi), encephalopathy (cerebral beriberi) — or heart failure (wet beriberi). Thiamine deficiency can be detected by the *in vitro* activation of erythrocyte transketolase by thiamine pyrophosphate, or by direct measurement of thiamine levels by microbiological, enzymatic, or chromatographic methods (McCormick and Green 1994).

Biochemical and clinical evidence of thiamine deficiency is commonly found in alcoholics (Wood *et al.* 1992; Joyce 1994; Kril 1996). The thiamine deficiency is due to a combination of poor intake, increased metabolic demands from alcohol consumption, and decreased intestinal absorption (Thomson and Majmuder 1981; Holzbach 1996). Furthermore, the folate deficiency and the general malnutrition seen in alcoholics may further aggravate the malabsorption of thiamine (Kril 1996).

Increased demands due to prolonged intravenous feeding with high-carbohydrate fluids can also lead to thiamine deficiency (Schiano *et al.* 1996; Nakasaki *et al.* 1997). A case of acute beriberi following liver transplantation has been reported (Cohen *et al.* 1997). A syndrome resembling the Wernicke–Korsakoff syndrome has been described in patients with colorectal carcinoma treated with high doses of the antitumour drugs doxifluridine and fluorouracil (Heier and Fossa 1986).

Long-term frusemide therapy in patients with congestive heart failure is associated with thiamine deficiency due to increased urinary loss (Seligmann *et al.* 1991) and this may contribute to impaired cardiac function. Thiamine supplementation could prevent this (Shimon *et al.* 1995). Evidence of thiamine deficiency — assessed by the *in vitro* effect of TPP on erythrocyte transketolase — was found in 90 per cent of these patients (Seligmann *et al.* 1991). Recent studies suggest that dietary deficiency may contribute to this (Brady *et al.* 1995).

Thiamine deficiency and Wernicke's encephalopathy are common in patients with AIDS (Butterworth *et al.* 1991; Baum *et al.* 1995; Davtyan and Vinters 1987). This is not related to treatment with zidovudine. A diabetic patient treated with tolazamide developed Wernicke's encephalopathy, and fibroblasts from these patients had abnormal transketolase (as shown by a high K_m for TPP) (Mukherjee *et al.* 1986). Wernicke's encephalopathy has also been described following lithium-induced diarrhoea (Epstein 1989), and after high doses of nitroglycerin (Shorey *et al.* 1984), possibly because of the high alcohol content of liquid formulations. Sulphates, which are added to some infusion solutions to prevent non-enzymic browning and decomposition during sterilization, have been suspected of causing destruction of thiamine which may have clinical consequences (Bassler and Heidenreich 1984). Thiamine status was reported not to be affected by long-term anticonvulsant treatment (Krause *et al.* 1988). However, low concentrations of thiamine have been reported in the cerebrospinal fluid of those on phenytoin treatment (Botez and Young 1991). Thiamine concentrations were also low in asthmatic children treated with theophylline (Shimizu *et al.* 1996).

Vitamin B₂ (riboflavine)

Riboflavine in the form of flavine nucleotides is required for the electron transport system, and deficiency causes rough scaly skin, angular stomatitis, cheilosis, glossitis, and stomatitis. Riboflavine deficiency can be detected by the measurement of erythrocyte glutathione reductase and its activation by *in vitro* addition of flavine adenine dinucleotide (FAD).

Many drugs such as chlorpromazine, imipramine, amitriptyline, and doxorubicin have been shown to cause riboflavine deficiency or depletion under experimental conditions (Pinto *et al.* 1981), but neither clinical or biochemical riboflavine deficiency has been demonstrated with these drugs. Biochemical evidence of riboflavine deficiency as shown by low erythrocyte glutathione reductase and increased *in vitro* activation by FAD may be found in 69 per cent of alcoholics (Wood *et al.* 1992). Reduced intake, reduced absorption, and increased requirement contribute to the deficiency. Oral contraceptive users have biochemical evidence of riboflavine deficiency (Sanpitak and Chayutimonkul 1974; Tyrer 1984). This could be important in areas of the world where riboflavine deficiency is common, due to poor nutrition. In a study in Thailand, however, riboflavine was found not to be affected by the use of oral contraceptives (Amatayakul *et al.* 1984). Riboflavine deficiency has been reported in up to 30–40 per cent of patients on long-term anticonvulsant therapy (Krause *et al.* 1988). The deficiency disappeared when the diet was changed, in spite of continued drug therapy. Thus the deficiency is probably a direct effect of poor nutrition rather than of the anticonvulsants.

Nicotinic acid

Nicotinamide, formed from nicotinic acid, is the active constituent of important co-factors (NAD and NADP) in oxidation–reduction reactions. Nicotinic acid deficiency leads to the syndrome of pellagra, which comprises dermatitis, diarrhoea, and dementia. Nicotinic acid status is assessed by the measurement of 24-hour excretion of the metabolites $N(1)$-methylnicotinamide and $N(1)$-methyl-3-carboxamide-6-pyridone or by measurement of fasting plasma tryptophan and other amino acids (McCormick and Greene 1994).

Nicotinic acid deficiency with pellagra-like features has been described in patients with tuberculosis undergoing treatment with isoniazid (Meyrick *et al.* 1981); the symptoms disappeared after treatment with nicotinic acid and pyridoxine. Isoniazid is a pyridoxine antagonist (see below) and pyridoxine is necessary for the synthesis of nicotinic acid from tryptophan. The extent of nicotinic acid deficiency in isoniazid treatment is illustrated by the finding of eight cases of pellagra in postmortem examinations of 106 tuberculosis patients (Ishii and Nishihara 1985). Pellagroid erythema caused by isoniazid has been reported (Schmutz *et al.* 1987). Sodium valproate (Gillman and Sandyk 1984), glibenclamide (Berova and Lazarova 1988), 5-fluorouracil (Stevens *et al.* 1993), and abuse of the analgesic morazone (Kingreen and Breger 1984), have all been reported to cause nicotinic acid deficiency. Pellagra-like encephalopathy following treatment of *Mycobacterium avium intracellulare* with several drugs has been reported (Brooks-Hill *et al.* 1985). A patient receiving long-term anticonvulsant treatment had pellagra which responded to vitamin therapy (Hebestreit *et al.* 1990). Pellagra has also been described in alcoholics (Vannucchi *et al.* 1991).

Vitamin B_6 (pyridoxine)

The vitamin pyridoxine exists in three forms, pyridoxal, pyridoxine, and pyridoxamine, which are converted to the active phosphate form. This vitamin is a co-factor for the transaminases and for decarboxylation of amino acids. Deficiency of pyridoxine leads to roughness of the skin, peripheral neuropathy, and sore tongue. Pyridoxine status can be assessed by the excretion of xanthuric acid after a tryptophan load or by the measurement of erythrocyte aspartate aminotransferase and its activation by pyridoxal phosphate. It can also be assessed by direct measurement of pyridoxine phosphate by an en-

zymatic or chromatographic method (McCormack and Greene 1994).

Isoniazid is an antagonist of pyridoxine that forms hydrazones with pyridoxal and pyridoxal phosphate, which are lost in the urine. These compounds inhibit pyridoxal kinase and pyridoxal phosphate-dependent enzymes (McCormick and Greene 1994). Measurement of erythrocyte aspartate aminotransferase activity showed evidence of pyridoxine deficiency in patients receiving isoniazid (Pellock *et al.* 1985). The incidence was dose related, and prophylactic pyridoxine was recommended. Hydralazine and phenelzine have been shown to reduce pyridoxine concentrations in experimental animals. Pyridoxine deficiency and peripheral neuropathy associated with phenelzine therapy have been described (Demers *et al.* 1984).

A number of studies have demonstrated abnormalities of tryptophan metabolism (as shown by the tryptophan load test) in women receiving oestrogens as oral contraceptives or menopausal hormone replacement therapy (Tyrer 1984; Amatayakul 1994), but others have found no difference in vitamin B_6 status between users and non-users of oral contraceptives (Brown *et al.* 1975). Some studies have shown that the tryptophan load test used in many studies may not be a valid index of pyridoxine status, as the oestrogen conjugates inhibit kynureninase independently of the pyridoxine status, thereby causing an abnormal result (Bender 1983). Using the erythrocyte aspartate aminotransferase activation index, however, and serum pyridoxal phosphate concentration, evidence of pyridoxine deficiency has been found in women taking oral contraceptives (Salih *et al.* 1986; Steegers Theunissen *et al.* 1992). The evidence for pyridoxine deficiency in oral contraceptive users may only be found in some groups, especially those who have marginal dietary deficiency to start with. Although oral contraceptives have been suggested to increase the metabolism of tryptophan through the nicotinic acid pathway, leading to an increase in the requirement of pyridoxine, it has not been possible to demonstrate an increase in the activity of tryptophan oxygenase (Bender 1983).

L-Penicillamine strongly inhibits pyridoxal-dependent enzymes and causes pyridoxine deficiency in animal studies. Although D-penicillamine is less active in this respect, polyneuropathy associated with D-penicillamine treatment has been described (Pedersen and Hogenhaven 1990).

Serum pyridoxal and pyridoxal phosphate concentrations were lower after dopamine (Weir *et al.* 1991) and theophylline (Hall *et al.* 1985; Reynolds and Natta 1985; Delport *et al.* 1988; Shimizu *et al.* 1996). Administration of theophylline to volunteers was shown to cause a reduction in plasma and erythrocyte pyridoxal phosphate concentrations. The decrease in pyridoxal phosphate was correlated with plasma theophylline concentrations (Ubbink *et al.* 1990). Long-term theophylline therapy is associated with deficiency of vitamin B_6 and may contribute to the toxicity of theophylline (Ubbink *et al.* 1989).

Vitamin B_6 status in patients taking anticonvulsants is poor, as shown by lower pyridoxal phosphate concentrations and higher activation of erythrocyte AST in epileptics. The plasma concentration of pyridoxal phosphate correlated with the dose and duration of treatment (Krause *et al.* 1988). Deficiency of pyridoxine can be demonstrated in nearly 25 per cent of alcoholics (Wood *et al.* 1992).

Vitamin B_{12}

A number of drugs are known to affect the absorption and utilization of vitamin B_{12} in man (Gluske 1995; Markle 1996). Malabsorption may be induced by colchicine, cholestyramine, ethanol, sodium aminosalicylate, metformin and phenformin, and trifluoperazine, (Lee 1993a). The malabsorption of vitamin B_{12} seen with cholestyramine is thought to be due to binding to intrinsic factor and interference with the formation of intrinsic factor–B_{12} complex. A similar mechanism has been proposed for neomycin. Colchicine interferes with absorption of vitamin B_{12} by altering the function of the ileal mucosa (Webb *et al.* 1968). In the case of sodium aminosalicylate, there is malabsorption of B_{12}, especially in subjects who have been treated with it for more than 6 weeks. The drug does not interfere with intrinsic factor, but probably acts by inhibiting some folate-dependent enzyme system in the gut. The absorptive defect disappears 2 weeks after stopping the drug (Lee 1993a).

Methotrexate treatment of rheumatoid arthritis and psoriasis caused a significant decrease in red cell B_{12} concentration (Leeb *et al.* 1995).

The biguanides metformin and phenformin cause malabsorption of vitamin B_{12} (Tomkin 1973), as shown by an abnormal Schilling test, and the malabsorption does not improve with addition of intrinsic factor; it is reversible within 2–8 weeks of stopping treatment. Megaloblastic anaemia has been reported to result from long-term treatment with metformin (Callaghan *et al.* 1980).

Malabsorption of B_{12} has been reported with methyldopa and allopurinol (Chen *et al.* 1982).

Ascorbic acid in high doses was associated with low serum B_{12} concentrations (Herbert *et al.* 1978), which were thought to be due to the destruction of B_{12} by the ascorbate (Herbert 1981), but this has not been confirmed (Rivers 1987). It is likely that only some forms of cobalamins not found in food are destroyed by ascorbic acid (Hogenkamp 1980).

Serum vitamin B_{12} concentrations were found to be significantly lowered in women taking oral contraceptives (Tyrer *et al.* 1984; Hjelt *et al.* 1985; Brattstrom *et al.* 1992). In postmenopausal women hormone replacement therapy had no effect on vitamin B_{12} status (Carmel *et al.* 1996).

Cimetidine, ranitidine, and omeprazole, and similar drugs, suppress intrinsic factor secretion and impair the absorpfion of B_{12} (Carmel 1995). Long-term treatment with omeprazole causes a decrease in B_{12} stores (Koop 1992) and a case of megaloblastic anaemia probably due to malabsorption of cobalamin has been reported (Bellou *et al.* 1996). Malabsorption of B_{12} has also been reported after use of the proprietary antacid Gelusil (Carmel 1995).

Malabsorption of B_{12} due to interference with binding of the intrinsic factor–B_{12} complex to the intestine can be demonstrated in up to 50 per cent of alcoholics, in the majority of alcoholics serum concentrations are normal probably due to the presence of liver damage, and frank B_{12} deficiency is relatively uncommon in alcoholics (Wood *et al.* 1992).

The high incidence of megaloblastic change seen in patients receiving nitrous oxide has been thought to be due to an acute B_{12} deficiency (Amess *et al.* 1978; Raeder 1996). This can be prevented by methionine and folinic acid (Weir and Scott 1995). Nitrous oxide inactivates the cobalamin-dependent enzyme methionine synthase (Weir and Scott 1995). Patients with subclinical cobalamin deficiency developed neuropathic symptoms on exposure to nitrous oxide anaesthesia (Kinsella and Green 1995). Prolonged anaesthesia with nitrous oxide in the presence of sepsis aggravates the effect on B_{12} (van Achterbergh *et al.* 1990). Exposure to nitrous oxide may cause B_{12} deficiency in bone marrow cells harvested for transplantation (Carmel *et al.* 1993).

Folate

Folate co-enzymes are essential for the transfer of single carbon units and one of the important examples of this is the synthesis of DNA. Drugs may cause folate deficiency in a number of different ways. They may interfere with the absorption of the vitamin by inhibiting the intestinal conjugase enzyme which reduces dietary polyglutamate to the monoglutamate form before absorption. Drugs such as methotrexate may inhibit the enzyme dihydrofolate reductase which catalyses the conversion of dihydrofolate to tetrahydrofolate, which is a co-factor necessary for the synthesis of DNA. Drugs which cause

B_{12} deficiency will affect the demethylation of methylfolate. Those which induce pyridoxine deficiency can also act on folate metabolism, as pyridoxine is involved in the demethylation of methylfolate (Lee 1993b).

Triamterene blocks dihydrofolate reductase and may cause folate deficiency and megaloblastic anaemia, especially in those with hepatic cirrhosis, in whom the clearance of the drug is reduced (McInnes 1996).

Co-trimoxazole is an effective antibacterial agent. The sulphonamide moiety blocks the utilization of p-aminobenzoic acid and thereby the synthesis of folate, while the trimethoprim acts as a spurious substrate for bacterial dihydrofolate reductase, preventing the reduction of any folate that may be formed. Treatment with co-trimoxazole might therefore be expected to cause folate deficiency, but in early studies no evidence of folate deficiency was found with conventional assays, though marginal deficiency was found using a sensitive deoxyuridine suppression test. Furthermore, several case reports of folate deficiency and megaloblastic anaemia have appeared in the literature (Chan et al. 1980). Considering the widespread use of co-trimoxazole, the incidence of folate deficiency is very low and folate status of some of those developing deficiency may have already been low before treatment (Lee 1993b). Another sulphonamide, sulphasalazine, has been reported to cause a decrease in red cell folate concentration (Longstretch and Green 1983) and macrocytic anaemia (Grieco et al. 1986; Prouse et al. 1987) and, using plasma total homocysteine as a sensitive marker of folate status, evidence of folate deficiency was found in rheumatoid arthritis patients taking it (Krogh Jensen et al. 1996). Supplementation with folinic acid to prevent folate deficiency has been recommended (Pironi et al. 1988). Megaloblastic anaemia may develop in patients treated with the antimalarial pyrimethamine.

Methotrexate (4-amino-10-methyl pteroylglutamic acid), which binds to dihydrofolate reductase, has been associated with megaloblastic anaemia and reduced red cell folate concentration (Hendel and Nyfords 1985; Reynolds 1996). Even with low-dose methotrexate therapy, fasting plasma homocysteine concentration, which is used as a sensitive indicator of antifolate status, was abnormal in patients with psoriasis (Refsum et al. 1989). Serum folate concentrations were found to be lower in patients with rheumatoid arthritis treated with low-dose methotrexate, and serum folate correlated with methotrexate concentrations (Leeb et al. 1995).

The association between anticonvulsant therapy and reduced concentration of serum and red cell folate is well recognized (Lee 1993b), and megaloblastic anaemia is seen in about 1 per cent of patients taking phenytoin, primidone, phenobarbitone, or a combination of these drugs (Rivey et al. 1984; O. Shalev et al. 1987; Lee 1993b). However, serum folate is reduced in a greater proportion of patients. Low red cell folate concentrations were found in 17 per cent of those taking carbamazepine, 13 per cent of those taking phenytoin, and 22 per cent of those taking more than one drug. The serum folate concentration was negatively correlated with the plasma phenytoin concentration (Goggin et al. 1987; Krause et al. 1988). Decreased serum folate concentrations during phenytoin therapy could be prevented by folate supplementation (Berg et al. 1995), which could also help to achieve better control of seizures (Lewis et al. 1995).

The effect of anticonvulsants on folate status is not fully understood. It may partly be due to reduced absorption of folate as a result of changes in pH in the gut induced by anticonvulsants. This may be responsible for decreased folate uptake either by direct inhibition of transport or indirectly by inhibiting folate conjugase activity. In animals, phenytoin given as the sodium salt had a greater effect on folate content of liver and brain than the free acid (Carl and Smith 1992). There is evidence, however, that anticonvulsants increase the metabolism of folate. Furthermore, phenytoin may have a direct effect on DNA synthesis, thereby contributing to the megaloblastic anaemia (Lee 1993b). Serum folate was lowered in those taking anticonvulsants that are enzyme inducers, such as phenobarbitone and carbamazepine, but not with those that are not, such as sodium valproate or zonisanide, suggesting that enzyme induction is an important reason for low folate concentrations (Kishi et al. 1997). Serum and red cell folate concentrations are not affected by lamotrigine (Sander and Patsalos 1992).

Serum and red cell folate concentrations are low in oral contraceptive users (Tyrer 1984; Steegers Theunissen et al. 1992; Harper et al. 1994), although overt folate deficiency is uncommon. Evidence of suboptimal folate status is further shown by higher plasma homocysteine concentration in the fasting state and after a methionine load. Similar findings were seen in men with prostatic carcinoma treated with oestrogens (Brattstrom et al. 1992). There is also concern that the low folate concentrations may predispose oral contraceptive users to cervical dysplasia and possibly malignancy (Butterworth et al. 1992). One possible mechanism of low folate concentration in oral contraceptive users is the increased metabolism of folate (Steegers Theunissen et al. 1993).

Folate deficiency, as shown by serum folate and plasma homocysteine concentrations, may be seen in a large proportion of alcoholics (Wood et al. 1992; Cravo *et al.* 1996). Factors contributing to this deficiency are poor diet, reduced absorption, decreased body stores due to liver damage, reduced enterohepatic circulation, an antagonistic effect of alcohol on the haemopoietic effects of folic acid and impaired ability to conserve 5-methyl tetrahydrofolate (Muldoon and McMartin 1994).

Acute folate deficiency has also been found in patients in an intensive care unit receiving intravenous nutrition (Tennant *et al.* 1981); this may have been due to the amino acid composition of the fluids used, as certain amino acids such as methionine may cause a decrease in serum folate.

Nitrous oxide was reported to cause folate deficiency 3 days after its use in anaesthesia, as shown by the deoxy-uridine suppression test (Amos *et al.* 1985). Urinary excretion of formic acid and formiminoglutamic acid are increased (Koblin *et al.* 1990). Other drugs associated with folate deficiency are allopurinol, cholestyramine, cycloserine, and methyldopa.

Although triamterene reduces absorption of folate in animals, serum folate concentrations in patients treated with triamterene are normal (Mason *et al.* 1991).

Latent folate deficiency may become clinically manifest during iron therapy because of the additional demand for this vitamin secondary to increased erythropoiesis (Scott 1963).

Red cell folate increased after zidovudine (Baum *et al.* 1991).

Ascorbic acid (vitamin C)

Ascorbic acid is essential for man but its function is not fully understood. Vitamin C is involved in hormone and neurotransmitter synthesis, is required for collagen synthesis, and acts as an antioxidant. Deficiency of ascorbate causes scurvy, but this is now rare. Low levels of ascorbate, however, may be harmful in other ways, such as affording poor protection against free radicals. Ascorbate status is assessed by the measurement of ascorbate concentration in plasma or leucocytes by a chemical method or by chromatography. There is still controversy, however, as to whether plasma, platelet, or leucocyte ascorbate gives the best assessment of vitamin C status (McCormick and Greene 1994).

Reduced concentrations of ascorbate have been observed in the plasma, leucocytes, platelets, and urine of users of oral contraceptives when compared with concentrations in non-users (Tyrer 1984). Possible explanations for the reduced concentrations include the stimulation by oral contraceptives of caeruloplasmin (which has ascorbate oxidase activity), decreased absorption, changes in tissue distribution, increased

excretion, and reduced concentrations of reducing compounds such as reduced glutathione (Tyrer 1984).

Low concentrations of ascorbate in leucocytes, to which reduced intake and malabsorption contribute, have been found in alcoholics (Wood *et al.* 1992), and low concentrations of ascorbate have been reported with the use of corticosteroids, cholestyramine, indomethacin, and tetracycline. Smokers have a lower intake of vitamin C and lower serum ascorbate concentrations than non-smokers, and even after adjustment for intake their serum concentrations are lower than those of non-smokers, suggesting an increased requirement. Deficiency of vitamin C, and of other vitamins, was reported in patients on long-term anticonvulsant therapy, though Krause and others (1988) found normal vitamin C concentrations in male patients and low concentrations that could not be attributed to drug treatment in female patients taking these drugs. Low vitamin C concentrations and increased urinary excretion were observed in women taking oral contraceptives. Decreased serum ascorbic acid concentration has been reported in vitamin A toxicity (Helsing 1996).

The relationship between intake of vitamin C and the plasma concentration of vitamin C is sigmoidal and, when large amounts of vitamin C are taken, high plasma concentrations are seen. 'Megadoses' of vitamin C are sometimes taken, as it has been suggested that vitamin C is effective in the treatment or prevention of a wide range of conditions including the common cold. A high intake of ascorbate can lead to increased excretion of urinary oxalate (Schmidt *et al.* 1981; Rivers 1987) and it increases the requirement for some vitamins such as vitamin E (Chen 1981). People who are susceptible to iron overload may be adversely affected by excess vitamin C (Rivers 1987). Recent evidence has failed to confirm the suggestion that vitamin C may cause destruction of vitamin B_{12} in food, or that vitamin C affects plasma uric acid concentrations (Rivers 1987).

Fat-soluble vitamins

Vitamin A

Vitamin A plays an important role in vision, stabilization of cellular and intracellular membranes, maintenance of the integrity of epithelial tissue, synthesis of glycoproteins, and spermatogenesis. Deficiency of vitamin A can lead to failure of normal growth, poor dark adaptation, keratomalacia, xerophthalmia, and follicular hyperkeratosis of the skin. Vitamin A has also been linked with cancer (Willett and Hunter 1994) and with immunity. There are three main forms of the vitamin: retinol, retinal, and retinoic acid. Each has a characteristic action on individual target organs. Vitamin A status is usually assessed by measurement of plasma retinol concentrations, although these only decrease when liver stores are depleted and increase when these are saturated. Vitamin A content of liver gives the best estimate of vitamin A status.

Malabsorption of vitamin A can occur whenever there is drug-induced malabsorption, such as that seen with cholestyramine, neomycin, and allopurinol. Low serum vitamin A and carotene concentrations and symptoms of vitamin A deficiency associated with steatorrhoea have been reported with the use of methyltestosterone. The symptoms and biochemical abnormalities reversed within 9 months of discontinuing the drug. Alcoholics may have lowered plasma retinol concentrations (Russell 1980). It must be pointed out, however, that an apparently low plasma retinol may result from changes in RBP, which is the specific transport protein of retinol. Plasma vitamin A concentrations may also be high in alcoholics, owing to hepatocellular damage. In a large series of patients receiving anticonvulsant therapy, significantly subnormal vitamin A concentrations were reported (Krause et al. 1988), but the concentrations did not correlate with variables in the anticonvulsant therapy and none of the patients had very low concentrations.

In women taking oral contraceptives, plasma concentrations of vitamin A are 30–80 per cent higher than in controls (Amatayakul et al. 1984, 1994; Tyrer 1984). The increased plasma concentration is due to an increase in RBP, and the concentrations of free vitamin A are unchanged, but hepatic stores may be depleted. Hypervitaminosis A can occur if there is excessive nutritional or therapeutic intake of the vitamin.

Vitamin D

Most of the vitamin D_3 (cholecalciferol) present in the body is formed in the skin by the action of ultraviolet light. Vitamin D_3 is transported in the plasma bound to a specific carrier protein and metabolised to its active form, 1,25-dihydroxycholecalciferol (1,25-DHCC) (Feldman et al. 1996). Deficiency of vitamin D leads to osteomalacia and rickets. Marginal vitamin D deficiency may increase the risk of osteoporosis (Heaney 1996). Vitamin D status is usually assessed by the measurement of its major circulating form, plasma 25-hydroxyvitamin D (25-OHD). Drugs may induce vitamin D deficiency by causing malabsorption or by interfering with its metabolism.

Drug-induced malabsorption (see Chapter 12) will lead to deficiency of vitamin D and of other fat-soluble vitamins. Neomycin and cholestyramine cause malab-

sorption by binding bile salts in the intestinal lumen. Low plasma 25-OHD has been reported in alcoholics, probably due to a combination of malabsorption, poor intake, reduced exposure to sunlight, and reduced storage. As a significant amount of the daily requirement of vitamin D comes from *in vivo* synthesis by the effect of sunlight, use of sunscreen agents may reduce vitamin D concentrations. Matsuoka and colleagues (1988) observed that in chronic users of the sunscreen agent *p*-aminobenzoic acid, plasma 25-OHD concentrations were lower than in normal subjects, and in one subject the concentration was in the deficiency range. Sunscreen cream completely blocks the vitamin D response to UV light (Matsuoka et al. 1990). In places where there is plenty of sunlight, however, such as Australia, regular use of sunscreen cream did not influence serum 25-OHD concentration, as sufficient UV radiation reaches the skin, creams notwithstanding (Marks et al. 1995).

Chronic anticonvulsant therapy is associated with a range of bone disease. Earlier reports showed that the predominant feature was osteomalacia or rickets with low serum calcium and phosphate concentrations (Shane 1996). However, recent studies have shown that anticonvulsant-induced bone disease is a high-bone-turnover state (see section on Bone Disease). Many of the anticonvulsants stimulate hepatic mixed-function oxidase activity (Jubiz et al. 1970). Metabolism of vitamin D and 25-OHD is increased two to threefold, and inactive metabolites of vitamin D appear in the urine and bile during anticonvulsant treatment (Hahn et al. 1972a). As a result, serum concentrations of 25-OHD have been reported to be low in patients taking anticonvulsants (Hahn et al. 1972b; Stamp et al. 1972) and this could result in secondary hyperparathyroidism. More recent studies, however, have shown conflicting results, some workers finding no differences from controls (Wark et al. 1979; Weinstein et al. 1984), while others again found the concentrations to be lowered (Valimaki et al. 1994). The discrepancy has been suggested to be due to geographic differences in the study populations. Thus, studies in which low serum 25-OHD concentrations were found were from more northern, less sunny, latitudes (Hahn 1993; Valimaki et al. 1994). This lack of vitamin D may contribute to the development of anticonvulsant bone disease in patients who are from Northern climates or who are institutionalized with little exposure to sunlight (Shane 1996).

Rifampicin has also been reported to accelerate the rate of degradation of vitamin D and its metabolites (Brodie et al. 1982).

Diphosphonate, clodronate, and etidronate cause a picture similar to that of osteomalacia, but this is due to the direct effect of the drugs on bone rather than to an effect on vitamin D metabolism.

Increased concentrations of vitamin D or its metabolites will occur when the intake of either is excessive (see Hypercalcaemia). Toxic effects include hypercalcaemia, renal impairment, mental change, and ectopic calcification. The commonest cause of increased intake of vitamin D or its metabolites is over-treatment. Vitamin D intoxication due to high concentrations in cooking oil has been reported (Down *et al.* 1979).

Treatment

Treatment of hypovitaminosis D is by supplementation with vitamin D or its analogues and, if practicable, withdrawal of the offending drug. Treatment of hypervitaminosis consists of withdrawal of the offending drug and treatment of the hypercalcaemia (see Hypercalcaemia).

Vitamin E

Vitamin E plays an important role in maintaining the integrity of plasma membranes and is an antioxidant, preventing lipid peroxidation and modulating the metabolism of the arachidonic acid cascade. It has been thought to play a role in the prevention of free-radical damage in many diseases, including cancer, arthritis, cataract and cardiovascular disease. Vitamin E status is usually assessed by the measurement of plasma vitamin E concentrations, but it is now recognized that these fluctuate in relation to plasma lipids, and vitamin E is best expressed as a ratio in relation to total lipids. Vitamin E status can also be assessed by red cell vitamin E concentrations and on the basis of peroxidizability of red cell ghosts and lipoprotein fractions exposed to oxidant stress. Features of vitamin E deficiency include haemolytic anaemia, increased erythrocyte fragility, and creatinuria. Vitamin E deficiency has also been associated with many other clinical entities (McCormick and Greene 1994).

Low vitamin E concentrations are found in malabsorption induced by drugs such as cholestyramine. Levels are normal in smokers, although erythrocytes from smokers have a greater tendency to peroxidization. Plasma α-tocopherol (the predominant form of vitamin E in plasma) has been reported to be reduced in patients taking anticonvulsant drugs (Kataoka *et al.* 1990). Reduced vitamin E concentrations were reported in children receiving anticonvulsant treatment, but in another study of over 500 epileptics the results were inconsistent (Krause *et al.* 1988). Experimental studies have shown a significant reduction in plasma α-tocopherol, as a result of contraceptives, but Tyrer (1984) found no association

between plasma concentrations and the use of oral contraceptives.

Plasma α-tocopherol concentrations fell during treatment with simvastatin but the ratio of α-tocopherol to cholesterol increased, suggesting that the decrease in vitman E concentration was due to reduction in cholesterol (Human *et al.* 1997).

Vitamin E is used commonly in paediatric practice and possible toxic effects associated with high plasma concentrations have been reported. These include inhibition of wound healing, fibrinolysis, platelet aggregation, a reduction in vitamin K-dependent coagulation, necrotizing enterocolitis, and sepsis. Intravenous use of tocopherol was associated with several deaths and with hepatic, renal, and haemopoietic toxicity. The exact cause of the toxicity is not known, but it has been suggested to be due to a contaminant. In the newborn, potentially toxic concentrations of vitamin E can arise with oral preparations owing to variations in intestinal absorption.

Vitamin K

Vitamin K is necessary for the hepatic synthesis of several plasma clotting factors, prothrombin (factor II), VII, IX, and X, and proteins C and S. It is present in two forms, K_1 (phylloquinone) and K_2 (menaquinone). K_1 comes from plants; K_2 is synthesized by bacterial flora in the colon and absorbed from there. Vitamin K is required for the γ-carboxylation of the glutamic acid residues of prothrombin and other proteins. The protein osteocalcin in bone is a vitamin K-dependent γ-carboxyglutamyl (Gla) protein and it may serve a regulatory function in mineralization. Vitamin K deficiency leads to a bleeding tendency, and vitamin K status is readily assessed indirectly by the measurement of prothrombin time. Other methods of assessing vitamin K status include a chromatographic method for measuring vitamin K concentration and an immunoassay (McCormick and Green 1994) of a protein (PIVKA II, an undercarboxylated prothrombin precursor) induced by the absence of vitamin K.

Vitamin K deficiency can arise as a result of reduction in intake, absorption, or utilization (Lipsky 1992). As bacterial synthesis of vitamin K contributes significantly to the daily requirement, drugs that inhibit the bacterial flora, such as sulphonamides and broad-spectrum antibiotics, can reduce the vitamin K status, leading to prolongation of prothrombin time (McCormick and Green 1994). In patients receiving anticoagulant therapy, administration of penicillin may reduce the amount of vitamin K and may make it difficult to control anticoagulant therapy. Some of the cephalosporins not only depress vitamin K synthesis in the gut, but also directly impair clotting factor synthesis.

Malabsorption induced by drugs such as neomycin, cathartics, and cholestyramine will lead to deficiency (Bithell 1993a). In alcoholics, vitamin K deficiency is common, as demonstrated by a prolonged prothrombin time that is rapidly correctable by vitamin K supplementation, showing that it is due to reduced intake or malabsorption, or both. In severe alcoholic liver disease vitamin K supplementation cannot correct the abnormal prothrombin time as there is a decrease in hepatic synthesis of coagulation factors. Drugs that cause cholestasis will lead to reduced vitamin K absorption together with malabsorption of fat and other fat-soluble vitamins.

Drugs that cause destruction of hepatic parenchymal cells, such as paracetamol (see Chapter 13), will lead to reduced synthesis of vitamin K-dependent clotting factors, and a prolonged prothrombin time will result.

Large amounts of vitamins A and E are known to antagonize vitamin K. In experimental animals, a close relationship between dietary vitamin A (when it is high) and prothrombin concentration has been shown. As the effect was not seen when vitamin A was given parenterally, it was thought that vitamin A prevents the absorption of vitamin K. Prolongation of prothrombin time as a result of large doses of vitamin E has been reported. It is not fully clear whether vitamin E affects the intestinal absorption or the metabolism of vitamin K. It is likely that the effect of vitamin E is due to inhibition of vitamin K-dependent carboxylase activity by α-tocopherol quinone (Bithell 1993a).

In newborns the plasma concentrations of prothrombin and other vitamin K-dependent proteins may be less than half those in later life. This is due to poor transfer of vitamin K across the placenta, absence of synthesis of vitamin K in the gut, which is sterile during the first few days of life, and decreased synthesis of clotting factor precursors (Kisker et al. 1988). Administration of warfarin anticoagulants to the mother may result in severe deficiency of vitamin K-dependent clotting factors in the neonate. Infants born to mothers treated with anticonvulsants such as phenobarbitone, primidone, and phenytoin are more prone than normal to vitamin K deficiency, and potentially fatal neonatal bleeding is seen in about 10 per cent of cases. Anticonvulsants may also cause subclinical vitamin K deficiency in pregnant women, as shown by raised serum concentrations of PIVKA II.

The anticoagulants bishydroxycoumarin and ethylbiscoumacetate, when given to pregnant women, may cause stillbirths and neonatal haemorrhages.

Patients on long-term parenteral nutrition may develop deficiency of vitamin K if supplements are not given.

The coumarin group of drugs, of which warfarin is the most popular, impairs the synthesis of vitamin K-dependent clotting factors (Olson 1984; Hirsh 1991) by interfering with the enzymatic reduction of vitamin K oxide and oxidized vitamin K (Bithell 1993b). Surreptitious abuse of anticoagulants (Weitzel et al. 1990) is not infrequent among medical and paramedical personnel, and this will prolong prothrombin times. This can be detected by the accumulation of vitamin K-2,3-epoxide. Accidental exposure to warfarin-containing products such as rodenticides (Grieff et al. 1987) or contaminated talc (Martin-Bouyer et al. 1983) may also occur.

The dose–response to warfarin varies widely between individuals but to a lesser extent in a given indiviudal, reflecting wide variations in the metabolism of the drug. The dose requirement of a fast metaboliser may be 10 times higher than that of a slow metaboliser, and older patients require less (Redwood et al. 1991). Apart from covert warfarin abuse, drug interactions are a common problem. Large numbers of drugs are known to alter warfarin action. Some, like phenylbutazone, inhibit albumin binding of vitamin K; others, like chloramphenicol, inhibit the metabolism of vitamin K; and yet others alter receptor site affinity. Drugs such as barbiturates and rifampicin induce the activity of the hepatic microsomal enzymes and increase the catabolism of warfarin (Bithell 1993b).

Cephalosporins, especially the second- and third-generation agents, may cause hypoprothrombinaemia which can be reversed by vitamin K administration (Sattler et al. 1988; Breen and St Peter 1991; Stork et al. 1994). These antibiotics cause a direct inhibition of γ-carboxylation by their N-methyl-thiotetrazole (NMTT) side chain or metabolites (Stork et al. 1994). Inhibition of vitamin K-dependent factors by cephalosporins appears to be unrelated to their bactericidal effects or to the presence of intestinal factors (Lipsky 1983; Shirakawa et al. 1990). Co-administration of glutathione may protect against this (Lipsky 1984). Hypoprothrombinaemia is most likely to occur in the elderly, and those with renal or hepatic impairment (Mueller et al. 1987; Vertoli et al. 1992; Stork et al. 1994).

Ivermectin, an anthelminthic drug, prolongs the prothrombin time when used in the treatment of onchocerciasis (Homeida et al. 1988) and has minor effects on vitamin K metabolism (Whitworth et al. 1992). Decreased concentration of several clotting factors and prolongation of prothrombin time was noted with use of interleukin-2, and the concomitant prophylactic use of vitamin K has been suggested to prevent this (Birchfield et al. 1992).

References

Aanderud, S., Myking, O.L., and Strandjord, R.E. (1981). The influence of carbamazepine on thyroid hormones and thyroxine binding globulin in hypothyroid patients substituted with thyroxine. *Clin. Endocrinol.* (Oxf.) 15, 247.

Aaron, J.E., Francis, R.M., Peacock, M., *et al.* (1989). Contrasting microanatomy of idiopathic and corticosteroid-induced osteoporosis. *Clin. Orthop.* 294.

Abdulla, M. (1979). Copper levels after oral zinc. *Lancet* i, 616.

Abero, K., Shelp, W.D., Kosseff, A., *et al.* (1982). Amoxapine-associated rhabdomyolysis and acute renal failure: a case report. *J. Clin. Psychiatry* 43, 426.

Abu-Hamdan, D.K., Desai, H., Sondheimer, J., *et al.* (1988). Taste acuity and zinc metabolism in captopril-treated hypertensive male patients. *Am. J. Hypertens.* 1, 303s.

Abu-Hamdan, D.K., Mahajan, S.K., Migdal, S.D., *et al.* (1986). Zinc tolerance test in uremia. Effect of ferrous sulfate and aluminum hydroxide. *Ann. Intern. Med.* 104, 50.

Abu Melha, A., Ahmed, N.A., and el Hassan, A.Y. (1987). Traditional remedies and lead intoxication. *Trop. Geogr. Med.* 39, 100.

Ackerman, B.H. and Kasbekar, N. (1997). Disturbances of taste and smell induced by drugs. *Pharmacotherapy* 17, 482.

Acomb, C., Hordon, L.D., Judd, A.T., *et al.* (1985). Metabolic alkalosis induced by 'Panadol Soluble'. *Lancet* ii, 614.

Adachi, J.D. (1997). Corticosteroid-induced osteoporosis. *Am. J. Med. Sci.* 313, 41.

Adachi, J., Bensen, W.G., Brown, J., *et al.* (1997). Intermittent etidronate therapy to prevent corticosteroid-induced osteoporosis. *N. Engl. J. Med.* 337, 382.

Adams, J.M., Hyde, W.H., Procianoy, R.S., *et al.* (1980). Hypochloremic metabolic alkalosis following tolazoline-induced gastric hypersecretion. *Pediatrics* 65, 298.

Adinoff, A.D. and Hollister, J.R. (1983). Steroid-induced fractures and bone loss in patients with asthma. *N. Engl. J. Med.* 309, 265.

Adrogué, H.J. and Madias, N.E. (1998*a*). Management of life-threatening acid–base disorders. Part 1. *N. Engl. J. Med.* 338, 26.

Adrogué, H.J. and Madias, N.E. (1998*b*). Management of life-threatening acid–base disorders. Part 2. *N. Engl. J. Med.* 338, 107.

Adu, D., Turney, J., Michael, J., *et al.* (1983). Hyperkalaemia in cyclosporin-treated renal allograft recipients. *Lancet* ii, 370.

Aggarwal, S.K. and Fadool, J.M. (1993). Cisplatin and carboplatin induced changes in the neurohypophysis and parathyroid, and their role in nephrotoxicity. *Anti-Cancer Drugs* 4, 149.

Aguilera, S., Deray, G., Desjobert, H., *et al.* (1992). Effects of cyclosporine on tubular acidification function in patients with idiopathic uveitis. *Am. J. Nephrol.* 12, 425.

Ahn, Y-H., and Goldman, J.M. (1985). Trimethoprim-sulfamethoxazole and hyponatremia. *Ann. Intern. Med.* 103, 161.

Aldenhovel, H.G. (1988). The influence of long-term anticonvulsant therapy with diphenylhydantoin and carbamazepine on serum gamma-glutamyltransferase, aspartate aminotransferase, alanine aminotransferase and alkaline phosphatase. *Eur. Arch. Psychiatry Neurol. Sci.* 237, 312.

Alderman, C.P., Rivera, G., and Richer, M. (1996). Adverse effects of the angiotensin-converting enzyme inhibitors. *Ann. Pharmacotherapy* 30, 55.

Alen, M. (1985). Androgenic steroid effects on liver and red cells. *Br. J. Sports Med.* 19, 15.

Alfrey, A.C. (1993). Aluminum toxicity in patients with chronic renal failure. *Ther. Drug Monit.* 15, 593.

al-Hemsi, B., McGory, R.W., Shepard, B., *et al.* (1996). Liver transplantation for hepatitis B cirrhosis: clinical sequela of passive immunization. *Clin. Transpl.* 10, 668.

Ali, B.H., Abdel Gayoum, A.A., and Bashir, A.A. (1992). Gentamicin nephrotoxicity in rat: some biochemical correlates. *Pharmacol. Toxicol.* 70, 419.

Alkhawajah, A.M. (1992). Alkohl use in Saudi Arabia. Extent of use and possible lead toxicity. *Trop. Geogr. Med.* 44, 373.

al-Khursany, I., Thomas, T.H., Harrison, K., *et al.* (1992). Reduced erythrocyte and leukocyte magnesium is associated with cyclosporin treatment and hypertension in renal transplant patients. *Nephrol. Dial. Transplant.* 7, 251.

Allred, J., Wong, W., and Kafetz, K. (1989). Elderly people taking non-steroidal anti-inflammatory drugs are unlikely to have excess renal impairment. *Postgrad. Med. J.* 65, 735.

AlMajed, S.A., Pandya, L., Alballa, S.R., *et al.* (1995). Hyperuricaemia during treatment for active pulmonary tuberculosis in a multi-racial population. *Saudi Med. J.* 16, 330.

Al-Mufti, H.I. and Arieff, A.I. (1985). Captopril-induced hyponatremia with irreversible neurologic damage. *Am. J. Med.* 79, 769.

Alun-Jones, E. and Williams, J. (1986). Hyponatremia and fluid retention in a neonate associated with maternal naproxen overdosage. *J. Toxicol. Clin. Toxicol.* 24, 257.

Amatayakul, K. (1994). Metabolism: vitamins and trace elements. In *Pharmacology of the Contraceptive Steroids* (ed. J.W. Goldzieher and K. Fotherby), p. 363. Raven Press, New York.

Amatayakul, K., Koottathep, S., Prapamontol, T., *et al.* (1994). The effect of oral contraceptives on protein metabolism. *J. Med. Assoc. Thai.* 77, 509.

Amatayakul, K., Uttaravichai, C., Singkamani, R., *et al.* (1984). Vitamin metabolism and the effects of multivitamin supplementation in oral contraceptive users. *Contraception* 30, 179.

Ambanelli, U., Ferraccioli, G.F., Serventi, G., *et al.* (1982). Changes in serum and urinary zinc induced by ASA and indomethacin. *Scand. J. Rheumatol.* 11, 63.

Amess, J.A., Burman, J.F., Rees, G.M., *et al.* (1978). Megaloblastic haemopoiesis in patients receiving nitrous oxide. *Lancet* ii, 339.

Amitai, Y. and Lovejoy, F.H., Jr. (1988). Hypokalemia in acute theophylline poisoning. *Am. J. Emerg. Med.* 6, 214.

Amos, R.J., Amess, J.A., Hinds, C.J., *et al.* (1985). Investigations into the effect of nitrous oxide anaesthesia on folate metabolism in patients receiving intensive care. *Chemotherapia* 4, 393.

Anderson, K.E. (1989). LHRH analogues for hormonal manipulation in acute intermittent porphyria. *Semin. Haematol.* 26, 10.

Anderson, K.E., Spitz, I.M., Bardin, C.W., *et al.* (1990). A gonadotropin releasing hormone analogue prevents cyclical attacks of porphyria. *Arch. Intern. Med.* 150, 1469.

Anderson, W., Youl, B., and Mackay, I.R. (1991). Acute theophylline intoxication. *Ann. Emerg. Med.* 20, 1143.

Andreasen, P.B., Lyngbye, J., and Trolle, E. (1973). Abnormalities in diphenylhydantoin therapy in epileptic outpatients. *Acta Med. Scand.* 194, 261.

Anelli, A., Brancaccio, D., Damasso, R., *et al.* (1989). Substitution of calcium carbonate for aluminum hydroxide in patients on hemodialysis. Effects on acidosis, on parathyroid function, and on calcemia. *Nephron* 52, 125.

Antman, K.H., Elias, A., and Ryan, L. (1990). Ifosfamide and mesna: response and toxicity at standard- and high-dose schedules. *Semin. Oncol.* 17, 68.

Antonini, G., Palmieri, G., Millefiorini, E., *et al.* (1989). Lead poisoning during heroin addiction. *Ital. J. Neurol. Sci.* 10, 105.

Antonios, T.F.T. and MacGregor, G.A. (1995). Angiotensin converting enzyme inhibitors in hypertension: potential problems. *J. Hypertens.* Suppl. 13, S11.

Apple, F.S. (1989). Diagnostic use of CK-MM, and CK-MB isoforms for detecting myocardial infarction. *Clin. Lab. Med.* 9, 643.

Appleby, L. (1984). Rapid development of hyponatraemia during low-dose carbamazepine therapy. *J. Neurol. Neurosurg. Psychiatry* 47, 1138.

Arafah, B.M. (1994). Decreased levothyroxine requirement in women with hypothyroidism during androgen therapy for breast cancer. *Ann. Intern. Med.* 121, 247.

Arellano, F. and Krupp, P. (1991). Muscular disorders associated with cyclosporin. *Lancet* 337, 915.

Argov, Z. and Mastaglia, F.L. (1988). Drug-induced neuromuscular disorders in man. In *Disorders of Voluntary Muscle* (5th edn) (ed. J.N. Walton), p. 981. Churchill Livingstone, London.

Ariceta, G., Rodriguez-Soriano, J., Vallo, A., *et al.* (1997). Acute and chronic effects of cisplatin therapy on renal magnesium homeostasis. *Med. Pediatr. Oncol.* 28, 35.

Arieff, A.I. (1986). Hyponatremia, convulsions, respiratory arrest, and permanent brain damage after elective surgery in a healthy woman. *N. Engl. J. Med.* 314, 1529.

Aroldi, A., Tarantino, A., Montagnino, G., *et al.* (1997). Effects of three immunosuppressive regimens on vertebral bone density in renal transplant recipients: a prospective study. *Transplantation* 63, 380.

Arrambide, K. and Toto, R.D. (1993). Tumor lysis syndrome. *Semin. Nephrol.* 13, 273.

Asch, M.J., White, M.G., and Pruitt, B.A. (1970). Acid base changes associated with topical sulfamylon therapy: retrospective study of 100 burn patients. *Ann. Surg.* 172, 946.

Ashraf, M., Chaudhary, K., Nelson, J., *et al.* (1995). Massive overdose of sustained-release verapamil: a case report and review of literature. *Am. J. Med. Sci.* 310, 258.

Ashraf, M., Scotchel, P.L., Krall, J.M., *et al.* (1983). cis-Platinum-induced hypomagnesemia and peripheral neuropathy. *Gynecol. Oncol.* 16, 309.

Ashraf, N., Locksley, R., and Arieff, A.I. (1981). Thiazide-induced hyponatremia associated with death or neurologic damage in outpatients. *Am. J. Med.* 70, 1163.

Ashton, M.G., Ball, S.G., Thomas, T.H., *et al.* (1977). Water intoxication associated with carbamazepine treatment. *BMJ* i, 1134.

Ashton, R.E., Hawk, J.L., and Magnus, I.A. (1984). Low dose oral chloroquine in the treatment of porphyria cutanea tarda. *Br. J. Dermatol.* 111, 609.

Assal, F. and Chauchot, F. (1994). Hyponatrémie d'origine thérapeutique. A propos d'un cas. *Encéphale* 20, 527.

Ataya, K., Abbasi, A., Mercado, A., *et al.* (1988). Bone density and reproductive hormones in patients with neuroleptic-induced hyperprolactinemia. *Fertil. Steril.* 50, 876.

Atkinson, S.A., Fraher, L., Gundberg, C.M., *et al.* (1989). Mineral homeostasis and bone mass in children treated for acute lymphoblastic leukaemia. *J. Pediatr.* 114, 793.

Aucamp, A.K., van Achterbergh, S.M., and Theron, E. (1981). Potential hazard of magnesium sulphate administration. *Lancet* ii, 1057.

Aull, L., Chao, H., and Coy, K. (1990). Heparin-induced hyperkalaemia. *DICP* 24, 244.

Aunsholt, N.A. (1989). Prolonged Q-T interval and hypokalemia caused by haloperidol. *Acta Psychiatr. Scand.* 79, 411.

Ayus, J.C. (1986). Diuretic-induced hyponatremia. *Arch. Intern. Med.* 146, 1295.

Bach, M.A., Blum, D.M., Rose, S.R., *et al.* (1992). Myalgia and elevated creatine kinase activity associated with subcutaneous injections of diluent. *J. Pediatr.* 121, 650.

Bachmeyer, C., Dhote, R., Sereni, D., *et al.* (1995). Hypercalcemia and parathyroid adenoma in patients on lithium therapy. Three cases and review of the literature. *Eur. J. Intern. Med.* 6, 223.

Bachynski, B.N., Flynn, J.T., Rodrigues, M.M., *et al.* (1986). Hyperglycemic acidotic coma and death in Kearns–Sayre syndrome. *Ophthalmology* 93, 391.

Baethge, B.A., Work, J., Landreneau, M.D., *et al.* (1993). Tophaceous gout in patients with renal transplants treated with cyclosporine A. *J. Rheumatol.* 20, 718.

Bagatell, C.J. and Bremner, W.J. (1996). Androgens in men — uses and abuses. *N. Engl. J. Med.* 334, 707.

Baglin, A., Boulard, J.C., Hanslik, T., *et al.* (1995). Metabolic adverse reactions to diuretics. Clinical relevance to elderly patients. *Drug Saf.* 12, 161.

Baglin, A., Prinseau, J., Aegerter, P., *et al.* (1992). Anomalies électrolytiques chez les personnes agées. Prévalence et relation avec le traitement médicamenteux. Étude multicentrique chez 631 sujets de 70 ans et plus. *Presse Méd.* 21, 1459.

Bailey, C.J. (1992). Biguanides and NIDDM. *Diabetes Care* 15, 755.

Bailey, C.J. and Turner, R.C. (1996). Metformin. *N. Engl. J. Med.* 334, 574.

Baker, E.J., Reed, K.D., and Dixon, S.L. (1989). Chlorthalidone-induced pseudoporphyria: clinical and microscopic findings of a case. *J. Am. Acad. Dermatol.* 21, 1026.

Bantle, J.P., Nath, K.A., Sutherland, D.E.R., *et al.* (1985). Effects of cyclosporine on the renin–angiotensin–aldosterone system and potassium excretion in renal transplant recipients. *Ann. Intern. Med.* 145, 505.

Bar, R.S., Wilson, H.E., Mazzaferri, E.L. (1975). Hypomagnesemic hypocalcemia secondary to renal magnesium wasting: a possible consequence of high dose gentamicin therapy. *Ann. Intern. Med.* 82, 646.

Barbosa, I., Coutinho, E., Athayde, C., *et al.* (1996). Androgen levels in women using a single implant of nomegestrol acetate. *Contraception* 53, 37.

Barbosa, J., Seal, U.S., and Doe, R.P. (1971). Effects of anabolic steroids on haptoglobin, orosomucoid, plasminogen, fibrinogen, transferrin, ceruloplasmin, α-1-antitrypsin, β-glucuronidase and total serum proteins. *J. Clin. Endocrinol. Metab.* 33, 388.

Barbour, L.A., Kick, S.D., Steiner, J.F., *et al.* (1994). A prospective study of heparin-induced osteoporosis in pregnancy using bone densitometry. *Am. J. Obstet. Gynecol.* 170, 862.

Bardin, T. and Lequesne, M. (1989). The osteoporosis of heparinotherapy and systemic mastocytosis. *Clin. Rheumatol.* 8 (Suppl.2), 119.

Barilla, D.E., Notz, C., Kennedy, D., *et al.* (1978). Renal oxalate excretion following oral oxalate loads in patients with ileal disease and with renal and absorptive hypercalciuria. Effect of calcium and magnesium. *Am. J. Med.* 64, 579.

Barnes, L.A. (1975). Safety considerations with high ascorbic acid dosage. *Ann. N.Y. Acad. Sci.* 258, 377.

Barrett-Connor, E., Chang, J.C., and Edelstein, S.L. (1994). Coffee-associated osteoporosis offset by daily milk consumption. The Rancho Bernardo Study. *JAMA* 271, 280.

Barton, C.H., Pahl, M., Vaziri, N.D., *et al.* (1984). Renal magnesium wasting associated with amphotericin B therapy. *Am. J. Med.* 77, 471.

Barton, C.H., Vaziri, N.D., Martin, D.C., *et al.* (1987). Hypomagnesemia and renal magnesium wasting in renal transplant recipients receiving cyclosporine. *Am. J. Med.* 83, 693.

Barton, C.H., Vaziri, N.D., Mina-Araghi, S., *et al.* (1989). Effects of cyclosporine on magnesium metabolism in rats. *J. Lab. Clin. Med.* 114, 232.

Baselga, J., Kris, M.G., Scher, H.I., *et al.* (1993). Phase II trial of gallium nitrate in previously treated patients with small cell lung cancer. *Invest. New Drugs* 11, 85.

Bashir, Y. and Tomson, C.R. (1988). Cardiac arrest associated with hypokalaemia in a patient receiving mithramycin. *Postgrad. Med. J.* 64, 228.

Bassler, K.H. and Heidenreich, O. (1984). Zur Problematik von Sulfitzusatz zu Infusionslösungen. *Infusionsther. Klin. Ernähr.* 11, 31.

Baum, M.K., Javier, J.J., Mantero-Atienza, E., *et al.* (1991). Zidovudine-associated adverse reactions in a longitudinal study of asymptomatic HIV-1-infected homosexual males. *J. Acquir. Immune Defic. Syndr.* 4, 1218.

Baum, M.K., ShorPosner, G., Lu, Y., *et al.* (1995). Micronutrients and HIV-1 disease progression. *AIDS* 9, 1051.

Baumann, G. (1979). Hyponatremia during adrenocorticotropin (ACTH) infusions. *Ann. Intern. Med.* 91, 499.

Baumann, R., Magos, A.L., Kay, J.D.S., *et al.* (1990). Absorption of glycine irrigating solution during transcervical resection of endometrium. *BMJ* 300, 304.

Bavoux, F. (1992). Nonsteroidal antiinflammatory drugs and fetal toxicity. *Presse Méd.* 21, 1909-1912.

Beall, D.P. and Scofield, R.H. (1995). Milk–alkali syndrome associated with calcium carbonate consumption. Report of 7 patients with parathyroid hormone levels and an estimate of prevalence among patients hospitalized with hypercalcemia. *Medicine* 74, 89.

Beastall, G.H., Cowan, R.A., Gray, J.M., *et al.* (1985). Hormone binding globulins and anticonvulsant therapy. *Scott Med. J.* 30, 101.

Beatty, O.L., Campbell, N.P., and Neely, R.D. (1989). Tetany in association with gentamicin therapy. *Ulster Med. J.* 58, 108.

Bechtel, U., Mucke, C., Feucht, H.E., *et al.* (1995). Limitations of pulse oral calcitriol therapy in continuous ambulatory peritoneal dialysis patients. *Am. J. Kidney Dis.* 25, 291.

Becker, M.A. and Roessler, B.J. (1995). Hyperuricaemia and gout. In *The Metabolic and Molecular Basis of Inherited Disease* (ed. C.R. Scriver, A.L. Beaudt, W.S. Sly, and D. Valle), p.1655. McGraw-Hill, New York.

Bedani, P.L., Perini, L., and Gilli, P. (1994). Acute rhabdomyolysis and hemoglobin reduction after bezafibrate overdose in hyperlipidemic patients on hemodialysis. *Nephron* 68, 512.

Behm, A.R. and Unger, W.P. (1974). Oral contraceptives and porphyria cutanea tarda. *Can. Med. Assoc. J.* 110, 1052.

Bei, L., Wood, R.J., and Rosenberg, I.H. (1986). Glucose polymer increases jejunal calcium, magnesium, and zinc absorption in humans. *Am. J. Clin. Nutr.* 44, 244.

Belaiche, J., Le Carrer, M., Krainik, F., *et al.* (1977). Clofibrate-induced increase in serum-creatine-phosphokinase level. *Lancet* i, 149.

Bellou, A., Aimone-Gastin, I., De Korwin, J.D., *et al.* (1996). Cobalamin deficiency with megaloblastic anaemia in one patient under long-term omeprazole therapy. *J. Intern. Med.* 240, 161.

Benhmida, M., Hachicha, J., Bahloul, Z., *et al.* (1995). Cyclosporine-induced hyperuricemia and gout in renal transplants. *Transplant Proc.* 27, 2722.

Bender, D.A. (1983). Effects of oestradiol and vitamin B_6 on tryptophan metabolism in the rat: implications for the interpretation of the tryptophan load test for vitamin B_6 nutritional status. *Br. J. Nutr.* 50, 33.

Bendz, H., Sjodin, I., Toss, G., *et al.* (1996). Hyperparathyroidism and long-term lithium therapy: a cross-sectional study and the effect of lithium withdrawal. *J. Intern. Med.* 240, 357.

Benjamin, N., Phillips, R.J., and Robinson, B.F. (1988). Verapamil and bendrofluazide in the treatment of hypertension: a controlled study of effectiveness alone and in combination. *Eur. J. Clin. Pharmacol.* 34, 249.

Bennett, C.L., Vogelzang, N.J., Ratain, M.J., *et al.* (1986). Hyponatremia and other toxic effects during a phase I trial of recombinant human gamma interferon and vinblastine. *Cancer Treat. Rep.* 70, 1081.

Bennett, I.C., Jr, Cary, F.H., Mitchell, G.I., *et al.* (1953). Acute methyl alcohol poisoning: a review based on experiences in an outbreak of 32 cases. *Medicine* 32, 431.

Bennett, W.M., Elzinga, L., and Kelley, V. (1988). Pathophysiology of cyclosporine nephrotoxicity: role of eicosanoids. *Transplant. Proc.* 20, 628.

Benowitz, N.L., Fitzgerald, G.A., Wilson, M., *et al.* (1993). Nicotine effects on eicosanoid formation and hemostatic function: comparison of transdermal nicotine and cigarette smoking. *J. Am. Coll. Cardiol.* 22, 1159-1167.

Berg, M.J., Stumbo, P.J., Chenard, C.A., *et al.* (1995). Folic acid improves phenytoin pharmacokinetics. *J. Am. Diet. Assoc.* 95, 352.

Berg, W., Bothor, C., Pirlich, W., *et al.* (1986). Influence of magnesium on the absorption and excretion of calcium and oxalate ions. *Eur. Urol.* 12, 274.

Berkelhammer, C.H., Wood, R.J., and Sitrin, M.D. (1988). Acetate and hypercalciuria during total parenteral nutrition. *Am. J. Clin. Nutr.* 48, 1482.

Berland, Y., Vacher Coponat, H., Durand, C., *et al.* (1991). Rhabdomyolysis with simvastatin use. *Nephron* 57, 365.

Bernard, S. (1991). Severe lactic acidosis following theophylline overdose. *Ann. Emerg. Med.* 20, 1135.

Berova, N., and Lazarova, A. (1988). Pellagra-ähnliche Veränderungen nach Glibenklamid-Behandlung bei einer Patientin mit Diabetes mellitus und Vitiligo. *Dermatol. Monatsschr.* 174, 50.

Berruti, A., Torta, M., Piovesan, A., *et al.* (1996). Serum and urinary profile of bone turn-over markers in a patient with tamoxifen-induced hypercalcaemia submitted to pamidronate therapy. *Breast* 5, 274.

Berth-Jones, J. and Hutchinson, P.E. (1992). Progress in self treatment for psoriasis vulgaris. *J. Clin. Pharmacol. Ther.* 17, 217.

Besunder, J.B. and Smith, P.G. (1991). Toxic effects of electrolyte and trace mineral administration in the intensive care unit. *Crit. Care Clin.* 7, 659.

Bevilacqua, M. (1994). Hyponatraemia in AIDS. *Baillière's Clin. Endocrinol. Metab.* 8, 837.

Bibler, M.R., Frame, P.T., Hagler, D.N., *et al.* (1987). Clinical evaluation of efficacy, pharmacokinetics, and safety of teicoplanin for serious gram-positive infections. *Antimicrob. Agents Chemother.* 31, 207.

Bikle, D.D., Halloran, B., Fong, L., *et al.* (1993). Elevated 1,25-dihydroxyvitamin D levels in patients with chronic obstructive pulmonary disease treated with prednisone. *J. Clin. Endocrinol. Metab.* 76, 456.

Birchfield, G.R., Rodgers, G.M., Girodias, K.W., *et al.* (1992). Hypoprothrombinemia associated with interleukin-2 therapy: correction with vitamin K. *J. Immunother.* 11, 71.

Biscarini, L. (1996). Anti-inflammatory analgesics and drugs used in gout. In *Meyler's Side Effects of Drugs* (13th edn) (ed. M.N.G. Dukes), p. 204. Elsevier, Amsterdam.

Bishop, N.J., Williams, D.M., Compston, J.C., *et al.* (1995). Osteoporosis in severe congenital neutropenia treated with granulocyte colony-stimulating factor. *Br. J. Haematol.* 89, 927.

Bithell, T.C. (1993a). Acquired coagulation disorders. In *Wintrobe's Clinical Haematology* (ed. C.R. Lee, T.C. Bithell, J. Forster, *et al.*), p. 1473. Lea and Febiger, Philadelphia.

Bithell, T.C. (1993b). Thrombosis and antithrombotic therapy. In *Wintrobe's Clinical Haematology* (ed. C.R. Lee, T.C. Bithell, J. Forster, *et al.*), p. 1515. Lea and Febiger, Philadelphia.

Blachley, J.D. and Knochel, J.P. (1980). Tobacco chewer's hypokalemia: licorice revisited. *N. Engl. J. Med.* 302, 784.

Blain, P.G., Lane, R.J., Bateman, D.N., *et al.* (1985). Opiate-induced rhabdomyolysis. *Hum. Toxicol.* 4, 71.

Blau, E.B. and Hoyman, S. (1997). Severe hypercalcemia, renal failure, and medullary nephrocalcinosis secondary to calcium carbonate ingestion. *Pediatr. Nephrol.* 11, 391.

Bleakley, P., Nichol, A.W., and Collins, A.G. (1979). Diazinon and porphyria cutanea tarda. *Med. J. Aust.* 1, 314.

Blom, H.J., and Monasch, E. (1983). Metabole acidose bij een patient met gestoorde nierfunctie na cholestyramine toediening. *Ned. Tijdschr. Geneeskd.* 127, 1446.

Blom, J.H., Kurth, K.H., and Splinter, T.A. (1985). Renal function, serum calcium and magnesium during treatment of advanced bladder carcinoma with *cis*-dichlorodiamineplatinum: impact of tumour site, patient age and magnesium suppletion. *Int. Urol. Nephrol.* 17, 331.

Blomfield, J., Dixon, S.R., and McCredie, D.A. (1971). Potential hepatotoxicity of copper in recurrent hemodialysis. *Arch. Intern. Med.* 128, 555.

Böhrer, H., Fleischer, F., and Krier, C. (1988). Hyperkalemic cardiac arrest after cardiac surgery following high-dose glucose-insulin-potassium infusion for inotropic support. *Anesthesiology* 69, 949.

Bond, G.R. and Van Zee, A. (1994). Overdosage of misoprostol in pregnancy. *Am. J. Obstet. Gynecol.* 171, 561.

Bonilla, M.A., Dale, D., Zeidler, C., *et al.* (1994). Long-term safety of treatment with recombinant human granulocyte colony-stimulating factor (r-metHuG-CSF) in patients with severe congenital neutropenias. *Br. J. Haematol.* 88, 723.

Bonkovsky, H.L. (1993). Advances in understanding and treating 'the little imitator,' acute porphyria. *Gastroenterology* 105, 590.

Boosalis, M.G., McCall, J.T., Ahrenholz, D.H., *et al.* (1987). Serum and urinary silver levels in thermal injury patients. *Surgery* 101, 40.

Booth, S.L. (1997). Skeletal functions of vitamin K dependent proteins: not just for clotting anymore. *Nutr. Rev.* 55, 282.

Borges, H.F., Hocks, J., and Kjellstrand, C.M. (1982). Mannitol intoxication in patients with renal failure. *Arch. Intern. Med.* 142, 63.

Bork, E. and Hansen, M. (1986). Severe hyponatremia following simultaneous administration of aminoglutethimide and diuretics. *Cancer Treat. Rep.* 70, 689.

Borron, S.W. and Baud, F.J. (1996). Acute cyanide poisoning: clinical spectrum, diagnosis, and treatment. *Arh. Hig. Rada Toksikol.* 47, 307.

Bory, M., Pierron, F., Panagides, D., *et al.* (1993). Severe hyperkalaemia induced by a non-cardioselective beta-adrenergic blocker and pheochromocytoma in a normotensive patient. *Eur. J. Med.* 2, 506.

Botez, M.I. and Young, S.N. (1991). Effects of anticonvulsant treatment and low levels of folate and thiamine on amine metabolites in cerebrospinal fluid. *Brain* 114, 333.

Boton, R., Gaviria, M., and Batlle, D.C. (1987). Prevalence, pathogenesis and treatment of renal dysfunction associated with chronic lithium therapy. *Am. J. Kidney Dis.* 10, 329.

Bouillon, T., Meineke, I., Port, R., *et al.* (1996). Concentration-effect relationship of the positive chronotropic and hypokalaemic effects of fenoterol in healthy women of childbearing age. *Eur. J. Clin. Pharmacol.* 51, 153.

Boulard, J.C., Hanslik, T., Alterescu, R., *et al.* (1994). Hypercalcémie symptomatique après association vitamin D–diuretiques thiazidiques. 2 cas chez des femmes agées. *Presse Méd.* 23, 96.

Bourke, J.F., Berth-Jones, J., and Hutchinson, P.E. (1993). Hypercalcaemia with topical calcipotriol. *BMJ* 306, 1344.

Boutsen, Y., Devogelaer, J.P., Malghem, J., *et al.* (1996). Antacid-induced osteomalacia. *Clin. Rheumatol.* 15, 75.

Braden, G., Von Oeyen, P., Smith, M., *et al.* (1985a). Mechanism of ritodrine and terbutaline-induced hypokalemia and pulmonary edema. *Kidney Int.* 27, 304.

Braden, G.L., Johnston, S.S., Germain, M.J., *et al.* (1985b). Lactic acidosis associated with the therapy of acute bronchospasm. *N. Engl. J. Med.* 313, 890.

Braden, G.L., Von Oeyen, P.T., Germain, M.J., *et al.* (1997). Ritodrine- and terbutaline-induced hypokalemia in preterm labor: mechanisms and consequences. *Kidney Int.* 51, 1867.

Bradford, R.H., Shear, C.L., Chremos, A.N., *et al.* (1994). Expanded Clinical Evaluation of Lovastatin (EXCEL) study results: two-year efficacy and safety follow-up. *Am. J. Cardiol.* 74, 667.

Brady, H.R., Goldberg, H., Lunski, C., and Uldall, P.R. (1988). Dialysis-induced hyperkalaemia presenting as profound muscle weakness. *Int. J. Artif. Org.* 11, 43.

Brady, H.R., Ryan, F., Cunningham, J., *et al.* (1989). Hypophosphatemia complicating bronchodilator therapy for acute severe asthma. *Arch. Intern. Med.* 149, 2367.

Brady, J.A., Rock, C.L., and Horneffer, M.R. (1995). Thiamin status, diuretic medications, and the management of congestive heart failure. *J. Am. Diet. Assoc.* 95, 541.

Brady, J.P. and Williams, H.C. (1967). Magnesium intoxication in a premature infant. *Pediatrics* 40, 100.

Braide, S.A. and Davies, T.J. (1987). Factors that affect the induction of gammaglutamyltransferase in epileptic patients receiving anti-convulsant drugs. *Ann. Clin. Biochem.* 24, 391.

Brand, J.M. and Greer, F.R. (1990). Hypermagnesemia and intestinal perforation following antacid administration in a premature infant. *Pediatrics* 85, 121.

Brattstrom, L., Israelsson, B., Olsson, A., *et al.* (1992). Plasma homocysteine in women on oral oestrogen-containing contraceptives and in men with oestrogen-treated prostatic carcinoma. *Scand. J. Clin. Lab. Invest.* 52, 283.

Breen, G.A. and St Peter, W.L. (1997). Hypoprothrombinemia associated with cefmetazole. *Ann. Pharmacother.* 31, 180.

Bremme, K., Eneroth, P., Nordstrom, L., *et al.* (1986). Effects of infusion of the beta-adrenoceptor agonist terbutaline on serum magnesium in pregnant women. *Magnesium* 5, 85.

Bressler, R.B. and Huston, D.P. (1985). Water intoxication following moderate-dose intravenous cyclophosphamide. *Arch. Intern. Med.* 145, 548.

Briceland, L.L. and Bailie, G.R. (1991). Pentamidine-associated nephrotoxicity and hyperkalemia in patients with AIDS. *DICP* 25, 1171.

Brimioulle, S., Berre, J., Dufaye, P., *et al.* (1989). Hydrochloric acid infusion for treatment of metabolic alkalosis associated with respiratory acidosis. *Crit. Care Med.* 17, 232.

Brivet, F.G., Naveau, S.H., Lemaigre, G.F., *et al.* (1994). Pancreatic lesions in HIV-infected patients. *Baillière's Clin. Endocrinol. Metab.* 8, 859.

Brock, P.R., Koliouskas, D.E., Barratt, T.M., *et al.* (1991). Partial reversibility of cisplatin toxicity in children. *J. Pediatr.* 118, 531.

Brocks, A.S., Reid, H., and Glazer, G. (1977). Acute intravenous zinc poisoning. *BMJ* i, 1390.

Brodie, M.J., Boobis, A.R., Hillyard, C.J., *et al.* (1982). Effect of rifampicin and isoniazid on vitamin D metabolism. *Clin. Pharmacol. Ther.* 32, 525.

Brooks, M.J. and Melnik, G. (1995). The refeeding syndrome: an approach to understanding its complications and preventing its occurrence. *Pharmacotherapy* 15, 713.

Brooks-Hill, P.W., Bishop, B.E., and Vellend, H. (1985). Pellagra-like encephalopathy complicating a multiple drug regimen for the treatment of pulmonary infection due to mycobacterium avium-intracellular. *Am. Rev. Respir. Dis.* 131, 476.

Brown, G.R. and Greenwood, J.K. (1994). Drug- and nutrition-induced hypophosphatemia: mechanisms and relevance in the critically ill. *Ann. Pharmacother.* 28, 626.

Brown, M.J., Brown, D.C., and Murphy, M.B. (1983). Hypokalemia from beta$_2$-receptor stimulation by circulating epinephrine. *N. Engl. J. Med.* 309, 1414.

Brown, R.O., Hamrick, K.D., Dickerson, R.N., *et al.* (1996). Hyperkalemia secondary to concurrent pharmacotherapy in a patient receiving home parenteral nutrition. *JPEN* 20, 429.

Brown, R.R., Rose, D.P., Leklem, J.E., *et al.* (1975). Urinary 4-pyridoxic acid, plasma pyridoxal phosphate, and erythrocyte aminotransferase levels in oral contraceptive users receiving controlled intakes of vitamin B$_6$. *Am. J. Clin. Nutr.* 28, 10.

Browning, J.J. and Channer, K.S. (1981). Hyperkalaemic cardiac arrhythmia caused by potassium citrate mixture. *BMJ* 282, 1366.

Brucato, A., Bonati, M., Gaspari, F., *et al.* (1993). Tetany and rhabdomyolysis due to surreptitious furosemide — importance of magnesium supplementation. *J. Toxicol Clin. Toxicol.* 31, 341.

Brunet, W.G., Hutton, L.C., and Henderson, A.R. (1989). The effect of nonionic radiographic contrast medium on serum electrolytes and proteins during intravenous urography. *Can. Assoc. Radiol. J.* 40, 139.

Brunner, J.E., Redmond, J.M., Haggar, A.M., *et al.* (1990). Central pontine myelinolysis and pontine lesions after rapid correction of hyponatraemia: a prospective magnetic resonance imaging study. *Ann. Neurol.* 27, 61.

Buchinsky, F.J., Ma, Y., Mann, G.N., *et al.* (1996). T lymphocytes play a critical role in the development of cyclosporin A-induced osteopenia. *Endocrinology* 137, 2278.

Bufano, G., Bellini, C., Cervellin, G., *et al.* (1990). Enteral nutrition in anorexia nervosa. *JPEN* 14, 404.

Bugge, J.F. (1996). Severe hyperkalaemia induced by trimethoprim in combination with an angiotensin-converting enzyme inhibitor in a patient with transplanted lungs. *J. Intern. Med.* 240, 249.

Burack, D.A., Griffith, B.P., Thompson, M.E., *et al.* (1992). Hyperuricemia and gout among heart transplant recipients receiving cyclosporine. *Am. J. Med.* 92, 141.

Burgess, C.D., Flatt, A., Siebers, R., *et al.* (1989). A comparison of the extent and duration of hypokalaemia following three nebulized beta$_2$-adrenoceptor agonists. *Eur. J. Clin. Pharmacol.* 36, 415.

Burnakis, T.G. and Mioduch, H.J. (1984). Combined therapy with captopril and potassium supplementation. A potential for hyperkalemia. *Arch. Intern. Med.* 144, 2371.

Burnett, R.J. and Reents, S.B. (1990). Severe hypomagnesemia induced by pentamidine. *DICP* 24, 239.

Burnier, M. and Brunner, H.R. (1992). Neurohormonal consequences of diuretics in different cardiovascular syndromes. *Eur. Heart J.* 13 Suppl. G, 28.

Burnier, M., Waeber, B., and Brunner, H.R. (1995). Clinical pharmacology of the angiotensin II receptor antagonist losartan potassium in healthy subjects. *J. Hypertens.* Suppl. 13, S23.

Burns, J. and Paterson, C.R. (1993). Effect of iron-folate supplementation on serum copper concentration in late pregnancy. *Acta Obstet. Gynecol. Scand.* 72, 616.

Burrell, L.M. (1997). A risk-benefit assessment of losartan potassium in the treatment of hypertension. *Drug Saf.* 16, 56.

Bush, M.E. and Dahms, B.B. (1984). Fatal hypervitaminosis A in a neonate. *Arch. Pathol. Lab. Med.* 108, 838.

Bushinsky, D.A. and Gennari, F.J. (1986). Life-threatening hyperkalemia induced by arginine. *Ann. Intern. Med.* 89, 632.

Bussien, J.P., d'More, T.F., Perret, L., *et al.* (1986). Single and repeated dosing of the converting enzyme inhibitor perindopril to normal subjects. *Clin. Pharmacol. Ther.* 39, 554.

Butterworth, C.E., Jr, Hatch, K., Cole, P., *et al.* (1988). Zinc concentration in plasma and erythrocytes of subjects receiving folic acid supplementation. *Am. J. Clin. Nutr.* 47, 484.

Butterworth C.E., Jr, Hatch, K.D., Macaluso, M., *et al.* (1992). Folate deficiency and cervical dysplasia. *JAMA* 267, 528.

Butterworth, R.F., Gaudreau, C., Vincelette, J., *et al.* (1991). Thiamine deficiency and Wernicke's encephalopathy in AIDS. *Metab. Brain Dis.* 6, 207.

Byatt, C.M., Millard, P.H., and Levin, G.E. (1990). Diuretics and electrolyte disturbances in 1000 consecutive geriatric admissions. *J. R. Soc. Med.* 83, 704.

Byrne, P.M., Freaney, R., and McKenna, M.J. (1995). Vitamin D supplementation in the elderly: review of safety and effectiveness of different regimes. *Calcif. Tissue Int.* 56, 518.

Caddell, J.L. and Olson, R.E. (1973). An evaluation of the electrolyte status of malnourished Thai children. *J. Pediatr.* 83, 124.

Caldwell, J.W., Nava, A.J., and de Haas D.D. (1987). Hypernatremia associated with cathartics in overdose management. *West. J. Med.* 147, 593.

Calic, R., Straus, B., and Cepelak, I. (1989). Changes of activities of some transferases, alkaline phosphatase and cholinesterase in the blood of women using oral contraceptives and *in vitro* influence of these agents on tissular enzyme levels in rat liver. *Z. Med. Lab. Diagn.* 30, 375.

Callaghan, T.S., Hadden, D.R., and Tomkin, G.H. (1980). Megaloblastic anaemia due to vitamin B$_{12}$ malabsorption associated with long-term metformin treatment. *BMJ* 280, 1214.

Callegari, P.E. (1997). Is there cyclosporine-induced bone disease? *J. Clin. Rheumatol.* 3, S93.

Calvert, G.M., Sweeney, M.H., Fingerhut, M.A., *et al.* (1994). Evaluation of porphyria cutanea tarda in U.S. workers exposed to 2,3,7,8-tetrachlorodibenzo-p-dioxin. *Am. J. Ind. Med.* 25, 559.

Campbell, I.W. (1985). Metformin and the sulphonylureas: the comparative risk. *Horm. Metab. Res.* Suppl. 15, 105.

Campbell, R.K., White, J.R., Jr, and Saulie, B.A. (1996). Metformin: a new oral biguanide. *Clin. Ther.* 18, 360.

Campbell, R.W. (1987). Mexiletine. *N. Engl. J. Med.* 316, 29.

Campfield, T. and Braden, G. (1989). Urinary oxalate excretion by very low birth weight infants receiving parenteral nutrition. *Pediatrics* 84, 860.

Canterall, M.C., Fort, J., Camps, J., *et al.* (1987). Acute intoxication due to topical application of diethyl glycol. *Ann. Intern. Med.* 106, 478.

Cantini, F., Niccoli, L., Bellandi, F., *et al.* (1995). Effects of short-term, high dose, heparin therapy on biochemical markers of bone metabolism. *Clin. Rheumatol.* 14, 663.

Caporali, R., Gentile, S., Caprotti, M., *et al.* (1991). Serum osteocalcin (bone Gla-protein) and steroid osteoporosis in rheumatoid arthritis. *J. Rheumatol.* 18, 148.

Capurso, A. (1991). Drugs affecting triglycerides. *Cardiology* 78, 218.

Carey, H.M. (1971). Principles of oral contraception: 2 side effects of oral contraceptives. *Med. J. Aust.* 2, 1242.

Carl, G.F. and Smith, M.L. (1992). Phenytoin-folate interactions: differing effects of the sodium salt and the free acid of phenytoin. *Epilepsia* 33, 372.

Carl, P., Crawford, M.E., Madsen, N.B., *et al.* (1987). Pain relief after major abdominal surgery: a double-blind controlled comparison of sublingual buprenorphine, intramuscular buprenorphine, and intramuscular meperidine. *Anesth. Analg.* 66, 142.

Carlisle, E.J., Donnelly, S.M., Vasuvattakul, S., *et al.* (1991). Glue-sniffing and distal renal tubular acidosis: sticking to the facts. *J. Am. Soc. Nephrol.* 1, 1019.

Carlsen, J.E., Kober, L., Torp-Pedersen, C., *et al.* (1990). Relation between dose of bendrofluazide, antihypertensive effect, and adverse biochemical effects. *BMJ* 300, 975.

Carlsson, E., Fellenius, E., Lundborg, P., *et al.* (1978). β-Adrenoceptor blockers, plasma potassium and exercise. *Lancet* ii, 424.

Carlsson, E.C., Rudolph, A., Stanger, P., *et al.* (1985). Pediatric angiocardiography with cohexol. *Invest. Radiol.* 20 (Suppl. 1), 575.

Carmel, R. (1995). Malabsorption of food cobalamin. *Baillière's Clin. Haematol.* 8, 639.

Carmel, R., Rabinowitz, A.P., and Mazumder, A. (1993). Metabolic evidence of cobalamin deficiency in bone marrow cells harvested for transplantation from donors given nitrous oxide. *Eur. J. Haematol.* 50, 228.

Carmel, R., Howard, J.M., Green, R., *et al.* (1996). Hormone replacement therapy and cobalamin status in elderly women. *Am. J. Clin. Nutr.* 64, 856.

Caron, J., Libersa, C., and Thomas, C. (1996). Drugs affecting blood clotting, fibrinolysis and hemostasis. In *Meyler's Side Effects of Drugs* (ed. M.N.G. Dukes), p. 1008. Elsevier, Amsterdam.

Castelbaum, A.R., Donofrio, P.D., Walker, F.O., *et al.* (1989). Laxative abuse causing hypermagnesemia, quadriparesis, and neuromuscular junction defect. *Neurology* 39, 746.

Castrillon, J.L., Mediavilla, A., Mendez, M.A., *et al.* (1993). Syndrome of inappropriate antidiuretic hormone secretion (SIADH) and enalapril. *J. Intern. Med.* 233, 89.

Cersosimo, R.J. and Lee, J.M. (1996). Creatine kinase elevation associated with 5-fluorouracil and levamisole therapy for carcinoma of the colon: a case report. *Cancer* 77, 1250.

Chakrabarti, R., Fearnley, G.R., and Evans, J.F. (1968). Effects of clofibrate on fibrinolysis, platelet stickiness, plasma-fibrinogen, and serum cholesterol. *Lancet* ii, 1007.

Chalmers, T.M. (1971). Clinical experience with ibuprofen in rheumatoid arthritis. *Schweiz. Med. Wochenschr.* 101, 280.

Chan, M.K., Beale, D., and Moorhead, J.F. (1980). Acute megaloblastosis due to cotrimoxazole. *Br. J. Clin. Pract.* 34, 187.

Chan, T.Y., Lee, K.K., Chan, A.Y., *et al.* (1995). Poisoning due to Chinese proprietary medicines. *Hum. Exp. Toxicol.* 14, 434.

Chanarin, I. (1980). Cobalamins and nitrous oxide: a review. *J. Clin. Pathol.* 33, 909.

Chapron, D.L., Gomolin, I.H., and Sweeney, K.R. (1989). Acetazolamide blood concentrations are excessive in the elderly: propensity for acidosis and relationship to renal function. *J. Clin. Pharmacol.* 29, 348.

Chapuy, M.C. and Meunier, P.J. (1990). Metabolic basis of vitamin D intoxication. In *The Metabolic and Molecular Basis of Acquired Disease* (ed. R.D. Cohen, B. Lewis,

K.G.M. Alberti and A.M. Denman), p. 1824. Baillière Tindall, London.

Chazan, R., Tadeusiak, W., Jaworski, A., *et al.* (1992). Creatine kinase (CK) and creatine kinase isoenzyme (CK-MB) acitivity in serum before and after intravenous salbutamol administration of patients with bronchial asthma. *Int. J. Clin. Pharmacol. Ther. Toxicol.* 30, 371.

Chazan, R., Jaworski, A., Tadeusiak, W., *et al.* (1994). Comparative study of the influence of ipratropium bromide versus salbutamol on the creatine kinase (CK) and creatine kinase isoenzyme CK-MB activity in serum of patients with bronchial asthma. *Pneumonologia i Allergologia Polska* 62, 70.

Chen, B., Shapira, J., Ravid, M., *et al.* (1982). Steatorrhoea induced by allopurinol. *BMJ* i, 1914.

Chen, L.H. (1981). An increase in vitamin E requirement induced by high supplementation of vitamin C in rats. *Am. J. Clin. Nutr.* 34, 1036.

Chertow, G.M., Seifter, J.L., Christiansen, C.L., *et al.* (1996). Trimethoprim-sulfamethoxazole and hypouricemia. *Clin. Nephrol.* 46, 193.

Chilvers, D.C., Jones, M.M., Selby, P.L., *et al.* (1985). Effects of oral ethinyl oestradiol and norethisterone on plasma copper and zinc complexes in post-menopausal women. *Horm. Metab. Res.* 17, 532.

Chimata, M., Masaoka, H., Fujimaki, M., *et al.* (1994). Low serum aminotransferase activity in patients undergoing regular hemodialysis. *Jpn J. Nephrol.* 36, 389.

Chin, L., Sievers, M.L., Herrier, R.N., *et al.* (1979). Convulsion as the etiology of lactic acidosis in acute isoniazid toxicity in dogs. *Toxicol. Appl. Pharmacol.* 49, 377.

Chines, A. and Pacifici, R. (1990). Antacid and sucralfate-induced hypophosphatemic osteomalacia: a case report and review of the literature. *Calcif. Tiss. Int.* 47, 291.

Chisolm, J.J. (1990). Evaluation of the potential role of chelation-therapy in treatment of low to moderate lead exposures. *Environ. Health Perspect.* 89, 67.

Choi, M.J., Fernandez, P.C., Patnaik, A., *et al.* (1993). Brief report: trimethoprim-induced hyperkalaemia in a patient with AIDS. *N. Engl. J. Med.* 328, 703.

Choudhary, P.P. and Hughes, R.A. (1995). Long-term treatment of chronic inflammatory demyelinating polyradiculo-neuropathy with plasma exchange or intravenous immuno-globulin. *Q. J. Med.* 88, 493.

Citrin, D.L., Wallemark, C.B., Nadler, R., *et al.* (1986). Estramustine affects bone mineral metabolism in metastatic prostate cancer. *Cancer* 58, 2208.

Clark, B.A. and Brown, R.S. (1992). Unsuspected morbid hypermagnesemia in elderly patients. *Am. J. Nephrol.* 12, 336.

Clemessy, J.L., Favier, C., Borron, S.W., *et al.* (1995). Hypokalaemia related to acute chloroquine ingestion. *Lancet* 346, 877.

Cohen, J., Shmueli, D., Keslin, J., *et al.* (1997). Acute beriberi following liver transplantation. *Clin. Nutr.* 16, 85.

Cohen, S.M., Wexner, S.D., Binderow, S.R., *et al.* (1994).

Prospective, randomized, endoscopic-blinded trial comparing precolonoscopy bowel cleansing methods. *Dis. Colon Rectum* 37, 689.

Cohn, J., Balk, R.A. and Bone, R.C. (1990). Dialysis-induced respiratory acidosis. *Chest* 98, 1285.

Connell, J.M., Rapeport, W.G., Gordon, S., *et al.* (1984*a*). Changes in circulating thyroid hormones during short-term hepatic enzyme induction with carbamazepine. *Eur. J. Clin. Pharmacol.* 26, 453.

Connell, J.M., Rapeport, W.G., Beastall, G.H., *et al.* (1984*b*). Changes in circulating androgens during short term carbamazepine therapy. *Br. J. Clin. Pharmacol.* 17, 347.

Connelly, D.M. (1970). Silver nitrate. Ideal burn wound therapy? *N.Y. State J. Med.* 70, 1642-1644.

Cooper, C., Coupland, C., and Mitchell, M. (1995). Rheumatoid arthritis, corticosteroid therapy and hip fracture. *Ann. Rheum. Dis.* 54, 49.

Copeland, P.M., Martin, J.B., and Ridgway, E.C. (1986). Cysteamine decreases prolactin responsiveness to thyrotropin-releasing hormone in normal men. *Am. J. Med. Sci.* 291, 16.

Corbett, J.J., Jacobson, D.M., Thompson, H.S., *et al.* (1989). Downbeating nystagmus and other ocular motor defects caused by lithium toxicity. *Neurology* 39, 481.

Coulson, I.H. and Misch, K. (1989). Fosfestrol-induced porphyria cutanea tarda. *Br. J. Urol.* 63, 648.

Cousins, M.J., Gourlay, G.K., Knights, K.M., *et al.* (1987). A randomized prospective controlled study of the metabolism and hepatotoxicity of halothane in humans. *Anesth. Analg.* 66, 299.

Cowan, R.A., Hartnell, G.G., Lowdell C.P., *et al.* (1984). Metabolic acidosis induced by carbonic anhydrase inhibitors and salicylates in patients with normal renal function. *BMJ* 289, 347.

Cowan, R.E. and Wright, J.T. (1981). Dapsone and severe hypoalbuminaemia in dermatitis herpetiformis. *Br. J. Dermatol.* 104, 201.

Crabb, D.W. (1990). Biological markers for increased risk of alcoholism and for quantitation of alcohol consumption. *J. Clin. Invest.* 85, 311.

Craig, J.C., Hodson, E.M. and Martin, H.C. (1994). Phosphate enema poisoning in children. *Med. J. Aust.* 160, 347.

Cravo, M.L., Gloria, L.M., Selhub, J., *et al.* (1996). Hyperhomocysteinemia in chronic alcoholism: correlation with folate, vitamin B-12, and vitamin B-6 status. *Am. J. Clin. Nutr.* 63, 220.

Creemers, M.C., Chang, A., Franssen, M.J., *et al.* (1995). Pseudoporphyria due to naproxen. A cluster of 3 cases. *Scand. J. Rheumatol.* 24, 185.

Crilly, R., Cawood, M., Marshall, D.H., *et al.* (1978). Hormonal status in normal, osteoporotic and corticosteroid-treated postmenopausal women. *J. R. Soc. Med.* 71, 733.

Crofford, O.B. (1995). Metformin. *N. Engl. J. Med.* 333, 588.

Cronin, J.W., Kroop, S.F., Diamond, J., *et al.* (1984). Alkalemia in diabetic ketoacidosis. *Am. J. Med.* 77, 192.

Crook, M.A. and Swaminathan, R. (1996). Disorders of plasma phosphate and indications for its measurement. *Ann. Clin. Biochem.* 33, 376.

Crook, M.A., Collins, D., and Swaminathan, R. (1996). Severe hypophosphataemia related to refeeding. *Nutrition* 12, 538.

Crozier, I.G., Ikram, H., Nicholls, M.G., *et al.* (1987). Acute hemodynamic, hormonal and electrolyte effects of ramipril in severe congestive heart failure. *Am. J. Cardiol.* 59, 155D.

Cullberg, C. (1974). Androgenic, anabolic, estrogenic and antiestrogenic effects of desogestrel and lynestrenol: effects on serum proteins and vaginal cytology. *Contraception* 30, 73.

Cummings, C.C. and McIvor, M.E. (1988). Fluoride-induced hyperkalemia: the role of Ca^{2+}-dependent K^+ channels. *Am. J. Emerg. Med.* 6, 1.

Cundy, T., Cornish, J., Evans, M.C., *et al.* (1994). Recovery of bone density in women who stop using medroxyprogesterone acetate. *BMJ* 308, 247.

Cunliffe, W.J., Berth-Jones, J., Claudy, A., *et al.* (1992). Comparative study of calcipotriol (MC 903) ointment and betamethasone 17-valerate ointment in patients with psoriasis vulgaris. *J. Am. Acad. Dermatol.* 26, 736.

Cunningham, S.K., Loughlin, T., Culliton, M., *et al.* (1985). The relationship between sex steroids and sex hormone-binding globulin in plasma in physiological and pathological conditions. *Ann. Clin. Biochem.* 22, 489.

Cutolo, M., Accardo, S., Cimmino, M.A., *et al.* (1982). Hypocupremia-related hypochromic anemia during D-penicillamine treatment. *Arthritis Rheum.* 25, 119.

Dahlman, T.C. (1993). Osteoporotic fractures and the recurrence of thromboembolism during pregnancy and the puerperium in 184 women undergoing thromboprophylaxis with heparin. *Am. J. Obstet. Gynecol.* 168, 1265.

Dahlman, T., Lindvall, N., and Hellgren, M. (1990). Osteopenia in pregnancy during long-term heparin treatment: a radiological study post partum. *Br. J. Obstet. Gynaecol.* 97, 221.

Dahlman, T.C., Sjoberg, H.E., and Ringertz, H. (1994). Bone mineral density during long-term prophylaxis with heparin in pregnancy. *Am. J. Obstet. Gynecol.* 170, 1315.

Dalton, T.A. and Berry, R.S. (1992). Hepatotoxicity associated with sustained-release niacin. *Am. J. Med.* 93, 102.

Dam, M. (1994). Practical aspects of oxcarbazepine treatment. *Epilepsia* 35 Suppl. 3, S23.

Daudon, M., Reveillaud, R.J., Normand, M., *et al.* (1987). Piridoxilate-induced calcium oxalate calculi: a new drug-induced metabolic nephrolithiasis. *J. Urol.* 138, 258.

Daugaard, G. (1990). Cisplatin nephrotoxicity: experimental and clinical studies. *Dan. Med. Bull.* 37, 1.

Daugaard, G. (1993). Tamoxifen and hypercalcaemia. *Ann. Oncol.* 4, 683.

Daugaard, G., Strandgaard, S., Holstein-Rathlou, N.H., *et al.* (1987). The renal handling of sodium and water is not affected by the standard-dose cisplatin treatment for testicular cancer. *Scand. J. Clin. Lab. Invest.* 47, 455.

Davey, P.G., Geddes, A.M., and Cowley, D.M. (1983). Study of alanine aminopeptidase excretion as a test of gentamicin nephrotoxicity. *J. Antimicrob. Chemother.* 11, 455.

Davidkova, T., Kikuchi, H., Fujii, K., *et al.* (1988). Biotransformation of isoflurane: Urinary and serum fluoride ion and organic fluorine. *Anesthesiology* 69, 218.

Davies, D.L. and Fraser, R. (1993). Do diuretics cause magnesium deficiency? *Br. J. Clin. Pharmacol.* 36, 1.

Davies, J.P. Bentley, P., and Ghose, R.R. (1989). Aminoglutethimide-induced hyperkalaemia. *Br. J. Clin. Pract.* 43, 263.

Davies, P.H. and Franklyn, J.A. (1991). The effects of drugs on tests of thyroid function. *Eur. J. Clin. Pharmacol.* 40, 439.

Davtyan, D.G., and Vinters H.V. (1987). Wernicke's encephalopathy in AIDS patient treated with zidovudine. *Lancet* i, 919.

Dawood, M.Y., Ramos, J., and Khan-Dawood, F.S. (1995). Depot leuprolide acetate versus danazol for treatment of pelvic endometriosis: changes in vertebral bone mass and serum estradiol and calcitonin. *Fertil. Steril.* 63, 1177.

Day, A.P., Feher, M.D., Chopra, R., *et al.* (1993). The effect of bezafibrate treatment on serum alkaline phosphatase isoenzyme activities. *Metabolism* 42, 839.

Day, N.P., Phu, N.H., Bethell, D.P., *et al.* (1996). The effects of dopamine and adrenaline infusions on acid-base balance and systemic haemodynamics in severe infection. *Lancet* 348, 219.

D'costa, D.F., Basu, S.K., and Gunasekera, N.P.R. (1990). ACE inhibitors and diuretics causing hypokalaemia. *Br. J. Clin. Pract.* 44, 26.

de Fronzo, R.A. and Goodman, A.M. (1995). Multicentre Metformin Study Group. Efficacy of metformin in patients with non-insulin-dependent diabetes mellitus. *N. Engl. J. Med.* 333, 541.

De Luca, F., Arrigo, T., Pandullo, E., *et al.* (1986). Changes in thyroid function tests induced by 2 month carbamazepine treatment in L-thyroxine-substituted hypothyroid children. *Eur. J. Pediatr.* 145, 77.

De Maat, M.P.M., Arnold, A.E.R., Van Buuren, S., *et al.* (1996). Modulation of plasma fibrinogen levels by ticlopidine in healthy volunteers and patients with stable angina pectoris. *Thromb. Haemost.* 76, 166.

De Maat, M.P.M., Knipscheer, H.C., Kastelein, J.J.P., *et al.* (1997). Modulation of plasma fibrinogen levels by ciprofibrate and gemfibrozil in primary hyperlipidaemia. *Thromb. Haemost.* 77, 75.

Dechant, K.L. and Goa, K.L. (1994). Calcitriol. A review of its use in the treatment of postmenopausal osteoporosis and its potential in corticosteroid-induced osteoporosis. *Drugs and Aging* 5, 300.

Degenring, F.H., Schatton, W., and Hotz, W. (1983). Atherosklerose-Behandlung mit Etofibrat retard. Neue Perspektiven. *Fortschr. Med.* 101, 1391.

del Giglio, A., Zukiwski, A.A., Ali, M.K., *et al.* (1991). Severe, symptomatic, dose-limiting hypophosphatemia induced by hepatic arterial infusion of recombinant tumor necrosis factor in patients with liver metastases. *Cancer* 67, 2459.

Delangre, T., Vernier, L., Moore, N., *et al.* (1990). Rhabdomyolyse aiguë au cours d'un traitement par le ciprofibrate. *Presse Méd.* 19, 1811.

Delany, A.M., Dong, Y., and Canalis, E. (1994). Mechanisms of glucocorticoid action in bone cells. *J. Cell. Biochem.* 56, 295.

Delport, R., Ubbink, J.B., Serfontein, W.J., *et al.* 1988). Vitamin B6 nutritional status in asthma. The effect of theophylline therapy on plasma pyridoxal-5-phosphate and pyridoxal levels. *Int. J. Vit. Nutr. Res.* 58, 67.

Delrio, F.G., Park, Y., Herzlich, B., *et al.* (1996). Case report: diclofenac-induced rhabdomyolysis. *Am. J. Med. Sci.* 312, 95.

Demedts, P., Theunis, L., Wauters, A., *et al.* (1994). Excess serum osmolality gap after ingestion of methanol: a methodology-associated phenomenon? *Clin. Chem.* 40, 1587.

Demers, R.G., McDonagh, P.H., and Moore, R.J. (1984). Pyridoxine deficiency with phenelzine. *South. Med. J.* 77, 641.

Demey, H.E., Daelemans, R.A., Verpooten, G.A., *et al.* (1988). Propylene-glycol induced side effects during intravenous nitroglycerin therapy. *Intens. Care Med.* 14, 221.

Deray, G., Benhmida, M., Hoang, P.L., *et al.* (1992). Renal function and blood pressure in patients receiving long-term, low- dose cyclosporine therapy for idiopathic autoimmune uveitis. *Ann. Intern. Med.* 117, 578.

Deslypere, J.P. and Vermeulen, A. (1991). Rhabdomyolysis and simvastatin. *Ann. Intern. Med.* 114, 342.

Devenport, M.H., Crook, D., Wynn, V., *et al.* (1989). Metabolic effects of low-dose fluconazole in healthy female users and non-users of oral contraceptives. *Br. J. Clin. Pharmacol.* 27, 851.

Deyssig, R. and Weissel, M. (1993). Ingestion of androgenic-anabolic steroids induces mild thyroidal impairment in male body builders. *J. Clin. Endocrinol. Metab.* 76, 1069.

Dhani, M.S., Drangova, R., Farkas, R., *et al.* (1979). Decreased aminotransferase activity of serum and various tissues in the rat after cefazolin treatment. *Clin. Chem.* 25, 1263.

Diamond, T., McGuigan, L., Barbagallo, S., *et al.* (1995). Cyclical etidronate plus ergocalciferol prevents glucocorticoid-induced bone loss in postmenopausal women. *Am. J. Med.* 98, 459.

DiBianco, R. (1986). Adverse reactions with angiotensin converting enzyme (ACE) inhibitors. *Med. Toxicol.* 1, 122.

Dickinson, R.J. and Swaminathan, R. (1978). Total body potassium depletion and renal tubular dysfunction following carbenoxolone therapy. *Postgrad. Med. J.* 54, 836.

Dietrichson, O. (1975). Chronic active hepatitis: aetiological considerations based on clinical and serological studies. *Scand. J. Gastroenterol.* 10, 617.

Diggory, P., Cassels-Brown, A., Vail, A., *et al.* (1995). Avoiding unsuspected respiratory side-effects of topical timolol with cardioselective or sympathomimetic agents. *Lancet* 345, 1604.

Dirix, L.Y., Moeremans, C., Fierens, H., *et al.* (1988). Symptomatic hyponatremia related to the use of propafenone. *Acta Clin. Belg.* 43, 143.

DiSilvio, T.V. (1978). Alcoholic myopathy and changes in serum enzyme activity. *Clin. Chem.* 24, 1653.

Doman, K., Perlmutter, J.A., Muhammedi, M., *et al.* (1993). Life-threatening hyperkalemia associated with captopril administration. *South. Med. J.* 86, 1269.

Dodig, S., Cepelak, I., Demirovic, J., *et al.* (1994). A study of some enzyme activities associated with theophylline administration. *Acta Pharmaceutica* 44, 45.

Domingo, P., Ferrer, S., Cruz, J., *et al.* (1995). Trimethoprim–sulfamethoxazole-induced renal tubular acidosis in a patient with AIDS. *Clin. Infect. Dis.* 20, 1435.

Dorup, I. (1994). Magnesium and potassium deficiency. Its diagnosis, occurrence and treatment in diuretic therapy and its consequences for growth, protein synthesis and growth factors. *Acta Physiologica Scand.* Suppl. 618, 1.

Dougados, M., Boumier, P., and Amor, B. (1987). Traitement de la spondylarthrite ankylosante par la salazosulfapyridine. Une étude en double aveugle controlée chez 60 malades. *Rev. Rhum. Mal. Ostéoartic.* 54, 255.

Douglas, A.S., Robins, S.P., Hutchison, J.D., *et al.* (1995). Carboxylation of osteocalcin in post-menopausal osteoporotic women following vitamin K and D supplementation. *Bone* 17, 15.

Douketis, J.D., Ginsberg, J.S., Burrows, R.F., *et al.* (1996). The effects of long-term heparin therapy during pregnancy on bone density. a prospective matched cohort study. *Thromb. Haemost.* 75, 254.

Down, P.F., Polak, A., and Regan, R.J. (1979). A family with massive acute vitamin D intoxication. *Postgrad. Med J.* 55, 897.

Downer, S., Joel, S., Allbright, A., *et al.* (1993). A double blind placebo controlled trial of medroxyprogesterone acetate (mpa) in cancer cachexia. *Br. J. Cancer* 67, 1102.

Druml, W., Kleinberger, G., Lenz, K., *et al.* (1986). Fructose-induced hyperlactemia in hyperosmolar syndromes. *Klin. Wochenschr.* 64, 615.

Dubick, M.A., Conteas, C.N., Billy, H.T., *et al.* (1987). Raised serum concentrations of pancreatic enzymes in cigarette smokers. *Gut* 28, 330.

DuBose, T.D., Jr, Cogan, M.G., and Rector, F.C., Jr. (1996). *Acid-Base Disorders. The Kidney* (ed. B.M. Brenner), p. 929. W.B.Saunders, Philadelphia.

Dujovne, C.A., Azarnoff, D.L., Huffman, D.H., *et al.* (1976). One-year trials with halofenate, clofibrate and placebo. *Clin. Pharmacol. Ther.* 19, 352.

Dukes, G.E., Sanders, S.W., Russo J.J., *et al.* (1984). Transaminase elevations in patients receiving bovine or porcine heparin. *Ann. Intern. Med.* 100, 646.

Dukes, M.N.G. (1996*a*). Metals. In *Meyler's Side Effects of Drugs* (ed. M.N.G. Dukes), p.583. Elsevier, Amsterdam.

Dukes, M.N.G. (1996*b*). Sex hormones. In *Meyler's Side Effects of Drugs* (ed. M.N.G. Dukes), p.1248. Elsevier, Amsterdam.

Dukes, M.N.G. (1996*c*). Anticonvulsants. In *Meyler's Side Effects of Drugs* (ed. M.N.G. Dukes), p. 136. Elsevier, Amsterdam.

Dunn, A.M. and Buckley, D.M. (1986). Non-steroidal anti-inflammatory drugs and the kidney. *BMJ* 293, 202.

Dwyer, C. and Chapman, R.S. (1991). Calcipotriol and hypercalcaemia. *Lancet* 338, 764.

Dyckner, T. (1990). Relation of cardiovascular disease to potassium and magnesium deficiencies. *Am. J. Cardiol.* 65, 44.

Dykman, T.R., Gluck, O.S., Murphy, W.A., *et al.* (1985). Evaluation of factors associated with glucocorticoid-induced osteopenia in patients with rheumatic diseases. *Arthritis Rheum.* 28, 361.

Earthman, T.P., Odom, L., and Mullins, C.A. (1991). Lactic acidosis associated with high-dose niacin therapy. *South. Med. J.* 84, 496.

Eastell, R. (1995). Management of corticosteroid-induced osteoporosis. UK Consensus Group Meeting on Osteoporosis. *J. Intern. Med.* 237, 439.

Eckford, S.D., Swami, K.S., Jackson, S.R., *et al.* (1994). Desmopressin in the treatment of nocturia and enuresis in patients with multiple sclerosis. *Br. J. Urol.* 74, 733.

Edelman, S. and Witztum, J.L. (1989). Hyperkalemia during treatment with HMG-CoA reductase inhibitor. *N. Engl. J. Med.* 320, 1219.

Einarson, T.R., Turchet, E.N., Goldstein, J.E., *et al.* (1985). Gout-like arthritis following cimetidine and ranitidine. *DICP* 19, 201.

Elder, G.H., Hift, R.J., and Meissner, P.N. (1997). The acute porphyrias. *Lancet* 349, 1613.

Elisaf, M., Merkouropoulos, M., Tsianos, E.V., *et al.* (1994). Acid-base and electrolyte abnormalities in alcoholic patients. *Miner. Electrolyte Metab.* 20, 274.

Elliott, H.L. (1996). Antihypertensive drugs. In *Meyler's Side Effects of Drugs* (ed. M.N.G. Dukes), p. 546. Elsevier, Amsterdam.

Ellis, C.N., Fradin, M.S., Messana, J.M., *et al.* (1991). Cyclosporine for plaque-type psoriasis. results of a multidose, double-blind trial. *N. Engl. J. Med.* 324, 277.

Ellis, P.M. and Tattersall, M.H.N. (1995). Tamoxifen flare — an unusual case of hypercalcaemia and transient rapidly progressive pancytopenia. *Aust. N.Z. J. Med.* 25, 375.

Emmerson, B.T. (1996). Drug therapy: the management of gout. *N. Engl. J. Med.* 334, 445.

Emmett, M., Sirmon, M.D., Kirkpatrick, W.G., *et al.* (1991). Calcium acetate control of serum phosphorus in hemodialysis patients. *Am. J. Kidney Dis.* 17, 544.

Epstein, R.S. (1989). Wernicke's encephalopathy following lithium-induced diarrhea. *Am. .J. Psychiatry* 146, 806.

Epstein, S. and Shane, E. (1996). Transplantation osteoporosis. In *Osteoporosis* (ed. R. Marcus, D. Feldman, and J. Kelsey), p. 947. Academic Press, California.

Epstein, S., Shane, E., and Bilezikian, J.P. (1995). Organ transplantation and osteoporosis. *Curr. Opin. Rheumatol.* 7, 255.

Ernst, E. (1992). Oral contraceptives, fibrinogen and cardiovascular risk. *Atherosclerosis* 93, 1.

Erramouspe, J., Galvez, R., and Fischel, D.R. (1996). Newborn renal tubular acidosis associated with prenatal maternal toluene sniffing. *J. Psychoactive Drugs* 28, 201.

Erstad, B.L., Campbell, D.J., Rollins, C.J., *et al.* (1994). Albumin and prealbumin concentrations in patients receiving postoperative parenteral nutrition. *Pharmacotherapy* 14, 458.

Eschbach, J.W., Abdulhadi, M.H., Browne, J.K., *et al.* (1989). Recombinant human erythropoietin in anemic patients with end-stage renal disease. Results of a phase III multicenter clinical trial. *Ann. Intern. Med.* 111, 992.

Ettinger, B., Tang, A., Citron, J.T., *et al.* (1986). Randomized trial of allopurinol in the prevention of calcium oxalate calculi. *N. Engl. J. Med.* 315, 1386.

Ettinger, L.J., Gaynon, P.S., Krailo, M.D., *et al.* (1994). A phase II study of carboplatin in children with recurrent or progressive solid tumors. A report from the Childrens Cancer Group. *Cancer* 73, 1297.

European Multicentre Trial. (1982). Cyclosporin A as sole immunosuppressive agent in recipients of kidney allografts from cadaver donors. *Lancet* ii, 57.

Evans, L.S., and Kleiman, M.B. (1986). Acidosis as a presenting feature of chloramphenicol toxicity. *J. Pediatr.* 108, 475.

Evans, R.T. (1986). Cholinesterase phenotyping: clinical aspects and laboratory applications. *Crit. Rev. Clin. Lab. Sci.* 23, 35.

Faller, J. and Fox, I.H. (1982). Ethanol induced hyperuricemia: evidence for increased urate production by activation of adenine nucleotide turn over. *N. Engl. J. Med.* 307, 1598.

Faraj, J.H. (1989). Hyperosmolality due to antacid treatment. *Anaesthesia* 44, 911.

Farese, R.V., Jr, Biglieri, E.G., Shackleton, C.H., *et al.* (1991). Licorice-induced hypermineralocorticoidism. *N. Engl. J. Med.* 325, 1223.

Farley, T.A. (1986). Severe hypernatremic dehydration after use of an activated charcoal–sorbitol suspension. *J. Pediatr.* 109, 719.

Farr, M., Symmons, D.P., and Bacon, P.A. (1985). Raised serum alkaline phosphatase and aspartate transaminase levels in two rheumatoid patients treated with sulphasalazine. *Ann. Rheum. Dis.* 44, 798.

Fass, R., Do, S., and Hixson, L.J. (1993). Fatal hyperphosphatemia following Fleet Phospo-Soda in a patient with colonic ileus. *Am. J. Gastroenterol.* 88, 929.

Fassler, C.A., Rodriguez, R.M., Badesch, D.B., *et al.* (1985). Magnesium toxicity as a cause of hypotension and hypoventilation. Occurrence in patients with normal renal function. *Arch. Intern. Med.* 145, 1604.

Feely, J. (1981). Propranolol and the hypercalcaemia of thyrotoxicosis. *Acta Endocrinol.* 98, 528.

Feinstein, E.I., Quion, V.H., Kaptein, E.M., *et al.* (1984). Severe hyperuricemia in patients with volume depletion. *Am. J. Nephrol.* 48, 77.

Feldman, D., Mallory, P.J., and Gross, C. (1996). Vitamin D: metabolism and action. In *Osteoporosis* (ed. R. Marcus, D. Feldman, and J. Kelsey), p. 205. Academic Press, California.

Fentiman, I.S. and Fogelman, I. (1993). Breast cancer and osteoporosis — a bridge at last. *Eur. J. Cancer* 29A, 485.

Fentiman, I.S., Caleffi, M., Rodin, A., *et al.* (1989). Bone mineral content of women receiving tamoxifen for mastalgia. *Br. J. Cancer* 60, 262.

Ferdinandus, J., Pederson, J.A., and Whang R. (1981). Hypermagnesemia as a cause of refractor hypotension, respiratory depression and coma. *Arch. Intern. Med.* 141, 669.

Ferrari, C., Testori, G., Scanni, A., *et al.* (1976). Reduction of serum alkaline phosphatase and gamma-glutamyl transpeptidase activities by short-term clofibrate. *N. Engl. J. Med.* 295, 449.

Fiaccadori, E., Coffrini, E., Fracchia, C., *et al.* (1994). Hypophosphatemia and phosphorus depletion in respiratory and peripheral muscles of patients with respiratory failure due to COPD. *Chest* 105, 1392.

Filejski, W., Kurowski, V., Batge, B., *et al.* (1993). Klinischer Verlauf und Therapie einer massiven Theophyllin-Intoxikation. *Dtsch. Med. Wochenschr.* 118, 1641.

Fishbane, S., Frei, G.L., Finger, M., *et al.* (1995). Hypervitaminosis A in two hemodialysis patients. *Am. J. Kidney Dis.* 25, 346.

Fiske, D.N., McCoy, H.E., and Kitchens, C.S. (1994). Zinc-induced sideroblastic anemia: report of a case, review of the literature, and description of the hematologic syndrome. *Am. J. Hematol.* 46, 147.

Fitzgerald, G.R., Delaney, E., Cushen, M., *et al.* (1989). Diuretic-associated hypokalaemia in hospital admissions. *Research Clinical Forums* 11, 49.

Fitzpatrick, J.M., Kasidas, G.P., and Rose, G.A. (1981). Hyperoxaluria following glycine irrigation for transurethral prostatectomy. *Br. J. Urol.* 53, 250.

Flack, J.M., Ryder, K.W., Strickland, D., *et al.* (1994). Metabolic correlates of theophylline therapy: a concentration-related phenomenon. *Ann. Pharmacother.* 28, 175.

Fogari, R., Zoppi, A., Malamani, G.D., *et al.* (1995). Effects of different antihypertensive drugs on plasma fibrinogen in hypertensive patients. *Br. J. Clin. Pharmacol.* 39, 471.

Fogelman, I. (1992). Gonadotropin-releasing hormone agonists and the skeleton. *Fertil. Steril.* 57, 715.

Folb, P.I. (1996). Cytostatics and immunsuppressive drugs. In *Meyler's Side Effects of Drugs* (ed. M.N.G. Dukes), p. 1336. Elsevier, Amsterdam.

Foldes, J., Balena, R., Ho, A., *et al.* (1991). Hypophosphatemic rickets with hypocalciuria following long-term treatment with aluminum-containing antacid. *Bone* 12, 67.

Foo, Y. and Konecny, P. (1997). Hyperamylasaemia in asymptomatic HIV patients. *Ann. Clin. Biochem.* 34, 259.

Forastiere, A.A., Belliveau, J.F., Goren, M.P., *et al.* (1988). Pharmacokinetic and toxicity evaluation of five-day continuous infusion versus intermittent bolus *cis*-diamminedichloroplatinum(II) in head and neck cancer patients. *Cancer Res.* 48, 3869.

Foster, J.E., Harpur, E.S., and Garland, H.O. (1992). An investigation of the acute effect of gentamicin on the renal handling of electrolytes in the rat. *J. Pharmacol. Exp. Ther.* 261, 38.

Franklyn, J.A., Wilkins, M.R., Wilkinson, R., *et al.* (1985a). The effect of propranolol on circulating thyroid hormone measurements in thyrotoxic and euthyroid subjects. *Acta Endocrinol.* 108, 351.

Franklyn, J.A., Davis, J.R., Gammage, M.D., *et al.* (1985b). Amiodarone and thyroid hormone action. *Clin. Endocrinol.* (Oxf.) 22, 257.

Frascino, J.A., Vanamee, P., and Rosen, P.P. (1970). Renal oxalosis and azotemia after methoxyflurane anaesthesia. *N. Engl. J. Med.* 283, 676.

Fraser, C.L. and Arieff, A.I. (1990). Fatal central diabetes mellitus and insipidus resulting from untreated hyponatremia: a new syndrome. *Ann. Intern. Med.* 112, 113.

Freed, M.I., Rastegar, A., and Bia, M.J. (1991). Effects of calcium channel blockers on potassium homeostasis. *Yale J. Biol. Med.* 64, 177.

Freimark, D., Leor, R., Hod, H., *et al.* (1991). Impaired hepatic function tests after thrombolysis for acute myocardial infarction. *Am. J. Cardiol.* 67, 535.

Friedman, E., Shadel, M., Halkin, H., *et al.* (1989). Thiazide-induced hyponatremia. Reproducibility by single dose rechallenge and an analysis of pathogenesis. *Ann. Intern. Med.* 110, 24.

Friis, M.L., Kristensen, O., Boas, J., *et al.* (1993). Therapeutic experiences with 947 epileptic out-patients in oxcarbazepine treatment. *Acta Neurol. Scand.* 87, 224.

Fritsch, C., Bolsen, K., Ruzicka, T., *et al.* (1997). Congenital erythropoietic porphyria. *J. Am. Acad. Dermatol.* 36, 594.

Frohlich, E.D. (1992). Current issues in hypertension. Old questions with new answers and new questions. *Med. Clin. North Am.* 76, 1043.

Frost, L., Danielsen, H., Dorup, I., *et al.* (1993). Skeletal muscle magnesium content during cyclosporin and azathioprine treatment in renal transplant recipients. *Nephrol. Dial. Transplant.* 8, 79.

Fruzzetti, F., De Lorenzo, D., Parrini, D., *et al.* (1994). Effects of finasteride, a 4 alpha-reductase inhibitor, on circulating androgens and gonadotrophin secretion in hirsute women. *J. Clin. Endocrinol. Metab.* 79, 831.

Fuentes, A. and Goldkrand, J.W. (1987). Angiotensin-converting enzyme activity in hypertensive subjects after magnesium sulfate therapy. *Am. J. Obstet. Gynecol.* 156, 1375.

Fuiano, G., Federico, S., Conte, G., *et al.* (1989). Uric acid and kidney. *Adv. Exp. Med. Biol.* 252, 107.

Fujimura, A., Ebihara, A., Hino, N., *et al.* (1989). Effects of traxanox sodium on blood pressure and serum uric acid in hypertensive patients: a preliminary study. *J. Clin. Pharmacol.* 29, 327.

Fujita, M., Itakura, T., Takagi, Y., *et al.* (1989). Copper deficiency during total parenteral nutrition: clinical analysis of three cases. *JPEN* 13, 421.

Fuller, K., Chambers, T.J., and Gallagher, A.C. (1991). Heparin augments osteoclast resorption-stimulating activity in serum. *J. Cell. Physiol.* 147, 208.

Fuller, N.J., Bates, C.J., Evans, P.H., *et al.* (1992). High folate intakes related to zinc status in preterm infants. *Eur. J. Pediatr.* 151, 51.

Fung, M.C., Weintraub, M., and Bowen, D.L. (1995). Hypermagnesemia. Elderly over-the-counter drug users at risk. *Arch. Fam. Med.* 4, 718.

Furie, B. and Furie, B.C. (1990). Molecular basis of vitamin K-dependent gamma-carboxylation. *Blood* 75, 1753.

Gabow, P.A., Hanson, T.J., Popovtzer, M.M., *et al.* (1977). Furosemide-induced reduction in ionized calcium in hypoparathyroid patients. *Ann. Intern. Med.* 86, 579.

Gabow, P.A., Anderson, R.J., Potts, D.E., *et al.* (1978). Acid–base disturbances in the salicylate-intoxicated adult. *Arch. Intern. Med.* 138, 1481.

Gafny, M., Silbergeld, A., Klinger, B., *et al.* (1994). Comparative effects of GH, IGF-I and insulin on serum sex hormone binding globulin. *Clin. Endocrinol.* (Oxf.) 41, 169.

Galante, A., De Luca, A., Pietroiusti, A., *et al.* (1994). Effects of opiates on blood rheology. *J. Toxicol. Clin. Toxicol.* 32, 411.

Gallery, E.D., Blomfield, J., and Dixon, S.R. (1972). Acute zinc toxicity in haemodialysis. *BMJ* iv, 331.

Gamstedt, A., Jarnerot, G., and Kagedal, B. (1981). Dose related effects of betamethasone on iodothyronines and thyroid hormone-binding protein. *Acta Endocrinol.* 96, 484.

Gan, S.C., Barr, J., Arieff, A.I., *et al.* (1992). Biguanide-associated lactic acidosis: case report and review of the literature. *Arch. Int. Med.* 152, 2333.

Gandelman, M.S. (1994). Review of carbamazepine-induced hyponatremia. *Prog. Neuro-Psychopharmacology Biol. Psychiatry* 18, 211.

Ganguli, P.C. and Mohamed, S.D. (1980). Long-term therapy with carbenoxolone in the prevention of recurrence of gastric ulcer. Natural history and evolution of important side-effects and measures to avoid them. *Scand. J. Gastroenterol.* 15, Suppl. 65, 63.

Gascon, N., Otal, C., Martinez-Bru, C., *et al.* (1993). Dipyrone interference on several common biochemical tests. *Clin. Chem.* 39, 1033.

Gaylord, M.S., Pittman, P.A., Bartness, J., *et al.* (1991). Release of benzalkonium chloride from a heparin-bonded umbilical catheter with resultant factitious hypernatremia and hyperkalemia. *Pediatrics* 87, 631.

Gearhart, M.O. and Sorg, T.B. (1993). Foscarnet-induced severe hypomagnesemia and other electrolyte disorders. *Ann. Pharmacother.* 27, 285.

Geissler, A.H., Turnlund, J.R., and Cohen, R.D. (1986). Effect of chlorthalidone on zinc levels, testosterone, and sexual function in man. *Drug Nutr. Interact.* 4, 275.

Georgieff, M.K., Chockalingam, U.M., Sasanow, S.R., *et al.* (1988). The effect of antenatal betamethasone on cord blood concentrations of retinol-binding protein, transthyretin, transferrin, retinol, and vitamin E. *J. Pediatr. Gastroenterol. Nutr.* 7, 713.

German, D.C. and Holmes, E.W. (1986). Hyperuricemia and gout. *Med. Clin. North Am.* 70, 419.

Germann, R., Schindera, I., Kuch, M., *et al.* (1996). Lebensbedrohliche Salicylatintoxikation durch perkutane Resorption bei einer schweren Ichthyosis vulgaris. *Hautarzt* 47, 624.

Gharavi, A.G., Diamond, J.A., Smith, D.A., *et al.* (1994). Niacin-induced myopathy. *Am. J. Cardiol.* 74, 841.

Ghose, R.R. (1985). Plasma arginine vasopressin in hyponatraemic patients receiving diuretics. *Postgrad. Med. J.* 61, 1043.

Giaccone, G., Donadio, M., Ferrati, P., *et al.* (1985). Disorders of serum electrolytes and renal function in patients treated with cis-platinum on an outpatient basis. *Eur. J. Cancer* 21, 433.

Gillman, M.A. and Sandyk, R. (1984). Nicotinic acid deficiency induced by sodium valproate. *S. Afr. Med. J.* 65, 986.

Gines, P. and Jimenez, W. (1996). Aquaretic agents: a new potential treatment of dilutional hyponatremia in cirrhosis. *J. Hepatol.* 24, 506.

Glazebrook, G.A. (1987). Effect of decicurie doses of radioactive iodine 131 on parathyroid function. *Am. J. Surg.* 154, 368.

Gluck, O.S., Murphy, W.A., Hahn, T.J., *et al.* (1981). Bone loss in adults receiving alternate day glucocorticoid therapy. A comparison with daily therapy. *Arthritis Rheum.* 24, 892.

Glueck, C.J., Speirs, J., and Tracy, T. (1990). Safety and efficacy of combined gemfibrozil-lovastatin therapy for primary dyslipoproteinemias. *J. Lab. Clin. Med.* 115, 603.

Glusker, J.P. (1995). Vitamin B_{12} and the B_{12} coenzymes. *Vitam. Horm.* 50, 1.

Godolphin, W., Cameron, E.C., Frohlich, J., *et al.* (1979). Spurious hypocalcemia in hemodialysis patients after heparinization. In-vitro formation of calcium soaps. *Am. J. Clin. Pathol.* 71, 215.

Goggin, T., Gough, H., Bissessar, A., *et al.* (1987). A comparative study of the relative effects of anticonvulsant drugs and dietary folate on the red cell folate status of patients with epilepsy. *Q. J. Med.* 65, 911.

Goldfarb, S., Walker, B.R., and Agus, Z.S. (1985). The uricosuric effect of oxaprozin in humans. *J. Clin. Pharmacol.* 25, 144.

Goldray, D., Weisman, Y., Jaccard, N., *et al.* (1993). Decreased bone density in elderly men treated with the gonadotropin-releasing hormone agonist decapeptyl (D-Trp6-GnRH). *J. Clin. Endocrinol. Metab.* 76, 288.

Goldwasser, H.D., Hooper, J.F., and Spears, N.M. (1989). Concomitant treatment of neuroleptic malignant syndrome and psychosis. *Br. J. Psychiatry* 154, 102.

Golik, A., Averbukh, Z., Cohn, M., *et al.* (1990a). Effects of diuretics on captopril-induced urinary zinc excretion. *Eur. J. Clin. Pharmacol.* 38, 359.

Golik, A., Modai, D., Averbukh, Z., *et al.* (1990b). Zinc metabolism in patients treated with captopril versus enalapril. *Metabolism* 39, 665.

Golub, M.S. and Domingo, J.L. (1996). What we know and what we need to know about developmental aluminum toxicity. *J. Toxicol. Environ. Health* 48, 585.

Golzarian, J., Scott, H.W., Jr, and Richards, W.O. (1994). Hypermagnesemia-induced paralytic ileus. *Dig. Dis. Sci.* 39, 1138.

Gonzalez, E.A. and Martin, K.J. (1992). Aluminum and renal osteodystrophy: a diminishing clinical problem. *Trends in Endocrinology and Metabolism* 3, 371.

Gonzalez, J. and Hogg, R.J. (1981). Metabolic alkalosis secondary to baking soda treatment of a diaper rash. *Pediatrics* 67, 820.

Gonzalez-Martin, G., Diaz-Molinas, M.S., Martinez, A.M., *et al.* (1991). Heparin-induced hyperkalemia: a prospective study. *Int. J. Clin. Pharmacol. Ther. Toxicol.* 29, 446.

Good, C.B., McDermott, L., and McCloskey, B. (1995). Diet and serum potassium in patients on ACE inhibitors. *JAMA* 274, 538.

Goodenough, G.K. and Lutz, L.J. (1988). Hyponatremic hypervolemia caused by a drug–drug interaction mistaken for syndrome of inappropriate ADH. *J. Am. Geriatr. Soc.* 36, 285.

Gordon, D., Beastall, G.H., McArdle, C.S., *et al.* (1986). The effect of tamoxifen therapy on thyroid function tests. *Cancer* 58, 1422.

Gosselink, A.T., Crijns, H.J., Wiesfeld, A.C., *et al.* (1993). Exercise-induced ventricular tachycardia: a rare manifestation of digitalis toxicity. *Clin. Cardiol.* 16, 270.

Gotjamanos, T. and Afonso, F. (1997). Unacceptably high levels of fluoride in commercial preparations of silver fluoride. *Aust. Dent. J.* 42, 52.

Goyer, R.A. (1989). Mechanisms of lead and cadmium nephrotoxicity. *Toxicol. Lett.* 46, 153.

Gradon, J.D., Fricchione, L., and Sepkowitz, D. (1991). Severe hypomagnesemia associated with pentamidine therapy. *Reviews on Infectious Diseases* 13, 511.

Granerus, A.K., Jagenburg, R., and Svanborg, A. (1977). Kaliuretic effect of L-dopa treatment in Parkinsonian patients. *Acta Med. Scand.* 201, 291.

Graninger, W., Pirich, K.R., Speiser, W., *et al.* (1986). Effect of thyroid hormones on plasma protein concentrations in man. *J. Clin. Endocrinol. Metab.* 63, 407.

Grant, S.M. and Heel, R.C. (1992). Recombinant granulocyte-macrophage colony-stimulating factor (rGM-CSF). A review of its pharmacological properties and prospective role in the management of myelosuppression. *Drugs* 43, 516.

Graves, J., Kenamond, T.G., and Whittier, F.C. (1988). Acute effects of nifedipine on renal electrolyte excretion in normal and hypertensive subjects. *Am. J. Med. Sci.* 296, 114.

Grayhack, J.T. (1984). Prostatic carcinoma: management. *J. Urol.* 132, 92.

Green, C.G., Doershuk, C.F., and Stern, R.C. (1985). Symptomatic hypomagnesemia in cystic fibrosis. *J. Pediatr.* 107, 425.

Greenberg, S., Reiser, I.W., Chou, S.Y., *et al.* (1993). Trimethoprim-sulfamethoxazole induces reversible hyperkalaemia. *Ann. Intern. Med.* 119, 291.

Gren, J. and Woolf, A. (1989). Hypermagnesemia associated with catharsis in a salicylate-intoxicated patient with anorexia nervosa. *Ann. Emerg. Med.* 18, 200.

Grieco, A., Caputo, S., Bertoli, A., *et al.* (1986). Megaloblastic anaemia due to sulphasalazine responding to drug withdrawal alone. *Postgrad. Med. J.* 62, 307.

Griffiths, K.D. and Parry, D.H. (1988). Hypomagnesaemia and hypocalcaemia after treatment with mitoxantrone. *BMJ* 297, 488.

Gudmundsson, J.A., Ljunghall, S., Bergquist, C., *et al.* (1987). Increased bone turnover during gonadotropin-releasing hormone superagonist-induced ovulation inhibition. *J. Clin. Endocrinol. Metab.* 65, 159.

Guevara, A., Labarca, J., and Gonzalez-Martin, G. (1993). Heparin-induced transaminase elevations: a prospective study. *Int. J. Clin. Pharmacol. Ther. Toxicol.* 31, 137.

Gunther, G., Mauz-Korholz, C., Korholz, D., *et al.* (1992). G-CSF and liver toxicity in a patient with neuroblastoma. *Lancet* 340, 1352.

Gunza, J.T., Pashayan, A.G., Mailliard, M.E., *et al.* (1992). Postoperative elevation of serum transaminases following isoflurane anesthesia. *J. Clin. Anesth.* 4, 336.

Guthrie, R.M. and Lott, J.A. (1986). Abnormal serum CK-MB following an aminotriptyline overdose. A case report and review of the literature. *J. Fam. Pract.* 22, 550.

Haag-Weber, M., Schollmeyer, P., and Horl, W.H. (1990). Failure to detect remarkable hypomagnesemia in renal transplant recipients receiving ciclosporin. *Miner. Electrolyte Metab.* 16, 66.

Haeney, M.R., Carter, G.F., Yeoman, W.B., *et al.* (1979). Long-term parenteral exposure to mercury in patients with hypogammaglobulinaemia. *BMJ* 11, 12.

Haenni, A. and Lithell, H. (1996). Urapidil treatment decreases plasma fibrinogen concentration in essential hypertension. *Metabolism* 45, 1221.

Haffner, C.A, and Kendall, M.J. (1992). Metabolic effects of β_2-agonists. *J. Clin. Pharm Ther.* 17, 155.

Hagley, M.T., Traeger, S.M., and Schuckman, H. (1994). Pronounced metabolic response to modest theophylline overdose. *Ann. Pharmacother.* 28, 195.

Hahn, T.J. (1993). Steroid and drug-induced osteopenia. In *Primer on Metabolic Bone Disease and Disorders of Mineral Metabolism* (ed. M.J. Favus), p. 252. Raven Press, New York.

Hahn, T.J., Birge, S.J., Scharp, C.R., *et al.* (1972*a*). Phenobarbital-induced alterations in vitamin D metabolism. *J. Clin. Invest.* 51, 741.

Hahn, T.J., Hendin, B.A., Scharp, C.R., *et al.* (1972*b*). Effect of chronic anticonvulsant therapy on serum 25-hydroxycalciferol levels in adults. *N. Engl. J. Med.* 287, 900.

Hall, M.A., Thom, H., and Russell, G. (1981). Erythrocyte aspartate aminotransferase activity in asthmatic and non-asthmatic children and its enhancement by vitamin B_6. *Ann. Allergy* 47, 464.

Hallen, J. (1996). K^+ balance in humans during exercise. *Acta Physiol. Scand.* 156, 279.

Halma, C., Jansen, J.B., Janssens, A.R., *et al.* (1987). Life-threatening water intoxication during somatostatin therapy. *Ann. Intern. Med.* 107, 518.

Halperin, M.L. and Scheich, A. (1994). Should we continue to recommend that a deficit of KCl be treated with NaCl? A fresh look at chloride-depletion metabolic alkalosis. *Nephron* 67, 263.

Hamed, M., Mitchell, H., and Clow, D.J. (1993). Hyponatraemic convulsion associated with desmopressin and imipramine treatment. *BMJ* 306, 1169.

Hamilton, W.F.D. and Robertson, G.S. (1974). Changes in serum uric acid related to the dose of methoxyflurane. *Br. J. Anaesth.* 46, 54.

Hankins, D.G., Saxena, K., Faville, R.J., Jr, *et al.* (1987). Profound acidosis caused by isoniazid ingestion. *Am. J. Emerg. Med.* 5, 165.

Hanlon, D.P. (1975). Interaction of thiamazole with zinc copper. *Lancet* i, 929.

Haq, I. and Asghar, M. (1989). Lead content of some traditional preparations — 'Kushtas'. *J. Ethnopharmacol.* 26, 287.

Hardin, T.C., Koeller, J.M., Kuhn, J.G., *et al.* (1993). Nutritional parameters observed during 28-day infusion of recombinant human tumor necrosis factor-alpha. *JPEN* 17, 541.

Hardman, K.A., Heath, D.A., and Nelson, H.M. (1993). Hypercalcaemia associated with calcipotriol (Dovonex) treatment. *BMJ* 306, 896.

Hardy, A.D., Sutherland, H.H., Vaishnav, R., *et al.* (1995). A report on the composition of mercurials used in traditional medicines in Oman. *J. Ethnopharmacol.* 49, 17.

Harlow, P.J., DeClerck, Y.A., Shore, N.A., *et al.* (1979). A fatal case of inappropriate ADH secretion induced by cyclophosphamide therapy. *Cancer* 44, 896.

Harper, J.M., Levine, A.J., Rosenthal, D.L., *et al.* (1994). Erythrocyte folate levels, oral contraceptive use and abnormal cervical cytology. *Acta Cytologica* 38, 324.

Harrison, A.R., Kasidas, G.P., and Rose, G.A. (1981). Hyperoxaluria and recurrent stone formation apparently cured by short courses of pyridoxine. *BMJ* 282, 2097.

Harrower, A.D. (1996). Pharmacokinetics of oral antihyperglycaemic agents in patients with renal insufficiency. *Clin. Pharmacokinet.* 31, 111.

Hautanen, A., Manttari, M., Manninen, V., *et al.* (1994). Gemfibrozil treatment is associated with elevated adrenal androgen, androstanediol glucuronide and cortisol levels in dyslipidemic men. *J. Steroid Biochem. Mol. Biol.* 51, 307.

Hawkins, D.F. and Benster, B. (1977). A comparative study of three low dose progestogens, chlormadinone acetate, megestrol acetate, and norethisterone, as oral contraceptives. *Br. J. Obstet. Gynaecol.* 84, 708.

Hazen, P.G. (1994). Pseudoporphyria in a patient receiving carisoprodol/aspirin therapy. *J. Am. Acad. Dermatol.* 31, 500.

Healy, M.A. and Aslam, M. (1986). Lead-containing preparations in the Asian community: a retrospective survey. *Public Health* 100, 149.

Heaney, R.P. (1996). Nutrition and risk for osteoporosis. In *Osteoporosis* (ed. R. Marcus, D. Feldman, and J. Kelsey), p. 483. Academic Press, California.

Heaney, R.P. and Recker, R.R. (1982). Effects of nitrogen, phosphorus, and caffeine on calcium balance in women. *J. Lab. Clin. Med.* 99, 46.

Heath, D.A., Palmer, J.S., and Aurbach, G.D. (1972). The hypocalcemic action of colchicine. *Endocrinology* 90, 1589.

Hebestreit, H., Pannenbecker, J., Mingers, A.M., *et al.* (1990). Pellagra unter antikonvulsiver Behandlung. *Monatsschr. Kinderheilk.* 138, 808.

Heckerling, P.S. (1987). Ethylene glycol poisoning with a normal anion gap due to occult bromide intoxication. *Ann. Emerg. Med.* 16, 1384.

Heckman, B.A. and Walsh, J.H. (1967). Hypernatremia complicating sodium sulphate therapy for hypercalcemic crisis. *N. Engl. J. Med.* 276, 1082.

Heier, M.S. and Fossa, S.D. (1986). Wernicke-Korsakoff-like syndrome in patients with colorectal carcinoma treated with high-dose doxifluridine (5'd-FUrd). *Acta Neurol. Scand.* 73, 449.

Helgeland, A. (1983). Double-bind comparison of trimazosin and propranolol in essential hypertension. *Am. Heart J.* 106, 1253.

Heller, I., Halevy, J., Cohen, S., *et al.* (1985). Significant metabolic acidosis induced by acetazolamide. Not a rare complication. *Arch. Intern. Med.* 145, 1815.

Helsing, E. (1996). Vitamins. In *Meyler's Side Effects of Drugs* (ed. M.N.G. Dukes), p. 1166. Elsevier, Amsterdam.

Hendel, J. and Nyfords, A. (1985). Impact of methotrexate therapy on the folate status of psoriatic patients. *Clin. Exp. Dermat.* 10, 30.

Hepburn, W.C., Abdul-Aziz, L.A.S., and Whiteoak, R. (1989). Danazol-induced hypercalcaemia in alphacalcidol-treated hypoparathyroidism. *Postgrad. Med. J.* 65, 849.

Herbert, V. (1981). Vitamin B_{12}. *Am. J. Clin. Nutr.* 34, 971.

Herbert, V., Jacob, E., Wong, K.T., *et al.* (1978). Low serum vitamin B_{12} levels in patients receiving ascorbic acid in megadoses: studies concerning the effect of ascorbate on radioisotope vitamin B_{12} assay. *Am. J. Clin. Nutr.* 31, 253.

Hermann, L.S. and Melander, A. (1992). Biguanides: basic aspects and clinical uses. In *International Textbook of Diabetes Mellitus*, Vol. 1 (ed. K.G.M. Alberti, A. De Herrmann, J.M., and Mayer, E.O. (1988). A long-term study of the effects of celiprolol on blood pressure and lipid-associated risk factors. *Am. Heart J.* 116, 1416.

Fronzor, H. Kelu, and P. Zimmet), p. 773. John Wiley, London.

Hespel, P., Lijnen, P., Fiocchi, R., *et al.* (1987). Effects of calcium antagonism on the resting and exercise-stimulated renin–aldosterone axis. *Methods Find. Exp. Clin. Pharmacol.* 9, 461.

Heyns, W., Drochmans, A., van der Schueren, E., *et al.* (1985). Endocrine effects of high-dose ketoconazole therapy in advanced prostatic cancer. *Acta Endocrinol.* 110, 276.

Higuchi, T., Komoda, T., Sugishita, M., *et al.* (1987). Certain neuroleptics reduce bone mineralization in schizophrenic patients. *Neuropsychobiology* 18, 185.

Hilbrands, L.B., Hoitsma, A.J., Wetzels, J.F.M., *et al.* (1996). Detailed study of changes in renal function after conversion from cyclosporine to azathioprine. *Clin. Nephrol.* 45, 230.

Hildebrandt, R., Weitzel, H.K., and Gundert-Remy, U. (1997). Hypokalaemia in pregnant women treated with the $beta_2$-mimetic drug fenoterol — a concentration and time dependent effect. *J. Perinat. Med.* 25, 173.

Hill, W.C., Gill, P.J., and Katz, M. (1985). Maternal paralytic ileus as a complication of magnesium sulfate tocolysis. *Am. J. Perinatol.* 2, 47.

Hirokawa, C.A. and Gray, D.R. (1992). Chlorpropamide-induced hyponatremia in the veteran population. *Ann. Pharmacother.* 26, 1243.

Hirsch, J. (1991). Drug therapy: Oral anticoagulant drugs. *N. Engl. J. Med.* 324, 1858.

Hjelt, K., Brynskov, J., Hippe, E., *et al.* (1985). Oral contraceptives and the cobalamin (Vitamin B_{12}) metabolism. *Acta Obstet. Gynecol. Scand.* 64, 59.

Hoeck, H.C., Laurberg, G., and Laurberg, P. (1994). Hypercalcaemic crisis after excessive topical use of a vitamin D derivative. *J. Intern. Med.* 235, 281.

Hogenkamp, H.P. (1980). The interaction between vitamin B_{12} and vitamin C. *Am. J. Clin. Nutr.* 33, 1.

Hoikka, V., Savolainen, K., Alhava, E.M., *et al.* (1982). Anticonvulsant osteomalacia in epileptic outpatients. *Ann. Clin. Res.* 14, 129.

Holick, M.F. (1995). Environmental factors that influence the cutaneous production of vitamin D. *Am. J. Clin. Nutr.* 61, 638S.

Hollenberg, N.K. and Mickiewicz, C. (1989). Hyperkalaemia in diabetes mellitus. Effect of a triamterene–hydrochlorothiazide combination. *Arch. Intern. Med.* 149, 1327.

Hollinger, M.A. (1996). Toxicological aspects of topical silver pharmaceuticals. *Crit. Rev. Toxicol.* 26 255.

Holmberg, L., Boman, G., and Bottiger, L.E. (1980). Adverse reactions to nitrofurantoin: analysis of 921 reports. *Am. J. Med.* 69, 733.

Holmes, R.P., Assimos, D.G., Leaf, C.D., *et al.* (1997). The effects of (1)-2-oxothiazolidine-4-carboxylate on urinary oxalate excretion. *J. Urol.* 158, 34.

Holzbach, E. (1996). Thiamine absorption in alcoholic delirium patients. *J. Stud. Alcohol* 57, 581),

Homeida, M.M., Bagi, I.A., Ghalib, H.W., *et al.* (1988). Prolongation of prothrombin time with ivermectin. *Lancet* i, 1346.

Honda, H. and Gindin, R.A. (1972). Gout while receiving levodopa for Parkinsonism. *JAMA* 219, 55.

Hood, M.A. and Finley, R.S. (1991). Fludarabine: a review. *DICP* 25, 518.

Horie, Y., Tanaka, K., Okano, J., *et al.* (1996). Cimetidine in the treatment of porphyria cutanea tarda. *Internal Medicine* 35, 717.

Horne, C.H.W., Howie, P.W., Weir, R.J., *et al.* (1970). Effect of estrogen–progestogen oral contraceptives on serum levels of $alpha_2$ macroglobulin, transferrin and IgG. *Lancet* i, 49.

Horowitz, J., Sukenik, S., and Altz-Smith, M. (1988). Recurrent hyperkalemia and acute renal failure following sulindac therapy. *Isr. J. Med. Sci.* 24, 433.

Howes, L.G. (1995). Which drugs affect potassium? *Drug Saf.* 12, 240.

Hruska, K.A. (1997). Renal osteodystrophy. *Baillière's Clin. Endocrinol. Metab.* 11, 165.

Huhtaniemi, I., Nikula, H., and Rannikko, S. (1985). Treatment of prostatic cancer with a gonadotrophin — releasing hormone agonist analog: acute and long term effects on endocrine functions of testis tissue. *J. Clin. Endocrinol. Metab.* 61, 698.

Human, J.A., Ubbink, J.B., Jerling, J.J., *et al.* (1997). The effect of simvastatin on the plasma antioxidant concentrations in patients with hypercholesterolaemia. *Clin. Chim. Acta* 263, 67.

Hume, A.L., Jack, B.W., and Levinson, P. (1990). Severe hyponatremia: an association with lisinopril? *DICP* 24, 1169.

Hunter, M.F., Ashton, M.R., Griffiths, D.M., *et al.* (1993). Hyperphosphataemia after enemas in childhood: prevention and treatment. *Arch. Dis. Child.* 68, 233.

Husband, D.J. and Watkin, S.W. (1988). Fatal hypokalaemia associated with ifosfamide/mesna chemotherapy. *Lancet* i, 1116.

Hutchison, F.N., Perez, E.A., Gandara, D.R., *et al.* (1988). Renal salt wasting in patients treated with cisplatin. *Ann. Intern. Med.* 108, 21.

Huynh, T., Vanner, S., and Paterson, W. (1995). Safety profile of 5-h oral sodium phosphate regimen for colonoscopy cleansing: lack of clinically significant hypocalcemia or hypovolemia. *Am. J. Gastroenterol.* 90, 104.

Ilberg, J.J., Turner, G.G., and Nultall, F.Q. (1978). Effect of phosphate or magnesium cathartics on serum calcium. *Arch. Intern. Med.* 138, 1114.

Ingrish, G. and Rietschel, R.L. (1996). Oxaprozin-induced pseudoporphyria. *Arch. Dermatol.* 132, 1519.

Innerfield, R.J. (1996). Metformin-associated mortality in U.S. studies. *N. Engl. J. Med.* 334, 1611.

Ishii, N. and Nishihara, Y. (1985). Pellagra encephalopathy among tuberculous patients: its relation to isoniazid therapy. *J. Neurol. Neurosurg. Psychiatry* 48, 628.

Ismail, A.A.A., Toppozada, M., Zahran, M., *et al.* (1992). Serum nickel, copper and zinc in Norplant® users. *Contraception* 45, 561.

Isojarvi, J.I.T., Pakarinen, A.J., and Myllyla, V.V. (1991). A prospective study of serum sex hormones during carbamazepine therapy. *Epilepsy Research* 9, 139.

Isojarvi, J.I.T., Repo, M., Pakarinen, A.J., *et al.* (1995). Carbamazepine, phenytoin, sex hormones, and sexual function in men with epilepsy. *Epilepsia* 36, 366.

Itoh, S., Yamaba, Y., Matsuo, S., *et al.* (1982). Sodium-valproate-induced liver injury. *Am. J. Gastroenterol.* 77, 875.

Ittel, T.H., Gladziwa, U., Muck, W., *et al.* (1991). Hyperaluminaemia in critically ill patients: role of antacid therapy and impaired renal function. *Eur. J. Clin. Invest.* 21, 96.

Iyengar, V., Chou, P.P., Costantino, A.G., *et al.* (1994). Excessive urinary excretion of zinc in drug addicts: a preliminary study during methadone detoxification. *Journal of Trace Elements and Electrolytes in Health and Disease* 8, 213.

Jackson, B. and Johnston, C.I. (1984). Angiotensin converting enzyme during acute and chronic enalapril therapy in essential hypertension. *Clin. Exp. Pharmacol. Physiol.* 11, 355.

Jacobson, M.A. (1992). Review of the toxicities of foscarnet. *J. Acquir. Immune Defic. Syndr.* 5 Suppl. 1, S11.

Jacobson, M.A. (1997). Drug therapy: Treatment of cytomegalovirus retinitis in patients with the acquired immune deficiency syndrome. *N. Engl. J. Med.* 337, 105.

Jacobson, M.A., Gambertoglio, J.G., Aweeka, F.T., *et al.* (1991). Foscarnet-induced hypocalcemia and effects of foscarnet on calcium metabolism. *J. Clin. Endocrinol. Metab.* 72, 1130.

Jaeger, A., Sauder, P., Kopferschmitt, J., *et al.* (1987). Clinical features and management of poisoning due to antimalarial drugs. *Medical Toxicology and Adverse Drug Experience* 2, 242.

Jansen, T., Megahed, M., Holzle, E., *et al.* (1995). Provocation of porphyria cutanea tarda by KUVA-therapy of vitiligo. *Acta Derm. Venereol.* (Stockh.) 75, 232.

Jeejeebhoy, K.N. (1984). Zinc and chromium in parenteral nutrition. *Bull. N.Y. Acad. Med.* 60, 118.

Jeffery, E.H., Abreo, K., Burgess, E., *et al.* (1996). Systemic aluminum toxicity: effects on bone, hematopoietic tissue, and kidney. *J. Toxicol. Environ. Health* 48, 649.

Jensen, E.J., Rungby, J., Hansen, J.C., *et al.* (1988). Serum concentrations and accumulation of silver in skin during three months treatment with an anti-smoking chewing gum containing silver acetate. *Hum. Toxicol.* 7, 535.

Jensen, I.W. (1985). Oestrogen-like effect of tamoxifen on concentration of thyroxin-binding globulin. *Lancet* ii, 1020.

Jeunemaitre, X., Chatellier, G., Kreft-Jais, C., *et al.* (1987). Efficacy and tolerance of spironolactone in essential hypertension. *Am. J. Cardiol.* 60, 820.

Jih, K.S., Wang, M.F., Chow, J.H., *et al.* (1996). Hypercapnic respiratory acidosis precipitated by hypercaloric carbohydrate infusion in resolving septic acute respiratory distress syndrome: a case report. *Chung-Hua I Hsueh Tsa Chih. (Chinese Medical Journal)* 58, 359.

Johnston, D.L., Humen, D.P., and Kostuk, W.J. (1984). Amrinone therapy in patients with heart failure. Lack of improvement in functional capacity and left ventricular function at rest and during exercise. *Chest* 86, 394.

Johnston, R.R., Cromwell, T.H., Eger, E.I., II, *et al.* (1973). The toxicity of fluroxene in animals and man. *Anesthesiology* 38, 313.

Jokubaitis, L.A., Knopp, R.H., and Frohlich, J. (1994). Efficacy and safety of fluvastatin in hyperlipidaemic patients with non-insulin-dependent diabetes mellitus. *J. Intern. Med.* Suppl. 236, 103.

Jone, C.M. and Wu, A.H. (1988). An unusual case of toluene-induced metabolic acidosis. *Clin. Chem.* 34, 2596.

Jones, A.F., Harvey, J.M., and Vale, J.A. (1989). Hypophosphataemia and phosphaturia in paracetamol poisoning. *Lancet* ii, 608.

Jones, D.P. and Chesney, R.W. (1995). Renal toxicity of cancer chemotherapeutic agents in children: ifosfamide and cisplatin. *Curr. Opin. Pediatr.* 7, 208.

Jones, M.G. and Swaminathan, R. (1990). The clinical biochemistry of creatine kinase. *Journal of the International Federation of Clinical Chemistry* 2, 108.

Jonsson, S., O'Meara, M., and Young, J.B. (1983). Acute cocaine poisoning. Importance of treating seizures and acidosis. *Am. J. Med.* 75, 1061.

Joyce, E.M. (1994). Aetiology of alcoholic brain damage: alcoholic neurotoxicity or thiamine malnutrition? *Br. Med. Bull.* 50, 99.

Juan, D. and Elrazak, M.A. (1979). Hypophosphataemia in hospitalized patients. *JAMA* 242, 163.

Jubiz, W., Meikle, A.W., Levinson, R.A., *et al.* (1970). Effect of diphenylhydantoin on the metabolism of dexamethasone. *N. Engl. J. Med.* 283, 11.

Judd, H.L. (1992). Gonadotropin-releasing hormone agonists: strategies for managing the hypoestrogenic effects of therapy. *Am. J. Obstet. Gynecol.* 166, 752.

Judd, L.E., Henderson, D.W., and Hill, D.C. (1986). Naproxen-induced pseudoporphyria. A clinical and ultrastructural study. *Arch. Dermatol.* 122, 451.

June, C.H., Thompson, C.B., Kennedy, M.S., *et al.* (1986). Correlation of hypomagnesemia with the onset of cyclosporine-associated hypertension in marrow transplant patients. *Transplantation* 41, 47.

Kaczmarski, R.S. and Mufti, G.J. (1990). Hypoalbuminaemia after prolonged treatment with recombinant granulocyte macrophage colony stimulating factor. *BMJ* 301, 1312.

Kadowaki, T., Hagura, R., Kajinuma, H., *et al.* (1983). Chlorpropamide-induced hyponatremia: incidence and risk factors. *Diabetes Care* 6, 468.

Kahan, B.D., Flechner, S.M., Lorber, M.I., *et al.* (1987). Complications of cyclosporine–prednisone immunosuppression in 402 renal allograft recipients exclusively followed at a single center for from one to five years. *Transplantation* 43, 197.

Kahn, A. and Blum, D. (1980). Hyperkalaemia and UNICEF type rehydration solution. *Lancet* i, 1082.

Kahn, A.M. (1988). Effect of diuretics on the renal handling of urate. *Semin. Nephrol.* 8, 305.

Kahn, A.M. (1989). Indirect coupling between sodium and urate transport in the proximal tubule. *Kidney Int.* 36, 378.

Kaji, M., Ito, M., Okuno, T., *et al.* (1992). Serum copper and zinc levels in epileptic children with valproate treatment. *Epilepsia* 33, 555.

Kajikawa, M., Nonami, T., Kurokawa, T., *et al.* (1993). Recombinant human erythropoietin and hypophosphatemia in patients with cirrhosis. *Lancet* 341, 503.

Kallner, G. and Petterson, U. (1995). Renal, thyroid and parathyroid function during lithium treatment — laboratory tests in 207 people treated for 1–30 years. *Acta Psychiatr. Scand.* 91, 48.

Kalsheker, N.A. and Hales, C.N. (1985). Insulin *in vivo* increases the *in vitro* fall of plasma potassium concentration in human venous blood. *Eur. J. Clin. Invest.* 15, 113.

Kamel, K.S., Ethier, J.H., Quaggin, S., *et al.* (1992). Studies to determine the basis for hyperkalemia in recipients of a renal transplant who are treated with cyclosporine. *J. Am. Soc. Nephrol.* 2, 1279-1284.

Kamel, K.S., Quaggin, S., Scheich, A., *et al.* (1994). Disorders of potassium homeostasis: an approach based on pathophysiology. *Am. J. Kidney Dis.* 24, 597.

Kamel, K.S., Halperin, M.L., Faber, M.D., *et al.* (1996). Disorders of potassium balance. In *The Kidney* (ed. B.M. Brenner), p. 999. W.B. Saunders, Philadelphia.

Kamoun, P.P., Bardet, J.I., Di Giulio, S., *et al.* (1982). Measurements of angiotensin converting enzyme in captopril-treated patients. *Clin. Chim. Acta* 118, 333.

Kang-Yum, E. and Oransky, S.H. (1992). Chinese patent medicine as a potential source of mercury poisoning. *Vet. Hum. Toxicol.* 34, 235.

Kanis, J.A. and Russell, R.G.G. (1977). Rate of reversal of hypercalcaemia and hypercalciuria induced by vitamin D and its 1-α-hydroxylated derivatives. *BMJ* i, 78.

Kappas, A., Sassa, S., Galbracth, R.A., *et al.* (1995). The prophyrias. In *The Metabolic Basis of Inherited Disease* (6th edn) (ed. C.R. Scriver, A.L. Beaudet, W.S. Sly, and D. Valle), p. 2103. McGraw-Hill, New York.

Kari, M.A., Raivio, K.O., Stenman, U.H., *et al.* (1996). Serum cortisol, dehydroepiandrosterone sulfate, and steroid-binding globulins in preterm neonates: effect of gestational age and dexamethasone therapy. *Pediatr. Res.* 40, 319.

Kariniemi, V. and Rosti, J. (1986). Intramuscular pethidine (meperidine) during labor associated with metabolic acidosis in the newborn. *J. Perinat. Med.* 14, 131.

Kashner, R.F. (1986). Total parenteral nutrition-associated metabolic acidosis. *JPEN* 10, 306.

Kataoka, K., Kanamori, N., Oishi, M., *et al.* (1990). Vitamin E status in pediatric patients receiving antiepileptic drugs. *Dev. Pharmacol. Ther.* 14, 96.

Katayama, S., Inaba, M., Maruno, Y., *et al.* (1987). Captopril-induced creatine kinase elevations: a possible role of the sulfhydryl group. *Hypertension* 10, 234.

Kaufman, M.B. and El-Chaar, G.M. (1996). Bone and tissue changes following prostaglandin therapy in neonates. *Ann. Pharmacother.* 30, 269.

Kauppinen, R. and Mustajoki, P. (1992). Prognosis of acute porphyria: occurrence of acute attacks, precipitating factors, and associated diseases. *Medicine* (Baltimore) 71, 1.

Kauwell, G.P.A., Bailey, L.B., Gregory J.F. III, *et al.* (1995). Zinc status is not adversely affected by folic acid supplementation and zinc intake does not impair folate utilization in human subjects. *J. Nutr.* 125, 66.

Kawarabayashi, T., Tsukamoto, T., Kishikawa, T., *et al.* (1989). Changes in serum calcium, magnesium, cyclic AMP and monoamine oxidase levels during pregnancy and under prolonged ritodrine treatment for preterm labor. *Gynecol. Obstet. Invest.* 28, 132.

Kay, R.G., Tasman-Jones, C., Pybus, J., *et al.* (1976). A syndrome of acute zinc deficiency during total parenteral alimentation in man. *Ann. Surg.* 183, 331.

Keating, J.N., Wada, L., Stokstad, E.L., *et al.* (1987). Folic acid: effect on zinc absorption in humans and in the rat. *Am. J. Clin. Nutr.* 46, 835.

Kedar, R.P., Bourne, T.H., Powles, T.J., *et al.* (1994). Effects of tamoxifen on uterus and ovaries of postmenopausal women in a randomised breast cancer prevention trial. *Lancet* 343, 1318.

Keen, R.W., Deacon, A.C., Delves, H.T., *et al.* (1994). Indian herbal remedies for diabetes as a cause of lead poisoning. *Postgrad. Med. J.* 70, 113.

Keilani, T., Schlueter, W., and Batlle, D. (1995). Selected aspects of ACE inhibitor therapy for patients with renal disease: impact on proteinuria, lipids and potassium. *J. Clin. Pharmacol.* 35, 87.

Keizer, S.E., Gibson, R.S., and O'Connor, D.L. (1995). Postpartum folic acid supplementation of adolescents: impact on maternal folate and zinc status and milk composition. *Am. J. Clin. Nutr.* 62, 377.

Keller, C., Zoller, W., Wolfram, G., *et al.* (1988). Unusual but reversible hepatic lesions following long-term treatment with pyridylcarbinol for familial hypercholesterolemia. *Klin. Wochenschr.* 66, 647.

Kelly, A.T., Short, B.L., Rains, T.C., *et al.* (1989). Aluminum toxicity and albumin. *ASAIO Trans.* 35, 674.

Kelner, M.J. and Bailey, D.N. (1985). Propylene glycol as a cause of lactic acidosis. *J. Anal. Toxicol.* 9, 40.

Kemp, S.F. and Canfield, M.E. (1983). Acute effects of growth hormone administration: vitamin A and visceral protein concentrations. *Acta Endocrinol.* 104, 390.

Kennedy, M.J., Shelley, R.K., and Daly, P.A. (1987). Potentiation of small cell lung cancer-related SIADH by trifluoperazine. *Eur. J. Respir. Dis.* 71, 450.

Kepes, J.J., Chen, W.Y., and Jim, Y.F. (1993). 'Mucoid dissolution' of bones and multiple pathologic fractures in a patient with past history of intravenous administration of polyvinylpyrrolidone (PVP). A case report. *Bone Miner.* 22, 33.

Kes, P. and Reiner, Z. (1990). Symptomatic hypomagnesemia associated with gentamicin therapy. *Magnes. Trace Elem.* 9, 54.

Khan, I.H. and Edward, N. (1993). Pancreatitis associated with diclofenac. *Postgrad. Med. J.* 69, 486.

Khanna, B.K. and Kumar, J. (1991). Hyperuricemic effect of ethambutol and pyrazinamide administered concomitantly. *Indian J. Tuberculosis* 38, 21.

Kharasch, E.D. (1995). Biotransformation of sevoflurane. *Anesth. Analg.* 81, S27.

Kharasch, E.D. (1996). Metabolism and toxicity of the new anesthetic agents. *Acta Anaesthesiol. Belg.* 47, 7.

Kimelman, N. and Albert, S.G. (1984). Phenothiazine-induced hyponatremia in the elderly. *Gerontology* 30, 132.

Kimura, T., Ota, K., Shoji, M., *et al.* (1995). Chlorpropamide-induced ADH release, hyponatremia and central pontine myelinolysis in diabetes mellitus. *Tohoku J. Exp. Med.* 177, 303.

King, W.D., Holloway, M., and Palmisano, P.A. (1992). Albuterol overdose: a case report and differential diagnosis. *Pediatr. Emerg. Care* 8, 268.

Kingreen, J.C. and Breger, G. (1984). Pellagra bei 'Morazon'-Abusus. *Zeitschrift für Hautkrankheiten* 59, 573.

Kinsella, L.J. and Green, R. (1995). 'Anesthesia paresthetica': nitrous oxide-induced cobalamin deficiency. *Neurology* 45, 1608.

Kirson, J.I., McQuiston, H.L., and Pierce, D.W. (1995). Severe elevations in serum creatine kinase associated with clozapine. *Clin. Psychopharmacol.* 15, 287.

Kishi, T., Fujita, N., Eguchi, T., *et al.* (1997). Mechanism for reduction of serum folate by antiepileptic drugs during prolonged therapy. *J. Neurol. Sci.* 145, 109.

Kisker, C.T., Perlman, S., Bohlken, D., *et al.* (1988). Measurement of prothrombin mRNA during gestation and early neonatal development. *J. Lab. Clin. Med.* 112, 407.

Kjaer, K., Hangaard, J., Petersen, N.E., *et al.* (1992). Effect of simvastatin in patients with type I (insulin-dependent) diabetes mellitus and hypercholesterolemia. *Acta Endocrinol.* 126, 229.

Klein, G.L. (1995). Aluminum in parenteral solutions revisited — again. *Am. J. Clin. Nutr.* 61, 449.

Klein, G.L. and Coburn, J.W. (1994). Total parenteral nutrition and its effects on bone metabolism. *Crit. Rev. Clin. Lab. Sci.* 31, 135.

Klein, G.L., Snodgrass, W.R., Griffin, M.P., *et al.* (1989). Hypocalcemia complicating defroxamine therapy in an infant with parenteral nutrition-associated aluminium overload. Evidence for a role of aluminium in the bone disease of infants. *J. Pediatr. Gastroenterol. Nutr.* 9, 400.

Klein, G.L., Herndon, D.N., Rutan, T.C., *et al.* (1990). Elevated serum aluminum levels in severely burned patients who are receiving large quantities of albumin. *J. Burn Care Rehabil.* 11, 526.

Kleinman, G.E., Rodriquez, H., Good, M.C., *et al.* (1991). Hypercalcemic crisis in pregnancy associated with excessive ingestion of calcium carbonate antacid (milk–alkali syndrome): successful treatment with hemodialysis. *Obstet. Gynecol.* 78, 496.

Kleyman, T.R., Roberts, C., and Ling, B.N. (1995). A mechanism for pentamidine-induced hyperkalemia: inhibition of distal nephron sodium transport. *Ann. Intern. Med.* 122, 103.

Kloppel, A. and Weiler, G. (1985). Erhöhte bis toxische Quecksilberkonzentrationen nach post-operativer Wundbehandlung mit Merbromin. *Beitr. Gerichtl. Med.* 43, 169.

Knochel, J.P. (1984). Diuretic-induced hypokalemia. *Am. J. Med.* 77, Suppl. 5A, 18.

Knochel, J.P. and Agarwal, R. (1996). Hypophosphataemia and hyperphosphataemia. In *The Kidney* (ed. B.M. Brenner), p. 1086. W.B. Saunders, Philadelphia.

Knopp, R.H., Illingworth, D.R., Stein, E.A., *et al.* (1996). Effect of pravastatin in the treatment of patients with type iii hyperlipoproteinemia. *American Journal of Therapeutics* 3, 755.

Knox, J.B., Demling, R.H., Wilmore, D.W., *et al.* (1995). Hypercalcemia associated with the use of human growth hormone in an adult surgical intensive care unit. *Arch. Surg.* 130, 442.

Knudsen, L. and Weisman, K. (1978). Taste dysfunction and changes in zinc and copper metabolism during penicillamine therapy for generalized scleroderma. *Acta Med. Scand.* 204, 75.

Knutsen, R., Bohmer, T., and Falch, J. (1994). Intravenous theophylline-induced excretion of calcium, magnesium and sodium in patients with recurrent asthmatic attacks. *Scand. J. Clin. Lab. Invest.* 54, 119.

Koblin, D.D. (1992). Characteristics and implications of desflurane metabolism and toxicity. *Anesth. Analg.* 75, S10.

Koblin, D.D., Tomerson, B.W., Waldman, F.M., *et al.* (1990). Effect of nitrous oxide on folate and vitamin B_{12} metabolism in patients. *Anesth. Analg.* 71, 610.

Koch, C. (1996). Blood, blood components, plasma and plasma products. In *Meyler's Side Effects of Drugs* (ed. M.N.G. Dukes), p. 962. Elsevier, Amsterdam.

Kofke, W.A., Young, R.S., Davis, P., *et al.* (1989). Isoflurane for refractory status epilepticus: a clinical series. *Anesthesiology* 71, 653.

Koide, H. (1991). [Three cases of hyponatremia during administration of pimozide]. [Japanese] *No To Hattatsu [Brain and Development]* 23, 502.

Koide, M. and Waud, B.E. (1972). Serum potassium concentrations after succinylcholine in patients with renal failure. *Anesthesiology* 36, 142.

Kolodzik, J.M., Eilers, M.A., and Angelos, M.G. (1990). Nonsteroidal anti-inflammatory drugs and coma: a case report of fenoprofen overdose. *Ann. Emerg. Med.* 19, 378.

Kolski, G.B., Cunningham, A.S., Niemec, P.W., Jr, *et al.* (1988). Hypokalemia and respiratory arrest in an infant with status asthmaticus. *J. Pediatr.* 112, 304.

Kone, B., Gimenez, L., and Watson, A.J. (1986). Thiazide-induced hyponatremia. *South. Med. J.* 79, 1456.

Kone, B.C., Whelton, A., Santos, G., *et al.* (1988). Hypertension and renal dysfunction in bone marrow transplant recipients. *Q. J. Med.* 69, 985.

Kontopoulos, A.G., Athyros, V.G., Papageorgiou, A.A., *et al.* (1996). Effects of simvastatin and ciprofibrate alone and in combination on lipid profile, plasma fibrinogen and low density lipoprotein particle structure and distribution in patients with familial combined hyperlipidaemia and coronary artery disease. *Coronary Artery Disease* 7, 843.

Koop, H. (1992). Review article: metabolic consequences of long-term inhibition of acid secretion by omeprazole. *Aliment. Pharmacol. Ther.* 6, 399.

Korttila, K., Grohn, P., Gordin, A., *et al.* (1984). Effect of hydroxyethyl starch and dextran on plasma volume and blood hemostasis and coagulation. *J. Clin. Pharmacol.* 24, 273.

Korzets, A., Dicker, D., Chaimoff, C., *et al.* (1992). Life-threatening hyperphosphatemia and hypocalcemic tetany following the use of Fleet enemas. *J. Am. Geriatr. Soc.* 40, 620.

Kostis, J.B., Lacy, C.R., Hall, W.D., *et al.* (1994). The effect of chlorthalidone on ventricular ectopic activity in patients with isolated systolic hypertension. The SHEP Study Group. *Am. J. Cardiol.* 74, 464.

Kotsaki-Kovatsi, V.P., Koehler-Samouilidis, G., Kovatsis, A., *et al.* (1997). Fluctuation of zinc, copper, magnesium and calcium concentrations in guinea pig tissues after administration of captopril (SQ 14225). *J. Trace Elem. Med. Biol.* 11, 32.

Kovacs, L., Pal, A., and Horvath, K. (1985). The effect of fenoterol on fetal metabolism: cord blood studies. *Acta Paediatr. Hung.* 26, 41.

Kozeny, G.A., Nicolas, J.D., Creekmore, S., *et al.* (1988). Effects of interleukin-2 immunotherapy on renal function. *J. Clin. Oncol.* 6, 1170.

Kozlowski, B.W., Taylor, M.L., Baer, M.T., *et al.* (1987). Anticonvulsant medication use and circulating levels of total thyroxine, retinol binding protein and vitamin A in children with delayed cognitive development. *Am. J. Clin. Nutr.* 46, 360.

Kragballe, K. and Iversen, L. (1993). Calcipotriol. A new topical antipsoriatic. *Dermatol. Clin.* 11, 137.

Krans, H.M.J. (1996). Insulin, glucagon and oral hypoglycaemic drugs. In *Meyler's Side Effects of Drugs* (ed. M.N.G. Dukes), p. 1290. Elsevier, Amsterdam.

Krapf, R., Schaffner, T., and Iten, P.X. (1992). Abuse of germanium associated with fatal lactic acidosis. *Nephron* 62, 351.

Kraus, R. and Flores-Suarez, L.F. (1995). Acute gout associated with omeprazole. *Lancet* 345, 461.

Krause, K.H., Berlit, P., Schmidt-Gayk, H., *et al.* (1987). Antiepileptic drugs reduce serum uric acid. *Epilepsy Res.* 1, 306.

Krause, K-H., Bonjour, J-P., Berlit, P., *et al.* (1988). Effects of long-term treatment with antiepileptic drugs on the vitamin status. *Drug and Nutrition Interactions* 5, 317.

Krebs, H.A., Woods, H.F., and Alberti, K.G.M. (1975). Hyperlactaemia and lactic acidosis. *Essays Biochem.* 1, 81.

Kreisberg, R.A. and Wood, B.C. (1983). Drugs and chemical-induced metabolic acidosis. *Clin. Endocrinol. Metab.* 12, 391.

Krentz, A.J., Ferner, R.E., and Bailey, C.J. (1994). Comparative tolerability profiles of oral antidiabetic agents. *Drug Saf.* 11, 223.

Kril, J.J. (1996). Neuropathology of thiamine deficiency disorders. *Metab. Brain Dis.* 11, 9.

Krishna, G.G., Riley, L.J., Jr, Deuter, G., *et al.* (1991). Natriuretic effect of calcium-channel blockers in hypertensives. *Am. J. Kidney Dis.* 18, 566.

Kroft, L.J.A., De Maat, M.P.M., and Brommer, E.J.P. (1993). The effect of ticlopidine upon plasma fibrinogen levels in patients undergoing suprapubic prostatectomy. *Thromb. Res.* 70, 349.

Krogh Jensen, M., Ekelund, S., and Svendsen, L. (1996). Folate and homocysteine status and haemolysis in patients treated with sulphasalazine for arthritis. *Scand. J. Clin. Lab. Invest.* 56, 421.

Krogsgaard, M.R., Thamsborg, G., and Lund, B. (1996). Changes in bone mass during low dose corticosteroid treatment in patients with polymyalgia rheumatica: a double blind, prospective comparison between prednisolone and deflazacort. *Ann. Rheum. Dis.* 55, 143.

Kruse, J.A. and Carlson, R.W. (1990). Rapid correction of hypokalemia using concentrated intravenous potassium chloride infusions. *Arch. Intern. Med.* 150, 613.

Kudoh, A., Sakai, T., and Matsuki, A. (1994). A marked elevation in serum CPK following sevoflurane anesthesia. *Jpn J. Anesthesiol.* 43, 246.

Kukreja, S.C., Bowser, E.N., Hargis, G.K., *et al.* (1976). Mechanisms of glucocorticoid-induced osteopenia: role of parathyroid glands. *Proc. Soc. Exp. Biol. Med.* 152, 358.

Kulkarni, P., Bhattacharya, S., and Petros, A.J. (1992). Torsade de pointes and long QT syndrome following major transfusion. *Anaesthesia* 47, 125.

Kuny, S. and Binswanger, U. (1989). Neuroleptic-induced extrapyramidal symptoms and serum calcium levels. Results of a pilot study. *Neuropsychobiology* 21, 67.

Kurnik, B.R., Singer, F., and Groh, W.C. (1991). Case report: dextran-induced acute anuric renal failure. *Am. J. Med. Sci.* 302, 28.

Kushner, R.F. and Sitrin, M.D. (1986). Metabolic acidosis. Development in two patients receiving a potassium-sparing diuretic and total parenteral nutrition. *Arch. Intern. Med.* 146, 343.

Kuzuya, T., Hasegawa, T., Shimizu, K., *et al.* (1993). Effect of antiepileptic drugs on serum zinc and copper concentrations in epileptic patients. *Int. J. Clin. Pharmacol. Ther.* 31, 61.

Laaksonen, R., Jokelainen, K., Sahi, T., *et al.* (1995). Decreases in serum ubiquinone concentrations do not result in reduced levels in muscle tissue during short-term simvastatin treatment in humans. *Clin. Pharmacol. Ther.* 57, 62.

Laaksonen, R., Ojala, J.P., Tikkanen, M.J., *et al.* (1994). Serum ubiquinone concentrations after short- and long-term treatment with HMG-CoA reductase inhibitors. *Eur. J. Clin. Pharmacol.* 46, 313.

Laan, R.F.J., Buijs, W.C.A., Van Erning, L.J.T., *et al.* (1993). Differential effects of glucocorticoids on cortical appendicular and cortical vertebral bone mineral content. *Calcif. Tissue Int.* 41, 52.

Lacroix, C., Guyonnaud, C., Chaou, M., *et al.* (1988). Interaction between allopurinol and pyrazinamide. *Eur. Respir. J.* 1, 807.

Lafforgue, P., Daver, L., Monties, J.R., *et al.* (1997). Bone mineral density in patients given oral vitamin K antagonists. *Rev. Rhum. Mal. Ostéoartic.* 64, 249.

Laine, J. and Holmberg, C. (1995). Renal and adrenal mechanisms in cyclosporine-induced hyperkalaemia after renal transplantation. *Eur. J. Clin. Invest.* 25, 670.

Laine, J. and Holmberg, C. (1996). Mechanisms of hyperuricemia in cyclosporine-treated renal transplanted children. *Nephron* 74, 318.

Lam, M., and Adelstein, D.J. (1986). Hypomagnesemia and renal magnesium wasting in patients treated with cisplatin. *Am. J. Kidney Dis.* 8, 164.

Lambert, M., Laterre, P.F., Leroy, C., *et al.* (1986). Modifications of liver enzymes during heparin therapy. *Acta Clin. Belg.* 41, 307.

Lambertus, M., Murthy, A.R., Nagami, P., *et al.* (1988). Diabetic keto-acidosis following pentamidine therapy in a patient with the acquired immunodeficiency syndrome. *West. J. Med.* 149, 602.

Lamm, C.I., Norton, K.I., Murphy, R.J.C., *et al.* (1988). Congenital rickets associated with magnesium sulfate infusion for tocolysis. *J. Pediatr.* 113, 1078.

Lammers, G.J. and Roos, R.A.C. (1993). Hyponatraemia due to amantadine hydrochloride and L-dopa/carbidopa. *Lancet* 342, 439.

Lane, S.J., Vaja, S., Swaminathan, R., *et al.* (1996). Effects of prednisolone on bone turnover in patients with corticosteroid resistant asthma. *Clin. Exp. Allergy* 26, 1197.

Langner, A., Verjans, H., Stapor, V., *et al.* (1993). Topical calcitriol in the treatment of chronic plaque psoriasis: a double-blind study. *Br. J. Dermatol.* 128, 566.

Laroche, M., Lamboley, V., Amigues, J.M., *et al.* (1997). Hyperparathyroidism during lithium therapy — two new cases. *Rev. Rhum. Mal. Ostéoartic.* 64, 132.

Larsen, P.R., Atkinson, A.J., and Wellman, H.N. (1970). The effect of diphenylhydantoin on thyroxine metabolism in man. *J. Clin. Invest.* 49, 1266.

Larsen, W., Fellowes, G., and Rickman, L.S. (1990). Life-threatening hypercalcemia and tamoxifen. *Am. J. Med.* 88, 440.

Laudignon, N., Ciampi, A., Coupal, L., *et al.* (1989). Frusemide and ethacrynic acid. Risk factors for the occurrence of serum electrolyte abnormalities and metabolic alkalosis in newborns and infant. *Acta Pediatr. Scand.* 78, 133.

Laurence, A.S. and McKean, J.F. (1990). Dantrolene and suxamethonium: myalgia, biochemical changes and serum dantrolene levels following oral dantrolene pre-treatment in laparoscopy patients. *Eur. J. Anaesthesiol.* 7, 493.

Laureno, R. and Karp, B.I. (1997). Myelinolysis after correction of hyponatraemia. *Ann. Intern. Med.* 126, 57.

Lauzurica, R., Bonal, J., Bonet, J., *et al.* (1988). Rhabdomyolysis, oedema and arterial hypertension: different syndromes related to topical use of 9-alpha-fluoroprednisolone. *J. Hum. Hypertens.* 2, 183.

Lawson, D.H., O'Connor, P.C., and Jick, H. (1982). Drug attributed alterations in potassium handling in congestive cardiac failure. *Eur. J. Clin. Pharmacol.* 23, 21.

Lawson, P.T., Lovaglio, J., and Lipkin, E.W. (1995). Osteopenia in rats supported by intravenous nutrition. *Am. J. Clin. Nutr.* 61, 346.

Le, H.T., Bosse, G.M., and Tsai, Y. (1994). Ibuprofen overdose complicated by renal failure, adult respiratory distress syndrome, and metabolic acidosis. *J. Toxicol. Clin. Toxicol.* 32, 315.

Le Meur, Y., Moesch, C., Rince, M., *et al.* (1995). Potential nephrotoxicity of intravenous infusions of naftidrofuryl oxalate. *Nephrol. Dial. Transplant.* 10, 1751.

Lee, G.R. (1993a). Megaloblastic and nonmegaloblastic macrocytic anaemia. In *Wintrobe's Clinical Haematology* (ed. C.R. Lee, T.C. Bithell, J. W. Forster, *et al.*), p. 745. Lea and Febinger, Philadelphia.

Lee, G.R. (1993b). Nutritional factors in the production and function of erythrocytes. In *Wintrobe's Clinical Haematology* (ed. C.R. Lee, T.C. Bithell, J. Forster, J.W., *et al.*), p. 158. Lea and Febinger, Philadelphia.

Lee, Y.K. and Shin, D.M. (1992). Renal salt wasting in patients treated with high-dose cisplatin, etoposide, and mitomycin in patients with advanced non-small cell lung cancer. *Korean J. Intern. Med.* 7, 118.

Leeb, B.F., Witzmann, G., Ogris, E., *et al.* (1995). Folic acid and cyanocobalamin levels in serum and erythrocytes during low-dose methotrexate therapy of rheumatoid arthritis and psoriatic arthritis patients. *Clin. Exp. Rheumatol.* 13, 459.

Lehot, J.J. (1989). Delayed respiratory depression following fentanyl anesthesia for cardiac surgery. *Crit. Care Med.* 17, 299.

Lei, K.I., Wickham, N.W., and Johnson, P.J. (1995). Severe hyponatremia due to syndrome of inappropriate secretion of antidiuretic hormone in a patient receiving interferon-alpha for chronic myeloid leukemia. *Am. J. Hematol.* 49, 100.

Leikin, J.B., Linowiecki, K.A., Soglin, D.F., *et al.* (1994). Hypokalemia after pediatric albuterol overdose: a case series. *Am. J. Emerg. Med.* 12, 64.

Leppik, I.E. (1992). Metabolism of antiepileptic medication — newborn to elderly. *Epilepsia* 33, S32.

Leson, C.L., McGuigan, M.A., and Bryson, S.M. (1988). Caffeine overdose in an adolescent male. *J. Toxicol. Clin. Toxicol.* 26, 407.

Leung, F.Y. (1995). Trace elements in parenteral micronutrition. *Clin. Biochem.* 28, 561.

Leuwer, M. and Motsch, J. (1996). Neuromuscular blocking agents and skeletal muscle relaxants. In *Meyler's Side Effects of Drugs* (ed. M.N.G. Dukes), p. 298. Elsevier, Amsterdam.

Levine, M.N. (1986). Nonhemorrhagic complications of anti-coagulant therapy. *Semin. Thromb. Hemost.* 12, 63.

Levy, M. (1995). Dental amalgam: toxicological evaluation and health risk assessment. *J. Can. Dent. Assoc.* 61, 667, 671.

Lewis, D.P., Van Dyke, D.C., Willhite, L.A., et al. (1995). Phenytoin–folic acid interaction. *Ann. Pharmacother.* 29, 726.

Li, M.K., Kavanagh, J.P., Prendiville, V., et al. (1986). Does sucrose damage kidneys? *Br. J. Urol.* 58, 353.

Lieberman, J. (1989). Enzymes in sarcoidosis: angiotensin-converting-enzyme (ACE). *Clin. Lab. Med.* 9, 745.

Lilijeqvist, J.A. and Edvardsson, N. (1989). Torsade de pointes tachycardias induced by overdosage of zimeldine. *J. Cardiovasc. Pharmacol.* 14, 666.

Lim, P.O. and MacDonald, T.M. (1996). Antianginal drugs and antitussives. In *Meyler's Side Effects of Drugs* (ed. M.N.G. Dukes), p. 488. Elsevier, Amsterdam.

Lin, H.Y., Rocher, L.L., McQuillan, M.A., et al. (1989). Cyclosporine-induced hyperuricemia and gout. *N. Engl. J. Med.* 321, 287.

Lindberg, J.S., Copley, J.B., Koenig, K.G., et al. (1993). Effect of citrate on serum aluminum concentrations in hemodialysis patients: a prospective study. *South. Med. J.* 86, 1385.

Linder, J., Levin, K., Saaf, J., et al. (1993). Influence of lithium treatment on calcium and magnesium in plasma and erythrocytes. *Lithium* 4, 115.

Linder, M.C. and Hazegh-Azam, M. (1996). Copper biochemistry and molecular biology. *Am. J. Clin. Nutr.* 63, 797S.

Lindinger, M.I. (1995). Potassium regulation during exercise and recovery in humans: implications for skeletal and cardiac muscle. *J. Mol. Cell. Cardiol.* 27, 1011.

Lindstedt, G., Lundberg, P-A., Hammond, G.L., et al. (1985). Sex hormone binding globulin — still many questions. *Scand. J. Clin. Lab. Invest.* 45, 1.

Linter, C.M. and Linter, S.P.K. (1986). Severe lactic acidosis following paraldehyde administration. *Br. J. Psychiatry* 149, 650.

Lipner, H.I., Ruzany, F., Dasgupta, M., et al. (1975). The behavior of carbenicillin as a nonreabsorbable anion. *J. Lab. Clin. Sci.* 86, 183.

Lipsky, J.J. (1983). N-methyl-thiotetrazole inhibition of the gamma carboxylation of glutamic acid: possible mechanism for antibiotic-associated hypoprothrombinaemia. *Lancet* ii, 192.

Lipsky, J.J. (1984). Mechanism of the inhibition of the gamma-carboxylation of glutamic acid by N-methylthiotetrazole-containing antibiotics. *Proc. Natl Acad. Sci. U.S.A.* 81, 2893.

Lipsky, J.J. (1992). Vitamin K deficiency. *Journal of Intensive Care Medicine* 7, 328.

Lipworth, B.J. (1992). Risks versus benefits of inhaled beta 2-agonists in the management of asthma. *Drug Saf.* 7, 54.

Lipworth, B.J., McDevitt, D.G., and Struthers, A.D. (1989). Prior treatment with diuretic augments the hypokalemic and electrocardiographic effects of inhaled albuterol. *Am. J. Med.* 86, 653.

Lisi, D.M. (1989). Muscle spasms and creatine kinase elevation following salbutamol administration. *Eur. Respir. J.* 2, 98.

Liu, B.A., Mittmann, N., Knowles, S.R., et al. (1996). Hyponatremia and the syndrome of inappropriate secretion of antidiuretic hormone associated with the use of selective serotonin reuptake inhibitors: a review of spontaneous reports. *Can. Med. Assoc. J.* 155, 519.

Liu, C.L., Mimouni, F., Ho, M., et al. (1988). *In vitro* effects of magnesium on ionized calcium concentration in serum. *Am. J. Dis. Child.* 142, 837.

Ljungstrom, K.G. and Renck, H. (1987). Metabolic acidosis in dextran-induced anaphylactic reactions. *Acta Anaesthesiol. Scand.* 31, 157.

LoCascio, V., Bonucci, E., Imbimbo, B., et al. (1984). Bone loss of glucocorticoid therapy. *Calcif. Tiss. Int.* 36, 435.

LoCascio, V., Bonucci, E., Imbimbo, B., et al. (1990). Bone loss in response to long-term glucocorticoid therapy. *Bone Miner.* 8, 39.

Lofaso, F., Baud, F.J., Halna du Frelay, X., et al. (1987). Hypokalémie au cours d'intoxications massives par la chloroquine. Deux cas. *Presse Méd.* 16, 22.

Longstretch, G.F. and Green, R. (1983). Folate status in patients receiving maintenance doses of sulfasalazine. *Arch. Intern. Med.* 143, 902.

Lonning, P.E., Bakke, P., Thorsen, T., et al. (1989). Plasma levels of estradiol, estrone, estrone sulfate and sex hormone binding globulin in patients receiving rifampicin. *J. Steroid Biochem.* 33, 631.

Lonning, P.E., Johannessen, D.C., Lien, E.A., et al. (1995). Influence of tamoxifen on sex hormones, gonadotrophins and sex hormone binding globulin in postmenopausal breast cancer patients. *J. Steroid Biochem. Mol. Biol.* 52, 491.

Lott, J.A. and Stang, J.M. (1989). Differential diagnosis of patient with abnormal serum creatine kinase isoenzymes. *Clin. Lab. Med.* 9, 627.

Lott, J.A. and Wolf, P.L. (eds) (1989). Creatine kinase. In *Clinical Enzymology. A Case-Oriented Approach*, p. 149. Field, Rich, New York.

Lott, J.A., Bond, L.W., Bobo, R.C., et al. (1990). Valproic acid-associated pancreatitis: report of three cases and a brief review. *Clin. Chem.* 36, 395.

Lukert, B.P. and Raisz, L.G. (1990). Glucocorticoid-induced osteoporosis: pathogenesis and management. *Ann. Intern. Med.* 112, 352.

Lukert, B.P., Johnson, B.E. and Robinson, R.G. (1992). Estrogen and progesterone replacement therapy reduces glucocorticoid-induced bone loss. *J. Bone Miner. Res.* 7, 1063.

Luscher, T.F., Siegenthaler-Zaber, G., and Kuhlmann, U. (1983). Severe hyponatremic coma due to diphenylhydantoin intoxication. *Clin. Nephrol.* 20, 268.

Lye, W.C. and Leong, S.O. (1994). Bilateral vocal cord paralysis secondary to treatment of severe hypophosphatemia in a continuous ambulatory peritoneal dialysis patient. *Am. J. Kidney Dis.* 23, 127.

Lyman, C.A. and Walsh, T.J. (1992). Systemically administered antifungal agents. A revew of their clinical pharmacology and therapeutic applications. *Drugs* 44, 9.

Maatman, T.J., Gupta, M.K., and Montie, J.E. (1984). The role of serum prostatic acid phosphatase as a tumor marker in men with advanced adenocarcinoma of the prostate. *J. Urol.* 132, 58.

McBurney, E.I. and Rosen, D.A. (1984). Elevated creatine phosphokinase with isotretinoin. *J. Am. Acad. Dermatol.* 10, 528.

McCarron, M., Wright, G.D., and Roberts, S.D. (1995). Water intoxication after low dose cyclophosphamide. *BMJ* 311, 292.

McCarthy, J.T., Milliner, D.S., and Johnson, W.J. (1990). Clinical experience with desferrioxamine in dialysis patients with aluminium toxicity. *Q. J. Med.* 74, 257.

McCaughan, D. (1984). Hazards of non-prescription potassium supplements. *Lancet* i, 513.

McColl, K.E.L., and Goldberg, A. (1980). Abnormal porphyrin metabolism in diseases other than porphyria. *Clin. Haematol.* 9, 427.

McColl, K.E.L., Dover, S., Fitzsimmons, E., et al. (1996). Porphyrins metabolism and the porphyrias. In *Oxford Textbook of Medicine* (3rd edn) (ed. D.J. Weatherall, J.G.G. Ledingham, and D.A. Warrell), p. 1388. Oxford University Press.

McConkey, B., Crockson, R.A., Crockson, A.P., et al. (1973). The effects of some antiinflammatory drugs on the acute phase proteins in rheumatoid arthritis. *Q. J. Med.* 42, 785.

McConnel, T.H. (1971). Fatal hypocalcemia from phosphate absoprtion from laxative preparation. *JAMA* 216, 147.

McCormick, D.B. and Greene, H.L. (1994). Vitamins. In *Teitz Textbook of Clinical Chemistry* (ed. C.A. Burtis and R. Ashwood), p. 1275. W.B. Saunders, Philadelphia.

McDiarmid, S.V. (1996). Renal function in pediatric liver transplant patients. *Kidney Int.* Suppl. 53, S77.

McDonagh, A.J. and Harrington C.I. (1989). Pseudoporphyria complicating etretinate therapy. *Clin. Exp. Dermatol.* 14, 437.

Macfarlane, D.G. and Dieppe, P.A. (1985). Diuretic-induced gout in elderly women. *Br. J. Rheumatol.* 24, 155.

McHenry, C.R. and Racke, F.K. (1993). Lithium effects on parathyroid function. *Lithium* 4, 87.

McInnes, G.T. (1996). Diuretics. In *Meyler's Side Effects of Drugs* (ed. M.N.G. Dukes), p. 558. Elsevier, Amsterdam.

McIntyre, J.W.R., Russell, J.C., and Chambers, M. (1973). Oxalemia following methoxyfluorane anesthesia in man. *Anaesth. Analg.* 52, 946.

McKenzie, R., Fried, M.W., Sallie, R., et al. (1995). Hepatic failure and lactic acidosis due to fialuridine (FIAU), an investigational nucleoside analogue for chronic hepatitis B. *N. Engl. J. Med.* 333, 1099.

Maclennan, A.C., Ahmad, N., and Lawrence, J.R. (1990). Activities of aminotransferases after treatment with streptokinase for acute myocardial infarction. *BMJ* 301, 321.

McMullen, J.K. (1977). Asystole and hypomagnesaemia during recovery from diabetic ketoacidosis. *BMJ* i, 690.

McPherson, M.L., Prince, S.R., Atamer, E.R., et al. (1986). Theophylline-induced hypercalcemia. *Ann. Intern. Med.* 105, 52.

Mactier, R.A. and Khanna, R. (1988). Hyperkalemia induced by indomethacin and naproxen and reversed by fluorocortisone. *South. Med. J.* 71, 799.

Magarian, G.J., Lucas, L.M., and Colley, C. (1991). Gemfibrozil-induced myopathy. *Arch. Intern. Med.* 151, 1873.

Magee, R. (1985). Chelation treatment of atherosclerosis. *Med. J. Aust.* 142, 514.

Maguire, J.F., Geha, R.S., and Umetsu, D.T. (1986). Myocardial specific creatine phosphokinase isoenzyme elevation in children with asthma treated with intravenous isoproterenol. *J. Allergy Clin. Immunol.* 78, 631.

Malas, K.L. and van Kammen, D.P. (1982). Markedly elevated creatine phosphokinase levels after neuroleptic withdrawal. *Am. J. Psychiatry* 139, 231.

Mallette, L.E. (1991). Acute and chronic effects of lithium on human calcium metabolism. *Lithium* 2, 209.

Mallette, L.E. and Eichhorn, E. (1986). Effects of lithium carbonate on human calcium metabolism. *Arch. Intern. Med.* 146, 770.

Mallette, L.E. and Gomez, L.S. (1983). Systemic hypocalcemia after clinical injections of radiographic contrast media: amelioration by omission of calcium chelating agents. *Radiology* 147, 677.

Mall-Haefeli, M., Darragh, A., and Werner-Zodrow, I. (1983). Effects of various combined oral contraceptives on sex steroids, gonadotropins and SHBG. *Ir. Med. J.* 76, 266.

Mantell, G., Burke, M.T., and Staggers, J. (1990). Extended clinical safety profile of lovastatin. *Am. J. Cardiol.* 66, 11B.

Manzione, N.C., Wolkoff, A.W., and Sassa, S. (1988). Development of porphyria cutanea tarda after treatment with cyclophosphamide. *Gastroenterology* 95, 1119.

Marais, G.E. and Larson, K.K. (1990). Rhabdomyolysis and acute renal failure induced by combination lovastatin and gemfibrozil therapy. *Ann. Intern. Med.* 112, 228.

Marasco, W.A., Gikas, P.W., Azziz-Baumgartner, R., et al. (1987). Ibuprofen-associated renal dysfunction. Pathophysiologic mechanisms of acute renal failure, hyperkalemia, tubular necrosis, and proteinuria. *Arch. Intern. Med.* 147, 2107.

Marin, F., Gonzalez Quintela, A., Moya, M., et al. (1989). Pseudohyperaldosteronism due to application of antihaemorrhoid cream. *Nephron* 52, 281.

Markell, M.S., Altura, B.T., Sarn, Y., et al. (1993). Relationship of ionized magnesium and cyclosporine level in renal transplant recipients. *Ann. N.Y. Acad. Sci.* 696, 408.

Markle, H.V. (1996). Cobalamin. *Crit. Rev. Clin. Lab. Sci.* 33, 247.

Markman, M., Cleary, S., and Howell, S.B. (1986). Hypomagnesemia following high-dose intracavitary cisplatin with systemically administered sodium thiosulfate. *Am. J. Clin. Oncol.* 9, 440.

Markman, M., Rottman, R., Reichman, B., et al. (1991). Persistent hypomagnesemia following cisplatin chemotherapy in patients with ovarian cancer. *J. Cancer Res. Clin. Oncol.* 117, 89.

Marks, R., Foley, P.A., Jolley, D., et al. (1995). The effect of regular sunscreen use on vitamin D levels in an Australian population: results of a randomized controlled trial. *Arch. Dermatol.* 131, 415.

Marks, V. and Chapple, P.A. (1967). Hepatic dysfunction in heroin and cocaine users. *Br. J. Addict.* 62, 189.

Marshall, A.W., Jakobovits, A.W., and Morgan, M.Y. (1982). Bromocriptine-associated hyponatraemia in cirrhosis. *BMJ* 285, 1534.

Marshall, J.C., Anderson, D.C., Burke, C.W., et al. (1972). Clomiphene citrate in man: increase in cortisol, luteinizing hormone, testosterone and steroid-binding globulin. *J. Endocrinol.* 53, 261.

Martin, B.J., McAlpine, J.K., and Devine, B.L. (1988). Hypomagnesaemia in elderly digitalised patients. *Scott. Med. J.* 33, 273.

Martin-Bouyer, G., Khanh, N.B., Linh, P.D., et al. (1983). Epidemic of haemorrhagic disease in Vietnamese infants caused by warfarin-contaminated talcs. *Lancet* i, 230.

Mason, J.B., Zimmerman, J., Otradovec, C.L., et al. (1991). Chronic diuretic therapy with moderate doses of triamterene is not associated with folate deficiency. *J. Lab. Clin. Med.* 117, 365.

Matsunaga, A., Handa, K., Mori, T., et al. (1992). Effects of niceritrol on levels of serum lipids, lipoprotein(a), and fibrinogen in patients with primary hypercholesterolemia. *Atherosclerosis* 94, 241.

Matsuoka, L.Y., Wortsman, J., Hanifan, N., et al. (1988). Chronic sunscreen use decreases circulating concentrations of 25-hydroxyvitamin D. A preliminary study. *Arch. Dermatol.* 124, 1802.

Matsuoka, L.Y., Wortsman, J., and Hollis, B.W. (1990). Use of topical sunscreen for the evaluation of regional synthesis of vitamin D3. *J. Am. Acad. Dermatol.* 22, 772.

Mattana, J., Perinbasekar, S., and Brod-Miller, C. (1997). Near-fatal but reversible acute renal failure after massive ibuprofen ingestion. *Am. J. Med. Sci.* 313, 117.

Mattar, J.A., Weil, M.H., Shubin, H., et al. (1974). Cardiac arrest in the critically ill. II. Hyperosmolal states following cardiac arrest. *Am. J. Med.* 56, 162.

Mavichak, V., Coppin, C.M., Wong, N.L., et al. (1988). Renal magnesium wasting and hypocalciuria in chronic cis-platinum nephropathy in man. *Clin. Sci.* 75, 203.

May, K.P., Mercill, D., McDermott, M.T., et al. (1996). The effect of methotrexate on mouse bone cells in culture. *Arthritis Rheum.* 39, 489.

Mazze, R.I. (1984). Fluorinated anaesthetic nephrotoxicity: an update. *Can. Anaesth. Soc. J.* 31, 16.

Meadow, R. (1993). Non-accidental salt poisoning. *Arch. Dis. Child.* 68, 448.

Medina, I., Mills, J., Leoung, G., et al. (1990). Oral therapy for Pneumocystis carinii pneumonia in the acquired immunodeficiency syndrome. A controlled trial of trimethoprim-sulfamethoxazole versus trimethoprim-dapsone. *N. Engl. J. Med.* 323, 776.

Meltzer, H.Y., Cola, P.A., and Parsa, M. (1996). Marked elevations of serum creatine kinase activity associated with antipsychotic drug treatment. *Neuropsychopharmacology* 15, 395.

Mendis, S. (1988). Serum aluminium concentration in subjects cooking in aluminium cookware using water containing fluoride. *Med. Sci. Res.* 16, 739.

Menkes, D.B. and Laverty, R. (1996). Hypnotics and sedatives. In *Meyler's Side Effects of Drugs* (ed. M.N.G. Dukes), p. 103. Elsevier, Amsterdam.

Mennen, M. and Slovis, C.M. (1988). Severe metabolic alkalosis in the emergency department. *Ann. Emerg. Med.* 17, 354.

Menon, P.A., Thach, B.T., Smith, C.H., et al. (1984). Benzyl alcohol toxicity in a neonatal intensive care unit. Incidence, symptomatology, and mortality. *Am. J. Perinatol.* 1, 288.

Menon, R.K., Mikhailidis, D.P., Bell, J.L., et al. (1986). Warfarin administration increases uric acid concentrations in plasma. *Clin. Chem.* 32, 1557.

Menon, R.K., Gill, D.S., Thomas, M., et al. (1987). Impaired carboxylation of oestocalcin in warfarin-treated patients. *J. Clin. Endocrinol. Metab.* 64, 59.

Menzies, D.G., Conn, A.G., Williamson, I.J., et al. (1989). Fulminant hyperkalaemia and multiple complications following ibuprofen overdose. *Medical Toxicology and Adverse Drug Experience* 4, 468.

Mercer, C.W. and Logic, J.R. (1973). Cardiac arrest due to hyperkalemia following intravenous penicillin administration. *Chest* 64, 358.

Meredith, T.J., Vale, J.A., and Proudfoot, A.T. (1996). Poisoning caused by analgesic drugs. In *Oxford Textbook of Medicine* (3rd edn) (ed. D.J. Weatherall, J.G.G. Ledingham, and D.A. Warrell), p. 1051. Oxford University Press.

Messina, O.D., Barreira, J.C., Zanchetta, J.R., et al. (1992). Effect of low doses of deflazacort vs prednisone on bone mineral content in premenopausal rheumatoid arthritis. *J. Rheumatol.* 19, 1520.

Meyboom, R.H.B. and Brodie-Meijer, C.C.E. (1996). Metal antagonists. In *Meyler's Side Effects of Drugs* (ed. M.N.G. Dukes), p. 605. Elsevier, Amsterdam.

Meyers, A.M., Feldman, C., Sonnekus, M.I., et al. (1990). Chronic laxative abusers with pseudo-idiopathic oedema and autonomous pseudo-Bartter's syndrome. A spectrum of metabolic madness, or new lights on an old disease? *S. Afr. Med. J.* 78, 631.

Meyrick, T.R.H., Payne, R.C.M., and Black, M.M. (1981). Isoniazid-induced pellagra. *BMJ* ii, 287.

Michel, B.A., Bloch, D.A., and Fries, J.F. (1991). Predictors of fractures in early rheumatoid arthritis. *J. Rheumatol.* 18, 804.

Michnovicz, J.J. and Galbraith, R.A. (1991). Cimetidine inhibits catechol estrogen metabolism in women. *Metabolism* 40, 170.

Milanino, R., Frigo, A., Bambara, L.M., et al. (1993). Copper and zinc status in rheumatoid arthritis — studies of plasma, erythrocytes, and urine, and their relationship to disease-activity markers and pharmacological treatment. *Clin. Exp. Rheumatol.* 11, 271.

Millane, T.A., Jennison, S.H., Mann, J.M., *et al.* (1992). Myocardial magnesium depletion associated with prolonged hypomagnesemia: a longitudinal study in heart transplant recipients. *J. Am. Coll. Cardiol.* 20, 806.

Millar, J.W. (1980). Rifampicin-induced porphyria cutanea tarda. *Br. J. Dis. Chest* 74, 405.

Miller, L.K., Sanchez, P.L., Berg, S.W., *et al.* (1983). Effectiveness of aztreonam, a new monobactam antibiotic, against penicillin-resistant gonococci. *J. Infect. Dis.* 148, 612.

Miller, V.A., Benedetti, F.M., Rigas, J.R., *et al.* (1997). Initial clinical trial of a selective retinoid X receptor ligand, LGD1069. *J. Clin. Oncol.* 15, 790.

Milligan, A., Graham-Brown, R.A., Sarkany, I., *et al.* (1988). Erythropoietic protoporphyria exacerbated by oral iron therapy. *Br. J. Dermatol.* 119, 63.

Milne, D.B. (1994). Trace elements. In *Teitz Textbook of Clinical Chemistry* (ed. C.A. Burtis and R. Ashwood), p. 1317. W.B. Saunders, Philadelphia.

Milne, D.B. and Johnson, P.E. (1993). Assessment of copper status: effect of age and gender on reference ranges in healthy adults. *Clin. Chem.* 39, 883.

Milne, D.B., Canfield, W.K., Mahalko, J.R., *et al.* (1984). Effect of oral folic acid supplements on zinc, copper, and iron absorption and excretion. *Am. J. Clin. Nutr.* 39, 535.

Milne, D.B., Lukaski, H.C., and Johnson, P.E. (1990). Effect of folic acid supplements on zinc balance and metabolism in men fed diets adequate in zinc. *J. Trace Elem. Exp. Med.* 3, 319.

Min, D.I. and Monaco, A.P. (1991). Complications associated with immunosuppressive therapy and their management. *Pharmacotherapy* 11, 119S.

Mitchell, S., Bayliff, C.D., and McCormack, D.G. (1993). Heparin induced hyperkalemia. *Can. J. Hosp. Pharm.* 46, 125.

MMWR (1983). Lead poisoning from Mexican folk remedies — California. *MMWR* 32, 554.

MMWR (1984). Lead poisoning-associated death from Asian Indian folk remedies — Florida. *MMWR* 33, 638, 643.

MMWR (1989). Lead poisoning associated with intravenous-methamphetamine use — Oregon, 1988. *MMWR* 38, 830.

Moder, K.G. and Hurley, D.L. (1990). Fatal hypernatremia from exogenous salt intake: report of a case and review of the literature. *Mayo Clin. Proc.* 65, 1587.

Modi, K.B., Horn, E.H., and Bryson, S.M. (1985). Theophylline poisoning and rhabdomyolysis. *Lancet* ii, 160.

Momblano, P., Pradere, B., Jarrige, N., *et al.* (1984). Metabolic acidosis induced by cetrimonium bromide. *Lancet* ii, 1045.

Momoi, T., Yamanaka, C., Tanaka, R., *et al.* (1995). Elevation of serum creatine phosphokinase during growth hormone treatment in patients with multiple pituitary hormone deficiency. *Eur. J. Pediatrics* 154, 886.

Monreal, M., Lafoz, E., Salvador, R., *et al.* (1989). Adverse effects of three different forms of heparin therapy: thrombocytopenia, increased transaminases, and hyperkalaemia. *Eur. J. Clin. Pharmacol.* 37, 415.

Monreal, M., Olive, A., Lafoz, E., *et al.* (1991). Heparins, coumarin and bone density. *Lancet* 338, 706.

Montemurro, L., Schiraldi, G., Fraioli, P., *et al.* (1991). Prevention of corticosteroid-induced osteoporosis with salmon calcitonin in sarcoid patients. *Calcif. Tissue Int.* 49, 71.

Moore, C.M. (1988). Hypernatremia after the use of an activated charcoal-sorbitol suspension. *J. Pediatr.* 112, 333.

Moore, M.R. (1993). Biochemistry of porphyria. *Int. J. Biochem.* 25, 1353.

Moratinos, J. and Reverte, M. (1993). Effects of catecholamines on plasma potassium: the role of alpha- and beta-adrenoceptors. *Fundam. Clin. Pharmacol.* 7, 143.

Morgan, D.B. and Davidson, C. (1980). Hypokalaemia and diuretics: An analysis of publications. *BMJ* 280, 905.

Morita, Y., Nishida, Y., Kamatani, N., *et al.* (1984). Theophylline increases serum uric acid levels. *J. Allergy Clin. Immunol.* 74, 707.

Morrison, D., Capewell, S., Reynolds, S.P., *et al.* (1994). Testosterone levels during systemic and inhaled corticosteroid therapy. *Respir. Med.* 88, 659.

Moser, M. (1990). Do different hemodynamic effects of antihypertensive drugs translate into different safety profiles?. *Eur. J. Clin. Pharmacol.* 38 Suppl. 2, S134.

Moser, M. (1992). Diuretics and cardiovascular risk factors. *Eur. Heart J.* 13 Suppl. G, 72.

Motley, R.J. (1990). Pseudoporphyria due to dyazide in a patient with vitiligo. *BMJ* 300, 1468.

Mountokalakis, T., Dourakis, S., Karatzas, N., *et al.* (1984). Zinc deficiency in mild hypertensive patients treated with diuretics. *J. Hypertens.* Suppl. 2, S571.

Mueller, R.J., Green, D., and Phair, J.P. (1987). Hypoprothrombinemia associated with cefoperazone therapy. *South. Med. J.* 80, 1360.

Muir, J.M., Hirsh, J., Weitz, J.I., *et al.* (1997). A histomorphometric comparison of the effects of heparin and low-molecular-weight heparin on cancellous bone in rats. *Blood* 89, 3236.

Mukherjee, A.B., Ghazanfari, A., Svoronos, S., *et al.* (1986). Transketolase abnormality in tolazamide-induced Wernicke's encephalopathy. *Neurology* 36, 1508.

Muldoon, R.T. and McMartin, K.E. (1994). Ethanol acutely impairs the renal conservation of 5-methyltetrahydrofolate in the isolated perfused rat kidney. *Alcohol Clin. Exp. Res.* 18, 333.

Murialdo, G., Galimberti, C.A., Fonzi, S., *et al.* (1994). Sex hormones, gonadotropins and prolactin in male epileptic subjects in remission: role of the epileptic syndrome and of antiepileptic drugs. *Neuropsychobiology* 30, 29.

Murphy, A., Cropp, C.S., Smith, B.S., *et al.* (1990). Effect of low-dose oral contraceptive on gonadotropins, androgens, and sex hormone binding globulin in nonhirsute women. *Fertil. Steril.* 53, 35.

Murphy, C.P., Cox, R.L., Harden, E.A., *et al.* (1992). Encephalopathy and seizures induced by intravesical alum irrigations. *Bone Marrow Transplant.* 10, 383.

Murphy, M.B., Scriven, A.J., Brown, M.J., *et al.* (1982). The effects of nifedipine and hydralazine induced hypotension on sympathetic activity. *Eur. J. Clin. Pharmacol.* 23, 479.

Murray, M.D. and Brater, D.C. (1993). Renal toxicity of the nonsteroidal anti-inflammatory drugs. *Ann. Rev. Pharmacol. Toxicol.* 33, 435.

Murray, W.J.G., Lindo, V.S., Kakkar, V.V., *et al.* (1995). Long-term administration of heparin and heparin fractions and osteoporosis in experimental animals. *Blood Coagul. Fibrinolysis* 6, 113.

Murthy, U.K., DeGregorio, F., Oates, R.P., *et al.* (1992). Hyperamylasemia in patients with the acquired immunodeficiency syndrome. *Am. J. Gastroenterol.* 87, 332.

Mustajoki, P. and Nordmann, Y. (1993). Early administration of heme arginate for acute porphyric attacks. *Arch. Intern. Med.* 153, 2004.

Myers, M.G. (1987). Hydrochlorothiazide with or without amiloride for hypertension in the elderly. A dose-titration study. *Arch. Intern. Med.* 147, 1026.

Nakasaki, H., Ohta, M., Soeda, J., *et al.* (1997). Clinical and biochemical aspects of thiamine treatment for metabolic acidosis during total parenteral nutrition. *Nutrition* 13, 110.

Nanji, A.A. and Denagri, J.F. (1984). Hypomagnesemia associated with gentamicin therapy. *DICP* 18, 596.

Nanji, A.A. and Lauener, R.W. (1984). Lactulose-induced hypernatremia. *DICP* 18, 70.

Navarro, J.F., Quereda, C., and Moreno, A. (1995). Renal tubular acidosis following treatment with foscarnet. *AIDS* 9, 1389.

Neaton, J.D., Grimm, R.J., Jr, Prineas, R.J., *et al.* (1993). Treatment of mild hypertension study. Final results. Treatment of mild hypertension study group. *JAMA* 270, 713.

Neil-Dwyer, G. and Marus, A. (1989). ACE inhibitors in hypertension: assessment of taste and smell function in clinical trials. *J. Hum. Hypertens.* 3, 169.

Nesher, G., Zimran, A., and Hershko, C. (1988). Reduced incidence of hyperkalemia and azotemia in patients receiving sulindac compared with indomethacin. *Nephron* 48, 291.

Newhouse, I.J., Clement, D.B., and Lai, C. (1993). Effects of iron supplementation and discontinuation on serum copper, zinc, calcium, and magnesium levels in women. *Med. Sci. Sports Exerc.* 25, 562.

Newmann, J.H., Neff, T.A., and Ziporin, P. (1977). Acute respiratory failure associated with hypophosphatemia. *N. Engl. J. Med.* 296, 1101.

Newnham, D.M., McDevitt, D.G., and Lipworth, B.J. (1991). The effects of frusemide and triamterene on the hypokalaemic and electrocardiographic responses to inhaled terbutaline. *Br. J. Clin. Pharmacol.* 32, 630.

Ng, R.H., Roe, C., Funt, D., *et al.* (1985). Increased activity of creatine kinase isoenzymes MB in a theophylline-intoxicated patient. *Clin. Chem.* 31, 1741.

Nicholls, M.G. (1987). Overview: angiotensin, angiotensin converting enzyme inhibition, and the kidney — congestive heart failure. *Kidney Int.* 31, Suppl. 20, S200.

Nieken, J., Mulder, N.H., Buter, J., *et al.* (1995). Recombinant human interleukin-6 induces a rapid and reversible anemia in cancer patients. *Blood* 86, 900.

Nilsson, O.S., Lindholm, T.S., Elmstedt, E., *et al.* (1986). Fracture incidence and bone disease in epileptics receiving long-term anticonvulsant drug treatment. *Arch. Orthop. Trauma Surg.* 105, 146.

Nilsson, T.K., Tomic, R., and Ljungberg, B. (1989). Effects of high dose medroxyprogesterone acetate treatment on antithrombin III and other plasma proteins in males with renal cell or prostatic carcinoma. *Scand. J. Urol. Nephrol.* 23, 11.

Nishiyama, M., Itoh, F., and Ujiie, A. (1997). Low-molecular-weight heparin (dalteparin) demonstrated a weaker effect on rat bone metabolism compared with heparin. *Jpn J. Pharmacol.* 74, 59.

Nomura, K., Noguchi, Y., Yoshikawa, T., *et al.* (1993). Long-term total parenteral nutrition and osteoporosis: report of a case. *Surgery Today* 23, 1027.

Noordzij, T.C., Leunissen, K.M.L., and Van Hooff, J.P. (1991). Renal handling of urate and the incidence of gouty arthritis during cyclosporine and diuretic use. *Transplantation* 52, 64.

Nordenstrom, J., Strigard, K., Perbeck, L., *et al.* (1992). Hyperparathyroidism associated with treatment of manic-depressive disorders by lithium. *Eur. J. Surgery* 158, 207.

Nordenstrom, J., Elvius, M., Bagedahl-Strindlund, M., *et al.* (1994). Biochemical hyperparathyroidism and bone mineral status in patients treated long-term with lithium. *Metabolism* 43, 1563.

Nordenvall, B., Backman, L., Larsson, L., *et al.* (1983). Effects of calcium, aluminum, magnesium and cholestyramine on hyperoxaluria in patients with jejunoileal bypass. *Acta Chir. Scand.* 149, 93.

Nordin, B.E.C. (1990). Calcium homeostasis. *Clin. Biochem.* 23, 3.

Nordin, B.E.C., Crilly, R.G., and Smith D.A. (1984). Osteoporosis. In *Metabolic Bone and Stone Disease* (ed. B.E.C. Nordin), p. 1. Churchill Livingstone, Edinburgh.

Nordt, S.P., Williams, S.R., Turchen, S., *et al.* (1996). Hypermagnesemia following an acute ingestion of Epsom salt in a patient with normal renal function. *J. Toxicol. Clin. Toxicol.* 34, 735.

Norgaard, A., Botker, H.E., Klitgaard, N.A., *et al.* (1991). Digitalis enhances exercise-induced hyperkalaemia. *Eur. J. Clin. Pharmacol.* 41, 609.

Norgaard, K., Snorgaard, O., Jensen, T., *et al.* (1990). Effects of octreotide on lipoproteins and endothelial function in type 1 (insulin-dependent) diabetic patients. *Diabetic Med.* 7, 909.

Novak, M.A., Roth, A.S., and Levine, M.R. (1988). Calcium oxalate retinopathy associated with methoxyflurane abuse. *Retina* 8, 230.

Nozue, T., Kobayashi, A., Kodama, T., *et al.* (1992). Pathogenesis of cyclosporine-induced hypomagnesemia. *J. Pediatr.* 120, 638.

Nozue, T., Kobayashi, A., Sako, A., *et al.* (1993). Evidence that cyclosporine causes both intracellular migration and inappropriate urinary excretion of magnesium in rats. *Transplantation* 55, 346.

Nussbaum, S.R., Younger, J., Vandepol, C.J., *et al.* (1993). Single-dose intravenous therapy with pamidronate for the treatment of hypercalcemia of malignancy: comparison of 30-, 60-, and 90-mg dosages. *Am. J. Med.* 95, 297.

Nuti, R., Vattimo, A., Turchetti, V., *et al.* (1984). 25-Hydroxy-cholecalciferol as an antagonist of adverse corticosteroid effects on phosphate and calcium metabolism in man. *J. Endocrinol. Invest.* 7, 445.

Nuttall, K.L. (1994). Porphyrins and disorders of porphyrin metabolism. In *Teitz Textbook of Clinical Chemistry* (ed. C.A. Burtis and R. Ashwood), p. 2073. W.B. Saunders, Philadelphia.

Oates, N.S., Shah, R.R., Idle, J.R., *et al.* (1983). Influence of oxidation polymorphism on phenformin kinetics and dynamics. *Clin. Pharmacol. Ther.* 34, 827.

O'Brien, J.G., Dong, B.J., Coleman, R.L., *et al.* (1997). A 5-year retrospective review of adverse drug reactions and their risk factors in human immunodeficiency virus-infected patients who were receiving intravenous pentamidine therapy for *Pneumocystis carinii* pneumonia. *Clin. Infect. Dis.* 24, 854.

O'Connell, J.E. and Colledge, N.R. (1993). Type IV renal tubular acidosis and spironolactone therapy in the elderly. *Postgrad. Med. J.* 69, 887.

O'Connor, D.T., Strause, L., Saltman, P., *et al.* (1987). Serum zinc is unaffected by effective captopril treatment of hypertension. *J. Clin. Hypertens.* 3, 405.

Odigwe, C.O., McCulloch, A.J., Williams, D.O., *et al.* (1986). A trial of the calcium antagonist nisoldipine in hypertensive non-insulin-dependent diabetic patients. *Diabetic Med.* 3, 463.

Oettgen, H.F., Stephenson, P.A., Schwartz, M.K., *et al.* (1970). Toxicity of *E. coli* L-asparaginase in man. *Cancer* 25, 253.

Ogonor, J.I. (1993). The effect of chloroquine on plasma albumin, bilirubin, amylase, alkaline phosphatase and blood urea in man. *J. Clin. Pharm. Ther.* 18, 209.

O'Gorman, M.A., Fivush, B., Wise, B., *et al.* (1995). Proximal renal tubular acidosis secondary to FK506 in pediatric liver transplant patients. *Clin. Transpl.* 9, 312.

Oikkonen, M. (1984). Isoflurane and enflurane in long anaesthesias for plastic microsurgery. *Acta Anaesthesiol. Scand.* 28, 412.

Oikkonen, M. and Meretoja, O. (1989). Serum fluoride in children anaesthetized with enflurane. *Eur. J. Anaesthesiol.* 6, 401.

Olano, J.P., Borucki, M.J., Wen, J.W., *et al.* (1995). Massive hepatic steatosis and lactic acidosis in a patient with AIDS who was receiving zidovudine. *Clin. Infect. Dis.* 21, 973.

Olbricht, T. and Benker, G. (1993). Glucocorticoid-induced osteoporosis: pathogenesis, prevention and treatment, with special regard to the rheumatic diseases. *J. Intern. Med.* 234, 237.

Olgaard, K., Storm, T., van Wowern, N., *et al.* (1992). Glucocorticoid-induced osteoporosis in the lumbar spine, forearm, and mandible of nephrotic patients: a double-blind study on the high-dose, long-term effects of prednisone versus deflazacort. *Calcif. Tissue Int.* 50, 490.

Olivares, M. and Uauy, R. (1996). Copper as an essential nutrient. *Am. J. Clin. Nutr.* 63, 791S.

Olveira Fuster, G., Mancha Doblas, I., Vazquez San Miguel, F., *et al.* (1996). Ingesta subreptica de diureticos como causa de pseudo-sindrome Bartter a propósito de un caso y diagnóstico diferencial. *Anales de Medicina Interna* 13, 496.

Ong, E.L., Ellis, M.E., McDowell, D., *et al.* (1988). Porphyria cutanea tarda in association with the human immunodeficiency virus infection. *Postgrad. Med. J.* 64, 956.

Orefice, G., Troisi, E., Selvaggio, M., *et al.* (1992). Effect of long-term mesoglycan treatment on fibrinogen plasma levels in patients with ischemic cerebrovascular disease. *Current Therapeutic Research — Clinical and Experimental* 52, 666.

Orwoll, E.S. (1982). The milk–alkali syndrome: current concepts. *Ann. Intern. Med.* 97, 242.

Oster, J.R., Singer, I., and Fishman, L.M. (1995). Heparin-induced aldosterone suppression and hyperkalemia. *Am. J. Med.* 98, 575.

Otsuka, F., Hayashi, Y., Ogura, T., *et al.* (1996). Syndrome of inappropriate secretion of antidiuretic hormone following intra-thoracic cisplatin. *Intern. Med.* 35, 290.

Packe, G.E., Robb, O., Robins, S.P., *et al.* (1996). Bone density in asthmatic patients taking inhaled steroids: comparison of budesonide and beclomethasone dipropionate. *J. R. Coll. Physicians Lond.* 30, 128.

Pahl, M.V., Vaziri, N.D., Ness, R., *et al.* (1984). Association of beta hydroxybutyrate acidosis with isoniazid intoxication. *J. Toxicol. Clin. Toxicol.* 22, 167.

Palestine, A.G., Austin, H.A., and Nussenblatt, R.B. (1986). Renal tubular function in cyclosporine-treated patients. *Am. J. Med.* 81, 419.

Palestine, A.G., Polis, M.A., De Smet, M.D., *et al.* (1991). A randomized, controlled trial of foscarnet in the treatment of cytomegalovirus retinitis in patients with AIDS. *Ann. Intern. Med.* 115, 665.

Panagakos, F.S., Jandinski, J.J., Feder, L., *et al.* (1995). Heparin fails to potentiate the effects of IL-1-beta-mediated bone resorption of fetal rat long bones *in vitro*. *Biochimie* 77, 915.

Pantuck, E.J., Pantuck, C.B., Ryan, D.E., *et al.* (1985). Inhibition and stimulation of enflurane metabolism in the rat following a single dose or chronic administration of ethanol. *Anesthesiology* 62, 255.

Papademetriou, V. (1994). Effect of diuretics on cardiac arrhythmias and left ventricular hypertrophy in hypertension. *Cardiology* 84 Suppl. 2, 43.

Pappas, N.J.J. (1989). Theoretical aspects of enzymes in diagnosis. Why do serum enzymes changes in hepatic, myocardial and other diseases? *Clin. Lab. Med.* 9, 595.

Pappas, A.A., Ackeman, B.H., Olsen, K.M., *et al.* (1991). Isopropanol ingestion: a report of six episodes with isopropanol and acetone serum concentration time data. *Clin. Toxicol.* 29, 11.

Parker, W.A. and Shearer, C.A. (1979). Phenytoin hepatotoxicity: A case report and review. *Neurology* 29, 175.

Parodi, A., Guarrera, M., and Rebora, A. (1988). Amiodarone-induced pseudoporphyria. *Photodermatology* 5, 146.

Parr, M.J., Anaes, F.C., Day, A.C., *et al.* (1990). Theophylline poisoning —a review of 64 cases. *Intensive Care Med.* 16, 394.

Pastoureau, P., Vergnaud, P., Meunier, P.J., *et al.* (1993). Osteopenia and bone-remodeling abnormalities in warfarin-treated lambs. *J. Bone Min. Res.* 8, 1417.

Patrono, C. and Dunn, M.J. (1987). The clinical significance of inhibition of renal prostaglandin synthesis. *Kidney Int.* 32, 1.

Patterson, W.P., Winkelmann, M., and Perry, M.C. (1985). Zinc-induced copper deficiency: megamineral sideroblastic anemia. *Ann. Intern. Med.* 103, 385.

Patwari, A.K., Aneja, S., Chandra, D., *et al.* (1996). Long-term anticonvulsant therapy in tuberculous meningitis — a four-year follow-up. *J. Trop. Pediatr.* 42, 98.

Payne, C.M., Bladin, C., Colchester, A.C., *et al.* (1992). Argyria from excessive use of topical silver sulphadiazine. *Lancet* 340, 126.

Pazzucconi, F., Mannucci, L., Mussoni, L., *et al.* (1992). Bezafibrate lowers plasma lipids, fibrinogen and platelet aggregability in hypertriglyceridaemia. *Eur. J. Clin. Pharmacol.* 43, 219.

Pearlman, C., Wheadon, D., and Epstein, S. (1988). Creatine kinase elevation after neuroleptic treatment. *Am. J. Psychiatry* 145, 1018.

Pearson, J.C., Dombrovskis, S., Dreyer, J., *et al.* (1983). Radio-immunoassay of serum prostatic acid phosphatase after prostatic massage. *Urology* 21, 37.

Peczkowska, M., Kabat, M., Janaszek-Sitkowska, H., *et al.* (1997). Zinc metabolism in essential hypertension and during angiotensin-converting enzyme inhibitor therapy — preliminary report. *Trace Elements and Electrolytes* 14, 82.

Pedersen, O.L. and Mikkelsen, E. (1979). Serum potassium and uric acid changes during treatment with timolol alone and in combination with a diuretic. *Clin. Pharmacol. Ther.* 26, 339.

Pedersen, P.B. and Hogenhaven, H. (1990). Penicillamine-induced neuropathy in rheumatoid arthritis. *Acta Neurol. Scand.* 81, 188.

Pegues, D.A., Hughes, B.J., and Woernle, C.H. (1993). Elevated blood lead levels associated with illegally distilled alcohol. *Arch. Intern. Med.* 153, 1501.

Pellock, J.M., Howell, J., Kendig, E.L., Jr, *et al.* (1985). Pyridoxine deficiency in children treated with isoniazid. *Chest* 87, 658.

Perazella, M.A. (1996). Hyperkalemia in the elderly: a group at high risk. *Conn. Med.* 60, 195.

Perazella, M. and Brown, E. (1993). Acute aluminum toxicity and alum bladder irrigation in patients with renal failure. *Am. J. Kidney Dis.* 21, 44.

Perez, A, Nere, T., and Famaly, I.P. (1989). Effects of chronic and acute corticosteroid therapy on zinc and copper status in rheumatoid arthritis patients. *Journal of Trace Elements and Electrolytes in Health and Disease* 3, 103.

Perrot, J.L., Guy, C., Bour Guichenez, G., *et al.* (1994). Porphyrie cutanée tardive induite par des inhibiteurs de l'HMG CoA reductase: simvastatine, pravastatine. *Ann. Derm. Venereol. (Stockh.)* 121, 817.

Petersen, L.R., Denis, D., Brown, D., *et al.* (1988). Community health effects of a municipal water supply hyperfluoridation accident. *Am. J. Public Health* 78, 711.

Petersson, I., Nilsson, G., Hansson, B.G., *et al.* (1987). Water intoxication associated with non-steroidal anti-inflammatory drug therapy. *Acta Med. Scand.* 221, 221.

Petren, S. and Vesterberg, O. (1987). Studies of transferrin in serum of workers exposed to organic solvents. *Br. J. Ind. Med.* 44, 566.

Pfeiffer, F.E., Homburger, H.A., Houser, O.W., *et al.* (1987). Elevation of serum creatine kinase B-subunit levels by radiographic contrast agents in patients with neurologic disorders. *Mayo Clin. Proc.* 62, 351.

Philip, W.J.U., Martin, J.C., Richardson, J.M., *et al.* (1995). Decreased axial and peripheral bone density in patients taking long-term warfarin. *Q. J. Med.* 88, 635.

Pierce, L.R., Wysowski, D.K., and Gross, T.P. (1990). Myopathy and rhabdomyolysis associated with lovastatin-gemfibrozil combination therapy. *JAMA* 264, 71.

Pierce, R.P., Gazewood, J., and Blake, R.L., Jr. (1991). Salicylate poisoning from enteric-coated aspirin. Delayed absorption may complicate management. *Postgrad. Med.* 89, 61, 64.

Pierides, A.M. and Alvasez-Ude, F. (1975). Clofibrate- induced muscle damage in patients with chronic renal failure. *Lancet* ii, 1279.

Pillans, P.I., Cowan, P., and Whitelaw, D. (1985). Hyponatraemia and confusion in a patient taking ketoconazole. *Lancet* i, 821.

Pineo, G.F. and Hull, R.D. (1993). Adverse effects of coumarin anticoagulants. *Drug Saf.* 9, 263.

Pinto, J., Huang, Y.P., and Rivlin, R.S. (1981). Inhibition of riboflavin metabolism in rat tissues by chlorpromazine, imipramine, and amitriptyline. *J. Clin. Invest.* 67, 1500.

Pironi, L., Cornia, G.L., Ursitti, M.A., *et al.* (1988). Evaluation of oral administration of folic acid and folinic acid to prevent folate deficiency in patients with inflammatory bowel disease treated with salicylazosulfapyridine. *Int. J. Clin. Pharmacol. Res.* 8, 143.

Pluskiewicz, W. and Nowakowska, J. (1997). Bone status after long-term anticonvulsant therapy in epileptic patients: evaluation using quantitative ultrasound of calcaneus and phalanges. *Ultrasound Med. Biol.* 23, 553.

Polan, M.L. and Barbieri, R.L. (1990). New treatment for endometriosis: synarel is a gonadotropin-releasing hormone agonist. *American Druggist* 201, 26.

Poole-Wilson, P.A. (1987). Diuretics, hypokalaemia and arrhythmias in hypertensive patients: still an unresolved problem. *J. Hypertens.* Suppl. 5, S51.

Poonguzhali, P.K. and Chegu, H. (1994). The influence of banana stem extract on urinary risk factors for stones in normal and hyperoxaluric rats. *Br. J. Urol.* 74, 23.

Pople, I.K. and Phillips, H. (1988). Bone cement and the liver. A dose-related effect? *J. Bone Joint Surg.* B-70, 364.

Pordy, R.C. (1994). Cilazapril plus hydrochlorothiazide: improved efficacy without reduced safety in mild to moderate hypertension. A double-blind placebo-controlled multicenter study of factorial design. *Cardiology* 85, 311.

Porter, K.G., McMaster, D., Elmes, M.E., *et al.* (1977). Anaemia and low serum-copper during zinc therapy. *Lancet* ii, 774.

Postlethwaite, A.E. and Kelley, W.N. (1971). Uricosuric effect of radiocontrast agents. A study in man of four commonly used preparations. *Ann. Intern. Med.* 74, 845.

Praga, M., Enriquez de Salamanca, R., Andres, A., *et al.* (1987). Treatment of hemodialysis-related porphyria cutanea tarda with deferoxamine. *N. Engl. J. Med.* 316, 547.

Prasad, A.S., Brewer, G.J., Schoomaker, E.B., *et al.* (1978). Hypocupremia induced by zinc therapy in adults. *JAMA* 240, 2166.

Preuss, H.G. and Burris, J.F. (1996). Adverse metabolic effects of antihypertensive drugs. Implications for treatment. *Drug Saf.* 14, 355.

Prichard, B.N.C., Owens, C.W.L., and Woolf, A.S. (1992). Adverse reactions to diuretics. *Eur. Heart J.* 13, 96.

Prince, R.L., Monk, K.J., Kent, G.N., *et al.* (1988). Effects of theophylline and salbutamol on phosphate and calcium metabolism in normal subjects. *Miner. Electrolyte Metab.* 14, 262.

Pritza, D.R., Bierman, M.H., and Hammeke, M.D. (1991). Acute toxic effects of sustained-release verapamil in chronic renal failure. *Arch. Intern. Med.* 151, 2081.

Prospert, F., Soupart, A., Brimioulle, S., *et al.* (1993). Evidence of defective tubular reabsorption and normal secretion of uric acid in the syndrome of inappropriate secretion of antidiuretic hormone. *Nephron* 64, 189.

Proudfoot, A.T., Vale, J.A. and Meredith, T.J. (1996). Poisoning caused by respiratory drugs. In *Oxford Textbook of Medicine* (3rd edn) (ed. D.J. Weatherall, J.G.G. Ledingham, and D.A. Warrell), p. 1068. Oxford University Press.

Prouse, P., Shawe, D., and Gumpel, J.M. (1987). Macrocytic anaemia in patients treated with sulfasalazine for rheumatoid arthritis. *BMJ* 294, 90.

Prystowsky, E.N. (1992). Effects of bepridil on cardiac electrophysiologic properties. *Am. J. Cardiol.* 69, 63D.

Przybylo, H.J., Stevenson, G.W., Schanbacher, P., *et al.* (1995). Sodium nitroprusside metabolism in children during hypothermic cardiopulmonary bypass. *Anesth. Analg.* 81, 952.

Purohit, O.P., Anthony, C., Radstone, C.R., *et al.* (1994). High-dose intravenous pamidronate for metastatic bone pain. *Br. J. Cancer* 70, 554.

Puttagunta, N.R., Gibby, W.A., and Smith, G.T. (1996). Human *in-vivo* comparative study of zinc and copper transmetalation after administration of magnetic-resonance-imaging contrast agents. *Invest. Radiol.* 31, 739.

Qureshi, A.R., Lindholm, B., Alvestrand, A., *et al.* (1994). Nutritional status, muscle composition and plasma and muscle free amino acids in renal transplant patients. *Clin. Nephrol.* 42, 237.

Qureshi, T. and Melonakos, T.K. (1996). Acute hypermagnesemia after laxative use. *Ann. Emerg. Med.* 28, 552.

Rado, J.P., Juhos, E., and Sawinsky, I. (1975). Dose–response relations in drug-induced inappropriate secretion of ADH: effects of clofibrate and carbamazepine. *Int. J. Clin. Pharmacol. Ther. Toxicol.* 12, 315.

Raeder, J.C. (1996). Nitrous oxide: Still a role in anaesthesia? *Current Opinion in Anaesthesiology* 9, 279.

Rahilly, G.T. and Berl, T. (1979). Severe metabolic alkalosis caused by administration of plasma protein fraction in end-stage renal failure. *N. Engl. J. Med.* 301, 824.

Rahman, A.R.A., McDevitt, D.G., Struthers, A.D., *et al.* (1992*a*). The effects of enalapril and spironolactone on terbutaline-induced hypokalemia. *Chest* 102, 91.

Rahman, A.R.A., McDevitt, D.G., Struthers, A.D., *et al.* (1992*b*). Sex differences in hypokalaemic and electrocardiographic effects of inhaled terbutaline. *Thorax* 47, 1056.

Ramsay, L.E., Yeo, W.W., and Jackson, P.R. (1994). Metabolic effects of diuretics. *Cardiology* 84 Suppl. 2, 48.

Randi, M.L., Mares, M., Fabris, F., *et al.* (1991). Decrease of fibrinogen in patients with peripheral atherosclerotic disease by ticlopidine. *Arzneimittelforschung* 41, 414.

Ranft, K. and Eibl-Eibesfeldt, B. (1990). Enterale Hyperoxalose bei Therapie mit Somatostatin-Analog. *Dtsch. Med. Wochenschr.* 115, 179.

Rao, K.J., Miller, M., and Moses, A.M. (1976). Hypocalcaemic tetany: result of a high-phosphate enema. *N.Y. State J. Med.* 76, 968.

Rao, M.L., Stefan, H., Scheid, C., *et al.* (1993). Serum amino acids, liver status, and antiepileptic drug therapy in epilepsy. *Epilepsia* 34, 347.

Rao, P.N. (1987). Fluid absorption during urological endoscopy. *Br. J. Urol.* 60, 93.

Ratcliffe, W.A., Hazelton, R.A., Thomson, J.A., *et al.* (1980). The effect of fenclofenac on thyroid function test *in vivo* and *in vitro*. *Clin. Endocrinol.* (Oxf.) 13, 569.

Rathbun, R.C. and Martin E.S. III. (1992). Didanosine therapy in patients intolerant of or failing zidovudine therapy. *Ann. Pharmacother.* 26, 1347.

Ratzmann, G.W. and Zollner, H. (1985). Hypomagnesiamie und Hypokaliamie während des Insulin-Hypoglykamietestes. *Z. Gesamte. Inn. Med.* 40, 567.

Rault, R.M. (1993). Hyponatremia associated with nonsteroidal antiinflammatory drugs. *Am. J. Med. Sci.* 305, 318.

Rauschning, W. and Pritchard, K.I. (1994). Droloxifene, a new antiestrogen: its role in metastatic breast cancer. *Breast Cancer Research and Treatment* 31, 83.

Reddig, S., Minnema, A.M., and Tandon, R. (1993). Neuroleptic malignant syndrome and clozapine. *Ann. Clin. Psychiatry* 5, 25.

Redwood, M., Taylor, C., Bain, B.J., *et al.* (1991). The association of age with dosage requirement for warfarin. *Age Ageing* 20, 217.

Refsum, H., Helland, S., and Ueland, P.M. (1989). Fasting plasma homocysteine as a sensitive parameter of antifolate effect: a study of psoriasis patients receiving-low-dose methotrexate treatment. *Clin. Pharmacol. Ther.* 46, 510.

Reid, D.J., Barr, S.I., and Leichter, J. (1992). Effects of folate and zinc supplementation on patients undergoing chronic hemodialysis. *J. Am. Diet. Assoc.* 92, 574.

Reid, D.M. and Harvie, J. (1997). Secondary osteoporosis. *Baillière's Clinical Endocrinology and Metabolism* (ed. I.R. Reid), p. 83. Baillière Tindall, London.

Reid, I.R. (1989). Pathogenesis and treatment of steroid osteoporosis. *Clin. Endocrinol.* (Oxf.) 30, 83.

Reid, I.R (1997). preventing glucorticoid-induced osteoporosis. *N. Engl. J. Med.* 337, 420.

Reid, I.R. and Ibbertson, H.K. (1987). Evidence for decreased tubular reabsorption of calcium in glucocorticoid-treated asthmatics. *Horm. Res.* 27, 200.

Reid, I.R. and Heap, S.W. (1990). Determinants of vertebral mineral density in patients receiving long-term glucocorticoid therapy. *Arch. Intern. Med.* 150, 2545.

Reid, I.R. and Grey, A.B. (1993). Corticosteroid osteoporosis. *Baillière's Clin. Rheumatol.* 7, 573.

Reid, I.R., Chapman, G.E., Fraser, T.R., *et al.* (1986). Low serum osteocalcin levels in glucocorticoid-treated asthmatics. *J. Clin. Endocrinol. Metab.* 62, 379.

Reid, I.R., Veale, A.G., and France, J.T. (1994). Glucocorticoid osteoporosis. *J. Asthma* 31, 7.

Reid, I.R., Wattie, D.J., Evans, M.C., *et al.* (1996). Testosterone therapy in glucocorticoid-treated men. *Arch. Intern. Med.* 156, 1173.

Reid, J.L., White, K.F., and Struthers, A.D. (1986). Epinephrine-induced hypokalemia: the role of beta adrenoceptors. *Am. J. Cardiol.* 57, 23F.

Rej, R. (1989). Aminotransferase in disease. *Clin. Lab. Med.* 9, 667.

Resnick, L.M., Nicholson, J.P., and Laragh, J.H. (1987). Calcium, the renin–aldosterone system, and the hypotensive response to nifedipine. *Hypertension* 10, 254.

Resnick, L.M., Nicholson, J.P., and Laragh, J.H. (1989). The effects of calcium channel blockade on blood pressure and calcium metabolism. *Am. J. Hypertens.* 2, 927.

Restuccio, A. (1992). Fatal hyperkalemia from a salt substitute. *Am. J. Emerg. Med.* 10, 171.

Reusz, G.S., Latta, K., Hoyer, P.F., *et al.* (1990). Evidence suggesting hyperoxaluria as a cause of nephrocalcinosis in phosphate-treated hypophosphataemic rickets. *Lancet* 335, 1240.

Rey, E., Luquel, L., Richard, M.O., *et al.* (1989). Pharmacokinetics of intravenous salbutamol in renal insufficiency and its biological effects. *Eur. J. Clin. Pharmacol.* 37, 387.

Reynolds, J.E.F. (ed.) (1996). *Martindale The Extra Pharmacopoeia* (31st edn). The Pharmaceutical Press, London.

Reynolds, R.D. and Natta, C.L. (1985). Depressed plasma pyridoxal phosphate concentrations in adult asthmatics. *Am. J. Clin. Nutr.* 41, 684.

Reynolds, T.B., Peters, R.L., and Yamada, S. (1971). Chronic active and lupoid hepatitis caused by a laxative oxyphenisatin. *N. Engl. J. Med.* 285, 813.

Reza, M.J., Kovick, R.B., Shine, K.I., *et al.* (1974). Massive intravenous digoxin overdosage. *N. Engl. J. Med.* 291, 777.

Rich, G.M., Mudge, G.H., Laffel, G.L., *et al.* (1992). Cyclosporine A and prednisone-associated osteoporosis in heart transplant recipients. *J. Heart Lung Transplant.* 11, 950.

Richens, A., McEwan, J.R., Deybach, J.C., *et al.* (1997). Evidence for both *in vivo* and *in vitro* interaction between vigabatrin and alanine transaminase. *Br. J. Clin. Pharmacol.* 43, 163.

Rigal, J., Furet, Y., Autret, E., *et al.* (1989). Hépatite mixte sévère au fénofibrate. Revue de la littérature à propos d'un cas. *Rev. Méd. Interne* 10, 65.

Riikonen, R., Simell, O., Jaaskelainen, J., *et al.* (1986). Disturbed calcium and phosphate homoeostasis during treatment with ACTH of infantile spasms. *Arch. Dis. Child.* 61, 671.

Riordan, C.A., Anstey, A., and Wojnarowska, F. (1993). Isotretinoin-associated pseudoporphyria. *Clin. Exp. Dermatol.* 18, 69.

Rivers, J.M. (1987). Safety of high-level vitamin C ingestion. *Ann. N.Y. Acad. Sci.* 498, 445.

Rivey, M.P., Schottelius, D.D., and Berg., M.J. (1984). Phenytoin-folic acid: a review. *DICP* 18, 292.

Robertshaw, M. and Swaminathan, R. (1993). Biochemical changes after a 100 km hill walk. *J. Med.* 24, 311.

Robertson, G.L. (1995). Diabetes insipidus. *Endocrinol. Metab. Clin. North Am.* 24, 549.

Robertson, G.L. and Berl, T. (1996). Pathophysiology of water metabolism. In *The Kidney* (ed. B.M. Brenner), p. 873. W.B. Saunders, Philadelphia.

Robertson, N.J. (1985). Fatal overdose from a sustained-release theophylline preparation. *Ann. Emerg. Med.* 14, 154.

Robertson, W.O. (1977). Danger of salt as an emetic. *BMJ* ii, 1022.

Robson, W.L. and Leung, A.K. (1994). Side effects and complications of treatment with desmopressin for enuresis. *J. Natl Med. Assoc.* 86, 775.

Rodriguez, M., Solanki, D.L., and Whang, R. (1989). Refractory potassium repletion due to cisplatin-induced magnesium depletion. *Arch. Intern. Med.* 149, 2592.

Roels, H., Lauwerys, R., Buchet, J.P., *et al.* (1987). Epidemiological survey among workers exposed to manganese: effects on lung, central nervous system, and some biological indices. *Am. J. Ind. Med.* 11, 307.

Rofe, A.M., Conyers, R.A.J., Bais, R., *et al.* (1979). Oxalate excretion in rats injected with xylitol or glycollate: stimulation by phenobarbitone pretreatment. *Aust. J. Exp. Biol. Med. Sci.* 57, 171.

Rogers, P.D. (1997). Cimetidine in the treatment of acute intermittent porphyria. *Ann. Pharmacother.* 31, 365.

Rogiers, P., Vermeier, W., Kesteloot, H., *et al.* (1989). Effect of the infusion of magnesium sulfate during atrial pacing on ECG intervals, serum electrolytes, and blood pressure. *Am. Heart J.* 117, 1278.

Rolla, G. and Bucca, C. (1988). Magnesium, beta-agonists, and asthma. *Lancet* i, 989.

Romer, F.K. and Jacobsen, F. (1982). The influence of prednisone on serum angiotensin-converting enzyme activity in patients with and without sarcoidosis. *Scand. J. Clin. Lab. Invest.* 42, 377.

Rosalki, S.B., Foo, A.Y., and Armtsen, K.W. (1989). Alkaline phosphatase of possible renal origin identified in plasma after colchicine overdose. *Clin. Chem.* 35, 702.

Rose, B.D. (1994). In *Clinical Physiology of Acid–base and Electrolyte Disorders* (4th edn). McGraw-Hill, New York.

Rosen, H.N., Maitland, L.A., Suttie, J.W., *et al.* (1993). Vitamin K and maintenance of skeletal integrity in adults. *Am. J. Med.* 94, 62.

Rosenmund, A., Camponovo, F., and Kochli, H.P. (1986). Der Einfluss hormoneller Kontrazeptiva und der Schwangerschaft auf Eisenstoffwechsel, Plasmalactoferrinkonzentration und Granulozytenzahl der Frau. *Schweiz. Med. Wochenschr.* 116, 1411.

Rossi, S.J., Schroeder, T.J., Hariharan, S., *et al.* (1993). Prevention and management of the adverse effects associated with immunosuppressive therapy. *Drug Saf.* 9, 104.

Rotenberg, F.A. and Giannini, V.S. (1992). Hyperkalemia associated with ketorolac. *Ann. Pharmacother.* 26, 778.

Roth, A., Miller, H.I., Belhassen, B., *et al.*. (1989). Slow-release verapamil and hyperglycemic metabolic acidosis. *Ann. Intern. Med.* 110, 171.

Roth, E., Valentini, L., Semsroth, M., *et al.* (1995). Resistance of nitrogen metabolism to growth hormone treatment in the early phase after injury of patients with multiple injuries. *J. Trauma* 38, 136.

Rubio-Luengo, M.A., Maldonado-Martin, A., Gil-Extremera, B., *et al.* (1995). Variations in magnesium and zinc in hypertensive patients receiving different treatments. *Am. J. Hypertens.* 8, 689.

Ruder, H., Corvol, P., Mahoudeau, J.A., *et al.* (1971). Effects of induced hyperthyroidism on steroid metabolism in man. *J. Clin. Endocrinol. Metab.* 33, 382.

Ruef, C., Blaser, J., Maurer, P., *et al.* (1996). Miscellaneous antibiotics. In *Meyler's Side Effects of Drugs* (ed. M.N.G. Dukes), p. 725. Elsevier, Amsterdam.

Ruegsegger, P., Medici, T.C., and Anliker, M. (1983). Corticosteroid-induced bone loss. A longitudinal study of alternate day therapy in patients with bronchial asthma using quantitative computed tomography. *Eur. J. Clin. Pharmacol.* 25, 615.

Ruff, M.E., Pincus, L.G., and Sampson, H.A. (1987). Phenytoin-induced IgA depression. *Am. J. Dis. Child.* 141, 858.

Russell, R.G.G., Smith, R., Preston, C., *et al.* (1974). Diphosphonate in Paget's disease. *Lancet* i, 894.

Russell, R.M. (1980). Vitamin A and zinc metabolism in alcoholism. *Am. J. Clin. Nutr.* 33, 2741.

Russell, S. and Young, M.J. (1994). Hypercalcaemia during treatment of psoriasis with calcipotriol. *Br. J. Dermatol.* 130, 795.

Rutten, J.M.J., Booij, L.H.D., Rulten, C.C.J., *et al.* (1980). The comparative neuromuscular blocking effects of some aminoglycoside antibiotics. *Acta Anaesthesiol. Belg.* 4, 293.

Ryan, M.F., Samy, A., and Young, J. (1996). Vigabatrin causes profound reduction in serum alanine transaminase activity. *Ann. Clin. Biochem.* 33, 257.

Ryan, M.P. (1987). Diuretics and potassium/magnesium depletion. Directions for treatment. *Am. J. Med.* 82, Suppl. 3A, 38.

Ryan, T., Coughlan, G., McGing, P., *et al.* (1989). Ketosis, a complication of theophylline toxicity. *J. Intern. Med.* 226, 227.

Ryder, R.E. (1987). The danger of high dose sodium bicarbonate in biguanide-induced lactic acidosis: the theory, the practice and alternative therapies. *Br. J. Clin. Pract.* 41, 730.

Ryffel, B., Weber, E., and Mihatsch, M.J. (1994). Nephrotoxicity of immunosuppressants in rats: comparison of macrolides with cyclosporin. *Experimental Nephrology* 2, 324.

Sadik, W., Kovacs, L., Pretnar-Darovec, A., *et al.* (1985). A randomized double-blind study of the effects of two low-dose combined oral contraceptives on biochemical aspects. *Contraception* 32, 223.

Sahin, G., Aydin, A., Isimer, A., *et al.* (1995). Aluminum content of infant formulas used in Turkey. *Biol. Trace Elem. Res.* 50, 87.

Sainsbury, S.J. (1991). Fatal salicylate toxicity from bismuth subsalicylate. *West. J. Med.* 155, 637.

Saitta, J.C., Ott, S.M., Sherrard, D.J., *et al.* (1993). Metabolic bone disease in adults receiving long-term parenteral nutrition: longitudinal study with regional densitometry and bone biopsy. *JPEN* 17, 214.

Sakhaee, K., Wabner, C.L., Zerwekh, J.E., *et al.* (1993). Calcium citrate without aluminum antacids does not cause aluminum retention in patients with functioning kidneys. *Bone Miner.* 20, 87.

Salem, P., Khalyl, M., Jabboury, K., *et al.* (1984). Cis-diamminedichloroplatinum (II) by 5-day continuous infusion. A new dose schedule with minimal toxicity. *Cancer* 53, 837.

Salih, E.S., Zein, A.A., and Bayoumi, R.A. (1986). The effect of oral contraceptives on the apparent vitamin B_6 status in some Sudanese women. *Br. J. Nutr.* 56, 363.

Salusky, I.B., Foley, J., Nelson, P., *et al.* (1991). Aluminum accumulation during treatment with aluminum hydroxide and dialysis in children and young adults with chronic renal disease. *N. Engl. J. Med.* 324, 527.

Salway, J.G. (1989). *Drug-test Interactions Handbook.* Chapman and Hall Medical, London.

Samani, N.J. (1991). Nifedipine and hypercalcaemia of primary hyperparathyroidism. *Lancet* 337, 372.

Sambrook, P. and Birmingham, J. (1993). Prevention of corticosteroid osteoporosis. A comparison of calcium, calcitriol and calcitonin. *N. Engl. J. Med.* 328, 1747.

Sambrook, P., Birmingham, J., Kempler, S., *et al.* (1990). Corticosteroid effects on proximal femur bone loss. *J. Bone Miner. Res.* 5, 1211.

Sambrook, P., Birmingham, J., Kelly, P., *et al.* (1993). Prevention of corticosteroid osteoporosis. A comparison of calcium, calcitriol and calcitonin. *N. Engl. J. Med.* 328, 1747.

Sander, J.W.A. and Patsalos, P.N. (1992). An assessment of serum and red blood cell folate concentrations in patients with epilepsy on lamotrigine therapy. *Epilepsy Res.* 13, 89.

Sang, G.W., Lorenzo, B., and Reidenberg, M.M. (1991). Inhibitory effects of gossypol on corticosteroid 11-beta-hydroxysteroid dehydrogenase from guinea pig kidney: a possible mechanism for causing hypokalemia. *J. Steroid Biochem. Mol. Biol.* 39, 169.

Sanpitak, N. and Chayutimonkul, L. (1974). Oral contraceptives and riboflavine nutrition. *Lancet* i, 836.

Santana, V.M., Schell, M.J., Williams, R., *et al.* (1992). Escalating sequential high-dose carboplatin and etoposide with autologous marrow support in children with relapsed solid tumors. *Bone Marrow Transplant.* 10, 457.

Sanwikarja, S., Kauffmann, R.H., te Velde, J., *et al.* (1989). Tubulointerstitial nephritis associated with pyrazinamide. *Neth. J. Med.* 34, 40.

Saruta, T., Suzuki, H., Kawamura, M., *et al.* (1985). Serum creatine phosphokinase levels during treatment with beta-adrenoreceptor blocking agents. *J. Cardiovasc. Pharmacol.* 7, 805.

Sato, K., Kondo, T., Iwao, H., *et al.* (1991). Sodium and potassium in red blood cells of premature infants during the first few days: risk of hyperkalaemia. *Acta Paediatr. Scand.* 80, 899.

Sattler, F.R., Weitekamp, M.R., Sayegh, A., *et al.* (1988). Impaired hemostasis caused by beta-lactam antibiotics. *Am. J. Surg.* 155, 30.

Sawhney, A.K. and Lott, J.A. (1986). Acetylcholinesterase and cholinesterase. In *Clinical Enzymology. A Case Orientation Approach* (ed. J.A. Lott and P.C. Wolf), p. 1. Field, Rich, New York.

Scheppach, W., Kortmann, B., Burghardt, *et al.* (1988). Effects of acetate during regular hemodialysis. *Clin. Nephrol.* 29, 19.

Schiano, T.D., Klang, M.G., Quesada, E., *et al.* (1996). Thiamine status in patients receiving long-term home parenteral nutrition. *Am. J. Gastroenterol.* 91, 2555.

Schindler, A.M. (1984). Isolated neonatal hypomagnesaemia associated with maternal overuse of stool softener. *Lancet* ii, 822.

Schindler, A.M. and Hines, L.B. (1988). Hypernatremic metabolic alkalosis in a two-month-old infant. *Hosp. Pract.* 23, 31.

Schmidt, K.H., Hagmaier, V., Hornig, D.H., *et al.* (1981). Urinary oxalate excretion after large intakes of ascrobic acid in man. *Am. J. Clin. Nutr.* 34, 305.

Schmidt, R.E. and Sesin, G.P. (1987). Hetastarch-induced hyperkalemia. *DICP* 12, 922.

Schmitt, K., Hausler, G., Blumel, P., *et al.* (1997). The influence of growth hormone monotherapy and growth hormone in combination with oxandrolone or testosterone on thyroxid hormone parameters and thyroxine binding globulin in patients with Ullrich–Turner syndrome. *Eur. J. Pediatr.* 156, 99.

Schmitz, B. and Trimble, M.R. (1995). Carbamazepine and PIP-syndrome in temporal lobe epilepsy. *Epilepsy Res.* 22, 215.

Schmutz, J.L., Cuny, J.F., Trechot, P., *et al.* (1987). Les erythèmes pellagroides médicamenteux. Une observation d'erythème pellagroïde secondaire à l'isoniazide. *Ann. Dermatol. Venereol.* 114, 569.

Schnabel, R., Rambeck, B., and Janssen, F. (1984). Fatal intoxication with sodium valproate. *Lancet* i, 221.

Schriber, J.R. and Negrin, R.S. (1993). Use and toxicity of the colony-stimulating factors. *Drug Saf.* 8, 457.

Schultz, R.E., Hanno, P.M., Levin, R.M., *et al.* (1983). Percutaneous ultrasonic lithotripsy: choice of irrigant. *J. Urol.* 130, 858.

Schwab, R.A. and Bachhuber, B.H. (1991). Delirium and lactic acidosis caused by ethanol and niacin co-ingestion. *Am. J. Emerg. Med.* 9, 363.

Schwartz, D.E., Kelly, B., Caldwell, J.E., *et al.* (1992). Succinylcholine-induced hyperkalemic arrest in a patient with severe metabolic acidosis and exsanguinating hemorrhage. *Anesth. Analg.* 75, 291.

Schwartz, R.H. and Jones, R.W.A. (1978). Transplacental hyponatraemia due to oxytocin. *BMJ* i, 152.

Schwinger, R.H.G. and Erdmann, E. (1992). Heart failure and electrolyte disturbances. *Methods Find. Exp. Clin. Pharmacol.* 14, 315.

Scoble, J.E., Freetone, A., Varghese, Z., *et al.* (1990). Cyclosporine-induced renal magnesium leak in renal transplant patients. *Nephrol. Dial. Transplant.* 5, 812.

Scoggin, C., McClellan, J.R., and Cary, J.M. (1977). Hyponatraemia and acidosis in association with topical treatment of burns. *Lancet* i, 959.

Scott, J.M. (1963). Iron-sorbitol-citrate in pregnancy anaemia. *BMJ* 2, 354.

Scott, J.T. (1991). Drug-induced gout. *Baillière's Clin. Rheumatol.* 5, 39.

Scott, J.T. and Higgens, C.S. (1992). Diuretic induced gout: a multifactorial condition. *Ann. Rheum. Dis.* 51, 259.

Screaton, G.R., Singer, M., Cairns, H.S., *et al.* (1992). Hyperpyrexia and rhabdomyolysis after MDMA ('ecstasy') abuse. *Lancet* 339, 677.

Seager, J. (1984). IgA deficiency during treatment of infantile hypothyroidism with thyroxine. *BMJ* 288, 1562.

Sedman, A. (1992). Aluminum toxicity in childhood. *Pediatr. Nephrol.* 6, 383.

Seely, E.W., LeBoff, M.S., Brown, E.M., *et al.* (1989). The calcium channel blocker diltiazem lowers serum parathyroid hormone levels *in vivo* and *in vitro*. *J. Clin. Endocrinol. Metab.* 68, 1007.

Selby, P.L. and Peacock, M. (1986). The effect of transdermal oestrogen on bone, calcium-regulating hormones and liver in postmenopausal women. *Clin. Endocrinol.* 25, 543.

Seligmann, H., Halkin, H., Rauchfleisch, S., *et al.* (1991). Thiamine deficiency in patients with congestive heart failure receiving long-term furosemide therapy: a pilot study. *Am. J. Med.* 91, 151.

Sevitt, L.H. and Wrong, O.M. (1968). Hypercalcaemia from calcium resin in patients with chronic renal failure. *Lancet* ii, 950.

Shaaban, M.M., Elewan, S.E., el-Sharkaway, M.M., *et al.* (1984). Effect of subdermal levonorgestrel contraceptive implants, Norplant, on liver functions. *Contraception* 30, 407.

Shah, G.M., Alvarado, P., and Kirschenbaum, M.A. (1990). Symptomatic hypocalcemia and hypomagnesemia with renal magnesium wasting associated with pentamidine therapy in a patient with AIDS. *Am. J. Med.* 89, 380.

Shalev, A., Hermesh, H., and Munitz, H. (1987). The hypouricemic effect of chlorprothixene. *Clin. Pharmacol. Ther.* 42, 562.

Shalev, O., Gilon, D., and Nubain, N.H. (1987). Masked phenytoin-induced megaloblastic anaemia in beta-thalassemia minor. *Acta Haematol.* 77, 186.

Shane, E. (1996). Osteoporosis associated with illness and medications. In *Osteoporosis* (ed. R. Marcus, D. Feldman, and J. Kelsey), p. 925. Academic Press, California.

Shannon, M. and Graef, J.W. (1989). Lead intoxication from lead-contaminated water used to reconstitute infant formula. *Clin. Pediatr.* 28, 380.

Shannon, M. and Lovejoy, F.H., Jr. (1989). Hypokalemia after theophylline intoxication. The effects of acute vs chronic poisoning. *Arch. Intern. Med.* 149, 2725.

Shaughnessy, S.G., Young, E., Deschamps, P., *et al.* (1995). The effects of low molecular weight and standard heparin on calcium loss from fetal rat calvaria. *Blood* 86, 1368.

Shek, C.C., Natkunam, A., Tsang, V., *et al.* (1990). Incidence causes and mechanism of hypercalcaemia in a hospital population in Hong Kong. *Q. J. Med.* 77, 1277.

Shelley, E.D., Shelley, W.B., and Burmeister, V. (1987). Naproxen-induced pseudoporphyria presenting a diagnostic dilemma. *Cutis* 40, 314.

Shelton, D. and Goulding, R. (1979). Silver poisoning associated with an antismoking lozenge. *BMJ* i, 267.

Sher, P.P. (1982). Drug interferences with clinical laboratory tests. *Drugs* 24, 24.

Shergy, W.J., Gilkeson, G.S., and German, D.C. (1988). Acute gouty arthritis and intravenous nitroglycerin. *Arch. Intern. Med.* 148, 2505.

Sherlock, S. (1971). Halothane hepatitis. *Gut* 12, 324.

Sheth, R.D., Wesolowski, C.A., Jacob, J.C., *et al.* (1995). Effect of carbamazepine and valproate on bone mineral density. *J. Pediatr.* 127, 256.

Shiah, C.J., Tsai, D.M., Liao, S.T., *et al.* (1994). Acute muscular paralysis in an adult with subclinical Bartter's syndrome associated with gentamicin administration. *Am. J. Kidney Dis.* 24, 932.

Shimizu, K. (1995). Aquaretic effects of the nonpeptide V2 antagonist OPC-31260 in hydropenic humans. *Kidney Int.* 48, 220.

Shimizu, T., Maeda, S., Arakawa, H., *et al.* (1996). Relation between theophylline and circulating vitamin levels in children with asthma. *Pharmacology* 53, 384.

Shimon, I., Almog, S., Vered, Z., *et al.* (1995). Improved left ventricular function after thiamine supplementation in patients with congestive heart failure receiving long-term furosemide therapy. *Am. J. Med.* 98, 485.

Shin, Y.K. and Kim, Y.D. (1988). Ventricular tachyarrhythmias during cesarean section after ritodrine therapy: interaction with anesthetics. *South. Med. J.* 81, 528.

Shionoiri, H. (1993). Pharmacokinetic drug interactions with ACE inhibitors. *Clin. Pharmacokinet.* 25, 20.

Shirakawa, H., Komai, M., and Kimura, S. (1990). Antibiotic-induced vitamin K deficiency and the role of the presence of intestinal flora. *Int. J. Vitam. Nutr. Res.* 60, 245.

Shorey, J., Bhardwaj, N., and Loscalzo, J. (1984). Acute Wernicke's encephalopathy after intravenous infusion of high-dose nitroglycerin. *Ann. Intern. Med.* 101, 500.

Shoskes, D.A., Radzinski, C.A., Struthers, N.W., *et al.* (1992). Aluminum toxicity and death following intravesical alum irrigation in a patient with renal impairment. *J. Urol.* 147, 697.

Shulman, K.L., Stadler, W.M., and Vogelzang, N.J. (1996). High-dose continuous intravenous infusion of interleukin-2 therapy for metastatic renal cell carcinoma: the University of Chicago experience. *Urology* 47, 194.

Siebels, M., Andrassy, K., Vecsei, P., *et al.* (1992). Dose dependent suppression of mineralocorticoid metabolism by different heparin fractions. *Thromb. Res.* 66, 467.

Siegel, D., Hulley, S.B., Black, D.M., *et al.* (1992). Diuretics, serum and intracellular electrolyte levels, and ventricular arrhythmias in hypertensive men. *JAMA* 267, 1083.

Siegler, E.L., Tamres, D., Berlin, J.A., *et al.* (1995). Risk factors for the development of hyponatremia in psychiatric inpatients. *Arch. Intern. Med.* 155, 953.

Siemes, H., Nau, H., Schultze, K., *et al.* (1993). Valproate (VPA) metabolites in various clinical conditions of probable VPA-associated hepatotoxicity. *Epilepsia* 34, 332.

Simmer, K., Iles, C.A., James, C., *et al.* (1987). Are iron-folate supplements harmful? *Am. J. Clin. Nutr.* 45, 122.

Simmer, K., Fudge, A., Teubner, J., *et al.* (1990). Aluminum concentrations in infant formulae. *J. Paediatr. Child Health* 26, 9.

Simmons, M.A., Adcock, E., III, Bard, H., *et al.* (1974). Hypernatremia and intracerebral hemorrhage and $NaHCO_3$ administration. *N. Engl. J. Med.* 291, 6.

Simons, M.L. and Goldman, E. (1988). Atypical malignant hyperthermia with persistent hyperkalaemia during renal transplantation. *Can. J. Anaesth.* 35, 409.

Singh, B.N. (1992). Bepridil therapy: guidelines for patient selection and monitoring of therapy. *Am. J. Cardiol.* 69, 79D.

Singhi, S.C., Jayashree, K., and Sarkar, B. (1996). Hypokalaemia following nebulized salbutamol in children with acute attack of bronchial asthma. *J. Paediatr. Child Health* 32, 495.

Sinzinger, H., Rauscha, F., Fitscha, P., *et al.* (1991). Calcium antagonists and hypercalcaemia. *Lancet* 337, 924.

Sipila, R., Skrifvars, B., and Tornroth, T. (1986). Reversible non-oliguric impairment of renal function during azapropazone treatment. *Scand. J. Rheumatol.* 15, 23.

Sivakumaran, M., Ghosh, K., Zaidi, Y., *et al.* (1996). Osteoporosis and vertebral collapse following low-dose, low molecular weight heparin therapy in a young patient. *Clin. Lab. Haematol.* 18, 55.

Sivasubramanian, K.N., Hoy, G., Davitt, M.K., *et al.* (1978). Zinc and copper changes after neonatal parenteral alimentation. *Lancet* i, 508.

Skinner, R., Pearson, A.D.J., Price, L., *et al.* (1989). Hypophosphataemic rickets after ifosfamide treatment in children. *BMJ* 298, 1560.

Skinner, R., Pearson, A.D., Price, L., *et al.* (1990). Nephrotoxicity after ifosfamide. *Arch. Dis. Child.* 65, 732.

Skinner, R., Pearson, A.D., English, M.W., *et al.* (1996). Risk factors for ifosfamide nephrotoxicity in children. *Lancet* 348, 578.

Skrede, S., Ro, J.S., and Mjolnerod, O. (1973). Effects of dextrans on the plasma protein changes during the postoperative period. *Clin. Chim. Acta* 48, 143.

Skrha, J., Sramkova, J., Rehak, F., *et al.* (1986). Serum iso-amylase activities during infusions of glucose and amino acids. *Eur. J. Clin. Invest.* 16, 35.

Sladen, G.E. (1972). Effects of chronic purgative abuse. *Proc. R. Soc. Med.* 65, 288.

Slayton, W., Anstine, D., Lakhdir, F., *et al.* (1996). Tetany in a child with AIDS receiving intravenous tobramycin. *South. Med. J.* 89, 1108.

Sloan, J.P., Wing, P., Dian, L., *et al.* (1992). A pilot study of anabolic steroids in elderly patients with hip fractures. *J. Am. Geriatr. Soc.* 40, 1105.

Smilkstein, M.J., Smolinske, S.C., Kulig, K.W., *et al.* (1988). Severe hypermagnesemia due to multiple-dose cathartic therapy. *West. J. Med.* 148, 208.

Smith, N.J. and Espir, M.L.E. (1977). Raised plasma arginine vasopressin concentration in carbamazepine-induced water intoxication. *BMJ* ii, 804.

Smith, S.R., Galloway, M.J., Reilly, J.T., *et al.* (1988). Amiloride prevents amphotericin B related hypokalaemia in neutropenic patients. *J. Clin. Pathol.* 41, 494.

Smith, T.J., Gill, J.C., Ambruso, D.R., *et al.* (1989). Hyponatremia and seizures in young children given DDAVP. *Am. J. Hematol.* 31, 199.

Smith, T.W. (1988). Digitalis: mechanisms of action and clinical use. *N. Engl. J. Med.* 318, 358.

Smolinske, S.C., Hall, A.H., Vandenberg, S.A., *et al.* (1990). Toxic effects of nonsteroidal anti-inflammatory drugs in overdose. An overview of recent evidence on clinical effects and dose–response relationships. *Drug Saf.* 5, 252.

Sobbrio, G.A., Granata, A., Granese, D., *et al.* (1991). Sex hormone binding globulin, cortisol binding globulin, thyroxine binding globulin, ceruloplasmin: changes in treatment with two oral contraceptives low in oestrogen. *Clin. Exp. Obstet. Gynecol.* 18, 43.

Soffer, B.A., Wright, J., Jr, Pratt, J.H., *et al.* (1995). Effects of losartan on a background of hydrochlorothiazide in patients with hypertension. *Hypertension* 26, 112.

Sola, R., Puig, L.L., Ballarin, J.A., *et al.* (1987). Pseudoporphyria cutanea tarda associated with cyclosporine therapy. *Transplantation* 43, 772.

Somani, P., Temesy-Armos, P.N., Leighton, R.F., *et al.* (1984). Hyponatremia in patients treated with lorcainide, a new antiarrhhythmic drug. *Am. Heart J.* 108, 1443.

Song, S., Chen, J.K., He, M.L., *et al.* (1989). Effect of some oral contraceptives on serum concentrations of sex hormone binding globulin and ceruloplasmin. *Contraception* 39, 385.

Sonino, N. (1987). The use of ketoconazole as an inhibitor of steroid production. *N. Engl. J. Med.* 317, 812.

Sonnenblick, M., Friedlander, Y., and Rosin, A.J. (1993). Diuretic-induced severe hyponatraemia. Review and analysis of 129 reported patients. *Chest* 103, 601.

Sozuer, D.T., Barutcu, U.B., Karakoc, Y., *et al.* (1995). The effects of antiepileptic drugs on serum zinc and copper levels in children. *J. Basic Clin. Physiol. Pharmacol.* 6, 265.

Specht-Leible, N., Schlierf, G., Lang, P.D., *et al.* (1993). Fibrinogen and bezafibrate — a pilot study in patients following percutaneous transluminal coronary angioplasty (PTCA). *Clinical Hemorheology* 13, 679.

Spector, T.D., Edwards, A.C., and Thompson, P.W. (1992). Use of a risk factor and dietary calcium questionnaire in predicting bone density and subsequent bone loss at the menopause. *Ann. Rheum. Dis.* 51, 1252.

Spector, T.D., Hall, G.M., McCloskey, E.V., *et al.* (1993). Risk of vertebral fracture in women with rheumatoid arthritis. *BMJ* 306, 558.

Speires, C.J., Dollery, C.T., Inman, W.H.W., *et al.* (1988). Postmarketing surveillance of enalapril II: Investigation of the potential role of enalapril in death with renal failure. *BMJ* 297, 830.

Spencer, H., Karamer, L., Osis, D., *et al.* (1985). Effects of aluminum hydroxide on fluoride and calcium metabolism. *J. Environ. Pathol. Toxicol. Oncol.* 6, 33.

Spigset, O. and Hedenmalm, K. (1995). Hyponatremia and the syndrome of inappropriate antidiuretic-hormone secretion (SIADH) induced by psychotropic-drugs. *Drug Saf.* 12, 209.

Spigset, O. and Hedenmalm, K. (1997). Hyponatremia in relation to treatment with antidepressants: a survey of reports in the World Health Organization data base for spontaneous reporting of adverse drug reactions. *Pharmacotherapy* 17, 348.

Spital, A. and Greenwell, R. (1991). Severe hyperkalaemia during magnesium sulfate therapy in two pregnant drug abusers. *South. Med. J.* 84, 919.

Sporn, A., Scothorn, D.M., and Terry, J.E. (1991). Metabolic acidosis induced by acetazolamide. *J. Am. Optom. Assoc.* 62, 934.

Sprague, S.M., Corwin, H.L., Wilson, R.S., *et al.* (1986). Encephalopathy in chronic renal failure responsive to deferoxamine therapy. Another manifestation of aluminum neurotoxicity. *Arch. Intern. Med.* 146, 2063.

Sprinkle, R.V. (1995). Leaded eye cosmetics: a cultural cause of elevated lead levels in children. *J. Fam. Pract.* 40, 358.

Stacpoole, P.W. (1993). Lactic acidosis. *Endocrinol. Metab. Clin. North Am.* 22, 221.

Stacpoole, P.W., Wright, E.C., Baumgartner, T.G., *et al.* (1992). A controlled clinical trial of dichloroacetate for treatment of lactic acidosis in adults. The Dichloroacetate-Lactic Acidosis Study Group. *N. Engl. J. Med.* 327, 1564.

Stahl, R.A., Kanz, L., Maier, B., *et al.* (1986). Hyperchloremic metabolic acidosis with high serum potassium in renal transplant recipients: a cyclosporine A associated side effect. *Clin. Nephrol.* 25, 245.

Stamp, T.C., Round, J.M., Rowe, D.J., *et al.* (1972). Plasma levels and therapeutic effect of 25-hydroxycholecalciferol in epileptic patients taking anticonvulsant drugs. *BMJ* 4, 9.

Stamvoll, M., Nurjham, N., Perriello, G., *et al.* (1995). Metabolic effects of metformin in non-insulin-dependent diabetes mellitus. *N. Engl. J. Med.* 333, 550.

Stanton, M.F. and Lowenstein, F.W. (1987). Serum magnesium in women during pregnancy, while taking oral contraceptives and after menopause. *J. Am. Coll. Nutr.* 6, 313.

Starzl, T., Fuing, J., Jordan, M., *et al.* (1990). Kidney transplantation under FK 506. *JAMA* 264, 63.

Steedman, D.J. (1988). Poisoning with sustained release potassium. *Arch. Emerg. Med.* 5, 206.

Steegers-Theunissen, R.P.M., Boers, G.H.J., Steegers, E.A.P., *et al.* (1992). Effects of sub-50 oral contraceptives on homocysteine metabolism: a preliminary study. *Contraception* 45, 129.

Steegers-Theunissen, R.P.M., Van Rossum, J.M., Steegers, E.A.P., *et al.* (1993). Sub 50 oral contraceptives affect folate kinetics. *Gynecol. Obstet. Invest.* 36, 230.

Steen, M. (1993). Review of the use of povidone-iodine (PVP-I) in the treatment of burns. *Postgrad. Med. J.* 69 Suppl. 3, S84.

Steidl, L., Tolde, I., and Svomova, V. (1987). Metabolism of magnesium and zinc in patients treated with antiepileptic drugs and with magnesium lactate. *Magnesium* 6, 284.

Sterns, R.H., Cox, M., Feig, P.U., *et al.* (1981). Internal potassium balance and the control of the plasma potassium concentration. *Medicine* 60, 339.

Stevens, H.P., Ostlere, L.S., Begent, R.H.J., *et al.* (1993). Pellagra secondary to 5-fluorouracil. *Br. J. Dermatol.* 128, 578.

Stevens, J.J., Griffin, R.M., and Stow, P.J. (1993). Prolonged use of isoflurane in a patient with tetanus. *Br. J. Anaesth.* 70, 107.

Stevenson, J.C. (1995). The impact of bone loss in women with endometriosis. *Int. J. Gynecol. Obstet.* 50, S11.

Stevenson, J.C., Lees, B., Gardner, R., *et al.* (1989). A comparison of the skeletal effects of goserelin and danazol in premenopausal women with endometriosis. *Horm. Res.* 32, 161.

Stomati, M., Hartmann, B., Spinetti, A., *et al.* (1996). Effects of hormonal replacement therapy on plasma sex hormone-binding globulin, androgen and insulin-like growth factor-1 levels in postmenopausal women. *J. Endocrinol. Invest.* 19, 535.

Stork, C., Etzel, J.V., Brocavich, J.M., *et al.* (1994). Cephalosporin-associated hypoprothrombinemia: case and review of the literature. *Journal of Pharmacy Technology* 10, 5.

Strandjord, R.E., Aanderud, S., Myking, O.L., *et al.* (1981). Influence of carbamazepine on serum thyroxine and triiodothyronine in patients with epilepsy. *Acta Neurol. Scand.* 63, 111.

Strong, P., Jewell, S., Rinker, J., *et al.* (1991). Thiazide therapy and severe hypercalcemia in a patient with hyperparathyroidism. *West. J. Med.* 154, 338.

Struwe, M., Kaempfer, S.H., Geiger, C.J., *et al.* (1993). Effect of dronabinol on nutritional status in HIV infection. *Ann. Pharmacother.* 27, 827.

Struys, A., Snelder, A.A., and Mulder, H. (1995). Cyclical etidronate reverses bone loss of the spine and proximal femur in patients with established corticosteroid-induced osteoporosis. *Am. J. Med.* 99, 235.

Subramanian, D. and Ayus, J.C. (1992). Case report: severe symptomatic hyponatremia associated with lisinopril therapy. *Am. J. Med. Sci.* 303, 177.

Sueblinvong, V. and Wilson, J.F. (1969). Myocardial damage due to imipramine intoxication. *J. Pediatr.* 74, 475.

Sullivan, P.A., Daly, B., and O'Connor, R. (1992). Enalapril versus combined enalapril and nadolol treatment: effects on blood pressure, heart rate, humoral variables, and plasma potassium at rest and during exercise in hypertensive patients. *Cardiovasc. Drugs Ther.* 6, 261.

Sunderam, M.B.M. and Swaminathan, R. (1981). Total body potassium depletion and severe myopathy induce to liquorice ingestion. *Postgrad. Med. J.* 57, 48.

Sunderrajan, S., Bauer, J.H., Vopat, R.L., *et al.* (1984). Post transurethral prostatic resection hyponatremic syndrome: case report and review of the literature. *Am. J. Kidney Dis.* 4, 80.

Sunderrajan, S., Brooks, C.S., and Sunderrajan, E.V. (1985). Nortriptyline-induced severe hyperventilation. *Arch. Intern. Med.* 145, 746.

Sussman, N.M. and McLain, L.W. (1979). A direct hepatotoxic effect of valproic acid. *JAMA* 242, 1173.

Sutton, R.A.L. and Dirks, J.H. (1996). Disturbances of calcium and magnesium metabolism. In *The Kidney* (ed. B.M. Brenner), p. 1038. W.B. Saunders, Philadelphia.

Suzuki, N., Nonaka, K., Kono, N., *et al.* (1986). Effects of the intravenous administration of magnesium sulphate on corrected serum calcium level and nephrogenous cyclic AMP excretion in normal human subjects. *Calcif. Tissue Int.* 39, 304.

Suzuki, Y. Ichikawa, Y., Saito, E., *et al.* (1988). Importance of increased urinary calcium excretion in the development of secondary hyperparathyroidism of patients under glucocorticoid therapy. *Metabolism* 32, 151.

Swainson, C.P., Colls, B.M., and Fitzharris, B.M. (1985). Cisplatinum and distal renal tubule toxicity. *N.Z. Med. J.* 98, 375.

Swales, J.D. (1991). Salt substitutes and potassium intake. *BMJ* 303, 1084.

Swaminathan, R. (1997). Biochemical markers for osteoporosis. In *Osteoporosis Illustrated* (ed. N.K. Arden and T.D. Spector), p. 71. Current Medical Literature, London.

Swaminathan, R. (1998). Hypo-hypermagnesaemia. *Oxford Textbook of Clinical Nephrology* (ed. J.S. Cameron, J.P. Greenfeld, D.N.S. Kerr, E. Ritz, and C.G. Winnearls), p. 271. Oxford University Press.

Swaminathan, R., Morgan, D.B., Ionescu, M., *et al.* (1978). Hypophosphataemia and its consequences in patients following open heart surgery. *Anaesthesia* 33, 601.

Swaminathan, R., Bradley, P., Morgan, D.B., *et al.* (1979). Hypophosphataemia in surgical patients. *Surgery* 148, 448.

Swaminathan, R., Chin, R.K., Lao, T.T.H., *et al.* (1989). Thyroid function in hyperemesis gravidarum. *Acta Endocrinol.* 120, 155.

Swash, M. and Schwarz, M.S. (eds) (1997). Drug-induced and toxic myopathies. In *Clinical Neurology*, p. 1331. Churchill Livingstone, Edinburgh.

Sweeney, J.D., Ziegler, P., Pruet, C., *et al.* (1989). Hyperzincuria and hypozincemia in patients treated with cisplatin. *Cancer* 63, 2093.

Sybrecht, G.W. (1983). Influence of brotizolam on the ventilatory and mouth-occlusion pressure response to hypercapnia in patients with chronic obstructive pulmonary disease. *Br. J. Clin. Pharmacol.* 16, 425S.

Sykes, A.P., Lawson, N., Finnegan, J.A., *et al.* (1991). Creatine kinase activity in patients with brittle asthma treated with long term subcutaneous terbutaline. *Thorax* 46, 580.

Taboulet, P., Baud, F.J., and Bismuth, C. (1993). Clinical features and management of digitalis poisoning — rationale for immunotherapy. *J. Toxicol. Clin. Toxicol.* 31, 247.

Taboulet, P., Clemessy, J.L., Freminet, A., *et al.* (1995). A case of life-threatening lactic acidosis after smoke inhalation — interference between beta-adrenergic agents and ethanol? *Intensive Care Med.* 21, 1039.

Tai, D.Y., Yeo, J.K., Eng, P.C., *et al.* (1996). Intentional overdosage with isoniazid: case report and review of literature. *Singapore Med. J.* 37, 222.

Taitel, H.F. and Kafrissen, M.E. (1995). Norethindrone — a review of therapeutic applications. *International Journal of Fertility and Menopausal Studies* 40, 207.

Takahashi, H., Fukuyama, M., Yoneda, S., *et al.* (1989). Comparison of nisoldipine and atenolol in the treatment of essential hypertension. *Arzneimittelforschung* 39, 379.

Takahashi. T., Minakami, H., Tamada, T., *et al.* (1997). Hyperamylasemia in response to ritodrine or ephedrine administered to pregnant women. *J. Am. Coll. Surg.* 184, 31.

Takeshita, N., Seino, Y., Ishida, H., *et al.* (1989). Increased circulating levels of gamma-carboxyglutamic acid-containing protein and decreased bone mass in children on anticonvulsant therapy. *Calcif. Tissue Int.* 44, 80.

Taylor, A. (1996). Detection and monitoring of disorders of essential trace elements. *Ann. Clin. Biochem.* 33, 486.

Taylor, D.R., Wilkins, G.T., Herbison, G.P., *et al.* (1992). Interaction between corticosteroid and beta-agonist drugs. Biochemical and cardiovascular effects in normal subjects. *Chest* 102, 519.

Taylor, D.R., Herbison, G.P., Sears, M.R., *et al.* (1993). Sex differences in hypokalaemic and electrocardiographic effects of inhaled terbutaline. *Thorax* 48, 776.

Taylor, J.W. and Bell, A.J. (1993). Lithium-induced parathyroid dysfunction — a case-report and review of the literature. *Ann. Pharmacother.* 27, 1040.

ten Holt, W.L., Klaassen, C.H., and Schrijver, G. (1994). [Severe hyponatremia, possibly due to inappropriate antidiuretic hormone secretion, during use of the antidepressant fluoxetine (see comments)]. *Ned. Tijdschr. Geneesk.* 138, 1181.

Tennant, G.B., Smith, R.C., Leinster, S.J., *et al.* (1981). Acute depression of serum folate in surgical patients during preoperative infusion of ethanol-free parenteral nutrition. *Scand. J. Haematol.* 27, 327.

Tester-Dalderup, C.B.M. (1996). Antifungal drugs. In *Meyler's Side Effects of Drugs* (ed. M.N.G. Dukes), p. 774. Elsevier, Amsterdam.

Texier, D., Chevallier, P., Perrotin, D., *et al.* (1982). Hypercalcaemia associated with resorbable haemostatic compresses. *Lancet* i, 688.

Thiebaud, D., Jaeger, P., and Jacquet, A.F. (1986). A single-day treatment of tumor-induced hypercalcemia by intravenous amino-hydroxypropylidene bisphosphonate. *J. Bone Miner. Res.* 1, 555.

Thijs, L., Staessen, J., Amery, A., *et al.* (1992). Determinants of serum zinc in a random population sample of four Belgian towns with different degrees of environmental exposure to cadmium. *Environ. Health Perspect.* 98, 251.

Thomas, A. and Verbalis, J.G. (1995). Hyponatremia and the syndrome of inappropriate antidiuretic hormone secretion associated with drug therapy in psychiatric patients. *CNS Drugs* 4, 357.

Thomas, S.H. and Stone, C.K. (1994). Acute toxicity from baking soda ingestion. *Am. J. Emerg. Med.* 12, 57.

Thomas, T.H., Ball, S.G., Wales, J.K., *et al.* (1978). Effect of carbamazepine on plasma and urine arginine — vasopressin. *Clin. Sci. Mol. Med.* 54, 419.

Thompson, C.B., June, C.H., Sullivan, K.M., *et al.* (1984). Association between cyclosporin neurotoxicity and hypomagnesaemia. *Lancet* ii, 1116.

Thompson, P.D., Gadaleta, P.A., Yurgalevitch, S., *et al.* (1991). Effects of exercise and lovastatin on serum creatine kinase activity. *Metabolism* 40, 1333.

Thomson, A.D. and Majumdar, S.K. (1981). The influence of ethanol on intestinal absorption and utilization of nutrients. *Clin. Gastroenterol.* 10, 263.

Thorkelsson, T. and Loughead, J.L. (1991). Long-term subcutaneous terbutaline tocolysis: report of possible neonatal toxicity. *J. Perinatol.* 11, 235.

Thorp, J.M., Mackenzie, I., and Simpson, E. (1987). Gross hypernatraemia associated with the use of antiseptic surgical packs. *Anaesthesia* 42, 750.

Tishler, M. and Armon, S. (1986). Nifedipine-induced hypokalaemia. *DICP* 20, 370.

Titanji, R. and Trofa, A. (1993). Hypokalaemia associated with ticarcillin-clavulanic acid. *Maryland Medical Journal* 42, 1013.

Tjellesen, L., Gotfredsen, A., and Christiansen, C. (1985). Different actions of vitamin D_2 and D_3 on bone metabolism in patients treated with phenobarbitone/phenytoin. *Calcif. Tissue Int.* 37, 218.

Tomkin, G.H. (1973). Malabsorption of vitamin B_{12} in diabetic patients treated with phenformin: a comparison with metformin. *BMJ* iii, 673.

Tomlinson, B., Cruickshank, J.M., Hayes, Y., *et al.* (1990). Selective beta-adrenoceptor partial agonist effects of pindolol and xamoterol on skeletal muscle assessed by plasma creatine kinase changes in healthy subjects. *Br. J. Clin. Pharmacol.* 30, 665.

Toone, B.K., Wheeler, M., and Fenwick, P.B. (1980). Sex hormone changes in male epileptics. *Clin. Endocrinol.* (Oxf.) 12, 391.

Travis, S.F., Sugerman, H.J., Ruberg, R.L., *et al.* (1971). Alterations of red-cell glycolytic intermediates and oxygen transport as a consequence of hypophosphataemia in patients receiving intravenous hyperalimetation. *N. Engl. J. Med.* 285, 763.

Trehan, R. and Clark, C.F. (1993). Valproic acid-induced truncal weakness and respiratory failure. *Am. J. Psychiatry* 150, 1271.

Tsai, J.C., Lai, Y.H., Shin, S.J., *et al.* (1987). [Rhabdomyolysis-induced acute tubular necrosis after the concomitant use of alcohol and pentazocine — a case report]. *Kao Hsiung I Hsueh Ko Hsueh Tsa Chih [Kaohsiung Journal of Medical Sciences]* 3, 299.

Tsao, C.Y., Wright, F.S., Genton, P., *et al.* (1993). Acute chemical pancreatitis associated with carbamazepine intoxication. *Epilepsia* 34, 174.

Tsipouras, N., Rix, C.J., and Brady, P.H. (1995). Solubility of silver sulfadiazine in physiological media and relevance to treatment of thermal burns with silver sulfadiazine cream. *Clin. Chem.* 41, 87.

Tsuda, Y., Satoh, K., Kitadai, M., *et al.* (1996). Effects of pravastatin sodium and simvastatin on plasma fibrinogen level and blood rheology in type II hyperlipoproteinemia. *Atherosclerosis* 122, 225.

Turetta, F., de Stefani, R., Milanesi, A., *et al.* (1985). Variation du calcium ionisé plasmatique au cours de l'angiographie en fluorescence. *J. Fr. Ophtalmol.* 8, 785.

Tuzhilin, S.A., Gonda, M., Carbonell, G., *et al.* (1982). Serum amylases and their inhibitors: 2, clinical and experimental observations — diet and steroid effects. *Am. J. Gastroenterol.* 77, 26.

Tyrer, L.B. (1984). Nutrition and the pill. *J. Reprod. Med.* 29 Suppl., 547.

Ubbink, J.B., Delport, R., Becker, P.J., *et al.* (1989). Evidence of a theophylline-induced vitamin B_6 deficiency caused by noncompetitive inhibition of pyridoxal kinase. *J. Lab. Clin. Med.* 113, 15.

Ubbink, J.B., Vermaak, W.J., Delport, R., *et al.* (1990). The relationship between vitamin B_6 metabolism, asthma, and theophylline therapy. *Ann. N.Y. Acad. Sci.* 585, 285.

Udezue, E., Dsouza, L., and Mahajan, M. (1995). Hypokalemia after normal doses of nebulized albuterol (salbutamol). *Am. J. Emerg. Med.* 13, 168.

Umekawa, T., Konya, E., Ishikawa, Y., *et al.* (1996). Verapamil reduces urinary oxalate excretion in hyperoxaluric stone formers. *Nishinihon J. Urology* 58, 267.

Umeki, S., Tsukiyama, K., Okimoto, N., *et al.* (1989). Urinastatin (Kunitz-type proteinase inhibitor) reducing cisplatin nephrotoxicity. *Am. J. Med. Sci.* 298, 221.

Umino, M., Miura, M., Kondo, T., *et al.* (1985). Effect of thiamylal and diazepam on release of myoglobin and creatine phosphokinase by succinylcholine chloride during halothane anesthesia. *Bull. Tokyo Med. Dent. Univ.* 32, 91.

Urbanek, R.W. and Cohen, D.J. (1994). Porphyria cutanea tarda: pregnancy versus estrogen effect. *J. Am. Acad. Dermatol.* 31, 390.

Urgert, P., Essed, N., van der Wag, C., *et al.* (1997). Separate effects of the coffee diterpenes cafestol and kahweol on serum lipids and liver aminotransferases. *Am. J. Clin. Nutr.* 65, 519.

Uribarri, J., Oh, M.S., and Carroll, H.J. (1990). Hyperkalemia in diabetes mellitus. *J. Diabet. Complications* 4, 3.

Usala, A.L., Madigan, T., Burguera, B., *et al.* (1994). High dose intravenous, but not low dose subcutaneous insulin-like growth factor-I therapy induces sustained insulin sensitivity in severely resistant type I diabetes mellitus. *J. Clin. Endocrinol. Metab.* 79, 435.

Vale, J.A., Proudfoot, A.T., and Meredith, T.J. (1996). Poisoning by alcohols and glycols. In *Oxford Textbook of Medicine* (3rd edn) (ed. D.J. Weatherall, J.G.G. Ledingham, and D.A. Warrell), p. 1079. Oxford University Press.

Valimaki, M.J., Tiihonen, M., Laitinen, K., *et al.* (1994). Bone mineral density measured by dual-energy x-ray absorptiometry and novel markers of bone formation and resorption in patients on antiepileptic drugs. *J. Bone Miner. Res.* 9, 631.

Valiquette, G., Herbert, J., and Meade-Dalisera, P. (1996). Desmopressin in the management of nocturia in patients with multiple sclerosis — a double-blind, crossover trial. *Arch. Neurol.* 53, 1270.

van Achterbergh, S.M., Vorster, B.J., and Heyns, A.D. (1990). The effect of sepsis and short-term exposure to nitrous oxide on the bone marrow and the metabolism of vitamin B_{12} and folate. *S. Afr. Med. J.* 78, 260.

van Amelsvoort, T., Bakshi, R., Devaux, C.B., *et al.* (1994). Hyponatremia associated with carbamazepine and oxcarbazepine therapy: a review. *Epilepsia* 35, 181.

van de Wiele, B., Rubinstein, E., Peacock, W., *et al.* (1995). Propylene glycol toxicity caused by prolonged infusion of etomidate. *J. Neurosurg. Anesthesiol.* 7, 259.

van der Meulen, J., Janssen, M.J., Langendijk, P.N., *et al.* (1992). Citrate anticoagulation and dialysate with reduced buffer content in chronic hemodialysis. *Clin. Nephrol.* 37, 36.

Van der Wiel, H.E., Lips, P., Huijgens, P.C., *et al.* (1993). Effects of short-term low-dose heparin administration on biochemical parameters of bone turnover. *Bone Miner.* 22, 27.

Van Dissel, J.T., Gerritsen, H.J., and Meinders, A.E. (1992). Severe hypophosphatemia in a patient with anorexia nervosa during oral feeding. *Miner. Electrolyte Metab.* 18, 365.

van Kalmthout, P.M., Engels, L.G., Bakker, H.H., *et al.* (1982). Severe copper deficiency due to excessive use of an antacid combined with pyloric stenosis. *Dig. Dis. Sci.* 27, 859.

Van Seters, A.P. and Moolenaar, A.J. (1991). Mitotane increases the blood levels of hormone-binding proteins. *Acta Endocrinol.* 124, 526.

Vannucchi, H., Moreno, F.S., Amarante, A.R., *et al.* (1991). Plasma amino acid patterns in alcoholic pellagra patients. *Alcohol Alcohol.* 26, 431.

Varkel, Y., Braester, A., Nusem, D., *et al.* (1988). Methyldopa-induced syndrome of inappropriate antidiuretic hormone secretion and bone marrow granulomatosis. *DICP* 22, 700.

Veech, R.L. and Gilmor, W.L. (1988). The medical and metabolic consequences of administration of sodium acetate. *Adv. Enzyme Regul.* 27, 313.

Velazquez, H., Perazella, M.A., Wright, F.S., *et al.* (1993). Renal mechanism of trimethoprim-induced hyperkalemia. *Ann. Intern. Med.* 119, 296.

Venkataraman, P.S., Tsang, R.C., Greer, F.R., *et al.* (1985). Late infantile tetany and secondary hyperparathyroidism in infants fed humanized cow milk formula. Longitudinal follow-up. *Am. J. Dis. Child.* 139, 664.

Verhage, A.H., Cheong, W.K., Allard, J.P., et al. (1995). Increase in lumbar spine bone mineral content in patients on long-term parenteral nutrition without vitamin D supplementation. *JPEN* 19, 431.

Vermeer, C., Jie, K.S.G., and Knapen, M.H.J. (1995). Role of vitamin K in bone metabolism. *Ann. Rev. Nutr.* 15, 1.

Vertoli, U., Vinci, C., and Naso, A. (1992). Hypoprothrombinemia and cephalosporins in uremics. *Nephron* 62, 239.

Veterans Administration Co-Operative Study Group on Antihypertensive Agents. (1984). Low dose captopril for the treatment of mild to moderate hypertension. I. Results of a 14-week trial. *Arch. Intern. Med.* 144, 1947.

Vial, T. and Descotes, J. (1996). Drugs acting on the immune system. In *Meyler's Side Effects of Drugs* (ed. M.N.G. Dukes), p. 1090. Elsevier, Amsterdam.

Viens, P., Thyss, A., Garnier, G., et al. (1989). GM-CSF treatment and hypokalaemia. *Ann. Intern. Med.* 111, 263.

Vieweg, V., Glick, J.L., Herring, S., et al. (1987). Absence of carbamazepine-induced hyponatremia among patients also given lithium. *Am. J. Psychiatry* 144, 943.

Villablanca, J.G., Khan, A.A., Avramis, V.I., et al. (1993). Hypercalcemia: a dose-limiting toxicity associated with 13-cis-retinoic acid. *Am. J. Pediatr. Hematol. Oncol.* 15, 410.

Villiger, L., Casez, J.P., Takkinen, R., et al. (1993). Diltiazem stimulates parathyroid hormone secretion *in vivo* whereas felodipine does not. *J. Clin. Endocrinol. Metab.* 76, 890.

Vincens, M., Mercier-Bodard, C., Mowszowicz, I., et al. (1989). Testosterone-estradiol binding globulin (TeBG) in hirsute patients treated with cyproterone acetate (CPA) and percutaneous estradiol. *J. Steroid Biochem.* 33, 531.

Vissers, R.J. and Pursell, R. (1996). Iatrogenic magnesium overdose: two case reports. *J. Emerg. Med.* 14, 187.

Vladutiu, O. and Reitz, M. (1980). Creatine kinase isoenzymes in aspirin intoxication. *Lancet* ii, 864.

Vlasses, P.H., Rotmensch, H.H., Swanson, B.N., et al. (1984). Indacrinone: natriuretic and uricosuric effects of various ratios of its enantiomers in healthy men. *Pharmacotherapy* 4, 272.

Von Wowern, N., Klausen, B., and Hylander, E. (1996). Bone loss and oral state in patients on home parenteral nutrition. *JPEN*, 20, 105.

Wagnerova, M., Wagner, V., Madlo, Z., et al. (1986). Seasonal variations in the level of immunoglobulins and serum proteins of children differing by exposure to air-borne lead. *J. Hyg. Epidemiol. Microbiol. Immunol.* 30, 127.

Wagnerova, M., Wagner, V., Znojemska, S., et al. (1988). Factors of humoral resistance in workers exposed to vinyl chloride with a view to smoking habits. *J. Hyg. Epidemiol. Microbiol. Immunol.* 32, 265.

Walden, C.E., Knopp, R..H., Johnson, J.L., et al. (1986). Effect of oestrogen/progestin potency on clinical chemistry measures. The Lipid Research Clinics Program Prevalence Study. *Am. J. Epidemiol.* 123, 517.

Walker, F.B., IV, Becker, D.M., Kowal-Nelley, B., et al. (1988). Lack of effect of warfarin on uric acid concentration. *Clin. Chem.* 34, 952.

Waller, P.C. and Ramsay, L.E. (1989). Predicting acute gout in diuretic-treated hypertensive patients. *J. Hum. Hypertens.* 3, 457.

Walsh, L.J., Wong, C.A., Pringle, M., et al. (1996). Use of oral corticosteroids in the community and the prevention of secondary osteoporosis: a cross sectional study. *BMJ* 313, 344.

Walter, G.F. and Maresch, W. (1987). Irrtümliche Kochsalzintoxikation bei Neugeborenen. Morphologische Befunde und pathogenetische Diskussion. *Klin. Pädiatr.* 199, 269.

Walter, U., Forthofer, R., and Witte, P.U. (1987). Dose–response relation of the angiotensin converting enzyme inhibitor ramipril in mild to moderate essential hypertension. *Am. J. Cardiol.* 59, 125D.

Walton, R.J., Russell, R.G.G., and Smith, R. (1975). Changes in the renal and extra renal handling of phosphate induced by sodium elidromate (EHDP) in man. *Clin. Sci.* 49, 45.

Wandrup, J. and Kancir, C. (1986). Complex biochemical syndrome of hypocalcemia and hypoparathyroidism during cytotoxic treatment of an infant with leukemia. *Clin. Chem.* 32, 706.

Warady, B.D., Lindsley, C.B., Robinson, F.G., et al. (1994). Effects of nutritional supplementation on bone mineral status of children with rheumatic diseases receiving corticosteroid therapy. *J. Rheumatol.* 21, 530.

Ward, M.J. and Routledge, P.A. (1988). Hypernatraemia and hyperchloraemic acidosis after bleach ingestion. *Hum. Toxicol.* 7, 37.

Wark, J.D., Larkins, R.G., Perry-Keene, D., et al. (1979). Chronic diphenylhydantoin therapy does not reduce plasma 25-hydroxy-vitamin D. *Clin. Endocrinol.* (Oxf.) 11, 267.

Warrell, R.P., Jr, Murphy, W.K., Schulman, P., et al. (1991). A randomized double-blind study of gallium nitrate compared with etidronate for acute control of cancer-related hypercalcemia. *J. Clin. Oncol.* 9, 1467.

Watkins, R.C., Hambrick, E.L., Benjamin, G., et al. (1990). Isoniazid toxicity presenting as seizures and metabolic acidosis. *J. Natl Med. Assoc.* 82, 57, 62, 64.

Watson, A.J., Watson, M.M., and Keogh, J.A. (1984). Metabolic abnormalities associated with tobramycin therapy. *Ir. J. Med. Sci.* 153, 96.

Watts, R.W.E. (1996). Disorders of oxalate metabolism. In *Oxford Textbook of Medicine* (3rd edn) (ed. D.J. Weatherall, J.G.G. Ledingham, and D.A. Warrell), p. 1444. Oxford University Press.

Webb, D.E., Austin, H.A., Belldegrun, A., et al. (1988). Metabolic and renal effects of interleukin-2 immunotherapy for metastatic cancer. *Clin. Nephrol.* 30, 141.

Webb, D.I., Chodos, R.B., Mahar, C.Q., et al. (1968). Mechanism of vitamin B_{12} malabsorption in patients receiving colchicine. *N. Engl. J. Med.* 279, 845.

Webberley, M.J. and Murray, J.A. (1989). Life-threatening acute hyponatraemia induced by low dose cyclophosphamide and indomethacin. *Post. Grad. Med. J.* 650, 950.

Weimar, V.M., Weimar, G.W., and Ceilley, R.J. (1978). Estrogen-induced porphyria cutanea tarda complicating treatment of prostatic carcinoma. *J. Urol.* 120, 643.

Weinstein, R.E., Bona, R.D., Altman, A.J., *et al.* (1989). Severe hyponatremia after repeated intravenous administration of desmopressin. *Am. J. Hematol.* 32, 258.

Weinstein, R.S., Bryce, G.F., Sappington, L.J., *et al.* (1984). Decreased serum ionized calcium and normal vitamin D metabolite levels with anticonvulsant drug treatment. *J. Clin. Endocrinol. Metab.* 58, 1003.

Weir, D.G. and Scott, J.M. (1995). The biochemical basis of neuropathy in cobalamin deficiency. *Baillière's Clin. Haematol.* 8, 479.

Weir, M.R., Keniston, R.C., Enriquez J.I., Sr, *et al.* (1991). Depression of vitamin B$_6$ levels due to dopamine. *Vet. Hum. Toxicol.* 33, 118.

Weir, M.R., Flack, J.M., and Applegate, W.B. (1996). Tolerability, safety, and quality of life and hypertensive therapy: the case for low-dose diuretics. *Am. J. Med.* 101, 83S.

Weiss, M., Hassin, D., Eisenstein, Z., *et al.* (1979). Elevated skeletal-muscle enzymes during quinidine therapy. *N. Engl. J. Med.* 300, 1218.

Weitzel, J.N., Sadowski, J.A., Furie, B.C., *et al.* (1990). Surreptitious ingestion of a long-acting vitamin K antagonist/rodenticide, brodifacoum: clinical and metabolic studies of three cases. *Blood* 76, 2555.

Welborn, J., Meyers, F.J., and O'Grady, L.F. (1988). Renal salt wasting and carboplatinum. *Ann. Intern. Med.* 108, 640.

Wen, S.F. (1997). Nephrotoxicities of nonsteroidal anti-inflammatory drugs. *Journal of the Formosan Medical Association* 96, 157.

Werther, C.A., Cloud, H., Ohtake, M., *et al.* (1986). Effect of long-term administration of anticonvulsants on copper, zinc, and ceruloplasmin levels. *Drug Nutr. Interact.* 4, 269.

West, C., Carpenter, B.J., and Hakala, T.R. (1987). The incidence of gout in renal transplant recipients. *Am. J. Kidney Dis.* 10, 369.

Wester, P.O. (1975). Zinc during diuretic treatment. *Lancet* i, 578.

Whang, R., Flink, E.B., Dyckner, T., *et al.* (1985). Magnesium depletion as a cause of refractory potassium depletion. *Arch. Intern. Med.* 145, 1686.

Wharton, J.M., Demopulos, P.A., and Goldschlager, N. (1987). Torsade de pointes during administration of pentamidine isethionate. *Am. J. Med.* 83, 571.

Wheat, J., Hafner, R., Wulfsohn, M., *et al.* (1993). Prevention of relapse of histoplasmosis with itraconazole in patients with the acquired immunodeficiency syndrome. The National Institute of Allergy and Infectious Diseases Clinical Trials and Mycoses Study Group. *Ann. Intern. Med.* 118, 610.

Wheeler, J.M., Knittle, J.D., and Miller, J.D. (1993). Depot leuprolide acetate versus danazol in the treatment of women with symptomatic endometriosis: a multicenter, double-blind randomized clinical trial. II. Assessment of safety. The Lupron Endometriosis Study Group. *Am. J. Obstet. Gynecol.* 169, 26.

Whelton, A. and Hamilton, C.W. (1991). Nonsteroidal anti-inflammatory drugs: effects on kidney function. *J. Clin. Pharmacol.* 31, 588.

Whitehead, R.P., Friedman, K.D., Clark, D.A., *et al.* (1995). Phase-I trial of simultaneous administration of interleukin-2 and interleukin-4 subcutaneously. *Clinical Cancer Research* 1, 1145.

Whiting, S.J. (1994). Safety of some calcium supplements questioned. *Nutr. Rev.* 52, 95.

Whitworth, J.A., Hay, C.R., McNicholas, A.M., *et al.* (1992). Coagulation abnormalities and ivermectin. *Ann. Trop. Med. Parasitol.* 86, 301.

Whorwood, C.B., Sheppard, M.C., and Stewart, P.M. (1993). Licorice inhibits 11 beta-hydroxysteroid dehydrogenase messenger ribonucleic acid levels and potentiates glucocorticoid hormone action. *Endocrinology* 132, 2287.

Whyte, K.F., Addis, G.J., Whitesmith, R., *et al.* (1987). Adrenergic control of plasma magnesium in man. *Clin. Sci.* 72, 135.

Whyte, K.F., Reid, C., Addis, G.J., *et al.* (1988). Salbutamol induced hypokalaemia: the effect of theophylline alone and in combination with adrenaline. *Br. J. Clin. Pharmacol.* 25, 571.

Widmer, P., Maibach, R., Kunzi, U.P., *et al.* (1995). Diuretic-related hypokalaemia: the role of diuretics, potassium supplements, glucocorticoids and beta 2-adrenoceptor agonists. Results from the comprehensive hospital drug monitoring programme, Berne (CHDM). *Eur. J. Clin. Pharmacol.* 49, 31.

Wilcox, J.C., McAllister, A.J., Sangster, G., *et al.* (1986). Effects of magnesium supplementation in testicular cancer patients receiving cis-platin: a randomised trial. *Br. J. Cancer* 54, 19.

Wilkinson, R., Lucas, G.L., Heath, D.A., *et al.* (1986). Hypomagnesaemic tetany associated with prolonged treatment with aminoglycosides. *BMJ* 292, 818,

Willett, W.C. and Hunter, D.J. (1994). Vitamin A and cancers of breast, large bowel and prostate: Epidemiological evidence. *Nutr. Rev.* 52, S53.

Williams, A. and Unwin, R. (1997). Prolonged elevation of serum creatine kinase (CK) without renal failure after ingestion of ecstasy. *Nephrol. Dial. Transplant.* 12, 361.

Williams, H.E. and Wandzilak, T.R. (1989). Oxalate synthesis, transport and the hyperoxaluric syndromes. *J. Urol.* 141, 742.

Williams, M.E. (1991). Endocrine crises. Hyperkalemia. *Crit. Care Clin.* 7, 155.

Williams, M.E. and Lewis, D. (1992). Hyperuricemic acute renal failure associated with FK506 nephrotoxicity. *Clin. Transplant.* 6, 194.

Willis, J.K., Tilton, A.H., Harkin, J.C., *et al.* (1990). Reversible myopathy due to labetalol. *Pediatr. Neurol.* 6, 275.

Wilson, C., Azmy, A.F., Beattie, T.J., *et al.* (1986). Hypermagnesemia and progression of renal failure associated with renacidin therapy. *Clin. Nephrol.* 25, 266.

Wilson, R.F., Dulchavsky, S.A., Soullier, G., *et al.* (1987). Problems with 20 or more blood transfusions in 24 hours. *Am. Surg.* 53, 410.

Witt, J.M., Koo, J.M., and Danielson, B.D. (1996). Effect of standard-dose trimethoprim/sulfamethoxazole on the serum potassium concentration in elderly men. *Ann. Pharmacother.* 30, 347.

Wolf, P.L., Williams, D., Coplon, N., *et al.* (1972). Low aspartate transaminase activity in serum of patients undergoing chronic hemodialysis. *Clin. Chem.* 18, 567.

Wolinsky-Friedland, M. (1995). Drug-induced metabolic bone disease. *Endocrinol. Metab. Clin. North Am.* 24, 395.

Wolpaw, T., Deal, C.L., Fleming-Brooks, S., *et al.* (1994). Factors influencing vertebral bone density after renal transplantation. *Transplantation* 58, 1186.

Wong, C.S., Pavord, I.D., Williams, J., *et al.* (1990). Bronchodilator, cardiovascular and hypokalaemic effects of fenoterol, salbutamol and terbutaline in asthma. *Lancet* 336, 1396.

Wood, B., Nicholls, K.M., and Breen, K.J. (1992). Nutritional status in alcoholism. *J. Hum. Nutr. Diet.* 5, 275.

Woodard, J.A., Shannon, M., and Lacouture, P.G. (1990). Serum magnesium concentration after repetitive magnesium cathartic administration. *Am. J. Emerg. Med.* 8, 297.

Woods, H.F. and Alberti, K.G.M. (1972). Dangers of intravenous fructose. *Lancet* ii, 1354.

Wright, A.J. and Wilkowske, C.J. (1987). The penicillins. *Mayo Clin. Proc.* 62, 806.

Wu, B., Atkinson, S.A., Halton, J.M., *et al.* (1996). Hypermagnesiuria and hypercalciuria in childhood leukemia: an effect of amikacin therapy. *Journal of Pediatric Hematology/Oncology* 18, 86.

Yamaki, M., Kusano, E., Tetsuka, T., *et al.* (1991). Cellular mechanism of lithium-induced nephrogenic diabetes insipidus in rats. *Am. J. Physiol.* 261, F505.

Yamamoto, T., Moriwaki, Y., Takahashi, S., *et al.* (1995). Xylitol-induced increase in the concentration of oxypurines and its mechanism. *Int. J. Clin. Pharmacol. Ther.* 33, 360.

Yamamoto, T., Moriwaki, Y., Takahashi, S., *et al.* (1997). Effect of ethanol and fructose on plasma uridine and purine bases. *Metabolism* 46, 544.

Yao, F.S., Seidman, S.F., and Artusio, J.G. (1980). Disturbance of consciousness and hypocalcemia after neomycin irrigation, and reversal by calcium and physostigmine. *Anaesthesiology* 53, 69.

Yassa, R., Iskandar, H., Nastase, C., *et al.* (1988). Carbamaz-epine and hyponatremia in patients with affective disorder. *Am. J. Psychiatry* 145, 339.

Yentis, S.M. (1990). Suxamethonium and hyperkalaemia. *Anaesth. Intensive Care* 18, 92.

Yip, L., Dart, R.C., and Gabow, P.A. (1994). Concepts and controversies in salicylate toxicity. *Emerg. Med. Clin. North Am.* 12, 351.

Young, D.S. (1995). Effects of drugs on clinical laboratory tests. (4th edn). AACC Press, Washington.

Yuen, W.C., Whiteoak, R., and Thompson, R.P.H. (1988). Zinc concentrations in leucocytes of patients receiving anti-epileptic drugs. *J. Clin. Pathol.* 41, 553.

Zalin, A.M., Hutchinson, C.E., Jong, M., *et al.* (1984). Hyponatraemia during treatment with chlorpropamide and Moduretic (amiloride plus hydrochlorothiazide). *BMJ* 289, 659.

Zaloga, G.P., Chernow, B., Pock, A., *et al.* (1984). Hypomagnesemia is a common complication of aminoglycoside therapy. *Surg. Gynecol. Obstet.* 158, 561.

Zanella, M.T., Maltei, J.E., Draibe, S.A., *et al.* (1985). Inadequate aldosterone response to hyperkalemia during angiotensin converting enzyme inhibition in chronic renal failure. *Clin. Pharmacol. Ther.* 38, 613.

Zantvoort, F.A., Derkx, F.H.M., Boomsma, F., *et al.* (1986). Theophylline and serum electrolytes. *Ann. Intern. Med.* 104, 134.

Zarrabi, M.H., Zucker, S., Miller, F., *et al.* (1979). Immunologic and coagulation disorders in chlorpromazine-treated patients. *Ann. Intern. Med.* 91, 194.

Zavagli, G., Ricci, G., Tataranni, G., *et al.* (1988). Life-threatening hyponatremia caused by vinblastine. *Med. Oncol. Tumor Pharmacother.* 5, 67.

Zeharia, A., Levy, Y., Rachmel, A., *et al.* (1987). Hyperkalemia as a late side effect of prolonged adrenocorticotrophic hormone therapy for infantile spasms. *Helv. Paediatr. Acta* 42, 433.

Zimran, A., Kramer, M., Plaskin, M., *et al.* (1985). Incidence of hyperkalaemia induced by indomethacin in a hospital population. *BMJ* 291, 107.

Zsigmond, E.K. and Robins, G. (1972). The effect of a series of anti-cancer drugs on plasma cholinesterase activity. *Can. Anaesth. Soc. J.* 19, 75.

18. Disorders of muscle, bone, and connective tissue

H. G. M. SHETTY, P. A. ROUTLEDGE, and D. M. DAVIES

Drugs may produce localized or diffuse disorders of muscle, bone, and connective tissue. These tissues may also be involved as a part of a more generalized drug-induced disease, and when this is the case they are more appropriately dealt with elsewhere in this book. Consequently, parts of this chapter serve mainly as signposts to other chapters, although they do also provide reminders that symptoms and signs involving bones, joints, tendons, and subcutaneous tissues may be the earliest or predominant indications of an adverse drug reaction.

Muscles

Myalgia and cramps

Myalgia, sometimes accompanied by muscle cramps, may be an early symptom of drug-induced polyneuropathy, myopathy, or disorders of the extrapyramidal system, but it is usually soon overshadowed by other features of these conditions (which are discussed in detail in Chapter 20). Drug-induced retroperitoneal fibrosis may similarly present with aching in legs and back in the early stages, because of vascular compression.

Myalgia affecting the calves only while walking is an uncommon complication of oral contraceptive therapy (Davies and Lund 1965) and may arouse suspicion of a vascular disorder when none is present. A syndrome of myalgia, arthralgia, and swelling affecting only the hands has been attributed to oral contraceptive therapy (Spiera and Plotz 1969), and in a patient with similar symptoms seen by one of us coldness and discolouration of the hands accompanied the attacks of pain. Slight muscular aching in patients taking oral contraceptives may be due to fluid retention caused by these compounds, and several other drugs can cause mild myalgia in this way.

Muscle cramps have also been described in association with diuretic, calcium antagonist, and β_2-agonist therapy. Diuretics may produce hyponatraemia, hypokalaemia, and hypomagnesaemia, which, in turn, cause muscle cramps. These and other adverse effects produced by diuretics are discussed in Chapter 17. In two patients who were not epileptic but had a history of idiopathic cramps, muscle pains and cramps, collapse, and seizures in the absence of electrolyte abnormalities have been attributed to metolazone therapy. The mechanism underlying this syndrome is unclear (Fitzgerald and Brennan 1976).

Oral salbutamol in doses of 4 mg thrice daily has been reported to cause muscle cramps in up to 45 per cent of patients (Palmer 1978). Terbutaline has also been shown to cause painful muscle cramps with persistent muscle twitching and tremor, and these signs and symptoms did not recur when the drug was replaced by orciprenaline (Zelman 1978), though Lotzof (1968) has reported that muscle cramps occur in about eight per cent of patients receiving orciprenaline and that they disappear when potassium is given concurrently.

Keidar and associates (1982) have described severe cramps with nifedipine in three patients, in two of whom rechallenge with the drug reproduced their symptoms; and in other cases described by MacDonald (1982) paraesthesiae accompanied the cramps. Doxazosin has been reported to cause muscle cramps in one per cent of patients (Young and Brogden 1988).

Suxamethonium has been reported to cause myalgia in about 50 per cent of patients on the day after surgery (Glauber 1966; McGloughlin et al. 1988; O'Sullivan et al. 1988). The pain occurs mainly in the neck, shoulders, back, and chest and in some cases has been likened to being 'driven over by a bus' (Glauber 1966). The aetiology of this adverse effect is unknown. It is commoner in women (Hegarty 1956; Leatherdale et al. 1959), and in non-pregnant than in pregnant women (Crawford 1971; Datta *et al.* 1977; Thind and Bryson 1983). Suxamethonium administration results in release of CK and myoglobin, but there is no obvious relationship between the pain and the extent of the biochemical changes (Laurence 1987). The intensity of pain is also unrelated to strength or even the presence of visible fasciculations (Newnam and Loudon 1966; O'Sullivan *et al.* 1988). Waters and Mapleson (1971) have observed that the pain appears to be worse in patients whose muscles do not appear to fasciculate or to fasciculate very little. Irreversible damage to muscle spindles (Rack and Westbury 1966), potassium flux (Mayrhofer 1959), lactic acid (Konig 1956), and serotonin (Kaniaris *et al.* 1973) have all been implicated in the causation of pain. Injection of small, non-paralysing doses of a non-depolarizing relaxant such as tubocurarine (Blitt *et al.* 1981) or gallamine, 2–3 minutes before suxamethonium, reduces the frequency of myalgia by about 20–30 per cent (White 1962; Glauber 1966; Erkola *et al.* 1983); but the disadvantages of non-depolarizing drugs are that they diminish or abolish the intensity of fasciculations, which are useful indicators of the drug effect for the anaesthetist, and impair the intensity of neuromuscular block, so that more suxamethonium is required to produce the desired effect (Cullen 1971; Masey *et al.* 1983). Soluble aspirin 600 mg given 1 hour preoperatively has been shown to reduce the frequency of myalgia to 21 per cent compared with 57 per cent in patients given suxamethonium alone and 36 per cent in a group who received tubocurarine 0.05 mg per kg 3 minutes before induction (McGloughlin *et al.* 1988). Aspirin does not impair the intensity of neuromuscular block or abolish the visible fasciculations, and its exact mechanism of action in relieving the myalgia is not known. Although it has been claimed that diazepam is effective in preventing myalgia (Fahmy *et al.* 1979), it has not been shown to be so in a study comparing its effect with that of tubocurarine (Manchikanti 1984).

The antimony compounds meglumine antimoniate and sodium stibogluconate, which are used for treatment of leishmaniasis, frequently cause myalgia (WHO technical report 1984). Danazol has been reported to cause myalgia, muscle cramps, muscle spasm, and elevation of CK (Buttram *et al.* 1985; Watts *et al.* 1985).

Severe myalgia, predominantly affecting the shoulder girdle and upper limbs, associated with elevation of CK, has occurred in hyperthyroid women treated with carbimazole for between 3 weeks and 3 months. Stopping the drug resulted in rapid resolution of symptoms and return of CK to normal concentrations (Page and Nussey 1989); it has been suggested that in such cases the cause

may be 'tissue hypothyroidism' rather than a direct adverse effect of the drug (O'Malley 1989).

Other drugs that have been described to cause myalgia include cimetidine (Burland 1978), enalapril (Cooper *et al.* 1987), guanethidine (Stocks and Robertson 1966), intramuscular iron injections (Ben-Ishay 1961), nalidixic acid (Gleckman *et al.* 1979), and transfer factor (Gibbon *et al.* 1983). Zidovudine therapy can cause myalgia; and also mitochondrial myopathy — resulting in muscle weakness; elevations of the serum creatine kinase (CK), blood lactate:pyruvate ratio; a myopathic pattern in the electromyogram; and 'ragged-red' fibres in a muscle biopsy (Mhiri *et al.* 1991; Chariot *et al.* 1994).

Topical minoxidil therapy has been associated with a reversible 'pseudopolymyalgia' syndrome of severe pain in the pelvic and shoulder girdles, fatigue, anorexia, weight loss, and a normal erythrocyte sedimentation rate. The symptoms cleared a few days after stopping the drug and recurred on rechallenge (Colamarino *et al.* 1990). A similar syndrome has complicated treatment with enalapril (Le Loët *et al.* 1989) and dipyridamole (Chassagne *et al.* 1990).

Severe and widespread myalgia and joint pains may occur in patients who have been taking daily doses of corticosteroids equivalent to 10 mg or more of prednisone for 30 days or longer when steroid therapy is withdrawn. In a few cases the illness progresses until it resembles systemic lupus erythematosus (SLE), and death may ensue (Kriegel and Müller 1972). Whether this type of case represents an unmasked spontaneous lupus erythematosus, previously controlled by the steroid therapy, is not clear. It would seem rational to treat these disorders by administering steroids again in the maximum dosage previously taken by the patient. The dose is then reduced by small amounts (1–2.5 mg of prednisone or its equivalent) at intervals of several days or longer, depending on the patient's condition.

Muscle damage

Drug-induced muscle injury may be primary, due to a direct action of the drug on muscle tissue, muscle metabolic enzymes, or neuromuscular transmitters; or secondary, when it follows hypokalaemia induced by the drug concerned. It is also a feature of polymyositis and dermatomyositis caused by drugs. Drug-induced myasthenia and myopathy are dealt with in Chapter 20.

Severe muscle damage can follow the intramuscular injection of chlorpromazine (O'Connor 1980) or diclofenac (Müller-Vahl 1984). This is rarely disabling, unless necrosis (rhabdomyolysis) is extensive or the site of injection becomes infected. It is usually of clinical importance only because it may cause a rise in the serum concentration of enzymes originating in muscle, which may be misleading if the possibility is overlooked (see Creatine kinase — Chapter 17). Repeated intramuscular injections of some drugs may cause severe fibrosis and contracture. The drugs most often implicated in western countries are the opiates (Mastaglia *et al.* 1971; Adams *et al.* 1983), but in India and South America the culprit is often an antibiotic (Blain and Lane 1983). Sterile abscesses and pain on injection have been described in between 18 and 75 per cent of patients treated with intramuscular pentamidine isethionate (Goa and Campoli-Richards 1987). Intramuscular injection of diclofenac has been shown to cause local myonecrosis and atrophy of the affected muscle (Stricker and van Kasteren 1992).

Rhabdomyolysis and myoglobinuria are very serious adverse effects of drugs. Rhabdomyolysis may result from a direct myotoxic effect of the drug; muscle ischaemia in drug overdose; or drug-induced malignant hyperthermia, neuroleptic malignant syndrome, central cholinergic syndrome, and polymyositis.

Treatment with lipid-lowering drugs has been associated with muscle damage and rhabdomyolysis, with an estimated incidence of one case per 100 000 treatment years (CSM 1995). The HMGCoA-reductase inhibitors (statins) lovastatin, pravastatin, and simvastatin have all been implicated (Corpier *et al.* 1988; Chariot *et al.* 1993; Hino *et al.* 1996). They are thought to inhibit mitochondrial adenosine triphosphate production, resulting in inadequate production of coenzyme-Q and haem A in the mitochondrial membrane, causing disturbed cellular energy production and cell death (Willis *et al.* 1990). Mibefradil, a calcium-channel blocker inhibits CYPP 3A4 which mediates the metabolism of simvastatin and lovastatin and if used concurrently with one of these may increase the risk of rhabdomyolysis. Pravastatin and fluvastatin, which have alternative metabolic pathways, can safely be combined with mibefradil (Roche Pharmaceuticals 1997). The risk of rhabdomyolysis with statins appears to be higher when they are given concurrently with cyclosporin, erythromycin, gemfibrozil, itraconazole, ketoconazole, levothyroxine, or nicotinic acid, or in the presence of renal impairment and possibly hyperthyroidism (Hino *et al.* 1996). They should be avoided in patients who are at risk of developing rhabdomyolysis, because of uncontrolled seizures, hypotension, or severe acute infections.

Ciprofibrate and gemfibrozil (Magarian *et al.* 1992) also cause rhabdomyolysis. The use of higher doses of ciprofibrate (e.g. 200 mg per day), is particularly likely to cause rhabdomyolysis; and concomitant use of ibuprofen was considered to have been a contributory factor in one patient with ciprofibrate-associated rhabdomyolysis (Ramachandran *et al.* 1997).

Myalgia, weakness, stiffness, malaise and elevation of CK is an uncommon adverse effect of clofibrate (Langer and Levy 1968; Sekowski and Samuel 1972) but asymptomatic elevation of muscle enzymes is frequent (Watermeyer *et al.* 1975). The dose of clofibrate should be reduced in patients with renal disease, who tend to develop myopathy most frequently (Goldberg *et al.* 1977). Bezafibrate has also been reported to cause muscle cramps, paresis, elevation of muscle enzymes, myoglobinaemia, and myoglobinuria, particularly in patients with impaired renal function (Rumpf *et al.* 1984). Nicotinic acid, when used on its own rather than with statins, can also cause myalgia, cramps, and an elevation of elevated CK and aspartate aminotransferase concentrations (Litin and Anderson 1989).

A number of other drugs, including aminocaproic acid, amphetamine, barbiturates, chloroquine, cocaine, colchicine, cyclosporin, diclofenac, diphenhydramine, diuretics, doxylamine, emetics, heroin, laxatives, methadone, pentazocine, phencyclidine, retinoids, suxamethonium, theophylline, and vincristine have been reported to cause rhabdomyolysis. For a detailed discussion of this disorder the reader is referred to a review by Köppel (1989).

Polymyositis and dermatomyositis

Penicillamine causes polymyositis, which may be mild, with elevation of muscle enzymes alone; moderately severe, with moderate muscular weakness; or severe, with marked muscular weakness, myolysis, and myocarditis, resulting in death (Wouters *et al.* 1982; Doyle *et al.* 1983). Polymyositis has also been attributed to cimetidine (Matthiesen 1979), in which case it has sometimes been accompanied by interstitial nephritis (Watson *et al.* 1983).

Death due to respiratory and renal failure has been reported in a young woman suffering from Chagas' disease who developed acute polymyositis, toxic erythema, and purpura while taking nifurtimox (Shaw *et al.* 1982).

Dermatomyositis has occurred in an 11-year-old boy a few days after injection of the local anaesthetic carticaine for tooth extraction, but a causal relationship has not been established (Rose *et al.* 1985). A dermatomyositis-like syndrome, with myopathic electromyogram, elevated lactic dehydrogenase and CK concentrations, developed in a 42-year-old woman given the nonsteroidal anti-inflammatory drug niflumic acid, resolving when it was stopped. The same patient had developed periorbital infiltrated erythematous oedema after receiving diclofenac for 3 months for treatment of arthralgia (Grob *et al.* 1989).

Dermatomyositis has been described in a 50-year-old man after 6 months of treatment with the HMGCoA-reductase inhibitor simvastatin (Khatak *et al.* 1994). Penicillamine is also known to cause dermatomyositis (Wouters *et al.* 1982).

Eosinophilia–myalgia syndrome

Over 1400 cases of the eosinophilia–myalgia syndrome (EMS) were reported in the USA between October 1989 and April 1990. In contrast, few cases have been enountered in Europe. A third of the American patients required hospitalization and 19 died (Medsger 1990). Almost all of them had taken over-the-counter dietary supplements containing L-tryptophan (LT). The median dose ingested was 1.5 g daily for periods of a few weeks to several years. In some patients the syndrome appeared only after they had stopped taking the supplements. The United States Centers for Disease Control and Prevention (CDC) set the following criteria for diagnosis of EMS: (1) a total peripheral blood eosinophil count of greater than 1×10^9 cells per L; (2) incapacitating myalgia; and (3) no evidence of infection or neoplasia that would account for eosinophilia or myalgia (CDC 1990; Kilbourne *et al.* 1990).

Most of the affected patients are women. In addition to myalgia, a number of other symptoms and signs may occur — fatigue, arthralgia, fever, cough, dyspnoea, oedema and induration of the extremities with a tendency to involve the lower limbs more than the upper limbs, alopecia, transient maculopapular or urticarial rashes in the early stages and morphoea-like lesions in the late stages, mouth ulcers, myocarditis, right ventricular strain, tricuspid insufficiency, muscle cramps, paraesthesiae, and ascending polyneuropathy resembling the Guillain–Barré syndrome (Kaufman *et al.* 1990; Medsger 1990). Eosinophilia is found in all cases. The erythrocyte sedimentation rate is normal or only slightly elevated and serum CK concentrations are rarely elevated. Histological examination of the muscles shows perivascular accumulation of lymphocytes and plasma cells, but no evidence of myofibrillar degeneration, indicating that the myalgia is likely to be due to damage to the peripheral sensory nerves. In fact, sensory and motor neurological symptoms and electrophysiological evidence of axonal degeneration have been described in some patients. Although dyspnoea and hypoxaemia are common, the chest X-ray is often clear and rarely

shows inflammatory infiltration (Kaufman *et al.* 1990; Medsger 1990).

The follow-up of EMS patients for almost 4 years has revealed that the age-matched and sex-matched mortality rate with EMS is more than three times higher than that of the general population. Most deaths (66 per cent) occurred within 18 months of the onset of symptoms. Although EMS survivors continued to have greater morbidity, the severity and numbers of symptoms diminished with time (Sullivan *et al.* 1996). After 18 to 24 months all symptoms, except cognitive changes, and nearly all physical findings were reported either to have resolved or improved in most patients. Worsening of cognitive function was noted in 32 per cent of patients. Prednisolone was beneficial in 79 per cent of patients who received it during the acute phase. No other treatment (including non-steroidal anti-inflammatory drugs, cyclosporin, methotrexate, hydroxychloroquine, azathioprine, diuretics, penicillamine, or plasmapheresis) was found to be consistently beneficial (Hertzman *et al.* 1995).

Between 1989 and 1990 in the USA, 96–100 per cent of patients with EMS were found to have consumed LT manufactured by Showa Denko KK (Belongia *et al.* 1990; Slutsker *et al.* 1990). Those who had consumed higher doses of the Showa Denko KK preparation were found to be more likely to develop EMS. Subsequent investigations revealed that the Showa Denko KK formulation of LT contained several abnormal constituents including 1,1-ethylidenebis-(L-tryptophan), also called EBT or peak E, and 3-phenylamino-alanine or peak 5. EBT has been shown to be a potent stimulator of fibroblast activation and collagen synthesis (Takagi *et al.* 1995). Some investigators reported EMS-like illness in animals fed on EBT but this could not be reproduced by several others. It is possible that other impurities in LT produced by Showa Denko and predisposing host factors may have contributed to its pathogenicity (Clauw and Pincus 1996).

Genetic polymorphism may play a role in the pathogenesis of EMS. It has been shown that the incidence of cytochrome P-450 CYP2D6 poor-metaboliser genotype for S-mephenytoin hydroxylation is higher in EMS patients than in control subjects (0.155 vs 0.061, $P = 0.007$). No difference in dapsone acetylation was detected between the two groups. Although these findings suggest that genetic polymorphism may be a factor in the pathogenesis of EMS, its precise role is unclear (Flockart *et al.* 1994).

Eosinophilia of between 1×10^9 and 30×10^9 per L has been noted in EMS patients and higher counts were found in fatal cases. EBT has been shown to upregulate interleukin-5 (IL-5) receptor expression on normodense eosinophils. It has been suggested that IL-5 may play an important role in the induction of eosinophilia and phenotypic conversion of eosinophils to hypodense state in acute EMS but the precise role of eosinophils, IL-5, IL-3, and granulocyte-monocyte-colony stimulating factor in the pathogenesis of EMS is unclear (Silver 1996).

Eosinophilia and a scleroderma-like syndrome have been observed in an individual with abnormal tryptophan metabolism (Sternberg *et al.* 1980) and alteration of bioavailability of tryptophan by a contaminant is thought to be the cause of 'fog fever' seen in cattle, which develop interstitial pneumonia with eosinophilic infiltrates (Blood and Radostits 1989). Plasma tryptophan levels before and after an oral dose in patients with the eosinophilia–myalgia syndrome and in normal subjects are similar, but the plasma concentrations of L-kynurenine and quinolinic acid, which are metabolites of tryptophan, are significantly higher in patients with active disease compared with those in whom eosinophilia has resolved and normal subjects. These findings suggest activation of the enzyme indoleamine-2,3-dioxygenase, which may have a pathogenetic role in the syndrome (Silver *et al.* 1990).

A small number of EMS cases have been reported in patients who had not consumed LT. Although there was an association between LT manufactured by Showa Denko KK and the EMS epidemic of late 1980s in the USA, in view of the continued occurrence of the disease it is likely that other factors may also be involved in its pathogenesis (Spitzer *et al.* 1995).

Bones

Osteoporosis and osteomalacia

Pain caused by drug-induced osteoporosis is usually acute in onset and commonly affects the back because of vertebral compression and collapse, but it may arise elsewhere due to spontaneous fractures of the ribs, pelvis, or other bones. Osteomalacia, too, may cause pain arising in the spine, though aching in other parts of the skeleton is likely, and spontaneous fractures are not uncommon. Sudden, or gradual and progressive, deformity of the spine may occur in either osteoporosis or osteomalacia. These disorders and their pathogeneses are discussed in Chapter 17.

Slipped epiphysis

It has been suspected for many years that slipping of the upper femoral epiphysis might have an endocrine basis. Harris (1950) concluded from experiments in rats that growth hormone decreases (while sex hormones increase) the shearing strength of the epiphyseal plate, thus predisposing to slipping of the epiphysis by altering the thickness of the third layer of the epiphyseal plate. He suggested that these findings might provide an explanation for the human disorder, especially when associated with the adiposogenital syndrome or with rapid adolescent growth. This hypothesis was supported by a case report (Rennie and Michell 1974) which described the development of a slipped femoral disc in a 15-year-old girl during treatment with growth hormone. Fidler and Brook (1974) reported similar occurrences in two younger children treated with the hormone.

Fractures and dislocations

Since patients with drug-induced osteomalacia may develop spontaneous fractures (see above), it is obvious that they are even more likely to sustain fractures from falls or other kinds of trauma. Ingestion of aluminium-containing antacids in large quantities for prolonged periods may result in phosphate depletion, osteomalacia, and pseudofractures in patients with normal renal function (Spencer and Kramer 1983). In patients with chronic renal failure who are on dialysis, exposure to excessive amounts of aluminium in the dialysate is believed to have a direct toxic effect on mineralization of bone and this may result in a high frequency of spontaneous fractures (Schneider *et al.* 1984; Malluche and Faugère 1985).

Methotrexate osteopathy, characterized by severe bone pain, pronounced osteoporosis, and spontaneous fractures of the lower limbs, has been described in children receiving long-term methotrexate therapy for acute lymphocytic anaemia (Râgab *et al.* 1970). It has also been described in adults given low-dose methotrexate for rheumatoid arthritis (Maenaut *et al.* 1996). The existence of methotrexate arthropathy in adults has been questioned by some investigators, because many patients with rheumatoid arthritis have other attributes predisposing to osteoporosis and fractures.

Fractures caused by falls are strongly associated with the use of barbiturates in the elderly (MacDonald and MacDonald 1977). Apart from causing impaired awareness and unsteadiness (a possible hazard of all hypnotics and sedatives in the elderly), barbiturates stimulate hepatic enzymes involved in the metabolism of vitamin D, and may thus induce or aggravate osteomalacia (Marshall 1977) (see also Chapter 17). The findings of MacDonald and MacDonald (1977) gained support from a case–control study involving 1021 elderly patients with hip fractures and 5606 elderly controls, which showed a significantly increased risk of hip fractures in association with hypnotics and anxiolytics that have long half-lives, tricyclic antidepressants, and antipsychotics. The risk increased with increasing doses of these drugs (Ray *et al.* 1987).

Patients taking levodopa plus benserazide for parkinsonism are more prone to fractures than those taking other antiparkinsonian drugs. This may partly be due to the increased mobility produced by the drugs and therefore an increased likelihood of accidental falls, but it is interesting to note that benserazide has caused skeletal changes in rats used for toxicity investigations (Barbeau and Roy 1976).

Repeated intramuscular injections into the deltoid may produce abduction deformity of the arm (Levin and Engel 1975) due to fibrosis of the muscle and contraction of fibrous tissue, which in extreme cases may lead to dislocation of the shoulder (Cozen 1977).

Muscle spasm severe enough to cause fracture–dislocation of the hips complicated myelography with meglumine iocarmate (Eastwood *et al.* 1978).

Aseptic (avascular, ischaemic) necrosis

Aseptic necrosis of bone is associated with certain types of drug therapy, as well as with trauma, a variety of natural disorders (Sutton 1968) or, very rarely, arteriography or radiotherapy (Kriegel and Müller 1972). The drug-induced disorder is almost always a complication of treatment with steroids (Cruess 1977) or ACTH and occurs too often to be coincidental, even in rheumatoid arthritis and systemic lupus erythematosus, which appear to predispose to aseptic necrosis. It may be, however, that only in certain conditions (of which rheumatoid arthritis and systemic lupus erythematosus may be examples) do steroids induce avascular necrosis, a possibility strengthened by the observation that while avascular necrosis may affect patients with renal disease under treatment with steroids and renal dialysis it is said not to occur in children with the nephrotic syndrome treated only with steroids (Gregg *et al.* 1980). The head of the femur is the commonest site of involvement (Solomon 1973) but the head of the humerus, the tibia, the condyle of the mandible, and the carpal bones may also be affected. In corticosteroid-induced cases, dose appears to be the major predictor of the risk of avascular necrosis (Felson and Anderson 1987). Large doses of prednisolone (60 mg) for 14 days every 6 weeks (Watkins and Williams 1982) have resulted in avascular necrosis of the head of the femur. In these cases prednisolone had been given with a number of cytotoxic drugs in the treatment of Hodgkin's disease. Even short courses of dexamethasone in large doses have caused the disease (McCluskey and Gutteridge 1982). The pathogenesis of steroid-induced aseptic necrosis is still unclear, but among the more plausible suggestions are a steroid-induced vasculitis of the small vessels supplying the affected portion of bone, or fat embolism, the fat emboli originating in a liver rendered excessively fatty by the action of steroids or ACTH (Sutton 1968). The fat embolism theory was not supported, however, by the histological studies of Solomon (1973), who examined 42 femoral heads removed from patients with avascular necrosis and concluded that the amount and the location of fat in the specimens was much the same as in specimens from patients with normal hips or from those suffering from other disorders of the femoral head. He proposed an alternative explanation for the disease, namely, that the diminished joint sensibility produced by the anti-inflammatory effect (and consequent analgesic effect) of steroids predisposes to microtrauma in osteoporotic bone, resulting in subarticular collapse of the femoral head.

Avascular necrosis is said to have complicated treatment with drugs of the 'phenylbutazone group' (Murray and Jacobson 1972), and has been caused by combination cancer chemotherapy (Harper *et al.* 1984).

Osteosclerosis, ectopic calcification, bone thickening, and bone destruction

Osteosclerosis may result from excessive doses of vitamin A or D, or fluorine, and is a rare feature of the milk–alkali syndrome. The bone changes of vitamin A excess are normally believed to be short-lasting, although a patient with hyperostosis induced by vitamin A has been found to have permanent deformity of long bones and scoliosis after 12 years of follow-up (Ruby and Mital 1974). Chronic vitamin D poisoning may result in ectopic calcification in the muscles, tendons, ligaments, subcutaneous tissue, and other parts of the body. Excessive intake of vitamin A or fluoride may result in calcification, usually confined to the tendons and periarticular tissues (Kriegel and Müller 1972). Calcification may rarely occur at the site of intramuscular or subcutaneous injections (Kriegel and Müller 1972).

Thickening of the skull, mainly the diploic space, with no abnormalities of other bones, has been observed in patients on long-term treatment with phenytoin, some of whom were also on other anticonvulsant drugs (Kattan 1970). Sodium valproate therapy has been reported to cause generalized skeletal pain and osteosclerosis affecting the distal metaphyses of femur, radius, and ulna (John 1981). The mechanism of these manifestations is unclear. Long-term isotretinoin therapy for ichthyosis has been shown to be associated with arthralgia or myalgia and an ossification disorder resembling diffuse idiopathic skeletal hyperostosis. Although lowering the dose or withdrawal of the drug resulted in clinical improvement, the radiological changes persisted over the observation period (Pittsley and Yoder 1983).

Asymptomatic skeletal fluorosis resulting in osteosclerosis, predominantly affecting the axial skeleton, has been observed in patients on long-term treatment with niflumic acid and flufenamic acid capsules containing fluoride (Del Favero 1984; Vrhovac 1988). The biochemical abnormalities included hypocalcaemia, hypocalciuria, high urinary fluoride, and raised serum alkaline phosphatase. Bone biopsy showed an increase in trabecular bone volume suggestive of bone fluorosis. The mechanism underlying the fluoride-induced changes in bone structure and the uneven distribution of osteosclerosis is unclear.

Clubbing of fingers associated with the ingestion of excessive doses of purgatives was described by Silk and others (1975), and other cases of this kind were subsequently described (Prior and White 1978; Malmquist et al. 1980), and a combination of clubbing of digits and hypertrophic osteoarthropathy due to purgative abuse has been described by Armstrong and others (1981). In the latter case the clubbing disappeared within 6 months of withdrawal of the purgative (senna in the form of Senokot), though at the time of the report the radiological abnormalities were still present.

Newman and Ling (1985) have shown a significant association between the use of non-steroidal anti-inflammatory drugs (NSAID) in patients with primary osteoarthrosis of the hip and acetabular destruction. The mechanism of this process is unclear, but it has been suggested that NSAID may inhibit the repair of necrotic bone, resulting in femoral head necrosis and trabecular microfractures (Newman and Ling 1985).

Joints

Arthralgia and arthritis

Mild arthralgia and arthritis may accompany almost any type of generalized skin eruption caused by drugs (discussed in Chapter 19); and more severe joint pains, with associated swelling, are an essential component of 'serum sickness', which can be induced by any one of a number of drugs (discussed in Chapter 27). A particularly severe example of arthropathy associated with a

reaction of this kind has been reported as an adverse reaction to carbimazole (Bethel 1979); and the crippling arthritis attributed to vaccination against swine influenza (Hasler v. United States 1981) may have had a similar cause.

The use of intradermal and intravesical BCG for immunotherapy in cancer patients has been reported to be associated with arthritis. Arthritis occurs in about 0.5 per cent of patients receiving intravesical BCG, and predominantly affects the lower limb joints, particularly the knee joints. Most of the reported cases have been in men, the majority of whom have HLA-B 27 (Lamm et al. 1986; Ochsenkühn et al. 1990; Jawad et al. 1993; Missioux et al. 1995). Following intradermal BCG, arthritis occurs after an average duration of 32 weeks and predominantly affects the hands (Torisu et al. 1978; Missioux et al. 1995).

Acute arthropathy, arthralgia, and chronic arthropathy have been described with rubella vaccine. Adult women (13–15 per cent) are more likely to develop arthritis or arthralgia than are children, and small peripheral joints are usually affected (Peters and Horowitz 1984; Tringle et al. 1986; Weibel and Benox 1996). Fluvirin (inactivated influenza vaccine; surface antigen) has been reported cause acute polyarthritis and arthralgia (Thurairajan 1997). Hepatitis B vaccination has also been shown to be associated with arthritis (Rogerson and Nye 1990; Gros et al. 1995).

Arthralgia and arthritis may be the early manifestation of systemic lupus erythematosus (SLE), and it is now recognized that some cases of this disorder can be attributed to drug treatment. The drugs implicated and the complex mechanisms involved are described later in this chapter. This disorder may also appear for the first time during the withdrawal of steroid therapy (see the section on Myalgia, under Muscles).

Vasculitis may present with polyarthralgia and polyarthritis. This uncommon disease may arise spontaneously or may be induced by drugs (Wokenstein and Revuz 1995; Jennette and Falk 1997).

Septic arthritis may occur as a result of faulty aseptic technique during intra-articular injections, or may complicate treatment with drugs that lower the body's resistance to infection, a subject which is discussed in detail in Chapter 25.

Quinolones have been shown to cause erosions of articular cartilage and permanent damage to weight-bearing joints in immature dogs when administered in very high doses for prolonged periods (Neu 1988). Joint disease has been described in association with quinolone therapy in human patients, involving norfloxacin (Jeandel et al. 1989), pefloxacin (Kesseler et al. 1989), and ciprofloxacin (Ball 1986; Alfaham *et al.* 1987). Nalidixic acid (the oldest of the quinolones) has also caused arthralgia and arthritis (Bailey *et al.* 1972; Gleckman *et al.* 1979).

Quinidine has been reported to cause symmetrical, reversible polyarthritis with no immunological abnormalities on three occasions in one patient (Kertes and Hunt 1982). Joint effusion, which recurred on rechallenge, has been attributed to practolol therapy (Fraser and Irvine 1976). Although it has been reported that arthralgia is a common adverse effect of β-blockers, particularly metoprolol (Savola 1983, 1984; Sills and Bosco 1986), a case–control study of 127 patients attending a hypertension clinic found no significant association (Walker and Ramsay 1985). An acute febrile polyarthritis has been reported with the antihypertensive drug prazosin (Cairns and Jordan 1976). Captopril has been reported to cause a migratory polyarthralgia with a false-positive test (VDRL) for syphilis, both of which resolved on discontinuation of the drug (Malnick and Schattner 1989).

Drug-induced gout is discussed in Chapter 17. Telescoping of the fingers and toes in a patient with chronic tophaceous gout has been attributed to treatment with allopurinol, and believed to have been due to rapid resorption of large and extensive osseous tophi without replacement by new bone (Gottlieb and Gray 1977).

Arthralgia may be a feature of the steroid-withdrawal syndrome but, paradoxically, steroids very rarely cause arthralgia and arthritis (Bailey and Armour 1974; Newmark *et al.* 1974; Bennett and Strong 1975). An unusual effect of steroids was reported by Tanenbaum (1972), who described a patient whose dermatitis of the distal phalanx of a finger was treated for 4 months with local applications of fluorinated steroids. The treatment resulted in disappearance of part of the underlying bone, which developed a 'pencil-sharpener' appearance that persisted during the 2 years of observation.

There is nothing to suggest that rheumatoid arthritis is ever induced by drugs, but iron–dextran complex (Imferon) when given by the 'total dose' method may cause an acute exacerbation of some of the symptoms and signs of this disorder, and this drug may cause arthralgia in patients not known to be suffering from rheumatoid arthritis. Sodium aurothiomalate has also been reported to cause exacerbation of rheumatoid arthritis at the start of treatment (Reynolds 1989). Levamisole (Dinai and Pras 1975) and interferon (Ferrazi *et al.* 1994) have been reported to worsen rheumatoid arthritis, and the former drug to have caused arthritis in two patients with Crohn's disease (Segal *et al.* 1977), and in a patient with Behçet's syndrome on two occasions when it was given (Siklos

1977). The NSAID meclofenamic acid bas been shown to aggravate psoriatic arthropathy (Meyerhoff 1983).

A polyarthritis has been described in association with clindamycin-induced colitis (Rollins and Moeller 1975). Painless deforming arthropathy has been reported with purgative abuse (Frier and Scott 1977) and is believed to be related to chronic purgative-induced bowel disease.

Arthritis has been attributed to treatment with interferon (Ching and Older 1997), gemfibrozil (Hammoudeh *et al.* 1995), methimazole (Hietarinta and Merilanti-Palo 1989), propylthiouracil (Oh *et al.* 1983), phenytoin (Stalnikowicz *et al.* 1982), simvastatin (McDonagh *et al.* 1993), tamoxifen (Creamer *et al.* 1994), cimetidine (CSM 1981), and ranitidine (SADRAC 1989).

Haemarthrosis

In patients who are on anticoagulant therapy, haemarthrosis has been described in the absence of obvious trauma (McLaughlin *et al.* 1966).

Shoulder–hand syndrome

A syndrome resembling the naturally occurring shoulder–hand syndrome, characterized by arthralgia affecting the shoulder and other joints of the upper limbs and sometimes accompanied by contractures and other changes, was first described many years ago as a complication of treatment with phenobarbitone (Maillard and Renard 1925). Subsequently, the barbiturates were implicated in similar cases reported in France (Maillard and Thomazi 1931; Bériel and Barber 1934; Castin and Gardien 1934; Arlet *et al.* 1967; Lequesne 1967), Scandinavia (Lövgren 1948), Holland (van der Korst *et al.* 1960) and Chile (Cuchacovich and Kappes 1987). In the cases attributed to phenobarbitone the drug had been given in daily doses of 100–300 mg for periods varying from a few weeks to more than 20 years, and the condition was usually, though not invariably, bilateral. The way in which phenobarbitone produced these changes was not apparent.

In many patients, particularly those with bilateral disease, acute symptoms of burning pain, oedematous swelling, and decreased sweating were followed after an interval of 3–9 months by dystrophic changes in the hand and contractures of the fingers (van der Korst *et al.* 1960).

In the 1960s a number of reports were published suggesting antituberculous therapy as a cause of the shoulder–hand syndrome, suspicion falling mainly on isoniazid (see Kriegel and Müller 1972). Typically, there was a sudden onset of pain, tenderness, and stiffness in the joints of the hand accompanied by severe pain in the shoulder. Most patients also experienced widespread myalgia and arthralgia, and some felt tired and depressed. Although paraesthesiae were felt by some patients, no convincing objective signs of neuropathy appeared. The disease was commonest in men aged 40–50 years. In some cases, restriction of movement of the shoulders and fingers became apparent within a few days of onset of symptoms, and after a few weeks the acute pain subsided to leave a 'frozen shoulder', flexion deformity of the elbow, and tendon contractures of the hand (Good et al. 1965). Similar deformities have occurred in the lower limbs (McKusick and Hsu 1961). In one series of cases (McKusick and Hsu 1961) isoniazid was the only antituberculous agent common to all the treatment regimens, and suspicion that this drug was to blame was strengthened by a fall in the incidence of the rheumatic syndrome in certain hospitals when the routine daily dosage of isoniazid was reduced from 600 mg to 300 mg (McKusick 1965).

The mechanism by which isoniazid produces rheumatic disorders is unclear, but it has been suggested (Good et al. 1965) that as isoniazid interferes with the metabolism of serotonin (Zarafonetis and Kalas 1960) an excess of this substance may produce fibrosis, as it has been shown to do when injected into the joints of animals, particularly those given isoniazid concurrently (Gum et al. 1960). There is no firm evidence that pyridoxine metabolism is involved in the production of the shoulder–hand syndrome, and prophylactic treatment with pyridoxine does not prevent the disorder (Good et al. 1965).

Complete immobility and severe pain of shoulder joint has been reported with antimony sodium tartrate injections. It occurred equally in the arm used for injection or in the other arm and the movement in the shoulder joint was regained 3–5 days after discontinuation of the drug (Davies 1968).

Disorders of growth

Corticosteroids

Long-term corticosteroid ('steroid') therapy in children inhibits hypophyseal growth hormone secretion and reduces the sensitivity of the peripheral tissues to the hormone, resulting in retardation of linear growth (Bondy 1985). It has been shown that the vitamin D_3 metabolites are reduced in the plasma of children on daily or intermittent long-term corticosteroid therapy for various disorders, and this may be the cause of inhibition of metabolism in cartilage and bone tissue rather than a direct effect of corticosteroids (Chesney et al. 1978; O'Reagan et al. 1979). Although corticotrophin (ACTH) is thought to produce less inhibition of growth than corticosteroids (Bondy 1985), it is recognized that it does inhibit growth hormone secretion and should therefore be used with caution in children if long-term therapy is required. It is difficult to assess objectively the contribution of corticosteroids and corticotrophin to growth retardation in many children who are taking them for serious systemic diseases that themselves may have a growth-suppressant effect. Withdrawal of corticosteroids before the end of puberty may result in normal growth in some children, but this may not be the case in all (Bondy 1985). Avoiding corticosteroids if at all possible and using them in smallest possible doses and intermittently are the best options in children to reduce the likelihood of growth impairment.

Tetracyclines

Tetracyclines are deposited in the growing bone and teeth of the fetus if administered during pregnancy and of the infant and young child if administered in infancy or early childhood. At doses of 7–25 mg (The Lancet 1963) they may produce an inhibition of linear growth by about 40 per cent (Cohlan et al. 1963). The effect of tetracyclines on teeth is described in Chapter 11. These drugs should be avoided in pregnancy and in children under the age of 12 years (British National Formulary 1997).

Central nervous system stimulants

Use of methylphenidate, amphetamine, and pemoline in prepubertal children with the hyperactive or attention-deficit syndrome has been shown to be associated with a retardation of growth in weight and stature that is related to the dose of the drugs and absence of 'drug holidays' (Safer and Allen 1973; Dickinson et al. 1979; Roche et al. 1979). It has been suggested that these drugs may interfere with the release of growth hormone that is normally produced by slow-wave sleep (Barter and Kammer 1978).

Cocaine

Cocaine abuse during pregnancy has been associated with significant growth retardation and a variety of other problems in infants, including congenital abnormalities, withdrawal symptoms, and an increased incidence of preterm delivery, perinatal mortality, and intrauterine fetal death (Fulroth et al. 1989; Neerhof et al. 1989).

Lead

Shukla and associates (1989) have reported that exposure to high concentrations of lead *in utero*, or relatively high concentrations in the neonatal period has a detrimental effect on growth in stature of infants, but Sachs and Moel (1989) found no correlation between growth and blood lead at any concentration.

Connective tissues

Tendons

Tendons may be affected in drug-induced gout, as in the natural disorder. They may also be involved in ectopic calcification, described earlier.

Spontaneous rupture of tendons may complicate treatment with steroid given by mouth or by local injection. The Achilles tendon is most often involved, but the patellar tendon can also rupture (Lee 1957; Cowan and Alexander 1961; Lee 1961; Smaill 1961; Melmed 1965; Ismail *et al.* 1969; Bedi and Ellis 1970). Cooney and others (1980) have claimed that rupture of tendons in patients taking corticosteroids is mainly due to natural connective tissue disorders affecting the tendons rather than to the steroids alone, and stated that no cases of tendon rupture had occurred in patients on high-dose steroid therapy for such diseases as asthma, skin disease, or lymphoproliferative conditions. Haines (1983), however, has described three patients who suffered bilateral rupture of the Achilles tendon while on systemic steroid therapy for chest diseases. He suggested that steroid therapy probably suppresses the repair of degenerated or partially ruptured tendons to such an extent that complete rupture can occur after minor strain.

There have been several reports of tendinitis and tendon rupture during treatment with the fluoroquinolones ciprofloxacin, ofloxacin, norfloxacin, and pefloxacin. The Achilles tendon is predominantly affected, but tendons of the quadriceps, extensor pollicis longus, peroneus brevis, and those of the rotator cuff are also known to be involved. The risk of tendon rupture appears to be high in the elderly, those on long-term steroid therapy, and those receiving fluoroquinolones for longer than 3 weeks. The mechanisms involved in fluoroquinolone-associated tendinopathy are unclear but ischaemia and mechanical forces (in view of the distribution of tendon involvement) are thought to be the likely contributory factors. An MRI scan is useful in diagnosing tendinopathy and tendon rupture. Treatment includes stopping the offending drug, rest, physiotherapy, and tendon repair if appropriate. Tendinitis usually resolves in about 3 weeks but can persist for 3 months. Tendon rupture may take 1 to 6 months to heal (McEwan and Davey 1985; Zabmniecki *et al.* 1996).

Adipose tissue

Atrophy and hypertrophy

Atrophy of subcutaneous fatty tissue may develop at the site of injection or topical application of corticosteroids (Johns and Bower 1970). There may be a genetic susceptibility to the corticosteroid-induced lipoatrophy. Three cases of severe lipoatrophy occurring within the same family after intramuscular injection of triamcinolone have been reported (von Eickstedt and Elsässer 1988). Hypertrophy of the adipose tissue may occur at the periphery of atrophic lesions, or may be the predominant reaction, when it leads to the formation of lipomata (Kriegel and Müller 1972). Lipomatosis affecting the mediastinal (Teates 1970), paraspinal (Streiter *et al.* 1982), and epidural (Bischoff 1988) regions has been attributed to corticosteroid therapy.

Atrophy and hypertrophy of subcutaneous fatty tissue may also develop with bovine and porcine insulins (McNally *et al.* 1988). Purified insulins appear to cause lipoatrophy less frequently than the conventional insulins. Injection of a purer animal insulin or human insulin into and around the atrophic tissue may result in the reversal of this adverse effect. Repeated injections of insulin to the same site may result in lipohypertrophy. This adverse effect can be averted by using different sites for injecting insulin, but the variability in insulin absorption from different anatomical sites should be kept in mind (Koivisto and Felig 1980; McNalley *et al.* 1988).

Nodular panniculitis

This disorder, characterized by subcutaneous nodules that may be tender and may later disappear leaving depressions at the affected sites, has occasionally followed the withdrawal of corticosteroid therapy (Taranta *et al.* 1958; Roenick *et al.* 1964; Jaffe *et al.* 1971; Saxena and Nigam 1988).

Fibrous tissue

Accelerated nodulosis, occurrence of multiple small nodules typically located on the fingers, has been described in about eight per cent of patients receiving low-dose methotrexate for rheumatoid arthritis (Kerstens *et al.* 1992). Fatal cardiac nodules have also been reported (Bruyn *et al.* 1993).

A number of migrainous patients under treatment with vasoconstrictor drugs have developed a disorder characterized by proliferation of fibrous tissue. Retroperitoneal fibrous tissue is mainly affected, but fibrotic changes have also been detected in the mediastinum, pleura, lungs, and pericardium. In most instances methysergide is believed to have been responsible for this disorder (Graham *et al.* 1964, 1968; Utz *et al.* 1965; Graham *et al.* 1966), but in a few cases ergotamine or dihydroergotamine are also suspected to have initiated fibrotic changes or to have reactivated fibrosis originally induced by methysergide (Graham *et al.* 1966). The symptoms and signs of retroperitoneal fibrosis include persistent pain in the loins and groins, oliguria, and pain on micturition, due to compression of one or both ureters by enveloping fibrous tissue, and myalgia, coldness, and oedema in the lower extremities, caused by involvement of the great vessels. The condition tends to regress when methysergide treatment is withdrawn (when it is as well also to withhold ergotamine compounds), but regression is not invariable (Schwartz and Dunea 1966).

In order to guard against this reaction it is wise to use the smallest effective dose of methysergide and the period of continuous treatment should never exceed 6 months. At the end of this time methysergide should be withheld for at least 1 month and whenever possible ergotamine compounds should also be withheld during the rest period (*The Lancet* 1966). Throughout treatment the patient should be seen regularly to ensure that any symptoms and signs suggestive of retroperitoneal fibrosis are detected as early as possible.

A number of β-adrenoceptor blocking drugs have been associated with retroperitoneal fibrosis, including atenolol (Doherty *et al.* 1978; Johnson and McFarland 1980); propranolol (Henri and Groleau 1981; Pierce *et al.* 1981); oxprenolol (McCluskey *et al.* 1980); metoprolol (Thompson and Julian 1982); sotalol (Laakso *et al.* 1982); and timolol (Rimmer *et al.* 1983); these multiple reports relating to a single pharmacological group have strengthened the belief that there may be a causal relationship. Pryor and colleagues (1983) disputed this, but Bullimore (1984), in turn, disputed their conclusions, and the question appears to remain unanswered at the present time.

There have also been isolated reports of retroperitoneal fibrosis developing in patients treated with a variety of other drugs, such as aspirin, phenacetin, and codeine (Lewis *et al.* 1975), bromocriptine (Herzog *et al.* 1989; Vermersch *et al.* 1989), haloperidol (Jeffries *et al.* 1982), lysergide (LSD) (Aptekar and Michinson 1970), methyldopa (Iversen *et al.* 1975; Ahmad 1983), and in patients abusing co-proxamol (Distalgesic — a mixture of propoxyphene and paracetamol) (Critchley *et al.* 1985), but

the evidence is insufficient to incriminate any of these drugs at the present time. It is interesting to note that lysergic acid LSD has structural similarity to methysergide, and bromocriptine is an ergot derivative.

Formaldehyde (1–10% solutions) used intravesically for the treatment of intractable haematuria has been reported to cause bladder wall fibrosis, ureteric fibrosis, and retroperitoneal fibrosis (Ferrie *et al.* 1983).

A fibrosing peritonitis has been recognized as one of the serious adverse reactions produced by the β-adrenoceptor blocking drug practolol as a part of the 'practolol syndrome' (Windsor *et al.* 1975; Eltringham *et al.* 1977; Marshall *et al.* 1977). This condition and the pericardial, pleural, skin, and eye disorders that may accompany it are discussed elsewhere in this book. Sclerosing peritonitis has also been described in association with propranolol (Ahmad 1981) and atenolol (Nillson and Pederson 1985).

The formation of fibrous plaques in the shaft of the penis, causing deformity and discomfort during erection are features of Peyronie's disease. This distressing condition has also been reported in patients under treatment with β-adrenoceptor blocking drugs, including labetalol (Kristensen 1979), metoprolol (Yudkin 1977), and propranolol (Coupland 1977; Osborne 1977; Wallis *et al.* 1977). Pryor and Kahn (1979) have reported a retrospective case–control study of 146 cases of Peyronie's disease, and Pryor and Castle (1982) a prospective study of 100 cases. It is now thought that atherosclerosis may be the aetiological factor in Peyronie's disease, and that the association of the latter with β-blocker therapy is coincidental (Chilton *et al.* 1982; Pryor and Castle 1982).

A case of rapidly progressive bilateral Dupuytren's contracture has been observed in a patient who had been under treatment with propranolol for some years (Coupland 1977) but this occurrence may well have been coincidental.

Cases of the carpal tunnel syndrome appear to have been precipitated by treatment with oestrogen–progestogen combinations or progestogens alone in high doses (Di Saia and Morrow 1977), danazol (Gray 1978; Sikka *et al.* 1983), and disulfiram (Howard 1982).

Drug-related systemic lupus erythematosus (D-RSLE)

A drug-related lupus-like syndrome attributed to sulphadiazine was first described by Hoffman (1945) and an SLE-like 'collagen disease' associated with hydralazine was reported by Morrow and others (1953). Several drugs are now known to cause D-RSLE. Drug-induced autoimmunity (DIA), in which drug therapy results in asymptomatic development of autoantibodies, elevated immunoglobulin levels, and other laboratory abnormalities, needs to be distinguished from D-RSLE. Although a large number of patients develop laboratory features of autoimmunity, such as antinuclear antibodies, for example, a very small proportion of them develop D-RSLE (Table 18.1).

Incidence of D-RSLE

In the United Stated of America 15–20 000 new cases of this condition are reported annually, procainamide being the drug most commonly implicated (Hess *et al.* 1993). The incidence in other countries is unknown. Factors such as the frequency of use of a particular drug and age of the population exposed to offending drugs may influence the incidence of the disease. Table 18.1 lists the varying incidences of D-RSLE with some of the drugs known to cause the disease.

TABLE 18.1

Incidence of D-RSLE and antinuclear antibodies with various drugs

Drug	Incidences (per cent) of		References
	D-RSLE	Antinuclear antibodies	
Procainamide	15–24	75	Blomgren *et al.* 1969
Hydralazine	5–10	15–45	Condemi *et al.* 1967 Litwin *et al.* 1981
Isoniazid	< 1	22	Rothfield *et al.* 1978
Methyldopa	< 2	19	Perry *et al.* 1971
Levodopa	<1.2	11	Henry *et al.* 1971
Oestrogen/ progestogen	< 1.2	< 1.2	Tarzy *et al.* 1972

Drugs involved in D-RSLE

Space precludes provision of a comprehensive list of references concerning drugs for which there is overwhelming evidence of culpability, and these references can be found in the following papers.

Hydralazine: Müller *et al.* 1955; Lee and Siegel 1968; Alarcón-Segovia 1969; Perry *et al.* 1970; Lee and Chase 1975. *Anticonvulsants:* Wilske *et al.* 1965; Lee and Siegel 1968; Alarcón-Segovia *et al.* 1972. *Antituberculous drugs:* Seligmann *et al.* 1965; Cannat and Seligmann 1966; Lee *et al.* 1966; Siegel *et al.* 1967; Alarcón-Segovia 1969; Rothfield *et al.* 1971. *Procainamide:* Dubois 1968; Fakhro *et al.* 1969; Hope and Bates 1972; Lee and Chase 1975; Bluestein *et al.* 1979. *Penicillamine:* Chalmers *et al.* 1982; Enzenauer *et al.* 1990;

Weinstein 1991; Donelly *et al.* 1993. *Sulphasalazine:* Griffiths and Kane 1977; Laversuch *et al.* 1995. *Minocycline:* Matsuura *et al.* 1992; Byrne *et al.* 1994; Gough *et al.* 1996; Masson *et al.* 1996.

Table 18.2 lists the drugs involved in reported cases of D-RSLE. Since, however, interpretation of a single case or only a small number of cases relating to a particular drug may be considered debatable, readers may wish to evaluate these cases and other relevant evidence for themselves, and the following references are provided for this purpose.

Acebutolol (Cody *et al.* 1979); *β-adrenoceptor blockers (in general)* (Wilson *et al.* 1978); *allopurinol* (Lee and Chase 1975); *ambenonium chloride* (Fries and Holman 1975); *aminoglutethimide* (McCracken *et al.* 1980); *atenolol* (Gouet *et al.* 1986); *captopril* (Pigott 1982; Reidenbeg *et al.* 1984; Sieber *et al.* 1990); *carbamazepine* (Alarcón-Segovia *et al.* 1972; Giorgio *et al.* 1991; Pacifici *et al.* 1991); *chlorpromazine* (Zarrabi *et al.* 1979); *chlorprothixene* (Haid 1964); *chlorthalidone* (Feltkamp *et al.* 1970); *clomiphene* (Ben-Chetrit and Ben-Chetrit 1994; Canvin and Capell 1995); *clonidine* (Witman and Davis 1981); *disopyramide* (Wanner and Irvin 1981); *enalapril* (Schwartz *et al.* 1990), *ethosuximide* (Livingston *et al.* 1968), *gold salts* (Castleman and Mandebaum 1950; Kapp *et al.* 1967; Goetz 1969); *griseofulvin* (Alexander 1962); *guanoxan* (Bordman *et al.* 1967; Cotton and Montuschi 1967; Alarcón-Segovia 1977); *hydrochlorothiazide* (Reed *et al.* 1985; Goodrich and Kohn 1993); *labetalol* (Griffiths and Richardson 1979); *levodopa* (Henry *et al.* 1971); *lithium* (Presley *et al.* 1976; Shukla and Borison 1982); *lovastatin* (Ahmad 1991); *methimazole* (Librik *et al.* 1970); *methoin* (Lindqvist 1957); *methyldopa* (Breckenridge *et al.* 1967; Sherman *et al.* 1967; Feltkamp *et al.* 1970; Harrington and Davis 1981; Dupont and Six 1982); *methysergide* (Racouchot *et al.* 1968); *minoxidil* (Tunkel *et al.* 1987); *nalidixic acid* (Rubinstein 1979); *nandrolone* (Radis and Callis 1997); *nitrofurantoin* (Selroos and Edgren 1975); *nomifensine* (Garcia-Morteo and Maldonado-Cocco 1983); *oral contraceptives* (Schleicher 1968; Bole *et al.* 1969; Kay *et al.* 1969; Elias 1973; Petri and Robinson 1997; Sanchez-Guerrero *et al.* 1997); *oxyphenbutazone* (Cameron 1975); *penicillin* (Walsh and Zimmerman 1953; Paull 1955; Finegold and Middleton 1971); *perphenazine* (Steen and Ramsey-Goldman 1988); *pheneturide* (Dorfmann *et al.* 1972); *phenylbutazone* (Ogryzlo 1956; Farid and Anderson 1971); *pindolol* (Bensaid *et al.* 1979); *practolol* (Raftery and Denman 1973; Jachuck *et al.* 1977); *prazosin* (Wilson *et al.* 1979; Marshall *et al.* 1979); *primidone* (Abuja and Schumacher 1966); *propafenone* (Guindo *et al.* 1986); *propranolol* (Harrison *et al.* 1976); *propylthiouracil* (Berkman *et al.* 1983; Best and Duncan 1964); *quinidine* (Kendall and Hawkins 1970); *spironolactone* (Uddin *et al.* 1979); *streptomycin* (Popkhristov and Kapnilov 1960); *sulphasalazine* (Crisp and Hoffbrand 1980; Carr-Locke 1982); *sulphonamides* (Hoffman 1945; Honey 1956; Rallison *et al.* 1961; Alarcón-Segovia *et al.* 1965); *tetracycline* (Domz *et al.* 1959); *timolol eye drops* (Zamber *et al.* 1992); *zinc salts* (aggravation of hydralazine-induced SLE) (Fjellner 1979).

TABLE 18.2
Drugs involved in reported cases of drug-related SLE

Group	Many or several reports and/or particularly convincing supporting evidence	Few or single reports and/or less convincing supporting evidence
Antiarrhythmic	procainamide	disopyramide quinidine
Anticonvulsant	ethosuximide methoin phenytoin primidone troxidone	carbamazepine pheneturide
Antihypertensive	hydralazine methyldopa	captopril chlorthalidone clonidine enalapril guanoxan hydrochlorothiazide minoxidil prazosin reserpine

Anti-infective	isoniazid
	minocycline
	sulphasalazine
		griseofulvin
		nalidixic acid
		nitrofurantoin
		penicillin
		sodium amino-
		  salicylate (PAS)
		streptomycin
		sulphonamides
		  (other than
		  sulphasalazine)
		tetracycline

Antithyroid	thiouracils	methimazole
β-Adrenoceptor blockers	practolol	acebutolol labetalol pindolol propranolol
Miscellaneous	chlorpromazine D-penicillamine	allopurinol ambenonium chloride aminoglutethimide chlorprothixene clomiphene gold salts α-interferon levodopa lithium lovastatin methysergide nomifensine oral contraceptives oxyphenbutazone perphenazine phenylbutazone propafenone spironolactone timolol eye drops zinc sulphate

Pathogenesis

The pathogenetic mechanisms are probably different for different drugs (Hughes *et al.* 1981). Slow acetylators are more likely to develop autoantibodies and D-RSLE more quickly than rapid acetylators during treatment with hydralazine and procainamide (Batchelor *et al.* 1980; Mansilla-Tinoco *et al.* 1982). No association between slow acetylator status and development of the disease has been observed with isoniazid and captopril. Therefore, slow acetylator status by itself may not be a predisposing factor for autoimmune reactions. The influence of rate of drug acetylation on the risk of development of some types of D-RSLE is discussed elsewhere, in Chapter 5. The frequency of HLA-DR4 has been shown to be between 70 and 73 per cent in patients with hydralazine-induced lupus. It has been suggested that this association may indeed be due to the null trait for complement protein C4 (genes for which are situated between HLA-B and LR loci) because in one study 76 per cent of patients compared with 43 per cent of normal controls have been shown to have one or more C4 null allele (Speirs *et al.* 1989). Other reported associations with histocompatibility antigens include: HLA-DR4 with penicillamine (Burns and Savkany 1979), HLA-Bw44 (Canoso *et al.* 1982) with chlorpromazine, and HLA-DQw7 with procainamide (Adams *et al.* 1993). The role of histocompatibility antigens and complement deficiency in the pathogenesis of D-RSLE needs further study.

Although the mechanisms involved in the pathogenesis of D-RSLE remain unclear, production of unstable but highly reactive oxidative metabolites of drugs which bind to cellular proteins might be involved in the development of autoimmunity. Among the pathogenetic mechanisms that have been suggested for one or other of a number of drugs are inhibition of enzymes; enhancement of formation of disulphide bonds; interference with cross-linkage of collagen and elastin; influence on the polymerization of macromolecular complexes; antagonism of some 'physiological' protective mechanisms or change in structure, antigenicity, or both, of DNA and soluble nucleic acid and cytoplasmic nucleoprotein (Harpey *et al.* 1972; Harpey 1973); and alteration of lymphocyte function (Raftery and Denman 1973; Bluestein *et al.* 1979; Hughes *et al.* 1981; Ochi *et al.* 1983). Procainamide and hydralazine inhibit DNA methylation and induce autoreactivity in human T lymphocytes. The autoreactive cells produce lupus-like illness *in vivo*. The autoreactivity has been shown to correlate with increase in lymphocyte-function-associated antigen-1 (Young *et al.* 1997).

TABLE 18.3
Clinical features of D-RSLE and naturally occurring SLE

Clinical features	Frequency (per cent)		
	Hydralazine	Procainamide	SLE
Arthralgia	84–95	77–91	92
Arthritis	0–50	18	–
Fever	50	45	84
Skin rash	25	5–18	72
Adenopathy	14	0–9	59
Myalgia	2–34	20–50	48
Pleuropulmonary	25–30	–	–
pleurisy	–	52	45
effusion	–	33	33
infiltrate	–	30	8
Pericarditis	2	14–18	31
Hepatosplenomegaly	8–75	20–33	5–10
CNS/seizures	0	0–2	16–25
Raynaud's phenomenon	–	5	23
Joint deformities	0	0	26
Renal involvement	2–20	0–5	46

(Based on the cases from Dubois and Tuffanelli 1964; Alarcón-Segovia 1969; Dubois 1969; Blomgren and associates 1972; Hahn and associates 1972; and Perry 1973)

Clinical features

The classical features of D-RSLE resemble those of naturally occurring systemic lupus erythematosus although there are some distinguishing features (Table 18.3). D-RSLE characteristically develops after a delay of 1 month to 5 years of treatment (Hughes 1987). There is a less pronounced female preponderance; only 48–61 per cent of cases induced by procainamide or hydralazine are females as against 89 per cent in naturally occurring SLE (Harpey 1974). Members of black races account for 30 per cent of cases of spontaneous SLE, but few develop D-RSLE (Dubois 1969; Perry 1973). The mean age of onset of D-RSLE is 55.2 years for procainamide and 52.8 years for hydralazine, as opposed to 27.5 years in spontaneous SLE (Alarcón-Sergovia 1969). Renal involvement has been reported in approximately 20 per cent of patients (Alarcón-Sergovia 1969; Björck *et al.* 1983). Central nervous system involvement is rare (Harmon and Portanova 1982), but pulmonary involvement may be commoner (Blomgren *et al.* 1972). D-RSLE associated with procainamide is more often accompanied by pericarditis than is the case with other drugs, and this may, rarely, cause cardiac tamponade and restrictive pericarditis (Browning *et al.* 1984).

Laboratory investigations

Antinuclear antibodies are invariably positive in D-RSLE and have been shown to be largely directed against nuclear histone (Fritzler and Tan 1978), predominantly histones H2A and H2B (Harmon and Portonova 1982). The non-complement-fixing nature of the antihistone antibodies may explain the low incidence of renal disease in D-RSLE (Fritzler and Tan 1978). The LE-cell phenomenon is quite marked in D-RSLE (Harmon and Portanova 1982). Unlike the situation in spontaneous SLE, D-RSLE is not usually associated with anti-double-stranded deoxyribonucleic acid (Winfield and Davis 1974). Complement levels are usually normal but hypocomplementaemia has been reported (Weinstein 1978). Anaemia, leucopenia, and hypergammaglobulinaemia may be present (Harmon and Portanova 1982). A circulating anticoagulant producing spontaneous abortion and deep vein thrombosis has been described in a 29-year-old woman who had D-RSLE associated with perphenazine (Steen and Ramsey-Goldman 1988). Evidence of circulating anticoagulant and elevation of IgM and a positive Coombs test has also been reported with D-RSLE involving chlorpromazine (Zarrabi *et al.* 1979).

Treatment and outcome

Withholding the offending drug usually results in resolution of symptoms in days or weeks, but they may persist for months or years in some patients (Alarcón-Segovia *et al.* 1967). Corticosteroid treatment may be necessary if there is pleuropericardial involvement (Harmon and Portanova 1982). Rarely, fatalities have been reported in patients with hydralazine-related (Sturman *et al.* 1988) and isoniazid-related SLE (Hoigné *et al.* 1975).

Drug-related pseudolupus

Venocuran, a proprietary preparation used in some European countries (but not in the UK) for the treatment of venous disorders, contains phenopyrazone, an extract of horse-chestnut (*Aesculus hippocastanum*), and glycosides derived from several plants, and has caused a syndrome in some ways resembling systemic lupus erythematosus but differing from it in that antinuclear antibodies are absent, though antimitochondrial antibodies are present in 90 per cent of cases (these antibodies are uncommon in SLE). About 30 per cent of affected patients experience such symptoms as myalgia and arthralgia, and more than 10 per cent develop the full pseudolupus syndrome. Symptoms regress on withdrawal of the drug, and corticosteroid therapy appears to be beneficial. It is not known which constituent of the drug is responsible for the disorder (Grob *et al.* 1975).

Types of reaction

Of the signs and symptoms described in this chapter, those due to venous thrombosis, fluid depletion, disturbances of electrolytes and of uric acid metabolism, osteomalacia, osteoporosis, and some cases of osteosclerosis can undoubtedly be classified as Type A (see Chapter 5), as also can the dental and bone disorders induced by ACTH and corticosteroids, and the haemarthrosis complicating anticoagulant therapy. A few of the remaining disorders that have been mentioned can be labelled Type B, but in most of them the underlying mechanisms are too poorly understood to make classification possible.

References

Abuja, G.K. and Schumacher, G.A. (1966). Drug-induced lupus erythematosus: primidone as a possible cause. *JAMA* 198, 669.

Adams, E.M., Horowitz, H.W., and Sundstrom, W.R. (1983). Fibrous myopathy in association with pentazocine. *Arch. Intern. Med.* 143, 2203.

Adams, L.E., Balakrishnan, K., Roberts, S.M., *et al.* (1993). Genetic, immunologic and biotransformation studies of patients on procainamide. *Lupus* 2, 89.

Ahmad, S. (1981). Sclerosing peritonitis and propranolol. *Chest* 79, 361.

Ahmad, S. (1983). Methyldopa and retroperitoneal fibrosis. *Am. Heart J.* 105, 1037.

Ahmad, S. (1991). Lovastatin-induced lupus erythematosus. *Arch. Intern. Med.* 151, 667.

Alarcón-Segovia, D. (1969). Drug-induced lupus syndromes. *Proc. Staff Meetings Mayo Clin.* 44, 664.

Alarcón-Segovia, D. (1977). Drug-induced antinuclear antibodies and lupus syndromes. *Curr. Ther.* 18, 85.

Alarcón-Segovia, D., Herskovic, T., Dearing, W.H., *et al.* (1965). Lupus erythematosus cell phenomenon in patients with chronic ulcerative colitis. *Gut* 6, 39.

Alarcón-Segovia, D., Wakim, K.G., Worthington, J.W., *et al.* (1967). Clinical and experimental studies on the hydralazine syndrome and its relationship to systemic lupus erythematosus. *Medicine* (Baltimore) 46, 1.

Alarcón-Segovia, D., Fishbein, E., Reyes, P.A., *et al.* (1972). Antinuclear antibodies in patients on anticonvulsant therapy. *Clin. Exp. Immunol.* 12, 39.

Alexander, S. (1962). Lupus erythematosus in two patients after griseofulvin treatment of *Trichophyton rubrum* infection. *Br. J. Dermatol.* 74, 72.

Alfaham, M., Holt, M.E., and Goodchild, M.C. (1987). Arthropathy in a patient with cystic fibrosis taking ciprofloxacin. *BMJ* 295, 699.

Amadori, G. and Fiore, D. (1984). Diagnostic problems in hydantoin immunotherapy. Review of literature and description of 3 cases. *Minerva Med.* 75, 2503.

Aptekar, R.G. and Michinson, J. (1970). Retroperitoneal fibrosis in two patients previously exposed to LSD. *Calif. Med.* 113, 77.

Arlet, J., Rascoul, A., Mole, J., and Roger, J.M. (1967). Observations de rhumatisme gardénalique. *Revue Rhum. Mal. Ostéo-artic.* 34, 193.

Armstrong, R.D., Crisp, A.J., Grahame, R., *et al.* (1981). Hypertrophic osteoarthropathy and purgative abuse. *BMJ* 282, 1836.

Bailey, R.R. and Armour, P. (1974). Acute arthralgia after high-dose intravenous methylprednisolone. *Lancet* ii, 1014.

Bailey, R.R., Natale, R., and Linton, A.L. (1972). Nalidixic acid arthralgia. *Can. Med. Assoc. J.* 107, 604.

Ball, A.P. (1986). Overview of clinical experience with ciprofloxacin. *Eur. J. Clin. Microbiol.* 5, 214.

Barbeau, A. and Roy, M. (1976). Six-year results of treatment with levodopa plus benserazide in Parkinson's disease. *Neurology* 26, 399.

Barter, M. and Kammer, H. (1978). Methylphenidate and growth retardation. *JAMA* 239, 1742.

Batchelor, J.R., Welsh, K.I., Mansilla-Tinoco, R., *et al.* (1980). Hydralazine-induced lupus erythematosus: influence of HLA-DR and sex on susceptibility. *Lancet* i, 1107.

Bedi, S.S. and Ellis, W. (1970). Spontaneous rupture of the calcaneal tendon in rheumatoid arthritis after local steroid injection. *Ann. Rheum. Dis.* 29, 494.

Belongia, E.A., Hedberg, C.W., Gleich, G.J., *et al.* (1990). An investigation of the cause of the eosinophilia–myalgia syndrome associated with tryptophan use. *N. Engl. J. Med.* 323, 357.

Ben-Chetrit, A. and Ben-Chetrit, E. (1994). Systemic lupus erythematosus induced by ovulation induction treatment. *Arthritis Rheum.* 37, 1614.

Ben-Ishay, D. (1961). Toxic reactions to intramuscular administration of iron–dextran. *Lancet* i, 476.

Bennett, W.M. and Strong, D. (1975). Arthralgia after high-dose steroids. *Lancet* i, 332.

Bensaid, J., Aldigier, J.C., and Gulde, N. (1979). Systemic lupus erythematosus syndrome induced by pindolol. *BMJ* i, 1603.

Bériel, M.M. and Barbier, J. (1934). Le rhumatisme gardénalique. *Presse Méd.* 42, 67.

Berkman, E.M, Orlin, J., Wolfsdorf, J. (1983). An antineutrophil antibody associated with propylthiouracil (PTU) induced lupus-like syndrome. *Transfusion* 23, 135.

Best, M.M. and Duncan, C.H. (1964). A lupus-like syndrome following propylthiouracil administration. *J. Ky Med. Assoc.* 62, 47.

Bethel, R.G.H. (1979). Carbimazole-induced arthropathy. *Br. J. Clin. Pract.* 33, 294.

Bischoff, C. (1988). Epidural lipomatosis as a complication of long term corticosteroid medication. *Dtsch. Med. Wochenschr.* 113, 1964.

Björck, S., Westberg, G., Svalander, C., *et al.* (1983). Rapidly progressive glomerulonephritis after hydralazine. *Lancet* ii, 42.

Blain, P.G. and Lane, R.J.M. (1983). Drugs and muscle. *Adverse Drug React. Acute Poisoning Rev.* 2, 1.

Blitt, C.D., Carlson, G.L., Rolling, G.D., *et al.* (1981). A comparative evaluation of pretreatment with non-depolarizing neuromuscular blockers prior to the administration of succinylcholine. *Anesthesiology* 55, 687.

Blomgren, S.E, Condemi, J.J., Bignall, M.C., *et al.* (1969). Antinuclear antibody induced by procainamide: a prospective study. *N. Engl. J. Med.* 281, 64.

Blomgren, S.E., Condemi, J.J., and Vaughan, J.H. (1972). Procainamide-induced lupus erythematosus. Clinical and laboratory observations. *Am. J. Med.* 52, 338.

Blood, D.C. and Radostits, O.M. (1989). Specific diseases of uncertain aetiology. In *Veterinary Medicine* (ed. D.C. Blood and O.M. Radostits), p. 1405. Baillière Tindall, London.

Bluestein, H.G., Zvaifler, N.J., Weisman, M.H., *et al.* (1979). Lymphocyte alteration by procainamide in relation to drug-induced lupus erythematosus. *Lancet* i, 816.

Bole, G.G., Friedlander, M.M., and Smith, C.K. (1969). Rheumatic symptoms and serological abnormalities induced by oral contraceptives. *Lancet* i, 323.

Bordman, P.L., Robinson, K.C., and Dudley Hart, F. (1967). Guanoxan and systemic lupus erythematosus. *BMJ* i, 111.

Breckenridge, A., Dollery, C.T., Worlledge, S.M., *et al.* (1967). Positive direct Coombs test and antinuclear factor in patients treated with methyldopa. *Lancet* ii, 1265.

British National Formulary Number 34 (1997). Tetracyclines. p .247. British Medical Association and the Royal Pharmaceutical Society of Great Britain.

Browning, C.A., Bishop, R.L., Heilpern, R.J., *et al.* (1984). Accelerated constrictive pericarditis in procainamide induced systemic lupus erythematosus. *Am. J. Cardiol.* 53, 376.

Bruyn, G.A.W., Essed, C.A., Houtman, P., *et al.* (1993). Fatal cardiac nodules in a patient with rheumatoid arthritis treated with low dose methotrexate. *J. Rheumatol.* 120, 912.

Bullimore, D.W. (1984). Do beta-adrenoceptor blocking drugs cause retroperitoneal fibrosis? *BMJ* 288, 719.

Burland, W.L. (1978). In *Proceedings of the Third International Symposium on Histamine H_2-receptor Antagonists* (ed. W. Creutzfeldt), p. 238. Excerpta Medica, Amsterdam.

Buttram, V.C., Reiter, R.C., and Ward, S. (1985). Treatment of endometriosis with danazol: report of a 6 year prospective study. *Fertil. Steril.* 43, 353.

Byrne, P.A.C., Williams, B.D., and Pritchard, M.H. (1994). Minocycline related lupus. *Br. J. Rheumatol.* 33, 674.

Cairns, S.A. and Jordan, S.C. (1976). Prazosin treatment complicated by acute febrile polyarthritis. *BMJ* ii, 1424.

Cameron, D.C. (1975). Diffuse pulmonary disorder caused by oxyphenbutazone. *BMJ* ii, 500.

Cannat, A. and Seligmann, M. (1966). Possible induction of antinuclear antibodies by isoniazid. *Lancet* i, 185.

Canoso, R.T., Lewis, M.E., and Yunis, E.J. (1982). Association of HLA-Bw44 with chlorpromazine-induced autoantibodies. *Clin. Immunol. Immunopathol.* 25, 278.

Canvin, J.M.G. and Capell, H.A. (1995). Clomiphene therapy and its potential role in rheumatic symptoms: Comment on the article by A. and E. Ben-Chetrit. *Arthritis Rheum.* 38, 1344.

Castin, P. and Gardien, P. (1934). Arthralgies et myalgies barbituriques. *Presse Méd.* 42, 1536.

Castleman, L. and Mandebaum, R.A. (1950). Gold poisoning and disseminated lupus erythematosus. *Am. Practit. Dig. Treat.* i, 561.

Centers for Disease Control (1990). Clinical spectrum of eosinophilia–myalgia syndrome — California. *MMWR* 39, 89.

Chalmers, A., Thompson D., and Stein, H.E (1982). Systemic lupus erythematosus during penicillamine therapy for rheumatoid arthritis. *Ann. Intern. Med.* 97, 659.

Chariot, P., Abadia, R., Agnus, D., *et al.* (1993). Simvastatin-induced rhabdomyolysis followed by MELAS syndrome. *Am. J. Med.* 94, 109.

Chariot, P., Monnet, I., Rohr, M., *et al.* (1994). Determination of the blood lactate: pyruvate ratio as a non-invasive test for the diagnosis of zidovudine myopathy. *Arthritis Rheum.* 7, 583.

Chassagne, P., Mejjad, O., Noblet, C., *et al.* (1990). Pseudo-polymyalgia rheumatica with dipyridamole. *BMJ* 301, 875.

Chesney, R.W., Mazess, R.B., Hamstra, A.J., *et al.* (1978). Reduction of serum 1,25-dihydroxy vitamin-D_3 in children receiving glucocorticoids. *Lancet* ii, 1123.

Chilton, C.P., Castle, W.M., Westwood, C.A., *et al.* (1982). Factors associated in the aetiology of Peyronie's disease. *Br. J. Urol.* 54, 748.

Clauw, D.J. and Pincus, T. (1996). The eosinophilia–myalgia syndrome : what we know, what we think we know, and what we need to know. *J. Rheumatol.* 23 (Suppl. 46), 2.

Cody, R.J. Jr, Calabrese, L.H., Clough, J.D., *et al.* (1979). Development of anti-nuclear antibodies during acebutolol therapy. *Clin. Pharmacol. Ther.* 25, 800.

Cohlan, S.Q., Bevelander, G., and Tiamsie, T. (1963). Growth inhibition of prematures receiving tetracycline: clinical and laboratory investigation. *Am. J. Dis. Child.* 105, 453.

Colamarino, R., Dubost, J.J., and Sauvezie, B. (1990). Poly-myalgia and minoxidil. *Ann. Intern. Med..* 113, 256.

Condemi J.J., Moore-Jones,D., Vaughan, J.H.,*et al.* (1967). Antinuclear antibodies following hydralazine toxicity. *N. Engl. J. Med.* 276, 486.

Cooney, L.M. Jr, Aversa, J.M., and Newman, J.H. (1980). Insidious bilateral intrapatellar tendon rupture in a patient with systemic lupus erythematosus. *Ann. Rheum. Dis.* 39, 592.

Cooper, W.D., Sheldon, D., Brown, D., *et al.* (1987). Post-marketing surveillance of enalapril: experience in 11 710 hypertensive patients in general practice. *J. R. Coll. Gen. Pract.* 37, 316.

Corpier, C.L., Jones, P.H., Suki, W.N., *et al.* (1988). Rhabdo-myolysis and renal injury with lovastatin use. Report of two cases in cardiac transplant recipients. *JAMA* 260, 239.

Cotton, S.G. and Montuschi, E. (1967). Guanoxan. *BMJ* iii, 174.

Coupland, W.W. (1977). Fibrosing conditions and propranolol. *Med. J. Aust.* ii, 137.

Cowan, M.A. and Alexander, S. (1961). Simultaneous bilateral rupture of Achilles tendons due to triamcinolone. *BMJ* i, 1658.

Cozen, L.N. (1977). Pentazocine injections as causative factor in dislocation of the shoulder. *J. Bone Joint Surg.* 59. 979.

Crawford, J.S. (1971). Suxamethonium muscle pains and pregnancy. *Br. J. Anaesth.* 43, 677.

Crisp, A.J. and Hoffbrand, B.I. (1980). Sulphasalazine-induced systemic lupus erythematosus in a patient with Sjögren's syndrome. *J. R. Soc. Med.* 73, 60.

Critchley, J.A.J., Smith, M.F., and Prescott, L.F. (1985). Distalgesic abuse and retroperitoneal fibrosis. *Br. J. Urol.* 57, 486.

Cruess, R.L. (1977). Cortisone-induced avascular necrosis of the femoral head. *J. Bone Joint Surg.* 59, 308.

CSM (Committee on Safety of Medicines) (1981). Cimetidine and arthropathy. *Current Problems No. 7.* HMSO, London.

CSM (Committee on Safety of Medicines) (1995). Rhab-domyolysis associated with lipid lowering drugs. *Current Problems in Pharmacovigilance 21*, p. 3. HMSO, London.

Cuchacovich, M.T. and Kappes, J.B. (1987) Shoulder–hand syndrome induced by phenobarbitone. *Rev. Med. Chil.* 115, 865.

Cullen, D.J. (1971). The effect of pretreatment with non-depolarizing muscle relaxants on the neuromuscular blocking action of succinylcholine. *Anesthesiology* 35, 572.

Dalakas, M.C., Illa, I., Pezeshkpour, G.H., *et al.* 1990. Mito-chondrial myopathy caused by long-term zidovudine therapy. *N. Engl. J. Med.* 322, 1098.

Datta, S., Crocker, J.S., and Alper, M.H. (1977). Muscle pain following administration of suxamethonium to pregnant and non-pregnant patients undergoing laparoscopic tubal ligation. *Br. J. Anaesth.* 49, 625.

Davies, A. (1968). Comparative trials of antimonial drugs in urinary schistosomiasis. *Bull. WHO* 38, 197.

Davies, D.M. and Lund, J.F. (1965). Myalgia and an oral contraceptive. *Lancet* ii, 1187.

Del Favero A. (1984). Antiinflammatory analgesics and drugs used in rheumatoid arthritis and gout. In *Side Effects of Drugs Annual 8* (ed. M.N.G. Dukes), p. 100. Elsevier Science Publishers, Amsterdam.

De Giorgio, C.M., Rabinowics, A.L., and Olivas, R.D. (1991). Carbamazepine-induced antinuclear antibodies and systemic lupus erythematosus-like syndrome. *Epilepsia* 32, 128.

Dickinson, L.D., Lee, J., Ringdahl, C., *et al.* (1979). Impaired growth in hyperkinetic children receiving pemoline. *J. Pediatr.* 94, 538.

Dinai, Y. and Pras, M. (1975). Levamisole in rheumatoid arthritis. *Lancet* ii, 556.

Di Saia, P.J. and Morrow, C.P. (1977). Unusual side-effects of megestrol acetate. *Am. J. Obstet. Gynecol.* 129, 460.

Doherty, C.G., McGeown, M.G., and Donaldson, R.A. (1978). Retroperitoneal fibrosis after treatment with atenolol. *BMJ* ii, 1786.

Donnelly, S., Levison D.A., and Doyle, D.V. (1993). Systemic lupus erythematosus-like syndrome with focal proliferative glomerulonephritis during D-penicillamine therapy. *Br. J. Rheumatol.* 32, 251.

Dorfmann, H., Kahn, M.F., and Deseze, S. (1972). Possibilité de lupus iatrogène induit par le phénéturide à propos de 2 observations. *Ann. Intern. Med.* 123, 331.

Doyle, D.R., McCurley, T.L., and Sergent, J.S. (1983). Fatal polymyositis in D-penicillamine treated rheumatoid arthritis. *Ann. Intern. Med.* 98, 327.

Dubois, E.L. (1969). Procainamide induction of a systemic lupus erythematosus-like syndrome. *Medicine* (Baltimore) 48, 217.

Dubois, E.L. and Tuffanelli, D.L. (1964). Clinical manifestations of systemic lupus erythematosus: computer analysis of 520 cases. *JAMA* 190, 104.

Dubois, E.L., Molina, J., Bilitch, M., *et al.* (1968). Procainamide-induced serological changes in asymptomatic patients. *Arthritis Rheum.* 11, 477.

Dupont, A. and Six, R. (1982). Lupus-like syndrome induced by methyldopa. *BMJ* 285, 696.

Eastwood, J.B., Parker, B., and Reid, B.R. (1978). Bilateral central fracture dislocation of hips after myelography with meglumine iocarmate (Dimer X). *BMJ* i, 692.

Elias, P.M. (1973). Erythema nodosum and serological lupus erythematosus. Simultaneous occurrence in a patient using oral contraceptives. *Arch. Dermatol.* 108, 716.

Eltringham, W.K., Espiner, H.J., Windsor, C.W.O., *et al.* (1977). Sclerosing peritonitis due to practolol: a report of 9 cases and their surgical management. *Br. J. Surg.* 64, 229.

Enzenauer, R.K., West, S.G., and Rubin, R.L. (1990). D-penicillamine-induced systemic lupus erythematosus. *Arthritis Rheum.* 33, 1582.

Erkola, O., Salmenperä, A., and Kuoppamäki, R. (1983). Five non-depolarizing muscle relaxants in precurarization. *Acta Anaesthesiol. Scand.* 27, 427.

Fahmy, N.R., Malek, N.S., and Lappas, D.G. (1979). Diazepam prevents some adverse effects of succinylcholine. *Clin. Pharmacol. Ther.* 26, 395.

Fakhro, A.M., Ritchie, R.F., and Lown, B. (1967). Lupus-like syndrome induced by procainamide. *Am. J. Cardiol.* 20, 367.

Farid, N. and Anderson, J. (1971). SLE-like reaction to phenylbutazone therapy. *Lancet* i, 1022.

Felson, D.T. and Anderson, J.J. (1987). A cross-study evaluation of association between steroid dose and bolus steroids and avascular necrosis of bone. *Lancet* i, 902.

Feltkamp, T.E.W., Dorhout, E.J., and Nieuwenhuis, M.G. (1970). Autoantibodies related to treatment with chlorthalidone and α-methyldopa. *Acta Med. Scand.* 187, 219.

Ferrie, B.G., Smith, P.J.B., and Kirk, D. (1983). Retroperitoneal fibrosis complicating intravesical formalin therapy. *J. R. Soc. Med.* 76, 831.

Fidler, M.W. and Brook, C.G.D. (1974). Slipped upper femoral epiphysis following treatment with human growth hormone. *J. Bone Joint Surg.* 56, 1719.

Finegold, I. and Middleton, E. Jr (1971). Positive lupus erythematosus preparations and penicillin sensitivity. *J. Allergy Immunol.* 48, 115.

Fitzgerald, M.X. and Brennan, M.J. (1976). Muscle cramps, collapse and seizures in two patients taking metolazone. *BMJ* i, 1381.

Fjellner, B. (1979). Drug-induced lupus erythematosus aggravated by oral zinc therapy. *Acta Derm. Venereol.* (Stockh.) 59, 368.

Flockhart, P.A., Clauw, D., Sale, E.B., *et al.* (1994). Pharmacogenetic characteristics of the eosinophilia–myalgia syndrome. *Clin. Pharmacol. Ther.* 56, 398.

Flores, A., Olive, A., Feliu, E., *et al.* (1994). Systemic lupus erythematosus following interferon therapy. *Br. J. Rheumatol.* 33, 787.

Fraser, D.M. and Irvine, N.A. (1976). Joint effusions and practolol. *Lancet* i, 89.

Frier, B.M. and Scott, R.D.M. (1977). Osteomalacia and arthropathy associated with prolonged abuse of purgatives. *Br. J. Clin. Pract.* 31, 17.

Fries, J.F. and Holman, H.R. (1975). SLE-like syndrome produced by drugs. In *Major Problems in Internal Medicine 6*, p. 134. W.B. Saunders, Philadelphia.

Fritzler, M.J. and Tan, E.M. (1978). Antibodies to histones in drug-induced and idiopathic erythematosus. *J. Clin. Invest.* 62, 560.

Fulroth, R., Phillips, B., and Durand, D.J. (1989). Perinatal outcome of infants exposed to cocaine and/or heroin in utero. *Am. J. Dis. Child.* 143, 905.

Garcia-Morteo, O. and Maldonado-Cocco, J.A. (1983). Lupus-like syndrome during treatment with nomifensine. *Arthritis Rheum.* 26, 936.

Gibson, J., Basten, A., and Van der Brink, C. (1983). Clinical use of transfer factor: 25 years on. *Clin. Immunol. Allergy* 3, 331.

Glauber, D. (1966). The incidence and severity of muscle pains after suxamethonium when preceded by gallamine. *Br. J. Anaesth.* 38, 541.

Gleckman, R., Alvarez, S., Joubert D.W., *et al.* (1979). Drug Therapy Reviews: Nalidixic acid. *Am. J. Hosp. Pharm.* 36, 1071.

Goa, K.L. and Campoli-Richards, D.M. (1987). Pentamidine isethionate. A review of its antiprotozoal activity, pharmacokinetic properties and therapeutic use in pneumocystis carinii pneumonia. *Drugs* 33, 242.

Goetz, G. (1969). Erythematodes-provokation durch Goldtherapie wegen primär-chronischer Polyarthritis. *Dtsch. Med. Wochenschr.* 94, 2045.

Goldberg, A.P., Sherrard, D.J., Hass, L.B., *et al.* (1977). Control of clofibrate toxicity in uraemic hypertriglyceridaemia. *Clin. Pharmacol. Ther.* 21, 317.

Good, A.E., Green, R.A., and Zarafonetis, C.J.D. (1965). Rheumatic symptoms during tuberculous therapy. A manifestation of isoniazid therapy. *Ann. Intern. Med.* 63, 800.

Goodrich, A.L. and Kohn, S.R. (1993). Hydrochlorothiazide induced lupus erythematosus: a new variant? *J. Am. Acad. Dermatol.* 28, 1001.

Gottlieb, N.L. and Gray, R.G. (1977). Allopurinol-associated hand and foot deformities in chronic tophaceous gout. *JAMA* 238, 1663.

Gouet, D., Marchaud, R., and Aucouturier, P. (1986). Atenolol induced systemic lupus erythematosus syndrome. *J. Rheumatol.* 13, 11.

Gough, A., Chapman, S., Wagstaff, K., *et al.* (1996). Minocycline induced autoimmune hepatitis and systemic lupus erythematosus-like syndrome. *BMJ* 312, 169.

Graham, J.R. (1964). Methysergide for prevention of headache (experience in five hundred patients over three years). *N. Engl. J. Med.* 270, 67.

Graham, J.R. (1968). Fibrosis associated with methysergide therapy. In *Drug-induced Diseases*, Vol. 3 (ed. L. Meyler and H.M. Peck). Associated Scientific Publishers, Amsterdam.

Graham, J.R., Suby, H.I., Le Compte, P.R., *et al.* (1966). Fibrotic disorders associated with methysergide therapy for headache. *N. Engl. J. Med.* 274, 359.

Gray, R.G. (1978). Bilateral carpal tunnel syndrome and arthritis associated with danazol administration. *Arthritis Rheum.* 21, 493.

Gregg, P.J., Barsoum, M.K., Soppitt, D., *et al.* (1980). Avascular necrosis of bone in children receiving high-dose steroid treatment. *BMJ* 281, 116.

Griffiths, I.D. and Richardson, J. (1979). Lupus-type illness associated with labetalol. *BMJ* ii, 496.

Grob, J.J., Collet, A.M., Bonerandi, J.J. (1989). Dermatomyositis-like syndrome induced by non-steroidal anti-inflammatory agents. *Dermatologica* 178, 58.

Grob, P.J., Müller-Schoop, J.W., Häcki, M.A., *et al.* (1975). Drug-induced pseudolupus. *Lancet* ii, 144.

Gros, K., Combe, C., and Kruger, K. (1995). Arthritis after hepatitis B vaccination. Report of three cases. *Scand. J. Rheumatol.* 24, 50.

Guindo, J., Rodriguez de la Serna, A., Borja, J., *et al.* (1986). Propafenone and a syndrome of the lupus erythematosus type. *Ann. Intern. Med.* 104, 589.

Gum, O.B., Smythe, C.J., Hamilton, S.K. Jr, *et al.* (1960). Effect of intra-articular serotonin and other amines on connective tissue proliferation of rabbit joints. *Arthritis Rheum.* 3, 447.

Hahn, B.H., Sharp, G.C., Irvin, W.S., *et al.* (1972). Immune responses to hydralazine and nuclear antigens in hydralazine-induced lupus erythematosus. *Ann. Intern. Med.* 76, 365.

Haid, A. (1964). Case of drug systemic lupus erythematosus from chlorprothixene ('Taractan'). *Ugeskr. Laeger* 126, 1112.

Haines, J.F. (1983). Bilateral rupture of the Achilles tendon in patients on steroid therapy. *Ann. Rheum. Dis.* 42, 652.

Harmon, C.E. and Portanova, J.P. (1982). Drug-induced lupus: clinical and serological studies. *Clin. Rheum. Dis.* 8, 121.

Harper, P.G., Trask, C., and Souhami, R.L. (1984). Avascular necrosis caused by combination chemotherapy without corticosteroids. *BMJ* 288, 267.

Harpey, J.P. (1973). Drugs and disseminated lupus erythematosus. *Adverse Drug React. Bull.* 43, 140.

Harpey, J.P. (1974). Lupus-like syndromes induced by drugs. *Ann. Allergy* 33, 256.

Harpey, J.P., Caille, B., Moulias, R., *et al.* (1972). Drug allergy and lupus-like syndrome (with special reference to penicillamine). In *Mechanisms in Drug Allergy* (ed. C.H. Dash and H.E.H. Jones), p. 51. Churchill Livingstone, Edinburgh.

Harrington, T.M. and Davis, D.E. (1981). Systemic lupus-like syndrome induced by methyldopa therapy. *Chest* 79, 696.

Harris, W.R. (1950). The endocrine basis for slipping of the upper femoral epiphysis. *J. Bone Joint Surg.* 32, 5.

Harrison, T., Sisca, T.S., and Wood, W.H. (1976). Propranolol-induced lupus erythematosus syndrome? *Postgrad. Med.*. 59, 241.

Hasler *v.* United States (517 F Supp. 1262-E. D. Mich. 1981). *Clin-Alert* 1981, item No. 251 B.

Hegarty, P. (1956). Postoperative muscle pains. *Br. J. Anaesth.* 28, 209.

Henri, L. and Groleau, M. (1981). Retroperitoneal fibrosis after treatment with propranolol. *Drug Intell. Clin. Pharm.* 15, 696.

Henry, R.E., Goldberg, L.E., Sturgeon, P., *et al.* (1971). Serological abnormalities associated with L-dopa therapy. *Vox Sang.* 20, 306.

Hertzman, P.A., Clauw, D.J., Kaufman, L.D., *et al.* (1995). The eosinophilia–myalgia syndrome: Status of 205 patients and results of treatment 2 years after onset. *Ann. Intern. Med.* 122, 851.

Herzog, A., Minne, H., and Ziegler, R. (1989). Retroperitoneal fibrosis in a patient with macroprolactinoma treated with bromocriptine. *BMJ* 298, 1315.

Hietarinta, M. and Merilanti-Palo, R. (1989). Methimazole-induced arthritis. *Scand. J. Rheumatol.* 18, 61.

Hino, I., Akama, H., Furuya, T., *et al.* (1996). Pravastatin-induced rhabdomyolysis in a patient with mixed connective tissue disease. *Arthritis Rheum.* 39, 1259.

Hoffman, B.J. (1945). Sensitivity to sulfadiazine resembling acute disseminated lupus erythematosus. *Arch. Dermatol. Syph.* 51, 190.

Hoigné, R., Biedermann, H.P., and Naegeli, H.R. (1975). INH-induzierter systemischer Lupus erythematodes: 2. Beobachtungen mit Reexposition. *Schweiz. Med. Wochenschr.* 105, 1726.

Honey, M. (1956). SLE presenting with sulphonamide hypersensitivity reaction. *BMJ* i, 1272.

Hope, R.R. and Bates, L.A. (1972). The frequency of procainamide-induced systemic lupus erythematosus. *Med. J. Aust.* ii, 298.

Howard, J.F. (1982). Arthritis and carpal tunnel syndrome associated with disulfiram (Antabuse) therapy. *Arthritis Rheum.* 25, 1484.

Hughes, G.R.V. (1987). Recent developments in drug-related systemic lupus erythematosus. *Adverse Drug React. Bull.* 123, 40.

Hughes, G.R.V., Rynes, R.I., Charavi, A., *et al.* (1981). The heterogenicity of serological findings and predisposing host factors in drug-induced lupus erythematosus. *Arthritis Rheum.* 24, 1070.

Ismail, A.M., Balakrishnan, R., and Rajakumar, M.K. (1969). Rupture of patellar ligament after steroid infiltration. Report of a case. *J. Bone Joint Surg.* 51, 503.

Iversen, B.M., Johannese, J.W., Nordahl, E., *et al.* (1975). Retroperitoneal fibrosis during treatment with methyldopa. *Lancet* ii, 302.

Jachuck, S.J., Stephenson, J., Bird, T., *et al.* (1977). Practolol-induced autoantibodies and their relation to oculo-cutaneous complication. *Postgrad. Med. J.* 53, 75.

Jaffe, N., Hie Won, L.H., and Vawter, G.F. (1971). Post-steroid panniculitis in acute leukaemia. *N. Engl. J. Med.* 284, 366.

Jawad, A.S.M., Kahn, L., and Copland, R.F.P. (1993). Reactive arthritis associated with Bacillus Calmette–Guérin immunotherapy for carcinoma of the bladder: a report of two cases. *Br. J. Rheumatol.* 32, 1018.

Jeandel, C., Manciaux, M.A., Bannwarth, B., *et al.* (1989). Arthritis induced by norfloxacin. *J. Rheumatol.* 16, 560.

Jeanette, J.C. and Falk, R.J. (1997). Small vessel vasculitis. *N. Engl. J. Med.* 337, 1512.

Jeffries, J.J., Lyall, W.A., Bezchlibnyk, K., *et al.* (1982). Retroperitoneal fibrosis and haloperidol. *Am. J. Psychiatry* 139, 1524.

John, G. (1981). Transient osteosclerosis associated with sodium valproate. *Dev. Med. Child Neurol.* 23, 234.

Johns, A.M. and Bower, B.D. (1970). Wasting of napkin area after repeated use of fluorinated steroid ointment. *BMJ* i, 347.

Johnson, J.N. and McFarland, J.B. (1980). Retroperitoneal fibrosis associated with atenolol. *BMJ* 280, 864.

Kaniaris, P., Galanopoulou, T., and Varnos, D. (1973). Effects of succinylcholine on plasma 5-HT levels. *Anaesth. Analg.* 52, 425.

Kapp, W., Klunker, W., and Fellman, N. (1967). Auslösung eines Lupus erythematodes durch Goldtherapie bei primär-chronischer Polyarthritis? *Dtsch. Med. Wochenschr.* 56, 1594.

Kattan, K.R. (1970). Calvarial thickening after Dilantin medication. *AJR* 110, 102.

Kaufman, L.D., Seidman, R.J., and Gruber, B.L. (1990). L-Tryptophan-associated eosinophilic perimyositis, neuritis and fasciitis. A clinicopathologic and laboratory study of 25 patients. *Medicine* (Baltimore) 69, 187.

Kay, D.R., Bole, G.G., and Ledger, W.J. (1969). The use of oral contraceptives and the occurrence of antinuclear antibodies and LE cells in women with early rheumatic disease. *Arthritis Rheum.* 12, 306.

Keidar, S., Binenboim, C., and Palant, A. (1982). Muscle cramps during treatment with nifedipine. *BMJ* 285, 1241.

Kendall, M.J. and Hawkins, C.F. (1970). Quinidine-induced lupus erythematosus. *Postgrad. Med. J.* 46, 729.

Kerstens, P.J.S., Boerbooms, A.M.T., Jeurissen, M.E.C., *et al.* (1992). Accelerated nodulosis during low dose methotrexate therapy for rheumatoid arthritis. An analysis of ten cases. *J. Rheumatol.* 19, 867.

Kertes, P. and Hunt, D. (1982). Polyarthritis complicating quinidine treatment. *BMJ* 284, 1373.

Kesseler, A., Lacassie, A., Hugot, J.P., *et al.* (1989). Pefloxacin induced joint disease in an adolescent with cystic fibrosis. *Ann. Pediatr.* 36, 275.

Khatak, F.H., Morris, I.M., Branford, W.A. (1994). Simvastatin-associated dermatomyositis. *Br. J. Rheumatol.* 33, 199.

Kilbourne, E.M., Swygert, L.A., and Philen, R.M. (1990). Interim guidance on the eosinophilia–myalgia syndrome. *Ann. Intern. Med.* 112, 85.

Koivisto, V.A. and Felig, P. (1980). Alterations in insulin absorption and in blood glucose control associated with varying insulin injection sites in diabetic patients. *Ann. Intern. Med.* 92, 59.

König, W. (1956). Über Beschwerden nach Anwendung von Succinylcholin. *Anaesthetist* 5, 50.

Köppel, C. (1989). Clinical features, pathogenesis and management of drug-induced rhabdomyolysis. *Med. Toxicol. Adverse Drug Experience* 4, 108.

Kristensen, B.O. (1979). Labetalol-induced Peyronie's disease. *Acta Med. Scand.* 206, 511.

Laakso, M., Arvala, I., Tervonen, S., *et al.* (1982). Retroperitoneal fibrosis associated with sotalol. *BMJ* 285, 1085.

Lamm, D.L., Stodgill, V.D., Stodgill, B.J., *et al.* (1986). Complications of BCG immunotherapy in 1278 patients with bladder cancer. *J. Urol.* 135, 272.

The Lancet (1963). Toxicity of tetracyclines. *Lancet* ii, 283.

The Lancet (1966). Drugs and retroperitoneal fibrosis. *Lancet* i, 969.

Lane, R.J.M. and Mastaglia, F.L. (1978). Drug-induced myopathies in man. *Lancet* ii, 562.

Langer, T. and Levy, R.I. (1968). Acute muscular syndrome associated with the administration of clofibrate. *N. Engl. J. Med.* 279, 856.

Laurence, A.S. (1987). Myalgia and biochemical changes following intermittent suxamethonium administration. *Anaesthesia* 42, 503.

Laversuch, C.J., Collins, D.A., Charles, P.J., *et al.* (1995). Sulphasalazine-induced autoimmune abnormalities in patients with rheumatic disease. *Br. J. Rheumatol.* 34, 435.

Leatherdale, R.A.L., Mayhew, R.A.J., and Hayton-Williams, D.S. (1959). Incidence of 'muscle pain' after short-acting relaxants: a comparison between suxamethonium chloride and suxamethonium bromide. *BMJ* i, 904.

Lee, H.B. (1957). Avulsion and rupture of the tendo calcaneus after injection of hydrocortisone. *BMJ* ii, 395.

Lee, M.L.H. (1961). Bilateral rupture of Achilles tendon. *BMJ* i, 1829.

Lee, S.L. and Chase, P.H. (1975). Drug-induced lupus erythematosus: a critical review. *Sem. Arthritis Rheum.* 5, 83.

Lee, S.L. and Siegel, M. (1968). Drug-induced lupus erythematosus. In *Drug-induced Diseases*, Vol. 3 (ed. L. Meyler and H.M. Peck), p. 239. Associated Scientific Publishers, Amsterdam.

Lee, S.L., Rivero, I., and Siegel, M. (1966). Activation of systemic lupus erythematosus by drugs. *Arch. Intern. Med.* 117, 620.

Le Loët, X., Moore, N., and Deshayes, P. (1989). Pseudopolymyalgia rheumatica during treatment with enalapril. *BMJ* 298, 325.

Lequesne, M. (1967). L'algo-dystrophie d'origine chimiothérapique. Pseudorhumatisme de l'isoniazide, de l'éthionamide du phénobarbital et de l'iode radioactive. *Sem. Hop. Paris* 43, 2581.

Levin, B.E. and Engel, W.K. (1975). Iatrogenic muscle fibrosis. Arm levitation as an initial sign. *JAMA* 234, 621.

Lewis, C.T., Molland, E.A., Marshall, V.R., *et al.* (1975). Analgesic abuse, ureteric obstruction and retroperitoneal fibrosis. *BMJ* ii, 76.

Librick, L., Sussman, L., Bejar, R., *et al.* (1970). Thyrotoxicosis and collagen-like disease in three sisters of American-Indian extraction. *J. Pediatr.* 76, 64.

Lindqvist, T. (1957). Lupus erythematosus disseminatus after administration of mesantoin. Report of two cases. *Acta Med. Scand.* 158, 131.

Litin, S.C. and Anderson, C.F. (1989). Nicotinic acid-associated myopathy: a report of three cases. *Am. J. Med.* 86, 481.

Livingstone, S., Rodriguez, H., Creen, C.A., *et al.* (1968). Systemic lupus erythematosus. Occurrence in association with ethosuximide therapy. *JAMA* 203, 731.

Lotzof, L. (1968). Orciprenaline in the treatment of asthma. *Med. J. Aust.* i, 1105.

Lövgren, O. (1948). Om s.k. barbitursyrereumatism. *Svenska Läkartidn.* 45, 234.

McCluskey, D.R., Donaldson, R.A., and McGeown, M.G. (1980). Oxprenolol and retroperitoneal fibrosis. *BMJ* 281, 1459.

McCluskey, J. and Gutteridge, D.H. (1982). Avascular necrosis of bone after high doses of dexamethasone during surgery. *BMJ* i, 333.

McCracken, M., Benson, E.A., and Hickling, P. (1980). Systemic lupus erythematosus induced by aminoglutethimide. *BMJ.* 281, 1254.

MacDonald, J.B. (1982). Muscle cramps during treatment with nifedipine. *BMJ* 285, 1744.

MacDonald, J.B. and MacDonald E.T. (1977). Nocturnal femoral fracture and continuing widespread use of barbiturate hypnotics. *BMJ* ii, 483.

McEwan, S.R. and Davey, P.G. (1988). Ciprofloxacin and tenosynovitis. *Lancet* ii, 900.

McGloughlin, C., Nesbitt, G.A., and Howe, J.P. (1988). Suxamethonium-induced myalgia and the effect of preoperative administration of oral aspirin. *Anaesthesia* 43, 565.

McKusick, A.B. (1965). Personal communication to Good *et al.* (1965).

McKusick, A.B. and Hsu, J.M. (1961). Clinical and metabolic studies of the shoulder–hand syndrome in tuberculous patients. In *Xth Congress of the International League against Rheumatism*, Vol. 2. Turin.

McLaughlin, G.E., McCarthy, D.J., and Segal, B.L. (1966). Hemarthrosis complicating anticoagulant therapy. *JAMA* 196, 1020.

McNally, P.G., Jowett, N.I., Kurinczuk, J.J., *et al.* (1988). Lipohypertrophy and lipoatrophy complicating treatment with highly purified bovine and porcine insulins. *Postgrad. Med. J.* 64, 850.

Maenaut, K., Westhovens, R., and Dequeker, J. (1996). Methotrexate osteopathy, does it exist? *J. Rheumatol.* 23, 2156.

Magarian, G.J., Lucas, L.M., and Colley, C. (1991). Gemfibrozil-induced myopathy. *Arch. Intern. Med.* 151, 1873.

Maillard, G. and Renard, G. (1925). Un nouveau traitement de l'épilepsie: la phénolyl-méthylmalonylurée (Rutonal). *Presse Méd.* 33, 315.

Maillard, G. and Thomazi, P. (1931). Douleurs provoquées par certains dérivés barbituriques au cours du traitement de l'épilepsie. *Presse Méd.* 39, 851.

Malluche, H.H. and Faugère, M.C. (1985). Aluminium: toxin or innocent bystander in renal osteodystrophy. *Am. J. Kidney Dis.* vi, 336.

Malmquist, J., Ericsson, B., Hulten-Nosslin, M.B., *et al.* (1980). Finger clubbing and aspartylglucosamine excretion in a laxative-abusing patient. *Postgrad. Med. J.* 56, 862.

Malnick, S.D.H. and Schattner, A. (1989). Arthralgia associated with captopril. *BMJ* 299, 394.

Manchikanti, L. (1984). Diazepam does not prevent succinylcholine-induced fasciculations and myalgia: a comparative evaluation of the effect of diazepam and d-tubocurarine pretreatments. *Acta Anaesthesiol. Scand.* 28, 523.

Mansilla-Tinoco, R., Harland, S.J., Ryan, P.J., *et al.* (1982). Hydralazine, antinuclear antibodies, and the lupus syndrome. *BMJ* 284, 936.

Marshall, A.J., Baddeley, H., Barrit, D.W., *et al.* (1977). Practolol peritonitis: a study of 16 cases and a survey of small bowel function in patients taking β-adrenergic blockers. *Q. J. Med.* 46, 135.

Marshall, A.J., McGraw, M.E., and Barritt, D.W. (1979). Positive antinuclear factor tests with prazosin. *BMJ* i, 165.

Marshall, W. (1977). Barbiturates and fractures. *BMJ* ii, 640.

Masey, S.A., Glazebrook, C.W., and Goat, V.A. (1983). Suxamethonium: a new look at pretreatment. *Br. J. Anaesth.* 55, 729.

Masson, C., Cherailler, A., Pascaretti, C., *et al.* (1996). Minocycline related lupus. *J. Rheumatol.* 23, 2160.

Mastaglia, F.L., Gardner-Medwin, D., and Hudgson, P. (1971). Muscle fibrosis and contracture in a pethidine addict. *BMJ* iv, 532.

Matsuura, T., Shimizu, Y., Fujimoto, H., *et al.* (1992). Minocycline-related lupus. *Lancet* 340, 1553.

Matthiesen, J. (1979). Polymyositis som en mulig bivirkning af cimetidin benhandling. *Ugeskr. Laeger* 141, 2762.

Mayrhofer, O. (1959). Die Wirksamkeit von d-Tubocurarin zur Verhütung der Muskelschmerzen nach Succinylcholin. *Anaesthetist* 8, 313.

Medsger, J.A., Jr. (1990). Tryptophan-induced eosinophilia–myalgia syndrome. *N. Engl. J. Med.* 322, 926.

Mehta, N.D., Hoberman, A.L., Vokes, E.E., *et al.* (1992). A 35 year old patient with chronic myelogenous leukemia developing systemic lupus erythematosus after alpha-interferon therapy. *Am. J. Hematol.* 41, 141.

Melmed, E.P. (1965). Spontaneous bilateral rupture of the calcaneal tendon during steroid therapy. *J. Bone Joint Surg.* 47, 104.

Meyerhoff, J.O. (1983). Exacerbation of psoriasis with meclofenamate. *N. Engl. J. Med.* 309, 496.

Mhiri, C., Baudrimont, M., Boone, G., *et al.* (1991). Zidovudine myopathy: a distinctive disorder associated with mitochondrial dysfunction. *Ann. Neurol.* 29, 606.

Missioux, D., Hermabessiere, J., and Sauvezie B. (1995). Arthritis and iritis after Bacillus Calmette–Guérin therapy. *J. Rheumatol.* 22, 2010.

Morrow, J.D., Schroeder, H.A., and Perry, H.M., Jr. (1953). Studies on the control of hypertension by hyphex II. Toxic reactions and side effects. *Circulation* 8, 829.

Muller, J.C., Rast, C.L. Jr, Pryor, W.W., *et al.* (1955). Late systemic complications of hydralazine (Apresoline) therapy. *JAMA* 157, 894.

Müller-Vahl, H. (1984). Aseptische Gewebsnekrose: eine schwerwiegende Komplikation nach intramuskulärer Injektion. *Dtsch. Med. Wochenschr.* 109, 786.

Murray, R.O. and Jacobson, H.G. (1972). *The Radiology of Skeletal Disorders*, Vol.1, pp. 553, 560. Churchill Livingstone, Edinburgh.

Neerhof, M.G., MacGregor, S.N., Retzky, S.S., *et al.* (1989). Cocaine abuse during pregnancy: peripartum prevalence and perinatal outcome. *Am. J. Obstet. Gynecol.* 161, 633.

Neu, H.C. (1988). Quinolones: a new class of antimicrobial agents with wide potential uses. *Med. Clin. North Am.* 72, 623.

Newman, N.M. and Ling, R.S.M. (1985). Acetabular bone destruction related to non-steroidal anti-inflammatory drugs. *Lancet* ii, 11.

Newmark, K.J., Mitra, S., and Berman, L.B. (1974). Acute arthralgia following high-dose intravenous methylprednisolone therapy. *Lancet* ii, 229.

Newnam, P.T.F. and Loudon, J.M. (1966). Muscle pain following administration of suxamethonium: the aetiological role of muscular fitness. *Br. J. Anaesth.* 38, 533.

Nillson, B.V. and Pederson, K.G. (1985). Sclerosing peritonitis associated with atenolol. *BMJ* 290, 518.

Oberg, K.E. (1989). Development of a SLE syndrome in a patient with malignant carcinoid tumour after treatment with alpha-interferon. *Interferon Cytokine* 12, 30.

Ochi, T., Goldings, E.A., Lipsky, P.E., *et al.* (1983). Immunomodulatory effect of procainamide in man: inhibition of human suppressor T-cell activity *in vitro*. *J. Clin. Invest.* 71, 36.

Ochsenkühn, T., Weber, M.M., and Caselmann, W.H. (1990). Arthritis after *Mycobacterium bovis* immunotherapy for bladder cancer. *Ann. Intern. Med..* 112, 882.

O'Connor, M. (1980). Muscle necrosis induced by intra-muscular chlorpromazine. *Med. J. Aust.* i, 36.

Ogryzlo, M.A. (1956). The LE (lupus erythematosus) cell reaction. *Can. Med. Assoc. J.* 75, 980.

Oh, B.K., Von Overveld, G.P., and Macfarlane, J.D. (1983). Polyarthritis induced by propylthiouracil. Case report. *Br. J. Rheumatol.* 22, 106.

O'Malley, B. (1989). Carbimazole-induced cramps. *Lancet* i, 1456.

O'Reagan, S., Chesney, R.W., Hamstra, A., *et al.* (1979). Reduced serum 1, 25(OH)$_2$-vitamin D$_3$ levels in prednisolone treated adolescents with systemic lupus erythematosus. *Acta Paediatr. Scand.* 68, 109.

Orth, D.N., Kovacs, W.J., and Debold, C.R. (1992). The adrenal cortex. In *Williams' Textbook of Endocrinology* (8th edn) (ed. J.D. Wilson and D.W. Foster), p. 519. W.B. Saunders, Philadelphia.

O'Sullivan, E.P., Williams, N.E., and Calvey, T.N. (1988). Differential effects of neuromuscular blocking agents on suxamethonium-induced fasciculations and myalgia. *Br. J. Anaesth.* 60, 367.

Osborne, D.R. (1977). Propranolol and Peyronie's disease. *Lancet* i, 131.

Pacifici, R., Paris L., Di Carlo, S., *et al.* (1991). Immunologic aspects of carbamazepine treatment in epileptic patients. *Epilepsia* 32, 122.

Page, S.R. and Nussey, S.S. (1989). Myositis in association with carbimazole therapy. *Lancet* i, 964.

Palmer, K.N.V. (1978). Muscle cramp and oral salbutamol. *BMJ* ii, 833.

Paull, A.M. (1955). Occurrence of the 'LE' phenomenon in a patient with a severe penicillin reaction. *N. Engl. J. Med.* 252, 128.

Perry, H.M. (1973). Late toxicity to hydralazine resembling systemic lupus erythematosus or rheumatoid arthritis. *Am. J. Med.* 54, 58.

Perry, H.M. Jr, Tan, E.M., Carmody, S., *et al.* (1970). Relationship of acetyl transferase activity to antinuclear antibodies and toxic symptoms in hypertensive patients treated with hydralazine. *J. Lab. Clin. Med.* 76, 114.

Perry, H.M. Jr, Chaplin, H. Jr, Carmody, S., *et al.* (1971). Immunologic findings in patients receiving methyldopa: a prospective study. *J. Lab. Clin. Med.* 78, 905.

Peters, M.E. and Horowitz, S. (1984). Bone changes after rubella vaccination. *AJR* 143, 27.

Petri, M. and Robinson, C. (1997). Oral contraceptives and systemic lupus erythematosus. *Arthritis Rheum.* 40, 797.

Pierce, J.R., Throstle, D.C., and Warner, J.J. (1981). Propranolol and retroperitoneal fibrosis. *Ann. Intern. Med.* 95, 244.

Piggott, P.V. (1982). Captopril and drug-induced lupus. *BMJ* 284, 1786.

Pittsley, R.A. and Yoder, F.W. (1983). Retinoid hyperostosis: skeletal toxicity associated with long-term administration of 13-cis-retinoic acid for refractory ichthyosis. *N. Engl. J. Med.* 308, 1012.

Popkhristov, P. and Kapnilov, S. (1960). Streptomycin as a factor producing and aggravating lupus erythematosus. *Vestn. Dermatol. Venerol.* 34, 10.

Presley, A.P., Kahn, A., and Williamson, N. (1976). Antinuclear antibodies in patients on lithium carbonate. *BMJ* ii, 280.

Prior, J. and White, I. (1978). Tetany and clubbing in a patient who ingested large quantities of senna. *Lancet* ii, 947.

Pryor, J.P. and Castle, W.M. (1982). Peyronie's disease associated with chronic degenerative arterial disease and not with beta-adrenoceptor blocking agents. *Lancet* i, 917.

Pryor, J.P. and Kahn, O. (1979). Beta-blockers and Peyronie's disease. *Lancet* i, 331.

Pryor, J.P., Castle, W.M., Dukes, D.C., *et al.* (1983). Do beta-adrenoceptor blocking drugs cause retroperitoneal fibrosis? *BMJ* 287, 639.

Rack, P.M.H. and Westbury, D.R. (1966). The effects of suxamethonium and acetylcholine on the behaviour of cat muscle spindles during dynamic stretching, and during fusimotor stimulation. *J. Physiol.* (Lond.) 186, 698.

Racouchot, J., Gaillard, L., and Guilane, J. (1968). Lupus erythémateux subaigu et méthysergide. *Lyon Méd.* 220, 1766.

Radis, C.D. and Callis, K.P. (1997). Systemic lupus erythematosus with membranous glomerulonephritis and transverse myelitis associated with anabolic steroid use. *Arthritis Rheum.* 40, 1899.

Raftery, E.B. and Denman, A.M. (1973). Systemic lupus erythematosus syndrome induced by practolol. *BMJ* ii, 452.

Râgab, A.H., Fresh, R.S., and Vetti, T.J. (1970). Osteoporotic fractures secondary to methotrexate therapy of acute leukaemia in remission. *Cancer* 25, 580.

Rallison, M.L., O'Brien, J., and Good, R.A. (1961). Severe reactions to long-acting sulfonamides: erythema multiforme exudativum and lupus erythematosus following administration of sulfamethoxypyridazone and sulfadimethodine. *Pediatrics* 28, 908.

Ramachandran, S., Giles, P.D., and Hartland, A. (1997). Acute renal failure due to rhabdomyolysis in presence of concurrent ciprofibrate and ibuprofen treatment. *BMJ* 314, 1593.

Ray, W.A., Griffin, M.R., Schaffner, W., *et al.* (1987). Psychotropic drug use and the risk of hip fracture. *N. Engl. J. Med.* 316, 363.

Reed, B.R., Huff, J.C., Jones, S.K., *et al.* (1985). Subacute cutaneous lupus erythematosus associated with hydrochlorothiazide therapy. *Ann. Intern. Med.* 103, 49.

Reidenberg, M.M., Case, D.B., Drayer, D.E., *et al.* (1984). Development of antinuclear antibody in patients treated with high doses of captopril. *Arthritis Rheum.* 27, 579.

Rennie, W. and Mitchell, N. (1974). Slipped femoral capital epiphysis occurring during growth hormone therapy. *J. Bone Joint Surg.* 56, 703.

Reynolds, J.E.F. (ed.) (1996). Analgesics and anti-inflammatory agents. In *Martindale The Extra Pharmacopoeia* (31st edn), p. 1. The Pharmaceutical Press, London.

Richman, D.D., Fischl, M.A., and Gvieco, M.H. (1987). The toxicity of azidothymidine (AZT) in the treatment of patients with AIDS and AIDS-related complex: double-blind, placebo-controlled trial. *N. Engl. J. Med.* 317, 192.

Rimmer, E., Richens, A., Forster, M.E., *et al.* (1983). Retroperitoneal fibrosis associated with timolol. *Lancet* i, 300.

Roche Pharmaceuticals (1997). Summary of product characteristics: Posicor.

Roche, A.F., Lipman, R.S., Overall, J.E., *et al.* (1979). The effects of stimulant medication on growth of hyperkinetic children. *Pediatrics* 63, 847.

Roenick, H.H., Haberic, J.R., and Arundell, F.D. (1964). Poststeroid panniculitis. *Arch. Dermatol.* 90, 387.

Rogerson, S.J. and Nye, F.J. (1990). Hepatitis B vaccine associated with erythema nodosum and polyarthritis. *BMJ* 301, 345.

Rollins, D.E. and Moeller, D. (1975). Polyarthritis associated with clindamycin-induced colitis. *JAMA* 231, 1228.

Rose, T., Nothjunge, J., and Schlote, W. (1985). Familial occurrence of dermatomyositis and progressive scleroderma after injection of a local anaesthetic for dental treatment. *Eur. J. Pediatr.* 143, 225.

Rothfield, N.F., Bierer, W.F., and Garfield, J.W. (1971). The induction of antinuclear antibodies by isoniazid: a prospective study. *Arthritis Rheum.* 14, 182.

Rothfield, N.F., Bierer, W.F., and Garfield, J.W. (1978). Isoniazid induction of antinuclear antibodies. A prospective study. *Ann. Intern. Med.* 88, 650.

Rubinstein, A. (1979). LE-like disease caused by nalidixic acid. *N. Engl. J. Med.* 301, 1288.

Ruby, L.K. and Mital, M.A. (1974). Skeletal deformities following chronic hypervitaminosis A. *J. Bone Joint Surg.* 56, 1283.

Rumpf, K.W., Barth, M., Blech, M., *et al.* (1984). Bezafibrat-induzierte Myolyse und Myoglobinurie bei Patienten mit eingeschränkter Nierenfunktion. *Klin. Wochenschr.* 62, 346.

Sachs, H.K. and Moel, D.I. (1989). Height and weight following lead poisoning in childhood. *Am. J. Dis. Child.* 143, 820.

SADRAC (Swedish Adverse Drug Reactions Advisory Committee) (1989). Ranitidine and arthralgia. *SADRAC Bull.* 55, 2.

Safer, D.J. and Allen, R.P. (1973). Factors influencing the suppressant effect of two stimulant drugs on the growth of hyperactive children. *Pediatrics* 51, 660.

Sanchez-Guerrero, J., Karlson, E.W., Liang, M.H., *et al.* (1997). Past use of oral contraceptives and the risk of developing systemic lupus erythematosus. *Arthritis Rheum.* 40, 804.

Savola, J. (1983). Arthropathy induced by beta blockade. *BMJ* 287, 1256.

Savola, J. (1984). Arthropathy induced by beta blockade. *BMJ* 288, 238.

Saxena, A.K. and Nigam, P.K. (1988). Panniculitis following steroid therapy. *Cutis* 42, 341.

Schilling, P.J., Jurzrock, R., Kantarjian, H., *et al.* (1991). Development of systemic lupus erythematosus after interferon therapy for chronic myelogenous leukemia. *Cancer* 68, 1536.

Schleicher, E. (1968). LE cells after oral contraceptives. *Lancet* i, 821.

Schneider, H., Kulbe, K.D., Weber, H., *et al.* (1984). Aluminium-free oral phosphate binder. *Trace Elem. Med.* 1, 76.

Schwartz, D., Pines, A., Averbuch, M., *et al.* (1990). Enalapril induced antinuclear antibodies. *Lancet* 336, 187.

Schwartz, F.D. and Dunea, G. (1966). Progression of retroperitoneal fibrosis despite cessation of treatment with methysergide. *Lancet* i, 955.

Segal, A.W., Pugh, S.F., Levi, A.J., *et al.* (1977). Levamisole-induced arthritis in Crohn's disease. *BMJ* ii, 555.

Sekowski, I. and Samuel, P. (1972). Clofibrate-induced acute muscular syndrome. *Am. J. Cardiol.* 30, 572.

Seligmann, M., Cannat, A., and Hamard, M. (1965). Studies on antinuclear antibodies. *Ann. N.Y. Acad. Sci.* 124, 816.

Selroos, O. and Edgren, J. (1975). Lupus-like syndrome associated with pulmonary reaction to nitrofurantoin. *Acta Med. Scand.* 197, 125.

Shaw, M., Petrone, J., Iglesias, D., *et al.* (1982). Polimiositis aguda por nifurtimox. *Arch. Argent. Dermatol.* 32, 191.

Sherman, J.D., Love, D.E., and Harrington, J.F. (1967). Anemia, positive lupus and rheumatoid factors with methyldopa. A report of 3 cases. *Arch. Intern. Med.* 120, 321.

Shukla, R., Bornschein, R.L., Dietrich, K.N., *et al.* (1989). Fetal and infant lead exposure: effects on growth in stature. *Pediatrics* 84, 604.

Shukla, V.R. and Borison, R.L. (1982). Lithium and lupus-like syndrome. *JAMA* 248, 921.

Shulman, L.E. (1975). Diffuse fasciitis with eosinophilia: a new syndrome? *Trans. Assoc. Am. Physicians* 88, 70.

Shulman, L.E. and Harvey, A.M. (1960). The nature of drug-induced systemic lupus erythematosus. *Arthritis Rheum.* 3, 464.

Sieber, C., Grimm, E., and Follath, F. (1990). Captopril and systemic lupus erythematosus syndrome. *BMJ* 301, 669.

Siegel, M., Lee, S.L., and Peress, N.S. (1967). The epidemiology of drug-induced systemic lupus erythematosus. *Arthritis Rheum.* 10, 407.

Sikka, A., Kemman, E., Vrabik, R.M., *et al.* (1983). Carpal tunnel syndrome associated with danazol therapy. *Am. J. Obstet. Gynecol.* 147, 103.

Siklos, P. (1977). Levamisole-induced arthritis. *BMJ* ii, 773.

Silk, D.B.A., Gibson, J.A., and Murray, C.R.H. (1975). Reversible finger clubbing in the case of purgative abuse. *Gastroenterology* 68, 790.

Sills, J.M. and Bosco, L. (1986). Arthralgia associated with beta-adrenergic blockade. *JAMA* 255, 198.

Silver, R.M. (1996). Pathophysiology of the eosinophilia–myalgia syndrome. *J. Rheumatol.* 23 (Suppl. 46), 26.

Silver, R.M., Heyes, M.P., Maize, J.C., *et al.* (1990). Scleroderma, fasciitis and eosinophilia associated with the ingestion of tryptophan. *N. Engl. J. Med.* 322, 874.

Slutsker, L., Hoesly, F.C., Miller, L., *et al.* (1990). Eosinophilia– myalgia syndrome associated with exposure to tryptophan from a single manufacturer. *JAMA* 264, 213.

Smaill, G.B. (1961). Bilateral rupture of Achilles tendons. *BMJ* i, 1657.

Smith, A.F., Macfie, W.G., and Oliver, M.F. (1970). Clofibrate, serum enzymes and muscle pain. *BMJ* ii, 86.

Solomon, L. (1973). Drug-induced arthropathy and necrosis of the femoral head. *J. Bone Joint Surg.* 55, 246.

Speirs, C., Chapel, H., Fielder, A.H.L., *et al.* (1989). Complement system protein C4 and susceptibility to hydralazine induced systemic lupus erythematosus. *Lancet* i, 922.

Spencer, H. and Kramer, L. (1983). Antacid-induced calcium loss. *Arch. Intern. Med.* 143, 657.

Spiera, H. and Plotz, C.M. (1969). Rheumatic symptoms and oral contraceptives. *Lancet* i, 571.

Spitzer, W.O., Haggerty, J.L., Berkson, L., *et al.* (1995). Continuing occurrence of eosinophilia myalgia syndrome in Canada. *Br. J. Rheumatol.* 34, 246.

Stalnikowicz, R., Mosseri, M., and Shalev, O. (1982). Phenytoin-induced arthritis. *Neurology* 32, 1317.

Steen, V.D. and Ramsey-Goldman, R. (1988). Phenothiazine-induced systemic lupus erythematosus with superior vena cava syndrome: case report and review of the literature. *Arthritis Rheum.* 31, 923.

Sternberg, E.M., van Woert, M.H., Young, S.M., *et al.* (1980). Development of a scleroderma-like illness during therapy with L-5-hydroxy tryptophan and carbidopa. *N. Engl. J. Med.* 303, 782.

Stocks, A.E. and Robertson, A. (1966). The long-term therapy of severe hypertension with guanethidine. *Med. J. Aust.* i, 893.

Streiter, M.L., Schneider, H.L., and Proto, A.V. (1982). Steroid-induced thoracic lipomatosis: paraspinal involvement. *AJR* 139, 679.

Stricker, B.H.Ch., and Van Kasteren, B.J. (1992). Diclofenac-induced isolated myonecrosis and Nicolau syndrome. *Ann. Intern. Med.* 117, 1058.

Sturman, S.G., Kumararatne, D., and Beevers, D.G. (1988). Fatal hydralazine-induced systemic lupus erythematosus. *Lancet* ii, 1304.

Sullivan, E.A., Kamb, M.L., Jones, L.J., *et al.* (1996). The natural history of eosinophilia–myalgia syndrome in a tryptophan-exposed cohort in South Carolina. *Arch. Intern. Med.* 156, 973.

Sutton, R.D. (1968). Aseptic necrosis of bone, a complication of corticosteroid therapy. In *Drug-induced Diseases*, Vol. 3 (ed. L. Meyler and H.M. Peck), p. 171. Associated Scientific Publishers, Amsterdam.

Takagi, H., Ochoa, M.S., Zhou, L., *et al.* (1995). Enhanced collagen synthesis and transcription by Peak E, a containment of L-tryptophan preparations associated with the eosinophilia myalgia syndrome epidemic. *J. Clin. Invest.* 96, 2120.

Tanenbaum, M.H. (1972). Topical steroid atrophy: a disappearing digit. *JAMA* 220, 126.

Taranta, A., Mack, H., Hass, R.G., *et al.* (1958). Nodular panniculitis after massive prednisone therapy. *Am. J. Med.* 25, 52.

Tarzy, B.J., Klallach, E.E., Garcia, C.R., *et al.* (1972). Rheumatic disease, abnormal serology and oral contraceptives. *Lancet* ii, 501.

Teates, C.D. (1970). Steroid-induced mediastinal lipomatosis. *Radiology* 96, 501.

Thind, G.S. and Bryson, T.H.L. (1983). Single-dose suxamethonium and muscle pain in pregnancy. *Br. J. Anaesth.* 55, 743.

Thompson, J. and Julian, D.G. (1982). Retroperitoneal fibrosis associated with metoprolol. *BMJ* 284, 83.

Thurairajan, G., Hope-Ross, W., Situnayake, R.D., *et al.* (1997). Polyarthropathy, orbital myositis and posterior scleritis: an unusual adverse reaction to influenza vaccine. *Br. J. Rheumatol.* 36, 120.

Tingle, A.J., Allen, M., Petty, R.E., *et al.* (1986). Rubella associated arthritis. Comparative study of joint manifestations associated with natural rubella infection and RA 27/3 rubella immunisation. *Ann. Rheum. Dis.* 45, 606.

Torisu, M., Miyahara, T., Shinohara, O., *et al.* (1978). A new side effect of BCG immunotherapy — BCG-induced arthritis in man. *Cancer Immunol. Immunother.* 5, 77.

Tunkel, A.R., Shuman, M., Popkin, M., *et al.* (1987). Minoxidil-induced systemic lupus erythematosus. *Arch. Intern. Med.* 147, 599.

Uddin, M.S., Lynfield, Y.L., Grosberg, S.J., *et al.* (1979). Cutaneous reaction to spironolactone resembling lupus erythematosus. *Cutis* 24, 198.

Utz, D.C., Rooke, E.D., Spittell, J.A., *et al.* (1965). Retroperitoneal fibrosis in patients taking methysergide. *JAMA* 191, 983.

van der Korst, J.K., Colenbrauer, H., and Cats, A. (1960). Phenobarbital and the shoulder–hand syndrome. *Ann. Rheum. Dis.* 25, 553.

Vermersch, P., Foissac-Gegoux, Ph., Caron, J., *et al.* (1989). Retroperitoneal fibrosis after treatment with bromocriptine. *Presse Méd.* 18, 841.

von Eickstedt, K.W. and Elsässer, W. (1988). Corticotrophins and corticosteroids. In *Meyler's Side Effects of Drugs* (11th edn) (ed. M.N.G. Dukes), p. 812. Elsevier Science Publishers, Amsterdam.

Vrhovac, B. (1988). Anti-inflammatory analgesics and drugs used in gout. In *Meyler's Side Effects of Drugs* (11th edn) (ed. M.N.G. Dukes), p. 170. Elsevier Science Publishers, Amsterdam.

Walker, F.J. (1989). Simvastatin: the clinical profile. *Am. J. Med.* 87 (Suppl. 4A), 44S.

Waller, P.C. and Ramsay, L.E. (1985). Do β-blockers cause arthropathy? A case control study. *BMJ* 291, 1684.

Wallis, A.A., Bell, R., and Sutherland, P.W. (1977). Propranolol and Peyronie's disease. *Lancet* ii, 980.

Walsh, J.R. and Zimmerman, J.H. (1953). The demonstration of the 'LE' phenomenon in patients with penicillin hypersensitivity. *Blood* 8, 65.

Wandl, U.B., Nagel-Hiemke, M., May, D., *et al.* (1992). Lupus-like autoimmune disease induced by interferon therapy for myeloproliferative disorders. *Clin. Immunol. Immunopathol.* 65, 70.

Wanner, W.R. and Irvin W.S. (1981). Disopyramide and antinuclear antibodies. *Am. Heart J.* 101, 687.

Watermeyer, G.S., Mann, J.I., Truswell, A.S., *et al.* (1975). Type IIa hyperlipoproteinaemia: an evaluation of four therapeutic regimens. *S. Afr. Med. J.* 49, 631.

Waters, D.J. and Mapleson, W.W. (1971). Suxamethonium pains: hypothesis and observation. *Anaesthesia* 26, 127.

Watkins, S.M. and Williams, J.R.B. (1982). Avascular necrosis of bone after high doses of dexamethasone during neurosurgery. *BMJ* 284, 742.

Watson, A.J.S., Dalbow, M.H., Stachura, I., *et al.* (1983). Immunological studies in cimetidine-induced nephropathy and polymyositis. *N. Engl. J. Med.* 308, 142.

Watts, J.F., Edwards, R.L., and Butt, W.R. (1985). Treatment of premenstrual syndrome using danazol: preliminary report of a placebo-controlled double-blind, dose-ranging study. *J. Int. Med. Res.* 13, 127.

Weibel, R.E. and Benor, D.E. (1996). Chronic arthropathy and musculo-skeletal symptoms associated with rubella vaccines. A review of 124 claims submitted to the National Vaccine Injury Compensation Program. *Arthritis Rheum.* 39, 1529.

Weinstein, A. (1991). D-penicillamine induced lupus erythematosus. *Arthritis Rheum.* 34, 1343.

Weinstein, J. (1978). Hypocomplementemia in hydralazine-induced systemic lupus erythematosus. *Am. J. Med.* 65, 553.

White, D.C. (1962). Observations on the prevention of muscle pain after suxamethonium. *Br. J. Anaesth.* 34, 332.

WHO technical report series 701 (1984). *Leishmaniasis.*

Willis, R.A., Folkers, K., Tucker, J.L., *et al.* (1991). Lovastatin decreases coenzyme Q levels in rats. *Proc. Natl Acad. Sci. USA* 87, 8928.

Wilske, K.R., Shalit, I.E., Willkens, R.F., *et al.* (1965). Findings suggestive of systemic lupus erythematosus in subjects on chronic anticonvulsant therapy. *Arthritis Rheum.* 8, 260.

Wilson, J.D., Bullock, J.Y., Sutherland, D.C., *et al.* (1978). Antinuclear antibodies in patients receiving non-practolol beta-blockers. *BMJ* i, 14.

Wilson, J.D., Booth, R.J., and Bullock, J.Y. (1979). Antinuclear factor in patients on prazosin. *BMJ* i, 553.

Windsor, W.O., Kurrein, F., and Dyer, N.H. (1975). Fibrous peritonitis a complication of practolol therapy. *BMJ* ii, 68.

Winfield, J.B. and Davis, J.S. (1974). Anti-DNA antibody in procaine-induced lupus erythematosus. Determinations using DNA fractionated by methylated albumin-kieselguhr chromatography. *Arthritis Rheum.* 17, 97.

Witman, G. and Davis, R. (1981). A lupus erythematosus syndrome induced by clonidine hydrochloride. *Rhode Island Med. J.* 64, 147.

Wolkenstein, P. and Revuz, J. (1995). Drug-induced severe skin reactions: incidence, management and prevention. *Drug Safety* 13, 56.

Wouters, J.M.G., van de Putte, L.B.A., Renier, W.O., *et al.* (1982). D-Penicillamine-induced polymyositis. *Neth. J. Med.* 25, 159.

Young, R.A. and Brogden, R.N. (1988). Doxazosin. A review of its pharmacodynamic and pharmacokinetic properties, and therapeutic efficacy in mild or moderate hypertension. *Drugs* 35, 525.

Yudkin, J.S. (1977). Peyronie's disease in association with metoprolol. *Lancet* ii, 1355.

Yung, R., Chang, S., Hemati, N., *et al.* (1997). Mechanisms of drug-induced lupus. *Arthritis Rheum.* 40, 1436.

Zabranieki, I., Negrier, I., Vergne, P., *et al.* (1996). Fluoroquinolone induced tendinopathy: report of 6 cases. *J. Rheumatol.* 23, 516.

Zamber, R.W., Starkebaum, G., Martens, H.F., *et al.* (1992). Drug induced lupus erythematosus due to ophthalmic timolol. *J. Rheumatol.* 19, 977.

Zarafonetis, C.J.D. and Kalas, J.P. (1960). Serotonin degradation by ceruloplasmin and its inhibition by isoniazid and iproniazid. *Am. J. Med. Sci.* 239, 203.

Zarrabi, M.H., Zucker, S., Miller, F., *et al.* (1979). Immunologic and coagulation disorders in chlorpromazine-treated patients. *Ann. Intern. Med.* 91, 194.

Zelman, S. (1978). Terbutaline and muscular symptoms. *JAMA* 239, 930.

19. Skin disorders

A. G. SMITH

Incidence

Adverse drug reactions more commonly affect the skin than any other organ, with approximately 30 per cent of reported drug reactions involving the skin. The contemporary pattern of reaction probably does not much differ from that reported by Kuokkanen (1972), of 46 per cent maculopapular, 23 per cent urticarial, 10 per cent fixed eruptions, 5 per cent erythema multiforme, 4 per cent Stevens–Johnson syndrome, 4 per cent exfoliative dermatitis and 3 per cent photosensitivity. A study of over 15 000 consecutive inpatients identified an overall reaction rate of 2.2 per cent (Bigby et al. 1986). The most commonly implicated drugs were amoxycillin (51 cases per 1000 courses), co-trimoxazole (34 per 1000), ampicillin (33 per 1000), cephalosporins (13 per 1000), and blood products. On the basis of this and other studies, such as that of Arndt and Jick (1976), the list of drugs unlikely ever to cause a rash is decidedly short: its members are digoxin; inorganic compounds like ferrous sulphate, potassium chloride, and milk of magnesia; and the various vitamins.

Significance

Some drug eruptions, such as toxic epidermal necrolysis, have a significant mortality. Others are part of a more widespread reaction. In the case of practolol (Felix et al. 1974), benoxaprofen (Halsey and Cardoe 1982), and amiodarone (McGovern et al. 1983) a high incidence of skin reaction was matched by a high incidence of internal organ involvement. In contrast to idiopathic urticaria and angioedema, that induced by ACE inhibitors carries a real risk of dyspnoea and laryngeal oedema (Sabroe and Kobza Black 1997). Pemphigus induced by penicillamine, unlike the idiopathic form, can be associated with minimal-change nephropathy (Savill et al. 1988).

Thus the frequent implication that drug rashes are trivial is to be deprecated.

Diagnosis

It is often difficult to establish that a drug has caused a particular rash. Frequently, the morphology corresponds with various idiopathic eruptions; more than one of the drugs a patient is receiving may be recognized as a possible cause of a rash; finally, it is rare for additional *in vivo* or *in vitro* tests to clarify the situation greatly.

Drug rashes, like other drug reactions, may be divided into Type A (augmented) and Type B (bizarre) (see Chapter 5). An example of a Type A reaction is the captopril eruption due to kinin potentiation (Wilkin et al. 1980); and of a Type B reaction, the practolol eruption (Felix et al. 1974). Type A reactions are easier to diagnose because they are predictable (especially with hindsight), occur in a high proportion of patients taking the drug, are dose related, and subside readily on drug withdrawal. In Type B reactions, diagnosis is complicated by low incidence rates, absence of dose-dependency, and even failure of resolution of the eruption on drug withdrawal, as in some cases of penicillamine-induced pemphigus (Santa Cruz et al. 1981).

In some instances the characteristics of the reaction make it difficult to maintain the Type A–Type B dichotomy. Examples of this are the high incidence of hydralazine-induced systemic lupus erythematosus in patients (especially females) who are slow acetylators and HLA DR4-positive (Batchelor et al. 1980); the 95 per cent incidence of eruption in patients with infectious mononucleosis treated with ampicillin (Puller et al. 1967); and the 10-fold increase in reaction rate to co-trimoxazole in AIDS patients (De Raeve et al. 1988). In other groups of patients these reactions would be designated Type B: here they might be termed augmentedly bizarre (Type AB).

In attempting to justify the diagnosis of a drug rash, the following points should be considered.

1. *History*   The interval between the initiation of drug therapy and the onset of the rash may be of value in diagnosis. Arndt and Jick (1972) found that most cutaneous reactions occur within one week of exposure to the drug. This early onset is especially probable in Type A reactions: for example, for the captopril eruption the mean ($\pm$ SD) latent period was 9 ± 4.4 days, whereas in the Type B practolol eruption it was 312 ± 240 days.

2. *Signs*   Few drug eruptions are pathognomonic of a particular drug. Historical exceptions are the scaly reticulated and lichenoid purpura produced by carbromal, and the embedded palmar–plantar warts combined with raindrop pigmentation caused by arsenic. The morphological pattern of the eruption may, however, be of great value in favouring a particular drug as being its cause. Thus a lichenoid eruption is commoner with thiazides than with penicillins, so although penicillins cause more rashes overall than do thiazides, a lichenoid eruption in a patient taking both types of drug is more likely to be due to the thiazide.

It is important to consider alternative aetiological candidates for any putative drug eruption. For example, most varieties of eczema are unrelated to systemic therapy; exceptions are the asteatotic eczema which may accompany retinoid therapy and the 'systemic contact dermatitis' which can complicate prior topical sensitization (see below). A recent study of rheumatological patients receiving systemic therapy found that many more skin problems were not drug related (mainly eczema, leucocytoclastic vasculitis, and capillaritis) than might relate to therapy (Wilkinson *et al.* 1993).

3. *Continuation and discontinuation (dechallenge) of therapy*   Most drug rashes will persist for as long as the drug is continued. There are some exceptions to this, as in the case of the transient maculopapular rash that may be produced by phenytoin (Wilson *et al.* 1978). The morbilliform eruption produced by penicillins may also fade with continued therapy.

The diagnostic value of continuation and discontinuation may be vitiated if the drug alone is not a sufficient cause of the eruption: thus, screening of ultraviolet light may abolish drug-induced photosensitivity. While the majority of eruptions will resolve when the initiating drug is withdrawn, there are exceptions to this. Thus in hyperpigmentation induced by oral contraceptives, antimalarials, or chlorpromazine, much of the pigment is bound in dermal macrophages, and it can persist for years. When drugs induce immunological changes, such as penicillamine pemphigus or hydralazine lupus

erythematosus, these also can persist long after drug withdrawal.

4. *Challenge*   The recurrence of a rash when a drug is readministered provides the best evidence of a causal relationship. Patients are often not enthusiastic about this procedure, and its use is contraindicated where the rash is part of an acute systemic disturbance, as with the nitrofurantoin exanthem, which may be accompanied by pulmonary oedema and eosinophilia. Another contraindication to challenge is in the more severe rashes such as toxic epidermal necrolysis, and the exanthems most likely to progress to erythroderma, such as those due to isoniazid and streptomycin.

5. *Special tests*   Epicutaneous and intracutaneous tests which suggest Type I hypersensitivity (Coombs and Gell classification) may be positive, especially in urticarial and maculopapular eruptions. Patch testing, indicating Type IV hypersensitivity, has been of value in the diagnosis of general eruptions due to diazepam, meprobamate, and practolol (Felix and Comaish 1974); carbamazepine (Houwerzijl *et al.* 1974); chloramphenicol (Rudzki *et al.* 1976); and in toxic epidermal necrolysis (Tagami *et al.* 1983). In a study of 242 patients with drug eruptions, Osawa *et al.* (1990) obtained positive intradermal tests in 89.7 per cent and positive patch tests in 31.5 per cent. Their overall positive rate of 62 per cent would seem to be higher than in most studies. Patch testing carries less risk of anaphylaxis than does prick testing but, rarely, systemic symptoms have occurred, as in a case of dyspnoea with piperazine patch testing (Fregert 1976).

Of *in vitro* tests, the radioallergosorbent (RAST) test has shown a good correlation with prick testing in penicillin allergy (Kraft and Wide 1976), but its use has not been widely extended to other drugs. The results of other *in vitro* tests have been disappointing. Lymphocyte transformation studies in a variety of drug reactions showed a positive response in only 13 per cent (Sarkany and Gaylarde 1978); macrophage migration inhibition tests (Halevy *et al.* 1990) produced a positive response in 70 per cent. Thus these tests neither verify nor falsify the diagnosis of a drug reaction. They do, however, when positive, increase the probability that the drug tested caused the eruption.

In practice, tests in which it is not sought to infer causation but to elicit differences between drug eruptions and their idiopathic simulators are often more helpful. For example, in differentiating between idiopathic and drug-related systemic lupus erythematosus, the absence of antibodies to double-stranded, and presence of antibodies to single-stranded, DNA will point to drug induction. There are, not infrequently, differences in histopathology between drug rashes and their idiopathic equivalents. These are discussed, where appropriate, under the different reaction patterns.

Exanthematous eruptions

Exanthematic drug rashes usually appear early in therapy; previously sensitized patients develop a rash at 1 to 3 days, and others most commonly between 7 and 13 days. This latency is variable, however, and eruptions may also appear up to 2 weeks after cessation of therapy. These eruptions are sometimes described as being scarlatiniform, rubelliform, or morbilliform, after the infections they mimic: they may also take on gyrate or reticular morphologies. However, these patterns are not specific to particular drugs. In common with the infections, the drug rash is generally symmetrical and of sudden onset, and may be accompanied by lymphadenopathy; but, in contrast, any fever tends to be mild, an enanthem absent, and eosinophilia more likely.

Exanthematic rashes may occur with most drugs. They are particularly common with the penicillins, especially ampicillin — which almost always causes a rash in cases of glandular fever and lymphatic leukaemia. Sulphonamides are a frequent cause, even more so in patients with AIDS (De Raeve et al. 1988). The incidence is slightly lower with pyrazolone derivatives (e.g. phenylbutazone), gold, phenytoin, carbamazepine, and captopril.

Drug exanthemata may be accompanied by acute alveolitis with excess of eosinophils in both the alveoli and peripheral blood. This is best recognised with nitrofurantoin (Holmberg et al. 1980), but also described in reactions to penicillin, sulphonamides, chlorpromazine and carbamazepine.

An increasing number of cases of an exanthematous eruption with added non-follicular pustulosis have been described in recent years. The eruption evolves and resolves acutely and is complicated by pyrexia and neutrophilia; the causal drugs are antibiotics, especially penicillins and macrolides, phenytoin, frusemide, hydroxychloroquine, naproxen, and diltiazem (Wakelin and James 1995). A similar syndrome with follicular pustules due to allopurinol was described by Fitzgerald et al. (1994).

Erythroderma

Widespread erythema (erythroderma), usually with severe desquamation (exfoliative dermatitis), may be caused by eczema, psoriasis, leukaemia, and lymphoma, as well as drugs. The condition is complicated by loss of temperature regulation, fluid and electrolyte loss, infection, cardiac failure, and venous thrombosis, and has a significant mortality. The commoner drug causes are sulphonamides, gold, p-aminosalicylic acid, isoniazid, streptomycin, phenytoin, and carbamazepine. The rash usually resolves when the drug is withdrawn, giving this group a better prognosis than those secondary to other conditions.

Hypersensitivity syndrome

The hypersensitivity syndrome is characterized by a maculopapular or erythrodermic rash in association with, variously, fever, lymphadenopathy, arthralgia, pneumonitis, myopathy, abnormal liver function tests, impaired renal function, eosinophilia, and atypical lymphocytosis. Mostly described in association with the anticonvulsants carbamazepine, phenytoin, and phenobarbitone, it can also occur with allopurinol and dapsone (Handfield-Jones et al. 1993).

Photosensitivity

Photosensitivity denotes reaction to normally harmless amounts of ultraviolet or visible radiation. Drugs may induce photosensitivity either by direct mechanisms in which the presence of the drug in the skin, in either altered or unaltered forms, is necessary, or by indirect effects on other organs. Examples of indirect photosensitivity are drug-associated lupus erythematosus, hepatic porphyria, and pellagra. Lupus erythematosus and porphyria are dealt with elsewhere. Pellagra can be induced by isoniazid acting as an antagonist of niacin, and also by chloramphenicol and the hydantoins, phenobarbitone, azathioprine, mercaptopurine, and fluorouracil (Stevens et al. 1993).

Direct photosensitivity may be divided into phototoxic (usually Type A) and photoallergic (Type B) mechanisms. Phototoxic reactions occur in a high proportion of those exposed, are dose dependent, may occur on first exposure, and have a short latency of minutes to a few hours; the opposite obtains in photoallergic reactions. Clinically, phototoxic reactions resemble sunburn and show the appropriate histology, with epidermal necrosis, dermoepidermal separation, and a sparse superficial lymphohistiocytic dermal infiltrate. Photoallergic reactions show a more varied morphology, which may be eczematous or papular and is less localized; the histological appearances are of epidermal spongiosis, oedema of the papillary dermis, and a deeper lympho-histiocytic dermal infiltrate. In practice, however, this distinction may be difficult to make.

The action spectrum of most drug photosensitizers is in the UVA range (320–400 nm) with some extension into UVB (290–320 nm), which is filtered off by window glass.

Predominantly phototoxic reactions

Amiodarone is structurally related to the psoralens and causes photosensitivity, which may persist for up to 6 months after stopping therapy, in nearly half of patients taking it (Ferguson et al. 1985). The drug's action spectrum is 334–460 nm.

The tetracyclines, especially demeclocycline, are more likely to cause photosensitivity than any other group of antibiotics. Their action spectrum is 320–420 nm. Sulphonamides, especially sulphamethoxazole, griseofulvin, and ciprofloxacin have also been implicated.

A number of the non-steroidal anti-inflammatory drugs are photosensitizers. Benoxaprofen produced a high incidence of phototoxicity (Ferguson et al. 1982). Of currently prescribed anti-inflammatory drugs, piroxicam (McKerrow and Greig 1986) has been most frequently cited; its reaction has features of both phototoxicity and photoallergy. The propionic acid derivatives aza-propazone and tiaprofenic acid are also recognized photosensitizers.

Other drugs with phototoxic potential include the thiazides, nalidixic acid and frusemide (both of which may produce blistering of exposed skin) and the ret-inoids (Ferguson and Johnson 1986).

Etretinate is more frequently implicated than isotreti-noin. It is suggested that a metabolite of etretinate is responsible for its phototoxicity. Variations in patient capacity for degradation of this and other drugs produc-ing phototoxicity may account for the comparative rarity of adverse reaction, which thus may have more affinity with Type B than Type A reactions.

Predominantly photoallergic reactions

Of the phenothiazines, chlorpromazine is the best recog-nized photosensitizer. It can cause both phototoxic and photoallergic reactions, with an action spectrum in the UVA range. Promethazine and thioridazine (Rohrborn and Brauninger 1987) are also photoallergens.

Quinine can induce photosensitivity in the form of oedema and erythema or a lichenoid eruption. Mono-chromator studies show delayed erythema induced by UVB, UVA, and visible radiation. Quinidine may in-duce either a lichenoid or eczematous UVA-induced photodermatosis, as well as a livedo reticularis type of eruption on light-exposed areas (Manzi et al. 1989).

Flushing and erythema

Ethanol-induced flushing in patients taking chlor-propamide or tolbutamide is well recognized. Similar reactions are described when ethanol is taken after griseofulvin, metronidazole, or a cephalosporin. These reactions are blocked both by the opiate antagonist naloxone and by prostaglandin-synthetase inhibitors such as indomethacin; the latter group also inhibit the flushing caused by nicotinic acid (Wilkin 1983). Flushing may occasionally be seen after administration of bromo-criptine, dacarbazine (DTIC), isoniazid, nitrofurantoin, and pentazocine and, rather more frequently, with cal-cium-channel blockers such as nifedipine and verapamil (Bork 1988a).

Erythromelalgia is burning pain, erythema, swelling, and warmth of the hands or feet, made worse by depen-dency, warming, and exercise, and eased by cooling or elevation. While the majority of cases are idiopathic or secondary to polycythaemia or hypertension, some have been associated with therapy with nicardipine, nifedipine, bromocriptine, and pergolide (Healsmith et al. 1991).

The induction of painful swollen and red hands and feet by cytotoxic drug therapy has also been described: the drug most frequently implicated has been cytara-bine, usually in combination with other cytotoxic drugs in the treatment of leukaemia (Shall et al. 1988), but other cases have occurred in the treatment of Hodgkin's disease and various cancers; and other drugs such as hydroxyurea, fluorouracil, methotrexate, and mercap-topurine have been cited. The reaction occurs 4 to 23 days after beginning treatment, with the development of sharply demarcated painful erythematous swellings, which may blister. Histological examination of affected skin shows necrotic keratinocytes, mild spongiosis, and a superficial perivascular lymphocytic infiltrate (Fitz-patrick 1992). The condition remits even if therapy is continued.

The use of the plasma expander hydroxyethylstarch may cause a persistent itchy erythema of the face and upper trunk associated with a dermal infiltrate of foamy macrophages (Cox and Popple 1996), but lone pro-longed pruritus, without erythema, appears to be more common.

Acneiform eruptions

Drugs may either exacerbate acne or precipitate its development in subjects without pre-existing acne. In the latter group the acne tends to be a more monomorphic papulo-pustular eruption, without conspicuous comedones, of sudden onset, and involving the extremities in addition to the face and trunk. The factors recognized as important in the aetiology of acne are: the sebum excretion rate (SER); follicular hyperkeratosis causing obstruction to sebum flow; the hormonal control of the sebaceous gland; and the bacteriology of the gland. Drugs influencing any of these may produce acne.

Androgens increase SER, and synthetic androgens such as danazol (Greenberg 1979) can cause acne in women, as can oral contraceptives that contain a progesterone component with significant androgenic activity, such as 19-norethisterone. Severe acne may be seen in athletes who take anabolic steroids (Kiraly *et al.* 1987). High doses of corticosteroids are recognized as a cause of monomorphic acne; inhaled corticosteroids are not exempt (Monk *et al.* 1993).

Isoniazid, especially in slow inactivators, may either induce or exacerbate acne by causing follicular hyperkeratosis (Oliwiecki and Burton 1988). Lithium (Yoder 1975), probably by the same mechanism, may also produce an acneiform eruption, which tends to be most severe on the limbs. Medicines containing bromides and iodides are now less frequently prescribed, but were recognized to cause acne, which might progress to bromoderma or iododerma. The potential acneogenic effect of halogens is emphasized by the occasional case report of halothane-induced acne (Guldager 1987).

PUVA therapy (the combination of psoralen with ultra-violet light A) may cause acne (Jones and Bleehan 1977). It was suggested that this might be a direct effect of heat and UVA; but the effect of PUVA on immune function and thus on bacterial sebaceous gland colonization may be more important, as is probably the case in the 15 per cent of patients treated with cyclosporin who develop acne (Bencini *et al.* 1986).

Alopecia

There are two patterns of drug-induced hair loss. In anagen effluvium drugs induce an abrupt cessation of the intense mitotic activity of anagen, and the hairs are shed within days or weeks as dystrophic anagen hairs with tapered and broken roots. In telogen effluvium, the follicle is precipitated into a premature resting phase, and the hairs are shed 2 to 4 months later as club hairs.

Anagen effluvium is a Type A effect of chemotherapeutic agents such as bleomycin, cyclophosphamide, cytarabine, dactinomycin, daunorubicin, doxorubicin, etoposide, fluorouracil, methotrexate, and the nitrosoureas (Kerker and Hood 1989). Colchicine (Haarms 1980) may produce a similar anagen effluvium. With both chemotherapeutic agents and colchicine an initial anagen loss may be complicated by subsequent telogen shedding.

Telogen effluvium can be caused by both heparin and the coumarin anticoagulants; lithium; β-blockers such as metoprolol, nadolol, and propranolol; and both interferon alpha and gamma — probably secondarily to the influenza-like symptoms (Tosti *et al.* 1994).

A degree of hair loss may occur in as many as 70 per cent of patients treated with either etretinate or acetretin; but it would seem to be a rarity with isotretinoin. There appears to be a continuing increased rate of telogen shedding, with a sustained decrease in duration of anagen, rather than the usual abrupt precipitation of anagen hairs into telogen (Berth-Jones and Hutchinson 1995). Full regrowth occurs on stopping therapy, or even on dose reduction. This regrowth may be associated with kinking of the hair shaft.

Most cases of telogen effluvium are secondary to a severe illness. It may therefore be difficult to establish whether the illness or its treatment is the cause of the hair loss. This problem has led to a number of instances in which the cause has been incorrectly attributed to one rather than the other.

Not surprisingly, drugs with androgenic activity such as stanozolol, danazol, metyrapone and anabolic steroids, oestrogen receptor antagonists such as tamoxifen, and inhibitors of oestrogen synthesis such as aminoglutethimide, may all cause androgenic alopecia. In men the pattern is the familiar one of bitemporal recession plus loss over the vertex; in women a diffuse thinning over the top of the scalp with preservation of the anterior hair line occurs.

Hirsutism and hypertrichosis

Hirsutism is an excessive growth of coarse hair of a male pattern in a female: it arises from the conversion of vellus (fine hair) to coarse terminal hair on the face, chest, and abdomen. Hypertrichosis is excessive hair growth in areas other than those influenced by androgens, such as the forehead and upper cheeks. In it vellus increases in length up to 3 cm, but shows little increase in diameter.

Hirsutism may be caused by any of drug with significant androgenic activity. Reversible hypertrichosis occurs in more than 80 per cent of patients receiving systemic minoxidil for a month or more. Cyclosporin may produce hypertrichosis in 50 per cent of transplant patients, but it rarely does so with the lower dosages used for dermatological conditions like psoriasis — 3–5 mg per kg per day as opposed to up to 15 mg per kg per day. Phenytoin, which like cyclosporin causes gingival hypertrophy, causes hypertrichosis in about 10 per cent of patients. The calcium-channel blockers nifedipine and verapamil may also cause these two side effects. Diazoxide (especially in children receiving it for idiopathic hypoglycaemia), penicillamine, erythropoietin, and the now withdrawn benoxaprofen may also cause hypertrichosis (Tosti *et al.* 1994).

Nail changes

A variety of nail-plate dystrophies may occur with retinoid therapy, especially etretinate and its successor acetretin rather than isotretinoin. The described changes include Beau's lines (transverse depressions of the nail plate); brittle nails and onychorrhexis (longitudinal superficial furrowing of the nail); onychoschizia (the distal nail splitting horizontally); and onychomadesis (separation of the nail plate from the matrix area with progression to shedding) (Baran *et al.* 1996). A number of chemotherapeutic agents may also induce a similar spectrum of nail changes. They have been described with bleomycin (including its intralesional use in periungual warts, with grooving and shedding of the nail), fluorouracil, hydroxyurea, and mercaptopurine (Daniel and Scher 1985).

Generalized drug eruptions may severely damage the nail. Thus shedding may occur with toxic epidermal necrolysis; subungual hyperkeratosis and pitting with psoriasiform drug eruptions due, for example, to practolol; and deformity and shedding with the lichenoid eruption of quinacrine (Bauer 1981), although nail dystrophy is in general rare in lichenoid drug eruptions.

Drug-induced onycholysis (separation of the nail plate from the nail bed) is best recognized in drugs which can produce phototoxicity, with the nail plate possibly acting as a convex lens which concentrates the light in the nail bed. This photo-onycholysis is described with the tetracyclines, chloramphenicol, chlorpromazine, thiazides, 8-methexypsoralen, and benoxaprofen. Various chemotherapeutic drugs such as bleomycin, fluorouracil, doxorubicin, and mitozantrone may also induce onycholysis by direct toxicity to the matrix (Creamer *et al.* 1995).

Abnormalities of nail pigmentation may result from both systemic and topical drugs. With systemic drugs the pigmentation tends to run parallel to the lunula and with topical drugs (such as dithranol) parallel to the proximal nail fold. Cytotoxic drugs such as bleomycin, cyclophosphamide, doxorubicin, fluorouracil, melphalan, and nitrogen mustard may induce a variety of changes such as diffuse pigmentation, transverse banding and longitudinal melanonychia (which has also been described with zidovudine and minocycline [Mellon and Dawber 1994]). Both the 9-aminoacridine (such as mepacrine) and the 4-aminoquinoline antimalarials (such as chloroquine and amodiaquine) may cause nail pigmentation; both diffuse blue-black colouration and longitudinal banding have been described.

Bullous dermatoses

A number of drugs may be associated with the development of pemphigus. In some cases the drug contains a thiol group, as with penicillamine and captopril; or the drug has a sulphur-containing ring as with piroxicam. Penicillin, ampicillin, and amoxycillin, which may generate penicillamine by metabolic degradation, and rifampicin and cephalexin have also been cited (Ruocco and Sacredoti 1991).

Drug-induced pemphigus may differ from the various forms of idiopathic pemphigus in a number of ways. There may be a prodromal maculopapular or urticarial rash; superficial lesions resembling pemphigus foliaceous are far commoner than those like pemphigus vulgaris. Histologically there may be different levels of intraepidermal splitting rather than just one; tissue-bound and circulating autoantibodies directed against epidermal cell surface antigens are less constantly present; but other circulating autoantibodies are sometimes present. Many cases settle following drug withdrawal alone; but others, in which the drug may have unmasked occult pemphigus, require systemic corticosteroid therapy.

Eruptions resembling bullous pemphigoid may be precipitated by a number of drugs: frusemide is the most frequently implicated followed by other sulphonamide-related drugs, and penicillamine, penicillin and PUVA (Ruocco and Sacredoti 1991). Again, many of the molecules of these drugs contain sulphur. Drug-induced pemphigoid differs from the idiopathic form in that it may occur in younger patients; there may be relative absence of eosinophils on routine histology; and tissue-bound and circulating antibasement-membrane-zone IgG antibodies may be absent, and others, such as intercellular antibodies, present.

Dermatitis herpetiformis, in which granular deposition of IgA along the dermo–epidermal junction occurs, may be exacerbated by iodides. The related linear

IgA disease is usually idiopathic, but may be caused by lithium, vancomycin, co-trimoxazole, diclofenac, and vigabatrin (Paul *et al.* 1997).

Fixed drug eruption

Sometimes a drug induces lesions that recur at the same site when it is given again. These fixed drug eruptions (FDE) have become increasingly common and now approximate in frequency to exanthematous eruptions (Alanko *et al.* 1989). The lesion is classically circular and may evolve through macular, raised, and blistered stages; it is bright or dusky red early on, and fades with pigmentation. The limbs are more frequently affected than the trunk, and involvement of the mouth and genitals is not rare. While the lesions may itch or burn, there are usually no constitutional symptoms. The time between taking the drug and the appearance of the FDE varies from a few to 24 hours.

Variants such as wandering, non-pigmenting, and linear FDE (Sigal-Nahum *et al.* 1988) are described, as is multifocal FDE (Sowden and Smith 1990) which may be difficult to distinguish from erythema multiforme and toxic epidermal necrolysis (Baird and De Villez 1988). In these cases the histology of intraepidermal vesiculation (sometimes in addition to dermo–epidermal separation), and a denser and more varied inflammatory infiltrate with eosinophils and neutrophils as well as lymphocytes, involving the deep as well as superficial dermal vessels, favours the diagnosis of FDE.

Of the great many drugs that may cause FDE the phenazone derivatives, sulphonamides, trimethoprim, barbiturates, tetracyclines, and carbamazepine are among the commonest (Alanko *et al.* 1989), and it is worth enquiring about the possibility of consumption of phenolphthalein in laxatives.

Oral challenge is a safe, reliable means of confirming the diagnosis, and patch testing at the site of the eruption, but not elsewhere, is often positive (Alanko 1994).

Skin malignancy

Drugs may facilitate the development of both pre-malignant and malignant skin lesions, and also give rise to cutaneous pseudomalignancies.

The role of the immune system in the inhibition of malignancy is reflected in the increased incidence of skin neoplasia in patients receiving immunosuppressive therapy. In renal transplant patients who were taking corticosteroids and azathioprine, many had warty or hyper-keratotic lesions, 25 per cent premalignant solar keratoses or Bowen's disease, and 12 per cent frankly malignant tumours — either squamous (SCC) or basal cell epitheliomata (BCC) (Shuttleworth *et al.* 1987). It has been suggested that the azathioprine metabolite 6-thioguanine is of aetiological significance, but as transplant patients who had been treated with cyclosporin and not azathioprine showed an even greater prevalence (20 per cent) of frank skin malignancy, this would appear to be mainly the result of immunosuppression (Shuttleworth *et al.* 1989).

Skin malignancy associated with immunosuppression differs from idiopathic skin malignancy in that there is a reversal of the ratio of SCC to BCC. This is normally 0.2:1.0; but in the transplant group it is 2.3:1.0 and the SCC is more aggressive than normal (Gupta *et al.* 1986). In this study of 523 patients there were also three with malignant melanoma and one with Kaposi's sarcoma, and a corresponding excess of internal malignancy, which included carcinoma of the cervix (suggesting the importance of papilloma virus common to both sites), lymphoma and reticulum cell sarcoma. Eruptive dysplastic naevi (which may dispose to malignant melanoma) are also described following renal transplantation (Barker and MacDonald 1988).

Hydroxyurea seems to dispose to the development of skin malignancy (Papi *et al.* 1993), as did arsenic, formerly used to suppress psoriasis (Evans 1977). The long latent period between exposure to arsenic and development of malignancy means that such cases are still being seen. The association of PUVA (psoralen plus UVA) therapy with the development of cutaneous SCC, is not surprising, but the apparent excess of internal malignancy is (Lindelof *et al.* 1991), and the possible excess of malignant melanoma is a further anxiety (Stern *et al.* 1997).

Drug-induced pseudolymphoma presents as papulonodules or infiltrated plaques, often associated with lymphadenopathy. Histological examination shows an upper dermal band-like lymphocytic infiltrate with atypical epidermotropism mimicking mycosis fungoides. The skin lesions generally appear within 6 months of starting therapy, and resolve in a month of stopping. The enlarged nodes, whose histology may also suggest a true lymphoma, resolve in 6 months. The drugs implicated include the anticonvulsants phenytoin and carbamazepine, and allopurinol, amiloride, diltiazem, clomipramine, and cyclosporin (Callot *et al.* 1996).

Lichenoid eruptions

Drug eruptions may resemble lichen planus either clinically or histologically. Clinically, drug-induced lichenoid eruptions may differ from idiopathic lichen planus in also having features of psoriasis, or eczema, or bullous pemphigoid — as in lichen planus pemphigoides (Ogg *et al.* 1997) or cutaneous lymphoma (Phillips *et al.* 1994). Histological features which favour a drug cause are: parakeratosis, a thinner epidermis with an interrupted granular layer, cytoid bodies in the cornified and granular layers, and a deeper dermal infiltrate rich in eosinophils (van den Haute *et al.* 1989). The drugs mainly implicated are the thiazides (lesions due to which may be preferentially distributed on areas exposed to light) and frusemide; the antimalarials mepacrine, chloroquine, and quinine; the antituberculous drugs *p*-aminosalicylic acid, streptomycin, and ethambutol; the antirheumatic drugs gold and penicillamine; the anticonvulsants carbamazepine and phenytoin; and antihypertensives, methyldopa, β-adrenoceptor antagonists, and ACE inhibitors such as captopril and enalapril (Rosen *et al.* 1995).

Thus the choice of which of a number of a patient's drugs to discontinue is frequently difficult; and the situation is further complicated by the often slow resolution of these eruptions; and the possibility of late malignancy in lichenoid eruptions (Bauer 1981).

Psoriasiform eruptions

Drugs may either produce psoriasiform eruptions in patients who have no disposition to idiopathic psoriasis, or exacerbate existing psoriasis. The former has been most notable, with β-adrenoceptor blocking drugs, of which practolol was the first to be recognized (Felix *et al.* 1974). Since then other β-blockers such as oxprenolol, propranolol, atenolol, and timolol have been incriminated (Gold *et al.* 1988). Macroscopically, the eruption consisted of patchy erythema and scaling worst over the knees and elbows, with more hyperkeratosis of palms and soles than is usual in idiopathic psoriasis; microscopically there were lichenoid as well as psoriasiform features. Importantly, the skin signs were sometimes a part of the oculocutaneous syndrome, which might also include keratitis, corneal ulcers, and fibrosis of lungs, pleura, pericardium, and peritoneum.

β-Adrenoceptor blockers may also exacerbate preexisting psoriasis, as may lithium (Lowe and Ridgway 1978), the 4-aminoquinoline antimalarials such as chloroquine, various non-steroidal anti-inflammatory agents and interferon alpha (Quesada and Gutterman 1986). Pharmacological explanations exist for some of these effects. Non-steroidal anti-inflammatory agents block the cyclo-oxygenase pathway of arachidonic acid metabolism, leading to synthesis of leukotrienes rather than prostaglandins; leukotrienes may be important in the pathogenesis of psoriasis. α-Interferon decreases the ratio of cyclic AMP to cyclic GMP, and lithium inhibits adenylate cyclase. These effects on cyclic nucleoside may also be of pathogenetic importance. While these mechanisms may suggest a Type A effect, their rarity in prospective studies with indomethacin (Sheehan-Dare *et al.* 1991) and chloroquine (Katugampola and Katugampola 1990) is more in keeping with Type B. Thus these drugs should not be regarded as contraindicated in psoriasis, though if they exacerbate the condition they might need to be withdrawn.

Skin necrosis

Skin necrosis may arise during therapy with either oral or parenteral anticoagulants. In oral therapy it has more often been recorded with warfarin than phenindione. Warfarin necrosis is said to occur in approximately one in every 1000 patients treated; obese women are most at risk and fatty areas the most susceptible. It mainly occurs between days 3 and 5 of therapy, especially after a loading dose. Erythema is followed by painful oedema and then blistering and infarction. Histological examination shows epidermal necrosis with platelet fibrin thrombi in dermal vessels and extravasation of red blood cells. Warfarin necrosis has been associated with the heterozygous state for deficiency of protein C (Bauer 1993). Resolution may occur with continuing therapy.

Heparin necrosis is similar clinically and histologically. It usually occurs at injection sites, but may be distant. The onset of necrosis (at 6–13 days) is later than with warfarin. The pathogenesis involves the production of antibodies to heparin–platelet complexes, with the production of thrombocytopenia and possibly systemic thrombosis. It is essential to stop the heparin in such cases (Yates and Jones 1993).

Cytotoxic drugs may produce skin necrosis in a number of ways. Most are vesicants and may irritate the vein through which they are being infused. If extravasation occurs, pain and erythema may be followed by necrosis and persistent ulceration (Bronner and Hood 1983). Lawrence and Dahl (1984) described two patterns of skin necrosis in the treatment of psoriasis with methotrexate. One occurs in the psoriatic plaques soon after starting therapy, and the other, which may occur at any time during therapy, in skin uninvolved by psoriasis, but the site of another disorder, such as venous stasis. The histological changes are of epidermal necrosis without significant vascular abnormality. Methotrexate may also produce the radiation-recall phenomenon (an inflammatory response at the site of previous irradiation during chemotherapy). This may be so severe as to produce cutaneous necrosis (Logan *et al.* 1988). The radiation-recall phenomenon is also described with cyclophosphamide, vincristine, bleomycin, and doxorubicin.

Cutaneous necrosis may be produced by vasoconstriction. This may be caused by noradrenaline added to local anaesthetics, so such preparations should not be used at acral sites. β-Adrenoceptor blocking drugs may so mpair cutaneous circulation as to cause necrosis (Hoffbrand 1979). Vasopressin, used to treat bleeding oesophageal varices, may rarely cause skin necrosis (Wormser *et al.* 1982).

A number of drugs such as penicillamine, bromocriptine, and bleomycin may produce a syndrome similar to systemic sclerosis. Especially in the case of bleomycin (Cohen *et al.* 1973), this may include gangrene of the finger tips.

Cutaneous vasculitis and panniculitis

The lesions of cutaneous vasculitis mainly involve the lower legs and evolve rapidly through red macules to urticated papules which become purpuric (palpable purpura), and in severe cases haemorrhagic blisters and ulcers may occur. The involvement of the skin may be part of a spectrum of systemic involvement, which may be life-threatening.

Histologically the lesions involve the postcapillary venules, which show fibrinoid necrosis of their walls and a perivascular infiltrate of mononuclear cells and neutrophils, the destruction of which (leucocytoclasis) produces the nuclear dust of leucocytoclastic vasculitis. It has been claimed that in drug-induced vasculitis mononuclear cells and eosinophils predominate and that leucocytoclasis and fibrinoid vascular lesions are inconspicuous (Mullick *et al.* 1979). Other reports do not, however, stress these discriminants, and suggest that there may be a change from neutrophilic and leucocytoclastic to mononuclear infiltration which is solely a function of time (Zax *et al.* 1990). The drugs implicated include the penicillins (especially ampicillin), sulphonamides, thiazides, and various non-steroidal anti-inflammatory drugs (Roujeau and Stern, 1994); radiographic contrast media (Kerdel *et al.* 1984); and retinoids (Dwyer *et al.* 1989).

Propylthiouracil may induce a clinically distinctive vasculitis initially involving the face and ear lobes and the production of antineutrophilic cytoplasmic antibodies, which are usually absent in drug-induced vasculitis (Dolman *et al.* 1993).

The term polyarteritis nodosa is best reserved for cases in which necrosis and vessel wall inflammation with leucocytoclasis occur in small to medium-sized arteries, corresponding to the occurrence of tender nodules along the course of a superficial artery. This pattern of vasculitis is generally not associated with drug therapy, but an association with abused drugs (especially methylamphetamine) has been described (Citron *et al.* 1970). Erythema nodosum is characterized clinically by tender cutaneous nodules and histologically by a septal panniculitis with sometimes a mild vasculitis. Various drugs have been incriminated including oral contraceptives, sulphonamides, penicillins, gold (Litt and Pawlak 1997) and minocycline in the case of which the erythema nodosum was associated with hyperpigmentation and neutrophilic alveolitis (Bridges *et al.* 1990).

Urticaria and angioedema

The lesions of urticaria consist of itchy circumscribed erythematous swellings of the skin, which resolve within hours. The pathological changes are oedema and perivascular inflammation of the superficial dermis. In angioedema the same changes are sited in the deep dermis, subcutis, and submucosa, producing deeper-set, skin-coloured, non-pruritic, and generally more persistent swellings. Importantly, both conditions may be associated with anaphylaxis. Urticaria and angioedema may occur together or independently and both conditions may be caused by the same drugs. The great majority of cases of urticaria/angioedema are, however, idiopathic and not drug related.

Urticaria or angioedema may be produced by direct pharmacological (predominantly Type A) reactions. Some drugs release mast-cell mediators directly. These include opiates, codeine, *d*-tubocurarine, amphetamines, hydralazine, quinine, and radiocontrast media (Bork 1988*b*). Aspirin and other non-steroidal anti-inflammatory drugs may produce urticaria by inhibiting cyclo-oxygenase, with enhanced biosynthesis of leukotrienes via the lipoxygenase pathway of arachidonic acid metabolism. Angiotensin-converting-enzyme inhibitors cause urticaria or angioedema via potentiation of bradykinin activity (Sabroe and Kobza Black 1997).

Allergic urticaria (Type B) may be caused by either Type I or Type III hypersensitivity and be precipitated by, especially, penicillin, but also pollen and mould extracts used for desensitization, chicken egg protein in vaccines, and blood transfusion products. Occasionally, food and drug additives may be implicated in urticaria — more in exacerbation than in the initial cause. Examples are the benzoates (E210–219), butylated hydroxyanisole (E320), butylated hydroxytoluene (E321), sulphites (E221–227), and the tartrazine dyes (E102) (Simon 1984). Thus tablets coloured yellow with tartrazine may not be the best choice for treating urticaria.

Erythema multiforme and Stevens–Johnson syndrome

Erythema multiforme

Erythema multiforme (EM) is a pleomorphic eruption of erythematous macules and papules which may become vesicular centrally, giving the characteristic target lesions. It tends to be symmetrical and acral, especially on the hands. In its mild form it is sometimes termed erythema multiforme minor to distinguish it from erythema multiforme major (Stevens–Johnson syndrome) in which ocular and oral lesions accompanied by fever and systemic upset occur. Toxic epidermal necrolysis, which might be considered as the extreme form of erythema multiforme, will be considered separately.

In all forms of EM the histology shows epidermal necrosis with ballooning degeneration of keratinocytes and dermo–epidermal splitting with a mild interface lymphocytic dermatitis. The stratum corneum is normal. Dermal inflammation is mild with a lymphocytic perivascular infiltrate of the superficial vessels.

About 10 per cent of EM minor is caused by drugs and 50 per cent of EM major. The main drugs implicated are: the sulphonamides, including combined trimethoprim and sulphamethoxazole (co-trimoxazole) and combined pyrimethamine and sulphadoxine (Fansidar), penicillins (especially ampicillin), various non-steroidal anti-inflammatory drugs, and the anticonvulsants carbamazepine and phenytoin. Less often implicated are the cephalosporins, rifampicin, allopurinol, and cyclophosphamide — and nearly 200 other drugs (Litt and Pawlak 1997).

A number of topical medications may, rarely, induce EM-like eruptions. These include sulphonamides and hyoscine used in ophthalmic preparations, mephenesin used for sports injuries, clioquinol, and neomycin (Fisher 1986).

Toxic epidermal necrolysis

The clinical criteria for toxic epidermal necrolysis (TEN) may include:

1. bullae or erosions covering 20 per cent or more of the body surface or involving three separate anatomical regions;
2. bullae or lesions developing on an erythematous base;
3. exclusion of staphylococcal scalded skin syndrome (SSSS);
4. appearance of such lesions on skin that has not been exposed to direct sunlight;
5. peeling of areas of skin larger than 3 square cm;
6. frequent involvement of mucous membranes;
7. appearance of tenderness within 48 hours of the onset of the rash;
8. fever; and
9. characteristic histology (Schopf *et al.* 1991).

The histological picture is much the same as in EM but with a sparser dermal inflammatory infiltrate. However, immunochemical studies show the dermal infiltrate in EM to be rich in T lymphocytes, and the sparser infiltrate of TEN to consist mainly of macrophages and dendrocytes, while tumour necrosis factor alpha is far more abundant in TEN (Paquet and Pierard 1997). Histology is of value in differentiating TEN from SSSS, in which condition the blister is just below the stratum corneum, epidermal cell necrosis is inconspicuous, and neutrophils (in addition to lymphocytes) are present in the dermal infiltrate.

Eighty per cent of cases of TEN are caused by drugs, generally the same drugs as cause EM, with the same relative frequency, and the condition usually becomes apparent 1 to 3 weeks after starting treatment with the causative drug. A higher incidence has been reported in patients with systemic lupus erythematosus and HIV infection, which hardly suggests that treatment by further immunosuppression with either corticosteroids or cyclosporin will be helpful. Indeed the data suggest that corticosteroids increase mortality, which is of the order of 34 per cent, compared with one per cent for Stevens–Johnson syndrome (Schopf *et al.* 1991).

Abnormalities of pigmentation

Abnormal pigmentation is mainly produced by either the deposition of drugs themselves in the skin, by their stimulation of melanogenesis, or by a combination of these two factors.

Drug deposition

Therapeutic use of compounds containing silver, bismuth, and mercury has declined and with it the incidence of the pigmentation they may produce (Granstein and Sober 1981). Wet dressings of silver nitrate solution, however, remain a popular treatment for leg ulcers and exudative dermatoses; and argyria may rarely follow this therapy (Marshall and Schneider 1977), and that of silver-containing antismoking lozenges (Shelton and Goulding 1979). The therapeutic use of gold salts may rarely be accompanied by the development of chrysiasis, in which there is a grey-blue pigmentation of areas of the skin exposed to light and of the sclerae. Gold particles are deposited in dermal macrophages and melanogenesis is increased (Smith *et al.* 1995). After long-term administration of systemic iron, a generalized haemochromatosis-like discolouration may appear (Pletcher *et al.* 1963).

Minocycline can produce a variety of patterns of skin hyperpigmentation, including diffuse pigmentation of areas exposed to sun, pigment limited to scars, and patchy pigmentation of the skin. More rarely, pigmentation of the sclerae and teeth may occur. Electron microscopy of affected skin demonstrates electron-dense cytoplasmic granules in dermal macrophages, which are probably deposits of the drug itself (Okada *et al.* 1989). Similar granules are also found in the involved skin of the photosensitivity-associated amiodarone pigmentation (Zachary *et al.* 1984), in which instance lipofuchsin deposition also occurs in dermal macrophages. Intracytoplasmic granules, which again probably consist largely of the drug itself, also occur in dermal macrophages in pigmentation due to chlorpromazine (Benning *et al.* 1988) and to mepacrine (Leigh *et al.* 1979). Similar pigmentation has been attributed to quinidine, which is structurally related to mepacrine (Mahler *et al.* 1986). Most patients taking mepacrine develop a yellowing of the skin, and in a minority a blue-black discolouration of the shins, nails, and hard palate occurs. As well as with the 9-amino-acridines (e.g. mepacrine), pigmentation may occur with the 4-aminoquinoline group (e.g. chloroquine, hydroxychloroquine, and amodiaquine). With the latter group, but not with mepacrine, there is a correlation between skin pigmentation and retinal damage.

Yellow discolouration of the skin may also be produced by β-carotene, which is used in the treatment of erythropoietic protoporphyria; as with mepacrine, and in contrast to jaundice, the sclerae are not discoloured. Clofazimine may directly stain the skin red within a few weeks of starting therapy. After 2–3 months of its use in leprosy, black-brown or violaceous-brown skin staining may develop, which may be due to complexes of the drug with fatty acids derived from the bacilli (Job *et al.* 1990).

Increased melanogenesis

Both corticotrophin (ACTH) and tetracosactrin contain the seven-amino-acid sequence common to peptides with melanocyte-stimulating activity, and their long-term administration leads to an Addisonian pattern of hyperpigmentation.

Chloasma (or melasma) due to epidermal (reversible) and dermal (relatively irreversible) pigmentation of the face occurs in about five per cent of women taking oral contraceptives. This appears to be due to a direct effect of oestrogens and progestogens on melanogenesis and not to stimulation of peptides related to melanocyte-stimulating hormone (MSH) (Smith *et al.* 1977). Similarly, no elevation of MSH was found in patients on phenytoin, of whom about 10 per cent may develop chloasma. Direct stimulation of melanocytes, as occurs with amphibian melanophores (Kuske and Krebs 1964) seems to be the likely mechanism. Likewise, no elevation of MSH has been demonstrated in the pigmentation of cytotoxic drug therapy (Kew *et al.* 1977). Busulphan may produce an Addisonian pattern of pigmentation in up to 20 per cent of those receiving it. Bleomycin produces a similar incidence of hyperpigmentation, but of a different pattern, with streaking on the trunk and heaviest pigmentation over the extensor surfaces of joints. Cyclophosphamide, melphalan, doxorubicin, fluorouracil, mustine hydrochloride, hydroxyurea, methotrexate, and mithramycin (Granstein and Sober 1981) may also produce hyperpigmentation. In common with these chemotherapeutic agents, zidovudine may cause Addisonian pigmentation of the skin (Merenich *et al.* 1989) although, like them, it more commonly causes nail hyperpigmentation.

Adverse reactions to topical medicaments

As with reactions to ingested drugs, reactions to topical preparations may be divided into Types A and B, of which Type B reactions in the form of allergic contact dermatitis are the more important. Sensitization is more readily induced percutaneously than by any other route, a fact which relates to the epidermal Langerhans cell's role in the afferent limb of the immune system. Thus, nearly all subjects can be sensitized by topical dinitrochlorobenzene (Friedmann *et al.* 1983), and penicillin and streptomycin produced so much contact dermatitis when applied locally as opposed to being given systemically that their topical use was abandoned.

Type A reactions

These may be divided into topical and systemic adverse effects. Drugs may be absorbed through the skin in sufficient amount to cause Type A systemic toxicity. This is most likely to occur with widespread diseased skin, in infants (with a high ratio of surface area to volume), in the thinned skin of old age, and when absorption is enhanced by the use of certain vehicles such as dimethylsulphoxide, or occlusive therapy. Toxicity from resorcinol (used in preparations for acne and causing impaired thyroid function and methaemoglobinaemia) and boric acid (a constituent of Eusol causing nephrotoxicity) has become a rarity as use of these preparations has declined. However, percutaneous salicylate poisoning from the numerous topical preparations which contain salicylic acid remains a possibility (Anderson and Ead 1979). The application of topical vitamin D analogues such as calcipotriol may be associated with elevation of serum calcium (Bourke et al. 1993). The use of coal-tar shampoos results in appreciable amounts of polycyclic aromatic hydrocarbons being absorbed (Schooten et al. 1995) — these are carcinogenic, but to date there is no epidemiological evidence that topical tar products cause skin or internal cancer.

Corticosteroids are the most widely prescribed topical preparations, and the commonest cause of Type A reactions. As a rule these reactions occur only with the more potent (usually fluorinated) preparations. The fluorine atom is not essential for these effects, as they occur with the more potent non-fluorinated preparations such as hydrocortisone butyrate 0.1%. Whilst mild expression of these effects has been described with 1% hydrocortisone (Guin 1981), it can to all intents and purposes be used safely.

When the most potent topical corticosteroids are used in large amounts (e.g. 300 g of clobetasol propionate per week) for long periods over large areas of diseased skin, hypothalamic–pituitary suppression with Cushingoid features can occur (Carruthers et al. 1975). Far more commonly troublesome are steroid-induced changes in the skin, of which the most prominent is thinning of both epidermis and dermis (Winter and Burton 1976). Dermal atrophy causes striae, telangiectasia, easy bruising, and fragile skin with poor wound healing.

Inappropriate corticosteroid treatment may result in the potentiation of infection, with masking of its expression. This may occur with bacteria (widespread folliculitis), viruses (e.g. disseminated molluscum contagiosum), arthropods (widespread and atypical scabies), and with fungal infections — the so-called 'tinea incognito' of Ive and Marks (1968).

If used on the face, the more potent steroids will induce rosacea and perioral dermatitis (Cotterill 1979) and their withdrawal may be associated with the conversion of plaque to pustular psoriasis (Boxley et al. 1975).

Primary irritant contact dermatitis

Primary irritant contact dermatitis provides an instance of Type A reaction occurring with topical drugs. While it is common with both tar and dithranol when used in psoriasis, it should not be forgotten that both may be allergens (Burden et al. 1994). The laxative co-danthrusate (danthron and docusate sodium) may cause a perianal irritant dermatitis; danthron is chemically very similar to dithranol (Harland and Mortimer 1992).

Phototoxic reactions may complicate therapy with tar (Diette et al. 1983) and, more commonly, with topical psoralens (Weber 1974). Photoallergy occurring with topical preparations may be caused by their content of hexachlorophane (Wennersten et al. 1984); and by the p-aminobenzoic acid esters (Mathias et al. 1978) which are used in sunscreens.

Type B reactions

Allergic contact dermatitis

Allergic contact dermatitis is the major complication of topical treatment. It may be caused not only by the active ingredient of a cream or ointment, but 'also by the base (e.g. lanolin), preservatives (e.g. parabens), emulsifiers (e.g. the span group), and various fragrances.

Incidence

Fourteen per cent of 4000 consecutive patients with eczema from five European skin clinics who were tested by the International Contact Dermatitis Research Group (ICDRG) were considered to have allergic contact dermatitis to medicaments. Neomycin and benzocaine were the most frequent sensitizers (four per cent each) (Cronin et al. 1970).

Predisposing factors

Patients with atopic eczema are no more likely to develop contact dermatitis than those with other forms of endogenous eczema (Bandmann et al. 1972). Certainly, contact sensitization is less readily induced experimentally in atopic subjects (Forsbeck et al. 1976). Any patient with longstanding eczema of any sort, however, is likely to have had prolonged treatment with medicaments and thus the opportunity to become sensitized. The prevalence of allergic contact dermatitis falls with advancing age (Hjorth and Fregert 1979); but it is wise to assume that the sensitized patient remains so for life.

It is probable that drugs delivered in an occlusive ointment base are more likely to be sensitive than when a cream base is used (Hjorth and Thomsen 1968). Creams, however, contain a greater number of potential sensitizers such as emulsifiers, humectants, and preservatives, which are not required in ointments.

Not surprisingly, the prevalence of medicament sensitivity relates to the prevalence of medicament usage. Thus, neomycin allergy occurred in 1.7 per cent of tested patients in Warsaw and 19 per cent in Finland (Macdonald and Beck 1983).

The most vulnerable site for acquisition of contact dermatitis is around chronic ulcers of the lower leg (Paramsothy *et al.* 1988), where medicament sensitivity occurs in excess of 50 per cent of patients tested, and in whom the development of one sensitivity may favour the development of more (ampliative medicament allergy). Other sites at risk, albeit less so, are the perianal and perineal areas (Lewis *et al.* 1994), and ears and eyelids (Wilkinson *et al.* 1987).

Patch tests

Patch testing is both a limited and comparatively safe form of challenge with the suspected allergen, and also the oldest (Jadassohn 1896) test of Type IV sensitivity.

The substances to be tested are applied to discs of filter paper stuck by heat to aluminium foil covered with polythene (the Al-test unit). The strips of foil are applied to the patient's back and left in place for two days, when they are removed and readings made. Positive patch tests are indicated by an eczematous reaction at the test site, but as 20 per cent of reactions finally judged positive may develop over the next 5 days (Mitchell 1978), late readings are important, especially with neomycin.

The ICDRG has developed a standard battery of patch test substances which can be obtained commercially. This includes neomycin 20%, benzocaine 5%, wool alcohols (lanolin) 30%, parabens 3%, balsam of Peru 25%, clioquinol 5%, and ethylenediamine 1%. All are found in many topical preparations and are common sensitizers. A battery of test substances is especially useful when the history is obscure. When the result of a test on a proprietary product is positive, it is desirable to retest with individual components of the preparation so that the allergen can be identified and the patient warned to avoid other products containing the allergen and other drugs which may cross-react with it.

The distinction between an irritant and allergic patch test may be difficult — just as the distinction between irritant and allergic dermatitis may be. The following points favour a true positive (allergic) patch test: positivity at low concentration; itching rather than soreness; eczematous morphology rather than an erosion; spread beyond the site of application; and continued evolution of response following removal of the patches (Cronin 1980*a*).

As an awareness of cross-reaction between topical sensitizers and systemically administered drugs is relevant to the safe prescription of both, medicament dermatitis will be discussed, with special emphasis on these cross-reactions. Most characteristically, when a patient has previously been sensitized to a topical drug and then receives the same or related drug systemically he develops a symmetrical eczematous eruption, with erythema, vesiculation, and desquamation — so-called 'systemic contact dermatitis'. Sometimes the rash is maximal around the eyelids and flexures; at other times it takes the form of palmar vesiculation. More rarely an EM-like or vasculitic eruption may occur.

Important sensitizers

Topical antibiotics and antibacterials   Topical antibiotics are indicated in the treatment of primary bacterial infections of the skin like impetigo and in combination with corticosteroids in the treatment of impetiginized eczema (Leyden and Kligman 1977*a*). They are best avoided in the treatment of potentially chronic conditions like leg ulcers, where the risk of sensitization is great. This is especially true of sodium fusidate (Verbov 1970) and gentamicin (Cronin 1980*b*), both of which may later have to be given systemically.

Neomycin remains the commonest topical sensitizer amongst the antibiotics and cross-reactions may occur with other aminoglycosides, such as framycetin, kanamycin, netilmicin, streptomycin, and tobramycin. Many patients sensitive to neomycin are also sensitive to bacitracin, but it is thought that the sensitization is simultaneous and independent. Systemic eczematization has been reported following the use of oral neomycin and the use of a bacitracin–neomycin dental preparation (Macdonald and Beck 1983).

Topical antibiotics are widely prescribed for acne. Clindamycin has been described as causing facial contact dermatitis (Coskey 1978) and also as producing allergy presenting as rosacea (de Kort and de Groot 1989). Actinac (containing chloramphenicol) is widely used in the United Kingdom, as are chloramphenicol eye drops and ointments. Although chloramphenicol sensitivity is rare (Cronin 1980*c*), it would seem prudent to avoid applying it topically in the long term. While sensitivity to benzoyl peroxide (Leyden and Kligman 1977*b*) may occur, this and retinoids are generally the most suitable topical treatments for acne.

Preparations containing clioquinol (iodochlorhydroxyquinoline, chinoform, Vioform) and chlorquinaldol are much used in combination with topical steroids and in medicated bandages (e.g. Quinaband). About two per cent of subjects routinely patch-tested are positive to clioquinol, and cross-reactions between topical clioquinol and chlorquinaldol and the quinoline anti-malarials may occur (Kernekamp and van Ketel 1980).

The imidazole topical antifungal preparations are weak sensitizers, but they have caused both localized contact dermatitis and systemic contact dermatitis when given as an oral solution (Fernandez *et al.* 1996).

Anti-inflammatory drugs   Hypersensitivity to topical corticosteroids has been increasingly recognized in recent years (Wilkinson 1994); it is usually detected by patch testing with tixocortol pivalate 1% in petrolatum and budesonide 1% in ethanol. Between two and five per cent of patch-test clinic patients currently produce positive reactions. However, intradermal testing may be necessary to demonstrate corticosteroid allergy (Wilkinson and English 1992), and this does carry a greater risk than patch testing of producing erythroderma or other severe reaction (Wilkinson *et al.* 1992). In general, the tendency for cross-reaction between corticosteroids is not great, in spite of their close chemical relationship. In addition to reaction to topical corticosteroids used in skin disease, contact dermatitis from budesonide in a nasal aerosol has been described (Jerez *et al.* 1990).

Topical non-steroidal anti-inflammatory drugs, such as piroxicam gel (used for musculoskeletal strains) (Green and Lowe 1992), and diclofenac drops (used for ocular inflammation) (Valsecchi *et al.* 1996) may cause contact dermatitis, with subsequent risk of reaction to systemic therapy.

Antihistamine creams   These are readily available 'over the counter' and carry the risk of sensitization without there being any good evidence of their efficacy. Diphenhydramine hydrochloride (contained, for example, in Caladryl cream) is well recognized as a cause of medicament dermatitis (Coskey 1983). Subsequent oral administration may cause a generalized eruption maximal at the site of previous sensitization (Shelley and Bennett 1972).

Local anaesthetics   The principal sensitizers are benzoic acid derivatives (benzocaine, amethocaine, procaine, and dibucaine). They are often contained in preparations for pruritus ani, where low-potency topical corticosteroids are more effective, and in many 'over the counter' preparations for sunburn, dermatitis, sore throats, and other minor ailments. Positive reactions to benzocaine are not necessarily due to direct topical use and may represent sensitization by compounds of similar chemical structure (sulphonamides, sulphonylureas, thiazide, diuretics, paraphenylenediamine hydrochloride, and azo dyes). In these cases benzocaine may be considered a detector of allergy to 'para group'

substances (substances containing a *p*-amino substituted benzene ring).

Cinchocaine (contained in Proctosedyl) is a quinoline derivative and does not cross-react with benzocaine, but may do so with clioquinol. It is well recognized as a sensitizer (Wilson 1966).

Lignocaine is an aminoacyl amide not chemically related to benzocaine or cinchocaine. It is widely used as a local anaesthetic and for cardiac arrhythmias and in some topical preparations (e.g. Betnovate rectal ointment). Contact allergy from lignocaine is very rare but has been described (Nurse and Rosner 1983).

Preservative and stabilizers   Preservatives and stabilizers are perhaps the commonest cause of medicament sensitization. Two per cent of patients patch tested to ethylenediamine (a stabilizer present in Tri-Adcortyl cream and also used as a solvent, corrosion inhibitor, and lubricant in industry) produce positive reactions (Eriksen 1975). Such patients are at risk of developing erythroderma if they later receive aminophylline (85% theophylline and 15% ethylenediamine) (Bernstein and Lorincz 1979).

A number of antihistamines (antazoline, chloropyrilene, methapyrilene, pyrilamine, promethazine and tripelennamine) are derivatives of ethylenediamine and should be avoided in patients sensitive to it. The risk of reaction, however, does not appear to be very great (King and Beck 1983).

Parabens (hydroxybenzoates) are effective preservatives for cosmetics, drugs and food. While they are not strong sensitizers, allergy to them is an especial problem in patients with leg ulcers, in contrast to their use in cosmetics, where a positive patch test is not incompatible with their continued use — part of the 'parabens paradox'. Systemic eczematization in patients sensitive to parabens has occurred as a consequence of the presence of parabens in preparations of lignocaine (Aeling and Nuss 1974) and ampicillin (Carradori *et al.* 1990). Sensitized patients have the potential to cross-react to the so-called 'para substances' discussed with benzocaine. Reports of such cross-reactions are, however, rare. There has been a tendency to replace parabens in creams with a concomitant increase in sensitivity to the substituted preservatives, such as sorbic acid (Coyle *et al.* 1981).

Contact urticaria

Contact urticaria refers to a weal-and-flare response elicited within a few minutes to an hour after the skin is exposed to certain rapidly absorbable agents (Odom and Maibach 1976). It may be divided into non-immunological (Type A) and immunological (Type B and IgE-mediated) categories; of these the non-immunological is the more common.

Type A contact urticaria may be caused by Trafuril (a nicotinic acid ester), dimethyl sulphoxide, sorbic acid, benzoic acid, and cinnamic acid (Fisher 1990).

Type B, immunological, contact urticaria is the more significant, as later systemic administration of the drug or its relatives may induce anaphylaxis. It has been described as being caused by the following drugs: bacitracin, cephalosporins, chloramphenicol, gentamicin, neomycin, penicillin, streptomycin, benzocaine, and mustine hydrochloride (Fisher 1990).

An important non-medicinal but medical problem is that of contact urticaria and generalized reaction, including anaphylaxis, to latex (the sap from the rubber tree, *Hevea brasiliensis*), which may be present in surgical gloves and be a cause of symptoms both to the operator and the operated upon (Tan *et al.* 1997).

References

Aeling, J.L, and Nuss, D.D. (1974). Systemic eczematous 'contact type'dermatitis medicamentosa caused by parabens. *Arch. Dermatol.* 110, 640.

Alanko, K. (1994). Topical provocation of fixed drug eruption: a study of 30 patients. *Contact Dermatitis* 31, 25.

Alanko, K., Stubb, S. and Kaupinnen, K. (1989). Cutaneous drug reactions: clinical types and causative agents. A five year study of in-patients (1981–1985). *Acta Derm. Venereol.* (Stockh.) 69, 223.

Anderson, J.A.R. and Ead, R.D. (1979). Percutaneous salicylate poisoning. *Clin. Exp. Dermatol.* 4, 349.

Arndt, K.A. and Jick, H. (1976). Rates of cutaneous reactions to drugs. A report of the Boston Collaborative Drug Surveillance Program. *JAMA* 235, 918.

Baird, B.J. and De Villez, R.L. (1988). Widespread bullous fixed drug eruption mimicking toxic epidermal necrolysis. *Int. J. Dermatol.* 27, 170.

Bandmann, H.J., Calman, C.D., Cronin, E. *et al.* (1972). Dermatitis from applied medicaments. *Arch. Dermatol.* 106, 335.

Baran, R., Dawber, R., Haneke, E. *et al.* (1996). In *A Text Atlas of Nail Disorders*, p. 72. Martin Dunitz, London.

Barker, J.N.W. and MacDonald, D.M. (1988). Eruptive dysplastic naevi following renal transplantation. *Clin. Exp. Dermatol.* 13, 123.

Batchelor, J.R., Welsh, K.I., Tinoco, R.M., *et al.* (1980). Hydralazine-induced systemic lupus erythematosus: influence of HLA-DR and sex on susceptibility. *Lancet* i, 1107.

Bauer, F. (1981). Quinacrine hydrochloride drug eruption (tropical lichenoid dermatitis): its early and late sequelae and its malignant potential. *J. Am. Acad. Dermatol.* 4, 239.

Bauer, K.A. (1993). Coumarin-induced skin necrosis. *Arch. Dermatol.* 129, 766.

Bencini, P.L., Montagnino, G., Sala, F., *et al.* (1986). Cutaneous lesions in 67 cyclosporin-treated renal transplant recipients. *Dermatologica* 172, 24.

Bernstein, J.E. and Lorincz, A.L. (1979). Ethylenediamine-induced exfoliative erythroderma. *Arch. Dermatol.* 115, 360.

Berth-Jones, J. and Hutchinson, P.E. (1995). Novel cycle changes in scalp hair are caused by etretinate therapy. *Br. J. Dermatol.* 132, 367.

Bigby, M., Jick, S., Jick, H., *et al.* (1986). Drug-induced cutaneous reactions: a report from the Boston Collaborative Drug Surveillance Program on 15,438 consecutive inpatients 1975 to 1982. *JAMA* 256, 3358.

Bork, K. (1988a). In *Cutaneous Side Effects of Drugs,* p. 318. W.B. Saunders, Philadelphia.

Bork, K. (1988b). In *Cutaneous Side Effects of Drugs*, p. 92. W.B. Saunders, Philadelphia.

Bourke, J.F., Berth-Jones, J., and Hutchinson, P.E. (1993). Hypercalcaemia with topical calcipotriol. *BMJ* 306, 1344.

Boxley, J.D., Dawber, R.P.R., and Summerly, R. (1975). Generalised pustular psoriasis on withdrawal of clobetasol propionate ointment. *BMJ* ii, 255.

Bridges, A.J., Graziano, F.M., Calhoun, W., *et al.* (1990). Hyperpigmentation, neutrophilic alveolitis and erythema nodosum resulting from minocycline. *J. Am. Acad. Dermatol.* 22, 959.

Bronner, A.K. and Hood, A.F. (1983). Cutaneous complications of chemotherapeutic agents. *J. Am. Acad. Dermatol.* 9, 645.

Burden, A.D., Muston, H., and Beck, M.H. (1994). Intolerance and contact allergy to tar and dithranol in psoriasis. *Contact Dermatitis* 31, 185.

Callot, V., Roùjeau, J.L., Bagot, M., *et al.* (1996). Drug-induced pseudolymphoma and hypersensitivity syndrome. *Arch. Dermatol.* 132, 1315.

Carradori, S., Peluso, A.M., and Faccioli, M. (1990). Systemic contact dermatitis due to parabens. *Contact Dermatitis* 22, 238.

Carruthers, R.J.G., August, P.J., and Staughton, R.C.D. (1975). Observations on the systemic effect of topical clobetasol propionate (Dermovate). *BMJ* iv, 203.

Citron, A.P., Halpern, M., McCarton, M., *et al.* (1970). Necrotizing angiitis associated with drug abuse. *N. Engl. J. Med.* 283, 1003.

Cohen, I.S., Mosher, M.B., and O'Keefe, E.J. *et al.* (1973). Cutaneous toxicity of bleomycin therapy. *Arch. Dermatol.* 107, 553.

Coskey, R.J. (1978). Contact dermatitis due to clindamycin. *Arch. Dermatol.* 114, 446.

Coskey, R.J. (1983). Contact dermatitis caused by diphenhydramine hydrochloride. *J. Am. Acad. Dermatol.* 8, 204.

Cotterill, J.A. (1979). Perioral dermatitis. *Br. J. Dermatol.* 101, 259.

Cox, N.H. and Popple, A.W. (1996). Persistent erythema and pruritus, with confluent histiocytic skin infiltrate, following the use of hydroxyethylstarch plasma expander. *Br. J. Dermatol.* 134, 353.

Coyle, H.E., Miller, E. and Chapman, R.S. (1981). Sorbic acid sensitivity from Unguentum Merck. *Contact Dermatitis* 7, 56.

Creamer, J.J., Mortimer, P.S., and Powles, T.J. (1995). Mitozantrone-induced onycholysis. A series of five cases. *Clin. Exp. Dermatol.* 20, 459.

Cronin, E. (1980*a*). *Contact Dermatitis,* p. 10. Churchill Livingstone, Edinburgh.

Cronin, E. (1980*b*). *Contact Dermatitis,* p. 209. Churchill Livingstone, Edinburgh.

Cronin, E. (1980*c*). *Contact Dermatitis,* p. 204. Churchill Livingstone, Edinburgh.

Daniel, C.R. and Scher, R.K. (1985). Nail changes caused by systemic drugs or ingestants. *Dermatol. Clin.* 5, 491.

De Kort, W.J.A. and de Groot, A.C. (1989). Clindamycin allergy presenting as rosacea. *Contact Dermatitis* 20, 72.

De Raeve, L., Song, M., and van Maldergem, L. (1988). Adverse cutaneous drug reactions in AIDS. *Br. J. Dermatol.* 119, 521.

Diette, K.M., Gange, R.W., Stern, R.S., *et al.* (1983). Coal tar phototoxicity: kinetics and exposure parameters. *J. Invest. Dermatol.* 81, 437.

Dolman, K.M., Gans R.O., Vervaat T. J. *et al.* (1993). Vasculitis and antineutrophil cytoplasmic autoantibodies associated with propylthiouracil therapy. *Lancet* 342, 651.

Dukes, M.N.G. (ed.) (1975). Blood and blood products. In *Meyler's Side Effects of Drugs,* Vol. 8, p. 725. Associated Scientific Publishers, Amsterdam.

Dwyer, J.M., Kenicer, K., Thompson, B.T. *et al.* (1989). Vasculitis and retinoids. *Lancet* ii, 494.

Eriksen, K.E. (1975). Allergy to ethylenediamine. *Arch. Dermatol.* 111, 791.

Evans, S. (1977). Arsenic and cancer. *Br. J. Dermatol.* 97 (Suppl. 15), 13.

Felix, R.H. and Comaish, J.S. (1974). The value of patch and other skin tests in drug eruptions. *Lancet* i, 1017.

Felix, R.H., Ive, F.A., and Dahl, M.C.G. (1974). Cutaneous and ocular reactions to practolol. *BMJ* iv, 321.

Ferguson, J. (1988). Drug induced photosensitivity. In *Dermatology in Five Continents,* p. 972. Springer-Verlag, Berlin.

Ferguson, J. and Johnson, B.E. (1986). Photosensitivity due to retinoids: clinical and laboratory studies. *Br. J. Dermatol.* 115, 275.

Ferguson, J., Addo, H.A., McGill, P.E., *et al.* (1982). A study of benoxaprofen-induced photosensitivity. *Br. J. Dermatol.* 107, 429.

Ferguson, J., Addo, H.A., Jones, S., *et al.* (1985). A study of cutaneous photosensitivity induced by amiodarone. *Br. J. Dermatol.* 113, 537.

Fernandez, L., Maquiera, E., Rodriguez, F., *et al.* (1996). Systemic contact dermatitis from miconazole. *Contact Dermatitis* 34, 217.

Fisher, A.A. (1986). Non eczematous contact dermatitis. In *Contact Dermatitis,* p. 100. Lea and Febiger, Philadelphia.

Fisher, A.A. (1990). Contact urticaria due to occupational exposures. In *Occupational Skin Disease* (ed. R.M. Adams), p. 113. W.B. Saunders, Philadelphia.

Fitzgerald, D.A., Heagerty, A.H.M., Stephens, M., *et al.* (1994). Follicular toxic pustuloderma associated with allopurinol. *Clin. Exp. Dermatol.* 19, 243.

Fitzpatrick, J.E. (1992). New histopathological findings in drug eruptions. *Dermatol. Clin.* 10, 19.

Forsheck, M., Hovmark, A., and Skog, E. (1976). Patch testing, tuberculin testing and sensitization with dinitrochlorobenzene and nitrosodimethylamine of patients with atopic dermatitis. *Acta Derm. Venereol.* (Stockh.) 56, 135.

Fregert, S. (1976). Respiratory symptoms with piperazine patch testing. *Contact Dermatitis* 2, 61.

Friedman, P.S., Moss, C., Shuster, S., *et al.* (1983). Quantitation of sensitization and responsiveness to dinitrochlorobenzene in normal subjects. *Br. J. Dermatol.* 109 (Suppl. 25), 86.

Gold, M.H., Holy, A.K., and Roenigk, H.H. Jr. (1988). Betablocking drugs and psoriasis. A review of cutaneous side effects and retrospective analysis of their effects on psoriasis. *J. Am. Acad. Dermatol.* 19, 837.

Granstein, R.D. and Sober, A.J. (1981). Drug and heavy metal induced hyperpigmentation. *J. Am. Acad. Dermatol.* 5, 1.

Green, C. and Lowe, J.G. (1992). Contact allergy to piroxicam gel. *Contact Dermatitis* 27, 261.

Greenberg, R.D. (1979). Acne vulgaris associated with antigonadotrophic (Danazol) therapy *Cutis* 24, 431.

Guin, J.D. (1981). Complications of topical hydrocortisone. *J. Am. Acad. Dermatol.* 4, 417.

Guldager, H. (1987). Halothane allergy as a cause of acne. *Lancet,* i, 1211.

Gupta, A.K., Cardella, C.J., and Haberman, H.F. (1986). Cutaneous malignant neoplasms in patients with renal transplants. *Arch. Dermatol.* 122, 1288.

Haarms, M. (1980). Haarausfall und Haarveränderungen nach Kolchizintherapie. *Hautarzt* 31, 161.

Halevy, S., Grunwald, M.H., Sandbank, M., *et al.* (1990). Macrophage migration inhibition factor (MIF) in drug eruption. *Arch. Dermatol.* 126, 48.

Halsey, J.P. and Cardoe, N. (1982). Benoxaprofen: side effect profile in 300 patients. *BMJ* 284, 1365.

Handfield-Jones, S.E., Jenkins, R.E., Whittaker, S.J., *et al.* (1993). The anticonvulsant hypersensitivity syndrome. *Br. J. Dermatol.* 129, 175.

Harland, C.C. and Mortimer, P.S. (1992). Laxative induced contact dermatitis. *Contact Dermatitis* 27, 268.

Healsmith, M.F., Graham-Brown, R.A.C., and Burns, D.A. (1991). Erythromelalgia. *Clin. Exp. Dermatol.* 16, 46.

Hjorth, N. and Fregert, S. (1979). In *Textbook of Dermatology* (ed. A. Rook, D.S. Wilkinson, and F.I.G. Ebling), p. 371. Blackwell Scientific, Oxford.

Hjorth, N. and Thomsen, K. (1968). Differences in the sensitizing capacity of neomycin in creams and ointments. *Br. J. Dermatol.* 80, 163.

Hoffbrand, B.I. (1979). Peripheral skin necrosis complicating beta-blockade. *BMJ* i, 1082.

Holmberg, L., Boman, G. and Bottiger, L.E. (1980). Adverse reactions to nitrofurantoin: an analysis of 921 cases *Am. J. Med.* 69, 733.

Houwerzijl, J., DeGast, G.C., and Nater, J.P. (1974). Tests for drug allergy. *Lancet*, ii, 655.

Ive, F.A. and Marks, R. (1968). Tinea incognito. *BMJ* iii, 149.

Jadassuhn, J. (1896). Zur Kenntnis der Arzneiexantheme. *Arch. Dermatol. Syphilol.* 34, 103.

Jerez, J., Rodriguez, F., Garces, M., *et al.* (1990). Allergic contact dermatitis from budesonide. *Contact Dermatitis* 22, 231.

Job, C.K., Yoder, L., Jacobsen, R.R., *et al.* (1990). Skin pigmentation from clofazimine therapy in leprosy patients: a reappraisal. *J. Am. Acad. Dermatol.* 23, 236.

Jones, C. and Bleehan, S.S. (1977). Acne induced by PUVA treatment. *BMJ* ii, 866.

Katugampola, G. and Katugampola, S. (1990). Chloroquine and psoriasis. *Int. J. Dermatol.* 29, 153.

Kerdel, F.A., Fraker, D.L., and Haynes, A. (1984). Necrotizing vasculitis from radiographic contrast media. *J. Am. Acad. Dermatol.* 10, 25.

Kerker, B.J. and Hood, A.F. (1989). Chemotherapy-induced cutaneous reactions. *Semin. Dermatol.* 8, 173.

Kernekamp, A.S. and van Ketel W.G. (1980). Persistence of patch test reactions to clioquinol (Vioform) and cross-sensitization. *Contact Dermatitis* 6, 455.

Kew, M.C., Mzamane, D., Smith, A.G., *et al.* (1977). MSH levels in doxorubicin-induced hyperpigmentation. *Lancet* i, 811.

King, C.M. and Beck, M. (1983). Oral promethazine hydrochloride in ethylenediamine sensitive patients. *Contact Dermatitis* 9, 444.

Kiraly, C.L., Collan, Y., and Alen, M. (1987). Effect of testosterone and anabolic steroids on the size of sebaceous glands in power athletes. *Am. J. Dermatopathol.* 9, 515.

Kraft, D. and Wide, L. (1976). Clinical patterns and results in radioallergosorbent tests (RAST) and skin tests in penicillin allergy. *Br. J. Dermatol.* 94, 593.

Kuokkanen, K. (1972). Drug eruptions: a series of 464 cases in the Department of Dermatology, University of Turku, Finland during 1966–70. *Acta Allergologica* 27, 407.

Kuske, H. and Krebs, A. (1964). Hyperpigmentierungen von Typus des Chloasmus nach Behandlung mit Hydrantoin Preparaten. *Dermatologica* 129, 121.

Lawrence, C.M. and Dahl, M.G.C. (1984). Two patterns of skin ulceration induced by methotrexate in patients with psoriasis. *J. Am. Acad. Dermatol.* 11, 1059.

Leigh, I.M., Kennedy, C.T.C., Ramsey, J.D., *et al.* (1979). Mepacrine pigmentation in systemic lupus erythematosus. *Br. J. Dermatol.* 101, 147.

Lewis, F.M., Harrington, C.I., and Gawkrodger, D.J. (1994). Contact sensitivity in pruritus vulvae: a common and manageable problem. *Contact Dermatitis* 31, 264.

Leyden, J.J. and Kligman, A.M. (1977a). The case for steroid-antibacterial combinations. *Br. J. Dermatol.* 96, 179.

Leyden, J.J. and Kligman, A.M. (1977b) Contact sensitivity to benzoyl peroxide. *Contact Dermatitis* 3, 273.

Lindelof, B., Sigurgeirsson, B., Tegner, E. *et al.* (1991). PUVA and cancer: a large scale epidemiological study. *Lancet*, 338, 91.

Litt, J.Z. and Pawlak, W.A. (1997). In *Drug Eruption Reference Manual,* p. 490. Parthenon Publishing Group, New York, London.

Logan, R.A., McFadden, J.P. and Eady, R.A.J. (1988). Reactivation of cutaneous radionecrosis associated with methotrexate therapy for psoriasis. *Clin. Exp. Dermatol.* 13, 350.

Lowe, N.J. and Ridgway, H.B. (1978). Generalised pustular psoriasis precipitated by lithium carbonate. *Arch. Dermatol.* 114, 1788.

Macdonald, R.H. and Beck, M. (1983). Neomycin: a review with particular reference to dermatological usage. *Clin. Exp. Dermatol.* 8, 249.

McGovern, B., Garan, H., Kelley, E., *et al.* (1983). Adverse reactions during treatment with amiodarone hydrochloride. *BMJ* 287, 175.

McKerrow, K.J. and Greig, D.E. (1986). Piroxicam induced photosensitive dermatitis. *J. Am. Acad. Dermatol.* 15, 1237.

Mahler, R., Sissons, W., and Watters, K. (1986). Pigmentation induced by quinidine therapy. *Arch. Dermatol.* 122, 1062.

Mallon, E. and Dawber, R.P.R. (1994). Longitudinal melanonychia induced by minocycline. *Br. J. Dermatol.* 130, 794.

Manzi, S., Kraus, V.B., and St. Clair, E.W. (1989). An unusual photoactivated skin eruption. Quinidine-induced livedo reticularis. *Arch. Dermatol.* 125, 417.

Marshall, I.P. and Schneider, R.P. (1977). Systemic argyria secondary to topical silver nitrate. *Arch. Dermatol.* 113, 1077.

Mathias, C.G.T., Maibach, H.I., and Epstein, J. (1978). Allergic contact dermatitis due to para-aminobenzoic acid. *Arch. Dermatol.* 114, 1665.

Merenich, J.A., Hannon, R.N., Gentry, R.H., *et al.* (1989). Azidothymidine-induced hyperpigmentation mimicking primary adrenal insufficiency. *Am. J. Med.* 86, 469.

Mitchell, J.C. (1978). Day 7 (D7) patch testing reading — valuable or not? *Contact Dermatitis* 4, 139.

Monk, B., Cunliffe, W.J., Layton, A.M., *et al.* (1993). Acne induced by inhaled corticosteroids. *Clin. Exp. Dermatol.* 18, 148.

Mullick, F.G., McAllister, H.A., Wagner, B.M., *et al.* (1979). Drug related vasculitis. *Hum. Pathol.* 10, 313.

Nurse, D.S. and Rosner, S.A. (1983). Contact dermatitis due to lignocaine. *Contact Dermatitis* 9, 513.

Odom R.B. and Maibach, H.I. (1976). Contact urticaria: a different contact dermatitis. *Cutis* 188, 672.

Ogg, G.S., Bhogal, B.S., Hashimoto, T., *et al.* (1997). Ramipril-associated lichen planus pemphigoides. *Br. J. Dermatol.* 136, 412.

Okada, N., Moriya, K., Nishida, K., *et al.* (1989). Skin pigmentation associated with minocycline therapy. *Br. J. Dermatol.* 121, 247.

Oliwiecki, S. and Burton, J.L. (1988). Severe acne due to isoniazid. *Clin. Exp. Dermatol.* 13, 276.

Osawa, J., Naiton, S., Aihara, M., *et al.* (1990). Evaluation of skin test reactions in patients with non-immediate type drug eruptions. *J. Dermatol.* (Tokyo) 17, 235.

Papi, M., Didona, B., De Pita, O., *et al.* (1993). Multiple skin tumours on light exposed areas during long-term treatment with hydroxyurea. *J. Am. Acad. Dermatol.* 28, 485.

Paquet, P. and Pierard, G.E. (1997). Erythema multiforme and toxic epidermal necrolysis: a comparative study. *Am. J. Dermatopathol.* 19, 127.

Paramsothy, Y., Collins, M., and Smith, A.G. (1988). Contact dermatitis in patients with leg ulcers. The prevalence of late positive reactions and evidence against systemic ampliative allergy. *Contact Dermatitis* 18, 30.

Paul, C., Wolkenstein, P., Prost, C., *et al.* (1997). Drug-induced linear IgA disease: target antigens are heterogeneous. *Br. J. Dermatol.* 136, 406.

Phillips, W.G., Vaughan-Jones, S., Jenkins, R., *et al.* (1994). Captopril-induced lichenoid eruption. *Clin. Exp. Dermatol.* 19, 317.

Pletcher, W.D., Brody, G.C., and Myers, M.C. (1963). Haemochromatosis following prolonged iron therapy in a patient with hereditary nonspherocytic hemolytic anemia. *Am. J. Med. Sci.* 246, 27.

Pullen, H., Wright, N., and Murdoch, J. McC. (1967). Hypersensitivity reactions to antibacterial drugs in infectious mononucleosis. *Lancet* ii, 1176.

Quesada, J.R. and Gutterman, J.U. (1986). Psoriasis and alpha-interferon. *Lancet* i, 1466.

Rohrhorn, W. and Brauninger, W. (1987). Thioridazine photoallergy. *Contact Dermatitis* 17, 241.

Roten, S.V., Mainetti, C., Donath, R., *et al.* (1995). Enalapril-induced lichen planus-like eruption. *J. Am. Acad. Dermatol.* 32, 293.

Roujeau, J.C. and Stern, R.S. (1994). Severe adverse cutaneous reactions to drugs. *N. Engl. J. Med.* 331, 1272.

Rudzki, E., Grzywa, Z., and Maciejowska, E. (1976). Drug reaction with positive patch tests to chloramphenicol. *Contact Dermatitis* 2, 181.

Ruocco, V. and Sacredoti, G. (1991). Pemphigus and bullous pemphigoid due to drugs. *Int. J. Dermatol.* 30, 307.

Sabroe, R.A. and Kobza Black, A. (1997). Angiotensin-converting enzyme (ACE) inhibitors and angio-oedema. *Br. J. Dermatol.* 136, 153.

Santa Cruz, D.J., Marcus, M.D., Prioleau, P.G., *et al.* (1981). Pemphigus-like lesions induced by D-penicillamine. *Am. J. Dermatopathol.* 3, 85.

Sarkany, I. and Gaylarde, P.M. (1978). Role of lymphocyte transformation in drug allergy. *Australas. J. Dermatol,* 19, 45.

Savill, J.S., Chia, Y., and Pusey, C.D. (1988). Minimal change nephropathy and pemphigus vulgaris associated with penicillamine treatment of rheumatoid arthritis. *Clin. Nephrol.* 29, 267.

Schopf, E., Sluhmer, A., Rzany, B., *et al.* (1991). Toxic epidermal necrolysis and Stevens–Johnson syndrome. An epidemiological study from West Germany. *Arch. Dermatol.* 127, 839.

Shall, L., Lucas, G.S., Whittaker, J.A., *et al.* (1988). Painful red hands: a side-effect of leukaemia therapy. *Br. J. Dermatol.* 119, 249.

Sheehan-Dare, R.A., Goodfield, M.J.D., and Rowell, N.R. (1991). The effect of oral indomethacin on psoriasis treated with the Ingram regime. *Br. J. Dermatol.* 125, 253.

Shelton, D. and Goulding, R. (1979). Silver poisoning associated with an anti-smoking lozenge. *BMJ* i, 267.

Shelley, W.B. and Bennett, R.G. (1972). Primary contact sensitization site: a determinant for the localisation of a diphenhydramine eruption. *Acta Derm. Venereol.* (Stockh.) 52, 376.

Shuttleworth, D., Marks, R., Griffin, P.J.A., *et al.* (1987). Dysplastic epidermal change in immunosuppressed patients with renal transplants. *Q. J. Med.* 64, 2609.

Shuttleworth, D., Marks, R., Griffin, P.J.A., *et al.* (1989). Epidermal dysplasia and cyclosporin therapy in renal transplant patients: a comparison with azathioprine. *Br. J. Dermatol.* 120, 551.

Sigal-Nahum, M., Konqui, A., Gauliet, A., *et al.* (1988). Linear fixed drug eruption. *Br. J. Dermatol.* 118, 849.

Simon, R.A. (1984). Adverse reactions to drug additives. *J. Allergy Clin. Immunol.* 74, 623.

Smith, A.G., Shuster, S., Thody, A.J., *et al.* (1977). Chloasma, oral contraceptives and plasma immunoreactive beta-MSH. *J. Invest. Dermatol.* 68,169.

Smith, R.W., Leppard, B., Barnett, N.L., *et al.* (1995). Chrysiasis revisited: a clinical and pathological study. *Br. J. Dermatol.* 133, 671.

Sowden, J.M. and Smith, A.G. (1990). Multifocal fixed drug eruption mimicking erythema multiforme. *Clin. Exp. Dermatol.* 15, 387.

Stern, R.S., Nichols, K.T. and Vakeva, L.H. (1997). Malignant melanoma in patients treated for psoriasis with methoxsalen (Psoralen) and ultraviolet A radiation (PUVA). *N. Engl. J. Med.* 336, 1041.

Stevens, H.P., Ostlere, I.S., Regent, R.H.J., *et al.* (1993). Pellagra secondary to 5-fluorouracil. *Br. J. Dermatol.* 128, 578.

Tagami, H., Tatsuta, K., Iwatski, K., *et al.* (1983). Delayed hypersensitivity in ampicillin-induced toxic epidermal necrolysis. *Arch. Dermatol.* 119, 910.

Tan, B.B., Lear, J.T., Watts, J., *et al.* (1997). Perioperative collapse: prevalence of latex allergy in patients sensitive to anaesthetic agents. *Contact Dermatitis* 36, 47.

Tosti, A., Misciali, C., Piraccini, B.M., *et al.* (1994). Drug-induced hair loss and hair growth: incidence, management and avoidance. *Drug Safety* 10, 310.

Valsecchi, R., Pansera, B., Leghissa, P., *et al.* (1996). Allergic contact dermatitis of the eyelids and conjunctivitis from diclofenac. *Contact Dermatitis* 34, 150.

Van den Haute, V., Antoine, J.L. and Lachapelle, J.M. (1989). Histological discriminant criteria between lichenoid drug eruption and idiopathic lichen planus: retrospective study on selected samples. *Dermatologica,* 179, 10.

van Schooten, F.J., Moonen, E.J.C., Rhijnsburger, E., *et al.* (1995). Dermal uptake of polycyclic aromatic hydrocarbons after hairwash with coal-tar shampoo. *Lancet* 344, 1505.

Verbov, J.L. (1970). Sensitivity to sodium fusidate. *Contact Dermatitis Newsletter* 7, 153.

Wakelin, S.H. and James, M.P. (1995). Diltiazem-induced acute generalised exanthematous pustulosis. *Clin. Exp. Dermatol.* 20, 341.

Weber, G. (1974). Combined 8-methoxypsoralen and black light therapy for psoriasis. *Br. J. Dermatol.* 90, 317.

Wennersten, G., Thume, P., Brodthagen, H., *et al.* (1984). The Scandinavian multicentre photopatch study: preliminary results. *Contact Dermatitis* 10, 305.

Wilkin, J.K. (1983). Flushing reaction. In *Recent Advances in Dermatology* (ed. A.J. Rook and H.I Maibach), Vol. 6, p. 157. Churchill Livingstone, Edinburgh.

Wilkin, J.K., Hammond, J.J., and Kirkendale, W.M. (1980). The captopril-induced eruption: a possible mechanism — cutaneous kinin potentiation. *Arch. Dermatol.* 116, 902.

Wilkinson, S.M. (1994). Hypersensitivity to topical corticosteroids. *Clin. Exp. Dermatol.*. 19, 1.

Wilkinson, S.M. and English, J.S.C. (1992). Patch tests are poor detectors of corticosteroid allergy. *Contact Dermatitis* 26, 67.

Wilkinson, S., Wilkinson, J.D., and Wilkinson, D.S. (1987). Medicament contact dermatitis: risk sites. *Boll. Dermatol. Allerg. Prof.* 2, 21.

Wilkinson, S.M., Smith, A.G., and English, J.S.C. (1992). Erythroderma following intradermal injection of the corticosteroid budesonide. *Contact Dermatitis* 27, 121.

Wilkinson, S.M., Smith, A.G., Davies, K.J., *et al.* (1993). Suspected cutaneous drug toxicity in rheumatoid arthritis — an evaluation. *Br. J. Rheumatol.* 32, 798.

Wilson, H.T.H. (1966). Dermatitis from anaesthetic ointments. *Practitioner* 197, 673.

Wilson, J.T., Hojer, B., Tomson, G., *et al.* (1978). High incidence of concentration-dependent skin reaction in children treated with phenytoin. *BMJ* i, 1583.

Winter, G.D. and Burton, J.L. (1976). Experimentally induced steroid atrophy in the domestic pig and man. *Br. J. Dermatol.* 94, 107.

Wormser, G.P., Kornblee, L.V., and Gottfried, E.B. (1982). Cutaneous necrosis following peripheral vasopressin therapy. *Cutis* 29, 249.

Yates, P. and Jones, S. (1993). Heparin skin necrosis — an important indicator of potentially fatal heparin sensitivity. *Clin. Exp. Dermatol.* 18, 138.

Yoder, F.W. (1975). Acneiform eruption due to lithium carbonate. *Arch. Dermatol.* 111, 396.

Zachary, C.B., Slater, D.N., Holt, D.W., *et al.* (1984). The pathogenesis of amiodarone-induced pigmentation and photosensitivity. *Br. J. Dermatol.* 110, 451.

Zax, R.H., Hodge, S.J., and Callen, J.P. (1990) Cutaneous leucocytoclastic vasculitis: serial histopathological evaluation demonstrates the dynamic nature of the infiltrate. *Arch. Dermatol.* 126, 69.

20. Neurological disorders

P. G. BLAIN and R. J. M. LANE

Introduction

When studying the neurotoxicity of drugs and other compounds it is sometimes useful to consider the nervous system as a federation of organ systems, each with different morphology and functional roles which are reflected in the predominant biochemical processes of the constituent cells. This heterogeneity affects the susceptibility of the individual cells or tracts to a specific toxic insult. Drugs may interfere with the functioning of neurones, neuroglia, and muscles at several levels so that neurological adverse effects have a broad spectrum of expression, from mild and possibly subtle changes in mental activity and behaviour to severe clinical neurological disorders.

Many of these adverse reactions can be classified as Type A (see Chapter 5) using our knowledge of the pharmacokinetics and pharmacodynamics of the drug. Such classification applies to adverse effects such as coma, syncope, seizures, some involuntary movement disorders, and many of the neuromuscular disorders. However, a significant number of neurological adverse reactions are not so classifiable, often because of ignorance of the underlying toxic mechanisms. As we increase understanding of the interaction between a drug's required and unwanted effects, and an individual's genetic and environmental background (see below), so many of the reactions currently classified as Type B may be seen to be Type A effects.

There is a natural decrement in both neuronal numbers and functional efficiency with age. Increasing evidence suggests that the effects of some neurotoxic chemicals and drugs may not become apparent unless neuronal numbers and function are below a critical threshold which then produce deficits that are apparent to both the individual and the clinician. In some cases of

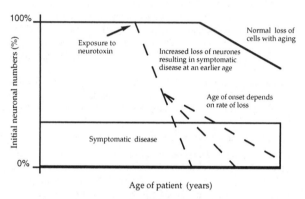

FIG. 20.1

Increased rate of loss of neurones following exposure to a neurotoxin, producing symptomatic neurological disease at an earlier age than normal

parkinsonism a genetic variation in the response of cells in the nigrostriatal tracts to neurotoxic oxidative stressmay exist. The adverse effects of exposure to a drug may not be apparent unless the functional activity and number of dopaminergic cells in these tracts has fallen below a critical threshold (Figure 20.1).

Genetic polymorphisms

Genetic polymorphisms in drug metabolism are increasingly being seen to also play a significant role in an individual's susceptibility to drug toxicity. The clinical consequences of slow acetylator phenotype include increased susceptibility to peripheral neuropathies produced by isoniazid, hydralazine, and dapsone. Similarly, following the administration of methoin, poor metabolisers of this drug have increased somnolence and intellectual impairment (Relling 1989). Phenotypic variation in plasma esterases, especially cholinesterases, may contribute to the toxicity of some anticholinesterases affecting not only the toxicity of these compounds directly, but also influencing their metabolism and elimination.

Genetic differences in the activity of a specific enzyme may be associated, in an individual, with an increased risk of developing certain neurological disorders. It is not yet clear how important these differences are for many drug-related adverse neurological effects, since experience to date has been principally with non-drug chemicals. Nevertheless, useful risk indicators can be derived.

Acetylator status

Acetylation is a conjugation reaction, usually for aromatic amines or hydrazines, where an acetyl group is transferred from acetyl co-enzyme A, by acetyltransferases, to receptor amines resulting in the formation of an amide. Many drugs and other chemicals are metabolised by this pathway and the slow gene frequency in a population varies from 20 to 90 per cent showing marked racial differences. Inheritance is as an autosomal recessive trait. Isoniazid is a potent irritant of the central nervous system, but an isoniazid-induced polyneuropathy was the first neurological adverse reaction to be recognized as associated with slow acetylation (Weber *et al.* 1983). The neurotoxic effect has been shown to be a consequence of isoniazid-induced vitamin B6 (pyridoxine) deficiency. A modest excess of slow acetylators in motor neurone disease and faster acetylators in Parkinson's disease, has been reported (Heathfield *et al.* 1990).

Debrisoquine-4-hydroxylase deficiency

Debrisoquine is metabolised by ring hydroxylation and polymorphic differences in metabolism have been established. The phenotype is determined from the ratio of the percentage of a dose excreted as unchanged debrisoquine to that excreted as the metabolite, 4-hydroxydebrisoquine (metabolic ratio). Family studies on the phenotype have indicated that it is an autosomal recessive trait with the enzyme deficiency present in approximately six to eight per cent of the UK population. Mutations in regulatory genes seem to be involved and at least four P-450 proteins are involved (Gonzalez *et al.* 1987, 1988, 1989). Cloning and sequencing of cDNAs from the livers of poor metabolisers have identified at least three variant RNAs, but as the products of intron mutants producing an incorrectly spliced P-450 pre-RNA.

Several studies of this phenotype have found no differences from the general population in the frequencies of Parkinson's disease, amyotrophic lateral sclerosis, or dementia. However, some studies do suggest a shift in the metabolic ratio in favour of poor metabolism in these patients, although the percentage of poor metabolisers is not significantly different from controls (Barbeau *et al.* 1985; Steventon *et al.* 1989*a*). Phenotype studies may not be the best predictors of abnormal genotypes since recent molecular studies suggest a modest but significant increase in poor metaboliser mutations in Parkinson's disease (Smith *et al.* 1992).

Sulphur metabolism

The phenotype for this oxidation polymorphism is determined by measuring sulphur oxides in urine following the administration of *S*-carboxymethyl-cysteine. The enzyme involved, cysteine dioxygenase, is the rate limiting step in the conversion of cysteine to sulphate. Patients with Parkinson's disease, amyotrophic lateral sclerosis, and presumed Alzheimer's disease are, as a group, very poor metabolisers. Cysteine dioxygenase has also been found to be deficient in Hallervorden–Spatz disease. The results suggest that individuals born with underactivity of this metabolic pathway are less capable of dealing with sulphur compounds used as drugs or found in the environment and food. *Brassica* vegetables (cabbages, etc.) have a high sulphur load and Parkinson's disease has been related to a high intake of raw vegetables. Sulphur availability may reduce the capacity to detoxify drugs and compounds, such as cyanide and heavy metals, and also be responsible for excess production of free radicals.

Monoamine oxidase B

MPTP (1-methyl-4-phenyl-1,2,3,6-tetrahydropyridine), a contaminant of illicit designer drugs, causes selective neuronal death, resulting in a neurological disorder similar to Parkinson's disease (Davis *et al.* 1979; Adams and Odunze 1991). The neurotoxic metabolite is the *N*-methyl-4-phenyl pyridinium ion (MPP+). Conversion, via the enzyme monoamine oxidase B (MAO-B), is an intoxication step when it occurs in the brain, but could be considered a detoxification if it occurs outside the brain, such as in the liver or gut, since MPP+ cannot cross the blood–brain barrier. MAO-B is found in platelets and there is evidence that the activity of this enzyme is closely related to that in the liver and brain. MPTP is a relatively simple chemical and similar compounds could be derived from tryptamine metabolism, endogenously or exogenously, or possibly from plants in food (Ramsden and Williams 1985). There is also the possibility that β-carbolines, tetrahydroisoquinolones, and trichlorethylene share the same pathway for metabolism and mechanism and site of toxicity with MPP+.

A study using phenylethylamine as substrate found an increased MAO-B activity in untreated patients with Parkinson's disease, although there was overlap with the normal range. When dopamine was used as substrate there was a much reduced activity. There may be several isoenzymes of MAO-B which could function as risk markers for screening, since inefficient enzymes may allow MPTP, or similar compounds, to reach the brain before conversion to MPP+. Alternatively, the reduced metabolism of dopamine in Parkinson's disease may produce a rise in dopamine levels, resulting in shunting down other metabolic pathways with the production of toxic metabolites, such as an orthohydroxylated derivative of dopamine, which has neuroexcitotoxic properties.

Methylation

The enzyme thiolmethyltransferase (TMT) carries out *S*-methylation, which masks functional chemical groups and reduces water solubility impairing further conjugation (Waring *et al.* 1989). TMT is involved in the detoxification of substances such as hydrogen sulphide and other free sulphydryl compounds including the thioesters of glutathione conjugates (a final common pathway for many toxic xenobiotics). Hydrogen sulphide has a similar toxic mechanism to cyanide, acting as a mitochondrial poison, and it may cause an acquired defect in mitochondrial function similar to that described in Parkinson's disease. Patients with amyotrophic lateral sclerosis have high activity of TMT, when assessed by *in vitro* test systems, but in Parkinson's disease and patients with Alzheimer's disease, low activity is found. The low enzyme activity has a high heritability, but it is possible for some individuals to have reduced activity of the normal enzyme or an isoenzyme. Heavy metals, such as mercury, form toxic derivatives with the enzyme and increased enzyme activity, such as that reported in the motor neurone diseases, might predispose to heavy metal poisoning.

N-methylation is carried out by *N*-methyltransferases, which can act on a number of different substrates, including substituted 4-phenyl pyridines, to form MPTP (Ansher *et al.* 1986). The level of enzyme activity can be determined by measurement of *N*-methylnicotinamide excretion in urine following administration of nicotinamide. In one study, patients with amyotrophic lateral sclerosis had normal excretion but those with Parkinson's disease excreted considerably increased amounts of this *N*-methyl derivative (Green *et al.* 1991).

Summary

Neurological adverse reactions are determined by the rates of absorption, distribution, biotransformation, and excretion as well as the toxicodynamics of a drug. The body's defences against toxic effects are complex and there are considerable interindividual, interracial, and interspecies variations in both toxicokinetics and toxicodynamics. Many of these variations will be dependent on genetic polymorphisms in the specific enzymes involved in the toxic mechanisms. Perhaps uniquely, in the nervous system early damage to neuronal function may not become clinically important until the natural decrease in neuronal numbers and function with age passes a critical threshold. This concept can explain why some neurodegenerative disorders may appear at an unusually early age in certain patients.

In this chapter some of the possible mechanisms underlying neurological adverse drug reactions will be discussed, although for many our knowledge of the pathogenesis is still minimal. It is convenient to classify drug-induced neurological disorders in terms of the presenting clinical syndromes and the neuroanatomical hierarchy, from cerebral cortex to muscle fibre (Lane and Routledge 1983).

Brain and meninges

Coma and encephalopathy

Coma implies bilateral cortical dysfunction or inhibition of the brainstem reticular formation. The clinical features of drug-induced coma are somewhat similar regardless of the drug or mechanisms involved. Typically, the pupillary and corneal reflexes are preserved while other brain-stem reflexes (e.g. the oculocephalic and oculovestibular [caloric] responses) are lost early (Cartlidge 1981; Ashton *et al.* 1989). In very deep coma, however, the pupillary and corneal reflexes may also be lost; indeed, drug overdosage must be excluded before a patient is said to be 'brain-dead'. Generalized flaccidity, with depressed or absent tendon reflexes, and flexor or equivocal plantar responses is typical, although some patients, particularly following tricyclic antidepressant poisoning or drug-induced hypoglycaemia, may have hyperreflexia and extensor plantar responses. Myoclonus and convulsions may also be seen.

Drug-induced coma and encephalopathy can arise in one of three ways: by a primary neurotoxic effect on the central nervous system through interference with synaptic transmission or cellular metabolism; by indirect effects on cerebral metabolism, for example in drug-induced hypoglycaemia, and in hepatic or renal failure; and through alterations in cerebral blood flow, resulting in ischaemic hypoxia. Drugs that produce sudden vasodilatation can cause syncope, due to the collapse of peripheral resistance, systemic and cerebral hypotension, and a diminished cerebral blood flow. Drug-induced hypotension is discussed in detail in Chapter 9.

Primary neurotoxic effects

The vast majority of cases of drug-induced coma are caused by overdose with drugs that are used therapeutically for their action on the central nervous system (Cartlidge 1981). They are principally psychoactive compounds, such as the benzodiazepines, phenothiazines, antidepressants, and narcotics. Coma of this kind can be regarded as a Type A reaction. Primary neurotoxic effects are generally dose related, and more likely to occur under circumstances in which drug elimination or metabolism is reduced. For example, cimetidine is excreted largely unchanged in the urine and its accumulation in renal failure may cause coma (McMillan *et al.* 1978). Lignocaine is predominantly metabolised by the liver, and coma followed administration of a standard dose of this drug to a patient with liver failure (Selden and Sasahara 1967).

Intravenous flumazenil has emerged as a useful therapeutic and diagnostic tool in reversal of coma due to overdose in which benzodiazepines might be implicated (even when a mixture of drugs has been taken) (Chern *et al.* 1993; Weinbroum *et al.* 1996), and flumazenil can also reverse seizures and encephalopathy induced by valproate; benzodiazepines and GABA receptors share functional characteristics (Steinhoff and Stodiek 1993). In opiate poisoning the pupils are markedly constricted, and a hand lens may be required to detect a preserved light reflex. It should be noted that opiates form the basis of many 'over-the-counter' cough suppressants (codeine, pholcodine, and dextromethorphan) and of some antidiarrhoeal agents. Naloxone is a very effective and specific opiate receptor antagonist, and should be administered to all cases of known or suspected opiate overdose. Since its half-life is only 1–2 hours, however, frequently repeated doses or an intravenous infusion may be required to reverse an opiate-induced coma (Blain and Lane 1983a). Recent studies have shown that intermittent cocaine usage may impair functions such as spatial memory, cognitive flexibility, and perceptual motor speed, but paradoxically may improve performance on some verbal functions (Hoff et al. 1996). Abusers also showed changes on EEG power spectral analysis, including paroxysmal alpha rhythms reminiscent of vertex waves in drowsiness (Roemer et al. 1995) (see also section on Seizures).

Recently, a new drug-induced encephalopathy, the 'serotonin syndrome', is being increasingly recognized. This may comprise a number of symptoms, including changes in mental status and behaviour (confusion, anxiety, and agitation), motor dysfunction (tremor, involuntary movements, myoclonus, weakness, hyperreflexia, dysarthria, and ataxia) and autonomic symptoms such as sweating, fever, chills, and diarrhoea (Kudo et al. 1997). In more severe cases, circulatory collapse and features of neuroleptic malignant syndrome (see below) may develop (François et al. 1997). The serotonin syndrome usually arises in patients taking combinations of drugs (and rarely single drugs) which include agents having specific or non-specfic agonist actions at serotonin receptors, including tricyclic antidepressants (particularly serotonin-reuptake inhibitors (SRI), such as fluoxetine, sertraline, and paroxetine). It occurs, therefore, most commonly in the treatment of psychiatric disorders but has also been reported in patients being treated with these drugs for depression in Parkinson's disease, in combination with selegiline (Richard et al. 1997), and in migraine prophylaxis, in combination with sumatriptan or ergot preparations (Mathew et al. 1996). Treatment is generally supportive, but dialysis (François et al. 1997), use of dantrolene (as in the malignant neuroleptic syndrome), and dopamine receptor agonists such as chlorpromazine (Graham 1997) may be required.

Coma and encephalopathy may also develop in association with drugs which might not be considered to have primary actions in the nervous system, and where the mechanisms involved are unclear (Type B reaction). There are literally dozens of reports of this type. Many of the drugs implicated have also been reported to cause seizures (see below). The drugs can be conveniently considered in pharmacological classes.

Anticancer drugs

The encephalopathic effects of certain cytotoxic drugs are being increasingly appreciated. Encephalopathic symptoms of confusion and drowsiness, sometimes accompanied by epileptic phenomena such as myoclonus, have been associated with the use of both established and newer antitumour and anticancer agents. There are reports implicating azacitidine, carmustine, cisplatin (Hitchins and Thomson 1988; Verschraegen et al. 1995), dimethyl sulphoxide, 5-fluorouracil (Takimoto et al. 1996), and paclitaxel (Taxol) (Perry and Warner 1996), while methotrexate can induce a severe demyelinating leucoencephalopathy (Gangi et al. 1980). Ifosfamide may cause a dose-related syndrome of mental dysfunction, ataxia, and seizures, with encephalographic evidence of a cortical abnormality, probably through its principal metabolite, chloroacetaldehyde (Goren et al. 1986). Pathological changes similar to experimental vincristine encephalopathy were observed on brain biopsy in a child with a reversible syndrome due to this drug (Hurwitz et al. 1988). Coma, unassociated with convulsions, may also occur following vincristine therapy (Whittaker et al. 1973).

A number of other drugs used as adjuvants in chemotherapy, and as immunosupressants, can also cause encephalopathy. The role of levamisole in this regard is debated but this drug appeared to precipitate a multifocal inflammatory leucoencephalopathy in a patient treated for melanoma; the cerebral lesions and clinical condition settled with steroids (Chastel and Mabin 1996). The use of OKT3 monoclonal antibodies (Muromonab CD3) has been associated with the development of paralysis, seizures, blindness, and psychotic episodes, notably at the initiation of treatment. The effects may be related to cytokine release induced by the drug (Min and Fallo 1993).

Considerable attention has been paid to the various neurotoxic effects of cyclosporin. Early reports linking this drug to the development of seizures, coma, encephalopathy, paresis, involuntary movements, and visual impairment were frequently obscured by additional drug-related and metabolic factors in bone marrow and organ transplant recipients, but the development of encephalopathy in cardiac transplant recipients, in whom such factors were not pertinent, has clearly demonstrated the drug's neurotoxic effects (Lane et al. 1988). The mechanism is controversial. Neurotoxicity is not clearly related to plasma concentrations of the whole drug, and cyclosporin metabolites (Kunzendorf et al.

1988) or even the drug's solvent (Hoefnagels *et al.* 1988) have been implicated. It is likely that damage to the blood–brain barrier, possibly through effects on endothelial cells, is important in the pathogenesis (Lane *et al.* 1988; Zaal *et al.* 1988). Several reports have described high-signal cortical lesions on MRI imaging, which resolved with clinical recovery after cyclosporin was withdrawn (Lane *et al.* 1988; Baulac *et al.* 1989). These lesions are thought to represent localized vasogenic oedema and cyclosporin neurotoxicity is recognized as one cause of the recently defined 'posterior leucoencephalopathy syndrome' (Hinchey *et al.* 1996). Rarely, the cerebral oedema in cyclosporin encephalopathy can be life-threatening; in one reported case emergency posterior fossa decompression was required for cerebellar oedema (Nussbaum *et al.* 1995).

Anticonvulsants

Anticonvulsants may not only sometimes cause a paradoxical increase in seizure frequency (see section on Seizures) but can also produce encephalopathy. This, again, is generally dose related, although young patients, those with mental retardation and complex epilepsy syndromes, patients on polytherapy, and those with highly epileptic electroencephalographic abnormalities appear to be at greatest risk (Baum 1996). The incidence of such complications has declined with the development of plasma drug concentration monitoring (Chadwick 1981), but paradoxical seizure activity, including non-convulsive status, can be caused by valproate, carbamazepine and vigabatrin, notably in patients with complex partial seizures (Bauer 1996). In coma associated with valproate poisoning, there may be associated gross cerebral oedema (Hintze *et al.* 1987), and the GABA agonist vigabatrin (Reynolds 1990) appears to have a propensity for causing disturbances in mood and behaviour in certain patients (Sander and Hart 1990), especially those with long-standing unstable epilepsy and pre-existing neuropsychiatric abnormalities (Dam 1990; Ring and Reynolds 1990; Robinson *et al.* 1990).

Anti-infectives

A number of anti-infective drugs can precipitate encephalopathy, as well as inducing seizures (see below). These include potent new antibiotics, notably β-lactams and the quinolines (Thomas 1994); most of the cephalosporins; antituberculous agents, particularly isoniazid (Siskind *et al.* 1993); antifungals such as amphotericin B (Walker and Rosenblum 1992); and antimalarials (see section on Seizures). Antiviral agents may also rarely be encephalopathic. Encephalopathy with confusion, immobility, and bradykinesia, sometimes with myoclonus, has been reported following treatment of herpes zoster with vidarabine (Vilter 1986), famiciclovir (Gales and Gales 1996), and aciclovir, in the presence of renal insufficiency (Beales *et al.* 1994).

Antiulcer drugs

The histamine H_2-receptor antagonists cimetidine, ranitidine, and nizatidine have all been reported to induce hallucinations and encephalopathy. Intravenous ranitidine also induced a temporary optic neuropathy in one reported case (Laniado *et al.* 1997).

Heavy metals

Heavy-metal poisoning, from industrial or environmental exposure to lead or mercury, may also cause encephalopathy and coma. Bismuth-containing compounds, such as the bismuth chelate (tripotassium dicitratobismuthate, De-Nol) for peptic ulcer, may be neurotoxic in patients with reduced renal function (Playford *et al.* 1990). Elimination of the drug shows complex kinetics due to storage and variable release rates from different tissues. Bismuth encephalopathy has occurred in epidemics in France. The clinical picture included a prodromal phase with changes in memory and behaviour, unsteadiness, cramps, and myalgia followed by the abrupt development of altered consciousness, myoclonus, and ataxia (Slikkerveer and de Wolff 1989).

A 68-year-old man with a low creatinine clearance who took twice the recommended dose of bismuth chelate daily for 2 months (equivalent to 864 mg bismuth per day), developed global cerebral dysfunction with hallucinations, ataxia, and an abnormal EEG. Whole-blood bismuth concentration was 880 μg per litre but fell to 46 μg per litre 50 days after the drug was withheld and treatment with dimercaprol given. His mental function also recovered (Playford *et al.* 1990).

Organic arsenicals, such as melarsoprol, can cause a severe encephalopathy with seizures and coma (Pialoux *et al.* 1988). The role of aluminium in the development of dialysis encephalopathy is well established. There is evidence that this complication can be reduced by the use of desferrioxamine, but there is a report that this drug can, paradoxically, exacerbate the problem on occasions (Swartz 1985).

Metabolic disturbances

Coma secondary to metabolic disturbances can be caused by drugs such as insulin and the oral antidiabetic drugs in therapeutic doses. Coma may be preceded by seizures in such cases, and hypoglycaemic coma due to sulphonylureas and biguanides is notoriously difficult to reverse, even with glucagon. The incidence of permanent cerebral damage in such cases is high. Severe electrolyte disturbances can rarely cause coma, independently of effects on electrical function of the heart and brain. Coma with severe hyperphosphataemia, hypocalcaemia, hypernatraemia, and hypokalaemia occurred in an elderly woman following an overdose and administration of hypertonic sodium phosphate enema (Knobel and Petchenko 1996). Too rapid a correction of hyponatraemia, arising from the use of the diuretic chlorthalidone, resulted in central pontine myelinolysis and a chronic parkinsonian syndrome (Sadeh and Goldhammer 1993). Coma related to drug-induced hepatic or renal damage is clinically similar to that occurring in hepatic or renal failure from other causes. Hyperreflexia and extensor plantar responses are common, as are rolling eye movements, in contrast to the paralysis of eye movements in coma directly due to drugs. In some situations it may be difficult to distinguish encephalopathy secondary to drug-induced hepatotoxicity from the primary neurotoxic effects of the hepatotoxin, as with cyclosporin (Menegaux *et al.* 1994).

Finally, it is important to bear in mind that drugs affecting neurotransmitters can have potent effects when an underlying neurodegenerative disease is present. For example, anticholinergic drugs used in Parkinson's disease can exacerbate a cholinergic deficit, producing a clinical picture of dementia (Kurlan and Como 1988).

Stroke

Drug-induced stroke is relatively rare, although drugs account for an increasing proportion of strokes in young people. Illicit drugs (cocaine and its derivatives, amphetamines, Ecstasy), appetite suppressants, decongestants, anabolic steroids, and oral contraceptives are most frequently implicated (Kelly *et al.* 1992; Kokkinos and Levine 1993*a*).

There is particular concern over the rapid growth in the use of cocaine as a recreational drug in recent years, and several studies have linked its use to an increased risk of stroke in the young (Daras *et al.* 1994; Lalouschek *et al.* 1995), although not all have confirmed such an association (Qureshi *et al.* 1997). Cocaine hydrochloride appears to cause intracerebral or subarachnoid haemorrhages almost exclusively (usually from pre-existing aneurysms or vascular malformations) while crack cocaine (alkaloidal cocaine) causes haemorrhages or infarcts with equal frequency. Haemorrhage probably results from the sudden increase in systemic arterial pressure induced by these drugs, while infarcts caused by crack cocaine may result from vasospasm of large arteries and secondary intravascular thrombosis (Konzen

et al. 1996). Symptoms typically begin about 3 hours after the drug has been taken.

Amphetamines and similar compounds, such as the anorexiants phenylpropanolamine and phentermine, can also cause stroke (Johnson *et al.* 1983; Maertens *et al.* 1987; Kelly *et al.* 1992; Kokkinos and Levine 1993*b*), either through sympathomimetic effects resulting in cerebral haemorrhages, or less commonly, through hypersensitivity angiitis (vasculitis), which can produce a 'beading' appearance of the intracerebral blood vessels on angiography (Ryu and Lin 1995). Other drugs that may induce hypertension and so predispose to cerebral vascular accidents are discussed in Chapter 9.

Conversely, there is also evidence that precipitate lowering of blood pressure by antihypertensive drugs, particularly in elderly patients with impaired cerebrovascular reserve, can precipitate ischaemic events, including watershed infarctions and 'misery perfusion' (Jansen *et al.* 1986; Hankey and Gubbay 1987). Cerebral perfusion in such patients becomes increasingly pressure dependent, and inappropriate lowering of blood pressure might contribute to the pathogenesis of dementia (Rogers *et al.* 1985; Lane 1991).

Cerebral venous thrombosis (Partziguian *et al.* 1996) and thrombotic strokes (Vessey 1973) have been described in patients taking oral contraceptives (Bickerstaff 1975). Retrospective studies by Vessey and Doll (1969) showed that the absolute risk to an individual woman is small. Inman and Vessey (1968) provided data suggesting that of every million women using oral contraceptives, about 100 would be admitted to hospital and about five would die each year from thrombotic stroke attributable to these agents. Inman and others (1970) suggested that the risk of thrombotic stroke is related to the oestrogen content of the oral contraceptive preparation and that low-dose preparations should be used when possible, but there is also evidence to suggest that the progestogen component of the contraceptive pill may play a part in some types of thromboembolic disease (Meade *et al.* 1980). Recent studies have also shown that activated protein C resistance, due to factor V Leiden and other undefined mechanisms, is an additional predisposing factor for cerebral venous thrombosis (Dulli *et al.* 1996; Zuber *et al.* 1996). Venous sinus thrombosis is discussed further in the section on Headache (see below).

Evidence has also accumulated to implicate oral contraceptives in subarachnoid haemorrhage, particularly in women who smoke (RCGP 1977; Petitti and Wingerd 1978). Oral contraceptives are a cause of hypertension (Weir *et al.* 1971), which may predispose to vascular disease and strokes in some women. Irey and others

(1978) described the pathological findings in three young women who developed strokes while taking oral contraceptives, and died. All three had thrombosis of major intracranial arteries with areas of focal intimal thickening, the latter presumably produced by the exogenous steroids. It is therefore important to ensure that women who are at risk of stroke, because of a history of thromboembolic disorders, hypertension, or migraine, do not use oral contraceptives (Bickerstaff 1975).

The use of other drugs has also been associated with thrombosis of cerebral vessels.

A 34-year-old body-builder who had been taking various anabolic steroids for over 4 years developed an acute right hemiparesis and speech difficulties. He had a simple partial seizure and an EEG showed abnormal slow activity consistent with a left hemisphere lesion. He made a slow recovery with residual weakness of the right upper limb. The authors suggested that there was an increased risk of stroke with the illicit use of anabolic steroids (Frankle *et al.* 1988).

Sclerotherapy for the treatment of varicose veins has been reported to cause reversible ischaemic neurological deficits (Trenkwalder and Lydtin 1994; Van der Plas *et al.* 1994).

Seizures

Drugs may precipitate seizures in epileptics, patients with a low seizure threshold due to cerebral or systemic disease, or in apparently healthy people (although they may have a family history of epilepsy, suggesting a genetic predisposition). Many drugs have been implicated (Chadwick 1981; Lane 1998), but for most the association is probably circumstantial.

Drug-induced seizures are uncommon. In a series of 12 617 medical inpatients, seizures attributed to drugs occurred in only 17 patients (0.13 per cent) (BCDSP 1972). In this study, the occurrence of seizures was greatest in patients receiving intravenous penicillin (four of 1245 patients), insulin (three of 763 patients, all of whom were hypoglycaemic), and infusions of lignocaine for cardiac arrhythmias (two of 349 cases). Seizures resulting from the use of 'recreational' drugs are probably now more common than iatrogenic seizures (Alldredge *et al.* 1989; Olsen *et al.* 1993). Drugs which cross the blood–brain barrier are most frequently implicated. Seizures can result from direct neurotoxic actions, or indirectly through adverse metabolic effects, such as anoxia (respiratory depressants), neuroglycopenia (insulin and oral hypoglycaemics), hypocalcaemia (steroids, phenytoin), hyperkalaemia (penicillins, particularly if given intrathecally), and water intoxication (oxytocin, vasopressin and carbamazepine).

Drugs causing seizures can be conveniently classified by pharmacological class, and are discussed here in roughly alphabetical order, for ease of reference (Lane 1998).

Anaesthetics can cause paradoxical neuronal excitation. This was well recognized in the days of ether anaesthesia, when signs of CNS excitation were commonly seen during induction. Most anaesthetics can precipitate seizures, although reports of anaesthetic agents causing seizures are infrequent. Halothane (Smith *et al.* 1966), methohexitone, propanidid (Barron 1974), ketamine (Thompson 1972), and the steroid anaesthetic agent Althesin (alphaxolone and alphadolone) (Evans and Keogh 1977) have been implicated, although the latter is sometimes used in the management of status epilepticus. Propofol seems to have particularly potent proconvulsive properties (Nowack and Jordan 1994), although, again, it has been used in the management of status epilepticus. High plasma concentrations of local anaesthetics, such as mepivacaine or lignocaine, can cause signs of cerebral irritation and convulsions (Arthur *et al.* 1988). Toxic plasma concentrations of lignocaine, given as an antiarrhythmic drug, can be achieved inadvertently with therapeutic infusions in patients with cardiac failure since there is often a decreased apparent volume of distribution of the drug in such patients. Rapid intravenous injection of lignocaine or theophylline may produce convulsions, most commonly in patients with liver disease.

Analeptics, such as the respiratory stimulant doxapram, may also produce seizures, and high doses of bronchodilators, such as terbutaline, may cause cerebral irritation and seizure activity (Friedman *et al.* 1982).

A number of analgesics can induce seizures. Induction of hepatic drug-metabolising enzymes increases the risk of convulsions caused by pethidine because of the increased plasma concentration of its metabolite norpethidine. There is a similar relationship between neurological symptoms, such as tremor, myoclonic jerks and seizures, and the plasma levels of the *N*-methylated metabolite of meperidine, normeperidine (Mauro *et al.* 1986). The mechanism by which the interaction of pethidine and monoamine oxidase inhibitors (MAOI) produces convulsions and hyperthermia is, however, not known.

Disopyramide and other antiarrythmics may occasionally cause seizures, and the β-adrenoceptor antagonist atenolol has been reported to precipitate them (Russell *et al.* 1979).

Most anti-infectives have, at some time, been associated with seizures. Antibiotics, notably penicillin and the newer synthetic and semisynthetic penicillins, including ampicillin (Serdaru *et al.* 1982), oxacillin, carbenicillin (Whelton *et al.* 1971), and ticarcillin (Kallay *et al.* 1979) are among the most common reported causes of iatrogenic seizures. Invariably the doses used were high; the patients had evidence of renal failure; or the drugs had been given intrathecally.

Some antibiotics, such as the β-lactams ceftazidine (Chetaille *et al.* 1994) and cefazolin (Bechtel *et al.* 1980) seem to cause seizures by direct neurotoxic actions in the presence of high plasma concentrations. In contrast, the proconvulsive actions of quinoline antibiotics, such as nalidixic acid and ciprofloxacin (Drug Intelligence and Clinical Pharmacy 1990) appear to be mediated through excitatory amino acid receptors (Williams and Helton 1991).

Several drugs now commonly used in the management of HIV infection can precipitate seizures, including pyrimethamine (for toxoplasmosis) and ganciclovir (for cytomegalovirus) (Ragab 1973; Barton *et al.* 1992).

Antituberculous therapy with cycloserine and isoniazid can also be associated with seizures, and slow acetylators of isoniazid may be at a greater risk. It was suggested many years ago that the mechanism was probably related to cerebral pyridoxine deficiency (Evans *et al.* 1960) and this is borne out by recent observations on isoniazid overdosage which can lead to profound metabolic acidosis, seizures, and obtundation. These seizures and the coma are reversed rapidly by intravenous pyridoxine (Brent *et al.* 1990).

Antimalarials can induce seizures and women appear particularly vulnerable to this adverse reaction (Fish and Espir 1988). Drugs such as chloroquine and mefloquine inhibit glutamate dehydrogenase, and thus GABAergic activity, causing either seizures in isolation (Ries and Pohlmann-Eden 1993) or as part of a toxic encephalopathy (Rouveix *et al.* 1989). The 'post-malarial neurological syndrome' of acute confusion or psychosis, often with associated seizures, occurred more commonly in patients treated with mefloquine than with quinine in one recent study (Mai *et al.* 1996).

Abrupt withdrawal of any anticonvulsant, particularly phenobarbitone, phenytoin, and benzodiazepines can precipitate seizures in epileptic patients. Paradoxically, anticonvulsant drugs, particularly carbamazepine (CBZ), can occasionally induce fits. The antidiuretic action of this drug can result in dilutional hyponatraemia, even at 'therapeutic' plasma levels; in one patient with refractory complex partial seizures demeclocycline corrected CBZ-induced water intoxication (Ringel and Brick 1986). Interestingly, CBZ overdosage causes a hierarchical decline in neurological function that is related to the plasma concentration of the drug, culminating in coma

and seizures (Weaver *et al.* 1988). Seizures were found to be an important indicator of a likely fatal outcome in overdosage in one study (Schmidt and Schmidt-Buhl 1995).

Antidepressants, particularly tricyclics such as imipramine and amitriptyline (Betts *et al.* 1968; Houghton 1971), may cause or precipitate seizures and should be used cautiously in epileptics. The subject of seizures in patients taking antidepressants (excluding MAOI) was reviewed by Trimble (1978), who regarded maprotiline, together with flupenthixol and nomifensine, as least likely to increase fit frequency in known epileptic patients. This opinion was, however, based largely on experimental data, and a later epidemiological study of reports to the Committee on Safety of Medicines of convulsions in patients taking antidepressants suggested that maprotiline is strongly epileptogenic and should be avoided in known epileptics (Edwards 1979; Parker and Lahmayer 1984). One study suggested that serotoninergic antidepressants, such as paroxetine, fluoxetine, and sertraline may be less epileptogenic than tricyclic compounds, and the highly selective serotonin re-uptake blocker fluvoxamine appeared almost devoid of this property (Harmant *et al.* 1990). However, a significant number of reports of seizures associated with all these drugs have accumulated (Lane 1998), although they may still be considered the drugs of choice for the treatment of depression in epileptics.

Lithium, used in the treatment of manic-depressive psychosis and cluster headache, can cause a number of neurological symptoms, including myoclonus and seizures, which are not invariably dose related, although they most often occur in patients with poor renal function (Demers *et al.* 1970). MAOI, such as phenelzine and tranylcypromine, may induce seizures independently of hypertensive reactions.

Seizures have been reported in association with several other classes of drugs, and with other miscellaneous medications. These include a variety of antihistamines, notably pheniramine (Buckley 1994) and anti-inflammatory drugs, such as indomethacin (Eeg-Olofsson *et al.* 1978) and mefenamic acid (Prescott *et al.* 1981). Hormone treatments can also cause seizures. The effect of hypoglycaemia, induced by insulin or oral antidiabetic drugs, is well recognized in this context; the profound and protracted hypoglycaemia caused by an overdose of sulphonyureas is particularly damaging. The relationship between seizures and the use of oral contraceptives and hormone replacement therapy (HRT) is more complex. In general, oestrogens are proconvulsive and progestogens anticonvulsive. Different studies have reported both increases and decreases in seizure frequency with oral contraceptives, and there is no good evidence that HRT will precipitate or exacerbate seizures.

Several immunosuppressants and cytotoxics have induced seizures. As discussed in the section on drug-induced encephalopathy, cyclosporin is particularly likely to cause neurological problems, including seizures, and cisplatin has been reported to induce an encephalopathy with seizures and visual disturbances, including cortical blindness (Hitchings and Thomson 1988).

Neuroleptics may cause seizures through direct neurotoxic effects. Phenothiazines, particularly chlorpromazine, prochlorperazine, and promazine, have been reported to cause seizures in non-epileptics (Jarvik 1970). Phenothiazines with a piperazine side-chain (e.g. fluphenazine and trifluoperazine) may be less likely to induce seizures than those with an aliphatic side-chain (e.g. chlorpromazine). More modern neuroleptics, such as haloperidol and clozapine can also induce seizures.

Intravenous and intrathecal water-soluble radiographic contrast media can cause seizures, although the increasing sophistication and availability of magnetic resonance imaging (MRI) in recent years has greatly reduced the incidence of such complications. Intrathecal metrizamide, in particular, was prone to induce seizures and if allowed into the cranium could cause significant EEG changes. The risk of seizure could be reduced by keeping the patient well hydrated and nursed in the upright position after the procedure (Chadwick 1981). Iopamidol was recently reported to cause seizures occasionally when used for outpatient investigation of lumbar radiculopathy (Ridge 1994), while in one case residual iophendylate, located in one site in the cranium, generated an epileptic focus on EEG more than 10 years after contrast myelography (Pascuzzi et al. 1988).

Seizures due to intravenous contrast media are less common and more likely to occur in the presence of underlying brain disease, especially glioma and metastases (Onada et al. 1987). They are usually of the convulsive form but non-convulsive seizures, presenting as lethargy and aphasia, have occurred following cerebral angiography with iothalamate (Vickrey and Bahls 1989). Inhibition of cerebral hexokinase activity has been suggested as the mechanism by which seizures are induced by this agent (Bertoni et al. 1981).

There are numerous reports of seizures associated with vaccines. These occur notably in infants and children with measles, mumps, and rubella (MMR), and pertussis vaccines, resulting in neonatal seizures and febrile convulsions. Seizures have occurred in older children following BCG inoculation, hepatitis B and influenza vaccination, and tetanus toxoid prophylaxis. Such seizures are presumably the result of an immune-system-mediated encephalitis.

Several classes of drugs taken for gastrointestinal disorders may cause fits. Proton-pump inhibitors, such as cimetidine and cisapride, can induce seizures, and histamine (H_2) antagonists may, rarely, cause reversible encephalopathic symptoms, including hallucinations, confusion, seizures, and, in one reported case, an acute optic neuropathy (Laniado et al. 1997). Such adverse effects are more likely in the elderly, or with intravenous use. Toxic effects of bismuth compounds used in the management of dyspepsia have already been mentioned in the context of an encephalopathy which may include myoclonus and seizures (Gordon et al. 1995).

There are many other reports of drug-associated seizures in which the mechanisms are unclear. For example, baclofen, used to spasticity, is said to induce seizures, particularly on withdrawal (Terrance and Fromm 1981; Barker and Grant 1982). However, animal studies suggest that baclofen has an anticonvulsant effect, and administration of the drug to epileptics in one controlled trial did not increase seizure frequency (Terrence et al. 1983).

Other drugs, for which more than 10 reports of an association with seizures have been made to the Committee on Safety of Medicines (CSM) in the UK since 1964, include bupivacaine, enflurane, aminophylline, salbutamol, pentazocine, fentanyl, tramadol, mexiletene, nifedipine, propranolol, erythromycin, co-trimoxazole, metronidazole, gabapentin, lamotrigine, valproate, vigabatrin, amoxapine, clomipramine, dothiepin, fluoxetine, lofepramine, mianserin, nortriptyline, paroxetine, trazodone, cetirizine, loratidine, terfenadine, diphenhydramine, diclofenac, ibuprofen, nefopam, clomiphene, desmopressin, mestranol, medroxyprogesterone, ifosfamide, methylprednisolone, vincristine, droperidol, risperidone, baclofen, bromocriptine, interferon, isotretinoin, metoclopramide, sumatriptan, streptokinase, diazepam, sulphasalazine, amoxycillin, ranitidine, danazol, atracurium, immunoglobulins and the vaccines for diphtheria, DTP, HIB, and polio (Lane 1998). Drugs cited by sources other than the CSM include mepivicaine, amiphenazole, dextropropoxyphene, cyclizine, doxylamine, phenylbutazone, and ergot.

Drug withdrawal

Drug-withdrawal seizures are far more common than seizures induced by drug use. This has already been mentioned in connection with anticonvulsants but it can occur following withdrawal of many other drugs, particularly alcohol, barbiturates, and benzodiazepines. Diazepam withdrawal as a cause of seizures was stressed by Vyas and Carney (1975) because of the ubiquitous use of the drug at that time. The withdrawal of other benzodiazepines carries the same risk (Ashton 1986), although the risk of seizures and status epilepticus seems greater with long-acting drugs, such as lorazepam and clorazepam (Laborde et al. 1987; Hauser et al. 1989).

Alcohol withdrawal seizures typically occur after 48–72 hours of abstinence. In one study of chronic alcoholics, the incidence of alcohol-withdrawal seizures was 15 per cent (Soyka *et al.* 1989). It appears to be more common in patients with cerebral atrophy or other underlying brain disease and in patients with a history of other drug dependencies, particularly to benzodiazepines (Pilke *et al.* 1984; Soyka *et al.* 1989; Koppel *et al.* 1992).

Finally, there is increasing concern over the problem of seizures associated with the use of recreational ('street') drugs. In one study, 98 of 945 cases of medical complications of cocaine use presented with seizures (Dhuna *et al.* 1991a). Generalized seizures were most common, and focal seizures were found to be frequently associated with underlying cocaine-related strokes or cerebral haemorrhage. In a subsequent report, these authors also suggested that habitual use of cocaine might induce independent epileptic activity (Dhuna *et al.* 1991b). Infants of addicted mothers appear particularly prone (Kramer *et al.* 1990). Seizures caused by other opiates seem less frequent; morphine appeared to have anticonvulsant properties in neonatal seizures (Wijberg *et al.* 1991). All the commonly used designer drugs, including the mescaline analogues (amphetamines, 'Ecstasy' (3,4-methylenedioxymethamphetamine, MDMA), synthetic opioids such as meperidine, and phencyclidine and derivatives) have been reported to cause seizures (Lane 1998). In some instances complex metabolic factors related to hyperthermia induced by such agents may be causative, but drugs such as MDMA, and hallucingens such as lysergic acid diethylamide (LSD), are strongly serotoninergic, and seizures have been precipitated by these drugs in the absence of other metabolic factors (Lehmann *et al.* 1995).

The relationship between cannabinoids and seizures is more complex. Marihuana contains a mixture of these compounds. Some, such as delta-tetrahydrocannabinol (THC), are generally proconvulsive, while others such as cannabidol are anticonvulsive. Not surprisingly, reports of both improvement (Consroe *et al.* 1975; Cuhna *et al.* 1980) and deterioration (Kesler and Reifer 1979) in seizure control in epileptics using marihuana have been reported, while seizures were rarely encountered in patients receiving THC for vomiting during cancer chemotherapy (Devine *et al.* 1987).

Headache

Drug-induced headache can be considered in two contexts: headache may occur in individuals who do not normally suffer recurrent or persistent primary headaches as a result of the pharmacological actions of certain drugs (Type A effects); and, paradoxically, headache can be caused by the drugs used to treat primary headache disorders (analgesic headache).

A survey of 10 506 reports to the WHO Collaboration Centre for International Drug Monitoring, from five countries, found that the drugs most frequently reported to cause non-specific headache included atenolol, cimetidine, glyceryl trinitrate, indomethacin, isosorbide dinitrate, nifedipine, ranitidine, sulphamethoxazole, and trimethoprim. Oral contraceptives were most commonly implicated with migraine, while isotretinoin, tetracyclines, and trimethoprim–sulphamethoxazole were associated with benign intracranial hypertension (BIH) (Asmark *et al.* 1989).

The most common mechanisms in the genesis of drug-induced headache included stretching of pain-sensitive cerebral blood vessel walls, by vasoconstriction or vasodilatation; intracranial fluid volume changes (including BIH); and chemical irritation of the meninges. Drug-induced hypertension may also be associated with headache.

Intracranial vascular causes

The vasodilator drugs most frequently implicated include amyl nitrite, bromocriptine, dopamine, glyceryl trinitrate, hydralazine, nifedipine, perhexilene, terbutaline, and theophylline. Headaches following administration of intravenous oestrogens and carmustine are associated with flushing, suggesting that they too may result from vasodilatation. Recreational use of cocaine can cause benign headaches with migrainous features in non-migraineurs. It has been suggested that the acute headache following ingestion results from vasoconstriction (which in some instances can lead to stroke — see above), while withdrawal headache might result from changes in central serotonin mechanisms (Dhuna *et al.* 1991). Acute withdrawal of drugs such as alcohol, amphetamines, caffeine, the ergots, and methysergide may also cause headache (*The Lancet* 1973).

Intracranial fluid changes

Headache may result from changes in intravascular or extravascular fluid volume in the intracranial compartment and can occur, for example, after the administration of osmotic agents such as glycerol. This explanation has also been given for the development of headaches at the start of treatment with non-steroidal anti-inflammatory analgesics (NSAID), notably indomethacin, which cause salt and water retention.

Benign intracranial hypertension (BIH, pseudotumour cerebri)

BIH is due to cerebral oedema and presents as headache associated with papilloedema, rarely without papilloedema, and sometimes complicated by diplopia due to VIth nerve paresis, visual blurring, and visual field defects. Drugs that give rise to the syndrome include the tetracyclines, nalidixic acid, corticosteroids, both oral and topical, nitrofurantoin, and the anaesthetic agents ketamine and nitrous oxide. Excess, as well as deficiency, of vitamin A and the use of etretinate (Bonnetblanc *et al.* 1983) may be associated also with the development of benign intracranial hypertension. Severe headache and papilloedema occurred in three patients treated with perhexilene maleate (Stephens *et al.* 1978). Cerebrospinal fluid pressures were not measured, but the results of other investigations suggested the diagnosis. BIH has been reported to follow therapy with the gonadotrophin analogue, lucoprotein acetate (Arbor *et al.* 1990).

Davidson (1971), reviewing the ocular complications of oral contraceptives (OC), described six patients with papilloedema, two of whom were diagnosed as cases of BIH. It was unclear whether this could be attributed to the OC, for the condition may occur spontaneously in young, often obese, women. Bickerstaff (1975) pointed out, however, that Davidson's affected patients were all slim. The mechanism by which OC cause BIH is unclear. It may involve salt and water retention and intracranial fluid redistribution, but there is increasing evidence that impairment of venous sinus drainage due to occult thrombosis, perhaps at microscopic level, may be important. Recent reports have supported an association between venous sinus thrombosis and OC (Partziguian *et al.* 1996), particularly in women with other prothrombotic conditions such as activated protein C resistance due, for example, to Factor V Leiden deficiency (Dulli *et al.* 1996; Zuber *et al.* 1996). This might also be relevant to the use of hormone relacement therapy (Strachan *et al.* 1995).

Raman and al-Tahan (1993) described a particularly graphic example of the likely association between BIH and venous sinus thrombosis.

A young woman presented with BIH, having taken OC for 3 years; 3 months later, she lapsed into coma, became decerebrate, and died within 48 hours. CT scanning revealed evidence of massive thrombosis of the deep venous system.

Aseptic meningitis

In addition to the ability to cause headache by intracranial volume changes, NSAID can also induce an aseptic meningitis, with a pleocytosis, raised protein, and low sugar in the CSF. In early reports, this complication with sulindac (Ballas and Donta 1982), tolmetin (Ruppert and Barth 1981), and ibuprofen (Giansiracusa *et al.* 1980) occurred in patients with lupus erythematosus, but it was also reported following treatment with co-trimoxazole in such a patient (Kremer *et al.* 1983). More recently an aseptic meningitis has been reported in otherwise healthy patients following the use of naproxen (Sylvia *et al.* 1988), and recurrent cases have been induced by ibuprofen therapy (Mifsud 1988; Chez *et al.* 1989). The latter authors reported increased intrathecal IgG synthesis in their cases, consistent with an antigen-specific immune response to the agent in the CNS.

Hypertension

Headache rarely results from hypertension but is a feature of the hypertensive crises induced by monoamine oxidase inhibitors when taken in combination with sympathetic agonists such as amphetamines, ephedrine, tricyclic antidepressants, or foods containing tyramine (see Chapter 9). The combination of amitriptyline, metoclopramide, and levodopa plus carbidopa (Sinemet) produced hypertension and headache in a patient with Parkinson's disease (Rampton 1977). Administration or sudden withdrawal of clonidine or propranolol may precipitate headache, as may that of labetalol, although the incidence of headache with this drug decreases with continuing use, suggesting the development of tolerance (Bayne *et al.* 1980).

Analgesic headache

The two commonest primary headache syndromes, migraine and tension headache, can usually be distinguished by their clinical characteristics. However, it is well recognized that there can be considerable overlap in manifestations in individual cases. In addition, the frequency of such headaches can increase to such an extent that a chronic daily headache develops. Various terms are used to describe this, depending on the manifestations, including chronic tension headache and 'migraine with interparoxysmal headache', but it is not clear that these are truly distinct entities. Indeed, many now believe that 'tension headache' may have similar central mechanisms to those involved in migraine. It is increasingly being recognized that the frequent and escalating use of 'instant relief' remedies for primary headaches plays an important part in the transformation of intermittent to chronic headache states (Diener and Wilkinson 1988; Olesen 1995).

Analgesic headache is essentially a Type B reaction; the offending drugs do not generally cause headache if taken for conditions other than primary headache

(Olesen 1995). Any drug used frequently for 'instant relief' appears to have this propensity, but ergot and its derivatives, narcotics, particularly codeine and dextropropoxyphene, and milder analgesics such as aspirin and paracetamol are most often implicated. Typically, patients begin to self-medicate with 'over-the-counter' preparations (or through repeat prescriptions without adequate supervision) and abuse develops over months or years. Compound preparations are notorious in this regard, and barbiturates may be included in the formulation, particularly in continental Europe (Olesen 1995).

Ergotamine has a short plasma half-life but frequent use can result in chronic vasoconstriction. Used daily it can cause a chronic headache of varying intensity, sometimes with migrainous features, while sudden withdrawal can result in severe and protracted migraine, leading to a vicious circle of persistent and recurrent vascular headache which may require hospital admission to break (Olesen 1995). It is not yet clear whether the newer selective serotonin receptor agonists, such as sumatriptan, zolmatriptan, and naratriptan, will prove less of a problem in this regard, but sumatriptan appears to ameliorate ergotamine headache and only rarely aggravates migraine. The mechanisms involved in analgesic headache are otherwise currently unclear.

Psychological factors in the precipitation of the primary headache and its relief by the drug, or drugs, may predispose to dependency in susceptible individuals. Once recognized, immediate withdrawal from the aggravating agent under careful supervision, coupled with diagnosis of the primary disorder and identification of aggravating or precipitating factors, is usually successful in stopping the headaches (Diener and Wilkinson 1988).

Extrapyramidal system

Although disorders of this system are usually referred to as drug-induced extrapyramidal syndromes, other neuronal tracts and systems in the brain stem and spinal cord are probably involved. Patients may have symptoms and signs similar to those of idiopathic Parkinson's disease or show involuntary movements now recognized to be characteristic effects of neuroleptic agents and some other drugs, including diazoxide, diphenhydramine and chlorprothixene, and the antimalarials amodiaquine and chloroquine. Several attempts have been made to classify the motor disorders (Duvoisin 1968) and a division into reversible and irreversible groups has been suggested (Lader 1970).

Drug-induced parkinsonism

This is probably the most common drug-induced disorder of involuntary movement. The clinical findings resemble classical paralysis agitans, except that a resting tremor is less prominent. Many drugs have been implicated, most frequently those antipsychotic drugs that antagonize dopaminergic neurotransmission. The clinical severity is variable and, paradoxically, patients suffering from naturally occurring Parkinson's disease do not appear to have increased sensitivity to these drugs (Dukes 1980).

A 74-year-old man with parkinsonism developed progressive cognitive and behavioural dysfunction suggestive of Alzheimer's disease but which resolved on withdrawal of his anticholinergic antiparkinsonian drugs (Kurlan and Como 1988).

Almost all the phenothiazines have been associated with the production of parkinsonism, which has also been induced by the butyrophenones (e.g. haloperidol) reserpine, methyldopa (Rosenblum and Montgomery 1980), lithium, metoclopramide (Indo and Ando 1982), the tricyclic antidepressants, and tetrabenazine. A reversible parkinsonism has been reported in an elderly woman taking perhexilene maleate (Gordon and Gordon 1981). Reduction of the dose of the drug usually produces a remission of symptoms and signs, although the administration of an anticholinergic drug can produce a rapid reversal of signs in acute severe drug-induced parkinsonism. There is no indication for concomitant prophylactic anticholinergic therapy in the treatment of an affective psychosis since there is strong evidence that this predisposes the patient to the development of an irreversible tardive dyskinesia; neither should levodopa be given since it frequently aggravates the underlying psychotic condition. The withdrawal of high-dose continuous intravenous haloperidol is reported to have been associated with a self-limited dyskinesia (Riker et al. 1997). Parkinsonism, associated with an irreversible orofacial dyskinesia, has been reported in a patient taking amoxapine (Lapierre and Anderson 1983). Sulpiride, a selective D_2-receptor antagonist with antipsychotic and antidepressant properties, has been reported to induce parkinsonism and a persistent segmental dystonia 2 months after starting the drug (Miller and Jankovic 1990). However, in general this drug seems to be less prone than others to produce this adverse effect.

The development of parkinsonism following exposure to a variety of neurotoxins has provided valuable insights into the pathogenesis of the idiopathic disorder. A severe parkinsonian syndrome developed in a 46-year-old man poisoned by cyanide. MRI showed multiple areas of low signal intensity in the globus pallidus and posterior putamen confirming the functional impairment of dopaminergic nigrostriatal neurones (Rosenberg et al. 1989).

Chronic manganese poisoning may cause a complex of symptoms and signs similar to those found in idiopathic Parkinson's disease and accompanied by similar neuropathological findings (Yamada *et al.* 1986). Gerlach and Riederer (1996) reviewed some of the current animal models of Parkinson's disease and compared the characteristic features with those of the disease in man.

The illicit synthesis and use of 'designer' drugs containing the contaminant 1-methyl-4-phenyl-1,2,5,6-tetrahydropyridine (MPTP) has been associated with the rapid development of extrapyramidal dysfunction. The administration of MPTP to man and animals results in the appearance of a parkinsonian syndrome, closely related to idiopathic Parkinson's disease. MPTP interacts with both the A and B forms of MAO but its main inhibitory effect results in an irreversible inhibition of MAO-B. The neurotoxicity of MPTP has been attributed to the formation of MPP+ from MPTP by MAO-B and the subsequent effects of MPP+ on mitochondrial respiration (Dostert and Strolin-Benedetti 1988). Parkinsonism induced by MPTP has been described as 'time-telescoped' Parkinson's disease and it is currently used as an animal model of the disease. MPP+ has been shown to be concentrated in neurones with a catecholamine uptake mechanism and this may explain the vulnerability of nigrostriatal dopaminergic neurones (Kopin and Markey 1988).

Several hypotheses about the mechanism of action of MPTP have been related to the pathogenesis of nigral cell death in Parkinson's disease. Changes in calcium influx have been implicated in both MPTP-induced parkinsonism and Parkinson's disease. Kupsch *et al.* (1996) reported that nimodipine, a blocker of L-type calcium channels, prevents dopaminergic MPTP-induced neurotoxicity in C57B1/6 black mice and in a non-human primate model of Parkinson's disease. They assessed the effects of nimodipine, continuously applied by pellet for 18 days, on behavioural, biochemical, and histological parameters, following systemic application of MPTP in marmosets. MPTP induced severe parkinsonian symptoms, with pronounced dopamine depletion in the caudate-putamen and a loss of tyrosine-hydroxylase-immunoreactive cells in the substantia nigra 7 days after MPTP-administration. Pretreatment with nimodipine did not antagonize the striatal dopamine depletion, but almost completely prevented MPTP-induced decrease of nigral tyrosine-hydroxylase-immunoreactive cells. These data suggest that nimodipine protects against MPTP-induced neurotoxicity at the cellular nigral level, but not at the synaptic striatal level. This suggests different mechanisms of actions of MPTP-induced neurotoxicity at the nigral versus the striatal level (Kupsch *et al.* 1996).

Other drugs of abuse may be associated directly with movement disorders. Seven patients are reported who developed cocaine-induced movement disorders, including choreoathetosis, akathisia, and parkinsonism with tremor (Daras *et al.* 1994). The cocaine-induced choreoathetoid movements were referred to as 'crack dancing'. Dopaminergic mechanisms are hypothesized to cause the euphoria, addiction, and abnormal movements.

The induction of an extrapyramidal syndrome by an exogenous chemical has given rise to speculation about the role of other environmental agents, such as pesticides, in the aetiology of chronic degenerative neurological diseases.

Akathisia

Akathisia is defined as involuntary continuous motor restlesness. The patient has a subjective desire to move about, pace the floor, alternately sit and stand, and stamp his feet. When the restlessness is confined to the feet it is termed tasikinesia. Although most commonly associated with levodopa therapy, it has apparently followed oxazepam withdrawal (Mendelsohn 1978) and can occur with the phenothiazines, butyrophenones (Weiner and Luby 1983), amoxapine (Ross *et al.* 1983), and paroxetine (Baldassano *et al.* 1996). Drug-induced akathisia has recently been reviewed (Blaisdell 1994; Lang 1995; Sachdev 1995*a,b*; Chung and Chiu 1996).

Acute dystonias

These dramatic and often alarming movement disorders are relatively common, particularly in children and young adults. The onset can be abrupt and may be mistaken for hysteria or even tetany. The muscles of the head and neck are mainly affected, with involuntary movement and spasm of the tongue, trismus, and facial grimacing and other orofacial dyskinesias. Oculogyric crises, torticollis and retrocollis, opisthotonus, axial dystonias, and a bizarre gait can occur, often accompanied by writhing movements of the limbs. The attacks are episodic and, although frightening to witness or experience, are usually painless. Between each episode muscle tone is normal, and during a subsequent attack different muscle groups may be affected.

A 32-year-old man with mental retardation and uncontrolled complex partial epilepsy developed frequent episodes of forced upward gaze after an increase in his daily divalproex sodium dosage. Reduction in the dose of co-administered carbamazepine resulted in prompt resolution but the upward gaze problem recurred several months later. The carbamazepine dose was decreased further with subsequent resolution of his signs. In this case an oculogyric crisis appeared to be induced by carbamazepine (Gorman and Barkley 1995).

Many of the antipsychotic drugs, such as the phenothiazines and butyrophenones, have been associated with acute dystonic reactions in the young. Other drugs include metoclopramide (Kerr 1996), tricyclic antidepressants, phenytoin (Chadwick *et al.* 1976), carbamazepine (Joyce and Gunderson 1980), and propranolol in high dosage (Crawford 1977). Spasmodic torticollis occurred in a patient treated with chlorzoxazone for back pain (Rosin 1981).

A case of acute dystonic reaction to methotrimeprazine is reported in a patient with untreated hypoparathyroidism (Gur *et al.* (1996). The authors note the potential for increased sensitivity of hypocalcaemic patients to the extrapyramidal adverse effects of antipsychotic drugs.

The patient was an 80-year-old man who had untreated hypoparathyroidism and chronic hypocalcaemia. He developed an acute dystonic reaction 20 minutes after ingestion of 25 mg methotrimeprazine. His disorientation, psychomotor restlessness, dystonic grimacing, protrusion of the tongue, and speech difficulties lasted for 4 days, despite a continuing hypocalcaemia. The authors suggest that striatal calmodulin-mediated adenylate cyclase activation is inhibited by the combined effects of the phenothiazine and hypocalcaemia. However, in this patient it was not possible to determine if the dystonic reaction was due to hypocalcaemia alone, the phenothiazine administration, or an interaction of the two. It is suggested that patients with hypocalcaemia may be more sensitive to the extrapyramidal adverse effects of antipsychotics and that acute and unexpected dystonic reactions to a small dose of an antipsychotic should indicate the need to measure the patient's serum calcium concentration.

The mechanism of action in some dystonias may relate to an increased release of dopamine and subsequent receptor hypersensitivity as the plasma concentration of the drug declines. Usually the dystonia remits once the drug is withdrawn. Intravenous benztropine or diazepam are useful in severe cases. Administration of another antipsychotic drug can sometimes be used to treat a severe dystonia.

The incidence of these reactions depends upon the patient population studied. The Boston Collaborative Drug Surveillance Program (BCDSP 1973) reported drug-induced extrapyramidal symptoms in 18 (0.8 per cent) of 2149 patients. These were all inpatients, mainly on short-term treatment, only one of them having been under treatment with one of the offending drugs at the time of admission. Of the 18 cases, trifluoperazine was the drug responsible for 14, another phenothiazine for one, and butyrophenones and tricyclic antidepressants for the other three. In all cases the symptoms disappeared when the drug was withdrawn. On the other hand, Ayd (1961) reported an overall incidence of approximately 39 per cent (with about 15 per cent drug-induced pseudoparkinsonism, 21 per cent akathisia, and 2.3 per cent acute dystonic reactions) in 3775 patients with major psychoses under treatment with phenothiazines. Obviously the epidemiology of this disorder warrants further study. About 2.5 per cent of a group

of patients treated with neuroleptic drugs developed acute dystonia within 48 hours of starting treatment (Rupniak *et al.* 1986).

Forty-seven railroad workers who were exposed to polychlorinated phenols, including the dioxin TCDD, while cleaning up a chemical spillage, were followed for over 6 years. There was a suggestion of an increase in action dystonias and postural intention tremor in a significant number of patients (Klawans 1987) although such an association has not been subsequently confirmed.

Chorea

Chorea usually presents as irregular, jerking, involuntary movements of the limbs. Often the slow writhing movements of athetosis or a dystonia are superimposed. The patient frequently attempts to disguise the movement by converting it into some reasonable action. There have been several reports of chorea occurring in patients taking the oral contraceptive pill (Riddoch *et al.* 1971; Bickerstaff 1975). This resolves within a couple of months of stopping the drug. Anabolic steroids (oxymethalone) have also been implicated (Tilzey *et al.* 1981). The most frequent association has been with the antipsychotic drugs and the anticonvulsants (especially phenytoin [Chadwick *et al.* 1976]). Choreoathetosis has been described in two patients intoxicated with phenytoin, with improvement after reduction of the dose (McLellan and Swash 1974).

An 80-year-old man had been treated with phenytoin for the management of his seizures (Sinard and Hedreen, 1995). Three years before his death he developed multiple neurological deficits, including bilateral chorea, ataxic gait, sensory neuropathy, and a progressive dementia. Postmortem examination of the patient's brain showed a marked but selective loss of neurons from both subthalamic nuclei, and Purkinje cell loss in the cerebellum. This pattern of injury is consistent with a toxic process and does not fit any characteristic pathological syndromes known to be associated with movement disorders or dementia. Phenytoin has been shown to cause choreiform movements, peripheral neuropathy, and cognitive decline in some patients, but the pathological basis for these changes has not been determined. The patient's chorea was probably related to neuronal loss in the subthalamic nuclei, but causes for his dementia and neuropathy were not found. The pathological findings may represent an unusual form of chronic phenytoin toxicity.

Long-term therapy with benzhexol caused choreiform movements that ceased on withdrawal and returned on direct challenge with the drug (Warne and Gubbay 1979). Amphetamines (Lundh and Tunving 1981), methadone (Wasserman and Yahr 1980), methylphenidate, amoxapine (Patterson 1983), and cimetidine (Kushner 1982) are also reputed to produce chorea.

Nine days after acute poisoning with carbon monoxide, a 24-year-old man developed choreoathetosis in the upper limbs and face. There were also memory disturbances that cleared within 6 months. A computed tomographic (CT) scan and nuclear magnetic resonance (NMR) showed symmetrical bilateral lesions in the globus pallidus (Meucci *et al.* 1989).

Pemoline, an indirectly acting sympathomimetic drug with actions similar to amphetamine, has been reported to cause choreoathetosis.

A 49-year-old man developed severe choreoathetosis with rhabdomyolysis and myoglobinuria after an increase in his dose of pemoline. This resolved after 48 hours (Briscoe *et al.* 1988).

Tremor

The problem of drug-induced tremor has been reviewed by Lane (1984). A large number of drugs can exacerbate physiological (postural) tremor, increasing both its frequency and amplitude. These include the tricyclic antidepressants, anticonvulsants (including sodium valproate), lithium, amiodarone, cimetidine (Bateman *et al.* 1981), and caffeine. Withdrawal of alcohol or benzodiazepines will also produce an increase in postural tremor. Paradoxically, both alcohol and primidone are effective in the treatment of benign (familial) essential tremor (Chakrabati and Pearace 1981).

Resting tremor is rarely drug induced, and is not a notable feature of parkinsonism, but it has been reported with amiodarone (Lustman and Moncou 1974). Action tremors may be seen as part of drug-induced postural tremor and are particularly a feature of lithium and valproate toxicity. Frank cerebellar signs, including tremor, may occur in phenytoin toxicity.

β-Adrenoceptor agonists, such as salbutamol, are well recognized to cause an increase in physiological tremor. The mechanism is not completely determined but probably involves an increase in the gain on the feedback loop which stimulates the tone in the antagonistic muscle groups used to maintain limb posture. A degree of tremor is inevitably seen after oral administration or high doses by nebulizer. Tolerance does develop with chronic usage and patients seem seldom to be inconvenienced by the tremor (Schaffler and Reeh 1987).

Anticonvulsants at toxic plasma concentrations may produce asterixis and myoclonus (Chadwick *et al.* 1976). The use of gabapentin has been associated with the development of both an oculogyric crisis and myoclonic movements (Reeves *et al.* 1996). Myoclonus has also been reported in a patient with renal disease taking metoclopramide (Hyser and Drake 1983).

Bharucha and Sethi (1996) reported two cases of complex movement disorders induced by fluoxetine.

A 72-year-old woman developed rhythmic palatal movements, myoclonus, chorea, and dystonia after 2 years of treatment with fluoxetine. The movements stopped 5 days after withdrawal of the drug. The second patient was a 58-year-old man who developed myoclonic jerking and rapid, stereotypic movements of his toes after a year on fluoxetine. Such complex movements had not been reported previously as an adverse effect of fluoxetine.

Wyllie and others (1997) reported the development of myoclonus in two patients with lymphoma treated with chlorambucil.

One, an 81-year-old man, developed jerking movements and stiffness that persisted for 3 days and was more intense at night. The dose of chlorambucil was reduced with a subsequent decrease in signs and resolution of the myoclonus occurred when the drug was stopped. Rechallenge evoked a return of tremors on the next day that later became constant but again resolved on discontinuation of the chlorambucil. The second case was a 75-year-old woman who developed jerking movements in her limbs, particularly in her arms and hip which were so severe that they prevented her from leaving home. All of her symptoms resolved within 2–3 days after the chlorambucil cycle was completed, so she was diagnosed as having had chlorambucil-induced myoclonus.

Chlorambucil-induced myoclonus has been described following overdose and in the treatment of the nephrotic syndrome in children. Three cases of reversible myoclonic activity associated with high-dose chlorambucil in adults have also been reported. In each case, the myoclonus resolved when the drug was withdrawn. Only one other conclusive case of low-dose myoclonus due to chlorambucil has been described in an adult. However, it does appear that myoclonus may be induced by normal therapeutic dosages in adults, and such patients should be observed closely and if drug-induced myoclonus develops the drug should be discontinued.

A 58-year-old man taking oral antidiabetic drugs and with chronic paranoid psychosis developed transient episodes of marked paranoid delusions, auditory hallucinations without confusion, shakiness of both upper extremities, tachycardia, and sweating. An EMG revealed many silent periods in postural active muscles with a maximum duration of 120 ms; blood glucose was 65–75 mg per dl. The patient noted some vibration in his outstretched hands and a drug-induced asterixis (clozapine, benperidol), amplified by the relative hypoglycaemia, was diagnosed. The symptoms disappeared after his oral antidiabetic dosage was reduced (Poersch *et al.* 1996).

Gilles de la Tourette syndrome

This rare, enigmatic syndrome has occurred after haloperidol withdrawal in a child with a congenital encephalopathy (Singer 1981). Paradoxically, it has also occurred in four children treated with the central nervous system stimulants dextroamphetamine, methylphenidate, or pemoline for hyperactivity (Lowe *et al.* 1982). In untreated Tourette's syndrome, movement disorders, such as tics, may be exacerbated by some drugs. Daniels and colleagues (1996) refer to cocaine-induced tics in untreated touretters. Prolonged neuroleptic treatment may induce motor and verbal tics thought to represent a tardive tourettism (Bharucha and Sethi 1995).

Tardive dyskinesia

This condition is most frequently seen in psychiatric hospitals in chronically ill patients treated with neuroleptic drugs. The extrapyramidal adverse effects of the neuroleptics include parkinsonism, dystonia, and akathisia (Stephen and Williamson 1984; Shaleve *et al.* 1987; Hatdie and Lees 1988), but these develop early in treatment and are mitigated by the concurrent administration of anticholinergic antiparkinsonian drugs. The condition of tardive dyskinesia develops much later in treatment, particularly after high doses of the drugs; it is estimated to occur in 10–20 per cent of those patients treated with neuroleptic drugs for more than one year.

A tardive dyskinesia is characterized by abnormal involuntary movements that most frequently start in the face with repetitive blinking and abnormal movements of the lips and tongue, but often extend to include a torticollis and choreoathetoid movements of the limbs and trunk. The only effective treatment is withdrawal of the neuroleptic drug, when an initial exacerbation is usually followed by gradual improvement over several months (Task Force 1980). Lesser measures, such as dose reduction or a change of drug, may be all that are possible in chronically psychotic patients. Antiparkinsonian drugs are believed to aggravate the condition and should therefore also be discontinued (Barnes 1988). Tardive dyskinesia is best prevented from developing by using the minimum effective doses of neuroleptics for the shortest possible time in the treatment of those conditions for which there are no alternative treatments.

The condition has long been regarded as due to a dopamine-receptor hypersensitivity. There is recent evidence that reduced gamma-aminobutyric acid (GABA) activity in striatal neurones may contribute to its development (Gerlach and Casey 1988). Tardive dyskinesia has been more extensively reviewed in articles by Barnes (1988), the American Psychiatric Association (Task Force 1980) and Latimer (1995).

Neuroleptic malignant syndrome (NMS)

This important and possibly underdiagnosed condition has been extensively reviewed (*The Lancet* 1984; Gibb and Lees 1985; Kellam 1987; Naganuma and Fujii 1994).

The essential clinical features of the syndrome are extrapyramidal rigidity, altered consciousness, and autonomic dysfunction with pyrexia, profuse sweating, tachycardia, and labile blood pressure. The serum creatine kinase (CK) is typically raised and a leucocytosis and abnormal liver function tests are often found. Patients rapidly become dehydrated with associated abnormalities in plasma electrolytes and, if untreated, progress to coma, often with seizures, and death in 20–30 per cent of cases, usually from hypoventilation or aspiration pneumonia. Myonecrosis and myoglobinaemic renal failure, hepatic necrosis, and cardiovascular failure may also develop (Velamoor *et al.* 1994). Disseminated intravascular failure can result in multiorgan failure and one case developed a peripheral neuropathy (Mesejo et al 1995).

The condition appears to result from a sudden reduction in central dopaminergic function in the striatum and hypothalamus (Henderson and Wooton 1981; Burke *et al.* 1981) usually related to treatment with dopamine-receptor blocking drugs such as haloperidol, fluphenazine, chlorpromazine, thiothixene, thioridazine, trimeprazine, trifluoroperazine, and prochlorperazine, and most commonly occurs in patients with presumed pre-existing central neurotransmitter dysfunction, including schizophrenia and other psychotic states, for which the neuroleptic medication is being prescribed. The condition has also, however, been described in many other non-psychotic conditions in relation to neuroleptic medication, including pre-operative sedation (Moyes 1973; Konikoff *et al.* 1984). Occasionally it may follow the withdrawal of neuroleptic drugs (Amore and Zazzeri 1995). The condition is also well described following abrupt reduction or withdrawal of the dopamine agonists levodopa and bromocriptine in Parkinson's disease, particularly in association with 'drug holidays', and with tetrabenazine and α-methyl-*p*-tyrosine, which deplete dopamine stores, in Huntington's chorea (Burke *et al.* 1981). It may occur with drug combinations that reduce dopamine receptor activity, such as dothiepin and phenelzine (Ritchie 1983) and amitriptyline and thioridazine (Eiser *et al.* 1982); and antipsychotic–anticholinergic combinations, the latter impairing the peripheral heat-loss mechanisms (Gibb and Lees 1985).

Lithium has been reported to provoke NMS in patients taking neuroleptic drugs, such as haloperidol (Loudon and Waring 1976; Goekoop and Carbaat 1982), and following its use in the management of off-period dystonia in Parkinson's disease (Pfeiffer and Sucha 1985; Koehler and Mirandolle 1988). NMS has rarely been reported in relation to isolated therapy with a tricyclic antidepressant (Grant 1984). It is also clear that relatively mild forms of NMS can occur under similar clinical circumstances and that the diagnosis may be missed (Clarke *et al.* 1988; Mezaki *et al.* 1989; Domingo *et al.* 1989). Neuroleptics can produce a *forme fruste* of NMS through their ability to interfere with central hypothalamic dopamine pathways and peripheral cholinergic and α-adrenergic thermoregulatory mechanisms. They also cause the release of calcium (Ca^{++})

from the sarcoplasmic reticulum, and raise serum creatine kinase levels (Meltzer and Moline 1970; Anderson 1972).

Cape (1994) warns that it is important to be vigilant about the neuroleptic malignant syndrome especially after prolonged exposure to neuroleptics.

In one case, NMS was diagnosed in a 29-year-old man who had been on fluphenazine decanoate for over a year, the onset coinciding with the cessation of his neuroleptic medication. Vigorous treatment, including assisted ventilation, was necessary and extended over 3 months. On recovery, his mental state and social functioning had undergone a marked improvement, sufficient for his release from hospital!

There is a considerable degree of overlap between the clinical characteristics of NMS and the syndromes of acute lethal catatonia and malignant hyperthermia (MH). NMS and MH have recently been contrasted and compared in a review by Keck *et al.* (1995).

Lethal catatonia is characterized by catatonia or stupor with waxy flexibility, occurring spontaneously in schizophrenia and other psychoses following a period of intensive agitation and hyperactivity. The typical extrapyramidal rigidity of NMS is not generally seen and the pyrexia tends to be a late phenomenon. It has been suggested that NMS is an iatrogenic form of lethal catatonia with the addition of the extrapyramidal effects of neuroleptic medication or underlying basal ganglia disease (Kellam 1987). Acute lethal catatonia has become rare since the introduction of electroconvulsive therapy (ECT) and the various neuroleptic drugs. Neuroleptic malignant syndrome may occur without muscle rigidity. Wong (1996) describes two patients with neuroleptic malignant syndrome who developed fever and altered consciousness while taking neuroleptics but who did not develop muscle rigidity. The symptoms subsided when the drugs was stopped but recurred on rechallenge. The report supports the concept of a spectrum of clinical severity of the neuroleptic malignant syndrome. Clozapine can induce a neuroleptic malignant syndrome that may have different features from classical NMS such as fewer extrapyramidal side effects and a lower rise in creatine kinase (Sachdev *et al.* 1995).

Dent (1995) described a 51-year-old man with a mild learning disability who was given chlorpromazine and thioridazine for sleeplessness and agitation. He developed the neuroleptic malignant syndrome which was treated successfully with intravenous diazepam. Without further exposure to neuroleptics, the patient became acutely unwell with signs of the catatonic syndrome which responded to oral diazepam. When the dose of diazepam was reduced the catatonic syndrome recurred and responded to an increase in his oral diazepam. In the past, the patient had been admitted to hospital with severe extrapyramidal symptoms and parkinsonism following prescription of neuroleptics for agitation. Patients with a susceptibility to

catatonic syndrome may be at increased risk of developing NMS, and therefore, should not be treated with neuroleptics.

Malignant hyperthermia (MH) shares with NMS the features of hyperpyrexia, its metabolic consequences, and muscular rigidity with release of CK and myoglobin, but is precipitated by anaesthetic agents (see below), and so the onset is generally more abrupt and the fever and increase in serum CK concentration more dramatic.

The pathogenesis of MH appears to be distinct, in that the muscular rigidity of NMS is relieved by centrally acting drugs such as diazepam and lorazepam, and by presynaptic blockade with pancuronium and curare, all of which are ineffective in MH. Both, however, may be relieved by dantrolene, which prevents calcium release at the sarcoplasmic reticulum, indicating a common final pathway for the muscular signs and symptoms, including myonecrosis. Furthermore, MH is known to have a dominant pattern of inheritance and to recur following re-exposure to anaesthetics while NMS occurs sporadically and rarely, if ever, recurs. It is interesting to note that muscle taken from an NMS survivor showed abnormal contracture on exposure to halothane (but not to caffeine as would be expected in MH [Caroff *et al.* 1983]), and that pigs with the porcine stress syndrome (clinically similar to human MH) had low striatal dopamine levels (Hallberg *et al.* 1983). A recent study also found increased intracellular Ca^{++} concentrations in NMS muscle fibres, as noted in patients with MH (Lopez *et al.* 1989).

Treatment of mild cases of NMS may require only supportive measures, removal of the neuroleptics, cooling, oxygen, intravenous hydration, and management of acidosis; but in most instances dantrolene sodium intravenously or orally, combined with bromocriptine orally, will be required and is generally rapidly effective (Gibb and Lees 1985). In refractory cases, intravenous benzodiazepines or even ECT may be required (Kellam 1987). NMS and MH are also discussed in Chapter 29.

Levodopa-induced movement disorders

These are typically Type A reactions that remit when the dose is reduced or the drug withdrawn. Orthostatic hypotension and syncope are also Type A reactions to levodopa. Two particular adverse effects deserve further discussion.

The 'on-off' phenomenon

This is usually a result of long-term levodopa therapy. Several times a day the patient goes through a cycle of benefit from levodopa, but accompanied by involuntary movements ('on'), which suddenly changes to a state of akinesia and severe rigidity ('off') (Marsden *et al.* 1973). Although this phenomenon is dose related it does not correspond to changes in blood concentrations of levodopa (Rosin *et al.* 1979). Smaller and more frequent doses of levodopa are often advocated to alleviate the condition and a change to bromocriptine is suggested

(Fahn *et al.* 1979). Bromocriptine, however, may produce marked mental changes and, indeed, can cause alteration in dopamine receptor sensitivity. Price and colleagues (1978) suggested that the dopamine antagonist tiapride can alleviate levodopa-induced dyskinesias without the necessity of a reduction in levodopa dosage.

Akinesia paradoxica

This adverse effect can be very difficult to distinguish from parkinsonian bradykinesia (Ambani and van Woert 1973). In akinesia paradoxica the patient experiences a sudden sensation of extreme heaviness of both feet, trembling, and a tendency to fall forwards but an inability to start walking. There is no rigidity and, once walking starts, the gait is fairly normal. The phenomenon is dose related and responds to a reduction in the dose of levodopa, unlike bradykinesia.

Other dyskinesias caused by levodopa

Oro-bucco-lingual-facial dyskinesias, which may progress to involve the trunk and limbs, can develop early in treatment with levodopa; fortunately they respond to a reduction in dose.

Neuropathies

Cranial neuropathies

The drugs that affect the functioning of the cranial nerves involved with vision and eye movements and with smell, taste, hearing, and balance, are discussed in greater detail in the relevant chapters on eye disorders (Chapter 21), and on ear, nose, and throat disorders (Chapter 22). Ackerman and Kasbekar (1997) have recently reviewed reports of disturbances of taste and smell induced by drugs, in particular anosmia, hyposmia, dysgeusia, parageusia, and ageusia. Seligmann *et al.* (1996) have reviewed drug-induced tinnitus and other drug-induced hearing disorders including possible mechanisms.

Visual evoked potentials (VEP) were studied in a patient who developed visual impairment during ethambutol treatment. The electroretinogram (ERG) and flash VEP were normal at the time of maximal visual loss, whereas pattern-reversal VEP at 2 and 5 months after the onset revealed evidence of severe bilateral optic nerve involvement, especially affecting macular fibres. Seven months after the onset, paramacular positive-negative-positive (PNP) complexes with a late positivity (scotomatous response) were recorded after pattern reversal and half-field stimulation, suggesting involvement of fibres subserving central vision. At a time when visual acuity was normal there was still electrophysiological evidence of a mild involvement of the anterior visual pathway. The papillomacular bundle seems

to be especially involved in ethambutol eye toxicity (Petrera *et al.* 1988). Optic neuropathy due to ethambutol may not always be reversible and two cases have been reported in which the toxic optic neuropathy was severe and irreversible despite prompt discontinuation of the drug (DeVita *et al.* 1987).

Kimura and co-workers (1996) described a 34-year-old man who had been receiving hemodialysis for 14 years, and who presented with a sudden onset of blurring of vision in both eyes after elcatonin therapy for hypercalcaemia. Fundoscopy showed normal discs, without swelling, and a normal retina in both eyes. Kinetic perimetry demonstrated central scotomas in both eyes. One month after discontinuing the elcatonin, his visual acuity returned to 20/20 in both eyes.

Visual and auditory neurotoxicity was reported in 42 out of 89 patients with transfusion-dependent anaemia receiving subcutaneous desferrioxamine. Seventy-one patients had abnormal visual evoked responses and 22 had abnormal audiograms with a high-frequency sensorineural deficit. The affected patients were younger, had lower serum ferritin levels, and were on higher doses of desferrioxamine (Freedman *et al.* 1988) than those unaffected.

Amiodarone has been implicated in the pathogenesis of optic neuropathy but the association has not been proven, although the incidence was significantly higher in patients treated with amiodarone than in an age-matched control group (Feiner *et al.* 1987). Lamellar inclusions were found in the large axons of the optic nerve from an asymptomatic subject and were interpreted as a drug-induced lipidosis (Mansour *et al.* 1988). Other reported neurotoxic effects of amiodarone include tremor, peripheral neuropathy, and ataxia. Some rarer effects include brain stem dysfunction with downbeat nystagmus, hemisensory loss and ataxia, dyskinesia, jaw tremor, and proximal myopathy. Electrophysiological examination showed a predominantly demyelinating peripheral neuropathy. These findings suggest that amiodarone neurotoxicity is not confined to the peripheral nervous system but also affects the central nervous system, including the basal ganglia and brain stem and their connections (Palakurthy *et al.* 1987). Amiodarone has been associated with mild visual loss secondary to a papilloedema and papillopathy.

A patient developed a bilateral toxic optic neuropathy 4 weeks after initiation of amiodarone therapy; 9 months later his vision was 20/50 in the right eye and 20/200 in the left (Nazarian and Jay 1988).

A 77-year-old man complained of 4 weeks of hearing loss and a progressive inability to walk. Previous treatment with a course of low-dose cytarabine was felt to be the cause of his acute cerebellar syndrome (Cersosimo *et al.* 1987).

Peripheral neuropathies

The pathological changes in a drug-induced peripheral neuropathy usually consist of axonal degeneration with secondary breakdown of the myelin sheath. Hypertrophy of Schwann cells occurs: the myelin debris undergoes phagocytosis; and eventually the axon regenerates along the existing basal laminal tubes of the Schwann cell. Neither the site of the damage nor its mechanism are known in most cases. A rarer pathological process in drug-induced neuropathy is segmental demyelination. This is more variable, affecting some Schwann cells but not others, the axons remaining intact. The internodal myelin degenerates and undergoes phagocytosis, with baring of the axon. Remyelination follows from Schwann cell replication.

Most neuropathies may be of a mixed nature with one of the pathological processes dominating (Bradley and Thomas 1974). Patients with underlying systemic diseases such as diabetes mellitus, alcoholism, and various deficiency states have a lower threshold for the development of a drug-induced neuropathy. Drug accumulation can occur in patients with impaired renal or hepatic function and when drug-metabolising enzymes are inhibited by other drugs (e.g. cimetidine). About half the population of the United Kingdom (in other parts of the world the proportion may be different) have an increased risk of developing a neuropathy if given isoniazid because they are slow to metabolise the drug by acetylation. Genetically determined slow inactivation of the drug may result in prolonged high serum drug concentrations that potentiate neurotoxic effects. Isoniazid interferes with pyridoxine metabolism and this may also be the mechanism of action in ethionamide and, possibly, pencillamine neuropathies.

Vincristine and colchicine are specific in their action on axonal neurotubular transport mechanisms. In a case with a very high dose of cisplatin, serious derangement of central and peripheral neurones with muscle atrophy and effects on other organs was seen (Maeda *et al.* 1987).

Although 2-chlorodeoxyadenosine (2-CdA) is neurotoxic at high doses, a 37-year-old man with lymphoplasmacytoid malignant lymphoma and pre-existing paraneoplastic neurological syndrome died of an rapidly progressive sensorimotor peripheral neuropathy after completing treatment with two courses of low-dose 2-CdA (Warzocha *et al.* 1996).

Chloramphenicol can produce a vitamin B_2 deficiency; while nitrofurantoin, especially in renal or hepatic failure, inhibits oxidative decarboxylation of pyruvate. Perhexiline maleate (Heathfield and Carabott 1982) and amiodarone (Martinez-Arizala *et al.* 1983) are unique in producing a pure segmental demyelination. Possibly their mechanism of action is through interference with glycolipid metabolism.

A summary of the drugs most commonly associated with a peripheral neuropathy and the predominant type of neuropathy produced is given in Table 20.1. It is probably more useful to consider the types of peripheral neuropathy produced and the drugs associated than simply to list the many drugs and their neurotoxic properties.

Mixed sensory and motor neuropathy

Sensory or sensorimotor distal polyneuropathy is probably the most commonly encountered drug-induced neuropathy. Patients present with the classical symptoms and signs of a mixed peripheral neuropathy. They complain of a symmetrical distal sensory loss, often more severe in the lower limbs and characterized by the classical glove-and-stocking distribution. There may be painful dysaesthesiae and depressed tendon reflexes. This is the classical type of neuropathy associated with isoniazid and ethionamide. These drugs are structurally related and, as previously stated, isoniazid interferes with pyridoxine metabolism, causing an axonal neuropathy that resembles Wallerian degeneration (Ochoa 1970). If the drug is withdrawn at the early stage of the neuropathy, then symptoms and signs remit. The neuropathy is associated with doses of isoniazid in excess of 300 mg daily, and it is recommended that pyridoxine should be given concurrently with isoniazid when large doses are used or when the patient is malnourished and likely to be suffering from a vitamin deficiency (Biehl and Vilter 1954).

McLachlan and Brown (1995) reported the case of a 18-year-old man who had been treated from birth with chronic high-dose pyridoxine for pyridoxine-dependent seizures. Within 2 years of starting treatment he developed a sensory neuropathy which did not progress over the following 16 years. Electrophysiological studies were consistent with a pure sensory neuronopathy due to centripetal degeneration of the processes of the dorsal root ganglion cells.

Nitrofurantoin, commonly used in the treatment of urinary tract infections, has caused peripheral neuropathy, particularly in patients with chronic renal failure (Toole and Parfish 1973). Lindholm (1967) reported an incidence of peripheral neuropathy of 62 per cent in patients with normal renal function and, indeed, a subclinical neuropathy was induced in normal volunteers given 400 mg of nitrofurantoin daily for 2 weeks (Toole *et al.* 1968). Ethambutol can also cause a sensorimotor neuropathy in addition to an optic neuropathy. Thalidomide was an important cause of a predominantly sensory neuropathy, the patients complaining of a painful burning sensation in the extremities with cramping pains in the calves. The symptoms persisted in up to half the patients after drug withdrawal (*The Lancet* 1969).

TABLE 20.1
Clinical syndromes of drug-induced neuropathy

Paraesthesiae only	Sensorimotor neuropathy	Predominantly motor
Colistin	Amiodarone	Amitriptyline
Cyatarabine	Amitriptyline	Amphotericin
Methysergide	Carbutamide	Cimetidine
Nalidixic acid	Chlorambucil	Dapsone
Phenelzine	Chloroquine	Imipramine
Propranolol	Chlorpropamide	Sulphonamides
Streptomycin	Clioquinol	
Sulthiame	Clofibrate	
	Colchicine	*Localized neuropathy*
	Disopyramide	
Sensory neuropathy	Disulfiram	Amphetamines
	Ethambutol	Amphotericin
Calcium carbimide	Glutethimide	Anticoagulants
Chloramphenicol	Gold	Ethoglucid
Diamines	Hydralazine	Mustine
Ergotamine	Indomethacin	Penicillin
Nitrofurazone	Isoniazid	
Procarbazine	Methaqualone	
Propylthiouracil	Methimazole	
Sulfoxone	Metronidazole	
Thiamphenicol	Nitrofurantoin	
	Penicillamine	
	Perhexiline	
	Phenylbutazone	
	Phenytoin	
	Podophyllin	
	Streptomycin	
	Thalidomide	
	Tolbutamide	
	Vinblastine	
	Vincristine	

(Adapted from Argov and Mastaglia 1979)

Follow-up of nine patients did not identify any reliable neurophysiological indicators of thalidomide-induced neuropathy, although a possible relationship with a slow acetylation polymorphism was suggested (Hess *et al.* 1986).

A 67-year-old man developed a peripheral neuropathy with glove-and-stocking sensory disturbances after the administration of metronidazole for hepatic amoebiasis. The clinical picture appeared to be that of myeloneuropathy and a sural nerve biopsy showed severe loss of myelinated fibres, a low density of unmyelinated fibres, and axonal degeneration (Takeuchi *et al.* 1988).

The cytotoxic drugs mustine hydrochloride, procarbazine, vincristine, and vinblastine, cause a predominantly sensory polyneuropathy (Weiss *et al.* 1974*a*,*b*). Vincristine neuropathy commonly develops after 2 months of treatment and may be more likely to occur in patients with lymphoma. Loss of tendon reflexes is accompanied by severe pain in proximal muscles. Paraesthesiae, sometimes with a definite sensory loss, can develop. The neuropathy is axonal in type and usually improves spontaneously on withdrawal of the drug (*The Lancet* 1973*a*). Some degree of sensorimotor neuropathy may occur in all patients on long-term treatment with this drug. When present, the motor weakness may be severe (Casey *et al.* 1973). A few patients also develop features of a painful proximal myopathy. Other neurological effects of cytotoxic drugs have been reviewed by Woodhouse and Blain (1983).

Over half of patients taking perhexiline maleate are found to have electrophysiological evidence of a neuropathy. A severe clinical neuropathy only develops after several months of treatment on daily doses of around 300 mg (Sebille 1978). In addition to dysaesthesiae and weakness, there may be evidence of cranial neuropathies, and a small number of patients develop intracranial hypertension. The neuropathy is slow to resolve following withdrawal of the drug and some degree of dysaesthesia may persist.

Patients on long-term phenytoin therapy (often 10 years or more) may develop a sensorimotor peripheral neuropathy (Lovelace and Horwitz 1968). These patients may have reduced vibration sense and depressed tendon reflexes, particularly if they have been on large doses of the drug (Dobkin 1977).

A sural nerve biopsy from a 47-year-old man on long-term phenytoin therapy and with peripheral neuropathy showed loss of large myelinated nerve fibres and a non-random clustered distribution of segmental demyelination and remyelination and axonal shrinkage. Sixteen months after stopping the phenytoin, the patient had improved on clinical and electrophysiological examination (Ramirez *et al.* 1986).

Irreversible cerebellar damage or an encephalopathy can also result from chronic phenytoin toxicity.

Chloroquine has been reported to cause a neuromyopathy, usually in patients taking 500 mg or more daily (Whisnant *et al.* 1963). A single case report has appeared of a neuropathy in a patient taking chloroquine as standard antimalarial therapy (Karstorp *et al.* 1973). A toxic myopathy and polyneuropathy may occur together with a cardiomyopathy (Estes *et al.* 1987). Rarely, a similar syndrome is caused by dapsone (Saqueton *et al.* 1969), disulfiram (Gardner-Thorpe and Benjamin 1971), and glutethimide (Haas and Marasigan 1968), the last drug being structurally related to thalidomide and also causing a cerebellar ataxia. Neuropathy is one of the most severe adverse effects of disulfiram. Frisoni and Di-Monda (1989) reviewed 37 cases of neuropathy reported since 1971. There was no numerical sex prevalence, although the incidence was higher in women. Symptom onset latency was longer and the neurological deficits were milder below a dose threshold of 250 mg daily or less, suggesting that the disulfiram neuropathy was dose dependent. In addition, chloral hydrate appeared to potentiate the neuropathy, but the mechanism is unknown.

Disulfiram is a rare cause of peripheral neuropathy in subjects being treated for chronic alcoholism. The pathogenesis is poorly understood but appears to be dose dependent and unlikely to occur below 250 mg per day. Dano and others (1996) reported the case of a 42-year-old man who presented with clinical features and electrophysiological and pathological findings consistent with a disulfiram-induced peripheral neuropathy.

Digitalis toxicity may be associated with paraesthesiae or shooting pains in the arms, back, and legs (Batterman and Gutner 1948). Lely and Van Enter (1970) described adverse effects from digitoxin intoxication occurring accidentally in 179 patients of whom two per cent complained of vague pains in the calves and arms. No paraesthesiae or neuralgic pains were noted.

A 62-year-old woman positive for hepatitis B surface antigen and with cirrhosis of the liver presented with distal weakness and paraesthesiae during treatment with adenine arabinoside 5′-monophosphate. She recovered several weeks after the drug was withdrawn. Electrophysiological and histological investigations demonstrated axonal neuropathy. The dose was relatively low (120 mg per kg), and age and advanced liver disease may have contributed to the neurotoxicity (Kanterewicz et al. 1990).

Rutkove (1997) described a patient who developed an unusual polyneuropathy after treatment with interferon α-2a for hepatitis C. The patient, a 46-year-old man with chronic hepatitis C, had an acute onset of an axonal polyneuropathy with prominent small-fibre involvement shortly after completing a 6-month course of therapy with low-dose interferon α-2a.

Twenty patients with AIDS or AIDS-related complex (ARC) received 2′,3′,dideoxycytidine in doses ranging from 0.03–0.25 mg per kg every 8 hours. Nine of the patients developed a mixed axonal neuropathy after between 9 and 12 weeks of treatment. The neuropathy differed from the slowly progressive painful neuropathy of AIDS in its sudden onset, motor involvement, and temporal relationship to the treatment (Dubinsky et al. 1989).

Almitrine dimesylate can induce a stereotypic sensory neuropathy associated with high plasma concentrations of the drug, but there is no evidence that these are due to slow oxidation of the parent compound (Belec et al. 1989). Almitrine is thought to cause a sensory neuropathy with sensory symptoms and signs confined to the distal parts of the lower limbs and involving large and small fibres with an axonal degeneration. Recovery is slow, taking 3 to 6 months after withdrawal of the drug (Bouche et al. 1989). A double-blind prospective study

of the effects of almitrine dimesylate on peripheral nerve function in patients with chronic bronchitis confirmed that the drug may be associated with the development of a peripheral neuropathy with slow resolution (Allen and Prowse 1989).

A longer follow-up of patients with clinical evidence of sensory peripheral neuropathy of the feet and lower legs found electrophysiological evidence of a distal axonopathy without denervation. The amplitudes of sensory potentials were reduced and conduction velocities were slightly decreased. On biopsy, mild neurogenic atrophy of muscles and a distal axonopathy were found, and light and electron microscopy confirmed axonal damage affecting myelinated fibres and to a lesser extent the unmyelinated fibres, and some degree of segmental demyelination (Gherardi et al. 1987). Clinical improvement was very slow and at 6 to 12 months many patients still had decreased vibration sensation and ankle reflexes and decreased motor nerve conduction velocities. In addition, there was evidence of subclinical disturbance of motor function in the upper limbs (Petit et al. 1987). Optic neuropathy has also been reported in a patient with sensorimotor neuropathy associated with almitrine that resolved completely 7 months after stopping the drug (Blondel et al. 1986).

Two cases of peripheral neuropathy were reported in patients treated with cyclosporin (Blin et al. 1989). Colchicine may produce a mixed picture of neuropathy and myopathy. Electrophysiological investigation was reported to show myopathic motor unit potentials, early recruitment in proximal and truncal muscles, fibrillation, and positive sharp waves or complex repetitive discharges that correlated with the course of the weakness, all of which resolved rapidly after discontinuation of the drug. The accompanying signs of axonal neuropathy persisted for longer but with little functional consequence (Kuncl et al. 1989).

The myopathy presents with proximal weakness and elevation of serum CK and an accompanying axonal polyneuropathy which slowly recovers. Electromyographic examination shows abnormal spontaneous activity. These features often result in a diagnosis of polymyositis or uraemic neuropathy, especially when there is decreased renal function and elevated serum colchicine. The myopathy is vacuolar, with marked accumulation of lysosomes and autophagic vacuoles. The pathogenesis probably involves disruption of the microtubular-dependent cytoskeletal network which interacts with lysosomes (Kuncl et al. 1987). (See also below under Vacuolar myopathy.)

De-Deyn and colleagues (1995) reported a 77-year-old man who had been taking colchicine for treatment of gout.

He complained of paraesthesiae in the lower limbs and neurological examination revealed a global muscular weakness, absent myotatic reflexes and diminished sensation. Serum CK levels were increased and electromyography showed spontaneous fibrillations and positive spikewaves. Motor and sensory conduction velocities were mildly reduced. Nerve histology was consistent with a chronic axonal neuropathy with a significant loss of myelinated axons. Combined neurogenic and myogenic features were found in skeletal muscle with focal myofibrillar disorganization and accumulation of autophagic vacuoles in muscle fibres. The features were consistent with the diagnosis of colchicine-induced myopathy and neuropathy and resolved after stopping of the colchicine therapy.

The development of a polyneuropathy with the radio-sensitizing drug misonidazole was found to be associated with a high peak plasma concentration and a large area under the clearance curve (Melgaard *et al.* 1988). Low doses of cisplatin (20 mg per m² weekly) have been reported to cause a primarily sensory neuropathy in patients with carcinomata and metastases and symptoms of painful paraesthesiae and numbness in a glove-and-stocking distribution. The neuropathy developed at a cumulative dose of between 100–640 mg per m² and recovery was incomplete despite withdrawal of the drug (Greenspan and Treat 1988). Cisplatin can also cause ototoxicity and has been reported to be associated with the clinical sign of Lhermitte, which is an indication of posterior column pathology and was considered to suggest spinal cord demyelination. The doses involved were high, and the sign resolved on cessation of the drug (Walther *et al.* 1987). The symptoms are those of a symmetrical, distal, predominantly sensory neuropathy of an axonal type with major involvement of propriocep-tion. A postmortem examination in one case showed a degeneration of the posterior column ganglia. Early clinical findings included distal paraesthesiae and de-creased tendon reflexes before the more serious findings of ataxia, pain, and Lhermitte's sign (Amiel *et al.* 1987).

Nerve biopsies from patients taking chloroquine for either connective tissue diseases or as antimalarial prophylaxis, who were suspected of having neuro-myopathy induced by chloroquine, showed segmental demyelination and remyelination. Cytoplasmic in-clusions were seen in Schwann cells, perineural and endothelial cells, and some interstitial cells, but never within axons themselves. Occasional curvilinear profiles were seen in perineural and Schwann cells with peri-neural calcification. These findings suggest that chloro-quine neuropathy is due to primary involvement of Schwann cells (Tegner *et al.* 1988). A peripheral neurop-athy in a patient with a psoriatic neuropathy was initially ascribed to hydroxychloroquine rather than naproxen but was shown to be related to therapeutic doses of naproxen on subsequent rechallenge (Rothenberg and Sufit 1987).

A case of painful legs and moving toes was reported as being due to a neuropathy caused by a combination of vincristine and metronidazole; the symptoms resolved within 6 weeks of withdrawal of the drugs (Gastaut 1986). A predominantly sensory peripheral neuropathy is caused by vincristine. Ocular palsies, hoarseness, autonomic neuropathy with postural hypotension, re-duced intestinal motility, and atony of the urinary blad-der can also occur. The neurotoxicity is dose related and cumulative with repeated doses up to 30–50 mg but recovery is slow (Legha 1986).

A 54-year-old man was reported to have developed lower limb paraesthesiae, mild distal global hypoaesthesia, and re-duced ankle reflexes after taking 150 mg amitriptyline daily for 2 years. An electromyogram (EMG) showed a sensorimotor pattern in all limbs, compatible with an axonal neuropathy. The clinical picture and electrophysiological changes resolved fol-lowing withdrawal of the drug (Zampollo *et al.* 1988).

Motor neuropathies

A predominantly motor neuropathy can be associated with the use of sulphonamides, dapsone, nitrofurantoin, or amphotericin. A combined motor and sensory per-ipheral neuropathy occurring in a man treated with dapsone for dermatitis herpetiformis resolved when sul-phapyridine was substituted for the dapsone (Ahrens *et al.* 1986). A motor neuropathy has also been reported with several tricyclic antidepressants, including amitrip-tyline and imipramine. An association between cimet-idine and a motor neuropathy has been described (Walls and Pearce 1980). Eade and others (1975) described a predominantly motor peripheral neuropathy associated with indomethacin, which regressed when the drug was stopped. A principally motor, but occasionally ascend-ing, sensorimotor neuropathy, similar clinically to the Guillain–Barré syndrome, can occur in patients treated with gold (Dick and Raman 1982). Painful paraesthesiae and fasciculations may be prominent and there may be an accompanying encephalopathy. Resolution is acceler-ated by chelating agents such as dimercaprol (Perry and Jacobsen 1984). The cerebrospinal fluid protein may be elevated in these patients. A patient was described who developed an acute peripheral neuropathy of Guillain–Barré type shortly after starting captopril for moderate hypertension; this resolved after stopping the drug (Chakraborty and Ruddell 1987). A similar syndrome was seen in two cases of amitriptyline overdose (Leys *et al.* 1987) and occurred so commonly with zimeldine that the drug was withdrawn (Fagius *et al.* 1985).

Subacute myelo-opticoneuropathy (SMON)

In 1973, Nakae and others reported the appearance in Japan of a new syndrome, subacute myelo-optic neurop-athy (SMON). Patients with this syndrome developed paraesthesiae in the limbs and an optic neuropathy. These symptoms were usually preceded by abdominal pain. The syndrome appeared to be associated with taking of large doses of between 1.1 and 1.3 g per day of clioquinol (Entero-Vioform). The number of cases reported has declined dramatically following a ban on the sale of clioquinol. The Japanese had taken particularly high doses of the drug, and although a case of dysaesthesiae following treatment with a preparation containing clioquinol has been reported in the United Kingdom (Terry 1971), the Japanese may have a genetic susceptibility to the development of this adverse effect.

Other neuropathies and radiculopathies

Facial numbness may occur with sulthiame treatment and has also been caused, together with a trigeminal neuropathy, by hydroxystilbamidine (Goldstein *et al.* 1963), trichloroethylene (Mitchell and Parsons-Smith 1969), and labetalol (Gabriel 1978). The mechanism of the cranial neuropathy associated with heavy trichloroethylene exposure is unknown but may involve contaminants or biotransformation to toxic metabolites. In severe cases there is destructive spread of the neuropathic process from the fifth cranial nerve nuclei up and down the brain stem. There is a suggestion also that the chemical reactivates latent orofacial herpes simplex (Cavanagh and Buxton 1989) (see also Chapter 25).

Batterman and Gutnor (1948) reported several patients under treatment with digitalis who developed aching in the lower third of the face, sometimes bilateral, together with a sharp stabbing pain reminiscent of trigeminal neuralgia.

An unusual sensory disturbance, in which patients developed discomfort, pain, and paraesthesiae in the perineal region following intravenous injections of hydrocortisone sodium phosphate, was described by Bartrop and Diba (1969). A similar syndrome is produced by intravenous injections of stilboestrol diphosphate (Honvan). Unilateral or bilateral sciatica and weakness of the legs (rarely progressing to paraplegia, as a result of chronic spinal arachnoiditis) may follow myelography (Shaw *et al.* 1978). This complication, although uncommon, is seen particularly after the use of iophendylate and less commonly with water-soluble contrast media such as methylglucamine iothalamate (meglumine iothalamate) (see also Chapter 28).

Beretta and co-workers (1996) described the case of a 30-year-old man with relapsed lymphoblastic lymphoma and CNS involvement who was treated by systemic chemotherapy and intrathecal injections of methotrexate, cytarabine, thiotepa, and hydrocortisone. He developed a persistent paraplegia with sensory and sphincteric insufficiency. Other causes, such as meningeal carcinomatosis, were excluded and the intrathecal chemotherapy was suspected as the likely cause.

Mielke-Ibrahim and others (1995) described a 25-year-old man who experienced pain, swelling and blistering in both arms together with a right brachial plexus paresis on the morning after taking alcohol in large amounts together with intranasal heroin.

His serum CK, acute-phase proteins, and IgE were raised. The pain was relieved by guanethidine block and the swelling and blisters responded to methylprednisolone. Function returned in the lower division of the brachial plexus within 10 days, but the upper division was still paretic 2 months later.

In another case, a 27-year-old man woke up with fever and proximal flaccid paralysis of the right arm the morning after injecting heroin. Creatine kinase was raised, as was pANCA titre (antineutrophil cytoplasm antibody : perinuclear fluorescence pattern). The cerebrospinal fluid showed an increase in cell count (15 per μL) ald protein (73 mg per dl). Acute renal failure supervened after 2 days but was successfully treated. The paresis was still present at 4 months.

A 21-year-old woman developed an upper brachial plexus lesion after attempting suicide with intravenous heroin accompanied by flunitrazepam and a bottle of whisky. She had raised levels of C-reactive protein and IgM. The paresis resolved within 6 weeks. In view of the immunological abnormalities it seems possible that the immune system was involved in the pathogenesis of the plexus lesions and the rhabdomyolysis.

Danazol has been reported to cause the carpal tunnel syndrome, probably as a result of fluid retention (Sikka *et al.* 1983). Finally, following injection with antitetanus serum, or vaccination against diphtheria, pertussis, rabies, or typhoid or paratyphoid fevers, a polyradiculitis similar to neuralgic amyotrophy may occur (Holliday and Bauer 1983). The patient usually experiences severe pain and then develops weakness and wasting of muscles, most often those innervated by the Vth and VIth cervical roots (Foster 1974). Less commonly a polyneuritis may be seen, sometimes taking the form of an acute ascending polyneuritis of the Guillain–Barré type (Miller and Stanton 1954). Ribera and Dutka (1983) report a case of the Guillain–Barré syndrome associated with the administration of hepatitis B vaccine.

A delayed distal axonopathy may occur with certain organophosphate compounds (Blain 1990). The original description of this syndrome involved triorthocresyl phosphate. The toxic effects were seen several weeks after acute exposure, and consisted of an ataxia and a mixed sensorimotor neuropathy principally affecting the lower limbs. Severe cases have shown marked motor effects resulting in a flaccid paralysis. The mechanism of this delayed neurotoxic effect is believed to be associated with the inhibition of a neuropathy target esterase (formerly called neurotoxic esterase). The neuropathological findings in this delayed neuropathy include a Wallerian degenertion rather than demyelination. Initially there is a focal lesion in large myelinated fibres that leads to axonal death distal to the lesion. Chronic effects following an acute single non-toxic exposure to organophosphates are less well defined and may be principally neuropsychological or behavioural. Neither delayed nor chronic toxic effects have been reported following exposure to carbamates, and both the plasma and red cell cholinesterases return rapidly to normal levels after acute poisoning with carbamates.

Neuromuscular junction

Drugs can block neuromuscular transmission by any one of four mechanisms (Argov and Mastaglia 1979):

1. presynaptic inhibition of propagation of the nerve action potential (local-anaesthetic-like effect);
2. postsynaptic curareform blockade of acetylcholine receptors;
3. combined presynaptic and postsynaptic effects, the presynaptic effect probably being due to impaired release of acetylcholine (membrane-stabilizing action) by inhibition of calcium movement through the nerve terminal membrane, and the postsynaptic effect due to a curareform blockade of acetylcholine receptors;
4. inhibition of ionic conductances across the muscle membrane, preventing generation of an end-plate potential.

Neuromuscular transmission is also compromised by compounds (such as the organophosphates) that inhibit acetylcholinesterase and increase the local concentration of acetylcholine at the neuromuscular junction (Blain 1990). Systemic cholinergic effects may even result from ocular instillation of an anticholinesterase. A patient developed a severe cholinergic syndrome following the use of echothiophate iodide ophthalmic drops (Manoguerra *et al.* 1995). There was profound muscle weakness that was initially diagnosed as myasthenia gravis. Red blood cell and serum cholinesterase levels were severely depressed and the symptoms resolved spontaneously following discontinuation of the eye drops.

The drugs producing clinical neuromuscular blockade can be classified in terms of the mechanisms involved, and although many exert both presynaptic and postsynaptic effects one action usually predominates at therapeutic doses. It is more useful, therefore, to consider the clinical syndromes that may occur and the classes of drugs most likely to be implicated.

Postoperative respiratory depression

This is probably the most common clinical manifestation of a drug-induced neuromuscular blockade. Drugs given before or during the operation or in the immediate postoperative period prevent re-establishment of spontaneous respiration. Occasionally, postoperative respiratory depression can follow an apparently normal recovery. due to an interaction between a drug and the muscle relaxants used during anaesthesia with potentiation of their effects and duration of action, a phenomenon termed 'recurarization'.

Postoperative respiratory depression is produced most commonly by the aminoglycoside antibiotics (streptomycin, neomycin, gentamicin, and kanamycin), the polymyxins (polymyxin B, colistin), tetracyclines, and lincomycin and its derivative clindamycin. It has also been encountered following instillation of chloroquine into the peritoneum to prevent the formation of adhesions (Jin-Yen 1971). Paralysis of respiratory muscles usually predominates, occasionally accompanied by generalized weakness. Treatment usually involves assisted respiration, although in the case of direct suppression of neuromuscular transmission by drugs an infusion of calcium gluconate to overcome the presynaptic component of the block and the use of parenteral neostigmine to antagonize a postsynaptic curare-like effect may be useful (Argov and Mastaglia 1979).

Postoperative respiratory depression must be distinguished from suxamethonium apnoea (*The Lancet* 1973b). Patients with an atypical serum pseudocholinesterase are unable to inactivate the muscle relaxant suxamethonium. Although the abnormality is usually genetically determined, an acquired cholinesterase deficiency can also occur in hepatic failure. Drugs such as phenelzine and the potent anticholinesterase ecothiopate (used in ophthalmological preparations) may reduce serum pseudocholinesterase activity. Cimetidine and ranitidine are both reported to inhibit cholinesterases (Hansen and Bertl 1983). A number of other drugs are known to potentiate the neuromuscular-blocking effect of suxamethonium and they may also precipitate postoperative apnoea.

The chemical agents used in 'nerve gases' are potent and irreversible inactivators of plasma cholinesterases. The organophosphate and carbamate insecticides can also inactivate cholinesterases but, in the case of the organophosphates, poisoning with these agents is reversible with pralidoxime if this drug is given rapidly after exposure. Both organophosphate insecticides and nerve gases are extensively absorbed through intact skin.

Activation or unmasking of myasthenia gravis

The safety factor for neuromuscular transmission is already reduced in myasthenia gravis, and drugs known to affect neuromuscular transmission, clinically or experimentally, should be used with extreme caution. Large doses of thyroxine or corticosteroids can produce a sudden deterioration in myasthenia gravis, although by what mechanism is unknown. Many of the drugs involved have a curare-like action on postsynaptic acetylcholine receptors. Withdrawal of the drug usually produces a remission of symptoms, but there are several reports of true myasthenia gravis being precipitated in predisposed patients. The drugs involved include the aminoglycoside antibiotics, chloroquine, procainamide, quinidine, β-adrenoceptor-blocking drugs, phenytoin, and lithium. A reversible drug-induced myasthenic syndrome is distinguishable from naturally occurring myasthenia gravis by the presence of acetylcholine receptor antibodies in the latter.

Ampicillin and erythromycin are commonly regarded as the antibiotics of choice in myasthenia gravis. There is, however, a single report of the electrophysiological characteristics of the Eaton–Lambert syndrome occurring in patients taking these two drugs (Herishanu and Taustein 1971).

Drug-induced myasthenic syndrome

This is a relatively uncommon disorder, since drugs known to inhibit neuromuscular transmission rarely do so at therapeutic doses in normal individuals because of the high safety factor inherent in the system. Adverse effects are usually only seen when this safety factor is compromised, as in electrolyte disturbances such as hyperkalaemia or hypocalcaemia. High plasma drug concentrations occurring with diminished renal function may also predispose a patient to these effects.

The clinical picture is that of myasthenia gravis with a rapid onset but prompt remission on withdrawal of the drug. A drug-induced myasthenic syndrome has been reported in association with many of the drugs already mentioned, particularly the aminoglycoside antibiotics and polymyxins (e.g. polymyxin B), β-adrenoceptor-blocking drugs, and the anticonvulsants phenytoin and troxidone. Carnitine has been reported to produce a myasthenic syndrome when given experimentally to reduce serum triglycerides in patients undergoing long-term haemodialysis (De Grandis et al. 1980). The metabolites of carnitine are structurally similar to acetylcholine and may compete at the receptor site. A myopathy with myasthenic features has been attributed to high doses of codeine linctus (Kilpatrick et al. 1982); the authors felt that the squill oxymel present in the linctus was responsible for the muscle weakness.

A 55-year-old man with idiopathic Parkinson's disease developed myasthenia gravis shortly after taking trihexyphenidyl. The myasthenic symptoms varied directly with the plasma trihexyphenidyl level but without any change in antiacetylcholine receptor antibody titre (Ueno et al. 1987).

Mechanism of action of specific drugs at the neuromuscular junction

Penicillamine

Penicillamine causes a myasthenic syndrome that is clinically and electrophysiologically identical to myasthenia gravis and is similarly characterized by the presence of acetylcholine receptor antibodies in nearly all affected patients (Alberb et al. 1980). Most reported cases have been in patients with rheumatoid arthritis, Wilson's disease, or primary biliary cirrhosis. The onset of myasthenia varies from 2 days to 8 years from the start of therapy although symptoms usually present after about 8 months. The doses involved have varied from 250–500 mg per day, with no clear association between cumulative dose and severity of symptoms. Why only a small number of patients develop the condition is not clear. The first symptoms are usually diplopia and ptosis. Although bulbar symptoms and signs may occur, when involvement is generalized it is usually mild and respiratory difficulty is unusual. The patients respond to edrophonium and in over 70 per cent of cases withdrawal of the drug results in a gradual remission of symptoms and signs. There is also a progressive fall of acetylcholine-receptor antibody titres, and electrophysiological improvement. In patients who fail to remit, an anticholinesterase drug (e.g. neostigmine) is useful.

It has been suggested that the drug unmasks latent myasthenia gravis in individuals possessing the HLA A1 B8 phenotype commonly found in the naturally occurring disease. The drug-induced condition differs in several respects, however, from the natural condition. The modal age of onset, mid-40s, is much later than in females with classical myasthenia gravis. The rate of fall of acetylcholine-receptor antibody titres and subsequent clinical and electrophysiological improvement is far more rapid following withdrawal of the drug than in the spontaneous disease. No association with thymoma has been reported, athough thymic hyperplasia and the presence of striated muscle antibodies are documented. Penicillamine therapy can result in generation of antibodies to platelets (causing thrombocytopenia), skin basement membrane (precipitating pemphigus), kidney (causing a nephritis and Goodpasture's syndrome), and nuclear constituents (causing systemic lupus erythematosus). The presence of striated muscle antibodies may be related to the development of thymic hyperplasia, and the increased frequency in patients with rheumatoid arthritis may reflect a non-specific effect of the drug on the immune system. Experimental work has shown that penicillamine binds covalently to a subunit of the acetylcholine receptor molecule and affects the affinity of the acetylcholine binding site (Bever et al. 1982). Such antigenic modulation could also act as a stimulus and result in acetylcholine-receptor antibody production. An identical clinical syndrome, including the production of acetylcholine-receptor antibodies, has been described in a patient with rheumatoid arthritis treated with chloroquine (Schumm et al. 1981).

β-Adrenoceptor-blocking drugs

β-Adrenoceptor-blocking drugs are associated with a number of subjective adverse effects, including muscle fatigue and peripheral coldness as well as neurological symptoms. In therapeutic doses, propranolol has a postsynaptic curare-like effect in vivo, competitively inhibiting the acetylcholine receptor and producing a rapid fall in the amplitude of miniature endplate potentials. Prolonged curarization due to propranolol has

TABLE 20.2
*Classification of drug-induced myopathies
(after Lane 1996)*

Type	Drugs	Pathology
I. *Focal myopathy*		
Acute	IM injections	'Needle myopathy'
Chronic	IM antibiotics	Fat, fibrous tissue, loss of muscle cells
II. *Acute and subacute painful myopathy*		
A. Myalgia	see text	Unknown
B. Myalgia with weakness and raised CK	see text	Unknown
C. Necrotizing myopathy	Alcohol, opiates, lipid-lowering drugs, IV steroids	Multifocal necrosis; phagocytosis; regeneration;
D. Vacuolar myopathy	Drugs causing hypokalaemia	Cytoplasmic vacuoles
E. Inflammatory myopathy	Penicillamine, phenytoin	Lymphocytic infiltration, necrosis
F. Mitochondrial myopathy	Zidovudine, germanium	Ragged red fibres; abnormal mito-chondria on EM
III. *Chronic painless proximal myopathy*		
A. With Type 2 fibre atrophy	Alcohol, steroids	Type 2 fibre atrophy
B. Vacuolar	Chloroquine, amiodarone, perhexilene, colchicine, vincristine	Lysosomes with myeloid bodies

been reported in postoperative patients (Rozen and Whan 1977). Practolol, pindolol, sotalol, and oxprenolol can also produce postsynaptic blockade. In doses far in excess of those commonly used, propranolol has a pre-synaptic effect (local anaesthetic action) on the propagation of the nerve action potential and inhibits neurotransmitter release. Chloroquine, lincomycin, and lithium have similar actions.

The symptoms of fatiguability and weakness, commonly found in hypertensive patients taking pro-pranolol, may be a result of its curare-like action. The drug has central effects and an action on peripheral blood flow, and these may contribute to this tiredness. Lipophilicity may be associated with an increased incidence of neurological symptoms (Lewis and McDevitt 1986). Skeletal muscle tremor, the most frequent dose-limiting adverse effect, may be reduced by changing the drug or starting at a low dose (Lulich *et al.* 1986).

Phenytoin

Phenytoin has both presynaptic and postsynaptic effects.

The presynaptic action is predominant at therapeutic doses and is believed to be due to a change in calcium flux across the nerve terminal membrane. Aggravation of myasthenia gravis and a myasthenic syndrome have been described in patients with phenytoin intoxication, and this may be due to a combination of decreased transmitter release and a postsynaptic curareform blockade.

Skeletal muscle

Complaints of weakness, cramps, and muscle aching are more commonly attributed to an underlying medical disorder than to drugs. However, although serious drug-induced myopathies are rare, it is likely that subclinical myotoxic effects are quite common. It is convenient to classify drug-induced myopathies on clinical and patho-logical findings (Lane 1996; Table 20.2) but it should be noted that a number of drugs can cause different clinical and pathological conditions depending on circumstances such as dosage and duration of administration.

Focal myopathy

The intramuscular injection of any drug can produce focal inflammation from traumatic necrosis, haematoma formation or low-grade infection, with an increase in serum CK level (acute focal myopathy, or 'needle myopathy'). Cephalothin, tetracycline, and paraldehyde injections are particularly likely to produce such damage (Greenblatt and Allen 1978). Repeated intramuscular injections over several months or years may produce severe fibrosis and contractures (chronic focal myopathy). In the West, drugs of abuse such as opiates (notably pentazocine) and tranquillizers are most commonly implicated (Oh *et al.* 1975), while on the Indian subcontinent repeated intramuscular injections of anti-biotics into the deltoid muscles of children have been reported to produce severe contractures (Shanmagasundaram 1980).

Acute and subacute painful proximal myopathy

Myalgia

Muscle pain and cramps are such common symptoms that they are often not investigated. Many unrelated drugs have been reported to cause myalgia without an increase in CK level, including: anticholinesterases, β-agonists, calcium antagonists, carbimazole, dipyrid-amole, danazol, diuretics, enalapril, niacin, and topical minoxidil (Litin and Anderson 1989; Lane 1996). Suxamethonium causes myalgia in about half the patients receiving it, on the day following surgery, sometimes with the release of CK and myoglobin (Laurence 1987) but there is no clear relationship between biochemical changes or the extent of fasciculation induced by the drug, and subsequent symptoms. It has been suggested that suxamethonium induces Ca^{++}-stimulated phospholipid hydrolysis, leading to myalgia mediated by prostanoids (*The Lancet* 1988) and to enzyme efflux due to membrane damage by free-radical-mediated peroxidation (Jackson *et al.* 1987). Treatment with soluble aspirin 600 mg per hour preoperatively appears to halve the incidence of this complication. Severe disabling myalgia within 3 days of starting high-dose alternate-day prednisolone, has been described in a patient with scleroderma with interstitial pulmonary fibrosis. The symptom resolved rapidly when the drug was withdrawn.

Myalgia with weakness and raised CK

Some drugs can cause an acute or subacute syndrome comprising myalgia, with muscle tenderness and weakness, particularly of proximal and axial muscles, and increasing CK levels. The symptoms and signs resolve rapidly on stopping the offending drug, but severe symptoms, including rhabdomyolysis, may ensue if the drug is not withdrawn. Muscle biopsy may demonstrate particular pathological changes with certain drugs (see below) but it is often not undertaken, although electromyographic changes suggesting a mild myopathy have been reported in some cases. This syndrome has been reported in patients treated with the diuretics bumetanide and metolazone, danazol (Spauding 1979), salbutamol (Palmer 1978), pyrazinamide (Fernandez-Sola *et al.* 1996), sulphasalazine (Norden *et al.* 1994), cytotoxic agents, cimetidine, clozapine (Scelsa *et al.* 1996), and lithium (Tyrer and Shopsin 1980). When muscle biopsy has been undertaken, four underlying pathogenetic mechanisms for drug-induced myopathy have been identified on histological grounds (Lane 1996).

Necrotizing myopathy

A considerable number of drugs can produce a necrotizing myopathy. The commonest causes are alcohol and opiates (Blain and Lane 1984). The myopathy induced by ε-aminocaproic acid (EACA) (Lane *et al.* 1979) is sudden in onset and usually occurs several weeks after starting the drug. Although doses in excess of 32 g per day have been taken by many patients without evidence of muscle damage, the myopathy usually occurs when the dose is greater than 18 g a day. In severe cases, rhabdomyolysis and myoglobinuria may develop (Brodkin 1980). The mechanism of action may be related to intravascular coagulation and ischaemic damage to the muscle, and biopsies from such patients may show capillary occlusion and fibrin deposits (Kennard *et al.* 1980), although this is exceptional (Britt *et al.* 1980). Withdrawal of the drug usually results in a rapid recovery.

α-Interferon can cause mild, self-limiting myalgia, but has also been reported to cause a necrotizing myopathy (Miglino *et al.* 1996), inflammatory myopathy (Matsuya *et al.* 1994), rhabdomyolysis (Greenfield *et al.* 1994), and myasthenia (Batocchi *et al.* 1995; see previous section). A painful proximal myopathy has also occurred in patients treated with propranolol (Forfar *et al.* 1979) and labetalol (Teicher *et al.* 1981), and with the vitamin A analogue isotretinoin (Hodak *et al.* 1986; Fiallo and Tagliapietra 1996). This drug can also cause apparently symptomless elevation of serum CK levels in occasional patients (Dicken 1984; Lane and Cream, personal observations).

Colchicine most often causes a neuromyopathy which develops after months or years of treatment (Kuncl *et al.* 1987; and see below), but occasional cases of more acute myopathy occur, usually in patients with impaired renal function (Schiff and Drislane 1992). Two groups of drugs have emerged recently as the commonest causes of iatrogenic necrotizing myopathy: cholesterol and lipid-lowering agents; and high-dose intravenous steroids, particularly in conjunction with neuromuscular paralysing agents (so-called 'critical illness myopathy' or 'acute myopathy of intensive care').

The fibric acid derivative clofibrate proved to be a particularly potent cause of myopathy. Although no longer widely prescribed in the United Kingdom, this drug was reported to produce a necrotizing myopathy, especially in patients with renal failure, the nephrotic syndrome, or hypothyroidism; 80 per cent of treated cases experienced myalgia within 3 weeks of starting the drug and significant weakness developed in over half (Rimon *et al.* 1984) with marked increases in CK in some (Rush *et al.* 1986). It has been demonstrated that patients developing this myopathy frequently have a raised plasma free fraction of chlorophenoxyisobutyric acid, the active metabolite of clofibrate. There has also been a report of reversible electrocardiographic changes of a cardiomyopathy in a young boy given clofibrate during the treatment of diabetes insipidus (Smals *et al.* 1977). The pathogenesis of clofibrate myopathy is not clear but it may be due to an interference in cholesterol synthesis that affects muscle membrane structure and function, impairment of lipid metabolism by inhibition of mitochondrial carnitine palmityl transferase leading to an increase in lipoprotein lipase activity resulting in muscle necrosis, or the local production of a toxic metabolite.

A number of new fibric acid derivatives have been introduced recently and some can, like clofibrate, cause raised CK levels and features of a painful proximal myopathy (Shetty and Routledge 1990). Bezafibrate, ciprofibrate (Betteridge and O'Bryan-Tear 1996), fenofibrate (Blane 1987), and gemfibrozil (Magarian et al. 1991) have all been reported to cause a similar myopathy, which may progress to rhabdomyolysis (Gorriz et al. 1996), and this seems particularly likely to occur when this class of drug is used in combination with an HMG-CoA reductase inhibitor, such as lovastatin, pravastatin, memvastatin, and simvastatin. These drugs, which convert HMG-CoA to mevalonic acid during cholesterol synthesis, cause myalgia with increased serum CK in about 0.5 per cent of treated cases, but the incidence is 10 times greater in combination with a fibric acid derivative and higher still in combination with cyclosporin (Corpier et al. 1988), which appears to impair biliary excretion of these drugs, resulting in higher plasma and tissue levels (Smith et al. 1991). Several reports have documented the development of rhabdomyolysis in patients treated with drugs of this type, including instances when these drugs were used in isolation (Bizzaro et al. 1992; Fernando-Zatarain et al. 1994). Recently, a case of simvastatin myopathy was reported in which biopsy changes typical of polymyositis were present (Giordano et al. 1997). This patient required treatment with methylprednisolone, in addition to withdrawal of the simvastatin, so it seems likely that simvastatin induced an immune-mediated myopathy, rather than acting as a direct myotoxin (see section on Inflammatory myopathy, below).

Nicotinic acid has been reported to cause a similar syndrome in this context (Litin and Anderson 1989). It has been suggested that lovastatin might inhibit production of mevalonic acid and thus ubiquinone formation, which is vital to mitochondrial oxidative phosphorylation (Maher et al. 1989).

Steroids commonly produce a chronic painless proximal myopathy (see below), but an acute painful myopathy has been observed in patients treated for severe asthma with large doses of intravenous hydrocortisone (MacFarlane and Rosenthal 1977; van Marie and Woods 1980) and in patients taking a 17-hydroxycorticosteroid (Perkoff et al. 1959). Similar cases of acute and subacute myopathy have been reported with high dose oral prednisone (Askari et al. 1976), and oral steroids can occasionally cause relatively selective respiratory muscle weakness (Janssens and Decramer 1989). Potent mineralo-

corticoids, such as fludrocortisone, can cause severe hypokalaemic myopathy (see below) (Rivera 1973). However, particular interest recently has concerned the origins of a syndrome of severe flaccid weakness, with areflexia and occasionally with extraocular muscle involvement, which typically develops in patients being treated with high-dose intravenous steroids, usually in an intensive care setting ('critical care myopathy', or 'acute myopathy of intensive care') (Lacomis et al. 1996). Such cases may be misdiagnosed as Guillain–Barré syndrome, or critical illness neuropathy, but the myopathy is characterized by increasing and often very high CK levels. Electromyography will identify myopathic changes and muscle biopsy usually reveals a necrotizing picture, with vacuolar change due to selective loss of myosin filaments (Lacomis et al. 1996; Lane 1996). This condition almost always arises in patients whose muscles are 'functionally denervated', usually through concomitant administration of neuromuscular blockers such as pancuronium, vecuronium, or doxacurium (Marik 1996). Such lesions have been reproduced experimentally in rats treated with dexamethasone after surgical denervation of muscles (Massa et al. 1992).

Cyclosporin has been implicated as a cause of necrotizing myopathy (Noppen et al. 1987; Goy et al. 1989; Grezard et al. 1990), and biopsy findings such as accumulations of subsarcolemmal mitochondria and increased amounts of glycogen and lipid in atrophic fibres have been reported (Goy et al. 1989). Concurrent administration of other drugs and somewhat inadequate documentation of these cases raised doubts regarding the association but a further carefully studied case has clearly established a relationship (Fernandez-Sola et al. 1990; Yamanishi et al. 1993).

One patient, a 65-year-old man, developed proximal myopathy 7 years after renal transplantation and was found to have 'ragged red' fibres on biopsy (Larner et al. 1994). This was attributed to cyclosporin-induced hypomagnesaemia, but the clinical presentation was atypical for cyclosporin-induced myopathy and such biopsy changes can sometimes be found in elderly subjects not taking this drug.

A patient who developed an acute painful proximal myopathy associated with the use of amiodarone has been reported. This was accompanied by hypothyroidism and a neuropathy, and the patient improved on drug withdrawal. Muscle biopsy demonstrated an acute necrotizing myopathy but the mechanism was unclear (Clouston and Donnelly 1989).

Myopathy caused by ipecacuanha and its active alkaloid emetine, is usually slowly progressive and but an acute, painful myopathy with degenerative changes on biopsy may also be seen (Sugie et al. 1984).

Finally, the current trend to self-medicate with large doses of Vitamin E as an 'antioxidant' has resulted in a number of cases of necrotizing myopathy. This is characterized by 'ragged red' fibres on Gomori trichrome staining of biopsies, but the sub-sarcolemmal accumulations comprise a variety of elements, including lysosomes (Bardosi and Dickmann 1987).

Vacuolar myopathy

Severe hypokalaemia can cause a myopathy that is often associated with prolonged use of diuretics such as chlorthalidone (Oh *et al.* 1971), purgatives, and licorice and glycyrrhizinic acid derivatives such as carbenoxolone (Lane and Mastaglia 1978). Amphotericin has also caused this type of myopathy (Drutz *et al.* 1970).

Hypokalaemic myopathy generally occurs when the serum potassium concentration is between 1–2 mmol per litre, especially if there is an accompanying hypochloraemic alkalosis. The clinical picture is similar to that seen during an attack of hypokalaemic periodic paralysis, with generalized weakness, often severe, and depressed tendon reflexes. Unlike periodic paralysis, however, the serum CK is often increased. Psychiatric symptoms such as dysphoria and hallucinations may occur. Electromyography shows evidence of muscle membrane damage, and the histological picture on biopsy is similar to that found in hypokalaemic periodic paralysis, except that the vacuoles, if present are not membrane bound (Bjorn Jensen *et al.* 1977). The syndrome may be superimposed on a drug-induced, chronic hypokalaemic myopathy (see below), in which case selective Type 2 fibre atrophy may also be seen. Return of the serum potassium concentration to normal usually results in a remission of clinical symptoms and signs, although serial muscle biopsies may show more persistent changes.

Colchicine taken in excess or in therapeutic doses in patients with renal or hepatic impairment may also produce myalgia, with proximal weakness and depressed or absent tendon reflexes and markedly raised serum CK levels. Muscle biopsy in such cases may also show a vacuolar myopathy, but this is due to an accumulation of lysosomes and autophagic vacuoles without fibre necrosis (Kuncl *et al.* 1987). However, this drug more commonly produces a complex neuromyopathy rather than a myopathy in isolation, and in such cases there is usually evidence of additional axonal neuropathy (*The Lancet* 1987) and defective neuromuscular transmission (Besana *et al.* 1987) (see below).

Myositis

A considerable number of drugs can induce an immune-mediated inflammatory myopathy. This can occur as part of a generalized hypersensitivity reaction to drugs such as penicillin and phenytoin (Harney and Glasberg 1983), and similar symptoms have been caused by levodopa, cromoglycate, propylthiouracil, cimetidine, vaccines, and α-interferon (Matsuya *et al.* 1994). Drugs such as hydralazine, procainamide (Fontiveros *et al.* 1980), sulphacetamide (Mackie and Mackie 1979), perhexilene (Tomlinson and Rosenthal 1977) and D-penicillamine (Fernandes *et al.* 1977; Morgan *et al.* 1981) can precipitate a syndrome similar to systemic lupus erythematosus, with raised ESR and positive double or single stranded DNA antibodies. This may be accompanied by a myositis and is probably more common in patients who are slow acetylators.

Eosinophilia–myalgia syndrome

An eosinophilic myositis, with eosinophilic perivasculitis and fasciitis, is a feature of the eosinophilia–myalgia syndrome. This syndrome, which comprises fatigue and intense myalgia, and often multisystem involvement, with arthralgia, fever, cough, dyspnoea, skin rash, and oedema, and evidence of myocarditis, pancreatitis, pneumonitis, and ascending polyneuritis, is characterized by an eosinophil count exceeding 2×10^9 cells per litre. The disorder is described in detail in Chapter 18.

Drug-induced mitochondrial myopathy

Confusion has surrounded the role of zidovudine in the production of myalgia and proximal myopathy in patients with AIDS and the AIDS-related complex (ARC). It was known that, prior to the introduction of zidovudine, HIV-infected patients could develop a necrotizing myopathy with little inflammatory infiltration ('HIV myopathy') in addition to a more commonly encountered inflammatory myopathy, but the incidence of this complication was greatly increased when use of the drug became widespread. Indeed, up to one-third of AIDS and ARC patients develop a myopathy after treatment for about one year, using 1–1.2 g of the drug daily, though this largely resolves on withdrawal of the drug (Lane *et al.* 1993).

The drug appears to act primarily by inhibiting mitochondrial function through inhibition of mitochondrial DNA polymerase, resulting in structural mitochondrial abnormalities and a characteristic microvacuolation and myofibrillary aggregation at light-microscopic level, with the development of the ragged red fibres of mitochondrial myopathy in more severe cases (Dalakas *et al.* 1990; Lane *et al.* 1993). This is associated with a reduction in mitochondrial DNA and respiratory-chain enzyme activities which is reversed when the drug is stopped (Arnaudo *et al.* 1991). However, zidovudine itself probably has only a mild intrinsic myotoxic action. A recent trial noted that, while myalgia was reported by almost half of all patients receiving the drug, compared with placebo, weakness was found with equal frequency in the two groups, although raised CK levels were more common in patients on active treatment (Simpson *et al.*

1997). Furthermore, withdrawal of zidovudine does not invariably result in resolution of symptoms and signs, and it now seems likely that the drug exacerbates an underlying low-grade HIV-related inflammatory myopathy (Dalakas *et al.* 1990; Lane *et al.* 1993). The incidence of this syndrome has reduced considerably since the maintenance dosage of zidovudine has been reduced.

Organic germanium compounds, used as antitumour agents, can produce a myopathy. Although this is a vacuolar myopathy (see Chronic painless proximal myopathies, below), there is evidence that this might arise through mitochondrial dysfunction (Higuchi *et al.* 1989).

Rhabdomyolysis

A more severe form of necrotizing myopathy, usually accompanied by extreme elevation of serum CK levels and myoglobinuria, may be caused by any of the drugs that produce an acute or subacute painful myopathy. The disorder is most often seen, however, with drugs of abuse such as opiates (Richter *et al.* 1971; Blain *et al.* 1985), amphetamines (Grossman *et al.* 1974), phencyclidine, ketamine, and alcohol (Lane 1996). Opiates and alcohol are directly myotoxic, while stimulants probably induce rhabdomyolysis by causing extreme motor excitation (Lane 1996).

Rhabdomyolysis has also been reported following accidental ingestion of paraphenylenediamine (Baud *et al.* 1983), and recently during administration of α-interferon for the treatment of hepatitis C (Greenfield *et al.* 1994).

The onset is acute with severe muscle pain, tenderness, and swelling. Generalized weakness is often found, the proximal muscles being more severely affected than the distal, and patients may be areflexic. Seizures and coma or depression of the level of consciousness may occur and about half the patients develop acute renal failure secondarily to acute tubular necrosis. Serum muscle enzymes and myoglobin levels are grossly elevated and electromyographic testing in the acute phase shows myopathic changes, frequently associated with increased spontaneous insertional activity due to surface-membrane damage. Biopsy at this stage may show severe necrosis, with nearly every muscle fibre in the section destroyed. In milder cases, however, the changes may be slight, with scattered focal necrosis, phagocytosis, and degeneration. Inflammatory infiltrates may also be seen.

Narcotics or alcohol are directly toxic to muscle, and the damage may accumulate through repeated use. Experimentally, narcotics alter membrane transport mechanisms and cellular energy production, and both narcotics and alcohol cause morphological changes in muscle cells when they are exposed to sublethal concentrations. The rhabdomyolysis associated with phencyclidine overdose may be secondary to extreme motor excitation rather than direct muscle toxicity.

The major complications of acute non-traumatic rhabdomyolysis are hyperkalaemia and acute renal failure. The acute tubular necrosis may be secondary to plugging of the renal tubules by an interaction between myoglobin and tubular proteins, or may result from a direct toxic action of myoglobin on the kidney (Grossman *et al.* 1974). Hyperkalaemia is common and may cause dangerous cardiac arrhythmias. There may also be characteristic changes in serum calcium and phosphate concentrations following release of phosphate from damaged muscle cells. Initially there is a paradoxical hypocalcaemia in the oliguric phase of the renal failure, followed by a rebound hypercalcaemia in the diuretic phase. The presence of pigment casts in the urine, a raised plasma CK, and myoglobinuria are diagnostic of rhabdomyolysis in a patient with acute renal failure (Grossman *et al.* 1974). The myoglobinuria may be transient but a raised serum myoglobin concentration as measured by radioimmunoassay is always found. Hypophosphataemia has been found to precipitate rhabdomyolysis in alcoholics and in patients undergoing treatment for diabetic ketoacidosis. It has also been caused by the administration of calcium supplements following parathyroidectomy (ane 1988).

Chronic painless proximal myopathy

This is probably the most common type of drug-induced muscle disease. Severe cases are uncommon but milder forms may be overlooked, particularly if the drug involved is a steroid and is used to treat a condition, such as polymyositis, in which muscle weakness and wasting may be interpreted as part of the clinical presentation of the disease.

The clinical features are typically of a slowly progressive, symmetrical proximal weakness, developing over months to years, with variable wasting, normal or depressed reflexes and normal CK. Biopsy changes may be of two types: selective Type 2 fibre atrophy, and vacuolar change.

Type 2 atrophy

This is most frequently seen in chronic alcohol-related myopathy, in steroid myopathy, and with drug-induced chronic hypokalaemia.

Steroid myopathy can be caused by any steroid, but fluorinated steroids such as triamcinolone, dexamethasone, and betamethasone are most often implicated. The myopathy is not clearly related to the dose or duration of treatment. Quantitative electromyography in patients treated with steroids for prolonged periods suggests that there is a high incidence of a subclinical myopathy (Yates 1970). Experimentally, steroids affect cell surface membranes and alter the resting membrane potential. There is experimental evidence that the effects on enzyme systems are secondary to an initial binding with a specific glucocorticoid receptor in the muscle cytosol. This complex binds to DNA in the cell nucleus and presumably affects RNA production. Glucocorticoids appear to initiate several important changes including a decrease in protein synthesis. The Type 2 fast-twitch, glycolytic muscle fibres are much more severely affected than the Type 1 slow-twitch, oxidative fibres. The highly selective involvement of Type 2b fibres in steroid myopathy may be related to inhibition of myophosphorylase activity in fibres that have a limited ability to utilize other energy sources in oxidative phosphorylation. Such biochemical changes may also explain the ultrastructural alterations in Cushing's disease and steroid myopathy, such as the development of intermyofibrillary vacuoles, excessive accumulation of cytoplasmic glycogen, and subsarcolemmal mitochondrial aggregation.

Vacuolar change

The syndrome may also be caused by a number of drugs that induce autophagic vacuoles containing membranous bodies: a lysosomal storage myopathy. In such cases, a drug-induced peripheral neuropathy is almost always present and this may play an important part in the clinical picture and pathological changes observed.

The drugs most commonly implicated are amphiphilic compounds such as chloroquine and its derivatives, used as anti-malarials and immunosuppressants in a variety of conditions. Chloroquine can also produce a clinical picture strongly reminiscent of myasthenia gravis, and other toxic manifestations such as retinopathy, radial corneal deposits, and skin and hair depigmentation may also be present (Ebringer and Colville 1967). Discontinuation of medication usually results in resolution of clinical and pathological changes over many months. These drugs appear to interact with phospholipid membrane systems in muscle fibres to produce myeloid bodies which are resistant to lysosomal degradation, resulting in fibre vacuolation and markedly increased lysosomal acid phosphatase activity.

As mentioned above, ipecacuanha, and emetine, can also cause a chronic, painless proximal myopathy; these drugs are also cardiotoxic (Mateer et al. 1985). Biopsy typically shows changes similar to those in experimental emetine myopathy, with targetoid fibres, cytoplasmic bodies, and many internalized fibres (Friedman 1987).

The neuromyopathy produced by amiodarone and perhexilene (Tomlinson and Rosenthal 1977) tends to be dominated by the neuropathic component; indeed, the neuropathy may occur in isolation. Colchicine and vincristine also cause a chronic vacuolar myopathy with membranous inclusions, but as a result of disruption of cytoskeletal architecture (Kuncl and Wiggins 1988). As mentioned above, colchicine can also cause an acute myopathy if plasma levels rise quickly, for example, in renal failure. Concomitant use of cyclosporin appears to increase this risk (Kuncl et al. 1987). Chronic myopathy related to the use of organic germanium compounds has been discussed previously as has also myopathy associated with rifampicin (Jenkins and Emerson 1989).

Myotonia

Myotonia is a clinical sign in which muscle fibres undergo prolonged contraction due to repetitive firing of action potentials by the muscle membrane. The muscle cannot relax properly after a voluntary contraction or mechanical or electrical stimulation.

Drug-induced myotonia in man occurs most commonly when a drug unmasks or aggravates the symptom in a patient with an undiagnosed myotonic disease, such as myotonic dystrophy or a congenital myotonia. This has been reported with β-blockers (Blessing and Walsh 1977), barbiturates, diuretics, and acetazolamide. The muscle pains, cramps, and weakness of which many patients complain when taking diuretics may result from the induction of a subclinical myotonia. Several agents are known to induce myotonia in animals but not necessarily in man. These include the lipid-lowering drugs triparanol and clofibrate (Kwiencinski 1978), propranolol, veratrum alkaloids, aconitine, 20,25-diazocholesterol, 2,4-dichlorphenoxyacetate, and several other monocarboxylic aromatic acids. Myotonia can also occur when there is a low extracellular chloride concentration. Depolarizing muscle relaxants (e.g. suxamethonium) can cause difficulties with intubation and ventilation during general anaesthesia in myotonic patients (Mitchell et al. 1978) but non-depolarizing agents (e.g. tubocurarine) do not have this effect.

Malignant hyperthermia (MH)

This is a serious and sometimes fatal response to various anaesthetic agents; in children it occurs in about 1 in 15 000, and overall in about 1 in 50 000 to 200 000 anaesthetics (Britt 1996). Predisposition to the condition is inherited as an autosomal dominant trait, with a gene frequency of about 1 in 200 of the population (Britt 1996). However, a number of different genes may confer susceptibility. MH in some families is linked to the ryanodine gene (RYR1, the sarcoplasmic-reticulum calcium-release channel) on 19q, but in others linkage is with the sodium-channel gene on chromosome 17, or no linkage has yet been established (Britt 1996).

MH is not strictly a drug-induced myopathy, but some affected individuals have an underlying myopathy, notably central core disease (which is due to a defect in RYR1), and a raised CK level may be found although this is not a sensitive indicator of predisposition. Many patients who develop hyperthermia with a particular anaesthetic may have undergone anaesthesia previously without complications. There is an *in vitro* test for the identification of susceptible individuals but it requires considerable expertise in interpretation (Ellis *et al.* 1978; Britt 1996). Platelet and red cell bioassays for screening patients also exist (Britt 1996).

Many anaesthetic agents can induce malignant hyperthermia, including suxamethonium, halothane, isoflurane, enflurane, methoxyflurane, trichloroethylene, ethylene, diethyl ether, cyclopropane, chloroform, and possibly ketamine (Page *et al.* 1972). It is also suspected that nitrous oxide and some local anaesthetics may induce the disorder.

MH usually occurs during anaesthesia but may begin immediately after operation. There is a severe pyrexia, metabolic acidosis, often general muscle rigidity, and myoglobinuria. The temperature may exceed 40°C (104°F). Apart from supportive measures, the specific emergency drug treatment consists of intravenous dantrolene.

A similar disorder affects the pig, which has been used as an animal model. There appears to be an abnormality in the control of the release of calcium and its reuptake by the sarcoplasmic reticulum. Excessive amounts of calcium within the muscle cytoplasm produce a sustained contraction that leads to hyperthermia, subsequent acidosis, hyperkalaemia, and muscle damage.

Disorders of bladder function

The bladder has a somatic nerve supply by the pudendal nerves, an autonomic nerve supply from sympathetic fibres carried in the hypogastric nerve, and parasympathetic fibres carried in the pelvic splanchnic nerves. The bladder base and neck and the proximal urethra are rich in α-adrenergic receptors while the bladder vault has β-adrenergic receptors. The act of micturition is a spinal reflex that can be inhibited by higher cortical centres. It is initiated by contraction of the detrusor muscle following parasympathetic stimulation. There is distension of the posterior part of the urethra, reflex relaxation of the external urethral sphincter, and voiding of urine.

Urinary retention

Inhibition of parasympathetic postganglionic cholin-

ergic neurones decreases bladder tone and can produce retention of urine, especially if there is already some degree of outflow obstruction from prostatic hypertrophy. This may be an adverse effect of drugs that are used therapeutically for their anticholinergic activity. This group includes atropine, benzhexol, benztropine, dicyclomine, hyoscine, methixene, orphenadrine, propantheline, and other derivatives of the belladonna alkaloids. Many compounds have an unwanted anticholinergic activity in addition to their intended therapeutic action, and can produce urinary retention. The major groups of drugs that have such an unwanted effect are the tricyclic antidepressants and the phenothiazines. Tricyclic antidepressants also stimulate α-adrenoceptors following blockade of neuronal reuptake of noradrenaline and produce constriction of the bladder neck. Monoamine oxidase inhibitors and disopyramide have also caused urinary retention. Oral and parenteral forms (but not preparations for inhalation) of β-adrenoceptor agonists, such as ephedrine, salbutamol, and terbutaline, have been associated with urinary retention. Theophylline preparations given intravenously (but not those given orally) have produced episodes of urinary retention associated with high plasma theophylline concentrations (Hassan 1983).

Urinary incontinence

Difficulty in the control of micturition, resulting in urinary incontinence, has been reported as a complication of treatment with prazosin (Thien *et al.* 1978), benoxaprofen, metoprolol, and the depot phenothiazines (Shaikh 1978). Kiruluta and others (1981) found that prazosin depressed the urethral pressure profile in urodynamic studies. The mechanism was thought to be by selective blockade of postsynaptic α-adrenoceptors in the proximal urethra. Total urinary incontinence occurred within 24 hours of the concurrent administration of phenoxybenzamine and methyldopa but not with either drug on its own. A subsequent challenge confirmed this interaction (Fernandez *et al.* 1981). Urinary incontinence was reported in two patients taking clonazepam. On discontinuing treatment normal bladder control was regained (Sandyk 1933).

Ureteric function

Ureteric activity is not affected by drugs acting on the autonomic nervous system since the ureteric muscle has no nerve supply. The initiation and propagation of peristaltic waves is an inherent property of ureteric muscle, controlled by a pacemaker focus in the calyces.

Conclusion

The nervous system is unique in its heterogeneity of structure and function, with consequent implications for the variation in biochemical mechanisms and the expression of toxic effects. The variability in susceptibility of the nervous system to exogenous toxins is due to a wide range of factors, although individual variations in pharmacokinetics and pharmacodynamics and the influence of age, sex, and disease are common to other organs. Finally, it must not be forgotten that the blood–brain barrier exists to control the entry of exogenous chemicals into the nervous system and the factors affecting the integrity and function of this barrier are still not clearly understood.

References

Ackerman, B.H. and Kasbekar, N. (1997). Disturbances of taste and smell induced by drugs. *Pharmacotherapy* 17, 482.

Adams, J.D. Jr and Odunze, I.N. (1991). Biochemical mechanisms of 1-methyl-4-phenyl-1,2,3,6-tetrahydropyridine toxicity: could oxidative stress be involved in the brain? *Biochem. Pharmacol.* 8, 1099.

Ahrens, E.M., Meckler, R.J., and Callen, J.P. (1986). Dapsone-induced peripheral neuropathy. *Int. J. Dermatol.* 25, 314.

Alberb, J.W., Hodach, R.J., Kimmel, D.W., et al. (1980). Penicillamine associated myasthenia gravis. *Neurology* 30, 1246.

Alldredge B.K., Lowenstein, D.H., and Simon, R.P. (1989). Seizures associated with recreational drug abuse. *Neurology* 39, 1037.

Allen, M.B. and Prowse, K. (1989). Peripheral nerve function in patients with chronic bronchitis receiving almitrine or placebo. *Thorax* 44, 292.

Ambani, L.M. and van Woert, M.H. (1973). Start hesitation — a side effect of long-term levodopa therapy. *N. Engl. J. Med.* 288, 1113.

Amiel, H., Gherardi, R., Giroux, C., et al. (1987). Neuropathy caused by cisplatin. 7 cases including one with an autopsy study. *Ann. Med. Intern.* (Paris) 138, 96.

Amore, M., Zazzeri, N. (1995). Neuroleptic malignant syndrome after neuroleptic discontinuation. *Prog. Neuropsychopharmacol. Biol. Psychiatry* 19, 1323.

Anderson, K.E. (1972). Effects of chlorpromazine, imipramine and quinidine on the mechanical activity of single skinned muscle fibres in the frog. *Acta Psychol. Scand.* 85, 532.

Ansher, S.S. Cadet, J.L., Jakoby, W.B., et al. (1986). Role of N-methyl-transferases in the neurotoxicity associated with the metabolites of 1-methyl-4-phenyl-1,2,3,6-tetrahydropyridine (MPTP) and other 4-substituted pyridines in the environment. *Biochem. Pharmacol.* 35, 3359.

Arber, N., Fadila, R., Pinkhas, J., et al. (1990). Pseudotumour cerebri associated with leuprorelin acetate. *Lancet* i, 668.

Argov, Z. and Mastaglia, F.L. (1979). Disorders of neuromuscular transmission caused by drugs. *N. Engl. J. Med.* 301, 409.

Arnaudo, E., Dalakas, M., Shanske, S., et al. (1991). Depletion of muscle mitochondrial DNA in AIDS patients with zidovudine-induced myopathy. *Lancet* 337, 508.

Arthur, G.R., Feldman, H.S., and Covino, B.G. (1988). Alterations in the pharmacokinetic properties of amide local anesthetics following local anesthetic induced convulsions. *Acta Anaesthesiol. Scand.* 132, 522.

Ashton, C.H. (1986). Adverse effects of prolonged benzodiazepine use. *Adverse Drug React. Bull.* No. 118, 440.

Ashton, C.H., Teoh, R., and Davies, D.M. (1989). Drug-induced stupor and coma: some physical signs and their pharmacological basis. *Adverse Drug React. Acute Poisoning Rev.* 8, 1.

Askari, A., Vignos, P.J. Jr, and Moskowitz, R.W. (1976). Steroid myopathy in connective tissue disease. *Am. J. Med.* 61, 435.

Asmark, H., Lundberg, P.O., and Olsson, S. (1989). Drug-related headache. *Headache* 29, 441.

Baldassano, C.F., Truman, C.J., Nierenberg, A., et al. 1996). Akathisia: a review and case report following paroxetine treatment. *Compr. Psychiatry* 37, 122.

Ballas, Z.K. and Donta, S.T. (1982). Sulindac-induced aseptic meningitis. *Arch. Intern. Med.* 142, 165.

Barbeau, A., Cloutier, Y., and Roy, M. (1985). Ecogenetics of Parkinson's disease: 4 Hydroxylation of debrisoquine. *Lancet* ii, 1213.

Bardosi, A., and Dickmann, U. (1987). Necrotising myopathy with paracrystalline inclulsion bodies in hypervitaminosis E. *Acta Neuropathol.* (Berl.) 75, 166.

Barker, I. and Grant, I.S. (1982). Convulsions after abrupt withdrawal of baclofen. *Lancet* ii, 556.

Barnes, T.R.E. (1988). Tardive dyskinesia. *Br. Med. J.* 296, 150.

Barnhart, E.R., Maggio, V.L., Alexander, L.R., et al. (1990). Bacitracin-associated peptides and contaminated L-tryptophan. *Lancet* 336, 742.

Barron, D.W. (1974). Propanidid in epilepsy. *Anaesthesia* 9, 445.

Barton, T.L., Roush, M.K., and Dever, L.L. (1992). Seizures associated with ganciclovir therapy. *Pharmacotherapy* 12, 413.

Bartrop, D. and Diba, Y.T. (1969). Paraesthesiae after intravenous efcortesol. *Lancet* i, 529.

Bateman, D.N., Bevan, P., Langley, B.P., et al. (1981). Cimetidine induced postural and action tremor. *J. Neurol. Neurosurg. Psychiatry* 44, 9.

Batocchi, A.P., Evoli, A., Servidei, S., et al. (1995). Myasthenia gravis during interferon alpha therapy. *J. Neurol. Neurosurg. Psychiatry* 58, 729.

Batterman, R.C. and Gutner, L.B. (1948). Hitherto undescribed neurological manifestations of digitalis toxicity. *Am. Heart J.* 36, 582.

Baud, F., Bismuth, C., Galliot, M., *et al.*. (1983). Rhabdomyolysis in para-phenylene diamine intoxication. *Lancet* ii, 514.

Bauer, J. (1996). Seizure-inducing effects of antiepileptic drugs: a review. *Acta Neurol. Scand.* 94, 367.

Baulac, M., Smadja, D., Cabrol, A., *et al.* (1989). Ciclosporin and convulsions in a series of heart transplant recipients. *Rev. Neurol.* (Paris) 145, 393.

Bayne, L., McLeod, P.J., and Ogilvie, R.I. (1980). Antihypertensive drugs. In *Meyler's Side Effects of Drugs* (9th edn) (ed. M.N.G. Dukes), p. 317. Excerpta Medica, Amsterdam.

BCDSP (Boston Collaborative Drug Surveillance Program) (1972). Drug-induced convulsions. *Lancet* ii, 677.

BCDSP (Boston Collaborative Drug Surveillance Program) (1973). Drug-induced extrapyramidal syndromes. *JAMA* 224, 889.

Beales, P., Almond, M.K., and Kwan, J.T. (1994). Acyclovir neurotoxicity following oral therapy: prevention and treatment in patients on haemodialysis. *Nephron* 66, 362.

Bechtel, T.P., Slaughter, R.L., and Moore, T.D. (1980). Seizures associated with high cerebrospinal fluid concentrations of cefazolin. *Am. J. Hosp. Pharm.* 37, 271.

Belec, L., Larrey, D., De-Cremoux, H., *et al.* (1989). Extensive oxidative metabolism of dextromethorphan in patients with almitrine neuropathy. *Br. J. Clin. Pharmacol.* 27, 387.

Beretta, F., Sanna, P., Ghielmini, M., *et al.* (1996). Paraplegie nach intrathekaler Chemotherapie. *Schweiz. Med. Wochenschr.* 126, 1107.

Bertoni, J.M., Schwartzman, R.J., van Horn, G., *et al.* (1981). Asterixis and encephalopathy following metrizamide myelography: investigations into possible mechanisms and review of the literature. *Ann. Neurol.* 9, 366.

Besana, C., Comi, G., Baldini, V., *et al.* (1987). Colchicine myoneuropathy. *Lancet* ii, 1271.

Betteridge, D.J. and O'Bryan-Tear, C.G. (1996). Comparative efficacy and safety of ciprofibrate and sustained-release bezafibrate in patients with type II hyperlipidaemia. *Postgrad. Med. J.* 72, 739.

Betts, T.A., Kalra, P.L., Cooper, R., *et al.* (1968). Epileptic fits as a probable side-effect of amitriptyline. *Lancet* i, 390.

Bever, C.T., Chang, H.W., Penn, A.S., *et al.* (1982). Penicillamine-induced myasthenia gravis: effects of penicillamine on acetylcholine receptor. *Neurology* (N.Y.) 32, 1077.

Bharucha, K.J. and Sethi, K.D. (1995). Tardive tourettism after exposure to neuroleptic therapy. *Mov. Disord.* 10, 791.

Bharucha, K.J. and Sethi, K.D. (1996). Complex movement disorders induced by fluoxetine. *Mov. Disord.* 11, 324.

Bickerstaff, E.R. (1975). *Neurological Complications of Oral Contraceptives.* Clarendon Press, Oxford.

Biehl, U.P. and Vilter, R.W. (1954). Effects of isoniazid on pyridoxine metabolism. *JAMA* 156, 1549.

Bizzarro, N., Bagolin, E., Milani, L., *et al.* (1992). Massive rhabdomyolysis and simvastatin. *Clin. Chem.* 38, 1504.

Bjorn Jensen, O., Mosdal, C., and Reske-Nielsen, E. (1977). Hypokalaemic myopathy during treatment with diuretics. *Acta Neurol. Scand.* 55/56, 455.

Blain, P.G. (1990). Aspects of pesticide toxicology. *Adverse Drug React. Acute Poisoning Rev.* 9, 37.

Blain, P.G. and Lane, R.J.M. (1983). Drugs and muscle. *Adverse Drug React. Acute Poisoning Rev.* 2, 1.

Blain, P.G. and Lane, R.J.M. (1984). Opiate induced rhabdomyolysis. *Br. Med. J.* 289, 228.

Blain, P.G., Lane, R.J.M., Bateman, D.N., *et al.* (1985). Opiate induced rhabdomyolysis. *Hum. Toxicol.* 4, 71.

Blane, G.F. (1987). Comparative toxicity and safety profile of fenofibrate and other fibric acid derivatives. *Am. J. Med.* 83 (Suppl. 5B), 26.

Blessing, W. and Walsh, J.C. (1977). Myotonia precipitated by propranolol therapy. *Lancet* i, 73.

Blin, O., Desnuelle, C., Pellissier, J.F., *et al.* (1989). Peripheral neuropathy and cyclosporin (apropos 2 cases). *Thérapie* 44, 55.

Blondel, M., Arnott, G., Defoort, S., *et al.* (1986). Eleven cases of neuropathy induced by almitrine, of which one had optic neuropathy. *Rev. Neurol.* 142, 683.

Bonnetblanc, J.M., Hugon, J., Dumas, M., *et al.* (1983). Intracranial hypertension with etretinate. *Lancet* ii, 974.

Bouche, P., Lacomblez, L., Leger, J.M., *et al. et al.* (1989). Peripheral neuropathies during treatment with almitrine: report of 46 cases. *J. Neurol.* 236, 29.

Bradley, W.G. and Thomas, P.K. (1974). The pathology of peripheral nerve disease. In *Diseases of Voluntary Muscle* (3rd edn) (ed. J.N. Walton), p. 234. Churchill Livingstone, Edinburgh.

Bradley, W.G., Fewings, J.D., Harris, J.B., *et al.* (1976). Emetine myopathy in the rat. *Br. J. Pharmacol.* 57, 29.

Brent, J., Vo, N., Kulig, K., *et al.* (1990). Reversal of prolonged isoniazid-induced coma by pyridoxine. *Arch. Intern. Med.* 150, 1751.

Briscoe, J.G., Curry, S.C., Gerkin, R.D., *et al.* (1988). Pemoline-induced choreoathetosis and rhabdomyolysis. *Med. Toxicol. Adverse Drug Exp.* 3, 72.

Britt, B.A. (1996). Malignant hyperthermia. In *Handbook of Muscle Disease* (ed. R.J.M. Lane), p. 451. Marcel Dekker, New York.

Britt, C.W., Light, R.R., Peters, B.H., *et al.* (1980). Rhabdomyolysis during treatment with epsilon-aminocaproic acid. *Arch. Neurol.* 37, 187.

Brodkin, H.M. (1980). Myoglobinuria following epsilon aminocaproic acid (EACA) therapy. Case report. *J. Neurosurg.* 53, 690.

Bruni, J., Gallo, J.M., Lee, C.S., *et al.* (1980). Interaction of valproic acid with phenytoin. *Neurology* (N.Y.) 30, 1233.

Buckley, N.A., Dawson, A.H., Whyte, I.M., *et al.* (1994). Pheniramine: a much abused drug. *Med. J. Aust.* 160, 188.

Burke, R.E., Fahn, S., Mayeux, R., *et al.* (1981). Neuroleptic malignant syndrome caused by dopamine-depleting drugs in the patient with Huntington's disease. *Neurology* (N.Y.) 31, 1022.

Cape, G. (1994). Neuroleptic malignant syndrome — a cautionary tale and a surprising outcome. *Br. J. Psychiatry* 164, 120.

Caroff, S., Rosenberg, H., and Gerber, J.C. (1983). Neuroleptic malignant syndrome and malignant hyperthermia. *Lancet* i, 244.

Cartlidge, N.E.F. (1981). Drug-induced coma. *Adverse Drug React. Bull.* No. 88.

Casey, E.G., Jelife, A.M., LeQuesne, P.M., *et al.* (1973). Vincristine neuropathy: Clinical and electrophysiological observations. *Brain* 96, 69.

Cavanagh, J.B. and Buxton, P.H. (1989). Trichloroethylene cranial neuropathy: is it really a toxic neuropathy or does it activate latent herpes virus? *J. Neurol. Neurosurg. Psychiatry* 52, 297.

Cersosimo, R.J., Carter, R.T., Matthews, S.J., *et al.* (1987). Acute cerebellar syndrome, conjunctivitis, and hearing loss associated with low-dose cytarabine administration. *Drug Intell. Clin. Pharmacol.* 21, 798.

Chadwick, D.W. (1981). Convulsions associated with drug therapy. *Adverse Drug React. Bull.* 87, 316.

Chadwick, D., Reynolds, E.H., and Marsden, C.D. (1976). Anticonvulsant-induced dyskinesias: A comparison with dyskinesias induced by neuroleptics. *J. Neurol. Neurosurg. Psychiatry* 39, 1210.

Chakrabati, A. and Pearace, J.M.S. (1981). Essential tremor: Response to primidone. *J. Neurol. Neurosurg. Psychiatry* 44, 650.

Chakraborty, T.K. and Ruddell, W.S. (1987). Guillain–Barré neuropathy during treatment with captopril. *Postgrad. Med. J.* 63, 221.

Chastel, C. and Mabin, D. (1996). Encephalopathies after levamisole therapy. *Neurology* 46, 288.

Chern, T.L. and Hu, S.C. (1993). Diagnostic and therapeutic utility of flumazenil in comatose patients with drug overdose. *Am. J. Emerg. Med.* 11, 122.

Chetaille, E., Masmoudi, K., Dimier-David, L., *et al.* (1994). Convulsions associated with excessive ceftazidine dosages in patients with renal failure. *Thérapie* 49, 435.

Chez, M., Gila, C.A., Ransohoff, R.M., *et al.* (1989). Ibuprofen-induced meningitis: detection of intrathecal IgG synthesis and immune complexes. *Neurology* 39, 1578.

Chung, W.S. and Chiu, H.P. (1996). Drug-induced akathisia revisited. *Br. J. Clin. Pract.* 50, 270.

Clarke, C.E., Shand, D., Yuill, G.M., *et al.* (1988). Clinical spectrum of neuroleptic malignant syndrome. *Lancet* ii, 969.

Clouston, P.D. and Donnelly, P.E. (1989). Acute necrotising myopathy associated with amiodarone therapy. *Aust. N.Z. J. Med.* 19, 483.

Consroe, P.F. (1975). Hallucinogenic agents, seizures, and drug antagonists. *Psychopharmacol. Bull.* 11, 56.

Corpier, C.L., Jones, F.H., Suki, W.N., *et al.* (1988). Rhabdomyolysis and renal injury with lovastatin use: report of two cases in cardiac transplant recipients. *JAMA* 260, 239.

Crawford, J.P. (1977). Dystonic reaction to high dose propranolol. *Br. Med. J.* iii, 1156.

Cunha, J.M., Carlini, E.A., Pereira, A.E., *et al.* (1980). Chronic administration of cannabidiol to healthy volunteers and epileptic patients. *Pharmacology* 21, 175.

Cyr, M., Laizure, S.C., and daCunha, C.M. (1997). Methazolamide-induced delirium. *Pharmacotherapy* 17, 387.

Dalakas, M.C., Illa, I., Pezeshkpour, G.H., *et al.* (1990). Mitochondrial myopathy caused by long-term zidovudine therapy. *N. Engl. J. Med.* 322, 1098.

Dam, M. (1990). Vigabatrin and behaviour disturbances. *Lancet* 335, 605.

Daniels, J., Baker, D.G., and Norman, A.B. (1996). Cocaine-induced tics in untreated Tourette's syndrome. *Am. J. Psychiatry* 153, 965.

Dano, P., Tammam, D., Brosset, C., *et al.* (1996). Les neuropathies périphériques dues au disulfirame. *Rev. Neurol.* (Paris) 152, 294.

Daras, M., Koppel, B.S., and Atos-Radzion, E. (1994). Cocaine-induced choreoathetoid movements ('crack dancing'). *Neurology* 44, 751.

Davidson, S.I. (1971). Reported adverse effects of oral contraceptives on the eye. *Trans. Ophthalmol. Soc. U.K.* 91, 561.

Davis, G.C., Williams, A.C., Markey, S.P. *et al.* (1979). Chronic Parkinsonism secondary to intravenous injection of meperidine analogues. *Psychiatry Res.* 1, 249.

De-Deyn, P.P., Ceuterick, C., Saxena, V., *et al.* (1995). Chronic colchicine-induced myopathy and neuropathy. *Acta Neurol. Belg.* 95, 29.

De Grandis, D., Mezzina, C., Fiaschi, A., *et al.* (1980). Myasthenia due to carnitine treatment. *J. Neurol. Sci.* 46, 365.

Demers, R., Lukesh, R., and Prichard, J. (1970). Convulsion during lithium therapy. *Lancet* ii, 315.

Dent, J. (1995). Catatonic syndrome following recovery from neuroleptic malignant syndrome. *J. Intellect. Disab. Res.* 39, 457.

Devine, M.L., Gow, G.F., Greenberg, B.R., *et al.* (1987). Adverse reactions to delta-9-tetrahydrocannabinol given as an antiemetic in a multicenter study. *Clin. Pharmacol.* 6, 319.

DeVita, E.G., Miao, M., and Sadun, A.A. (1987). Optic neuropathy in ethambutol-treated renal tuberculosis. *Eur. J. Clin. Ophthalmol.* 7, 77.

Dhuna, A., Pascual-Leone, A., and Belgrade, M. (1991). *J. Neurol. Neurosurg. Psychiatry* 54, 803.

Dick, D.J. and Raman, D. (1982). The Guillain–Barré syndrome following gold therapy. *Scand. J. Rheumatol.* 1, 119.

Dicken, C.H. (1984). Retinoids: a review. *J. Am. Acad. Dermatol.* 11, 541.

Diener, H.C. and Wilkinson, M. (1988). *Drug-induced Headache.* Springer-Verlag, Berlin.

Dobkin, B.H. (1977). Reversible subacute peripheral neuropathy induced by phenytoin. *Arch. Neurol.* 34, 189.

Domingo, P., Munoz, J., Bonastre, M., *et al.* (1989). Benign type of malignant syndrome. *Lancet* i, 50.

Dostert, P. and Strolin-Benedetti, M. (1988). The bases of MPTP neurotoxicity. *Encéphale* 14, 399.

Douglas, C.R. and Harms, R.H. (1990). An evaluation of a stepdown amino-acid feeding program for commercial pullets to 20 weeks of age. *Poult. Sci.* 69, 763.

Drug Intelligence and Clinical Pharmacy (1990). Potential neurologic toxicity related to ciprofloxacin. *Drug Intell. Clin. Pharm.* 24, 138.

Drutz, D.J., Fan, J.H., Tai, T.Y., *et al.* (1970). Hypokalemic rhabdomyolysis and myoglobinuria following amphotericin B therapy. *JAMA* 211, 824.

Dubinsky, R.M., Yarchoan, R., Dalakas, M., *et al.* (1989). Reversible axonal neuropathy from the treatment of AIDS and related disorders with 2',3'-dideoxycytidine (ddC). *Muscle–Nerve* 12, 856.

Dukes, M.N.G. (ed.) (1980). *Meyler's Side Effects of Drugs* (9th edn). Excerpta Medica, Amsterdam.

Dulli, D.A., Luzzio, C.C., Williams, E.C., *et al.* (1996). Cerebral venous thrombosis and activated protein C resistance. *Stroke* 27, 1731.

Duvoisin, R.C. (1968). Neurological reactions to psychotropic drugs. In *Psychopharmacology: a Review of Progress 1957–1967*, p. 111. U.S. Government Printing Office, Washington.

Eade, O.E., Acheson, E.D., Cuthbert, M.F., *et al.* (1975). Peripheral neuropathy and indomethacin. *BMJ* ii, 66.

Ebringer, A. and Colville, P. (1967). Chloroquine neuromyopathy associated with keratopathy and retinopathy. *BMJ* ii, 219.

Edwards, J.G. (1979). Antidepressants and convulsions. *Lancet* ii, 1368.

Eeg-Olofsson, O., Malmros, I., Elwin, C.E., *et al.* (1978). Convulsions in a breast-fed infant after maternal indomethacin. *Lancet* ii, 215.

Eiser, R., Neff, M.S., and Slifkin, R.F. (1982). Acute myoglobinuric renal failure, a consequence of the neuroleptic malignant syndrome. *Arch. Intern. Med.* 142, 601.

Ellis, F.R., Harriman, D.G.F., and Currie, S. (1978). Screening for malignant hyperthermia in susceptible patients. In *Second International Symposium on Malignant Hyperthermia* (ed. J.A. Aldreta and B.A. Britt), p. 273. Grune and Stratton, New York.

Estes, M.L., Ewing-Wilson, D., Chou, S.M., *et al.* (1987). Chloroquine neuromyotoxicity. Clinical and pathologic perspective. *Am. J. Med.* 82, 447.

Evans, D.A.P., Manley, K.A., and McKusick, V.A. (1960). Genetic control of isoniazid metabolism in man. *BMJ* ii, 485.

Evans, J.M. and Keogh, J.A.M. (1977). Adverse reactions to intravenous anaesthetic induction agents. *BMJ* ii, 735.

Fahn, S., Cote, L.J., Snider, S.R., *et al.* (1979). The role of bromocriptine in the treatment of parkinsonism. *Neurology* (N.Y.) 29, 1077.

Feiner, L.A., Younge, B.R., Kazmier, F.J., *et al.* (1987). Optic neuropathy and amiodarone therapy. *Mayo Clin. Proc.* 62, 702.

Fernandes, L., Swinson, D.R., and Hamilton, E.B.D. (1977). Dermatomyositis complicating penicillamine treatment. *Ann. Rheum. Dis.* 36, 94.

Fernandez, P.G., Sahni, S., Galway, B.A., *et al.* (1981). Urinary incontinence due to interaction of phenoxy-benzamine and alpha-methyldopa. *Can. Med. Assoc. J.* 124, 174.

Fernandez-Sola, J., Campistol, J., Casademont, J., *et al.* (1990). Reversible cyclosporin myopathy. *Lancet* 335, 362.

Fernandez-Sola, J., Campistol, J.M., Miro, O., *et al.* (1996). Acute toxic myopathy due to pyrazinamide in a patient with renal transplantation and cyclosporine therapy. *Nephrol. Dial. Transplant.* 11, 1850.

Fernando-Zatarain, G., Navarro, V., Garcia, H., *et al.* (1994). Rhabdomyolysis and acute renal failure asociated with lovastatin. *Nephron* 66, 483.

Fewings, J.D., Burns, R.J., and Kakulas, B.A. (1973). A case of acute emetine myopathy. In *Clinical Studies in Myology* (ed. B.A. Kakulas), p. 594. Excerpta Medica, Amsterdam.

Fiallo, P. and Tagliapietra, A.G. (1996). Severe acute myopathy induced by isotretinoin. *Arch. Dermatol.* 132, 1521.

Fish, D.R. and Espir, M.L.E. (1988). Convulsions associated with anti-malarial drugs: implications for people with epilepsy. *BMJ* 297, 526.

Fontiveros, E.S., Cumming, W.J.K., and Hudgson, P. (1980). Procainamide-induced myositis. *J. Neurol. Sci.* 45, 143.

Forfar, J.C., Brown, G.J., and Cull, R.E. (1979). Proximal myopathy after beta-blockade. *BMJ* ii, 1331.

Foster, J.B. (1974). Clinical features of some miscellaneous neuromuscular disorders. In *Diseases of Voluntary Muscle* (3rd edn) (ed. J.N. Walton), p. 890. Churchill Livingstone, Edinburgh .

François, B., Marquet, P., Desachy, A., *et al.* (1997). Serotonin syndrome due to an overdose of moclobemide and clomipramine. *Intens. Care Med.* 23, 122.

Frankle, M.A., Eichbert, R., and Zachariah, S.B. (1988). Anabolic androgenic steroids and a stroke in an athlete: case report. *Arch. Phys. Med. Rehabil.* 69, 623.

Freedman, M.H., Boyden, M., Taylor, M., *et al.* (1988). Neurotoxicity associated with deferoxamine therapy. *Toxicology* 49, 283.

Friedman, E.J. 1984). Death from ipecac intoxication in a patient with anorexia nervosa. *Am. J. Psychiatry* 141, 702.

Friedman, R., Zitelli, B., Jardine, B., *et al.* (1982). Seizures in a patient receiving terbutaline. *AJDC* 136, 1091.

Frisoni, G.B. and Di-Monda, V. (1989). Disulfiram neuropathy: a review and report of a case. *Alcohol Alcohol.* 24, 429.

Gabriel, R. (1978). Circumoral paraesthesiae and labetalol. *BMJ* i, 580.

Gales, B.J. and Gales, M.A. (1996). Confusion and bradykinesia associated with famciclovir therapy for herpes zoster. *American Journal of Health-System Pharmacy* 53, 1454.

Gangji, D, Reaman, G.H., Cohen S.R., *et al.* (1980). Leucoencephalopathy and elevated levels of myselin basic protein in the cerebrospinal fluid of patients with actue lymphoblastic leukemia. *N. Engl. J. Med.* 303, 19.

Gardner-Thorpe, C. and Benjamin, S. (1971). Peripheral neuropathy after disulfiram administration. *J. Neurol. Neurosurg. Psychiatry* 34, 253.

Gastaut, J.L. (1986). Painful legs and moving toes. A drug-induced case. *Rev. Neurol.* 142, 641.

Gerlach, J. and Casey, D.E. (1988). Tardive dyskinesia. *Acta Psychiatr. Scand.* 77, 369.

Gerlach, M. and Riederer, P. (1996). Animal models of Parkinson's disease: an empirical comparison with the phenomenology of the disease in man. *J. Neurol. Transm.* 103, 987.

Gherardi, R., Baudrimont, M., Gray, F., *et al.* (1987). Almitrine neuropathy. A nerve biopsy study of 8 cases. *Acta Neuropathol.* 73, 202.

Giansiracusa, D.F., Blumberg, S., and Kantrowitz, F.G. (1980). Aseptic meningitis associated with ibuprofen. *Arch. Intern. Med.* 140, 1553.

Gibb, W.R.G. and Lees, A.J. (1985). The neuroleptic malignant syndrome — a review. *Q. J. Med.* 56, 421.

Giordano, N., Senesi, M., Matti, G., *et al.* (1997). Polymyositis associated with simvastatin. *Lancet* 349, 1600.

Glazer, W.M., Bower, M.B., Charney, D.S., *et al.* (1989). The effect of neuroleptic discontinuation on psychopathology, involuntary movements, and biochemical measures in patients with persistent tardive dyskinesia. *Biol. Psychiatry* 26, 224.

Goekoop, J.G. and Carbaat, P.A.T. (1982). Treatment of neuroleptic malignant syndrome with dantrolene. *Lancet* ii, 49.

Goldstein, N.P., Gibilisco, J.A., and Rushton, J.G. (1963). Trigeminal neuropathy and neuritis. *JAMA* 184, 458.

Gonzalez, F.J. (1988). The molecular biology of cytochrome P450s. *Pharmacol. Rev.* 40, 243.

Gonzalez, F.J., Matsunaga, T., Nagata, K., *et al.* (1987). Debrisoquine-4-hydroxylase: Characterisation of a new F450 gene subfamily regulation, chromosomal mapping and molecular analysis of the DA rate polymorphism. *DNA* 6, 149.

Gonzalez, F.J., Skoda, R.C., Kimura, S. *et al.* (1988). Characterisation of the common genetic defect in humans deficient in debrisoquine metabolism. *Nature* 331, 442.

Gordon, M. and Gordon, A.S. (1981). Perhexiline maleate as a cause of reversible parkinsonism and peripheral neuropathy. *J. Am. Geriatr. Soc.* 29, 259.

Gordon, M.F., Abrams, R.I., Rubin, D.B., *et al.* (1995). Bismuth subsalicylate toxicity as a cause of prolonged encephalopathy with myoclonus. *Mov. Disord.* 10, 220.

Goren, M.P., Wright, R.K., Pratt, C.B., *et al.* (1986). Dechlorethylation of ifosfamide and neurotoxicity. *Lancet* ii, 1219.

Gorman, M. and Barkley, G.L. (1995). Oculogyric crisis induced by carbamazepine. *Epilepsia* 36, 1158.

Gorriz, J.L., Sancho, A., Lopez-Martin, J.M., *et al.* (1996). Rhabdomyolysis and acute renal failure associated with gemfibrozil therapy. *Nephron* 74, 437.

Goy, J.J., Stauffer, J.C., Deruaz, J.P., *et al.* (1989). Myopathy as possible side-effect of cyclosporin. *Lancet* i, 1446.

Graham, P.M. (1997). Successful treatment of the toxic serotonin syndrome with chlorpromazine. *Med. J. Aust.* 166(3), 166.

Grant, R. (1984). Neuroleptic malignant syndrome. *BMJ* 288, 1690.

Green, S., Buttrum, S., Molloy, H., *et al.* (1991). N-methylation of pyridines in Parkinson's disease. *Lancet* 338, 120.

Greenblatt, D.J. and Allen, M.D. (1978). Intramuscular injection site complications. *JAMA* 240, 542.

Greenfield, S.M, Harvey, R.S., and Thompson, R.F.H. (1994). Rhabdomyolysis after treatment with interferon alpha. *BMJ* 309, 512.

Greensplan, A. and Treat, J. (1988). Peripheral neuropathy and low dose cisplatin. *Am. J. Clin. Oncol.* 11, 660.

Grezard, O., Lebranchuy, Y., Birmele, B., *et al.* (1990). Cyclosporin-induced muscular toxicity. *Lancet* 335, 177.

Grossman, R.A., Hamilton, R.W., Morse, B.M., *et al.* (1974). Nontraumatic rhabdomyolysis and acute renal failure. *N. Engl. J. Med.* 291, 807.

Gur, H., Paz, Y., and Sidi, Y. (1996). Acute dystonic reaction to methotrimeprazine in hypoparathyroidism. *Ann. Pharmacother.* 30, 957.

Haas, D.C. and Marasigan, A. (1968). Neurological effects of glutethimide. *J. Neurol. Neurosurg. Psychiatry* 31, 561.

Hallberg, J.W., Draper, D.D., Topel, D.G., *et al.* (1983). Neural catecholamine deficiencies in the porcine stress syndrome. *Am. J. Vet. Res.* 44, 368.

Hankey, G.J. and Gubbay, S.S. (1987). Focal cerebral ischaemia and infarction due to antihypertensive therapy. *Med. J. Aust.* 146, 412.

Hansen, W.E. and Bertl, S. (1983). Inhibition of cholinesterases by ranitidine. *Lancet* i, 235.

Hardie, R.J. and Lees, A.J. (1988). Neuroleptic-induced Parkinson's syndrome: clinical features and results of treatment with levodopa. *J. Neurol. Neurosurg. Psychiatry* 51, 850.

Harmant J., van Ryckevorsel-Harmant, K., de Barsy, Th., *et al.* (1983). Myopathy and hypersensitivity to phenytoin. *Neurology* 33, 790.

Hassan, S.N. (1983). Urinary retention with theophylline. *South. Med. J.* 76, 408.

Hauser, P.O., Devinsky, M., de Bellis, W.H., *et al.* (1989). Post-benzodiazepine withdrawal delerium with catatonic features. *Arch. Neurol.* 46, 696.

Heafield, M.T.E., Waring, R.H., Sturman, S.G., *et al.* (1990). N-acetylator status in neurodegenerative disease. *Med. Sci. Res.* 18, 963.

Heathfield, K.W.G. and Carabott, F. (1982). Adverse effects of perhexiline. *Lancet* i, 507.

Henderson, V.W. and Wooton, G.F. (1981). Neuroleptic malignant syndrome: a pathogenetic role for dopamine receptor blockade? *Neurology* (N.Y.) 31, 132.

Hendrickx, B. (1990). Fluvoxamine: an antidepressant with low (or no) epileptogenic effect. *Lancet* 336, 386.

Herishanu, Y. and Taustein, I. (1971). The electromyographic changes induced by antibiotics: a preliminary study. *Confin. Neurol.* 33 41.

Hess, C.W., Hunziker, T., Kupfer, A., *et al.* (1986). Thalidomide-induced peripheral neuropathy. A prospective clinical, neurophysiological and pharmacogenetic evaluation. *J. Neurol.* 233, 83.

Higuchi, I., Izumo, S., Kuriyama, M., *et al.* (1989). Germanium myopathy: clinical and experimental pathological studies. *Acta Neuropathol.* (Berlin) 79, 300.

Hinchey, J., Chaves, C., Appignani, B., *et al.* (1996). A reversible posterior leukoencephalopathy syndrome. *N. Engl. J. Med.* 334, 494.

Hintze, G., Klein, H.H., Prange, H., *et al.* (1987). A case of valproate intoxication with extensive brain oedema. *Klin. Wochenschr.* 65, 424.

Hitchins, R.N. and Thomson, D.B. (1988). Encephalopathy following cisplatin, bleomycin and vinblastine therapy for non-seminomatous germ cell tumour of testis. *Aust. N.Z. J. Med.* 18, 67.

Hodak, E., Gadoth, N., David, M., *et al.* (1986). Muscle damage induced by isotretinoin. *BMJ* 293, 435.

Hoefnagels, W.A.J., Gerritsen, E.J.A., Brouver, O.F., *et al.* (1988). Cyclosporin encephalopathy associated with fat embolism induced by the drug's solvent. *Lancet* ii, 901.

Hoff, A.L., Riordan, H., Morris, L., *et al.* (1996). Effects of crack cocaine on neurocognitive function. *Psychiatry Res.* 60, 167.

Holliday, P.L. and Bauer, R.B. (1983). Polyradiculoneuritis secondary to immunization with tetanus and diphtheria toxoids. *Arch. Neurol.* 40, 56.

Houghton, A.W.S. (1971). Convulsions precipitated by amitriptyline. *Lancet* i, 138.

Hurwitz, R.L., Mahoney, D.H., Armstrong, D.L., *et al.* (1988). Reversible encephalopathy and seizures as a result of conventional vincristine administration. *Med. Pediatr. Oncol.* 16, 216.

Hyser, C.L. and Drake. M.E. (1983). Myoclonus induced by metoclopramide therapy. *Arch. Intern. Med.* 143, 2201.

Indo, T. and Ando, K. (1982). Metoclopramide-induced parkinsonism. Clinical characteristics of ten cases. *Arch. Neurol.* 39, 494.

Inman, W.H.W. and Vessey, M.P. (1968). Investigation of deaths from pulmonary, coronary and cerebral thrombosis and embolism in women of childbearing age. *BMJ* ii, 193.

Inman, W.H.W., Westerholm, B., and Engelund, A. (1970). Thromboembolic disease and the steroidal content of oral contraceptives: a report to the Committee on Safety of Drugs. *BMJ* ii, 203.

Irey, N.S., McAllister, H.A., and Henry, J.M. (1978). Oral contraceptives and stroke in young women: a clinicopathologic correlation. *Neurology* 28, 1216.

Jackson, M.J., Wagenmakers, A.J.M., and Edwards, R.H.T. (1987). The effects of inhibitors of arachidonic acid metabolism on efflux of intracellular enzymes from skeletal muscle following experimental damage. *Biochem. J.* 241, 403.

Jansen, P.A.F., Gribnau, F.W.F., Schulte, B.P.M. *et al.* (1986). Contribution of inappropriate treatment for hypertension to pathogenesis of stroke in the elderly. *BMJ* 293, 914.

Janssens, S. and Decramer, M. (1989). Corticosteroid-induced myopathy and the respiratory muscles. Report of two cases. *Chest* 95, 1160.

Jarvik, M.E. (1970). Drugs used in the treatment of psychiatric disorders. In *The Pharmacological Basis of Therapeutics* (4th edn) (ed. L.S. Goodman and A. Gilman), p. 189. Macmillan, London.

Jenkins, P. and Emerson, P.A. (1981). Myopathy induced by rifampicin. *BMJ* 283, 105.

Jin-Yen, T. (1971). Clinical and experimental studies on mechanism of neuromuscular blockade by chloroquine diorotate. *Jpn J. Anesth.* 20, 491.

Johnson, D.A., Etter, H.S., and Reeves, D.M. (1983). Stroke and phenylpropanolamine use. *Lancet* ii, 970.

Joyce, R.P. and Gunderson, C.H. (1980). Carbamazepine-induced orofacial dyskinesia. *Neurology* (N.Y.) 30, 1333.

Kallay, M.C., Tabechian, H., Riley, G.R., *et al.* (1979). Neurotoxicity due to ticarcillin in patient with renal failure. *Lancet* i, 608.

Kane, J.M. and Smith J.M. (1982). Tardive dyskinesia. *Arch. Gen. Psychiatry* 39, 473.

Kanterewicz, E., Bruguera, M., Viola, C., *et al.* (1990). Toxic neuropathy after adenine arabinoside treatment in chronic HBsAg-positive liver disease. *J. Clin. Gastroenterol.* 12, 90.

Karstorp, A., Ferngren, H., Lundbergh, P., *et al.* (1973). Neuromyopathy during malaria suppression with chloroquine. *BMJ* iv, 736.

Keck, P.E., Jr, Caroff, S.N., and McElroy, S.L. (1995). Neuroleptic malignant syndrome and malignant hyperthermia: end of a controversy? *J. Neuropsychiatry Clin. Neurosci.* 7, 135.

Kellam, A.M.P. (1987). The neuroleptic malignant syndrome, so called. *Br. J. Psychiatry* 150, 752.

Kelly, M.A., Gorelick, P.B., and Mirza, D. (1992). The role of drugs in the etiology of stroke. *Clin. Neuropharmacol.* 151, 249.

Kennard, C., Swash, M., Henson., R.A. (1980). EACA myopathy — myopathy due to epsilon amino-caproic acid. *Muscle Nerve* 3, 202.

Kerr, G.W. (1996). Dystonic reactions: two case reports. *J. Accid. Emerg. Med.* 13, 221.

Kessler, G.F., Demers, L.M., and Berlin, C. (1974). Phencyclidine and fatal status epilepticus. *N. Engl. J. Med.* 291, 979.

Kilpatrick, C., Braund, W., and Burns, R. (1982). Myopathy with myasthenic features possibly induced by codeine linctus. *Med. J. Aust.* ii, 410.

Kimura, H., Masai, H., and Kashii, S. (1996). Optic neuropathy following elcatonin therapy. *J. Neurophthalmol.* 16, 134.

Kiruluta, G.H., Mercer, A.R., and Winsor, G.M. (1981). Prazosin as cause of urinary incontinence. *Urology* 18, 618.

Klawans, H.L.K. (1987). Dystonia and tremor following exposure to 2,3,7,8-tetrachlorodibenzo-*p*-dioxin. *Mov. Disord.* 2, 255.

Koehler, P.J. and Mirandolle, J.F.M. (1988). Neuroleptic malignant-like syndrome and lithium. *Lancet* ii, 1499.

Kokkinos, J. and Levine, S.R. (1993*a*). Stroke. *Neurol. Clin.* 11, 577.

Kokkinos, J. and Levine, S.R. (1993*b*). Possible association of ischaemic stroke with phentermine. *Stroke* 24, 310.

Konikoff, F., Kuritzky A., Jerushahmi, Y., *et al.* (1984). Neuroleptic malignant syndrome induced by a single injection of haloperidol. *BMJ* 289, 1228.

Konzen, J.P., Levine, S.R., and Garcia, J.H. (1996). Vasospasm and thrombus formation as possible mechanisms of stroke related to alkaloidal cocaine. *Stroke* 27, 147.

Kopin, I.J. and Markey, S.P. (1988). MPTP toxicity: implications for research in Parkinson's disease. *Annu. Rev. Neurosci.* 11, 81.

Koppel, B.S., Daras, M., Tuchman, A.J., *et al.* (1992). Relationship between alcohol and seizures in a city hospital population. *Epilepsy* 5, 31.

Kornowski, R., Fines, A., and Levo, Y. (1995). Ischemic stroke following an intramuscular injection of diclofenac. Case report. *Angiology* 46, 1145.

Kramer, L.D., Locke, G.E., Ogunyemi, A., *et al.* (1990). Neonatal cocaine-related seizures. *J. Child Neurol.* 5, 60.

Kremer, I., Ritz, R., and Brummer, F. (1983). Aseptic meningitis as an adverse effect of co-trimoxazole. *N. Engl. J. Med.* 308, 1481.

Kudo, K., Sasaki, I., Tsuchiyama, K., *et al.* (1987). Serotonin syndrome during clomipramine monotherapy: comparison of two diagnostic criteria. *Psychiatry Clin. Neurosci.* 51, 43.

Kuncl, R.W. and Wiggins, W.W. (1988). Toxic myopathies. *Neurol. Clin.* 6, 593.

Kuncl, R.W., Duncan, G., Watson, D., *et al.* (1987). Colchicine myopathy and neuropathy. *N. Engl. J. Med.* 316, 1562.

Kuncl, R.W., Cronblath, D.R., Avila, O., *et al.* (1989). Electrodiagnosis of human colchicine myoneuropathy. *Muscle Nerve* 12, 360.

Kunzendorf, V., Brockmoller, J., Jochinsen, F., *et al.* (1988). Cyclosporin metabolites and central nervous system toxicity. *Lancet* i, 1223.

Kupsch, A., Sautter, J., Schwarz, J.R., *et al.* (1996). 1-Methyl - 4 - phenyl - 1,2,3,6 - tetrahydropyridine - induced neurotoxicity in non-human primates is antagonized by pretreatment with nimodipine at the nigral, but not at the striatal level. *Brain Res.* 741, 185.

Kurlan, R. and Como, P. (1988). Drug-induced alzheimerism. *Arch. Neurol.* 45, 356.

Kushner, M.J. (1982). Chorea and cimetidine. *Ann. Intern. Med.* 96, 126.

Kwiencinski, H. (1978). Myotonia induced with clofibrate in rats. *J. Neurol.* 219, 107.

Laborde, A., Nogue, S., Munne, P., *et al.* (1987). Status epilepticus caused by abstinence from lorazepam. *Med. Clin.* 89, 885.

Lacomis, D., Giuliani, M.J., Van Gott, A., *et al.* (1996). Acute myopathy of intensive care: clinical, electromyographic, and pathological aspects. *Ann. Neurol.* 40, 645.

Lader, M.H. (1970). Drug-induced extrapyramidal syndromes. *J.R. Coll. Physicians Lond.* 5, 87.

Lalouschek, W., Schneider, F., Aull, S., *et al.* (1995). Cocaine abuse — with special reference to cerebrovascular complications. *Wien. Klin. Wochenschr.* 107, 516.

Lancer, J.W. (1973). *The Mechanism and Management of Headache* (2nd edn), p. 49. Butterworth, London.

The Lancet (1969). Thalidomide neuropathy. *Lancet* ii, 713.

The Lancet (1973*a*). Neurotoxicity of vincristine. *Lancet* i, 980.

The Lancet (1973*b*). Suxamethonium apnoea. *Lancet* i, 246.

The Lancet (1976). Diagnosis of brain death. A paper endorsed by the Conference of the Royal Colleges and Faculties of the U.K. *Lancet* ii, 1069.

The Lancet (1984). Neuroleptic malignant syndrome. *Lancet* i, 545.

The Lancet (1987). Colchicine myoneuropathy. *Lancet* ii, 668.

The Lancet (1988). Suxamethonium myalgia. *Lancet* ii, 944.

Lane, R.J.M. (1984). Drugs and tremor. *Adverse Drug React. Bull.* 106, 392.

Lane, R.J.M. (1991). Cardiogenic dementia revisited. *J.R. Soc. Med.* 84, 577.

Lane, R.J.M. (1996). Toxic and drug-induced myopathies. In *Handbook of Muscle Disease* (ed.R.J.M. Lane), p. 379. Marcel Dekker, New York.

Lane, R.J.M. (1998). The Epilepsies. Aetiological factors — Toxic. In *Handbook of Clinical Neurology* (ed. P.J. Vinken and G.W. Bruyn). Elsevier, Amsterdam (in press).

Lane, R.J.M. and Routledge, P.A. (1983). Drug-induced neurological disorders. *Drugs* 26, 124.

Lane, R.J.M., McLelland, N.J., Martin, A.M., *et al.* (1979). Epsilon-aminocaproic acid (EACA) myopathy. *Postgrad. Med. J.* 55, 282.

Lane, R.J.M., Roche, S.W., Leung, A.A.W., *et al.* (1988). Cyclosporin neurotoxicity in cardiac transplant recipients. *J. Neurol. Neurosurg. Psychiatry* 51, 1434.

Lane, R.J.M., McLean, K.A., Moss, J., *et al.* (1993). Myopathy in HIV infection: the role of zidovudine and the significance of tubuloreticular inclusions. *Neuropatholgy and Applied Neurobiology* 19, 406.

Lang, A.E. (1994). Withdrawal akathisia: case reports and a proposed classification of chronic akathisia. *Move. Disord.* 9, 188; Comment (1995). *Ibid.* 10, 235.

Lapierre, Y.D. and Anderson, K. (1983). Dyskinesia associated with amoxapine antidepressant therapy: A case report. *Am. J. Psychiatry* 140, 493.

Larner, A.J., Sturman, S.G., Hawkins, J.B., *et al.* (1994). Myopathy with ragged red fibres following renal transplantation: possible role of cyclosporin-induced hypomagnesaemia. *Acta Neuropathol.* (Berlin) 88, 189.

Latimer, P.R. (1995). Tardive dyskinesia: a review. *Can. J. Psychiatry* 40 (7 Suppl. 2), 49.

Laurence, A.S. (1987). Myalgia and biochemical changes following intermittent suxamethonium administration. *Anaesthesia* 42, 503.

Legha, S.S. (1986). Vincristine neurotoxicity. Pathophysiology and management. *Med. Toxicol.* 1, 421.

Lehmann, E., Thom, C.H., and Croft, D.N. (1995). Delayed severe rhabdomyolysis after taking "ecstasy". *Postgrad. Med. J.* 71, 186.

Lely, A.H. and van Enter, C.H.J. (1970). Large-scale digitoxin intoxication. *BMJ* iii, 737.

Lewis, R.V. and McDevitt, D.G. (1986). Adverse reactions and interactions with beta-adrenoceptor blocking drugs. *Med. Toxicol.* 1, 343.

Lindholm, T. (1967). Electromyographic changes after nitrofurantoin (Furadantin) therapy in non-uraemic patients. *Neurology* (N.Y.) 17, 1017.

Litin, S.C. and Anderson, C.F. (1989). Nicotinic acid-associated myopathy: a report of three cases. *Am. J. Med.* 86, 481.

Lopez, J.R., Sanchez, V., and Lopez, M.J. (1989). Sarcoplasmic ionic calcium concentration in neuroleptic malignant syndrome. *Cell Calcium* 10, 223.

Loudon, J.B. and Waring, H. (1976). Toxic reactions to lithium and haloperidol. *Lancet* ii, 1088.

Lovelace, R.E. and Horwitz, S.J. (1968). Peripheral neuropathy in long-term diphenylhydantoin therapy. *Arch. Neurol.* 18, 69.

Lowe, T.L., Cohen, D.J., Detlor, J., *et al.* (1982). Stimulant medications precipitate Tourette's syndrome. *JAMA* 247, 1168.

Lulich, K.M., Goldie, R.G., Ryan, G., *et al.* (1986). Adverse reactions to beta-2 agonist bronchodilators. *Med. Toxicol.* 1, 286.

Lundh, H. and Tunving, K. (1981). An extrapyramidal choreiform syndrome caused by amphetamine addiction. *J. Neurol. Neurosurg. Psychiatry* 44, 728.

Lustman, F. and Moncu, G. (1974). Amiodarone and neurological side-effects. *Lancet* i, 568.

Macdonald, J.B. (1982). Muscle cramps during treatment with nifedipine. *BMJ* 285, 1744.

MacDonald, R.D. and Engel, A.G. (1970). Experimental chloroquine myopathy. *J. Neuropathol. Exp. Neurol.* 29, 479.

MacFarlane, I.A. and Rosenthal, F.D. (1977). Severe myopathy after status asthmaticus. *Lancet* ii, 615.

Mackie, B.S. and Mackie, L.E. (1979). Systemic lupus erythematosus–dermatomyositis induced by sulphacetamide eye drops. *Australas. J. Dermatol.* 29, 49.

McLachlan, R.S. and Brown, W.F. (1995). Pyridoxine dependent epilepsy with iatrogenic sensory neuronopathy. *Can. J. Neurol. Sci.* 22, 50.

McLellan, D.L. and Swash, M. (1974). Choreoathetosis and encephalopathy induced by phenytoin. *BMJ* ii, 204.

McMillan, M.A., Ambis, D., and Siegel, J.H. (1978). Cimetidine and mental confusion. *N. Engl. J. Med.* 298, 284.

Maeda, K., Ueda, M., Ohtaka, H., *et al.* (1987). A massive dose of vincristine. *Jpn J. Clin. Oncol.* 17, 247.

Maertens, P., Lum, G., Williams, J.P., *et al.* (1987). Intracranial haemorrhage and cerebral angiopathic changes in a suicidal phenylpropanolamine poisoning. *South. Med. J.* 80, 1584.

Magarian, G.J., Lucas, L.M., and Colley, C. (1991). Gemfibrozil-induced myopathy. *Arch. Intern. Med.* 151, 1873.

Maher, V.M.G., Pappu, A., Illingworth, D.R., *et al.* (1989). Plasma mevalonate response in lovastatin-related myopathy. *Lancet* ii, 1098.

Mal, N.T.H., Day, N.P.J., and Chuong, L.V., *et al.* (1996). Post-malaria neurological syndrome. *Lancet* 348, 917.

Manoguerra, A., Whitney, C., Clark, R.F., *et al.* (1995). Cholinergic toxicity resulting from ocular instillation of echothiophate iodide eye drops. *J. Toxicol. Clin. Toxicol.* 33, 463.

Mansour, A.M., Puklin, J.E., and O'Grady, R. (1988). Optic nerve ultrastructure following amiodarone therapy. *J. Clin. Neurol. Ophthalmol.* 8, 231.

Marik, P. (1996). Doxacurium-corticosteroid acute myopathy: another piece to the puzzle. *Crit. Care Med.* 24, 1266.

Marsden, C.D., Parkes, J.D., and Rees. J.E. (1973). A year's comparison of treatment of patients with Parkinson's disease with levodopa combined with carbidopa versus treatment with levodopa alone. *Lancet* ii, 1459.

Martinez-Arizala, A., Sobol, S.M., McCarty, G.E., *et al.* (1983). Amiodarone neuropathy. *Neurology* 33, 643.

Massa, R., Carpenter, S., Holland, P., *et al.* (1992). Loss and renewal of thick myofilaments in glucocorticoid-treated rat soleus after denervation and reinnervation. *Muscle Nerve* 15, 1290.

Mathew, N.T., Tietjen, G.E., and Lucker, C. (1996). Serotonin syndrome complicating migraine pharmacotherapy. *Cephalalgia* 161, 323.

Matsuya, M., Abe, T., Tosaka, M., *et al.* (1994). The first case of polymyositis associated with interferon therapy. *Internal Medicine* (Kushiro Hospital, Japan) 33, 806.

Mauro, V.F., Bonfiglio, M.F., and Spunt, A.L. (1986). Meperidine-induced seizure in a patient without renal dysfunction or sickle cell anaemia. *Clin. Pharm.* 5, 837.

Meade, T.W., Greenberg, G., and Thompson, S.G. (1980). Progestogens and cardiovascular reactions associated with oral contraceptives and a comparison of the safety of 50- and 30 µg oestrogen preparations. *BMJ* 280, 1157.

Melgaard, B., Kohler, O., Sand-Hansen, H., *et al.* (1988). Misonidazole neuropathy. A prospective study. *J. Neuro-oncol.* 6, 227.

Meltzer, H.Y. and Moline, R. (1970). Plasma enzymatic activity after exercise. Study of psychiatric patients and their relatives. *Arch. Gen. Psychiatry* 22, 390.

Mendelsohn, G. (1978). Withdrawal reactions after oxazepam. *Lancet* i, 565.

Menegaux, F., Keeffe, E.B., Andrews, B.T., *et al.* (1994). Neurological complications of liver transplantation in adult versus pediatric patients. *Transplantation* 58, 447.

Mesejo, A., Nunez, C., Simo, M., *et al.* (1995). Neuroleptic malignant syndrome, multiorgan failure and peripheral polyneuropathy. *Revista de Neurologia* 23, 136.

Meucci, G., Rossi, G., and Mazzoni, M. (1989). A case of transient choreoathetosis with amnesic syndrome after acute monoxide poisoning. *Ital. J. Neurol. Sci.* 10, 513.

Mezaki, T., Ohtani, S.I., Abe, K., *et al.* (1989). Benign type of malignant syndrome. *Lancet* i, 49.

Mielke, I.R., Deppe, W., and Lucking, C.H. (1995). Armplexusläsionen und Rhabdomyolysen nach Heroinabusus. Hinweise auf eine immunologische Genese. *Dtsch. Med. Wochenschr.* 120, 55.

Mifsud, A.J. (1988). Drug-related recurrent meningitis. *J. Infect.* 17, 151.

Miglino, M., Fierri, I., Canepa, L., *et al.* (1993). An unusual reaction to alpha interferon in a case of non-Hodgkin's lymphoma. *Haematologica* 78, 411.

Miller, H.G. and Stanton, J.B. (1954). Neurological sequelae of prophylactic inoculation. *Q. J. Med.* 23, 1.

Miller, L.G. and Jankovic, J. (1990). Sulpiride-induced tardive dystonia. *Mov. Disord.* 5, 83.

Min, D.I. and Fallo, S.A. (1993). Encephalopathy associated with muromonab-CD3. *Clin. Pharmacol.* 12, 601.

Mitchell, A.B.S. and Parsons-Smith, B.G. (1969). Trichloroethylene neuropathy. *BMJ* i, 422.

Mitchell, M.M., Ali, H.H., and Savarese, J.J. (1978). Myotonia and neuromuscular blocking agents. *Anesthesiology* 49, 44.

Morgan, G.J., McGuire, J.H., and Ochoa, J. (1981). Penicillamine induced myositis in rheumatoid arthritis. *Muscle Nerve* 4, 127.

Moyes, D.G. (1973). Malignant hyperpyrexia caused by trimeprazine. *Br. J. Anaesth.* 45, 1163.

Naganuma, H. and Fujii, I. (1994). Incidence and risk factors in neuroleptic malignant syndrome. *Pharmacopsychiatry* 27, 139.

Nakae, K., Yamamoto, S., and Shigematsu, I. (1973). Relation between subacute myelo-optic neuropathy (SMON) and clioquinol: nation-wide survey. *Lancet* i, 171.

Nazarian, S.M. and Jay, W.M. (1988). Bilateral optic neuropathy associated with amiodarone therapy. *J. Clin. Neurol. Ophthalmol.* 8, 25.

Noppen, M., Velkeniers, B., Dierckx, R., *et al.* (1987). Cyclosporin and myopathy. *Ann. Intern. Med.* 107, 945.

Norden, D.K., Lichenstein, G.R., and Williams, W.V. (1994). Sulphasalazine-induced myopathy. *Am. J. Gastroenterol.* 89, 801.

Nowack, W.J. and Jordan, R. (1994). Propofol, seizures and generalised paroxysmal fast activity in the EEG. *Clin. Electroencephalog.* 25, 110.

Nussbaum, E.S., Maxwell, R.E., Bitterman, P.B., *et al.* (1995). Cyclosporin A toxicity presenting with acute cerebellar edema and brainstem compression. *J. Neurosurg.* 82, 1068.

Ochoa, J. (1970). Isoniazid neuropathy in man. Quantitative electron microscopy study. *Brain* 93, 831.

Oh, S.J., Douglas, J.E., and Brown, R.A. (1971). Hypokalaemic vacuolar myopathy associated with chlorthalidone treatment. *JAMA* 216, 1858.

Oh, S.J., Rollins, J.L., and Lewis, I. (1975). Pentazocine-induced fibrous myopathy. *JAMA* 231, 271.

Ohta, S., Tachikama, O., Makino, Y., *et al.* (1990). Metabolism and brain accumulation of tetrahydro-isoquinoline (TIQ), a possible Parkinsonism-inducing substance, in an animal model of a poor debrisoquine metaboliser. *Life Sci.* 46, 599.

Olesen, J. (1995). Analgesic headache. *BMJ* 310, 479.

Olson, K.R., Kearney, T.E., Dyer, J.E., *et al.* (1993). Seizures associated with poisoning and drug overdose. *Am. J. Emerg. Med.* 11, 565.

Onda, K., Tekada, N., and Tanaka, R. (1987). Clinical course and CT findings in patients with contrast media associated figures. *No-To-Shinkei* 39, 331.

Page, P., Morgan, M., and Loh, L. (1972). Ketamine anaesthesia in paediatric procedures. *Acta Anaesthesiol. Scand.* 16, 155.

Palakurthy, P.R., Iyer, V., and Mecker, R.J. (1987). Unusual neurotoxicity associated with amiodarone therapy. *Arch. Intern. Med.* 147, 881.

Palmer, K.N.V. (1978). Muscle cramp and oral salbutamol. *BMJ* ii, 833.

Parker, J. and Lahmeyer, H. (1984). Maprotiline poisoning: a case of cardiotoxicity and myoclonic seizures. *J. Clin. Psychiatry* 45, 312.

Partziguian, T., Camerlingo, M., Castro, L., *et al.* (1996). Cerebral venous thrombosis in young adults. Experience in a stroke unit, 1988–1994. *Ital. J. Neurol. Sci.* 17, 419.

Pascuzzi, R.M., Roos, K.L., and Scott, J.A. (1988). Chronic focal seizure disorder as a manifestation of intracranial iophendylate. *Epilepsia* 29, 294.

Patterson, J.F. (1983). Amoxapine-induced chorea. *South. Med. J.* 76, 1077.

Perkoff, G.T., Silber, T., and Tyler, F.H. (1959). Studies in disorders of muscle. Xll. Myopathy due to the administration of therapeutic amounts of 17-hydroxycorticosteroids. *Am. J. Med.* 26, 1891.

Perry, J.R. and Warner, E. (1996). Transient encephalopathy after paclitaxel (Taxol) infusion. *Neurology* 46, 1596.

Perry, R. and Jacobsen, E.S. (1984). Gold-induced encephalopathy. Case report. *J. Rheumatol.* 11, 233.

Petit, H., Leys, D., Hurtevent, J.F., *et al.* (1987). Neuropathies and almitrine. 14 cases. *Rev. Neurol.* 143, 510.

Petitti, D.B. and Wingerd, J. (1978). Use of oral contraceptives, cigarette smoking and risk of subarachnoid haemorrhage. *Lancet* ii, 234.

Petrera, J.E., Fledelius, H.C., and Trojaborg, W. (1988). Serial pattern evoked potential recording in a case of toxic optic neuropathy due to ethambutol. *Electroencephalogr. Clin. Neurophysiol.* 71, 146.

Pfeiffer, R.F. and Sucha, E.L. (1985). On–off induced malignant hyperthermia. *Ann. Neurol.* 18, 138.

Pialoux, G., Kernbaum, S., and Vachon, F. (1988). Arsenical-induced encephalopathy during the treatment of African trypanosomiasis. *Bull. Soc. Pathol. Exot. Filiales* 81, 555.

Pilke, A., Partinen, M., and Kovanen, J. (1984). Status epilepticus and alcohol abuse: an analysis of 82 status epilepticus admissions. *Acta Neurol. Scand.* 70, 443.

Playford, R.J., Matthews, C.H., Campbell, M.J., *et al.* (1990). Bismuth induced encephalopathy caused by tripotassium dicitrato bismuthate in a patient with chronic renal failure. *Gut* 31, 359.

Poersch, M., Hufnagel, A., and Smolenski, C. (1996). Medikamente induzierte Asterixis verstärkt durch relative Hypoglykämie. *Nervenarzt* 67, 323.

Prescott, L.F., Balali-Mood, M., Critchley, J.A.J., *et al.* (1981). Avoidance of mefenamic acid in epilepsy. *Lancet* ii, 418.

Price. P., Parkes, J.D., and Marsden, C.D. (1978). Tiapride in Parkinson's disease. *Lancet* ii, 1106.

Qureshi, A.I., Akbar, M.S., Czander, E.S., *et al.* (1997). Crack cocaine use and stroke in young patients. *Neurology* 48, 341.

Ragab, A.H. (1973). Pyrimethamine in central nervous system leukaemia. *Lancet* i, 1061.

Rahman, N.U. and Al-Tahan, A.R. (1993). Computer tomographic evidence of an extensive thrombosis and infarction of the deep venous system. *Stroke* 24, 744.

Ramirez, J.A., Mendell, J.R., Warmolts, J.R., *et al.* (1986). Phenytoin neuropathy: structural changes in the sural nerve. *Ann. Neurol.* 19, 162.

Rampton, D.S. (1977). Hypertensive crisis in a patient given Sinemet, metoclopramide, and amitriptyline. *BMJ* ii, 607.

Ramsden, D.B. and Williams, A.C. (1985). Production in nature of compound resembling methylphenyltetrahydropyridine, a possible cause of Parkinson's disease. *Lancet* i, 215.

RCGP (1977). Royal College of General Practitioners Oral Contraceptive Study. *Lancet* ii, 727.

Reeves, A.L., So, E.L., Sharbrough, F.W ., *et al.* (1996). Movement disorders associated with the use of gabapentin. *Epilepsia* 37, 988.

Relling, M.V. (1989). Polymorphic drug metabolism. *Clin. Pharm.* 8, 852.

Reynolds, E.H. (1990). Vigabatrin: rational treatment for chronic epilepsy. *BMJ* 300, 277.

Ribera, E.F. and Dutka, A.J. (1983). Polyneuropathy associated with administration of hepatitis B vaccine. *N. Engl. J. Med.* 309, 614.

Richard, I.H., Kurlan, R., Tanner, C., *et al.* (1997). Serotonin syndrome and the combined use of deprenyl and an antidepressant in Parkinson's disease. *Neurology* 48, 1070.

Richter, R.W., Challener, Y.B., Pearson, J., *et al.* (1971). Acute myoglobinuria associated with heroin addiction. *JAMA* 216, 1172.

Riddoch, D., Jefferson, M., and Bickerstaff, E.R. (1971). Chorea and the oral contraceptives. *BMJ* iv, 217.

Ridge, I.L. (1994). Seizures after myelography with iopamidol. *Am. J. Emerg. Med.* 12, 329

Ries, S. and Fohlmann-Ede, B. (1993). Zerebrale Kraupfenfelle während einer Malaria Prophylaxae mit Mefloquin. *Dtsch. Med. Wochenschr.* 113, 1911.

Riker, R.R., Fraser, G.L., and Richen, P. (1997). Movement disorders associated with withdrawal from high-dose intravenous haloperidol therapy in delirious ICU patients. *Chest* 111, 1778.

Rimon, D., Ludatsher, R., and Cohen, L. (1984). Clofibrate-induced muscular syndrome: case report with ultrastructure findings and review of the literature. *Isr. J. Med. Sci.* 20, 1082.

Ring, H.A. and Reynolds, E.H. (1990). Vigabatrin and behaviour disturbance. *Lancet* i, 970.

Ringel, R.A. and Brick, J.F. (1986). Perspective on carbamazepine-induced water intoxication: reversal by demeclocycline. *Neurology* 36, 1506.

Ritchie, P. (1983). Neuroleptioc malignant syndrome. *BMJ* 287, 561.

Rivera, V.M. (1973). Interpretation of serum creatine phosphokinase. *JAMA* 225, 993.

Roberts, W.C. (1989). Safety of fenofibrate. US and worldwide experience. *Cardiology* 76, 169.

Robinson, M.K., Richens, A., and Oxley, R. (1990). Vigabatrin and behaviour disturbances. *Lancet* 336, 504.

Roemer, R.A., Cornwell, A., Dewart, D., *et al.* (1995). Quantitative electroencephalographic analyses in cocaine-preferring polysubstance abusers during abstinence. *Psychiatry Res.* 58, 247.

Rogers, R.L., Meyer, J.S., Mortel, K.F., *et al.* (1985). Age-related reductions in cerebral vasomotor reactivity and the law of initial value: a 4-year prospective, longitudinal study. *J. Cereb. Blood Flow Metab.* 5, 79.

Rosenberg, N.L., Myers, J.A., and Martin, W.R. (1989). Cyanide-induced Parkinsonism: clinical, MRI and 6-fluorodopa PET studies. *Neurology* (N.Y.) 39, 142.

Rosenblum, A.M. and Montgomery, E.B. (1980). Exacerbation of parkinsonism by methyldopa. *JAMA* 244, 2727.

Rosin, A.J., DeVereux, D., Eng, N., *et al.* (1979). Parkinsonism with 'on–off' phenomena. *Arch. Neurol.* 36, 32.

Rosin, M.A. (1981). Chlorzoxazone-induced spasmodic torticollis. *JAMA* 246, 2575.

Ross, D.R., Walker, J.I., and Peterson, J. (1983). Akathisia induced by amoxapine. *Am. J. Psychiatry* 140, 115.

Rothenberg, R.J. and Sufit, R.L. (1987). Drug-induced peripheral neuropathy in a patient with psoriatic arthritis. *Arthritis Rheum.* 30, 221.

Rouveix, B., Bricaire, C., Michon, G.F., *et al.* (1989). Mefloquin and an acute brain syndrome. *Ann. Intern. Med.* 110, 577.

Rozen, M.S. and Whan, R.McK. (1977). Prolonged curarisation associated with propranolol therapy. *Lancet* i, 73.

Rupniak, N.M., Jenner, P., and Marsden, C.D. (1986). Acute dystonia induced by neuroleptic drugs. *Psychopharmacology* 88, 403.

Ruppert, G.B. and Barth, W.F. (1981). Tolmetin-induced aseptic meningitis. *JAMA* 245, 67.

Rush, P., Baron, M., and Kaputsa, M. (1986). Clofibrate-myopathy: a case report and review of the literature. *Sem. Arthritis Rheum.* 15, 226.

Russell, D., Veger, J., Bunae, U. B., *et al.* (1979). Epileptic seizures precipitated by atenolol. *J. Neurol. Neurosurg. Psychiatry* 42, 484.

Rutkove, S.B. (1997). An unusual axonal polyneuropathy induced by low-dose interferon alfa-2a. *Arch. Neurol.* 54, 907.

Ryu, S.J. and Lin, S.K. (1995). Cerebral arteritis associated with oral use of phenylpropolamine: report of a case.

Taiwan I Hsueh Hui Tsa Chih [J. Formosan Med. Assoc.] 94, 53.

Sachdev, P. (1995a). The epidemiology of drug-induced akathisia: Part I. Acute akathisia. *Schizophr. Bull.* 21, 431.

Sachdev, P. (1995b). The epidemiology of drug-induced akathisia: Part II. Chronic, tardive, and withdrawal akathisia. *Schizophr. Bull.* 21, 451.

Sachdev, P., Kruk, J., Kneebone, M., *et al.* (1995). Clozapine-induced neuroleptic malignant syndrome: review and report of new cases. *J. Clin. Psychopharmacol.* 15, 365.

Sadeh, M. and Goldhammer, Y. (1993). Extrapyramidal syndrome responsive to dopaminergic treatment following recovery from central pontine myelinolysis. *Eur. Neurol.* 33, 48.

Sander, J.W. and Hart, Y.M. (1990). Vigabatrin and behaviour disturbances. *Lancet* 335, 57.

Sandyk, R. (1983). Urinary incontinence associated with clonazepam therapy. *S. Afr. Med. J.* 64, 230.

Saqueton, A.C., Lonnez, A.L., Vick, N.A., *et al.* (1969). Dapsone and peripheral motor neuropathy. *Arch. Dermatol.* 100, 214.

Scelsa, S.N., Simpson, D.M., and McQuistion, H.L. (1996). Clozapine-induced myotoxicity in patients with chronic psychotic disorders. *Neurology* 47, 1513.

Schiff, D. and Drislane, F.W. (1992). Rapid-onset colchicine myoneuropathy. *Arthr. Rheum.* 35,1535.

Schmidt, S. and Schmitz-Buhl, M. (1995). Signs and symptoms of carbamazepine overdose. *J. Neurol.* 242, 169.

Schumm, F., Wietholter, H., and Fateh-Moghadam, A. (1981). Myasthenie-syndrom unter Chloroquin-therapie. *Dtsch. Med. Wochenschr.* 52, 1715.

Sebille, A. (1978). Prevalence of latent perhexilene neuropathy. *BMJ* i, 1321.

Selden, R., and Sasahara, A.A. (1967). Central nervous system toxicity induced by lidocaine. Reports of a case in a patient with liver disease. *JAMA* 202, 908.

Seligmann, H., Podoshin, L., Ben-David, J., *et al.* (1996). Drug-induced tinnitus and other hearing disorders. *Drug Saf.* 14, 198.

Serdaru, M., Diquet, B., and Lhermitte, F. (1982). Generalised seizures and ampicillin. *Lancet* ii, 617.

Shaikh, A. (1978). Urinary incontinence during treatment with depot phenothiazines. *BMJ* i, 1698.

Shalev, A., Hermesh, H., and Munitz, H. (1987). Severe akathisia causing neuroleptic failure. *Acta Psychiatr. Scand.* 76, 715.

Shanmagasundaram, T.K. (1980). Post-injection fibrosis of skeletal muscle: a clinical problem. *Int. Orthop.* 4, 31.

Shaw, M.D.M., Russell, J.A., and Grossart, K.W. (1978). The changing pattern of spinal arachnoiditis. *J. Neurol. Neurosurg. Psychiatry* 41, 97.

Shetty, H.G.M. and Routledge, P.A. (1990). Adverse effects of hypolipidaemic drugs. *Adverse Drug React. Bull.* 142, 532.

Sikka, A., Keramann, E., Vrablek, R.M., *et al.* (1983). Carpal tunnel syndrome associated with danazol therapy. *Am. J. Obstet. Gynecol.* 147, 102.

Simpson, D.M., Slasor, P., Dafni, U., *et al.* (1997). Analysis of myopathy in a placebo-controlled zidovudine trial. *Muscle Nerve* 20, 382.

Sinard, J.H. and Hedreen, J.C. (1995). Neuronal loss from the subthalamic nuclei in a patient with progressive chorea. *Mov. Disord.* 10, 305.

Singer, W.D. (1981). Transient Gilles de la Tourette syndrome after chronic neuroleptic withdrawal. *Dev. Med. Child Neurol.* 23, 518.

Siskind, M.S., Thienemann, D., and Kirlin, L. (1993). Isoniazid-induced neurotoxicity in chronic dialysis patients: report of three cases and a review of the literature. *Nephron* 64, 303.

Slikkerveer, A. and de Wolff, F.A. (1989). Pharmacokinetics and toxicity of bismuth compounds. *Med. Toxicol. Adverse Drug Exp.* 4, 303.

Smals, A.G.H., Beex, L.V.A., and Kloppenborg, P.W.C. (1977). Clofibrate-induced muscle damage with myoglobinuria and cardiomyopathy. *N. Engl. J. Med.* 296, 942.

Smith, C.A.D., Gough, A.C., Leigh, P.N., *et al.* (1992). Debrisoquine hydroxylase gene polymorphism and susceptibility to Parkinson's disease. *Lancet* 339, 1375.

Smith, P.A., Macdonald, T.R., and Jones, C.S. (1966). Convulsions associated with halothane anaesthesia. *Anesthesia* 21, 229.

Smith, F.F., Eydelloth, R.S., Grossman, S.J., *et al.*(1991). HMG-CoA reductase inhibitor-induced myopathy in the rat; cyclosporine A interaction and mechanism studies. *J. Pharmacol. Exp. Ther.* 257, 1225.

Soyka, M., Lutz, W., Kauert G., *et al.* (1989). Epileptic seizures and alcohol withdrawal: significance of additional use (and misuse) of drugs and electroencephalographic findings. *J. Epilepsy* 2, 109.

Spaulding, W.B. (1979). Myalgia and elevated creatine phosphokinase with danazol in hereditary angioedema. *Ann. Intern. Med.* 90, 854.

Steinhoff, B.J. and Stodieck, S.R. (1993). Temporary abolition of seizure activity by flumazenil in a case of valproate-induced non-convulsive status epilepticus. *Seizure* 2, 261.

Stephen, P.J. and Williamson, J. (1984). Drug-induced Parkinsonism in the elderly. *Lancet* ii, 1082.

Stephens, W.P., Eddy, J.D., Parsons, L.M., *et al.* (1978). Raised intracranial pressure due to perhexiline maleate. *BMJ* i, 21.

Steventon, G.B., Sturman, S.G., Heafield, M.T.E., *et al.* (1989). Platelet monoamine oxidase-B activity in Parkinson's disease. *J. Neurol. Transm.* 1, 255.

Strachan, R., Hughes, D., and Cowie, R. (1995). Thrombosis of the straight sinus complicating hormone replacement therapy. *Br. J. Neurosurg.* 9, 805.

Sugie, H., Russin, R., and Verity, M.A. (1984). Emetine myopathy: two case reports with pathobiochemical analysis. *Muscle Nerve* 7, 54.

Swartz, R.D. (1985). Desferoxamine and aluminium removal. *Am. J. Kidney Dis.* 6, 358.

Sylvia, L.M., Forlenza, S.W., and Brocavich, J.M. (1988). Aseptic meningitis associated with naproxen. *Drug Intell. Clin. Pharm.* 22, 399.

Takeuchi, H., Yamada, A., Touge, T., *et al.* (1988). Metronidazole neuropathy: a case report. *Jpn J. Psychiatry Neurol.* 42, 291.

Takimoto, C.H., Zhi-Hong, L., and Zhang, R. (1996). Severe neurotoxicity following 5-fluorouracil-based chemotherapy in a patient with dihydropyrimidine dehydrogenase deficiency. *Clin. Cancer Res.* 2, 477.

Task Force (1980). Task Force on late neurological effects of antipsychotic drugs. Tardive dyskinesia: summary of a task force report of the American Psychiatric Association. *Am. J. Psychiatry* 137, 1163.

Tegner, R., Tome, F.M., Godeau, P., *et al.* (1988). Morphological study of peripheral nerve changes induced by chloroquine treatment. *Acta Neuropathol.* 75, 253.

Teicher, A., Rosenthal, T., Kissin, E., *et al.* (1981). Labetalol-induced toxic myopathy. *BMJ* 282, 1824.

Terrence, C.G. and Fromm, G.H. (1981). Complications of baclofen withdrawal. *Arch. Neurol.* 38, 588.

Terry, S.I. (1971). Transient dysaesthesiae and persistent leucocytosis after clioquinol therapy. *BMJ* iii, 745.

Thien, T.H., Delaere, K.R.J., Debruyne, F.M.J., *et al.* (1978). Urinary incontinence caused by prazosin. *BMJ* i, 622.

Thompson, G.E. (1972). Ketamine-induced convulsions. *Anesthesiology* 37, 662.

Tilzey, A., Heptonstall, J., and Hamblin, T. (1981). Toxic confusional state and choreiform movements after treatment with anabolic steroids. *BMJ* 283, 349.

Tomlinson, I.W.K. and Rosenthal, F.D. (1977). Proximal myopathy after perhexiline maleate treatment. *BMJ* ii, 1319.

Toole, J.F. and Parrish, M.L. (1973). Nitrofurantoin polyneuropathy. *Neurology* (N.Y.) 23, 554.

Toole, J.F., Gergen, J.A., Hayes, D.M., *et al.* (1968). Neural effects of nitrofurantoin. *Arch. Neurol.* 18, 680.

Trenkwater, F. and Lydtin, H. (1994). Ischaemic neurological deficit after sclerotherapy. *Lancet* 343, 428.

Trimble, M. (1978). Non-monoamine oxidase inhibitor antidepressants and epilepsy: A review. *Epilepsia* 19, 241.

Tyrer, S. and Shopsin, B. (1980). Neural and neuromuscular side-effects of lithium. In *Handbook of Lithium Therapy* (ed. F.N. Johnson), p. 289. MTP Press, Lancaster.

Ueno, S., Takahashi, M., Kajiyama, K., *et al.* (1987). Parkinson's disease and myasthenia gravis: adverse effect of trihexyphenidyl on neuromusclar transmission. *Neurology* (N.Y.) 37, 832.

Van der Plas, J.P., Lambers, J.C., Van Wersch, J.W., *et al.* (1994). Reversible ischaemic neurological deficit after sclerotherapy of varicose veins. *Lancet* 343, 428.

van Marle, W. and Woods, K. L. (1980). Acute hydrocortisone myopathy. *BMJ* 281, 271.

Velamoor, V.R., Norman, R.M., Caroff, S.N., *et al.* (1994). Progression of symptoms in neuroleptic malignant syndrome. *J. Nerv. Ment. Dis.* 182, 168.

Verschraegen, C., Conrad, C.A., and Hong, W.K. (1995). Subacute encephalopathic toxicity of cisplatin. *Lung Cancer* 13, 305.

Vessey, M.P. (1973). Oral contraceptives and stroke. *N. Engl. J. Med.* 288, 906.

Vessey, M.P. and Doll, R. (1969). Investigation of relation between use of oral contraceptives and thromboembolic disease: a further report. *BMJ* ii, 651.

Vickrey, B.G. and Bahls, F.H. (1989). Non-convulsive status epilepticus following cerebral angiography. *Ann. Neurol.* 25, 199.

Vilter, R.W. (1986). Vidarabine-associated encephalopathy and myoclonus. *Antimicrob. Agents Chemother.* 29, 933.

Vyas, I. and Carney, M.W.P. (1975). Diazepam and withdrawal fits. *BMJ* ii, 44.

Walker, R.W. and Rosenblum, M.K. (1992). Amphotericin B-associated leukoencephalopathy *Neurology* 42, 2005.

Walls, T.J. and Pearce, S.J. (1980). Motor neuropathy associated with cimetidine. *BMJ* 281, 974.

Walther, P.J., Rossitch, E. Jr, and Bullard, D.E. (1987). The development of Lhermitte's sign during cisplatin chemotherapy. Possible drug-induced toxicity causing spinal cord demyelination. *Cancer* 60, 2170.

Waring, R.H., Steventon, G., Heafield, M.T.E., *et al.* (1989). S-Methylation in Parkinson's disease and motor neurone disease. *Lancet* ii, 356.

Warne, R.W. and Gubbay, S.S. (1979). Choreiform movements induced by anticholinergic therapy. *Med. J. Aust.* i, 465.

Warzocha, K., Krykowksi, E., Gora Tybor, J., *et al.* (1996). Fulminant 2-chlorodeoxyadenosine-related peripheral neuropathy in a patient with paraneoplastic neurological syndrome associated with lymphoma. *Leuk. Lymphoma* 21, 343.

Wasserman, S. and Yahr, M.D. (1980). Choreic movements induced by the use of methadone. *Arch. Neurol.* 37, 727.

Weaver, D.F., Camfield, F., and Fraser A. (1988). Massive carbamazepine overdose: Clinical and pharmacological observations in five episodes. *Neurology* 38, 755.

Weber, W.W., Hein, D.W., Litwin, A., *et al.* (1983). Relationship of acetylator status to isoniazid toxicity, lupus erythematosus, and bladder cancer. *Fed. Proc.* 42, 3086.

Weinbroum, A., Rudick, V., Sorkine, P., *et al.*. (1996). Use of flumazenil in the treatment of drug overdose: a double-blind and open clinical study in 110 patients. *Crit. Care Med.* 24, 199.

Weiner, W.J. and Luby, E.D. (1983). Persistent akathisia following neuroleptic withdrawal. *Ann. Neurol.* 13, 466.

Weinstein, L. (1970). Drugs used in the chemotherapy of leprosy and tuberculosis. In *The Pharmacological Basis of Therapeutics* (4th edn) (ed. L.S. Goodman and A. Gilman), p. 1311. Macmillan, London.

Weir, R.J., Briggs, E., Browning, J., *et al.* (1971). Blood pressure in women after one year of oral contraception. *Lancet* i, 467.

Weiss, H.D., Walker, M.D., and Wiernik, P.H. (1974a).

Neurotoxicity of commonly used antineoplastic agents. *N. Engl. J. Med.* 291, 75.

Weiss, H.D., Walker, M.D., and Wiernik, P.H. (1974*b*). Neurotoxicity of commonly used antineoplastic agents. *N. Engl. J. Med.* 291, 127.

Whelton, A., Carter, G.G., Garth, M.A., *et al.* (1971). Carbenicillin-induced acidosis and seizures. *JAMA* 218, 1942.

Whisnant, J.P., Espinosa, R.E., Kierland. R.R., *et al.* (1963). Chloroquine neuromyopathy. *Proc. Staff Meet. Mayo Clin.* 38, 501.

Whittaker, J.A., Parry, D.H., Bunch, C., *et al.* (1973). Coma associated with vincristine therapy. *BMJ* iii, 335.

Wong, M.M. (1996). Neuroleptic malignant syndrome: two cases without muscle rigidity. *Aust N.Z. J. Psychiatry* 30, 415.

Woodhouse, K.W. and Blain, P.G. (1983). Some organ-specific adverse reactions to cytotoxic drugs. *Adverse Drug React. Acute Poisoning Rev.* 2, 123.

Wyllie, A.R., Bayliff, C.D., and Kovacs, M.J. (1997). Myo-clonus due to chlorambucil in two adults with lymphoma. *Ann. Pharmacother.* 31, 171.

Yamada, M., Ohno, S., Okayasu, I., *et al.* (1986). Chronic manganese poisoning: a neuropathological study with determination of manganese distribution in the brain. *Acta Neuropathol.* 70, 273.

Yamanishi, Y., Ishibe, Y., Taooka, Y., *et al.* (1993). A case of cyclosporin-induced myopathy. *Ryumachi* 33, 63.

Yates, D.A.H. (1970). Steroid myopathy. In *Muscle Diseases* (ed. J.N. Walton, N. Canal, and G. Scarlato), p. 482. Excerpta Medica, Amsterdam.

Zaal, M.J.W., de Vries, J., and Boen-Tan, Y.T.N. (1988). Is cyclosporin toxic to endothelial cells? *Lancet* ii, 956.

Zampollo, A., Sozzi, G., and Basso, F. (1988). Amitriptyline related peripheral neuropathy. Case report. *Ital. J. Neurol. Sci.* 9, 89.

Zuber, M., Toulon, F., Marnet, L., *et al.* (1996). Factor V Leiden mutation in cerebral venous thrombosis. *Stroke* 27, 1721.

21. Eye disorders

R. J. HARRISON

Introduction

The essential function of the eye is to bring incoming light to a focus on the retinal photoreceptors and to transmit the resultant electrical impulses through the optic nerve and visual pathway to the visual cortex. Although all the ocular structures contribute to this process, the irreducibly necessary elements are a clear, regularly refracting cornea at the front of the eye and a healthy retina and optic nerve at the back. Many drugs can have adverse effects on the eye and ocular adnexa and in this chapter discussion will concentrate on the more serious effects of commonly prescribed drugs and the means by which they can cause ocular damage.

Eyelids and periorbital tissues

Almost any eye-drop or ointment can cause allergic contact dermatitis of the eyelids. Of the antibiotics, neomycin is the most likely to cause an allergic response, and atropine is the most sensitizing of the other topical ocular preparations. Allergic responses can also occur to preservatives in topical preparations (a Type B response) (Wilson 1979; Kruyswijk et al. 1980).

Drugs which discolour or alter pigmentation of the skin can affect the eyelids as elsewhere in the body. These include amiodarone, chlorpromazine, quinidine, and the 4-aminoquinolone group (e.g. chloroquine, hydroxychloroquine, and amodiaquine), and gold- and silver-containing compounds that are now rarely prescribed. The 4-aminoquinolones may also cause whitening of the eyelashes and eyebrows (poliosis). Interferon can cause growth of thick, curly eyelashes up to 6.5 cm in length (Foon 1984). Eyelid skin can be involved in phototoxic (Type A) reactions to thiazides, retinoids, some antibiotics including tetracyclines, sulphonamides, and ciprofloxacin, and intravenous fluorescein administered for fluorescein angiography. Photoallergic (Type B) reactions can occur with the phenothiazines and quinine.

The initial treatment of hyperthyroidism with antithyroid drugs may cause acute periorbital oedema and induce or exacerbate exophthalmos (Gwinup et al. 1982; Sridama and DeGroot 1989). Lithium carbonate, long-term high-dosage corticosteroids, and vitamin A may also give rise to exophthalmos (Lazarus et al. 1981).

Lacrimal apparatus, conjunctiva, and cornea

The cornea is continually lubricated with aqueous tears from the lacrimal gland, mucin from the conjunctival goblet cells, and an oily secretion from the Meibomian glands in the eyelids. These secretions are spread across the cornea by regular blinking, and maintenance of the precorneal tear film is essential for normal corneal function. Decreased tear production or abnormality of the eyelids can cause symptoms of ocular discomfort, and, if severe, can give rise to corneal ulceration, scarring, and vascularization.

The secretion of tears from the lacrimal glands is controlled by the parasympathetic nervous system, and drugs with cholinergic or anticholinergic actions may respectively increase or decrease aqueous tears. Cholinergic drugs such as methacholine and carbachol, and anticholinesterase agents such as neostigmine can increase tear production but this is unlikely to cause epiphora unless there is obstruction of lacrimal drainage. Reduction of tear secretion by drugs with anticholinergic action, for example antispasmodics and tricyclic antidepressants, may give rise to symptoms of ocular irritation, burning and itching, but symptoms can be controlled if necessary with artificial tears. These Type A adverse effects cease when the drug is stopped.

Isotretinoin can cause blepharoconjunctivitis and subjective complaints of dry eyes (Blackman et al. 1979).

The drug is probably secreted in the tears, but the signs and symptoms may also be secondary to the reduction in Meibomian gland secretion with resultant increased tear evaporation and osmolarity (Mathers *et al.* 1991). An increase in *Staphylococcus aureus* infection has been noted (Blackman *et al.* 1979). Steroids are used widely for their anti-inflammatory and immunosuppressive effects. In addition to glaucoma and cataract formation, discussed below, latent herpes simplex keratitis may be reactivated (Kaufman and Rayfield 1988).

Eye-drops containing silver or mercury compounds are now rarely used, but in the past caused conjunctival deposition of the metal concerned that gave the conjunctiva a blue-grey or even black appearance. Administration of adrenaline eye-drops for glaucoma can cause discrete black or brown deposits containing a melanin-like pigment (Wilson 1979).

A severe sight-threatening, dry-eye syndrome can occur with drugs that cause structural damage to the lacrimal apparatus or conjunctiva. Subconjunctival scarring can obstruct the small ductules through which tears pass from the lacrimal glands to the subconjunctival sac, and conjunctival mucin production will be reduced or eliminated if conjunctival goblet cells are destroyed.

One of the most devastating ocular complications of systemic therapy is the Stevens–Johnson syndrome. This is an acute inflammatory vesiculobullous reaction of the skin and mucous membranes, most commonly affecting children and young adults. Ocular involvement occurs in 43–81 per cent of patients, with 35 per cent experiencing permanent visual sequelae (Robin and Dugel 1988). While the inflammation is self-limiting and non-progressive, the subsequent conjunctival scarring, with attendant obstruction of lacrimal ductules and loss of goblet cells, can give rise to an intractable and sight-threatening dry-eye syndrome. This can be further complicated by trichiasis (in-turning eye lashes that rub the cornea), and the outcome of these processes frequently involves varying degrees of corneal opacification, vascularization, keratinization, and thinning. At least 200 drugs have been reported to give rise to the Stevens–Johnson syndrome, including sulphonamides (the most common culprits), penicillin, ampicillin, isoniazid, anticonvulsants, salicylates, and phenylbutazone. Fortunately, the syndrome is a rare idiosyncratic response to treatment. Patients with the syndrome are significantly more likely than controls to have HLA-Bw44 antigen.

A number of other drugs can cause subconjunctival scarring with synblepharon (fibrotic bands between the conjunctiva of the eyeball and eyelid), and mild to severe dry-eye syndrome ('sicca syndrome'). These include

systemically administered practolol, now withdrawn from general use (Rahi *et al.* 1976), cyclophosphamide (Al-Tweigeri *et al.* 1996), and penicillamine (Marti-Huguet *et al.* 1989). Several antineoplastic agents are secreted in tears and can cause blepharitis and punctate keratitis, which normally resolves with discontinuation of the drug. Cicatricial ectropion and punctal-canalicular stenosis with epiphora have been reported as a late complication of 5-fluorouracil therapy (Straus *et al.* 1997). Topically administered drugs causing sicca syndrome include idoxuridine (Lass *et al.* 1983), adrenaline, dipivefrin (Blanchard 1987), and ecothiopate iodide (Patten *et al.* 1976).

Many topical ophthalmic drugs or the accompanying preservative can cause damage to the conjunctival and corneal epithelium, as can the active ingredients and preservatives in contact-lens cleaning solutions (Wilson 1979; Mondino *et al.* 1982). Concentrations of benzalkonium as low as 0.01% may cause emulsification of the cell wall lipids, and may damage corneal epithelial microvilli and prevent adherence of the mucoid layer of the tear film to the cornea (Fraunfelder 1996). Medications used topically whilst wearing soft contact lenses can accumulate in the contact lens material, whence it can be slowly released, achieving a much higher and therefore possibly toxic concentration in the tear film than would otherwise be the case (Silbert 1996). Systemic medications may be secreted by the lacrimal gland in tears and by this means also accumulate in soft contact lenses. For example, rifampicin can stain them orange (Lyons 1979). Patients with dry-eye syndrome or other ocular surface disease are particularly vulnerable to toxic effects of topical drugs (Burstein 1985). It can be difficult to distinguish clinically between the original condition and the adverse effect of the drug or preservative. Preservative-free formulations of some ophthalmic drugs, including β-blockers for glaucoma, prednisolone, and some antibiotics and ocular lubricants, are now available.

Long-term use of topically administered medications can have subclinical effects on the conjunctiva and ocular surface (Sherwood *et al.* 1989; Baudouin *et al.* 1994). Studies have shown that glaucoma surgery is more likely to fail due to fibrosis of the filtering bleb (the surgically created fistula) in patients who have received multiple topical therapy (Broadway *et al.* 1994), although this has not been confirmed by other investigators (Johnson *et al.* 1994; Detry-Morel *et al.* 1995). To overcome problems of fistula closure in trabeculectomy and recurrence of pterygium, mitomycin C and 5-fluorouracil have been used intra- and postoperatively to reduce subconjunctival scarring. Serious complications include ocular hypotony, corneal ulceration, and scleral melting (Stamper *et al.* 1992; Costa *et al.* 1993; Ticho *et al.* 1993).

Drugs are frequently administered subconjunctivally in ophthalmic practice, particularly antibiotics and corticosteroids. Gentamicin can cause capillary closure (Jenkins *et al.* 1990). Depot injections of corticosteroids can have prolonged adverse effects necessitating surgical removal of the depot (Mills *et al.* 1986; Akduman *et al.* 1996).

Drugs that give rise to corneal deposits generally cause few symptoms. Regularly arranged, and hence transparent, collagen fibrils make up 90 per cent of the cornea. The anterior surface is lined by the five- to six-layered corneal epithelium and the posterior surface by the single layered corneal endothelium. Like epithelium elsewhere, corneal epithelium is constantly replicating, the cells dividing at the corneal periphery (the limbus) and migrating towards the centre. Epithelial cells migrating from the superior and inferior limbus meet at the junction of the superior two-thirds and inferior one-third of the cornea, to form an often microscopically visible linear opacity called the Hudson–Stähli line. A number of drugs, notably chloroquine, amodiaquine, amiodarone, and clofazimine can give rise to fine deposits scattered throughout the corneal epithelium, and when these cause increased prominence of the Hudson–Stähli line the condition is called cornea verticillata (Walinder *et al.* 1976; D'Amico *et al.* 1981; Neilsen *et al.* 1983). These deposits rarely interfere with vision, but can occasionally give rise to symptoms of haloes around lights. They disappear without long-term ill effect if the drug is discontinued. Deposits in the corneal stroma rarely affect vision and are much rarer than epithelial deposits, but may occur with systemic gold therapy, chlorpromazine, topical organomercurials used as antiseptics, indomethacin, and clofazimine (Rasmussen *et al.* 1976; Gottlieb and Major 1978; McCormick *et al.* 1985; Font *et al.* 1989).

Abuse of anaesthetic eye-drops can cause a neurotrophic keratitis, features of which include reduced or absent corneal sensation and a typical chronic corneal epithelial defect and ulcer (Wilson 1979).

Smoking free-base ('crack') cocaine may also cause a neurotrophic keratitis, described as 'crack cornea' (Sachs *et al.* 1993). Keratitis has also been described in methamphetamine abusers (Poulsen *et al.* 1996).

The lens, iris, and ciliary body

The lens consists of a lens capsule composed of a thickened basement membrane, and regularly arranged transparent lens fibres. The lens is metabolically active, and new lens fibres are made throughout life, although much more slowly after the age of 30 years. The lens is attached by a series of fine fibres, called zonules, to a ring of smooth muscle, called the ciliary body, lying behind the root of the iris. The iris has sympathetic and parasympathetic innervation which respectively dilates and constricts the pupil; the ciliary body is innervated by the parasympathetic nervous system only. Accommodation (focusing on near objects) is achieved by contraction of the ciliary body, which decreases the tension the zonules exert on the lens capsule, allowing the lens to assume a more spherical shape and thus increasing its focusing power.

Drugs that adversely affect the lens can be considered in four categories:

1. drugs that cause lens opacities due to disruption of lens fibres and accumulation of fluid, that is, cataract;
2. drugs that cause lens deposits without damaging lens structure;
3. drugs that affect lens hydration; and
4. drugs that affect the parasympathetic innervation of the ciliary body.

Cataract formation is the most serious toxic effect of drugs on the lens, as it is irreversible, and can necessitate cataract extraction (Sundmark 1966). Glucocorticoids are by far the most important cause of drug-induced cataract, although research so far has failed to elucidate fully the mechanism for cataract formation (Urban and Cotlier 1986; Jacob *et al.* 1987). Cataract can occur after topical ocular, oral, or parenteral administration, but most studies have found no association with inhaled steroids (Donshik *et al.* 1981; Simons *et al.* 1993; Toogood *et al.* 1993; Abuekteish *et al.* 1995; Barenholtz 1996). There appears to be a degree of variability in individual susceptibility to cataract formation. Several studies have found no correlation between daily and total dose of corticosteroids and cataract formation but both positive and negative HLA associations have been reported (Skalka and Prchal 1980; Adhikary *et al.* 1982; Kollaritis *et al.* 1982; Debnath *et al.* 1987; Fournier *et al.* 1990; Tripathi *et al.* 1992). If cataract is detected at an early stage and steroid therapy stopped, the cataract may not progress and may sometimes regress. Other toxic causes of cataract include antineoplastic agents such as busulphan (Hamming *et al.* 1976; Al-Tweigeri *et al.* 1996) and nitrogen mustards (François and Van Oye 1977), phenytoin (Bar *et al.* 1983; Mathers *et al.* 1987), isotretinoin (Lerman 1992; Heuberger and Buchi 1994), and sodium cyanate used to treat sickle cell haemoglobinopathy (Nicholson *et al.* 1976). Allopurinol was reported to cause cataract, but this was not confirmed by a controlled study (Fraunfelder *et al.* 1982; Clair *et al.*

1989). Topical cholinesterase inhibitors can cause cataract, the onset being usually more rapid in patients aged over 60 years. These drugs, which include ecothiopate, demecarium, and isoflurophate, were formerly used to treat glaucoma and strabismus but are now rarely prescribed.

As with the cornea, systemically administered gold, chlorpromazine, and amiodarone can give rise to deposits under the anterior lens capsule (Gottlieb and Major 1978; Flach *et al.* 1983; McCormick *et al.* 1985; Alexander *et al.* 1985). These deposits rarely interfere with vision, and do not appear to lead to cataract formation. One patient with a unilateral ptosis who had taken chlorpromazine for 10 years had much more marked changes in the exposed eye, suggesting that chlorpromazine-induced ocular toxicity is a result of drug interaction with sunlight (Deluise and Flynn 1981).

Drugs with anticholinergic effects, such as benztropine, the phenothiazines, and tricyclic antidepressants, will reduce accommodation, while cholinergic agents and cholinesterase inhibitors will induce accommodation, making the patient myopic and thus blurring the vision for distance. There may also be a concurrent effect on pupil size that can contribute to the visual disturbance. Some drugs that have no effect on the ciliary body can induce myopia by increasing lens hydration and thus the curvature of the lens. These include oral contraceptives, prochlorperazine, sulphonamides and tetracyclines, and thiazides and related diuretics. The visual disturbance resolves with discontinuation of the drug (Fraunfelder 1996).

The uvea is the vascular tunic of the eye, comprising the iris, ciliary body, and choroid. Uveitis (inflammation of the uvea) may be subclassified as iritis, cyclitis, and choroiditis, according to its site. Uveitis has occurred in a small number of patients treated with disodium pamidronate, used in the management of hypercalcaemia of malignancy and Paget's disease (Macarol and Fraunfelder 1994). Uveitis may occur after starting oral sulphonamides, most commonly with co-trimoxazole (Tilden *et al.* 1991). Topical ocular amphotericin B has, rarely, been reported to cause a severe uveitis. Severe uveitis can also occur after treatment of onchocerciasis but this may be a reaction to the release of foreign protein from dead microfilariae, rather than a toxic drug reaction (Fraunfelder 1996).

Pupillary constriction (miosis) is an inevitable consequence of topically applied cholinergic drugs, such as pilocarpine, and cholinesterase inhibitors. Although these drugs are effective in lowering the intraocular pressure in patients with glaucoma, the reduction in light entering the eye through the constricted pupil can cause difficulties for the patient, particularly in dim light and when driving at night. With the advent of alternative treatments for glaucoma, miotics are used much less frequently. Miosis from systemic therapy is uncommon, but occurs with morphine and other opiates that act as central disinhibitors of the parasympathetic neurons of the third nerve nucleus. Latanoprost, a recently introduced prostaglandin analogue used topically for treating glaucoma, can increase melanogenesis in iris melanocytes and so change eye colour (Wistrand *et al.* 1997).

Intraocular pressure and glaucoma

The corneo-scleral envelope of the eye has the consistency of the leather of a football, and like a football requires internal pressure above atmospheric to maintain a constant shape and thus stable refraction. Normal intraocular pressure lies between 10 and 22 mm Hg, and is maintained by continuous flow of aqueous, a serumlike fluid produced by the ciliary body. The aqueous circulates between lens and iris into the anterior chamber, the cavity between cornea and iris–lens diaphragm, where it drains through the trabecular meshwork near the iris root, and thence into the venous circulation.

The term glaucoma encompasses a number of conditions characterized by loss of retinal nerve fibres, clinically manifested as pathological cupping of the optic disc and visual field defect, and usually accompanied by raised intraocular pressure. By far the commonest type of glaucoma is chronic open-angle glaucoma, in which the trabecular meshwork appears normal but aqueous outflow through it is reduced. Narrow-angle glaucoma (acute and chronic angle-closure glaucoma) is much less common, and is caused by anatomical shallowness of the anterior chamber such that the iris touches the anterior surface of the cornea, preventing aqueous access to the trabecular meshwork. Narrow-angle glaucoma normally has an acute onset with pain and visual loss which may be precipitated by dilatation of the pupil (Brooks *et al.* 1986). It is treated with surgical or laser iridotomy.

Drugs with anticholinergic, sympathetic, and possibly serotoninergic actions will dilate the pupil (Fraunfelder 1996; Eke and Bates 1997). This can precipitate angle closure, but only in those individuals who already have shallow anterior chambers. Prescription of tricyclic antidepressants for patients already known to have glaucoma carries minimal risk, as the great majority will have open angles and will not be at risk of angle closure, and the small group of patients diagnosed as having angle-closure glaucoma will have been treated with iridotomy. Patients who unknowingly have a predisposition to angle closure are at greater risk, and all patients treated with tricyclic antidepressants or other anticholinergics should be advised to seek attention if they develop ocular symptoms.

The capacity of topical ocular corticosteroids to raise intraocular pressure by reducing the outflow of aqueous through the trabecular meshwork has been very well documented: up to 30 per cent of patients develop raised pressures after using topical corticosteroids for several weeks (Alward 1990). Raised intraocular pressure also occurs, but less frequently, with systemic corticosteroids, high doses of inhaled corticosteroids, and topical dermal corticosteroids, particularly when applied to the face (François 1977; Ticho *et al.* 1977; Aggarwal *et al.* 1993; Garbe *et al.* 1997). The intraocular pressure usually falls if the corticosteroid is withdrawn or the dosage reduced. As corticosteroid-induced glaucoma is usually asymptomatic until irreversible visual field loss is well advanced, it is to be recommended that patients on long-term corticosteroid therapy should have regular intraocular pressure measurements. Accumulation of histologically distinct material in the trabecular meshwork has been found in eyes with corticosteroid-induced glaucoma (Johnson *et al.* 1997).

The retina

Light is received by the sensory retina and transformed photochemically into an electric impulse which passes through the optic nerve to the visual centres of the central nervous system. The vertebrate retina is oriented so that the photoreceptors are located in the outermost portions of the retina, directly adjacent to the retinal pigment epithelium (RPE). Microvilli protrude from the apical surface of the retinal pigment epithelial cells to surround the outer segment of the photoreceptors. The photoreceptors undergo a continuous, physiological cyclic degeneration, and discarded outer segments are phagocytosed by intracellular lysosomes within the pigment epithelium. Increasing numbers of lipofuscin granules are found in the RPE with age, and they may represent lysosomal products of the phagocytosed photoreceptor outer segments. Many drugs exhibit a high binding capacity for melanin, and, because of the biochemical interdependence of the RPE and the photoreceptors, drugs that are toxic to the one may also destroy the other. The photoreceptors and all the other neural elements of the retina and optic nerve are part of the central nervous system and, when destroyed, are incapable of regeneration, so loss of vision is irreversible.

Chloroquine administered in doses used for malaria does not cause retinal toxicity, but the much higher doses of chloroquine and hydroxychloroquine used in treating patients with systemic lupus erythematosus and rheumatoid arthritis are toxic to the retina, and the risk of retinopathy increases with total dose. Very few cases have been reported in patients receiving less than 300 g chloroquine, and even patients who received a cumulative dose of over 1 kg chloroquine did not develop retinopathy provided the daily dose was kept below 250 mg per day or 4.4 mg per kg per day for chloroquine and 400 mg per day or 7.7 mg per kg per day for hydroxychloroquine.

The British Royal College of Ophthalmologists recommends a maximum dose of 4 mg per kg lean body-weight per day of chloroquine phosphate (equivalent to approximately 2.5 mg of chloroquine base per kg), and 6.5 mg per day of hydroxychloroquine (Royal College of Ophthalmologists 1993) — the substantial difference between doses expressed in terms of chloroquine base and its salts should be noted. Chloroquine accumulates in tissue over a long period of time; chloroquine and its metabolites have been detected in plasma, red blood cells, and urine as long as 5 years after discontinuation of the drug (Easterbrook 1988; Grant *et al.* 1990).

The characteristic features of chloroquine toxicity are found in the central retina, that is the macula and fovea. The fovea is the concave depression in the centre of the macula and when light is shone into the eye by the ophthalmoscope it behaves like a concave mirror, producing a bright spot of light in front of the retina called the foveal reflex. Initially there is loss of foveal reflex and increased pigmentation in the macula, with later development of a ring of depigmentation surrounded by a ring of increased pigmentation, referred to as the bull's-eye lesion. The patient experiences loss of visual acuity, and central, paracentral, and peripheral scotomata (blind spots in the visual field) may also be present. Colour vision may also be abnormal. There may be some recovery of vision if chloroquine is withdrawn in the very early stages of chloroquine toxicity, but unfortunately ocular toxicity, once established, usually does not regress, and it may even progress despite the drug no longer being taken (Brinkley *et al.* 1979; Ogawa *et al.* 1979). There is no effective treatment for chloroquine toxicity, and the clinician should be aware that the danger of toxicity increases as the cumulative dose increases. There is no simple test for early chloroquine toxicity, and the prescribing physician may feel insufficiently skilled to detect the subtle changes of foveal reflex and macular pigmentation, but if daily and total recommended dosages are not exceeded, the risks of visual loss are small (Mark 1982).

Tamoxifen is a non-steroidal anti-oestrogen used since 1970 in the treatment of breast cancer. In 1978 Kaiser-Kupfer and Lippman reported retinal toxicity in four patients in whom tamoxifen was used in relatively high doses. Since then there have been reports of ocular toxicity at doses of 20 to 30 mg a day (Vinding and Vestinielsen 1983; Pavlidis et al. 1992). Most patients in whom toxicity was reported had been taking the drug for at least one year. Clinically, patients have numerous tiny white refractile retinal lesions in the macular and paramacular areas. White superficial corneal opacities may also be present. Cystoid macular oedema with associated reduction of visual acuity is a common component of the toxicity. Histologically, small spherical lesions containing glycosaminoglycans have been found in nerve fibre and inner plexiform layers of the retina; these have been interpreted as possibly representing axonal degenerative products (Nayfield and Gorin 1996).

Vigabatrin is a selective, irreversible inhibitor of gamma-aminobutyric acid used for treating epilepsy. It was released on the market in 1989, and in 1997 three patients with severe, irreversible loss of field of vision after taking the drug for 2 to 3 years were reported by Eke and colleagues (1997). Abnormalities on fundoscopy were minimal, but electrodiagnostic tests suggested damage to the outer retina. As patients are often unaware of loss of peripheral field of vision until it is far advanced, the incidence of this adverse effect remains to be established. All patients so far reported were taking other medication for epilepsy, and it is unknown whether this is a sole effect or a result of drug interaction. Too little is known at this stage to classify this reaction as type A or B.

Digitalis has been known since the 18th century to cause a variety of reversible visual symptoms, from shimmering or flickering of lights to temporary blindness, and these symptoms are now considered to result from toxic effects on the photoreceptors (Weleber and Shults 1981; Butler et al. 1995). The phenothiazines have a particular affinity for melanin, but only thioridazine is known to produce a symptomatic pigmentary retinopathy, and the effect is dose dependent, occurring rarely at dosages below 600 mg a day (Meredith et al. 1978; Godel et al. 1990). Visual acuity is affected little, if at all, but defects in visual field are more common. The oxazolidinediones (e.g. troxidone) used for treating epilepsy can cause a prolonged 'dazzle effect' when the eyes are exposed to light, a toxic effect that seems to be specific to the retinal cones (Fraunfelder 1996). There are a number of reports of retinal toxicity from the chelating drug desferrioxamine. Visual symptoms and signs include reduction of visual acuity, abnormalities of colour vision, retinal pigment epithelial changes, and tortuosity and dilatation of retinal vessels (Cases et al. 1990; Cohen et al. 1990). Quinine is toxic to the outer layers of the retina and pigment epithelium, and also possibly to the retinal ganglion cells and optic nerve fibres, but seldom causes ocular adverse effects unless an overdose is taken. Visual loss may be profound, but there is usually some return of vision (Boland et al. 1985; Grant and Schuman 1993). Toxic effects from these drugs could be considered type A responses. Retinal vascular occlusion has been reported in women taking oral contraceptives, but there is little evidence that the incidence is greater than in women not taking oral contraceptives (Grant and Schuman 1993).

Retinal detachment has occurred after treatment with topical miotics, particularly the cholinesterase inhibitors, but cause and effect has not yet been established (Beasley and Fraunfelder 1979). Macular oedema with visual loss in aphakic eyes (i.e. eyes after cataract surgery) is a well-established complication of use of topical adrenaline for treating glaucoma (Kolker and Becker 1968). Experiments on rabbits and cats showed that topical adrenaline reaches the retina in higher concentrations when the lens is removed (Kramer 1980). Vision nearly always returned to normal or near-normal levels within months of stopping the treatment.

Severe ocular bacterial and fungal infections (endophthalmitis and panophthalmitis) and viral retinitis are frequently treated with antimicrobial drugs administered directly into the posterior segment of the eye. Cases of macular infarction have been reported, particularly with the use of aminoglycosides (Campochiaro and Conway 1991). Periocular depot corticosteroids inadvertently injected into the eye are highly toxic, and the visual outcome is usually very poor (Zinn 1981; Jain et al. 1992).

The optic nerve

Both ethambutol and isoniazid, used in the treatment of tuberculosis, can cause a retrobulbar neuritis. Toxic ocular effects of ethambutol are uncommon at dosages below 15 mg per kg, but at higher levels occur in one to two per cent of patients. Clinical symptoms and signs include reduced visual acuity, colour vision defects, and visual field loss, and generally occur 3 to 6 months after starting the drug. Vision usually improves within 3 to 12 months after stopping the drug, but optic atrophy with permanent loss of vision may occur (Barron *et al.* 1974; Kumar *et al.* 1993; Woung *et al.* 1995; Fraunfelder 1996). Toxic retrobulbar neuritis from isoniazid is not common, and can respond to treatment with pyridoxine (Grant and Schuman 1993). Several cases of optic neuritis have been reported in patients taking disulfiram for chronic alcoholism. They usually occurred after several months' treatment, when the patient was no longer taking alcohol but still smoking. In most cases vision returned to normal within a few weeks of discontinuing the disulfiram (Norton and Walsh 1972; Acheson and Howard 1988). Chloramphenicol has been reported to cause bilateral optic disc swelling with central visual loss and paracentral scotomata, and subsequent optic atrophy (Kittel and Cornelius 1969; Harley *et al.* 1970). Anterior ischaemic optic neuropathy has been reported with intravenous omeprazole (Schönhöfer and Werner 1997) and amiodarone (Krieg and Schipper 1992; Sedwick 1992). Clioquinol, formerly widely used to treat diarrhoea, is selectively toxic to the axons of the optic nerves and to tracts of the spinal cord (Gran and Schuman 1993). The effect on vision has varied from disturbance of colour vision to blindness from optic atrophy (Boergen 1973).

Many drugs, including corticosteroids, the tetracyclines, nalidixic acid, the quinolones, vitamin A, all-trans retinoic acid, cyclosporin, lithium, amiodarone, phenytoin, thyroxine, growth hormone, danazol, β-human chorionic gonadotrophin, and hormonal contraceptives can cause benign intracranial hypertension with papilloedema (Griffin 1992; Grant and Schuman 1993; Fraunfelder 1996). Vision is not usually affected in the early stages, but secondary optic atrophy with reduced vision can occur if papilloedema is prolonged. Patients can experience transient obscuration of vision and sixth nerve palsies with diplopia.

Disturbances of ocular movement

As with voluntary motor function elsewhere in the body, disorders of eye movement can be due to upper motor neurone or lower motor neurone lesions. Upper motor neurone control of ocular movement is achieved by a number of complex and interrelated reflex systems that include gaze-holding fixation and refixation reflexes that keep the object of interest focused on the macula, pursuit reflexes controlling smooth and saccadic eye movements that track an object of interest as it moves across the visual field, vestibulo-ocular reflexes that maintain fixation despite movements of the head, and vergence reflexes that move the eyes disjunctively so that near objects are focused on both maculae. Disturbance of ocular movement can result from toxic effects on reflex pathways, extrapyramidal and cerebellar systems contributing to motor control, the IIIrd, IVth, and VIth cranial nerves and their nuclei, the neuromuscular junction, and the extraocular muscles.

Drug-induced disorders of higher visuomotor centres give rise to nystagmus, with or without symptoms of oscillopsia (illusory movement of the visual environment), oculogyric crises (sudden uncontrollable elevation of both eyes accompanied by neck retraction and twitching of the shoulder girdle muscles), slow or absent saccadic movements with or without reduction in smooth pursuit, and paresis and paralysis of convergence causing symptoms of diplopia for near vision. Disruption of communication between the IIIrd, IVth, and VIth nerve nuclei (internuclear ophthalmoplegia) can also occur, causing characteristic patterns of restriction of eye movement with diplopia. Lower motor neurone disorders affecting the IIIrd, IVth, and VIth cranial nerves give rise to extraocular muscle pareses with diplopia that varies according to the direction of gaze. Some drugs can have a myasthenic neuromuscular blocking effect, causing ptosis and restricted ocular movement with diplopia.

Many drugs can give rise to nystagmus, usually reversible on withdrawal of the precipitating agent. Nystagmus due to phenytoin is dose related, and is the first sign of systemic toxicity. The nystagmus resolves on withdrawal or reduction in dosage, but may take many months (Fraunfelder 1996). Downbeat nystagmus can be caused by carbamazepine and lithium, and horizontal and vertical nystagmus may occur with barbiturate poisoning. (Chrousos *et al.* 1987; Halmagyi *et al.* 1989; Grant and Schuman 1993). Vestibular nystagmus can follow from the toxic effects of streptomycin on the vestibular apparatus (Marra *et al.* 1988). Oculogyric crises can be produced by the phenothiazines, lithium, levodopa, and tricyclic antidepressants. These are extrapyramidal changes and are dose related (Sandyk 1984). Tardive oculogyric crises can occur as part of tardive dyskinesia from long-term phenothiazine therapy (FitzGerald and Jankovic 1989). The benzodiazepines, phenothiazines, risperidone, carbamazepine, and phenobarbitone can affect the speed and velocity of saccadic eye movements, although symptoms are not usually experienced by the patient (Tedeschi *et al.* 1989; Remler *et al.* 1990; King 1994; Fafrowicz *et al.* 1995; Sweeny *et al.* 1997). Patients taking phenytoin and carbamazepine have increased incidences of vertical and horizontal diplopia which appears to be a central effect on the vergence centres or the vestibulo-ocular reflex, or both of these (Remler *et al.* 1990). These effects could be considered type A reactions.

Several different classes of drugs can cause a syndrome clinically similar to myasthenia gravis, the first signs of which may involve the eyes, with ptosis and extraocular muscle pareses. These drugs include many antibiotics: the aminoglycosides, the penicillins, the tetracyclines, erythromycin, polymyxin, and bacitracin; chloroquine; the heavy metals (for example, gold, lead, and thallium); and penicillamine. High doses of phenytoin have been reported to cause temporary total external ophthalmoplegia and two cases of temporary unilateral superior oblique paresis have been attributed to digitoxin (Grant and Schuman 1993). Bilateral ptosis and blepharoclonus (rapid fluttering of the eyelids) induced by tapping the glabellar area are features of chronic barbiturate intoxication (Grant and Schuman 1993).

Vincristine is neurotoxic and has been reported to cause facial pareses, ptosis, and extraocular muscle pareses. It is also toxic to retinal ganglion cells and the optic nerve, and in a few instance in children has caused transient cortical blindness.

Higher visual centres

More than 300 drugs have been reported to cause visual hallucinations which resolve on reduction of dose or withdrawal of the drug (Fraunfelder 1996). Women taking oral contraceptives have an increased incidence of migraine, occasionally with irreversible ischaemia of the visual cortex with resultant homonymous field defects (Eicholtz 1975). Ibuprofen has been reported to cause visual disturbances, possibly the result of transient multifocal lesions of the visual pathway (Ridder and Tomlinson 1992). Nicastro (1990) reported three cases of visual disturbance with ibuprofen, but macular oedema was suspected in two. Fraunfelder (1993) concluded that there may be a rare idiosyncratic optic nerve response associated with ibuprofen. There are a number of reports of temporary visual loss associated with bladder irrigation with glycine solution during transurethral resection of the prostate. This may be due to oedema of the occipital cortex, or a toxic effect on the retina (Grant and Schuman 1993).

Cisplatin has been reported to cause transient cortical blindess in adults (Al-Tweigeri *et al.* 1996).

Fetal abnormalities

Optic nerve hypoplasia is a well-recognized manifestation of the fetal alcohol syndrome, but many other ocular abnormalities can occur (Strömland and Hellström 1996). The eye is the second most commonly affected organ in thalidomide embryopathy, only surpassed by the upper limbs (Strömland and Miller 1993). Other ocular teratogens include busulfan, chlorambucil, lysergide, lithium, troxidone, isotretinoin, and warfarin (Fraunfelder 1996). Possible teratogens include phenytoin, primidone, cyclophosphamide, and ethambutol (Hampton and Drepostman 1981; Kirshon *et al.* 1988; Fraunfelder 1996). Cocaine and lysergide (LSD) have also been reported as possible causes of fetal abnormalities (Chan *et al.* 1978; Margolis and Martin 1980; Good *et al.* 1992). (See also Chapter 7.)

Systemic effects of topical ophthalmic therapy

Significant systemic absorption of topical therapy occurs not from the conjunctiva or anterior segment of the eye, but from the nasal mucosa after the drug has passed through the nasolacrimal passages with the tears. Systemic absorption is less when medicines are prescribed as ointments or gels, and pressure applied to the nasolacrimal sac after instillation of drops can reduce flow into the nasolacrimal passages.

Topical β-adrenergic antagonists used to treat glaucoma can cause systemic effects, and these are contraindicated in patients with bronchoconstriction and conduction defects of the heart. Betaxolol, which is β_1-selective, and carteolol, which has intrinsic sympathomimetic activity (ISA), may have fewer systemic effects (Zimmerman 1993). The parasympathomimetic substance pilocarpine, also used to treat glaucoma, can cause headache, sweating, nausea, vomiting, diarrhoea, increased salivation and other parasympathetic effects. Phospholine iodide, an anticholinesterase now rarely used for glaucoma, can have similar effects, and may cause cardiac arrest if suxamethonium is used in general anaesthesia (Grant and Schuman 1993; Fraunfelder 1996).

The anticholinergic mydriatics cyclopentolate, tropicamide, and atropine can cause somnolence, hyperactivity, disorientation, tachycardia, vasodilatation with facial flushing, vasomotor collapse, seizures, and even death. Children are particularly vulnerable; reduced-strength cyclopentolate and tropicamide drops are used for infants, and atropine for children is prescribed as ointment rather than drops. The sympathomimetic phenylephrine, also used to dilate the pupil, can cause increased blood pressure, headache, tremor, and sweating (Leroy *et al.* 1989; Grant and Schuman 1993; Wheatcroft *et al.* 1993).

Topical and subconjunctival corticosteroids can cause adrenal suppression particularly in children. Two cases of Cushing's syndrome (one fatal) have been reported (Romano *et al.* 1977). A few cases of aplastic anaemia have been attributed to topical ocular chloramphenicol therapy, but it has been argued that this may be chance association and not cause and effect. The risk, if any, is extremely small (Abrams *et al.* 1980; Doona and Walsh 1995; McGhee and Anastas 1996).

Ophthalmic dyes

Topically applied fluorescein and rose bengal are used routinely in ophthalmic practice for diagnostic purposes, and, apart from stinging and burning sensations, the adverse effects are minimal (Fraunfelder 1996). Fluorescein inactivates the preservatives found in most ophthalmic solutions and they can become contaminated with *Pseudomonas* (Richards *et al.* 1969). For this reason fluorescein is incorporated in dry paper strips or, in soluble form, in single-dose sterile units. Intravenous fluorescein is used regularly to investigate circulation to the retina and choroid and, less frequently, to the sclera, conjunctiva, and iris. Mild systemic adverse effects of nausea, vomiting, and discolouration of the urine are common and transient (Kwiterovich *et al.* 1991; Fraunfelder 1996). More severe systemic adverse effects include phototoxic skin reactions, haemolytic anaemia, urticaria, seizures, and anaphylactic shock, but fortunately are rare (Kwiterovich *et al.* 1991; Munizza *et al.* 1993; Danis and Stephens 1997). Extravasation of fluorescein at the injection site can cause skin necrosis (Elman *et al.* 1987). Indocyanine green is particularly useful in the investigation of the choroidal circulation, and has a lower incidence of adverse effects than fluorescein (Fraunfelder 1996).

Conclusion

A large number of different drugs has been reported to cause ocular adverse effects, but the majority of these are reversible and of little clinical importance. A few drugs, most notably corticosteroids and chloroquine, are known to cause irreversible ocular damage with attendant loss of vision in a significant proportion of patients, and suitable arrangements should be made to monitor patients taking them for these toxic effects. The rare but severe complication of drug-induced Stevens–Johnson syndrome is idiosyncratic and unpredictable, and therefore not amenable to preventive measures, except in the general context of prescribing drugs only when necessary and appropriate.

Further reading

Fraunfelder, F.T. (ed.) (1996). *Drug-induced Ocular Side Effects*. Williams & Wilkins, Baltimore.
Grant, W.M. and Schuman. J.S. (eds) (1993). *Toxicology of the Eye*. Charles Thomas, Springfield, Illinois.

References

Abrams, S.M., Degnan, T.J., and Vinciguerra, V. (1980). Marrow aplasia following topical application of chloramphenicol eye ointment. *Arch. Intern. Med.* 140, 576.
Abuekteish, F., Kirkpatrick, J.N., and Russell, G. (1995). Posterior subcapsular cataract and inhaled corticosteroid therapy. *Thorax* 50, 674.
Acheson, J.F. and Howard, R.S. (1988). Reversible optic neuropathy associated with disulfiram. A clinical and electrophysiological report. *Neuro-Ophthalmology* 8, 175.
Adhikary, H.P., Sells, R.A., and Basu, P.K. (1982). Ocular complications of systemic steroid after renal transplantation and their association with HLA. *Br. J. Ophthalmol.* 66, 290.
Adukman, L., Kolker, A.E., Black, D.L., *et al.* (1996). Treatment of persistent glaucoma secondary to periocular steroids. *Am. J. Ophthalmol.* 122, 275.
Aggarwal, R.K., Potamitis, T., Chong, N.H., *et al.* (1993). Extensive visual loss with topical facial steroids. *Eye* 7, 664.
Alexander, L.J., Bowerman, L., and Thompson, L.R. (1985). The prevalence of the ocular side-effects of chlorpromazine in the Tuscaloosa Veterans Administration patient population. *J. Am. Optom. Assoc.* 56, 872.
Al-Tweigeri, T., Nabholtz, J., and Mackey, J.R. (1996). Ocular toxicity and cancer chemotherapy. A review. *Cancer* 78, 1359.
Alward, W.L.M. (1990). Corticosteroid induced glaucoma. In *Duane's Clinical Ophthalmology* (section ed. R.K. Parrish), p. 7. J.B. Lippincott, London.
Bar, S., Feller, N., and Savir, H. (1983). Presenile cataract in phenytoin-treated epileptic patients. *Arch. Ophthalmol.* 101, 422.
Barenholtz, H. (1996). Effect of inhaled corticosteroids on the risk of cataract formation in patients with steroid-dependent asthma. *Ann. Pharmacother.* 30, 1324.
Barron, C.J., Tepper, L., and Iovine, G. (1974). Ocular toxicity from ethambutol. *Am. J. Ophthalmol.* 77, 256.
Baudouin, C., Garcher, C., Haouat, N., *et al.* (1994). Expression of inflammatory membrane markers by conjunctival cells in chronically treated patients with glaucoma. *Ophthalmology* 101, 454.
Beasley, H. and Fraunfelder, F.T. (1979). Retinal detachment and topical ocular miotics. *Ophthalmology* 86, 95.
Blackman, H.J., Peck, G.L, Olsen, T.G., *et al.* (1979). Blepharoconjunctivitis: a side effect of 13-cis-retinoic acid therapy for dermatologic diseases. *Ophthalmology* 86, 753.
Blanchard, D.L. (1987). Adrenergic-associated symblepharon. *Glaucoma* 9, 18.
Boergen, K.P. (1973). Optic nerve damage through antidiarrhoeal preparations. *Klin. Monatbl. Augenheilkd.* 76, 312.

Boland, M.E., Roper, S.M., and Henry, J.A. (1985). Complications of quinine poisoning. *Lancet* i, 384.

Brinkley, J.R., Dubois, E.L., and Ryan, S.J. (1979). Long-term course of chloroquine retinopathy after cessation of medication. *Am. J. Ophthalmol.* 88, 1.

Broadway, D.C., Grierson, I., O'Brien, C., *et al.* (1994). Adverse effects of topical antiglaucoma medication. II. The outcome of filtration surgery. *Arch. Ophthalmol.* 112, 1446.

Brooks, A.M., West, R.H., and Gillies, W.E. (1986). The risks of precipitating acute angle-closure glaucoma with the clinical use of mydriatic agents. *Med. J. Aust.* 145, 34.

Burns, C.A. (1973). Indomethacin-induced ocular toxicity. *Am. J. Ophthalmol.* 76, 312.

Burstein, N.L. (1985). The effects of topical drugs and preservatives on the tears and corneal epithelium in dry eye. *Trans. Ophthalmol. Soc. U.K.* 104, 402.

Butler, V.P. Jr., Odel, J.G., Rath, E., *et al.* (1995). Digitalis-induced visual disturbances with therapeutic serum digitalis concentrations. *Ann. Intern. Med.* 123, 676.

Campochiaro, P.A. and Conway, B.P. (1991). Aminoglycoside toxicity — a survey of retinal specialists. Implications for ocular use. *Arch. Ophthalmol.* 109, 946.

Cases, A., Kelly, J., Sabater, F., *et al.* (1990). Ocular and auditory toxicity in hemodialyzed patients receiving desferrioxamine. *Nephron* 56, 19.

Chan, C.C., Fishman, M., and Egbert, P.R. (1978). Multiple ocular abnormalities associated with maternal LSD ingestion. *Arch. Ophthalmol.* 96, 282.

Chrousos, G.A., Cowdry, R., Schuelein, M., *et al.* (1987). Two cases of downbeat nystagmus and oscillopsia associated with carbamazepine. *Am. J. Ophthalmol.* 103, 221.

Cohen, A., Martin, M., Mizanin, J., *et al.* (1990). Vision and hearing during deferoxamine therapy. *J. Pediatr.* 117 (2 Pt 1), 826.

Costa, V.P., Wilson, R.P., Moster, M.R., *et al.* (1993). Hypotony maculopathy following the use of topical mitomycin C in glaucoma filtration surgery. *Ophthalmic Surg.* 24, 389.

D'Amico, D.J., Kenyon, K.R., and Ruskin, J.N. (1981). Amiodarone keratopathy: drug induced lipid storage disease. *Arch. Ophthalmol.* 99, 257.

Danis, R.P. and Stephens, T. (1997). Photoxic reactions caused by sodium fluorescein. *Am. J. Ophthalmol.* 123, 694.

Debnath, S.C., Abomelha, M.S., Jawdat, M., *et al.* (1987). Ocular side effects of systemic steroid therapy in renal transplant patients. *Ann. Ophthalmol.* 19, 435.

Deluise, V.P. and Flynn, J.T. (1981). Asymmetric anterior segment changes induced by chlorpromazine. *Ann. Ophthalmol.* 13, 953.

Detry-Morel, M., Boschi, A., Sempoux, P., *et al.* (1995). Effects of local medications on intraocular pressure control following trabeculectomy. *Bull. Soc. Belge Ophtalmol.* 259, 135.

Donshik, P.C., Cavanaugh, H.D., Boruchoff, S.A., *et al.* (1981). Posterior subcapsular cataracts induced by topical corticosteroids following keratoplasty for keratoconus. *Ann. Ophthalmol.* 13, 29.

Doona, M. and Walsh, J.B. (1995). Use of chloramphenicol as topical eye medication: time to cry halt?. *BMJ* 310, 1217.

Easterbrook, M. (1988). Ocular effects and safety of antimalarial agents. *Am. J. Med.* 85 (Suppl. 4A), 23.

Eicholtz, W. (1975). Striking accumulation of vascular-induced homonymous defects of the visual field in young women. *Münch. Med. Wochenschr.* 117, 571.

Eke, T. and Bates, A.K. (1997). Acute angle closure glaucoma associated with paroxetine. *BMJ* 314, 1387.

Eke, T., Talbot, J.F., and Lawden, M.C. (1997). Severe persistent visual field constriction associated with vigabatrin. *BMJ* 314, 180.

Elman, M.J., Fine, S.L., Sorenson, J., *et al.* (1987). Skin necrosis following fluorescein extravasation. A survey of the Macula Society. *Retina* 7, 89.

Fafrowicz, M., Unrug, A., Marek, T., *et al.* (1995). Effects of diazepam and buspirone on reaction time of saccadic eye movements. *Neuropsychobiology* 32, 156.

FitzGerald, P.M. and Jankovic, J. (1989). Tardive oculogyric crises. *Neurology* 39, 1434.

Flach, A.J., Dolan, B.J., Sudduth, B., *et al.* (1983). Amiodarone-induced lens opacities. *Arch. Ophthalmol.* 101, 1554.

Font, R.L., Sobol, W., and Matoba, A. (1989). Polychromatic corneal and conjunctival crystals secondary to clofazimine in a leper. *Ophthalmology* 96, 311.

Foon, K.A. (1984). Increased growth of eyelashes in a patient given leukocyte A interferon. *N. Engl. J. Med.* 311, 1259.

Fournier, C., Milot, J.A., Clermont, M.J., *et al.* (1990). The concept of corticosteroid cataractogenic factor revisited. *Can. J. Ophthalmol.* 25, 345.

François, J. (1977). Corticosteroid glaucoma. *Ann. Ophthalmol.* 9, 1075.

François, J. and Van Oye, R. (1977). Immunodepressors in ophthalmology. *Ann. Oculist* 210, 89.

Fraunfelder, F.T. (1996). *Drug-induced Ocular Side Effects* (4th edn). Lea & Febiger, Philadelphia.

Fraunfelder, F.T., Hanna, C., Dreis, M.W., *et al.* (1992). Cataracts associated with allopurinol therapy. *Am. J. Ophthalmol.* 94, 137.

Garbe, E., LeLorier, J., Boivin, J.F., *et al.* (1997). Inhaled and nasal glucocorticoids and the risks of ocular hypertension or open-angle glaucoma. *JAMA* 277, 722.

Godel, V., Loewenstein, A., and Lazar, M. (1990). Spectral electroretinography in thioridazine toxicity. *Ann. Ophthalmol.* 22, 293.

Good, W.V., Ferriero, D.M., Golabi, M., *et al.* (1992). Abnormalities of the visual system in infants exposed to cocaine. *Ophthalmology* 99, 341.

Gottlieb, N.L. and Major, J.C. (1978). Ocular chrysiasis correlated with gold concentrations in the crystalline lens during chrysotherapy. *Arthritis Rheum.* 21, 704.

Grant, W.M. and Schuman, J.S. (1993). *Toxicology of the Eye* (4th edn). Charles Thomas, Springfield, Illinois.

Grant, S., Greenseid, D.Z., and Leopold, I.H. (1990). Toxic retinopathies. In *Duane's Clinical Ophthalmology* (section ed. W.E. Benson), p. 2. J.B. Lippincott, London.

Griffin, J.P. (1992). A review of the literature on benign intracranial hypertension associated with medication. *Adverse Drug React. Toxicol. Rev.* 11, 41.

Gwinup, G., Elias, A.N., and Ascher, M.S. (1982). Effect on exophthalmos of various methods of treatment of Graves' disease. *JAMA* 247, 2135.

Halmagyi, G.M., Lessell, I., Curthoys, I.S., *et al.* (1989). Lithium-induced downbeat nystagmus. *Am. J. Ophthalmol.* 107, 664.

Hamming, N.A., Apple, D.J., and Goldberg, M.F. (1976). Histopathology and ultrastructure of busulfan-induced cataract. *Graefes Arch. Clin. Exp. Ophthalmol.* 200, 139.

Hampton, G.R. and Drepostman, J.I. (1981). Ocular manifestations of the fetal hydantoin syndrome. *Clin. Pediatr.* (Phila.) 20, 475.

Harley, R.D., Huang, N.N., Macri, C.H., *et al.* (1970). Optic neuritis and optic atrophy following chloramphenicol in cystic fibrosis patients. *Trans. Am. Ophthalmol. Soc.* 74, 1011.

Heuberger, A. and Buchi, E.R. (1994). Irreversible cataract as a possible side effect of isotretinoin. *Klin. Monatsbl. Augenheilkd.* 204, 465.

Jacob, T.J., Karim, A.K., and Thompson, G.M. (1987). The effects of steroids on human lens epithelium. *Eye* 1, 722.

Jain, V.K., Mames, R.N., McGorray, S., *et al.* (1992). Inadvertent penetrating injury to the globe with periocular corticosteroid injection. *Ophthalmic Surg.* 22, 508.

Jenkins, C.D., McDonnell, P.J., and Spalton, D.J. (1990). Randomised single blind trial to compare the toxicity of subconjunctival gentamicin and cefuroxime in cataract surgery. *Br. J. Ophthalmol.* 74, 734.

Johnson, D., Gottanka, J., Flugel, C., *et al.* (1997). Ultrastructural changes in the trabecular meshwork of human eyes treated with corticosteroids. *Arch. Ophthalmol.* 115, 375.

Johnson, D.H., Yoshikawa, K., Brubaker, R.F *et al.* (1994). The effect of long-term medical therapy on the outcome of filtration surgery. *Am. J. Ophthalmol.* 117, 139.

Kaiser-Kupfer, M.I. and Lippman, M.E. (1978). Tamoxifen retinopathy. *Cancer Treat. Rep.* 62, 315.

Kaufman, H.E. and Rayfield, M.A. (1988). Viral conjunctivitis and keratitis. In *The Cornea* (ed. H.E. Kaufman, B.A. Barron, M.B. McDonald, and S.R. Waltman), p. 299. Heinemann, Oxford.

King, D.J. (1994). Psychomotor impairment and cognitive disturbances induced by neuroleptics. *Acta Psychiatr. Scand.* (Suppl. 380), 53.

Kirshon, B., Wasserstrum, N., Willis, R., *et al.* (1988). Teratogenic effects of first-trimester cyclophosphamide therapy. *Obstet. Gynecol.* 72, 462.

Kittel, V. and Cornelius, C. (1969). Optic nerve injury by chloramphenicol. *Klin. Monatsbl. Augenheilkd.* 155, 83.

Kolker, A.E. and Becker, B. (1968) Epinephrine maculopathy. *Arch. Ophthalmol.* 79, 552.

Kollaritis, C.R., Swann, E.R., Shapiro, R.S., *et al.* (1982). HLA A1 and steroid-induced cataracts in renal transplant patients. *Ann. Ophthalmol.* 14, 1116.

Kramer, S.G. (1980). Epinephrine distribution after topical administration to phakic and aphakic eyes. *Trans. Am. Ophthalmol. Soc.* 78, 947.

Krieg, P. and Schipper, I. (1992). Bilateral optic neuropathy following amiodarone therapy. *Klin. Monatsbl. Augenheilkd.* 200, 128.

Kruyswijk, M.R., van Driel, L.M., Polak, B.C., *et al.* (1980). Contact allergy following administration of eye drops and eye ointments. *Doc. Ophthalmol.* 48, 251.

Kumar, A., Sandramouli, S., Verma, L., *et al.* (1993). Ocular ethambutol toxicity: is it reversible? *J. Clin. Neuro Ophthalmol.* 13, 15.

Kwiterovich, K.A., Maguire, M.G., Murphy, R.P., *et al.* (1991). Frequency of adverse systemic reactions after fluorescein angiography. Results of a prospective study. *Ophthalmology* 98, 1139.

Lass, J.H., Thoft, R.A., and Dohlman, C.H. (1983). Idoxuridine-induced conjunctival cicatrization. *Arch. Ophthalmol.* 101, 747.

Lazarus, J.H., John, R., Bennie, E.H., *et al.* (1981). Lithium therapy and thyroid function: a long term study. *Psychol. Med.* 11, 85.

Lerman, S. (1992). Ocular side effects of Accutane therapy. *Lens Eye Toxic. Res.* 9, 429.

Leroy, M.P., Cantineau, D., Brasdefer, D., *et al.* (1989). Adverse effects of neosynephrine. *Bull. Soc. Ophtalmol. France* 89, 234.

Lyns, R.W. (1979). Orange contact lenses from rifampicin. *N. Engl. J. Med.* 174, 586.

Macarol, V. and Fraunfelder, F.T. (1994). Pamidronate disodium and possible ocular adverse drug reactions. *Am. J. Ophthalmol.* 118, 220.

Margolis, S. and Martin, L. (1980). Anophthalmos in an infant of parents using LSD. *Ann. Ophthalmol.* 12, 1378.

Mark, J.S. (1982). Chloroquine retinopathy: is there a safe daily dose? *Ann. Rheum. Dis.* 41, 52.

Marra, T.R., Reynolds, N.C. Jr., and Stoddard J.J. (1988). Subjective oscillopsia ('jiggling' vision) presumably due to aminoglycoside ototoxicity. A report of two cases. *J. Clin. Neuro Ophthalmol.* 8, 35.

Marti-Huguet, T., Quintana, M., and Cabiro, I. (1989). Cicatricial pemphigoid associated with D-penicillamine treatment. *Arch. Ophthalmol.* 1107, 115.

Mathers, W., Kattan, H., Earll, J., *et al.* (1987). Development of presenile cataract in association with high serum levels of phenytoin. *Ann. Ophthalmol.* 19, 291.

Mathers, W.D., Shields, W.J., Sachdev, M.S., *et al.* (1991). Meibomian gland morphology and tear osmolarity: changes with Accutane therapy. *Cornea* 10, 286.

McCormick, S.A., DiBartolomeo, A.G., Raju, V.K., *et al.* (1985). Ocular chrysiasis. *Ophthalmology* 92, 1432.

McGhee, C.N.J. and Anastas, C. (1996). Widespread ocular use of topical chloramphenicol: is there justifiable concern regarding idiosyncratic aplastic anaemia? *Br. J. Ophthalmol.* 80, 182.

Meredith, T.A., Aaberg, T.M., and Willerson D. (1978). Progressive chorioretinopathy after receiving thioridazine. *Arch. Ophthalmol.* 96, 1172.

Mills, E.W., Siebert, L.F., and Climenhaga, D.B. (1986). Depot triamcinolone-induced glaucoma. *Can. J. Ophthalmology* 21, 150.

Mondino, B.J., Salamon, G.W., and Zaidman, G.W. (1982). Allergic and toxic reactions of soft contact lens wearers. *Surv. Ophthalmol.* 26, 337.

Munizza, M., Kavitsky, D., Schainker, B.A *et al.* (1993). Hemolytic anaemia associated with injection of fluorescein. *Transfusion* 33, 689.

Nayfield, S.G. and Gorin, M.B. (1996). Tamoxifen-associated eye disease. *J. Clin. Oncol.* 14, 1018.

Neilsen, C.E., Andreasen, F., and Bjerregaard, P. (1983). Amiodarone induced cornea verticillata. *Acta Ophthalmol.* 61, 474.

Nicastro, N.J. (1990). Visual disturbances associated with over-the-counter ibuprofen in three patients. *Ann. Ophthalmol.* 22, 447.

Nicholson, D.H., Harkness, D.R., Benson, W.E., *et al.* (1976). Cyanate-induced cataracts in patients with sickle-cell hemoglobinopathies. *Arch. Ophthalmol.* 94, 927.

Norton, A.L. and Walsh, F.B. (1972). Disulfiram-induced optic neuritis. *Trans. Am. Acad. Ophthalmol. Otol.* 76, 1263.

Ogawa, S., Kurumatani, N., Shibaike, N., *et al.* (1979). Progression of retinopathy long after cessation of chloroquine therapy. *Lancet* i, 1408.

Patten, J.T., Cavanagh, H.D., and Allansmith, M.R. (1976). Induced ocular pseudopemphigoid. *Am. J. Ophthalmol.* 82, 272.

Pavlidis, N.A., Petris, C., Briassoulis, E., *et al.* (1992). Clear evidence that long-term, low-dose tamoxifen can induce ocular toxicity: a prospective study of 63 patients. *Cancer* 69, 2961.

Poulsen, E.J., Mannis, M.J., and Chang, S.D. (1996). Keratitis in methamphetamine abusers. *Cornea* 15, 477.

Rahi, A.H., Chapman, C.M., Garner, A., *et al.* (1976). Pathology of practolol-induced ocular toxicity. *Br. J. Ophthalmol.* 60, 312.

Rasmussen, K., Kirk, L., and Faurbye, A. (1976). Deposits in the lens and cornea of the eye during long-term chlorpromazine medication. *Acta Psychiatr. Scand.* 53, 1.

Remler, B.F., Leigh, R.J., Osorio, I., *et al.* (1990). The characteristics and mechanisms of visual disturbance associated with anticonvulsant therapy. *Neurology* 40, 791.

Richards, R.M.E., Suwanprakorn, P., Neawbanij, S., *et al.* (1969). Preservation of fluorescein solutions against contamination with *Pseudomonas aeruginosa*. *J. Pharm. Pharmacol.* 21, 681.

Ridder, W.H. and Tomlinson, A. (1992). Effect of ibuprofen on contrast sensitivity. *Optom. Vis. Sci.* 69, 652.

Robin, J.B. and Dugel, R. (1988). Immunologic disorders of the cornea and conjunctiva. In *The Cornea* (ed. H.E. Kaufman, B.A. Barron, M.B. McDonald, and S.R. Waltman), p. 529. Heinemann, Oxford.

Romano, P.E., Traisman, H.S., and Green, O.C. (1977). Fluorinated corticosteroid toxicity in infants. *Am. J. Ophthalmol.* 84, 247.

Sandyk, R. (1984). Oculogyric crisis induced by lithium carbonate. *Eur. Neurol.* 23, 92.

Sedwick, L.A. (1992). Getting to the heart of visual loss: when cardiac medication may be dangerous to the optic nerves. *Surv. Ophthalmol.* 36, 366.

Schönhöfer, P.S. and Werner, B. (1997). Ocular damage associated with proton pump inhibitors. *BMJ* 314, 1805.

Sherwood, M.B., Grierson, I., Millar, L., *et al.* (1989). Long-term morphologic effects of antiglaucoma drugs on the conjunctiva and Tenon's capsule in glaucomatous patients. *Ophthalmology* 96, 327.

Silbert, J.A. (1996). A review of therapeutic agents and contact lens wear. *J. Am. Optom. Assoc.* 67, 165.

Simons, F.E., Persaud, M.P., Gillespie, C.A., *et al.* (1993). Absence of posterior subcapsular cataracts in young patients treated with inhaled glucocorticoids. *Lancet* 342, 776.

Skalka, H.W. and Prchal, J.T. (1980). Effect of corticosteroids on cataract formation. *Arch. Ophthalmol.* 98,1773.

Sridama, V. and DeGroot, L.J. (1989). Treatment of Graves' disease and the course of ophthalmolopathy. *Am. J. Med.* 87, 70.

Stamper, R.L., McMenemy, M.G., and Lieberman, M.F. (1992). Hypotonous maculopathy after trabeculectomy with subconjunctival 5-fluorouracil. *Am. J. Ophthalmol.* 114, 544.

Straus, D.J., Masouf, F.A.. Ellerby, R.A., *et al.* (1977). Cicatricial ectropion secondary to 5-fluorouracil therapy. *Med. Pediatr. Oncol.* 3, 15.

Strömland, K. and Hellström, A. (1996). Fetal alcohol syndrome — an ophthalmological and socioeducational prospective study. *Pediatrics* 97, 845.

Strömland, K. and Miller, M.T. (1993). Thalidomide embryopathy: revisited 27 years later. *Acta Ophthalmol.* 71, 238.

Sundmark, E. (1966). The cataract-inducing effect of systemic corticosteroid therapy. *Acta Ophthalmol.* 44, 291.

Sweeny, J.A., Bauer, K.S., Keshavan, M.S., *et al.* (1997). Adverse effects of risperidone on eye movement activity: a comparison of risperidone and haloperidol in antipsychotic-naive schizophrenic patients. *Neuropsychopharmacology* 16, 217.

Tedeschi, G., Casucci, G., Allocca, S., *et al.* (1989). Neuroocular side effects of carbamazepine and phenobarbital in epileptic patients as measured by saccadic eye movement analysis. *Epilepsia* 30, 62.

Ticho, U. and Ophir, A. (1993). Late complications after glaucoma filtering surgery with adjunctive 5-fluorouracil. *Am. J. Ophthalmol.* 115, 506.

Ticho, U., Durst, A., Licht, A., *et al.* (1977). Steroid-induced glaucoma in renal transplant recipients. *Israel J. Med. Sci.* 13, 871.

Tilden, M., Rosenbaum, J.T., and Fraunfelder, F.T. (1991). Systemic sulfonamides as a cause of bilateral anterior uveitis. *Arch. Ophthalmol.* 109, 67.

Toogood, J.H., Markov, A.E., Baskerville, J., *et al.* (1993). Association of ocular cataracts with inhaled and oral steroid therapy during long-term treatment of asthma. *J. Allergy Clin. Immunol.* 91, 571.

Tripathi, R.C., Kipp, M.A., Tripathi, B.J., *et al.* (1992). Ocular toxicity of prednisone in paediatric patients with inflammatory bowel disease. *Lens Eye Toxic. Res.* 9, 469.

Urban, R.C. Jr and Cotlier, E. (1986). Corticosteroid-induced cataracts. *Surv. Ophthalmol.* 31, 102.

Vinding, T. and Nielsen, N.V. (1983). Retinopathy caused by treatment with tamoxifen in low dosage. *Acta Ophthalmol.* 61, 45.

Walinder, P.E., Gip, L., and Sempa, M. (1976). Corneal changes in patients treated with clofazimine. *Br. J. Ophthalmol.* 60, 526.

Weleber, R.G. and Shults, W.T. (1981). Digoxin retinal toxicity. Clinical and electrophysiological evaluation of cone dysfunction syndrome. *Arch. Ophthalmol.* 99, 1568.

Wheatcroft, S., Sharma, A., and McAllister, J. (1993). Reduction in mydriatic drop size in premature infants. *Br. J. Ophthalmol.* 77, 364.

Wilson, F.M. (1979). Adverse external ocular effects of topical ophthalmic medications. *Surv. Ophthalmol.* 24. 57.

Wistrand, P.J., Stjernschantz, J., and Olsson, K. (1997). The incidence and time-course of latanoprost-induced iridial pigmentation as a function of eye colour. *Surv. Ophthalmol.* 41 (Suppl. 2), S129.

Woung, L.C, Jou, J.R., and Liaw, S.L. (1995). Visual function in recovered ethambutol optic neuropathy. *J. Ocul. Pharmacol.* 11, 411.

Zimmerman, T.J. (1993). Topical ophthalmic beta blockers: a comparative review. *J. Ocul. Pharmacol.* 9, 373.

Zinn, K.M. (1981). Iatrogenic intraocular injection of depot corticosteroid and its surgical removal using the pars plana approach. *Ophthalmology* 88, 13.

22. Ear, nose, and throat disorders

C. DIAMOND

The ear

The study of adverse drug reactions affecting the ear, nose, and throat system has had both an expected and an unexpected benefit. As expected, awareness of possible adverse effects has enabled the medical profession to prevent harm coming to patients and thereby to fulfil its primary obligation: *primum non nocere*. The unexpected benefit has been the new knowledge gained concerning the normal physiological mechanisms of hearing and, to a lesser extent, of taste and smell. Search for the mechanism of the adverse reaction has often illuminated the mechanism of the normal physiological process. This may be illustrated by a single example at this stage. Streptomycin was first introduced into clinical medicine in 1945 by Hinshaw and Feldman. They treated 34 tubercular patients with this new drug and noted a striking response to therapy in some of them. The preliminary report (Hinshaw and Feldman 1945) is a model of good practice. They made modest claims for the benefits of the drug. They recorded that one of their patients had transient deafness and three of their patients had apparent disturbance of vestibular function when large doses were administered for prolonged periods. Having recorded the adverse effect, they pondered about the mechanism of the adverse reaction and tentatively suggested it might be caused by a selective neurotoxic effect on the eighth cranial nerve. The quest for the ototoxic mechanism has led to a great deal of animal and clinical research, as a result of which it is now known that streptomycin damages the hair cells of the cochlea and the hair cells of the vestibular apparatus and does not damage the eighth nerve itself. The knowledge gained by this research has resolved a problem of cochlear physiology, namely, the source of the cochlear microphonic electrical potential. There are two main cochlear electrical potentials evoked by auditory stimuli: the cochlear microphonic (CM) and the eighth nerve compound action potential (AP). When the eighth nerve is severed AP disappears, as one would expect, but CM persists. The source of CM was initially a mystery. Animal and human studies have shown that when the cochlear hair cells are destroyed by aminoglycoside antibiotics CM disappears while AP persists. It has thus been demonstrated that CM is generated by the cochlear hair cells.

Ototoxic adverse reactions were known for a long time before streptomycin was introduced. Hawkins (1967) has suggested that the Shamans, priest doctors of the Incas in ancient Peru, were aware of the ototoxic effects of wormseed, source of the anthelmintic chenopodium oil, and of Peruvian bark, source of the antimalarial cinchona alkaloids. Peruvian bark was introduced into Spain in 1632 by Jesuit missionaries returning from South America. In England in 1692 Richard Morton, Physician in Ordinary to King William III, wrote in his *Pyretologia* — a book of fevers — of his experience of the bark and of its temporary ototoxic effect, '. . . I have never known anyone suffer a misfortune as a result of using the Bark, other than to experience a distressing type of hearing loss at the time of use. . . .' (quoted by Stephens 1982); thus the fact that certain drugs can have an ototoxic effect has been known for centuries.

Deafness has been reported in association with a number of medications that are no longer in use, for example, arsenic (Salvarsan), strychnine, and valerian (Mawson 1967). In this chapter, however, consideration will only be given to drugs and therapeutic substances that are in current use. Ototoxic industrial compounds will not be considered, although some of these compounds can harm people who do not encounter them as industrial hazards. For example, some individuals have suffered deafness and vertigo after using hair dyes containing paraphenylenediamine, which is a recognized labyrinthine poison (Lumsden and McDowell 1968); also the organophosphorus insecticide malathion is reported to have produced profound permanent sensorineural deafness in a young man who used a spray

TABLE 22.1
Major ototoxic drugs in order of decreasing incidence of toxicity [Friedlander 1979]

Drug	Cochlear toxicity	Vestibular toxicity
Minocycline		+ + + +
Kanamycin	+ + +	+
Amikacin	+ + + +	
Neomycin	+ + +	+
Streptomycin	+	+ + +
Viomycin	+ +	+ +
Gentamicin	+	+ + +
Tobramycin	+	+ + +
Ethacrynic acid	+ + +	+
Frusemide	+ + + +	
Vancomycin	+ + + +	
Quinine	+ + + +	
Salicylates	+ + + +	
Polymyxin B†		+ + + +
Colistin†		+ + + +

* ototoxicity is indicated on a scale of 0 to + + + +
† applied topically
After I.R. Friedlander (1979). Reprinted by permission of the *New England Journal of Medicine* 301, 213.

containing this chemical in his father's orchard (Harell *et al.* 1978*a*). In the latter example the reaction appears to have been a Type B reaction.

Friedlander (1979) has compiled a table of the major ototoxic drugs showing their relative incidence and listing their cochlear and vestibular toxicity under separate columns (Table 22.1).

Ototoxic antibiotics

Aminoglycoside antibiotics

The number of aminoglycoside antibiotics with ototoxic properties has grown steadily since streptomycin was first used in patients in 1945. The list includes capreomycin, dihydrostreptomycin, framycetin, gentamicin, kanamycin, neomycin, paromomycin, tobramycin, and viomycin. Although they do not belong to the group, it is convenient to consider polymyxin B and polymyxin E (colistin), vancomycin, and ristocetin with the aminoglycoside antibiotics. All these drugs can damage both the auditory and vestibular parts of the inner ear but they do tend to cause preferential damage to one or the other. This is illustrated by Table 22.1. In addition, all the aminoglycosides are nephrotoxic. The search for less toxic aminoglycosides has led to the production of the semisynthetic aminoglycosides amikacin and netilmicin. In equipotent dosages amikacin and gentamicin have an equivalent degree of auditory toxicity (Smith *et al.* 1977). The potential margin of safety of netilmicin appears to be much greater than that of gentamicin and amikacin. Netilmicin and gentamicin are equipotent in their antibacterial action, yet 150 mg per kg of netilmicin produces less cochlear damage than 50 mg per kg of gentamicin in guinea-pigs (Brummet *et al.* 1978). If a new drug appears to be less ototoxic than others in animals, it does not necessarily follow that it will be less ototoxic in humans. Tjernstrom (1980) carried out a prospective evaluation of both auditory and vestibular function in 76 patients receiving treatment with netilmicin. Audiometry and electronystagmography were performed before, during, and after treatment. Only one patient showed any ototoxic effect and the adverse reaction in this patient was a subclinical reversible disturbance of vestibular function. There have been several other trials that suggest that netilmicin is significantly less ototoxic in humans than gentamicin and amikacin and is also less ototoxic than tobramycin (Lerner *et al.* 1983).

Nature and mechanism of aminoglycoside antibiotic ototoxicity

It has been repeatedly demonstrated in animal and human studies that the principal structural lesion produced by these drugs is a degeneration of the sensory (hair) cells. The hair cells of the cochlea are confined to the organ of Corti. The vestibular hair cells are found in the macula of the saccule, the macula of the utricle, and the ampullae of the three semicircular canals. Kohonen (1965) and many other investigators have shown that, although these drugs differ in the degree of cochlear damage they cause, the pattern of cochlear hair cell injury is common to all members of the group. Damage is greatest in the outer hair cells at the base of the cochlea (which respond to high-frequency sound) and diminishes progressively towards the apex and helicotrema. This is reflected in the audiogram, which reveals a high tone sensorineural deafness with lesser impairment of the hearing for the middle and lower sound frequencies (Fig. 22.1). Severe damage results in total deafness in all frequencies. Hair cell degeneration is irreversible and the deafness produced by it is therefore permanent. The vestibular disturbance produced by the aminoglycosides does not cause acute vertigo such as is seen in patients with Menière's disease. Instead, an unusual and highly characteristic type of disequilibrium is produced, in which the patient experiences a vertical oscillation of his surroundings every time he moves. The patient seldom has symptoms while he is confined to bed but when he is able to walk he does so with the feet wide apart and has great difficulty walking in a straight line. Objects in his visual field appear to bounce up and down in time with

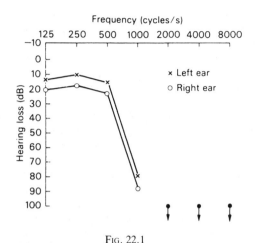

FIG. 22.1

Bilateral high-tone deafness following daily neomycin irrigation of the pleural cavity after removal of a mesothelioma in a 47-year-old man: total loss of hearing at 8000, 4000, and 2000Hz, severe loss at 1000Hz, and normal hearing at 500, 250, and 125Hz.

each footfall. As soon as the patient stops moving the bouncing of his surroundings ceases. The term 'bobbing oscillopsia' has been applied to this symptom. This pattern of disequilibrium was described shortly after the introduction of streptomycin (Brown and Hinshaw 1946; Wallner 1949), and has also been described in patients receiving gentamicin (Ramsden and Ackrill 1982). True rotational vertigo is rare in aminoglycoside vestibulotoxicity. Caloric tests and rotational tests show a loss of labyrinthine function. Frequently nystagmus is not detectable clinically. It can often be demonstrated by electronystagmography, however. Although the hair cell damage in the vestibule is permanent, as it is in the cochlea, the patient's balance steadily improves after a few months and improvement can sometimes continue for up to 2 years. This is the result of adaptive changes in the central mechanisms of balance control and these adaptive changes develop more readily in younger than in older patients.

The mechanism of aminoglycoside ototoxicity has not yet been fully explained. It was previously considered that the ototoxic mechanism might be explained on a pharmacokinetic basis by the prolonged high concentration of these drugs in the inner ear fluids. Doubt has been cast on this explanation because, although the perilymph concentration may be high, the concentration in the inner ear tissue (as opposed to the perilymph) does not appear to be significantly higher than the concentration in the liver (Toyoda and Tachibana 1978) or in the heart, lung, and spleen (Desrochers and

Schacht 1982). It has been pointed out that the concentration of aminoglycosides in perilymph associated with complete hair cell loss following chronic drug administration was only 0.5 per cent of the cytotoxic drug concentration *in vitro* (Brummet and Fox 1982). It has therefore been suggested that the hair cells of the inner ear may be intrinsically more sensitive or more susceptible to damage by aminoglycosides than are the cells of the liver, lung, heart, and spleen. Spoendlin (1966) has suggested that the aminoglycosides may produce their ototoxic effect on the hair cells in the same way that they exert their antibacterial activity, namely, by inhibition of protein synthesis. It has been suggested more recently that there is a specific interaction between aminoglycosides and cell membrane lipids with disturbance of calcium ion binding and phosphorylation processes (Fee 1980; Schacht 1986). A molecular and cellular hypothesis of aminoglycoside ototoxicity based on human genetic studies has been proposed by Cortopassi and Hutchin (1994). A rare maternally inherited genetic susceptibility to aminoglycoside-induced hearing loss has been demonstrated in certain Asian families. The genetic defect involved has been identified as an A-to-G nucleotide substitution at the 1555 position within the 125 ribosomal RNA gene. This mutation occurs at an elevated frequency among sporadic cases of aminoglycoside-induced hearing loss. The theory proposed by these authors is that a microsomal dysfunction could lead to a drop in APT levels with defective ion-pump function and, as a result, Ca^{++} could accumulate in the cytosol. Ion pumps are essential to maintain the balance of K^+, Na^+, and Ca^{++} ions in the hair cells as well as in the stria vascularis. Since the report of Cortopassi and Hutchin, other workers have identified this mutation in several families in China and Mongolia who have suffered from aminoglycoside ototoxicity (Pandya *et al.* 1997). In the USA the nucleotide 1555 A-G mutation was identified in seven of 41 individuals (17 per cent) with hearing loss after aminoglycoside exposure. The ethnic origin of the individuals with the predisposing mutations included Caucasians, Hispanics, and Asians. Four of the seven patients with the 1555 A-G mutation had had a family history of aminoglycoside ototoxicity (Fischel Ghodsian *et al.* 1997). The authors suggest that the mutation may not be as rare as previously thought and that a significant proportion of patients with aminoglycoside deafness may harbour it. They recommend that a family history enquiry should be made before starting patients on aminoglycosides.

One of the most puzzling features of aminoglycoside ototoxicity is the latency of onset of the damage in some cases. Deafness has often been noticed within a few days of starting an aminoglycoside in low dosage and such an occurrence suggests a direct assault on the cochlear hair cells by the antibiotic, leading to hair cell degeneration. It has frequently been reported, however, that deafness or vertigo began some time after administration of the drug had ceased and thereafter progressed remorselessly. This appears to be incompatible with a mechanism of direct injury to the hair cells. Wilson and Ramsden (1977) have thrown considerable light on this problem by demonstrating the changes produced by intravenous tobramycin on the electrocochleogram of three patients. When peak serum levels exceeded the accepted maximum safe level of 8–10 mg per litre, an immediate dramatic reduction in the electrical output of the cochlea was observed. This recovered fully as the serum tobramycin level fell. Although electrocochleography revealed objective measurable reduction of hearing acuity, none of the three patients noticed any subjective auditory or vestibular symptoms. Yung and Dorman (1986) also showed diminished electrical output of the cochlea by electrocochleography in three patients receiving tobramycin. The speed of onset and recovery of the electrical changes produced by the aminoglycoside is so rapid that the changes cannot be explained by a process of structural damage followed by tissue repair. It is possible to speculate that the electrical changes are due to alterations in the ionic composition of the hair cell that are initially reversible. Damage to the stria vascularis would, after a latent period, render it unable to maintain endolymph homoeostasis and would therefore cause hair cell damage of delayed onset. It should be emphasized that this is only one speculation in a field where many speculations abound.

Topical administration (non-aural) of aminoglycoside antibiotics

The risk of ototoxic damage from the topical use of neomycin was the subject of a leading article in the *British Medical Journal* (1969) and is now widely recognized. It has been repeatedly shown that absorption, and therefore ototoxicity, can occur after oral, peritoneal, or intrabronchial administration, as well as after wound irrigation (Fig. 22.1). There still appears, however, to be a tendency to regard the aminoglycosides as 'the non-absorbable' antibiotics. Weinstein and others (1977) illustrated their absorption very clearly. They studied 10 patients undergoing total hip-replacement surgery who received intraoperative wound irrigation with a 1% neomycin solution. The serum concentration of neomycin was estimated during the first 4 hours of the postoperative period. All 10 patients showed striking systemic absorption of neomycin. Ototoxicity following the use of

0.1% gentamicin cream to a fairly small area of skin was reported by Drake (1974). The patient applied the cream four times daily to a paronychial infection of her great toes. After 2 days of treatment she developed bilateral tinnitus. The medication was stopped for 2 days and the tinnitus subsided, but recurred when she resumed topical application of the drug.

Little and Lynn (1975) reported a case of deafness in a 20-year-old man suffering from burns covering 10 per cent of the body surface. His burned area of skin was repeatedly sprayed with an antibiotic aerosol containing neomycin, bacitracin, and polymyxin. On the fifteenth day of treatment he complained of mild hearing loss and within the following 48 hours he developed severe permanent bilateral sensorineural deafness. The ototoxicity of topical antibiotics can be overlooked in young children who have not developed speech. Bamford and Jones (1978) studied six young boys who received burns covering 10–22 per cent of their body surfaces. Their ages at the time of the burns were between 8 and 16 months. The burns were treated with sprays containing neomycin, bacitracin, and polymyxin. All six suffered a retardation of speech and language development, and audiometry (when they were old enough for this test) showed quite severe hearing losses. The occurrence of such case reports prompted the Committee on Safety of Medicines (1977) to send a notice to all doctors in the UK warning them of the ototoxic potential of aerosols containing neomycin. Unfortunately deafness due to topical administration of neomycin continues to occur. Gerharz and others (1995) reported a series of three patients with end-stage renal disease who had undergone bladder irrigation with neomycin sulphate solution. All three patients suffered severe progressive hearing loss with characteristic changes in the audiogram. Complete irreversible deafness occurred after 3, 4, and 10 months and two of the patients also developed vestibular dysfunction together with spontaneous nystagmus.

Other ototoxic antibiotics

Apart from minocycline, few of the other antibiotics commonly cause ototoxic damage when they are administered systemically.

Minocycline

This antibiotic inflicts its ototoxic damage almost exclusively upon the vestibule and causes severe vertigo and a powerful suppression of the normal caloric responses of the ear. Early reports gave conflicting accounts of the incidence of adverse reactions. Gould and

Brockler (1972) recorded a 30 per cent incidence of vertigo in a small series of patients and Yeadon and Garratt (1975) recorded a seven per cent incidence of vestibular upset in a large-scale trial in general practice. In a series of 19 patients, Williams and others (1975) reported that treatment with minocycline had to be abandoned in 17 patients (89 per cent) because of severe vertigo. In an important review article, Allen (1976) concluded that the average reported incidence of vestibular adverse effects was in the region of 76 per cent and felt, therefore, that minocycline should not be recommended for general use. There have been no convincing reports of hearing loss due to minocycline, and guinea-pig studies have shown no histological damage to the ear by this drug. It has been suggested that minocycline may act centrally on the pontomedullary region of the brain and that it may not have a direct peripheral action on the ear.

Erythromycin

Ototoxic adverse reactions occur rarely with this drug but they are particularly interesting because they develop with dramatic suddenness, and swift recovery usually takes place when the drug is stopped. Erythromycin has been in clinical use since the 1950s but there are probably only about 50 reported cases of ototoxic damage in the English-language literature. The typical symptoms exhibited by the patients are tinnitus, subjective hearing loss, and sometimes an impairment of balance. The hearing loss is sensorineural and usually affects the low, middle, and high frequencies, producing a flat audiometric pattern unlike the principally high-tone hearing loss seen with aminoglycoside toxicity. Seven patients developed reversible deafness while receiving intravenous erythromycin (Mintz et al. 1973; Karmody and Weinstein 1977; Quinnan and McCabe 1978). Three patients suffered transient deafness following oral erythromycin in dosages ranging between 2 and 4 g daily. One of these patients had severe diabetic nephropathy (Eckman et al. 1975) and the other two suffered from both hepatic disease and azotaemia (van Marion et al. 1978). Only two to five per cent of orally administered erythromycin is excreted in the urine, while the rest is concentrated in the liver and excreted in the bile. Advanced renal failure, however, causes a two-fold prolongation of the half-life of erythromycin in the body (Lee et al. 1955). It seems reasonable to conclude that, in all 10 cases, ototoxicity was the result of very high peak blood concentrations of erythromycin. Mery and Kanfer (1979) reported three elderly patients with severe renal insufficiency who received total doses of 7–12 g of erythromycin over 4–6 days. They developed bilateral

symmetrical sensorineural deafness which recovered within 2 weeks of stopping the drug. The authors concluded that the daily dosage of erythromycin should not exceed 1.5 g in patients with a raised serum creatinine. In two patients on continuous ambulatory peritoneal dialysis, erythromycin caused an approximately 60 decibel sensorineural hearing loss which recovered shortly after the drug was discontinued (Taylor et al. 1981). The authors pointed out that, although liver function tests were normal in both patients, excretion of erythromycin is delayed in patients with end-stage renal failure. This has been emphasized by a report from Kroboth and others (1983) of a 52-year-old woman on home dialysis for polycystic disease of the kidneys. She was given 1 g of erythromycin lactobionate intravenously every 6 hours and developed deafness on the second day. The drug was stopped and her hearing improved. Erythromycin ototoxicity has been described in renal transplant patients, and more recently Moral and others (1994) have reported three liver transplant patients who developed erythromycin-related toxicity. Miller (1982) reported the case of a 71-year-old lady without renal or hepatic disease who was given 1 g of erythromycin lactobionate 6-hourly intravenously. After three doses she noticed deafness and her audiogram showed a 60 decibel hearing loss across the frequency range in both ears. Her hearing recovered quickly after the drug was discontinued. It is important to emphasize that the ototoxic reaction is seen with any salt or ester of the drug. It is an event to be expected at very high serum concentrations. The mechanism of ototoxicity of erythromycin is not known and animal studies have not proved helpful. From a clinical standpoint the ototoxic reaction bears a close resemblance to salicylate ototoxicity and is quite different from aminoglycoside ototoxicity.

Chloramphenicol

This drug is reputed to be ototoxic when given systemically. For many years this reputation was based on a single case report by Gargye and Dutta (1959), who attributed bilateral sensorineural deafness in a child to treatment with an excessive dosage of chloramphenicol (estimated as 125 mg per kg body-weight daily for 26 days). The child received the medication from an unqualified practitioner, however, and was not seen by the authors until 10 months after receiving the drug. The child was 20 months old at the time of this treatment and, understandably enough, no formal assessment of his hearing ability before the chloramphenicol therapy is recorded, and the possibility of congenital deafness cannot be ruled out. Iqbal and Srivatsav (1984) added a second case to the literature when they reported an

18-year-old Indian girl who was given a 17-day course of chloramphenicol for typhoid fever. About one month after completion of treatment she developed tinnitus and deafness in one ear. Investigation revealed a high-tone hearing loss and a reduced caloric response in the affected ear. A few months later she developed fever again and was given a 7-day course of chloramphenicol. About a month after her second course of chloramphenicol she developed bilateral tinnitus and deafness and over the following 5 months she progressed to a complete bilateral deafness with bilateral loss of caloric responses. There have been other reports of partial hearing loss in patients receiving chloramphenicol and ampicillin for treatment of meningitis but little weight can be given to them because meningitis itself frequently causes partial or complete deafness. The paucity of reports of ototoxicity after systemic administration of a drug that has been in widespread use since 1948 casts doubt upon the ototoxic reputation of systemic chloramphenicol.

Cephalexin

The cephalosporins have not been regarded as potentially ototoxic drugs. Sennesael and others (1982), however, reported two patients with renal disease who developed dizziness and vertigo while taking cephalexin. The drug was stopped and the dizziness disappeared within 4 weeks in both patients. Audiometry was normal in both patients but electronystagmography demonstrated a temporary unilateral labyrinthine dysfunction.

Ampicillin

There is no convincing evidence that this drug is ototoxic although, on several occasions, it has been reported to cause deafness when used in the treatment of patients with meningitis. As has been already mentioned, deafness is a well-recognized complication of meningitis. Nadol (1978) has reported that partial or complete hearing loss as a sequel of bacterial meningitis occurred in 21 per cent of patients over the age of 2½ years who survived the illness. A search of the literature has failed to find any reports of deafness following treatment with ampicillin for extracranial infections.

Teicoplanin

This glycopeptide antibiotic is structurally and antigenically similar to vancomycin and may have similar adverse effects. Maher and others (1986) record the case of a 39-year-old man with Down's syndrome who received teicoplanin for infective endocarditis. An audiogram on the eighth day of treatment was normal. An audiogram on the 31st day of treatment showed a 60 decibel sensorineural hearing loss at the 8 kHz frequency in both ears. The hearing for the other frequencies was normal. The drug was stopped and serial audiograms over the following 5 months showed that the high-tone hearing loss persisted. A study of the comparative ototoxicity of teicoplanin and tobramycin in guinea pigs demonstrated that both drugs were equally ototoxic to the vestibule but that teicoplanin was somewhat less toxic to the cochlea than tobramycin (Cazals et al. 1987).

Antibiotic ear-drops and antiseptics

The use of ototoxic antibiotics in ear-drops and powders is the subject of considerable controversy and further work needs to be done to establish the degree of risk involved. It has been demonstrated that gentamicin, neomycin, polymyxin, streptomycin, chloramphenicol, and erythromycin can cause inner-ear damage in guinea-pigs after instillation into the middle-ear cleft (Stupp et al. 1973). Many other workers have shown this effect after placing various antibiotic solutions and powders into the middle ears of different experimental animals. In addition, propylene glycol, the vehicle used in chloramphenicol ear-drops and other aural preparations, has been suspected of ototoxicity. Morizono and Johnstone (1975) studied the effects of placing solutions of propylene glycol into the middle ears of guinea-pigs. They reported that propylene glycol in concentrations of 10% or more always caused irreversible inner-ear deafness. Their experiments were repeated by Vernon and others (1978) with certain modifications, and diametrically opposite results were obtained. Vernon's group found no adverse effects on the middle ear or inner ear with 10% propylene glycol solutions placed in the middle ear. In addition, when they instilled 90% propylene glycol into the middle ear they found no inner-ear damage, though some middle-ear dysfunction was produced by this high concentration. The use of topical chloramphenicol in ears has largely been abandoned by otologists in Great Britain, but ear-drops containing aminoglycoside antibiotics and polymyxin are used frequently in otitis media. Chronic forms of tubotympanic otitis media often fail to respond to treatment when antibiotic therapy is given solely by the systemic route. Chronic suppurative otitis media is, of course, an ototoxic disease and is associated with an insidious inner-ear deafness. Most otologists believe that pus in the middle ear is more dangerous than antibiotic solution in the middle ear. Although antibiotic solutions diffuse easily into the inner ear from the healthy middle ears of experimental animals, similar diffusion does not appear to take place often in infected human middle ears with the dilute antibiotic solutions used in clinical practice. Nevertheless, there are a few scattered reports in the literature of sudden deterioration in hearing immediately after the instillation of topical drops containing a solution of a single antibiotic or a mixture of antibiotics and steroids. In the majority of these reports there was some recovery of hearing provided the ear-drops were discontinued. Editorials in the *Medical Journal of Australia* (1975) and in *The Lancet* (1976) expressed concern about the possible toxicity of antibiotic ear-drops. Kohonen and Tarkkanen (1969), writing on the use of antibiotic ear-drops in otitis media, stated: 'Widespread clinical use with very few known complications suggests that the risk cannot be very large, but it is, on the other hand, possible that moderate hearing losses in chronically infected ears have been unduly attributed to infection only'.

There is a need, however, for prospective, double-blind, controlled trials to assess the validity of these clinical impressions or assumptions. One such trial has been reported by McKelvie and others (1975). They carried out repeated audiometric testing on patients with chronic middle-ear infections over a 4-year period. Half of the ears were treated with gentamicin ear-drops and the other half with placebo drops. The placebo used was the vehicle for the gentamicin ear-drops. They found no adverse effect of gentamicin ear-drops on the cochlea. A smaller trial by Browning and others (1988) found no incidence of ototoxic inner- ear damage in patients using ear-drops containing gentamicin over a 4–6-week period. However, in a series of 124 patients with otitis media treated with antibiotic ear-drops over a 12–24-month period, Podoshin and others (1989) concluded that a small degree of sensorineural hearing loss (approximately 2–11 decibels) might be attributable to the ear-drops. In an article reviewing the literature, Roland (1994) could only find four cases of severe deafness following the use of ear-drops in English-language sources, and 37 cases in the non-English literature. The majority of otologists in Great Britain and the USA feel that clinical expediency justifies the use of antibiotic ear-drops in chronic otitis media. They consider that the risk of ototoxicity is small but recommend that the drops should be stopped immediately if the patient notices any loss of hearing. Two more recent reports give rise to anxiety that ototoxicity from ear-drops may have been under-reported in the past and may be more common than has hitherto been realized. Hui and others (1997) describe two patients who had suffered from chronic otitis media for many years and had perforations of the tympanic membranes. Both had prolonged treatment with aminoglycoside ear-drops and both developed a marked sensorineural deafness which the authors

thought was much more likely to be due to the ear-drops than to the ear disease. Wong and Rutka (1997) reported five cases of ototoxic damage from ear-drops containing gentamicin seen in their department. Four of the patients had pre-existing perforations and one had patent ventilation tubes in the tympanic membranes when they were treated with the ear-drops. All had quite prolonged treatment and all well-documented vestibular dysfunction after treatment. Two showed deterioration of hearing from their pretreatment audiograms. The other three showed some deafness but no pretreatment audiograms were available to assess the deafness due to treatment.

For many years the Committee on Safety of Medicines has warned that there is an increased risk of drug-induced deafness when ear-drops containing aminoglycosides and polymyxins are used in patients who have a perforation of the tympanic membrane. The *British National Formulary* (September 1997) repeats the Committee's warning but points out that many specialists use these drops if the otitis media fails to settle with systemic antibiotics, on the grounds that the unresolved infection carries a higher risk of ototoxicity than the drops themselves. It would seem impossible, on the basis of the currently available information, to quantify the degree of risk accurately. At present most specialists believe that there is a real risk in the use of these ear-drops in chronic otitis media but they believe that it is a small risk.

Some patients have suffered unexplained inner-ear deafness following myringoplasty procedures to repair tympanic membrane perforations. Suspicion has fallen on chlorhexidine antiseptic solution used to cleanse the skin of the pinna and external auditory canal preoperatively. Many surgeons now pack the external canal to prevent any possible diffusion of antiseptic solution through the middle ear to the inner ear. Bismuth–iodoform–paraffin paste (BIPP) is a standard postoperative dressing in ENT surgery. Iodoform intoxication has been reported when large amounts of this substance are used to pack the sizeable cavities created by maxillary sinus surgery. Fortunately, iodoform intoxication is not a problem when BIPP packs are used in the relatively small cavities associated with middle-ear and mastoid operations (O'Connor *et al.* 1977).

Ototoxic diuretics

There have been several reports of both transient and permanent deafness following treatment with ethacrynic acid and frusemide (Pillay *et al.* 1969; Schwartz *et al.* 1970; Lloyd-Mostyn and Lord 1971), and it is clear from the reports that impaired renal function enhances the ototoxic effect of these diuretics. The speed of onset of deafness can be quite startling, especially when the diuretics are administered by rapid intravenous injection. Hanzelik and Peppercorn (1969) record one patient with previously normal hearing who complained of tinnitus and hearing loss within 5 minutes of receiving 10 mg of ethacrynic acid intravenously. Examination 10 minutes later confirmed her deafness. The hearing returned to normal after 8 hours.

Vestibular damage with disturbance of balance appears to be rare. Gomolin and Garshick (1980) reported the unusual case of a 40-year-old man who developed deafness and dizziness accompanied by fine nystagmus in all directions during an intravenous infusion of ethacrynic acid. The hearing returned to normal and the nystagmus disappeared within an hour of stopping the drug.

Two other loop diuretics, bumetanide and piretanide, are ototoxic. In animal studies, they have a similar degree of ototoxicity (Rybak and Whitworth 1986). Ethacrynic acid is more ototoxic than frusemide in humans. The ototoxic potential of bumetanide is similar to that of ethacrynic acid but its diuretic potential is 40 times greater. Thus, a lower dose of bumetanide may be expected to have the same diuretic effect but a lower ototoxic effect (Oliveira 1989*a*).

Nature and mechanism of diuretic ototoxicity

Although there are many reports of permanent deafness from diuretics, the majority of patients suffering from diuretic-induced ototoxicity experience immediate and short-lived deafness. Vestibular damage with disturbance of balance occurs rarely. This contrasts markedly with aminoglycoside-induced ototoxicity, in which deafness is more often delayed and permanent deafness and vestibular disturbance is a common finding. Despite the marked difference in their clinical features, there are striking similarities between the two types of ototoxicity.

Mathog and others (1970) have shown that both ethacrynic acid and frusemide produce a primary depression of the electrical output of the cochlea with almost complete recovery in one hour in experimental animals. This bears a strong resemblance to the changes in the electrocochleograms following intravenous tobramycin reported by Wilson and Ramsden (1977) (see above). Mathog and others (1970) also showed that ethacrynic acid in doses above 10 mg per kg produced a delayed severe secondary depression of cochlear electrical output with evidence of outer hair-cell degeneration in the basal and middle turns of the cochlea. Matz and others (1969), reporting on the temporal bone of a patient with permanent deafness due to ethacrynic acid, showed that the structural lesion produced was outer

hair-cell damage, most marked in the basal turn of the cochlea. It seems possible, therefore, that the reversible deafness may be due to short-term alterations in the composition of the endolymph and that long-term changes in the endolymph cause hair-cell damage and permanent deafness. Cohn and his co-workers (1971) reported complete reversal of the K^+/Na^+ ratio in the endolymph 10 minutes after the intravenous administration of ethacrynic acid in dogs. Frusemide and ethacrynic acid are chemically dissimilar, but they have a similar diuretic action and a similar ototoxic action. It has therefore been suggested that their ototoxic action is due to their diuretic properties, which alter the ionic composition of the inner-ear fluids. It would seem unwise, however, to extrapolate the results from experiments in the dog to the human cochlea because this reversal of relative endolymph concentrations of sodium and potassium appears to be species dependent. Bosher (1980) has shown that ethacrynic acid administered intravenously to guinea-pigs and rats caused only small changes in the concentrations of sodium and potassium in the endolymph. The mechanism of ototoxicity caused by diuretics in humans is unknown and remains the subject of interesting speculation.

Salicylate ototoxicity

In general, ototoxicity caused by salicylates is not serious, provided that the drug is withdrawn as soon as symptoms appear, because the damage is usually reversible. Large amounts of salicylates are consumed and therefore ototoxic effects are commonly encountered. Ototoxic symptoms can occur with all salicylates and with salicylate compounds, for example, Benorylate (salicylate and paracetamol) and sulphasalazine (salicylate and sulphonamide). Tinnitus and deafness are prominent symptoms and vertigo is also experienced sometimes when the serum salicylate concentration reaches toxic levels. The therapeutic serum level of salicylate is 200–300 mg per litre and symptoms of salicylism occur as the concentration approaches 300 mg per litre. Effective dosage, therefore, must be close to toxic dosage. Since symptoms appear promptly with peak serum salicylate levels, one would expect aspirin deafness to be strongly dependent on the unit dosage used. This is confirmed in a report by the Boston Collaborative Drug Study Program, which records an overall incidence of salicylate-induced deafness of 11 per 1000 patients exposed. With unit dosage of 600–899 mg, however, the rate was only 1 per 1000 and, with 900–1199 mg, 45 per 1000, rising to 150 per 1000 when unit doses larger than 1200 mg were used (Porter and Jick 1977). Pearlman

(1966) records that two women suffered from deafness as a result of the application of an ointment containing 5% salicylic acid to the skin. Both women had psoriasis involving more than 90 per cent of the skin surface. Serum salicylate levels of 350 mg per litre and 240 mg per litre were achieved.

In humans, the hearing loss from salicylate toxicity is a reversible sensorineural hearing loss affecting all frequencies fairly evenly. There may perhaps be a tendency for the upper frequencies to be slightly more susceptible to damage than the lower frequencies in some patients (Waltner 1955; Myers et al. 1965; McCabe and Day 1965; Ramsden et al. 1985). Tinnitus frequently precedes the onset of deafness. Imbalance is much less commonly reported. There is considerable evidence from animal experiments to show that salicylate ototoxicity is not associated with hair cell damage. Electrophysiological studies in guinea-pigs (Mitchell et al. 1973) and in adult cats (Stypulkowski 1990) have shown that the cochlear microphonic potential (CM) is not decreased by salicylate administration but the compound nerve action potential (AP) is temporarily diminished by the drug. Similar preservation of the CM and reversible diminution of the AP has been recorded in two patients suffering from salicylate overdosage (Ramsden et al. 1985). de Moura and Hayden (1968), in a temporal bone examination of a woman affected by salicylate ototoxicity, found no evidence of hair cell damage or other structural abnormality attributable to salicylates. It has been suggested that the ototoxic effects of salicylates are due to a temporary metabolic blockade at the hair cell/neural interface, the chemical transmitter at which is as yet unidentified (Ramsden et al. 1985). This biochemical mechanism is consistent with the classification of salicylate ototoxicity as a Type A reaction.

Ototoxicity of quinine and chloroquine

Both these drugs are used in the treatment of malaria, and both have been responsible for inner-ear damage.

Quinine has been given in large doses to a multitude of patients without causing any deafness. Individual susceptibility or idiosyncrasy seems to be an important factor. The hearing loss is predominantly in the low tones. Tinnitus is an early symptom. The deafness is not usually severe and is reversible in the majority of patients if the drug is withdrawn early.

Chloroquine has been observed to cause tinnitus and perceptive deafness. The deafness tends to occur after prolonged high dosage and is usually irreversible. Its onset may take place after the drug has been discontinued (Toone et al. 1965), exhibiting the same peculiar latency so frequently noted with the aminoglycoside antibiotics. Chloroquine has a strong affinity for melanin and therefore tends to accumulate in melanin-containing cells. If labelled chloroquine is injected into pigmented rats it accumulates in the melanin-rich cells of the stria vascularis and is retained there for a prolonged period. It is not found in the endolymph or perilymph. In albino rats, no accumulation of chloroquine takes place in any part of the inner ear (Dencker and Lindquist 1975). This again suggests that the primary ototoxic injury is likely to be to the stria vascularis and that damage to this tissue causes a gradual change in the composition of the endolymph, which damages the hair cells. Melanin-rich cells are present in retina and in the inner ear. Patients with deafness and vertigo following chloroquine therapy may also suffer from visual disturbances (Dwivedi and Mehra 1978). Chloroquine deafness is uncommon in Western Europe and the USA, but Obiako (1979) reported a series of 50 patients seen in the University of Nigeria teaching hospital during a period of less than 2 years who had suffered deafness after treatment with chloroquine phosphate injections. Chloroquine is very frequently prescribed in the west, and other, malarious regions of Africa because practically every complaint is provisionally blamed on malaria; and, because of a widespread faith in and willingness to pay extra for injections, it is often quite unnecessarily given parenterally — with obvious dangers when the re-use of needles is common.

Ototoxicity of cytotoxic drugs

Mustine hydrochloride (nitrogen mustard) is now acknowledged to be an ototoxic drug. Deafness is most common in patients who have had a regional perfusion that included the circulation to the ear. This produces a correspondingly higher blood level in the area of the cochlear blood supply. Deafness seldom follows intravenous administration, but Schuknecht (1964) described a 30-year-old woman who received mustine hydrochloride for Hodgkin's disease in a dose of 0.8 mg per kg body-weight by injection while fully alert. Immediately afterwards she noticed tinnitus, a bilateral decrease in hearing, and vertigo. An audiogram showed a bilateral symmetrical perceptive deafness. Cummings (1968) demonstrated in cats that mustine hydrochloride produced structural damage in the hair cells of the organ of Corti. Bleomycin may produce ototoxic damage when given in high dosage, whether administered systemically or topically to the middle ear (Ballantyne 1973).

Cisplatin (cis-platinum) is an inorganic heavy metal with antineoplastic properties which has been used in the chemotherapy of tumours of the testis, prostate, bladder, ovary, cervix, and breast. Although its more prominent adverse effects involve the gastrointestinal and renal systems, auditory symptoms have also been produced. Temporary tinnitus and high-tone deafness were noted in 20 per cent of a series of patients by Higby and his colleagues (1974). Since then, numerous other papers showing that ototoxic damage by this drug is not just an occasional occurrence have been published. Rybak (1981) reviewed the literature and noted that the published incidence of ototoxicity varied from nine to 90 per cent in the series he surveyed. Schaefer and others (1981) recorded a case of a man with vestibular damage as well as cochlear hearing loss attributed to the use of this drug. In their series of 24 patients treated with cisplatin, Strauss and colleagues (1983) reported that 25 per cent of their patients suffered ototoxic injury. They stated that the treatment factors that appear to increase the ototoxic effect are: high dose per treatment, prolonged therapy, total cumulative dosage, and bolus administration. In common with most other authors, they reported that the effect was a high-tone sensorineural deafness and that the maximal loss at any single frequency did not exceed 25 decibels. Van der Hulst and colleagues (1988) used special high-frequency audiometers to measure the hearing loss between 8 kHz and 20 kHz. The hearing thresholds routinely tested in clinical practice are those in the 0.125 kHz–8 kHz range. These authors demonstrated that in the majority of patients with cisplatin deafness, the hearing loss began between 10 kHz and 18 kHz. Hearing loss at these high frequencies would not be noticed by the patient and would not be recordable with standard clinical audiometers. Laurell and Jungnelius (1990) carefully assessed the ototoxic effect of high-dose (100–120 mg per m² body-surface) cisplatin on 54 patients. In this series 81 per cent showed significant high-frequency hearing loss while 41 per cent also showed significant loss of hearing for the middle frequencies used in human speech. They found the ototoxic effect was determined more by the amount of the single dose than by the accumulated dose. No ototoxic effects were seen below a peak plasma concentration of 1 μg per litre. The ototoxic effect was not increased by pre-existing hearing loss *per se* but was slightly increased by age. They calculated a risk factor that could be applied for second and subsequent courses of cisplatin therapy. They estimated that after each course of high-dosage cisplatin 25 per cent of patients would sustain a 25 per cent deterioration of their remaining high-frequency (3 kHz–8 kHz) hearing threshold. In the majority of patients the hearing loss is permanent, but some cases of partial and even of complete recovery have been reported. Human and animal histopathological studies have demonstrated severe destruction of the outer hair cells in the basal turn of the cochlea similar to that seen in aminoglycoside ototoxicity (Kopelman *et al.* 1988; Hinojossa *et al.* 1995).

Vincristine is a cytotoxic drug known to have neurotoxic properties. Mahajan and others (1981) reported the first recorded case of sensorineural deafness after treatment with this drug. Their patient was a 73-year-old woman who had two acute episodes of deafness following vincristine therapy. After the first episode of deafness her hearing recovered completely within 2 months. Later she had a recurrence of her tumour and was given a second course of treatment. Once again she became deaf and recovered her hearing over a period of 2 months.

Misonidazole is a potent antitumour agent that selectively increases the effect of ionizing radiations on poorly oxygenated tumour cells. It was used as a radiosensitizer in a series of 21 patients by Waltzman and Cooper (1981). Hearing loss secondary to the drug developed in 11 (52 per cent) of the patients. The hearing loss was sensorineural and all the affected patients experienced complete or partial recovery of hearing within a few weeks. The authors found no relationship between the degree of hearing loss and the age, sex, and previous hearing status of the patient, with the dose of the drug used, or with the anatomical site of the tumour.

Ototoxicity of β-adrenoceptor blockers

Initially these drugs were considered to be relatively free from adverse effects in the ear, though propranolol was known to cause mild reversible inner ear disturbance occasionally (Lloyd Mostyn 1969). Practolol, however, had some totally unexpected adverse effects, including deafness, following long-term use (Wright 1975). The type of deafness caused by practolol differs from any other known type of drug-induced deafness. In addition to inducing a sensorineural deafness, it can cause conductive deafness. The conductive deafness is due to a sterile effusion into the middle-ear cleft (serous otitis media) and responds to myringotomy and the insertion of a tympanostomy tube. The sensorineural deafness either improves or remains static when the drug is withdrawn (Jones *et al.* 1977). The ototoxic mechanism is unknown. Practolol was withdrawn from general use and is now reserved for short-term use in hospitals only. Up to the end of 1977 a total of 1878 cases of adverse reactions to practolol had been reported to the Committee on Safety of Medicines. In 150 of these, deafness was noted to have occurred but in only 36 was it the main complaint (Committee on Safety of Medicines 1978, personal communication).

Miscellaneous ototoxic drugs and vaccines

Desferrioxamine

Desferrioxamine is a chelating agent introduced in 1963 for treatment of iron overload resulting from long-term blood transfusion therapy. Deafness was recorded in patients with thalassaemia receiving treatment with desferrioxamine but initially the deafness was attributed to the thalassaemia (De Virgiliis *et al.* 1979). Serious auditory and visual disturbances attributable to the use of desferrioxamine were, however, reported by Olivieri and colleagues (1986) and have been confirmed by others (Cases *et al.* 1988; Wonke *et al.* 1989; Styles and Vichinsky 1996). The drug causes a sensorineural hearing loss maximal in the higher sound frequencies. In severe cases, the deafness extends into the middle and lower sound frequencies. Partial and sometimes complete recovery of hearing may occur when the drug is stopped. Some patients show no recovery and have required hearing aids to ameliorate the permanent deafness. The incidence of damage to the hearing was almost 25 per cent in the 89 patients treated by Olivieri and colleagues (1986). They stopped treatment and approximately one-third of affected patients regained normal or next to normal hearing within 3 weeks. Desferrioxamine treatment was restarted after a rest period of some months with a lower dosage of the drug without causing any further hearing loss. There was a 26 per cent incidence of damage to the hearing in the 50 patients reported by Wonke and others (1989). Five of these patients (10 per cent) had severe hearing loss. Treatment with desferrioxamine was stopped in these five patients and was replaced by chelation with Ca-DTPA (calcium diethylene triamine pentacetic acid) with zinc supplements. Hearing recovered completely within 19 months in one patient and improved substantially in the other four patients while chelation with Ca-DTPA was being administered.

Propoxyphene hydrochloride

This mild analgesic, which is used fairly widely in North America, is reported to have caused a moderate degree of sensorineural deafness and vestibular disturbance in a young man who mistakenly took approximately four times the recommended dosage for a period of 6 days (Lupin and Harley 1976). A case of total permanent deafness following chronic propoxyphene abuse has been recorded by Harell and his colleagues (1978*b*). These authors believe that ototoxicity is often overlooked because severe propoxyphene intoxication is frequently fatal.

Naproxen

Chapman (1982) reported the case of a patient who developed permanent bilateral sensorineural deafness and acute renal failure from treatment with the non-steroidal anti-inflammatory drug naproxen. His report draws attention to the possibility of other prostaglandin-synthetase-inhibiting drugs being ototoxic. Since then there have been occasional reports of auditory complications caused by mefenamic acid (Morris and Fletcher 1986).

Nortriptyline

This may produce deafness not detectable by routine pure-tone audiometry. Smith and others (1972) described an 8-year-old enuretic who received the drug for 9 months. Although his pure-tone thresholds were normal, his tone-decay and speech-discrimination tests were depressed. These recovered after the drug was stopped, suggesting that the drug had produced a more subtle type of ototoxic damage.

Imipramine

Racy and Ward-Racy (1980) reported four patients who received imipramine for depression and developed tinnitus as an adverse reaction. The tinnitus was reduced or abolished by reducing the dosage of imipramine. This is a helpful report, because many tinnitus sufferers are treated with imipramine for depression caused by tinnitus.

Propylthiouracil

Both unilateral sensorineural deafness and systemic lupus erythematosus were produced by this drug in a patient described by Smith and Spalding (1972). Fortunately, termination of the drug led to recovery both from the lupus erythematosus and from the hearing impairment.

Bromocriptine

This drug has been implicated as the cause of deafness in three patients suffering from hepatic encephalopathy (Lanthier *et al.* 1984). A high-tone hearing loss was produced, which improved when the dosage was reduced, suggesting that the ototoxicity is reversible.

Indomethacin

Vertigo and tinnitus have been recorded in patients given this drug, together with vomiting, confusion, and ataxia (Hart and Boardman 1965; Rothermich 1966). It is uncertain whether all of these symptoms are of central origin.

Quinidine

The adverse effects of quinidine therapy (cinchonism) include tinnitus and deafness. Rosketh and Storstein (1963) quote the occurrence of vertigo and tinnitus in 24 of a series of 274 patients treated with quinidine.

Dantrolene

The possibility that this skeletal muscle relaxant may have ototoxic potential has been raised by Pace-Balsan and Ramsden (1988). They reported the case of a 19-year-old girl with athetoid cerebral palsy. She was known to have normal hearing in the left ear and a longstanding, non-progressive, sensorineural deafness of 70 decibels in the right ear, the cause of which had never been positively identified. On the fifth day of dantrolene treatment she suddenly developed a 70 decibel hearing loss in the previously normal left ear and lost all her remaining hearing in the previously partially deaf right ear. There was no associated tinnitus or vertigo and no recovery of hearing took place. The authors stated that it is only by reporting such possible cases of ototoxic damage that suspicion may be aroused.

Vaccines

Sudden hearing loss following vaccination or the therapeutic use of antisera is, fortunately, a rare event. The majority of reported cases have occurred following the administration of tetanus antitoxin, and a few have occurred after vaccinations against whooping cough and rabies. Mair and Elverland (1977) recorded the case of a young girl who developed a local hypersensitivity reaction on her arm at the site of a routine revaccination against tetanus and diphtheria. She also developed a unilateral, irreversible, total hearing loss at the same time. The authors reviewed the literature and suggested that a hypersensitivity reaction accounts for the deafness in these patients. Healy (1972) postulated that mumps vaccine was responsible for a unilateral perceptive deafness found on routine audiological screening in a boy whose hearing had been normal on screening one year earlier. In the intervening year he had been given the mumps virus vaccine, but had suffered no illness.

Relative frequency of ototoxic damage

It is difficult to give more than a rough estimate of the incidence of ototoxic damage. The Boston Collaborative Drug Surveillance Program monitors adverse reactions in a continuing series of patients admitted to medical wards, and therefore reports on a highly selected sample. In 1973, it reported that 32 out of 11 526 medical in-

TABLE 22.2
Incidence of ototoxic damage

Drug	Incidence per 1000 patients exposed	
	In 1973 report	In 1977 report
Aspirin (plain, buffered, and enteric coated)	11	11
Aminoglycoside antibiotics	13	7
Ethacrynic acid	7	10
Quinidine	3	1

patients (three per 1000) developed deafness attributed to drugs. In 1977, the numbers monitored had risen to 32 812 and the number of patients with deafness attributed to drugs was 53 (1.6 per 1000) (Porter and Jick 1977). The principal drugs implicated are indicated in Table 22.2.

Arcieri and others (1970) studied the records of 1327 patients treated with gentamicin and found significant ototoxicity in 31 cases (2.3 per cent). Gailiunas and others (1978) estimated that the incidence of gentamicin ototoxicity was 1.8 per cent in the general population of patients receiving the drug, but 30 per cent among patients on long-term haemodialysis.

Brummet and Morrison (1990) have suggested that the reported incidence of hearing loss due to aminoglycoside drugs may be exaggerated. They point out that the definition of ototoxicity in most clinical studies of aminoglycosides is an increase in pure-tone threshold, from a base-line audiogram, of either 15 decibels or more at two frequencies, or 20 decibels or more at a single frequency. In their study of 20 volunteers who were not taking any known ototoxic drugs, they found test–retest differences of 15 decibels or more at two frequencies in 33 per cent, and of 20 decibels or more at a single frequency, in 20 per cent of the volunteers. They concluded that many of the audiometric threshold changes reported to represent aminoglycoside ototoxicity may actually represent the normal variation in audiometric threshold movements found in normal individuals.

Factors influencing ototoxicity

Drug concentration in the inner ear

This is probably the most important single factor in the production of ototoxic damage. It will be affected by the dose of the drug given, by the route of administration, and by the rate of excretion.

Intolerance

There is no doubt that some individuals show a markedly heightened sensitivity to ototoxic drugs. In an interesting clinical experiment, Meyer zum Guttesberge and Stupp (1969) gave 26 otosclerotic patients a standard dose of streptomycin preoperatively and took perilymph samples at stapedectomy. Five hours after injection, the average level of streptomycin in the perilymph was $260 \mu g$ per litre. Very large variations in the level, however, were found among the 26 patients, and in some cases the level in the perilymph was many times higher than that in the serum. It is tempting to speculate that intolerance may sometimes be due to abnormally high ability of an individual to accumulate the drug in the inner ear. As previously mentioned, a rare genetic susceptibility to aminoglycoside-induced hearing loss has been reported by Cortopassi and Hutchin (1994).

Renal and hepatic disease

Many ototoxic drugs (for example, the aminoglycoside antibiotics) are excreted by the kidney. If renal function is impaired, the serum level and inner-ear concentration of the drug can increase alarmingly. Since many ototoxic drugs are also nephrotoxic, it is unwise to assume that if renal function is normal at the beginning of treatment it will remain so throughout. Berk and Chalmers (1970) reported five cases of ototoxic damage by oral neomycin in patients with hepatic cirrhosis. Two of these patients had normal renal function throughout treatment, while two others had relatively low serum antibiotic levels despite the presence of renal failure. All five received large total doses of neomycin (750–2500 g) over periods ranging from 8 to 24 months before ototoxic damage became apparent. The authors emphasize that, despite minimal absorption of the drug from the gut and correspondingly low serum levels, and even in the presence of normal renal function, oral neomycin can be harmful.

Ballantyne (1970) also reported sensorineural hearing loss in six of 13 patients treated with oral neomycin for hepatic failure; four had no ascites and were treated with neomycin alone, while two had ascites and received diuretics as well.

Placental transport

The developing otocyst is most vulnerable to damage by drugs and viral infections during the first 3 months of fetal life. Mature development is achieved by the sixth fetal month.

Thalidomide

Livingstone (1965) reported 14 children with congenital bilateral meatal atresia due to their mothers being given thalidomide; three had perceptive deafness in addition to outer and middle-ear damage.

Isotretinoin

This vitamin A derivative is a well known teratogen. John and Ganti (1987) reported two infants with microtia and anotia and associated nervous systems malformations, born to mothers who had used isotretinoin during pregnancy for severe acne.

Chloroquine and quinine

Matz and Naunton (1968) reported on the temporal bone of a child whose mother had taken 250 mg chloroquine twice daily during the first trimester. The specimen showed complete cochlear damage. In this family, two siblings also developed profound sensorineural hearing loss following their mother's taking chloroquine during pregnancy. In three other pregnancies she did not take chloroquine and these had resulted in three children with normal hearing.

McKinna (1966) reported two cases of congenital deafness in infants whose mothers had taken a high dose of quinine during pregnancy in an effort to induce abortion. Histological examination of the temporal bone revealed degenerative changes in the spiral ganglion cells of the inner ear.

Streptomycin

Conway and Birt (1965) reported on 17 children whose mothers had received streptomycin during pregnancy. Four of the children showed a mild unilateral high-tone hearing loss. These authors concluded that the risk of fetal ear damage with streptomycin therefore appears to be small.

Ototoxic synergism

Mutual potentiation of ototoxicity seems to be possible when, for example, an ototoxic antibiotic and diuretic are used simultaneously. Meriwether and others (1971) recorded two patients who were receiving non-toxic doses of an aminoglycoside antibiotic and who developed deafness following a standard intravenous dose of ethacrynic acid. Both had normal renal function. West and others (1973) showed particularly severe cochlear damage in guinea-pigs exposed to kanamycin and ethacrynic acid. Ototoxic synergism between gentamicin and frusemide was suspected in a group of patients reported by Thomsen and colleagues (1976). A possible explanation of the ototoxic synergism experienced with aminoglycoside antibiotics and loop diuretics has been suggested by Ohtani and others (1978a,b). They found that the kanamycin concentration in rabbit serum, cerebrospinal fluid, and perilymph was much higher after a single injection of kanamycin with frusemide than after a single injection of kanamycin alone. They obtained a similar result when they substituted the newer loop diuretic bumetanide for frusemide. They concluded that the ototoxic interaction is caused by the inhibiting effect of the diuretic on the excretion of the aminoglycoside. Thus, the enhancement of the ototoxicity is related to the diuretic potency of the diuretic used. (This subject is also discussed in Chapter 33.)

There is also some evidence to suggest increased sensitivity to drug-induced deafness in patients with diminished cochlear function from any cause such as, for example, presbyacusis, previous otitis media, or acoustic trauma. Dayal and others (1971) showed that guinea-pigs exposed to a combination of kanamycin and the noise generated by children's incubators sustained hair cell damage. Neither agent produced hair cell damage when acting alone. Since premature children are often given aminoglycoside antibiotics while being nursed in incubators, the work of these authors may be of practical importance. It appears that, in guinea-pigs, kanamycin in small dosages increases the susceptibility of hair cells to noise and that this increased susceptibility lingers for 20 days after the drug has been stopped (Gannon et al. 1979).

Prevention of ototoxicity

A great variety of ingenious attempts have been made to reduce the ototoxicity of aminoglycosides and cisplatin by biochemical methods. It was hoped that giving vitamin A, or vitamin B complex, or vitamin C with aminoglycosides would reduce ototoxicity but these have been found to be ineffective. Some experimental evidence suggests that administering an aminoglycoside in the form of its pantothenic or glucuronate salt might decrease ototoxicity but this has not been substantiated in practice. It has been proposed that calcium ions might reduce the ototoxic effect of streptomycin by competing for receptor sites in the inner ear. It has also been suggested that glycosaminoglycan acids might exert a protective role against ototoxicity. Similarly, substances that inhibit the production of free radicals by aminoglycosides have also been considered to be helpful in reducing ototoxicity. For reasons not fully understood, hyperglycaemia appears to reduce the toxic effects of kanamycin on the guinea-pig cochlea. The possibility of combining glucose administration with aminoglycoside

therapy has therefore been considered. There is evidence giving more reason for hope that fosfomycin, a phosphonic acid antibiotic may ameliorate the toxic effects of aminoglycosides and cisplatin. A number of trials have shown that fosfomycin reduced the ototoxicity of aminoglycosides both in experimental animals and humans. Fosfomycin has also been shown to exert a protective effect against the ototoxic and nephrotoxic effects of cisplatin in a number of experimental animals (Oliveira 1989b).

Recent Phase II and Phase III clinical trials have demonstrated that amifostine reduces neurotoxicity (including ototoxicity), nephrotoxicity, and the haematological toxicity of cytotoxic drugs without reduction in antitumour efficacy (Albert and Bleyer 1996). The mechanism of protection is thought to be related to the selective uptake of amifostine into normal tissue compared with tumour tissue, with intracellular binding and detoxification of anticancer drugs.

It has been standard practice to monitor the serum concentration of ototoxic drugs to prevent the occurrence of high, toxic levels. In the past many clinical workers have emphasized the value of daily estimation of serum peak and trough levels of drugs when aminoglycosides are being administered. In day-to-day control of dosage levels they found trough levels more helpful than peak levels. However, in recent years there has been a minor revolution in the administration of the daily dosage of aminoglycosides. In patients without pre-existing renal impairment, the drug is now often given in a single undivided dose once daily instead of the traditional divided dose every 8 or 12 hours. Once-daily dosage results in higher serum peak levels and lower trough levels. In a meta-analysis of 21 randomized trials Barza and others (1996) concluded that once-daily administration of aminoglycosides is as effective as multiple daily dosing and has a lower risk of nephrotoxicity and no greater risk of ototoxicity.

In the last two decades the measurement of otoacoustic emissions has become a valuable investigation in otolaryngological practice. These emissions are acoustical (mechanical, non-electrical) signals which originate from the contractile movement of outer hair cells in the cochlea. The signals are transmitted from the inner ear to the external ear canal via the middle-ear conduction apparatus and can be picked up from the external ear canal by a suitable microphone. With appropriate equipment, measuring otoacoustic emissions in the external ear canal is a quick, non-invasive, painless, and objective method of measuring the activity of the outer hair cells of the cochlea. Reduction in otoacoustic emission can be detected before any hearing loss is measurable by pure-tone audiometry in patients receiving aminoglycosides (Hotz *et al.* 1994) and in patients receiving cisplatin (Ozturan *et al.* 1996). Monitoring otoacoustic emissions has been proposed as a method of early identification and consequent prevention of aminoglycoside and cisplatin ototoxicity.

Jolicoeur (1972) made a number of recommendations which are still valid and which may be summarized as follows:

1. the dose of ototoxic drug used should be determined by the weight of the patient and should be the smallest dose compatible with efficient treatment;
2. treatment should not be unduly prolonged, and patients should be questioned daily regarding tinnitus, vertigo, and diminution of hearing;
3. hearing should be measured before, during, and some weeks after treatment;
4. in a patient with renal disease, the dose of the ototoxic compound should be reduced;
5. renal function should be checked throughout treatment, and it should be borne in mind that in elderly patients there is an increased likelihood of impaired renal function;
6. it should be remembered that patients who already have some sensorineural damage will be more vulnerable to the effects of ototoxic drugs; and
7. patients should be kept in a proper state of hydration.

As in so many other fields, awareness of the danger is the most important single factor in prevention.

The nose

It is well recognized that drugs can produce nasal obstruction, nasal bleeding, and anosmia.

Nasal obstruction

Rhinitis medicamentosa caused by the prolonged use of vasoconstrictor drops and sprays in the nose is probably still the commonest form of iatrogenic nasal obstruction.

Hypersensitivity reactions

Topical antibiotics used in the nose may cause hypersensitivity reactions and are not recommended. Nasal allergy caused by drugs and foods is well recognized, and aspirin, for example, can produce nasal obstruction and profuse rhinorrhoea in allergic individuals. Asthma, nasal polyps, and aspirin allergy form a familiar triad in ENT practice. Presley (1988) reported an interesting case of severe rhinitis with profuse rhinorrhoea and grossly oedematous swelling of the nasal mucosa in a 76-year-old man receiving penicillamine. He also had cutaneous lesions and a skin biopsy was compatible with penicillamine-induced pemphigus foliaceus. Penicillamine was stopped and all symptoms cleared rapidly.

Nasal drops and sprays

Ephedrine, amphetamine, and privine all lose vasoconstrictor efficacy if used over a long period, and produce an increasing amount of after-congestion (Wilson and Schild 1968). The chronic and often severe mucosal swelling thus produced can cause extreme narrowing of the nasal passages. It is fortunate that so many patients obtain relief from their obstruction within a short time of stopping the drug. Neonates are particularly at risk from the excessive use of these drops because they are obligate nasal breathers and do not develop oral breathing until some time between the ages of 2–6 months. Nasal obstruction in neonates can cause severe respiratory distress. Osguthorpe and Shirley (1987) record the case of a child started on phenylephrine nasal drops at birth. The parents instilled the drops before each feed (every 3–4 hours). At the age of 3 weeks the infant was having multiple daily episodes of apnoea and cyanosis. Clinical examination, blood tests, and radiological investigations revealed oedematous obstructing turbinates, polycythaemia, cardiomegaly, and prominence of the pulmonary vasculature. Most paediatricians advocate limiting the therapy in children to 5–7 days in order to avoid rhinitis medicamentosa. Several studies have shown that oxymetazoline and xylometazoline cause rhinitis medicamentosa if used for a few weeks. In prospective trials involving healthy adult volunteers, all the subjects had developed well-established rhinitis medicamentosa after 30 days' treatment but none had developed it before the 10th day. This reinforces the standard advice that decongestant nasal drops should not be taken for more than 10 days in adults. In addition it has been shown that benzalkonium chloride, a preservative commonly added to xylometazoline and other decongestant solutions, increases the severity of rhinitis medicamentosa (Garf and Juto 1994; Grat *et al.* 1995).

Nasal preparations of sodium cromoglycate and beclomethasone dipropionate are now available for the treatment of allergic rhinitis. These drugs were first introduced for intrabronchial administration in patients with asthma, and a few complications from their use in this way have been reported. There have been no reports so far of serious adverse effects with the intranasal use of these drugs in standard dosage. Minor symptoms of sneezing, stinging, and some blood-stained nasal discharge are sometimes encountered but are not serious.

Although oropharyngeal candidiasis is a well-recognized complication of inhalation of corticosteroids in asthmatic patients, no cases of nasal candidiasis due to the long-term use of intranasal corticosteroids have been recorded in the literature (Webb 1993).

Block (1975) reported some degree of nasal congestion in three patients using intranasal sodium cromoglycate. Mygind and others (1978) followed up a group of 33 patients who had prolonged treatment lasting from 9–36 months with beclomethasone dipropionate. They found no adverse effects with a daily dose of 200–400 μg. Heroman and co-workers (1980), however, recorded the disturbing case of a 4-year-old girl who developed adrenal suppression and cushingoid changes following treatment with 0.1% dexamethasone nasal drops. She suffered from chronic serous otitis media and was given 3 drops in each nostril 4 times daily for 8 weeks. The short corticotrophin stimulation test confirmed the adrenal suppression. The drops were stopped and eventually her appearance returned to normal and her adrenal function was adequate on retesting. It is clear that topical nasal steroids must be used with great caution in children until a safe dosage has been established.

A case of Cushing's syndrome due to the abuse of betamethasone nasal drops is reported by Stevens (1988) in a young man who took them in excessive dosage (approximately 130 ml in 10 weeks). Stevens calculated that this dose was equivalent to 20 mg of prednisolone daily.

The anticholinergic drug ipratropium bromide has been used intrabronchially for its bronchodilator effect for many years. It has recently become available in the form of an intranasal aerosol for the treatment of watery rhinorrhoea and perennial rhinitis and has proved very effective. No significant systemic effects were noted in a trial of 40 patients on long-term treatment. Mild nasal adverse effects occurred but usually resolved during the trial as patients adjusted the dosage (Milford *et al.* 1990).

Antihypertensives

Drugs such as methyldopa, reserpine, and guanethidine, which inhibit adrenergic function, give rise to nasal congestion and obstruction due to their unopposed parasympathetic activity. This is usually a fairly minor symptom that patients tolerate quite well once the cause is explained to them. This is clearly a Type A reaction. The angiotensin-converting-enzyme (ACE) inhibitor enalapril was reported as the cause of severe nasal obstruction in a 45-year-old woman with a history suggestive of mild allergic rhinitis (Finnerty *et al.* 1986). After 4 weeks' treatment she developed severe nasal obstruction that was not relieved by intranasal sodium cromoglycate,

nasal steroids, or oral antihistamines. Enalapril was stopped and the nasal blockage cleared within 2 days. Enalapril was restarted a fortnight later and nasal obstruction recurred within 2 days. This seems likely to have been a Type B reaction typical of drug allergy.

Oral contraceptives

These drugs have been blamed for the occurrence of nasal congestion, together with a plugged feeling in the ear and a distortion of sound (presumably due to obstruction of the Eustachian tube), in a number of patients (Banovetz 1972). In some cases, changing from a sequential to a concomitant contraceptive or vice versa relieves the problem. In the *Interim Report on Oral Contraceptives and health* by the Royal College of General Practitioners (1974), which covered 46 000 women in 1400 practices observed over 4 years, there was a well-marked increase in the incidence of nasal catarrh and allergic rhinitis in women taking these drugs.

Epistaxis

Nasal bleeding in patients receiving long-term anticoagulant therapy is a frequent cause of referral to an ENT clinic and warfarin is probably the drug most commonly implicated. Dipyridamole, which inhibits platelet aggregation and adhesion, is another well-documented cause of epistaxis.

More recently attention has been drawn to the effect of aspirin and other non-steroidal anti-inflammatory drugs, which also alter platelet function. In a study of 53 patients admitted to an ENT ward for epistaxis, Watson and Shenoi (1990) found that four times as many of the patients were taking non-steroidal anti-inflammatory drugs as in a matched control group admitted to the same ward with other diagnoses. The authors recommended that doctors and their patients should be warned of the possible risk of epistaxis as well as of gastrointestinal haemorrhage before beginning treatment with non-steroidal anti-inflammatory drugs.

Anosmia and disturbances of taste

It is common practice to consider these two subjects separately. However, this is another area where the search for the mechanism of the adverse reaction has yielded new information about the normal physiological process. As a result, it has been demonstrated that certain drugs cause loss of both smell and taste by the same mechanism. Some drugs impair the function of only one of these two senses and different mechanisms of drug-induced loss of smell or taste do exist. In addition, the mechanisms of the adverse reaction of a number of drugs on the senses of taste and smell still remain unknown. None the less there is some benefit to be gained from studying the loss of the sense of smell and taste together.

Although chemically induced anosmia is an occupational hazard in workers exposed to carbon dioxide, carbon disulphide, and phosphorus oxychloride (MacIntyre 1971), it is rarely caused by drugs. The application of cocaine, the repeated use of vasoconstrictor drops, and the use of topical neomycin have been held responsible for anosmia (Rebattu *et al.* 1972). Kerekovic and Curkovic (1971) have pointed out that the aminoglycoside antibiotics can be olfactotoxic as well as ototoxic. In a series of 300 patients treated with streptomycin they found eight cases of complete anosmia and 13 of hyposmia attributable to the antibiotic. Several lipid-lowering drugs have been reported to cause a reduction in smell function. The list includes cholestyramine, clofibrate, gemfibrozil, and pravastatin (Henkin 1994). As a general rule drugs cause a reduced or a distorted sense of smell more commonly than a complete smell loss. Fortunately the disturbance of smell function caused by drugs is often reversible.

Many medicaments cause abnormalities of taste by processes not yet properly understood, for example, gold salts, levodopa, biguanides, oxyfedrine, lincomycin, ethambutol, and aspirin (Rollin 1978; Guerrier and Uziel 1979). Minor taste disturbances have been reported in patients receiving griseofulvin (Fogan 1971), metronidazole (Powell 1968), and lithium carbonate (Duffield 1973). Transient taste loss has been reported with the use of etidronate, one of the diphosphonate group of drugs used in the treatment of hypercalcaemia found in various disease states (Jones *et al.* 1987), and also as a remedy for senile osteoporosis and Paget's disease. Transitory disturbance of taste has also been reported during the intravenous injection of the antihypertensive drug diazoxide and the cytotoxic drug carmustine. The antibiotic carbenicillin, the antihistamine azelastine, and the antiarrhythmic drug propafenone have been reported to cause a transient bitter or altered taste sensation. Interest in drug-induced disorders of taste was sparked by the classic paper by Henkin and others (1967), who studied the effect of the chelating agent penicillamine on taste sensation. They found that the drug caused a loss of taste sensation in only four per cent of patients with Wilson's disease, in which the body stores an excessive amount of copper. In diseases, however, in which the body stores copper normally, for example, rheumatoid arthritis, scleroderma, cysteinuria,

and idiopathic pulmonary fibrosis, they found that penicillamine caused a loss of taste sensation in 32 per cent of patients. Further studies led Henkin and Bradley (1969) to the conclusion that a deficiency of copper and zinc ions and an excess of the thiol group brought about a decrease in taste sensitivity. This prompted the authors to recommend oral administration of copper and zinc in the treatment of abnormalities of taste (Henkin and Bradley 1970). Day and Golding (1974) found that taste disturbance was dose related. If the dosage of penicillamine is below 900 mg daily, there is a 25 per cent incidence of taste disturbance in patients with Wilson's disease. The incidence climbs to 50 per cent when the daily dosage exceeds 900 mg. It would appear that taste disturbance is reversible within a period of 8–10 weeks, whether or not penicillamine is discontinued (Jaffe 1968). Topronin and pyritinol, which have therapeutic actions similar to penicillamine, have also been reported to cause a similar taste disturbance.

There has been considerable controversy in the past on whether drug-induced taste disorders were due to a central selective action on taste sensation or to a peripheral effect on the taste buds themselves. The results of research into this matter have been very thoroughly described by Henkin (1994). In his words, an ancillary result of understanding the effects of drugs on taste and smell '. . . may be the furnishing of sufficient clues to unlock some of the mysteries underlying taste and smell function'. There is now agreement that the vast majority of drug-induced taste and smell disorders are due to an adverse effect on the peripheral taste and smell receptors. It has been shown that zinc metalloproteins are critically important in the maintenance of both taste and smell receptor integrity. Taste buds and olfactory receptors do not contain, and therefore are not dependent upon, blood vessels and lymphatics for nutrition and support. Instead they are primarily dependent on salivary proteins and nasal mucus proteins to maintain their structural and functional integrity. Any drug that alters these maintenance proteins can alter taste and smell function. In particular, any drug that interferes with zinc metabolism can adversely affect the function of zinc metalloproteins and thereby alter the function of taste and smell receptors.

The taste disturbance caused by penicillamine is thought to be due to a chelation of zinc from the zinc metalloproteins in salivary mucus. Treatment with zinc alone has been reported to be successful in relieving the taste disturbance caused by penicillamine both in Wilson's disease and in other diseases. In patients with Wilson's disease it is believed that copper–zinc interactions may lead to a greater chelation of copper with a lesser chelation of zinc and a lesser degree of taste disturbance.

The ACE inhibitors captopril and enalapril both cause taste disturbance and less often a disturbance of smell. ACE is a zinc-dependent enzyme and it is thought that inhibition of this enzyme may result in chelation of zinc at the taste and smell receptors. Estimates of the incidence of taste disturbance with captopril vary between one per cent and 20 per cent. Taste function usually recovers after cessation of treatment but recovery is sometimes delayed for many months. Several diuretics have been found to cause taste disturbance. The thiazide diuretics are known to produce hyperzincuria, especially when taken for prolonged periods. Frusemide, ethacrynic acid, and spironolactone also produce taste disturbance by a variety of mechanisms which result in zinc chelation. The calcium-channel blockers nifedipine, amlodipine, and diltiazem cause disturbances of taste and smell and it is thought that they possibly do so by inhibiting calcium-channel activity necessary for normal function of taste and smell receptors. Therefore it would appear that the adverse effects of penicillamine, ACE inhibitors, diuretics, and calcium-channel blockers on taste and smell are Type A reactions.

Some drugs have a selective action on the sense of taste in that they depress the taste sensation of salty substances without diminishing the taste of sweet, sour, or bitter items. Acetazolamide, a carbonic anhydrase inhibitor, has been shown to alter the taste sensation of carbonated drinks and to eliminate the tingle associated with carbonation. Graber and Kelleher (1988) reported that when acetazolamide was taken as a prophylactic against mountain sickness it abolished the carbonated tingle of beer and soda water and gave these drinks an unpleasant taste. They included in their report a translation of a Scandinavian study by Hansson (1961) demonstrating that both the systemic use of acetazolamide and the use of mouth rinses containing carbonic anhydrase inhibitors reduced the taste of salt and enhanced the taste of sweetness. It would seem likely that the drug exerts its effect by causing a local change in the normal working environment of taste receptor buds and is the consequence of inhibition of carbonic anhydrase. This would represent a Type A reaction. Support is given to the theory of a peripheral rather than a central selective action on taste sensation in a study by Lang and others (1988). They reported on the effect of chlorhexidine 0.2% mouth rinses taken by a group of 24 volunteers, who noted a significant and selective impairment in taste perception for salt but not for sucrose (sweet), citric acid (sour), or quinine (bitter). The altered taste sensation began on the first day of using chlorhexidine rinses and

continued until the last day of use of the rinse, returning to normal when the mouth rinses were discontinued. (This subject is also discussed in Chapter 11.)

Buccal cavity and salivary glands
(see also Chapter 11)

A very large number of drugs are known to cause stomatitis, and the list grows yearly. Mercurial diuretics, now seldom used, remain a well-remembered cause. Oral antibiotics, particularly the tetracyclines and chloramphenicol, can induce a vitamin B deficiency and also a monilial infection of the oral cavity, both well-recognized factors in the development of glossitis, stomatitis, and pharyngitis. Fortunately the monilial infection will respond quickly to treatment with nystatin.

It is less well known that a wide variety of modern cytotoxic drugs can produce stomatitis. Mention may be made of the oral ulceration caused by cyclophosphamide, chlorambucil, and bleomycin. Although oral or intramuscular methotrexate fairly often causes stomatitis, it is strikingly rare after intravenous administration. Mercaptopurine, colaspase (asparaginase), actinomycin D, azotomycin, plicamycin (mithramycin), mitomycin, fluorouracil, and bendamustine (Imet 3393) are all recognized causes of stomatitis, while the antileukaemic drug daunorubicin is reported to have caused oropharyngeal ulceration in 12 of 38 children treated by Holton and others (1968).

Dentists are familiar with the oral lesions caused by the local application of salicylates, but the unsuspecting physician may be confused by this kind of ulceration. Even the aspirin-fortified chewing gum used for relief of throat discomfort after tonsillectomy has been known to produce these ulcers. It is interesting that sublingual isoprenaline not uncommonly causes buccal ulceration, and pancreatic extract can cause severe oral ulceration, presumably by enzymic digestion of the mucous membrane because of the patient's failure to swallow quickly enough.

There have been a small number of reports of buccal ulceration caused by chloroquine, griseofulvin, barbiturates, the indanedione group of anticoagulants, and more recently by gold therapy (Glenert 1984) and by proguanil (Daniels 1986).

Xerostomia and sialorrhoea

Dryness of the mouth and throat is a very well known adverse effect of drugs with anticholinergic or atropine-like activity. The list of such drugs is extensive and includes:

1. antihistamines, e.g. diphenhydramine and deptropine;
2. antihypertensives, e.g. methyldopa, guanethidine, clonidine, and the rauwolfia alkaloids;
3. anorectic agents, e.g. fenfluramine and diethylpropion;
4. antiarrhythmic drugs, e.g. disopyramide;
5. benzodiazepine hypnotics, e.g. flurazepam;
6. butyrophenones, e.g. haloperidol.

The major tranquillizer loxapine, the vasodilator guancidine, and the pituitary inhibitor bromocriptine also produce xerostomia as an unwanted effect.

By way of contrast, drugs that have cholinergic effects will produce an excessive flow of saliva. In addition, their cholinergic action on the nasal and bronchial mucosa will cause excessive nasal and bronchial secretion. Deanol (2-dimethylaminoethanol) is used in the management of several neurological disorders and is thought to be effective through its conversion in the body to choline and acetylcholine. Nesse and Carroll (1976) report the case of a woman who received deanol therapy for 3 weeks and developed sialorrhoea, rhinorrhoea, and dyspnoea due to increased bronchial secretion. When the drug was discontinued, symptomatic improvement was apparent within 16 hours, and by the second day the lungs were clear and the rhinorrhoea and sialorrhoea had ceased. Certain drugs are capable of causing xerostomia in some patients and sialorrhoea in others. Breier and others (1994) compared the effect of the two neuroleptic drugs clozapine and haloperidol on their patients. They found clozapine caused excess salivation in 74 per cent of cases and a dry mouth in 11 per cent. Haloperidol on the other hand caused excess salivation in 15 per cent of cases and a dry mouth in 65 per cent. The cholinergic and anticholinergic adverse effects are clearly Type A reactions.

In 1988 the WHO record file contained five cases of hypersalivation and also 10 cases of gynaecomastia attributed to the ACE inhibitor captopril (Adverse Drug Reactions Advisory Committee 1988). The mechanism of captopril-induced sialorrhoea is unknown at present.

Hyperplasia and hypertrophy of the gums

This seems a somewhat bizarre complication of drug treatment, but its occurrence after the use of phenytoin was well documented by Bergmann (1967) and also by Livingston and Livingston (1969), who estimated the incidence to be as high as 40 per cent in the 15 000 patients they surveyed. Neither the occurrence nor the degree of hyperplasia is related to the dosage, and it may be due to a hypersensitivity reaction. In most cases the gums return to normal within a year of stopping the drug. It is suggested that phenytoin should not be used as the drug of first choice in epileptic children receiving orthodontic treatment, or for female epileptics, especially during adolescence.

A great deal has been written about the possible adverse effects of oral contraceptives. Hypertrophic gingivitis has been recorded (Lynn 1967; Lindhe and Bjorn 1968; El-Ashiry et al. 1970) as a complication of these drugs, but the incidence appears to be low. Giustiniani and co-workers (1987) reported a case of gingival hyperplasia in a patient receiving verapamil. The drug was stopped and the hyperplasia settled. Treatment with diltiazem was started after an interval and the gingival hyperplasia recurred. In a series of 107 patients who had had renal transplants, Slavin and Taylor (1987) recorded that 51 per cent of the patients treated with nifedipine and cyclosporin, but only eight per cent of those receiving cyclosporin alone developed hyperplasia. Bowman and others (1988) recorded gingival hyperplasia in a 72-year-old man who received diltiazem. They pointed out that calcium is known to be involved in the control of tissue growth and suggested that the calcium-blocking effect of these agents may be part of the common pathogenesis of drug-induced gingival hyperplasia. There now seems to be an increased awareness of the association of gingival hyperplasia with calcium-channel blockers. In a series of 115 men treated at a veterans' hospital, nifedipine was found to cause more cases of gingival hyperplasia (38%) than diltiazem (21%) and verapamil (19%) (Steel et al. 1994). (See also Chapter 11.)

Salivary gland disorders

Salivary gland swelling has been reported as an adverse effect of insulin, phenylbutazone, oxyphenbutazone, iodides, and also occasionally of some antihypertensive drugs. Shaper (1966) reported that three to five per cent of his diabetic patients in Uganda developed parotid gland enlargement when started on insulin therapy or after an increase in dosage, while Lawrence (1965) mentioned that this had occurred in 20 of his patients. The swelling can be painful, and a number of these patients were referred to an ENT specialist on account of 'earache'. Salivary gland swelling caused by phenylbutazone and oxyphenbutazone has been mistaken for mumps (Gross 1969; Mirsky 1970). In the patient described by Chen and colleagues (1977), the oxyphenbutazone-induced swelling of parotid and submandibular salivary glands was accompanied by pyrexia and transient eosinophilia. They suggested that the reaction was an allergic response (Type B reaction) producing oedema and spasm of the smooth muscle in the salivary ducts.

Harden (1968) proved beyond doubt that the salivary gland swelling caused by iodides was dose dependent. He described a patient who developed bilateral submandibular salivary gland tenderness and swelling after taking the equivalent of 6 g of iodine per day for 36 hours in the form of a cough medicine. The medicine was discontinued, and 48 hours later the swelling had disappeared. The medicine was restarted 14 days later and once more the swelling occurred, but again it disappeared 3 days after stopping the drug. Harden demonstrated that whenever the plasma iodine concentration rose above 11 mg per 100 ml, the glandular swelling reappeared. He stated that the true incidence of salivary gland enlargement resulting from iodine administration was uncertain, and reports in the literature are few. It is important none the less to consider iodide administration in the differential diagnosis of painful salivary gland enlargement, as extensive investigation may be avoided and rapid cure achieved by withdrawal of the drug. Either the submandibular or the parotid glands may be affected. The pathogenesis is uncertain. It is well known that iodide is concentrated in saliva to many times the plasma level. The drug is also concentrated in the thyroid, stomach, and breasts. (This subject is also discussed in Chapter 11.)

The throat

The oesophagus

Drugs pass from the mouth to the stomach through the oesophagus so rapidly that adverse drug reactions in this organ are seldom seen. If the passage of drugs through the oesophagus is delayed, however, the risk of local damage appears to be increased.

McCall (1975) attributed a case of oesophageal ulceration with fatal haemorrhage to the use of slow-release potassium chloride (Slow-K) tablets. The patient had an aneurysmal dilatation of the left atrium sufficient to impede the passage of oesophageal contents.

Howie and Strachan (1975) first drew attention to the hold-up of Slow-K in the oesophagus after cardiac surgery in patients with enlarged hearts, and observed that this delayed passage of the drug produced oesophageal ulceration and stricture formation. Their barium studies showed a Slow-K tablet lodged in a compressed segment of the oesophagus, and they pointed out that the risk of taking this drug would be increased in those patients who required a prolonged period of recumbency.

There have been a number of reports of oesophageal ulceration due to emepronium bromide, a drug used for urinary incontinence and nocturia. The drug is frequently taken without water before going to bed. It is a parasympatholytic agent with peripheral actions similar to those of atropine. Although oral ulceration has been described in confused elderly patients who may have had difficulty in swallowing, oesophageal ulceration by this drug has also been reported in fit, young people who have no known oesophageal problems (Strouthidis *et al*. 1972; Puhakka 1978). Because of these and other problems emepronium bromide is no longer used. Similar oesophageal ulcers have been found in people who have no oesophageal obstruction after swallowing tetracycline (Crowson *et al*. 1976), doxycycline (Schneider 1977), clindamycin (Sutton and Gosnold 1977), co-trimoxazole (Bjarnason and Bjornsson 1981), theophylline (Enzenauer *et al*. 1984), and also bacampicillin and clorazepate.

Carlborg and others (1983) have documented a series of 40 patients with endoscopically proven oesophageal ulcers following ingestion of tablets or capsules containing oxytetracycline, doxycycline, or limecycline. In their series, doxycycline in capsule form caused most of the ulcers. This suggests that capsules are more prone to lodge and dissolve in the oesophagus than tablets. After recommendations from the Swedish Adverse Reaction Committee in 1979, doxycycline capsule preparations were withdrawn from the Swedish market. The number of doxycycline-induced ulcers in Sweden appears to have diminished as a result of this decision.

Evans and Roberts (1976) studied the passage through the oesophagus of barium sulphate tablets (made to the size and shape of aspirin tablets) in 98 consecutive patients during routine radiological screening. In 57 patients, the tablets remained in the oesophagus for longer than 5 minutes. One patient, with no radiological abnormality of the oesophagus, retained a tablet for 45 minutes. The incidence of retention of the tablets in the oesophagus was found to be increased more than twofold in those patients with radiologically demonstrated oesophageal abnormalities. Oesophageal irritation with stenosis or ulceration has been reported with fluorouracil, large doses of chloral hydrate, or very large doses of aspirin. A single tablet of ferrous sulphate that lodged in the hypopharynx caused severe swelling and ulceration of the hypopharynx and cervical oesophagus (Abbarah *et al*. 1976). The lesson of these reports is that tablets or capsules should always be washed down with a glass of water, preferably in the erect position, especially if they are taken after meals. Special precautions must be taken with patients who are recumbent or who have any degree of oesophageal obstruction. The recently introduced drug alendronate, an aminobiphosphate approved for use in postmenopausal osteoporosis, has been shown to cause oesophageal ulcers. In premarketing surveillance studies of more than 1300 patients taking alendronate 10 mg four times daily, oesophageal ulcers were reported in 1.5 per cent; early indications suggest that the postmarketing incidence may prove to be higher than this (Colina *et al.* 1997).

The larynx

Glottic oedema is the most dangerous element of angioedema (angioneurotic oedema), and is seen more commonly in the hereditary form of this disease than in the sporadic form due to food and drug allergies. The dangers of X-ray contrast media in iodine-sensitive individuals have been known for a long time. Seymour (1969) reported a case of glottic oedema during angiography which required an emergency laryngostomy. This occurred despite the fact that the patient was given an antihistamine and hydrocortisone before the injection of the contrast medium. When the reaction began, adrenaline was administered but failed to influence significantly the development of tissue oedema. Glottic oedema has also been reported following treatment with colaspase (L-asparaginase) (Storti and Quaglino 1970) and with penicillin (Dunn 1967).

Laryngospasm resulting from the use of barbiturates is well known to anaesthetists, and intravenous thiopentone is notorious in this respect. The anaesthetic agents desflurane, isoflurane, and propofol have also been found to cause laryngospasm. Doxapram and ethamivan are central nervous stimulants and non-specific analeptics. They can cause muscle twitching, and both have been known to cause laryngospasm.

Although the laryngeal changes in myxoedema are very well recognized by ENT specialists, it is surprising to find that no cases of hoarseness following treatment with antithyroid drugs are described in recent literature. Virilization of the larynx after treatment with testosterone or anabolic steroids was, however, very well documented by Kambic and Lenart (1969) and by Johanson and others (1969). They point out that many anabolic agents are included in low dosage in various combination preparations under names that do not indicate the presence of an androgen. Whenever a woman complains of a change in her voice, one should carefully enquire about any drugs she may be taking. The use of drostanolone propionate in hormone-dependent breast cancer was a fairly common cause of virilization of the larynx in the UK.

The introduction of inhaled steroids has been a major advance in the treatment of patients with asthma. Adverse effects have been few, consisting mainly of mild sore throats, oropharyngeal candidiasis, and hoarseness. Williams and others (1983) studied a group of 14 patients with hoarseness who were receiving inhaled steroids. Incomplete adduction of the vocal cords on phonation was found in nine of these 14 patients, and the authors postulated that this was the cause of the hoarseness and was due to steroid-induced myopathy of the adductor muscles. They found that the muscle weakness was related to the dose and potency of the inhaled steroid and that the weakness and dysphonia were reversed when the inhaled steroid was stopped. Resolution sometimes took a few weeks to be complete. This is an unexpected adverse reaction and the theory of causation is ingenious. *The Lancet* (1984) expressed the opinion that the steroid myopathy explanation was plausible but unproven. It certainly cannot account for all the cases of hoarseness in patients taking inhaled steroids. In five of the 14 patients in the series mentioned, no vocal cord abnormality was present. Candidiasis was thought to be the sole cause of hoarseness in three of these five patients, and in the remaining two there was neither candidiasis nor vocal cord abnormality, and no organic cause for the hoarseness was found. Although steroid inhalers are commonly prescribed, the incidence of hoarseness associated with their use is small. The hoarseness is generally mild and reversible. The reason for the hoarseness in some cases remains obscure and the steroid myopathy theory has still to be proven.

The ACE inhibitor-associated cough may be mentioned in this section since the vocal cords and their motor nerve supply from the vagus constitute the efferent arm of the cough reflex. The majority of the afferent sensory fibres of the reflex run in the vagus nerve also. The cough occurs in about 25 per cent of patients taking ACE inhibitors, and enalapril is thought to be worse than lisinopril for this adverse effect. The cough is characteristically dry and tickly. Inhaled sodium cromoglycate was found to reduce coughing in most of the patients studied by Hargreaves and Benson (1995) but did not completely suppress it in any individual. ACE inhibitors are known to have a vagotonic action and the cough may therefore be regarded as a Type A reaction.

References

Abbarah, T.R., Fredell, J.E., and Ellenz, G.B. (1976). Ulceration by oral ferrous sulphate. *JAMA* 236, 2320.

Adverse Drug Reactions Advisory Committee (1988). Hypersalivation and gynaecomastia associated with captopril. *Adverse Reactions Newsletter, No. 1.* WHO Collaborating Centre for International Drug Monitoring, Uppsala.

Albert, D. S. and Bleyer, W.A. (1996). Future development of amifostine in cancer treatment. *Semin. Oncol.* 23, 90.

Allen, T.C. (1976). Minocycline. *Ann. Intern. Med.* 84, 482.

Arcieri, G.M., Falco, F.G., Smith, H.M., *et al.* (1970). Clinical research experience with gentamicin: incidence of adverse reactions. *Med. J. Aust.* i (Suppl.), 30.

Ballantyne, J. (1970). Iatrogenic deafness. *J. Laryngol. Otol.* 84, 967.

Ballantyne, J. (1973). Ototoxicity: a clinical review. *Audiology* 12, 325.

Bamford, M.F.M. and Jones, L.F. (1978). Deafness and biochemical imbalance after burns treatment with topical antibiotics in young children. Report of 6 cases. *Arch. Dis. Child.* 53, 326.

Banovetz, J.D. (1972). In *Drugs of Choice* (ed. W. Modell), p. 645. C.V. Mosby, St Louis.

Barza, M., Ionnidis, J.P., Cappelleri, J.C., *et al.* (1996). Single or multiple daily doses of aminoglycosides: a meta-analysis. *BMJ* 312, 338.

Bergmann, C.L. (1967). Dilantin (diphenylhydantoin): its effect on the gingival tissues. *Dent. Dig.* 73, 63.

Berk, D.P. and Chalmers, T. (1970). Deafness complicating antibiotic therapy of hepatic encephalopathy. *Ann. Intern. Med.* 73, 393.

Berman, J.L. (1985). Dysomnia, dysgeusia and diltiazem. *Ann. Intern. Med.* 102, 717.

Bjarnason, I. and Bjornsson, S. (1981). Oesophageal ulcers. An adverse reaction to co-trimoxazole. *Acta Med. Scand.* 209, 431.

Block. S.H. (1975). Side effects of cromolyn sodium therapy. *J. Pediatr.* 87, 502.

Bosher, S.K. (1980). The nature of the ototoxic actions of ethacrynic acid upon the mammalian endolymph system. 1. Functional aspects. *Acta Otolaryngol.* 89, 407.

Boston Collaborative Drug Surveillance Program (1973). Drug-induced deafness. *JAMA* 224, 515.

Bowman, J.M., Levy, B.A., and Grubb, R.V. (1988). Gingival overgrowth induced by diltiazem. *Oral Surg. Oral Med. Oral Pathol.* 65, 183.

Breier, A., Buchanan, R.W., Kirkpatrick, B., *et al.* (1994). Effects of clozapine on positive and negative symptoms in outpatients with schizophrenia. *Am. J. Psychiatry* 151, 20.

British Medical Journal (1969). Deafness after topical neomycin. *BMJ* iv, 181.

Brown, H.A. and Hinshaw, H.C. (1946). Toxic reaction of streptomycin on the eighth nerve apparatus. *Proc. Staff Meet. Mayo Clin.* 21, 347.

Browning, G.G., Gatehouse, S. and Calder, I.T. (1988) Medical management of active chronic otitis media: a controlled study. *J. Laryngol. Otol.* 102, 491.

Brummett, R.E. and Fox, K.E. (1982). Studies of aminoglycoside ototoxicity in animal models. In *The Aminoglycosides. Microbiology, Clinical Use and Toxicology* (ed. A. Whelton and H.C. Neu), p. 419. Marcel Dekker, New York.

Brummett, R.E., Fox, K.E., Brown R.T., *et al.* (1978). Comparative ototoxic liability of netilmicin and gentamicin. *Arch. Otolaryngol.* 104, 579.

Brummett, R.E. and Morrison, M. S. (1990). The incidence of aminoglycoside antibiotic induced hearing loss. *Arch. Otolaryngol. Head Neck Surg.* 116, 406.

Carlborg, B., Densert, O., and Lindquist, C. (1983). Tetracycline induced oesophageal ulcers. A clinical and experimental study. *Laryngoscope* 93, 184.

Cases, A., Kelly, J., Sabater, J., *et al.* (1988). Acute visual and auditory neurotoxicity in patients with end-stage renal disease receiving desferrioxamine. *Clin. Nephrol.* 29, 176.

Cazals, Y., Erre, J.P., Aurousseau, C., *et al.* (1987). Ototoxicity of teicoplanin in the guinea pig. *Br. J. Audiol.* 21, 27.

Chapman, P. (1982) . Naproxen and sudden hearing loss. *J. Laryngol. Otol.* 96, 163.

Chen, J.H., Ottolenghi, P., and Distenfeld, H. (1977). Oxyphenbutazone-induced sialadenitis. *JAMA* 238, 1399.

Cohn, E.S., Gordes, E.H., and Brusilow, S.W. (1971). Ethacrynic acid effect on the composition of cochlear fluids. *Science* 171, 910.

Colina, R.E., Smith, M., Kikendall, J.W., *et al.* (1997). New probable increasing cause of esophageal ulceration: alendronate. *Am. J. Gastroenterol.* 92, 704.

Committee on Safety of Medicines (1977). *Adverse Reactions Series No. 14*, London.

Conway, N. and Birt, B.D. (1965). Streptomycin in pregnancy; effect on the foetal ear. *BMJ* ii, 260.

Cortopassi, G. and Hutchin, T. (1994). A molecular and cellular hypothesis for aminoglycoside-induced deafness. *Hear. Res.* 78, 27.

Crowson, T.D., Head, L.H., and Ferrante, W.A. (1976). Esophageal ulcers associated with tetracycline therapy. *JAMA* 235, 2747.

Cummings, C.W. (1968). Experimental observations on the ototoxicity of nitrogen mustard. *Laryngoscope* 78, 530.

Daniels, A.M. (1986). Mouth ulceration: incidence study. *Lancet* i, 269.

Day, A.T. and Golding, J. (1974). Hazards of penicillamine therapy in the treatment of rheumatoid arthritis. *Postgrad. Med. J.* 50 (Suppl.), 71.

Dayal, V.S., Kokshanian, A., and Mitchell, D.P. (1971). Combined effects of noise and kanamycin. *Ann. Otol. Rhinol. Laryngol.* 80, 897.

de Moura, L.E.P. and Hayden, R.C. (1968). Salicylate ototoxicity: a human temporal bone report. *Arch. Otolaryngol.* 87, 368.

Dencker, L. and Lindquist, N.G. (1975). Distribution of labelled chloroquine in the inner ear. *Arch. Otolaryngol.* 101, 185.

Desrochers, C.S. and Schacht, J. (1982). Neomycin concentrations in inner ear tissues and other organs of the guinea pig after chronic drug administration. *Acta Otolaryngol.* 93, 233.

De Virgiliis, S., Argiolu, F., Sanna, G., *et al.* (1979). Auditory involvement in thalassemia major. *Acta Haematol.* 61, 209.

Drake, T.E. (1974). Reaction to gentamicin sulfate cream. *Arch. Dermatol.* 110, 638.

Duffield, J.E. (1973). Side effects of lithium carbonate. *BMJ* i, 491.

Dunn, J.H. (1967). Oral penicillin and anaphylactoid reactions. *JAMA* 202, 552.

Dwivedi, G.S. and Mehra, Y.N. (1978). Ototoxicity of chloroquine phosphate. *J. Laryngol. Otol.* 92, 701.

Eckman, M.R., Johnson, T., and Riess, R. (1975). Partial deafness after erythromycin. *N. Engl. J. Med.* 292, 649.

El-Ashiry, G.M., El-Karfawy, A.H., Nasr, M.F., *et al.* (1970). Comparative study of the influence of pregnancy and oral contraceptives on the gingivae. *Oral Surg.* 30, 472.

Enzenauer, R.W., Bass, J.W., and McDonnell, J.T. (1984). Oesophageal ulceration associated with oral theophylline. *N. Engl. J. Med.* 310, 261.

Evans, K.T. and Roberts, G.M. (1976). Where do all the tablets go? *Lancet* ii, 1237.

Fee, W.E. (1980). Aminoglycoside ototoxicity in the human. *Laryngoscope* 90 (Suppl.), 24.

Finnerty, A., Littley, M., and Reid, P. (1986). Enalapril-induced nasal blockage. *Lancet* ii, 1395.

Fischel Ghodsian, N., Prezant, T.R., Chaltraw, W .E. *et al.* (1997). Mitochondrial gene mutation is a significant predisposing factor in aminoglycoside ototoxicity. *Am. J. Otolaryngol. Head and Neck Med. Surg.* 18, 173.

Fogan, L. (1971). Griseofulvin and dysgeusia: implications? *Ann. Intern. Med.* 74, 795.

Friedlander, I.R. (1979). Ototoxic drugs and the detection of ototoxicity. *N. Engl. J. Med.* 301, 213.

Gailiunas, J. Jr, Dominguez-Moreno, M., Lazarus, J.M., *et al.* (1978). Vestibular toxicity of gentamicin. *Arch. Intern. Med.* 138, 1621.

Gannon, R.P., Tso, S.S., and Chung, D.Y. (1979). Interaction of kanamycin and noise exposure. *J. Laryngol. Otol.* 93, 341.

Gargye, A.K. and Dutta, D.V. (1959). Nerve deafness following chloromycetin therapy. *Indian J. Pediatr.* 26, 265.

Gerharz, E.W., Weingartner, K., Melekos, M.D., *et al.* (1995). Neomycin-induced perception deafness followimg bladder irrigation in patients with end-stage renal disease. *Br. J. Urol.* 76, 479.

Giustiniani, S., Robustelli della Cuna, F., and Marieni, M. (1987). Hyperplastic gingivitis during diltiazem therapy. *Int. J. Cardiol.* 15, 247.

Glenert, U. (1984). Drug stomatitis due to gold therapy. *Oral Surg. Oral Med. Oral Pathol.* 58, 52.

Gomolin, I.H. and Garshick, E. (1980). Ethacrynic acid-induced deafness accompanied by nystagmus. *N. Engl. J. Med.* 303, 702.

Gould, W.J. and Brockler, K.H. (1972). Minocycline therapy. *Arch. Otolaryngol.* 96, 291.

Graber, M. and Kelleher, S. (1988). Side effects of acetazolamide: the champagne blues. *Am. J. Med.* 84, 979.

Graf, P. and Juto, J.E. (1994). Decongestion effect and rebound swelling of the nasal mucosa during 4-week use of xylometazoline. *ORL J. Otorhinolaryngol. Relat. Spec.* 56, 157.

Graf, P., Hallen, H. and Juto, J.E. (1995). Benzalkonium chloride in a decongestant nasal spray aggravates rhinitis medicamentosa in healthy volunteers. *Clin. Exp. Allergy* 25, 395.

Gross, L. (1969). Oxyphenbutazone-induced parotitis. *Ann. Intern. Med.* 70, 1229.

Guerrier, Y. and Uziel, A. (1979). Clinical aspects of taste disorders. *Acta Otolaryngol.* 87, 232.

Hansson, H.P.J. (1961). On the effect of carbonic anhydrase inhibition on the sense of taste: an unusual side effect of a medication (trans. D. Vigertz). *Nord. Med.* 65, 566.

Hanzelik, E. and Peppercorn, M. (1969). Deafness after ethacrynic acid. *Lancet* i, 416.

Harden, R.McG. (1968). Submandibular adenitis due to iodide administration. *BMJ* i, 160.

Harell, M., Shea, J.J., and Emmett, J.R. (1978a). Bilateral sudden deafness following combined insecticide poisoning. *Laryngoscope* 88, 1348.

Harell M., Shea, J.J., and Emmett, J.R. (1978b). Total deafness with propoxyphene abuse. *Laryngoscope* 88, 1518.

Hargreaves, M.R. and Benson, M.K. (1995). Inhaled sodium cromoglycate in angiotensin-converting enzyme inhibitor cough. *Lancet* 345, 13.

Hart, F.D. and Boardman, P.L. (1965). Indomethacin and phenylbutazone: a comparison. *BMJ* ii, 1281.

Hawkins, E. Jr (1967). In *Deafness in Childhood* (ed. F. McConnell and P.H. Ward). Vanderbilt University Press, Nashville.

Healy, C.E. (1972). Mumps vaccine and nerve deafness. *Am. J. Dis. Child.* 123, 612.

Henkin, R.I. (1994). Drug-induced taste and smell disorders. Incidence, mechanisms and management related primarily to sensory receptor dysfunction. *Drug Safety* 11, 318.

Henkin, R.I. and Bradley, D.F. (1969). Regulation of taste acuity by thiols and metal ions. *Proc. Nat. Acad. Sci. USA* 62, 30.

Henkin, R.I. and Bradley, D.F. (1970). Hypogeusia corrected by Ni^{++} and Zn^{++}. *Life Sci.* 9, 701.

Henkin, R.I., Keiser, H.R., Jaffe, I.A., *et al.* (1967). Decreased taste sensitivity after D-penicillamine reversed by copper administration. *Lancet* ii, 1268.

Heroman, W.M., Bybee, D.E., Cardin, J., *et al.* (1980). Adrenal suppression and cushingoid changes secondary to dexamethasone nose drops. *J. Pediatr.* 96, 500.

Higby, D.J., Wallace, H.J., Albert, D., *et al.* (1974). Diamminodichloroplatinum in the chemotherapy of testicular tumours. *J. Urol.* 112, 100.

Hinojossa, R., Riggs, L.C., Strauss, M., *et al.* (1995). Temporal bone histopathology of cisplatin ototoxicity. *Am. J. Otol.* 16, 31.

Hinshaw, H.C. and Feldman, W.H. (1945). Streptomycin in the treatment of clinical tuberculosis: a preliminary report. *Proc. Staff Meet. Mayo Clin.* 20, 313.

Holton, C.P., Lonsdale, D., Nora, A.H., *et al.* (1968). Clinical study of daunomycin (NSC-82151) in children with acute leukemia. *Cancer* 22, 1014.

Hotz, M.A., Harris, F.P. and Probst, R. (1994). Otoacoustic emissions: an approach for monitoring aminoglycoside-induced ototoxicity. *Laryngoscope* 104, 1130.

Howie, A.D. and Strachan, R.W. (1975). Slow release potassium chloride treatment. *BMJ* ii, 176.

Hui, Y., Park, A., Crysdale, W.S., *et al.* (1997). Ototoxicity from ototopical aminoglycosides. *J. Otolaryngol.* 26, 53.

Iqbal, S. and Srivatsav, C.B.P. (1984). Chloramphenicol toxicity: a case report. *J. Laryngol. Otol.* 98, 523.

Jaffe, I.A. (1968). Effects of penicillamine on the kidney and taste. *Postgrad. Med. J.* 44 (Suppl.), 15.

Jahn, A.F. and Ganti, K. (1987). Major auricular malformations due to accutane (isotretinoin). *Laryngoscope* 97, 832.

Johanson, A.J., Brasel, J.A., and Blizzard, R.M. (1969). Growth in patients with gonadal dysgenesis receiving fluoxymesterone. *J. Pediatr.* 75, 1015.

Jolicoeur, G. (1972). Ototoxic changes due to drugs. In *Drug-induced Diseases*, Vol. 4 (ed. L. Meyler and H.M. Peck), p. 540. Associated Scientific Publishers, Amsterdam.

Jones, P.B.B., McCloskey, E.V., and Kanis, J.A. (1987). Transient taste loss during treatment with etidronate. *Lancet* ii, 637.

Jones, R.F.McN., Wright, H.D., and Ballantyne, J.C. (1977). Practolol and deafness. *J. Laryngol. Otol.* 91, 963.

Kambic, V. and Lenart, I. (1969). Modifications cliniques et histologiques de la muqueuse laryngienne des femmes après le traitement par la testostérone. *J. Fr. Otorhinolaryngol.* 18, 97.

Karmody, C.S. and Weinstein, L. (1977). Reversible sensorineural hearing loss with intravenous erythromycin lactobionate. *Ann. Otol. Rhinol. Laryngol.* 86, 9.

Kerekovic, M. and Curkovic, M. (1971). Olfactotoxicity of streptomycin. *Int. Rhinol.* 9, 97.

Kohonen, A. (1965). Effect of some ototoxic drugs upon the pattern and innervation of cochlear sensory cells in the guinea pig. *Acta Otolaryngol.* (Suppl.) 208, 1.

Kohonen, A. and Tarkkanen, J. (1969). Cochlear damage from ototoxic antibiotics by intratympanic application. *Acta Otolaryngol.* 68, 90.

Kopelman, J., Budnick, A.S., Sessions, R.B., et al. (1988). Ototoxicity of high dose cisplatin by bolus administration in patients with advanced cancers and normal hearing. *Laryngoscope* 98, 858.

Kroboth, P.D., McNeil, M.A., Kreeger, A., et al. (1983). Hearing loss and erythromycin pharmacokinetics in a patient receiving haemodialysis. *Arch. Intern. Med.* 143, 1263.

The Lancet (1976). Ear-drops. *Lancet* i, 896.

The Lancet (1984). Inhaled steroids and dysphonia. *Lancet* i, 375.

Lang, N.P., Catalanotto, F.A., Knöpfli, R.U., et al. (1988). Quality-specific taste impairment following the application of chlorhexidine digluconate mouth rinses. *J. Clin. Periodontol.* 15, 43.

Lanthier, P.L., Morgan, M.Y., and Ballantyne, J. (1984). Bromocriptine associated ototoxicity. *J. Laryngol. Otol.* 98, 399.

Laurell, G. and Jungnelius, U. (1990). High dose cisplatin treatment: hearing loss and plasma concentrations. *Laryngoscope* 100, 724.

Lawrence, R.D. (1965). Evanescent parotitis in diabetes. *BMJ* ii, 1432.

Lee, C.C., Anderson, R.C., and Chen, K.K. (1955). Renal clearance of erythromycin. *Proc. Soc. Exp. Biol. Med.* 88, 584.

Lerner, A.M., Cone, L.A., Jansen, W., et al. (1983). Randomised controlled trial of the comparative efficiency, auditory toxicity, and nephrotoxicity of tobramycin and netilmicin. *Lancet* i, 1123.

Levenson, J.L. and Kennedy, K. (1985). Dysomnia, dysgeusia and nifedipine. *Ann. Intern. Med.* 102, 135.

Lindhe, J. and Bjorn, A.L. (1968). Influence of hormonal contraceptives on gingiva of women. *Dent. Dig.* 74, 389.

Little, P.J. and Lynn, K.L. (1975). Neomycin toxicity. *N.Z. Med. J.* 81, 445.

Livingston, S. and Livingston, H.L. (1969). Diphenylhydantoin gingival hyperplasia. *Am. J. Dis. Child.* 117, 265.

Livingstone, G. (1965). Congenital ear abnormalities due to thalidomide. *Proc. R. Soc. Med.* 58, 493.

Lloyd-Mostyn, R.H. (1969). Tinnitus and propranolol. *BMJ* ii, 766.

Lloyd-Mostyn, R.H. and Lord, I.J. (1971). Ototoxicity of intravenous frusemide. *Lancet* ii, 1156.

Lumsden, R.B. and McDowell, G.D. (1968). In *Logan Turner's Diseases of the Nose, Throat, and Ear* (7th edn) (ed. J.P. Stewart and J.F. Birrell), p. 533. Wright, Bristol.

Lupin, A.J. and Harley, C.H. (1976). Inner ear damage related to propoxyphene ingestion. *Can. Med. Assoc. J.* 114, 596.

Lynn, B.D. (1967). The 'pill' as an etiologic agent in hypertrophic gingivitis. *Oral Surg.* 24, 333.

McCabe, P.A. and Day, F.L. (1965). The effect of aspirin on auditory sensitivity. *Ann. Otol. Rhinol. Laryngol.* 74, 312.

McCall, A.J. (1975). Slow-K ulceration of oesophagus with aneurysmal left atrium. *BMJ* iii, 230.

MacIntyre, I. (1971). Prolonged anosmia. *BMJ* ii, 709.

McKelvie, P., Johnstone, I. Jamieson, I., et al. (1975). The effect of gentamicin ear drops on the cochlea. *Br. J. Audiol.* 9, 45.

McKinna, A.J. (1966). Quinine-induced hypoplasia of the optic nerve. *Can. J. Ophthalmol.* 1, 261.

Mahajan, S.L., Ikeda, Y., Myers, T.J., et al. (1981). Acute acoustic nerve palsy associated with vincristine therapy. *Cancer* 47, 2404.

Maher, E.R., Hollman, A., and Gruneberg, R.N. (1986). Teicoplanin induced ototoxicity in Down's syndrome. *Lancet* i, 613.

Mair, I.W.S. and Elverland, H.H. (1977). Sudden deafness and vaccination. *J. Laryngol. Otol.* 91, 323.

Mathog, R.H., Thomas, W.G., and Hudson, W.R. (1970). Ototoxicity of new and potent diuretics. *Arch. Otolaryngol.* 92, 7.

Matz, G.J. and Naunton, R.F. (1968). Ototoxicity of chloroquine. *Arch. Otolaryngol.* 88, 370.

Matz, G.J., Beal, D.D., and Krames, L. (1969). Ototoxicity of ethacrynic acid demonstrated in a human temporal bone. *Arch. Otolaryngol.* 90, 152.

Mawson, S.R. (1967). *Diseases of the Ear*, p. 441. Edward Arnold, London.

Medical Journal of Australia (1975). Ear drops and iatrogenic deafness. *Med. J. Aust.* ii, 626.

Meriwether, W.D., Mangi, R.J., and Serpick, A.A. (1971). Deafness following standard intravenous dose of ethacrynic acid. *JAMA* 216, 795.

Mery, J.P. and Kanfer, A. (1979), Ototoxicity of erythromycin in patients with renal insufficiency. *N. Engl. J. Med.* 301, 944.

Meyer zum Guttesberge, A. and Stupp, H.F. (1969). Streptomycin spiegel in der Perilymphe des Menschen. *Acta Otolaryngol.* 67, 171.

Milford, C.A., Mugliston, T.A., Lund, V.J., *et al.* (1990). Long-term safety and efficacy study of intranasal ipratropium bromide. *J. Laryngol. Otol.* 104, 123.

Miller, S.M. (1982). Erythromycin ototoxicity. *Med. J. Aust.* ii, 242.

Mintz, U., Amir, J., Pinkhas, J., *et al.* (1973). Transient perceptive deafness due to erythromycin lactobionate. *JAMA* 255, 1122.

Mirsky, S. (1970). Salivary gland reaction to phenylbutazone. *Can. Med. Assoc. J.* 102, 91.

Mitchell, C., Brummet, R.E., Himes, D., *et al.* (1973). Electrophysiological study of the effect of sodium salicylate upon the cochlea. *Arch. Otolaryngol.* 98, 297.

Moral, A., Navasa, M., Rimola, A., *et al.* (1994). Erythromycin ototoxicity in liver transplant patients. *Transpl. Int.* 7, 62.

Morizono, T. and Johnstone, B.M. (1975). Ototoxicity of chloramphenicol ear drops with propylene glycol as solvent. *Med. J. Aust.* ii, 634.

Morris, D.L. and Fletcher, A. (1986). Hyperacusis after treatment with mefenamic acid. *BMJ* 293, 823.

Morton, R. (1692). *Pyretologia: seu Exercitationes de Morbus Universalis Acutis.* Samuel Smith, London (quoted by Stephens, S.D.G. 1982).

Myers, E.N., Bernstein, J.M., and Fosriporolous, G. (1965). Salicylate ototoxicity, a clinical study. *N. Engl. J. Med.* 273, 587.

Mygind, N., Sørensen, H., and Pedersen, C.B. (1978). The nasal mucosa during long-term treatment with beclomethasone dipropionate aerosol. *Acta Otolaryngol.* 85, 437.

Nadol, J.B. (1978). Hearing loss as a sequela of meningitis. *Laryngoscope* 88, 739.

Nesse, R. and Carroll, B.J. (1976). Cholinergic side-effects associated with deanol. *Lancet* ii, 50.

Obiako, M.N. (1979). Chloroquine ototoxicity: an iatrogenic tragedy. *Ghana Med. J.* 18, 179. Quoted in *Side Effects of Drugs annual 7 — 1983* (ed. M.N.G. Dukes), p. 295. Associated Scientific Publishers, Amsterdam.

O'Connor, A.F.F., Freeland, A.P., Heal, D.J., *et al.* (1977). Iodoform toxicity following the use of BIPP: a potential hazard. *J. Laryngol. Otol.* 91, 903.

Ohtani, I., Ohtsuki, K., Omata, T., *et al.* (1978a). Potentiation and its mechanisms of cochlear damage resulting from furosemide and aminoglycoside antibiotics. *Otorhinolaryngol.* (Fukuoka) 40, 53.

Ohtani, I., Ohtsuki, K., Omata, T., *et al.* (1978b). Interaction of bumetanide and kanamycin. *Otorhinolaryngol.* (Fukuoka) 40, 216.

Oliveira, J.A.A. (1989a). *Audiovestibular toxicity of drugs*, Vol. 2, p. 140. CRC Press Inc., Boca Raton, Florida.

Oliveira, J.A.A. (1989b). *Audiovestibular toxicity of drugs*, Vol. 1, p. 138. CRC Press Inc., Boca Raton, Florida.

Olivieri, N.F., Buncic, J. R., Chew, E., *et al.* (1986). Visual and auditory neurotoxicity in patients receiving subcutaneous deferoxamine infusions. *N. Engl. J. Med.* 314, 869.

Osguthorpe, J.D. and Shirley, R. (1987). Neonatal respiratory distress from rhinitis medicamentosa. *Laryngoscope* 97, 829.

Ozturan, O., Jerger, J., Lew, H., *et al.* (1996). Monitoring of cisplatin ototoxicity by distortion-product otoacoustic emissions. *Auris, Nasis, Larynx* 23, 147.

Pace-Balzan, A. and Ramsden, R.T. (1988). Sudden bilateral sensorineural hearing loss during treatment with dantrolene sodium (dantrium). *J. Laryngol. Otol.* 102, 57.

Pandya, A., Xia, X., Radnaabazar, J., *et al.* (1997). Mutation in the mitochondrial 12S rRNA gene in two families from Mongolia with matrilineal aminoglycoside ototoxicity. *J. Med. Genet.* 34, 169.

Pearlman, L.V. (1966). Salicylate intoxication from skin application. *N. Engl. J. Med.* 274, 164.

Pillay, V.K.G., Schwartz, F.D., Aimi, K., *et al.* (1969). Transient and permanent deafness following treatment with ethacrynic acid in renal failure. *Lancet* i, 77.

Podoshin, L., Fradis, M., and Ben-David, J. (1989). Ototoxicity of ear drops in patients suffering from chronic otitis media. *J. Laryngol. Otol.* 103, 46.

Porter, J. and Jick, H. (1977). Drug-induced anaphylaxis, convulsions, deafness, and extrapyramidal symptoms. *Lancet* i, 587.

Powell, S.J. (1968). Metronidazole. An anti-infective agent of growing importance. *Medicine Today* 2, 44.

Presley, A.P. (1988). Penicillamine-induced rhinitis. *BMJ* 296, 1332.

Puhakka, H.J. (1978). Drug-induced corrosive injury of the oesophagus. *J. Laryngol. Otol.* 42, 927.

Quinnan, G.U. and McCabe, W.R. (1978). Ototoxicity of erythromycin. *Lancet* i, 1160.

Racy, J. and Ward-Racy, A. (1980). Tinnitus in imipramine therapy. *Am. J. Psychiatry* 137, 854.

Ramsden, R.T. and Ackrill, P. (1982). Bobbing oscillopsia from gentamicin toxicity. *Br. J. Audiology* 16, 147.

Ramsden, R.T., Latif, A., and O'Malley, S. (1985). Electrocochleographic changes in acute salicylate overdosage. *J. Laryngol. Otol.* 99, 1269.

Rebattu, J.P., Lafon, H., and Cajgfinger, H. (1972). La pathologie iatrogène en oto-rhino-laryngologie. *Lyon Méd.* 118, 787.

Roland, P.S. (1994). Clinical ototoxicity of topical antibiotic drops. *Otolaryngol. Head and Neck Surg.* 110, 598.

Rollin, H. (1978). Drug related gustatory disorders. *Ann. Otol. Rhinol. Laryngol.* 87, 1.

Rosketh, R. and Storstein, O. (1963). Quinidine therapy of chronic auricular fibrillation. *Arch. Intern. Med.* 111, 184.

Rothermich, N.O. (1966). An extended study of indomethacin. *JAMA* 195, 531.

Royal College of General Practitioners (1974). *Interim Report on Oral Contraceptives and Health.* London.

Rybak, L.P. (1981). Cis-platinum associated hearing loss. *J. Laryngol. Otol.* 95, 745.

Rybak, L.P and Whitworth, C. (1986). Comparative ototoxicity of furosemide and piretamide. *Acta Otolaryngol.* 101, 59.

Schacht, J. (1986). Molecular mechanisms of drug-induced hearing loss. *Hear. Res.* 22, 297.

Schaefer, S.D., Wright, C.G., Post, J.D., *et al.* (1981). Cisplatinum vestibular toxicity. *Cancer* 47, 857.

Schneider, R. (1977). Doxycycline esophageal ulcers. *Am. J. Digest. Dis.* 22, 805.

Schuknecht, H.F. (1964). The pathology of several disorders of the inner ear which cause vertigo. *South. Med. J.* 57, 1161.

Schwartz, G.H., David, D.S., Riggio, R.R., *et al.* (1970). Ototoxicity induced by furosemide. *N. Engl. J. Med.* 282, 1413.

Sennasael, J. Verbeelen, D., and Lauwers, S. (1982). Ototoxicity associated with cephalexin in 2 patients with renal failure. *Lancet* ii, 1154.

Seymour, J. (1969). Severe laryngeal oedema during injection with sodium metrizoate (Triosil). *Br. Heart J.* 31, 529.

Shaper, A.G. (1966). Parotid gland enlargement and the insulin–oedema syndrome. *BMJ* i, 803.

Slavin, J. and Taylor, J. (1987). Cyclosporin, nifedipine and gingival hyperplasia. *Lancet* ii, 739.

Smith, C.R., Baughman, K.L., Edwards, C.Q., *et al.* (1977). Controlled comparison of amikacin and gentamicin. *N. Engl. J. Med.* 296, 349.

Smith, K.E. and Spaulding, J.S. (1972). Ototoxic reaction to propylthiouracil. *Arch. Otolaryngol.* 96, 368.

Smith, K.E., Reece, C.A., and Kauffman, R. (1972). Ototoxic reaction associated with the use of nortriptyline hydrochloride. *J. Pediatr.* 80, 1046.

Spoendlin, H. (1966). Zur Ototoxizität des Streptomyzins. *Practica Otorhinolaryngol.* 28, 305.

Steele, R.M., Schuna, A.A., and Schreiber, R.T. (1994). Calcium antagonist induced gingival hyperplasia. *Ann. Intern. Med.* 120, 663.

Stephens, S.D.G. (1982). Some historical aspects of ototoxicity. *Br. J. Audiol.* 16, 76.

Stevens, D.J. (1988). Cushing's syndrome due to abuse of betamethasone nasal drops. *J. Laryngol. Otol.* 102, 219.

Storti, E. and Quaglino, D. (1970). Dysmetabolic and neurological complications in leukaemic patients treated with L-asparaginase. *Recent Results Cancer Res.* 33, 344.

Strauss, M., Towfighi, J., Lord, S., *et al.* (1983). Cis-platinum ototoxicity: clinical experience and temporal bone histopathology. *Laryngoscope* 93, 1554.

Strouthidis, T.M., Mankikar, G.D., and Irvine, R.E. (1972). Ulceration of the mouth due to emepronium bromide. *Lancet* i, 72.

Styles, L.A. and Vichinsky, E.P. (1996). Ototoxicity in haemoglobinopathy patients chelated with desferrioxamine. *J. Paediatr. Haematol. Oncol.* 18, 42.

Stypulkowski, P.H. (1990). Mechanisms of salicylate ototoxicity. *Hear. Res.* 46, 113.

Sutton, D.R. and Gosnold, J.K. (1977). Oesophageal ulceration due to clindamycin. *BMJ* i, 1598.

Taylor, R., Schofield, I.S., Ramos, J.M., *et al.* (1981). Ototoxicity of erythromycin in peritoneal dialysis patients. *Lancet* ii, 935.

Thomsen, J., Bech, P., and Szpirt, W. (1976). Otologic symptoms in chronic renal failure. The possible role of aminoglycoside–furosemide interaction. *Arch. Otorhinolaryngol.* 214, 71.

Tjernstrom, O. (1980). Prospective evaluation of vestibular and auditory function in 76 patients treated with netilmicin. *Scand. J. Infect. Dis.* (Suppl. 23), 122.

Toone, E.C., Hayden, G.D., and Ellman, H.M. (1965). Ototoxicity of chloroquine. *Arthritis. Rheum.* 8, 475.

Toyoda, Y. and Tachibana, M. (1978). Tissue levels of kanamycin in correlation with oto and nephrotoxicity. *Acta Otolaryngol.* 86, 9.

van der Hulst, R.J.A., Dreschler, W.A., and Uranus, N.A.M. (1988). High frequency audiometry in prospective clinical research of ototoxicity due to platinum derivatives. *Ann. Otol. Rhinol. Laryngol.* 97, 133.

van Marion, W.F., van der Meer, J.W.M., Kalff, M.W., *et al.* (1978). Ototoxicity of erythromycin. *Lancet* ii, 214.

Vernon, J., Brummett, R., and Walsh, T. (1978). The ototoxic potential of propylene glycol in guinea pigs. *Arch. Otolaryngol.* 104, 726.

Wallner, L.J. (1949). The otologic effects of streptomycin therapy. *Ann. Otol. Rhinol. Laryngol.* 58, 111.

Waltner, J.G. (1955). The effect of salicylates on the inner ear. *Ann. Otol.* 64, 617.

Waltzman, S.B.G. and Cooper, J.S. (1981). Nature and incidence of misonidazole-produced ototoxicity. *Arch. Otolaryngol.* 107, 52.

Watson, M.G. and Shenoi, P.M. (1990). Drug-induced epistaxis. *J. R. Soc. Med.* 83, 162.

Webb, E.L. (1993). Nasal candidiasis in a patient on long term intranasal corticosteroid therapy. *J. Allergy Clin. Immunol.* 91, 680.

Weinstein, A.J., McHenry, M.C., and Gavan, T.L. (1977). Systemic absorption of neomycin irrigation solution. *JAMA* 238, 152.

West, B.A., Brummett, R.E., and Himes, D.L. (1973). Interaction of kanamycin and ethacrynic acid. *Arch. Otolaryngol.* 98, 32.

Williams, A.J., Baghat, M.S., Stableforth, D.E., *et al.* (1983). Dysphonia caused by inhaled steroids: recognition of a characteristic laryngeal abnormality. *Thorax* 38, 813.

Williams, D.N., Laughlin, L.W., and Yhu-Hsiung Lee (1975). Minocycline: possible vestibular side effects. *Lancet* ii, 744.

Wilson, A. and Schild, H.O. (1968). *Applied Pharmacology*, p. 150. Churchill, London.

Wilson, P. and Ramsden, R.T. (1977). Immediate effects of tobramycin on human cochlea and correlation with serum tobramycin levels. *BMJ* i, 259.

Wong, D.L. and Rutka, J.A. (1997). Do aminoglycoside otic preparations cause ototoxicity in the presence of tympanic membrane perforations? *Otolaryngol. Head Neck Surg.* 116, 404.

Wonke, B., Hoffbrand, A.V., Aldouri, M., *et al.* (1989). Reversal of desferrioxamine induced auditory neurotoxicity during treatment with Ca-DTPA. *Arch. Dis. Child.* 64, 77.

Wright, P. (1975). Untoward effects associated with practolol administration: oculomucocutaneous syndrome. *BMJ* i, 595.

Yeadon, A. and Garratt, P.R. (1975). Minocycline (Minocin): a large-scale assessment in general practice. *Clin. Trials J.* 12, 3.

Yung, M.W. and Dorman, E.B. (1986). Electrocochleography during intravenous infusion of cisplatin. *Arch. Otolaryngol. Head Neck Surg.* 112, 823.

23. Drug-induced psychiatric disorders

C. H. ASHTON and A. H. YOUNG

Introduction

Neuropsychiatric reactions accounted for 30 per cent of adverse drug reactions in general practice in 1979 (Martys 1979) and the incidence may be increasing as the number of available drugs and the awareness of adverse drug reactions increases. Such reactions not only occur with psychotropic and non-psychotropic drugs administered therapeutically but also, increasingly, with recreational drugs.

Problems of ascertainment

Psychiatric symptoms are common and it is often difficult to establish whether they are caused by a particular drug or by other factors such as intercurrent or underlying illness. Association with drug use is further confounded by the fact that psychiatric symptoms may be delayed in onset and may persist for weeks or months after drug withdrawal. The relation of such symptoms to a particular drug must be assessed on the basis of such factors as frequency and consistency, temporal association, relation to drug plasma concentrations, and the response to rechallenge with the drug. A further problem is that of recognition: drug-induced psychiatric symptoms may be both overlooked and overdiagnosed. Consistent application of recognized diagnostic systems and terminology (see below) would help in the classification of drug-induced psychiatric reactions. A good discussion of the often confused and ambiguous use of the term 'drug-nduced psychosis' is provided by Poole and Brabbins (1996).

Predisposing factors

Metabolic status

There is great interindividual variability in the rates of metabolism of certain drugs, especially those metabolised by cytochrome P-450 systems, which show genetic polymorphism. Many drugs which can cause psychiatric symptoms are substrates for the cytochrome P-450 CYP2D6 (Sjöqvist 1989; Cholerton et al. 1992; Dahl and Bertilsson 1993). Poor metabolisers of such drugs (5–10 per cent of Caucasian populations) are especially vulnerable to psychiatric and other adverse effects (Preskorn 1993). Differences in the rate of hydroxylation by S-mephenytoin hydroxylase may greatly alter the plasma concentration of diazepam (Bertilsson et al. 1990) and poor metabolisers are at increased risk of adverse effects such as oversedation. Similar degrees of metabolic variability occur with other psychotropic drugs including monoamine oxidase inhibitors (MAOI), trazodone, and buproprion (Preskorn 1993). Ethnic origin is another contributor to metabolic variability. In Asian populations, deficiency of the CYP2D6 enzyme is extremely rare although the average activity of this enzyme is less than in Caucasians (Lee and Jeyaseelan 1994). However, there is a high incidence of poor hydroxylators of S-mephenytoin in Asians (Bertilsson et al. 1990).

Drug interactions

The use of drug combinations greatly increases the risk of adverse reactions (Hurwitz and Wade 1969). Such effects are due to drug interactions which may be pharmacodynamic or pharmacokinetic. Pharmacodynamic interactions are often due to additive effects at the site of drug action. A recent example is the 'serotonin syndrome' characterized by neurological, mental, gastrointestinal, and cardiovascular effects (Sternbach 1991a), which has occurred in patients taking combinations of MAOI with tricyclic antidepressants or selective serotonin reuptake inhibitors (SSRI) (Neuvonen et al. 1993; Nierenberg and Semprebon 1993) and sometimes combinations of SSRI and lithium (CSM 1989; Serfaty et al.

1995) or carbamazepine (Dursun 1993). Combinations of antidepressants may also produce adverse pharmacokinetic interactions. Selective serotonin reuptake inhibitors, including paroxetine, fluoxetine, sertraline, fluvoxamine, and citalopram all inhibit CYP2D6 activity (Crewe *et al.* 1992) and combination with other drugs, metabolised by the same P-450 enzyme system can result in toxic serum concentrations of either or both drugs (Grundemar 1995).

Age

The elderly are particularly susceptible to the effects of central nervous system depressants. This is due to both pharmacokinetic factors, such as decreased metabolic efficiency and reduced renal function, and pharmacodynamic factors including increased tissue sensitivity and perhaps reduced receptor plasticity. For example, oxidation of benzodiazepines is impaired in elderly persons. Thus, benzodiazepines which are metabolised by oxidation (e.g. diazepam, nitrazepam) are more likely to accumulate and cause oversedation than benzodiazepines which are metabolised by conjugation (e.g. temazepam, lormetazepam), since the latter pathway is relatively spared in age (Greenblatt *et al.* 1983). The elderly are also more sensitive than younger subjects to cognitive impairment caused by benzodiazepines (Castleden *et al.* 1977; Cook *et al.* 1983). The metabolism of antidepressants is also impaired in the elderly.

Similar differences in drug metabolism occur in young children and infants, in whom hepatic drug-metabolising enzyme systems are not fully developed. Thus, for example, diazepam metabolism is impaired in neonates and intrauterine exposure to benzodiazepines may result in the 'floppy infant syndrome' with oversedation and other features (see Chapter 7).

Personality

Personality variables, especially the level of anxiety, are important in determining responses to both central nervous system stimulants and depressants. Patients with anxiety disorders have an increased sensitivity to the stimulant and anxiogenic effects of caffeine (Greden 1974; Boulenger and Uhde 1982; Boulenger *et al.* 1984; Charney *et al.* 1985; Bruce *et al.* 1992). Such patients are also prone to an exacerbation of anxiety symptoms when starting treatment with tricyclic antidepressants (Westenberg and den Boer 1993) and are more likely to suffer withdrawal symptoms on cessation of antidepressants (Tyrer 1984). In some anxious patients benzodiazepines cause an increase in anxiety, insomnia, hypnogogic hallucinations, nightmares, and irritability (Baldessarini

1980; Rogers *et al.* 1981), and paradoxical excitatory effects of benzodiazepines appear to be more common in anxious patients (Lader and Petursson 1981).

Somatic and psychiatric disease

Adverse psychiatric reactions are increased in the presence of disease especially in those with pre-existing impairment of brain function. Some patients are particularly sensitive to certain types of drugs or psychiatric effects. Thus, patients with Lewy body dementia are prone to adverse psychiatric and physical effects from even small doses of neuroleptics. (McKeith *et al.* 1992). A family history of affective disorder may predispose to drug-induced precipitation of depression or mania (Whitlock and Evans 1978); constitutional susceptibility to schizophrenia appears to increase the risk of its precipitation by cannabis (McGuire *et al.* 1995) and possibly by amphetamines and LSD. Nevertheless, as Davison and Hassanyeh (1991, p. 601) remark even 'those with unblemished psychiatric records are by no means immune' from drug-induced psychiatric disorders.

Environment, expectation, and placebo effects

Environment, expectation, and placebo effects can all affect susceptibility to adverse psychiatric drug reactions. Stressful environments, isolation, and the sensory isolation sometimes induced by eye surgery or deafness are well known to encourage such reactions (Linn *et al.* 1953; Zuckerman 1964; Hammeke *et al.* 1983; Davison 1989*a*). Expectations of patients, nurses, and doctors can all affect responses to both drugs and placebo (Melzack 1973). Adverse effects from antidepressants are readily reported in patients who have been dependent on prescribed benzodiazepines, a susceptibility undoubtedly partially based on the fear of becoming 'addicted' again.

Expectation also plays a large part in the response to recreational drugs (Ashton *et al.* 1981) and influences the type of 'trip' experienced with recreational drugs such as cannabis, lysergide (LSD), and *N*-methyl-*d*-methamphetamine (MDMA, 'Ecstasy'). The usual effects are enhancement of the prevailing mood (Hollister 1982; Jaffe 1980; Nahas and Paton 1979) and in congenial social gatherings euphoria is commonly experienced. If, however, the surroundings are threatening, severe dysphoria and other effects including flashbacks may result.

Multifactorial causation of psychiatric drug reactions

Psychiatric drug reactions usually result from a multiplicity of causes and for this reason they are often unpredictable; they may sometimes occur on one occasion yet fail to recur on later exposure to the same drug.

Type A and B reactions

Type A (augmented) and B (bizarre) reactions are defined in Chapter 5. Most adverse psychiatric drug reactions are of Type A in that they are dose dependent or recognizably related to the known pharmacological properties of the drug. However, individual susceptibility to particular doses and drug effects is variable. Nevertheless, even reactions described as 'paradoxical', such as excitement and aggression in response to benzodiazepines, are probably directly related to the pharmacological effects of the drug, including disinhibition or acute toxic delirium. Some drug effects appear to be unpredictable but this may be because the full range of a drug's pharmacological effect is not known or the pathology of the illness being treated is not understood.

Classification

The classification of adverse psychiatric reactions to drugs used in this chapter is based on that of the Diagnostic and Statistical Manual of Mental Disorders (DSM IV) (American Psychiatric Association 1994) and includes:

1. Substance-induced delirium
2. Substance-induced dementia and associated states
3. Substance-induced mood disorder
   a. depression
   b. mania, hypomania
4. Substance-induced psychotic disorder
   a. psychosis
   b. isolated hallucinations, circumscribed hallucinatory states
   c. persisting perception disorder (flashbacks)
5. Substance-induced anxiety disorder
6. Other substance-induced states
   a. sleep disorders
   b. drug withdrawal reactions.

The clinical manifestations of these disorders are described in DSM IV, which also lists a number of specific substance-related disorders induced by nicotine, cocaine, hypnotics, and anxiolytics and other substances not described here. However, in general, there is nothing specific about the psychiatric disorders that a drug can cause. Thus, the same drugs may appear under several different headings. Furthermore, so many drugs have been reported to produce psychiatric reactions that it is impossible to give an exhaustive account or to list all possible references. Some selection has therefore been inevitable in this chapter.

Delirium

Delirium is the most commonly encountered psychiatric effect of drug overdose (Evans 1980) but may occur at usual therapeutic doses. It may result from direct toxic effects of a drug on cerebral function, or from indirect effects on cerebral metabolism — for example, hypoglycaemia with insulin or electrolyte abnormality with diuretics. The risk of drug-induced delirium is greatly increased by the presence of underlying cerebral dysfunction, such as hepatic encephalopathy, head injury, visual encephalitis, or hypoxia. Elderly patients are particularly susceptible, and in them, especially, anxiety and delirium can merge under environmental stress, for instance in an intensive care unit (Shader et al. 1987).

Lipowski (1975) distinguished between two clinical variants, hyperactive and hypoactive delirium. The hyperactive form is marked by psychomotor overactivity, excitability, high behavioural and autonomic arousal, and a tendency to hallucinations and persecutory delusions. This variant is typified by the withdrawal syndrome from alcohol, delirium tremens. In hypoactive delirium there is reduced psychomotor activity, even to the point of stupor, with apathy, daytime somnolence, slowed and impoverished thought processes, and less likelihood of hallucinations. This type may be seen with a number of central nervous system depressant drugs. Lipowski (1975) regarded the two clinical variants of delirium as the opposite poles of a continuum with common mixed forms in between.

The mechanisms of delirium, like those of most psychiatric disorders, are imperfectly understood. Maintenance of a clear consciousness with orientation of self in time and space requires accurate co-ordination between neural activity in many cortical and subcortical structures, including those involved in learning, memory, and many types of information processing. It also requires a degree of background cortical excitation sufficient to maintain arousal (Routenberg 1968; Mountcastle 1974; Webster 1978). Many neurotransmitters are involved in these interneuronal activities. Furthermore, the cortical neurones themselves must be adequately supplied with essential nutrients, such as oxygen, glucose, and electrolytes, in order to carry out their functions. It is clear that this elaborate system is susceptible to disruption by various direct and indirect actions of many drugs.

Anticholinergic drugs

Drugs with anticholinergic (antimuscarinic) properties are the commonest pharmacological group able to induce delirium. This effect is dose related and regularly occurs on overdose, though it has not infrequently occurred in clinical practice. The 'central anticholinergic syndrome' (Longo 1966) includes excitement, sometimes preceded by sedation, with disturbance of consciousness, hallucinations (usually visual), and ataxia with characteristic systemic features of dry mouth, hot dry skin, dilated pupils, and tachycardia.

Atropine, hyoscine, scopolamine

These drugs, used for preoperative medication, can induce both preanaesthetic (Smiler *et al.* 1973) and postanaesthetic delirious excitement. Scopolamine (hyoscine), sold in proprietary hypnotics in the USA, has caused an excited, delirious state (Baile *et al.* 1977), though this may follow initial sedation (Korolenko *et al.* 1969). The administration of atropine to control cardiac arrhythmia after cardiac infarction has induced delirium with slow cerebration, somnolence, and inattention, especially in patients over 60 years of age (Erikssen 1969).

The use of mydriatric eye-drops containing atropine and homatropine (Hoefnagel 1961), hyoscine (Freund and Merin 1970), or cyclopentolate (Shihab 1980; Khurana *et al.* 1988) has been associated with delirium, accompanied by auditory and visual hallucinations and subsequent amnesia. Such preparations are sometimes introduced into drinks for criminal purposes, the delirious victim being more easily robbed (Brizer and Manning 1982).

Abuse of stramonium, which contains atropine and hyoscine, for hallucinogenic purposes, alone or in various forms including preparations from the flowers of *Datura stramonium* (Jimson weed) (Dean 1963; DiGiacoma 1968; Goldsmith *et al.* 1968; Hall *et al.* 1977) has not infrequently precipitated the central anticholinergic syndrome. Gowdy (1972) reviewed 212 cases of toxicity following such abuse and reported visual hallucinations, disorientation, hyperactivity, and amnesia in nearly 50 per cent, together with characteristic anticholinergic physical effects.

Some antidiarrhoeal drugs contain atropine or propantheline and, if taken in overdose, may cause delirium of the central anticholinergic type (Proudfoot 1982).

Antiparkinsonian drugs

Anticholinergic drugs used for treating Parkinson's disease and for controlling extrapyramidal effects of antipsychotics can induce excited delirium with visual hallucinations in therapeutic doses (Porteous and Ross 1956; Stephens 1967; McClelland 1985). These drugs include benzhexol, benztropine, procyclidine, orphenadrine, biperiden, and others. In addition, these drugs may cause delirium when abused for their euphoriant and hallucinogenic effects (Pullen *et al.* 1984; Kaminer *et al.* 1982; Crawshaw and Mullen 1984). When used in combination with neuroleptics with anticholinergic properties (for example, thioridazine), the effects may be additive (McClelland 1985).

Antipsychotic drugs

Some phenothiazines, including chlorpromazine, promazine, promethazine, methotrimeprazine, pericyazine, thioridazine, and pipothiazine, have marked anticholinergic effects. These drugs, particularly after parenteral administration, can precipitate a hyperactive delirium of the central anticholinergic type, preceded by restlessness and agitation (Mariani 1988). They can also induce a hypoactive delirium soon after taking of an overdose (Evans 1980). The butyrophenone haloperidol, which has little anticholinergic activity, can also induce delirium when used either alone or in combination with anticholinergic drugs (Evans 1980). Delirium has also occurred with oral metoclopramide, although it is neither antipsychotic nor anticholinergic (Fishbain and Rogers 1987).

Antihistamines

Some antihistamines (H_1-receptor antagonists), including diphenhydramine, cyclizine, pheniramine, and chlorpheniramine, have significant anticholinergic actions, and all the above have been reported to produce delirium of the central cholinergic type (Davidson and Hickey-Dwyer 1991).

Antidepressants

Many tricyclic antidepressants (imipramine, amitriptyline, clomipramine, nortriptyline, desipramine, protriptyline, doxepin, and dothiepin) have significant anticholinergic actions and can cause toxic delirium, delusions, visual hallucinations, and other features of the central anticholinergic syndrome (Schmidt *et al.* 1986). Delirium occurred in 13 per cent of 150 patients with adverse reactions to antidepressants reviewed by Davies and colleagues (1971); in patients over the age of 40 the incidence was 35 per cent. The central nervous system toxicity of antidepressants is dose dependent. Burke and Preskorn (1995) state that the relative risk for delirium from tricyclic antidepressants which are tertiary amines increases 14- and 38-fold above plasma concentrations of 300 ng and 450 ng per ml respectively. Additive anticholinergic effects of concomitant neuroleptic treatment increase the toxicity of tricyclics, and neuroleptics also increase tricyclic blood concentrations (Linnoila *et al.* 1982; Siris *et al.* 1982). Patients recovering from tricyclic antidepressant poisoning after overdose may develop a hyperactive delirium as consciousness returns; their condition may last for some hours (Evans 1980).

Delirium due to the central anticholinergic syndrome produced by the above drugs usually abates rapidly after withdrawal of the offending drug, but if necessary it can be very quickly terminated by intravenous preparations of physostigmine, an anticholinesterase which enters the brain (Proudfoot 1982). Antipsychotic drugs with anticholinergic effects should not be used, since they may exacerbate the condition (Shader and Greenblatt 1972).

Sympathomimetic drugs

Although mania and paranoid psychoses are more common adverse psychiatric effects of sympathomimetic drugs, hyperactive delirium with excitement, hallucinations, and paranoid delusions can occur. Such delirium is described after overdose of amphetamine, methylphenidate, phenmetrazine, or ephedrine (Kane and Florenzano 1971; Evans 1980). Phenylpropanolamine can also cause a hyperactive delirium (Norvenius *et al.* 1979), which has also been described after overdose of the related drugs theophylline, aminophylline, and fenfluramine (Evans 1980; SADRAC 1987). These reactions are presumably due to extreme over-arousal mediated by central monoaminergic systems.

Dopaminergic drugs

Cocaine

Delirium may be one of the manifestations of acute cocaine intoxication (Manschreck *et al.* 1987; O'Brien and Woody 1991; Lacayo 1995), although mania, paranoid psychoses and other psychiatric symptoms are more common. 'Drug smuggler's delirium' (Ramnakha and Barton 1993) has occurred in couriers when the contents of packages of cocaine, concealed in the rectum or vagina, have accidentally leached out. When this occurs the couriers may take benzodiazepines to stop themselves getting too 'high' or agitated. Nevertheless, the outcome may be fatal from cardiovascular and central nervous system complications.

Levodopa

Hyperactive delirium may also be provoked by levodopa, and appears to be closely dose related. Celesia and Barr (1970) and Damasio and colleagues (1971) reported a prodromal phase of insomnia and increasing anxiety, progressing to delirium; withholding or reducing the dose of levodopa or giving tranquillizers rapidly brought the delirium under control. Delirious states and other psychiatric reactions were often delayed for some months after starting treatment, their development often coinciding with an increase in dose. In one study (O'Brien *et al.* 1971) of 20 parkinsonian patients whose dosage of levodopa was carefully titrated against psychiatric symptoms, no confusional states developed although there were three cases of hypomania. In another study of 100 patients over a period of 6 years (Sweet *et al.* 1976), however, an episode of agitated delirium developed in 60 per cent of patients; the authors claimed that this high incidence was due to increasing brain vulnerability to levodopa from the advancing dementia produced by the underlying parkinsonian disorder. In another study, nearly half of 88 patients with Parkinson's disease who were treated with levodopa developed vivid dreams, hallucinations, illusions, and confusion (Moskowitz *et al.* 1978). Goodwin (1971) reviewed 908 patients receiving levodopa for Parkinson's disease. Of these, 20 per cent had psychiatric complications, the most common of which were delirium (4.4 per cent), followed by depression (4.2 per cent), agitation (3.6 per cent), paranoid psychosis (3.6 per cent), and hypomania (1.5 per cent).

Bromocriptine, amantadine

Both bromocriptine, a dopamine-receptor agonist, and amantadine, which stimulates neuronal dopamine release, can cause delirium and other psychiatric symptoms similar to those induced by levodopa (Calne *et al.* 1978; Pearce and Pearce 1978; Hollister 1986). Amantadine-induced delirium can be reversed by physostigmine (Casey 1978), suggesting that amantadine has actions other than dopamine release.

Antidepressants

Tetracyclic compounds

Antidepressant drugs with significant anticholinergic effects (mostly tricyclic antidepressants) can produce delirium of the central anticholinergic type. In addition, the tetracyclic maprotiline, which has relatively little anticholinergic action but is a potent inhibitor of synaptic noradrenaline reuptake, can cause delirium in overdose. This develops within 1–2 hours of ingestion, when an initial hyporeflexia is followed by hyperreflexia; disturbance of consciousness with confusion and hallucinations may last for up to 48 hours (Evans 1980). The mechanism in this case is possibly central noradrenergic overactivity, similar to the delirium caused by sympathomimetic drugs, but may include anticholinergic actions (Proudfoot 1982).

Specific serotonin reuptake inhibitors

The commonest psychiatric adverse effects of these drugs are stimulation or sedation of the central nervous system, but serious toxic reactions with delirium can arise when specific serotonin-reuptake inhibitors (SSRI) are taken in combination with other drugs which increase central serotonin activity. Known as the 'serotonin syndrome', this reaction consists of excitation, restlessness, fluctuations in consciousness, and delirium, with tremor, rigidity, myoclonus, sweating, flushing, pyrexia, shivering, cardiovascular changes, and, rarely, coma and death (Sternbach 1991; Edwards 1992, 1994). The syndrome has been reported when specific serotonin-reuptake inhibitors have been combined with irreversible MAOI, lithium, L-tryptophan, or, occasionally, tricyclics and other drugs (Sternbach 1991; Edwards 1994). Edwards (1994) recommends that, because of this potential interaction, at least 2 weeks should elapse between stopping an irreversible MAOI and introducing an SSRI, or between discontinuing the latter and starting an MAOI. In the case of fluoxetine, at least 6 weeks should elapse, because of its slow elimination, and its metabolite norfluoxetine.

No treatment methods for the serotonin syndrome have been established, but cyproheptadine, a serotonin antagonist, and dantrolene, a muscle relaxant, have been recommended (Szabadi and Bradshaw 1995). Other symptomatic treatment measures (cold blankets, sedatives, anticonvulsants, antihypertensives, and β-adrenoceptor antagonists) are described by Sternbach (1991).

MAOI

MAOI, when taken alone in overdose, or in combination with other drugs such as other MAOI, tricyclic antidepressants, or foods rich in tyramine or dopamine, can cause a toxic delirium leading to severe cerebral excitation and loss of consciousness. Central nervous system toxicity caused by phenelzine has been successfully treated by chlorpromazine and possibly results particularly from central dopaminergic overactivity. Drug interactions with monoamine oxidase inhibitors which may cause central nervous system toxicity are described by Edwards (1995). (See also Chapter 20.)

Lithium

Lithium toxicity is not uncommon and occurs after overdose and sometimes during therapeutic usage. Toxicity is most likely when the serum lithium concentration is above the therapeutic range, now considered to be between 0.5 and

1.0 mmol per litre in blood specimens taken 12 hours after the last dose (Tyrer 1996). Severe toxicity is unusual below levels of 2.0 mmol per litre but can occur below this level and even within the therapeutic range (Evans 1980). Delirium — which can be hyperactive or hypoactive — may occur, associated with psychotic features and sometimes with convulsions (Evans 1980). Long-term psychiatric and neurological sequelae have been reported following lithium toxicity, and withdrawal of lithium has also been reported to cause delirium (Wilkinson 1979).

The incidence of lithium toxicity in clinical use is not known. Shopsin and colleagues (1970) reported that 80 per cent of their patients treated with lithium showed some evidence of behavioural toxicity at serum concentrations between 1.16 and 1.9 mmol per litre. However, the incidence has declined as risk factors have become more widely known; a survey in the USA cited by Tyrer (1996) showed that of patients having some form of lithium toxicity, moderate to severe reactions occurred in about 15 per cent, but the morbidity rate was less than one per cent. Apart from excessive dosage, risk factors for lithium toxicity include sodium depletion or dehydration from any cause, impaired renal excretion, and interactions with other drugs (Aronson and Reynolds 1992; Edwards 1995; Tyrer 1996). Drugs which may increase lithium toxicity by reducing lithium clearance include diuretics (especially thiazides), non-steroidal anti-inflammatory drugs (NSAID), and some antihypertensive drugs (e.g. angiotensin-converting-enzyme inhibitors). Drugs that increase lithium toxicity without increasing serum lithium concentration include calcium channel antagonists (diltiazem, verapamil), anticonvulsants (phenytoin, carbamazepine), haloperidol, SSRI, and others listed by Tyrer (1996) and Edwards (1995).

Mechanisms of lithium toxicity are discussed by Tyrer (1996) and appear to involve the accumulation of high concentrations of lithium in the brain, from which it is slow to clear because of progressive reduction in the activity of the lithium pump responsible for the efflux of lithium from cells. Cellular excretion of lithium decreases progressively as toxicity develops. In profound cases of lithium toxicity diffuse encephalopathy occurs causing neurological and cognitive abnormalities. With concomitant drugs, particularly haloperidol and tricyclic antidepressants, a syndrome similar to the neuroleptic malignant syndrome may develop. Treatment of lithium toxicity is described by Tyrer (1996) and may include gastric lavage, saline diuresis, and haemodialysis.

Anticonvulsants

Many anticonvulsants can produce delirium, which is usually dose related. However, epileptic patients have an increased risk of developing a psychiatric disorder, and combinations of drugs are often employed, so that psychiatric reactions can occur when plasma concentrations are at subtherapeutic levels and sometimes in the absence of physical signs such as ataxia and nystagmus (Davison and Hasasanyeh 1991). Phenobarbitone, primidone, phenytoin, sodium valproate, and carbamazepine can all cause a hypoactive delirium with

drowsiness, sometimes preceded by an initial period of stimulation and euphoria similar to alcohol intoxication (Evans 1980; Tollefson 1980; Reynolds 1981). A hyperactive delirium also occurs as part of the phenobarbitone abstinence syndrome following phenobarbitone intoxication (Evans 1980).

Hypnotics and anxiolytics

Intoxication with hypnotics and anxiolytics, including barbiturates, benzodiazepines, chlormethiazole, and chloral derivatives can cause drowsiness and delirium, often accompanied by ataxia, dysarthria, and nystagmus. Occasionally there is an initial hyperactive phase, but in overdose a hypoactive delirium with clouded consciousness proceeding to coma occurs (Evans 1980). In elderly subjects even normal therapeutic doses can induce delirium, which may lead to bizarre behaviour, falls, and fractures (Evans 1980; Jarvis 1981). Withdrawal reactions of sedatives and hypnotics in dependent subjects may include a hyperactive delirium.

Muscle relaxants

The muscle relaxant baclofen, an agonist at $GABA_B$ receptors in the spinal cord, also has central actions and can produce delirium as well as a schizophreniform psychosis in overdose and can cause an abstinence syndrome (Evans 1980).

Analgesic and anti-inflammatory drugs

Opioids

All opioids have central nervous system depressant actions and in overdose can cause severe disturbances of consciousness leading to coma and convulsions, but delirious states appear to be relatively rare. However, dextropropoxyphene has produced hypoactive delirium with hallucinations, ataxia, and vertigo (Evans 1980). Pethidine has induced delirium (Eisendrath *et al.* 1987), and morphine, pentazocine, pethidine, and dihydrocodeine have all caused paranoid–hallucinatory psychoses (Davison and Hassanyeh 1991).

Salicylates

Self-poisoning with aspirin, and accidental overdose of the drug in children, are not uncommon and can produce delirious states. Early signs of central nervous system toxicity are tinnitus, deafness, nausea, and vomiting. In severe cases there may be progression to delirium with extreme agitation, confusion, and finally coma and convulsions. Loss of consciousness is rare in adults and children over 2 years old, but is encountered after overdose in children under 2 years. The psychiatric features are largely due to derangements of acid–base and electrolyte balance and dehydration resulting from hyperventilation, vasodilatation, sweating, vomiting, and hyperpyrexia. Salicylates may also reduce brain glucose levels (Proudfoot 1982). Toxic symptoms start at plasma concentrations above 300 mg per litre, but values as high as 1700 mg per litre have been observed after overdose (Proudfoot 1982).

NSAID

Overdose of indomethacin produces dizziness, lightheadedness, and vertigo, leading to delirium, which is seen quite frequently (Evans 1980). The related drug sulindac has also induced delirium (Thornton 1980).

Recreational drugs

Alcohol

Delirious states, either hyper- or hypoactive, can occur during acute alcohol intoxication and, with increasing doses, lead to coma. Delirium tremens is described with other drug withdrawal syndromes later in this chapter. It appears on about the third day of untreated total abstinence in dependent alcoholics when such subjects become disorientated, severely agitated, and prey to terrifying hallucinations, accompanied by signs of autonomic overactivity including tremor. Delirium tremens occurs in about 20 per cent of alcohol-dependent individuals who present to inner-city hospitals in the USA and Australia, and in these the mortality is about eight per cent (Hall and Zador 1997). However, in patients admitted to detoxification units, delirium tremens occurs in less than five per cent (Schultz 1991). The picture may be complicated by alcoholic hepatic encephalopathy (Benzer 1991).

Disulfiram, used to prevent relapses in alcoholics after detoxification, can itself cause delirium (as well as schizophreniform and manic reactions in the absence of alcohol ingestion (Liddon and Satran 1967). Concurrent ingestion of metronidazole increases the risk of a psychiatric reaction (Rothstein and Clancy 1969).

Hallucinogens

The primary effect of hallucinogenic drugs such as LSD and MDMA ('Ecstasy') is to produce changes in perception, thought, and mood. However, acute intoxication with high doses can induce a hyperactive delirium with florid hallucinations and extreme agitation, which can occasionally persist for some weeks (Evans 1980; Hollister 1986). The main psychiatric adverse effects and mechanisms of action of these drugs are discussed later in this chapter.

Phencyclidine, ketamine

Phencyclidine and ketamine can cause a combination of psychiatric symptoms, stimulant and sedative, psychotomimetic and catatonic. With phencyclidine intoxication the commonest pattern seen in individuals referred for treatment is that of delirium (Gorelick and Balster 1995), which can proceed through stages from behavioural toxicity to stupor or light coma and finally deep coma with unresponsiveness to pain. Delirium lasting several days is quite common during recovery after phencyclidine-induced coma, and may occur transiently as the final phase of an episode of intoxication (Gorelick and Balster 1995).

Ketamine has similar effects when abused for recreational purposes, a practice which appears to be increasing (Awounda 1996). When used as an anaesthetic in adults it can produce delirium on emergence from anaesthesia, the incidence depending on the dosage used (Dundee et al. 1970). Halothane and isoflurane can also produce postanaesthetic delirium (Davison et al. 1975). The multiple mechanisms of action of phencyclidine and ketamine are described later in this chapter.

Cannabis

Acute intoxication with cannabis can produce delirium (Talbot and Teague 1969; Chopra and Smith 1974; Tennant and Groesbeck 1972; Nahas 1984). This has been uncommon in the UK but may be becoming more frequent with the widespread use of potent preparations such as Skunkweed (Cohen and Johnson 1988; Wylie et al. 1995). Episodes are usually self-limiting over a few days; they can occur in individuals with no history of psychiatric illness. The mechanisms of action of cannabis are discussed further on.

Volatile solvents

Inhalation of volatile solvents is a recreational pastime pursued mainly by the young, with a peak prevalence between the ages of 13–15 years. Clinical effects have been reviewed by Sourindrhin (1985), Herzberg and Wolkind (1983), and Ashton (1990). Features of acute intoxication are similar to those of alcohol intoxication; a delirious state with clouding of consciousness, illusions, and hallucinations is less common. The period of intoxication is usually brief, with recovery within an hour, sometimes with amnesia for the entire episode. However, experienced users can maintain a 'high' for up to 12 hours by judicious, repeated sniffing (Black 1982). Chronic users often report transient symptoms of toxic psychosis, usually with an affective component, and self-destructive and antisocial acts may be carried out under the influence of solvents. In severe intoxication, convulsions, status epilepticus, and coma may occur. Sudden death may occur from anoxia, vagal inhibition, cardiac arrhythmia, or trauma (accident or suicide) (Shepherd 1989), and solvent abuse accounts for about 120–150 deaths per year in the UK (Taylor et al. 1993). Chronic solvent abuse can cause neurological, renal, cardiac, and respiratory damage (Marjot and McLeod 1989).

Abused solvents are obtained from a large number of easily available products and commonly contain organic solvents (toluene, benzene, n-hexane, amyl acetate, butane) or aerosol products containing freons (Black 1982; Meredith et al. 1989). These substances are fat soluble, easily absorbed, and have central nervous system depressant effects like general anaesthetics. Amyl and butyl nitrites are sometimes inhaled for their vasodilator properties in homosexual encounters (Sigell et al. 1978). Delirium can occur after abuse of volatile anaesthetics such as nitrous oxide; Sterman and Coyle (1983) reported a long-lasting delirium which cleared slowly over 3 weeks following heavy use of this gas. Addiction to salbutamol inhalers has frequently been reported and is thought to be due, at least partly, to the fluorinated hydrocarbon propellant (Thompson et al. 1983; Prasher and Corbett 1990).

Management of acute solvent toxicity consists of standard measures, with cardiorespiratory resuscitation when necessary, conventional treatment of cardiac arrhythmias, and intensive supportive treatment (Richardson 1989).

Corticosteroids

Psychiatric complications are reported to occur in up to five per cent of patients receiving systemic corticosteroids (Hollister 1986). These cover a spectrum with symptoms ranging from affective through schizophreniform disorders to delirium, the symptoms sometimes alternating in individual patients (Hall et al. 1979). Children appear to be particularly susceptible (Rutgers et al. 1988). There have been numerous reports of cases of clear-cut delirium (cited in Evans 1980; McClelland 1985). Other psychiatric disturbances associated with corticosteroids and other hormones are described later.

Cardiovascular drugs

Digitalis preparations

Toxic effects associated with digitalis preparations are still quite common in hospital inpatients (Hoffman and Bigger 1990). Psychiatric effects usually occur at the same dosage as cardiotoxic effects but can occur at normal therapeutic concentrations (Eisendrath and Sweeney 1987). 'Digitalis delirium' has long been recognized and can include paranoid delusions and coloured hallucinations (King 1950; Church and Marriott 1959). The risk of developing digitalis toxicity is increased by older age, myocardial ischaemia or infarction, hypoxaemia, hypothyroidism, potassium or magnesium deficiency, renal insufficiency, and interaction with other drugs (Wamboldt et al. 1986). The most frequent cause is concurrent administration of a diuretic that causes potassium loss (Hoffman and Bigger 1990). Mechanisms of delirium include electrolyte disturbance and cerebral hypoxia as well as possible catecholamine release by digitalis (Saxena and Bhargara 1975).

β-Adrenoceptor antagonists

Delirium, associated with visual and tactile hallucinations, has been reported both during propranolol therapy (Topliss and Bond 1977; Helson and Duque 1978; Paykel et al. 1982; Hollister 1986) and after its abrupt withdrawal (Patterson 1985; Golden et al. 1989). Atenolol has also provoked delirium with visual hallucinations and paranoid ideation in an 85-year-old man when dosage was increased from 100 to 200 mg daily (Arber 1988). Nightmares, nocturnal hallucinations, and depression are more common adverse psychiatric effects of this group of drugs. The α-adrenoceptor antagonist prazosin has provoked delirium in patients with renal failure (Chin et al. 1986).

Antiarrhythmic drugs

Delirium has been associated with a number of antiarrhythmic drugs related to cocaine, including intravenous lignocaine (Graham et al. 1981; Turner 1982; Saravary et al.

1987), tocainide (Currie and Ramsdale 1984), and mexiletine (CSM 1986). These drugs can also produce hallucinations and paranoid psychoses. Delirium has also been reported with the calcium-channel antagonist verapamil (Jacobson et al. 1987) and with disopyramide (Evans 1980). It can also occur with quinidine (Evans 1980).

Gastrointestinal drugs

The histamine H_2-receptor antagonists cimetidine and ranitidine can both cause delirium (Kinnell and Webb 1979; Hughes et al. 1983; Mandal 1986; MacDermott et al. 1987), as well as paranoid psychoses, mania, hallucinations, and depression. Early reports involved elderly patients, often with renal or hepatic impairment and elevated serum concentrations (Davison and Hassanyeh 1991), but psychiatric reactions can occur at any age and at therapeutic blood levels (Papp and Curtis 1984). Delirium usually develops within 2 days of starting cimetidine therapy and remits within 2–3 days of discontinuation (Sonnenblick et al. 1982); delirium is not usually associated with long-term use (Hollister 1986). Cimetidine, but not other histamine H_2-receptor antagonists, inhibits the cytochrome oxidase P-450 CYP2D6 and therefore slows the metabolism of other substrates for this enzyme, including tricyclic antidepressants; an interaction between imipramine and cimetidine may provoke psychiatric symptoms (Miller et al. 1987).

Anti-infective and antineoplastic drugs

Antibacterial agents

Delirium has been reported with streptomycin (Porot and Destaing 1950), chloramphenicol (Pereau and Maurice 1950), intravenous erythromycin (Umstead and Neumann 1986), gentamicin (Kane and Byrd 1975), and griseofulvin (Hollister 1986). Paranoid–hallucinatory psychoses have also been reported with streptomycin, erythromycin, and griseofulvin. Cefuroxime and other cephalosporins have been associated with delirium, but usually in severely ill elderly patients (Hollister 1986). Hyperactive delirium may sometimes accompany the extreme anxiety reaction which occasionally occurs after injection of benzylpenicillin (Evans 1980). 4-quinolones have neuropsychiatric effects including confusion, and, occasionally, delirium, hallucinations, and psychotic reactions (Evans 1980; Ball 1989). Convulsions may occur when quinolones are combined with NSAID.

High doses of the antituberculous drugs isoniazid and cycloserine have both caused delirium, both singly and in combination (Wallach and Gershon 1972; Evans 1980), and delirium is one of the many neuropsychiatric effects of cycloserine (Wallach and Gershon 1972; Evans 1980). Sodium aminosalicylate (PAS) can also cause a delirium when taken in high doses (Evans 1980). Rifampicin occasionally causes confusion and drowsiness (Mandell and Petri 1996), and an acute toxic confusional state with disorientation, agitation, incoherence, hallucinations, and delusions has been reported in a 60-year-old man receiving rifampicin daily (Martindale

1982). The antifungal drug amphotericin has precipitated acute delirium when administered intrathecally (Winn *et al.* 1979).

Antiviral agents

Of antiviral drugs, aciclovir has provoked delirium and visual hallucinations (Jones and Beier-Hanratty 1986), and ganciclovir provoked delirium in three per cent of subjects of clinical trials (Davey 1990).

Antiparasitic agents

Quinine (and its isomer quinidine used for cardiac arrhythmias) can cause a hyperactive delirium leading to coma when used in excessive dosage (Evans 1980). Chloroquine, mepacrine, amodiaquine, and niridazole can produce delirium and confusional states (Evans 1980; Hollister 1986). Mefloquine produces a range of adverse psychiatric effects, among which alterations in the level of consciousness and disorientation are sometimes seen, more frequently during therapeutic rather than prophylactic use (Palmer *et al.* 1993).

Antineoplastic agents

In cancer chemotherapy, the alkylating agents dacarbazine and hexamethylmelamine have been reported to cause delirium with an incidence of five per cent and 20 per cent respectively (Peterson and Popkin 1980). Colaspase has also produced delirium (Peterson and Popkin 1980), and as many as 50 per cent of 44 patients with metastatic cancer treated with interleukin-2 became delirious (Denicoff *et al.* 1987).

Mechanisms

The mechanisms by which these agents produce their adverse psychiatric effects are clearly various, and they are largely unknown. In many cases the drugs are used for severe illnesses in debilitated patients in whom other factors such as dehydration and pyrexia may predispose to delirium. In the case of isoniazid two other factors may be involved. Isoniazid is structurally related both to nicotinamide, vitamin B_3, and to iproniazid, a monoamine oxidase inhibitor. It inhibits the conversion of tryptophan to niacin by inducing a deficiency of pyridoxine coenzymes and can evoke manifestations of niacin deficiency, including pellagra, especially in malnourished patients. Treatment with niacin is effective in reversing such symptoms (Wallach and Gershon 1972). The inhibition of monoamine oxidase may also contribute to delirium by increasing central monoaminergic activity. In the case of 4-quinolones, these compounds have been shown to interact with the GABA/benzodiazepine receptor complex, displacing benzodiazepines from their binding sites (Unseld *et al.* 1990). A consequent decrease in GABA-ergic activity may contribute to the neurotoxic effects of these antibiotics. Other antibacterial and antiviral agents (e.g. streptomycin, aciclovir) are known to have direct neurotoxic effects but the exact mechanism by which they produce delirium is not understood. Drug withdrawal reactions, including delirium, are discussed on later in this chapter.

Dementia and associated states

Most forms of dementia caused by drugs are reversible and drug toxicity is the commonest cause of reversible dementia, accounting for approximately a third of such conditions (Bennett 1992). Elderly patients are the most susceptible. The reasons are partly pharmacokinetic, such as decreased efficiency of drug metabolism and elimination, and partly pharmacodynamic — a greater sensitivity to central nervous system depressants probably related to neuronal loss. An added factor is polypharmacy; because of the increased incidence of physical illnesses, elderly patients often accumulate multiple drug prescriptions over the years.

Dementia induced by drugs may be slow to resolve, continuing for weeks or months after discontinuation of the drug. Sometimes (e.g. after alcoholic detoxication) it does not resolve completely and the patient is left with some degree of cognitive impairment or personality change, presumably due to irreversible brain damage (Lipowski 1975). Lipowski (1975) also stressed that dementia, like any other syndrome, has degrees of severity. Sometimes it may cause mild impairments manifest only in situations that require a high level of intellectual performance; at the other extreme it may interfere with the basic necessities of living (Cummings 1995).

There are considerable methodological difficulties in studying drug-induced cognitive impairment, especially if the impairment develops insidiously and is mild and without obvious clinical signs. There have been few, if any, long-term prospective randomized trials which have adequately controlled for other variables which may affect cognitive performance, such as co-morbidity, use of other drugs, or cognitive level before drug use. Ethical considerations may add to the problems of devising such investigations. This section considers drugs that have been reported to produce any clinically significant cognitive impairment, especially of learning and memory — reversible, partially reversible, or irreversible.

Alcohol

The best known of drug-induced dementias is that caused by alcohol, which is the second most common adult dementia after Alzheimer's disease (Nace and Isbell 1991). The classical florid form is Korsakoff's syndrome, which consists of a retrograde amnesia combined with inability to form new memories, especially to recall the temporal sequence of events, and an apathetic loss of insight into the disability (Lancet 1990*a*). The full-blown Wernicke–Korsakoff syndrome is now rare, as it responds to treatment with thiamine and other vitamins. Wernicke's encephalopathy resolves readily with thiamine treatment but recovery of the Korsakoff state may be only partial: McEvoy (1982) estimated that 20 per cent of patients recover completely over a period of months to years; 60 per cent show some improvement, and 20 per cent improve only minimally. Eckardt and Martin (1986) reported that approximately nine per cent of alcoholics develop a degree of dementia, although some improvement occurs with abstinence. In some cases, global decrements in intelligence and of both episodic and semantic memory occur, giving a picture similar to Alzheimer's disease (Martin et al. 1989). In addition, Korsakoff's dementia may develop without prior overt Wernicke's encephalopathy (Lishman 1990). Lesser degrees of cognitive impairment are also commonly detected in alcoholics and moderate to heavy drinkers (Robertson 1984).

Acute alcohol intoxication can also have serious effects on memory. Alcoholic 'blackouts' — periods of retrograde amnesia — are associated with high blood alcohol concentrations and may occur in those not dependent on alcohol as well as at any time in the course of alcoholism (Nace and Isbell 1991). Memory impairment at blood alcohol concentrations of about 50 mg per 100 ml or more has also been demonstrated in numerous studies of normal subjects (e.g. Jones 1973).

Mechanisms

Several mechanisms combine to produce alcoholic dementia. Wernicke's encephalopathy is due to thiamine deficiency, associated with poor diet and reduced food absorption in alcoholism. There may also be a hereditary susceptibility related to genetic polymorphism for the transketolase enzyme which requires thiamine as a co-factor (Thomas 1986). This condition is treatable with thiamine but may sometimes go unrecognized. In a series of 51 cases diagnosed at necropsy, only seven had been recognized during life (Harper 1979). A pellagra-like state may also occur due to nicotinic acid deficiency.

Korsakoff's psychosis probably results from a combination of thiamine deficiency and direct neurotoxic effects of alcohol (Lishman et al. 1987; Lishman 1990). The latter effects may be due to accumulation of toxic metabolites which require the coenzyme nicotinamide adenine dinucleotide (NAD) for their metabolism (Rogers et al. 1981). In addition, a genetic deficiency of the cytochrome P-450 enzyme CYP2D6 may lead to the formation of a neurotoxic tetrahydroisoquinolone (J.R. Idle, personal communication). Korsakoff's dementia is associated with bilateral damage to diencephalic structures including the thalamus, mammillary bodies, and terminal portions of the fornix (Brierley 1977; Mair et al. 1979). Damage to the hippocampus, septal region, and cortex is sometimes found, and frontal-lobe lesions appear to be associated with confabulation. In Wernicke's encephalopathy the cerebellum is affected, accounting for the ataxia. Histological changes include demyelinization and neuronal loss, with proliferation of microglia and fibrous astrocytes. Vascular changes secondary to alcohol consumption may add to the brain pathology.

The reasons for the localized neuropathological damage associated with alcoholism are not clear (Thompson et al. 1988). However, brain imaging studies have shown that diffuse cerebral atrophy, both cortical and subcortical, is common in chronic alcoholics, even in the absence of Korsakoff's syndrome (Lishman 1990). It is estimated that one in 10 patients seen in alcohol treatment units have clinically obvious organic brain damage, and over half the remaining 90 per cent have demonstrable brain shrinkage and cognitive impairments on formal testing, although slight improvement in both structural and functional changes occurs after abstinence (Lee et al. 1979; *British Medical Journal* 1981). Neuropathological evidence suggests that the reversible changes are due to loss of synapses, while the irreversible component is due to loss of neurones (Thompson et al. 1988).

Acute alcohol intoxication can cause functional impairment of memory and cognitive performance by effects on a number of neuronal systems (reviewed by Lishman et al. 1987; Lishman 1990; Tabakoff and Hoffman 1990; Gonzales and Hoffman 1991; Peoples et al. 1996), including effects on cell membranes, synaptic transmission and GABA and NMDA receptor activity. Alcohol also affects the release and turnover of acetylcholine and monoamines, and pathological changes may involve neurones in the nucleus basalis and locus coeruleus (Lishman 1990).

Benzodiazepines

Benzodiazepines produce an anterograde amnesia, a property utilized, along with the sedative and anxiolytic actions, when the drugs are employed as premedication before surgery or for anaesthesia. The amnesic effect of normal doses has been investigated in several studies (Wolkowitz et al. 1987; Danion et al. 1989; Curran 1992; File et al. 1992; Weingartner et al. 1992; Vidailhet et al. 1996). Acquisition of new information is deficient, an effect that may be partly due to sedative actions, but there appear also to be specific amnesic effects which are separate from sedation. Episodic memory (the remembering of recent events), is particularly impaired, while semantic memory (memory for words), intermediate memory (the ability to recall digits over a few seconds), and retrieval are relatively unaffected. Zolpidem and zopiclone may have similar but less marked effects (Mendelson and Jain 1995). The effects on memory are more marked in heavy consumers of alcohol and the memory impairment is similar to that seen in alcoholic Korsakoff's syndrome.

The impairment of recent memory by benzodiazepines (e.g. triazolam) may lead to memory lapses (transient global amnesia) many hours after the drug has been taken (Morris and Estes 1987; Bixler et al. 1991; Woods et al. 1992; Rush et al. 1993) and it has sometimes led to charges of shoplifting (McClelland 1990). The elderly are particularly vulnerable to the amnesic effects of benzodiazepines, and forgetfulness, amnesic episodes, or confusion may resemble dementia in older patients taking benzodiazepines (Evans and Jarvis 1972).

Significant cognitive impairment also occurs in those taking benzodiazepines regularly for prolonged periods. Memory deficits were observed by Curran (1992) in patients who had taken benzodiazepines regularly for a mean of 10 years, and controlled studies have shown a variety of cognitive deficits in such patients (Hendler *et al.* 1980; Petursson *et al.* 1983; Brosan *et al.* 1986; Lucki *et al.* 1986; Golombok *et al.* 1988; Tata *et al.* 1994; Gorenstein *et al.* 1995). There is some evidence to suggest that cognitive impairment persists after benzodiazepine withdrawal (Borg 1987). Bergman and colleagues (1989) found slight but incomplete neuropsychological improvement in high-dose benzodiazepine abusers 4 to 6 years after stopping drug use and many ex-users of benzodiazepines complain that their intellectual functions have been permanently affected by them.

Mechanisms

The primary action of benzodiazepines is enhancement of GABA activity by an interaction with specific binding sites on $GABA_A$ receptors which increases the affinity of these receptors for GABA (Mohler and Okada 1977; Squires and Braestrup 1977; Costa 1981). GABA neurones consist of small interneurones forming widely distributed local circuits which exert a powerful inhibitory influence on the excitability of neighbouring neurones, and decrease the release of acetylcholine, noradrenaline, dopamine, and serotonin (Haefely *et al.* 1981). These neurotransmitters, especially acetylcholine, are crucially involved in memory systems, and it is possibly by such secondary effects that benzodiazepines exert their amnesic actions. Furthermore, GABA/benzodiazepine receptors in the human brain are found in high density in cerebral structures associated with memory processes (Eymin *et al.* 1992).

Some studies employing computerized tomography have suggested that benzodiazepine use is associated with enlarged cerebral ventricles or increased ventricular/brain ratio compared with controls (Lader *et al.* 1984; Schmauss and Krieg 1987; Uhde and Killner 1987; Bergman *et al.* 1989), although other studies have not agreed (Poser *et al.* 1983; Perera *et al.* 1987; Moodley *et al.* 1993). It remains unclear whether chronic benzodiazepine use causes cortical atrophy or other brain lesions, and, if so, whether the changes are reversible, but such changes if present might be associated with persisting cognitive impairment.

Anticonvulsant drugs

Some anticonvulsants can impair cognitive function, especially in patients receiving polytherapy. Effects are generally related to serum drug concentrations but cognitive impairments can occur at serum levels within the therapeutic range and without clinical signs of neurotoxicity (nystagmus, ataxia, etc.), and patients on anticonvulsants commonly complain of poor memory and mental slowing. The degree of cognitive impairment produced by drugs has been underestimated in the past (Reynolds 1978); it is important because the drugs are often taken for prolonged periods. Thus, patients may be subjected to years of drug-related intellectual dulling that might be amenable to reduction of dosage or the use of monotherapy. The effects of anticonvulsant drugs on cognitive function were reviewed by Trimble (1987), Vining (1987), and Smith and Beck (1992). Phenobarbitone, primidone, phenytoin, and benzodiazepines have been shown to impair cognitive function, while

carbamazepine, sodium valproate, and the newer anticonvulsants (e.g. gabapentin) produce relatively little impairment.

Mechanisms

The mechanisms of action of anticonvulsants are various. Phenobarbitone enhances the actions of GABA by interacting at a specific site on the $GABA_A$ receptor (Haefely 1990), and its mode of action on cognitive performance is probably similar to that of benzodiazepines. Phenytoin inhibits sodium-channel and T-type calcium-channel activity on neuronal membranes and may decrease calcium-mediated neurotransmitter release (Bleck and Klawans 1992). Phenobarbitone, primidone, and especially phenytoin, interfere with folic acid metabolism, and folic acid deficiency may possibly contribute to cognitive impairment during long-term treatment with these drugs (Trimble *et al.* 1980). Carbamazepine also inhibits sodium channels and may increase potassium-channel currents (Schmutz *et al.* 1992); in addition, it enhances GABA-ergic neurotransmission (Goodwin and Jamison 1990). The actions on ion channels are thought to be mainly responsible for the anticonvulsant and membrane-stabilizing activity of phenytoin and carbamazepine, but it is not clear whether they also account for the effects on cognitive function.

Lithium

Many patients taking lithium complain of memory problems. In pooled data from 12 investigations, memory problems were the third most frequently (28.2 per cent) reported subjective adverse effect of lithium, behind excessive thirst and polyuria (Goodwin and Jamison 1990), and were also the most important reason given by patients for non-compliance with lithium therapy. The effect was reported by euthymic patients and was not due to depression. Formal studies of the cognitive effects of lithium at usual therapeutic doses in normal subjects were reviewed by Judd and colleagues (1987). Lithium produces small but significant decrements in a wide range of cognitive tests, including memory tests, probably resulting from a slowing in rate of central information processing.

Results from studies of lithium effects on cognitive performance in patients have been conflicting: both detrimental effects and lack of significant effects have been reported in large numbers of studies (reviewed by Goodwin and Jamison 1990). The latter authors believe, however, that adverse cognitive effects from lithium are far from rare, and that they are too often dismissed as being secondary to the primary illness. The degree of cognitive impairment is usually dose related — another reason for keeping serum lithium concentrations at the lowest effective level. Hatcher and colleagues (1990) stress that patients treated with lithium should be warned that their ability to drive may be affected: these authors found that psychiatric outpatients on lithium had significantly slower reaction times than controls on a driving-simulator test.

Some patients may develop early signs of neurotoxicity at lithium serum concentrations of 1.3–2 mmol per litre or even at normal therapeutic serum concentrations; these include reversible confusion, cognitive impairment, lassitude, disorientation, slurred speech, restlessness, and irritability (Goodwin and Jamison 1990). More severe and incompletely reversible memory impairment may occur at higher serum concentrations (Saxena and Mallikarjuna 1988). A severe and sometimes irreversible encephalopathy can result from the combination of lithium and haloperidol (Cohen and Cohen 1974; Loudon and Waring 1976; Thomas 1979; Donaldson and Cunningham 1983; Goodwin and Jamison 1990). Similar reactions are described in combination with thioridazine (Spring 1979), thiothixene (Fetzer *et al.* 1981), and fluphenazine (Singh 1982).

Anticholinergic drugs

Anticholinergic drugs have marked and specific effects on memory. Drachman (1978) and Caine *et al.* (1981) showed in normal subjects that central cholinergic blockade with scopolamine (hyoscine) did not affect immediate memory (digit span) but selectively impaired the ability to store new information and to retrieve old information. The amnesic properties of hyoscine and atropine are a useful addition to their other anticholinergic effects when the drugs are administered as preoperative medication. Benzhexol, an anticholinergic drug widely used for its antiparkinsonian effects, has also been shown to impair memory functions in non-demented geriatric patients at a dose of 2 mg (Potamianos and Kellett 1982) and in normal subjects (King and Henry 1992). It is possible that the use of anticholinergic agents may contribute to cognitive impairment in patients with Parkinson's disease or in those taking neuroleptic drugs.

Mechanisms

Abundant evidence indicates that it is in cholinergic synapses that specific alterations vital to learning and memory occur (Deutsch 1971; Drachman 1978; Squire and Davis 1981). Both muscarinic and nicotinic receptors are involved in cholinergic transmission at cortical and subcortical levels in the brain. The amnesic effects of hyoscine and atropine are ascribed to muscarinic receptors, but drugs which act on nicotinic receptors (e.g. nicotine) also affect memory. The memory deficits produced by anticholinergic drugs resemble those which develop in Alzheimer's disease, and this observation led to the search for cholinergic loss and the use of cholinergic drugs (e.g. tacrine) in this condition. It is also suggested (Drachman 1978) that a degree of central acetylcholine depletion occurs in normal ageing and this may account for the increased susceptibility of the elderly to the amnesic effects of anticholinergic drugs.

Neuroleptics

The effects of neuroleptics on memory and cognitive performance have been reviewed by King (1990), King and Henry (1992), and Judd and colleagues (1987). Although many of these drugs have anticholinergic actions, they generally have only mild effects on learning and memory in normal subjects. Sedative effects with chlorpromazine and thioridazine may depress psychomotor function and sustained attention, but higher cognitive functions appear to be relatively unaffected.

Haloperidol actually improved performance in some tests, such as choice reaction time and selective attention in normal subjects (King and Henry 1992; Williams *et al.* 1996). In schizophrenic patients, trifluoperazine and haloperidol improved short-term memory, while chlorpromazine and thioridazine slightly impaired short-term verbal memory but not immediate, long-term, or visual short-term memory (Eitan *et al.* 1992). It is suggested that haloperidol improves the filtering of irrelevant stimuli (latent inhibition) in schizophrenics (Williams *et al.* 1996).

However, there is evidence suggesting that neuroleptic drugs may hasten cognitive deterioration in patients with dementia (Holmes *et al.* 1997; McShane *et al.* 1997). Both authors found that an increased rate of cognitive decline in patients with dementia was significantly associated with the use of neuroleptics. In patients with Alzheimer's disease, the combination of neuroleptic use and the apolipoprotein E ε4 allele carried greater risk of rapid cognitive decline (Holmes *et al.* 1997). It is clearly important to investigate which neuroleptics increase the risk, and whether drugs with lesser anticholinergic activity, such as haloperidol, or the newer antipsychotic drugs, such as sulpiride, clozapine, olanzepine and others, carry a lower risk (Bentham *et al.* 1997; Tobiansky and Blanchard 1997).

Antidepressants

Many tricyclic antidepressant drugs have prominent anticholinergic as well as sedative effects and may cause memory and other cognitive impairments. The effects of antidepressants with different sedative and anticholinergic profiles on memory and psychomotor functions have been investigated in normal subjects (Louwerens *et al.* 1986; Judd *et al.* 1987; Curran *et al.* 1988). Imipramine, amitriptyline, and also trazodone have all produced cognitive impairments following acute or long-term administration.

In psychiatric patients receiving antidepressants (mainly imipramine which has definite anticholinergic effects), Davies and colleagues (1977) reported a high incidence of 'confusional episodes' defined as a behavioural change characterized by impaired orientation or memory, or other evidence of acute intellectual impairment. Such episodes occurred in 13 per cent of the total sample of 150 patients but increased to 35 per cent in those over 40 years of age. Of the 20 patients who developed this syndrome (16 with depressive disorder, three with schizophrenia, one with character disorder), 11 were also receiving the anticholinergic agent benztropine along with perphenazine. It would appear that older age increases susceptibility to cognitive impairment especially when a combination of anticholinergic drugs is administered.

A study of patients with depression successfully treated with amitriptyline showed slight slowing of reaction time and minimal impairment of performance in a divided attention task compared with controls (Gerhard and Hobi 1986). These authors commented that the changes were not sufficient to rule out safe car driving.

Cannabis

Acute effects of cannabis include significant cognitive and

psychomotor impairments with marked disruption of memory, short-term memory being particularly susceptible. Research in this area has been reviewed by Golding (1992). In general, cannabis has been shown to impair immediate memory with little impairment of recall of previously stored information. In addition, a frequent error is the intrusion of unrelated material, suggesting a failure to filter out irrelevant information during the memory encoding process. The effects on memory may persist for more than 24 hours after the last dose and seriously impair performance in complicated tasks such as piloting in a flight simulator (Leirer *et al.* 1991).

Chronic cannabis users are also cognitively impaired even when not 'high'. This may be due to the very slow elimination of cannabinoids and their active metabolites which are stored in fatty tissues (tissue elimination half-life approximately 7 days) so that regular cannabis users may be chronically intoxicated. Such individuals have been shown in many studies to perform less well than controls, particularly in tasks involving attention, memory, and complex information processing (Schwartz *et al.* 1991; Fletcher *et al.* 1996; Pope and Yurgelun Todd 1996; and others reviewed by Golding 1992; Hall *et al.* 1994). The question of whether cognitive impairment is a permanent sequela of chronic cannabis use has been much debated (Schwartz 1991; Hall *et al.* 1994; Solowij 1995) although the evidence suggests that increasing duration of use leads to progressively greater impairment. It is not known to what extent such impairment may recover with prolonged abstinence.

Mechanisms

The psychological effects of cannabis are exerted by cannabinoids, particularly Δ^9-tetrahydrocannabinol, acting on central cannabinoid receptors (Devane *et al.* 1988; Matsuda *et al.* 1990). High densities of these receptors are found in the hippocampus and cerebral cortex, suggesting a role in cognitive function. Central cannabinoid receptors belong to a family of G-protein-coupled receptors which act through second-messenger systems. Cannabinoids have been shown to exert powerful inhibitory effects on adenylate cyclase, thus decreasing the responsiveness of neurones by inhibiting calcium and possibly potassium ion conductance (Howlett *et al.* 1990; Deadwyler *et al.* 1995; Pertwee 1995). Interactions with other neurotransmitters, including cholinergic and monoaminergic systems, are not yet fully understood but may be involved in the cognitive effects of cannabis.

Cocaine and amphetamine

Permanent cognitive deficits, including dementia, can result from chronic high-dose cocaine and amphetamine abuse (Fischman 1987; Manschreck *et al.* 1987; Pascual-Leone *et al.* 1991; Lacayo 1995). These abnormalities are probably secondary to drug-induced cardiovascular pathology including cerebrovascular accidents, transient ischaemic episodes, and necrotizing angiitis (Fischman 1987; Lacayo 1995). Multifocal areas of hypoperfusion in the frontal and temporal regions in chronic cocaine abusers without a history of cerebrovascular accidents have been shown in single-positron-emission computed tomography (SPECT) studies (Tumeh *et al.* 1990).

3,4-methylenedioxymethamphetamine (MDMA, 'Ecstasy')

Cognitive impairment has been demonstrated in chronic MDMA users (Krystal and Price 1992; Curran and Travill 1997; Parrott *et al.* 1997). Conclusions from these studies are limited by the fact that most of the MDMA users also took other recreational drugs, including alcohol and cannabis. Nevertheless, the results suggest that MDMA may cause cognitive damage which may not always be reversible. MDMA is known to cause degeneration of serotonergic neurones. Serotonergic systems are involved in normal memory function, and it is suggested that memory problems in MDMA users may be caused by serotonergic degeneration in the hipocampus and/or frontal cortex (Parrott *et al.* 1997).

Phencyclidine

Chronic use of phencyclidine has been reported to cause loss of memory (*British Medical Journal* 1980) and persisting neuropsychological damage (Russ and Wong 1979; Gorelick and Balster 1995). Although phencyclidine use has declined in recent years, ketamine is increasing in popularity as a recreational drug and may have similar effects. Other effects and mechanisms of action of phencyclidine and ketamine are discussed later in this chapter.

Organic solvents

Chronic exposure to organic solvents can occur in many occupations, such as dry cleaning, the paint industry, and mechanical and engineering occupations involving degreasing. White and Proctor (1997) have reviewed the hazards of such exposure. Mild cases show cognitive deficits, attentional impairment, motor slowing or inco-ordination, visuospatial deficits, and short-term memory loss. Permanent mild cognitive deficits may ensue. Severe cases may resemble multiple sclerosis or cerebrovascular dementia, and a chronic toxic encephalopathy with dementia may develop. Acute toxic encephalopathy may be seen in recreational solvent abusers and repeated abuse over a long period may also lead to permanent cognitive impairment. The exact mechanism of toxicity varies with different solvents, but the agents, being lipid soluble, tend to accumulate in the brain and exert direct neurotoxic effects.

Organophosphates

Organophosphates are irreversible inhibitors of the enzyme acetylcholinesterase and lead to excessive accumulation of acetylcholine followed by overstimulation of cholinergic neurones. High-dose exposure, as in the case of nerve gases used in chemical warfare, leads to a cascade of events recently illuminated by Solberg and Belkin (1997). Convulsions due to excessive cholinergic activity cause excessive glutamate release, NMDA (*N*-methyl-D-aspartate) receptor activation, calcium accumulation, and cell death. Less dramatic sequelae may follow chronic or repeated exposure to organophosphates used as pesticides or sheep dips. Such exposure may cause insomnia, nightmares, anxiety, tremor, depression, drowsiness, poly-neuropathy, impairment of concentration, decreased speed of information processing, and other delayed neurobehavioural effects (Stephens et al. 1995; Lader 1997; O'Malley 1997). The cognitive impairments may be long-lasting and perhaps contribute to the neuropsychological complaints associated with the 'Gulf War syndrome' in exposed military personnel. Chronic neurotoxic effects including memory impairment associated with chronic low-level exposure to the organochloride insecticide chlordane have also been reported (O'Malley 1997).

Depression

Many psychoactive drugs can cause both depressive and manic reactions. The degree of drug-induced mood changes is variable and may not necessarily constitute a major psychiatric disorder. Some drugs are actively sought out for their euphoric effects (e.g. recreational drugs); others are prescribed as treatments for various disorders (therapeutic drugs). In the latter case, attribution of mood change to a particular drug can be difficult, since the condition may be due to the illness being treated, to drug combinations, or to other adverse effects of the drug such as apathy, anorexia, or insomnia that may be mistakenly interpreted as depression. Problems of diagnosis are discussed by Edwards (1989a).

Cardiovascular drugs

Older antihypertensive drugs

Reserpine, methyldopa, guanethidine, debrisoquine, beth-anidine, and clonidine cause central depletion of monoamines or interference with monoamine neurotransmission, and depression was a known risk of their use (Paykel et al. 1982; Edwards 1989a).

β-Adrenoreceptor antagonists

β-Adrenoceptor antagonists are still widely used for hypertension, angina, and cardiac arrhythmias, and all of them have been associated with depression. The incidence of depression was estimated, after review of over 30 studies, to be about one per cent with propranolol (Paykel et al. 1982). Propranolol was followed by the introduction of less lipophilic congeners which enter the brain less readily, and which appear less likely to cause depression (Paykel 1982). Nevertheless, mild depression has been reported with oxprenolol (Paykel 1982), nadolol (Russell and Shuckit 1982), metoprolol (Assayheen and Michell 1982), and practolol (Wiseman 1971), and psychiatric symptoms have been reported with atenolol (Arber 1988). Mild depression has also been reported with pindolol (Morgan et al. 1974; Paykel et al. 1982). In addition, topical application of timolol and betax-olol eye drops have provoked suicidal depression (Nolan 1982; Orlando 1986).

Many of these drugs cause fatigue, sleep disturbances, and dysphoria which may be interpreted as depression, and Edwards (1989a) concluded that true depression is not common but may be more likely in those with a positive family or past history. Guidelines for the management of the depressed hypertensive patient were provided by Paykel and colleagues (1982). Mechanisms by which β-receptor antagonists may produce depression include interference with central adrenergic neuro-transmission and central serotonin-antagonism, which has been shown for propranolol (Middlemiss et al. 1977). In addition, pindolol directly antagonizes the 5-HT$_{1A}$ receptor (Pérez et al. 1997).

Calcium-channel blockers

Calcium-channel blockers, used for angina and hypertension, have been associated with depression. For example, treatment resistance in established cases of severe depression has been related to concurrent nifedipine therapy (Eccleston and Cole 1990), and eight cases of severe depression apparently resulting from diltiazem therapy have been reported (Biriell et al. 1989). The mechanism of the effect may be interference with intra-neuronal calcium homoeostasis, affecting the synthesis and release of neurotransmitters (Turner and Goldin 1985; Hullett et al. 1988).

Other cardiovascular drugs

Psychiatric adverse effects sometimes occur with diuretics; cases of depression have been reported but these are probably due to indirect effects including hyponatraemia, hypokalaemia, concomitant drugs, or the underlying illness (Paykel 1982; Edwards 1989a). Depression has classically been associated with digitalis preparations, but it is usually part of a more generalized toxic state or due to the cardiac disease rather than the drug (Edwards 1989a). There have been reports of depression with the α-adrenoceptor-blocker prazosin (Edwards et al. 1987) and the antiarrhythmic drug flecainide (Drerup 1988) and possibly intravenous lignocaine (Saravay et al. 1987).

Cholesterol-lowering agents

Several reports have suggested a linkage between cholesterol lowering and mortality from non-cardiac causes, mainly sui-cides, violence, and accidents (Muldoon et al. 1990; Chen et al. 1991). There is considerable doubt concerning the reality of this association and whether any linkage is causal (Wysowski and Gross 1990; Betteridge 1993; Kassler-Taub et al. 1993). However, some studies have shown an increased rate of suicide (Lindberg et al. 1992), alcohol-related disease (Neaton et al. 1992), and depression (Morgan et al. 1993) in subjects with low plasma cholesterol levels. A suggested mechanism is that lowered blood cholesterol concentration could cause alterations in central transmitter function leading to depression (Engelberg 1992). However, a meta-analysis showed that the increase in violent deaths related only to patients who had been treated by drugs rather than by low cholesterol diets (Schmidt 1992), and the possibility arose that cholesterol-lowering drugs may directly affect brain function. Experiments to date have not confirmed this relationship, at least for brain 5-HT function (Delva *et al.* 1996).

Depressive symptoms have occurred in patients treated with pravastatin (Leichleitner *et al.* 1992) and simvastatin (Duits and Bos 1993) for hypercholesterolaemia, and sleep disturbance has been reported with simvastatin (Barth *et al.* 1990) and lovostatin (Sinzinger *et al.* 1994). In general, however, it is unlikely that any of the cholesterol-lowering agents directly cause depression (Shetty and Routledge 1990; Elliott 1992; Harrison and Ashton 1994; Cutler *et al.* 1995). It remains possible that acute lowering of serum cholesterol or alteration of plasma triglycerides (Fowkes *et al.* 1992) may cause depression with violent tendencies in some subjects.

Hormones

Glucocorticoids

Depression is common in Cushing's disease, occurring in 15–20 per cent of cases. Severe depression with risk of suicide can also occur as an adverse reaction to glucocorticoid therapy, although it is less common than euphoria. The Boston Collaborative Drug Surveillance Program (BCDSP 1971) noted that steroids were the commonest cause of serious psychiatric reactions in medical wards. Analysis of 718 consecutive admissions receiving prednisone (BCDSP 1972) found 21 patients with acute psychiatric reactions; six patients were manic and two seriously depressed; others had paranoid delusions, hallucinations, violent behaviour, and other symptoms. A definite dose-related effect was identified, the incidence of psychiatric disorder rising from 1.3 per cent on doses of prednisone below 40 mg daily to 18.4 per cent on doses over 80 mg daily. However, psychiatric reactions can also appear at low doses (Greeves 1984). Underlying conditions, such as multiple sclerosis, or a positive family history, may increase vulnerability in some patients (Hollister 1986). Prolonged glucocorticoid treatment may lead to pituitary–adrenal suppression with psychiatric symptoms, including depression on withdrawal.

Steroid psychoses have been relieved by spacing out the daily dosage or switching to an enteric-coated formulation, both of which reduce peak blood concentrations (Glynne-Jones *et al.* 1986). Successful treatment or prophylaxis of steroid psychoses with lithium has also been reported (Falk *et al.* 1979; Goggans *et al.* 1983; Terao *et al.* 1997): Brown and colleagues (1997) note that the adverse psychiatric effects of corticosteroids and their treatment responses are strikingly similar to those of bipolar affective disorder. The mechanism is not clear, but many brain neurones contain corticosteroid receptors (McEwen 1995) which interact with central serotonin receptors. This interaction may in part explain the effects on mood (Young *et al.* 1994).

Oestrogens and progestogens

There has been controversy on whether oestrogens or progestogens, or both, used for oral contraception or as hormone replacement therapy can cause depression. Several large studies, reviewed by Edwards (1989*a*), gave conflicting results. One (Vessey *et al.* 1985) found no difference in the incidence of depressive neurosis or affective psychosis in 9504 women taking oral contraceptives compared with 7242 women using other contraceptive methods; in another study, of 23 000 women on oral contraceptives, Kay (1984) reported a significant relationship between the strength of the oestrogen component of the preparation used and the prevalence of depression (but not suicide). It was not possible to demonstrate a relationship with the progestogen content. The overall results of many studies suggest a slight increase in depressive symptoms in women taking high oestrogen formulations, but this risk is probably minimal with the present use of lower-oestrogen contraceptives.

Women with a previous history of depression may be more likely to develop depressive symptoms with oral contraceptives, but in some women the symptoms are the same as in premenstrual tension present before oral contraceptive use. In contrast, other women obtain relief from premenstrual tension, and some report an increased sense of well-being when taking oral contraceptives or hormone-replacement therapy. In the *British National Formulary* (1997) depression is listed as an adverse effect of oestrogen hormone-replacement therapy, and depression, insomnia, and somnolence are listed as ill effects of progestogens. Suggested mechanisms of depression with oral contraception are that progestogens enhance MAO activity (Grant and Pryse-Davies 1968) and that oestrogens in high doses reduce serotonin synthesis by causing pyridoxine deficiency (Edwards 1989*a*). However, pyridoxine was not effective in depression occurring in women on oral contraceptives (Adams 1980). Oestrogens also modulate 5-HT$_{1A}$ receptor function (Young *et al.* 1993).

Testosterone and derivatives; anabolic steroids

Depression is common in withdrawal of anabolic steroids from dependent subjects but depression with suicidal ideation can also occur during use, especially of high doses (Pope and Katz 1987; Brower *et al.* 1989). Psychiatric effects of anabolic–androgenic steroids have been reviewed by Williamson and Young (1992), Brower (1991), Pope and Katz (1988), and Karch (1996).

Other anabolic steroids including nandrolone, occasionally used in aplastic anaemia and osteoporosis in postmenopausal women, and stanozolol, used for vascular manifestations of Beçhet's disease and hereditary angioedema, can also cause depression (*British National Formulary* 1997).

Anxiolytics, hypnotics, sedatives

Long-term use of benzodiazepines can induce depression, aggravate pre-existing depression, and provoke suicide (Lader and Petursson 1981; Priest and Montgomery 1987; Ashton 1987, 1995*a*; CSM 1988). Depression was also described with long-term use of barbiturates (Tollefson 1980) and bromides (Davison and Hassanyeh 1991), and is a common feature of alcoholism (Hollister 1986). Depression which can be severe, protracted, and lead to suicide, also occurs in benzodiazepine withdrawal in dependent patients (Petursson and Lader 1981; Olajide and Lader 1984; Busto *et al.* 1986; Ashton 1987, 1995*b*). The mechanisms are not known but probably involve disturbances of central monoamine activity (Nutt 1996).

Antipsychotic drugs

The question of whether antipsychotic drugs can cause depression is still somewhat controversial. By 1980 more than 30 publications (reviewed by Ananth and Chadirian 1980) had noted an association between depression and the use of all types of neuroleptics in schizophrenic and manic patients. Even recently Willner (1995) stated that depression is frequently encountered as an adverse effect of neuroleptic therapy in schizophrenia, while the *British National Formulary* (1997) lists depression as an adverse effect of chlorpromazine and advises that fluphenazine should be avoided in depression.

Critical analysis of the evidence, however, reviewed by Hirsch (1982), Siris (1991), and Edwards (1989a), indicates that depressive symptoms occurring in schizophrenia are generally not due to antipsychotic treatment. First, many studies show that such symptoms usually improve during antipsychotic therapy, and depressive symptoms may increase if antipsychotics are withdrawn (Wistedt and Palmstierna 1983). Secondly, a comparison of 74 schizophrenic patients on placebo or depot fluphenazine showed that symptoms of depression were as common in the placebo group as in the active-treatment group (Hirsch et al. 1973). Thirdly, several studies found no relationship between dosage, or plasma or cerebrospinal fluid concentrations of neuroleptics and the presence of depressive symptoms in schizophrenia. Finally, neuroleptics with antidepressants are effective as treatments for psychotic or agitated depression (Robertson and Trimble 1983).

Thus the weight of evidence suggests that antipsychotics are an unlikely cause of depression. On the other hand, some adverse effects of neuroleptic drugs, such as akinesia, akathisia, lethargy, and sedation may be mistakenly diagnosed as depression (Siris 1991). In addition, negative symptoms of schizophrenia such as apathy, affective flattening, and impaired volition may be revealed by treatment with some antipsychotics. Furthermore, changes in affect may be part of the schizophrenic illness itself and some studies suggest that these changes may respond to antidepressant drugs.

Nevertheless, a few case reports suggest that metoclopramide, a dopamine-receptor antagonist without antipsychotic properties except in high dosage, can precipitate a depressive syndrome (Weddington and Banner 1986; Feder 1987).

Antidepressant drugs

Somewhat paradoxically, increases in some depressive symptoms have sometimes been linked with the therapeutic use of antidepressant drugs in patients with depression. For example, some studies have suggested that fluoxetine might cause an increase in suicidal ideation in a subgroup of depressed patients (Daluji and Ferguson 1988; Dasgupta 1990; Hoover 1990; Teicher et al. 1990; Masand et al. 1991; and others cited by Beasley et al. 1991). However, a comprehensive meta-analysis of pooled data from 17 double-blind clinical trials (Beasley et al. 1991) found no excess risk of suicidal acts or emergence of substantial suicidal thoughts associated with fluoxetine, and it seems unlikely that antidepressants in general have this effect.

A second observation is that some depressed patients, after an initial positive response, apparently become unresponsive to antidepressants. Donaldson (1989) described three patients with major depression who were treated with phenelzine. After an excellent early response, each patient relapsed while still on treatment and developed a depression which was more severe than before, and which was chronic and refractory to all other drug treatments or ECT. Mann (1983) described four other cases. Similar apparent tolerance has been described with tricyclic antidepressants (Zetin et al. 1983; Cohen and Baldessarini 1985). The mechanism of these effects is not clear but it was suggested that they could be due to lasting receptor or transmitter changes.

There are several reports of long-lasting depression after long-term repeated or high-dose use of MDMA (Benazzi and Mazzoli 1991; McGuire et al. 1994a), and Green and Goodwin (1996) suggest that neurotoxicity in humans may occur slowly and insidiously, causing depression after a delay of several years. Other effects of this drug and possible mechanisms are given elsewhere in this chapter. Depression is also a feature of many drug-withdrawal reactions, described later in this chapter.

Appetite suppressants

Depression, sometimes severe, has also been observed both in withdrawal and during treatment with appetite suppressants including fenfluramine, dexfenfluramine, diethylproprion, and phentermine (Edwards 1989a; McTavish and Heel 1992; Silverstone 1992; CSM 1993a). Fenfluramine and dexfenfluramine have now been withdrawn because of cardiac complications (CSM 1997).

Drugs used in Parkinson's disease

Depression has been reported as an adverse effect of levodopa in patients with Parkinson's disease (Edwards 1989a). Pearce (1984), states that depression occurs in half of all patients given levodopa and responds to antidepressant drugs, although confusion and psychostimulant effects are also common psychiatric reactions. It is not always clear whether depression is due to the drug or the disease (in which depression is an integral feature). In some patients depression may be associated with the 'off' phase of the 'on-off' phenomenon associated with levodopa treatment of Parkinson's disease (Nissenbaum et al. 1987). Depression has also been associated with the use of amantadine and other drugs in Parkinson's disease, usually as part of a more generalized psychiatric disturbance.

Anticonvulsants

Several anticonvulsant drugs have been associated with depression in epileptic patients. However, such patients are already at increased risk of psychiatric disorders and anticonvulsant drugs are not uncommonly used in combination. Thus the contribution of any particular drug or dosage to the development of depression may be difficult to ascertain. Phenobarbitone, primidone, and phenytoin can cause depression

(Tollefson 1980; *Drug and Therapeutics Bulletin* 1994). Depression has also been described with carbamazepine (Gardner and Cowdry 1986) and ethosuximide (Buchanan 1972), and as an adverse effect of vigabatrin and topiramide it is cited in the *British National Formulary* (1997).

Analgesics

Pure opioid agonists such as morphine may cause dysphoria in one to two per cent of patients treated for chronic pain, but the incidence of dysphoria is much higher (10 per cent) with mixed agonists/antagonists such as pentazocine, nalbuphine, and butanorphol (Twycross andc McQuay 1989). Of the commonly used NSAID, the incidence of adverse effects, both somatic and psychiatric, is greatest with indomethacin, which may aggravate depression or other psychiatric disorders, epilepsy, and Parkinson's disease (Sunshine and Olsen 1989). Depression may also be encountered during treatment with phenylbutazone' (Edwards 1989a).

Anti-infective drugs

Antibacterial agents

Depression is not a commonly reported adverse effect of antibacterial agents. However, among the adverse psychiatric effects of antituberculous agents, mental depression, drowsiness and asthenia, along with restlessness and tremor, are common with ethionamide, and a number of neuropsychiatric effects are associated with cycloserine (Mandell and Petri 1996). These appear within the first 2 weeks of therapy, stopping on withdrawal, and include somnolence, headache, tremor, dysarthria, confusion, nervousness, irritability, psychotic states with suicidal tendencies, and catatonic and depressive reactions.

Antimalarial agents

Mefloquine can produce a variety of neuropsychiatric effects which may include anxiety, depression, and dysphoria but more usually features psychotic manifestations or hallucinations (Palmer *et al.* 1993). Other antimalarials rarely produce psychiatric effects.

Antifungal agents

Only griseofulvin has been reported to be associated with adverse psychiatric effects (Bennett 1996), which include lethargy, mental confusion, psychomotor impairment, fatigue, depression, and augmentation of the depressant effects of alcohol. Headache, which may be severe, occurs in 15 per cent of cases.

Antiviral agents

These agents have been reviewed by Hayden (1996). Neurotoxic effects and other physical symptoms are common but do not usually include depression. Somnolence and lethargy occur with combinations of zidovudine and aciclovir; behavioural disturbances with ganciclovir and vidarabine; insomnia with zidovudine, didanosine, and amantadine. Amantadine, however, has induced depression and other psychological disturbances (Flaherty and Bellur 1981).

Antineoplastic drugs

Interferons are used in the treatment of malignant disease and severe viral infections. Dose-related psychiatric effects include impaired concentration, anxiety, depression, and fatigue (Adams *et al.* 1984; Renault *et al.* 1987; Hayden 1996). Alkylating agents such as dacarbazine may also induce depression (Peterson and Popkin 1980). Of the antimetabolites, intravenous fluouracil may cause mood lability (Peterson and Popkin 1980), and when used topically for actinic keratosis has been reported to cause depression in 25 per cent of cases (Milstein 1980). Vincristine, vinblastine, and colaspase have also induced depression (Peterson and Popkin 1980). These are all extremely toxic drugs and depressed mood may result from other unpleasant effects such as nausea, vomiting, and alopecia.

Miscellaneous

Both cimetidine (Jefferson 1979) and ranitidine (Billings and Stein 1986) have been reported to cause depression. There have been reports of severe depression following the use of oral etritinate and isoretinoin for psoriasis and acne (Hazen *et al.* 1983; Borbujo *et al.* 1987; Henderson and Highet 1989). Depression is listed as an adverse effect of baclofen (*British National Formulary* 1997), and depression lasting several weeks is reported as a postanaesthetic effect of halothane and isoflurane (Davison *et al.* 1975). There are isolated reports of depression associated with the use of other drugs (Edwards 1989a) but , as with several of the drugs mentioned here, it is not clear whether such reactions are due to the drug or the disease. Severe depression has been described as a chronic effect of hallucinogenic drugs (Seymour and Smith 1991).

Mania and hypomania

Dopaminergic drugs

Cocaine, amphetamine

There is strong evidence that dopamine is involved in reward pathways in the brain (Nutt 1996) and many drugs that enhance central dopaminergic activity produce euphoria in normal subjects. Although most of these drugs also increase noradrenergic activity, the euphoric effect appears to be mediated through dopaminergic pathways since it is antagonized by dopamine receptor antagonists but not by adrenoceptor antagonists (Willner 1995). In some doses and in some subjects the initial euphoria induced by dopaminergic agents can escalate to psychiatric states which closely resemble mania or hypomania. For example, acute intoxication with cocaine or amphetamine is characterized by euphoria, impulsiveness, rapid thoughts, hyperactivity, irritability, and suspiciousness (Cocores *et al.* 1991). The result in both cases can be a florid manic or hypomanic state which responds to dopamine-receptor-blocking antipsychotic drugs.

Drugs used in Parkinson's disease

The dopamine precursor, levodopa, can induce dose-related hypomania or mania in patients with Parkinson's disease; the incidence appears to be only about 1.5 per cent, while other psychiatric complications (including delirium, depression, agitation, and paranoid psychosis) are more common (Goodwin 1971). Levodopa may also precipitate hypomanic episodes in patients with bipolar affective disorder (Bunney *et al.* 1972). The dopamine-receptor agonist bromocriptine, and amantadine, which is thought to increase dopamine release, have also precipitated mania in patients with Parkinson's disease. Mania has rarely been reported in patients treated with bromocriptine for suppression of lactation (Brook and Cookson 1978; Vlissides *et al.* 1978) or pituitary tumours (Turner *et al.* 1984). Other dopaminergic drugs used in Parkinson's disease including the dopamine-receptor stimulants apomorphine, lysuride, and pergolide, and the monoamine oxidase B inhibitor selegeline can produce psychiatric effects including euphoria, restlessness, confusion, and psychosis.

Mechanisms

Exactly why these drugs should produce mania, or what relationship mania bears to their euphoric effects, is not clear, but it is notable that the same drugs also produce other psychiatric effects, including paranoid psychoses and in some cases depression. By different mechanisms, they all increase central dopaminergic activity (cocaine by reuptake block; amphetamine by increased dopamine release; levodopa by increased synthesis; and bromocriptine by receptor stimulation), and dopamine activation in mesolimbic pathways, especially the nucleus accumbens, appears to be important for euphoriant effects. Many of these drugs, including cocaine, amphetamine, other psychostimulants, and bromocriptine (Ross and Ward 1992), are subject to abuse because of their euphoriant effects. Possibly, excessive dopaminergic stimulation and spread of activation to other pathways may produce a range of abnormal psychiatric states ranging through hypomania to mania and other psychoses. Supersensitivity of dopamine receptors has been suggested to account for mania which sometimes occurs on amphetamine withdrawal (Miller 1991).

Sympathomimetic agents

Drugs which by various mechanisms increase adrenergic activity (and in some cases also dopaminergic activity) can also produce mania or hypomania, which has been described with pseudoephedrine (Wood 1994), phenylpropanolamine (Grieger *et al.* 1990), phenylephrine, and ephedrine (Waters and Lapierre 1981). Mania or hypomania has also been described with aminophylline, theophylline, and caffeine (Davison and Hassanyeh 1991). In addition, the bronchodilator salbutamol, a β-adrenoceptor agonist, can cause euphoria and mania (Jacquot and Bottari 1981) and is sometimes abused for its euphoric effects.

Antidepressant drugs

Manic or hypomanic reactions have been attributed to all types of antidepressant drugs including monoamine oxidase inhibitors, tricyclics, SSRI, and atypical antidepressant agents. Some

monoamine oxidase inhibitors, especially tranylcypromine, but also to some extent phenelzine, have amphetamine-like actions and are sometimes abused for their euphoric effects (Tyrer 1982; Varzopoulos and Krull 1991). Hypomania has been precipitated in depressed patients by tranylcypromine and phenelzine (Remick *et al.* 1989), and also by pargyline used to treat both depression and hypertension (Folks and Arnold 1983). Procarbazine, a monoamine oxidase inhibitor used to treat Hodgkin's disease, was reported to aggravate mania in a patient also receiving prednisolone (Carney *et al.* 1982). Cases of mania apparently precipitated by withdrawal from isocarboxazid and during treatment with isoniazid have also been described (Rothschild 1985; Stasick and Zatin 1985).

Tricyclic antidepressants can also precipitate mania, especially in patients with bipolar depression (Tyrer 1993). The risk is much lower in unipolar depression; about 2.5 per cent of patients with recurrent unipolar depression developed hypomania during continuing treatment with imipramine (Kupfer *et al.* 1988). Rapid cycling of mood in manic-depressive patients has been attributed to tricyclic antidepressants (Wehr and Goodwin 1979), and mania is sometimes provoked by tricyclic withdrawal (Mirin *et al.* 1981; Nelson *et al.* 1983; Gupta and Narang 1986). Mania has also been described in children (aged 6–12 years) treated for depression with nortriptyline for 25 weeks or more (Bunney and Garland 1982).

Drugs which enhance serotonergic activity can also provoke mania, which has been reported with SSRI, including fluoxetine (Lebegue 1987), citalopram (White *et al.* 1986), and sertraline (Laporta *et al.* 1987). Mania has also been reported with trazodone (Knobler *et al.* 1986; Jabeen and Fisher 1991). There are also numerous reports of hypomania or mania following administration of the serotonin precursors L-tryptophan or 5-hydroxytryptophan, in both psychiatric and non-psychiatric patients (Meltzer and Lowy 1987); fenfluramine has also been implicated (Stasick and Zetin 1985).

Alprazolam, a benzodiazepine reputed to have antidepressant activity (Feighner 1982), shares with other antidepressants the ability to cause mania, which has been reported in a few case studies (France and Krishnan 1984; Arana *et al.* 1985; Burke 1987; Goodman and Charney 1987; Cole and Kando 1993). Discontinuation or reduction of dosage of lithium in patients with bipolar affective disorder is liable to lead to manic relapse (Margo and McMahon 1982; Mander and Loudon 1988; Goodwin 1994); the risk is less in patients with unipolar depression, who are more likely to have a relapse of depression (Tyrer *et al.* 1983).

Mechanisms

Antidepressants in general increase synaptic concentrations of monoamines (by inhibition of monoamine oxidase or of monoamine reuptake systems). Monoamine oxidase inhibitors increase synaptic concentrations of dopamine, noradrenaline, and serotonin; the antidepressant reuptake inhibitors increase concentrations mainly of noradrenaline or serotonin with varying degrees of selectivity. All have been used as drugs of abuse; monoamine oxidase inhibitors (Tyrer 1982), tricyclics (Cohen *et al.* 1978; Cantor 1979; Dorman *et al.* 1995), and SSRI (Singh and Catalan 1996), apparently for their euphoriant effects.

However, as stated above, the relation between drug-induced euphoria and the ability to provoke hypomania or mania is not clear. Furthermore, the extent to which the drugs uncover a latent manic-depressive disorder remains debatable; the risk of manic reactions is greatly increased in bipolar affective disorder.

Anticholinergic drugs

Anticholinergic drugs used to counteract extrapyramidal effects of neuroleptics, such as benztropine, benzhexol, biperiden, procyclidine, and orphenadrine, can produce euphoriant effects and are frequently abused for this purpose, especially among schizophrenics but also by non-psychiatric patients (Woody and O'Brien 1974; Marriott 1976; Kaminer *et al.* 1982; Crawshaw and Mullen 1984; Coid and Strang 1982; Pullen *et al.* 1984; Janowsky and Risch 1987). These drugs in overdose usually cause delirium and hallucinations but can provoke mania.

Mechanisms

In many brain systems there is a mutually inhibitory balance between dopaminergic and cholinergic activity and the mechanism for anticholinergic-induced mania and euphoria may be a release of dopaminergic activity. As discussed by Janowsky and Risch (1987), cholinomimetic drugs tend to have depressive effects, and mania can occur as a rebound effect from the cholinomimetic drug physostigmine.

Hormones

Glucocorticoids

Euphoria is common during treatment with glucocorticoids and elevation of mood may in some patients progress to mania, which is more common than depression (see above) with these drugs. Hall and colleagues (1979) described steroid psychoses as 'spectrum' disorders with symptoms ranging from affective, through schizophreniform, to those of an organic brain syndrome, individual patients being differently affected. Psychiatric reactions are dose related and are more common on doses above 40 mg prednisone or equivalent daily. Manic or hypomanic reactions can occur in patients with no previous psychiatric history (for example, see Mullen and Romans-Clarkson 1993), and can also appear as part of a corticosteroid withdrawal reaction.

Anabolic steroids

Anabolic steroids are not uncommonly abused in high dosage. Psychiatric effects include euphoria, aggression, irritability, nervous tension, changes in libido, hypomania, mania, and psychosis (Brower *et al.* 1989; Williamson and Young 1992; Karch 1996). Pope and Katz (1988) interviewed 41 steroid abusers and found that five subjects (12.2 per cent) met DSM IIIR criteria for a manic episode during steroid exposure and eight others (19.5 per cent) were classed as 'subthreshold manic', fulfilling all but one of the diagnostic criteria. In studies on normal volunteers who were not abusers (reported by Karch 1996), subjects taking high doses (240 mg per day) of methyl-testosterone reported euphoria, irritability, and mood swings, and two out of 20 experienced an acute manic or hypomanic episode. Mania has also been reported as a withdrawal reaction to high-dose steroid abuse (Pope and Katz 1988).

Other drugs

Cardiovascular drugs

Nifedipine (Tacke 1987), diltiazem, captopril (Zubenko and Nixon 1984; McMahon 1985), and procainamide (McCrum and Guidry 1978; Rice *et al.* 1988) have been reported to induce mania.

Gastrointestinal drugs

The histamine H_2-receptor antagonists cimetidine (Hollister 1986) and ranitidine (Patterson 1987; Delerue *et al.* 1988) can cause mania.

Anti-infective agents

Mania has been reported with the antimalarials mepacrine (James *et al.* 1987), chloroquine (Torrey 1968; Bhatia 1991), and quinine (Verghese 1988), the antituberculous agent cycloserine (Wallach and Gershon 1972), and with zidovudine used in the treatment of HIV- ated illness (Evans and Perkins 1990).

Miscellaneous

There are case reports of manic or hypomanic reactions to baclofen (Arnold *et al.* 1980), buspirone, (McIvor and Sinanan 1990), metoclopramide, a dopamine-receptor antagonist (Ritchie and Preskorn 1994); carbamazepine (Hollister 1986), indomethacin (Hollister 1986), and disulfiram (Usdin and Robinson 1951).

Psychotic disorders

There is some confusion concerning the definition of drug-induced psychoses (Poole and Brabbins 1996). In this section, drug-associated disorders characterized by prominent hallucinations or delusions occurring in a clear consciousness (DSM IV) (American Psychiatric Association 1994), sometimes accompanied by incoherent thought and changes of affect, giving a 'schizophreniform' picture, are included. Such disorders are usually associated with drug intoxication or withdrawal but may in some cases persist beyond the elimination of the drug. Drugs may cause this picture in previously healthy people, but may also aggravate a pre-existing psychosis, or be taken because of a psychotic relapse, and it is not always easy to define the cause. Furthermore, such reactions increasingly occur in the context of polydrug abuse, so it may not be possible to incriminate a particular drug, let alone disentangle drug effects from previous or underlying functional psychosis.

Amphetamines and related agents

Amphetamine has long been considered the archetype of drugs

that can induce a schizophreniform psychosis; indeed 'amphetamine psychosis' has been used as a model for schizophrenia (Bell 1965; Segal and Janowsky 1978), and the dopaminergic actions of amphetamine have been used as an argument for the dopamine theory of schizophrenia (Snyder 1982). Despite this, psychosis is not an inevitable consequence of acute or even chronic amphetamine use. However, amphetamines can induce psychosis in individuals with no previous history or family history of psychosis and also aggravate symptoms in pre-existing schizophrenia. The drug-induced psychosis may persist for several days after amphetamine withdrawal, and amphetamine can be detected in the urine for up to 48 hours after a single dose (Poole and Brabbins 1996). Amphetamine psychosis responds to dopamine-receptor-blocking antipsychotic drugs such as haloperidol.

Drugs related to amphetamine, including benzamphetamine, dexamphetamine, methamphetamine, diethylproprion, phentermine, methylphenidate, phenmetrazine, ephedrine, phenylpropanolamine, and possibly the appetite suppressants fenfluramine and dexfenfluramine, can all produce schizophrenia-like reactions (Shannon *et al.* 1974; Davison 1976; Hollister 1986; Murphy and Watters 1986; Watters and Le Ridant 1986; SADRAC 1987; Davison and Hassanyeh 1991; Miller 1991). The psychiatric effects of agents are usually ascribed to increased central dopaminergic activity but probably also involve increased noradrenergic and serotonergic activity.

Cocaine

Acute intoxication with cocaine is generally characterized by euphoria which may lead on to hypomania or mania, although features of paranoid psychosis are sometimes present (Cocores *et al.* 1991). However, cocaine is very rapidly eliminated, with a plasma elimination half-life of about 1 hour (Fischman 1987; Strang and Edwards 1989). For this reason, its effects, unlike those of amphetamine, are of very brief duration (lasting only some 15–20 minutes after smoking free-base cocaine or 'crack'), followed by a withdrawal 'crash'. Chronic, repeated use of large doses of cocaine can produce a schizophreniform psychosis similar to that of amphetamine, with paranoid ideation, thought disturbance, stereotyped movements, and hallucinations which may be visual, auditory, or tactile. Formication (not often seen in schizophrenia), a feeling of pricking or crawling under the skin which may lead to picking and excoriation and delusions of parasitosis is typical (Brecher 1972; Jaffe 1980; Fischman 1987; O'Brien and Woody 1991). Largely because of cocaine's short duration of action, most addicts are also polydrug users (Cocores *et al.* 1991) and the clinical effects may be confused and prolonged by the actions of other drugs. The mechanisms of the psychotic reaction to cocaine are probably similar to those of amphetamine. Cocaine inhibits synaptic reuptake of dopamine, noradrenaline, and serotonin and high doses undoubtedly cause gross disruption of these systems in the brain.

Levodopa

The dopamine precursor levodopa has caused psychotic reactions in patients with Parkinson's disease. Paranoid delusional psychosis was reported in 3.6 per cent of 908 such patients reviewed by Goodwin (1971). Similar observations have been made in other series (Celesia and Barr 1970; Murphy 1973). These disturbances appear to be dose related and the onset of psychosis may be delayed for several months after the start of levodopa treatment (Celesia and Barr 1970). Levodopa not surprisingly exacerbates psychiatric symptoms in schizophrenia if used to treat extrapyramidal effects of neuroleptic drugs (Yaryura-Tobias *et al.* 1970, 1972). Adverse psychiatric effects of levodopa usually occur during therapeutic use, but the drug is occasionally abused for its hallucinogenic effects (Evans 1980).

Bromocriptine

The dopamine receptor agonist bromocriptine can provoke reactions similar to those seen with levodopa, but psychosis is more severe and may be protracted despite withdrawal of the drug (Pearce 1984). Bromocriptine is also used for postpartum suppression of lactation, and manic or schizomanic psychosis has been reported after doses of 7.5–30 mg daily, with recovery after 1–7 days (Brooke and Cookson 1978; Vlissides *et al.* 1978). Turner and colleagues (1984) reported similar reactions with larger doses used to treat pituitary tumours.

Like other dopaminergic drugs, bromocriptine exacerbates schizophrenia (Proctor *et al.* 1983). It is sometimes used as a treatment to reduce craving in cocaine and amphetamine withdrawal, but is occasionally abused, adding to the paranoid psychoses resulting from these drugs (Ross and Ward 1992). Similar psychotic reactions have been associated with related drugs, including piribedil (Gerner *et al.* 1976) and lysuride (Turner *et al.* 1984), and psychoses sometimes develop when bromocriptine is withdrawn (Lipper 1976; Shukla *et al.* 1985).

Lysergide (LSD)

LSD is an hallucinogenic agent which has agonist actions on serotonin 5-HT$_{1A}$ and 5-HT$_2$ receptors. Its effects, like those of amphetamine, have been proposed as a model for schizophrenia (Claridge 1978) and have suggested that serotonergic systems are involved in schizophrenia (Van Kammen and Gelertner 1987*a*). The psychological and psychiatric effects of LSD have been described by many authors (Brecher 1972; Davison 1976; Jaffe 1980; Hollister 1982; Davison and Hassanyeh 1991).

Acute reactions to LSD can be elicited by doses as small as 100 μg and can last 2–10 hours. Psychological symptoms include alterations in mood, and hallucinations. A prolonged psychotic reaction can be provoked in vulnerable individuals or by larger doses. This reaction lasts for more than 48 hours and includes paranoid delusions, schizophreniform auditory hallucinations, and overwhelming panic. This type of reaction, which closely resembles naturally occurring schizophrenia (Davison 1976), occurred in about one to two per cent of patients given LSD for psychotherapeutic purposes (Cohen 1960; Smart and Bateman 1967; Malleson 1971). Medical use of LSD is now obsolete but similar psychoses are seen in recreational users (Seymour and Smith 1991). Psychotic reactions rarely last more than a few hours in these users (Hollister 1986) but prolonged and persistent reactions have been reported, sometimes occurring after a delay (Hatrick and Dewhurst 1970). Whether or not these are due to an underlying schizophrenic disorder is still not clear.

The mechanisms of LSD-induced psychiatric disorders are thought to be related to its potent agonist actions on 5-HT$_2$ receptors located in the temporal and prefrontal cortex (Aghajanian et al. 1987; Sadzot et al. 1989). In addition, LSD has both agonist and antagonist activity at dopamine and noradrenergic receptors, which may also be involved (Freedman and Boggan 1982).

MDMA, 'Ecstasy'

MDMA, as its chemical structure suggests, combines some of the properties of amphetamine and LSD, and it is therefore not surprising that it causes psychiatric effects. These have been reviewed by Seymour and Smith (1991), Krystal and colleagues (1992), and Green and others (1995). MDMA is taken recreationally in the 'rave' youth culture for its relatively gentle euphoric effects, combined with a feeling of social empathy, and stimulant and antifatigue properties. Unwanted psychiatric effects are dose related (Seymour and Smith 1991). Acute low-dose (50–150 mg) effects are mild, but high doses (300–400 mg) may cause severe anxiety, panic, paranoid psychosis, suicidal thoughts, and violence. Prolonged repeated use of MDMA is usually combined with polydrug abuse, especially of amphetamines, and these users may display a variety of psychiatric syndromes, including an MDMA-associated schizophreniform psychosis clinically similar to that seen in psychiatric patients with no history of substance abuse (McGuire et al. 1994a). Other cases of psychosis apparently related to repeated use of MDMA have been reported (McGuire and Fahy 1991; Schifano 1991; Winstock 1991; McCann and Ricaurte 1993). Some of these patients developed a chronic psychosis lasting several months or more after cessation of MDMA use and some were non-responsive or only partially responsive to antipsychotic drugs (McGuire and Fahy 1991; Schifano 1991; McGuire et al. 1994a).

Mechanisms

The acute effects of MDMA are probably due to release of serotonin (and possibly dopamine) from nerve terminals in the brain, but the longer-lasting psychosis and depression may result from neurotoxic effects on serotonergic, and possibly dopaminergic neurones (Rattray 1992; Green et al. 1995; Green and Goodwin 1996). In rats and in several species of non-human primates, MDMA in doses comparable to those used by humans causes degeneration of fine serotonergic nerve terminals and loss of serotonergic neurones as well as decreased concentrations of serotonin and its metabolite 5-HIAA in several brain regions and in cerebrospinal fluid (Wilson et al. 1989; Ricaurte et al. 1990). It seems likely that MDMA can cause similar effects in humans: although there is still no unequivocal evidence of brain damage, decreased concentrations of the serotonin metabolite 5-HIAA were found in the cerebrospinal fluid of 30 regular users of MDMA (Ricaurte et al. 1990; McCann et al. 1994). Neurodegeneration seems to result from the metabolites

of MDMA rather than the parent compound. It has been proposed that the metabolites oxidize to form free radicals which cause tissue damage (Rattray 1992; Green and Goodwin 1996), and are in turn inactivated via the CYP2D6 cytochrome oxidase (Tucker et al. 1994). Thus it is likely that subjects who are poor metabolisers of MDMA due to genetic deficiency of CYP2D6 are more susceptible to psychiatric and other toxic effects of MDMA. Another line of evidence suggests that the MDMA neurotoxin may be a metabolite of dopamine (Rattray 1992), and dopamine appears to be involved in the degenerative process since development of lesions of dopaminergic pathways and blockade of dopamine receptors prevents long-term neurotoxicity in animals while the dopamine precursor levodopa enhances the process (Green et al. 1995).

It is interesting that SSRI prevent the MDMA-induced release of serotonin and block MDMA neurotoxicity in the laboratory (Singh 1995). Some recreational MDMA users have found that fluoxetine does not block the euphoric effect of MDMA but in fact prolongs the 'high', and the fashion is growing to take the drugs in combination — a practice which may incidentally mitigate the toxic effects of MDMA (Singh 1995). Unfortunately 'Ecstasy' tablets sold on the market are often contaminated with other drugs which may increase their toxicity. These include ephedrine (Shewan and King 1996), amphetamine, LSD, amphetamine analogues of mescaline related to MDMA (MDEA, MDA, MBDB), caffeine, phenylethylamine (Winstock and King 1996), and γ-hydroxybutyrate (also known as GBH or liquid ecstasy), a compound that can cause coma and convulsions (Stell and Ryan 1996). Other related hallucinogenic drugs which have sometimes enjoyed recreational popularity include peyote, mescaline, psilocybin, and DMT (*N,N*-dimethyltryptamine).

Cannabis

The most common adverse psychiatric effects of acute cannabis use are panic attacks and anxiety symptoms (Thomas 1993) but heavy cannabis use can also lead to an acute psychosis resembling schizophrenia. Such reactions have been described in many studies (Thacore and Shukla 1976; Tennant and Groesbeck 1977; Rottanborg et al. 1982; Carney et al. 1984; Mathers and Ghodse 1992; McGuire et al. 1994b) which indicate that cannabis can produce a functional psychosis in individuals with no history of psychiatric illness. The reaction may be schizophreniform, with persecutory and religious delusions, or hypomanic in nature; it appears to be dose related and is probably more common in those who use the present preparations of cannabis such as 'skunk' which contains high concentrations of tetrahydrocannabinol (THC) (Wylie et al. 1995). The psychosis usually resolves within a week but may be severe enough to require treatment with antipsychotic drugs and may sometimes be prolonged for several weeks (Carney et al. 1984). Prolonged effects may be due to the slow elimination of cannabinoids, which are sequestrated in fatty tissues; the tissue elimination half-life of tetrahydrocannabinol is about 7 days and complete elimination of a single dose can take up to 30 days (Maykut 1985).

While a cannabis-related schizophreniform reaction can occur in patients with no psychiatric history, those with mental illness may be more vulnerable. Rates of cannabis use among psychiatric patients are known to be high, probably over 40 per cent (Meuser *et al.* 1990; Menezes *et al.* 1996). It has been suggested that cannabis may precipitate schizophrenia (Andreasson *et al.* 1987) and that a familial disposition to schizophrenia may predispose to cannabis-induced psychosis (McGuire *et al.* 1995), but this question is still debated. However, there is a greater consensus that cannabis can aggravate the symptoms of schizophrenia and sometimes antagonize the controlling effects of antipsychotic drugs (Treffert 1978; Tunving 1985; Negrete *et al.* 1986; Weller and Halikas 1985; Cleghorn *et al.* 1991; Allebeck *et al.* 1993; Thomas 1993; Linszman *et al.* 1994; Martinez-Arevelo *et al.* 1994; Baigent *et al.* 1995). On the other hand, some schizophrenic patients claim that they take cannabis as a form of self-medication because it makes them 'feel better' (Dixon *et al.* 1990; Peralta and Cuesta 1992).

Mechanisms

The psychiatric effects of cannabis are due to the presence of psychoactive cannabinoids of which the most potent is tetrahydrocannabinol (THC). These cannabinoids interact with specific cannabinoid receptors in the brain (Devane *et al.* 1988; Matsuda *et al.* 1990). The function of these receptors is not known, but high concentrations are present in limbic system 'reward' centres, including the nucleus accumbens and amygdala, and activaiton of these by cannabinoids is thought to account for the euphoric effects of cannabis. THC has been shown to increase dopamine release from the nucleus accumbens and frontal cortex (Miller and Gold 1993), a property in common with cocaine and amphetamines and other addictive drugs.

Phencyclidine and ketamine

Phencyclidine was introduced as an anaesthetic agent which produced an unusual type of dissociative anaesthesia in which patients were unresponsive, analgesic, and amnesic for surgery. However, a high risk of unpredictable adverse effects, including dysphoria, confusion, delirium, and psychosis, precluded its general use and in 1965 it was relegated to veterinary use until 1978 when it was withdrawn in the USA. Nevertheless, it was widely used as a recreational drug in the US and the UK in the mid-seventies and is still used illicitly to some extent, usually in a polydrug context with cannabis, cocaine, alcohol, and other drugs. Ketamine, which is chemically and pharmacologically similar to phencyclidine, was introduced instead; it has a lower incidence of adverse effects in anaesthetic practice. However, recreational abuse of ketamine ('Super K') is now increasing, often in tablets mixed with ephedrine, selegiline, or procaine — designed to mimic 'Ecstasy' tablets (Jansen 1993; Shewan and King 1996).

The psychiatric effects of phencyclidine and ketamine, which are distinct from all other classes of street drugs, were reviewed by Giannini (1991), Gorelick and Balster (1995), Balster (1987), and Jaffe (1980). Phencyclidine was studied with particular interest because some of its psychiatric effects are similar to schizophrenia; it was reported to exacerbate symptoms in schizophrenia, and chronic users sometimes developed schizophreniform disorders. For these reasons, like amphetamine and LSD, phencyclidine was proposed as a model for schizophrenia (Snyder 1982; Balster 1987; Krystal *et al.* 1993; Lahti *et al.* 1993).

Clinically, phencyclidine and ketamine have a curious mixture of effects which combine many of the effects of amphetamines, sedative/anxiolytics, and atypical opioids such as cyclozocine and dextrorphan, which are agonists of opioid/phencyclidine sigma receptors and can produce hallucinations. Amphetamine-like effects include euphoria, anxiety, insomnia, and anorexia. Sedative effects include calmness, psychic numbing, anergia, and depression. Hallucinogenic and psychotomimetic effects include time distortion, distortion of body image, synaesthesia, and schizophreniform psychosis with hallucinations and paranoid delusions in an alert and orientated consciousness. This state may be associated with violence, although patients may later be amnesic for the period of intoxication. A catatonic state with negativism, mutism, a blank stare, and catalepsy, combined with anaesthesia, may also occur.

Phencyclidine is usually taken orally or by intranasal insufflation. The onset of effects occur 20–40 minutes after oral use, peaking at 90 minutes. The period of acute intoxication usually lasts 4–8 hours but may continue up to 48 hours, since the drugs are sequestered in fatty tissues from which they are slowly released over several days. Delirium lasting several days has been described. Chronic phencyclidine usage appears to produce an organic brain disorder with long-term neuropsychological damage. Chronic abusers become aggressive; suffer loss of recent memory, dysphasia, and difficulty in time estimation; and develop personality disorders with anxiety and a schizophreniform psychosis which can last 6–12 months after stopping the drug.

Mechanisms

The mechanisms of action of phencyclidine and ketamine are complex; they have been reviewed by Gianini (1991) and Gorelick and Balster (1995). The drugs are non-competitive antagonists at NMDA receptors, and also bind to associated phencyclidine/sigma receptors. They also have agonist actions at dopamine receptors, complex interactions with both nicotinic and muscarinic acetylcholine receptors, and poorly understood interactions with noradrenergic and serotonergic systems. These multiple actions may combine to produce delirium and psychosis.

Antidepressant drugs

Tricyclic antidepressants and MAOI may occasionally precipitate a paranoid psychosis, thought to be due to activation of latent schizophrenia (McClelland 1985). Psychoses have also been reported as rare adverse effects of MAOI (Murphy 1979; AMA Drug Evaluation 1980; Dubovsky 1987) and Aizenberg and colleagues (1991) reported a case of delusional parasitosis associated with phenelzine. Schizophreniform psychosis is seen rarely in tricyclic antidepressant withdrawal (Halle *et al.* 1991) and paranoid delusions with hallucinations have occurred in withdrawal from MAOI (Halle and Dilsaver 1993). A case of Capgras syndrome (a delusion that someone familiar — in this case her husband — has been replaced by an impostor) in an elderly patient with severe depression was attributed to her lithium treatment (Canagasabey and Katona 1991).

Anticholinergic drugs

Abuse of anticholinergic drugs in high doses can cause toxic psychoses, and these have been reported with benztropine (Woody and O'Brien 1974), benzhexol (Marriott 1976; Crawshaw and Mullen 1984), and procyclidine (Coid and Strang 1982). Toxic psychoses have also been reported with some antihistamines which have significant antimuscarinic properties including diphenhydramine (Lambert 1987; Schreiber *et al.* 1988), cyclizine (Gott 1968), and pheniramine (Yapalater and Rockwell 1950). One case report describes a psychosis in a patient taking a proprietary antidiarrhoeal medicine containing belladonna (Buckley *et al.* 1990).

Hormones

Corticosteroids

Corticosteroids can cause both depression and mania. They can also cause a schizophreniform paranoid psychosis, usually with marked affective loading (Davison 1976). Paranoid symptoms include auditory hallucinations, paranoid delusions and violent behaviour (BCDSP 1972). Corticosteroids may also aggravate symptoms in schizophrenic patients (Hollister 1986).

Androgenic anabolic steroids

Anabolic steroids were reported to induce psychotic symptoms in five (12.2 per cent) of 41 abusers interviewed by Pope and Katz (1988). Of these five subjects, one had auditory hallucinations of voices, lasting 5 weeks; a second developed a paranoid delusion that friends were stealing from him; two had delusions of reference; and the fifth had the grandiose delusion that he could pick up a car and turn it over. Four other subjects had mild psychotic symptoms during periods of steroid exposure. Annitto and Leymam (1980) also reported an acute schizophrenic episode in a young athlete who was taking anabolic steroids surreptitiously. Increases in aggression (' 'roid rage') are also frequently reported in users of anabolic steroids (Barker 1987; Pope and Katz 1988; Williamson and Young 1992; Kennedy 1994).

Cardiovascular drugs

Psychotic reactions have rarely been associated with propranolol in high and in normal dosage, and on withdrawal (Koehler and Gath 1977; Gershon *et al.* 1979; Steinert and Pugh 1979; Thompson 1979; Hollister 1986), and on withdrawal of clonidine (Adler *et al.* 1982). Paranoid psychosis has been reported with digitalis preparations (Gorelich *et al.* 1978).

Antiarrhythmic drugs may also cause paranoid psychoses, which have been reported with intravenous lignocaine (Graham *et al.* 1981; Turner 1982; Saravay *et al.* 1987), tocainide (Currie and Ramsdale 1984; CSM 1986), mexiletine (CSM 1986), disopyramide (Padfield *et al.* 1977; Ahmad *et al.* 1979), and quinidine (Deleu and Schmedding 1987). Of the calcium-channel blockers, nifedipine and diltiazem have been reported to cause paranoid-hallucinatory psychoses (Palat *et al.* 1984; Kahn 1986). A case of psychosis has recently been noted with doxazosin, an antihypertensive drug related to prazosin (Evans *et al.* 1997).

The β-adrenergic stimulant salbutamol, used as a bronchodilator, can cause psychotic reactions with disturbed behaviour, hallucinations, and persecutory delusions (Prasher 1993), and addiction to prescribed aerosols for their hedonic effects has been described (Gluckman 1974; Pratt 1982; Prasher and Corbett 1990).

Anti-infective agents

Paranoid–hallucinatory psychoses have been reported in association with several antibiotics including streptomycin (Porot and Destaing 1950), chloramphenicol (Pereau and Maurice 1950), intravenous erythromycin (Umstead and Neumann 1986), ofloxacin (Zaudig and von Bose 1987), isoniazid (Wallach and Gershon 1972; Ball and Rosser 1989), cycloserine (Wallach and Gershon 1972), and dapsone (Garrett 1971). Cycloserine is also reported to exacerbate symptoms in schizophrenic patients (Simeon *et al.* 1970), and acute schizophreniform psychoses have occurred with cephaloridine and cephalothin (Evans 1980).

Of the antimalarial drugs, chloroquine and mepacrine have been associated with paranoid-hallucinatory psychoses (Kabir 1969; James *et al.* 1987) and psychotic manifestations are also reported with mefloquine (Palmer *et al.* 1993).

The antiviral drug amantadine has caused acute psychotic exacerbation in schizophrenic patients (Hausner 1980; Nestelbaum *et al.* 1986) and aciclovir has caused paranoid delusions and hallucinations (Jones and Beier-Hanratty 1986).

Opioids

Morphine can occasionally cause paranoid thinking and hallucinations (D'Souza 1987; Leipzig *et al.* 1987; Jellema 1987; Kalso and Vainio 1988), but psychiatric effects including paranoid-hallucinatory psychoses are more common with pentazocine (Blazer and Haller 1975; Goldstein 1985) and also occur with dihydrocodeine (Taylor *et al.* 1978), while buprenorphine and methadone have caused hallucinations (Jellema 1987; McEvilly and O'Carroll 1989). These effects are possibly due to actions at sigma opioid receptors.

NSAID

Indomethacin, sulindac, and ibuprofen have caused paranoid-hallucinatory psychoses (Carney 1977; Kruis and Barger 1980; Griffith *et al.* 1982), and fenbufen was reported to have caused visual hallucinations in one patient (Morris and Hardway 1985),

TABLE 23.1
Drugs that can induce hallucinations
(visual, auditory, tactile, or other, not necessarily
associated with delirium or psychosis)

Drug	References
Analgesics/anaesthetics	
Indomethacin, fenbufen	Morris and Hardway 1985; Braddock and Heard 1986
Ketamine*	Jansen 1993
Opiates, opioids*	Bruera *et al.* 1992
Opioid agonists/antagonists* (pentazocine, nalorphine, naloxone, buprenorphine)	Woods 1956; Alexander and Spence 1974; Wood *et al.* 1974
Refopam	Piercy *et al.* 1981; Johnson *et al.* 1993
Salicylates	Greer *et al.* 1965
Antibacterial/antiviral/antiparasitic drugs	
Aciclovir	British National Formulary 1997
Cephalosporins	Al-Zahawi and Sprott 1988
Chloramphenicol	Pereau and Morris 1950
Chloroquine, mefloquine, mepacrine	Kabir 1969; Croft and World 1996; van Riemsdijk *et al.* 1997
Cycloserine	Wallach and Gershon 1972
Dapsone	Jarrett 1971
Erythromycin	Umstead and Neumann 1986
Isoniazid	Ball and Rosser 1989
Procaine penicillin	Ilechukwu 1990
Streptomycin	Porot and Destaing 1950
Sulphonamides	Frisch 1973
Anticonvulsants	
Ethosuximide	Buchanan 1972
Phenytoin	Glaser and Reynolds 1972
Sodium valproate	Trimble and Reynolds 1976
Anticholinergic drugs	
Atropine, hyoscine	Gowdy 1972; Perry and Perry 1995
Atropine, hyoscine, tropicamide, cyclopentolate eye-drops	Davidson and Hickey-Dwyer 1991
Benztropine, benzhexol, orphenadrine, procyclidine	Woody and O'Brien 1974; Coid and Strang 1982; Crawshaw and Mullen 1984
Antidepressants	
Lithium	Ferrier *et al.* 1995
MAOI	White 1987
SSRI	Price *et al.* 1996; Fava and Gardi 1995 Dorman *et al.* 1995
Tricyclic antidepressants	
Antihistamines *	
Cyclizine, dimenhydrinate diphenhydramine, pheniramine	Malcolm and Miller 1972; Jones *et al.* 1973; Schreiber *et al.* 1988

*also used as drugs of abuse

(Table 23.1 continued)

Antineoplastic drugs	
Cyclosporin	Steg and Garoia 1991
Vincristine	Gosh *et al.* 1994
Antiparkinsonian drugs	
Amantadine	Forssman *et al.* 1972
Bromocriptine	Turner *et al.* 1984
levodopa	Celesia and Barr 1970; Gilbert 1976
Cardiovascular and respiratory drugs	
Aminophylline	Prescott 1978
Antiarrhythmics	
amiodarone	Coumel and Fidelle 1980
disopyramide	Padfield *et al.* 1977
flecainide	Ramhamadany *et al.* 1986
lignocaine (IV)	Saravay *et al.* 1987
quinidine	Deleu and Schmedding 1987
tocainide	CSM 1986
β-Adrenoceptor agonists (salbutamol*)	Whitehouse and Novosel 1989; Prasher 1993
β-Adrenoceptor antagonists	Fleming *et al.* 1982; Paykel *et al.* 1982
Calcium-channel blockers	
diltiazem	Bushe 1988
nifedipine	Kahn 1986
Digoxin, digitalis preparations	Gorelick *et al.* 1978; Closson 1983; Eisendrath and Sweeney 1987
Diuretics	Paykel *et al.* 1982
Isosorbide dinitrate	Rosenthal 1987
Prazosin	Patterson 1988
Hypnotics/sedatives/anxiolytics *	
Benzodiazepines (high doses or withdrawal)	Hallstrom and Lader 1981 Owen and Tyrer 1983; Ashton 1984, 1987, 1997
Zopiclone, zolpidem	CSM 1990
Other therapeutic agents	
Anabolic steroids*	Pope and Katz 1987
Baclofen (withdrawal)	Swigar and Bowers 1986
Cimetidine, ranitidine	Agarwal 1978; Adler *et al.* 1980; Price *et al.* 1985; Lesser *et al.* 1987
Clonidine	Brown *et al.* 1980
Corticosteroids*	BCDSP
Oral contraceptives	Kane 1968; Daly *et al.* 1967
Tacrine (?)	Davis and Powchik 1995
Recreational drugs *	
Alcohol (acute toxicity and withdrawal	Jaffe 1980; Gelder *et al. 1983*
Amphetamine and related drugs also used therapeutically (ephedrine, mephentermine, phenylpropanolamine, mazindol, methylphenidate, cathine, diethylpropion, fenfluramine)	Lucas and Weiss 1971; Norvenius *et al.* 1979; Petursson 1979; Angrist 1983; CSM 1985; Whitehouse and Duncan 1987; Brooke *et al.* 1988; Carney 1988; Devan 1990; CSM 1993*a*; Sullivan 1996

(continued)

(Table 23.1 continued)

(Recreational drugs*)

Cannabis	Nahas and Paton 1979
Cocaine	Siegel 1978
LSD and related drugs	Davison 1976; Hollister 1982; Jaffe 1980
MDMA, 'Ecstasy'	McGuire *et al.* 1994*a*
NDMA and related drugs	Peroutka *et al.* 1988; McGuire and Fahy 1991; McGuire *et al.* 1994*a*
Organic solvents	Black 1982
Phencyclidine	Giannini 1991

*also used as drugs of abuse

although this reaction appears to be rare (Brook and Jackson 1982).

Anticonvulsants

Phenytoin can produce a number of psychiatric symptoms including hallucinations, delusions, and paranoid and schizophreniform psychoses (Franks and Richter 1979). Exacerbation of both acute and chronic schizophrenia has been reported with sodium valproate (Lautin *et al.* 1980; Meldrum 1982). Carbamazepine can induce schizophreniform psychoses (Franks and Richter 1979; Matthews 1988), as can ethosuximide (Roger *et al.* 1968; Buchanan 1972) and occasionally clonazepam (White *et al.* 1982; Jaffe and Gibson 1986). Psychosis is listed in the British National Formulary (1997) as an adverse effect of vigabatrin, while abnormal thinking and emotional lability with abnormal behaviour are listed for topiramide.

Disulfiram

Disulfiram, sometimes used to prevent relapses in abstinent alcoholics, inhibits the enzyme dopamine β-hydroxylase, thus increasing brain dopamine concentrations; like other dopaminergic drugs, it can induce psychotic reactions (Rothstein and Clancy 1969). Most adverse reactions to disulfiram are associated with delirium, but psychosis in a clear consciousness has also been reported (Knee and Razani 1974; Ewing *et al.* 1977; Quail and Karelse 1980; Rossiter 1992). A case of Capgras syndrome has been reported after 500 mg of disulfiram daily for 2 weeks (Daniel *et al.* 1987). Established schizophrenia is also aggravated by disulfiram (Heath *et al.* 1965).

Baclofen

Baclofen, a muscle relaxant which is an agonist of GABA$_B$ receptors but may also have some dopaminergic activity (Wolf *et al.* 1982), has been associated with various psychiatric symptoms including catatonia and mutism (Pauker and Brown 1986) and paranoid-hallucinatory psychoses (Jones and Lance 1976; Swigar and Bowers 1986; Yassa and Iskander 1988). Baclofen was found to aggravate schizophrenia when tried as a treatment for this disorder (Hollister 1986).

Hallucinatory states

Hallucinations may be part of a drug-induced delirium or psychotic state. Hypnagogic or hypnopompic hallucinations may be part of a drug-induced sleep disorder. Hallucinations may also occur in several drug withdrawal syndromes or as delayed 'flashbacks' after certain recreational drugs. Occasionally, isolated hallucinations occur in the setting of a clear consciousness.

Drug-induced visual hallucinations may start as unformed images, such as abstract shapes or flashes of light, progressing to complex forms of animals or people and scenes in vivid colours (Barodawala and Mulley 1997). The form of the hallucinations may to some extent be characteristic of the drug involved. Thus, the hallucinations of alcoholic delirium tremens are classically of rodents, while those induced by cocaine and amphetamine intoxication or by benzodiazepine withdrawal are typically of insects and sometimes associated with formication. Some hallucinations seem to merge into illusions or misperceptions, so that a coat hanging on the door takes the form of a person. Hallucinations caused by hallucinogens, such as LSD or cannabis, are commonly synaesthetic along with time and space distortions and general heightening of sensory perceptions, so that details are perceived with singular clarity.

Auditory hallucinations induced by drugs may be unformed, grading from tinnitus, hissing, and whistles, to bangs or thumps, but are occasionally formed (e.g. singing voices) and may be associated with deafness. Chronic alcoholism (alcoholic hallucinosis) may also characterized by auditory hallucinations, often of voices uttering insults or threats, occurring in a clear consciousness. Drugs which affect cerebellar function, such as alcohol, benzodiazepines, and cannabis may cause proprioceptive or kinaesthetic hallucinations with feelings of falling, imbalance, movement, inner vibration, or of the environment moving. A very large number of drugs can induce any of these types of hallucinations (Table 23.1).

The mechanisms of drug-induced hallucinations are unclear. In many cases they appear to result from excess cortical excitation caused by CNS stimulants or withdrawal from CNS depressants. Other drugs, such as cannabinoids and LSD, are known to have preferential actions in brain sensory areas. Sensory deprivation with secondary cortical hypersensitivity may contribute to drug effects in some cases such as auditory hallucinations in partial deafness and visual hallucinations after cataract operation (Barodawala and Mulley 1997). Since hallucinations can be triggered by such a range of drugs, it appears that imbalanced activity of any one of a large number of neurotransmitters may be involved. It is of interest that preliminary functional MRI (fMRI) studies (in schizophrenia) suggest that cerebral blood flow changes during formed hallucinations are similar to those occurring during the relevant external stimuli (Woodruff *et al.* 1994). In most cases hallucinations quickly resolve when the causative drug is removed or the acute stage of a withdrawal reaction is passed, although occasionally they may be persistent.

Persisting perception disorder (flashbacks)

Flashbacks are transient recurrences of some aspect of an hallucinogenic drug experience occurring after a period of normality following the original intoxication. Flashbacks have been described after LSD and related drugs, phencyclidine, ketamine, cannabis, and MDMA. They can occur after a single ingestion but more commonly occur after multiple drug exposures. They usually consist of perceptual disturbances but can include emotional and somatic reactions. Flashbacks may occur spontaneously and episodically or they may be self-induced by thinking about them or triggered by entry into a dark environment, various other drugs (especially cannabis), anxiety, fatigue or stress. They may last several months or continue episodically for over five years. The subject is aware of their unreality.

Flashbacks may have multiple aetiologies and have been reported in people who have never ingested a hallucinogenic drug: for example in post-traumatic stress disorder. It has been suggested that drug-related flashbacks may be due to a residue of the drug being released into the brain at a later time. While this may conceivably occur with slowly eliminated drugs such as cannabis and phencyclidine, there is no direct evidence of retention and prolonged storage of LSD and related drugs (Seymour and Smith 1991) and it would not account for the persistence of flashbacks over periods of years. Emotional and accompanying somatic experiences can recur and may lead to prolonged anxiety states or psychoses following a frightening flashback (Seymour and Smith 1991).

Lysergide (LSD)

The visual phenomenology of the LSD flashback was described by Abraham (1983) who interviewed 123 LSD users (drawn largely from an acute psychiatric outpatient population) and 40 matched control subjects who had never used hallucinogens. Visual flashbacks included colour confusion, difficulty in reading, flashes of bright colour, haloes around objects, illusions of movement, intensifications of colour, positive and negative after-images, macropsia and micropsia, and trailing phenomena (apparent trails following moving objects), and many other manifestations. Over 50 per cent of the hallucinogen users reported flashback symptoms occurring a week or more after the last exposure to the drug, and in half of these they had lasted for five years or more. Control subjects reported some similar visual symptoms but with significantly (P<0.001) lower frequency. Similar delayed visual disturbances after hallucinogen exposure have been reported by many other authors (Frosch et al. 1965; Robbins 1967; Woody 1970; Asher 1971; Woody 1971; Abraham 1983; Kaminer et al. 1991).

Mechanisms of hallucinogen-induced flashbacks were discussed by Abraham (1983). One of the most common precipitants is entry into a dark environment, suggesting a failure of function of an inhibitory system in the visual pathway. Failure of inhibition could also explain diverse manifestations such as trailing, colour intensifications and confusions and after-images. The visual disturbances may be mediated in the lateral geniculate nucleus which (in the macaque monkey) contains on-off colour neurones with receptive fields similar to those described in flashbacks. Although there is no direct evidence that hallucinogens exert localized toxic effects at this site, it has been suggested that flashbacks could represent episodes of visual seizures generated from the lateral geniculate nucleus. Abraham's (1983) observations that flashbacks were reduced in intensity and frequency by benzodiazepines but exacerbated by phenothiazines are consistent with this suggestion. Cognitive factors and genetic susceptibility may also influence the occurrence of hallucinogen-induced flashbacks.

Cannabis

Cannabis can precipitate visual flashbacks in LSD users (Abraham 1983) and flashbacks have also been reported with cannabis, apparently without usage of other hallucinogens (Paton et al. 1973; Brown and Stickgold 1976; Stanton et al. 1976; Edwards 1983). The flashbacks with cannabis appear to be emotionally charged and Paton et al. (1973) suggest that the whole perception of a 'bad trip', like an intense emotional experience, enters the memory stores at the time of intoxication, presumably to re-emerge as in post-traumatic stress disorder. Persistent visual changes following cannabis use have also been reported (Levi and Miller 1990; Laffi and Saffran 1993).

Ketamine and phencyclidine

There is surprisingly little reference in the literature to flashbacks with phencyclidine. However, ketamine has been associated with recurring phenomena or flashbacks (Fine and Finestone 1973; Perel and Davidson 1976; Siegel 1978; Jansen 1990; Jansen 1993). It is not clear whether these phenomena result from drug-induced physiological changes or represent a functional response in predisposed personalities. They do not usually show the clear and marked perceptual features of LSD flashbacks.

MDMA, 'Ecstasy'

MDMA can produce flashbacks (Creighton et al. 1991; McGuire and Fahy 1992; McGuire et al. 1994). In these cases it is difficult to separate apparent flashbacks from associated psychotic or anxiety reactions and the use of other drugs, but it does appear that recurrence of symptoms, including perceptual distortions, can occur several weeks after the last exposure to MDMA.

Anxiety disorders

Anxiety symptoms are common in the general population. They are present to some extent in almost all psychiatric disorders, frequently accompany somatic illness, and may often be precipitated or exacerbated by drugs. Drug-related anxiety symptoms vary in type and intensity from feelings of tension, restlessness, and agitation to severe and overwhelming panic with fear of imminent death. The onset of anxiety may be during drug treatment or during withdrawal after regular use, sometimes after a delay of days or even weeks. In general any drug which activates brain arousal systems can cause anxiety symptoms if the dose is high enough. Thus central nervous system stimulants readily cause anxiety during use, while withdrawal from central nervous system depressant drugs has similar effects. The mechanisms of action of most of these drugs have been described in other sections.

Caffeine and theophylline

Caffeine produces a dose-related central nervous system stimulation which may include anxiety, jitteriness, nervousness, shakiness, and tremor, as well as insomnia in normal subjects at doses around 200–500 mg (Shanahan and Hughes 1986; Lader and Bruce 1989). This syndrome of 'caffeinism' may be indistinguishable from an anxiety disorder. There is considerable individual variation in this response, which may partly be due to differences in metabolic rate, but subjects with high trait anxiety, generalized anxiety, or phobic or panic disorder appear to be particularly sensitive to the anxiogenic effects of caffeine (Greden 1974; Greden et al. 1978; Boulenger and Uhde 1982; Bruce et al. 1992) and their symptoms improve if caffeine intake is decreased (Greden 1974).

Theophylline has possibly even more potent central nervous system stimulant effects than caffeine (Lader and Bruce 1989) and its adverse effects include anxiety, tension, irritability, and insomnia (Schraa and Dirks 1982; Hollister 1986) and, at high concentrations, convulsions (Andersson and Persson 1980). The anxiogenic effects have been less studied than those of caffeine, but clinical observations indicate that the use of theophylline preparations may add to the anxiogenic effects of hypoxia in patients with obstructive respiratory disease.

The anxiogenic effects of caffeine and theophylline, like the effects on sleep, are thought to be due to blockade of central adenosine A_1 receptors (Lader and Bruce 1989; Stradling 1993; Jain et al. 1995; Jacobsen 1996).

Amphetamines and related drugs

Acute intoxication with amphetamine typically causes anxiety and restlessness along with the initial euphoria; with increasing doses mood becomes predominantly anxious and may progress to psychosis. Anxiety and fear usually accompany the delusions and hallucinations of amphetamine psychosis (Miller 1991). Anxiety disorder may also occur with compounds related to amphetamine including diethylproprion, phentermine, methylphenidate, phenmetrazine, mazindol, and phenylpropanolamine (Miller 1991). β-Adrenoceptor agonists such as isoprenaline and salbutamol may also provoke anxiety, restlessness, nervousness, tremor, irritability, insomnia, and emotional lability (Hollister 1986; Prasher 1993).

Lysergide (LSD)

Acute intoxication with LSD may produce a dysphoric reaction or 'bad trip' in as many as 20 per cent of drug exposures (Jaffe 1980). Such reactions usually consist of panic attacks and feelings of loss of control or of becoming insane. They are influenced by the prevailing mood and personality of the taker and by the environmental setting, but sometimes occur in users who have previously experienced 'good trips'. While relatively low doses may exacerbate anxiety, higher doses are more likely to cause psychosis with hallucinations and paranoia (Parliamentary Office of Science and Technology 1996)

MDMA, 'Ecstasy'

MDMA can produce autonomic hyperarousal associated with feelings of restlessness and anxiety (Krystal and Price 1992; McGuire et al. 1994). Panic attacks and anxiety, insomnia, and depression can last for months or even years after discontinuation (Green et al. 1995).

Phencyclidine

Intoxication with phencyclidine can cause excitement and agitation, amongst other psychiatric symptoms, and chronic use may be associated with anxiety as well as psychosis, depression, and neuropsychological impairment (Giannini 1991; Gorelick and Balster 1995).

Cannabis

Anxiety is one of the commonest adverse psychiatric effects of cannabis (Paton et al. 1973). It can be severe with panic attacks and is most likely to occur in anxious or drug-naive subjects and in those who take cannabis in an unfavourable environment (Brill and Nahas 1984). In a New Zealand survey (Thomas 1996) 22 per cent of people who completed a questionnaire about problems they experienced with cannabis use reported panic attacks or anxiety. Acute anxiety reactions may include restlessness, depersonalization, derealization, a feeling of loss of control, fear of dying, and panic, and may last for several hours after cannabis use (Thomas 1993). Similar reactions can occur with nabilone, a synthetic cannabinoid used therapeutically for the control of vomiting caused by antineoplastic drugs. Anxiety is also a feature of cannabis withdrawal.

Cocaine

Acute intoxication with cocaine, as well as sometimes causing mania and psychotic reactions, not uncommonly produces anxiety following the initial euphoria, and anxiety may also be associated with the 'crash' following acute intoxication, and with the more prolonged withdrawal syndrome. Cocaine-associated panic is a well-established consequence of chronic use (Cocores et al. 1991; Lacayo 1995). The prevalence of panic attacks is reported to be as high as 64 per cent in cocaine users (Anthony et al. 1989) and the association remains strong even after adjustment for pre-existing psychiatric conditions, use of alcohol and cannabis, and sociodemographic risk factors (Lacayo 1995).

Dopaminergic drugs

Levodopa produced overactivity, restlessness, and agitation in 3.6 per cent of 908 patients receiving the drug for Parkinson's disease (Goodwin 1971) and increasing anxiety was observed as a prodromal symptom in patients who developed psychoses during levodopa treatment for Parkinson's disease (Celesia and Barr 1970). Bromocriptine, piribedil, and lysuride can produce similar symptoms (Gerner *et al.* 1976; Calne *et al.* 1978; Pearce and Pearce 1978; Turner *et al.* 1984).

Phenothiazines, metoclopramide

Phenothiazines with antimuscarinic effects can precipitate delirium of the central anticholinergic type, which is often preceded by restlessness and agitation, particularly after parenteral administration (Mariani 1988); oral metoclopramide can precipitate a similar reaction (Fishbain and Rogers 1987).

Antidepressant drugs

Anxiety, agitation, and insomnia are recognized adverse effects of the tricyclic antidepressant protriptyline, SSRI, venlafaxine, and MAOI, and anxiety is a common feature of antidepressant withdrawal reactions. However, antidepressant drugs (including tricyclics, SSRI, and MAOI) also have therapeutic effects, usually after a delay of 2–3 weeks, in anxiety disorders (Tyrer 1989; Westenberg and Den Boer 1993; Montgomery 1995). Nevertheless, these drugs may cause an initial aggravation of anxiety symptoms and agitation early in treatment. Westenberg and Den Boer (1993) suggested that the anxiogenic effect may be due to an initial increase in serotonergic function (e.g. resulting from reuptake inhibition), while later down-regulation of postsynaptic 5-HT receptors may account for the delayed anxiolytic effects. Among the SSRI, increased anxiety is reported most frequently with fluoxetine (Tyrer 1993), and Montgomery (1995) suggests that this may be related to its 5-HT$_{1C}$ agonist properties.

Benzodiazepines

Anxiety is a well-recognized feature of the benzodiazepine withdrawal syndrome but can also occur as an adverse effect of acute or chronic usage. Severe anxiety reactions with depersonalization and derealization, fear of going insane, restlessness, and other symptoms caused by the potent and short-acting benzodiazepine triazolam were described by Van der Kroef (1979). Anxiety between doses and daytime anxiety after nighttime use can also occur with triazolam and other short-acting benzodiazepines such as alprazolam (Morgan and Oswald 1982; Ashton 1987; Drug and Therapeutics Bulletin 1991). Increased anxiety may also occur as an acute 'paradoxical' excitatory effect of benzodiazepines (Lader and Peturson 1981). In addition, increasing anxiety with the onset of panic attacks, agoraphobia, and other phobias, may develop during long-term benzodiazepine usage (as with alcohol), possibly as a result of drug tolerance (Ashton 1987; Cohen 1992). Worsening of post-traumatic stress disorder has been reported with alprazolam (Cole and Kando 1993).

Benzodiazepine antagonists and inverse agonists

While benzodiazepine receptor agonists (such as diazepam) are mainly anxiolytic, inverse agonists at the same receptors (such as β-carbolines) have the opposite effect and are anxiogenic (Braestrup *et al.* 1983). Flumazenil is a competetive antagonist of both benzodiazepine agonists and inverse agonists. It can induce panic, anxiety, dysphoria, and other benzodiazepine withdrawal symptoms in patients dependent on benzodiazepines (Harrison-Read *et al.* 1996) and in patients who have taken a benzodiazepine overdose (Ashton 1985). Conversely, flumazenil can alleviate some protracted withdrawal symptoms in patients who have stopped benzodiazepines after long-term use (Lader and Morton 1992). In addition, flumazenil precipitates panic in patients with panic disorder who are not taking benzodiazepines; it appears to be not markedly anxiogenic in patients with generalized anxiety disorder, and its psychological effects in normal control subjects are not significant (Nutt *et al.* 1993). These observations have led to the suggestion that in panic disorder and in benzodiazepine dependence there is a functional shift of the benzodiazepine receptor towards the inverse agonist position.

Buspirone

Although buspirone has anxiolytic properties, after a delay of 2–3 weeks it can acutely produce a marked dysphoria with anxiety, nervousness, excitement, and restlessness (Lader 1989; Deakin 1993) and panic at high doses (Coplan *et al.* 1995).

Baclofen

Anxiety has been reported as an adverse effect of the muscle relaxant (GABA$_B$-receptor agonist) baclofen (Jones and Lance 1976) as well as depression, paranoia, and hallucinations. Severe anxiety, agitation, insomnia, hallucinations, and paranoid delusions have been described in baclofen withdrawal (Swigar and Bowers 1986).

Anticonvulsants

Anxiety and restlessness occur occasionally as adverse effects of carbamazepine (Tollefson 1980) and ethosuximide (Roger *et al.* 1968; Buchanan 1972). However, sedation and drowsiness are more common adverse effects of anticonvulsants.

General anaesthetics

Postanaesthetic excitement with anxiety and tension is described after several general anaesthetics, particularly cyclopropane, ether, halothane, isoflurane, and ketamine (Dundee *et al.* 1970; Davison and Hassanyeh 1991).

Corticosteroids

Mental disturbances caused by glucocorticoids usually consist of depression or paranoia, but withdrawal of steroids after long-term therapy may be associated with anxiety, depersonalization, irritability, emotional lability, and fatigue, as well as depression (Wolkowitz and Rapaport 1989). These authors attributed the effects to pituitary–adrenal suppression resulting from steroid use. Anabolic steroid abuse is sometimes associated with panic disorders, anxiety and depression, hyperactivity, irritability, and other psychiatric disorders (Karch 1996). Withdrawal reactions are described elsewhere.

Other hormones

Thyroxine may cause anxiety with palpitations, and hypoglycaemic symptoms from excessive insulin dosage may include anxiety.

Anti-infective drugs

An acute non-anaphylactic reaction with psychiatric features occurring after intramuscular injection of aqueous procaine penicillin is termed Hoigné's syndrome (Hoigné 1962). It occurs within a minute of injection and includes extreme apprehension or fear of death, kinaesthetic disturbances, illusions and hallucinations, and depersonalization along with physical symptoms (Ilechukwu 1990). It can occasionally develop, in susceptible people, into a chronic neurosis or post-traumatic stress syndrome. This reaction is attributed to the effects of procaine being inadvertently injected intravascularly and reaching limbic areas in the brain (Ilechukwu 1990), but similar reactions have been reported with other depot penicillins (Hoigné et al. 1984). Cycloserine may cause a number of psychiatric symptoms, including anxiety and agitation (Wallach and Gershon 1972; Simeon et al. 1970). Interferons can also cause anxiety and depression (Adams et al. 1984; Renault et al. 1987).

Severe neuropsychiatric reactions to prophylactic doses of the antimalarial drug mefloquine occur at a frequency of about one in 10 000 to 20 000 patients (CSM 1996), although the incidence of mild adverse psychiatric effects may be much greater (Van Riemsdijk et al. 1997). These effects include anxiety and panic as well as hallucinations and paranoid delusions. Of 132 neuropsychiatric effects reported to the Drug Safety Unit of the Inspectorate of Health Care in the Netherlands between 1992 and 1995 (Van Riemsdijk et al. 1997), there were 50 reports of anxiety, 31 of agitation, six of depersonalization, and 25 of insomnia or nightmares. Anxiety varied from a tense feeling and nervousness to severe panic disorders. Symptoms usually appeared within 3 weeks of starting mefloquine. Most subjects had no previous psychiatric history and had not used other drugs. Anxiety has also been reported with chloroquine (Bhatia 1991). The mechanism for these reactions is not known.

Withdrawal syndromes

Anxiety, which may be severe, is a feature of the withdrawal syndrome of many drugs.

Sleep disorders

Drug-induced sleep disorders may take the form of insomnia (difficulty in initiating or maintaining sleep, or a feeling of non-restorative sleep), hypersomnia (excessive nocturnal sleep or daytime somnolence), or parasomnia (usually in the form of disturbing dreams or nightmares). Many sleep disorders are mixed. Drug-induced sleep disorders have been reviewed by Buysse (1991) and Ashton (1994a).

Anxiolytics, sedatives, hypnotics

All drugs in this group can cause oversedation with daytime drowsiness and hangover effects the day after night-time use. All of them have profound effects on sleep stages. In addition, all have additive effects with alcohol and other central nervous system depressants.

Benzodiazepines

The effects of benzodiazepines and other sedative/hypnotics on sleep have been reviewed by Ashton (1994a). In short-term use benzodiazepines generally hasten onset of sleep, decrease nocturnal awakenings, increase total sleeping time, and often impart a sense of deep and refreshing sleep. However, they produce alterations in the duration of the various sleep stages. Light sleep (Stage 2) is prolonged and mainly accounts for the increased sleeping time. By contrast, the duration of both deep slow-wave sleep (SWS) and rapid-eye-movement sleep (REMS) may be considerably reduced. Dreaming is diminished. Tolerance to these effects develops rapidly, within a few days or weeks of regular use, and may lead to decreased hypnotic efficacy and escalation of dosage. Sleep latency, Stage 2 sleep, SWS, REMS, and intrasleep awakenings all tend to return to pretreatment levels after a few weeks on the same dose, and dreaming may return. Increase in dosage may lead to hangover effects with daytime oversedation and drowsiness, particularly with slowly eliminated benzodiazepines (e.g. diazepam, nitrazepam). Occasionally, benzodiazepines produce paradoxical, apparently stimulant, effects, particularly in anxious patients, including increased anxiety, insomnia, hypnagogic hallucinations, and nightmares.

On benzodiazepine withdrawal after chronic use, the effects on sleep are reversed and a withdrawal syndrome which includes rebound insomnia, frequent awakenings, vivid dreams, and nightmares is common and may be long-lasting. With rapidly eliminated benzodiazepines (e.g. triazolam, now withdrawn in the UK) this rebound may occur in the latter part of the night, even on continued administration.

The effects of benzodiazepines result from their interaction with benzodiazepine binding sites on the $GABA_A$ receptor complex, causing enhancement of GABA activity in the brain (Haefely 1990). There are copious GABA/benzodiazepine receptors in the reticular formation, limbic system, and cerebral cortex and GABA enhancement in these areas is thought to account for the hypnotic and sedative effects. Secondary effects on monoamine or cholinergic systems may cause the changes in REMS. With chronic use, down-regulation of GABA receptors occurs (probably due to changes in affinity for GABA), and on withdrawal a state of GABA underactivity is exposed and leads to the withdrawal syndrome.

Barbiturates

Barbiturates have many similarities to benzodiazepines and their effects on sleep are similar. Daytime somnolence may occur, owing to slow elimination and tolerance, and rebound effects with insomnia and nightmares occur as with benzodiazepines, as also may paradoxical excitement. Barbiturates bind to the GABA/benzodiazepine receptor and enhance the actions of GABA, but at high doses they exert a GABA-mimetic effect and cause prolonged opening of chloride channels in the neuronal membrane (Haefely 1990). This latter action accounts for the more generalized central nervous system depression and greater toxicity of barbiturates compared with benzodiazepines.

Chloral derivatives

These drugs have effects on sleep similar to benzodiazepines and barbiturates and can produce daytime somnolence (hangover effects), drug dependence, and an abstinence syndrome on withdrawal (Ashton 1994a).

Chlormethiazole

This drug has hypnotic properties similar to barbiturates but because of its fairly rapid elimination (elimination half-life 1–4 hours) daytime hangover effects are less common. Tolerance, dependence, and withdrawal effects occur. The combination of chlormethiazole and alcohol can result in coma and fatal respiratory depression. This complication is due partly to additive central nervous system effects but alcohol also increases the bioavailability of chlormethiazole by impairing first-pass metabolism, particularly in alcoholic cirrhosis (McInnes 1987; Drug Interactions 1996; Duncan and Taylor 1996).

Zopiclone

Zopiclone, a cyclopyrrolone, is a non-benzodiazepine hypnotic which binds to two subtypes of the GABA$_A$/benzodiazepine receptor (benzodiazepines bind to three subtypes). It has properties similar to benzodiazepines and the same potential for adverse psychiatric reactions including dependence (CSM 1990; The Lancet 1990b). Four cases of dependence on zopiclone, prescribed for insomnia, were reported by Jones and O'Sullivan (1998). Sleepiness and morning hangover have been described although these may be less frequent and severe than with benzodiazepines; nightmares may also occur (Hallstrom 1994). Nevertheless, zopiclone appears to cause lesser changes in sleep stages than benzodiazepines and less rebound insomnia, although transient worsening of sleep does occur on withdrawal (Chaudoir et al. 1990; Elie et al. 1990; Fleming et al. 1990).

Zolpidem

Zolpidem, an imidazopyridine, also acts on GABA/benzodiazepine receptors, but at low doses is relatively specific for one subtype, the omega-1 receptor. It is rapidly eliminated (half-life 2 hours), and at therapeutic dosage (5–10 mg) does not appear to cause hangover effects, although daytime drowsiness does occur with 30 mg doses (Drug and Therapeutics Bulletin 1995). It is not clear whether doses of 5–10 mg doses cause early-morning waking like alcohol and short-acting benzodiazepines

such as triazolam, which has a similar half-life (Ashton 1997a), but tolerance and waking after 3 hours has been reported with 20 mg doses (Cavallero et al. 1993), and night-time restlessness is listed in the data sheet. Nightmares, depression, and episodes of confusion and memory disturbance are reported in one to two per cent of patients; hallucinations or hypnagogic hallucinations have been reported (Drug and Therapeutics Bulletin 1995). The effects on sleep stages have been investigated in a number of studies (Brunner et al. 1991; Declerk et al. 1992; Monti et al. 1994; Mendelson and Jain 1995; Salva and Costa 1995). Zolpidem appears to have lesser effects than benzodiazepines, but can decrease REMS and possibly increase SWS with little evidence of rebound insomnia (measured next day) after 3–4 weeks' use.

Buspirone

Buspirone has anxiolytic effects but does not act on GABA/benzodiazepine receptors. It is a mixed agonist/antagonist at serotonin 5HT$_{1A}$ receptors and also has antagonistic actions at dopamine receptors (Eison et al. 1986; Traber and Glaser 1987; Lader 1991). Its metabolite 1-PP is an α_2-receptor antagonist (Deakin 1993). Buspirone can produce restlessness, anxiety, and insomnia and may aggravate panic (Deakin 1993).

Alcohol

Alcohol, although a central nervous system depressant, is a common cause of insomnia. Its acute and chronic effects on sleep are described by Rall (1990), Ashton (1994a), and Stradling (1993). In normal adults, acute use of alcohol at bedtime reduces sleep latency, reduces REMS, and increases SWS. Later in the night, following metabolism of the alcohol, rebound effects occur with frequent arousals, increased REMS, and vivid dreams or nightmares accompanied by tachycardia and sweating. In chronic alcoholics, sleep is markedly fragmented and punctuated by frequent awakenings. Alcohol withdrawal further disrupts sleep, with dreams and nightmares and light fragmented sleep which may continue for weeks or years. Alcohol acts similarly to benzodiazepines and barbiturates by augmenting GABA-mediated synaptic inhibition through interaction with GABA$_A$ receptors controlling chloride channels. Its effects on sleep are thought to be related to this effect.

Amphetamine and related compounds

Amphetamines and related compounds (dexamphetamine, methylphenidate, ephedrine, pseudoephedrine, and others) are psychostimulant drugs which possess sympathomimetic activity and produce a state of behavioural arousal and activation (Pulvirenti and Koob 1994). These drugs enhance noradrenergic, dopaminergic, and serotonergic transmission in the central and peripheral nervous system, mainly by increasing the release of transmitter. Pemoline, an oxazolidine derivative, has similar, though weaker, psychostimulant properties (Eisen et al. 1993), and cocaine is a potent psychostimulant which acts by inhibiting monoamine reuptake. MDMA ('Ecstasy') has some amphetamine-like properties, including central stimulant and antifatigue effects. This drug can cause insomnia that can last months or years after cessation of drug use (Green *et al.* 1995). β-Adrenoceptor agonists such as salbutamol also have central stimulant effects and are sometimes abused (Prasher 1993).

All these drugs reduce sleep duration, decrease REMS and SWS, increase sleep latency, and increase sleep fragmentation (Buysse 1991; Eisen *et al.* 1993; Prasher 1993). They can cause a dose-related insomnia during use, and daytime somnolence and hypersomnia with increased dreaming and nightmares on withdrawal after long-term use, especially after high-dose recreational abuse.

Appetite suppressants

Diethylproprion, mazindol, and phentermine may, like amphetamine, cause insomnia. *d*- and *d,l*-dexfenfluramine, though chemically related to amphetamine, mainly increase central serotonergic activity by increased release and reuptake inhibition. These drugs have little psychostimulant activity but can cause both daytime sedation and disturbed sleep (McTavish and Heel 1992; Silverstone 1992; Idzikowski and Shapiro 1993). They decrease the duration of REMS, and sleep is fragmented with periods of drowsiness and increased wakefulness (Lewis *et al.* 1971). Several authors have reported increased dreaming and nightmares associated with fenfluramine (Mullen and Wilson 1974; Innes *et al.* 1977; Mullen *et al.* 1977). Dreaming appears to be positively related to plasma concentrations, and increased awareness of dreaming despite reduced REMS may be due to intrasleep wakefulness.

Caffeine, theophylline

Caffeine, the well-known stimulant present in coffee, tea, cocoa, cola drinks, chocolate, and some over-the-counter analgesics, is a common cause of insomnia. It increases sleep latency (Zwyghuizen-Doorenbos *et al.* 1990), decreases total sleep time, decreases the time spent in REMS and Stages 3 and 4 SWS, and increases the number of intrasleep arousals in a dose-related manner in normal volunteers (Lader and Bruce 1989; Stradling 1993). There is wide individual variation in sensitivity to the stimulant effects of caffeine and also in rates of caffeine metabolism. Levy and Zylber Katz (1983) found that some poor sleepers have prolonged caffeine elimination half-lives and Tiffin and colleagues (1995) found that otherwise healthy poor sleepers had significantly greater variance in caffeine clearance and elimination rates than normal sleepers. Caffeine-induced insomnia can lead to sleep deprivation. The ensuing daytime sleepiness is reduced by further caffeine and a cycle may be established of poor sleep combated by increased daytime caffeine consumption (Stradling 1993). Withdrawal of caffeine then leads to daytime sleepiness, increased slow-wave activity (delta) on the EEG, and headaches (Griffiths *et al.* 1986; Lader *et al.* 1996).

Theophylline, a methylxanthine related to caffeine and present in several bronchodilator preparations, may also cause insomnia, and nightmares have been reported (*Drugs Newsletter* 1986). The mechanism of action of caffeine and theophyl-line appears to be antagonism of central adenosine A_1 and A_2 receptors which normally exert a central nervous system depressant action (Stradling 1993; Jain *et al.* 1995; Jacobson 1996).

Antidepressant drugs

Many antidepressant drugs have pronounced effects on sleep (reviewed by Hartmann 1976; Kay *et al.* 1976; Buysse 1991; Ashton 1992, 1994*a*, and summarized by Eisen *et al.* 1993). Several of the tricyclic and related compounds have sedative actions and may cause daytime drowsiness, to which tolerance usually develops rapidly. Those with sedative effects include amitriptyline, clomipramine, dothiepin, doxepin, maprotiline, mianserin, trazodone, nefazodone, and trimipramine. Other related compounds (imipramine, amoxapine, desipramine, lofepramine, nortriptyline, and viloxazine) are less sedative, and protriptyline is stimulant. MAOI (phenelzine, tranyl-cypromine, isocarboxazid, moclobemide) have central stimulant effects and often cause insomnia, although they can occasionally cause somnolence. SSRI and venlafaxine, which inhibits both serotonin and noradrenaline reuptake, can all cause insomnia (especially if taken at night) and occasionally daytime drowsiness (Preskorn 1996). Nightmares have been reported during treatment with fluoxetine 20–30 mg daily (Lepkifker *et al.* 1995) and buproprion (Balon 1996).

Nearly all antidepressants that have been studied appear to share the property of suppressing REMS, and this has been shown for both tricyclics and MAOI. Since REMS is increased in depression this action tends to normalize sleep in depressed patients. However, suppression of REMS does not necessarily coincide with improvement in mood, and REMS is also decreased in normal volunteers. A rebound of REMS occurs on drug withdrawal after long-term use of antidepressants, with increased dreaming, nightmares, and insomnia. Most antidepressants, although they alleviate early morning waking in depressed patients, have little effect on SWS. Trazodone and nefazodone, however, are reported to increase SWS in both patients and normal subjects, with an increase in sleep latency but little decrease or even an increase in total REMS time (Scharf *et al.* 1990; Goodwin 1996).

The mechanisms of the sleep changes induced by antidepressants include effects on monoaminergic activity affecting sleep and arousal systems. The sedative effects of tricyclics may be partly due to additional anticholinergic activity, but some sedative antidepressants (mianserin, trazodone) have little anticholinergic action; both these compounds inhibit α_2-adrenoceptors. Antihistamine effects may also be related to sedation.

Mood stabilizers

Lithium can cause daytime sleepiness to which some tolerance occurs. Sleep studies show that it increases SWS and total sleep time, and delays and reduces REMS in patients with depressive disorders and in normal controls (Tyrer and Shopsin 1980; Friston *et al.* 1989; Buysse 1991; Eisen *et al.* 1993). Insomnia and anxiety, as well as relapse of the underlying disorder, may occur on lithium withdrawal (Klein *et al.* 1981). Carbamazepine and, less commonly, sodium valproate may cause daytime sedation. Carbamazepine has been shown, like lithium, to augment SWS and suppress REMS (Eisen *et al.* 1993).

Antipsychotic drugs

Many antipsychotic drugs have sedative effects and can produce subjective sleepiness. This effect occurs with phenothiazines, butyrophenones, thioxanthines, and pimozide, and with clozapine and sulpiride. These drugs tend to normalize the disrupted and fragmented sleep pattern of schizophrenic patients. They decrease wakefulness, increase total sleep time, and increase SWS. REMS is increased with low doses and decreased with higher doses (Kay 1976; Buysse 1991; Eisen *et al.* 1993). Insomnia may occur on antipsychotic withdrawal. The mechanism of action of these drugs is probably complex and includes antagonistic effects on monoaminergic systems as well as anticholinergic and antihistamine effects.

Dopamine agonists

While low doses of levodopa may improve subjective sleep quality in patients with Parkinson's disease, nightmares and hallucinations are early symptoms of levodopa intolerance and, later, daytime agitation and confusion may be added (Pearce 1984). Sleep studies with levodopa have given conflicting results with equivocal changes in REMS and SWS (Buysse 1991). Other dopaminergic drugs used in Parkinson's disease including bromocriptine, apomorphine, and selegeline (also used in narcolepsy) can also cause insomnia, while amantidine, lysuride, and pergolide may cause insomnia or drowsiness (McEvoy 1987; British National Formulary 1997), and amantadine (also used as an antiviral agent) has been associated with nightmares and night terrors (Flaherty and Beller 1981).

Anticholinergic and cholinomimetic drugs

Cholinergic agonists and anticholinesterases (arecoline, pilocarpine, physostigmine, carbachol, tacrine, aricept, and organophosphates) increase wakefulness and arousal. Effects on sleep include nightmares in high doses, insomnia, decreased SWS, and increased REMS (Wyatt and Gillin 1976; Buysse 1991; Berger *et al.* 1996). Conversely, anticholinergic agents (atropine, scopolamine, benztropine, and antipsychotic or antidepressant drugs with anticholinergic effects) generally cause sedation with increased sleepiness, although toxic doses of atropine lead to arousal and agitation. Effects on sleep stages include decreased REMS and sometimes increased SWS (Wyatt and Gillin 1976; Buysse 1991). These effects are due to interference with cholinergic mechanisms involved in arousal and sleep; cholinergic activity is associated with arousal and with the induction or facilitation of REMS.

Anticonvulsants

Most anticonvulsants have some sedative actions, although the degree of this effect is considerably less with the newer compounds. Barbiturates (see above) can cause drowsiness and somnolence, to which tolerance soon develops, and rebound insomnia and nightmares (as well as convulsions) on withdrawal. Phenytoin also causes sleepiness, although it can also cause transient nervousness and insomnia (*British National Formulary* 1997). Sleep studies show that it reduces REMS and may increase SWS (Buysse 1991). Bizarre and severe nightmares have been reported with this drug in elderly patients (Solomon *et al.* 1993). Carbamazepine causes sleepiness and decreases sleep latency. Sodium valproate is less sedative and has little effect on sleep stages although it may decrease REMS (Buysse 1991). Clonazepam and clobazam have effects similar to other benzodiazepines (see above), including sedation and sometimes paradoxical excitement. Ethosuximide can cause drowsiness, and night terrors are also reported (*British National Formulary* 1997).

Newer anticonvulsants have been reviewed by Upton (1994). Vigabatrin can cause drowsiness and, rarely, marked sedation with stupor as well as psychosis in vulnerable patients. Adverse effects of gabapentin and lamotrigine are usually mild but can include somnolence and fatigue. Felbamate can cause somnolence or insomnia and topiramate can cause somnolence, agitation, emotional changes, and depression (*British National Formulary* 1997).

The mechanism of action of several anticonvulsants involves alterations, by various routes, in either GABA or excitatory amino acid activity. Barbiturates and benzodiazepines enhance the inhibitory actions of GABA by actions at or near the GABA/benzodiazepine receptor complex. Carbamazepine, phenytoin, and sodium valproate block voltage-dependent Na^+ channels, preventing the release of excitatory amino acids, particularly glutamate. The mechanism of action of ethosuximide is unknown (Rall and Schleifer 1990).

The mechanisms of action of the newer agents are imperfectly understood and are discussed by Upton (1994a). Vigabatrin irreversibly inhibits the enzyme GABA aminotransferase, preventing the breakdown of GABA and increasing brain GABA concentrations. However, a decrease in brain levels of excitatory amino acids (glutamate and aspartate) may also be involved in its anticonvulsant (and sedative) effects. Gabapentin was originally designed to facilitate GABA activity, and has a similar structure to GABA, but paradoxically it does not seem to have a GABA-mimetic action. It reacts with specific binding sites linked to Ca^{++} ion channels in the brain but how this interaction leads to anticonvulsant properties is unknown. Lamotrigine appears to act primarily by blockade of voltage-dependent Na^+ channels, preventing excessive release of excitatory neurotransmitters, especially glutamate. Felbamate also blocks Na^+ channels and may additionally modulate the function of NMDA receptors and enhance GABA-mediated responses.

Opioids

Opioids have sedative effects, and drowsiness commonly occurs with morphine, heroin, methadone, pethidine, and similar compounds, although tolerance develops with prolonged use. These effects are probably due to agonist activity at opioid

μ-receptors in the limbic system and locus coeruleus (Jaffe and Martin 1980). The partial opioid agonist pentazocine can cause insomnia and nightmares (Alexander and Spence 1974), possibly because of its agonist action on sigma opioid receptors. Opioids decrease REMS and SWS (Buysse 1991) and rebound insomnia occurs on withdrawal.

Antihistamines

Histamine H_1-receptor antagonists which enter the brain have sedative actions and can cause drowsiness, although paradoxical stimulation may rarely occur with high dosage and in children. These agents include the older antihistamines, such as diphenhydramine, promethazine, triprolidine, chlorpheniramine, and others. Promethazine, which is available over-the-counter as a hypnotic and is sometimes used for sedation in children, has a slow onset of action and slow elimination (half-life 12 hours). Polysomnographic measures have shown that these drugs suppress REMS and modestly increase SWS (Nicholson et al. 1985; Roth et al. 1987). Suppression of REMS is sometimes associated with REMS rebound on discontinuation (Buysse 1991).

In contrast, newer histamine H_1-receptor antagonists, such as astemizole, terfenadine, loratidine, and others, penetrate the brain only minimally and do not cause sedation. Nevertheless, insomnia and nightmares have been reported with terfenadine (Data Sheet Compendium 1995–6). Histamine H_2-antagonists do not usually cause sedation, although cimetidine, but not ranitidine, has been shown to increase SWS (Nicholson et al. 1985) and to be associated occasionally with confusional states.

Histamine acts as a central neurotransmitter and several subtypes of histamine receptors (H_1, H_2, H_3) have been identified in the brain (Nicholson 1987; Pollard and Schwartz 1987). Stimulation of H_1- and H_2-receptors markedly potentiates excitatory signals produced by excitatory amino acids and synaptically evoked spikes, and it has been suggested that histamine acts as a 'waking amine' (Schwartz et al. 1986). The sedative actions of antihistamines which enter the brain follow from antagonism of these actions.

Drugs used in anaesthesia

Dreaming is well known to occur under anaesthesia, particularly with nitrous oxide, ether, and cyclopropane (Dillon 1970). Dreams after ketamine seem to be different, being brightly coloured and of a hallucinatory nature, more like the effects described with hallucinogenic drugs. They typically occur during recovery, sometimes accompanied by delirium (British Medical Journal 1971). Perioperative dreaming was described in 16.7 per cent of 72 paediatric patients aged 5–14 years who received suxamethonium as a muscle relaxant (O'Sullivan et al. 1988). The incidence was only 2.8 per cent in 72 patients who were pretreated with tubocurarine, a non-depolarizing agent. The effect of suxamethonium was attributed to the production of an arousal-type EEG, possibly due to muscle-spindle discharge produced by this drug.

Antihypertensive drugs

The effects of antihypertensive drugs in use up to 1982 were extensively reviewed by Paykel and colleagues (1982).

β-Adrenergic-receptor antagonists

Several of these drugs, especially the more lipophilic, can cause drowsiness, insomnia, vivid dreams, and nightmares, as well as hallucinations. With propranolol the mean incidence of lethargy, drowsiness, and fatigue was 3.8 per cent in 33 studies involving 1773 patients treated for hypertension, angina, or arrhythmias (Paykel et al. 1982); insomnia was much less common (incidence 0.7 per cent in published studies). There were several reports of bizarre and distressing dreams and nightmares, with an incidence of 1.6 per cent. The distinction between nighmares and hypnagogic or hypnopompic hallucinations is not always clear. Fleminger (1978) found that 17.5 per cent of 63 patients taking a mean daily dose of 254 mg of propranolol experienced vivid hallucinations or illusions at the onset of sleep or the moment of waking, which were sometimes reported as dreams.

Other β-blockers may also affect sleep. Sleep disturbances, including drowsiness, bizarre dreams, and nightmares, have been reported with oxprenolol, pindolol, sotalol, bisoprolol, metoprolol, alprenolol, and atenolol (Collins and King 1972; Zacharias 1973; Morgan et al. 1974; Waal-Manning and Simpson 1974; Paykel et al. 1982; Kuriama 1994; Data Sheet Compendium 1995–6). Topical ocular timolol caused somnolence in 1.9 per cent and insomnia in seven per cent of 1721 patients with adverse reactions to this agent reported to the National Registry of Drug-Induced Ocular Side-Effects between 1978 and 1985 (Shore et al. 1987). Somnolence is listed as an adverse effect of celiprolol in the British National Formulary (1997) and fatigue and sleep disturbances are listed for carvedilol.

The mechanisms involved in the effects of β-blockers on sleep are not clear but presumably involve the complex and ill-understood role of noradrenaline in arousal and sleep systems (discussed by Zoltoski and Gillin 1994). Drugs that increase monoamine activity (tricyclic antidepressants, MAOI, amphetamines, and others) decrease REMS. Possibly the nightmares associated with β-blockers are due to blockade of central β-adrenergic receptors causing an increase in REMS. Noradrenergic systems are also involved in arousal, and the function of these systems may be impaired by β-blockers that enter the central nervous system, resulting in drowsiness. Strangely, sleep EEG studies in man have failed to show any effect of these agents in normal human subjects (Dunleavy et al. 1971).

Methyldopa

Methyldopa produces dose-related sedation with drowsiness and fatigue in over 38 per cent of patients; bad dreams and nightmares are also reported but at much lower frequency (Paykel et al. 1982). Sleep EEGs in normal volunteers given methyldopa showed increased REMS and decreased SWS, an effect attributed to central serotonin depletion (Baekeland and Lundwall 1971).

Clonidine

Sedation is frequent with clonidine, with an incidence of 68 per cent overall, and patients taking clonidine tend to sleep more heavily than usual (Paykel *et al.* 1982). Disturbances of sleep, nightmares, early morning waking, and insomnia have also been reported by several authors (cited by Paykel *et al.* 1982). Vivid dreams and insomnia also occur as part of the clonidine-withdrawal syndrome. Clonidine is an α-adrenergic agonist and has been shown to decrease both REMS and orthodox sleep while causing drowsiness (Zoltoski and Gillin 1994).

α-adrenoceptor antagonists

These drugs block postsynaptic α-adrenoceptors, both peripherally and centrally. Doxazosin, indoramin, and prazosin may all cause sedation and drowsiness (*British National Formulary* 1997).

Angiotensin-converting-enzyme (ACE) inhibitors

These drugs may cause sleep disturbance, and nightmares have been reported with captopril (Haffner *et al.* 1993).

Other cardiovascular drugs

Nightmares and sleeplessness are reported adverse effects of amiodarone (*Data Sheet Compendium* 1995–6); nightmares and vivid dreams may occasionally occur with the calcium-channel blockers verapamil (Kumar and Hodges 1988) and nifedipine, and the antiarrhythmic drug flecainide (*Drugs Newsletter* 1986). Nightmares and somnolence are common in digitalis intoxication (Lely and Van Enter 1970).

Corticosteroids and NSAID

Corticosteroids have stimulant effects which may increase subjective wakefulness and cause insomnia (Idzikowski and Shapiro 1993). They may decrease both SWS and REMS (Buysse 1991; Young *et al.* 1994). Indomethacin and diclofenac can cause drowsiness or insomnia, and nightmares have been reported with naproxen (Bakht and Miller 1991), nabumetone (Inman *et al.* 1990), and diclofenac (*Data Sheet Compendium* 1995–6).

Anti-infective and antineoplastic agents

Sleep disorders have occasionally been reported after various antibiotics, including insomnia with amoxycillin and ampicillin (Beal *et al.* 1986), nightmares with oral erythromycin (Black and Dawson 1988; Williams 1988), severe sleep disorders and nightmares with ofloxacin (Upton 1994*b*; *Data Sheet Compendium* 1995–6), and anxiety, drowsiness, and insomnia with cycloserine (Wallach and Gershon 1972). Griseofulvin has caused insomnia (Tester-Dalderup 1984). The antimalarial agent mefloquine, a quinolone derivative, has been associated with a large range of neuropsychiatric adverse effects in which insomnia and nightmares are prominent, even at prophylactic doses (250 mg weekly) (van Riemsdijk *et al.* 1997).

Various antineoplastic agents produce neuropsychiatric effects including sleep disturbance. Somnolence, as well as de-lirium, has been associated with methotrexate (Kay *et al.* 1972), and interleukin-2 can provoke psychiatric disturbance in which somnolence is prominent (Denicoff *et al.* 1987).

Drug-withdrawal reactions

Drug-withdrawal reactions are described below. Insomnia or nightmares, or both, may accompany withdrawal of drugs with depressant activity, while somnolence occurs after withdrawal of central nervous system stimulants.

Drug-withdrawal reactions

Many, if not all, drugs that cause adaptive receptor changes on prolonged administration are liable to be associated with withdrawal symptoms if the drug is abruptly discontinued, and sometimes if dosage is reduced. Drug withdrawal reactions are important because they can be misdiagnosed as psychiatric or physical illness if a careful drug history is not obtained. In general, withdrawal syndromes tend to consist of mirror images of the drug's initial effects. Thus abrupt withdrawal from long-term usage of β-blockers (e.g. propranolol) can give rise to tachycardia, palpitations, hypertension, anxiety, and other signs of increased sympathetic activity, with a picture that may be mistaken for an anxiety state. On sudden cessation of benzodiazepines after prolonged use, anticonvulsant effects may be replaced by epileptic seizures, muscle relaxation by increased muscle tension, hypnotic effects by insomnia or nightmares, and anxiolytic effects by increased anxiety. Conversely, with stimulant and euphoriant drugs such as cocaine and amphetamine, withdrawal reactions may consist of depression and lethargy.

Not all these symptoms are inevitable in any individual patient. The particular features of a withdrawal syndrome, the time of onset, duration, and intensity are modified by many other factors. Such factors include pharmacokinetic variables, especially drug half-life, type of drug, dosage and duration of use, rate of withdrawal, personality characteristics, psychiatric state, and others. Withdrawal reactions are most likely to occur with drugs that have been taken regularly for some time (months or more) in relatively high dosage. They tend to be more acute in onset with relatively rapidly eliminated drugs (e.g. lorazepam, paroxetine), and attenuated with longer-acting drugs (e.g. diazepam, fluoxetine). Although withdrawal symptoms from different drug groups have several features in common, characteristic substance-specific withdrawal symptoms also occur, such as perceptual disturbances with benzodiazepines and severe gastrointestinal symptoms with opiates. Withdrawal effects are promptly reversed by an appropriate dose of the drug concerned.

Mechanisms of withdrawal reactions

The development of pharmacodynamic tolerance to a drug sets the scene for the withdrawal syndrome. Such tolerance results from a series of homoeostatic responses which tend to restore normal function despite the presence of the drug. These responses usually involve up- or down-regulation of receptors upon which the drug acts, and often secondary changes in other neurotransmitter systems. Cessation of the drug exposes all the adaptations which have accrued to counteract its presence, releasing a rebound of unopposed activity. This state is manifested clinically as a withdrawal syndrome.

Management of withdrawal

Withdrawal reactions from prescribed drugs can be attenuated and often prevented by slow, tapered withdrawal, a process which may require several weeks or months, and may be combined with psychological support (Schatzberg *et al.* 1997a; Ashton 1994; Lejoyeux *et al.* 1996). Sometimes it is possible to substitute a more slowly eliminated drug from the same drug group (e.g. diazepam for lorazepam) and then taper the second drug.

With alcohol and recreational drugs, supervised detoxification is the usual treatment, complemented by substitution of an alternative drug to counteract severe withdrawal effects (e.g. benzodiazepines for alcohol detoxification). Other drugs with specific effects on particular symptoms are sometimes helpful, such as clonidine in opiate withdrawal, and carbamazepine to prevent seizures in high-dose benzodiazepine abusers.

Antidepressants

Withdrawal symptoms have been associated with virtually all antidepressant drugs, including tricyclic and heterocyclic compounds, MAOI, SSRI, and the serotonin/noradrenaline reuptake inhibitor venlafaxine. The characteristics of the withdrawal reaction differ somewhat between the drug groups, and are considered separately.

Tricyclic and heterocyclic antidepressants

It has been known for over 30 years that withdrawal symptoms can follow discontinuation of tricyclic antidepressants (e.g. Kramer *et al.* 1961). Subsequent literature has been reviewed by Dilsaver and Greden (1984), Tyrer (1984), *Drug and Therapeutics Bulletin* (1986), Dilsaver (1989, 1994), Garner and others (1993), and Lejoyeux and co-workers (1996), and withdrawal syndromes have been reported not only for the older tricyclic antidepressants such as imipramine and amitriptyline but also for newer related compounds such as trazodone. Four main categories of symptoms are described: (1) gastrointestinal and somatic distress symptoms; (2) sleep disturbances; (3) movement disorders; and (4) psychological disturbances. Sleep disturbance is characterized by initial and middle insomnia and excessive, vivid, and often frightening dreams. Of the psychological disturbances, anxiety and agitation are the most common.

Withdrawal symptoms can appear not only after abrupt cessation of tricyclic antidepressants but also during dosage tapering and even after a few missed doses (Garner *et al.* 1993). They usually emerge within the first 2 weeks of drug withdrawal (Ayd 1986) and subside over the next few weeks. The incidence of the syndrome varied between 0 and 100 per cent in 12 different studies between 1959 and 1994 (Lejoyeux *et al.* 1996); Tyrer (1984) found an incidence of about 30 per cent in patients with neurotic depression and phobic neuroses. There are few reports of withdrawal symptoms associated with the more recently introduced antidepressants such as lofepramine, maprotiline, mianserin, and viloxazine, but trazodone, a relatively selective but weak serotonin reuptake inhibitor which also antagonizes 5-HT$_2$ and α_2-adrenoceptors, can produce a withdrawal syndrome (Otani *et al.* 1994) similar to that of other selective inhibitors (see below).

MAOI

Withdrawal reactions associated with MAOI are of much greater severity than those precipitated by tricyclic antidepressant withdrawal (Dilsaver 1994; Lejoyeux *et al.* 1996). In particular, tranylcypromine, which is related to amphetamine and is potentially a drug of abuse (Le Gassicke *et al.* 1965; Pagliaro and Pagliaro 1993; Lejoyeux 1995), can produce a withdrawal syndrome similar to that of amphetamine. In addition, both phenelzine and tranylcypromine are associated with a characteristic withdrawal syndrome which usually appears within days of discontinuation. The incidence in one series of patients on phenelzine was 32.2 per cent (Tyrer 1984); symptoms include panic, headache, shaking, sweating, nausea, and perceptual disturbances. Cognitive impairment, a feature not usually seen in tricyclic antidepressant disorder, may include disorientation in space and time, disorganization of thought processes, and incapacity to recognize familiar faces (Lejoyeux *et al.* 1996). Depression induced by withdrawal may exceed the severity of the disorder for which the drug was originally prescribed (Halle and Dilsaver 1993). Paranoid delusions and hallucinations may also occur. In addition, motor symptoms, including ataxia, athetosis, catatonia, and myoclonic jerks, have been reported. A marked feature after high dosage is severe sleep disturbance with somnolence, rebound of REMS, and nightmares (Le Gassicke *et al.* 1965). There appear to be no reports in the literature of withdrawal effects from the recently introduced reversible and short-acting MAOI moclobemide.

SSRI

The characteristic withdrawal symptoms that follow withdrawal of SSRI are the subject of several reviews (Coupland *et al.* 1996; Lane 1996; Lejoyeux *et al.* 1996; Preskorn *et al.* 1996; Price *et al.* 1996; and Schatzberg *et al.* 1997a). Symptoms, which are usually mild, appear 1–10 days after stopping or, occasionally, after reducing the dosage of an SSRI that has been taken regularly for a few months or more; the time of appearance depends on the elimination half-life of the individual drug. Somatic symptoms include disequilibrium, gastrointestinal symptoms, influenza-like symptoms, sensory disturbances, and occasionally extrapyramidal effects (Stoukides and Stoukides

1991). Psychological symptoms include anxiety, crying spells, confusion, memory problems, aggression, and irritability.

Such symptoms have been reported after withdrawal of all the SSRI, and also with trazodone (Otani *et al*. 1994), although this is a weak serotonin reuptake inhibitor. The true incidence is not known but the risk appears to be greatest with the relatively rapidly eliminated SSRI paroxetine (plasma elimination half-life of 21 hours on multiple dosage) and least with the slowly eliminated fluoxetine which has a plasma elimination half-life of 5–7 days and an active metabolite (norfluoxetine) with a half-life of 7–15 days (Preskorn *et al*. 1996; Price *et al*. 1996; Young and Ashton 1997). In small clinical studies the incidence of withdrawal reactions was variously reported as 38.5 per cent and 50 per cent for paroxetine (Barr *et al*. 1994; Keuthen *et al*. 1994) and 28 per cent for fluvoxamine (Mallya *et al*. 1993), while Oehrberg and colleagues (1995) reported a 34.5 per cent incidence in 55 patients with panic disorder when paroxetine was withdrawn after 12 weeks' treatment.

Venlafaxine

Venlafaxine is a recently introduced antidepressant which is a combined inhibitor of synaptic serotonin and noradrenaline reuptake. Clinical studies on 1060 patients showed a 15 per cent incidence of dizziness, 20 per cent headache, and 19 per cent nausea following significant dosage reduction or abrupt discontinuation of this drug. Corresponding figures for placebo were two per cent dizziness, eight per cent headache, and three per cent nausea (Data on file, Wyeth 1997). Three apparent withdrawal reactions were reported by Louie (1996). These included auditory hallucinations, gastrointestinal symptoms, and bizarre dreams in one case; nausea, dizziness, shock-like sensations, and increased dreaming in another; and nausea, diarrhoea, and dizziness in a third. In all cases the symptoms remitted when venlafaxine was resumed. The withdrawal symptoms reported with this drug appear to be similar to those described on withdrawal of SSRI.

Lithium

Anxiety, insomnia, and irritability (Klein *et al*. 1981) and delirium (Wilkinson 1979) have been reported on withdrawal of lithium. However, Schou (1993) argues that the evidence for abstinence phenomena after lithium discontinuation is weak, and that the symptoms may be confused with recurrence of manic-depressive illness. Recurrence of mania in patients with bipolar affective disorder on discontinuation of lithium is well documented (Margo and McMahon 1982; Tyrer *et al*. 1983; Mander and Loudon 1988; Goodwin 1994).

Mechanisms of antidepressant withdrawal syndromes

Several mechanisms have been proposed to account for antidepressant-withdrawal syndromes (Dilsaver *et al*. 1987, 1989, 1994; Coupland *et al*. 1996; Lane 1996; Lejoyeux *et al*. 1996; Preskorn *et al*. 1996; Schatzberg *et al*. 1997*b*). Some symptoms may be at least partially due to cholinergic over-activity resulting from the upregulation of muscarinic receptors which occurs in response to long-term use of drugs with anticholinergic effects, an action shared by many tricyclics, MAOI, and some SSRI. Withdrawal of the drug reveals the consequent hyperexcitability of cholinergic systems. The cholin-

ergic hypothesis is supported by the findings that tricyclic antidepressant withdrawal symptoms have been relieved by anticholinergic agents (Dilsaver *et al*. 1983), and that paroxetine, the SSRI with the highest incidence of withdrawal effects, has the greatest affinity for muscarinic receptors (Richelson 1994).

Perturbations of monoaminergic systems have also been proposed to account for some antidepressant withdrawal symptoms. In the case of antidepressants which block serotonin reuptake (some tricyclics, MAOI, SSRI, and venlafaxine) it has been proposed that a sudden drop of serotonergic activity on withdrawal might account for some symptoms such as sleep disorders and anxiety (Coupland *et al*. 1996; Lejoyeux *et al*. 1996; Schatzberg *et al*. 1997*b*). Rebound of noradrenergic activity on tricyclic antidepressant withdrawal has also been proposed to account for some symptoms such as anxiety (Charney *et al*. 1982). Similarly, rebound of dopaminergic activity has been proposed to account for the psychotic features of MAOI withdrawal (Dilsaver 1994).

Pharmacokinetic factors may explain the increased risk of a withdrawal syndrome with some antidepressants. For example, the SSRI paroxetine and fluvoxamine have relatively short elimination half-lives (21 or 14 hours on multiple dosing, Preskorn *et al*. 1996), and at high plasma concentrations inhibit their own metabolism by the cytochrome P-450 enzyme CYP2D6. As plasma levels fall following discontinuation, their elimination becomes more rapid and may bring about an acute state of cholinergic and serotonergic dysregulation. Slower elimination (e.g. with fluoxetine) may allow time for intrinsic receptor readjustments and therefore attenuate withdrawal symptoms.

Hypnotics and anxiolytics

Benzodiazepines

A characteristic benzodiazepine withdrawal syndrome has been recognized for many years; it can occur on cessation or re-duction of drug use, not only after high doses but also after prolonged therapeutic dosage. The features have been de-scribed by numerous authors (Petursson and Lader 1981; Owen and Tyrer 1983; Ashton 1984, 1987, 1991, 1995*b*; Busto *et al*. 1986; Tyrer *et al*. 1989; Seivewright and Dougal 1993). Many of the symptoms are common to all anxiety states including panics, tremor, insomnia, and autonomic symptoms, but there are also some less usual features, such as sensory hypersensitivity, per-ceptual disturbances, hallucinations, muscle cramps, twitches and fasiculation, and formication. Abrupt withdrawal from relatively high doses can result in convulsions, delirium, and psychotic reactions. A withdrawal syndrome can also occur in neonates whose mothers have taken benzodiazepines regularly during pregnancy (see Chapter 7).

Withdrawal symptoms appear within 1–3 days of stopping short-acting benzodiazepines (e.g. lorazepam) and about 7 days after withdrawal of longer-acting ones (e.g. diazepam). With rapidly eliminated benzodiazepines (e.g. alprazolam, tri-azolam), symptoms may appear between doses. The acute withdrawal syndrome is classically described as lasting 5–28 days with a peak of severity around 2 weeks post-withdrawal after which most symptoms return to prewithdrawal levels. However, some symptoms may be protracted, lasting many months (Higgitt *et al.* 1990; Ashton 1991, 1995*b*; Tyrer 1991). Protracted symptoms may include anxiety, insomnia, depression, perceptual and motor symptoms, and gastrointestinal disturbances (Olajide and Lader 1984; Ashton 1995).

The reported incidence of the withdrawal syndrome for benzodiazepines varies between nil and 100 per cent in different studies, depending on the patient population and the definition of withdrawal, but is probably over 40 per cent in patients withdrawing from therapeutic doses (Tyrer *et al.* 1983). Prolonged use, high dosage, certain personality types, and possibly potent relatively short-acting benzodiazepines may be predisposing factors (Marriott and Tyrer, 1993; Tyrer 1993b). Treatment in patients who have been taking therapeutic doses consists mainly of slow dosage tapering combined with psychological support (Ashton 1994*b*). Antidepressants may be needed to combat depression, which can be severe (Ashton 1987). For high-dose recreational benzodiazepine abusers a more rapid controlled schedule of inpatient detoxification is preferable; several methods are reviewed by Ashton (in press).

Mechanisms

Long-term use of benzodiazepines causes compensatory changes in GABA/benzodiazepine receptors, including decreased density and decreased affinity for $GABA_A$ (Cowen and Nutt 1982; Nutt 1996). There may also be secondary changes in other receptor systems normally inhibited by GABA, resulting in increased sensitivity to or output of excitatory neurotransmitters. Withdrawal of benzodiazepines exposes the individual to a state of relative GABA underactivity with a resulting rebound of central nervous system excitation. The affinity of GABA receptors for GABA is slow to reverse and may account for some of the protracted symptoms. This possibility is supported by the finding that flumazenil, a benzodiazepine antagonist, can reverse some longstanding withdrawal symptoms, possibly by 'resetting' GABA receptors to their normal affinity state (Lader and Morton 1992).

Other hypnotics and anxiolytics

Zopiclone and zolpidem, which have been introduced relatively recently as hypnotics, are not benzodiazepines but nevertheless act on GABA/benzodiazepine receptors. If used regularly for more than a few weeks zopiclone, and possibly zolpidem, can produce similar withdrawal effects to benzodiazepines (Dorian *et al.* 1983; CSM 1990; *The Lancet* 1990*b*; Cavallaro *et al.* 1993; Ashton 1997*a*). Of the older hypnotics, barbiturates are now obsolete (though still used by some). They can produce a severe abstinence syndrome with anxiety, hallucinations, delirium, and convulsions (Jaffe 1980). Chlormethiazole and chloral derivatives also act on GABA/benzodiazepine receptors, and they can induce dependence and an abstinence syndrome similar to that of barbiturates and benzodiazepines. The anxiolytic drug buspirone appears to be relatively free of withdrawal effects (Lader 1991; Murphy *et al.* 1989).

Opioids

Opioid dependence and withdrawal reactions are rarely a problem when the drugs are used clinically for pain relief (Hollister 1985; Twycross and McQuay 1989) and descriptions of opioid-withdrawal syndromes mostly refer to high-dose abusers (Farrell 1994; Hollister 1985; Gossop *et al.* 1987; Jaffe and Martin 1990; Belkin and Gold 1991).

An acute withdrawal syndrome can be precipitated within minutes by the opioid antagonist naloxone in dependent subjects. Without naloxone, the time of onset depends on the duration of action of the opioid used. A marked early and continuing feature is an intense craving for further opioids, often leading to drug-seeking behaviour. Craving begins at about the time the next dose is usually due, 4–6 hrs after the last dose of heroin; 12–24 hrs for the longer-acting methadone. If the drug is not available, an influenza-like syndrome is heralded by aches in the muscles and bones, usually involving the back and legs, followed by lachrymation, rhinorrhoea, gastrointestinal disturbances, agitation, and other symptoms.

A feature relatively peculiar to opioid withdrawal is frequent yawning; pupillary dilatation may also be more marked than in most other withdrawal states, and increased sensitivity to pain is noted in DSM IV. Hot and cold flushes combined with piloerection in severe cases engendered the expression 'cold turkey', while muscle jerks in the legs ares referred to in the phrase 'kicking the habit'. Hallucinations, delirium, and psychotic reactions are rare compared with hypnotic and alcohol withdrawal. Life-threatening symptoms, such as convulsions, are not usual in opioid withdrawal, which is described as subjectively severe but objectively mild (Gossop *et al.* 1987).

Withdrawal symptoms peak about 3 days after abrupt opioid withdrawal and subside over the next week. The onset of symptoms is delayed by tapered withdrawal and giving methadone, but still occurs following the last methadone dose (Gossop *et al.* 1989). Protracted withdrawal symptoms may continue for weeks or months and include anxiety, dysphoria, anhedonia, insomnia, and continued craving; the latter symptom no doubt accounts largely for the high relapse rate after detoxification.

A typical withdrawal syndrome can occur with all synthetic and natural opioids including codeine, dihydrocodeine, and the mixed opioid agonists/antagonists such as pentazocine and buprenorphine. A paranoid-hallucinatory psychosis after withdrawal of dextropropoxyphene has been described (Harris and Harper 1979). The incidence of the syndrome appears to be high, affecting almost all those presenting at drug dependence units (West and Gossop 1994). A neonatal withdrawal syndrome occurs in the babies of opioid-dependent mothers (Zelsen *et al.* 1973).

Mechanisms

The exact mechanisms of the opioid withdrawal syndrome are unclear but it may be due partly to a decreased output of endogenous opioids resulting from chronic exposure to the drugs. In human heroin addicts, Herz (1981) found reduced cerebrospinal fluid and plasma concentrations of β-endorphin and metenkephalin, a finding borne out by animal work (Herz and Holt 1982). The main site of action of narcotic analgesics is the μ opioid receptor, activation of which is thought to be responsible for analgesia, euphoria, drowsiness, and other effects reviewed by Thompson (1984). Activation of μ receptors also inhibits the release of other neurotransmitters, including monoamines, acetylcholine, and substance P (Henderson 1983; North and Williams 1983). Rebound release of these substances in withdrawal could account for the tachycardia, influenza-like symptoms, and increased pain sensitivity. In particular, opioids depress the firing rate and release of noradrenaline from the locus coeruleus. The resulting rebound rise in noradrenergic activity during withdrawal (Simonato 1996) undoubtedly contributes to the anxiety and hyperexcitability of the abstinence syndrome. This effect can be counteracted by α_2-adrenergic agonists such as clonidine and lofexidine which are well known to reduce opioid-withdrawal symptoms (Farrell 1994).

The craving which is so prominent in opioid withdrawal probably involves the important actions of opioids in limbic system reward mechanisms (Di Chiara and North 1992; Simonato 1996; Di Chiara 1997). Endogenous opioids, possibly acting through a dopaminergic link (Wise and Bozarth 1987), are vital to the normal operation of these systems. Opioid withdrawal decreases dopamine output in the nucleus accumbens, and decreased dopaminergic transmission in the mesolimbic system is thought to be responsible for the aversive aspects (Di Chiara and North 1992). This aversive stimulus may account for the intense desire for further opioids, leading to drug-seeking behaviour.

The management of opioid withdrawal has been reviewed by Johns (1994), Farrell (1994) and Boyer and Feighner (1996).

Antipsychotics

Withdrawal reactions after chronic treatment with antipsychotic drugs have been recognized for many years (Hollister *et al.* 1960; Lacoursiere *et al.* 1976). Three main types of reaction are described: generalized symptoms of cholinergic and dopaminergic overactivity, and symptoms thought to result from drug-induced dopamine-receptor hypersensitivity ('disuse supersensitivity') in the nigrostriatal system (withdrawal dyskinesias) or limbic system (withdrawal psychosis). Generalized withdrawal symptoms are described by Dilsaver (1994) and include nausea, vomiting, diarrhoea, rhinorrhoea, sweating, myalgias, paraesthesias, anxiety, agitation, restlessness, tremor, vertigo, and insomnia. These symptoms are most marked after chronic use of agents with pronounced anticholinergic activity (Luchins *et al.* 1980; Chouinard *et al.* 1984) and have been described following discontinuation of phenothiazines, thioxanthenes, and butyrophenones. Simultaneous withdrawal of antimuscarinic drugs increases the likelihood of these symptoms. The reaction generally appears 1–4 days after the drug is stopped and abates gradually over 7–14 days. It is not confined to schizophrenic patients and has been noted in non-psychotic tuberculous patients treated with chlorpromazine 300 mg per day for 9–12 months (Hollister 1964).

Withdrawal dyskinesias are also common when antipsychotics, especially those which carry a high risk of inducing extrapyramidal effects, are withdrawn after long-term treatment (Gardos *et al.* 1978; Chouinard *et al.* 1984; Gualtieri *et al.* 1984; Perényi *et al.* 1985; Baldessarini 1996*a*), usually consisting of choreoathetosis or tardive dyskinesia. Withdrawal psychoses of the schizophreniform type can also occur, with or without dyskinesia, and not only in schizophrenic patients (Chouinard and Jones 1980; Witschy *et al.* 1984; Perényi *et al.* 1985). These symptoms usually develop within a week of drug discontinuation, but respond within days to reinstatement. If withdrawal is indicated, drug dosage should be gradually tapered over a period of months.

Anticholinergic drugs prescribed for extrapyramidal effects of antipsychotics are also sometimes abused, mainly by psychiatric patients (McInnis and Petursson 1984; Pullen *et al.* 1984). Withdrawal reactions, which last 2 weeks or more, consist of signs of cholinergic overactivity including sweating, tachycardia, photophobia, headaches, anxiety, and irritability. Such reactions have been reported with benzhexol, orphenadrine, biperiden, procyclidine, and benztropine, in patients with schizophrenia, bipolar affective disorder, and personality disorder, and anticholinergic drugs are often combined with other drugs of abuse (Pullen *et al.* 1984).

Alcohol

The clinical manifestations of alcohol withdrawal are well known and were reviewed by Schultz 1991) and Hall and Zador (1997). They vary in severity from mild symptoms accompanying the familiar alcohol hangover to the full-blown picture of delirium tremens, depending on the degree and duration of drinking. Symptoms appear about 6 hours after a substantial fall in the blood alcohol concentration and at first consist of tremulousness, malaise, nausea or vomiting, sweating, and other autonomic symptoms, combined with anxiety, depression, or irritability. These symptoms peak between 24–36 hours and may subside after 48 hours.

In more severe cases, the syndrome proceeds at its peak to hallucinations which occur in 3–10 per cent of alcoholic patients during withdrawal. These are most commonly visual although they may involve any of the senses and can occur without delirium. They usually last only hours but may persist for weeks. Generalized tonic–clonic withdrawal seizures occur in 5–15 per cent of alcoholic patients, with a maximum incidence 24 hours after the last drink. They occur singly, or in short bursts over 6–12 hours, and rarely develop into status epilepticus. The EEG shows sharp waves, spikes, and paroxysmal changes at this stage but reverts to normal as the convulsions pass.

If untreated, about 30 per cent of patients with convulsions may develop delirium tremens, but this occurs in less than five per cent of patients hospitalized for alcohol withdrawal. The onset of delirium tremens is generally delayed, occurring between 72 and 96 hours after cessation of drinking, sometimes after the transient hallucinatory phase has subsided. Delirium tremens is characterized by gross tremors, agitation, delirium with hallucinations, increased autonomic activity, including copious sweating and sometimes incontinence, and hyperpyrexia. Delirium tremens may coexist with hepatic encephalopathy (see Chapter 13), and it is important to exclude this possibility, as central nervous system depressants which may be indicated for the agitation of delirium tremens are likely to worsen hepatic encephalopathy. The mean duration of delirium tremens is 56 hours, with a range of 10–150 hours (Schultz 1991). This condition can cause death from cardiovascular, metabolic, or infectious complications; the mortality rate with good hospital care is about two per cent (Schultz 1991).

Craving for alcohol is a major component of the alcohol withdrawal syndrome and is highly correlated with the degree of both physical and affective withdrawal symptoms (Stockwell 1994). Mild withdrawal symptoms, particularly anxiety, especially when combined with the conditioning effects of alcohol-related cues, are also important contributors to loss of control over alcohol consumption and to relapse after alcohol detoxification (Stockwell *et al.* 1994). A protracted alcohol withdrawal syndrome includes continued craving, depression, and weakness.

A neonatal withdrawal syndrome occurs in the babies of chronic alcoholic mothers. This occurs within 48 hours of birth and includes sleep disturbances, tremor, hyper-reflexia, and feeding difficulties (see Chapter 7).

Mechanisms
The mechanisms of the alcohol withdrawal syndrome are complex and there is evidence that many neurotransmitter systems are involved. Chronic alcohol use causes down-regulation of (inhibitory) GABA$_A$ receptors and up-regulation of (excitatory) glutamate NMDA receptors (Schultz 1991; Littleton and Little 1994; Nutt 1996; O'Brien 1996; Spanagel and Zieglgänsberger 1997): exposure of these changes on cessation of alcohol probably accounts for the generalized central nervous system excitability and autonomic overactivity seen in withdrawal. The anticholinesterase physostigmine has been used successfully in the management of selected cases of delirium tremens (Powers *et al.* 1981). In addition there is evidence that alcohol interacts with endogenous opioid systems and a deficiency in endogenous opioid concentrations may contribute to the withdrawal syndrome (Schultz *et al.* 1980). Thirdly, the euphoric effect of alcohol may be at least partly due to stimulation of dopamine release in the nucleus accumbens (Nutt 1996), and as with opioid withdrawal, decreased dopaminergic activity in limbic system reward systems may be the essential factor in the craving and drug-seeking behaviour associated with alcohol withdrawal. Paradoxically, however, delirium tremens appears to be associated with increased dopaminergic activity, since it responds to dopamine-receptor blocking agents such as haloperidol. Changes in serotonergic and related neuroendocrine effects may be further contributory factors to

protracted abstinence symptoms (Schultz 1991). Activation of the cholecystokinin CCKB-receptor may also be involved in alcohol withdrawal (Nutt 1996).

Methods of alcohol detoxification and longer-term management have been discussed by Schultz (1991), Tollefson (1991), Sellers and colleagues (1992), Hodgson (1996), Nutt 1996, and Spanagel and Zieglgänsberger (1997).

Cannabis

A cannabis withdrawal syndrome has been unequivocally demonstrated in placebo-controlled studies (Mendelson *et al.* 1984; Nahas 1984; Mendelson 1987; Pertwee 1991). The syndrome has similarities to both alcohol and opiate withdrawal states, and includes restlessness, anxiety, dysphoria, irritability, insomnia, anorexia, tremor, and autonomic effects such as sweating, salivation, and gastrointestinal disturbances. The syndrome appears about 6–10 hours after cessation of regular cannabis use and usually lasts several days, although some subjects report disturbed sleep for several weeks. A daily dose of 180 mg of Δ^9-tetrahydrocannabinol (THC) a day (one or two modern 'good quality' joints) for 11–21 days has been shown in laboratory studies to be sufficient to produce a well-defined withdrawal syndrome (Jones 1983).

It is claimed that the cannabis withdrawal syndrome is mild and short-lived (Hollister 1986; Abood and Martin 1992). The physical symptoms may be cushioned by the slow elimination of THC, which has a tissue elimination half-life of about 7 days, but some psychological symptoms are protracted and there is increasing evidence that people are seeking professional help with withdrawal (Roffman and Barnhart 1987; Roffman *et al.* 1988; Stephens *et al.* 1993; Kuhar and Pilotte 1996; Thomas 1996). The mechanism of the withdrawal symptoms is not clear but may involve changes in endogenous cannabinoid receptors in the brain (Matsuda *et al.* 1990), many of which are situated in limbic system reward areas.

Cocaine, amphetamines, and related psychostimulants

Gawin and Kleber (1986) described three phases of abstinence symptoms in 30 outpatient cocaine abusers: the 'crash', the 'withdrawal', and the 'extinction'. The 'crash', which is familiar to cocaine abusers, develops rapidly (within 15–30 min) after heavy cocaine use and consists of extreme dysphoria, anhedonia, insomnia but desire to sleep, irritability, anxiety, and craving for more cocaine. Many cocaine abusers take other drugs including heroin, benzodiazepines, alcohol, and cannabis to allay these unpleasant symptoms. Hence most cocaine addicts are polydrug abusers and may be dependent on several drugs (Cocores *et al.* 1991). The acute 'crash' merges into a dysphoric lethargy and anergia followed by hypersomnolence and hyperphagia, the whole phase lasting up to 4 days. During the second withdrawal phase, subjects become euthymic but feelings of anhedonia, dysphoria, anxiety, and irritability, along with increasing craving, return over the next several weeks, usually culminating in a return to cocaine use. The extinction phase only occurs in those who remain abstinent; subjects are generally euthymic but experience intense episodic cocaine craving triggered by environmental cues, and relapse is likely. Protracted withdrawal, with anhedonia, anergia, and craving lasting for years, has been reported in a few subjects (Strang *et al.* 1993).

These clearly demarcated phases were not evident in two inpatient studies of cocaine addicts who were not polydrug users reviewed by Lago and Kosten (1994). In these patients abstinence symptoms, including craving, declined smoothly over 21–28 days of observation. However, the initial 'crash' may have been missed if it occurred before hospitalization. Most studies emphasize the relative absence of physical signs such as increased autonomic activity in cocaine withdrawal: heart rate is in fact usually decreased (O'Brien 1996). There appear to be no physical life-threatening consequences of cocaine withdrawal, the main features of which are the severe and often irresistible craving combined with lethargy, anhedonia, and somnolence.

Amphetamine has many similarities to cocaine. It has a high addictive potential (Miller 1991) but rather less than cocaine (Hollister 1985). As with cocaine, many amphetamine abusers are also polydrug abusers, employing 'downers' such as heroin, barbiturates, benzodiazepines, and alcohol to overcome the stimulant effects of amphetamine (Miller 1991). Amphetamine abusers who quit after a bout of high-dosage use are protected from the 'crash' of cocaine abstinence by the longer elimination half-life of amphetamine which is 10–15 hours compared with about 1 hour for cocaine (Lago and Kosten 1994). However, cessation from heavy use of amphetamines produces an abstinence syndrome similar to that of cocaine. An initial period of hypersomnolence is followed by a protracted period of lethargy, hunger, sleep disturbance with rebound of REM sleep and vivid dreaming, mood lability, depression, confusion and perceptual abnormalities, paranoid ideation, and craving. Stereotypic behaviours and movements are also reported (Miller 1991). Other sympathomimetic amines including dextroamphetamine, methamphetamine, phenmetrazine, methylphenidate, diethylproprion, and over-the-counter Do-Do tablets containing ephedrine (Loosmore and Armstrong 1990) may produce similar abstinence effects. Fenfluramine, phenylpropanolamine, and mazindol have relatively little abuse potential (O'Brien 1996).

Mechanisms

Both cocaine and amphetamines increase central dopaminergic activity: cocaine inhibits synaptic reuptake of dopamine as well as noradrenaline and serotonin, while amphetamine stimulates presynaptic release of dopamine and other monoamines. The euphoriant effect of these drugs is thought to result from increased dopamine activity in rewarding brain areas, such as the nucleus accumbens and prefrontal cortex (Wise and Bozarth 1987; Miller 1994). A rebound decrease in dopaminergic activity in these areas during withdrawal is thought to account for the anhedonia and craving in abstinence (Nutt 1996), and the prolonged abstinence syndrome may be due to a protracted decrease in dopaminergic tone (Lago and Kosten 1994). Prolonged use of both cocaine and amphetamine use may result in dopamine depletion with compensatory development of postsynaptic dopamine receptor supersensitivity. Such supersensitivity in the caudate nucleus may underlie the stereotypic movements sometimes seen in amphetamine abstinence. Both cocaine and amphetamines inhibit sleep and decrease REM sleep. Rebound effects, probably involving perturbations of several monoamines, may account for the somnolence and vivid dreaming. Neurochemical changes in cocaine withdrawal are further discussed by Schenk and colleagues (1993), Holman (1994), and Kuhar and Pilotte (1996).

Acute cocaine or amphetamine detoxification is not usually associated with significant alterations in vital signs, withdrawal seizures, or delirium (Cocores *et al.* 1991), although there is a risk of suicide at this stage (Strang *et al.* 1993). Symptoms subside gradually over a period of days and initial management involves mainly supervision and psychological support. The greatest problem is prevention of relapse after detoxification, due to continued craving. Management of this phase has been reviewed by several authors (Cocores *et al.* 1991; Schuckit 1994; Strang *et al.* 1993; Pulvirenti and Koob 1994; Berger *et al.* 1996; Halikas *et al.* 1989).

Anabolic/androgenic steroids, glucocorticoids, and oestrogens

Anabolic/androgenic steroids are increasingly being abused, not only by competitive athletes to increase performance and aggression, but also by aesthetes who wish to improve their appearance (Lukas 1996). A large range of such steroids is available for oral ingestion or injection, including testosterone, testosterone derivatives, and modified testosterone analogues. Steroid abusers may take several different preparations at once or in cycles, often in excessively high dosage, and may combine them with other drugs, such as alcohol, cannabis, or cocaine, with which they may interact (Lukas 1996). Abuse of anabolic/androgenic steroids produces numerous adverse physical and psychiatric effects (Williamson and Young 1992) and can also produce physical dependence and an abstinence syndrome on withdrawal.

Withdrawal effects were described by Brower (1991), Brower and others (1990), and Pope and Katz (1988). There appear to be two phases of withdrawal: an initial phase of symptoms similar to those of opioid withdrawal, starting 1–2 days after the last dose and lasting about a week, and a prolonged phase consisting of depressive symptoms and craving which may continue for several months. Depression may be severe and lead to suicide. Brower and others (1990) found that 84 per cent of steroid abusers reported withdrawal symptoms, and 50 per cent reported craving. Other symptoms included fatigue, depressed mood, restlessness, anorexia, headaches, insomnia, and decreased libido. Pope and Katz (1988) interviewed 41 steroid abusers of whom five developed major depression while withdrawing and two within 3 months of stopping steroids; only one of these had a history of major depression before steroid use.

Mechanisms

The mechanisms of the withdrawal syndrome are not clear, but steroids are known to act both at intracellular receptors, which then affect gene expression, and to alter membrane ion permability affecting the release of neurotransmitters and neurohormones (McEwen 1991). Management of anabolic steroid withdrawal consists of supportive measures and symptomatic treatment, such as antidepressant drugs for depression. Steroid-induced hypogonadism and other hormonal disorders may require specialized endocrinological treatment. Some subjects take human chorionic gonadotrophin, a hormone which is available illicitly, to restimulate their endogenous testosterone production (Pope and Katz 1988).

Glucocorticoids are also sometimes abused in high dosage (Hollister 1985). Rapid withdrawal produces a syndrome of anorexia, nausea, lethargy, joint and muscle pain, weakness, and skin desquamation (Bacon et al. 1966; Hargreave et al. 1969; Schimmer and Parker 1996). Withdrawal psychoses of manic or schizophrenic types also occur (Judd et al. 1983; Venkatarangan et al. 1988). Wolkowitz and Rapaport (1989) described psychiatric symptoms including anxiety, depression, depersonalization, irritability, emotional lability, fatigue, and memory difficulties following prednisolone withdrawal, and attributed these to pituitary–adrenal suppression caused by the drug.

Rare cases of schizophreniform psychosis have been reported after abrupt withdrawal of oestrogens and clomiphene (Keeler et al. 1964; Altmark et al. 1987; Faulk 1989; Mallet et al. 1989).

Other withdrawal syndromes

DSM IV specifies other withdrawal syndromes, including that from nicotine, and a number of other substance abuse disorders (caffeine, hallucinogens, phencyclidine, nitrite inhalants), each of which may produce withdrawal reactions; these are not discussed here.

References

Abood, M.E. and Martin, B.M. (1992). Neurobiology of marijuana abuse. Trends Neurosci. 13, 201.

Abraham, H.D. (1982). Chronic impairment of colour vision in users of LSD. Br. J. Psychiatry 140, 518.

Abraham, H.D. (1983). Visual phenomenology of the LSD flashback. Arch. Gen. Psychiatry 40, 884.

Adams, P.W. (1980). Pyridoxine, the pill and depression. J. Pharmacother. 3, 20.

Adams, F., Quesada, J.R., and Gutterman, J.U. (1984). Neuropsychiatric manifestations of human leukocyte interferon therapy in patients with cancer. JAMA 252, 938.

Adler, L.E., Sadja, L., and Wilets, G. (1980). Cimetidine toxicity manifested as paranoia and hallucinations. Am. J. Psychiatry 137, 1112.

Adler, L.E., Bell, J., Kirch, D., et al. (1982). Psychosis associated with clonidine withdrawal. Am. J. Psychiatry 139, 110.

Agarwal, S.K. (1978). Cimetidine and visual hallucinations. JAMA 240, 214.

Aghajanian, G.K., Sprouse, J.S., and Rasmussen, K. (1987). Physiology of the midbrain serotonin system. In Psychopharmacology: The Third Generation of Progress. (ed. H.Y. Meltzer), p. 141. Raven Press, New York.

Ahmad, S., Sheikh, A.I., and Meeran M.K. (1979). Disopyramide-induced acute psychosis. Chest 76, 712.

Aizenberg, D., Schwartz, B., and Zemishlany, Z. (1991). Delusional parasitosis associated with phenelzine. Br. J. Psychiatry 159, 716.

Alexander, J.I. and Spence, A. (1974). CNS effects of pentazocine. BMJ ii, 224.

Allebeck, P., Adamson, C., and Engstrom, A. (1993). Cannabis and schizophrenia: a longitudinal study of cases treated in Stockholm County. Acta Psychiatr. Scand. 88, 21.

Altmark, D., Tomer, R., and Segal, M. (1987). Psychotic episode induced by ovulation-initiating treatment. Israel J. Med. Sci. 23, 1156.

Al-Zahawi, M.F. and Sprott, M.S. (1988). Hallucinations in association with ceftazidime. BMJ 297, 858.

AMA Drug Evaluation (1980). Drugs used in affective disorders. In AMA Drug Evaluation, p. 187. American Medical Association, Chicago.

American Psychiatric Association (1994). Diagnostic and Statistical Manual of Mental Disorders (4th edn). Washington, DC.

Ananth, J. and Chadiri, A.M. (1980). Drug-induced mood disorders. Int. Pharmacopsychiatry 15, 59.

Andersson, K. and Persson, C.G.A. (1980). Extrapulmonary effects of theophylline. Eur. J. Respir. Dis. (Suppl.) 61, 17.

Andreasson, S., Allebeck, A., Engstrom, A., et al. (1987). Cannabis and schizophrenia: a longitudinal study of Swedish conscripts. Lancet 2, 1483.

Angrist, B. (1983). Psychoses induced by CNS stimulants and related drugs. In Stimulants: Neurochemical, Behavioral and Clinical Perspectives (ed. I. Creese), p. 1. Raven Press, New York.

Annito, W.J. and Leyman, W.A. (1980). Anabolic steroids and acute schizophrenic episode. J. Clin. Psychiatry 41, 143.

Anthony, J.C., Tien, A.Y., and Petronis, K.R. (1989). Epidemiologic evidence on cocaine use and panic attacks. Am. J. Epidemiol. 129, 543.

Arana, G.W., Wilens, T.E., and Baldessarini, R.J. (1985). Plasma corticosterone and cortisol following dexamethasone in psychiatric patients. Psychoneuroendocrinology 10, 49.

Arber, N. (1988). Delirium induced by atenolol. BMJ 297, 1048.

Arnold, E.S., Rudd, S.M., and Kirshner, H. (1980). Manic psychosis following rapid withdrawal from baclofen. Am. J. Psychiatry 137, 1466.

Aronson, J.K. and Reynolds, D.J.M. (1992). Lithium. BMJ 305, 1273.

Asher, H. (1971). Trailing phenomena — a long-lasting LSD side effect. Am. J. Psychiatry 127, 1233.

Ashton, H. (1984). Benzodiazepine withdrawal: an unfinished story. BMJ 288,1135.

Ashton, C.H. (1985). Benzodiazepine overdose: are specific antagonists useful? BMJ 290, 805.

Ashton, H. (1987). Benzodiazepine withdrawal: outcome in 50 patients. Br. J. Addict. 83, 665.

Ashton, C.H. (1990). Solvent abuse: Little progress after 20 years. *BMJ* 300, 135.

Ashton, H. (1991). Protracted withdrawal syndromes from benzodiazepines. *Journal of Substance Abuse Treatment* 8, 19.

Ashton, H. (1992). *Brain Function and Psychotropic Drugs.* Oxford University Press.

Ashton, H. (1994a). The effect of drugs on sleep. In *Sleep* (ed.R. Cooper), p. 175. Chapman & Hall Medical, London.

Ashton, H. (1994b). The treatment of benzodiazepine dependence. *Addiction* 89, 1535.

Ashton, H. (1995a). Toxicity and adverse consequences of benzodiazepine use. *Psychiatric Annals* 25, 158

Ashton, H. (1995b). Protracted withdrawal from benzodiazepines: The post-withdrawal syndrome. *Psychiatric Annals* 25, 174.

Ashton, C.H (1997). Management of insomnia. *Prescribers' Journal* 37, 1

Ashton, H. (1998). Benzodiazepine abuse. In *All You Need to Know about Drink, Drugs and Dependence* (ed. J. de Belleroche). Harwood Academic Press, Reading, Berks (in press).

Ashton, H., Golding, J.F., Marsh, V.R., *et al.* (1981). The seed and the soil: effect of dosage, personality and starting state on the response to D9-tetrahydrocannabinol in man. *Br. J. Clin. Pharmacol.* 12, 705.

Assayheen, T.A. and Michell, G. (1982). Metoprolol in hypertension. *Med. J. Aust.* i, 73.

Awuonda, M. (1996). Swedes alarmed at ketamine misuse. *Lancet* 348, 122.

Ayd, F.J. (1986). Five to fifteen years' maintenance doxepin therapy. *Int. Clin. Psychopharmacol.* 1, 53.

Bacon, P.A., Myles, A.B., Beardwell, C.G., *et al.* (1966). Corticosteroid withdrawal in rheumatoid arthritis. *Lancet,* ii, 935.

Baekeland, F. and Lundwall, L. (1971). Effects of methyldopa on sleep patterns in man. *Electroencephalogr. Clin. Neurophysiol.* 31, 269.

Baigent, M., Holme, G., and Hafner, R.J. (1985). Self reports of the interaction between substance abuse and schizophrenia. *Aust. N.Z. J. Psychiatry* 29, 69.

Baile, W.F., De Paulo, J.R., and Schmidt, C.W. Jr. (1977). Emergency room management of organic brain syndromes caused by over-the-counter hypnotics. *Maryland State Med. J.* 26, 61.

Bakht, F.R. and Miller, L.G. (1991). Naproxen-associated nightmares. *South. Med. J.* 84, 1271.

Baldessarini, R.J. (1980). Drugs and the treatment of psychiatric disorders. In *The Pharmacological Basis of Therapeutics* (ed. A.G. Gilman, L.S. Goodman, and A. Gilman), p. 391. Macmillan, New York.

Baldessarini, R.J. (1996). Drugs and the treatment of psychiatric disorders: Psychosis and anxiety. In *Goodman and Gilman's The Pharmacological Basis of Therapeutics* (ed. J.G. Hardman and L.E. Limbird), p. 399. McGraw-Hill, New York.

Ball, P. (1989). Adverse reactions and interactions of fluoroquinolones. *Clin. Invest. Med.* 12, 28.

Ball, R. and Rosser, R. (1989). Psychosis and anti-tuberculosis therapy. *Lancet* ii, 205.

Balon, R. (1996). Bupropion and nightmares. *Am. J. Psychiatry* 153, 579.

Balster, R.L. (1987). The behavioural pharmacology of phencyclidine. In *Psychopharmacology: The Third Generation of Progress* (ed. H.Y. Meltzer), p. 1573. Raven Press, New York

Barker, S. (1987). Oxymethalone and aggression. *Br. J. Psychiatry* 151, 564.

Barodawala, S. and Mulley, G.P. (1997). Visual hallucinations. *J. R. Coll. Phys.* 31, 42.

Barr, L.C, Goodman, W.K., and Price, L.H. (1994). Physical symptoms associated with paroxetine discontinuation. *Am. J. Psychiatry* 151, 289.

Barth, J.D., Kruisbring, O.A.E., and Van Dijk, A.I. (1990). Inhibitors of hydroxymethylglutaryl coenzyme A reductase for treating hypercholesterolaemia. *BMJ* 301, 669.

BCDSP (Boston Collaborative Drug Surveillance Program) (1971). Psychiatric side-effects of non-psychiatric drugs. *Semin. Psychiatry* 3, 435.

BCDSP (Boston Collaborative Drug Surveillance Program) (1972). Acute adverse reactions to prednisone in relation to dosage. *Clin. Pharmacol. Ther.* 13, 694.

Beal, D.M., Hudson, B., and Zaiaic, M. (1986). Amoxicillin-induced psychosis. *Am. J. Psychiatry* 143, 255.

Beasley, C.M., Dornseif, B.E., Bosomworth, J.C., *et al.* (1991). Fluoxetine and suicide: a meta-analysis of controlled trials of treatment for depression. *BMJ* 303, 685.

Belkin, B.M. and Gold, M.S. (1991). Opioids. In *Comprehensive Handbook of Drug and Alcohol Addiction* (ed. N.S. Miller), p. 537. Marcel Dekker, New York.

Bell, D.S. (1965). Comparison of amphetamine psychosis and schizophrenia. *Br. J. Psychiatry* 3, 701.

Benazzi, F. and Mazzoli, M. (1991). Psychiatric illness associated with 'ecstasy'. *BMJ* 338, 1520.

Bennett, D.A. (1992). Dementia. In *Textbook of Clinical Neuropharmacology and Therapeutics* (2nd edn) (ed. H.L. Klawans, C.G. Goetz, and C.M. Tanner), p. 271. Raven Press, New York.

Bennett, J.E. (1996). Antimicrobial agents: antifungal agents. In *Goodman and Gilman's The Pharmacological Basis of Therapeutics* (ed. J.G. Hardman and L.E. Limbird), p. 1175. McGraw Hill, New York.

Bentham, P.W., Goh, S.E., Gregg, E.M., *et al.* (1997). Authors have not proved their argument. *BMJ* 314, 1412.

Benzer, D.G. (1991). Medical consequences of alcohol addiction. In *Comprehensive Handbook of Drug and Alcohol Addiction* (ed. N.S. Miller), p. 551. Marcel Dekker, New York.

Berger, S.P., Hall, S., Mickalian, J.D., *et al.* (1996). Haloperidol antagonism of cue-elicited cocaine craving. *Lancet* 347, 504.

Bergman, H., Borg, S., Engelbrektson, K., *et al.* (1989). Dependence on sedative-hypnotics: neuropsychological impairment, field dependence and clinical course in a 5-year follow-up study. *Br. J. Addict.* 84, 547.

Bertilsson, L., Ballie, T.A., and Reviriego, J. (1990). Factors influencing the metabolism of diazepam. *Pharmacol. Ther.* 45, 85.

Betteridge, D.J. (1993). The cholesterol reduction controversy. *'Risk' The Journal of Coronary Risk Factors* 1, 15.

Bhatia, M.S. (1991). Chloroquine-induced psychiatric complications. *Br. J. Psychiatry* 159, 735.

Billings, R.F. and Stein, M.B. (1986). Depression associated with ranitidine. *Br. J. Psychiatry* 143, 915.

Biriell, C., McEwen, J., and Sanz, E. (1989). Depression associated with diltiazem. *BMJ* 299, 796.

Bixler, E.O., Kales, A., Manfredi, R.L., *et al.* (1991). Next-day memory impairment with triazolam use. *Lancet* 337, 827.

Black, D. (1982). Misuse of solvents. *Health Trends* 14, 27.

Black, R.J. and Dawson, T.A.J. (1988). Erythromycin and nightmares. *BMJ*, 296, 1070.

Blazer, D.G. and Haller, L. (1975). Pentazocine psychosis. A case of persistent delusions. *Dis. Nerv. Syst.* 36, 404.

Bleck, T.P. and Klawans, H.L. (1992). Convulsive disorders: mechanisms of epilepsy and anticonvulsant action. In *Textbook of Clinical Neuropharmacology and Therapeutics* (2nd edn) (ed. H.L. Klawans, C.G. Goetz, and C.M. Tanner), p. 23. Raven Press, New York.

Borbujo, M.J.M., Casado, J.Z.M., Garijo, L.M.B., *et al.* (1987). Etretinate. Depression and behavioral changes: case report. *Med. Clin.* 89, 577.

Borg, S. (1987). Sedative hypnotic dependence: neuropsychological changes and clinical course. *Nord. Psykiatr. Tidsskr.* 41 (Suppl.), 17.

Boulenger, J-P. and Uhde, T.W. (1982). Caffeine consumption and anxiety: preliminary results of a survey comparing patients with anxiety disorders and normal controls. *Psychopharmacol. Bull.* 18, 53.

Boulenger, J-P., Uhde, T.W., Wolff, E.A., *et al.* (1984). Increased sensitivity to caffeine in patients with panic disorders. *Arch. Gen. Psychiatry* 41, 1067.

Boyer, W.F. and Feighner, J.P. (eds) (1996). Other uses of the selective serotonin reuptake inhibitors. In *Selective Serotonin Reuptake Inhibitors* (2nd edn) p. 267. John Wiley and Sons, Chichester.

Braddock, L.E. and Heard, R.N.S. (1986). Visual hallucinations due to indomethacin: a case report. *Clin. Psychopharmacol.* 1, 263.

Braestrup, C., Nielsen, M., Honore, T., *et al.* (1983). Benzodiazepine receptor ligands with positive and negative efficacy. *Neuropharmacology* 22, 1451.

Brecher, E.M. (1972). *Licit and Illicit Drugs.* Consumers Union, Mount Vernon, New York.

Brierley, J.B. (1977). Neuropathology of amnesic states. In *Amnesia* (ed. C.W.M. Whitby and O.L. Zangwill), p. 199. Butterworth, London.

Brill, H. and Nahas, G.G. (1984). Cannabis intoxication and mental illness. In *Marihuana in Science and Medicine* (ed. G.G. Nahas), p. 263. Raven Press, New York.

British Medical Journal (1971). Ketamine — a new anaesthetic. *BMJ* 2, 666

British Medical Journal (1980). Phencyclidine: the new American street drug. *BMJ* 281, 1511.

British Medical Journal (1981). Minor brain damage and alcoholism. *BMJ* 283, 455.

British National Formulary (1997) (No. 31)

Brizer, D.A. and Manning, D.W. (1982). Delirium induced by poisoning with anti-cholinergic agents. *Am. J. Psychiatry* 139, 1343.

Brook, P.G. and Jackson, D. (1982). UK general practice experience of fenbufen in elderly patients. *Eur. J. Rheumatol. Inflamm.* 2, 326.

Brooke, D., Kerwin, R., and Lloyd, K. (1988). Di-ethylpropion hydrochloride-induced psychosis. *Br. J. Psychiatry* 152, 572.

Brooke, N.M. and Cookson, I.B. (1978). Bromocriptine-induced mania? *BMJ* i, 790.

Brosan, L., Broadbent, D., Nutt, D., *et al.*. (1986). Performance effects of diazepam during and after prolonged administration. *Psychol. Med.* 16, 561.

Brower, K.J., Blow, F.C., Beresford, T.P., *et al.* (1989). Anabolic-androgenic steroid dependence. *J. Clin. Psychiatry* 50, 31.

Brower, K.J., Eliopolis, G.A., Blow, F.C., *et al.* (1990). Evidence for physical and psychological dependence on anabolic androgenic steroids in eight weight lifters. *Am. J. Psychiatry* 147, 510.

Brower, K.J. (1991). Anabolic-androgenic steroids. In *Comprehensive Handbook of Drug and Alcohol Addiction* (ed. N.S. Miller), p. 521. Marcel Dekker, New York.

Brown, M.J., Salmon, D., and Rendell, M. (1980). Clonidine hallucinations. *Ann. Intern. Med.* 93, 456.

Brown, A. and Stickgold, A. (1976). Marijuana flashback phenomena. *Journal of Psychedelic Drugs* 8, 275.

Brown, E.S., Suppes, T., and Khan, D.A. (1997). Affective symptoms from corticosteroids: a hypothesis for bipolar disorder. *Abstract of 150th Annual Meeting of American Psychiatric Association, Sandiego, California* 131, 101.

Bruce, M., Scott, N., Shine, P., *et al.* (1992). Anxiogenic effects of caffeine in patients with anxiety disorders. *Arch. Gen. Psychiatry* 49, 867.

Bruera, E., Schoeller, T., and Montejo, T. (1992). Organic hallucinosis in patients receiving high doses of opiates for cancer pain. *Pain*, 48, 397.

Brunner, D.P., Dijk, D-J., Münch, M., *et al.* (1991). Effect of zolpidem on sleep and sleep EEG spectra in healthy young men. *Psychopharmacology* 104, 1.

Buchanan, R.A. (1972). Ethosuximide toxicity. In *Antiepileptic drugs* (ed. D.M. Woodbury, J.K. Penry, and R.P. Schmidt). Raven Press, New York.

Buckley, P., Larkin, C., and O'Callaghan, E. (1990). Psychosis following use of proprietary antidiarrhoeal medicines. *Br. J. Psychiatry* 157, 758.

Bunney, W.E., Goodwin, F.K., Murphy, D.L., *et al.* (1972). The 'switch-process' in manic-depressive illness. *Arch. Gen. Psychiatry* 27, 304.

Bunney, W.E. Jr and Garland, B.L. (1982). A second generation catecholamine hypothesis. *Pharmacopsychiatria* 15, 111.

Burke, W.J. (1987). Benzodiazepine-induced hypomania. *J. Clin. Psychopharmacol.* 7, 356.

Burke, M.J. and Preskorn, S.H. (1995). Short-term treatment of mood disorders with standard antidepressants. In *Psychopharmacology: The Fourth Generation of Progress* (ed. F.E. Bloom and D.J. Kupfer), p. 1053. Raven Press, New York.

Bushe, C.J. (1988). Organic psychosis caused by diltiazem. *J. R. Soc. Med.* 81, 296.

Busto, U., Sellers, E.M., Naranjo, C.A., *et al.* (1986). Patterns of benzodiazepine abuse and dependence. *Br. J. Addict.* 81, 87.

Buysse, D.J. (1991). Drugs affecting sleep, sleepiness and performance. In *Sleep, Sleepiness and Performance* (ed. T.H. Monk), p. 249. John Wiley, Chichester.

Caine, E.D., Weingartner, H., Ludlow, C.L., *et al.* (1981). Qualitative analysis of scopolamine-induced amnesia. *Psychopharmacology* 74, 74.

Calne, D.B., Plotkin, C., Williams, A.C., *et al.* (1978). Long-term treatment of parkinsonism with bromocriptine. *Lancet* i, 735.

Canagasabey, B. and Katona, C.L.E. (1991). Capgras syndrome in association with lithium toxicity. *Br. J. Psychiatry* 159, 879.

Cantor, R. (1979). Methadone maintenance and amitriptyline. *JAMA* 241, 2378.

Carney, M.W.P. (1977). Paranoid psychosis with indomethacin. *BMJ* ii, 994.

Carney, M.W.P. (1988). Diethylpropion and psychosis. *Br. J. Psychiatry* 152, 146.

Carney, M.W.P., Ravindran, A., and Lewis, D.S. (1982). Manic psychosis associated with procarbazine. *BMJ* 284, 82.

Carney, M.W.P., Bacelle, L., and Robinson, B. (1984). Psychosis after cannabis abuse. *BMJ* 288, 1047.

Casey, D.E. (1978). Amantadine intoxication reversed by physostigmine. *N. Engl. J. Med.* 9, 298.

Castleden, C.M., George, C.F., Marcer, D., *et al.* (1977). Increased sensitivity to nitrazepam in old age. *BMJ* 1, 10.

Cavallaro, R., Regazzetti, M.G., and Smeralid, E. (1993). Tolerance and withdrawal with zolpidem. *Lancet* 342, 374.

Celesia, G.C. and Barr, A.N. (1970). Psychosis and other psychiatric manifestations of levodopa therapy. *Arch. Neurol.* 23, 193.

Charney, D.S., Heninger, G.R., Sternberg, D.E., *et al.* (1982). Abrupt discontinuation of tricyclic antidepressant drugs: evidence for noradrenergic hyperactivity. *Br. J. Psychiatry* 141, 377.

Charney, D.S., Heninger, G.R., and Jatlow, P.I. (1985). Increased anxiogenic effects of caffeine in panic disorder. *Arch. Gen. Psychiatry* 42, 233.

Chaudoir, P.J., Bodkin, N.L., O'Donnell, J., *et al.* (1990). A comparative study of zopiclone and triazolam in patients with insomnia. In *Zopiclone in Clinical Practice* (ed. I. Hindmarch and B. Musch), p. 21. CNS (Clinical Neuroscience) Publishers, London.

Chen, Z., Peto, R., Collins, R., *et al.* (1991). Serum cholesterol concentrations and coronary heart disease in a population with low cholesterol concentrations. *BMJ* 303, 276.

Chin, D.K.F., Ho, A.K.C., and Tse, C.Y. (1986). Neuropsychiatric complications related to use of prazosin in patients with renal failure. *BMJ* 293, 1347.

Cholerton, S., Daly, A.K., and Idle, J.R. (1992). The role of individual human cytochromes P450 in drug metabolism and clinical response. *Trends Pharmacol. Sci.* 13, 434.

Chopra, G.S. and Smith, J.W. (1974). Psychotic reactions following cannabis use in East Indians. *Arch. Gen. Psychiatry* 30, 24.

Chouinard, G., Bradwein, J., Annable, L., *et al.* (1984). Withdrawal symptoms after long-term treatment with low-potency neuroleptics. *J. Clin. Psychiatry* 45, 500.

Chouinard, G. and Jones, B.D. (1980). Neuroleptic-induced supersensitivity psychosis: clinical and pharmacological characteristics. *Am. J. Psychiatry* 137, 16.

Church, G. and Marriott, J.H.L. (1959). Digitalis delirium: a report on three cases. *Circulation* 20, 549.

Claridge, G. (1978). Animal models of schizophrenia: the case for LSD-25. *Schizophr. Bull.* 4, 186.

Cleghorn, J.M., Kaplan, R.D., Szechtman, B., *et al.* (1991). Substance abuse and schizophrenia: effect on symptoms but not on neurocognitive function. *J. Clin. Psychiatry* 52, 26.

Closson, R.G. (1983). Visual hallucinations as the earliest symptom of digoxin intoxication. *Arch. Neurol.* 40, 386.

Cocores, J., Pottash, A.C., and Gold, M.S. (1991). Cocaine. In *Comprehensive Handbook of Drug and Alcohol Addiction* (ed. N.S. Miller), p. 341. Marcel Dekker, New York.

Cohen, S. (1960). Lysergic acid diethylamide: side effects and complications. *J. Nerv. Ment. Dis.* 139, 30.

Cohen, S.I. (1992). Phobic disorders and benzodiazepines in the elderly. *Br. J. Psychiatry* 160, 135.

Cohen, K.J., Harburg, R., and Stimmel, B. (1978). Abuse of amitriptyline. *JAMA* 240, 1372.

Cohen, B.M. and Baldessarini, R.J. (1985). Tolerance to the therapeutic effects of antidepressants. *Am. J. Psychiatry* 142, 489.

Cohen, J.W. and Cohen, N.H. (1974). Lithium carbonate, haloperidol and irreversible brain damage. *JAMA* 230, 1283.

Cohen, S.I. and Johnson, B.A. (1988). Psychosis from alcohol or drug abuse. *BMJ* 297, 1270.

Coid, J. and Strang, H. (1982). Mania secondary to procyclidine ('Kemadrin') abuse. *Br. J. Psychiatry* 141, 81.

Cole, J.O. and Kando, J.C. (1993). Adverse behavioral events reported in patients taking alprazolam and other benzodiazepines. *J. Clin. Psychiatry* 10 (Suppl.), 49.

Collins, I.S. and King, I.W. (1972). Pindolol (Visken, LB46), a new treatment for hypertension: report of a multicentre open study. *Curr. Ther. Res.* 14, 185.

Cook, P.J., Huggett, A., Graham-Pole, R., *et al.* (1983). Hypnotic accumulation and hangover in elderly inpatients: a controlled double-blind study of temazepam and nitrazepam. *BMJ* 286, 100.

Coplan, J.D., Wolk, S.I., and Klein, D.F. (1995). Anxiety and serotonin 1A receptors. In *Psychopharmacology: The Fourth Generation of Progress* (ed. F.E. Bloom and D.J. Kupfer), p. 301. Raven Press, New York.

Costa, E. (1981). The role of gamma-aminobutyric acid in the action of 1,4 benzodiazepines. In *Towards Understanding Receptors* (ed. J.W. Lamble), p. 176. Elsevier/North-Holland, Amsterdam.

Coumel, P. and Fidelle, J. (1980). Amiodarone in the treatment of cardiac arrhythmias in children: 135 cases. *Am. Heart J.* 100, 1063.

Coupland, N.J., Bell, C.J., and Potokar, J.P. (1996). Serotonin reuptake inhibitor withdrawal. *J. Clin. Psychopharmacol.* 16, 356.

Cowen, P.J. and Nutt, D.J. (1982). Abstinence symptoms after withdrawal from tranquillising drugs: is there a common neurochemical mechanism? *Lancet* ii, 360.

Crawshaw, J.A. and Mullen, P.E. (1984). A study of benzhexol abuse. *Br. J. Psychiatry* 145, 300.

Creighton, F.J., Black, D.L., and Hyde, C.E. (1991). 'Ecstasy' psychosis and flashbacks. *Br. J. Psychiatry* 159, 713.

Crewe, H.K., Lennard, M.S., Tucker, G.T., et al. (1992). The effect of selective serotonin re-uptake inhibitors on cytochrome P4502D6 (CYP2D6) activity in human liver microsomes. *Br. J. Clin. Pharmacol.* 34, 262.

Croft, A.M.J. and World, M.J. (1996). Neuropsychiatric side-effects of mefloquine. *Lancet* 347, 326.

CSM (Committee on Safety of Medicines) (1985). Actifed syrup and hallucinations in children. *Current Problems* 14, 2. HMSO, London.

CSM (Committee on Safety of Medicines) (1986). Update: recurrent ventricular tachycardia: adverse drug reactions. *BMJ* 292, 50.

CSM (Committee on Safety of Medicines) (1988). Benzodiazepines: dependence and withdrawal symptoms. *Current Problems* 21, 1. HMSO, London.

CSM (Committee on Safety of Medicines) (1989). Fluvoxamine and fluoxetine — interaction with monoamine oxidase inhibitors, lithium and tryptophan. *Current Problems* 26. HMSO, London.

CSM (Committee on Safety of Medicines) (1990). Zopiclone (Zimovane) and neuro-psychiatric reactions. *Current Problems* 30, 2. HMSO, London.

CSM (Committee on Safety of Medicines) (1993). Neuro-psychiatric adverse reactions associated with fenfluramines. *Current Problems in Pharmacovigilance* 19, 8, HMSO, London.

CSM (Committee on Safety of Medicines) (1994). Neuroleptic sensitivity in patients with dementia. *Current Problems in Pharmacovigilance* 20, 6. HMSO, London.

CSM (Committee on Safety of Medicines) (1996). Mefloquine (Lariam) and neuropsychiatric reactions. *Current Problems in Pharmacovigilance* 22, 6. HMSO, London.

CSM (Committee on Safety of Medicines) (1997). Fenfluramine and dexfenfluramine withdrawn. Further cases of valvular heart disease. *Current Problems in Pharmacovigilance* 23, 13. HMSO, London.

Cummings, J.L. (1995). Dementia: the failing brain. *Lancet* 345, 1481.

Curran, V. (1992). Memory functions, alertness and mood of long-term benzodiazepine users: a preliminary investigation of the effects of a normal daily dose. *J. Psychopharmacol.* 6, 69.

Curran, H.V. and Travill, R.A. (1997). Mood and cognitive effects of 3,4-methylenedioxymethamphetamine (MDMA, 'ecstasy'): week-end 'high' followed by mid-week low. *Addiction* 92, 821.

Curran, H.V., Sakulsriprong, M., and Lader, M. (1988). Antidepressants and human memory: an investigation of four drugs with different sedative and anticholinergic profiles. *Psychopharmacology* 95, 520.

Currie, P. and Ramsdale, D.R. (1984). Paranoid psychosis induced by tocainamide. *BMJ* 288, 606.

Cutler, N., Sramek, J., Veroff, A., et al. (1995). Effects of treatment with simvastatin and pravastatin on cognitive function in patients with hypercholesterolaemia. *Br. J. Clin. Pharmacol.* 39, 333.

Dahl, M-L. and Bertilsson, L. (1993). Genetically variable metabolism of antidepressants and neuroleptic drugs in man. *Pharmacogenetics* 3, 61.

Daly, R.J., Kane, F.J., and Ewing, J.A. (1967). Psychosis associated with the use of a sequential oral contraceptive. *Lancet* ii, 444.

Damasio, A.R., Lobo-Antunes, J., and Macedo, C. (1971). Psychiatric aspects in parkinsonism treated with L-dopa. *J. Neurol. Neurosurg. Psychiatry* 34, 502.

Damluji, N.F. and Ferguson, J.M. (1988). Paradoxical worsening of depressive symptomatology caused by antidepressants. *J. Clin. Psychopharmacol.* 8, 347.

Daniel, D.G., Swallows, A., and Wolff, F. (1987). Capgras delusions and seizures in association with therapeutic doses of disulfiram. *South. Med. J.* 80, 1577.

Danion, J-M., Zimmermann, M-A., Willard-Schroeder, D., et al. (1989). Diazepam induces a dissociation between explicit and implicit memory. *Psychopharmacology* 99, 238.

Dasgupta, K. (1990). Additional cases of suicidal ideation associated with fluoxetine. *Am. J. Psychiatry* 147, 1570.

Data Sheet Compendium 1995/6. Datapharm Publications, London.

Davey, P.G. (1990). New anti-viral and anti-fungal drugs. *BMJ* 300, 793.

Davidson, S.I. and Hickey-Dwyer, M. (1991). Eye disorders. In *Textbook of Adverse Drug Reactions* (4th edn) (ed. D.M. Davies), p. 567. Oxford University Press.

Davies, R.K., Tucker, G.J., Harrow, M., et al. (1971). Confusional episodes and anti-depressant medication. *Am. J. Psychiatry* 128, 95.

Davis, K.L. and Powchik, P. (1995). Tacrine. *Lancet* 345, 625.

Davison, A.N. (1982). Ageing research matures. *Trends Neurosci.* 5, 217

Davison, K. (1976). Drug-induced psychoses and their relationship to schizophrenia. In *Schizophrenia Today* (ed. D. Kemali, G. Bartholini, and D. Richter), p. 105. Pergamon Press, Oxford.

Davison, K. (1989a). Adverse psychiatric reactions to drugs used in the ITU. *Care of the Critically Ill* 5, 9.

Davison, K. (1989b). Acute organic brain syndromes. *Br. J. Hosp. Med.* 41, 89.

Davison, K. and Hassanyeh, F. (1991). Psychiatric Disorders. In *Textbook of Adverse Drug Reactions* (4th edn) (ed. D.M. Davies), p. 601. Oxford University Press.

Davison, L.A., Steinhelber, J.C., and Eger, E.I. (1975). Psychological effects of halothane and isoflurane anesthesia. *Anesthesiology* 43, 313.

Deadwyler, S.A., Hampson, R.E., and Childers, S.R. (1995). Functional significance of cannabinoid receptors in brain. In *Cannabinoid Receptors* (ed. R. Pertwee), p. 205. Academic Press, New York.

Deakin, J.F.W. (1993). A review of clinical efficacy of 5-HT1A agonists in anxiety and depression. *J. Psychopharmacol.* 7, 283.

Dean, E.S. (1963). Self-induced stramonium intoxication. *JAMA* 185, 882.

Declerck, A.C., Ruwe, F., O'Hanlon, J.F., *et al.* (1992). Effects of zolpidem and flunitrazepam on nocturnal sleep of women subjectively complaining of insomnia. *Psychopharmacology* 106, 497.

Delerue, O., Muller, J-P., Destee, A., *et al.* (1988). Mania-like episodes associated with ranitidine. *Am. J. Psychiatry* 145, 271.

Deleu, D. and Schmedding, E. (1987). Acute psychosis as idiosyncratic reaction to quinidine: report of two cases. *BMJ* 294, 1001.

Delva, N.J., Matthews, D.R., and Cowen, P.J. (1996). Brain serotonin (5-HT) neuroendocrine function in patients taking cholesterol-lowering drugs. *Biol. Psychiatry* 39, 100.

Denicoff, K.D., Rubinon, D.R., and Papa, M.Z. (1987). The neuropsychiatric effects of treatment with interleukin-2 and lymphokine-activated killer cells. *Ann. Intern. Med.* 107, 293.

Deutsch, J.A. (1971). The cholinergic synapse and the site of memory. *Science* 174, 788.

Devan, G.S. (1990). Phentermine and psychosis. *Br. J. Psychiatry* 156, 442.

Devane, W.A., Dysarz, F.A., Johnson, M.R., *et al.* (1988). Determination and characterisation of a cannabinoid receptor in ratbrain. *Mol. Pharmacol.* 34, 605.

Di Chiara, G. (1997). Cortical and limbic dopamine (on opiate addiction): do not mix before use! *Trends Pharmacol. Sci.* 18, 77.

Di Chiara, G. and North, R.A. (1992). Neurobiology of opiate abuse. *Trends Pharmacol. Sci.* 13, 185.

DiGiacomo, J.N. (1968). Toxic effect of stramonium simulating LSD trip. *JAMA* 204, 265.

Dillon, J.B. (1970). Ketamine. *Lancet* ii, 310.

Dilsaver, S.C. (1989). Antidepressant withdrawal syndromes: phenomenology and pathophysiology. *Acta Psychiatr. Scand.* 79, 113.

Dilsaver, S.C. (1994). Withdrawal phenomena associated with antidepressant and antipsychotic agents. *Drug Saf.* 10, 103.

Dilsaver, S.C. and Greden, J.F. (1984). Antidepressant withdrawal phenomena. *Biol. Psychiatry* 19, 237.

Dilsaver, S.C., Kronfol, Z., Sackellares, J.C., *et al.* (1983). Antidepressant withdrawal syndromes: evidence supporting the cholinergic overdrive hypothesis. *J. Clin. Psychopharmacol.* 3, 157.

Dilsaver, S.C., Feinberg, M., and Greden, J.F. (1983). Antidepressant withdrawal symptoms treated with anticholinergic agents. *Am. J. Psychiatry* 140, 249.

Dilsaver, S.C., Greden, J.F., and Snider, R.M. (1987). Antidepressant withdrawal syndromes: phenomenology and physiopathology. *Int. Clin. Psychopharmacol.* 2, 1.

Dixon, L., Haas, G., Wedien, P.J., *et al.* (1990). Acute effects of drug abuse in schizophrenic patients: clinical observations and patients' self-reports. *Schizophrenia Bulletin* 16, 69.

Donaldson, S.R. (1989). Tolerance to phenelzine and subsequent refractory depression: three cases. *J. Clin. Psychiatry* 50, 33.

Donaldson, I.M.G. and Cunningham, J. (1983). Persisting neurologic sequelae of lithium carbonate therapy. *Arch. Neurol.* 40, 747.

Dorian, P., Sellers, E.M., Kaplan, H., *et al.* (1983). Evaluation of zopiclone physical dependence liability in normal volunteers. *Pharmacology* 27 (Suppl. 2), 228.

Dorman, A.. Talbot, D., Byrne, P., *et al.* (1995). Misuse of dothiepin. *BMJ* 311, 1502.

Drachman, D.A. (1978). Central cholinergic system and memory. In *Psychopharmacology: a Generation of Progress* (ed. M.A. Lipton, A. DiMascio, and K.F. Killam), p. 651. Raven Press, New York.

Drerup, U. (1988). Zentral nervose Nebenwirkungen unter antiarrhythmika-Therapie. Psychotische Depression unter Flecainid. *Dtsch. Med. Wochenschr.* 113, 386.

Drug Interactions (1996). *A Source Book of Adverse Interactions, their Mechanisms, Clinical Importance and Management* (4th edn) (ed. I.H. Stockley), p. 27. The Pharmaceutical Press, London.

Drug Newsletter (1986). From the Region's yellow cards . . . drugs and nightmares. *Drug Newsletter* 38, 155.

Drug and Therapeutics Bulletin (1986). Problems when withdrawing antidepressives. *Drug Ther. Bull.* 24, 29.

Drug and Therapeutics Bulletin (1991). The sudden withdrawal of triazolam — reasons and consequences. *Drug Ther. Bull.* 29, 89.

Drug and Therapeutics Bulletin (1994). Drug treatment of epilepsy. *Drug Ther. Bull.* 32, 45.

Drug and Therapeutics Bulletin (1995). Zolpidem — a hypnotic with a difference? *Drug Ther. Bull.* 33, 37.

D'Souza, M. (1987). Unusual reaction to morphine. *Lancet* ii, 98.

Dubovsky, S.L. (1987). Psychopharmacologic treatment in neuropsychiatry. In *Textbook of Neuropsychiatry* (ed. R.E. Hales and S.C. Dubovsky), p. 417. American Psychiatric Press, Washington DC.

Duits, N. and Bos, F. (1993). Depressive symptoms and cholesterol-lowering drugs. *Lancet* 341, 114.

Duncan, N. and Taylor, D. (1996). Chlormethiazole or chlordiazepoxide in alcohol detoxification. *Psychol. Bull.* 20, 599.

Dundee, J.W., Bovill, J., Knox, J.W.D., *et al.* (1970). Ketamine as an induction agent in anaesthetics. *Lancet* i, 1370.

Dunleavy, D.L.F., MacLean, A.W., and Oswald, I. (1971). Debrisoquine, guanethidine, propranolol and human sleep. *Psychopharmacologia* 21, 101.

Dursun, S.M. (1993). Toxic serotonin syndrome after fluoxetine plus carbamazepine. *Lancet* 342, 442.

Eccleston, D. and Cole, A.J. (1990). Calcium channel blockade and depressive illness. *Br. J. Psychiatry* 156, 889.

Eckardt, M.J. and Martin, P.R. (1986). Clinical assessment of cognition in alcoholism. *Alcohol. Clin. Exp. Res.* 10, 128.

Edwards, G. (1983). Psychopathology of a drug experience. *Br. J. Psychiatry* 143, 509.

Edwards, J.G. (1989). Drug-related depression: clinical and epidemiological aspects. In *Depression: An Integrated Approach* (ed. K. Herbst and E. Paykel), p. 81. Heinemann, Oxford.

Edwards, J.G. (1992). Selective serotonin reuptake inhibitors. *BMJ* 304, 1644.

Edwards, J.G (1994). Drugs in focus: 14. Selective serotonin reuptake inhibitors in the treatment of depression. *Prescribers' Journal* 34, 197.

Edwards, J.G. (1995). Adverse reactions to and interactions with psychotropic drugs: mechanisms, methods of assessment, and medicolegal considerations. In *Seminars in Clinical Psychopharmacology* (ed. D.J. King), p. 480. Royal College of Physicians, London.

Einerson, T.R. and Yoder, E.S. (1982). Triazolam psychosis — a syndrome? *Drug Intell. Clin. Pharmacol.* 16, 330.

Eisen, J., MacFarlane, J., and Shapiro, C.M. (1993). Psychotropic drugs and sleep. *BMJ* 306, 1331.

Eisendrath, S.J. and Sweeney, M.A. (1987). Toxic neuropsychiatric effects of digoxin at therapeutic serum concentrations. *Am. J. Psychiatry* 144, 506.

Eisendrath, S.J., Goldman, B., Douglas, J., *et al.* (1987). Meperidine-induced delirium *Am. J. Psychiatry* 144, 1062.

Eison, A.S., Eison, M.S., Stanley, M., *et al.* (1986). Serotonergic mechanisms in the behavioural effects of buspirone and gepirone. *Pharmacol. Biochem. Behav.* 24, 701.

Eitan, N., Levin, Y., Ben-Artzi, E., *et al.* (1992). Effects of antipsychotic drugs on memory functions of schizophrenic patients. *Acta Psychiatr. Scand.* 85, 74.

Elie, R., Frenay, M., Le Morvan, P., *et al.* (1990). Efficacy and safety of zopiclone and triazolam in the treatment of geriatric insomniacs. In *Zopiclone in Clinical Practice* (ed. I. Hindmarch and B. Musch), p. 39. CNS (Clinical Neuroscience) Publishers, London.

Elliott, H. (1992). Choosing an appropriate lipid-lowering treatment. *Prescriber* 3, 40.

Engelberg, H. (1992). Low serum cholesterol and suicide. *Lancet* 339, 727.

Erikssen, J. (1969). Atropine psychosis. *Lancet* i, 53.

Evans, L. (1980). Psychological effects caused by drugs in overdose. *Drugs* 19, 220.

Evans, M., Perera, P.W., and Donoghue, J. (1997). Drug induced psychosis with doxazosin. *BMJ* 314, 1869.

Evans, J.G. and Jarvis, E.H. (1972). Nitrazepam and the elderly. *BMJ* iv, 487.

Evans, D.L. and Perkins, D.O. (1990). The clinical psychiatry of AIDS. *Curr. Opin. Psychiatry* 3, 96.

Ewing, J., Mueller, R., Rouse, P., *et al.* (1977). Low levels of dopamine β-hydroxylase and psychosis. *Am. J. Psychiatry* 134, 927.

Eymin, C., Koppp, N., Laurent, B., *et al.* (1992). Central benzodiazepine-binding sites in human cerebral structures associated with memory processes. *Dementia* 3, 232.

Falk, W.E., Mahnke, M.W., and Poskanzer, D.C. (1979). Lithium prophylaxis of corticotrophin-induced psychosis. *JAMA* 241, 1011.

Farrell, M. (1994). Opiate withdrawal. *Addiction* 89, 1471.

Farwell, J.R., Lee, Y.J., Hirtz, D.G., *et al.* (1990). Phenobarbital for febrile seizures — effects on intelligence and on seizure recurrence. *N. Engl. J. Med.* 322, 364.

Faulk, M. (1989). Psychosis in a transsexual. *Br. J. Psychiatry* 155, 285.

Fava, G.A. and Gardi, S. (1995). Withdrawal syndrome after paroxetine and sertraline discontinuation. *J. Clin. Psychopharmacol.* 15, 374.

Feder, R. (1987). Metoclopramide and depression. *J. Clin. Psychiatry* 48, 38.

Feighner, J.P. (1982). Benzodiazepines as antidepressants. In *Modern Problems of Pharmacopsychiatry* (ed. T.A. Ban), p. 196. Karger, Basel.

Ferrier, I.N., Tyrer, S.P., and Bell, A.J. (1995). Lithium therapy. *Adv. Psychiatric Treatment* 1, 102.

Fetzer, J., Kader, G., and Danahy, S. (1981). Lithium encephalopathy: a clinical, psychiatric and EEG evaluation. *Am. J. Psychiatry* 138, 1622.

File, S.E., Sharma, R., and Shaffer, J. (1992). Is lorazepam-induced amnesia specific to the type of memory or to the task used to assess it? *J. Psychopharmacol.* 6, 76.

Fine, J. and Finestone, E.C. (1973). Sensory disturbances following ketamine. anaesthesia: recurrent hallucinations. *Anesth. Analg.* 52, 428.

Fischman, M.W. (1987). Cocaine and the amphetamines. In *Psychopharmacology: The Third Generation of Progress* (ed. H.Y. Meltzer), p. 1543. Raven Press, New York.

Fishbain, D.A. and Rogers, A. (1987). Delirium secondary to metoclopramide. *J. Clin. Psychopharmacol.* 7, 281.

Flaherty, J. and Bellur, S. (1981). Mental side effects of amantadine therapy. *Clin. Psychiatry* 42, 344.

Fleming, J.A., McClure, D.J., Mayes, C., *et al.* (1990). A comparison of the efficacy, safety and withdrawal effects of zopiclone and triazolam, in the treatment of insomnia.In *Zopiclone in Clinical Practice* (ed. I. Hindmarch and B. Musch), p. 29. CNS (Clinical Neuroscience) Publishers, London.

Fleminger, R. (1978). Visual hallucinations and illusions with propranolol. *BMJ* i, 1182.

Fletcher, J.M., Page, J.B., Francis, D.J., *et al.* (1996). Cognitive correlates of long-term cannabis use in Costa-Rican men. *Arch. Gen. Psychiatry* 53, 1051.

Folks, D. and Arnold, E.S. (1983). Pargyline-induced mania in primary affective disorder. *J. Clin. Psychiatry* 44, 25.

Forssman, B., Kihlstrand, S., Larson, L.E. (1972). Amantadine therapy in parkinsonism. *Acta Neurol. Scand.* 48, 1.

Fowkes, F.G., Leng, G.C., Donnan, P.T., *et al.* (1992). Serum cholesterol, triglycerides and aggression in the general population. *Lancet* 340, 995.

France, R.D. and Krishnan, K.P. (1984). Alprazolam-induced manic reaction. *Am. J. Psychiatry* 141, 1127.

Franks, R.D. and Richter, A.J. (1979). Schizophrenia-like psychosis associated with anticonvulsant toxicity. *Am. J. Psychiatry* 136, 973.

Freedman, D.X. and Boggan, W.O. (1982). Biochemical pharmacology of psychotomimetics. In *Psychotropic Agents Part III* (ed. F. Hoffmeister and S. Stille), p. 57. Springer-Verlag, Heidelberg.

Freund, M. and Merin, S. (1970). Toxic effects of scopolamine eye drops. *Am. J. Ophthalmol.* 70, 637.

Frisch, J.M. (1973). Clinical experience with adverse reactions to trimethoprim-sulfamethoxazole. *J. Infect. Dis.* 128 (Suppl.), 607.

Friston, K.J., Sharpley, A.L., Solomon, R.A., *et al.* (1989). Lithium increases slow wave sleep: possible mediation by brain 5-HT2 receptors? *Psychopharmacology* 98, 139.

Frosch, W.A., Robbins, E.S., and Stern M. (1965). Untoward reactions to lysergic acid diethylamide (LSD) resulting in hospitalisation. *N. Engl. J. Med.* 273, 1235.

Gardner, D.L. and Cowdry, R.W. (1986). Development of melancholia during carbamazepine treatment in borderline personality disorder. *J. Clin. Psychopharmacol.* 6, 236.

Gardos, G., Cole, J.O., and Tarsy, D. (1978). Withdrawal syndromes associated with anti-psychotic drugs. *Am. J. Psychiatry* 135, 1321.

Garner, E.M., Kelly, M.W., and Thompson, D.F. (1993). Tricyclic antidepressant withdrawal syndrome. *Ann. Pharmacother.* 27, 1068.

Garrett, A.S. (1971). Anti-leprosy drugs. *BMJ* iv, 300.

Gawin, F.H. and Kleber, H.D. (1986). Abstinence symptomatology and psychiatric diagnosis in cocaine abusers: clinical observations. *Arch. Gen. Psychiatry* 43, 107.

Gelder, M., Gath, D., and Mayou, R. (1983). Dependence on alcohol and drugs. In *Oxford Textbook of Psychiatry* (ed. M. Gelder, D. Goth, and R. Mayou), p. 422. Oxford University Press.

Gerhard, U. and Hobi, V. (1986). Is the depressive patient under adequate pharmacological treatment fit for driving? In *Drugs and Driving* (ed. J.F. O'Hanlon and J.J. de Gier), p. 221. Taylor and Francis, London and Philadelphia.

Gerner, R.H., Post, R.M., and Bunney, W.E. (1976). A dopaminergic mechanism in mania. *Am. J. Psychiatry* 133, 1177.

Gershon, E.S., Goldstein, R.E., and Moss, A.J. (1979). Psychosis with ordinary doses of propranolol. *Ann. Intern. Med.* 90, 938.

Giannini, A.J. (1991). Phencyclidine. In *Comprehensive Handbook of Drug and Alcohol Addiction* (ed. N.S. Miller), p. 383. Marcel Dekker, New York.

Gilbert, R.M. (1976). Caffeine as a drug of abuse. In *Research Advances in Alcohol and Drug Problems* (ed. R.J. Gibbons, Y. Israel, H. Kalant, *et al.*), p. 49. John Wiley, New York.

Glaser, G.H. (1972). Diphenylhydantoin toxicity. In *Antiepileptic Drugs* (ed. D.M. Woodbury, J.K. Penry, and R.P. Schmidt), p. 219. Raven Press, New York.

Gluckman, L. (1974). Ventolin psychosis. *N.Z. Med. J.* 80, 411.

Glynne-Jones, R., Vernon, C.C., and Bell, G. (1986). Is steroid psychosis preventable by divided doses? *Lancet* ii, 1404.

Goggans, F.C., Weisberg, L.J., and Koran, L.M. (1983). Lithium prophylaxis of prednisolone psychosis: a case report. *Clin. Psychiatry J.* 44, 111.

Golden, R.N., Hoffman, J., Falk, D., *et al.* (1989). Psychoses associated with propranolol withdrawal. *Biol. Psychiatry* 25, 351.

Golding, J.F. (1992). Cannabis. In *Handbook of Human Performance* (ed. D. Swann), p. 169. Academic Press, London.

Goldsmith, S.R., Frank, I., and Ungerleider, J.T. (1968). Poisoning from ingestion of a stramonium–belladonna mixture: Asthmador. *JAMA* 204, 169.

Goldstein, G. (1985). Pentazocine. *Drug Alcohol Depend.* 14, 313.

Golombok, S., Moodley, P., and Lader, M. (1988). Cognitive impairment in long-term benzodiazepine users. *Psychol. Med.* 18, 365.

Gonzales, R.A. and Hoffman, P.L. (1991). Receptor gated channels may be selective CNS targets for ethanol. *Trends Pharmacol. Sci.* 12, 1.

Goodman, W.K. and Charney, D.S. (1987). A case of alprazolam, but not lorazepam, inducing manic symptoms. *J. Clin. Psychiatry* 48, 117.

Goodwin, F.K. (1971). Psychiatric side-effects of levodopa in man. *JAMA* 218, 1915.

Goodwin, G.M. (1994). Recurrence of mania after lithium withdrawal. *Br. J. Psychiatry* 164, 149.

Goodwin, G.M. (1996). How do antidepressants affect serotonin receptors? The role of serotonin receptors in therapeutic and side effect profile of the SSRIs. *J. Clin. Psychiatry* 57 (Suppl.), 49.

Goodwin, F.K. and Jamison, K.R. (1990). *Manic Depressive Illness.* Oxford University Press.

Gorelick, D.A., Kussin, S.Z., and Kahn, I. (1978). Paranoid delusions and auditory hallucinations associated with dignoxin intoxication. *J. Nerv. Ment. Dis.* 166, 817.

Gorelick, D.A. and Balster, R.L. (1995). Phencyclidine. In *Psychopharmacology: The Fourth Generation of Progress* (ed. H.Y. Meltzer), p. 1767. Raven Press, New York.

Gorenstein, C., Bernik, M.A., Pompéias, A., *et al.* (1995). Impairment of performance associated with long-term use of benzodiazepines. *J. Psychopharmacol.* 9, 313.

Gosh, K., Sivakumaran, M., Murphy, P., *et al..* (1994). Visual hallucinations following treatment with vincristine. *Clin. Lab. Haematol.* 16, 355.

Gossop, M., Bradley, B., and Phillip, G.T. (1987). An investigation of withdrawal effects shown by opiate addicts during and subsequent to a 21-day in-patient methadone detoxification procedure. *Addict. Behav.* 12, 1.

Gossop, M., Green, L., Phillips, G., *et al.* (1989). Lapse, relapse and survival among opiate addicts after treatment. *Br. J. Psychiatry* 154, 348.

Gott, P.H. (1968). Cyclizine toxicity. International abuse of a proprietary anti-histamine. *N. Engl. J. Med.* 279, 596.

Gowdy, J.M. (1972). Stramonium intoxication. Review of symptomatology in 212 cases. *JAMA* 221, 585.

Graham, C.F., Turner, W.M., and Jones, J.K. (1981). Lidocaine-propranolol interactions. *N. Engl. J. Med.* 304, 1301.

Grant, R.H.E. and Pryse-Davies, J. (1968). Effect of oral contraceptives on depressive mood changes and on endometrial monoamine oxidase and phosphatases. *BMJ* iii, 777.

Greden, J.F. (1974). Anxiety or caffeinism: a diagnostic dilemma. *Am. J. Psychiatry* 131, 1089.

Greden, J.F., Fontaine, P., Lubetsky, M., *et al.* (1978). Anxiety and depression associated with caffeinism among psychiatric inpatients. *Am. J. Psychiatry* 135, 963.

Green, A.R., Cross, A.J., and Goodwin, G.M. (1995). Review of the pharmacology and clinical pharmacology of 3,4-methylenedioxymethamphetamine (MDMA or 'Ecstasy'). *Psychopharmacology* 119, 247.

Green, A.R. and Goodwin, G.M. (1996). Ecstasy and neurodegeneration. *BMJ* 312, 1493.

Greenblatt, D.J., Divoll, M., Abernethy, D.R., *et al.* (1972). Benzodiazepine: hypnotics: kinetic and therapeutic options. *Sleep* 5, S 18.

Greenblatt, D.J., Divoll, M., Abernethy, D.R., *et al.* (1983). Clinical pharmacokinetics of the newer benzodiazepines. *Clin. Pharmacokinet.* 8, 233.

Greer, H.D., Ward, H.P., and Corbrin, K.B. (1965). Chronic salicylate intoxication in adults. *JAMA* 193, 555.

Greeves, J.A. (1984). Rapid-onset steroid psychosis with very low dose of prenisolone. *Lancet* i, 1119.

Grieger, T.A., Clayton, A.H., and Goyer, P.F. (1990). Affective disorder following use of phenylpropanolamine. *Am.J. Psychiatry* 147, 367.

Griffiths, R.R., Bigelow, G.E., and Liebson, I.A. (1986). Human coffee drinking: reinforcing and physical dependence producing effects of caffeine. *J. Pharmacol. Exp. Ther.* 239, 416.

Griffith, J.D., Smith, C.H., and Smith, R.C. (1982). Paranoid psychosis in a patient receiving ibuprofen, a prostaglandin synthesis inhibitor: case report. *J. Clin. Psychiatry* 43, 499.

Grundemar, L. (1995). Risks in combination therapy of antidepressant drugs. *Trends Pharmacol. Sci.* 16, 17.

Gualtieri, C.T., Quade, D., Hicks, R.E., *et al.* (1984). Tardive dyskinesia and other clinical consequences of neuroleptic treatment in children and adolescents. *Am. J. Psychiatry* 141, 20.

Gupta, R. and Narang, R.L. (1986). Mania induced by gradual withdrawal from long-term treatment with imipramine. *Am. J. Psychiatry* 143, 260.

Haefley, W., Pieri, L., Pole, P., *et al.* (1981). General pharmacology and neuropharmacology of benzodiazepine derivatives. In *Handbook of Experimental Pharmacology,* Vol. 55, II (ed. H. Hoffmeister and G. Stille), p. 13. Springer-Verlag, Berlin.

Haefley, W. (1990). Benzodiazepine receptor and ligands: structural and functional differences. In *Benzodiazepines: Current Concepts* (ed. I. Hindmarch, G. Beaumont, S. Brandon, and B.E. Leonard), p. 1. John Wiley, Chichester.

Haffner, C.A., Smith, B.S., and Pepper, C. (1993). Hallucinations as an adverse effect of angiotensin in converting enzyme inhibition. *Postgrad. Med. J.* 69, 240.

Halikas, J., Kemp, K., Kuhn, K., *et al.* (1989). Carbamazepine for cocaine addiction. *Lancet* i, 623.

Hall, R.C.W., Popkion, M.K., and McHenry, L.E. (1977). Angel's trumpet psychosis: a CNS anti-cholinergic syndrome. *Am. J. Psychiatry* 134, 312.

Hall, T.C.W., Popkin, M.K., Stickney, S.K., *et al.* (1979). Presentation of the steroid psychoses. *J. Nerv. Ment. Dis.* 167, 229.

Hall, W., Solowij, N., and Lemon, J. (1994). *National Drug Monograph Series No. 27.* Australian Government Publishing Service, Canberra.

Hall, W. and Zador, D. (1997). The alcohol withdrawal syndrome. *Lancet* 349, 1897.

Halle, M.H., Del Medico, V.J., and Dilsaver, S.C. (1991). Symptoms of major depression: acute effect of withdrawing antidepressants. *Acta Psychiatr. Scand.* 83, 238.

Halle, M.H. and Dilsaver, S.C. (1993). Tranylcypromine withdrawal phenomena. *J. Psychiatry Neurosci.* 18, 49.

Hallstrom, C.O. (1994). Drugs in focus: 12. Zopiclone. *Prescribers' Journal* 34, 115.

Hallstrom, C. and Lader, M. (1981). Benzodiazepine withdrawal phenomena. *Int. Pharmacopsychiatry* 16, 235.

Hammeke, T.A., McQuillen, M.P., and Cohen, B.A. (1983). Musical hallucinations associated with acquired deafness. *J. Neurol. Neurosurg. Psychiatry* 4, 570.

Hargreave, F.E., McCarthy, D.S., and Pepys, J. (1969). Steroid 'pseudorheumatism' in asthma. *BMJ* i, 443.

Harper, C. (1979). Wernicke's encephalopathy: a more common disease than realised. A neuropathological study of 51 cases. *J. Neurol. Neurosurg. Psychiatry* 42, 226.

Harris, B. and Harper, M. (1979). Psychosis after dextropropoxyphene. *Lancet* ii, 743.

Harrison, R.W.S. and Ashton, C.H. (1994). Do cholesterol-lowering agents affect brain activity? A comparison of simvastatin, pravastatin, and placebo in healthy volunteers. *Br. J. Clin. Pharmacol.* 37, 231.

Harrison-Read, P.E., Tyrer, P., Lawson, C., *et al.* (1996). Flumazenil-precipitated panic and dysphoria in patients dependent on benzodiazepines: a possible aid to abstinence. *J. Psychopharmacol.* 10, 89.

Hartmann, E. (1976). Long-term administration of psychotropic drugs: effects on human sleep. In *Pharmacology of Sleep* (ed. R.L. Williams and I. Karacan), p. 211. John Wiley, New York.

Hatcher, S., Sims, R., and Thompson, D. (1990). The effects of chronic lithium treatment on psychomotor performance related to driving. *Br. J. Psychiatry* 157, 275.

Hatrick, J.A. and Dewhurst, K. (1970). Delayed psychosis due to LSD. *Lancet* ii, 742.

Hatsukami ,D., Keenan, R., Halikas, J., *et al.* (1991). Effects of carbamazepine on acute responses to smoked cocaine-base in human cocaine users. *Psychopharmacology* 104, 120.

Hausner, R.S. (1980). Amantadine-associated recurrence of psychosis. *Am. J. Psychiatry* 137, 240.

Hayden, F.G. (1996). Antimicrobial agents: antiviral agents. In *Goodman and Gilman's The Pharmacological Basis of Therapeutics* (9th edn) (ed. J.G. Hardman and L.E. Limbird), p. 1191. McGraw-Hill, New York.

Hazen, P.G., Carney, J.F., Walker, A.E., *et al.* (1983). Depression: a side effect of 13-cis-retinoic acid therapy. *J. Am. Acad. Dermatol.* 9, 278.

Heath, R.G., Nesselhof, W., Bishop, M.P., *et al.* (1965). Behavioral and metabolic changes associated with administration of tetraethylthiuram disulfide (Antabuse). *Dis. Nerv. Syst.* 26, 99.

Helson, L. and Duque, L. (1978). Acute brain syndrome after propranolol. *Lancet* i, 98.

Henderson, G. (1983). Electrophysiological analysis of opioid action. *Br. Med. Bull.* 39, 59.

Henderson, C.A. and Highet, A.S. (1989). Depression induced by etretinate. *BMJ* 298, 964.

Hendler, N., Cimini, C., Ma, T., *et al.* (1980). A comparison of cognitive impairment due to benzodiazepines and to narcotics. *Am. J. Psychiatry* 137, 828.

Herz, A. (1981). Role of endorphins in addiction. *Mod. Probl. Pharmacopsychiatry* 17, 175.

Herz, A. and Holt, V. (1982). On the role of endorphins in addiction. In *Advances in Pharmacology and Therapeutics II.* Vol. 1. *CNS Pharmacology — Neuropeptides* (ed. H. Yoshida, Y. Hagihara, and S. Ebashi), p. 67. Pergamon Press, Oxford.

Herzberg, J.L. and Wolkind, S.N. (1983). Solvent sniffing in perspective. *Br. J. Hosp. Med.* January, 72.

Higgitt, A., Fonagy, P., Toone, B., *et al.* (1990). The prolonged benzodiazepine withdrawal syndrome: anxiety or hysteria? *Acta Psychiatr. Scand.* 82, 165.

Hirsch, S.R. (1982). Depression 'revealed' in schizophrenia. *Br. J. Psychiatry* 140, 421.

Hirsch, S.R., Gaind, R., Rohde, P.D., *et al.* (1973). Outpatient maintenance of chronic schizophrenic patients with long-acting fluphenazine: A double-blind placebo trial. *BMJ* i, 633.

Hodgson, R. (1994). The treatment of alcohol problems. *Addiction* 89, 1529.

Hoefnagel, D. (1961). Toxic effects of atropine and homatropine eyedrops in children. *N. Engl. J. Med.* 264, 168.

Hoffman, B.F. and Biggar, J.T. (1990). Digitalis and allied cardiac glycosides. In *Goodman and Gilman's The Pharmacological Basis of Therapeutics* (8th edn) (ed. A.G. Gilman, T.W. Rall, A.S. Nies, and P. Taylor), p. 814. Pergamon Press, Oxford.

Hoigné, R. (1962). Acute side-reactions to penicilin. *Acta Med. Scand.* 171, 201.

Hoigné, R., Keller, H., and Sonntag, R. (1984). Penicillins, cephalosporins and tetracyclines. In *Meyler's Side Effects of Drugs* (10th edn) (ed. M.N.G. Dukes), p. 146. Elsevier, Amsterdam.

Hollister, L.E., Elkenberry, D.T., and Raffel, S. (1960). Chlorpromazine in nonpsychotic patients with pulmonary tuberculosis. *Am. Rev. Respir. Dis.* 81, 562.

Hollister, L.E. (1964). Complications from psychotherapeutic drugs. *Clin. Pharmacol. Ther.* 5, 322.

Hollister, L.E. (1982). Pharmacology and toxicology of psychotomimetics. In *Psychotropic Agents Part III. Alcohol and Psychotomimetics, Psychotropic Effects of Central Acting Drugs* (ed. F. Hoffmeister and G. Stille), p. 321. Springer-Verlag, Berlin.

Hollister, L.E. (1985). *Drug Tolerance, Dependence, and Abuse.* Upjohn.

Hollister, L.E. (1986). Drug-induced psychiatric disorders and their management. *Med. Toxicol.* 1, 428.

Holman, R.B. (1994). Biological effects of central nervous system stimulants. *Addiction*, 89, 1435.

Holmes, C., Fortenza, O., Powell, J., *et al.* (1997). Carriers of apolipoprotein E e4 allele seem particularly susceptible to their effects. *BMJ* 314, 1411.

Hoover, C.E. (1990). Additional cases of suicidal ideation associated with fluoxetine. *Am. J. Psychiatry* 147, 1570.

Howlet, A.C., Bidaut-Russell, M., Devane, W.A., *et al.* (1990). The cannabinoid receptor: biochemical, anatomical and behavioral characterization. *Trends Neurosci.* 13, 420.

Hughes, J.D., Reed, W.D., and Serjeant, C.S. (1983). Mental confusion associated with ranitidine. *Med. J. Aust.* ii, 12.

Hullett, F.J., Potkin, S.G., Levy, A.B., *et al.* (1988). Depression associated with nifedipine-induced calcium channel blockade. *Am. J. Psychiatry* 145, 1277.

Hurwitz, N. and Wade, O.L. (1969). Intensive hospital monitoring of adverse reactions to drugs. *BMJ* i, 531.

Idzikowski, C. and Shapiro, C.M. (1993). Non-psychotic drugs and sleep. *BMJ* 306, 1118.

Ilechukwu, S.T.C. (1990). Acute psychotic reactions and stress response syndromes following intramuscular aqueous procaine penicillin. *Br. J. Psychiatry* 156, 554.

Inman, W.H.W., Wilton, L.V., Pearce GL., *et al.* (1990). Prescription-event monitoring of nabumetone. *Pharmacol. Med.* 4, 309.

Innes, J.A., Watson, M.L., Ford, M.J., *et al.* (1977). Plasma fenfluramine levels, weight loss, and side effects. *BMJ* ii, 1322.

Jabeen, S. and Fisher, C.J. (1991). Trazodone-induced transient hypomanic symptoms and their management. *Br. J. Psychiatry* 158, 275.

Jacobsen, F.M., Sack, D., and James, S.P. (1987). Delirium induced by verapamil. *Am. J. Psychiatry* 144, 248.

Jacobson, K.A. (1996). Specific ligands for the adenosine receptor family. *Neurotransmissions* XII, 1.

Jacquot, M. and Bottari, R. (1981). Etat maniaque ayant été déclenché par la prise orale de salbutamol. *Encéphale* 7, 45.

Jaffe, J.H. (1980). Drug addiction and drug abuse. In *The Pharmacological Basis of Therapeutics* (ed. A.G. Gilman, L.S. Goodman, and A. Gilman), p. 535. Macmillan, New York.

Jaffe, R. and Gibson, E. (1986). Clonazepam withdrawal psychosis. *J. Clin. Psychopharmacol.* 6, 193.

Jaffe, J.H. and Martin, W.R. (1980). Opioid analgesics and antagonists. In *The Pharmacological Basis of Therapeutics* (6th edn) (ed. A.G. Gilman, L.S. Goodman, and A. Gilman), p. 494. Macmillan, New York.

Jaffe, J.H. and Martin, W.T. (1990). Opioid analgesics and antagonists. In *Goodman and Gilman's The Pharmacological Basis of Therapeutics* (8th edn) (ed. A.G. Gilman, T.W. Rall, A.S. Nies, and P. Taylor), p. 485. Pergamon Press, Oxford.

Jain, N., Kemp, N., Edeyemo, O., *et al.* (1995). Anxiolytic activity of adenosine receptor activation in mice. *J. Psychopharmacol.* 116, 2127.

JAMA (1996). Does heavy marijuana use impair human cognition and brain function? *JAMA* 275, 560.

James, J.J., James, N.S., Morgenstern, M., *et al.* (1987). Quinacrine-induced toxic psychosis in a child. *Pediatr. Infect. Dis.* 6, 427.

Janowsky, D.S. and Risch, S.C. (1987). Role of acetylcholine mechanisms in the affective disorders. In *Psychopharmacology: The Third Generation of Progress* (ed. H.Y. Meltzer), p. 527. Raven Press, New York.

Jansen, K.L.R. (1990). Ketamine — can chronic use impair memory? *Int. J. Addiction* 25, 133.

Jansen, K.L.R. (1993). Non-medical use of ketamine. Dissociative states in unprotected settings may be harmful. *BMJ* 306, 601.

Jarvis, E.H. (1981). Drugs and the elderly patients. *Adverse Drug Reaction Bulletin* 86, 312.

Jefferson, J.W. (1979). Central nervous system toxicity of cimetidine: a case of depression. *Am. J. Psychiatry* 136, 346.

Jellema, J.G. (1987). Hallucinations during sustained-release morphine and methadone administration. *Lancet* ii, 392.

Johns, A. (1994). Opiate treatments. *Addiction* 89, 1551.

Johnson, K.M. (1987). Neurochemistry and neurophysiology of phencyclidine. In *Psychopharmacology: The third generation of progress* (ed. H.Y. Meltzer), p. 1581. Raven Press, New York.

Johnson, M., Ashton, H., Marsh, R., *et al.* (1993). Songs, rockets and whistling kettles: electroencephalographic changes in drug related auditory disturbances and treatment with acupuncture and transcutaneous electrical nerve stimulation. *Acupuncture in Medicine* 11, 98.

Jones, B.M. (1973). Memory impairment on the ascending and descending limbs of the blood alcohol curve. *J. Abnormal Psychol.* 82, 24.

Jones, P.G. and Beier-Hanratty, S.A. (1986). Acyclovir: neurologic and renal toxicity. *Ann. Intern. Med.* 104, 892.

Jones, R.F. and Lance, J.W. (1976). Baclofen (Lioresal) in the long-term management of spasticity. *Med. J. Aust.* i, 654.

Jones, R.T. (1983). Cannabis tolerance and dependence. In *Cannabis and Health Hazards* (ed. K.. Fehr. and H. Kalant). Toronto Addiction Research Foundation.

Jones, I.R. and Sullivan, G. (1988). Physical dependence on zopiclone: case reports. *BMJ* 316, 117.

Judd, F.K., Burrows, G.D., and Norman, T.R. (1983). Psychosis after withdrawal of steroid therapy. *Med. J. Aust.* ii, 350.

Judd, L.L., Squire, L.R., Butters, N., *et al.* (1987). Effects of psychotropic drugs on cognition and memory in normal humans and animals. In *Psychopharmacology: The third generation of progress* (ed. H.Y. Meltzer), p. 1467. Raven Press, New York.

Kabir, S.M.A. (1969). Chloroquine psychosis. *Trans. R. Soc. Trop. Med. Hyg.* 63, 549.

Kahn, J.K. (1986). Nifedipine-associated acute psychosis. *Am. J. Med.* 81, 705.

Kalso, E. and Vainio, A. (1988). Hallucinations during morphine but not during oxycodone treatment. *Lancet* ii, 912.

Kaminer, Y., Munitz, H., and Wijsenbeek, H. (1982). Trihexyphenidyl ('Artane') abuse — euphoriant and anxiolytic. *Br. J. Psychiatry* 140, 473.

Kaminer, Y. and Hrecznyj, B. (1991). Lysergic acid diethylamide-induced chronic visual disturbance in an adolescent. *J. Nerv. Ment. Dis.* 179, 173.

Kane, F.J. (1968). Psychiatric reactions to oral contraceptives. *Am. J. Obstet. Gynecol.* 102, 1053.

Kane, F.J. and Byrd, G. (1975). Acute toxosis associated with gentamicin therapy. *South. Med. J.* 68, 1283.

Kane, F.J. and Florezano, R. (1971). Psychosis accompanying use of bronchodilator compound. *JAMA* 215, 2116.

Karch, S.B. (1996). Anabolic steroids. In *The Pathology of Drug Abuse* (2nd edn), p. 409. CRC Press, London.

Kassler-Taub, K.B., Woodward, T., and Markowitz, J.S. (1993). Depressive symptoms and pravastatin. *Lancet* 341, 371.

Kay, H.E.M., Knapton, P.J., and O'Sullivan, J.P. (1972). Encephalopathy in acute leukemia associated with methotrexate therapy. *Arch. Dis. Child.* 47, 344.

Kay, D.C., Blackburn, A.B., Buckingham, J.A., *et al.* (1976). Human pharmacology of sleep. In *Pharmacology of sleep* (ed. R.L. Williams and I. Karacan), p. 83. John Wiley, New York.

Kay, C.R. (1984). The Royal College of General Practitioners' oral contraception study: some recent observations. *Clin. Obstet. Gynecol.* 11, 759.

Keeler, M.H., Kane, F., and Daly, R. (1964). An acute schizophrenic episode following abrupt withdrawal of Enovid in a patient with previous post-partum psychiatric disorder. *Am. J. Psychiatry* 120, 1123.

Kennedy. M. (1994). Drugs and athletes — an update. *Adverse Drug Reaction Bulletin* 169, 639.

Keuthen, N.J., Cyr, P., Ricciardi, J.A., *et al.* (1994). Medication withdrawal symptoms in obsessive-compulsive disorder patients treated with paroxetine. *J. Clin. Psychopharmacol.* 14, 206.

Khurana, A.K., Ahluwalia, B.K., Rajan, C., *et al.* (1988). Acute psychosis associated with topical cyclopentolate hydrochloride. *Am. J. Ophthalmol.* 105, 91.

King, J.T. (1950). Digitalis delirium. *Ann. Intern. Med.* 33, 1360.

King, D.J. (1990). The effect of neuroleptics on cognitive and psychomotor function. *Br. J. Psychiatry* 157, 799.

King, D.J. and Henry, G. (1992). The effects of neuroleptics on cognitive and psychomotor function: A preliminary study in healthy volunteers. *Br. J. Psychiatry* 160, 647.

Kinnell, H.G. and Webb, A. (1979). Confusion associated with cimetidine. *BMJ* ii, 1438.

Klein, H.E., Broucek, B., and Greil, W. (1981). Lithium withdrawal triggers psychotic states. *Br. J. Psychiatry* 139, 255.

Knee, S. and Razani, J. (1974). Acute organic brain syndrome: a complication of disulfiram therapy. *Am. J. Psychiatry* 131, 1281.

Knobler, H.Y., Emanuel, D., Mester, R., *et al.* (1986). Trazadone-induced mania. *Br. J. Psychiatry* 149, 787.

Koehler, K. and Guth, W. (1977). Schizophrenie-ähnliche Psychose nach einnahme von Propranolol. *Münch. Med. Wochenschr.* 119, 443.

Korolenko, C.P., Yevseyeva, T.A., and Volkov, P.P. (1969). Data for a comparative account of toxic psychoses of various aetiologies. *Br. J. Psychiatry* 115, 273.

Kramer, J.C., Klein, D.F., and Fink, M. (1961). Withdrawal symptoms following discontinuation of imipramine therapy. *Am. J. Psychiatry* 118, 549.

Kruis, R. and Barger, R. (1980). Paranoid psychosis with sulindac. *JAMA* 243, 1420.

Krystal, J.H. and Price, L.H. (1992). Chronic 3,4-methylenedioxymethamphetamine (MDMA) use: effects on mood and neuropsychological function? *Am. J. Drug Alcohol Abuse* 18, 331.

Krystal, J.H., Karper, L.P., Seibyl, J.P., *et al.* (1993). Dose-related effects of the NMDA antagonist, ketamine, in healthy humans. *Schizophr. Res.* 9, 240.

Kuhar, M.J. and Pilotte, N.S. (1996). Neurochemical changes in cocaine withdrawal. *Trends Pharmacol. Sci.* 17, 260.

Kumar, K.L. and Hodges, M. (1988). Disturbing dreams with long-acting verapamil. *N. Engl. J. Med.* 318, 929.

Kupfer, D.J., Carpenter, L.L., and Frank, E. (1988). Possible role of antidepressants in precipitating mania and hypomania in recurrent depression. *Am. J. Psychiatry* 145, 804.

Kuriama, S. (1994). Bisoprodol-induced nightmares. *J. Hum. Hypertens.* 8, 731.

Lacayo, A. (1995). Neurologic and psychiatric complications of cocaine abuse. *Neuropsychiatry Neuropsychol. Behav. Neurol.* 8, 53.

Lacousiere, R.B., Spohn, H.E., and Thompson, K. (1976). Medical effects of abrupt neuroleptic withdrawal. *Comp. Psychiatry* 17, 285.

Lader, M. (1988). The psychopharmacology of addiction — benzodiazepine tolerance and dependence. In *Psychopharmacology of Addiction* (ed. M. Lader), p. 1. Oxford University Press.

Lader, M.H. (1989). Newer anti-anxiety drugs. In *Psychopharmacology of Anxiety* (ed. P. Tyrer), p. 243. Oxford University Press.

Lader, M. (1991). Can buspirone induce rebound, dependence or abuse? *Br. J. Psychiatry* 159, 45.

Lader, M.H. (1997). The psychopharmacology of toxic substances. *J. Psychopharmacol.* 11 (Suppl.) A4, 13.

Lader, M. and Bruce, M. (1986). States of anxiety and their induction by drugs. *Br. J. Clin. Pharmacol.* 22, 251.

Lader, M. and Bruce, M.S. (1989). The human pharmacology of the methylxanthines: In *Human Psychopharmacology: Measures and Methods*, Vol. 2 (ed. I. Hindmarsh and P.D. Storer), p. 179. John Wiley, London.

Lader, M.H. and Morton, S.V. (1992). A pilot study of the effects of flumazenil on symptoms persisting after benzodiazepine withdrawal. *J. Psychopharmacol.* 6, 357.

Lader, M. and Petursson, H. (1981). Benzodiazepine derivatives — side effects and dangers. *Biol. Psychiatry* 16, 1195.

Lader, M.H., Ron, M., and Petursson, H. (1984). Computed axial brain tomography in long-term benzodiazepine users. *Psychol. Med.* 14, 203.

Lader, M., Cardwell, C., Shine, P., *et al.* (1996). Caffeine withdrawal symptoms and rate of metabolism. *J. Psychopharmacol.* 10, 110.

Laffi, G.L. and Safran, A.B. (1993). Persistent visual changes following hashish consumption. *Br. J. Ophthalmol.* 77, 601.

Lago, J.A. and Kosten, T.R. (1994). Stimulant withdrawal. *Addiction* 89, 1477.

Lahti, A.C., Gao, X.M., Cascella, N.G., *et al.* (1993). Can NMDA antagonists help us understand the psychosis mechanism in schizophrenia? *Schizophr. Res.* 9, 241.

Lambert, M.T. (1987). Paranoid psychoses after abuse of proprietary cold remedies. *Br. J. Psychiatry* 151, 548.

The Lancet (1990a). Korsakoff's syndrome. *Lancet* 336, 912.

The Lancet (1990b). Zopiclone: another carriage on the tranquilliser train. *Lancet* 335, 507.

Lane, R.M. (1996). Withdrawal symptoms after discontinuation of selective serotonin reuptake inhibitors (SSRIs). *Journal of Serotonin Research* 3, 75.

Laporta, M., Chouinard, G., Goldbloom, D., *et al.* (1987). Hypomania induced by sertraline, a new serotonin re-uptake inhibitor. *Am. J. Psychiatry* 144, 1513.

Lautin, A., Angrist, B., Stanley, M., *et al.* (1980). Sodium valproate in schizophrenia. Some biochemical correlates. *Br. J. Psychiatry* 137, 240.

Lebegue, B. (1987). Mania precipitated by fluoxetine. *Am. J. Psychiatry* 144, 1620.

Lee, E.J.D. and Jeyaseelan, K. (1994). Frequency of human CYP2D6 mutant alleles in a normal Chinese population. *Br. J. Clin. Pharmacol.* 37, 605.

Lee, K., Moller, L., Hardt, F., *et al.* (1979). Alcohol-induced brain damage and liver damage in young males. *Lancet* ii, 759.

Le Gassicke, J., Ashcroft, G.W., Eccleston, D., *et al.* (1965). The clinical state, sleep and amine metabolism of a tranylcypromine (Parnate) addict. *Br. J. Psychiatry* 3, 357.

Leichleitner, M., Hoppichler, F., Kanwalinka, G., *et al.* (1992). Depressive symptoms in hypercholesterolaemic patients treated with pravastatin. *Lancet* 340, 910.

Leipzig, R.M., Goodman, H., Gray, G., *et al.* (1987). Reversible narcotic-induced mental status impairment in patients with metastatic cancer. *Pharmacology* 35, 47.

Leirer, V.O., Yesavage, J.A., and Morrow, D.G. (1991). Marijuana carry-over effects on aircraft pilot performance. *Aviat. Space Environ. Med.* 62, 221.

Lejoyeux, M., Adàs, J., Mourad, I., *et al.* (1996). Antidepressant withdrawal syndrome. Recognition, prevention and management. *CNS Drugs* 5, 278.

Lely, A.H. and van Enter, C.H.J. (1970). Large scale digoxin intoxication. *BMJ* iii, 737.

Lepkifker, E., Dannon, P.N., Iancu, I., *et al.* (1995). Nightmares related to fluoxetine treatment. *Clin. Neuropharmacol.* 18, 90.

Lesser, I.M., Miller, B.L., Boone, K., *et al.* (1987). Delusions in a patient treated with histamine H2 receptor antagonists. *Psychosomatics* 28, 501.

Levi, L. and Miller, N.R. (1990). Visual illusions associated with previous drug abuse. *J. Clin. Neuro-ophthalmol.* 10, 103.

Levy, M. and Zylber-Katz, E. (1983). Caffeine metabolism and coffee-attributed sleep disturbances. *Clin. Pharmacol. Ther.* 33, 770.

Lewis, S.A., Oswald, I., and Dunleavy, D.L.F. (1971). Chronic fenfluramine administration: some cerebral effects. *BMJ* 3, 67.

Liddon, S.C. and Satran, R. (1967). Disulfiram (Antabuse) psychosis. *Am. J. Psychiatry* 123, 1284.

Lindberg, G., Råstam, L., Gullberg, B., *et al.* (1992). Low serum cholesterol concentration and short term mortality from injuries in men and women. *BMJ* 305, 277.

Linn, I., Kahn, R.L., Coles, R., *et al.* (1953). Patterns of behaviour disturbance following cataract extraction. *Am. J. Psychiatry* 110, 281.

Linnoila, M., George, L., and Guthrie, S. (1982). Interaction between antidepressants and perphenazine in psychiatric patients. *Am. J. Psychiatry* 139, 1329.

Linszman, D.H., Dingemans, P.M., and Lenior, M.E. (1994). Cannabis abuse and the course of recent-onset schizophrenic disorders. *Arch. Gen. Psychiatry* 51, 273.

Lipowski, Z.J. (1975). Delirium clouding of consciousness and confusion. *J. Nerv. Ment. Dis.* 145, 227.

Lipper, S. (1976). Psychosis in patient on bromocriptine and levodopa with carbidopa. *Lancet* ii, 571.

Lishman, W.A., Jacobson, R.R., and Acker, C. (1987). Brain damage in alcoholism: current concepts. *Acta Med. Scand.* (Suppl.) 717, 5.

Lishman, W.A. (1990). Alcohol and the brain. *Br. J. Psychiatry* 156, 635.

Littleton, J. and Little, H. (1994). Current concepts of ethanol dependence. *Addiction* 89, 1397.

Longo, V.G. (1966). Behavioural and EEG effects of atropine and related compounds. *Pharmacol. Rev.* 18, 965.

Loosmore, S. and Armstrong, D. (1990). Do-Do abuse. *Br. J. Psychiatry* 157, 278.

Loudon, J. and Waring, H. (1976). Toxic reactions to lithium and haloperidol. *Lancet* ii, 1088.

Louie, A.K., Lannon, R.A. Kirsch, M.A., *et al.* (1996). Venlafaxine withdrawal reactions. *Am. J. Psychiatry* 153, 1652.

Louwerens, J.W., Brookhuis, K.A., and O'Hanlon, J.F. (1986). Several antidepressants' acute effects upon actual driving performance and subjective mental activation. In *Drugs and Driving* (ed. J.F. O'Hanlon and J.J. de Gier), p. 203. Taylor and Francis, London and Philadelphia.

Lucas, A.T. and Weiss, M. (1971). Methylphenidate hallucinosis. *JAMA* 217, 1079.

Luchins, D.J., Freed, W.J., and Wyatt, R.J. (1980). The role of cholinergic supersensitivity in the medical symptoms associated with withdrawal of antipsychotic drugs. *Am. J. Psychiatry* 137, 1395.

Lucki, I., Rickels, K., and Geller, A.M. (1986). Chronic use of benzodiazepines and psychomotor and cognitive test performance. *Psychopharmacology* 88, 426.

Lukas, S.E. (1996). CNS effects and abuse liability of anabolic-androgenic steroids. *Annu. Rev. Pharmacol. Toxicol.* 36, 333

McCann, U.D. and Ricaurte, G.A. (1993). Reinforcing subjective effects of (+)-3,4-methylenedioxymethamphetamine ('ecstasy') may be separable for its neurotoxic actions: clinical evidence. *J. Clin. Psychopharmacol.* 13, 214.

McCann, U.D., Ridenour, A., Shaham, Y., *et al.* (1994). Serotonergic neurotoxicity after (±) 3,4-methylenedioxymetamphetamine (MDMA; 'Ecstasy'): a controlled study in humans. *Neuropsychopharmacology* 10, 129.

McClelland, H.A. (1985). Psychiatric disorders. In *Textbook of Adverse Drug Reactions* (3rd edn) (ed. D.M. Davies), p. 550. Oxford University Press.

McClelland, H.A. (1990). The forensic implications of benzodiazepine usage. In *Benzodiazepines: Current Concepts* (ed. I. Hindmarch, G. Beaumont, S. Brandon, and B.E. Leonard), p. 227. John Wiley, Chichester.

McCrum, I.D. and Guidry, J.R. (1978). Procainamide-induced psychosis. *JAMA* 240, 1265.

MacDermott, A.J., Insole, J., and Kaufman, B. (1987). Acute confusional episodes during treatment with ranitidine. *BMJ* 294, 1616.

MacEvilly, M. and O'Carroll, C. (1989). Hallucinations after epidural buprenorphine. *BMJ* 298, 928.

McEvoy, J.P. (1982). The chronic neuropsychiatric disorders associated with alcoholism. In *Encyclopedic Handbook of Alcoholism* (ed. E.M. Pattison and E. Kaufman), p. 167. Gardner Press, New York.

McEvoy, J.P. (1987). A double-blind crossover comparison of antiparkinsonian drug therapy: amantadine versus anticholinergic in 90 normal volunteers, with an emphasis on differential effects on memory function. *J. Clin. Psychiatry* 48, 20.

McEwen, B.S. (1991). Non-genomic and genomic effects of steroids on neural activity. *Trends Pharmacol. Sci.* 12, 141.

McEwen, B.S. (1995). Neuroendocrine interactions. In *Psychopharmacology: The Fourth Generation of Progress* (ed. F.E. Bloom and D.J. Kupfer), p. 705. Raven Press, New York.

McGuire, P. and Fahy, T. (1991). Chronic paranoid psychosis after misuse of MDMA ('ecstasy'). *BMJ* 302, 697.

McGuire, P. and Fahy, T. (1992). Flashbacks following MDMA. *Br. J. Psychiatry* 160, 276.

McGuire, P.K., Cope, H., and Fahy, T. (1994*a*). Diversity of psychopathology associated with use of 3,4-methylenedioxymethamphetamine ('Ecstasy'). *Br. J. Addict.* 165, 391.

McGuire, P.K., Jones, P., Harvey, I., *et al.* (1994*b*). Cannabis and acute psychosis. *Schizophr. Res.* 13, 161.

McGuire, P.K., Jones, P., Harvey, I., *et al.* (1995). Morbid risk of schizophrenia for relatives of patients with cannabis-associated psychosis. *Schizophr. Res.* 15, 277.

McInnes, G.T. (1987). Chlormethiazole and alcohol: a lethal cocktail. *BMJ*, 294, 592.

McInnis, M. and Petursson, H. (1984). Trihexyphenidyl dependence. *Acta Psychiatr. Scand.* 69, 538.

McIvor, R.J. and Sinanan, K. (1991). Buspirone-induced mania. *Br. J. Psychiatry* 158, 136.

McKeith, I., Fairburn, A., Perry, R., et al. (1992). Neuroleptic sensitivity in patients with senile dementia of Lewy body type. *BMJ* 305, 673.

McMahon, T. (1985). Bipolar affective symptoms associated with use of captopril and abrupt withdrawal of pargyline and propranolol. *Am. J. Psychiatry* 142, 759.

McShane, R., Keene, J., Gedling, K., et al. (1997). Do neuroleptic drugs hasten cognitive decline in dementia? Prospective study with necropsy follow up. *BMJ* 314, 266.

McTavish, D. and Heel, R.C. (1992). Dexfluramine. A review of its pharmacological properties and therapeutic potential in obesity. *Drugs* 43, 713.

Mair, W.G.P., Warrington, E.K., and Weiskrantz, L. (1979). Memory disorder in Korsakoff's psychosis. *Brain* 102, 749.

Malcolm, R. and Miller, W.C. (1972). Dimenhydrinate (Dramamine) abuse: hallucinogenic experiences with a proprietary anti-histamine. *Am. J. Psychiatry* 128, 1012.

Malleson, N. (1971). Acute adverse reactions to LSD in clinical and experimental use in the UK. *Br. J. Psychiatry* 118, 229.

Mallett, P., Marshall, E.J., and Blacker, C.V.R. (1989). 'Puerperal psychosis' following male to female sex reassignment. *Br. J. Psychiatry* 155, 257.

Mallya, G., White, K., and Gunderson, C. (1993). Is there a serotonergic withdrawal syndrome? *Biol. Psychiatry* 33, 851.

Mandal, S.K. (1986). Psychiatric side-effects of ranitidine. *Br. J. Clin. Pract.* 40, 260.

Mandell, G.L. and Petrie, W.A. (1996). Antimicrobial agents: Drugs used in the chemotherapy of tuberculosis and leprosy. In *Goodman and Gilman's The Pharmacological Basis for Therapeutics* (9th edn) (ed. J.G. Hardman and L.E. Limbird), p. 1155. McGraw-Hill, New York.

Mander, A. and Loudon, J. (1988). Rapid recurrence of mania following abrupt discontinuation of lithium. *Lancet* 2, 15.

Mann, J.J. (1983). Loss of antidepressant effect with long-term monoamine oxidase inhibition. *J. Clin. Psychopharmacol.* 3, 363.

Manschreck, T.C., Allen, D.F., and Neville, M. (1987). Freebase psychosis: cases from a Bahamanian epidemic of cocaine abuse. *Comp. Psychiatry* 28, 555.

Margo, A. and McMahon, P. (1982). Lithium withdrawal triggers psychosis. *Br. J. Psychiatry* 141, 407 and 431.

Mariani, P.J. (1988). Adverse reactions to chlorpromazine in the treatment of migraine. *Ann. Emerg. Med.* 17, 380.

Marjot, R. and McLeod, A.A. (1989). Chronic non-neurological toxicity from volatile substance abuse. *Hum. Toxicol.* 8, 301.

Martin, P.R., Adinoff, B., Eckhardt, M., et al. (1989). Effective pharmacotherapy of alcoholic amnestic disorder with fluvoxamine. *Arch. Gen. Psychiatry* 46, 617.

Marriott, P. (1976). Dependence on antiparkinsonian drugs. *BMJ* i, 152.

Marriott, S. and Tyrer, P. (1993). Benzodiazepine dependence: avoidance and withdrawal. *Drug Saf.* 9, 93.

Martindale: The Extra Pharmacopoeia (1982). (ed. J.E.F. Reynolds and B. Prasad). Pharmaceutical Press, London.

Martinez-Arevelo, M.J., Calcedo-Ordonez, A., and Varo-Prieto, J.R. (1994). Cannabis consumption as a prognostic factor in schizophrenia. *Br. J. Psychiatry* 164, 679.

Martys, C.R. (1979). Adverse reactions to drugs. *BMJ* ii, 1194.

Masand, P., Gupta, S., and Dewan M. (1991). Suicidal ideation associated with fluoxetine treatment. *N. Engl. J. Med.* 324, 420.

Mason, S.T. and Fibiger, H.C. (1979). Possible behavioural function for noradrenaline-acetylcholine interaction in brain. *Nature* 277, 396.

Mathers, D.C. and Ghodse, A.H. (1992). Cannabis and psychotic illness. *Br. J. Psychiatry* 161, 648.

Matsuda, L.A., Lolait, S.J., Brownstein, M.J., et al. (1990). Structure of cannabinoid receptor and functional expression of the cloned cDNA. *Nature* 346, 561.

Matthew, G. (1988). Psychiatric symptoms associated with carbamazepine. *BMJ* 296, 1071.

Maykutt, M.O. (1985). Health consequences of acute and chronic marihuana use. *Prog. Neuropsychopharmacol. Biol. Psychiatry* 9, 209.

Mayo, K.M., Falkowski, W., and Jones, C.A.H. (1993). Caffeine: use and effects in long-stay psychiatric patients. *Br. J. Psychiatry* 162, 543.

Medawar, C. and Rassaby, E. (1991). Triazolam overdose, alcohol, and manslaughter. *Lancet* 338, 1515.

Meldrum, B. (1982). GABA and acute psychoses. *Psychol. Med.* 12, 1.

Meltzer, H.Y. and Lowy, M.T. (1987). The serotonin hypothesis of depression. In *Psychopharmacology: The Third Generation of Progress* (ed. H.Y. Meltzer), p. 513. Raven Press, New York.

Melzack, R. (1973). *The Puzzle of Pain*. Penguin, Harmondsworth.

Mendelson, J.H. (1987). Marihuana. In *Psychopharmacology: The Third Generation of Progress* (ed. H.Y. Meltzer), p. 1565. Raven Press, New York.

Mendelson, J.H., Mellow, N.K., Lex, B.W.E., et al. (1984). Marijuana withdrawal syndrome in a woman. *Am. J. Psychiatry* 141, 1289.

Mendelson, W.B. and Jain, B. (1995). An assessment of short-acting hypnotics. *Drug Saf.* 13, 257.

Menezes, P.R., Johnson, S., Thornicroft, G., et al. (1996). Drug and alcohol problems among individuals with severe mental illness in South London. *Br. J. Psychiatry* 168, 612.

Meredith, T.J., Ruprah, M., Liddle, A., et al. (1989). Diagnosis and treatment of acute poisoning with volatile substances. *Hum. Toxicol.* 8, 277.

Meuser, K.T., Yarnold, P.R., Levinson, D.F., et al. (1990). Prevalence of drug abuse in schizophrenia: Demographic and social correlates. *Schizophr. Bull.* 16, 31.

Middlemiss, D.N., Blakeborough, L., and Leather, S.R. (1977). Direct evidence for an interaction of beta-adrenergic blockers with 5-HT receptor. *Nature* 267, 289.

Mikkelson, E.J. (1978). Caffeine and schizophrenia. *J. Clin. Psychiatry* 39, 732.

Miller, M.E., Perry, C.J., and Siris, S.G. (1987). Psychosis in association with combined cimetidine and imipramine treatment. *Psychosomatics* 28, 217.

Miller, N.S. (1991). Amphetamines. In *Comprehensive Handbook of Drug and Alcohol Abuse* (ed. N.S. Miller), p. 427. Marcel Dekker, New York.

Miller, N.S. and Gold, M.S. (1993). A hypothesis for a common neurochemical basis for alcohol and drug disorders. *Psychiatr. Clin. North Am.* 16, 105.

Miller, M.E., Perry, C.J., and Siris, S.G. (1987). Psychosis in association with combined cimetidine and imipramine treatment. *Psychosomatics* 28, 1688.

Milstein, H.G. (1980). Mental depression secondary to fluorouracil therapy for actinic keratoses. *Arch. Dermatol.* 116, 1100.

Mirin, S.M., Schatzberg. A.F., and Creasey, D.E. (1981). Hypomania and mania after withdrawal of tricyclic antidepressants. *Am. J. Psychiatry* 138, 87.

Mohler, H. and Okada, R. (1977). Benzodiazepine receptors: Demonstration in the central nervous system. *Science* 198, 849.

Montgomery, S.A. (1995). Selective serotonin reuptake inhibitors in the acute treatment of depression. In *Psychopharmacology: The Fourth Generation of Progress* (ed. F.E. Bloomn and D.J. Kupfer), p. 1043. Raven Press, New York.

Monti, J.M., Attali, P., Monti, D., *et al.* (1994). Zolpidem and rebound insomnia — a double-blind, controlled polysomnographic study in chronic insomniac patients. *Pharmacopsychiatry* 27, 166.

Moodley, P., Golombok, S., Shine, P., *et al.* (1993). Computed axial brain tomograms in long-term benzodiazepine users. *Psychiatry Res.* 48, 135.

Morgan, K. and Oswald, I. (1982). Anxiety caused by short-life hypnotic. *BMJ* 284, 942

Morgan, T.O., Sabto, J., Anavekar, S.N., *et al.* (1974). A comparison of beta adrenergic blocking drugs in the treatment of hypertension. *Postgrad. Med. J.* 50, 253.

Morgan, R.E., Palinkas, L., Barrett-Connor, E.L., *et al.* (1993). Plasma cholesterol and depressive symptoms in older men. *Lancet* 341, 75.

Morris, H.H. and Estes, M.L. (1987). Traveler's amnesia: transient global amnesia secondary to triazolam. *JAMA* 258, 945.

Morris, D.E. and Hardway, R.L. (1985). Visual hallucinations induced by fenbufen. *BMJ* 290, 822.

Moruzzi, G. and Magoun, H.W. (1949). Brain stem reticular formation and evolution of the EEG. *Electroenceph. Clin. Neurophysiol.* 1, 455.

Moskocvitz, C., Moses, R., and Klawans, H.L. (1978). Levodopa-induced psychosis: a kindling phenomenon. *Am. J. Psychiatry* 135, 669.

Mountcastle, V.B. (1974). Sleep wakefulness and the conscious state: intrinsic regulatory mechanisms of the brain. In *Medical Physiology* (ed. V.B. Mountcastle), p. 254. C.V. Mosby, St. Louis.

Muldoon, M.F., Manuck, S.B., and Matthews, K.A. (1990). Lowering cholesterol concentrations and mortality: a quantitative review of primary prevention trials. *BMJ* 301, 309.

Mullen, A. and Wilson, C.W.M. (1974). Fenfluramine and dreaming. *Lancet* ii, 594.

Mullen, A., Wilson, C.W.M., and Wilson, B.P.M. (1977). Dreaming, fenfluramine, and vitamin C. *BMJ* 1, 70.

Mullen, R.S. and Romans-Clarkson, S.E. (1993). Behavioural sensitisation and steroid-induced psychosis. *Br. J. Psychiatry* 162, 549.

Murphy, D.D. (1973). Mental effects of L-dopa. *Annu. Rev. Med.* 24, 209.

Murphy, D.L. (1979). The behavioral toxicity of monoamine oxidase inhibiting antidepressants. *Adv. Pharmacol. Chemother.* 14, 71.

Murphy, D. and Watters, J. (1986). Psychosis induced by fenfluramine. *BMJ* 292, 992.

Murphy, S.M., Owen, R., and Tyrer, P. (1989). Comparative assessment of efficacy and withdrawal symptoms after six and twelve weeks treatment with diazepam or buspirone. *Br. J. Psychiatry* 154, 529.

Nace, E.P. and Isbell, P.G. (1991). Alcohol. In *Clinical Textbook of Addictive Disorders* (ed. R.J. Frances and S.I. Miller), p. 43. Guildford Press, New York.

Nahas, G.G. (ed.) (1984). Toxicology and pharmacology. In *Marihuana in Science and Medicine,* p. 109. Raven Press, New York.

Nahas, G.G. and Paton, W.D.M. (1979). *Marihuana: Biological Effects.* Pergamon Press, Oxford.

Neaton, J.D., Blackburn, H., Jacobs, D., *et al.* (1992). The Multiple Risk Factor Intervention Trial Research Group. Serum cholesterol level and mortality findings for men screened in the Multiple Risk Factor Intervention Trial. *Ann. Intern. Med.* 152, 1490.

Negrete, J.C., Knapp, W.P., Douglas, D.E., *et al.* (1986). Cannabis affects the severity of schizophrenic symptoms: results of a clinical survey. *Psychological Medicine* 16, 515.

Nelson, J.C., Schottenfeld, R.S., and Conrad, C.D. (1983). Hypomania after disipramine withdrawal. *Am. J. Psychiatry* 40, 624.

Nestelbaum, Z., Siris, S.G., Rifkin, A., *et al.* (1986). Exacerbation of schizophrenia associated with amantadine. *Am. J. Psychiatry* 143, 1170.

Neuvonen, P.J., Pohjola-Sintonen, S., Tacke, U., *et al.* (1993). Five fatal cases of serotonin syndrome after moclobemide-citalopram or moclobemide–clomipramine overdoses. *Lancet* 342, 1419.

Nicholson, A.N. (1987). New antihistamines free of sedative side effects. *Trends Pharmacol. Sci.* 8, 247.

Nicholson, A.N., Pascoe, P.A., and Stone, B.M. (1985). Histaminergic systems and sleep studies in man with H1 and H2 antagonists. *Neuropharmacology* 24, 245.

Nierenberg, D.W. and Semprebon, M. (1993). The central nervous system serotonin syndrome. *Clin. Pharmacol. Ther.* 53, 84.

Nissenbaum, H., Quinn, N.P., Brown, R.G., *et al.* (1987). Mood swings with the 'on–off' phenomenon in Parkinson's disease. *Psychol. Med.* 17, 899.

Nolan, B.Y. (1982) Acute suicidal depression associated with the use of timolol. *JAMA* 247, 1567.

North, R.A. and Williams, J.T. (1983). How do opiates inhibit neurotransmitter release? *Trends Neurosci.* 6, 337.

Norvenius, G., Widerlov, E., and Lonnerholm, G. (1979). Phenylpropanolamine and mental disturbances. *Lancet* ii, 1367.

Nutt, D.J. (1996) Addiction: brain mechanisms and their treatment implications. *Lancet* 347, 31.

Nutt, D.J., Glue, P., Lawson, C., *et al.* (1993). Do benzodiazepine receptors have a causal role in panic disorder? In *Psychopharmacology of Panic* (ed. S.A. Montgomery), p. 74. Oxford University Press.

O'Brien, C.P., DiGiacomo, J.N., Fahn, S., *et al.* (1971). Mental effects of high dosage levodopa. *Arch. Gen. Psychiatry* 24, 61.

O'Brien, C.P. (1996) Drug addiction and drug abuse. In *Goodman & Gilman's The Pharmacological Basis of Therapeutics* (9th edn) (ed. J.G. Hardman and L.E. Limbird), p. 557. McGraw-Hill, New York.

O'Brien, C.P. and Woody, G.E. (1991). Psychiatric syndromes produced by cocaine. In *Physiopathology of Illicit Drugs: Cannabis, Cocaine, Opiates* (ed. G.G. Nahas and C. Latour), p. 219. Pergamon Press, Oxford.

O'Malley, M. (1997). Clinical evaluation of pesticide exposure and poisonings. *Lancet* 349, 1161.

Oehrberg, S., Christiansen, P.E., Behnke, K., *et al.* (1995). Paroxetine in the treatment of panic disorder. *Br. J. Psychiatry* 167, 374.

Olajide, D. and Lader, M. (1984). Depression following withdrawal from long-term benzodiazepine use: a report of four cases. *Psychol. Med.* 14. 937.

Orlando, R.G. (1986). Clinical depression associated with betaxolol. *Am. J. Ophthalmol.* 102, 275.

Oswald, I. (1982). Anxiety caused by a short-life hypnotic. *BMJ* 285, 511.

O'Sullivan, E.P., Childs, D., and Bush, G.H. (1988). Perioperative dreaming in paediatric patients who receive suxamethonium. *Anaesthesia* 43, 104.

Otani, K., Tanaka, O., Kaneko, S., *et al.* (1994). Mechanisms of the development of trazodone withdrawal symptoms. *Int. Clin. Psychopharmacol.* 9, 131.

Owen, R.T. and Tyrer, P. (1983). Benzodiazepine dependence. A review of the evidence. *Drugs* 25, 385.

Padfield, P.L., Smith, D.A., Fitzsimons, E.J., *et al.* (1977). Disopyramide and acute psychosis. *Lancet* i, 1152.

Pagliaro, L.A. and Pagliaro, A.M. (1993). The phenomenon of abusable psychotropic use among North American youth. *J. Clin. Pharmacol.* 33, 676.

Palat, G.K., Hooker, E.A., and Movahed, A. (1984). Secondary mania associated with diltiazem. *Clin. Cardiol.* 7, 611.

Palmer, K.J., Holliday, S.M., and Brogden, R.N. (1993). Mefloquine: a review of its antimalarial activity, pharmacokinetic properties and therapeutic efficacy. *Drugs* 45, 430.

Papp, K.A. and Curtis, R.M. (1984). Cimetidine-induced psychosis in a 14-year old girl. *Can. Med. Assoc. J.* 131, 1081.

Parliamentary Office of Science and Technology (1996). *Common Illegal Drugs and their Effects — Cannabis, Ecstasy, Amphetamines and LSD.* HMSO, London.

Parrott, A.C. and Kentridge, R. (1982). Personal constructs of anxiety under the 1,5-benzodiazepine derivative clobazam related to trait anxiety levels of the personality. *Psychopharmacology* 75, 353.

Parrott, A.C., Lees, D., Ross, C., *et al.* (1997). Memory impairments in recreational users of MDMA (Ecstasy). *J. Psychopharmacol.* 11 (Suppl.), 335.

Pascual-Leone, A., Dhuna, A., and Anderson D.C. (1991). Longterm neurological complications of chronic habitual cocaine abuse. *Neurotoxicology* 12, 393.

Paton, W.D.M., Pertwee, R.G., and Tylden, E. (1973). Clinical aspects of cannabis action. In *Marijuana* (ed. R. Mechoulam), p. 335. Academic Press, London/New York.

Patterson, J.F. (1985). Psychosis following discontinuation of a long-acting propranolol preparation. *J. Clin. Psychopharmacol.* 5, 125.

Patterson, J.F. (1987). Triazolam syndrome in the elderly. *South. Med. J.* 80, 1425.

Patterson, J.F. (1988). Auditory hallucinations induced by prazosin. *J. Clin. Psychopharmacol.* 8, 228.

Pauker, S.L. and Brown, R. (1986). Baclofen-induced catatonia. *J. Clin. Psychopharmacol.* 6, 387.

Paykel, E.S., Fleminger, R., and Watson, J.P. (1982). Psychiatric side-effects of anti-hypertensive drugs other than reserpine. *J. Clin. Psychopharmacol.* 2, 14.

Pearce, J.M.S. (1984). Drug treatment in Parkinson's disease. *BMJ* 288, 1777.

Pearce, I. and Pearce, J.M.S. (1978). Bromocriptine in Parkinsonism. *BMJ* i, 1402.

Peoples, R.W., Li Chaoying, and Weight F.F. (1996). Lipid vs. protein theories of alcohol action in the nervous system. *Annu. Rev. Pharmacol. Toxicol.* 36, 185.

Peralta, V. and Cuesta, M.J. (1992). Influence of cannabis abuse on schizophrenic psychopathology. *Acta Psychiatr. Scand.* 85, 127.

Pereau, O. and Maurice, H. (1950). Les troubles psychiques au cours de la fièvre typhoïde traitée par la chloromycétine. *Sem. Hôp. Paris* 26, 1060.

Perel, A. and Davidson, J.T. (1976). Recurrent hallucinations following ketamine. *Anaesthesia* 31, 1081.

Perényi, A., Frecska, E., Bagdy, G., *et al.* (1985). Changes in mental condition, hyperkinesias and biochemical parameters after withdrawal of chronic neuroleptic treatment. *Acta Psychiatr. Scand.* 72, 430.

Perera, K.M.H., Powell, T., and Jenner, F.A. (1987). Computerized axial tomographic studies following long-term use of benzodiazepines. *Psychol. Med.* 17, 775.

Pérez, V., Gilaberte, I., Faries, D., *et al.* (1997). Randomised, double-blind, placebo-controlled trial of pindolol in combination with fluoxetine antidepressant treatment. *Lancet* 349, 1594.

Pertwee, R.G. (1991). Tolerance to and dependence on psychotropic cannabinoids. In *The Biological Basis of Drug Tolerance and Dependence* (ed. J.A. Pratt), p. 232. Academic Press, London/New York.

Pertwee, R.G. (ed.) (1995). Pharmacological, physiological and clinical implications of the discovery of cannabinoid receptors: an overview. In *Cannabinoid Receptors*, p. 1. Academic Press, London/New York.

Peterson, L.G. and Popkin, M.K. (1980). Neuropsychiatric effects of chemotherapeutic agents for cancer. *Psychosomatics* 21, 141.

Petursson, H., Gudjonsson, G.H., and Lader, M.H. (1983). Psychometric performance during withdrawal from long-term benzodiazepine treatment. *Psychopharmacology* 81, 345.

Petursson, H. and Lader, M.H. (1981). Benzodiazepine dependence. *Br. J. Addict.* 76, 13.

Piercy, D.M., Cumming, J.A., Dawling, S., *et al.* (1981). Death due to overdose of nefopam. *BMJ* 283, 1508.

Pollard, H. and Schwartz, J-C. (1987). Histamine pathways and their functions. *Trends Neurosci.* 10, 86.

Poole, R. and Brabbins, C. (1996). Drug induced psychosis. *Br. J. Psychiatry* 168, 135.

Pope, H.G. and Katz, D.L. (1987). Bodybuilder's psychosis. *Lancet* i, 863.

Pope, H.G. and Katz, D.L. (1988). Affective and psychotic symptoms associated with anabolic steroid use. *Am. J. Psychiatry* 145, 487.

Pope, H.G. and Yurgelin-Todd, D. (1996). The residual cognitive effects of heavy marijuana use in college students. *JAMA* 275, 521.

Porot, M. and Destaing, F. (1950). Stréptomycine et troubles mentaux. *Ann. Med. Psychol.* 108, 47.

Porteous, H.B. and Ross, D.N. (1956). Mental symptoms in Parkinsonism following benzhexol therapy. *BMJ* ii, 138.

Poser, W., Poser, S., Roscher, D., *et al.* (1983). Do benzodiazepines cause cerebral atrophy? *Lancet* i, 715.

Postma, J.U. and van Tilburg, W. (1975). Visual hallucinations and delirium during treatment with amantadine (Symmetrel). *J. Am. Geriatr. Soc.* 23, 212.

Potamianos, G. and Kellett, J.M. (1982). Anticholinergic drugs and memory: The effects of benzhexol on memory in a group of geriatric patients. *Br. J. Psychiatry* 140, 470.

Powers, J.S., Decoskey, D., and Kahrilas, P.J. (1981). Physostigmine for treatment of delirium tremens. *J. Clin. Pharmacol.* 21, 57.

Prasher, V.P. and Corbett, J.A. (1990). Aerosol addiction. *Br. J. Psychiatry* 157, 922.

Prasher, V.P. (1993). The current debate concerning β-agonists in asthma. *J. R. Soc. Med.* 86, 743.

Pratt, H.F. (1982). Abuse of salbutamol inhalers in young people. *Clin. Allergy* 12, 203.

Prescott, L.F. (1978). Anti-inflammatory agents and drugs used in rheumatism and gout. In *Side Effects of Drugs, Annual 2* (ed. M.N.G. Dukes), p. 94. Associated Scientific Publishers, Amsterdam.

Preskorn, S.H. (1993). Pharmacokinetics of antidepressants: Why and how they are relevant to treatment. *J. Clin. Psychiatry* 54, 14.

Preskorn, S., Lane, R., and Magnus, R. (1996). The SSRI withdrawal syndrome. Abstract: Collegium Internationale Neuro-psychopharmacologium, June 1996.

Price, J.S., Waller, P.C., Wood, S.M., *et al.* (1985). A comparison of the post-marketing of four selective serotonin re-uptake inhibitors including the investigation of symptoms occurring on withdrawal. *Br. J. Clin. Pharmacol.* 42, 757.

Price, J.S., Waller, P.C., Wood, S.M., *et al.* (1996). A comparison of the post-marketing safety of four selective serotonin re-uptake inhibitors including the investigation of symptoms occurring on withdrawal. *Br. J. Clin. Pharmacol.* 42, 757.

Priest, R.G. and Montgomery, S.A. (1987). Benzodiazepines and dependence: A College Statement. *Bull. R. Coll. Psychiatrists* 12, 107.

Proctor, A.W., Littlewood, R., and Fry, AH. (1983). Bromocriptine-induced psychosis in acromegaly. *BMJ* 286, 50.

Proudfoot, A. (1982). *Diagnosis and Management of Acute Poisoning*. Blackwell Scientific Publications, Oxford.

Pullen, G.P., Best, N.R., and Maguire, J. (1984). Anticholinergic drug abuse: a common problem? *BMJ* 289, 612.

Pulvirenti, L. and Koob, G.F. (1994). Dopamine receptor agonists, partial agonists and psychostimulant addiction. *Trends Pharmacol. Sci.* 15, 374.

Quail, M. and Karelse, R. (1980). Disulfiram psychosis. *S. Afr. Med. J.* 57, 551.

Rall, T. (1990). Hypnotics and sedatives: Ethanol. In *Goodman and Gilman's The Pharmacological Basis of Therapeutics* (8th edn) (ed. A.G. Gilman, T.W. Rall, A.S. Nies, and P. Taylor), p. 345. Pergamon Press, Oxford.

Rall, T.W. and Schleifer, L.S. (1990). Drugs effective in the therapy of the epilepsies. In *Goodman and Gilman's The Pharmacological Basis of Therapeutics.* (8th edn) (ed. A.G. Gilman, T.W. Rall, A.S. Nies, and P. Taylor), p. 436. Pergamon Press, Oxford.

Ramhamadany, E., Mackenzie, S., and Ramsdale, D.R. (1986). Dysarthria and visual hallucinations due to flecainide toxicity. *Postgrad. Med. J.* 62, 61.

Ramnakha, P.S. and Barton, I. (1993). Drug smuggler's delirium. *BMJ* 306, 470.

Rattray, M. (1992). Ecstasy: rave now, pay later? *The Biochemist,* Nov. 3.

Remick, R.A., Froese, C., and Keller, F.D. (1989). Common side-effects associated with monoamine oxidase inhibitors. *Prog. Neuropsychopharmacol. Biol. Psychiatry* 13, 497.

Renault, P.F., Hoofnagle, J.H., Park, Y., *et al.* (1987). Psychiatric complications of long-term interferon alfa therapy. *Arch. Intern. Med.* 147, 1577.

Reynolds, E.H. (1978). Drug treatment of epilepsy. *Lancet* ii, 721.

Reynolds, E.H. (1981). Biological factors in psychological disorders associated with epilepsy. In *Epilepsy and Psychiatry* (ed. E.H. Reynolds and M.R. Trimble), p. 264. Churchill Livingstone, Edinburgh.

Ricaurte, G.A., Finnegan, K.T., DeLanney, L.E., *et al.* (1990). Aminergic metabolites in cerebrospinal fluid of humans previously exposed to MDMA: preliminary observations. *Ann. N.Y. Acad. Sci.* 600, 699.

Rice, H., Haltzman, S., and Tucek, C. (1988). Mania associated with procainamide. *Am. J. Psychiatry* 145, 129.

Richardson, H. (1989). Volatile substance abuse. *Hum. Toxicol.* 8, 319.

Richelson, E. (1994). The pharmacology of antidepressants at the synapse: focus on the newer compounds. *J. Clin. Psychiatry* 55 (Suppl. 9), 34.

Ritchie, K.S. and Preskorn, S.H. (1994). Mania induced by metoclopramide: case report. *J. Clin. Psychiatry* 45, 180.

Robbins, E. and Frosch, W.A. (1967). Further observations on untoward reactions to LSD. *Am. J. Psychiatry* 124, 393.

Robertson, I. (1984). Does moderate drinking cause mental impairment? *BMJ* 289, 711.

Robertson, M.N. and Trimble, M.R. (1983). Depressive illness in patients with epilepsy: a review. *Epilepsia* 24 (Suppl. 2), 109.

Roffman, R.A. and Barnhart, R. (1987). Assessing need for marijuana dependence treatment through an anonymous telephone interview. *Int. J. Addict.* 22, 639.

Roffman, R.A., Stephens, R.S., Simpson, E.E., *et al.* (1988). Treatment of marijuana dependence: Preliminary results. *J. Psychoactive Drugs* 20, 129.

Roger, J., Grangeon, H., Guey, J., *et al.* (1968). Psychological and psychiatric symptoms in treatment of epileptics with ethosuximide. *Encéphale* 57, 407.

Rogers, H.J., Spector, R.G., and Trounce, J.R. (1981). *A Textbook of Clinical Pharmacology.* Hodder and Stoughton, Tunbridge Wells.

Rosenthal, R. (1987). Visual hallucinations and suicidal ideation attributed to isosorbide dinitrate. *Psychosomatics* 28, 555.

Ross, R.G. and Ward, N.G. (1992). Bromocriptine abuse. *Biol. Psychiatry* 31, 404.

Rossiter, S.K. (1992). Psychosis with disulfiram prescribed under probation order. *BMJ* 305, 763.

Roth, T., Roehrs, T., Koshorek, J., *et al.* (1987). Sedative effects of antihistamines. *J. Allergy Clin. Immunol.* 80, 94.

Rothschild, A.J. (1985). Mania after withdrawal of isocarboxacid. *J. Clin. Psychopharmacol.* 5, 340.

Rothstein, E. and Clancy, D. (1969). Toxicity of disulfiram combined with metronidazole. *N. Engl. J. Med.* 280, 1006.

Rottenburg, D.R., Robins, A.H., Ben-Arie, O., *et al.* (1982). Cannabis-associated psychosis with hypomanic features. *Lancet* 2, 1364.

Routtenberg, A. (1968). The two arousal hypothesis: reticular formation and limbic system. *Psychol. Rev.* 75, 51.

Rush, C.R., Higgins, S.T., Hughes, J.R., *et al.* (1993). A comparison of the acute behavioral effects of triazolam and temazepam in normal volunteers. *Psychopharmacology* 112, 407.

Russ, C. and Wong, D. (1979). Diagnosis and treatment of the phencyclidine psychosis: clinical considerations. *Ann. Intern. Med.* 88, 210.

Russell, J.W. and Shuckit, M.A. (1982). Anxiety and depression in patients on nadolol. *Lancet* ii, 1286.

Rutgers, A.W.F., Links, T.P., Cioultre, R.L., *et al.* (1988). Behavioural disturbances after effective ACTH treatment of the dancing-eyes syndrome. *Dev. Med. Child Neurol.* 30, 408.

SADRAC (Swedish Adverse Drug Reactions Advisory Committee) (1987). Fenfluramine — psychiatric reactions. *SADRAC Bull.* No. 49.

Sadzot, B., Baraban, J.M., Glennon, R.A., *et al.* (1989). Hallucinogenic drug interactions at human brain 5-HT$_2$ receptors: implications for treating LSD-induced hallucinogenesis. *Psychopharmacology* 98, 495.

Salvà, P. and Costa J. (1995). Clinical pharmacokinetics and pharmacodynamics of zolpidem. *Clin. Pharmacokinet.* 19, 142.

Saravay, S.M., Marke, J., Steinberg, M.D., *et al.* (1987). Doom anxiety and delirium in lidocaine toxicity. *Am. J. Psychiatry* 144, 159.

Saxena, P.T. and Bhargara, K.P. (1975). The importance of a central adrenergic mechanism in the cardiovascular responses to ouabain. *Eur. J. Pharmacol.* 31, 332.

Saxena, S. and Mallikarjuna, P. (1988). Severe memory impairment with acute overdose lithium toxicity. A case report. *Br. J. Psychiatry* 152, 853.

Scharf, M.B., Roth, P.B., Dominguez, R.A., *et al.* (1990). Estazolam and flurazepam: a multicenter, placebo-controlled comparative study in outpatients with insomnia. *J. Clin. Pharmacol.* 30, 461.

Schatzberg, A.F., Haddad, P., Kaplan, E., *et al.* (1997a). Serotonin reuptake inhibitor discontinuation syndrome: a hypothetical definition. *J. Clin. Psychiatry* 58, 5.

Schatzberg, A.F., Haddad, P., Kaplan, E., *et al.* (1997b). Possible biological mechanisms of the serotonin reuptake inhibitor discontinuation syndrome. *J. Clin. Psychiatry* 58, 23.

Schenk, S., Valadez, A., McNamara, C., *et al.* (1993). Development and expression of sensitization to cocaine's reinforcing properties: role of NMDA receptors. *Psychopharmacology* 111, 332.

Schifano, F. (1991). Chronic atypical psychosis associated with MDMA ("ecstasy") abuse. *Lancet* 338, 1335.

Schimmer, B.P. and Parker, K.L. (1996). Adrenocorticotrophic hormone; adrenocortical steroids and their synthetic analogs; inhibitors of synthesis and actions of adrenocortical hormones. In *Goodman and Gilman's The Pharmacological Basis of Therapeutics* (9th edn) (ed. J.G. Hardman and L.E. Limbird), p. 1459. McGraw-Hill, New York.

Schmauss, C. and Krieg, J-C. (1987). Enlargement of cerebrospinal fluid spaces in long-term benzodiazepine abusers. *Psychol. Med.* 17, 869.

Schmidt, J.G. (1992). Cholesterol lowering treatment and mortality. *BMJ* 305, 1226.

Schmidt, L.G., Grohmann, R., Muller-Oerlinghausen, B., *et al.* (1986). Adverse drug reactions to first and second-generation antidepressants. A critical evaluation of drug surveillance data. *Br. J. Psychiatry* 148, 38.

Schmutz, M., Brugger, F., Bürki, H., *et al.* (1992). Antiepileptics and the hippocampus. In *The Temporal Lobes and the Limbic System* (ed. M.R. Trimble and T.G. Bolwig), p. 91. Wrightson Biomedical Publishing, Petersfield.

Schou, M. (1993). Is there a lithium withdrawal syndrome? An examination of the evidence. *Br. J. Psychiatry* 163, 514.

Schraa, J.C. and Dirks, J.F. (1982). The influence of corticosteroids and theophylline on cerebral function. *Chest* 82, 181.

Schreiber, W., Pauls, A.M., and Kreig, J.C. (1988). Toxische Psychose als Akutmanifestation der Diphenydramin-vergiftung. *Dtsch. Med. Wochenschr.* 113, 180.

Schuckit, M.A. (1994). The treatment of stimulant dependence. *Addiction* 89, 1559.

Schultz, R., Wuster, M., Duka, T., *et al.* (1980). Acute and chronic ethanol treatment changes endorphin levels in brain and pituitary. *Psychopharmacology* 68, 221.

Schultz, R. (1991). Alcohol withdrawal syndrome. In *Comprehensive Handbook of Drug and Alcohol Addiction* (ed. N.S. Miller), p. 1091. Marcel Dekker, New York.

Schwartz, R.H. (1991). Heavy marijuana use and recent memory impairment. In *Physiopathology of Illicit Drugs* (ed. G.G. Nahas and C. Latour). *Advances in the Biosciences*, Vol. 80, p. 13. Pergamon Press, Oxford.

Schwartz, J.C., Amarg, J.M., and Jasbarg, M. (1986). Three classes of histamine receptors in brain. *Trends Pharmacol. Sci.* 7, 24.

Segal, D.S. and Janowsky, D.S. (1978). Psychostimulant-induced behavioral effects: Possible models of schizophrenia. In *Psychopharmacology: A Generation of Progress* (ed. M.A. Lipton, A. DiMascok, and K.F. Killan), p. 461. Raven Press, New York.

Seivewright, N. and Dougal, W. (1993). Withdrawal symptoms from high dose benzodiazepines in poly drug users. *Drug Alcohol Depend.* 32, 15.

Sellers, E.M., Higgins, G.A., and Sobell, M.B. (1992). 5-HT and alcohol abuse. *Trends Pharmacol. Sci.* 13, 69.

Serfaty, M.A., McCluskey, S., and Eccleston, D. (1995). Extreme suicidality following serotonin syndrome. *Br. J. Psychiatry* 167, 410.

Seymour, R.B. and Smith, D.E. (1991). Hallucinogens. In *Comprehensive Handbook of Drug and Alcohol Addiction* (ed. N.S. Miller), p. 455. Marcel Dekker, New York.

Shader, R.I. and Greenblatt, D.J. (1972). Belladonna alkaloids and synthetic anticholinergics: Uses and toxicity. In *Psychiatric Complications of Medical Drugs* (ed. R.I. Shader), p. 93. Raven Press, New York.

Shader, R.I., Kennedy, J.S., and Greenblatt, D.J. (1987). The treatment of anxiety in the elderly. In *Psychopharmacology: The Third Generation of Progress* (ed. H.Y. Meltzer), p. 1141. Raven Press, New York.

Shanahan, M.P. and Hughes, R.N. (1986). Potentiation of performance-induced anxiety by caffeine in coffee. *Psychol. Rep.* 59, 83.

Shannon, P.J., Leonard, D., and Kidson, A. (1974). Fenfluramine and psychosis. *BMJ* 2, 576.

Shepherd, R.T. (1989). Mechanism of sudden death associated with volatile substance abuse. *Hum. Toxicol.* 8, 287.

Shetty, H.G.M. and Routledge, P.A. (1990). Adverse effects of hypolipidaemic drugs. *Adverse Drug Reaction Bulletin* 142, 532.

Shewan, D. and Dalgarno, P. (1996). Ecstasy and neurodegeneration. . . . such as ketamine. *BMJ* 313, 424.

Shihab, Z.M. (1980). Psychotic reaction in an adult after topical cyclopentolate. *Ophthalmologica* 181, 228.

Shopsin, B., Johnson, G., and Gershon, S. (1970). Neurotoxicity with lithium: Differential drug responsiveness. *Int. Pharmacopsychiatry* 5, 170.

Shore, J.H., Fraunfelder, F.T., and Meyer, S.M. (1987). Psychiatric side-effects from topical ocular timolol, a beta-adrenergic blocker. *J. Clin. Psychopharmacol.* 7, 264.

Shukla, S., Turner, W.J., and Newman, G. (1985). Bromocriptine-related psychosis and treatment. *Biol. Psychiatry* 20, 326.

Sigell, L.T., Kapp, F.T., Fusaro, G.A., *et al.* (1978). Popping and snorting volatile nitrites: a current fad for getting high. *Am. J. Psychiatry* 135, 1216.

Siegel, R.K. (1978). Phencyclidine and ketamine intoxication: a study of four populations of recreational users. In *Phencyclidine Abuse: an Appraisal* (ed. R.C. Peterson and R.C. Stillman). National Institute of Drug Research Monograph Series 21. National Institute on Drug Abuse, Rockville, Maryland.

Silverstone, T. (1992). Appetite suppressants. A review. *Drugs* 43, 820.

Simeon, J., Fink, M., Itil, T.M., *et al.* (1970). D-cycloserine therapy of psychosis by symptom provocation. *Comp. Psychiatry* 11, 80.

Simonato, M. (1996). The neurochemistry of morphine addiction in the neocortex. *Trends Pharmacol. Sci.* 17, 410.

Singh, A. (1995). Ecstasy and prozac. *New Scientist* October 14, 51.

Singh, A.N. and Catalan, J. (1996). The misuse potential of antidepressants. *J. Psychopharmacol.* 10 (Suppl.) Abstract 122.

Singh, S.V. (1982). Lithium carbonate and fluphenazine decanoate producing irreversible brain damage. *Lancet* ii, 278.

Sinzinger, H., Mayr, F., Schmid, P., *et al.* (1994). Sleep disturbance and appetite loss after lovastatin. *Lancet* 343, 973.

Siris, S.G., Cooper, T.B., Riofkin, A.E., *et al.* (1982). Plasma imipramine concentrations in patients receiving concomitant fluphenazine decanoate. *Am. J. Psychiatry* 139, 104.

Siris, S. (1991). Diagnosis of secondary depression in schizophrenia. Implications for DSM IV. *Schizophr. Bull.* 17, 75.

Sjækvist, F. (1989). Pharmacogenetics of antidepressants. In *Clinical Pharmacology in Psychiatry* (eds. S.G. Dahl and L.F. Gram), p. 181. Springer-Verlag, Berlin.

Smart, R.G. and Bateman, K. (1967). Unfavourable reactions to LSD: a review and analysis of the available case reports. *Can. Med. Assoc. J.* 97, 1214.

Smiler, B.G, Bartholomew, E.G., Sivak, B.J., *et al.* (1973). Physostigmine reversal of scopolamine delirium in obstetric patients. *Am. J. Obstet. Gynecol.* 116, 326.

Smith, M.C. and Bleck, T.P. (1992). Convulsive disorders: toxicity of anticonvulsants. In *Textbook of Clinical Neuropharmacology and Therapeutics* (2nd edn) (ed. H.L. Klawans, C.G. Goetz, and C.M. Tanner), p. 45. Raven Press, New York.

Snyder, S.H. (1982). Schizophrenia. *Lancet* ii, 970.

Solberg, Y. and Belkin, M. (1997). The role of excitotoxicity in organophosphorous nerve agents central poisoning. *Trends Pharmacol. Sci.*, 18, 183.

Solomon, K. and Bonsack, B.A. (1993). Bizarre nightmares associated with valproic acid: a rare side-effect in the elderly. *Clinical Gerontologist* 14, 31.

Solowij, N. (1995). Do cognitive impairments recover following cessation of cannabis use? *Life Sci.* 56, 2119.

Sonnenblick, M., Rosin, A.J., and Weissberg, N. (1982). Neurological and psychiatric side-effects of cimetidine — report of 3 cases with review of literature. *Postgrad. Med. J.* 58, 415.

Sourindrhin, I. (1985). Solvent misuse. *BMJ* 290, 94.

Spanagel, R. and Zieglgänsberger, W. (1997). Anti-craving compounds for ethanol: new pharmacological tools to study addictive processes. *Trends Pharmacol. Sci.* 18, 54.

Spring, G.K. (1979). Neurotoxicity with combined use of lithium and thioridazine. *J. Clin. Psychiatry* 40, 135.

Squire, L.R. and Davis, H.P. (1981). The pharmacology of memory: a neurobiological perspective. *Annu. Rev. Pharmacol. Toxicol.* 21, 323.

Squires, R.F. and Braestrup, C. (1977). Benzodiazepine receptors in the rat brain. *Nature* 266, 732.

Stanton, J.D., Mintz, J., and Franklin, R.M. (1976). Drug flashbacks II. Some additional findings. *Am. J. Psychiatry* 129, 751.

Stasick, C. and Zetin, M. (1985). Organic manic disorders. *Psychosomatics* 29, 394.

Steg, R.E. and Garcia, E.G. (1991). Complex visual hallucinations and cyclosporine neurotoxicity. *Neurology* 41, 1156.

Steinert, J. and Pugh, C.R. (1979). Two patients with schizophrenic-like psychoses after treatment with beta-adrenergic blockers. *BMJ* i, 790.

Stell, I.M. and Ryan, J.M. (1996). γ-Hydroxybutyrate is a new recreational drug that may lead to loss of consciousness. *BMJ* 313, 424.

Stephens, D.A. (1967). Psychotoxic effects of benzhexol hydrochloride. *Br. J. Psychiatry* 16, 987.

Stephens, R.S., Roffman, R.A., and Simpson, E.E. (1993). Adult marijuana users seeking treatment. *J. Consult. Clin. Psychol.* 61, 1100.

Stephens, R., Spurgeon, A., Calvert, I.A., et al. (1995). Neuropsychological effects of long-term exposure to organophosphates in sheep dip. *Lancet* 345, 1135.

Sterman, A.B. and Coyle, P.K. (1983). Subacute toxic delirium following nitrous oxide abuse. *Arch. Neurol.* 40, 446.

Sternbach, H. (1991). The serotonin syndrome. *Am. J. Psychiatry* 148, 705.

Stockwell, T. (1994). Alcohol withdrawal: an adaptation to heavy drinking of no practical significance. *Addiction* 89, 1447.

Stockwell, T., Sitharthan, T., McGrath, D., et al. (1994). The measurement of alcohol dependence and impaired control in community samples. *Addiction* 89, 167.

Stoukides, J.A. and Stoukides, C.A. (1991). Extrapyramidal symptoms upon discontinuation of fluoxetine. *Am. J. Psychiatry* 148, 1263.

Stradling, J.R. (1993). Recreational drugs and sleep. *BMJ* 306, 573.

Strang, J. and Edwards, G. (1989). Cocaine and crack. *BMJ* 299, 337.

Strang, J., Johns, A., and Caan, W. (1993). Cocaine in the UK — 1991. *Br. J. Psychiatry* 162, 1.

Sullivan, G. (1996). Acute psychosis following intravenous abuse of pseudoephedrine: a case report. *J. Psychopharmacol.* 10, 324.

Sunshine, A. and Olsen, N.Z. (1989). Non-narcotic analgesics. In *Textbook of Pain* (2nd edn) (ed. P.D. Wall and R. Melzack), p. 679. Churchill Livingstone, Edinburgh.

Sweet, R.D., McDowell, F.H., Fiegenson, J.S., et al. (1976). Mental symptoms in Parkinson's disease during chronic treatment with levodopa. *Neurology* (Minneapolis) 26, 305.

Swigar, M.E. and Bowers, M.B. (1986). Baclofen withdrawal and neuropsychiatric symptoms: a case report and review of other case literature. *Comp. Psychiatry* 27, 396.

Szabadi, E. and Bradshaw, C.M. (1995). Affective disorders: 1. Antidepressants. In *Seminars in Clinical Psychopharmacology* (ed. D.J. King), p. 138. Royal College of Physicians, London.

Tabakoff, B. and Hoffman, P.L. (1990). Neurochemical effects of alcohol. In *Clinical Textbook of Addictive Disorders* (ed. F.J. Frances and S.I. Miller), p. 501. Guildford Press, New York.

Tacke, U. (1987). Mania induced by biochemical imbalance. *BMJ* 295, 1485.

Talbot, J.A. and Teague, J.W. (1969). Marijuana psychosis. *JAMA* 210, 299.

Tata, P.R., Rollings, M.J., Collins, M., et al. (1994). Lack of cognitive recovery following withdrawal from long-term benzodiazepine use. *Psychol. Med.* 24, 203.

Taylor, J.C., Normal, C.L., Griffiths, J.M., et al. (1993). *Trends in Deaths Associated with Abuse of Volatile Substances 1971–1991.* St George's Hospital Medical School, London.

Taylor, M., Galloway, D.B., Petrie, J.C., et al. (1978). Psychotomimetic effects of pentazocine and dihydrocodeine tartrate. *BMJ* ii, 1198.

Teicher, M.H., Glod, C., and Cole, J.O. (1990). Emergence of intense suicidal preoccupation during fluoxetine treatment. *Am. J. Psychiatry* 147, 207.

Tennant, F.S. and Groesbeck, C.J. (1972). Psychiatric effects of hashish. *Arch. Gen. Psychiatry* 27, 133.

Terao, T., Yopshimura, R., Shiratuchi, T., et al. (1997). Effects of lithium on steroid-induced depression. *Biol. Psychiatry* 41, 1225.

Tester-Daldrup, C.B.M. (1984). Anti-fungal drugs. In *Meyler's Side Effects of Drugs* (10th edn) (ed. M.N.G. Dukes), p. 516. Elsevier, Amsterdam.

Thacore, V.R. and Shukla, S.R.P. (1976). Cannabis psychosis and paranoid schizophrenia. *Arch. Gen. Psychiatry* 33, 383.

Thomas, C.J. (1979). Brain damage with lithium and haloperidol. *Br. J. Psychiatry* 134, 552.

Thomas, P.K. (1986). Brain atrophy and alcoholism. *BMJ* 292, 787.

Thomas, H. (1993). Psychiatric symptoms in cannabis users. *Br. J. Psychiatry* 163, 141.

Thomas, H. (1996). A community survey of adverse effects of cannabis use. *Drug Alcohol Depend.* 42, 201.

Thompson, M.K. (1979). Schizophrenia-like psychosis after treatment with beta-blockers. *BMJ* i, 1084.

Thompson, J.W. (1984). Opioid peptides. *BMJ* 288, 259.

Thompson, P.J., Dhillon, P., and Cole, P. (1983). Addiction to aerosol treatment: the asthmatic alternative to glue sniffing. *BMJ* 287, 1515.

Thomson, A.D., Pratt, O.E., Jeyasingham, M., *et al.* (1988). Alcohol and brain damage. *Hum. Toxicol.* 7, 455.

Thornton, T.L. (1980). Dementia induced by methyldopa with haloperidol. *N. Engl. J. Med.* 294, 1222.

Tiffin, P., Ashton, H., Marsh, R., *et al.* (1995). Pharmacokinetic and pharmacodynamic responses to caffeine in poor and normal sleepers. *Psychopharmacology* 121, 494.

Tobiansky, R. and Blanchard, M. (1997). Trials must determine which neuroleptics are best in dementia. *BMJ* 314, 1411.

Tollefson, G. (1980). Psychiatric implications of anti-convulsant drugs. *J. Clin. Psychiatry* 41, 295.

Tollefson, G.D. (1991). Anxiety and alcoholism: a serotonin link. *Br. J. Psychiatry* 159 (Suppl. 12), 34.

Topliss, D. and Bond, R. (1977). Acute organic brain syndrome after propranolol treatment. *Lancet* ii, 1133.

Torrey, E.F. (1968). Chloroquine seizures: report of four cases. *JAMA* 204, 115.

Traber, J. and Glaser, J. (1987). 5-HT$_{1A}$ receptor-related anxiolytics. *Trends Pharmacol. Sci.* 8, 432.

Treffert, D.A. (1978). Marijuana use in schizophrenia: A clear hazard. *Am. J. Psychiatry* 135, 1213.

Trimble, M. and Reynolds, E.H. (1976). Anti-convulsant drugs and mental symptoms. A review. *Psychol. Med.* 6, 169.

Trimble, M.R., Corbett, J.A., and Donaldson, D. (1980). Folic acid and mental symptoms in children with epilepsy. *J. Neurol. Neurosurg. Psychiatry* 43, 1030.

Trimble, M.R. (1987). Anticonvulsant drugs and cognitive function: a review of the literature. *Epilepsia* 28 (Suppl. 3), S37.

Tucker, G.T., Lennard, M.S., Ellis, S.W., *et al.* (1994). The demethylation of methylenedioxymethamphetamine ('Ecstasy') by debrisoquine hydroxylase (CYP2D6). *Biochem. Pharmacol.* 47, 1151.

Tumeh, S.S., Nagel, J.S., English, R.J., *et al.* (1990). Cerebral abnormalities in cocaine abusers: Demonstration by SPECT perfusion brain scintigraphy. *Radiology* 176, 821.

Tunving, K. (1985). Psychiatric effects of cannabis use. *Acta Psychiatr. Scand.* 72, 209.

Turner, T.H., Cookson, J.C., Wass, J.A.H., *et al.* (1984). Psychotic reactions during treatment of pituitary tumours with dopamine agonists. *BMJ* 289, 1101.

Turner, T.J. and Goldin, S.M. (1985). Calcium channels in rat brain synaptosomes: identification and pharmacological characterization: high affinity blockade by organic Ca channel blockers. *J. Neurosci.* 5, 841.

Turner, W.M. (1982). Lidocaine and psychotic reactions. *Ann. Intern. Med.* 97, 149.

Twycross, R.G. and McQuay, H.J. (1989). Opioids. In *Textbook of Pain* (2nd edn) (ed. P.D. Wall and R. Melzack), p. 686. Churchill Livingstone, Edinburgh.

Tyrer, P.J. (1982). Monoamine oxidase inhibitors and amine precursors. In *Drugs in Psychiatric Practice* (ed. P.J. Tyrer), p. 249. Butterworth, London.

Tyrer, P. (1984). Clinical effects of abrupt withdrawal from tricyclic antidepressants and monoamine oxidase inhibitors after long-term treatment. *J. Affect. Disord.* 6, 1.

Tyrer, P. (1989). Choice of treatment in anxiety. In *Psychopharmacology of Anxiety* (ed. P. Tyrer), p. 255. British Association for Psychopharmacology Monograph. Oxford Medical Publications.

Tyrer, P. (1991). The benzodiazepine post-withdrawal syndrome. *Stress Medicine* 7, 1.

Tyrer, S.P. (1993a). Adverse reactions to drugs used in the treatment and prophylaxis of depression and mania. *Adverse Drug Reaction Bulletin* (No. 160), 603.

Tyrer, P. (1993b). Pharmacological differences in the dependence potential of benzodiazepines. In *Benzodiazepine Dependence* (ed. C. Hallstrom), p. 221. Oxford University Press.

Tyrer, S.P. (1996). Lithium intoxication: Appropriate treatment. *CNS Drugs* 6, 426.

Tyrer, S. and Shopsin, B. (1980). Neural and neuromuscular side-effects of lithium. In *Handbook of Lithium Therapy* (ed. F.N. Johnson), p. 289. MTP Press, Lancaster.

Tyrer, P., Owen, R., and Dawling, S. (1983). Gradual withdrawal of diazepam after long-term therapy. *Lancet* i, 1402.

Tyrer, S.P., Shopsin, B., and Aronson, M. (1983). Dangers of reducing lithium. *Br. J. Psychiatry* 142, 427.

Tyrer, P., Murphy, S., and Riley, P. (1989). The benzodiazepine withdrawal symptom questionnaire. *J. Affect. Disord.* 19, 53.

Uhde, T.W. and Kellner, C.H. (1987). Cerebral ventricular size in panic disorder. *J. Affect. Disord.* 12, 175.

Umstead, G.S. and Neumann, K.H. (1986). Erythromycin ototoxicity and acute psychotic reaction in cancer patients with hepatic dysfunction. *Arch. Intern. Med.* 146, 897.

Unseld, E., Ziegler, G., Gemeirhardt, A., *et al.* (1990). Possible interaction of fluoroquinolones with the benzodiazepine-GABA$_A$-receptor complex. *Br. J. Clin. Pharmacol.* 30, 63.

Upton N. (1994a). Mechanisms of action of new antiepileptic drugs: rational design and serendipitous findings. *Trends Pharmacol. Sci.* 15, 456.

Upton, C. (1994b). Sleep disturbances in children treated with ofloxacin. *BMJ* 309, 1411.

Usdin, G. and Robinson, K.E. (1951). Psychosis during Antabuse administration. *Arch. Neurol. Psychiatry* 66, 38.

Van Der Kroef, C. (1979). Reactions to triazolam. *Lancet* ii, 526.

Van Kammen, D.P. and Gelertner, J. (1987a). Biochemical instability in schizophrenia. I. The norepinephrine system. In *Psychopharmacology: The Third Generation of Progress* (ed. H.Y. Meltzer), p. 745. Raven Press, New York.

Van Kammen, D.P. and Gelertner, J. (1987b). Biochemical instability in schizophrenia. II. The serotonin and γ-aminobutyric acid systems. In *Psychopharmacology: The Third Generation of Progress* (ed. H.Y. Meltzer), p. 753. Raven Press, New York.

Van Riemsdijk, M.M., Van Der Klauw, M.M., Pepplinkhuizen, L., *et al.* (1997). Spontaneous reports of psychiatric adverse effects to mefloquine in the Netherlands. *Br. J. Clin. Pharmacol.* 44, 105.

Varzopoulos, D. and Krull F. (1991). Dependence on mono-amine oxidase inhibitors in high dose. *Br. J. Psychiatry* 158, 856.

Venkatarangan, S.H.M., Kutcher, S.P., and Notkin, R.M. (1988). Secondary mania with steroid withdrawal. *Can. J. Psychiatry* 33, 631.

Verghese, C. (1988). Quinine psychosis. *Br. J. Psychiatry* 153, 575.

Vessey, M.P., McPherson, K., Lawless, M., *et al.* (1985). Oral contraceptives and serious psychiatric illness: absence of an association. *Br. J. Psychiatry* 146, 45.

Vidailhet, P., Kazœs, M., Danion, J-M., *et al.* (1996). Effects of lorazepam and diazepam on conscious and automatic memory processes. *Psychopharmacology* 127, 63.

Vining, E.P.G. (1987). Cognitive dysfunction associated with antiepileptic drug therapy. *Epilepsia* 28 (Suppl. 2), S18.

Vlissides, D.N., Gill, D., and Castelow, J. (1978). Bromocriptine-induced mania? *BMJ* i, 510.

Waal-Manning, H.J. and Simpson, F.O. (1974). Pindolol: a comparison with other antihypertensive drugs and a double-blind placebo trial. *N.Z. Med. J.* 80, 151.

Wallach, M.B. and Gershon, S. (1972). Psychiatric sequelae to tuberculous chemotherapy. In *Psychiatric Complications of Medical Drugs* (ed. R.I. Shader), p. 201, Raven Press, New York.

Wamboldt, F.S., Jefferson, J.W., and Wamboldt, M.Z. (1986). Digitalis intoxication misdiagnosed as depression by primary care physicians. *Am. J. Psychiatry* 143, 219.

Waters, B.G.H. and Lapierre, Y.D. (1981). Secondary mania associated with sympathomimetic drug use. *Am. J. Psychiatry* 138, 837.

Watters, K. and Le Ridant, A. (1986). Psychosis induced by fenfluramine. *BMJ* 292, 1465.

Webster, K.E. (1978). The brainstem reticular formation. In *The Biological Basis of Schizophrenia* (ed. G. Hemmings and W.A. Hemmings), p. 3. MTP Press, Lancaster.

Weddington, W.W. and Banner, A. (1986). Organic affective syndrome associated with metoclopramide: Case report. *J. Clin. Psychiatry* 47, 208.

Wehr, T.A. and Goodwin, F.K. (1979). Rapid cycling in manic-depressives induced by tricyclic anti-depressants. *Arch. Gen. Psychiatry* 36, 555.

Weingartner, H.J., Hommer, D., Lister, R.G., *et al.* (1992). Selective effects of triazolam on memory. *Psychopharmacology* 106, 341.

Weller, R.A. and Hallikas, J.A. (1985). Marijuana and psychiatric illness: a follow-up study. *Am. J. Psychiatry* 142, 848.

West, R. and Gossop, M. (1994). Overview: A comparison of withdrawal symptoms from different drug classes. *Addiction* 89, 1483.

Westenberg, H.G.M. and Den Boer, J.A. (1993). Serotonergic basis of panic disorder. In *Psychopharmacology of Panic* (ed. S.A. Montogmery), p. 91. Oxford University Press.

White, M.C., Silverman, J.J., and Harrison, J.W. (1982). Psychosis associated with clonazepam therapy for blepharospasm. *J. Nerv. Ment. Dis.* 170, 117.

White, K., Keck, P.E., and Lipinski, J. (1986). Serotonin-uptake inhibitors in obsessive-compulsive disorder: a case report. *Comp. Psychiatry* 27, 211.

White, P.D. (1987). Myclonus and episodic delirium associated with phenelzine: a case report. *J. Clin. Psychiatry* 48, 340.

White, R.F. and Proctor, S.P. (1997). Solvents and neurotoxicity. *Lancet* 349, 1239.

Whitehouse, A.M. and Duncan, J.M. (1987). Ephedrine psychosis rediscovered. *Br. J. Psychiatry* 150, 258.

Whitehouse, A.M. and Novesel, S. (1989). Salbutamol psychosis. *Biol. Psychiatry* 26, 631.

Whitlock, F.A. and Evans, L.E.J. (1978). Drugs and depression. *Drugs* 15, 53.

Wilkinson, D.G. (1979). Difficulty in stopping lithium prophylaxis. *BMJ* i, 235.

Williams, N.R. (1988). Erythromycin: a case of nightmares. *BMJ* 296, 214.

Williams, J.H., Wellman, N.A., Geaney, D.P., *et al.* (1996). Antipsychotic drug effects in a model of schizophrenic attentional disorder: a randomized controlled trial of the effects of haloperidol on latent inhibition in healthy people. *Biol. Psychiatry* 40, 1135.

Williamson, D.J. and Young, A.H. (1992). Psychiatric effects of androgenic and anabolic-androgenic steroid abuse in men: a brief review of the literature. *J. Psychopharmacol.* 6, 20.

Willner P. (1995). Dopaminergic mechanisms in depression and mania. In *Psychopharmacology: The Fourth Generation of Progress* (ed. F.E. Bloom and D.J. Kupfer), p. 921. Raven Press, New York.

Wilson, M.A., Ricaurte, G.A., and Molliver, M.E. (1989). Distinct morphologic classes of serotonergic axons in primates exhibit differential vulnerability to the psychotropic drug 3,4-methylenedioxymethamphetamine. *Neuroscience* 28, 121.

Winn, R.E., Bower, M.J., and Richards, M.J. (1979). Acute toxic delirium: neurotoxicity of intrathecal amphotericin B. *Arch. Intern. Med.* 139, 706.

Winstock, A.R. (1991). Chronic paranoid psychosis after misuse of MDMA. *BMJ* 302, 1150.

Winstock, A.R. and King, L.A. (1996). Tablets often contains substances in addition to, or instead of, ecstasy. *BMJ* 313, 423.

Wise, R.A. and Bozarth, M.A. (1987). The psychomotor stimulant theory of addiction. *Psychol. Rev.* 94, 469.

Wiseman, R.A. (1971). Practolol: accumulated data on unwanted effects. *Postgrad. Med. J.* (Suppl.) 47, 68.

Wistedt, B. and Palmstierna, T. (1983). Depressive symptoms in chronic schizophrenic patients after withdrawal of long-acting neuroleptics. *J. Clin. Psychiatry* 44, 369.

Witschy, J.K., Malone, G.L., and Holden, L.D. (1984). Psychosis after neuroleptic withdrawal in a manic-depressive patient. *Am. J. Psychiatry* 141, 105.

Wolf, M.E., Almy, G., Toll, M., *et al.* (1982). Mania associated with the use of baclofen. *Biol. Psychiatry* 17, 757.

Wolkowitz, O.M. and Rapaport, M. (1989). Longstanding behavioral changes following prednisolone withdrawal. *JAMA* 261, 1731.

Wolkowitz, O.M., Weingartner, H., Thompson, K., *et al.* (1987). Diazepam-induced amnesia: a neuropharmacological model of an 'organic amnestic syndrome'. *Am. J. Psychiatry* 144, 25.

Wood, A.J.J., More, D.C., Campbell, C., *et al.* (1974). CNS effects of pentoazocine. *BMJ* i, 305.

Wood, K.A. (1994). Nasal decongestant and psychiatric disturbance. *Br. J. Psychiatry* 164, 566.

Woodruff, P., Brammer, M., Mellers, J., *et al.* (1994). Auditory hallucinations and perception of external speech. *Lancet* 346, 1035.

Woods, J.F., Katz, J.L., and Winger, G. (1992). Benzodiazepines: use, abuse, and consequences. *Pharmacol. Rev.* 44, 151.

Woods, L.A. (1956). The pharmacology of nalorphine. *Pharmacol. Rev.* 8, 175.

Woody, G.E. (1970). Visual disturbance experienced by hallucinogenic drug abusers while driving. *Am. J. Psychiatry* 127, 683.

Woody, G.E. and O'Brien, C.P. (1974). Anticholinergic toxic psychosis in drug abusers treated with benztropine. *Comp. Psychiatry* 15, 439.

Wyatt, R.J. and Gillin, J.C. (1976). Biochemistry of human sleep. In *Pharmacology of Sleep* (ed. R.L. Williams, I. Karacan, and J.H. Masserman), p. 239. John Wiley, New York.

Wyeth (1997). Data on file, NDA 20-151.

Wylie, A., Scott, R.T.A., and Burnett, S.J. (1995). Psychosis due to 'skunk'. *BMJ* 311, 125.

Wysowski, D.K. and Gross, T.P. (1990). Deaths due to accidents and violence in two recent trials of cholesterol-lowering drugs. *Arch. Intern. Med.* 150, 2169.

Yapalater, A.R. and Rockwell, F.V. (1950). Toxic psychosis due to prophenpyridamine (Trimeton). Report of a case. *JAMA* 143, 428.

Yaryura-Tobias, J., Wolpert, A., Dana, L., *et al.* (1970). Action of L-dopa in drug-induced extra-pyramidalism. *Dis. Nerv. Syst.* 31, 60.

Yaryura-Tobias, J.A., Diamond, B., and Merlis, S. (1972). Psychiatric manifestations of levodopa. *Can. Psychiatr. Assoc. J.* 17 (Suppl. II), 123.

Yassa, R.Y. and Iskander, H.L. (1988). Baclofen-induced psychosis: two cases. *J. Clin. Psychiatry* 49, 318.

Young, A.H. and Ashton, C.H. (1997). Pharmacokinetics of fluoxetine. *Trends Pharmacol. Sci.* 17, 400.

Young, A.H., Dow, R.C., Goodwin, G.M., *et al.* (1993). The effects of adrenalectomy and ovariectomy on the behavioural and hypothermic responses of rats to 8-hydroxy-2(DI-*n*-propylamino)tetralin (8-OH-DPAT). *Neuropharmacology* 32, 653.

Young, A.H., Sharpley, G.M., Campling, G.M., *et al.* (1994). Effects of hydrocortisone on brain 5-HT function and sleep. *J. Affect. Disord.* 32, 139.

Zacharias, F.J. (1973). Beta-blockers in hypertension. *Brux. Med.* 111, 46.

Zaudig, M. and von Bose, M. (1987). Oxoflavin-induced psychosis. *Br. J. Psychiatry* 151, 563.

Zelsen, C., Lee, S.J., and Casalino, M. (1973). Comparative effects of maternal intake of heroin and methadone. *N. Engl. J. Med.* 289, 1216.

Zetin, M., Aden, G., and Moldowsky, R. (1983). Tolerance to amoxapine antidepressant effects. *Clin. Ther.* 5, 638.

Zoltoski, R.K. and Gillin, J.C. (1994). The neurochemistry of sleep. In *Sleep* (ed. R. Cooper), p.135. Chapman & Hall Medical, London.

Zubenko, G.S. and Nixon, R.A. (1984). Mood-elevating effect of captopril in depressed patients. *Am. J. Psychiatry* 141, 110.

Zuckerman, M. (1964). Perceptual isolation as a stress situation. *Arch. Gen. Psychiatry* 11, 255.

Zwyghuizen-Doorenbos, A., Roehrs, T.A., Lipschutz, L., *et al.* (1990). Effects of caffeine on alertness. *Psychopharmacology* 100, 36.

24. Disorders of blood cells and haemostasis

Part 1 Disorders of blood cells

G. H. JACKSON, J. CAVET, and S. J. PROCTOR

Introduction

As the number of pharmacological agents in use increases, and the understanding of the biology of the haemopoietic system improves, the nature of the adverse effects of drugs on the haemopoietic system becomes a more fertile area for research. It is the intention in this chapter to attempt to relate such effects to possible mechanisms. For many interactions this is not possible and only speculative unproven mechanisms can be considered. For drug reactions which are well known in the literature, the simple expedient of tabulating them has been used and the reader is referred to the original paper or reviews on the subject.

In order to understand fully the effects of drugs on the developing blood elements, a short résumé of the biology of blood cell development and the growth factors involved in normal marrow activity has been given. As many of these growth factors have been cloned and produced in recombinant form for clinical use, a brief summary of the potential clinical use of such factors will also be included, as such agents, like other drugs, also have some deleterious effects on haemopoiesis.

Biology of blood cell development

The human bone marrow is a large vascular organ comprising some four per cent of lean body-weight in the mature adult. The relative size of the haemopoietic marrow in infancy and childhood is greater, and in the ageing adult the relative size of the haemopoietic marrow declines. Thus the adverse effects of drugs on paediatric and geriatric patients can be different. Throughout life the marrow is the site of normal haemopoiesis, a finely controlled process that allows the production of all circulating blood cells at a rate determined by the body's variable demand, in which a small undifferentiated self-renewing population of pluripotent stem cells gives rise to large numbers of fully mature cells including erythrocytes, granulocytes, platelets, macrophages, and T and B lymphocytes. The production of mature cells is complex and strictly regulated, so that stable blood cell counts are maintained in health and yet these can alter swiftly in response to trauma or infection. Normally 4×10^8 white cells and 1×10^{10} red cells are replaced per hour (Metcalf 1987). The neutrophil count can increase 10-fold, however, in response to severe infection within a matter of 24 hours. Clearly, to allow such an amplification of cell numbers during differentiation there must be a number of stages between the stem cell and the fully differentiated end cell. Each stage is associated with a gradual loss of potential and a decline in proliferative capacity such that the mature granulocyte has only a life span of some 48 hours and mature platelets of some 5 days.

Cell culture systems that allow investigation of proliferation and differentiation of cells from the bone marrow have been developed and refined, so that it is possible to analyse not only haemopoietic progeny but also bone marrow stromal cells. The control of the haemopoietic system to allow the production of large numbers of cells at a rate depending on variable demand is extremely complex, and it is only recently that the regulation of the system has begun to be unravelled. Interest has centred on a group of glycoproteins which have been shown to stimulate the growth of intermediate cells in the haemopoietic system (Fig. 24.1) (Balkwill 1989). These include stem-cell factor (SCF or c-kit ligand), erythropoietin (EPO), granulocyte–macrophage colony-stimulating factor (GM-CSF), granulocyte colony-stimulating factor (G-CSF), macrophage colony-stimulating factor (M-CSF), thrombopoietin (TPO) and multi-CSF, often referred to as interleukin-3 (IL-3). The

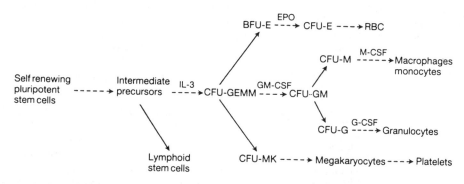

Fɪɢ. 24.1.

Model of haemopoiesis, from pluripotent self-renewing stem cell to non-dividing end cell, showing some sites of action of some of the haemopoietic growth factors.

CFU–GEMM	colony-forming unit, granulocyte–erythroid–macrophage–megakaryocyte
CFU–GM	colony-forming unit, granulocyte–macrophage
BFU–E	burst-forming unit, erythroid
CFU–E	colony-forming unit, erythroid
CFU–G	colony-forming unit, granulocyte
CFU–M	colony-forming unit, macrophage
CFU–MK	colony-forming unit, megakaryocyte

IL–3	interleukin-3
GM–CSF	granulocyte–macrophage colony-stimulating factor
G–CSF	granulocyte colony-stimulating factor
M–CSF	macrophage colony-stimulating factor
EPO	erythropoietin
TPO	thrombopoietin

haemopoietic lineages affected by these agents are diagrammatically demonstrated in Figure 24.1. Chromosomal localization of the above biological response modifiers is now known and most have been cloned; and recombinant DNA technology has allowed their development for clinical use. The bone marrow microenvironment and the interactions of the above growth factors with all elements and/or production by elements of the bone marrow stroma is, at the present time, being dissected, but there is little doubt that the bone marrow, stroma, and matrix are critically involved in the regulation of haemopoiesis (Dexter 1987). It is thus evident that drugs that induce bone marrow failure may affect haemopoiesis through effects on the stem cell, the bone marrow micro-environment, or any of the intermediate stages between stem cell and the mature end cell.

Bone marrow failure

Peripheral blood cytopenia arising primarily as a result of a specific failure of bone marrow precursor cells, rather than the production of abnormal cells or the production of normal cells that are subjected to an abnormal environment, is termed bone marrow hypoplasia or aplasia. The remaining cells within the bone marrow appear normal and the marrow stroma does not seem to be altered.

Bone marrow hypoplasia can take two forms: aplastic anaemia, in which the pluripotent stem cell is damaged,

leading to pancytopenia, and single-cell cytopenias where the failure lies in one or other of the committed cell lines, the other cell lines being unaffected.

Aplastic anaemia

Aplastic anaemia is usually defined as peripheral blood pancytopenia associated with a hypocellular marrow. The remaining cells within the marrow and the marrow architecture are normal, and the finding of abnormal cells or excess fibrosis within the marrow excludes a diagnosis of aplastic anaemia (Gordon-Smith 1989; Adamson and Erslev 1990).

The presenting features are those of bone marrow failure, including anaemia, neutropenia, and thrombocytopenia; the onset of symptoms may be insidious. The reader is directed to haematological texts (Gordon-Smith and Lewis 1989; Adamson and Erslev 1990) for a review of diagnosis and treatment options.

Drug-induced aplastic anaemia constitutes approximately 25 per cent of all aplasia and can be divided into two forms: (a) inevitable, and (b) idiosyncratic. These two categories may be regarded as Type A and Type B reactions respectively (see Chapter 5).

Inevitable (dose-dependent, Type A) drug-induced aplastic anaemia

Many cytotoxic chemotherapeutic agents have a low therapeutic index and are toxic to normal dividing cells

TABLE 24.1
*Cytotoxic agents that regularly induce
bone marrow aplasia*

Actinomycin D	Fludarabine
Amsacrine	Fluorouracil
Azathioprine	Hydroxyurea
Busulphan	Idarubicin
Carboplatin	Ifosfamide
Carmustine (BCNU)	Lomustine (CCNU)
Chlorambucil	Melphalan
Cisplatin	Mercaptopurine
Cyclophosphamide/	Methotrexate
ifosfamide	Mitomycin
Cytarabine	Mitozantrone
(cytosine arabinoside)	Plicamycin (mithramycin)
Daunorubicin	Procarbazine
Deoxycoformycin	Taxols
Doxorubicin	Thioguanine
(Adriamycin)	Thiotepa
Epirubicin	
Etoposide	

as well as malignant cells. The effects of such drugs are mediated via action upon DNA replication, with action in certain cases upon RNA transcription, protein synthesis, or mitotic mechanisms. As the haemopoietic system is constantly 'turning over' it is, therefore, not-surprising that temporary hypoplasia is frequently encountered with many forms of cytotoxic chemotherapy. Indeed, bone marrow hypoplasia is the dose-limiting toxicity of a large number of these agents (Table 24.1). This is largely predictable and, with careful attention to dosage, is usually reversible. Autologous bone marrow transplantation has been developed to avoid the prolonged aplasia induced by these agents in the therapy of haematological malignancy. This allows doses of drugs to be increased when marrow toxicity would otherwise have limited them. Occasionally, repeated or prolonged courses of therapy, particularly with alkylating agents (especially busulphan), can produce prolonged and unpredictable aplasia. Aplasia can also develop as part of the evolution of many haematological disorders, thus complicating the relevance of a particular therapeutic agent in this context.

Severe prolonged pancytopenia following standard doses of azathioprine and mercaptopurine (MP) is a rare but well described adverse effect and appears to be related to an inherited abnormality of drug metabolism. One of the key enzymes in the metabolism and inactivation of azathioprine and MP is thiopurine methyltransferase (TPMT). Deficiency of this enzyme is inherited as an autosomal recessive trait with around one in 300 of most populations studied having no detectable enzyme activity. Individuals with this deficiency suffer

no known harm unless treated with MP or azathioprine, when they develop severe prolonged hypoplasia which usually recovers provided the patient receives intensive haematological support.

Idiosyncratic (dose-independent, Type B) aplastic anaemia

The association between aplastic anaemia and drug therapy has long been recognized. The relative rarity of aplastic anaemia and the absence of appropriate tests mean that a causal association between aplastic anaemia and drug therapy is not easy to prove. Investigation of the aetiology of aplastic anaemia is complicated by the observation that there can be a delay of 1–6 months between exposure to the supposed causative drug or agent and the development of the anaemia. The slow onset of symptoms often leads to symptomatic treatment that may further complicate retrospective analysis of the drug history. The literature is littered with case reports of aplastic anaemia developing in patients taking any one of a number of drugs, but clearly this does not prove cause and effect and only careful case–control studies will yield valuable data.

TABLE 24.2
Drugs strongly linked with aplastic anaemia

Antibacterials	Chloramphenicol
	Co-trimoxazole
	Sulphonamides
	Tetracyclines
Anti-inflammatory agents	Benoxaprofen
	Fenbufen
	Gold
	Indomethacin
	Oxyphenbutazone
	Penicillamine
	Phenylbutazone
	Piroxicam
Antithyroid drugs	Carbimazole
	Thiouracils
Antimalarials	Amodiaquine
	Mepacrine
	Pyrimethamine
Anticonvulsants	Phenytoin
Antidepressants	Chlorpromazine
	Dothiepin
	MDMA
	('Ecstasy')
Antihypertensives	Lisinopril
Antidiabetics	Chlorpropamide
	Tolbutamide
Other	Acetazolamide
	Ticlopidine

There are only a few therapeutic compounds for which the link between a drug and aplastic anaemia is strong (Table 24.2). The idiosyncratic induction of aplastic anaemia by these compounds has made it difficult to study mechanisms, and it is still not known if these drugs are toxic to the pluripotential stem cell population, either directly or via the immune system, or whether their toxicity is exerted via another mechanism such as the induction of damage to the bone marrow stroma. It is possible that individual susceptibility to drug-induced aplasia is mediated by metabolic pathways that are genetically determined. A possible role has been mooted for concomitant infections, particularly those of viral origin (Levy 1997).

Chloramphenicol

Chloramphenicol, an early antibiotic which is still widely used, particularly in the third world, was one of the first agents to be associated with the development of aplastic anaemia.

Its antimicrobial action depends upon the binding to the rRNA of bacterial ribosomes and the inhibition of bacterial protein synthesis. It does not inhibit eukaryotic ribosomes, although it may bind to the ribosomal RNA found within mitochondria. This may prove to be the basis for chloramphenicol-induced aplasia, but another factor, possibly genetic, may be involved.

Aplasia can be dose related particularly with high serum levels $>25 \mu g$ per ml (Yunis 1973), and more likely with extended therapy (Oski 1979). Inhibition of mitochondrial ferrochelatase results in diminished iron uptake by erythroid precursors causing anaemia. Thrombocytopenia and agranulocytosis may follow, but are reversible within 2–3 weeks of stopping the drug (Oski 1979).

The idiosyncratic aplasia is irreversible, often fatal, but very rare, occurring in only one case per $25–40 \times 10^3$ courses of treatment (Wallerstein *et al.* 1969). Often slight delay in presentation occurs, and prognosis is poor in those developing aplasia up to 2 months after stopping the drug (Polak *et al.* 1972). There is a suspicion that the risk of aplasia is greater with the oral use of the drug, but this is uncertain (Ristuccia 1985). Liver dysfunction and aplasia have also been linked (Casale *et al.* 1982). Monitoring blood levels will not predict aplasia and the risk must be put into perspective: it is less than that from anaphylaxis due to penicillin (Rudolph and Price 1973). Cases have been ascribed to ocular administration (Carpenter 1975; Stevens and Mission 1987) but the link is controversial and the subject of much debate (McGhee and Anastas 1996; Rayner and Buckley 1996). Chloramphenicol is a very cheap and useful drug and the presently accepted uses have been reviewed by Smyth and Pallet (1988).

Non-steroidal anti-inflammatory drugs

Non-steroidal anti-inflammatory drugs (NSAID) have been associated with the development of agranulocytosis and aplastic anaemia. Phenylbutazone and oxyphenbutazone, both pyrazole derivatives, either had their indications restricted or, in some countries, were withdrawn from the market because of their association with the development of aplastic anaemia or agranulocytosis (Inman 1977). Other NSAID associated with aplastic anaemia or agranulocytosis include benoxaprofen, indomethacin, piroxicam, and sulindac. A number of other NSAID, including aspirin, have been linked with aplastic anaemia, but purely anecdotally.

Gold and penicillamine

Gold and penicillamine, both second-line agents in the treatment of patients with rheumatoid arthritis, have been linked with the development of aplastic anaemia. Again the exact mechanisms are not understood, but high concentrations of gold salts inhibit haemopoietic colony formation *in vitro*. Both gold and penicillamine therapy usually induce thrombocytopenia or neutropenia, or both of these, before aplastic anaemia, so regular blood count monitoring is valuable in patients taking these second-line agents. Cessation of therapy is advised if a patient's platelet or white cell count falls. Gold may be removed from the body in patients with gold-induced aplastic anaemia using the agent dimercaprol, although there is no evidence that this therapy will hasten recovery. Gold-induced aplastic anaemia has been successfully treated by immunosuppression (Doney *et al.* 1988) and marrow transplantation (Baldwin *et al.* 1977). Confirmatory reports on aplasia and gold therapy (Williams *et al.* 1987) continue to appear.

Other drugs

Additional agents implicated in the development of pancytopenia include zidovudine (Mir and Costello 1988), which is used in the treatment of HIV-positive patients, and this effect may be potentiated by the addition of ganciclovir (Jacobson *et al.* 1988). Additional anecdotal cases have involved lorazepam (El Sayed and Symonds 1988) and methazolamide, a carbonic anhydrase inhibitor (Mogk and Cyrlin 1988).

Red cell aplasia

Pure red cell aplasia (PRCA) is a haematological disorder characterized by anaemia, reticulocytopenia, and

TABLE 24.3
Drugs reported to induce pure red blood cell aplasia

Azathioprine	Old *et al.* 1978
Carbamazepine	Medberry *et al.* 1987
Chloramphenicol	Alter *et al.* 1978
Chlorpropamide	Planas *et al.* 1980; Gill *et al.* 1980
Co-trimoxazole	Ammus and Yunis 1987
Dapsone—*see* Maloprim	
Fenoprofen	Ammus and Yunis 1987
Fludarabine	Leporrier *et al.* 1993
FK506	Suzuki *et al.*1996
Gold (sodium aurothiomalate)	Reid and Patterson 1977
Halothane	Ammus and Yunis 1987
Isoniazid	Ammus and Yunis 1987
Maloprim (dapsone/pyrimethamine)	Ammus and Yunis 1987
Penicillin	Ammus and Yunis 1987
Pentachlorophenol	Ammus and Yunis 1987
Phenobarbitone	Ammus and Yunis 1987
Phenylbutazone	Alter *et al.* 1978
Phenytoin	Alter *et al.* 1978
Pyrimethamine—*see* Maloprim	
Sulphasalazine	Ammus and Yunis 1987
Sulphathiazide	Ammus and Yunis 1987
Sulphonamides	Alter *et al.* 1978
Sulphonylureas	Alter *et al.* 1978
Thiamphenicol	Ammus and Yunis 1987
Tolbutamide	Ammus and Yunis 1987
Valproate sodium	Macdougall-Lorna 1982

TABLE 24.4
Drugs reported to induce agranulocytosis

Acetazolamide	Meprobamate
Allopurinol	Methimazole
Amitriptyline	Methyldopa
Amodiaquine	Oxyphenbutazone
Benzodiazepines	Paracetamol
Captopril	Penicillamine
Carbamazepine	Penicillins and
Carbimazole	semi-synthetic
Cephalosporins	penicillins
Chloramphenicol	Pentazocine
Chloroquine	Phenacetin
Chlorothiazide	Phenothiazines
Chlorpromazine	Phenylbutazone
Chlorpropamide	Phenytoin
Chlorthalidone	Procainamide
Clindamycin	Propranolol
Cimetidine	Propylthiouracil
Co-trimoxazole	Pyrimethamine
Dapsone	Quinidine
Desipramine	Quinine
Disopyramide	Ranitidine
Ethacrynic acid	Rifampicin
Fansidar	Sodium aminosalicylate
(pyrimethamine/sulfadoxine)	(*p*-aminosalicylic acid)
Gentamicin	Streptomycin
Gold	Sulphadoxine
Hydralazine	Sulphonamides
Hydrochlorothiazide	Tetracyclines
Imipramine	Tocainide
Indomethacin	Tolbutamide
Isoniazid	Vancomycin
Levamisole	

erythroid hypoplasia or aplasia. The marrow is usually cellular and the myeloid and megakaryocytic lines are normal. PRCA has been reported in association with a number of drugs (see Table 24.3). In most cases the mechanism of drug-induced PRCA is unknown. Phenytoin-induced PRCA may involve more than one possible mechanism — direct toxic effects on DNA synthesis by erythroid cells have been suggested (Yunis *et al.* 1967) but humoral effects are thought to be important also. Patients' immunoglobulin has been shown to markedly inhibit BFU-E and CFU-E only in the presence of phenytoin (Dessypris *et al.* 1985). There is no specific indication that the drugs act by modifying erythropoietin release or activity.

The acquired variety of this disorder is usually of immune origin and may be associated with a tumour of the thymus (Krantz 1976). This form of the disorder is rare but can be treated effectively by removal of the thymus. PRCA is often seen in settings of disordered immunity such as SLE, AIDS, autoimmune haemolysis, and plasma cell dyscrasias; interestingly, it has arisen after treatment with the cytotoxic drug fludarabine, which causes a decrease in CD4 T-helper lymphocytes (Jaccard *et al.* 1993).

A report from Itoh and others (1988) suggests that methyldopa might cause red cell aplasia by suppression of erythroid colony-forming units.

Drug-induced granulocytopenia

Agranulocytosis or neutropenia, although rare, can be severe and even life-threatening. Adverse drug reactions are thought to be a common cause of neutropenia (see *Drug and Therapeutics Bulletin* 1997 for review), although study of drug-induced neutropenia is difficult because it is not predictable, numerous agents have been implicated (Table 24.4), and there is no ideal animal model for study. Clearly there are a number of drugs, particularly cytotoxic agents, that produce predictable and usually reversible bone marrow aplasia which can particularly affect the granulocyte count, and these agents have been discussed earlier in the section on Aplastic anaemia.

Idiosyncratic drug-induced agranulocytoses usually fall into two main categories. First, immune-mediated agranulocytosis can result from antibody-mediated or complement-mediated damage to granulocytic precursors (Levitt 1983) or peripheral neutrophil destruction (Heimpel 1988). This type of reaction is more common in the older female patient and it generally occurs early in a course of treatment to which the patient has previously been exposed. The second type of reaction usually involves dose-related toxicity from the effects of the drug on protein synthesis or cell replication. This interaction is often non-selective, and other haemopoietic and non-haemopoietic tissues may be involved. Antithyroid drugs and phenothiazines are particular examples of drugs that act in this way; thus monitoring of blood counts in the first months of treatment is important with these agents.

Platelet–drug interactions

Thrombocytopenia due to reduced platelet production

Platelets are derived from megakaryocytes, which are non-proliferative cells. Study of megakaryocytes is complicated by the fact that the precursors are capable of cell division and endomitosis (nuclear reduplication so that diploid and polydiploid forms exist). In spite of the problems, clonogenic assays of megakaryocyte progenitors do exist (Nakeff and Bryan 1978). Unfortunately, the exact mechanisms of drug actions on the megakaryocyte progenitors remain unknown. This phenomenon is rare, though alcohol (Levine et al. 1986), α-interferon (Talpaz et al. 1987), oestrogens (Cooper and Bigelow 1960), and thiazide diuretics (Bottiger and Westerholm 1972) have all been implicated. Thrombocytopenia has also been described after ganciclovir treatment in a patient with chronic myeloid leukaemia after bone marrow transplantation (Grosso and Grosso 1996).

Drug-induced autoimmune thrombocytopenia

Large numbers of compounds (Table 24.5) have been reported to induce autoimmune thrombocytopenia, although only a few have been consistently linked with this disorder. These include gold (Walker et al. 1986), heparin (Warkentin et al. 1990), methyldopa (Manohitharajah et al. 1971), quinidine and quinine (Shulman 1972), rifampicin (Blajchman et al. 1970), and sulphonamides (Hamilton and Sheets 1978).

Immunologically mediated thrombocytopenia occurs by at least two mechanisms: the first is exemplified by quinine and quinidine. The Fab portion of immunoglobulin G binds to a complex formed by the drug (or its metabolite) and a platelet membrane component (typically GP1B or GP2b/3a) (Visentin et al. 1991.)

TABLE 24.5
Drugs reported to induce autoimmune thrombocytopenia

Acetazolamide	Bertino et al. 1957
Actinomycin	Hodder et al. 1985
Allopurinol	Rosenbloom and Gilbert 1981
Alpha-interferon	Abdi et al. 1986
Amiodarone	Weinberger et al. 1987
Amitriptyline	Taniguchi and Hamada 1996
Ampicillin	Brooks 1974
Aspirin	Garg and Sarker 1974
Carbamazepine	Ponte 1983
Carbenicillin	Conti et al. 1984
Cephalosporins	Lown and Barr 1987
Chenodeoxycholic acid	Conti et al. 1984
Chloroquine	Nieweg et al. 1963
Chlorothiazide	Bottiger and Westerholm 1972
Chlorpheniramine	Eisner et al. 1975
Chlorpropamide	Bottiger and Westerholm 1972
Chlorthalidone	Bottiger and Westerholm 1972
Cimetidine	Glotzback 1982
Clozapine	Assion et al. 1996
Co-trimoxazole	Claas et al. 1979
Cyclophosphamide	Mueller-Eckhardt et al. 1983
Danazol	Arrowsmith and Dreis 1986
Desferrioxamine	Walker et al. 1985
Diazepam	Conti and Gandolfo 1983
Diazoxide	Wales and Wolff 1967
Diclofenac	Kramer et al. 1986
Digoxin	Pirovino et al. 1981
Diltiazem	Baggott 1987
Frusemide	Bottiger and Westerholm 1972
Gentamicin	Chen et al. 1980
Glymidine	Von dem Borne et al. 1986
Gold	Bottiger and Westerholm 1972
Hydrochlorothiazide	Okafor et al. 1986
Imipramine	Karpatkin et al. 1977
Isoniazid	Zorab 1960
Levamisole	El-Ghobari and Capella 1977
Meprobamate	Karpatkin et al. 1977
Methyldopa	Pai and Pai 1988
Mianserin	Stricker et al. 1985
Minoxidil	Peitzman and Martin 1980
Morphine	Cimo et al. 1982
Muromonab-CD3 (OKT3)	Bottiger and Westerholm 1972
Nitrofurantoin	Bottiger and Westerholm 1972
Oxprenolol	Hare and Hicks 1979
Oxyphenbutazone	Handley 1971
Penicillamine	Harrison and Hickman 1975
Penicillin	Conti et al. 1984
Phenylbutazone	Tolot et al. 1976
Phenytoin	Cimo et al. 1977
Piroxicam	Meisner et al. 1985
Procainamide	Giordano et al. 1987
Quinidine	Christie et al. 1985
Quinine	Christie et al. 1985
Ranitidine	Gafter et al. 1987
Rifampicin	Pau and Fisher 1987
Risperidone	Pau and Fisher 1987

(continued overleaf)

Table 24.5 continued

Sodium aminosalicylate (*p*-aminosalicylic acid)	Eisner and Kasper 1972
Sodium valproate	Barr *et al.* 1982
Sulphasalazine	Pena *et al.* 1985
Sulphonamides	Hamilton and Sheets 1978
Teicoplanin	Veldman *et al.* 1996
Thioguanine	Karpatkin *et al.* 1977
Valproate—*see* Sodium valproate	
Vancomycin	Walker and Heaton 1985
Vitamin A (isotretinoin)	Johnson and Rapini 1987

The Fc portion of the IgG is free and hence available to phagocytic cell Fc-receptor-mediated binding and subsequent destruction (Smith 1987).

Heparin is of particular interest in that it commonly produces a mild thrombocytopenia, possibly by inducing platelet aggregation, and it can also, rarely, induce a severe thrombocytopenia that is immunologically mediated. Heparin-associated immune thrombocytopenia (HIT) usually begins within 3 to 15 days of commencing therapy although it may occur more rapidly if the patient has been previously exposed to heparin. It is caused by IgG binding via its Fab portion to a complex made up of heparin and platelet factor four (Kelton *et al.* 1994). The Fc portion of the antibody can bind to the platelet Fc receptor, triggering platelet activation and aggregation (Horsewood *et al.* 1991). Heparin-induced thrombocytopenia is strongly associated with thrombosis, particularly arterial occlusions, and has a high morbidity and mortality (see also Chapter 9).

A rapid switch to oral anticoagulation will avoid this complication, but if heparin is to be continued for some time then the platelet count should be regularly monitored and if it falls significantly an alternative antithrombotic therapy should be used (Warkentin *et al.* 1990). Low-molecular-weight heparin has been associated with HIT and thrombosis, albeit at a lower rate than unfractionated heparin; hence it cannot be used as a substitute (Warkentin and Kelton 1989; Walterns 1996). Drugs used successfully in HIT include ancrod, a defibrinogenating snake venom (Demers *et al.* 1991), iloprost, and heparinoids such as Org 10172 (Magnani 1993), although *in vitro* cross-reactivity with heparinoids occurs in around 10 per cent of cases.

In any patient with acute thrombocytopenia of unknown aetiology, all treatment should be stopped or, if this is not possible, the drugs should be changed. Usually the platelet count rises within 7 days, although it is occasionally delayed, and the patient should be managed in the standard way. Once a patient has demon-

strated drug sensitivity in this way then the drug should be carefully avoided in the future.

Red cell–drug interactions

Immune-mediated red cell destruction

Drug-induced haemolytic anaemia has been recognized for some time; it is usually a relatively benign process although severe and even fatal cases may occur. It must be distinguished from spontaneous forms of autoimmune haemolytic anaemia and other types of drug-induced non-immune red cell destruction, which usually occur upon exposure of inherently defective red cells to a drug or its metabolites. The incidence of immune haemolytic anaemia appears to be increasing, possibly due to the introduction of numerous new drugs and escalation in numbers of drug prescriptions.

There are four major mechanisms of drug-induced immune haemolysis, although it is not always easy in individual cases to be certain that the haemolysis is drug induced or to be sure of the mechanisms involved.

Hapten-induced haemolysis

Most drugs are substances of low molecular weight that are unable to stimulate an immune response on their own. In hapten-induced immune haemolysis the drug binds to the red cell membrane and the drug–red cell complex stimulates an immune response, sometimes called the 'planted antigen' mechanism. Penicillins (White *et al.* 1968), cephalosporins (Gralnick *et al.* 1971), and tetracyclines (Wenz *et al.* 1974) can induce this type of immune response when given in high doses for long periods. Usually an IgG antibody is responsible for this type of haemolysis, which will be detected in a direct antiglobulin test. If the antibody is eluted from the patient's red blood cells then it will not react with other red cells unless they have been preincubated with the drug or are drug-coated (indirect antiglobulin test negative unless drug is included in the test system). Interestingly, while a number of patients on high doses of penicillin develop a positive direct antiglobulin reaction very few develop haemolytic anaemia.

Cephalosporins and semi-synthetic penicillins also cross-react with penicillin and can bind to the red cell membrane and in some instances induce immune haemolytic anaemia.

Tetracycline and tolbutamide may also bind to red cell membranes and thus act as haptens for an immune response, as may cisplatin, teniposide, melphalan, and methotrexate.

Drug-induced autoantibody production

Certain drugs, particularly methyldopa, levodopa, and mefenamic acid (Breckenridge *et al.* 1967; Scott *et al.* 1968; Bernstein 1979; Beutler 1985), are capable of inducing autoantibodies against red blood cells. In this situation the drug does not act as a hapten but may act to suppress the normal controls on the immune system, allowing the expression of autoantibodies against normally occurring red cell antigens. Alternatively, the drug may alter the red cell membrane so that one or more of the membrane proteins appear foreign, hence inducing an autoantibody against the red cell. Usually this type of haemolysis is slow in onset and generally mild, and the IgG-coated red cells are sequestered in the spleen. The IgG will be detectable on both the red cell and also in the serum, and will react with a number of different red cells without preincubation with the offending drug. A number of patients receiving methyldopa will develop a positive direct antiglobulin test, but few will develop clinically significant haemolysis. Induction of autoantibody production is thought to involve alteration to immunoregulatory T cells, as is seen with fludarabine (Byrd *et al.* 1995), deoxycoformycin, α-interferon (Takase *et al.* 1995) and immunoglobulin (Schiavotto *et al.* 1993).

Immune complex mechanisms

In this type of reaction there is formation of a complex between the drug, an immunoglobulin, and a drug-membrane binding site. Usually, red blood cell destruction is intravascular following completion of the complement cascade, although there may be some destruction in the liver and spleen. This type of haemolysis can be fairly brisk. The process is largely IgM-mediated, but the direct antiglobulin reaction is usually only positive to components of the complement cascade. Drugs implicated are shown in Table 24.6.

Non-immunological protein absorption

Cephalosporin antibiotics can induce the non-specific absorption of plasma proteins to the red blood cell membrane, which may produce a positive direct antiglobulin reaction; but haemolysis has not been seen. This type of interaction may, however, interfere with blood cross-matching in patients receiving cephalosporin therapy.

Non-immune red cell damage

Oxidation damage to red cells

As oxygen is transferred from the haemoglobin molecule in the tissues, highly reactive oxygen species such as the superoxide anion can be generated (Carrell *et al.* 1975), which are capable of denaturing haemoglobin and inactivating vital red blood cell enzymes. The red cell has a number of antioxidant defence mechanisms, which include catalase and reduced glutathione working through the enzymes glutathione peroxidase and glutathione transferase. The most important red cell enzyme that protects against oxidant stress is glucose-6-phosphate dehydrogenase (G6PD) (Beutler 1978).

Drugs that act as oxidants *in vivo* or which increase the generation of activated oxygen species may produce high levels of oxidative stress in the red cell. Red cells that have a lowered reducing capacity due to enzyme deficiency, such as G6PD deficiency, cannot operate effective reduction pathways to prevent haemolysis.

Extensive lists of drugs that can be given safely to G6PD-deficient individuals are available and readers are referred to the excellent text produced by Beutler (1978) for details.

Table 24.7 lists the drugs that have clearly been associated with significant haemolysis in G6PD-deficient patients (Beutler 1985). Interestingly, deficiency of the enzymes glutathione reductase and glutathione peroxidase is not associated with haemolytic anaemia (Beutler

TABLE 24.6
Drugs reported to induce haemolysis following formation of an immune complex

Antimony (stibophen)	Harris 1956
Chlorpropamide	Logue *et al.* 1970
Isoniazid	Schwartz *et al.* 1995
Melphalan	Schwartz *et al.* 1995
Methotrexate	Woolley *et al.* 1983
Quinidine	Croft *et al.* 1968
Quinine	Muirhead *et al.* 1958
Rifampicin	Lakshminarayan *et al.* 1973
Sulphonamides	Schwartz *et al.* 1995
Tetracyclines	Schwartz *et al.* 1995
Thiazides	Schwartz *et al.* 1995

TABLE 24.7
Drugs that have been clearly shown to cause clinically significant haemolytic anaemia in G6PD deficiency

Acetanilide	Phenylhydrazine
Doxorubicin	Primaquine
Glibenclamide	Succimer
Methylene blue	Sulphacetamide
Nalidixic acid	Sulphamethoxazole
Naphthalene	Sulphanilamide
Niridazole	Sulphapyridine
Nitrofurantoin	Thiazolesulphone
Pamaquine	Toluidine blue
Phenazopyridine	

1985). Antioxidants have been used to treat oxidative cyclosporin-induced haemolysis (Azuma *et al.* 1993).

Haemolysis due to non-oxidative drugs

Many chemicals have been associated with non-immune, non-oxidative red cell destruction (Table 24.8). Beutler (1985) has discussed the varying mechanisms. Lead, for example, shortens the life-span of red cells probably by inhibiting the enzyme pyrimidine 5'-nucleotidase producing basophilic stippling of red cells. Lead also inhibits several enzymes involved in the synthesis of haem. Copper can cause haemolysis, which can be seen in Wilson's syndrome, but the mechanism is unclear. Among commonly used drugs, cisplatin (Getaz *et al.* 1980; Levi *et al.* 1981), carboplatin (Maloisel *et al.* 1995), and penicillamine (Harrison and Hickman 1976) are most frequently associated with non-oxidative red cell destruction. The exact mechanisms of destruction are not known.

TABLE 24.8
Agents that may cause haemolysis by non-oxidative mechanism

Aniline	Nitrobenzene
Arsine	Penicillamine
Chlorate	Phenazopyridine
Cisplatin	Resorcin
Copper	Sodium
Formaldehyde	aminosalicylate
Lead	(*p*-aminosalicylic
Mephenesin	acid)
	Sulphasalazine
	Zinc ethylene *bis*
	(dithiocarbamate)

Drug-induced megaloblastic anaemia

Megaloblastic anaemia is a disorder with characteristic abnormalities of the blood and bone marrow induced by impaired DNA synthesis. RNA and protein synthesis continue normally giving rise to the well-recognized morphological changes of megaloblastic anaemia.

Drugs can impair DNA synthesis in a number of ways (listed in Table 24.9) and will eventually produce a megaloblastic anaemia (Stibbins and Bertino 1976; Scott and Weir 1980; Ammus and Yunis 1989).

Zidovudine (AZT), a thymidine analogue, inhibits the retroviral enzyme reverse transcriptase and has been shown to be a potent inhibitor of the HIV virus. It is, however, a toxic drug inducing macrocytosis in most patients, and in some cases produces a severe megaloblastic anaemia often associated with neutropenia. B_{12} and folate levels are usually normal (Mir and Costello

TABLE 24.9
Drugs that may induce megaloblastic anaemia

Drugs that interfere with vitamin B_{12} metabolism

  Alcohol
  Colchicine
  Metformin
  Neomycin
  Nitrous oxide (if prolonged)
  Omeprazole
  Phenformin
  Sodium aminosalicylate (*p*-aminosalicylic acid)
  Vitamin C (in large doses)

Drugs that interfere with folate metabolism

(a) Dihydrofolate reductase inhibitors

  Aminopterin
  Methotrexate
  Pentamidine
  Proguanil
  Pyrimethamine
  Triamterene
  Trimethoprim

(b) Impaired folate absorption/utilization

  Alcohol
  Cholestyramine
  Cycloserine
  Metformin
  Nitrofurantoin
  Oral contraceptive agents
  Phenobarbitone
  Phenytoin
  Potassium (slow-release)
  Primidone
  Sulphasalazine

Drugs that interfere with DNA synthesis directly

  Aciclovir
  Azathioprine
  Cytarabine
  Floxuridine
  Fluorouracil
  Hydroxyurea
  Mercaptopurine
  Thioguanine
  Zidovudine

Mechanism unknown

  Benzene
  Tetracycline
  Vinblastine
  Vitamin A

1988; Youle and Gazzard 1990). These adverse effects can limit or even preclude the drug's use. In a double-blind, randomized, placebo-controlled trial, a 25 per cent or greater fall in haemoglobin was observed in 40 per cent of patients given AZT. The correct approach to patients who develop severe red cell aplasia on AZT is not known, although these patients seem to have a poor prognosis.

Drug-induced sideroblastic anaemia

Sideroblastic anaemia results from disordered haem synthesis and is associated with the accumulation of iron in mitochondria, forming typical ring sideroblasts. Usually the red blood cells are hypochromic, although a dimorphic picture is commonly seen. The reticulocyte count is low or normal and bone marrow aspiration usually reveals erythroid hyperplasia with numerous basophilic normoblasts and plentiful ring sideroblasts. These changes have been described in association with a number of drugs (see Table 24.10). The anaemia may be quite severe, necessitating transfusion. Removal of the drug in question and/or pyridoxine therapy usually results in reversal of the changes and resolution of the associated anaemia.

TABLE 24.10
Drugs that may induce sideroblastic anaemia

Alcohol	Hines 1960
Chloramphenicol	Beck *et al.* 1967
Cycloserine	Haden 1967; Tomlin 1973
Isoniazid	Verwilghen *et al.* 1965
Penicillamine	Ramselaar *et al.* 1987
Phenacetin	Popovic *et al.* 1973
Progesterone	Brodsky *et al.* 1994
Pyrazinamide	McCurdy *et al.* 1966
Zinc	Ramaduai *et al.* 1993

Antituberculous drugs, including isoniazid and pyrazinamide, are associated with the development of sideroblastic anaemia. Isoniazid probably interferes with the synthesis of δ-aminolaevulinic acid, an important precursor in haem synthesis. Pyrazinamide may interfere with vitamin B_6 metabolism.

Chloramphenicol also interferes with haem synthesis, producing anaemia which is distinct from the rarer aplastic anaemia. This production of sideroblastic anaemia only occurs when chloramphenicol is given in high doses (over 2 g per day) and is thought to be due to suppression of mitochondrial respiratory pathways.

Copper depletion secondary to chelation (as used to treat Wilson's disease) can lead to sideroblastic anaemia (Condamine *et al.* 1993; Perry *et al.* 1996). Zinc can cause sideroblastic change as a result of interference with copper absorption and handling (Patterson *et al.* 1985; Ramadurai *et al.* 1993).

Methaemoglobinaemia

The iron of haem in red cells normally stays in the divalent form. The loss of an additional electron can create a trivalent form of iron known as methaemoglobin. Normally the cell copes with this stress through the NADH reducing system via the enzyme NADH diaphorase. Certain drugs and chemicals have the capacity to increase greatly the rate at which this occurs, and it is a more common occurrence in children than in adults. Details of the agents involved are discussed by Beutler (1985) and Benz (1995). Additions to the list of agents that cause methaemoglobinaemia are metoclopramide (Kearns and Fisher 1988) and prilocaine, a local anaesthetic (Menahem 1988). Both reactions were seen in children. The observation has been confirmed recently when prilocaine–lignocaine cream used as local skin anaesthetic in children aged 1–6 years caused an increase in levels of methaemoglobin (Frayling *et al.* 1990). This caused no clinical symptoms, but users are warned against frequent use in paediatric patients.

Drug-induced haematological tumours

Drug-induced myelodysplasia and leukaemia

Cytotoxic drugs

A number of studies have demonstrated that long-term survivors of certain malignancies, such as Hodgkin's disease (Tucker *et al.* 1988), ovarian carcinoma (Einhorn *et al.* 1982), and childhood malignancies (Tucker *et al.* 1987) treated with cytotoxic chemotherapy and radiotherapy are at risk of developing myelodysplasia and acute non-lymphocytic leukaemia. Alkylating agents, in particular, have been implicated in most studies as being leukaemogenic. The additional toxicity of radiotherapy when used in conjunction with chemotherapy is disputed, and the incidence varies in different series. In the United Kingdom, for example, secondary leukaemia after therapy for Hodgkin's disease therapy occurs in less than one per cent of cases (Proctor and Evans 1985), whereas in series from North America the incidence has been as high as seven per cent. Carcinogenic mechanisms of cytotoxic chemotherapy have been difficult to study. Direct DNA damage or prolonged immunosuppression have been suggested as possible mechanisms.

In those developing secondary AML after treatment for ALL there is an association with prolonged administration of epidophyllotoxins (etoposide and teniposide) (Pui *et al.* 1989, 1991). Blasts from secondary leukaemias after epipodophyllotoxin treatment can often be shown to have cytogenetic abnormalities of the 11q23 chromosomal region, which has been linked to malignant transformation of pluripotential stem cells. A specific translocation, t(9;11)(p21;q23) has been identified in patients developing secondary AML (especially those with monocytic differentiation) after treatment of solid tumours involving epipodophyllotoxins (Web *et al.* 1986; Ratain *et al.* 1987; Pedersen-Bjergaard *et al.* 1988).

The risk of secondary leukaemia remains small and clearly should not restrict the use of chemotherapy essential for cure or prolonged survival in those with otherwise incurable disease. As improvements in treatment regimens continue, however, and cure rates increase, careful consideration of the long-term adverse effects of cytotoxic chemotherapy will be important (see also Chapter 26).

Drug-induced non-Hodgkin's lymphoma (NHL) and solid tumours

Cytotoxic drugs

Following the successful therapy of Hodgkin's disease the problems of secondary non-Hodgkin's lymphoma or other solid tumours have emerged. The cumulative risk of developing a secondary NHL at 10 years is approximately 1.8 per cent and of secondary cancer 8.8 per cent (Cosset *et al.* 1990). Alkylating agents used in primary chemotherapy are regarded as being involved in this process (see also Chapter 26).

Secondary malignancies reported after successful treatment of ALL in children include malignant gliomas (Ochs and Mulhern 1988) and thyroid and parotid carcinomas (Tefft *et al.* 1968; Tang *et al.* 1980).

References

Abdi, E.A., Brien, W., and Venner, P.M. (1986). Auto-immune thrombocytopenia related to interferon therapy. *Scand. J. Haematol.* 36, 515.

Adamson, J.W. and Erslev, A.J. (1990). Aplastic anaemia. In *Hematology* (4th edn) (ed. W.J. Williams, E. Beutler, A.J. Erslev, and M.A. Lichtman), p. 158. McGraw-Hill, New York.

Alter, B.P., Potter, N.U., and Li, F.P. (1978). Classification and aetiology of the aplastic anaemias. *Clin. Haematol.* 7, 431.

Ammus, S.S. and Yunis, A.A. (1987). Acquired pure red cell aplasia. *Am. J. Haematol.* 24, 311.

Ammus, S.S. and Yunis, A.A. (1989). Drug-induced red cell dyscrasias. *Blood Reviews* 3, 71.

Arrowsmith, J.B. and Dreis, M. (1986). Thrombocytopenia after treatment with danazol. *N. Engl. J. Med.* 315, 585.

Assion, H.J., Kolbinger, H.M., Rao, M.L., *et al.* (1996). Lymphocytopenia and thrombocytopenia during treatment with risperidone or clozapine. *Pharmacopsychiatry* 29, 227.

Azuma, E., Hirayama, M., Nakano, T., *et al.* (1995). Acute haemolysis during cyclosporin therapy successfully treated with vitamin E. *Bone Marrow Transplant.* 16, 321.

Baggott, L.A. (1987). Diltiazem-associated immune thrombocytopenia. *Mt Sinai J. Med.* 54, 500.

Baldwin, J.L., Storb, R., Thomas, E.D., *et al.* (1977). Bone marrow transplantation in patients with gold-induced marrow aplasia. *Arthritis Rheum.* 20, 1043.

Balkwill, F.R. (1989). The colony-stimulating factors. In *Cytokines in Cancer Therapy* (ed. F.R. Balkwill), p. 114. Oxford University Press.

Ballin, A., Brown, E.J., Koren, G., *et al.* (1988). Vitamin C-induced erythrocyte damage in premature infants. *J. Pediatr.* 113, 114.

Barr, R.D., Copeland, S.A., Stockwell, M.L., *et al.* (1982). Valproic acid and immune thrombocytopenia. *Arch. Dis. Child.* 57, 681.

Beck, E.A., Ziegler, G., Schmid, R., *et al.* (1967). Reversible sideroblastic anaemia caused by chloramphenicol. *Acta Haematol.* (Basel) 38, 1.

Benz, E.J. Jr (1995). Hemoglobin variants associated with hemolytic anaemia, altered oxygen affinity and methemaglobinemias. In *Hematology: Basic Principles and Practice* (2nd edn) (ed. R. Hoffman, E.J. Benz Jr, S.J. Shattil, *et al.*), p. 653. Churchill Livingstone, New York.

Bernstein, R.M. (1979). Reversible haemolytic anaemia after levodopa–carbidopa. *BMJ* i, 1461.

Bertino, J.E., Rodman, T., and Myerson, R.M. (1957). Thrombocytopenia and renal lesions associated with acetazolamide (Diamox) therapy. *Arch. Intern. Med.* 99, 1006.

Beutler, E. (1978). *Hemolytic Anaemia in Disorders of Red Cell Metabolism.* Plenum Press, New York.

Beutler, E. (1985). Chemical toxicity of the erythrocyte. In *Toxicology of the Blood and Bone Marrow* (ed. R.D. Irons), p. 39. Raven Press, New York.

Blajchman, M.A., Lowry, R.C., Pettit, J.E., *et al.* (1970). Rifampicin-induced immune thrombocytopenia. *BMJ* iii, 24.

Bottiger, L.E. and Westerholm, B. (1972). Drug-induced thrombocytopenia. *Acta Med. Scand.* 191, 541.

Breckenridge, A., Dollery, C.T., Worlledge, S.M., *et al.* (1967). Positive direct Coombs tests and antinuclear factor in patients treated with methyldopa. *Lancet* ii, 1265.

Brodsky, R.A., Hasegawa, S., Fibach, E., *et al.* (1994). Acquired sideroblastic anaemia following progesterone treatment. *Br. J. Haematol.* 87, 859.

Brooks, A.P. (1974). Thrombocytopenia during treatment with ampicillin. *Lancet* ii, 723.

Byrd, J.C., Hertler, A.A., Weiss, R.B., *et al.* (1995). Fatal recurrence of autoimmune haemolytic anaemia following pentostatin treatment in a patient with a history of fludarabine-associated haemolytic anaemia. *Ann. Oncol.* 6, 300.

Carpenter, G. (1975). Chloramphenicol eye drops and marrow aplasia. *Lancet* ii, 326.

Carrell, R.W., Winterbourn, C.C., and Rachmilewitz, E.A. (1975). Activated oxygen and haemolysis. *Br. J. Haematol.* 30, 259.

Casale, T.B., Macher, A.M., and Fauci, A.S. (1982). Complete hematologic and hepatic recovery in a patient with chloramphenicol hepatitis–pancytopenia syndrome. *J. Pediatr.* 101, 1025.

Chen, J-H., Wiener, L., and Distenfeld, A. (1980). Immunologic thrombocytopenia induced by gentamicin. *N.Y. State J. Med.* 80, 1134.

Christie, D.J., Mullen, P.C., and Aster, R.H. (1985). Fab-mediated binding of drug-dependent antibodies to platelets in quinidine- and quinine-induced thrombocytopenia. *J. Clin. Invest.* 75, 310.

Cimo, P.L., Pisciotta, A.V., Desai, R.G., *et al.* (1977). Detection of drug-dependent antibodies by the ^{51}Cr platelet lysis test: documentation of immune thrombocytopenia induced by diphenylhydantoin, diazepam, and sulfisoxazole. *Am. J. Haematol.* 2, 65.

Cimo, P.L., Hammond, J.J., and Moake, J.L. (1982). Morphine-induced immune thrombocytopenia. *Arch. Intern. Med.* 142, 832.

Claas, F.H., van der Meer, J.W.M., and Langerak, J. (1979). Immunological effect of co-trimoxazole on platelets. *BMJ* ii, 898.

Condamine, L., Hermine, O., Alvin, P., *et al.* (1993). Acquired sideroblastic anaemia during treatment of Wilson's disease with triethylene tetramine hydrochloride. *Br. J. Haematol.* 83, 166.

Conti, L. and Gandolfo, G.M. (1983). Benzodiazepine-induced thrombocytopenia. Demonstration of drug-dependent platelet antibodies in two cases. *Acta Haematol.* 70, 386.

Conti, L., Fidani, P., Christolini, A., *et al.* (1984). Detection of drug-dependent IgG antibodies with anti-platelet activity by the antiglobulin consumption assay. *Haemostasis* 14, 480.

Cooper, B.A. and Bigelow, F.S. (1960). Thrombocytopenia associated with the administration of diethylstilbestrol in man. *Ann. Intern. Med.* 52, 907.

Cosset, J.M., Henry-Amar, M., and Meerwaldt, J.H. (1990). Long term toxicity of Hodgkin's disease treatment. *4th International Conference on Malignant Lymphoma, Lugano* 12, (Abstract).

Croft, J.D., Swisher, S.N. Jr, Gilliland, B.C., *et al.* (1968). Coombs test positivity induced by drugs: mechanisms of immunologic reactions and red cell destruction. *Ann. Intern. Med.* 68, 176.

Demers, C., Ginsberg, J.S., Brilledwards, P., *et al.* (1991). Rapid anticoagulation using ancrod for heparin-induced thrombocytopenia. *Blood* 78, 2194.

Dessypris, E.N. (1988). *Pure Red Cell Aplasia*. Johns Hopkins University Press, Baltimore.

Dessypris, E.N., Redline, S., Harris, J.W., *et al.* (1985). Diphenylhydantoin-induced pure red cell aplasia. *Blood* 65, 789.

Dexter, T.M. (1987). Stem cells in normal growth and disease. *BMJ* 295, 1192.

Doney, K., Storb, R., Buckner, C.D., *et al.* (1988). Treatment of gold-induced aplastic anaemia with immunosuppressive therapy. *Br. J. Haematol.* 68, 469.

Drug and Therapeutics Bulletin (1997). Drug-induced agranulocytosis. *Drug Ther. Bull.* 35, 49.

Einhorn, N., Eklund, G., Frazen, S., *et al.* (1982). Late side effects of chemotherapy in ovarian carcinoma: a cytogenetic, hematologic and statistical study. *Cancer* 49, 2234.

Eisner, E.V. and Kasper, K. (1972). Immune thrombocytopenia due to a metabolite of para-aminosalicylic acid. *Am. J. Med.* 53, 790.

Eisner, E.V., LaBocki, N.L., and Pinkney, L. (1975). Chlorpheniramine dependent thrombocytopenia. *JAMA* 231, 735.

El-Ghobari, A.F. and Capella, H.A. (1977). Levamisole-induced thrombocytopenia. *BMJ* ii, 555.

El Sayed, S. and Symonds, R.P. (1988). Lorazepam induced pancytopenia. *BMJ* 296, 1332.

Frayling, I.M., Addison, G.M., Chattergee, K., *et al.* (1990). Methaemoglobinaemia in children treated with prilocaine–lignocaine cream. *BMJ* 301, 153.

Gafter, U., Komlos, L., Weinstein, T., *et al.* (1987). Thrombocytopenia, eosinophilia, and ranitidine. *Ann. Intern. Med.* 106, 477.

Gardner, L. and Grosso, L.E. (1996). Gancyclovir-induced megakaryocyte loss in chronic myeloid leukaemia post bone marrow transplantation. *Am. J. Haematol.* 53, 204.

Garg, S.K. and Sarker, C.R. (1974). Aspirin-induced thrombocytopenia on an immune basis. *Am. J. Med. Sci.* 267, 129.

Getaz, E.P., Beckley, S., Fitzpatrick, J., *et al.* (1980). Cisplatin-induced hemolysis. *N. Engl. J. Med.* 302, 334.

Gill, M.J., Ratliff, D.A., and Harding, L.K. (1980). Hypoglycaemic coma, jaundice and pure red blood cell aplasia following chlorpropamide therapy. *Arch. Intern. Med.* 140, 714.

Giordano, N., Sancasciani, S., Cantore, M., *et al.* (1987). Thrombocytopenic purpura associated with piroxicam. *Clin. Exp. Rheumatol.* 5, 298.

Glotzback, R.E. (1982). Cimetidine-induced thrombocytopenia. *South. Med. J.* 75, 232.

Gordon-Smith, E.C. (1989). Aplastic anaemia — aetiology and clinical features. In *Clinical Haematology*, Vol. 2 (ed. E.C. Gordon-Smith), p. 1. Baillière, London.

Gordon-Smith, E.C. and Lewis, S.M. (1989). Aplastic anaemia and other types of bone marrow failure. In *Postgraduate Haematology* (3rd edn) (ed. A.V. Hoffbrand and S.M. Lewis), p. 83. Heinemann, London.

Gralnick, H.R., McGinniss, M., Elton, W., *et al.* (1971). Hemolytic anemia associated with cephalothin. *JAMA* 217, 1193.

Haden, H.T. (1967). Pyridoxine-responsive sideroblastic anemia due to antituberculous drugs. *Arch. Intern. Med.* 20, 602.

Hamilton, H.E. and Sheets, R.F. (1978). Sulfisoxazole-induced thrombocytopenic purpura. *JAMA* 239, 2586.

Handley, A.J. (1971). Thrombocytopenia and LE cells after oxyphenbutazone. *Lancet* i, 245.

Hare, D.L. and Hicks, B.H. (1979). Thrombocytopenia due to oxprenolol. *Med. J. Aust.* ii, 259.

Harris, J.W. (1956). Studies on the mechanism of drug induced hemolytic anaemia. *J. Lab. Clin. Med.* 47, 760.

Harrison, E.E. and Hickman, J.W. (1975). Hemolytic anemia and thrombocytopenia associated with penicillamine ingestion. *South. Med. J.* 68, 113.

Harrison, E.E. and Hickman, J.W. (1976). D-penicillamine and haemolytic anaemia. *Lancet* i, 38.

Heimpel, H. (1988). Drug-induced agranulocytosis. *Medical Toxicology and Adverse Drug Experience* 3, 449.

Hines, J. (1960). Reversible megaloblastic and sideroblastic abnormalities in alcoholic patients. *Br. J. Haematol.* 16, 87.

Hodder, F.S., Kempert, P., McCormack, S., *et al.* (1985). Immune thrombocytopenia following actinomycin-D therapy. *J. Pediatr.* 107, 611.

Horsewood, P., Hayward, C.P.M., Warkentin, T.E., et al. (1991). Investigation of mechanisms of monoclonal antibody-induced platelet activation. *Blood* 78, 1019.

Inman, W.H.W. (1977). Study of fatal bone marrow depression with special reference to phenylbutazone and oxyphenbutazone. *BMJ* i, 1500.

Itoh, K., Wong, P., Asai, T., *et al.* (1988). Pure red cell aplasia induced by α-methyldopa. *Am. J. Med.* 84, 1088.

Jaccard, A., Oksendendler, E., and Clauvel, J.P. (1993). Cytopenia and fludarabine. *Lancet* 342, 555.

Jacobson, M.A., Miranda, P.D., Gordon, S.M., *et al.* (1988). Prolonged pancytopenia due to combined gancyclovir and zidovudine therapy. *J. Infect. Dis.* 158, 489.

Johnson, T.M. and Rapini, R.P. (1987). Isotretinoin-induced thrombocytopenia. *J. Am. Acad. Dermatol.* 17, 838.

Karpatkin, M., Siskind, G.W., and Karpatkin, S. (1977). The platelet factor 3 immuno injury technique re-evaluated: development of a rapid test for antiplatelet antibody: detection in various clinical disorders, including immunologic drug-induced and neonatal thrombocytopenias. *J. Lab. Clin. Med.* 82, 400.

Kearns, G.L. and Fisher, D.H. (1988). Metoclopramide induced methemoglobinemia. *Pediatrics* 82, 364.

Kelton, J.G., Smith, J.W., Warkentin, T.E., *et al.* (1994). Immunoglobulin G from patients with heparin-induced thrombocytopenia binds to complex of heparin and platelet factor 4. *Blood* 83, 3232.

Kramer, M.R., Levene, C., and Hershko, C. (1986). Severe reversible autoimmune haemolytic anaemia and thrombocytopenia associated with diclofenac therapy. Case report. *Scand. J. Haematol.* 36, 118.

Krantz, S.B. (1976). Diagnosis and treatment of pure red cell aplasia. *Med. Clin. North Am.* 60, 945.

Kurtzman, G.J., Ozawa, K., Cohen, B., *et al.* (1987). Chronic bone marrow failure due to persistent B19 parvovirus infection. *N. Engl. J. Med.* 317, 287.

Lakshminarayan, S., Sahn, S.A., and Hudson, L.D. (1973). Massive haemolysis caused by rifampicin. *BMJ* 282, 2003.

Leporrier, M., Reman, O., and Troussard, X. (1993). Pure red cell aplasia with fludarabine for C.L.L. *Lancet* 342, 1049.

Levi, J.A., Aroney, R.S., and Dalley, D.N. (1981). Haemolytic anaemia after cisplatin treatment. *BMJ* 282, 2003.

Levine, R.F., Spivak, J.L., and Meagher, R.C. (1986). Effect of ethanol on thrombopoiesis. *Br. J. Haematol.* 62, 345.

Levy, M. (1997). Role of viral infections in the induction of adverse drug reactions. *Drug Safety* 16, 1.

Logue, G.L., Boyd, A.E., and Rosse, W.F. (1970). Chlorpropamide induced immune hemolytic anaemia. *N. Engl. J. Med.* 283, 900.

Lown, J.A. and Barr, A. (1987). Immune thrombocytopenia induced by cephalosporins specific for thiomethyltetrazole side chain. *J. Clin. Pathol.* 40, 700.

McCurdy, P.R., Donohoe, R.F., and Magovern, M. (1966). Reversible anemia caused by pyrazinoic acid (pyrazinamide). *Ann. Intern. Med.* 64, 1280.

Macdougall-Lorna, G. (1982). Pure red cell aplasia associated with sodium valproate therapy. *JAMA* 247, 53.

McGhee, C.N. and Anastas, C.N. (1996). Widespread ocular use of topical chloramphenicol: is there justifiable concern regarding aplastic anaemia? *Br. J. Ophthalmol.* 80, 182.

Mackie, F., Verran, D., Horvath, J., *et al.* (1996). Severe thrombocytopenia with OKT3 use for steroid-resistant rejection in a cadaveric renal transplant recipient. *Nephrol. Dial. Transplant.* 11, 2378.

Magnani, H.N. (1993). Heparin-induced thrombocytopenia: an overview of 230 patients treated with orgaran. *Thromb. Haemost.* 70, 554.

Maloisel, F., Kurtz, J.E., Andres, E., *et al.* (1995). Platin salts-induced haemolytic anaemia: cisplatin and the first case of carboplatin-induced haemolysis. *Anticancer Drugs* 6, 324.

Manohitharajah, S.M., Jenkins, W.J., Roberts, P.D., *et al.* (1971). Methyldopa and associated thrombocytopenia. *BMJ* i, 494.

Medberry, C.A., Pappas, A., and Ackerman, B.H. (1987). Carbamazepine and erythroid arrest. *Drug Intell. Clin. Pharm.* 21, 439.

Meisner, D.J., Carlson, R.J., and Gottlieb, A.J. (1985). Thrombocytopenia following sustained-release procainamide. *Arch. Intern. Med.* 145, 700.

Menahem, S. (1988). Prilocaine hydrochloride and neonatal methaemoglobinaemia. *Aust. N.Z. J. Obstet. Gynaecol.* 28, 76.

Metcalf, D. (1987). The molecular control of normal and leukaemic granulocytes and macrophages. *Proc. R. Soc. Lond. (Biol.)* 230, 389.

Mir, N. and Costello, C. (1988). Zidovudine and bone marrow. *Lancet* ii, 1195.

Mogk, L.G. and Cyrlin, M.M. (1988). Blood dyscrasias and carbonic anhydrase inhibitors. *Ophthalmology* (Rochester) 95, 768.

Mueller-Eckhardt, C., Küenzlen, E., Kiefel, V., *et al.* (1983). Cyclophosphamide-induced immune thrombocytopenia in a patient with ovarian carcinoma successfully treated with intravenous gamma globulin. *Blut* 46, 165.

Muirhead, E.E., Halden, E.R., and Groves, M. (1958). Drug dependent Coombs (antiglobulin) test and anemia. Observations on quinine and acetophenetidine. *Arch. Intern. Med.* 101, 87.

Nakeff, A. and Bryan, J. E. (1978). Megakaryocyte proliferation and its regulation as revealed by CFU-M analysis. In *Hemopoetic Cell Differentiation* (ed. D.W. Golde, M.J. Cline, D. Metcalf, and C.F. Fox), p. 241. Academic Press, New York.

Nieweg, H.O., Bouma, H.G., DeVries, K., *et al.* (1963). Haematological side effects of some antirheumatic drugs. *Ann. Rheum. Dis.* 22, 440.

Ochs, J. and Mulhern, R.K. (1988). Late effects of anti-leukaemic treatment. *Pediatr. Clin. North Am.* 35, 815.

Okafor, K.C., Griffin, C., and Ngole, P.M. (1986). Hydro-chlorothiazide-induced thrombocytopenic purpura. *Drug Intell. Clin. Pharm.* 20, 60.

Old, C.W., Flannery, E.P., Grogan, T.M., *et al.* (1978). Azathioprine-induced pure red cell aplasia. *JAMA* 240, 552.

Oski, F.A. (1979). Hematological consequences of chloramphenicol therapy. *J. Pediatr.* 94, 515.

Pai, R.G. and Pai, S.M. (1988). Methyldopa-induced reversible immune thrombocytopenia. *Am. J. Med.* 85, 123.

Patterson, W.P., Winkelman, M., and Perry, M.C. (1985). Zinc-induced copper deficiency: megamineral sideroblastic anaemia. *Ann. Intern. Med.* 103, 385.

Pau, A.K. and Fisher, M.A. (1987). Severe thrombocytopenia associated with once-daily rifampin therapy. *Drug Intell. Clin. Pharm.* 21, 882.

Pedersen-Bjergaard, J., Philip, P., Ravn, V., *et al.* (1988). Therapy-related acute non-lymphocytic leukaemia of FAB type M4 or 5 with early onset and t(9;11)(q21;Q23) or a normal karyotype: a separate entity? *J. Clin. Oncol.* 6, 395.

Peitzman, S.J. and Martin, C. (1980). Thrombocytopenia and minoxidil. *Ann. Intern. Med.* 92, 874.

Pena, J.M., Gonzalez, J.J., Garciaal, J., *et al.* (1985). Thrombo-cytopenia and sulfasalazine. *Ann. Intern. Med.* 102, 277.

Perry, A.R., Pagliuca, A., Fitzsimmons, E.J., *et al.* (1981). Digoxin-associated thrombocytopenia. *Eur. J. Clin. Pharmacol.* 19, 205.

Planas, A.T., Kranwinkel, R.N., Solitsky, H.B., *et al.* (1980). Chlorpropamide induced pure red blood cell aplasia. *Arch. Intern. Med.* 140, 707.

Polak, B.C.P., Wesseling, H., Schut, D., *et al.* (1972). Blood dyscrasias attributed to chloramphenicol. *Acta Med. Scand.* 192, 409.

Ponte, C.D. (1983). Carbamazepine-induced thrombocyto-penia, rash and hepatic dysfunction. *Drug Intell. Clin. Pharm.* 17, 642.

Popovic, K., Sknulovic, D., and Sknulovic, M. (1973). Sidero-blastic anemia in chronic phenacetin misuse. *Clin. Toxicol.* 6, 585.

Proctor, S.J. and Evans, R.G.B. (1985). Recognition of a chronic relapsing form of Hodgkin's disease in a population of patients demonstrating no second tumours. *Clin. Radiol.* 36, 461.

Pui, C.H., Behm, F.G., Raimondi, S.C., *et al.* (1989). Second-ary AML in children treated for ALL. *N. Engl. J. Med.* 321, 136.

Pui, C.H., Ribeiro, R.C., Hancock, M.L., *et al.* (1991). AML in children treated with epipodophyllotoxins for ALL. *N. Engl. J. Med.* 325, 1682.

Ramadurai, J., Shapiro, C., Kozloff, M., *et al.* (1993). Zinc abuse and sideroblastic anaemia. *Am. J. Haematol.* 42, 227.

Ramselaar, A.C., Pekker, A.W., Huber-Bruning, O., *et al.* (1987). Acquired sideroblastic anaemia after aplastic anaemia caused by D-penicillamine therapy for rheumatoid arthritis. *Ann. Rheum. Dis.* 46, 156.

Ratain, M.J., Kaminer, I.S., Bitran, J.D., *et al.* (1987). Acute non-lymphocytic leukaemia following etoposide and cisplatin combination chemotherapy for advanced non-small cell carcinoma of the lung. *Blood* 70, 1412.

Rayner, S.A. and Buckley, R.J. (1996). Ocular chlor-amphenicol and aplastic anaemia — is there a link? *Drug Safety* 14, 273.

Reid, G. and Patterson, A.C. (1977). Pure red cell aplasia after gold treatment. *BMJ* ii, 1457.

Retsagi, G., Kelly, J.P., and Kaufman, D.W. (1988). Risk of agranulocytosis and aplastic anaemia in relation to use of antithyroid drugs. *BMJ* 297, 262.

Ristuccia, A.M. (1985). Chloramphenicol: clinical pharma-cology in pediatrics. *Ther. Drug Monit.* 7, 159.

Rosenbloom, D. and Gilbert, R. (1981). Reversible flu-like syndrome, leukopenia, and thrombocytopenia induced by allopurinol. *Drug Intell. Clin. Pharm.* 15, 286.

Rudolph, A.E. and Price, E.V. (1973). Penicillin reactions among patients in venereal disease clinics: a national survey. *JAMA* 223, 499.

Schiavotto, C., Ruggeri, M., and Rodegheiro, F. (1993). Ad-verse reactions after high-dose intravenous immu-noglobulin: incidence in 83 patients treated for ITP and a review of the literature. *Haematologica* 78 (Suppl. 2), 35.

Schwartz, R.S. (1995). Autoimmune haemolytic anaemias. In *Hematology: Basic Practice* (2nd edn) (ed. R. Hoffman, E.J. Benz Jr, *et al.*), p. 710. Churchill Livingstone, New York

Scott, G.L., Myles, A.B., and Bacon, P.A. (1968). Auto-immune haemolytic anaemia and mefenamic acid therapy. *BMJ* iii, 534.

Scott, J.M. and Weir, D.G. (1980). Drug induced megaloblastic change. *Clin. Haematol.* 9, 587.

Shulman, N.R. (1972). Immunologic reactions to drugs. *N. Engl. J. Med.* 287, 408.

Smith, M.E., Reid, D.M., Jones, C.E., *et al.* (1987). Binding of quinine- and quinidine-dependent antibodies to platelets is mediated by the Fab domain of immunoglobulin G and is not Fc dependent. *J. Clin. Invest.* 79, 912.

Smyth, E.G. and Pallett, A.P. (1988). Clinician's guide to antibiotics. Chloramphenicol. *Br. J. Hosp. Med.* 39, 424.

Stevens, J.D. and Mission, G.P. (1987). Ophthalmic use of chloramphenicol. *Lancet* ii, 1456.

Stibbins, R. and Bertino, J.R. (1976). Megaloblastic anaemia produced by drugs. *Clin. Haematol.* 5, 619.

Stricker, B.H., Barendregt, J.N., and Claas, F.H. (1985). Thrombocytopenia and leucopenia with mianserin-depend-ent antibodies. *Br. J. Clin. Pharmacol.* 19, 102.

Suhrland, L.G. and Weisberger, A.S. (1969). Delayed clear-ance of chloramphenicol from serum in patients with hae-matological toxicity. *Blood* 34, 466.

Suzuki, S., Osalka, Y., Nakai, I., *et al.* (1996). Pure red cell aplasia induced by FK506. *Transplantation* 61, 831.

Takase, K., Nakano, T., Hamada, M., *et al.* (1993). Haemolytic anaemia provoked by recombinant alpha-interferon. *J. Gastroenterol.* 30, 795.

Talpaz, M., Kantarijan, H.M., McCredie, K.B., *et al.* (1987). Clinical investigation of human alpha-interferon in chronic myelogenous leukaemia. *Blood* 69, 1280.

Tang, T.T., Holcenberg, J.S., Duck, S.C., *et al.* (1993). Thyroid cancer following treatment for ALL. *Cancer* 45, 1572.

Taniguchi, S. and Hamada, T. (1996). Photosensitivity and thrombocytopenia due to amitriptyline. *Am. J. Haematol.* 53, 49.

Tefft, M., Vawter, G.F., and Mitus, A. (1968). Secondary primary neoplasms in children. *AJR* 103, 800.

Tolot, F., Prost, G., Guignot, B., *et al.* (1976). Manifestations multiples d'intolérance à une association d'anti-inflammatoires. Rôle de la phénylbutazone. *Sémin. Hop. Paris* 52, 185.

Tomlin, G.H. (1973). Isoniazid as a cause of neuropathy and sideroblastic anaemia. *Practitioner* 211, 773.

Tucker, M.A., Meadows, A.T., Boice, J.D. Jr, *et al.* (1987). Leukemia after therapy with alkylating agents for childhood cancer. *J. Natl Cancer Inst.* 78, 459.

Tucker, M.A., Coleman, C.A., Cox, R.S., *et al.* (1988). Risk of second cancers after treatment for Hodgkin's disease. *N. Engl. J. Med.* 318, 76.

Veldman, R.G., Vanderpijl, J.W., and Claas, F.H.J. (1996). Teicoplanin induced thrombocytopenia. *Nephron* 73, 721.

Verwilghen, R., Reybrouk, G., Callens, L., *et al.* (1965). Antituberculous drugs and sideroblastic anaemia. *Br. J. Haematol.* 11, 92.

Visentin, G.P., Newman, P.J., and Aster, R.H. (1991). Characteristics of quinine- and quinidine-induced antibodies specific for platelet glycoproteins IIb and IIIa. *Blood* 77, 2668.

von dem Borne, A.E.G., Pegels, J.G., van der Stadt, R.J., *et al.* (1986). Thrombocytopenia associated with gold therapy: a drug induced autoimmune disease?. *Br. J. Haematol.* 63, 509.

Wales, J. and Wolff, F. (1967). Haematological side effects of diazoxide. *Lancet* i, 53.

Walker, D.J., Saunders, P., and Griffiths, I.D. (1986). Gold induced thrombocytopenia. *J. Rheumatol.* 13, 225.

Walker, J.A., Sherman, R.A., and Eisinger, R.P. (1985). Thrombocytopenia associated with intravenous deferoxamine. *Am. J. Kidney Dis.* 6, 254.

Walker, R.W. and Heaton, A. (1985). Thrombocytopenia due to vancomycin. *Lancet* i, 932.

Wallerstein, R.O., Condit, P.K., Kasper, C.K., *et al.* (1969). State-wide study of chloramphenicol therapy and fatal aplastic anemia. *JAMA* 208, 2045.

Walterns, M. (1996) Enoxaparin heparin-induced thrombocytopenia syndrome. *Anaesth. Intens. Care* 24, 616.

Warkentin, T.E. and Kelton, J.G. (1989). Heparin-induced thrombocytopenia. *Annu. Rev. Med.* 40, 31.

Warkentin, T.E. and Kelton, J.G. (1990). Heparin and platelets. *Hematol. Oncol. Clin. North Am.* 4, 243.

Weh, H.J., Kabisch, H., Landbeck, G., *et al.* (1986). Translocation (9;11)(p21;q23) in a child with acute monoblastic leukaemia following two and a half years after successful chemotherapy for neuroblastoma. *J. Clin. Oncol.* 4, 1518.

Weinberger, I., Rotenberg, Z., Fuchs, J., *et al.* (1987). Amiodarone-induced thrombocytopenia. *Arch. Intern. Med.* 147, 735.

Wenz, B., Klein, R.L., and Lacezari, P. (1974). Tetracycline-induced immune hemolytic anemia. *Transfusion* 14, 265.

White, J.M., Brown, D.L., Hepner, G.W., *et al.* (1968). Penicillin induced haemolytic anaemia. *BMJ* iii, 26.

Wiholm, B.E. and Emanuelsson, S. (1996). Drug-related blood dyscrasias in a Swedish reporting system 1985–1994. *Eur. J. Haematol.* 57 (Suppl. 60), 42.

Williams, L.M.E., Joos, R., Proot, F., *et al.* (1987). Gold induced aplastic anaemia. *Clin. Rheumatol.* 6, 600.

Woolley, P.V.III, Sacher, R.A., Priego, V.M., *et al.* (1983). Methotrexate-induced immune haemolytic anaemia. *Br. J. Haematol.* 54, 543.

Youle, M. and Gazzard, B. (1990). The treatment of HIV disease. In *Clinical Haematology*, Vol. 3 (ed. C. Costello), p. 153. Baillière, London.

Yunis, A.A. (1973). Chloramphenicol induced bone marrow suppression. *Sem. Hematol.* 10, 225.

Yunis, A.A., Arimura, G.K., Lutcher, C.L., *et al.* (1967). Biochemical lesion in dilantin-induced erythroid aplasia. *Blood* 30, 587.

Zorab, P.A. (1960). Fulminating purpura during antituberculosis drug treatment. *Tubercle* 41, 219.

24. Part 2 Disorders of haemostasis

A. C. WOOD, P. J. CAREY, and S. J. PROCTOR

Introduction

In health, haemostasis is maintained by a complex series of dynamically interacting mechanisms involving vascular endothelium, platelets, plasma coagulation proteins and enzymes and their inhibitors, and the components of the fibrinolytic system. Drugs may affect this delicate balance in a wide variety of ways. Groups of drugs, such as oral and parenteral anticoagulants, and thrombolytic, antiplatelet, and antifibrinolytic agents are used to manipulate haemostatic mechanisms in the management of thromboembolic disease and haemorrhage. Haemorrhagic adverse reactions to these agents may result from overdosage, abnormal sensitivity in individuals to usual dosage, interactions with other drugs or agents, or idiosyncratic reactions. These drugs may also cause non-haemostatic adverse effects, which are discussed elsewhere in this book. Adverse haemostatic effects of other drugs usually occur because of a predominant effect on particular components of the normal haemostatic system.

This section will briefly review the physiological mechanisms of haemostasis, and then consider haemorrhagic adverse reactions to those agents that are used deliberately to manipulate those mechanisms, dealing mainly with haemostatic and adverse effects of antithrombotic and haemostatic agents. Lastly, adverse haemostatic effects of other drugs will be reviewed according to which component of the coagulation system is predominantly affected. The adverse reaction of thrombocytopenia has been dealt with in Part 1 of this chapter and is not further considered in detail.

Normal haemostasis

The major components of this dynamically interactive order are described here separately and briefly in order to clarify the causes of the adverse drug reactions discussed.

Platelets

These are non-nucleated discoid structures that circulate in the blood at a level of $150-400 \times 10^9$ per litre. Their outer membrane is extensively invaginated to form an interconnecting canalicular system of tubules which provide a large phospholipid surface that facilitates many plasma coagulation reactions. Several different types of glycoprotein molecule, including glycoprotein IIb IIIa project from the membrane surface, acting as receptors for other coagulation proteins, including thrombin, fibrinogen, and von Willebrand factor (VWF). These variously facilitate calcium release within the platelet, aggregation to other platelets, and attachment to damaged endothelium. Calcium release causes contractile proteins inside the outer membrane to effect shape changes in the activated platelet encouraging irreversibility of the aggregation phenomenon and forming a stable platelet plug at the site of injury. Activation is associated with release of inclusion-body contents. Dense bodies within the platelet contain vasoactive substances, such as 5-hydroxytryptamine, and aggregation stimulators including ADP, ATP, and adrenaline; α-granules contain coagulation proteins such as fibrinogen, factor V, factor VIII, β-thromboglobulin, thrombospondin, and multimerin. Calcium also stimulate the production of the potent vasoconstrictor thromboxane A_2 (TXA_2) from arachidonic acid available from the platelet membrane via the pathway shown in Fig. 24.2.

The amount of free calcium ion (Ca^{++}) available is heavily influenced by cyclic adenosine monophosphate (c-AMP). In general, high levels of c-AMP are associated with low levels of Ca^{++}, and vice versa.

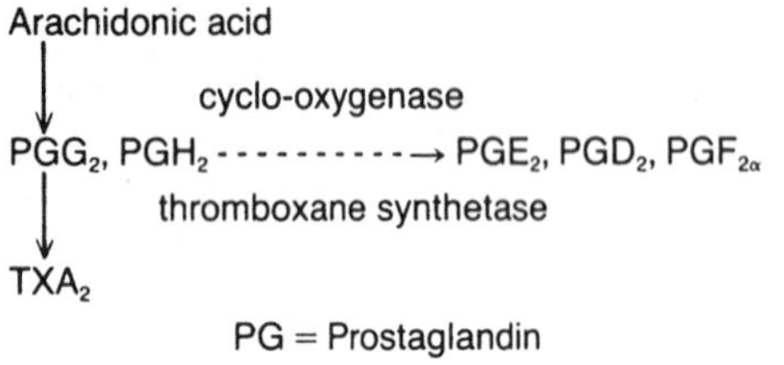

Arachidonic acid

$$\downarrow \quad \text{cyclo-oxygenase}$$

$$PGG_2, PGH_2 \dashrightarrow PGE_2, PGD_2, PGF_{2\alpha}$$

$$\downarrow \quad \text{thromboxane synthetase}$$

$$TXA_2$$

PG = Prostaglandin

FIG. 24.2.

Drugs may thus affect platelet function by several mechanisms, including interference with surface receptors, calcium availability, and prostaglandin metabolism.

Plasma coagulation

The formation of a stable fibrin clot from circulating soluble fibrinogen is mediated by a sequence of enzymatic reactions, depicted in simplified form in Fig. 24.3. The intrinsic pathway is activated by damaged endothelium, and the extrinsic pathway by exposure to extravascular tissue thromboplastins. After pathway activation, circulating inactive polypeptide factors are sequentially converted to active serine proteases which in turn activate the next in sequence, providing an amplifying cascade of molecular activation. The reactions occur on a phospholipid surface and require Ca^{++}. The generation of thrombin is central in this series of reactions in that it has both pro- and anticoagulant properties. Under normal circumstances initiation of the anticoagulant pathway provides a controlled coagulation cascade and clot formation at the site of injury. A series of feedback mechanisms initiate the anticoagulant side of the pathway.

The co-factors factor V and factor VIII catalyse, respectively, the activation of factor X by factor IX_a and the activation of prothrombin by factor X_a, enabling these reactions to occur many times faster. These co-factors are inhibited by protein C and its co-factor protein S, which are vitamin K-dependent and thus affected by oral anticoagulation in addition to factors II, VII, IX, and X. The inhibitor antithrombin III (AT III) inhibits factor X_a and also IX_a, XI_a, and XII_a. Heparin acts as a co-factor for this inhibitor.

Fibrinolysis

Once a haemostatic plug has formed and maintained the integrity of the vessel, the prevention of its propagation and its eventual removal occur by fibrinolysis. This is not a separate process, but is continuously interacting with coagulation. Fibrin is digested by the enzyme plasmin. Plasminogen is the inert precursor of plasmin and circulates in the blood. Activation of plasminogen to form plasmin is brought about by tissue plasminogen activator (tPA), produced by vascular endothelium. tPA also has a binding site for fibrin, thus localizing the activation of plasminogen to the site of clot. α_2-Antiplasmin and α_2-macroglobulin inhibit excess circulating plasmin. Plasminogen activator inhibitor, also produced by vascular endothelium, is a rapid inactivator of non-fibrin-bound tPA, preventing unwanted plasminogen activation in the circulation. In addition to fibrinolysis, plasminogen activation causes the cleavage of platelet and endothelial glycoprotein receptors for VWF and fibrinogen, thus impairing aggregation, a decrease in factors V and VIII, and an increase in fibrin degradation products (FDP) which inhibit plasma coagulation. Drugs that cause plasminogen activation are used in thrombolytic therapy.

Vascular endothelium

The balance between coagulation and fibrinolysis is regulated to a large extent by the endothelial cell lining of the circulation.

Against clot formation it provides a barrier protecting the blood from extravascular procoagulant stimuli, inhibits platelet aggregation, and encourages vasodilatation by producing prostacyclin, inhibits plasma coagulation by producing AT III and thrombomodulin (which binds thrombin and causes activation of protein C), and encourages fibrinolysis by producing tPA.

On the other hand, the endothelium expresses VWF, encouraging platelet adhesion, producing plasminogen activator inhibitor and, when damaged, initiating the intrinsic coagulation cascade.

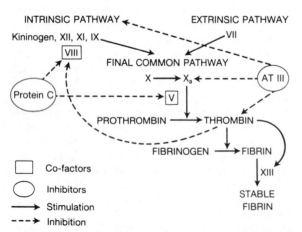

FIG. 24.3

Adverse reactions to antithrombotic drugs

Oral anticoagulants

These agents are widely used for the prophylaxis and treatment of venous thrombosis, the prevention of arterial thromboembolism, especially following prosthetic valvular replacement and myocardial infarction.

They are classified, according to their structure, into the coumarins, which include warfarin, the single most widely used agent; and the indanediones, of which phenindione is the most commonly prescribed example. They work by antagonizing the action of vitamin K, thus inhibiting production by the liver of functional forms of factors II, VII, IX, and X. They also inhibit the production of the co-factor inhibitor protein C.

Dosage requirements vary between individuals. Maintenance of an adequate therapeutic anticoagulant effect while minimizing the risk of haemorrhagic complications requires regular laboratory monitoring and appropriate dose adjustment. The most widely accepted control method uses the prothrombin time test performed with a thromboplastin reagent that has been standardized directly or indirectly against an international standard reference material. Test result times are expressed as a ratio of 'normal', standardized for the particular thromboplastin reagent used, and expressed as an international normalized ratio (INR). Therapeutic ranges for the INR lie within the limits of 2.0–4.5 and vary according to the indication for anticoagulation (British Society for Haematology 1990).

The dose required to maintain an individual within the therapeutic range may vary with time. Interaction with other concomitantly administered drugs is a major cause of difficulty with control (see below).

Haemorrhage

Bleeding is the major complication of anticoagulant therapy. Spontaneous bleeding, including bruising, subconjunctival haemorrhage, epistaxis, haemoptysis, haematemesis, melaena, haematuria, menorrhagia, and intracranial bleeding, are more common in patients taking oral anticoagulants, especially when control is poor.

In increased incidence of spontaneous splenic rupture has also been reported (Blankenship and Indeck 1993). Haemorrhagic risk appears to be highest during initial therapy with the monthly risk of major bleeding falling from 3 per cent in the first month to 0.3 per cent after the first year of treatment (Landefeld and Goldman 1989).

Specific patient-related risk factors include the presence of other serious pathology, especially renal, gastrointestinal, cerebrovascular and cardiovascular disease, increasing age, trauma, invasive procedures, and the use of other antithrombotic agents. Intensity of anticoagulation is a significant factor. Randomized trials have shown that less intense therapy is associated with a lower risk of clinically significant bleeding (Landefeld and Beyth 1993; Levine et al. 1995) Landefeld and colleagues (1990) developed a bleeding risk index to estimate the likelihood of major bleeding in the hospitalized patient commencing long-term anticoagulation.

Apart from drug interactions, poor control may result from lack of compliance, intercurrent infection, alcohol ingestion, and other dietary factors.

Drug interactions affecting control of oral anticoagulant therapy

Drugs may affect oral anticoagulation in several ways. Those which reduce the intestinal absorption of vitamin K will potentiate the anticoagulant effect. Potentiation may also occur as a result of displacement of the anticoagulant from plasma albumin binding, increasing the level of active free drug. Agents may affect the metabolism of anticoagulants by the microsomal enzymes in the liver either by inducing these enzymes, enhancing drug elimination and reducing anticoagulant effect, or by inhibiting enzymes and potentiating anticoagulation. Warfarin exists as a mixture of the R and S optical isomers, the latter being some five times more active than the former in terms of anticoagulant effect. There are differences in the microsomal metabolism of the two isomers, and in the presence of some drugs effects may occur because of preferential metabolism of one isomer. Table 24.11 lists some drugs that may have an important interaction with oral anticoagulant treatment.

Changes in, or short-term intermittent courses of, concomitant therapy are much more likely to cause difficulty with anticoagulant control than stable long-term therapy with a constant dose of another agent.

Skin necrosis

An important non-haemorrhagic adverse effect of warfarin is the occasional occurrence of a necrotic skin rash during the induction phase of therapy. Pathogenesis is not fully understood but diffuse thrombosis in small vessels has been found, initially described in patients with heterozygous protein C deficiency (Broekmans et al. 1983; McGehee et al. 1983;. Samama et al. 1984). This coagulation inhibitor is also Vitamin K dependent and has a half vitamin K dependent and has a half-life of 6 hours, similar to that of factor VII, but shorter than those of the other vitamin K-dependent factors (Weiss et

TABLE 24.11
Drugs that may affect oral anticoagulation

Drugs that may potentiate oral anticoagulants

Amitriptyline	Ciprofloxacin	Metronidazole
Aspirin	Clofibrate	Nalidixic acid
Allopurinol	Danazol	Norfloxacin
Aminoglycosides	Disulfiram	Omeprazole
Amiodarone	Erythromycin	Oxyphenbutazone
Androgenic steroids	Fluoxetine	Paracetamol
Azapropazone	Glucagon	Piroxicam
Bezafibrate	α-Interferon	Quinidine
Cephalosporins	Itraconazole	Sulphonamides
Chloral hydrate	Ketoconazole	Tetracyclines
Chloramphenicol	Mefenamic acid	Tamoxifen
Cimetidine		

Drugs that may reduce the effect of oral anticoagulants

Azathioprine	Dichloral-	Mercaptopurine
Barbiturates	phenazone	Vitamin K
Carbimazole	Glutethimide	Phenytoin
Cholestyramine	Griseofulvin	Rifampicin
Cyclophosphamide	Haloperidol	Thiouracils
Cyclosporin		

al. 1987). Thus, during the early stages of oral anticoagulation there is a state of increased tendency to thrombosis, especially when protein C levels are already low. It has also been described in protein S and AT III deficiency and, rarely, in individuals who are not deficient.

Warfarin resistance

The commonest reason for failure to achieve anticoagulation with oral agents is poor patient compliance. Occasionally, however, a patient may be genuinely resistant to anticoagulation with warfarin. Satisfactory control can then usually be achieved with an indanedione.

Rebound hypercoagulability

The sudden termination of therapy with coumarin anticoagulants has previously been thought to increase the risk of further thromboembolism but controlled trials do not substantiate this theory. Sudden or gradual withdrawal of therapy is associated with the same risk unless withdrawal is on account of severe bleeding complications (Sixty Plus Reinfarction Group 1980).

Heparin

This parenteral anticoagulant is widely used for the initial treatment and for the prevention of venous and arterial thrombosis and for maintaining blood fluidity in vascular catheters and extracorporeal circulations.

Standard unfractionated heparin (UFH) is a naturally occurring sulphated glycosaminoglycan usually derived from bovine or porcine lung and intestinal mucosa. It has a heterogeneous molecular weight varying from 5000 to 30 000. A specific tetrasaccharide sequence binds to AT III, enhancing this molecule's inhibition of thrombin and activated factors X, XI, and XII. Heparin also binds directly to thrombin, exerting an important anticoagulant effect. This is greater for the higher-molecular-weight forms, which bind to both AT III and thrombin in a ternary complex. Lower-molecular weight forms more specifically inhibit X_a activity. UFH is unable to inhibit thrombin bound to fibrin and X_a bound to platelets.

Heparin has a short half-life in the circulation of about 90 minutes. It may be given by intermittent bolus or continuous intravenous infusion; the latter method avoids wide fluctuations and is associated with fewer haemorrhagic complications (Salzman et al. 1975; Glazier and Crowell 1976). Subcutaneous administration is usually used for low-dose prophylaxis but can also be used to deliver full-dose anticoagulation (Walker et al. 1987).

Maintenance of adequate anticoagulation while minimizing the risk of haemorrhage requires dosage adjustment according to results of laboratory control tests. Conventionally, the partial thromboplastin time (PTT) test is used. This has a more useful response curve over the therapeutic range than the thrombin time, though the latter is more sensitive to small amounts of heparin. Alternatively, an indirect assay of heparin may be performed, usually by assessing X_a inactivation with a chromogenic substrate.

Low-molecular-weight heparins (LMWH)

LMWH are prepared by the depolymerisation of unfractionated heparin (molecular weight 4000–5000). These heparin fragments with smaller saccharide units catalyse the inhibition of anti-X_a including platelet bound X_a. with less antithrombin activity than UFH. Compared with UFH, the various LMWH available all have increased bioavailability, longer half-life, and much less variation in dose response, so that weight adjusted dosing is possible. Monitoring is not routinely required hut as the APTT is not prolonged by LMWH the anti-X_a assay is used. Reduced interaction with platelet function and vascular permeability potentially reduces adverse effects especially those due to microvascular bleeding. LMWH are increasingly used for prophylaxis and treatment of thrombosis, and controlled trials confirm equal or greater efficacy compared with UFH, with fewer adverse effects (Turpie et al. 1986; Pineo and Hull 1997).

Haemorrhage

Spontaneous haemorrhage, particularly soft-tissue bleeding such as wound haemorrhage following surgery, cannula insertions, and intramuscular injections, and including the potentially dangerous complication of retroperitoneal bleeding, may occur. Risk increases with heparin dose and with patient age, particularly in women (Holm *et al.* 1985); severity of concomitant illness, especially renal failure ; administration of other agents interfering with coagulation, such as aspirin (Walker and Jick 1980); and a previous bleeding tendency (Salzman *et al.* 1975).

The relatively reduced antithrombin effect compared with anti-factor X_a activity of low-molecular-weight LMWH fractions suggested the theoretical possibility of a more favourable ratio of antithrombotic effect to haemorrhagic risk for these agents, and this has now been borne out in clinical trials.

Rebound hypercoagulability may occur if protamine sulphate is used to reverse the effects of heparin.

Thrombocytopenia

Heparin-induced thrombocytopenia (HIT) with its thromboembolic complications is a serious adverse reaction that is less common with LMWH and is discussed in Part 1 of this chapter.

Heparinoids

Danaparoid sodium (Orgaran) is a mixture of heparan sulphate, dermatan sulphate, and chondroitin sulphate and has high anti-X_a activity. As there is little cross-reactivity with UFH and LMWH its main use is as an anticoagulant in HIT.

Antithrombin agents

Direct inhibitors of thrombin such as hirudin, hirudin analogues, factor X_a inhibitors, and recombinant versions of endogenous anticoagulants have been under increasing investigation over the last few years.

Hirudin is a 65-amino-acid polypeptide isolated from the salivary gland of the leech *Hirudo medicinalis*. It is a potent inhibitor of thrombin and is now available in recombinant form. Hirudin and its derivatives inhibit clot-bound and fluid-phase thrombin, and adrenaline-induced platelet aggregation. Although clinical trials indicate a predictable response, a fine balance exists with an increased risk of intracranial haemorrhage following thrombolysis with higher doses of hirudin (GUSTO-II 1994; TIMI 9A 1990). Age, hypertension and low body-

weight also increase the risk of intracranial haemorrhage (Armstrong and Mant 1995; Hirsh *et al.* 1995). Use of lower doses in conjunction with thrombolytic therapy is being evaluated. Bleeding may be reversed by prothrombinase-complex concentrates (PCC). Ancrod is a purified defibrinating agent derived from the Malayan pit viper which cleaves fibrinopeptide A from fibrinogen to produce non-cross-linked fibrin. It provides an alternative therapy if heparin is contraindicated, and has been successfully used in patients with HIT (Cole *et al.* 1993; Soutar and Ginsberg 1993).

Thrombolytic therapy

Thrombolytic agents are used in the management of peripheral arterial thromboembolic disease, massive pulmonary embolism, severe proximal deep-vein thrombosis, and for the unblocking of vascular catheters.

The agents available all act directly or indirectly as activators of plasminogen, reacting more or less selectively with fibrin-bound plasminogen. Streptokinase (SK) is a protein derived from β-haemolytic streptococcal culture. Urokinase (UK) is a trypsin-like protease derived from human urine, with similar thrombolytic properties but avoiding the problem of inactivation by antistreptococcal antibodies. Recombinant DNA technology yielded the further agents acylated plasminogen–streptokinase complex (APSAC), recombinant single-chain and double-chain tissue plasminogen activator (tPA), and recombinant single-chain urokinase plasminogen activator (scuPA) (Marder and Sherry 1988). Thrombolytic agents produce maximal activation of fibrin-bound plasminogen, but the various agents differ in their propensity to activate plasma plasminogen, resulting in fibrinogen proteolysis and a so-called lytic state. This effect is minimal with r-tPA and r-scuPA, which are more fibrin-selective, moderate with UK, and greatest with SK and APSAC (Marder and Sherry 1988). Large randomized trials in the 1980s demonstrated impressive results in terms of mortality reduction and limitation of ventricular damage when these agents were used early in myocardial infarction, especially when sequential aspirin treatment followed the initial thrombolysis (ISIS-2 1988; GISSI 1987; AIMS 1988; Van der Werf and Arnold 1988).

Haemorrhage

The relatively hypocoagulable state which may result from thrombolytic therapy is remarkably well tolerated by an intact vascular system. Bleeding complications therefore most frequently arise at sites of vascular injury or tissue damage. The incidence of major bleeding complications is thus relatively low, provided that these agents are not used inappropriately in patients with recent trauma or surgery, peptic ulceration, hypertension, or pre-existing coagulation impairment. This incidence is not related to the degree of hypofibrinogenaemia (TIMI-9A 1987), but is related to the duration and intensity of therapy. For example prolonged treatment with SK followed by heparin anticoagulation for deep-vein thrombosis (DVT) is associated with an incidence of serious bleeding (intracranial or requiring transfusion) of about 5 per cent (Goldhaber *et al.* 1984). Short-term use of this agent in AMI produces rates for example, of haemorrhagic stroke of O.1 per cent, bleeding requiring transfusion 0.5 per cent, and minor bleeds in 2 per cent (ISIS-2 1988).

Because most bleeding episodes are associated with sites of existing tissue injury, rather than caused by the so-called lytic state. the newer fibrin-selective agents have not been associated with a lower incidence of these adverse effects. The first extensive studies to address this compared SK with tPA. SK was associated with a greater degree of hypofibrinogenaemia than tPA in the 1988 TIMI study (Rao *et al.* 1988), but no greater incidence of haemorrhagic complications.

The subsequent GISSI-2 study (GISSI 1990), comparing tPA and SK in a randomized study of 12 490 patients, found a slightly but significantly higher incidence of major bleeds in the SK group (1 per cent) compared with the tPA group (0.5 per cent), although this was more marked in patients receiving sequential heparin (half the patients in each group) and the heparin at their dosage did not improve the therapeutic end points (mortality and severe left ventricular damage). Also the incidence of stroke was higher in the tPA group (1.1 per cent vs. 0.9 per cent in the SK group) although this was not statistically significant.

The GUSTO study (GUSTO Investigators 1993) compared four therapeutic strategies: SK with SC heparin, SK with IV heparin, 'accelerated' (rapid administration) tPA with IV heparin, and SK plus tPA with IV heparin. The rates of haemorrhagic stroke in the four groups respectively were 0.49 per cent, 0.54 per cent, 0.72 per cent, and 0.94 per cent, representing a significant excess for the tPA-containing regimens. The combined end point of death or disabling stroke was, however, significantly lower in the accelerated tPA group than the SK groups, indicating superior cardiovascular efficacy at the expense of a smaller increase in this haemorrhagic complication.

The risk of haemorrhage for an individual must be weighed against the likely benefit of thrombolysis, depending on the severity of the thromboembolic problem. For thrombolytic therapy in AMI, a strategy of individual risk assessment for intracranial haemorrhage was developed using data from several international databases (Simoons *et al.* 1993). These workers found four independent predictors by multivariate analysis: age over 65 years; body weight below 70kg; hypertension on hospital admission; and administration of tPA.

For proximal DVT, despite evidence that thrombolytic therapy may be more effective than heparin alone at preventing late post-phlebitic sequelae (Rogers and Lutcher 1990), it is arguable that the risk of potentially serious haemorrhage should preclude its use in this situation (O'Meara *et al.* 1994).

Allergic/hypotensive reactions

Probably because of previous exposure to streptococcal antigens, acute allergic reactions to SK (3.6 per cent) and APSAC (5.1 per cent) are more common than with tPA (0.8 per cent) (ISIS-3 1992). They include fever, angioedema, bronchospasm, and anaphylaxis, but most are minor and only 10 per cent give rise to persistent symptoms. Their incidence was not influenced by prophylactic steroids (ISIS-2 I988).

Treatment with SK or APSAC may produce a rise in anti-SK antibody titres that may persist for 6–12 months (Jalihal and Morris 1990). For this reason, if further thrombolytic treatment is required within this time, a non-antigenic recombinant agent is recommended.

Antiplatelet agents

A number of drugs with antiplatelet effects, such as aspirin, dipyridamole, prostacyclin, ticlopidine, and dextran are used in the treatment or secondary prevention of such arterial thromboembolic diseases as myocardial infarction, transient ischaemic attacks, and peripheral vascular disease.

Many other drugs may have incidental unwanted effects on platelet function mediated by similar mechanisms and these are discussed in the next section.

Antiplatelet effects of drugs may only become apparent as abnormalities on *in vitro* testing, or may cause prolongation of the bleeding time, purpura or mucocutaneous bleeding, or haemorrhagic problems following trauma or surgery. Difficulties are more frequently encountered if there is an underlying haemorrhagic disorder or concomitant anticoagulant therapy.

Aspirin acts as an inhibitor of cyclo-oxygenase (Roth and Majerus 1975) thereby inhibiting platelet production of TXA_2. Prostacyclin production by endothelial cells is also inhibited, but because endothelial cells are able to synthesize cyclo-oxygenase the antiplatelet effect is greater (Kallmann *et al.* 1987). Randomised trials have confirmed that it is an effective antithrombotic agent in doses ranging from 75 mg to 1.2 g daily, the lower doses being associated with fewer adverse events. No increase in major haemorrhage has been reported when used in conjunction with coumarins or thrombolytics but there is an excess of minor bleeding. The small increased incidence of haemorrhagic stroke is masked by patients at risk of thromboembolic events but is an important consideration if contemplating primary prevention in a low-risk population (Hirsh *et al.* 1995).

Dipyridamole inhibits platelet phosphodiesterase, causing a rise in platelet c-AMP and hence reduced Ca^{++} availability. It has no proven antithrombotic effect when used as a single agent and when combined with aspirin is no more effective than aspirin alone. Systemic embolism in patients already on warfarin may be reduced.

Prostacyclin, in addition to being a potent vasodilator, is an inhibitor of platelet aggregation as it also causes an increase in c-AMP.

Ticlopidine is a thienopyridine derivative. It is useful if aspirin cannot be tolerated or if it has failed to prevent recurrent thromboembolism. Adverse effects include neutropenia and thrombocytopenia, as described in the previous chapter. More recently TTP has been described (Ariyoshi *et al.* 1995). The overall risk of minor bleeding can be estimated at 10 per cent of all patients, with an increased bleeding time if used in combination with aspirin. Concomitant corticosteroids reduce bleeding.

Dextran is a neutral polysaccharide with a large molecular mass (40–70 kDaltons). Molecules are absorbed onto the platelet surface impairing aggregation and adhesion.

Anagrelide is a powerful anti-aggregating agent belonging to the imidazoquinazone series of compounds. Its major use is in the treatment of thrombocytosis.

Glycoprotein IIb–IIIa antagonists

The platelet IIb–IIIa membrane receptor is pivotal in platelet aggregation through fibrinogen binding. New agents, for example, integrelin, abciximab, bind to this receptor thus preventing aggregation. Clinical trials reported assess their efficacy in acute platelet-dependent ischaemic syndromes such as unstable angina and post-coronary angioplasty (Epic study 1994). Major bleeding events are variable but appear to be related to dose and weight (Ohman *et al.* 1995; Tcheng and Durham 1995).

Adverse reactions to haemostatic drugs

Antifibrinolytic agents

These drugs inhibit plasminogen activation. Amino-caproic acid and tranexamic acid bind to plasminogen by its lysine binding site and prevent association with fibrin so that activation cannot occur. They are useful systemically for troublesome mucosal bleeding such as epistaxis and menorrhagia, especially in haemophilia and von Willebrand's disease. They may also be used to treat systemic fibrinolysis and, if necessary, to attempt to reverse the effect of thrombolytic therapy. Tranexamic acid is also used as a topical agent.

These agents may precipitate ureteric obstruction by formation of a clot if there is haematuria, which is therefore a contraindication to their use. They should not be given to patients with recent thromboembolic disease.

Desmopressin

Deamino-D-arginine vasopressin (DDAVP, Desmopressin) is a synthetic neuropeptide developed for the management of diabetes insipidus. In addition to its antidiuretic effects it increases endogenous levels of factor VIII and von Willebrand factor. It is used in the management of mild haemophilia and von Willebrand's disease, allowing avoidance of exposure to blood products, and has also been effective in bleeding due to platelet dysfunction in uraemia and in cardiac surgery. It causes thrombocytopenia in patients with type IIb von Willebrand's disease, in which it is therefore contraindicated. It may cause water retention and hypernatraemia. Fluid balance monitoring and avoidance of excess intake are necessary precautions.

Factor concentrates

There is an increased incidence of thromboembolic complications with the use of factor IX and prothrombin complex concentrates (Kasper 1975). These are used for treating bleeding episodes in congenital factor IX deficiency, and to supplement replacement treatment in other haemorrhagic states such as liver disease, oral anticoagulant overdosage, and disseminated intravascular coagulation (DIC). Factor VIII inhibitor bypass agent (FEIBA) is used to treat haemorrhage in patients with antibodies to factor VIII, and is also associated with thrombotic complications.

Adverse haemostatic reactions to other drugs

Drugs interfering with platelet function

Cyclo-oxygenase inhibitors

Aspirin has been discussed above. Many non-steroidal anti-inflammatory drugs, such as ibuprofen, indomethacin, naproxen, and phenylbutazone, and the uricosuric sulphinpyrazone, have a similar effect (Simon and Mills 1980). In some cases this effect is reversible, whereas in the case of aspirin the effect on the bleeding time lasts for 5–7 days (i.e. for the life of the affected platelets, rather than the half-life in the circulation of the drug).

Drugs increasing platelet c-AMP levels

In addition to dipyridamole and prostacyclin (see above), theophylline and caffeine have this effect, and may prolong the bleeding time.

Drugs interfering with the platelet surface

Dextran (see above) is used therapeutically for this purpose, but if it or hydroxyethyl starch are used as plasma expanders the antiplatelet effect may be an unwanted adverse reaction.

High doses of a penicillin can cause prolongation of the bleeding time in normal volunteers and may cause bleeding problems in patients (Sattler *et al.* 1986). The proposed mechanism of action is via binding to the platelet membrane and interference with adhesion (Cazenave *et al.* 1973). Similar effects have been reported with moxalactam, some cephalosporins, and nitrofurantoin.

Non-thrombocytopenic purpura

The clinical manifestation of purpura is most often due to thrombocytopenia or to defective platelet function. A similar picture can, however, be caused by damage to small blood vessels either by immunological mechanisms or by changes in vascular permeability. A list of drugs that have been associated with this phenomenon is given in Table 24.12 (Bloom and Thomas 1987).

Drugs affecting plasma coagulation

Hypoprothrombinaemia

Reduction in the vitamin K-dependent clotting factors has been mentioned above in connection with oral anticoagulation. Depletion of these factors with prolongation of the prothrombin time is a recognized adverse

TABLE 24.12
Drugs associated with non-thrombocytopenic purpura

Aspirin	Digoxin	Oestrogens
Allopurinol	Frusemide	Penicillins
Arsenicals	Gold salts	Phenacetin
Atropine	Iodides	Piperazine
Barbiturates	Indomethacin	Procaine
Belladonna	Isoniazid	Quinine
Chloral hydrate	Meprobamate	Quinidine
Chloramphenicol	Mercury	Reserpine
Chlorothiazide	Methyldopa	Sulphonamides
Chlorpropamide	Nifedipine	Tolbutamide
Coumarins		

effect of cephalosporin antibiotic therapy (Betchold 1984 *et al.* 1984; Conjera *et al.* 1988).

Factor X deficiency

Acquired factor X deficiency with an associated clinical bleeding disorder has been reported as a complication of treatment with the cytotoxic drug amsacrine (Carter and Winfield 1988).

Disseminated intravascular coagulation

This widespread inappropriate deposition of fibrin in the circulation occurs secondarily to a wide variety of causes involving extensive tissue damage. The cytotoxic drug colaspase (asparaginase), commonly used in the treatment of acute lymphoblastic leukaemia, is recognized occasionally to cause this phenomenon (Legnani *et al.* 1988). This may be due to acquired low antithrombin III levels.

Thrombotic thrombocytopenic purpura (TTP)

This rare disorder is characterized by the inappropriate deposition of platelet plugs in the microcirculation; it manifests as thrombocytopenia and a microangiopathic haemolytic anaemia associated with fever, renal failure, and neurological abnormalities. The aetiology is thought to be due to endothelial damage. Cyclosporin A, ticlopidine, FK506, Norplant contraceptive system, and H$_2$-antagonist therapy have all been implicated as potential causes (Dzik *et al.* 1987; Holman *et al.* 1993; Kallal and Lee 1996; Fraser *et al.* 1996).

Thrombosis
(See also Chapter 9)

Many interacting factors, including drug therapy, have been recognized to be associated with an increased risk of arterial or venous thromboembolic disease. As well as the classical risk factors, inherited abnormalities have become increasingly recognized as important predisposing risk factors.

Oral contraceptive pill

There has been a long-established association between use of the oral contraceptive pill (OC) and a four- to ninefold increased incidence of venous thromboembolic disease. This risk is considerably greater if other thrombotic risk factors are present, as illustrated by the increased incidence of thromboembolism in women with inherited thrombophilia who take OC. This is recognized especially with the more frequent abnormalities such as activated protein C resistance (APCR) due to factor V Leiden. Epidemiological studies confirm that the use of third-generation OC containing desgestrel, gestodene, or norgestimate have a higher risk of venous thrombosis than that associated with second-generation OC containing levonorgestrel. Recent evidence suggests that this may be due to a form of acquired APCR (Rosing *et al.* 1997). Hormone replacement therapy is also associated with an increased incidence of venous thromboembolism, albeit smaller (two- to threefold). No difference between the different preparations has been reported. The use of 'emergency contraception' has not been associated with an increase in thrombosis (Webb and Tabener 1993).

Lupus anticoagulant

This acquired anticardiolipin antibody, first detected in systemic lupus erythematosus, interferes with plasma coagulation *in vitro*, causing prolongation of the partial thromboplastin time, but associated clinically with a predisposition to thrombosis rather than a bleeding diathesis. It has also been found in patients receiving treatment with procainamide (Heyman *et al.* 1988) or with α-interferon.

Type of reaction

Most of the adverse reactions described above are of Type A, the exceptions being immune thrombocytopenia and, possibly, osteoporosis, disseminated intravascular coagulation, thrombotic thrombocytopenic purpura, and thrombosis due to lupus anticoagulant, which are Type B (see Chapter 5).

References

AIMS Trial Study Group (1988). Effect of intravenous APSAC on toxicity after acute myocardial infarction: Preliminary report of a placebo-controlled clinical trial. *Lancet* i, 545.

Armstrong, P.W. and Mant, M.]. (1995). Bleeding risks, risk factors and management of bleeding complications after treatment with anticoagulants, specific antithrombins, or IIb–IIIa receptor blockers. *Eur. Heart J.* 161, 75.

Ariyoshi, K., Shinohara, K., and Ruirong, X. (1997). Thrombotic thrombocytopenic purpura caused by ticlopidine, successfully treated by plasmapheresis. *Am. J. Hematol.* 54, 175.

Betchold, H., Andrassy, K., and Jahnchen, E. (1984). Evidence for impaired hepatic vitamin K metabolism in patients treated with *N*-methyl thiotetrazole cephalosporins. *Thromb. Haemost.* 51, 358.

Blankenship, J.C. and Indeck, M. (1993). Spontaneous splenic rupture complicating anticoagulant or thrombolytic therapy. *Am. J. Med.* 94, 433.

Bloom, A.L. and Thomas, D. P. (1987). *Haemostasis and Thrombosis* (2nd edn). Churchill Livingstone, Edinburgh.

British Society for Haematology (1990). Guidelines on oral anticoagulant control.

Broekmans, A.W. and Bertina, R.M. (1990). Protein C. In *Recent Advances in Blood Coagulation 4* (ed. L. Poller), p. 117. Churchill Livingstone, Edinburgh.

Carter, C. and Winfield, D.A. (1988). Factor X deficiency during treatment of relapsed acute myeloid leukaemia with amsacrine. *Clin. Lab. Haematol.* 10, 225.

Cazenave, J.P., Packman, M.A., Guccione, M.A., *et al.* (1973). Effects of penicillin G on platelet aggregation release and adherence to collagen. *Proc. Soc. Exp. Biol. Med.* 142, 159.

Cole, C.W., Bormanis, J., Luna, G.K., *et al.* (1993). Ancrod versus heparin for anticoagulation during vascular surgical procedures. *J. Vasc. Surg.* 17, 288.

Conjera, A., Bell, W., and Lipsky, J.J. (1988). Cefotetan and hypoprothrombinemia. *Ann. Intern. Med.* 108, 643.

Dzik, W.H., Georgi, B.A., Khettry, V., *et al.* (1987). Cyclosporin associated thrombotic thrombocytopenic purpura following liver transplantation: successful treatment with plasma exchange. *Transplantation* 44, 570.

Epic Investigators (1994). Use of a monoclonal antibody against the glycoprotein IIb/IIIa receptor in high risk coronary angioplasty. *N. Engl. J. Med.* 330, 956.

Fraser, J.L., Millenson, M., Malynn, E.R., *et al.* (1996). Possible association between Norplant contraceptive system and thrombotic thrombocytopenic purpura. *Obstet. Gynecol.* 87, 860.

GISSI (Gruppo Italiano per lo studio della streptochinasi nell 'infarto miocardico') (1987). Long-term effects of intravenous thrombolysis in acute myocardial infarction: final report of the GISSI study. *Lancet* ii, 871.

GISSI-2 (Gruppo Italiano per lo studio della sopravvivenza nell 'infarto miocardico') (1990). A factorial randomized trial of alteplase versus streptokinase and heparin versus no heparin among 12 490 patients with acute myocardial infarction. *Lancet* ii, 65.

Glazier, R.L. and Crowell, E.B. (1976). Randomised prospective trial of continuous vs intermittent heparin therapy. *JAMA* 236, 1365.

Goldhaber, S.Z., Buring, J.E., Lipnick, R.J., *et al.* (1984). Pooled analyses of randomized trials of streptokinase and heparin in phlebographically documented acute deep vein thrombosis. *Am. J. Med.* 76, 393.

GUSTO (Global Utilization of Streptokinase and Tissue plasminogen activator for Occluded coronary arteries) Investigators (1993). An international randomized trial comparing four thrombolytic strategies for acute myocardial infarction. *N. Engl. J. Med.* 329, 673.

GUSTO-II (1994). Randomized trial of intravenous heparin versus recombinant hirudin for acute coronary syndromes. *Circulation* 90, 1631.

Hall, J.D., Pavli, R.M., and Wilson, K.M. (1980). Maternal and fetal sequelae of anticoagulation during pregnancy. *Am. J. Med.* 68, 122.

Heyman, M.R., Flores, R.M., Edelman, B.B., *et al.* (1988). Procainamide induced lupus anticoagulant. *South. Med. J.* 81, 934.

Hirsh, J., Dalen, J.E., Fuster, V., *et al.* (1995). Aspirin and other platelet active drugs. *Chest* 1O8, 247.

Holm, H.A., Abildgaard, U., and Kalvenes, S. (1985). Heparin assays and bleeding complications in treatment of deep vein thrombosis with particular reference to retroperitoneal bleeding. *Thromb. Haemost.* 53, 278.

ISIS-2 (Second International Study of Infarct Survival) and Collaborative Group) (1988). Randomized trial of intravenous streptokinase, oral aspirin, both or neither among 17 187 cases of suspected acute myocardial infarction. *Lancet* ii, 349.

ISIS-3 (Third International Study of Infarct Survival) (1992). A randomized comparison of streptokinase vs. anistreplase and of aspirin plus heparin vs. aspirin alone among 41 299 cases of suspected acute myocardial infarction. *Lancet* 339, 753.

Jalihal, S. and Morris, G.K. (1990). Antistreptokinase titres after intravenous streptokinase. *Lancet* 335, 184.

Kallal, K.M., and Lee M/ (1996). Thrombotic thrombocytopenic purpura associated with histamine H2 receptor antagonist therapy. *West. J. Med.* 164, 446.

Kallmann, R., Niewenhuis, H.K., de Groot, P.G., *et al.* (1987). Effects of low doses of aspirin, 10 mg and 30 mg daily, on bleeding time, thromboxane production and 6-keto-PGF$_{1\alpha}$ excretion in healthy subjects. *Thromb. Res.* 45, 355.

Kasper, C.K. (1975). Factor IX concentrates: thromboembolic complications. *Thromb. Haemost.* 33, 640.

Landefeld, C.S. and Goldman, L. (1989). Major bleeding in outpatients treated with warfarin: incidence and prediction by factors known at the start of outpatient therapy. *Am. J. Med.* 87, 144.

Landefeld, C.S. and Beyth, J.R. (1993). Anticoagulant-related bleeding: Clinical epidemiology, prediction, and prevention. *Am. J. Med.* 95, 315.

Landefeld, C.S., Mcquire, E., and Rosenblatt, M.W. (1990). A bleeding risk index for estimating the probability of major bleeding in hospitalised patients starting anticoagulant therapy. *Am. J. Med.* 89, 569.

Legnani, C., Paleredi, G., Pession, A., Poggi, M., and Vecchi, V. (1988). Intravascular coagulation phenomenon associated with prevalent fall in fibrinogen and plasminogen during L-asparaginase treatment in leukaemic children. *Haemostasis* 18, 179.

Levine, M., Raskob, G.E., Landefeld, C.S. *et al.* (1995). Haemorrhagic complications of anticoagulant treatment. *Chest* 108, 276S.

Marder, V. and Sherry, S. (1988). Thrombolytic therapy: current status. *N. Engl. J. Med.* 23, 1512.

McGehee, W.G., Klotz, T.A., Epstein, D.J., *et al.* (1983). Coumarin induced necrosis in a patient with familial protein C deficiency. *Blood* 62 (Suppl.), 304(a).

Ohman, E.M., Harrington, R.A., Lincoff, A.M., *et al.* (1995). Early clinical experience with integrelin, an inhibitor of the platelet glycoprotein IIb/IIIa integrin receptor. *Eur. Heart J.* 16 (Suppl. L), 50.

O'Meara J.J., McNutt R.A., Evans A.T., *et al.* (1994). A decision analysis of streptokinase plus heparin as compared with heparin alone for deep vein thrombosis. *N. Engl. J. Med.* 330, 1864.

Pineo, G.F. and Hull, R.D. (1997). Low molecular weight heparin: Prophylaxis and treatment of venous thromboembolism. *Annu. Rev. Med.* 48, 79.

Rao, A.K., Pratt, C., and Berke, A. (1988). Thrombolysis in myocardial infarction (TIMI) trial phase 1: hemorrhagic complications and changes in plasma fibrinogen and fibrinolytic system in patients treated with recombinant tissue plasminogen activator and streptokinase. *J. Am. Coll. Cardiol.* 11, 1.

Rogers L.Q. and Lutcher L.L. (1990). Streptokinase therapy for deep vein thrombosis: a comprehensive review of the English literature. *Am. J. Med.* 88, 389.

Rosing, J., Tans, G., Nicholaes, G.A.F., *et al.* (1997). Oral contraceptives and venous thrombosis: different sensitivities to activated protein C in women using second and third generation oral contraceptives. *Br. J. Haematol.* 97, 233.

Roth, D.J. and Majerus, P.W. (1975). The mechanism of the effect of aspirin on human platelets: acetylation of a particulate fraction protein. *J. Clin. Invest.* 56, 624.

Sachs, B.P., Masterton, T., Jewett, J.F., *et al.* (1984). Reproductive mortality in Massachusetts in 1981. *N. Engl. J. Med.* 311, 1667.

Salzman, E.W., Deykin, D., Shapiro, R.M., *et al.* (1975). The management of heparin therapy. Controlled prospective trial. *N. Engl. J. Med.* 191, 1046.

Samama, M., Horrelou, M.H., Soria, J., *et al.* (1984). Successful programme of anticoagulation in severe protein C deficiency and skin necrosis at the initiation of oral anticoagulant treatment. *Thromb. Haemost.* 51, 132.

Sattler, F.R., Weittekamp, M.R., and Ballard, J.O. (1986). Potential for bleeding with the new beta lactam antibiotics. *Ann. Intern. Med.* 105, 924.

Simon, L.S. and Mills, J.A. (1980). Non-steroidal anti-inflammatory drugs. *N. Engl. J. Med.* 302, 1179.

Simoons M.L., Maggioni A.P., Knatterud G., *et al.* (1993). Individual risk assessment for intracranial haemorrhage during thrombolytic therapy. *Lancet* 342, 1523.

Sixty-plus Reinfarction Group (1980). A double-blind trial to assess long term oral anticoagulant therapy in elderly patients with myocardial infarction. *Lancet* ii, 989.

Soutar, R.L. and Ginsberg, J.S. (1993). Anticoagulant therapy with Ancrod. *Crit. Rev. Oncol. Haematol.* 15, 23.

Tcheng, J.E. and Durham, N.C.(1995). Enhancing safety and outcomes with the newer antithrombotic and antiplatelet agents. *Am. Heart J.* 130, 573.

Thrombolysis in Myocardial Infarction (TIMI) trial, phase I (1987). A comparison between intravenous tissue plasminogen activator and intravenous streptokinase. *Circulation* 76, 142.

TIMI-9A Trial — Antman, E.M. for the TIMI-9A Investigators (1990). Hirudin in acute myocardial infarction. Safety report from the Thrombolysis and thrombin Inhibition in Myocardial Infarction (TIMI) 9A trial. *Circulation* 89, 1545.

Turpie, A.G.G., Levine, M.N., Hirsch, J., *et al.* (1986). A randomized controlled trial of a low molecular weight heparin (enoxaparin) to prevent deep vein thrombosis in patients undergoing elective hip surgery. *N. Engl. J. Med.* 315, 925.

van der Werf, F. and Arnold, A.E.R. (1988). The European Co-operative Study Group for recombinant tissue type plasminogen activator: Intravenous tissue plasminogen activator and size of infarct, left ventricular function and survival in acute myocardial infarction. *Br. Med. J.* 297, 1374.

Walker, A.M. and Jick, H. (1980). Predictors of bleeding during heparin therapy. *JAMA* 244, 1209.

Walker, M.G., Shaw, J.W., Thomson, G.J.L., *et al.* (1987). Subcutaneous calcium heparin versus intravenous sodium heparin in treatment of established acute deep vein thrombosis of the legs: a multicentre prospective randomised trial. *Br. Med. J.*294, 1189.

Webb, A. and Tabener, D. (1993). Clotting factors after emergency contraception. *Advances in Contraception* 9, 75.

Weiss, P., Soff, G.A., Halkin, M., *et al.* (1987). Decline of proteins C and S and factor II, VII, IX and X during initiation of warfarin therapy. *Thromb. Res.* 45, 783.

25. Effects of drugs on infections

D. M. DAVIES

Introduction

Some drugs can aggravate, reactivate, or predispose to certain infections. They do this by weakening host defences against the micro-organisms; changing the environment of the organisms, so facilitating their multiplication; encouraging the emergence of more virulent organisms; or by making treatment with antimicrobial drugs less effective.

The host is protected against infection by the barriers presented to micro-organisms by properly functioning organs, and by intact skin and mucosal surfaces and the antimicrobial properties of the secretions produced by these. Other defences include active white blood cells and tissue macrophages; a lymphatic system of adequate mass and function; and effective inflammatory and immune responses. Drugs can undermine these defences in several ways. Some diminish the mass of lymphoid tissue, change the number and behaviour of white blood cells, reduce the intensity of the inflammatory reaction, and alter the immune response. A variety of drugs may damage blood-forming tissues, so reducing the number of circulating polymorphonuclear cells, while other agents induce changes in the function or response of these cells or of macrophages. Preparations of sex hormones may cause alterations in bodily structure and biochemistry that appear to predispose to infection. Antibacterial therapy alters the pattern of the body's bacterial flora, and this may lead to multiplication of drug-resistant organisms normally kept in check by force of numbers of their drug-susceptible fellows. Treatment with antibacterial drugs may also be responsible for changes within bacterial species, whereby resistant organisms flourish while drug-sensitive strains die out; and the survivors may possibly be more invasive than were the dead; and some resistant organisms are capable of transferring their powers of resistance to previously vulnerable neighbours.

Some of these actions deserve further consideration. Corticotrophin (ACTH) and adrenal glucocorticoids (but not deoxycorticosterone) damage lymphocytes and reduce the mass of lymphoid tissue (Sayers and Travis 1970). Under the influence of steroid therapy the number of circulating eosinophils diminishes and the migration and activity of phagocytes are impeded. The inflammatory process, characterized by oedema and capillary dilatation followed by capillary and fibroblast proliferation, collagen deposition and, finally, scar formation, is inhibited (Spain 1961).

Although corticosteroids are capable of reducing plasma concentrations of some immunoglobulins (Butler and Rosen 1973; Bond 1977; Christensen et al. 1985), in man when the drugs are given in ordinary therapeutic doses antibody production is not inhibited, as it is in some animal species, and response to antigen is normal (Butler 1975). Other elements of the immune process, including the complement system, also remain unimpaired, but delayed hypersensitivity is suppressed (Sayers and Travis 1970).

Most antineoplastic agents act, by various mechanisms, on cell growth; and some that are used for immunosuppression are particularly active in preventing lymphocyte proliferation and function. Such actions explain why these drugs suppress bone marrow activity, damage immunologically competent cells, and impair the immune response, so making patients more susceptible to infections of all kinds. These infections are not necessarily prevented by nursing such patients in a sterile environment, since the infecting organisms often come from the patient's own respiratory tract or gut (Lessof 1972).

In addition to corticosteroids, a variety of drugs can reduce serum concentrations of one or more of the immunoglobulins. Such drugs include the immunosuppressants, particularly azathioprine and cyclosporin; the antirheumatoid drugs gold and penicillamine; the anticonvulsants carbamazepine and phenytoin; dextrans;

and, in infants, thyroxine (Sorrell *et al.* 1971; Skrede *et al.* 1973; Gilhus *et al.* 1982; Bardana *et al.* 1984; van Reil *et al.* 1984; Seager 1984; Christensen *et al.* 1985; Webster 1987). However, this effect is not necessarily the main factor, or even a contributory one, in the aggravation, reactivation, or precipitation of the infections with which some of these drugs have been associated.

It has been suggested that the immune response can be impaired by a combination of the antimalarial drugs dapsone and pyrimethamine (Lee and Lau 1988); the antipsychotic drug clozapine (König *et al.* 1993); and the anticonvulsant zonisamide (Aitani *et al.* 1996).

Some drugs change certain elements of the inflammatory response in tissues. As examples: povidone–iodine, applied locally, may inhibit leucocyte migration and fibroblast aggregation in wounds (Vilijanto 1980); nitrogen mustard interferes with the release of lactic acid by phagocytes (Walter and Israel 1974), so diminishing their effectiveness against some micro-organisms; indomethacin impairs the mobility of polymorphonuclear leucocytes, while diclofenac aggravates the impairment of bactericidal activity present in rheumatoid arthritis (Youinou and Le Goff 1987); cimetidine reduces the number of suppressor/cytotoxic lymphocytes in mice (Osband *et al.* 1981), an observation that may have implications in human disease; Intralipid, a lipid emulsion used for parenteral nutrition, has been shown to impair the clearance of bacteria from the circulation and to enhance the virulence of bacteria in animals, and to inhibit the chemotaxis of human neutrophil leucocytes *in vitro*, and these findings suggest that the emulsion may increase the risk of bacterial infection in some patients (Fischer *et al.* 1980), as well as fungal infections (see below); iron–dextran appears to have an effect on macrophage activity, possibly because of the large dextran complexes present in the plasma (Becroft *et al.* 1977).

The relationship between infection and iron and desferrioxamine is a complex and fascinating one. Some workers have claimed that iron-deficient human infants have an increased susceptibility to infection (Arbeter *et al.* 1971), possibly because of impaired cellular immunity (Joynson *et al.* 1972; MacDougall *et al.* 1975) and disturbances in granulocyte function (Chandra 1944; Likhite *et al.* 1976; Yetgin *et al.* 1979; Swarup-Mitra and Sinha 1982). Lymphocyte function and the immune response may also be impaired in iron deficiency; but Masawe and others (1974) pointed out that, paradoxically, iron deficiency appears to protect against some infections. To complicate matters further, Masawe and colleagues (1974) drew attention to experiments *in vitro* and in laboratory animals (e.g. Fletcher and Goldstein 1970) demonstrating that elemental iron promotes the

growth, multiplication, and virulence of many micro-organisms; and it is well recognized that patients with iron overload are more susceptible than normal subjects to a variety of infections. The implications of these relationships as regards medical treatment are considered further under some of the specific infections discussed below.

It has long been known that tears, saliva, and nasal secretions have antibacterial properties (Wilson and Miles 1955). It has also been observed that nasal secretions carry antibodies to certain viruses (Allison 1972). It would not therefore be surprising if impaired secretion of tears predisposed to infection of the eyes, and reduced production of saliva to infection of the buccal mucosa and salivary glands, and clinical experience suggests that this is so. Elderly patients under treatment with drugs with anticholinergic properties (for example, tricyclic antidepressants) are prone to develop oral and lingual ulcers (Hall 1972), and it may be that these are infective in origin; but as yet there is no evidence that treatment with drugs that reduce nasal secretion predisposes to viral infections.

Antimicrobial properties have also long been attributed to another bodily secretion, gastric juice. In 1933 Kemps presented evidence to show that certain infections occur more commonly in people with hypochlorhydria than in those with normal gastric acid secretion, and in the following year Hurst, physician to Guy's Hospital, suggested that British servicemen due to be posted to the tropics should have gastric test meals and not be sent abroad if they had achlorhydria, which would make them vulnerable to certain tropical infections. The question of whether or not the reduction of gastric acidity produced by drugs used for this purpose may predispose to infection by ingested organisms normally destroyed by gastric acid has been the subject of much discussion. Some workers (Ruddell *et al.* 1980; Stockbrugger *et al.* 1981; Deane *et al.* 1982) have found significant alteration in the pattern of gastric microflora during cimetidine treatment, while others (Milton-Thompson *et al.* 1982) detected no such change. When the bacterial population of the small intestine was investigated, it was shown that the use of omeprazole promotes bacterial overgrowth, as does, to a lesser degree, ranitidine (Carulli *et al.* 1995). Clinical observations relating to this subject are discussed below under specific infections.

Almost all the adverse effects described in this chapter are the result of either the normal pharmacological action or the known chemical properties of the drugs concerned and can therefore be regarded as Type A reactions (see Chapter 5).

Bacterial infections

Some years after the introduction of the antibiotics, the emergence and spread of organisms (particularly staphylococci) resistant to many or all of the antibiotics available at the time became a serious problem. It has been observed that a high incidence of antibiotic-resistant organisms is often related to usage of a particular antibiotic and that a reduction in the use of an antibiotic is often followed by a reduction in the frequency with which resistant strains are isolated. If the use of antibiotics brings about an increase in population of resistant organisms, then this effect can be regarded as a drug reaction, though not an *adverse* reaction unless it can be shown that resistant organisms are more invasive (that is, more likely to cause new cases of infection) than non-resistant strains. Some studies have suggested that this may be the case.

An interesting change in bacterial metabolism following prolonged antibacterial therapy has been reported (Maskell *et al.* 1976). Patients given long-term, low-dose treatment with co-trimoxazole (sulphamethoxazole–trimethoprim) have occasionally been found to have become infected with bacteria dependent on thymine or thymidine for growth and resistant to co-trimoxazole. The organisms may survive *in vivo* because of the availability of thymine in the infected tissues; but they may not grow on culture media deficient in thymine, and this fact may be misinterpreted as meaning that the organisms are fully sensitive to the antibacterial agents against which they are being tested.

The factors that determine the emergence of strains of micro-organisms resistant to one or more antibacterial drugs are very complex, and for further information the reader is referred to comprehensive reviews (Brumfitt and Hamilton-Miller 1987), but there seems little doubt that excessive and inappropriate use of these drugs, particularly those with a very broad spectrum of activity, aggravates the situation and has led to the emergence of resistant organisms not only of familiar species but also those rarely encountered as pathogens in earlier times (e.g. *Acinetobacter* spp., *Corynebacterium jeikeium*, *Pseudomonas maltophila*, *Serratia* spp., and *Staphylococcus epidermidis*) which are now responsible for serious infections at a variety of sites (Midtvedt 1989). In the case of *Staphylococcus epidermidis*, its ability rapidly to become resistant to ciprofloxacin has been attributed to excretion of this drug in sweat, and other fluoroquinolones and some other antibacterial drugs that are excreted in this way might also develop resistance to skin bacteria for this reason (Høiby *et al.* 1997). Restricted and circumspect administration tends to reduce the development of resistant organisms.

It has been known for some time that there is an increased incidence of complications during and after surgical operations in patients undergoing long-term steroid therapy and that operations performed under 'steroid cover' are more likely to be followed by wound infection than operations on patients not so treated. Steroids, and also non-steroidal anti-inflammatory drugs, have also been shown to increase the risk of serious complications of operative treatment for diverticular disease of the colon, so that caution should be exercised when prescribing such drugs for patients with a history of diverticulosis (Corder 1987), and it was suggested that these drugs impair the ability of the colon to limit or terminate inflammatory processes occurring within diverticula or, alternatively or in addition, may mask symptoms, so that patients present with more advanced disease.

Staphylococcal infections

Broad-spectrum antibiotics, notably the tetracyclines, so alter the normal flora of the gut that pathogenic organisms resistant to the drugs may multiply inordinately for want of competition from their absent friends. Staphylococcal infection was once considered to be the main cause of the severe diarrhoea and enterocolitis that occasionally complicates treatment with broad-spectrum antibacterial drugs, not only when these drugs are given orally but also when they are given parenterally (Lundsgaard-Hansen *et al.* 1960) if some of the drug is excreted into the gut (as is the case with the tetracyclines). The disorder is a very serious one, the mortality rate in the past having been as high as 60 per cent (Spaulding 1962). In more recent times a diagnosis of staphylococcal enterocolitis has become very rare, the most recent case to be reported (which followed the prophylactic use of a cephalosporin) being complicated by hypochlorhydria resulting from subtotal gastrectomy (Morita *et al.* 1991); and it has been suggested that some of the cases attributed to *Staphylococcus aureus* may have been caused by *Clostridium difficile* (Phillips and Eykyn 1987). It should still, however, be included in the differential diagnosis (though less likely than infection with *Cl. difficile* — see below) when the condition of a patient who was previously making good progress deteriorates abruptly and anorexia, and abdominal pain or distension develop or worsen. Other infections due to resistant staphylococci that may follow antibacterial therapy include acute arthritis, osteomyelitis, parotitis, pneumonia, endocarditis, and septicaemia.

Staphylococcal infections may also complicate treatment with corticosteroids, immunosuppressive drugs, and the immunostimulant aldesleukin (recombinant interleukin-2) (Richards1991; Siegel and Puri 1991) and have followed the use of indomethacin for closure of patent ductus arteriosus in premature infants (Hersen *et al.* 1988). A most unusual case of staphylococcal septicaemia and the toxic shock syndrome occurred in a patient with hypogammaglobulinaemia complicated by a severe adverse reaction to carbamazepine (Bahamdan *et al.* 1995). During treatment of acne vulgaris with isotretinoin, marked changes occur in the skin, including almost total suppression of sebum production which, in turn, leads to dryness, inflammatory changes, and alteration in the bacterial population. The organism present in acne, *Propionibacterium acnes*, falls significantly in number, together with Gram-negative commensals. Colonization of the skin and anterior nares with *Staphylococcus aureus* follows in most patients, of whom a relatively small proportion develop folliculitis, furuncles, or even cellulitis, usually during or shortly after a course of treatment (Leyden and James 1987). Paronychia and pyogenic granuloma-like lesions may also arise (Blumenthal 1984).

Streptococcal infections

In animal experiments it has been shown that streptococcal infection of blood and tissues is markedly enhanced following cortisone injections (Mogabgab and Thomas 1950). Streptococcal infection commonly arises in patients suffering from drug-induced agranulocytosis, and may complicate treatment with steroids or with cytotoxic drugs, of which cytarabine has been implicated as a major risk factor for *Streptococcus viridans* septicaemia following its use in conjunction with bone marrow transplantation (Englehard *et al.* 1995). Unlike staphylococcal infection, it can rarely, if ever, be attributed to antibacterial therapy.

Infection with *E. coli* and other Gram-negative organisms

These bacteria have always been less susceptible to antibacterial drugs than Gram-positive organisms, but whether there has been any great increase in resistant strains is uncertain, and there is little evidence to suggest that resistant Gram-negative organisms are essentially more virulent than the drug-sensitive strains. It does seem, however, that with the increasing use of broad-spectrum antibiotics there has been an increase in the prevalence of serious infections caused by Gram-negative organisms. Treatment with an antibacterial drug may occasionally be complicated by infection with coliform organisms resistant to this and other drugs. Septicaemia may occur and has a high mortality rate. Coliform infections may also complicate long-term treatment with corticosteroid drugs and immunosuppressive agents; and an unusual case of coliform septicaemia has occurred in an elderly patient following a barium enema (Schwartz *et al.* 1994).

Ureteric dilatation analogous to that occurring in pregnancy is seen in some patients taking oral contraceptives (Marshall *et al.* 1966; Guyer and Delany 1970), and in some cases this appears to predispose to infection with coliform organisms.

Other Gram-negative organisms causing septicaemia in association with treatment with antibacterial agents, cytotoxic drugs, immunosuppressants, or indomethacin (in premature infants given it for closure of a patent ductus arteriosus) (Hersen *et al.* 1988), are *Klebsiella* spp., *Pseudomonas* spp., *Paracolon* bacteria, *Proteus* spp., and *Neisseria subflava* (Domingo *et al.* 1996). *Pseudomonas* bacteraemia has accompanied neutropenia induced by the antiplatelet drug ticlopidine (Geleto *et al.* 1996).

It has been observed that when corticosteroid creams, ointments, or sprays are used to treat varicose ulcers, these often increase rapidly in size and depth and commonly become severely infected with *Ps. aeruginosa (Ps. pyocyanea)*. Antibiotics or antibacterial substances contained in some preparations of this kind fail to prevent these secondary infections. While topical corticosteroids can be valuable in the treatment of stasis eczema, it is most important to prevent the medicament from entering any abrasion or ulcer within the treated area.

Barry and Reeve (1974) observed a high incidence of Gram-negative sepsis in Polynesian babies given injections of iron-dextran soon after birth as prophylactic or curative treatment for iron-deficiency anaemia. When this treatment was abandoned there was a dramatic fall in the incidence of infection. These workers suggested that iron given in this way might overcome immune mechanisms and promote infection (see earlier), and they advise against this method of treatment.

Chlamydial infections

Meta-analysis of 29 case–control studies supported the view that oral contraceptives increase susceptibility to *Chlamydia trachomatis* infection of the genital tract (Cottingham and Hunter 1992).

Salmonellosis, shigellosis, and *Campylobacter* gastroenteritis

The suggestion that a reduction in gastric acid might predispose patients to infection by ingested pathogens has been mentioned earlier, and further evidence supports this view. Thus Wingate (1990) suspected that omeprazole had precipitated recurrent enteric infections in some patients; Nwokolo and others (1994) blamed cimetidine, ranitidine, and omeprazole for a number of cases of diarrhoea caused by *Campylobacter,* salmonellae, or shigellae; and Neal and colleagues (1994; 1996) considered omeprazole to have predisposed to *Campylobacter* enteritis and H_2-antagonists to salmonellosis; but Scott and co-workers (1994), while agreeing that omeprazole increased susceptibility to *Campylobacter* infection, exonerated the H_2-antagonists in this respect.

Other drugs believed to have precipitated the infection are antibiotic therapy (Neal *et al.* 1994), antidiarrhoeal agents (Smith *et al.* 1990; Huppertz *et al.* 1991), antilymphocytic globulin combined with corticosteroids (Allard *et al.* 1992), and corticosteroids combined with radiotherapy (Cortes *et al.* 1992).

Cholera

The possibility that patients taking drugs that reduce gastric acidity might be more susceptible to infection by swallowed organisms has been mentioned earlier. It was for this reason that, while studying cholera in 1892, Max von Pettenkofer, professor of hygiene at Munich, took sodium bicarbonate to neutralize gastric acid when he ingested a culture of *Vibrio cholerae* (Cohen and van Everdingen 1990, cited by Köhler and Speelman 1992).

V. cholerae is known to be highly susceptible to destruction by gastric acid, which would explain the observation that people with total or subtotal gastrectomy were especially liable to infection during epidemics of cholera infection which occurred in Israel and Italy (Carpenter 1987). It would seem to follow that those taking antacids are at greater risk of contracting the disease, and Köhler and Speelman (1992) stated that mineral antacids, cimetidine, ranitidine, and omeprazole have such an effect, though they did not provide detailed evidence to support this claim.

Helicobacter pylori infection

It is now generally accepted that infection with this curved or spiral Gram-negative bacterium is a major aetiological factor in duodenal or gastric ulceration (see reviews by Heatley [1995] and Penman *et al.* [1997].

One of the treatment regimens that have been used to eradicate this infection is the so-called bismuth triple therapy, in which tripotassium bismuthate is combined with two or more antibacterial drugs, and the observation that some effects of the bismuth compound are abolished by aspirin might well be important clinically, though this has not yet been firmly established.

Clostridial infections

Pseudomembranous colitis is an infection of the colon caused by *Clostridium difficile*. As a natural disease it may, rarely, occur in otherwise healthy people or, more often, in patients already suffering from some predisposing condition such as chronic colonic obstruction or carcinoma, leukaemia, or uraemia (Larson 1987). Most frequently, however, it complicates treatment with antimicrobial drugs: clindamycin and lincomycin are the commonest culprits, followed by ampicillin and amoxycillin; but almost all commonly used antimicrobial agents have been implicated at times, including, paradoxically, vancomycin (Miller and Ringler 1987; Hecht and Olinger 1989; Schenfeld and Pote 1995) and metronidazole (Daly and Chowdary 1983), which are the drugs of first and second choice, respectively, for the treatment of the condition.

It has been suggested that cases of severe enterocolitis attributed to drug-induced staphylococcal infection (see earlier) in the past were in fact due to *Clostridium difficile* infection.

Drugs other than antimicrobials that have been suspected of having induced *Cl. difficile* colitis are cytarabine (Roda 1987) and combinations of cytotoxic agents (Satin *et al.* 1989; Iveson and Chan 1992; Kamthan *et al.* 1992; Nielsen *et al.* 1992; Sriuanpong and Voravud 1995).

A case of pseudomembranous colitis without evidence of *Cl. difficile* infection but firmly diagnosed by colonoscopy and biopsy has been attributed to the antidiabetic drug chlorpropamide (Gupta and Sachar 1985); and diclofenac given intramuscularly (Gentric and Pennee 1996) has been suspected as a cause.

An Australian study has drawn attention to the very considerable cost of the increased stay in hospital resuling from the diarrhoea caused by this disorder (Riley *et al.* 1995). This subject is also discussed in Chapter 12.

Yersinia enterocolitica infections

It is known that patients with iron overload are prone to systemic yersiniosis (Robins-Browne *et al.* 1978; Hoen *et al.* 1988), a condition that rarely, if ever, occurs in patients with normal iron stores, and long-term iron therapy has been associated with infection caused by this organism (Leighton and MacSween 1987), as has accidental acute poisoning with ferrous sulphate (Milteer *et al.* 1989). But, paradoxically, the treatment of iron overload with desferrioxamine also appears to predispose to this disorder (Robins-Browne and Prpic 1983; Nouel *et al.* 1991), the suggested explanation being that the supply of exogenous siderophores, such as desferrioxamine, enables the organism to overcome the handicap of being unable to synthesize iron-binding components (Robins-Browne and Prpic 1983).

Legionella infections

Legionella pneumophila, the cause of Legionnaires' disease, has been found to be the infecting organism in more than a third of patients who develop bacterial pneumonia following treatment with the immunosuppressive drug tacrolimus after liver transplantation (Singh *et al.* 1996). The infection has also been attributed to treatment with cyclosporin (Pillemer *et al.* 1989) or corticosteroids (Jivà *et al.* 1993).

Brucellosis

It was suggested some time ago that the risk of contracting brucellosis might be increased during treatment with the older antacids and later a case was described in which a young man taking cimetidine contracted brucellosis (*Br. melitensis*) by eating infected cheese that proved harmless to other members of his family (Cristiano and Paradisi 1982). Presumably, treatment with other drugs that reduce gastric acidity might also predispose to this disorder, as well as to such serious intestinal infections as cholera and salmonellosis; and omeprazole has certainly been suspected to have precipitated recurrent enteric infection (Wingate 1990). It should, however, be noted that as far as brucellosis and cimetidine are concerned an explanation not involving reduction of gastric acidity has been put forward by Thorne (1982), namely that cimetidine lowers the number of suppressor/cytotoxic T lymphocytes with consequent acute exacerbation of latent or chronic brucellosis.

Listeriosis

Infection with *Listeria monocytogenes* has been attributed to treatment with antilymphocyte globulin (Girmenia *et al.* 1988); chlordeoxyadenosine (Spielberger *et al.* 1993); fludarabine (Cleveland and Gelfand 1993); low-dose methotrexate (McCambridge *et al.*

1995; Hayem *et al.* 1996); and corticosteroids alone (Sobrevilla *et al.* 1962) or in combination wih fludarabine (Anaissie *et al.* 1992) or with cyclophosphamide and methotrexate (Giunta and Piazza 1992).

Nocardiosis

This disorder, a systemic infection caused by a Gram-positive filamentous bacterium, has been associated with a variety of malignant and autoimmune diseases, chronic lung conditions, diabetes, plasma protein abnormalities, and certain rare diseases of other types. In some cases, treatment with cytotoxic drugs, corticosteroids, immunosuppressive agents, or combinations of these appears to have increased the risk of infection, and cases in which low-dose methotrexate for rheumatoid arthritis was considered to be the cause have been reported (Keegan and Byrd 1988; Cornelissen *et al.* 1991).

Tuberculosis

Experiments in animals demonstrated that tuberculosis infection worsened when the infected animal was given adrenal corticosteroids in large doses, and subsequent studies suggested that the disease in man could be induced, reactivated, or aggravated by corticosteroid therapy. This risk came to be regarded as a considerable one, but after analysing data supplied by 50 chest physicians in England, Scotland, and Wales for the years 1959 and 1960, Mayfield (1962) concluded that in this country during the years under review corticosteroid therapy had not made any significant contribution either to the incidence of new cases of tuberculosis or to the relapse rate of old cases, and he failed to find any striking evidence of especially acute or insidious disease. Nevertheless, he admitted that British experience might not reflect exactly the situation elsewhere, and he suggested that a careful search (including a chest X-ray) should be made for past or present tuberculosis before corticosteroid treatment is started; that chest X-rays should be repeated periodically throughout treatment and for a year thereafter; and that in some cases, notably when old tuberculosis lesions are present, cover of corticosteroid treatment by antituberculous drugs should be considered.

Following a later study, in a population with a high prevalence of tuberculosis (Cowie and King 1987), it was concluded that the risk of tuberculosis in asthmatics, attributable to corticosteroid therapy, is not great enough to justify the routine use of antituberculosis prophylaxis.

In renal transplant recipients mycobacterial infection

is more likely to occur in those given high-dose cyclosporin therapy than in those receiving other types of immunosuppressive drugs or low-dose cyclosporin (John *et al.* 1994).

BCG

Vaccination against tuberculosis using the live Bacillus Calmette–Guérin has been followed by progressive lupus vulgaris (Izumi and Matsunaga 1982), disseminated tuberculous infection (Mackay *et al.* 1980; Morugasu *et al.* 1988), tuberculous meningitis (Morrison *et al.* 1988; Tardieu *et al.* 1988), and osteomyelitis (Nishi *et al.* 1997) but such cases have been rare. Very much more common have been cases that have followed intravesical instillation of the vaccine into the bladder as immunological therapy for cancer of that organ, particularly when operations on the bladder or prostate have been performed at the same time or soon afterwards. In most instances bacteraemia has resulted in disseminated miliary lesons, but in a few the infection has been localized, causing osteomyelitis (Hoppe *et al.* 1992; Katz *et al.* 1992; Civen *et al.* 1994; Morgan and Iseman 1996), hepatic granulomata (Proctor *et al.* 1993; Arzt and Forouhar 1995), prostatic granuloma (Sai *et al.* 1990; LaFontaine *et al.* 1997), epididymo-orchitis (Truelson *et al.* 1992), or mycotic aneurysm of the aorta (Izes *et al.* 1993; Hellinger *et al.* 1995); in one case a tuberculous granuloma of the penis followed spillage of BCG during intravesical instillation (Ribera *et al.* 1995). Except for a small number of cases, immunological suppression by corticosteroids or the human immunodeficiency virus has not been a factor in these complications.

Mixed bacterial infections

Respiratory infections

The risk of non-specific respiratory tract infections among previously healthy recruits to the Singapore armed services increased during prophylactic antimalarial therapy with a combination of dapsone and pyrimethamine (Maloprim), particularly while they were engaged in strenuous physical activity, and it was suggested that the antimalarial combination caused some degree of immunosuppression (Lee and Lau 1988).

Hidradenitis suppurativa

Some cases of hidradenitis suppurativa, the term applied to recurrent boils affecting the axillary apocrine sweat glands, anogenital area, and breasts, and caused by a variety of anaerobic bacteria, have been attributed, fairly convincingly, to the use of combined oral contraceptives (Stellon and Wakeling 1989); other cases have been blamed on lithium treatment (Gupta *et al.* 1995).

Abscesses

Abscesses, some sterile and some containing mixed organisms, have long been known to follow the intramuscular injection of such irritant drugs as paraldehyde and quinine, and more recent examples have involved chloroquine (Ahmed and Fahal 1989), diclofenac (Ali and Mathias 1991), and aurothioglucose (Sowa 1993).

Formation of an extradural abscess has followed extradural injection of a combination of a local anaesthetic and a corticosteroid (Goucke and Graziotti 1990) and an epidural abscess after a local anaesthetic alone (Borum *et al.* 1995).

Pyoderma

Atypical pyoderma of the nose, caused by a mixture of staphylococci and streptococci has occurred in a patient under treatment with isotretinoin (Helpern 1985).

Viral infections

The defences against viral infection include the natural resistance of cells at the primary site of infection, the activity of macrophages, and the effects of circulating antibody and cell-mediated immunity (Allison 1972). Drugs may interfere with one or more of these protective mechanisms.

Animal experiments

In monkeys infected with smallpox, viraemia persisted longer in those concurrently treated with steroids than in those not so treated, and deaths from the infection were confined to the steroid-treated animals, three-quarters of which died (Rao *et al.* 1968). In mice, the severity of viral hepatitis is increased by treatment with corticosteroids (Datta and Isselbacher 1969). In other experiments it was shown that the multiplication of Coxsackie virus and the viruses of poliomyelitis, Rift Valley fever, and encephalomyelitis was enhanced by corticosteroids or ACTH (Findley and Howard 1952). Immunosuppression by cyclophosphamide potentiated the infectivity and ill-effects of some members of the arborvirus, enterovirus, and herpesvirus groups (Allison 1972).

Human infections

Herpes viruses

The five viruses in this group that are most likely to cause human disease are herpes simplex, varicella–zoster, the

Epstein–Barr virus, human herpes virus type 6, and cytomegalovirus. In some instances, these infections appear to be aggravated, reactivated, or precipitated by certain drugs. As far as herpes simplex, herpes zoster, and varicella are concerned, an association between the disease and treatment with corticosteroids, immunosuppressive drugs, or antineoplastic agents is now well established, and the number of published cases has become to large for them to be listed here. Reactivation of herpes simplex is an unusual complication of intrathecal administration of morphine (Pennant and Wallace 1991; Duffy 1993; Rose and Hill 1993) or epidural injection of fentanyl (Valley *et al.* 1992). It has also been attributed to antidepressive treatment with fluoxetine (Reed and Glick 1991) and, in an isolated case, to ingestion of a Chinese herbal preparation (Jones 1991).

Infection with the Epstein–Barr virus appears to have been precipitated by the immunosuppressive drug muromonab-CD3 (OKT3) in transplant recipients (Ren and Chan 1988; Junker *et al.* 1989).

Cytomegalovirus infection has been attributed to treatment with the following drugs and drug combinations: corticosteroids alone (Wiest *et al.* 1989; Nelson *et al.* 1993) or combined with cyclophosphamide (Mayer *et al.* 1988), or methotrexate (Wallace and Luchi 1996), or methotrexate and ketoprofen (Salinier 1992); methotrexate alone (Aglas *et al.* 1995) or combined with hydroxychloroquine and folic acid (Bowman and Mowat 1995). Gold therapy (Wong *et al.* 1993) and some combinations of antineoplastic drugs (Baker *et al.* 1994; Theodossiou *et al.* 1995) have also been implicated. Some observers have suggested that the immunosuppressive drug muromonab-CT3 (OKT3) increases the incidence of cytomegalovirus infection in transplant recipients (Costanzo-Nordin *et al.* 1992), but others (Lake *et al.* 1993) dispute this.

It has been known for years that exposure to trichloroethylene, in industry or during general anaesthesia, is occasionally followed by neuropathy of the trigeminal nerve. It had been generally accepted that the cause is a direct toxic effect of the chemical on some part of the nerve tract, though as far back as 1944 Humphrey and McClelland suspected that the lesion might be due to an indirect effect of the chemical in reactivating latent herpes simplex infection of the nerve; but they were not able to prove their hypothesis because of the inadequacy of investigative methods available at that time. Much more recently the problem was readdressed by Cavanagh and Buxton (1989), who presented detailed and very convincing evidence of the involvement of the virus in the induction of trigeminal palsies following trichloroethylene exposure.

Poliomyelitis

Very rarely (about one case in 2.5 million doses), paralytic poliomyelitis has followed oral administration of the live attenuated poliomyelitis vaccine (Querfurth and Swanson 1990; Beausoleil *et al.* 1994); in one case the affected child was already infected with the human immunodeficiency virus (Ion-Nedelcu *et al.* 1994) and in another case (fatal) the patient had hypogammaglobulinaemia (Groom *et al.* 1994). The disease has also occurred in an unvaccinated contact of a vaccinated patient (Sullivan *et al.* 1995) and in a vaccinated child's father who himself had been vaccinated against poliomyelitis in childhood (Mermel *et al.* 1993).

According to Wiest and others (1989), corticosteroids are capable of precipitating poliomyelitis.

Other viruses

Immunosuppressive therapy has been complicated by measles (Meadow *et al.* 1969; *British Medical Journal* 1976; Pullan *et al.* 1976) and influenza A pneumonia (Embrey and Geist 1995); and antineoplastic treatment has been held responsible for parvovirus infection (Rao *et al.* 1994) and also for reactivation of hepatitis B in carriers of that organism (Ohtsu *et al.* 1991). The use of alfa-interferon for chronic hepatitis C has caused an exacerbation of the disease (Shindo *et al.* 1992).

Vaccination against smallpox is no longer required in the general population but it may still be advisable in those few laboratory workers who may be exposed to pox viruses, and it should be remembered that corticosteroids may precipitate and greatly increase the severity of vaccinia (Levy 1969; MacKenzie *et al.* 1969).

Virus–drug interactions

In some viral infections the use of certain drugs appears to predispose to other disorders. Examples are the characteristic rash induced by ampicillin (and, less often, by other penicillins — see Chapter 27 on *Drug Allergy*) in the presence of the Epstein–Barr virus, the combination of hypersensitivity rashes and fever in patients with AIDS when given prophylactic or curative treatment with co-trimoxazole for *Pneumocystis carinii* infection, and Reye's syndrome in patients with virus infections treated with salicylates; and it has been claimed that AIDS patients who misuse inhaled nitrates are particularly liable to develop Kaposi's sarcoma, but this claim has been the subject of much controversy. A case has been reported in which general anaesthesia in a child suffering from an upper respiratory tract infection was suspected to have induced viral myocarditis (Jones 1993).

Several aspects of this interesting subject have been reviewed by Haverkos and colleagues (1991).

Fungal infections

Aspergillosis

Infection with one of the *Aspergillus* species, usually affecting the lungs but very occasionally the oesophagus, has complicated treatment with ACTH or corticosteroids (Nabarro 1960; Sidranski and Pearl 1961; Wiest *et al.* 1989; Crean *et al.* 1992; Hongou *et al.* 1992; Jivà *et al.* 1993), cytotoxic drugs (Kluin-Nelemans *et al.* 1991; Niimi *et al.* 1991), or immunosuppressants, sometimes given with corticosteroids for such disorders as Crohn's disease (Scalzini *et al.* 1995) or in association with organ transplantation (Gelpi *et al.* 1994; Singh *et al.* 1996). The infection has also been encountered in a diabetic patient who developed ketoacidosis after treatment with pentamidine for AIDS, and in another given low-dose methotrexate for rheumatoid arthritis (O'Reilly *et al.* 1994).

Candidiasis

Candida infections of mouth, oesophagus, gut, and anus may occur during treatment with antibiotics, usually, but not invariably, those with a broad antibacterial spectrum, and some observers believe that such infections remain confined to the mucosal surfaces unless the patient is also being treated with corticosteroids. Other workers have observed, however, that systemic candidiasis can be precipitated by antibiotics alone in debilitated patients. According to Symmers (1966), broad-spectrum antibiotics have little effect on susceptibility to fungal infections other than candidiasis or, more rarely, geotrichosis.

Oral and oesophageal or laryngeal candidiasis may complicate treatment with ACTH or corticosteroids when they are given systemically, or may occur when aerosol sprays containing such steroids as dexamethasone, beclomethasone, and triamcinolone are used for the treatment of asthma, but it has been claimed that children are relatively immune to this complication (Godfrey *et al.* 1974). Patients taking omeprazole have developed oral or oesophageal candidiasis (Larner and Lendrum 1992; Carro *et al.* 1993; Mosiman 1993). Acute disseminated candidiasis has complicated both short-term (Botas and Sola 1994) and long-term (Boyd and Chappel 1961) corticosteroid therapy, combined treatment with corticosteroids and antibiotics (Bendel and Rade 1961), immunosuppressive therapy (Tomietto *et al.* 1995), and cytotoxic treatment in connection with bone marrow transplantation (Mudad *et al.* 1994).

Patients treated for oropharyngeal candidiasis with fluconazole (Akova *et al.* 1991) or given the drug prophylactically when undergoing bone marrow transplantation (Wingard *et al.* 1991) have developed infection with the somewhat unfamiliar *Candida krusei*.

There has been controversy over the role of oral contraceptives in genital candidiasis. Yaffee and Grots (1965) suggested that these drugs predisposed to vulval and vaginal candidiasis, often resistant to treatment, but this was disputed by Morris and Morris (1969) and Lazan (1971), and by Davidson and Oates (1985), who studied patients from three different centres over a period of 8 years and found no correlation between oral contraceptive use and genital candidal infection, a view supported by the observations of MacDonald and others (1993). However, Spinillo and colleagues (1995) found that while oral contraceptive use was not related to initial attacks of vulvovaginal candidiasis, it did increase the risk of recurrent infection. The debate continues.

Recurrent vulvovaginal candidiasis has complicated treatment with tamoxifen (Sobel *et al.* 1996); and the oral retinoid drug acetretin has been suspeced of predisposing patients to the condition (Middelbeek *et al.* 1993), though the evidence is not yet conclusive.

Stark and others (1978) suggested that previous treatment with cimetidine predisposes to *Candida* peritonitis in patients with perforated ulcer, but Hassan and Browne (1978) disputed this. Triger and colleagues (1981) commented that suppression of gastric acid production may permit overgrowth of *Candida* within the gastrointestinal tract, and they described three cases of systemic candidiasis complicating acute hepatic failure in patients treated with cimetidine.

Kochar and others (1988) described a patient whose duodenal ulcer, which had failed to heal after treatment with cimetidine for 3 months, was found to have been infiltrated with *Candida albicans*. The lesion began to heal satisfactorily when ranitidine was substituted for cimetidine and the antifungal drug nystatin was added to the treatment regimen. The authors postulated that in this case the reduction of gastric acidity together with the effects of cimetidine on the immune system and on leucocyte function were responsible for invasive candidiasis. Earlier, Minoli and colleagues (1987) had claimed that short-term cimetidine therapy is not complicated by invasive candidiasis.

A number of cases have been reported in which patients receiving prolonged intravenous infusions of nutrients such as amino acids and lipids ('intravenous hyperalimentation') developed *Candida* septicaemia (Curry and Quie 1971; Vogel *et al.* 1972). This type of treatment probably predisposes to infection because of the long duration of intravenous cannulation, but why in these circumstances the risk of fungal infection is much greater than that of bacterial infection is uncertain.

Cryptococcosis

Patients with various diseases have developed cryptococcosis when treated with corticosteroids (Goldstein and Rambo 1962; Bennington *et al.* 1964; Jacobs 1993; Bernstein *et al.* 1994), cytotoxic drugs (Frieden *et al.* 1993; Leenders *et al.* 1995), and immunosuppressive agents (Singh *et al.* 1996), including low-dose methotrexate therapy for rheumatoid arthritis (Altz-Smith 1987).

Mucormycosis (phycomycosis, zygomycosis)

This infection has been encountered during corticosteroid therapy (Hutter 1959; Rex *et al.* 1988; Sane *et al.* 1989), as well as in patients treated with desferrioxamine during long-term haemodialysis (Veis *et al.* 1987; Sombolos *et al.* 1988; Daley *et al.* 1989; Seeverens *et al.* 1992) or given the drug for iatrogenic iron overload (Slade and MacNab 1991; Ammon *et al.* 1992; Murray *et al.* 1996).

Other fungal infections

Alternariosis (cutaneous) (Macher *et al.* 1995), coccidiomycosis (Aguardo *et al.* 1988; Mahaffrey *et al.* 1993), histoplasmosis (Dismukes *et al.* 1978; Perez and Wilking 1992; Fucci and Nightengale 1997), and sporotrichosis (Kaufman 1962) have been attributed to treatment with ACTH or corticosteroids. Histoplasmosis has also been blamed on low-dose methotrexate therapy (Witty *et al.* 1992).

Application of steroids to the skin, particularly under occlusive dressings, may predispose to local fungal infections (Gill *et al.* 1963), sometimes atypical in appearance and size (Ive and Marks 1968; Peterkin and Khan 1969), or the steroid may aggravate existing fungal infection even when combined with a topical antifungal drug (Reynolds *et al.* 1991).

Protozoal infections

Experiments in animals have demonstrated that the effects of protozoal infections are aggravated by corticosteroid therapy (Kass and Finland 1953). In man, amoebiasis has been attributed to steroid therapy (Eisert *et al.* 1959) and activation of latent amoebic infections has also been described (Mody 1959; Amin 1978; Stuiver and Goud 1978). Indeed, in countries in which amoebiasis is endemic, it is now considered prudent to endeavour to exclude occult intestinal amoebiasis before using steroids more than briefly (de Glanville, personal communication). An association between various kinds of drug treatment and infection with *Pneumocystis carinii* has now become firmly established, as witnessed by the spate of published reports in the last few years — again too numerous to be listed here. The drugs that have been involved are ACTH or tetracosactrin; corticosteroids, including preparations for inhalation; single or combined immunosuppressive agents, including those used for rheumatoid arthritis; and desferrioxamine (Koudies *et al.* 1988).

Prophylactic treatment with pentamidine by inhalation in AIDS patients does not always prevent either pulmonary (Stien and Weems 1991) or disseminated (De Roux 1991) infection with this organism.

As far as some of the immunosuppressive agents are concerned, findings in patients infected with the human immunodeficiency virus may be relevant: it has been shown that the risk of these patients developing *Pneumocystis carinii* pneumonia is closely linked to the absolute count of CD4 cells in the blood, a count of less than 200 cells per mm^3 making infection very likely (Phair *et al.* 1990). The use of antilymphocyte globulin, antithymocyte globulin and, particularly, muromonab-CD3 (OKT3) will produce a similar effect and may explain differing incidences of this infection in different populations of transplant recipients.

Reactivation of latent cryptosporidial infection has been attributed to diarrhoea induced by the laxative docusate calcium and the antibiotic erythromycin in a diabetic patient (Holley and Thiers 1986). The erythromycin was replaced by cephalexin, and the patient was also given prednisone and azathioprine, so it is difficult to decide which of these drugs was the culprit.

Toxoplasmosis may complicate treatment with immunosuppressive drugs (Cohen 1970; Slavin *et al.* 1994), and it has occurred in patients taking pentamidine as prophylaxis against *Pneumocystis carinii* infection (Zangerle and Allerberger 1991). It may be due to reactivation of organisms lying dormant in the patient's own tissues; this possibility is supported by the finding that nine out of 19 patients with AIDS who had positive serological tests for *Toxoplasma gondii* developed cerebral toxoplasmosis when given pentamidine or co-trimoxazole as prophylactic treatment for *P. carinii* infection, whereas only one out of 22 patients without toxoplasma antibodies suffered this complication (Zangerle and Allerberger 1991).

Toxoplasmosis should be suspected when unexplained fever or focal neurological signs appear in patients under treatment with one of these drugs (Cohen 1970).

Szanto (1971) reported a case in which *Trichomonas vaginalis* infection appeared to follow systemic administration of oxytetracycline, and responded to treatment with metronidazole only after the oxytetracycline was withheld. He suggested that oxytetracycline might have interfered in some way with the action of metronidazole.

It now seems firmly established that there is a relationship between iron and amoebiasis. It has been shown experimentally (Latour and Reeves 1965; Diamond *et al.* 1978) that *Entamoeba histolytica* needs iron for growth, has a high requirement for the element, and obtains it from the host. It might therefore be expected that an excess of body iron would increase susceptibility to amoebiasis, while iron deficiency would protect against infection (unless outweighed by the impairment of certain bodily defences against infection, thought to occur in iron deficiency — see earlier); and these expectations appear to have been fulfilled. Iron overload was found to be commoner in black Africans who had died of amoebiasis than in the general population (Bothwell *et al.* 1984). Iron deficiency, on the other hand, appeared to protect against amoebiasis in milk-drinking African nomads, and when some of these subjects were treated with oral iron the infection rate rose sharply, but this did not happen when the iron was given by injection (Murray *et al.* 1980), and it was concluded that it is the intestinal content of iron rather than the iron state of the body as a whole that is important in controlling the growth of *Entamoeba histolytica*.

It has also been observed that there is a tendency for malarial infections to occur or flare up when iron deficiency anaemia is treated (Masawe *et al.* 1974; Murray *et al.* 1975; Murray *et al.* 1978), and injections of iron–dextran (Imferon) in infants appeared to increase their chances of contracting malaria (Oppenheimer *et al.* 1984). (See also above under Infection with *E. coli* and other Gram-negative organisms.)

Nematode infections

Infection with *Strongyloides stercoralis* is encouraged by treatment with corticosteroids and immunosuppressive drugs (Cruz *et al.* 1966; Purtilo *et al.* 1974; Yamori *et al.* 1979; Kaslow *et al.* 1990), corticosteroids alone (Higenbottam and Heard 1976), or chemotherapy with or without radiotherapy (Ayden *et al* 1994); and a case has been described in which an existing infection was thought to have been aggravated by treatment with cimetidine in a patient undergoing chemotherapy for lymphoma (Ainley *et al.* 1986). The disease may manifest itself by gastrointestinal discomfort, diarrhoea, pruritus, urticaria, pneumonia, and pulmonary infarction with haemoptysis, and widespread dissemination of larvae may prove fatal.

A case of severe trichinosis has been attributed to treatment with thiabendazole, a drug used in the treatment of protozoal infections (de Vedia *et al.* 1995).

Colonization of the gastric mucosa by trophozoites of *Giardia lamblia* in two patients taking omeprazole for peptic ulceration has been reported by Reynaert and others (1995), who commented that, while intestinal giardiasis is common, gastric infection by the organism is rare, occurring usually in patients with hypochlorhydria and achlorhydria. The authors suggested that reduction of gastric acidity by omeprazole might have been responsible for the atypical infestation in these cases.

Arthropod infestation

Of several members of a family suffering from Norwegian scabies, only one proved refractory to benzyl benzoate therapy. This patient was also under treatment with etretinate, and it was postulated that reduction of skin sebum, a recognized effect of etretinate, enhanced susceptibility to the infestation, since it is known that *Sarcoptes scabiei* favours areas of skin in which sebum secretion is minimal (Zlotogorski and Leibovici 1987).

Interference with the efficacy of antimicrobial therapy

Some drugs may harm patients suffering from infections by reducing the effectiveness of other drugs being used in treatment. (See also Chapters 5 and 33.)

Antibiotic combinations

Chloramphenicol, a bacteriostatic drug, weakens the bactericidal action of penicillin in pneumococcal meningitis in animals (Wallace *et al.* 1965), and tetracycline has the same effect on the disease in man (Lepper and Dowling 1951). Staphylococci sensitive to lincomycin but resistant to erythromycin become less susceptible to the first of these drugs when the second is administered concurrently (Griffith *et al.* 1965). In streptococcal infections, penicillin has been found to be more effective than erythromycin, while a combination of these drugs was the least successful form of treatment (Strom 1955). Neomycin and kanamycin reduce the absorption of orally administered penicillin (Cheng and White 1962).

The antibacterial effect of gentamicin is reduced by benzylpenicillin and by carbenicillin (McLaughlin and Reeves 1971), which has the same effect on kanamycin (Stockley 1974) and ticarcillin (Bint and Burtt 1980), but it has been suggested that this interaction is not likely to be clinically significant except in patients with severe renal impairment in whom prolonged high concentrations of the penicillin would be expected and doses would be given infrequently (Bint and Burtt 1980). In laboratory experiments nitrofurantoin reduces the antibacterial effect of nalidixic acid on a variety of Gram-negative bacteria (Stille and Ostner 1966; Piguet 1969).

Other drug combinations

When phenobarbitone is given at the same time as griseofulvin, the serum concentrations of the antifungal drug may be lower than when it is given alone (Busfield *et al.* 1963; Riegelman *et al.* 1970), and its therapeutic effect may be impaired (Lorenc 1967). It has been postulated that an increased rate of metabolism of griseofulvin by hepatic microsomal enzymes stimulated (induced) by phenobarbitone is to blame, but an alternative explanation is that phenobarbitone decreases absorption of griseofulvin by stimulating bile secretion, which in turn stimulates peristalsis (Stockley 1974).

The absorption of tetracyclines is reduced by antacids containing bismuth, calcium, magnesium, or aluminium salts, and by calcium-containing foods. This effect is probably due to tight chemical binding of the antibiotic to the antacid (chelation), but it is possible that alteration in gastrointestinal pH plays a part (Stockley 1974), since sodium bicarbonate also markedly reduces absorption of tetracyclines (Barr *et al.* 1971). Aluminium compounds also impair the absorption of isoniazid when they are given concurrently, so an interval should be left between the administration of the two medicines; and both aluminium and magnesium antacids impair absorption of 4-quinolone antibacterial drugs (especially ciprofloxacin), so that these groups of drugs should not be given within 2–4 hours of each other. Ferrous sulphate has a similar effect on tetracycline absorption (Neuvonen *et al.* 1970), due to chelation, but the clinical importance of this interaction has been questioned (Bateman 1970), and further doubt about its clinical relevance has been raised by retrospective studies of the efficacy of tetracyclines in patients who were taking iron tablets (Crooks *et al.* 1977). Some of these interactions can be avoided if the drugs are given separately at an interval of 3 hours or more (Gothoni *et al.* 1972).

The bioavailabiliy of ciprofloxacin is decreased when didanosine is given concurrently, but when the first of these drugs is administered before the second the interaction is not considered to be clinically significant (Knupp and Barbhaiya 1997).

The efficacy of the antifungal drug fluconazole appears to be impaired by concurrent administration of combinations of the antituberculous drugs rifampicin and pyrazinamide with either isoniazid or ethambutol (Parkin *et al.* 1990).

It has been shown experimentally that cyclamates, present as sweetening agents in a variety of food and drink, reduce the absorption of lincomycin (Wagner 1969), but whether or not this is clinically relevant is uncertain (Stockley 1974). The absorption of lincomycin is also impaired by kaolin (Wagner 1961), which might well be prescribed for symptomatic treatment at the same time as the antibiotic is being used as a specific remedy. An interval of 2 hours, however, between the administration of the drugs prevented the interaction (Wagner 1968) (see also Bint and Burtt 1980, and Chapter 33).

Sulphonamides inhibit bacterial growth by interference with the uptake by the bacteria of *p*-aminobenzoic acid, but enough of this substance is provided by the metabolic products of the local anaesthetics procaine and benzocaine, and of the 'antifibrotic' drug potassium *p*-aminobenzoate, to overcome this inhibitory effect. Fortunately, the occasions on which this situation is likely to arise are few and far between; nevertheless, the potential interaction should be kept in mind.

Interactions of antimicrobial drugs in infusion solutions

A number of antibacterial agents may be inactivated when dissolved in infusion fluids, either by the fluids themselves or by other drugs added to them. Information on the stability of antibacterial drugs in infusion solutions and possible adverse interactions between drugs added to these fluids is provided by the current *British National Formulary*. (See also Chapter 33.)

Masking of infection by drugs

This subject is discussed fully in Chapter 32.

References

Aglas, F., Rainer, F., Hermann, J., *et al.* (1995). Interstitial pneumonia due to cytomegalovirus following low-dose methotrexate treatment for rheumatoid arthritis. *Arthritis Rheum.* 38, 291.

Aguardo, J.L., Greaves, T., Hutchinson, H.T., *et al.* (1988). Pneumonia in infants given adrenocorticotropic hormone for infantile spasms. *J. Pediatr.* 112, 508.

Ahmed, M.E. and Fahal, A.H. (1989). Acute gluteal abscesses: injectable chloroquine as a cause. *J. Trop. Med. Hyg.* 92, 317.

Ainley, C.C., Clarke, D.G., Timothy, A.R., *et al.* (1986). *Strongyloides stercoralis* hyperinfection associated with cimetidine in an immunosuppressed patient: diagnosis by endoscopic biopsy. *Gut* 27, 337.

Aitani, M., Kawabata, S., Kimura, K., *et al.* (1996). A case of pneumonia associated with antiepileptic drug-induced immunodeficiency. *Nippon Kyobi Rinsho* 55, 679.

Akova, M., Akalin, H.E., Uzun, O., *et al.* (1991). Emergence of *Candida krusei* infections after therapy of oropharyngeal candidiasis with fluconazole. *Eur. J. Clin. Microbiol. Infect. Dis.* 10, 58.

Ali, M.T. and Mathias, I.M. (1991). Continued problems with diclofenac. *Anaesthesia* 46, 1089.

Allard, S., O'Driscoll, J., and Laurie, A. (1992). Salmonella osteitis in aplastic anaemia after antilymphocyte globulin and steroid treatment. *J. Clin. Path.* 45, 174.

Allison, A.C. (1972). Immunity against viruses. In *The Scientific Basis of Medicine, Annual Reviews* (ed. I. Gilliland and J. Francis), p. 51. Athlone, London.

Altz-Smith, M., Kendall, L.G., and Stamm, A.M. (1987). Cryptococcosis associated with low-dose methotrexate for arthritis. *Am. J. Med.* 83, 179.

Amin, N. (1978). Amoebiasis and corticosteroids. *BMJ* ii, 1084.

Ammon, A., Rumpf, K.W., Hommerich, C.P., *et al.* (1992). Rhinocerebral mucormycosis during deferoxamine treatment. *Dtsch. Med. Wochenschr.* 117, 1434.

Anaissie, E., Kontoyannis, D.P., Kantarjian, H., *et al.* (1992). Listeriosis in patients with chronic lymphatic leukaemia treated with fludarabine and prednisolone. *Ann. Intern. Med.* 117, 466.

Arbeter, A., Echeverri, L., Fraco, D., *et al.* (1971). Nutrition and infection. *Fed. Proc.* 30, 1421.

Arzt, M.R. and Farouhar, F. (1995). Granulomatous hepatitis as a complication of bacillus Calmette–Guérin therapy for bladder cancer. *Ann. Clin. Lab. Sci.* 25, 409.

Ayden, H., Doppl, W., Battman, A., *et al.* (1994). Opportunistic *Strongyloides stercoralis* hyperinfection in lymphoma patients undergoing chemotherapy and/or radiotherapy: report of a case. *Acta Oncol.* 33, 78.

Bahamdan, K.A., Quazi, F.M., Khare, A.K., *et al.* (1995). Toxic shock syndrome complicating an adverse drug reaction in a man. *Int. J. Dermatol.* 34, 661.

Baker, J.L., Gosland, M.P., and Herrington, J.D. (1994). Cytomegalovirus colitis after 5-fluorouracil and interferon-alpha therapy. *Pharmacotherapy* 14, 246.

Bardana, E.J., Jr, Gabourel, J.D., Davies, G.H., *et al.* (1984). Effects of phenytoin on man's immunity: Evaluation of changes in serum immunoglobulins, complement, and antinuclear antibody. *Am. J. Med.* 64, 579.

Barr, W.H., Adir, J., and Garrettson, L. (1971). Decrease of tetracycline absorption in man by sodium bicarbonate. *Clin. Pharmacol. Ther.* 12, 779.

Barry, D.M.J. and Reeve, A.W. (1974). Iron and infection in the newborn. *Lancet* ii, 1385.

Bateman, F.J.A. (1970). Effects of tetracyclines. *BMJ* iv, 802.

Beausoleil, J.L., Nordgren, R.E., and Modlin, J.F. (1994). Vaccine-associated paralytic poliomyelitis. *J. Child Neurol.* 9, 334.

Becroft, D.M.O., Dix, M.R., and Farmer, K. (1977). Intramuscular iron–dextran and susceptibility of neonates to bacterial infections. *In vitro* studies. *Arch. Dis. Child.* 52, 778.

Bendel, W.L. and Rade, G.J. (1961). Acute disseminated candidiasis in aplastic anaemia. Potentiation by antibiotics and steroids. *Arch. Intern. Med.* 108, 916.

Bennington, J.L., Haber, S.L., and Morgenstern, N.L. (1964). Increased susceptibility to cryptococcosis following steroid therapy. *Dis. Chest* 45, 262.

Bernstein, S., Flomenberg, P., Letzer, O. *et al.* (1994). Disseminated crytococcal disease complicating steroid therapy for *Pneumocystis carinii* pneumonia in a patient with AIDS. *South. Med. J.* 87, 537.

Bint, A.J. and Burtt, I. (1980). Adverse antibiotic drug interactions. *Drugs* 20, 57.

Block, S.H. (1972). Indomethacin. *JAMA* 222, 1062.

Blumenthal, G. (1984). Paronychia and pyogenic granuloma-like lesions with isotretinoin. *J. Am. Acad. Derm.* 10, 677.

Bond, W.S. (1977). Toxic reactions and side effects of glucocorticoids in man. *Am. J. Hosp. Pharm.* 34, 479.

Borum, S.E., McLeskey, C.H., Williams, J.B., *et al.* (1995). Epidural abscess after obstetric epidural analgesia. *Anesthesiology* 82, 1523.

Botas, C. and Sola, A. (1994). *Candida* sepsis associated with hydrocortisone use in preterm infants. *Clin. Res.* 42, 90A.

Bothwell, T.H., Adams, E.B., Simon, M., *et al.* (1984). The iron status of black subjects with amoebiasis. *S. Afr. Med. J.* 65, 601.

Bowman, S. and Mowat, A. (1995). Cytomegalovirus in methotrexate-treated patients: comment on the concise communication by Aglas *et al.* (1995). *Arthritis Rheum.* 38, 1861.

Boyd, J.F. and Chappell, A.G. (1961). Fatal mycetosis due to *Candida albicans* after combined steroid and antibiotic therapy. *Lancet* ii, 19.

British Medical Journal (1976). Measles encephalitis during immunosuppressive therapy. *BMJ* i, 1552.

Brumfitt, W. and Hamilton-Miller, J.M.T. (1987). Principles and practice of antimicrobial chemotherapy. In *Avery's Drug Treatment* (3rd edn) (ed. T.M. Speight), p. 1216. Churchill Livingstone, Edinburgh.

Busfield, D., Child, K.J., Atkinson, R.M., *et al.* (1963). An effect of phenobarbitone on blood levels of griseofulvin in man. *Lancet* ii, 1042.

Butler, W.T. (1975). Corticosteroids and immunoglobulin synthesis. *Transplant Proc.* 7, 49.

Butler, W.T. and Rosen, R.D. (1973). Effect of corticosteroids on immunity in man, I. Decreased serum IgG concentration caused by 3 or 5 days of high doses of methylprednisolone. *J. Clin. Invest.* 52, 2629.

Carpenter, C.C.J. (1987). Cholera. In *Oxford Textbook of Medicine* (2nd edn) (ed. D.J. Weatherall, J.G.G. Ledingham, and D.A. Warrell), p. 5.231. Oxford University Press.

Carro, P.G., Toro, H., Balanzo, J., *et al.* (1993). Esophagic candidiasis in a patient treated with omeprazole. *Med. Clin.* (Barc.) 100, 639.

Carulli, M.T., Epstein, O., and Black, C.M. (1995). Small bowel bacterial overgrowth and omeprazole in a patient with systemic sclerosis. *Br. J. Rheumatol.* 34 (suppl. 1).

Cavanagh, J.B. and Buxton, P.H. (1989). Trichloroethylene cranial neuropathy: is it really a toxic neuropathy or does it activate latent herpes virus? *J. Neurol. Neurosurg. Psychiatry* 52, 297.

Chandra, R.K. (1944). Reduced bactericidal capacity of polymorphs in iron deficiency. *Arch. Dis. Child.* 48, 864.

Cheng, S.H. and White, A. (1962). Effect of orally administered neomycin on the absorption of penicillin V. *N. Engl. J. Med.* 267, 1296.

Christensen, E., Schlichting, P., Fauerholdt, L., *et al.* (1985). Changes of laboratory variables wih time in cirrhosis: prognostic and therapeutic significance. *Hepatology* 5, 843.

Civen, R., Berlin, G., and Panosian, C. (1994). Vertebral osteomyelitis after intravesical administration of bacille Calmette–Guérin. *Clin. Infect. Dis.* 18, 1013.

Cleveland, K.O. and Gelfand, M.S. (1993). Listerial brain abscess in a patient treated with chronic lymphocytic leukaemia treated with fludarabine. *Clin. Infect. Dis.* 17, 816.

Cohen, A.F. and van Everdingen, J.J.E. (1990). De arts als proefkonijn. In *De Openbaringen van Hippocrates.* Belvédère Publishers, Overveen.

Cohen, S.N. (1970). Toxoplasmosis in patients receiving immunosuppressive therapy. *JAMA* 211, 657.

Corder, A. (1987). Steroids, non-steroidal anti-inflammatory drugs, and serious septic complications of diverticular disease. *BMJ* 295, 1238.

Cornelissen, J.J., Bakker, L.J., Van der Veen, M.J., *et al.* (1991). *Nocardia asteroides* pneumonia complicating low-dose methotrexate treatment of refractory rheumatoid arthritis. *Ann. Rheum. Dis.* 50, 642.

Cortes, E., Zuckerman, M.J., and Ho, H. (1992). Recurrent *Salmonella arizona* infection after treatment for metastatic carcinoma. *J. Clin. Gastroenterol.* 14, 157.

Costanzo-Nordin, M.R., Swinnen, L.J., Fisher, S.G., *et al.* (1992). Cytomegalovirus infection in heart transplant recipients — relationship to immunosuppression. *J. Heart Lung Transplant.* 11, 837.

Cottingham, J. and Hunter, O. (1992). *Chlamydia trachomatis* and oral contraceptive use: a quantitative review. *Genitourin. Med.* 68, 209.

Cowie, R.L. and King, R.M. (1987). Pulmonary tuberculosis in corticosteroid-treated asthmatics. *S. Afr. Med. J.* 72, 849.

Crean, J.M., Niederman, M.S., Fein, A.M. *et al.* (1992). Rapidly progressive respiratory failure due to *Aspergillus* pneumonia: a complication of short-term corticosteroid therapy. *Crit. Care Med.* 20, 148.

Cristiano, P. and Paradisi, F. (1982). Can cimetidine facilitate infections by oral route? *Lancet* ii, 45.

Crooks, J., Stevenson, I.H., Shepherd, A.M.M., *et al.* (1977). In *Drug Interactions* (ed. D. Grahame-Smith), p. 3. Macmillan, London.

Cruz, T., Reboucas, G., and Rochas, H. (1966). Fatal strongyloidiasis in patients receiving corticosteroids. *N. Engl. J. Med.* 275, 1093.

Curry, C.R. and Quie, P.G. (1971). Fungal septicaemia in patients receiving parenteral hyperalimentation. *N. Engl. J. Med.* 285, 1221.

Daly, A.L., Velaquez, L.A., Bradley, S.F., *et al.* (1989). Mucormycosis: association with deferoxamine therapy. *Am. J. Med.* 87, 768.

Daly, J.J. and Chowdary, K.V.S. (1983). Pseudomembranous colitis secondary to metronidazole. *Dig. Dis. Sci.* 28, 573.

Datta, D.V. and Isselbacher, K.J. (1969). Effects of corticosteroids on mouse hepatitis virus infection. *Gut* 10, 522.

Davidson, F. and Oates, J.K. (1985). The pill does not cause 'thrush'. *Br. J. Obstet. Gynaecol.* 92, 1265.

De Roux, S., Adsay, V., and Iaochim, H.L. (1991). Disseminated infection with *Pneumocystis carinii* related to administration of pentamidine aerosol. *Arch. Int. Med.* 151, 1672.

de Vedia, L., Prieto R., Orduna, T., *et al.* (1995). Severe case of trichinosis secondary to thiabendazole therapy. *Prensa Med. Argentina* 82, 968.

Deane, S., Youngs, D., Poxon, V., *et al.* (1982). Cimetidine and gastric microflora. *Br. J. Surg.* 67, 371 (abstr. 51).

Diamond, L.S., Harlow, D.R., Phillips, B.P., *et al.* (1978). *Entamoeba histolytica*: iron and nutritional immunity. *Arch. Invest. Med.* (*Mex.*) Suppl.1, 9, 329.

Dismukes, W.E., Royal, S.A., and Tynes, B.S. (1978). Disseminated histoplasmosis in corticosteroid-treated patients. Report of five cases. *JAMA* 240, 1495.

Domingo, P., Coll, P., Maroto, P., *et al.* (1996). *Neisseria subflava* bateremia in a neutropenic patient. *Arch. Intern. Med.* 156, 1762.

Duffy, B.L. (1993). Intrathecal morphine and herpes reactivation. *Anaesth. Intensive Care* 21, 377.

Eisert, J., Hannibal, J.E. Jr, and Sanders, S.L. (1959). Fatal amebiasis complicating corticosteroid management of pemphigus vulgaris. *N. Engl. J. Med.* 261, 843.

Embrey, R.P. and Geist, L.J. (1995). Influenza A pneumonia following treatment of acute cardiac allograft reaction with murine anti-CD3 antibody (OKT3). *Chest* 108, 1456.

Engelhard, D., Elishoov, H., Or, N., *et al.* (1995). Cytosine arabinase as a major risk factor for *Streptococcus viridans* septicemia following bone marrow transplantation: a 5-year prospective study. *Bone Marrow Transplant.* 16, 565.

Findley, G.M. and Howard, E.M. (1952). The effects of cortisone and adrenocorticotrophic hormone on poliomyelitis and other virus infections. *J. Pharm. Pharmacol.* 4, 37.

Fischer, G.W., Hunter, K.W., Wilson, S.R., *et al.* (1980). Diminished bacterial defences with Intralipid. *Lancet* ii, 819.

Fletcher, J. and Goldstein, E. (1970). The effect of parenteral iron preparations on experimental pyelonephritis. *Br. J. Exp. Pathol.* 51, 280.

Fred, L., Rivo, J.B., and Barrett, T.F. (1951). Development of active pulmonary tuberculosis during ACTH and cortisone therapy. *JAMA* 147, 242.

Frieden, T.R., Bia, F.J., Heald, P.W., *et al.* (1993). Cutaneous cryptococcosis in a patient with cutaneous T cell lymphoma receiving therapy with photophoresis and methotrexate. *Clin. Infect. Dis.* 17, 776.

Fucci, J.C. and Nightengale, M.L. (1997). Primary esophageal histoplasmosis. *Am. J. Gastroenterol.* 92, 530.

Geleto, S.M., Melbourne, K.M., and Mikolich, D.J. (1996). *Pseudomonas* bacteremia precipitated by ticlopidine-induced neutropenia. *Ann Pharmacother.* 30, 346.

Gelpi J., Chernoff, A., Snydman, D., *et al.* (1994). A brain abscess after liver transplantation with long-term survival. *Transplantation* 57, 1669.

Gentric, A. and Pennee, Y.L. (1996). Diclofenac-induced pseudomembranous colitis. *Lancet* 340, 126.

Gill, K.A. Jr, Katz, H.I., and Baxter. D.L. (1963). Fungus infections occurring under occlusive dressings. *Arch. Dermatol.* 88, 348.

Gilhus, N.E., Strandjord, R.E., and Arli, J.A. (1982). The effect of carbamazepine on serum immunoglobulin concentrations. *Acta Neurol. Scand.* 66, 172.

Girmenia, C., Iori, A.P., Arcese, W., *et al.* (1988). Fatal listeria meningitis in immunosuppressed patients. *Lancet* i, 794.

Giunta, G. and Piazza, I. (1992). Fatal septicaemia due to *Listeria monocytogenes* in a patient with systemic lupus erythematosus receiving cyclosporin and high prednisone doses. *Neth. J. Med.* 40, 197.

Godfrey, S., Hambleton, G., and König, P. (1974). Steroid aerosols and candidiasis. *BMJ* ii, 387.

Goldstein, E. and Rambo, O.N. (1962). Cryptococcal infection following steroid therapy. *Ann. Intern. Med.* 56, 114.

Gothoni, G., Neuvonen, P.J., Mattila, M., *et al.* (1972). Iron–tetracycline interaction: effect of time interval between the drugs. *Acta Med. Scand.* 191, 409.

Goucke, C.R. and Graziotti, P. (1990). Extradural abscess following local anaesthetic and steroid injection for chronic low back pain. *Br. J. Anaesth.* 65, 427.

Griffith, L.J., Ostrander, W.E., Mullins, C.G., *et al.* (1965). Drug antagonism between lincomycin and erythromycin. *Science* 147, 746.

Groom, S.N., Clewley, J., Litton, P.A., *et al.* (1994). Vaccine-associated poliomyelitis. *Lancet* 343, 609.

Gupta A.K., Knowles, S.R., Gupta M.A., *et al.* (1995). Lithium therapy associated with hidradenitis suppurativa: case report and review of the dermatologic side effects of lithium. *J. Am. Acad. Dermatol.* 32, 382.

Gupta, R. and Sachar, D.B. (1985). Chlorpropamide-induced cholestatic jaundice and pseudomembranous colitis. *Am. J. Gastroenterol.* 78, 811.

Guyer, P.B. and Delany, D. (1970). Urinary tract dilatation and oral contraceptives. *BMJ* iv, 588.

Hall, M.R.P. (1972). Drugs and the elderly. *Adverse Drug React. Bull.* 35, 108.

Hassan, K.E. and Browne, M.K. (1978). Candida peritonitis and cimetidine. *Lancet* ii, 1054.

Haverkos, H.W., Amsel, Z., and Drotman, D.P. (1991). Adverse virus–drug interactions. *Rev. Infect. Dis.* 13, 697.

Hayem, G., Meyer, O., and Kahn, M-F. (1996). *Listeria monocytogenes* infection in a patient treated with methotrexate for rheumatoid arthritis. *J. Rheumatol.* 23, 198.

Heatley, R.V. (1995). *The Helicobacter Handbook*. Blackwell, London.

Hecht, J.R. and Olinger, E.J. (1989). *Clostridium difficile* colitis secondary to intravenous vancomycin. *Dig. Dis. Sci.* 34, 148.

Hellinger, W.C., Oldenburgh, W.A., and Alvarez, S. (1995). Vascular and other serious infection with *Mycobacterium bovis* after Bacillus of Calmette–Guérin therapy for bladder cancer. *South. Med. J.* 88, 1212.

Helpern, D.J. (1985). Atypical pyoderma as a side effect of isotretinoin. *J. Am. Acad. Derm.* 13, 1045.

Hersen, V.C., Krause, P.J., Eisenfeld, L.I., *et al.* (1988). Indomethacin-associated sepsis in very-low-birthweight infants. *AJDC* 142, 555.

Higenbottam, T.W. and Heard, B.E. (1976). Opportunistic pulmonary strongyloidiasis complicating asthma treated with steroids. *Thorax* 31, 226.

Hoen, B., Renoult, E., Jonon, B., *et al.* (1988). Septicaemia due to *Yersinia enterocolitica* in a long-term haemodialysis patient after a single desferrioxamine administration. *Nephron* 50, 378.

Høiby, N., Jarløv, J.O., Kemp, M., *et al.* (1997). Excretion of ciprofloxacin in sweat and multiresistant *Staphylococcus epidermidis*. *Lancet* 349, 167.

Holley, H.P. and Thiers, B.H. (1986). Cryptosporidiosis in a patient receiving immunosuppressive therapy: possible reactivation of latent infection. *Dig. Dis. Sci.* 31, 1004.

Hongou,M., Yamane, M., Igishi, T., *et al.* (1992). Fatal case of invasive pulmonary aspergillosis (septic type) during treatment for status asthmaticus. *Kokyu To Junkan* 11, 344.

Hoppe, J.E., Orlikowski, T., Klingebiel, T., *et al.* (1992). Costal B.C.G. osteomyelitis presenting as a bone tumour. *Infection* 20, 94.

Humphrey, J.H.C. and McClelland, M. (1944). Cranial nerve palsies with herpes following general anaesthesia. *BMJ* i, 315.

Huppertz, H-I. and Scheurlen, W. (1991). *Salmonella* septic arthritis presenting as reactive arthritis. *J. Rheumatol.* 18, 1112.

Hutter, R.V.P. (1959). Phycomycetous infection (mucormycosis) in cancer patients: a complication of therapy. *Cancer* 12, 330.

Ion-Nedelcu, N., Dobrescu, A., Strebel, P.M., *et al.* (1994). Vaccine-associated paralytic poliomyelitis and HIV infection. *Lancet* 343, 51.

Ive, F.A. and Marks, R. (1968). Tinea incognita. *BMJ* iii, 149.

Iveson, T.J. and Chan, A. (1992). Pseudomembranous colitis complicating chemotherapy. *Lancet* 339, 192.

Izes, J.K., Birle III, W., and Thomas, C.B. (1993). Corticosteroid-associated fatal mycobacterial sepsis occurring 3 years after instillation of intravesical bacillus Calmette-Guérin. *J. Urol.* 150, 1498.

Izumi, A.K. and Matsunaga, J. (1992). BCG vaccine-induced lupus vulgaris. *Arch. Dermatol.* 118, 171.

Jacobs, H.W. (1963). Unusual fatal infectious complications of steroid-treated liver disease. *Gastroenterology* 44, 519.

Jivà, T.M., Kallau, M.C., Marin, M.G., *et al.* (1993). Simultaneous legionellosis and invasive aspergillosis in an immunocompetent patient newly treated wih corticosteroids. *Chest* 104, 1929.

John, G.T., Vincent, L., Jayaseelani, L., *et al.* (1994). Cyclosporin immunosuppression and mycobacterial infection. *Transplantation* 58, 247.

Jones, A.G. (1993). Anaesthetic death of a child with a cold. *Anaesthesia* 48, 642.

Jones, R.R. (1991). Recurrent facial herpes associated with Chinese herbal remedy. *Lancet* 337, 55.

Joynson, D.H.M., Jacobs, A., Walker, D.M., *et al.* (1972). Defect of cell-mediated immunity in patients with iron-deficiency anaemia. *Lancet* ii, 1058.

Junker, A.K., Chan, K.W., and Lirenman, D.S. (1989). Epstein–Barr virus infections following OKT3 treatment. *Transplantation* 47, 574.

Kamthan, A.G., Bruckner, H.W., Hirschman, S.Z., *et al.* (1992). *Clostridium difficile* diarrhea induced by cancer chemotherapy. *Arch. Intern. Med.* 15, 1715.

Kaslow, J.E., Novey, H.S., Zich, R.H., *et al.* (1990). Disseminated strongyloidiasis: an unheralded risk of corticosteroid therapy. *J Allergy. Clin. Immunol.* 86, 138.

Kass, E.H. and Finland, M. (1953). Adrenocortical hormones in infection and immunity. *Annu. Rev. Microbiol.* 7, 361.

Katz, D.S., Wogalter, H., D'Esposito, R.F., *et al.* (1992). *Mycobacterium bovis* vertebral osteomyelitis and psoas abscess after intravesical B.C.G. therapy for bladder carcinoma. *Urology* 40, 63.

Kaufman, J.H. (1962). Cutaneous sporotrichosis and candidiasis occurring in a patient on prolonged steroid therapy. *J. Mich. State Med. Assoc.* 61, 190.

Keegan, J. and Byrd, J.W. (1988). Nocardiosis associated with low-dose methotrexate for rheumatoid arthritis. *J. Rheumatol.* 15, 1585.

Kluin-Nelemans, J.C., Koelma, J.A., van der Merwe, P.C., *et al.* (1991). Fulminant pulmonary *Aspergillus* infection occluding the aortic arch after high-dose antileukemic chemotherapy. *Cancer* 67, 3123.

Knupp, C.A. and Barbhaiya, R.H. (1997). A multiple-dose pharmacokinetic interaction study between didanosine (Videx®) and ciprofloxacin (Cipro®) in male subjects seropositive for HIV but asymptomatic. *Biopharm. Drug. Dispos.* 18, 65.

Kochar, R., Talwar, P., Singh, S., *et al.* (1988). Invasive candidiasis following cimetidine therapy. *Am. J. Gastroenterol.* 83, 102.

Köhler, W. and Speelman, P. (1992). A time of cholera. In *The Beast in Man,* Part 1 (ed. A van Everdingen), pp. 115, 123. Belvédère Publishers, Overveen.

König, F., Stumpp. W., Kohler, T., *et al.* (1993). Bacterial infection during high dosage therapy with clozapine. *Nervenarzt* 64, 681.

Kouides, P.A., Slapak, C.A., Rosenwasser, L.J., *et al.* (1988). *Pneumocystis carinii* pneumonia as a complication of desferrioxamine therapy. *Br. J. Haematol.* 70, 383.

LaFontaine, P.D., Middleman, B.R., Graham Jr, S.D., *et al.* (1997). Incidence of granulomatous prostatitis and acid-fast bacilli after intra-vesical BCG therapy. *Urology* 49, 363.

Lake, K., Anderson, D., Milford, S., *et al.* (1993). The incidence of cytomegalovirus disease is not increased after OKT3 induction therapy. *J. Heart Lung Transplant.* 12, 5378.

Larner, A.J. and Lendrum, R. (1992). Oesophageal candidiasis after omeprazole. *Gut* 33, 860.

Larson, H.E. (1987). Clostridial infection of gastrointestinal tract — pseudomembranous colitis. In *Oxford Textbook of Medicine* (2nd edn) (ed. D.J. Weatherall, J.G.G. Ledingham, and D.A. Warrell), p. 5.274. Oxford University Press.

Latour, N.G. and Reeves, R.E. (1965). An iron requirement for growth of *Entamoeba histolytica* in culture; and the anti-amoebal activity of 7-iodo-8-hydroxy-quinoline-5-sulfonic acid. *Exp. Parasitol.* 17, 203.

Lazan, A. (1971). Gynecologic moniliasis: incidence with various contraceptive methods. *J. Med. Soc. N.J.* 68, 37.

Lee, P.S. and Lau, E.Y.L. (1988). Risk of acute non-specific respiratory tract infection in healthy men taking dapsone–pyrimethamine for prophylaxis against malaria. *BMJ* 296, 893.

Leenders, A., Sonneveld, P., and de Maie, S. (1995). Cryptococcal meningitis following fludarabine treatment for chronic lymphatic leukaemia. *Eur. J. Microbiol. Infect. Dis.* 14, 826.

Leighton, P.M. and MacSween, H.M. (1987). *Yersinia* hepatic abscesses subsequent to long-term iron therapy. *JAMA* 257, 964.

Lepper, M.H. and Dowling. H.F. (1951). Treatment of pneumococcic meningitis with penicillin compared with penicillin plus aureomycin. *Arch. Intern. Med.* 88, 489.

Lessof, M.H. (1972). The current status of transplantation immunology. In *The Scientific Basis of Medicine: Annual Reviews, 1972* (ed. I. Gilliland and J. Francis), p. 122. Athlone, London.

Levy, J.S. (1969). Vaccinia gangrenosum; rare complication of smallpox vaccination. *South. Med. J.* 62, 1408.

Leyden, J.J. and James, W.D. (1987). *Staphylococcus aureus* infection as a complication of isotretinoin. *Arch. Dermatol.* 123, 606.

Likhite, V., Rodvein, R., and Crosby, W.H. (1976). Depressed phagocytic function exhibited by polymorphonuclear leucocytes from chronically iron-deficient rabbits. *Br. J. Haematol.* 34, 251.

Lorenc, E. (1967). A new factor in griseofulvin treatment failures: case report. *Mo. Med.* 64, 32.

McCambridge, M.A., Vogelsang, S.A., and Ockenhouse, C.F. (1995). *Listeria monocytogenes* infection in a patient treated with methotrexate for rheumatoid arthritis. *J. Rheumatol.* 22, 786.

MacDonald, T.M., Beardon, P.H.G., McGilchrist, M.M., *et al.* (1993). The risks of symptomatic vaginal candidiasis. *Q. J. Med.* 86, 419.

MacDougall, L.G., Anderson, R., MacNab, G.M., *et al.* (1975). The immune response in iron-deficient children:

impaired cellular defense mechanisms with altered humoral components. *J. Pediatr.* 86, 833.

Mackay, A., Macloud, T., Alcorn, M.J., *et al.* (1980). Fatal disseminated BCG infection in an eighteen-year-old boy. *Lancet* ii, 1332.

MacKenzie, N.G., Chapman, O.W., and Middleton, P.J. (1969). Progressive vaccinia with chronic lymphatic leukaemia. *N.Z. Med. J.* 70. 324.

McLaughlin, J.E. and Reeves, D.S. (1971). Clinical and laboratory evidence for inactivation of gentamicin by carbenicillin. *Lancet* i, 261.

Macher, L., Machet, M-C., Maillot, F., *et al.* (1995). Cutaneous alternariosis occurring in a patient treated with local intra-rectal steroids. *Acta Derm. Venereol.* 75, 328.

Mahaffey, K.W., Hippenmyer, C.L., Mandel, R., *et al.* (1993). Unrecognized coccidiomycosis complicating *Pneumocystis carinii* pneumonia in patients infected with the human immunodeficiency virus and treated wih steroids. A report of two cases. *Arch. Intern. Med.* 153, 1496.

Marshall, S., Lyon, R.P., and Minkler, D. (1966). Ureteral dilatation following use of oral contraceptives. *JAMA* 198, 782.

Masawe, A.E.J., Muindi, J.M., and Swai, G.B.R. (1974). Infections in iron deficiency and other types of anaemia in the tropics. *Lancet* ii, 314.

Maskell, R., Okubadejo, O.A., and Payne, R.H. (1976). Thymine-requiring bacteria associated with co-trimoxazole therapy. *Lancet* i, 834.

Mayer, G., Watschinger, B., Pohanka, E., *et al.* (1988). Cytomegalovirus infection after kidney transplantation using cyclosporin A and low-dose prednisolone immunosuppression. *Nephrol. Dial. Transplant.* 3, 464.

Mayfield, R.B. (1962). Tuberculosis occurring in association with corticosteroid treatment. *Tubercle* 43, 55.

Meadow, S.R., Weller. R.O., and Archibald, R.W.R. (1969). Fatal systemic measles in a child receiving cyclophosphamide for nephrotic syndrome. *Lancet* ii, 876.

Mermel, L., Sanchez de Moa, D., Sutter, R.W., *et al.* (1993). Vaccine-associated paralytic poliomyelitis. *N. Engl. J. Med.* 329, 810.

Middelbeek, A., Sturkenboom, M.C., and de Jong-van den Berg, L.T.W. (1993). Vaginal candidiasis associated with acetretin? *Pharm. World Sci.* 15 (Suppl. K), 10.

Midtvedt, T. (1989). Penicillins, cephalosporins, and tetracyclines. In *Side Effects of Drugs — Annual 13* (ed. M.N.G. Dukes and L. Beeley), p. 210. Elsevier, Amsterdam.

Miller, S.N. and Ringler, R.P. (1987). Vancomycin-induced pseudomembranous colitis. *J. Clin. Gastroenterol.* 9, 114.

Milteer, R.M., Sarpong, S., and Poydras, U. (1989). *Yersinia enterocolitica* septicemia after accidental oral overdose. *Pediatr. Infect. Dis. J.* 8, 537.

Milton-Thompson, G.J., Lightfoot, N.F., Ahmet, Z., *et al.* (1982). Intragastric acidity, bacteria, nitrite, and *N*-nitroso compounds before, during, and after cimetidine treatment. *Lancet* i, 1091.

Minoli, G., Teruzzi, V., Butti, G.C., *et al.* (1987). Invasive candidiasis does not complicate short-term treatment of duodenal ulcer. *Gastrointest. Endosc.* 33, 227.

Mody, V.R. (1959). Corticosteroids in latent amoebiasis. *BMJ* ii, 1399.

Mogabgab, W.J. and Thomas, L. (1950). Quoted by Fred *et al.* (1951) (see above).

Morgan, M.B. and Iseman, M.D. (1996). *Mycobacterium bovis* vertebral osteomyelitis as a complication of intravesical bacille Calmette–Guérin. *Am. J. Med.* 100, 372.

Morita H., Tani, M., Adaci, H., *et al.* (1991). Methicillin-resistant *Staphylococcus aureus* (MRSA) enteritis associated with prophylactic cephalosporin administration and hypochlorhydria after subtotal gastrectomy. *Am. J. Gastroenterol.* 86, 791.

Morris, C.A. and Morris, D.F. (1969). 'Normal' vaginal microbiology of women of childbearing age in relation to use of oral contraceptives and vaginal tampons. *J. Clin. Pathol.* 20, 636.

Morrison, W.L., Webb, W.J.S., Aldred, J., *et al.* (1988). Meningitis after BCG vaccination. *Lancet* i, 654.

Morugasu, B. Quah, T.C., Quack, S.H., *et al.* (1988). Disseminated BCG infection — a case report. *J. Singapore Pediatr. Soc.* 30, 139

Mosiman, F. (1993). Esophageal candidiasis, omeprazole and organ transplantation — a word of caution. *Transplantation* 56, 492.

Mudad, R., Vredenburgh, J., Paulson, E.K., *et al.* (1994). A radiologic syndrome after high-dose chemotherapy and autologous bone marrow transplantation, with clinical and pathologic features of systemic candidiasis. *Cancer* 74, 1360.

Murray, M.F., Galetta, S.L., Raops, E.C., *et al.* (1996). Deferoxamine-associated mucormycosis in a non-dialysis patient. *Infect. Dis. Clin. Pract.* 5, 395.

Murray, M.J., Murray, A.B., and Murray, C.J. (1980). The salutary effect of milk on amoebiasis and its reversal by iron. *BMJ* i, 1351.

Murray, M.J., Murray, A.B., Murray, N.J., *et al.* (1975). Refeeding-malaria and hyperferraemia. *Lancet* i, 636.

Murray, M.J., Murray, A.B., Murray, M.B., *et al.* (1978). The adverse effects of iron repletion on the course of certain infections. *BMJ* ii, 1113.

Nabarro, J.D.N. (1960). The pituitary and adrenal cortex in general medicine. *BMJ* ii, 625.

Neal, K.R., Brij, S.O., Slack, R.C.B., *et al.* (1994). Recent treatment with H$_2$-antagonists and antibiotics and gastric surgery as risk factors for salmonella infection. *BMJ* 308, 176.

Neal, K.R., Scott, H.M., Slack, R.C.B., *et al.* (1996). Omeprazole as a risk factor for campylobacter gastroenteritis: a case–control study. *BMJ* 312, 414.

Nelson, M.R., Erskine, D., Hawkins, D.A., *et al.* (1993). Treatmen with corticosteroids — a risk factor for the development of clinical cytomegalovirus disease in AIDS. *AIDS* 7, 375.

Neuvonen, P.J., Gothoni, G., Hackman, R., *et al.* (1970). Interference of iron with the absorption of tetracyclines in man. *BMJ* iv, 532.

Nielsen, H., Daugaard, M., Tvede, M., *et al.* (1992). High incidence of *Clostridium difficile* during intensive chemotherapy for disseminated germ cell cancer. *Br. J. Cancer* 66, 666.

Niimi, T., Kajita, M., and Saito, H. (1991). Necrotizing aspergillosis in a patient receiving neoadjuvant chemotherapy for non-small cell lung carcinoma. *Chest* 100, 277.

Nishi, J-I., Kamenosono, A., and Pada Sarker, K. (1997). Bacille Calmette–Guérin osteomyelitis. *Pediatr. Infect. Dis.* 16, 32.

Nouel, O., Voisin, P.M., Vaucel, J., *et al.* (1991). *Yersinia enterocolitica* septicemia associated with idiopathic haemochromatosis and desferrioxamine therapy. A case report. *Presse Méd.* 20, 1494.

Nwokolo. C.U., Loft, D.E., Vaucel, J., *et al.* (1994). Increased incidence of bacterial diarrhoea in patients taking gastric acid antisecretory drugs. *Eur. J. Gastroenterol. Hepatol.* 6, 697.

Ohtsu, T., Sai, T., Oka, M., *et al.* (1991). Activation of hepatitis virus B by chemotherapy containing glucocorticoid in hepatitis B virus carriers with hematologic malignancies. *Jpn J. Clin. Oncol.* 21, 360.

Oppenheimer, S.J., Gibson, F.D., Macfarlane, S.B., *et al.* (1984). Iron supplementation and malaria. *Lancet* i, 389.

O'Reilly, S., Hartley, P., Jeffers, M., *et al.* (1994). Invasive pulmonary aspergillosis associated with low-dose methotrexate therapy for rheumatoid arthritis: a case report of treatment with itraconazole. *Tubercle Lung Dis.* 75, 153.

Osband, M.E., Shen, T.J., Shlesinger, M., *et al.* (1981). Successful tumour immunotherapy with cimetidine in mice. *Lancet* i, 636.

Parkin, J., Tomlinson, D.R., and Pinching, A.J. (1990). Interaction between fluconazole and rifampicin. *BMJ* 301, 818.

Penman, I.D., Palmer, K.P., and Blackwell, C.C. (1997). *Helicobacter pylori:* the story so far. *J. R. Coll. Physicians Edinb.* 27, 37.

Pennant, J.H. and Wallace, D. (1991). Intrathecal morphine and reactivation of oral herpes simplex. *Anesthesiology* 75, 167.

Perez, M.D. and Wilking, A.P. (1992). Disseminated histoplasmosis in pediatric rheumatic disease patients treated with corticosteroids. *J. Rheumatol.* (suppl. 33), 112.

Peterkin, G.A.G. and Khan, S.A. (1969). Iatrogenic skin disease. *Practitioner* 202, 117.

Phair, J., Munoz, A., Detels, R., and the Multicenter AIDS Cohort Study Group (1990). The risk of *Pneumocystis carinii* pneumonia among men infected with human immunodeficiency virus type I. *N. Engl. J. Med.* 322, 161.

Phillips, I. and Eykyn, S.J. (1987). Staphylococci. In *Oxford Textbook of Medicine* (2nd edn) (ed. D.J. Weatherall, J.G.G. Ledingham, and D.A. Warrell), p. 5.191. Oxford University Press.

Piguet, D. (1969). *In vitro* inhibitive action of nitrofurantoin on the bacteriostatic activity of nalidixic acid. *Ann. Inst. Pasteur* (Paris) 116, 43.

Pillemer, S.R., Webb, D., and Yocum, D.E. (1989). Legionnaires' disease in a patient with rheumatoid arthritis treated with cyclosporine. *J. Rheumatol.* 16, 117.

Proctor, D.D., Chopra, S., Rubenstein, S.C., *et al.* (1993). Mycobacteremia and granulomatous hepatitis following initial intravesicular bacillus Calmette–Guérin instillation for bladder carcinoma. *Am. J. Gastroenterol.* 88, 1112.

Pullan, C.R., Noble, T.C., Scott, D.J., *et al.* (1976). Atypical measles infections in leukaemic children on immunosuppressive treatment. *BMJ* i, 1562.

Purtilo, D.T., Meyers, D.M., and Connor, D.H. (1974). Fatal strongyloidiasis in immunosuppressed patients. *Am. J. Med.* 56, 488.

Querfurth, H. and Swanson, P.D. (1990). Vaccine-associated paralytic poliomyelitis. Regional case series and review. *Arch. Neurol.* 47, 541.

Rao, A.R., Sukumar, M.S., Kamalakshi, S., *et al.* (1968). Experimental variola in monkeys. *Indian J. Med. Res.* 56, 1855.

Rao, S.P.P., Miller, S.T., and Cohen, B.J. (1994). B19 parvovirus infection in children with malignant solid tumours. *Med. Pediatr. Oncol.* 22, 255.

Reed, S.M. and Glick, J.W. (1991). Fluoxetine and reactivation of the herpes simplex virus. *Am. J. Psychiatry* 148, 949.

Ren, E.C. and Chan, S.H. (1988). Possible enhancement of Epstein–Barr infections by the use of OKT3 in transplant recipients. *Transplantation* 45, 988.

Rex, J.H., Ginsberg, A.M., Fries, L.F., *et al.* (1988). *Cunninghamella bertholletiae* infection associated with deferoxamine therapy. *Rev. Infect. Dis.* 10, 1187.

Reynaert, H., Fernandes, E., Bourgain, C., *et al.* (1995). Proton pump inhibition and gastric giardiasis: a causal or casual association? *J. Gastroenterol.* 30, 775.

Reynolds, R.D., Boiko, S., and Lucky, A.W. (1991). Exacerbation of tinea corporis during treatment with 1% clotrimazole/0.05% betamethasone dipropionate (Lotrison). *Am. J. Dis. Child.* 145, 1224.

Ribera, M., Bielsa, J., Materola, J.M., *et al.* (1995). Mycobacterium B.C.G. infection of the glans penis: a complication of intravesical adminisration of bacillus Calmette–Guérin. *Br. J. Dermatol.* 132, 307.

Richards, J.M., Gilewski, T.A., and Vogelzang, N.J. (1991). Association of interleukin-2 therapy with staphylococcal bacteremia. *Cancer* 67, 1570.

Riegelman, S., Rowland, M., and Epstein, W.L. (1970). Griseofulvin-phenobarbital interaction in man. *JAMA* 213, 426.

Riley, T.V., Codde, J.P., and Rouge, I.L. (1995). Increased length of stay in hospital due to *Clostridium difficile*-associated diarrhoea. *Lancet* 345, 455.

Robins-Browne, R.M. and Prpic, J.K. (1983). Desferrioxamine and systemic yersiniosis. *Lancet* ii, 1372.

Robins-Browne, R.M., Rabson, A.R., and Koornhof, H. (1979). Generalized infection with *Yersinia enterocolitica* and the role of iron. *Contrib. Microbiol. Immunol.* 5, 277.

Roda, P. (1987). *Clostridium difficile* colitis induced by cytarabine. *Am. J. Clin. Oncol.* 10, 451.

Rose, A. and Hill, A. (1993). Intrathecal morphine and herpes reactivation. *Anaesth. Intensive Care* 21, 126.

Ruddell, W.S.J., Axon, A.T.R., Findlay, J.M., *et al.* (1980). Effect of cimetidine on gastric bacterial flora. *Lancet* i, 672.

Sai, S., Sakakibara, T., Takashi, M., *et al.* (1990). Granulomatous prostatitis after intravesical B.C.G. immunotherapy: a case report. *Hinyokika Kiyo* 36, 953.

Salinier, L., de Jaureguiberry, J.P., Carlos, E., *et al.* (1992). Cytomegalovirus pneumopathy during rheumatoid arthritis treated with low-dose methotrexate. *Rev. Med. Interne* 13 (Suppl. 6), 223.

Sane, A., Manzi, S., Perfect, J., *et al.* (1989). Deferoxamine treatment as a risk factor for zygomycete infection. *J. Infect. Dis.* 159, 151.

Satin, A.J., Harrison, C.R., Hancock, K.C., *et al.* (1989). Relapsing *Clostridium difficile* toxin-associated colitis in ovarian cancer patients treated with chemotherapy. *Obstet. Gynecol.* 74, 487.

Sayers, G. and Travis, R.H. (1970). Adrenocorticotropic hormone, adrenocortical steroids and their synthetic analogs. In *The Pharmacological Basis of Therapeutics* (4th edn) (ed. L.S. Goodman and A. Gilman), pp. 1622, 1624. Macmillan, New York.

Scalzini, A., Barni, C., Stellini, R., *et al.* (1995). Fatal invasive aspergillosis during cyclosporine and steroids treatment for Crohn's disease. *Dig. Dis. Sci.* 40, 528.

Schenfeld, L.A. and Pote, H.H., Jr. (1995). Diarrhea associated with parenteral vancomycin therapy. *Clin. Infect. Dis.* 20, 1578.

Schwartz, J., Rosenfeld, V., Rafael, C., *et al.* (1994). Septicemia associated with barium enema. *J. Am. Geriatr. Soc.* 42, 570.

Scott, H.M., Neal, K.R., Slack, R.C.B., *et al.* (1994). Omeprazole treatment, a patient risk factor for Campylobacter gastroenteritis. *Gastroenterology* 106 (suppl.), 1049.

Seager, J. (1984). IgA deficiency during treatment of infantile hypothyroidism with thyroxine. *BMJ* 288, 1562.

Seeverens, H.J.T., Tijhuis, G.J., Ruijs, G.J., *et al.* (1992). Dialysis-associated mucormycosis and desferrioxamine treatment: a case report with review of the role of oxygen radicles. *Neth. J. Med.* 41, 275.

Shindo, M., Di Bascelie, A.M., and Hoofnagel, J.H. (1992). Acute exacerbation of liver disease during interferon-alpha therapy for chronic hepatitis C. *Gastroenterology* 102, 1406.

Sidransky, H. and Pearl, M.A. (1961). Pulmonary fungus infections associated with steroid and antibiotic therapy. *Dis. Chest* 39, 630.

Siegel, J.P. and Puri, R.K. (1991). Interleukin-2 toxicity. *J. Clin. Oncol.* 9, 694.

Singh. N., Gayowski, T., Wagener, M., *et al.* (1996). Pulmonary infection in liver transplant recipients receiving tacrolimus: changing patterns of microbial etiologies. *Transplantation* 61, 396.

Skrede, S., Ro, J.S., and Mjolnerod, O. (1973). Effects of dextrans on the plasma proteins changes during the postoperative period. *Clin. Chim. Acta* 48, 143.

Slade, M.P. and McNab, A.A. (1991). Fatal mucormycosis associated wtih deferoxamine. *Am. J. Ophthalmol.* 112, 594.

Slavin, M.A., Meyers, J.D., Remington J.S., *et al.* (1994). *Toxoplasma gondii* infection in marrow transplant recipients: a 20-year experience. *Bone Marrow Transpl.* 13, 549.

Smith, D.F., Smith, C.C., Douglas, J.G., *et al.* (1990). Severe salmonellosis related to oral administration of antidiarrhoeals. *Scot. Med. J.* 35, 176.

Sobel, J.D., Chaim, W., and Leaman, D. (1996). Recurrent vulvovaginal candidiasis associated with long-term tamoxifen treatment in postmenopausal women. *Obstet. Gynecol.* 88, 704.

Sobrevilla, L.A., Tedeschi, L.G., Cronin, J.F., *et al.* (1962). *Listeria monocytogenes* meningitis as a complication of steroid therapy. *Boston Med. Q.* 13, 62.

Sombolos, K., Kalekou, H., Barboutis, K., *et al.* (1988). Fatal phycomycosis in a haemodialysed patient receiving deferoxamine. *Nephron* 49, 169.

Sorrell, T.C., Forbes, I.J., Burness, F.R., *et al.* (1971). Depression of immunoglobulin function in patients treated with phenytoin sodium (sodium diphenylhydantoin). *Lancet* ii, 1233.

Sowa, J.M. (1993). Sterile oily abscess from gold therapy. *Arthritis Rheum.* 36, 1632.

Spain, D.M. (1961). Steroid alterations in the histopathology of chemically induced inflammation. In *Inflammation and Diseases of Connective Tissue* (ed. L.C. Mills and J.W. Mayer). Saunders, Philadelphia.

Spaulding, W.B. (1962). Dangers in the use of some potent drugs. *Can. Med. Assoc. J.* 87, 1275.

Spielberger, R.T., Stock, W., and Larson, R.A. (1993). Listeriosis after 2-chlordeoxyadenosine treatment. *N. Engl. J. Med.* 328, 813.

Spinillo, A., Capuzzo, E., Nicola, S., *et al.* (1995). The impact of oral contraception on vulvovaginal candidiasis. *Contraception* 51, 293.

Sriuanpong, V. and Voravud, N. (1995). Antineoplastic-associated colitis in Chulalongkorn University Hospital. *J. Med. Assoc. Thai.* 78, 424.

Stark, F.R., Ninos, N., Hutton, J., *et al.* (1978). *Candida* peritonitis and cimetidine. *Lancet* ii, 744.

Stellon, A.J. and Wakeling, M. (1989). Hidradenitis suppurativa associated with oral contraceptives. *BMJ* 298, 28.

Stien, D.S. and Weems, J.J. (1991). Cavitary *Pneumocystis carinii* pneumonia in patients receiving aerosol pentamidine prophylaxis. *South. Med. J.* 84, 273.

Stille, W. and Ostner, K.H. (1966). Antagonismus Nitrofurantoin–Nalidixinsäure. *Klin. Wochenschr.* 44, 155.

Stockbrugger, R.W., Eugenidis, N., Bartholomew, B.A., *et al.* (1981). Cimetidine treatment, intragastric bacterial overgrowth and its consequences. *Gastroenterology* 80, 1295.

Stockley, I. (1974). *Drug Interactions and their Mechanisms*, p. 35. Pharmaceutical Press, London.

Strom, J. (1955). The question of antagonism between penicillin and chlortetracycline, illustrated by therapeutical experiments in scarlatina. *Antibiotic Med.* 1, 6.

Stuiver, P.C. and Goud, Th.J. (1978). Corticosteroids and liver amoebiasis. *BMJ* ii, 394.

Sullivan, A-A., Boyle, R.S., and Whitby, R.M. (1995). Vaccine-associated paralytic poliomyelitis. *Med. J. Aust.* 163, 423.

Swarup-Mitra, S. and Sinha, A.K. (1982). PMN function in

nutritional anaemias: phagocytosis and bacterial killing. *Indian J. Med. Res.* 75, 259.

Symmers, W.St.C. (1966). Septicaemia candidosis. In *Symposium on Candida infections* (ed. H.I. Winner and R. Hurley), p. 208. Churchill Livingstone, Edinburgh.

Szanto, S. (1971). *Trichomonas* and oxytetracycline. *BMJ* ii, 467.

Tardieu, M., Truffot-Pernot, C., Carriere, J.P., *et al.* (1988). Tuberculous meningitis due to BCG in two patients. *Lancet* i, 440.

Theodossiou, C., Temeck, B., Vargas, H., *et al.* (1995). Cytomegalovirus enteritis after treatment with 5-fluorouracil, leukovorin, cisplatin, and alpha-interferon. *Am. J. Gastroenterol.* 90, 1174.

Thorne, R.D. (1982). Cimetidine and brucellosis. *Lancet* ii, 217.

Tomietto, F., Ramondi, C., Frasca, G.M., *et al.* (1995). Disseminated candidiasis in a lupus nephritis patient under long-term immunosuppression. *Nephrol. Dialysis Transplant.* 10, 896.

Triger, D.R., Goepel, J.R., Slater, D.N., *et al.* (1981). Systemic candidiasis complicating acute hepatic failure in patients treated with cimetidine. *Lancet* ii, 837.

Truelson, T., Wishnow, K.I., and Johnson, D.E. (1992). Epididymo-orchitis developing as a late manifestation of intravesicular bacillus Calmette–Guérin and masquerading as a primary testicular malignancy: a report of two cases. *J. Urol.* 148, 1534.

Valley, M.A., Rourke, D.L., and McKenzie, A.M. (1992). Recurrence of thoracic and labial herpes simplex infection in a patient receiving epidural fentanyl. *Anesthesiology* 76, 1056.

van Riel, P.L., Van de Putte, L.B., Gribnau, F.W., *et al.* (1984). Serum IgA and gold-induced toxic effects in patients with rheumatoid arthritis. *Arch. Intern. Med.* 144, 1401.

Veis, J.H., Contigulia, R., Klein, M., *et al.* (1987). Mucormycosis in deferoxamine-treated patients on dialysis. *Ann. Intern. Med.* 107, 258.

Viljanto, J. (1980). Disinfection of surgical wounds without inhibition of normal wound healing. *Arch. Surg.* 115, 253.

Vogel, C.M., Kingsburg, R.J., and Baue, A.E. (1972). Intravenous hyperalimentation: a review of two and one-half years' experience. *Arch. Surg.* 105, 414.

Wagner, J.G. (1961). Biopharmaceutics: absorption aspects. *J. Pharm. Sci.* 50, 359.

Wagner, J.G. (1968). Aspects of pharmacokinetics and biopharmaceutics in relation to drug activity. *Am. J. Pharmacol.* 141, 5.

Wagner, J.G. (1969). Cyclamates antagonistic to antibiotics. *J. Am. Diet. Assoc.* 54, 121.

Wallace, J.F., Smith, R.H., Garcia, M., *et al.* (1965). Antagonism between penicillin and chloramphenicol in experimental pneumococcal meningitis. *Antimicrob. Ag. Chemother.* 5, 439.

Wallace, J.R. and Luchi, M. (1996). Fatal Cytomegalovirus pneumonia in a patient receiving corticosteroids for mixed connective tissue disease. *South. Med. J.* 89, 726.

Walter, J.B. and Israel, M.S. (eds) (1974). *General Pathology*, p. 96. Churchill Livingstone, Edinburgh.

Webster, A.D.B. (1987). Immune deficiency. In *Oxford Textbook of Medicine* (2nd edn) (ed. D.J. Weatherall, J.G.G. Ledingham, and D.A. Warrell), p. 4.80. Oxford University Press.

Wiest, P.M., Flanigan, T., Salata, R.A., *et al.* (1989). Serious infectious complications of corticosteroid therapy for COPD. *Chest* 95, 1180.

Wilson, G.S. and Miles, A.A. (1955). *Topley and Wilson's Principles of Bacteriology and Immunity* (4th edn), pp. 1163, 1167. Arnold, London.

Wingard, J.R., Merz, W.G., Rinaldi, M.G., *et al.* (1991). Increase in *Candida krusei* infection among patients with bone marrow transplantation and neutropenia treated prophylactically with fluconazole. *N. Engl. J. Med.* 325, 1274.

Wingate, D.L. (1990). Acid reduction and recurrent enteritis. *Lancet* 335, 222.

Witty, I.A., Steiner, F., Curtmen, M., *et al.* (1992). Disseminated histoplasmosis in patients receiving low-dose methotrexate therapy for psoriasis. *Arch. Dermatol.* 128, 91.

Wong, V., Wyatt, J., Lewis, F., *et al.* (1993). Gold-induced enterocolitis complicated by Cytomegalovirus infection: a previously unrecognized association. *Gut* 34, 1002.

Yaffee, H.S. and Grots, I. (1965). Moniliasis due to norethynodrel with mestranol. *N. Engl. J. Med.* 272, 647.

Yamori, S., Yamamoto, M., Kawabata, A., *et al.* (1989). Strongyloidiasis following long-term corticosteroid therapy. *Nippon Kyobu Shikkan Gakkai Zasshi* 27, 1228.

Yetgin, S., Altay, C., Ciliv, G., *et al.* (1979). Myeloperoxide activity and bactericidal function of PMN in iron deficiency. *Acta Haematol.* 61, 10.

Youinou, P. and Le Goff, P. (1987). Drug-induced impairment of polymorphonuclear bactericidal ability in rheumatoid arthritis. *Ann. Rheum. Dis.* 46, 50.

Zangerle, R. and Allerberger, F. (1991). Effect of prophylaxis against *Pneumocystis carinii* on toxoplasma encephalitis. *Lancet* 337, 1232.

Zlotogorski, A. and Liebovici, V. (1987). Does etretinate exacerbate scabies? *Br. J. Dermatol.* 116, 882.

26. Neoplastic disorders

J. S. MALPAS and D. M. DAVIES

The role of hormones, immunosuppressants, and cytotoxic agents in the causation of neoplasia is now well established. As a result, some agents have been withdrawn, and others such as stilboestrol are no longer used. The degree of risk associated with the use of oestrogen replacement therapy in causing breast cancer, the relationship of the contraceptive pill to the causation of cancer of the breast, or its possible protective effect in reducing the incidence of cancer of the ovary, are now major concerns in the field of public health. One of the most striking recent advances has been the publication of studies of large numbers of adults and children followed up over a considerable period of time following cancer therapy, in whom second malignant neoplasms (SMN) have been identified (Draper et al. 1986; Falkson et al. 1989; Meadows et al. 1989; van Leeuwen et al. 1989; Devereux et al. 1990; Lokich 1990; Petru and Schmähl 1991; Henry-Amar 1992; Swerdlow et al. 1992; van Leeuwen et al. 1994a; Boivin et al. 1995). In addition, some large series have now been the subject of case controls (Kaldor et al. 1990a,b), which have enabled the relative risks for individual chemotherapeutic agents to be calculated. An account of these findings and an examination of the factors influencing the occurrence of drug-associated neoplasia is the subject of this chapter.

In 1979, the International Agency for Research on Cancer (IARC) published a list of chemical substances including drugs in the order of certainty that they might be carcinogenic to man. An abbreviated list referring to the drugs presently in use is given in Table 26.1. Group 1 comprised drugs for which there was strong evidence of a causal association between exposure and cancer in man. Group 2 included drugs that were probably carcinogens, with those most likely to be so included in the A category. Groups 2B and 3 contained drugs of undecided or unlikely potential. Since then many more agents, particularly those used for treating cancer, could be added to the list, and agents such as chlorambucil would probably now feature in Group 1.

TABLE 26.1
Drugs that are carcinogenic to man

Group 1
Diethylstilboestrol
Melphalan
Mustine hydrochloride (mechlorethamine, nitrogen mustard)

Group 2A
Chorambucil
Cyclophosphamide

Groups 2B and 3
Isoniazid
Phenytoin

(Modified from IARC.)

Hormones as carcinogens

Herbst and Scully (1970) reported seven cases of adenocarcinoma of the vagina in adolescent girls in the Eastern United States. This clustering of cases alerted Herbst to the finding in the eighth case that the mother had been treated with diethylstilboestrol during the first trimester of pregnancy. A retrospective analysis showed some of the other seven mothers had also been treated in this way. Greenwald and others (1971) confirmed this association, and eventually 333 cases of clear-cell carcinoma were found to be associated with stilboestrol therapy. This unequivocal demonstration of the carcinogenicity of stilboestrol not only alerted doctors to the possible hazards of short-term intensive administration, but also to the possibility that long-term low-dose hormonal therapy, such as that used in oral contraception or in hormonal replacement therapy after the menopause, might be hazardous.

Oral contraceptives

The role of oral contraceptives in the induction of breast cancer is still the subject of debate. It should be remembered that combination oral contraceptives which contain a synthetic oestrogen (usually ethinyl oestradiol) and a synthetic progestogen effectively stop ovarian function. This should therefore mimic the effect of the menopause and theoretically reduce the risk of breast cancer (Pike 1986). Epidemiological studies have found little evidence that this occurs and, indeed, reanalysis (CGHFBC 1996) of data from 54 epidemiological studies of the use of oral contraceptives (OC) by 53 279 women with breast cancer and 100 239 women without the disease suggested that there is a small but significant risk of breast cancer in women during the use of OC and up to 10 years after cessation of the drugs, but not thereafter. The relative risk for current users of OC compared with women who had never used the drugs was 1.2 (95 per cent CI 1.15–1.33), falling, after stopping the treatment for 1–4 years, or 5–9 years, to 1.16 (CI 1.08–1.23) and 1.07 (CI 1.02–1.13) respectively. The relative risk was highest (1.22) in women who began using OC before the age of 20 years. There was no significant association between breast cancer and the doses or types of hormones contained in the OC taken by the women. The authors of the report were uncertain whether the increased risk calculated for OC users reflected the earlier diagnosis, the effect of the drugs, or a combination of both factors.

The role of oral contraception in other gynaecological cancer is less clear. The results of a study on behalf of the Oxford Family Planning Association (Vessey *et al.* 1983) suggested that invasive carcinoma of the cervix was increased in patients on oral contraceptives, and further studies from the same source (Zondervan *et al.* 1996) strengthened the original conclusions. In the Oxford Family Planning Association study 13 cases were found in users of 'the pill', and none in users of intrauterine devices. Since the association with virus infection has become established, it may be possible that this is not an independent factor but related to sexual behaviour.

There is now good evidence of a reduction in the risk of endometrial carcinoma when oestrogen and progestogens are given together (CASH study 1983*a,b*), and a reduced risk of ovarian cancer in the case–control studies of Rosenberg and colleagues (1982), Cramer and others (1982), and Pike (1986), when long-term contraceptive agents were used. The risk of developing endometrial cancer was approximately halved in those women taking the pill, and it appeared that the protection lasted for at least 10 years after stopping the treatment.

Oestrogen replacement

The increasing use of oestrogen replacement therapy in women in an attempt to prevent menopausal symptoms and osteoporosis has produced concern that this might be provoking an increase in the incidence of carcinoma of the breast. Kendall and Horton (1990) concluded that there was no evidence that hormone replacement therapy caused an increase in breast cancer, but concern arose from the results of a Swedish study by Bergkvist and co-workers (1989). This was a prospective study of over 23 000 Swedish women on hormone replacement therapy, comparing them with a group in the same geographical area. The study found no increased risk of breast cancer in the population as a whole, but subgroup analysis revealed major differences. In those treated with oestradiol for 9 years, there was an increased risk of 1.8 times that of the control population with regard to the development of breast cancer. The risk rose to fourfold in those treated with oestradiol and progestogen for 4 years. This study conflicts with the finding of Gambrell and colleagues (1983), who found that the incidence of carcinoma was less in those women taking a combined oestrogen and progestogen preparation.

A reanalysis of about 90 per cent of previously published epidemiological studies relating to the use of hormone replacement therapy has been carried out (BCGHFBC 1997). The studies provided data on 52 705 women with breast cancer and 108 411 women without the disease. From the reanalysis it was concluded that there was an increased relative risk of breast cancer among women who were currently using, or had recently used HRT, for more than 5 years and that the risk was associated with the length of exposure to the treatment. The findings in respect of long-term users of HRT amounted to an extra 12 cases of breast cancer by the age of 70 years for every 1000 women who began treatment at the age of 50 years and continued it for 20 years (LaCroix and Burke 1997). The study did not, however, provide adequate information on whether the effects of oestrogen-only HRT differed from those of oestrogen–progestogen HRT as far as the risk of breast cancer is concerned, and this question remains to be answered.

Endometrial carcinoma was found to be increased by Smith and others (1975) and Ziel and Finkel (1975), in studies in which they determined the incidence in menopausal and postmenopausal women who were given oestrogen alone. The risk of 'unopposed' oestrogen therapy was 4.5 times greater in those on therapy than in controls. The risk increased the longer the duration of therapy, rising to nearly 14-fold after 7 years. Other studies (Gray *et al.* 1977; McDonald *et al.* 1977) confirmed this.

Elwood (1981) found that patients presenting with endometrial carcinoma had a far better survival when they had had oestrogen, the non-users having a death rate some five times that of those women who had used oestrogens.

The question of whether it is safe to give unopposed oestrogen therapy to women who have had a hysterectomy for such a condition as endometriosis and endometrial malignancies has been raised by a case of endometrial stromal sarcoma (McCluggage *et al.* 1996) and one of endometrial carcinoma (Carr *et al.* 1996), which occurred 23 years and 1 year after hysterectomy and 5 years and 1 year after starting oestrogen replacement treatment, respectively.

Oestrogen replacement therapy does not appear to increase the risk of cancer of the cervix (Parazzini *et al.* 1997 — but see Oral contraceptives above) or ovarian cancer (Hempling *et al.* 1997).

In conclusion, hormones may be shown to play an aetiological role in the production of cancer. Paradoxically, while promoting it in one organ, they can protect against it in another, and the administration of mixtures of hormones, as in the use of low-dose oral contraceptives, may negate any carcinogenic activity. Furthermore, the aggressiveness of the cancer produced seems to be modified by the nature of the hormonal stimulus.

Immunosuppressive drugs as carcinogens

This section will deal with those drugs that are specifically used to depress immune reactions and have been employed, for example, to prevent rejection of marrow or kidney grafts. Many drugs have an immunosuppressive effect, but are not used for that purpose therapeutically, and will not therefore be considered.

The first reports of a greater than expected incidence of malignant disease following renal or bone marrow transplantation started to appear in the late 1970s (Calne *et al.* 1979; Kinlen *et al.* 1979). At that time, immunosuppression was usually achieved with a combination of drugs, such as steroids and azathioprine or steroids and cyclophosphamide. Another agent that was commonly added was methotrexate. A major feature was the incidence of lymphoid malignancy (Kinlen *et al.* 1979). It was unusual for other malignancies to occur, and if this happened they were usually rare mesenchymal sarcomas. There was also a definite time relationship to the onset of the lymphoma. Another notable feature was the predilection for the central nervous system.

At that time the hypothesis was that in some way 'immune surveillance' of the body, which inhibited the growth of clones of malignant cells, was disturbed, possibly by reducing specific cells in the lymphoid system

called 'natural killer cells'. This hypothesis is less favoured now, and it seems to us that the carcinogenic effect of the immunosuppressants is as likely to be due to a direct effect on the genome. However, the mechanism remains to be established.

Azathioprine

This drug has been shown to induce an increased number of lymphoid, mesenchymal, and skin malignancies following organ transplantation (Kinlen *et al.* 1979; Shell *et al.* 1991; Nachbauer *et al.* 1994); in the control of autoimmune diseases, such as rheumatoid arthritis (Isomaki *et al.* 1982; Csuka and Banson 1996; Aguilar *et al.* 1997); or in the treatment of multiple sclerosis (Confavreux *et al.* 1996). Skin malignancies have occurred in patients treated with azathioprine following kidney or liver transplantation (Shell *et al.* 1991; Taylor and Shuster 1992); or for chronic skin disorders (Nachbar *et al.* 1993; Bottomley *et al.* 1995); or multiple sclerosis (Goodkin *et al.* 1992). Interestingly, the use of the drug in inflammatory bowel disease was not found to increase the incidence of cancer above that of the population at large (Connell *et al.* 1994). The increased incidence over that observed in a control population is related to the dose and length of treatment.

Cyclosporin

Calne and colleagues (1979) first reported the occurrence of lymphoma in three transplant patients receiving cyclosporin. Evidence of this association has since been strengthened by epidemiological studies (Gruber *et al.* 1991; Shiel *et al.* 1991; Villardell *et al.* 1992; Gruber *et al.* 1994) and a number of individual case reports (e.g. Zanke *et al.* 1989; Fric *et al.* 1990; Brown 1991; Delbello *et al.* 1991; Koo *et al.* 1992; Zijlmans *et al.* 1992; Masouye *et al.* 1993; Wiles *et al.* 1994), though in some of these cases the association could have been coincidental.

Other neoplasms attributed to treatment with cyclosporin include squamous carcinoma of the skin (Bos and Meincardi 1989), acute myeloid leukaemia (Butler *et al.* 1990), malignant melanoma (Mérot *et al.* 1990), cancer of the lung (Klein *et al.* 1991); Kaposi's sarcoma (Villadell *et al.* 1992), cancer of the penis (Piepkorn *et al.* 1993), adenocarcinoma of the mouth (Yamamoto *et al.* 1996), and carcinoma of the cervix (Grossman *et al.* 1996).

Cyclophosphamide

Cyclophosphamide has been found to increase the incidence of bladder, lymphoproliferative, and myeloproliferative tumours. Elliot *et al.* (1982) reported the development of bladder cancer in two women treated with cyclophosphamide for lupus nephritis, and Baltus and others (1983) showed that the risk of malignancy in 81 patients with rheumatoid arthritis treated with cyclophosphamide was 4.1 times as great as in 81 control subjects. Travis and colleagues reported a case–control study involving 6171 patients who had been treated with cyclophosphamide for non-Hodgkin's lymphoma. Those treated had a 4.5-fold greater risk of developing bladder cancer than controls, the risk depending on the cumulative dose; while Talar-Williams and co-workers (1996) found that eight of 1445 patients treated with cyclophosphamide for Wegener's granulomatosis developed bladder cancer, an incidence 31 times higher than in the general population. A number of other cases of bladder cancer attributed to cyclophosphamide have been reported (Thrasher *et al*. 1990; Cannon *et al*. 1992; Ortiz *et al*. 1992; Radis *et al*. 1993; Pedersen-Bjergaard *et al*. 1995).

Other malignancies believed to have been caused by the drug include acute myelocytic leukaemia (Escalante *et al*. 1989), squamous cell cancer of the skin (Choy *et al*. 1989), carcinoma of lung (Choy *et al*. 1989), leiomyosarcoma of the ethmoid sinus (Reich *et al*. 1995), and renal cell carcinoma (Oden 1996).

Methotrexate

This drug has been suspected of causing lymphoma in patients treated for rheumatoid arthritis (Flipo and Delaporte 1997; Siekenik *et al*. 1997), but Bologna and others (1997) found no increase in cancer risk in 426 patients treated with the drug for this disease, and Rustin and colleagues (1996) found a low cancer risk in patients treated for gestational trophoblastic tumours with methotrexate and calcium folinate; a medium risk in those given a combination of methotrexate, calcium folinate, hydroxycarbamide, dactinomycin, mercaptopurine, and either etoposide or declomycin; and a high risk with a combination of methotrexate, calcium folinate, etoposide, dactinomycin, vincristine, and cyclophosphamide. Urothelial cancer was reported to have occurred during treatment of rheumatoid arthritis with methotrexate (Bréchignac *et al*. 1996), though the authors commented that the association might have been a coincidence.

Cytotoxic agents and second malignant tumours
(See also Chapter 24)

By far the greatest number of second malignant tumours

(SMN) occur in patients who are treated for cancer with cytotoxic agents. The exponential rise of SMN in patients who are surviving for 5, 10, or more years is a major cause for concern, especially in those tumours like Hodgkin's disease or Wilms' tumour, where cure is probable. It is true that the phenomenon is being seen only as the price of success, and it must be kept in perspective as a relatively rare occurrence, but given that there might be a propensity to form malignant tumours in a particular person, there is no doubt that it is important to study these patients and to try and identify which are the cytotoxic drugs responsible, and what host factors put a patient particularly at risk.

Several methods have been used to study SMN. Individual case reports have been important to establish risk, but have been little use in quantifying it. The two most useful methods have been cohort and case–control studies. In cohort studies, specific groups of patients are observed for a number of years to identify specific malignancies. The person–years of observation are calculated from the start of observation to last follow-up, death, or diagnosis of SMN, whichever is the first. Tumour incidence rates from the general population specific for age, sex, race, and calendar year are multiplied by the accumulated person–years to decide the number of expected tumours. The observed number is then divided by the expected number to get the relative risk. The 95 per cent confidence interval is then calculated, and the degree of significance of the finding can be stated. Although there are a number of criticisms of this method, this type of study has been informative.

Another type of analysis is the case–control study, in which the exposure to chemotherapy of individuals who develop SMN (cases) and those who do not (controls) is compared. The controls are matched as closely as possible, and ideally the largest number possible is obtained, although it is important that they be collected without bias.

These two methods have been used in most of the studies described below, and have enabled not only the time scale of production of SMN to be studied, but more recently have identified the causative agents.

Evidence from studies on Hodgkin's disease

A number of reports have demonstrated that survivors of Hodgkin's disease treated with chemotherapy develop SMN (Arsenau *et al*. 1972; Coltman and Dixon 1982; Boivin *et al*. 1984; Tucker *et al*. 1988; Devereux *et al*. 1990; Lokich 1990; Petru and Schmähl 1991; Henry-Amar 1992; Swerdlow *et al*. 1992; Van Leeuwen *et al*.

TABLE 26.2
Distribution of cases of acute non-lymphocytic leukaemia according to chemotherapy

Chemotherapy	Cases (n)	Controls (n)
Combinations		
Mustine hydrochloride (mechlorethamine, nitrogen mustard) + prednisolone	115	187
Chlorambucil + procarbazine	7	9
Cyclophosphamide + procarbazine	17	21
Doxorubicin + dacarbazine	19	19
Other combinations containing an alkylating agent	45	59
Combinations with no alkylating agent	9	12
Single agents		
Carmustine	3	3
Bleomycin	5	3
Chlorambucil	16	10
Cyclophosphamide	8	19
Cytarabine	1	6
Lomustine	9	5
Mustine hydrochloride	9	5
Procarbazine	7	9
Thiotepa	3	3
Vinblastine	26	41
Vincristine	3	6

(After Kaldor *et al.* 1990 *a,b*)

TABLE 26.3
Relative risk of acute non-lymphocytic leukaemia for patients with selected chemotherapy histories, irrespective of radiotherapy received

Chemotherapy history	Cases (n)	Controls (n)	Relative risk
MP only			
<6 cycles	30	89	4.7 (2.2–10)
>6 cycles	20	28	14.0 (5.1–37)
Any	50	117	6.4 (3.0–13)
CP only			
<6 cycles	1	4	3.3 (0.33–33)
>6 cycles	3	1	38.0 (3.6–410)
Any	4	5	11.0 (2.6–48)
ChP only	1	5	2.8 (0.29–27)
Chlorambucil only	3	1	27.0 (2.5–300)
MP + CP only	1	2	7.3 (0.59–90)
MP + DD only	2	8	4.1 (0.65–26)
MP + lomustine only	3	2	12.0 (1.5–91)
MP + vinblastine only	4	11	4.7 (1.2–19)

MP = mustine hydrochloride (mechlorethamine, nitrogen mustard)+procarbazine and no other alkylating agent
CP=cyclophosphamide+procarbazine and no other alkylating agent
ChP = combinations including chlorambucil+procarbazine and no other alkylating agent
DD includes doxorubicin and dacarbazine and no other alkylating agent
Figures in brackets are 95 per cent confidence intervals
(After Kaldor *et al.* 1990 *a,b*)

1994*a*; Boivin *et al.* 1995). Among the first reports of a greater than expected number of SMN in Hodgkin's disease was that of Arsenau and others (1972), who noted an increase in non-lymphomatous malignant tumours, and related this to the non-intensive chemotherapy being given at that time.

Subsequent studies showed that this increase particularly took the form of myeloblastic leukaemia (Tucker *et al.* 1988; Devereux *et al.* 1990; Van Leeuwen *et al.* 1994*a,b*) though in one study solid tumours predominated.

The evidence has come from either single institution or collaborative trial groups. Although most groups have reported a dozen or more leukaemias, these numbers have been insufficient in themselves to allow for an examination of risk factors. In adult Hodgkin's disease, Kaldor and colleagues (1990*b*) have combined the data for 12 population-based cancer registries in Europe and Canada, and six large hospitals in Europe. They have carried out a case–control study on 163 cases of leukaemia following treatment. They show that there was a relative risk of leukaemia of nine (95 per cent confidence intervals 4.1–20), as compared with patients treated with

radiotherapy alone. Table 26.2 shows the distribution of acute non-lymphocytic leukaemia according to type of chemotherapy in the series given.

Table 26.3 gives estimates of the relative risk of acute non-lymphocytic leukaemia for patients with selected chemotherapy regardless of radiotherapy received. With these data it is only possible to calculate the relative rates for combinations of drugs used frequently, that is, mustine hydrochloride (chlorethezine, chlormethine, mechlorethamine, nitrogen mustard), and procarbazine, cyclophosphamide and procarbazine, and doxorubicin and dacarbazine. Relatively few patients received single agents. In 55 patients who received mustine hydrochloride and procarbazine, the relative risk was 6.4; for cyclophosphamide and procarbazine, 11; and for chlorambucil, over 27, although in this case the number of patients receiving the agent was small. Van Leeuwen and colleagues (1994*a*) studied a cohort of 1939 patients treated for Hodgkin's disease over a 20-year period and found that those treated with mustine hydrochloride were at the greatest risk of developing leukaemia, followed by those treated with a combination of lomustine and teniposide.

TABLE 26.4
Alkylating agent dose and risk of leukaemia or non-Hodgkin lymphoma

AAD score	Leukaemia/NHL risk
1	0.02
2	0.02
4	0.03
6	0.06
8	0.10
10	0.10

(After Meadows *et al.* 1989)

In children with Hodgkin's disease, Meadows and colleagues (1989) have recorded second neoplasms in series from 11 major hospitals. Solid tumours, non-lymphocytic leukaemia, and non-Hodgkin lymphoma developed in 18, 17, and three patients respectively in the 979 children at risk. The study proposed an alkylating agent dose (AAD) risk for each patient. The score was calculated as follows: a single alkylating agent of at least 6 months' duration was assigned a score of 1; for double alkylating agents given for 6 months, a score of 2 was given. Thus, 6 months' MOPP or COPP were given a score of 2 because these contain two alkylating agents. The AAD scores were calculated for each individual patient. The study shows a close correlation between total alkylating agent received, the AAD score, and the risk for leukaemia and non-Hodgkin lymphoma (Table 26.4).

These adult and paediatric studies go a long way to indicate that alkylating agents (in particular mustine hydrochloride, cyclophosphamide, chlorambucil, and procarbazine) can be placed in the IARC's Group 1. Does Hodgkin's disease reveal anything more about the drugs used in its treatment? The vinca alkaloids vinblastine and vincristine have formed part of treatment programmes over many years, and have been used relatively infrequently as single agents. Van Leeuwen and others (1989) reviewed the relative risk for various combinations of cytotoxic agents used in treating 744 patients with Hodgkin's disease admitted to the Netherlands Cancer Institute from 1966 to 1983. No excess risk was observed in Hodgkin's patients treated with vinblastine alone, so that this suggests that vinblastine does not play an important role in increasing leukaemia risk.

Evidence from studies on ovarian cancer

Corroboration of these findings in alkylating agents can be found in the study of other cancers, and in particular ovarian cancer. Green and co-workers (1986) estimated the cumulative 10-year risk of contracting leukaemia for 333 women treated with cyclophosphamide as 5.4 per cent. The incidence peaked at 5–6 years, and subsequently declined. Kaldor and colleagues (1990*a*), again using a case–control method, studied the incidence of acute leukaemia in patients following chemotherapy for ovarian cancer. The data were taken from 11 population-based registries in Europe and Canada, and two large hospitals in Europe. One hundred and fourteen cases of leukaemia were identified, and matched in the manner previously described. Because single agents are given more frequently in ovarian cancer than in other conditions such as Hodgkin's disease, the patient-years of observation were considerably greater for single agents, and allowed the order of risk to be ranked (Table 26.5).

Carcinogenicity of cytotoxic agents

It can be seen from the above studies that chlorambucil, melphalan, and thiotepa present a high relative risk

TABLE 26.5
Distribution of cases and controls with acute non-lymphocytic leukaemia according to type of chemotherapy, with relative risks according to type and dose, among patients who received only one form of chemotherapy

Drug	Low dose				High dose			
	Cases	Controls	Median dose (mg) (controls)	Relative risk	Cases	Controls	Median dose (mg) (controls)	Relative risk
Chlorambucil	2	2	170	14.0	5	2	3200	23.0
Cyclophosphamide	4	14	1200	2.2	8	15	22 500	4.1
Melphalan	9	18	170	12.0	17	18	400	23.0
Thiotepa	4	5	30	8.3	5	6	600	9.7
Treosulfan	1	3	64 000	3.6	7	2	260 000	33.0

Low and high doses were defined with respect to median dose in the controls.
(After Kaldor *et al.* 1990*a,b*)

TABLE 26.6
Leukaemogenicity of cytotoxic agents in order of potential, based on reported relative risks

1. Chlorambucil
2. Melphalan
3. Procarbazine
4. Thiotepa
5. Mustine hydrochloride (mechlorethamine, nitrogen mustard)
6. Cyclophosphamide
7. Vinblastine

Note. Etoposide is now a well-recognized leukaemogenic chemotherapeutic agent, and this needs to be considered when it is used in multidrug regimens.

while treosulfan and cyclophosphamide rank rather lower. Cyclophosphamide was also found to be less leukaemogenic in children than other agents (de Vathaire *et al.* 1989) in a study of 634 children treated between 1942 and 1969, which showed that in 280 children treated with non-alkylating agents or cyclophosphamide the relative risk was 2.9, whereas with all other alkylating agents the relative risk was 7.4. Further evidence of the relative safety of cyclophosphamide has come in a study from Curtis and others (1990), who found 24 cases of acute myeloid leukaemia in 13 734 women treated for breast cancer with chemotherapy. When compared with another group of 7974 women who had received no chemotherapy, the relative risk was 11.5 per cent (95 per cent confidence interval 7.4–17.1). In a case–control study the relative risk for melphalan in the women with breast cancer was 44.6 (95 per cent confidence interval 4.9–409), and for cyclophosphamide 1.3 (95 per cent confidence interval 0.3–6.6), once again emphasizing the different potential of different alkylating agents for producing SMN. A study by Falkson and others (1989) showed that 23 of 1460 patients receiving mitolactol (dibromodulcitol, DBD) for adjuvant treatment of breast cancer developed leukaemia or myelodysplasia. The authors concluded that DBD is one of the most potent leukaemogenic agents in use, and recommended that it should no longer be employed as an adjuvant. This study did not, however, calculate a relative risk for the drug, so that its exact place in the order of carcinogenicity is difficult to determine.

It ought to be possible now to assign an order of leukaemogenicity to commonly used chemotherapeutic agents; this would be of importance in the planning of treatment programmes. As an approximation, on evidence so far, it is suggested that the order is that shown in Table 26.6.

Anticonvulsant hydantoins and malignant lymphoma

Members of the hydantoin group of drugs, particularly phenytoin, are known to produce changes in lymphoid tissue (Rosenfeld *et al.* 1961; Anthony 1970; *The Lancet* 1971; Tashima and de los Santos 1974; Li *et al.* 1975; Wilden and Scott 1978). Sometimes the disorder presents as a syndrome comprising fever, rash, lymphadenopathy and, occasionally, enlargement of the liver and spleen. In some instances histological changes have been interpreted as indicative of malignant lymphoma, but have resolved after withdrawal of the drug suspected of causing the reaction. Classical Hodgkin's disease and non-Hodgkin's lymphoma have also been attributed to these drugs, and the latter condition was the subject of a report by Garcia-Suarez and others (1996) who described a patient on long-term treatment with phenytoin who developed such a tumour, together with biopsy evidence of infection with the Epstein–Barr virus. However, the current opinion is that the causal association suggested is probably not valid.

Calcium antagonists

The question of whether or not calcium-channel blocking drugs (e.g. diltiazem, nifedipine, verapamil) can cause cancer has been the subject of much controversy. Evidence suggesting such an association has been presented by a number of investigators (Hardell *et al.* 1996; Pahor *et al.* 1996a,b; Fitzpatrick *et al.* 1997), and a suggested mechanism is that these drugs inhibit apoptosis (programmed cell death) (Daling 1996). Such inhibition could result in the survival of cells that accumulate genetic changes which render them premalignant. Others, however, have been unable to confirm that these drugs are carcinogenic (Borhani *et al.* 1996; Braun *et al.* 1996; Jick *et al.* 1997; Olsen *et al.* 1997), and the view of an *ad hoc* subcommittee of the World Health Organisation and the International Society of Hypertension (WHO–ISH 1997) is that available evidence does not validate the claim that treatment with calcium antagonists increases the risk of cancer. The conclusions of the subcommittee, however, have themselves been questioned (Psaty and Furberg 1997) but supported by others (Howes and Edwards 1998).

Phenacetin abuse and carcinoma

Long-continued abuse of analgesic drug combination containing phenacetin is likely to have been responsible for some cases of transitional cell carcinoma of the renal pelvis (*British Medical Journal* 1969; *The Lancet* 1969; Bengtsson and Angervall 1970). Fortunately, in most countries phenacetin is no longer used.

Other drugs

Various unrelated drugs have been suspected of causing neoplastic disease, but the evidence is as yet insuffient to confirm a causal relationship. Some of these drugs and the tumours they are reported to have caused are listed in Table 26.7.

Host-related factors

It is increasingly important to recognize the role of chemotherapy and host interaction, especially when assessing the safety of chemotherapeutic drug regimens. The role of immunological status has been referred to above. More recently the importance of genetic abnormalities or tumour cell phenotype has become apparent. Draper and colleagues (1986), in a follow-up study of 882 retinoblastoma patients treated with surgery, radiotherapy, or chemotherapy, compared the outcome of these treatments in 384 children known to have the genetic form of the disease with that in 498 others who had the non-genetic form. Comparing the incidence of SMN in children with genetic disease treated by radiotherapy and chemotherapy, or chemotherapy alone, a total of 10 patients had a second malignancy, while none were noted in the non-genetic group, showing that there was an increased susceptibility of SMN there was already an underlying genetic defect.

Pui and others (1989) studied the risk of development of acute myeloid leukaemia during initial remission of 733 consecutive children treated with intensive chemotherapy for acute lymphoblastic leukaemia. In the study, 13 patients developed myelogenous leukaemia. While there was a wide variation in the karyotype at diagnosis of the acute lymphoblastic patients who eventually developed AML, an unusual finding was the frequency with which a T cell phenotype was found. Of 98 patients with T cell phenotypes, five developed AML, while in 635 without the phenotype, eight developed AML. This is significant (P=0.004), and in a multivariate analysis of risk factors remains highly significant (P=0.001). Thus genetic and phenotype changes may produce susceptibility to the action of cytotoxic drugs.

TABLE 26.7

Other drugs and types of tumour involved in some recently reported suspected cases of iatrogenic malignancy (single or few reports, the evidence being as yet insufficient to suggest a causal relationship)

Drug	Tumour	Reference
5-Aminolaevulinic acid (topical)	malignant melanoma	Wolf *et al.* 1997
Antacids (Bisodol)	papillary tumours of bladder and renal pelvis	Vella *et al.* 1996
Corticosteroids (betamethasone, prednisone)	Kaposi's sarcoma	Corda *et al.* 1996 Stazucki *et al.* 1997
Epoetin	acute leukaemia	Mazarello *et al.* 1997
Granulocyte-colony stimulating factor	acute leukaemia	Corey *et al.* 1996
Hydroxyurea	skin cancer	Callott-Mellot *et al.* 1996
Isotretinoin	myxoid liposarcoma	Butt *et al.* 1996
Platinum compounds	acute leukaemia	Colontero *et al.* 1993 Philpott *et al.* 1996
PUVA (methoxsalen and UVA)	skin cancer	Stern and Nichols 1996
Tacrolimus	skin cancer	Rezeig *et al.* 1997
Tamoxifen	uterine malignancies	Chew *et al.* 1996 Cuenca *et al.* 1996 Peters-Engl *et al.* 1996; McCluggage *et al.* 1997
Testosterone	prostate cancer	Loughlin and Richie 1997
Vitamin A (high-dose)	lung cancer	Albanes *et al.* 1996 Omenn *et al.* 1996

Conclusion

It has become apparent that hormones, immunosuppressants, and chemotherapeutic agents can induce malignancy, and that it is now possible to arrange these last in an order of the risk that malignancy may occur. This must be increasingly important to the medical oncologist designing curative therapies. It is also necessary to remember that underlying genetic abnormalities or surface phenotypes of the tumour being treated will influence susceptibility, and this is likely to be of increasing importance.

References

Aguilar, H.I., Burgart, L.J., and Geller, A. (1997). Azathioprine-induced lymphoma manifesting as fulminant hepatic failure. *Mayo Clin. Proc.* 72, 643.

Albanes, D., Heinonen, P.O., Taylor, P.R., *et al.* (1996). α-Tocopherol and β-carotene prevention study: effects of base-line characteristics and study compliance. *J. Natl Cancer Inst.* 88, 1560.

Anthony, J.J. (1970). Malignant lymphoma associated with hydantoin drugs. *Arch. Neurol.* 22, 450.

Arsenau, J.C., Sponzo, R.W., Levin, D.L., *et al.* (1972). Nonlymphomatous malignant tumours complicating Hodgkin's disease. Possible association with intensive therapy. *N. Engl. J. Med.* 287, 1119.

Baltus, J.A., Boersma, J.W., Hartman, A.P., *et al.* (1983). The occurrence of malignancies in patients with rheumatoid arthritis treated with cyclophosphamide: a controlled retrospective follow-up. *Ann. Rheum. Dis.* 42, 368.

Bengtsson, U. and Angervall, L. (1970). Analgesic abuse and tumours of the renal pelvis. *Lancet* i, 305.

Bergkvist, L., Adami, H.O., Persson, I., *et al.* (1989). The risk of breast cancer after oestrogen and oestrogen–progestogen replacement. *N. Engl. J. Med.* 321, 293.

Boivin, J-F., Hutchison, G.B., Lyden, M., *et al.* (1984). Second primary cancers following treatment of Hodgkin's disease. *J. Natl Cancer Inst.* 72, 233.

Boivin, J-F., Hutchison, G.B., Zauber, A.G., *et al.* (1995). Incidence of second cancers in patients treated for Hodgkin's disease. *J. Natl Cancer Inst.* 87, 732.

Bologna, C., Picot, M.C., Jorgensen, C., *et al.* (1997). Study of eight cases of cancer in 426 rheumatoid arthritis patients treated with methotrexate. *Ann. Rheum. Dis.* 56, 97.

Borhani, N.O., Mercuri, M., Borhani, P.A., *et al.* (1996). Final outcome results of the Multicentre Isradipine Diuretic Atherosclerosis Study (MIDAS). A randomized controlled trial. *JAMA* 276, 785.

Bos, J.D. and Meinardi, M.M.H. (1989). Two distinct squamous-cell carcinomas in a psoriatic patient receiving low-dose cyclosporine maintenance treatment. *J. Am. Acad. Dermatol.* 122 (Suppl. 36), 4.

Bottomley, W.W., Ford, G., and Cunliffe, W.J. (1995). Aggressive squamous carcinomas developing in patients receiving long-term azathioprine. *Br. J. Dermatol.* 133, 460.

Braun, S., Boykov, V., Behar, F., *et al.* (1996). Calcium antagonists and mortality in patients with coronary artery disease: a cohort study of 11 575 patients. *J. Am. Coll. Cardiol.* 28, 7.

Bréchignac, X., Desmurs, H., de Wazières, B., *et al.* (1996). Urothelial cancer during rheumatoid polyarthritis treated with methotrexate: is this relationship a coincidence? *Rev. Med. Interne* 17 (Suppl. 3), 458.

British Medical Journal (1969). Phenacetin and bladder cancer. *BMJ* iv, 701.

Brown, L.A., Wiselke, M., Campbell, A., *et al.* (1991). High-grade T-cell lymphoma following treatment with cyclosporin-A. *Histopathology* 19, 225.

Butler, J., Korb, S., and Light, J. (1990). Acute myelogenous leukaemia in a renal allograft recipient receiving cyclosporine therapy. *Transplantation* 49, 813.

Butt, A., Roberts, D.L., and Schenolikar, A. (1996). Soft tissue sarcoma in association with isotretinoin therapy. *J. Dermatol. Treat.* 7, 266.

Callott-Mellot, C., Bodmeyer, C., Chosidow, O., *et al.* (1996). Cutaneous carcinoma during long-term hydroxyurea therapy: a report of 5 cases. *Arch. Dermatol.* 132, 1395.

Calne, R.Y., Rolles, K., White, D.J., *et al.* (1979). Cyclosporin A initially as the only immunosuppressant in 34 recipients of cadaveric organs — 33 kidneys, 2 pancreases and 2 livers. *Lancet* ii, 1033.

Cannon, J., Linke, C.A., and Cos, L.R. (1992). Cyclophosphamide-associated carcinoma of urothelium: modalities for prevention. *Urology* 38, 413.

Carr, J.A., Schoon, P.A., and Look, K.Y. (1996). An atypical recurrence of endometrial carcinoma following estrogen replacement therapy. *Gynecol. Oncol.* 60, 498.

CASH (Centers for Disease Control: Cancer and steroid hormone study) (1983a). *JAMA* 249, 1596.

CASH (Centers for Disease Control: Cancer and steroid hormone study) (1983b). *JAMA* 249, 1600.

CGHFBC (Collaborative Group on Hormonal Factors in Breast Cancer) (1996). Breast cancer and hormonal contraceptives: collaborative reanalysis of individual data on 53 297 women with breast cancer and 100 239 women without breast cancer from 554 epidemiological studies. *Lancet* 347, 713.

CGHFBC (Collaborative Group on Hormonal Factors in Breast Cancer) (1997). Breast cancer and hormone replacement therapy: collaborative reanalysis from 51 epidemiological studies of 52 705 women with breast cancer and 108 411 women without breast cancer. *Lancet* 350, 1047.

Chew, S.B., Carmalt, H., Gillett, D. (1997). Leiomyoma of the uterus in a woman on adjuvant tamoxifen therapy. *Breast* 5, 429.

Choy, D.S.J., Gearhart, R.P., Gould, W.J. *et al.* (1989). Development of multiple carcinomas in a long-term survivor of Wegener's granulomatosis treated with immunosuppressive drugs. *N.Y. State J. Med.* 89, 680.

Colontero, G., Malkasian, G.D., and Edmondson, J.H. (1993). Secondary myelodysplasia and acute leukemia. *J. Natl Cancer Inst.* 85, 1858.

Coltman, C.A. and Dixon, D.O. (1982). Second malignancies complicating Hodgkin's disease — the National Cancer Institute experience. *Cancer Treat. Rep.* 66, 1023.

Confavreux, C., Saddler, P., Grimaud, J., *et al.* (1996). Risk of cancer from azathioprine therapy in multiple sclerosis: case-control study. *Neurology* 46, 1607.

Connell, W.R., Kinlen, L.J., Ritchie, J.K., *et al.* (1994). Cancer risk from azathioprine in inflammatory bowel disease. *Gastroenterology* 106 (Suppl.), 667.

Corda, L., Benerecetti, D., Ungari, M., *et al.* (1996). Kaposi's disease and sarcoidosis. *Eur. J. Resp. Dis.* 9, 383.

Corey, S.J., Wollman, M.R., and Deshpande, R.V. (1996). Granulocyte colony-stimulating factor and congenital neutropenia — risk of leukemia. *J. Pediatr.* 129, 187.

Cramer, D.W., Hutchison, G.B., Welch, W.R., *et al.* (1982). Factors affecting the association of oral contraceptives and ovarian cancer. *N. Engl. J. Med.* 307, 1047.

Csuka, H.E. and Hanson, G.A. (1996). Resolution of a soft-tissue sarcoma after discontinuation of azathioprine therapy. *Arch. Intern. Med.* 156, 1573.

Cuenca, R.E., Giachino, J., Arrendondo, M.A., *et al.* (1996). Endometrial carcinoma associated with breast carcinoma: low incidence with tamoxifen use. *Cancer* 77, 2058.

Curtis, R.E., Boice, J.D., Moloney, W.C., *et al.* (1990). Leukaemia following chemotherapy for breast cancer. *Cancer Res.* 50, 2741.

Daling, J.R. (1996). Calcium channel blockers and cancer: is an association biologically plausible? *Am. J. Hypertens.* 9, 713.

Delbello, H.W., Dick, W.H., Carter, C.B., *et al.* (1991). Polyclonal B cell lymphoma of renal transplant ureter induced by cyclosporin: case report. *J. Urol.* 146, 1613.

De Vathaire, F., Schweisguth, O., Rodary, C., *et al.* (1989). Long term risk of second malignant neoplasm after a cancer in childhood. *Br. J. Cancer* 59, 448.

Devereux, S., Selassie, T.G., Hudson, G.V., *et al.* (1990). Leukaemia complicating treatment for Hodgkin's disease: the experience of the British National Lymphoma Investigation. *BMJ* 301, 1077.

Draper, G.J., Sanders, B.M., and Kingston, J.E. (1986). Second primary neoplasms in patients with retinoblastoma. *Br. J. Cancer* 53, 661.

Elliott, R.W., Essenhigh, D.M., and Morvey, A.R. (1982). Cyclophosphamide treatment of systemic lupus erythematosus: risk of bladder cancer exceeds benefit. *BMJ* 284, 1160.

Elwood, J.M. (1981). Estrogens and endometrial cancer: some answers and further questions. *Can. Med. Assoc. J.* 124, 1129.

Escalante, A., Kaufman, R.L., and Beardmore, T.D. (1989). Acute myelocytic leukemia after the use of cyclophosphamide in the treatment of polyarteritis nodosa. *J. Rheumatol.* 16, 1147.

Falkson, G., Gelman, R.S., Dreicer, R., *et al.* (1989). Myelodysplastic syndrome and acute nonlymphocytic leukaemia secondary to mitolactol treatment in patients with cancer. *J. Clin. Oncol.* 9, 1252.

Fitzpatrick, A.L., Dating, J.R., Furberg, C.D., *et al.* (1997). Use of calcium channel blockers and breast cancer risks in postmenopausal women. *Cancer* 80, 1435.

Flipo, R-M. and Delaporte, E. (1997). Cutaneous pseudolymphoma occurring during methotrexate therapy for rheumatoid arthritis. *J. Rheumatol.* 24, 809.

Fric, H., Hartman, A., and Klehr, H.U. (1990). Regression of cerebral lymphoma due to transplantation following cyclosporin reduction. *Klin. Wochenschr.* 68, 1189.

Gambrell, R.D., Maier, R.C., and Sanders, B.I. (1983). Decreased incidence of breast cancer in postmenopausal estrogen–progestogen users. *Obstet. Gynecol.* 62, 435.

Garcia-Suarez, J., Dominguez-Franjo, P., Del Campo, J.F. *et al.* (1996). EBV-positive non-Hodgkin's lymphoma developing after phenytoin therapy. *Br. J. Haematol.* 95, 376.

Goodkin, D.E., Daughtry, M.M., and Vanderbrug-Medendorp, S.V. (1992). Incidence of malignancy following cyclophosphamide or azathioprine treatment of multiple sclerosis. *Ann. Neurol.* 32, 257.

Gray, L.A., Christopherson, W.M., and Hoover, R.N. (1977). Estrogen and endometrial cancer. *Obstet. Gynecol.* 49, 385.

Greene, M.H., Harris, E.L., and Gershenson, D.M. (1986). Melphalan may be a more potent leukaemogen than is cyclophosphamide. *Ann. Intern. Med.* 105, 360.

Greenwald, P., Barlow, J.J., Nasca, P.C., *et al.* (1971). Vaginal cancer after maternal treatment with synthetic oestrogens. *N. Engl. J. Med.* 285, 390.

Grossman, R.H., Haugee, E., and Dubertret, L. (1996). Cervical intraepithelial neoplasm in a patient receiving long-term cyclosporin for the treatment of severe plaque psoriasis. *Br. J. Dermatol.* 135, 147.

Gruber, S.A., Skjei, K.L., Sothern, R.B., *et al.* (1991). Cancer development in renal allograft recipients treated with conventional and cyclosporin immunosuppression. *Transplant. Proc.* 23, 1104.

Gruber, S.A., Gillingham, K., Sothern, R.B., *et al.* (1994). De novo cancer in cyclosporin-treated and non-cyclosporin treated adult primary renal allograft recipients. *Clin. Transplantation* 8, 388.

Hardell, L., Axelson, O., and Fredrikson, H. (1996). Antihypertensive drugs and risks of malignant disease. *Lancet* 348, 542.

Hempling, R.E., Wong, C., Piver, S., *et al.* (1997). Hormone replacement therapy as a risk factor for epithelial ovarian cancer: results of a case–control study. *Obstet. Gynecol.* 89, 1012.

Henry-Amar, H. (1992). Second cancer after the treatment for Hodgkin's disease: a report from the International Database on Hodgkin's disease. *Ann. Oncol.* 3 (Suppl. 4), 117.

Herbst, A.L. and Scully, R.E. (1970). Adenocarcinoma of the vagina in adolescence; a report of 7 cases including 6 clear cell carcinomas (so-called mesonephromas). *Cancer* 25, 745.

International Agency for Research on Cancer (1979). *Evaluation of the Carcinogenic Risk of Chemicals to Humans.* Howes, L.G. and Edwards, C.T. (1998). Calcium antagonists and cancer: is there really a link? *Drug Saf.* 18, 1.

IARC Monographs, Supplement 1. IARC, Lyon, France.

Isomaki, H.I.A., Hakulinen, T., and Joutsenlahti U. (1982). Excess risk of lymphomas, leukaemia and myeloma in patients with rheumatoid arthritis. *Ann. Rheum. Dis.* 41, (Suppl. 1), 34.

Jick, H., Jick, S., Derby, L.E., *et al.* (1997). Calcium-channel blockers and risk of cancer. *Lancet* 349, 525.

Kaldor, J.M., Day, N.E., Pettersson, F., *et al.* (1990*a*). Leukaemia following chemotherapy for ovarian cancer. *N. Engl. J. Med.* 322, 1.

Kaldor, J.M., Day, N.E., Clarke, A., *et al.* (1990*b*). Leukaemia following Hodgkin's disease. *N. Engl. J. Med.* 322, 7.

Kendall, M.J. and Horton, R.C. (1990). Clinical pharmacology and therapeutics: reviews in medicine. *Postgrad. Med. J.* 66, 166.

Kinlen, L.J., Sheil, A.G.R., Peto, J., *et al.* (1979). Collaborative United Kingdom–Australasian study of cancer in patients treated with immunosuppressive drugs. *BMJ* ii, 1461.

Klein, J.S., Goldin, H.M., Keegan, C., *et al.* (1991). Clear-cell carcinoma of the lung in a patient treated with cyclosporine for epidermolysis bullosa acquisita. *J. Am. Acad. Dermatol.* 24, 297.

LaCroix, A.Z and Burke, W. (1997). Breast cancer and hormone replacement therapy (commentary on the CGHFBC study). *Lancet* 350, 1042.

The Lancet (1969). Analgesic abuse and tumours of the renal pelvis. *Lancet* i, 1233.

The Lancet (1971). Is phenytoin carcinogenic? *Lancet* ii, 1071.

Li, F.P., Willard, D.R., Goodman, R., *et al.* (1975). Malignant lymphoma after diphenylhydantoin (Dilantin) therapy. *Cancer* 36, 1359.

Lokich, J.J. (1990). Secondary uncommon solid neoplasms in cured Hodgkin's disease and follow-up of the original B-DOPA chemotherapy patient group. *Am. J. Clin. Oncol. — Cancer Clin. Trials* 13, 247.

Loughlin, K.R. and Richie, J.P. (1997). Prostate cancer after exogenous testosterone treatment for impotence. *J. Urol.* 157, 1845.

McCluggage, W.G., Bailie, C., Weir, P., *et al.* (1996). Endometrial stromal sarcoma arising in pelvic endometriosis in a patient receiving unopposed oestrogen therapy. *Br. J. Obstet. Gynaecol.* 103, 1252.

McCluggage, W.G., McManus, D.T., Lioe, T.F., *et al.* (1991). Uterine carcinosarcoma in association with tamoxifen therapy. *Br. J. Obstet. Gynaecol.* 104, 748.

McDonald, T.W., Annegers, J.F., O'Fallow, W.M., *et al.* (1977). Exogenous estrogen and endometrial carcinoma — a case controlled study. *Am. J. Obstet. Gynecol.* 127, 572.

Masouy, I., Salomon, D., and Saurat, J-H. (1993). B-cell lymphoma after cyclosporine for keratosis lichenoides chronica. *Arch. Dermatol.* 129, 914.

Mazarella, V., Spleniani, G., Tozzo, C., *et al.* (1997). Acute leukemia in an uremic patient undergoing erythropoetin treatment. *Nephron* 76, 361.

Meadows, A.T., Obringer, A.C., Marrero, O., *et al.* (1989). Second malignant neoplasms following childhood Hodgkin's disease; treatment and splenectomy as risk factors. *Med. Pediatr. Oncol.* 17, 477.

Mérot, Y., Miescher, P.A., Balsiger, F., *et al.* (1990). Cutaneous malignant melanoma occurring under cyclosporin-A therapy: a report of two cases. *Br. J. Dermatol.* 123, 237.

Nachbar, F., Stolz, W., Volkenardt, M., *et al.* (1993). Squamous-cell carcinoma in localised scleroderma following immunosuppressive therapy with azathioprine. *Acta Derm. Venereol.* (Stockh.) 73, 217.

Nachbauer, K., Feichtinger, H., Fend, F., *et al.* (1994). EBV-associated Hodgkin's disease after cyclosporin A therapy following liver transplantation. *Z. Gastroenterol.* 32, 269.

Oden, H. (1996). Renal cell carcinoma associated with cyclophosphamide therapy for Wegener's granulomatosis. *Scand. J. Rheumatol.* 25, 391.

Olson, J.H., Sørensen, H.T., Friis, S., *et al.* (1997). Cancer risk in users of calcium channel blockers. *Hypertension* 29, 1091.

Omenn, G.S., Goodman, G.S., and Thornquist M.D., *et al.* (1996). Risk factors for lung cancer and for intervention effects in CARET, the Beta-carotene and Retinol Efficacy Trial. *J. Natl Cancer Inst.* 88, 1550.

Ortiz, A., Gonzalez-Parra, E., Alvarez-Costa, G., *et al.* (1992). Bladder cancer after cyclophosphamide therapy for lupus nephritis. *Nephron* 60, 378.

Pahor, H., Guralnik, J.H., Ferrucci L., *et al.* (1996a). Calcium-channel blockade and the incidence of cancer in aged populations. *Lancet* 348, 493.

Pahor, H., Guralnik, J.H., Salive, H.E., *et al.* (1996b). Do calcium channel blockers increase the risk of cancer? *Am. J. Hypertens.* 9, 695.

Parazini, F., La Veccia, C., Negri, E., *et al.* (1997). Case-control study of oestrogen replacement therapy and risk of cervical cancer. *BMJ* 315, 85.

Pedersen-Bjergaard, J., Jønsson, V., Pedersen, M., *et al.* (1995). Leiomyosarcoma of urinary bladder after cyclophosphamide. *J. Clin. Oncol.* 3, 532.

Peters-Engl, C., Hedl, H., Danmayr, E., *et al.* (1996). Endometrial cancer after tamoxifen treatment: a descriptive study of 25 breast cancer patients who subsequently developed endometrial cancer. *Anticancer Res.* 16 (5B), 3241.

Petru, E. and Schmähl, D. (1991). Cytotoxic chemotherapy-induced second neoplasms: clinical aspects. *Neoplasma* 38, 147.

Pfatzner, W. and Przybilla, B. (1997). Malignant melanoma and levodopa: is there a relationship? *J. Am. Acad. Dermatol.* 37, 332.

Philpott, N.J., Elebute, M.O., Powler, R., *et al.* (1996). Platinum agents and secondary myeloid leukaemia. *Br. J. Haematol.* 93, 884.

Piepkorn, H., Kumasaka, B.N., Krieger, J.N., *et al.* (1995). Development of human papillovirus-associated Buschke–Lawenstein penile carcinoma during cyclosporine therapy for generalized pustular psoriasis. *J. Am. Acad. Dermatol.* 29, 321.

Psaty, B.H. and Furberg, C.D. (1997). Clinical implications of the World Health Organisation — International Society statement on calcium antagonists. *J. Hypertens.* 15, 1197.

Pui, C.H., Behm, F.G., Raimondi, S.C., *et al.* (1989). Secondary acute myeloid leukaemia in children treated for acute lymphoid leukaemia. *N. Engl. J. Med.* 321, 136.

Radis, C.D., Kwoh, C.K., Morgan, M.C., *et al.* (1993). Risk of malignancy in cyclophosphamide-treated patients with rheumatoid arthritis: a 20-year follow-up study. *Arthritis Rheum.* 36 (Suppl.) R19.

Reich, D.S., Palmer, C.A., and Peters, G.E. (1995). Ethmoid sinus leiomyosarcoma after cyclophosphamide treatment. *Otolaryngol. Head Neck Surg.* 113, 495.

Rezeig, M.A., Fashir, B.M., Hainau, B., *et al.* (1997). Kaposi's sarcoma in liver transplant recipients of FK506: two case reports. *Transplantation* 63, 1520.

Rosenberg, L., Shapiro, S., Slone, D., *et al.* (1982). Epithelial ovarian cancer and combination oral contraceptives. *JAMA* 247, 2310.

Rosenfeld, S., Swiller, A.I., Shenoy, Y.M.V., *et al.* (1961). Syndrome simulating lymphosarcoma induced by diphenylhydantoin. *JAMA* 176, 491.

Rustin, G.J.S., Newlands, E.S., and Luts, J.M. (1996). Combination but not single agent methotrexate chemotherapy for gestational trophoblastic tumours increases the incidence of secondary tumours. *J. Clin. Oncol.* 14, 2769.

Sheil, A.G.R., Disney, A.P.S., and Amiss, M.N. (1991). Cancer development in cadaveric donor renal allograft recipients treated with azathioprine (AZA) or cyclosporine (CyA) or AZA/CyA. *Transplant. Proc.* 23, 1111.

Siekenik, S., Ariad, S., and Flusser, D. (1997). Malignancy in a patient with rheumatoid arthritis treated with methotrexate. *J. Rheumatol.* 24, 806.

Smith, D.C., Ross, P., Thompson, D.J., *et al.* (1975). Association of exogenous estrogen and endometrial carcinoma. *N. Engl. J. Med.* 293, 1164.

Starzycki, Z., Bogdaszewska-Czabanowska, J., Zeman, J., *et al.* (1997). Disseminated Kaposi's sarcoma after long-term prednisone therapy. *Eur. J. Dermatol.* 7, 307.

Stein, J.P., Skinner, E.C., Boyd, S.D., *et al.* (1993). Squamous carcinoma of the bladder associated with cyclophosphamide therapy for Wegener's granulomatosis. *J. Urol.* 149, 588.

Stern, R.S. and Nichols, K.T. PUVA Follow-up Study. (1996). Therapy with orally administered methoxysalen and ultraviolet A radiation during childhood increases the risk of basal cell carcinoma. *J. Pediatr.* 129, 915.

Swerdlow, A.J., Douglas, A.J., Vaughan Hudson, G. (1992). Risk of second primary cancers after Hodgkin's disease by type of treatment: analysis of 2846 patients in the British National Lymphoma Investigation. *BMJ* 304, 1137.

Talar-Williams, C., Hijazi, Y.M., Walther, H.H., *et al.* (1996). Cyclophosphamide-induced cystitis and bladder cancer in patients with Wegener granulomatosis. *Ann. Intern. Med.* 124, 477.

Tashima, C.K. and de los Santos, R. (1974). Lymphoma and anticonvulsive therapy. *JAMA* 228, 286.

Taylor, A.E.H. and Shuster, S. (1992). Skin cancer after renal transplantation: the causal role of azathioprine. *Acta Derm. Venereol.* (Stockh.) 72, 115.

Thrasher, J.B., Miller, G.J., and Wettlaufer, J.N. (1990). Bladder leiomyosarcoma following cyclophosphamide therapy for lupus nephritis. *J. Urol.* 143, 119.

Travis, L.B., Curtis, R.E., Glimelius, B. *et al.* (1995). Bladder and kidney cancer following cyclophosphamide therapy for non-Hodgkin's lymphoma. *J. Natl Cancer Inst.* 87, 524.

Tucker, M.A., Coleman, C.N., Cox, R.S., *et al.* (1988). Risk of second cancers after treatment for Hodgkin's disease. *N. Engl. J. Med.* 318, 76.

Van Leeuwen, F.E., Somers, R., Taal, B.G., *et al.* (1989). Increased risk of lung cancer, non-Hodgkin's lymphoma, and leukaemia following Hodgkin's disease. *J. Clin. Oncol.* 7, 1046.

Van Leeuwen, F.E., Chorus, A.M.J., Van den Belt-Dusebout, A.W., *et al.* (1994*a*). Leukemia risk following Hodgkin's disease: relation to cumulative dose of alkylating agents, treatment with tenoposide combinations, number of episodes of chemotherapy, and bone marrow damage. *J. Clin. Oncol.* 12, 1063.

Van Leeuwen, F.E., Klokman, W.J., Hagenbeek, A., *et al.* (1994*b*). Second cancer risk following Hodgkin's disease: a 20-year follow-up study. *J. Clin. Oncol.* 12, 312.

Vella, J.P., Doyle, G.D., and Carmody, M. (1996). Metachronous transitional cell carcinoma and tubulointerstitial nephritis after chronic ingestion of antacids: a novel disease association. *Nephrol. Dial. Transplant.* 11, 2367.

Vessey, M.P., Lawless, M., McPherson, K., *et al.* (1983). Neoplasm of the cervix uteri and contraception: a possible adverse effect of the Pill. *Lancet* ii, 392.

Villadell, J., Oppenheim, F., Talhot-Wright, R., *et al.* (1992). Increased risk of malignant tumors in renal transplant recipients receiving cyclosporine. *Transplant. Proc.* 24, 1948.

WHO–ISH (Ad Hoc Subcommittee of the Liaison Committee of the World Health Organisation and the International Society of Hypertension) (1997). Effects of calcium antagonists on the risks of coronary heart disease, cancer and bleeding. *J. Hypertens.* 15, 105.

Wilden, J.N. and Scott, C.A. (1978). A pseudolymphomatous reaction in soft tissue associated with phenytoin sodium. *J. Clin. Pathol.* 31, 761.

Wiles, H.B., Laver, J., and Baum, D. (1994). T-cell lymphoma in a child after heart transplantation. *J. Heart Lung Transplant.* 13, 1019.

Wolf, P., Fink-Puches, R., Reimann-Weber, A., *et al.* (1997). Development of malignant melanoma after repeated photodynamic therapy with 5-aminolevulinic acid at the exposed site. *Dermatology* 194, 53.

Yamamoto, T., Katayama, I., and Nishioka, K. (1996). Adenocarcinoma of the mouth in a patient with psoriasis under short-term cyclosporine therapy. *Dermatology* 193, 72.

Zanke, B.W., Rush, D.N., Jeffery, J.R. *et al.* (1989). HTLV-I T-cell lymphoma in a cyclosporine-treated renal transplant patient. *Transplantation* 48, 695.

Ziel, H.K. and Finkel, W.D. (1975). Increased risk of endometrial carcinoma among users of conjugated estrogens. *N. Engl. J. Med.* 293, 1167.

Zijlmans, J.M.J., van Rijthoven, A.W.A., Kluin, P.H., *et al.* (1992). Epstein–Barr virus-associated lymphoma in a patient with rheumatoid arthritis treated with cyclosporine. *N. Engl. J. Med.* 326, 1363.

Zondervan, K.T., Carpenter, L.M., Painter, R., *et al.* (1996). Oral contraceptives and cervical cancer — further findings from the Oxford Family Planning Association contraceptive study. *Br. J. Cancer* 73, 1291.

27. Drug allergy and tests for its detection

E-S. K. ASSEM

Part 1 Drug allergy

Introduction

Drug allergy continues to present an immense challenge both as a special type of adverse drug reaction (ADR) and as a special discipline of allergy. By definition 'drug allergy' is mediated by immunological mechanisms. The term 'hypersensitivity', used as an alternative to 'allergy' in other parts of this book and elsewhere, lacks precision and will not be used in this chapter. Allergic drug reactions are of Type B (see Chapter 5).

Epidemiology

Though well appreciated, allergic and other ADR may be grossly under-reported (reporting procedures are voluntary in most countries; see comparison with the event-monitoring method [Fletcher 1991]), and a high proportion may be unrecognized or misdiagnosed, for instance anaesthetic reactions (Youngman *et al.* 1983; Dundee 1986; Nimmo 1988). Allergy constitutes a small proportion of all ADR, approximately 20 per cent Lakshmanan *et al.* 1986; Laurence and Bennett 1992). In a large study in USA, 1.7 per cent of a total of 36 653 admissions were due to drug toxicity/reactions and 10 per cent of these were allergic (Classen *et al.* 1991). One of the reasons for misdiagnosis is the occurrence of an unrecognized or unusual manifestation.

Although drug allergy is a rare cause of death, it may contribute significantly to patient morbidity. To support this statement, the author wishes to refer to a relatively well-defined (and not so subtle as other types) reaction, anaphylaxis. Anaesthetics are among the many causes of anaphylactic reaction (AR). Around 3.5 million general anaesthetics (GA) are given in the UK every year and according to conservative estimates between 175 and 800 AR occur (Assem 1990*b*). A four per cent mortality suggests seven to 32 deaths per annum. Frequencies of reactions are available for other groups of drugs, for example, β-lactam antibiotics, non-steroidal anti-inflammatory drugs (NSAID), and iodinated radiocontrast media (Assem 1984*b*), and extension of these calculations would certainly point to the magnitude of the problem.

Distinctive features of allergic drug reactions

1. They have no correlation with known pharmacological properties of the drug (unlike toxic reactions).
2. There is no linear relationship with drug dosage (unlike toxic reactions).
3. They often include a rash, angioedema, the serum sickness syndrome, anaphylaxis, and asthma, which are reactions similar to those of classical protein allergy.
4. They require an induction period on primary exposure but not on readministration.
5. They disappear on cessation of therapy and reappear after readministration of a small dose.
6. They usually occur in a minority of persons receiving the drug.
7. Desensitization may be possible.

Some, if not all, of these criteria are not specific; for example, the reaction to a small dose may be due to idiosyncrasy. There are also instances of drug allergy that do not fulfil the above criteria. The lack of history of a sensitizing dose of penicillin is not uncommon, and in this case previous exposure may have been to penicillin-like compounds that may be present in many natural substances. Another example is the occasional persistence of, or even the appearance of fresh, symptoms and signs after the cessation of therapy. Hyposensitization may not be possible, because of the development of reactions during this process.

Factors affecting the incidence of allergic reactions

There are several factors predisposing to allergy during drug therapy: (1) the drug; (2) the patient (the so-called constitutional factors); and (3) the disease for which the drug is given.

The drug as an allergen

An antigen is an agent capable of inducing antibody formation or a cell (lymphocyte)-mediated immune response. Antigens may or may not produce allergy.

Effect of molecular size

Drugs that are themselves macromolecules, such as protein or peptide hormones and dextrans, which are polysaccharides, act as complete antigens, while simple chemicals cannot do so. Simple chemicals may be arbitrarily defined as those having a molecular weight less than 500–1000. Macromolecular contaminants, which may result from the production processes or storage of simple chemicals, may be a cause of allergic reactions to these preparations.

It has been suggested that standard preparations of benzylpenicillin contain high-molecular-weight contaminants (macromolecular fractions [MMF], separable by dextran gel 'Sephadex' chromatography) that evoke reactions in allergic subjects (Batchelor *et al.* 1967; Knudsen *et al.* 1967; Stewart 1967). This fact has not turned out, however, to be as important as was thought. On the other hand, macromolecular contaminants are important in the allergenicity of semisynthetic penicillins such as ampicillin (Knudsen *et al.* 1970).

Formation of antigens from simple chemicals

Simple chemicals that are incomplete antigens are called 'haptens'. The fact that simple chemicals may induce antibody formation and hypersensitivity of immediate or delayed type, or both, was established many years ago (Landsteiner 1945; Gell *et al.* 1948).

Hapten–protein conjugates of many chemicals, which can now be prepared *in vitro*, can be shown to be antigenic. Irreversible conjugation of the simple chemical with proteins by covalent bonds seems to be essential for the formation of a complete antigen. There is evidence suggesting that a similar mechanism occurs *in vivo*. Reversible binding, which frequently occurs between drugs and plasma proteins, is generally inadequate for the sensitization process.

Having stated the prerequisites for formation of proper antigens from simple chemicals, and having assumed

that conjugation of metabolites of chemically simple drugs takes place *in vivo* prior to the immune response, it still remains to be seen if exceptions to these rules can emerge. One such possible exception is the group of neuromuscular blockers (NMB) with a bis-quaternary ammonium structure. These compounds are certainly allergenic, and seem to behave like 'proper' antigens in eliciting histamine release from basophil leucocytes of allergic individuals (Assem 1977*b*, 1983*b*, 1984*a*; Didier *et al.* 1987).

Simple chemicals vary greatly in their ability to induce allergy. Some rarely, if ever, do so; others can cause an immunological response in virtually every subject, and allergy in many of those receiving them. It is important to stress the fact that the presence of an immunological response does not necessarily mean allergy. A drug may induce an immunological response, as evidenced by the formation of hapten-specific antibodies, without the production of clinical manifestations of allergy. Probably everyone who receives penicillin develops antibodies against the penicilloyl group, which is the 'major' haptenic determinant derived from penicillin. It has also been reported that penicillin antibodies were found in almost all subjects who denied ever having received penicillin therapy during their lifetime (Levine *et al.* 1966), and it was suggested that these antibodies represented an immunological response to penicillins in foods such as milk and dairy products. Moreover, a review by Dewdney and co-workers (1991) of the literature on penicillin allergy revealed a very small number of individuals in whom there is reasonable clinical and documentary evidence that penicillin residues in milk triggered an allergic reaction. A naturally occurring immunoglobulin-G (IgG) antibody-like substance, capable of binding to the quaternary ammonium group and to NMB, was also detected in human and animal sera (Assem 1990*a*). If confirmed, this preliminary finding could have some importance, both as an 'immunological' phenomenon and as a clue as to how 'spontaneous' sensitization to NMB could occur (see Part 2 for technical detail and alternative explanation).

The importance of drug metabolites

The ability of simple chemicals to react covalently with proteins *in vitro* can be correlated with their immunogenicity *in vivo* in experimental animals, as shown by the frequency of induction of contact sensitivity and anaphylactic reactions (Eisen 1959). There are many simple chemicals, however, including most of the drugs that are currently used for therapeutic purposes, that do not react with protein *in vitro* but which are capable of inducing antibody formation *in vivo*. The ability of some of these compounds to produce allergic reactions and induce antibody formation may be explained by the formation *in vivo* of metabolites that react with proteins. Since our knowledge about the various metabolites of most drugs is limited, little is known about the various haptenic determinant groups that are derived from the drugs that are capable of inducing an immunological response.

In theory, any of the various degradation products of any compound, whether arising from metabolic processes in the body or by non-metabolic processes that may even take place before the drug is administered, may be capable of becoming an antigen and inducing allergy.

In instances where a drug gives rise to more than one allergen, the relative importance of each allergen may vary in different patients; but, on the whole, one of these is likely to be the main allergen in most allergic patients. The best-known example is penicillin allergy, which will be discussed at length later in this chapter.

The various ways in which a drug (a simple chemical) can become antigenic are shown in Fig. 27.1.

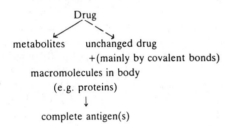

FIG. 27.1 Formation of antigens from simple chemicals.

Most drugs are metabolised by cytochrome P-450-dependent enzymes to highly reactive compounds. In fact, this principle has been applied in devising some of the new *in vitro* allergy tests, to be discussed in Part 2 of this chapter.

Alternatives to the above-mentioned conventional view have been suggested by various workers (e.g. de Weck 1977). It has also now emerged that the process of antigen formation described above is involved in one of two main pathways (de Weck 1996) of T-lymphocyte stimulation. The drug/hapten-protein thus formed is then digested by the antigen-presenting cells and presented to T lymphocytes in the form of drug-peptide fragments set in the groove of a class II major histocompatibility complex (MHC). In the other pathway the drug/hapten binds directly to the MHC complex of the antigen-presenting cell. Further details are given below, under the relevant variety of immune response.

Allergy to 'inactive' ingredients of drug preparations

Ingredients (such as vehicles and excipients) other than the active drug(s) in any preparation may themselves be responsible for an allergic reaction to a medicinal preparation.

Allergenicity of different preparations of the same drug or closely related derivatives

It has been found in the case of penicillin that, in general, allergic reactions to semisynthetic compounds are much more frequent than reactions to natural penicillins (benzylpenicillin and phenoxymethylpenicillin; Idsøe *et al.* 1968). This is probably due in part to the previously mentioned 'contamination' with antigenic macromolecules. Such contaminants could be (1) polymers of the drug; (2) enzymes (i.e. bacterial amidase) used to cleave side chains of natural penicillins prior to their replacement with new side chains; (3) contaminants of the enzyme; or (4) penicilloylated enzyme or contaminants.

It seems likely that additives or formulations that are used to prolong the action of penicillin (e.g. procaine) may themselves be allergens; or may increase the antigenicity and allergenicity of penicillin; that is, they may act as 'adjuvants'. The effect of adding a β-lactamase inhibitor (e.g. clavulanic acid) to certain penicillin preparations (e.g. amoxycillin) on the occurrence of allergic reactions has not been properly evaluated. We have only examined the effect of β-lactamase inhibitors in *in vitro* tests for penicillin allergy (see Part 2 — Tests for drug allergy).

Route of administration

The severity and manifestations of allergy depend to some extent on the route of administration; thus, for example, anaphylactic reactions are usually more dramatic when the drug is given by injection than when it is given orally. Oral administration of drugs, for example, oral penicillin preparations, however, can occasionally cause as rapid and severe a reaction as that produced by injection (Simmonds *et al.* 1978).

Coincidental drug therapy

It has been reported (BCDSP 1972) that patients suffering from gout and treated with allopurinol have a significantly raised incidence of 'reaction' (skin rash) to ampicillin, which is probably allergic in nature. It is tempting to speculate that drug interactions, apart from producing changes in the pharmacological or toxic effects, might also enhance or reduce the allergic reaction to a drug.

The patient

The permissive role played by the host in producing an allergic reaction is the subject of much speculation but only a few facts are known. In view of the several steps involved in the production of an allergic response to a simple chemical, many variables may be considered as contributory host factors.

Genetic predisposition

Association with other allergies

Patients with a history of allergic disease such as 'atopic' disease (eczema, hay fever, or asthma) or drug reactions, whether definitely allergic or due to an unidentified mechanism, have a significantly higher incidence of allergic drug reactions. This fact, although previously disputed, is becoming more generally accepted, and surveys or proper epidemiological studies support it (e.g. the survey by Hurwitz [1969]). Penicillin allergy occurs more often in atopic than in non-atopic patients (Levine *et al.* 1966).

In my experience, this is true of allergy to many other drugs (Assem 1977a,b, 1983a,b), and not only of allergic drug reactions but also of reactions simulating allergy but apparently not mediated by immunological mechanisms, for example, asthma induced by aspirin and other NSAID (non-immunological anaphylactic-like ['anaphylactoid'] reactions, described later). Another example is the anaphylactic-like reaction produced by narcotic analgesics (Assem 1976). Caution should, however, be exercised since we do not clearly understand the mechanism of anaphylactoid reactions and some of them may eventually turn out to be immunological in nature, as has already happened in the case of anaphylactoid reactions to neuromuscular blockers, as explained below.

Definitive genetic studies

Correlation with HLA serotypes   One of the recent approaches to the question of genetic aspects of allergy is to study its possible association with the major histocompatibility (HLA) antigens. This has been carried out in patients with reagin- (mainly IgE) mediated allergy to ragweed pollen, using highly purified preparations of various pollen allergens (Marsh *et al.* 1973). Quantitative prick-in skin tests were used to classify patients according to the intensity of skin response to each allergen. The results suggested a significant correlation between a particular HLA serotype and the ability to develop reagin-mediated allergy to a particular allergen (as detected by skin testing). This correlation was highly significant, firstly in the case of allergens that were of relatively simple chemical structure, and secondly where

the individual differences in response, particularly when judged by the concentration of allergen required to elicit a response, were clearly distinguishable. Thus, these two conditions may be necessary in order to show a marked association in a population as genetically polymorphic as man.

It should be pointed out that the skin response to an allergen may be influenced by several factors other than the amount of reagin (or IgE) present in the skin; it is the net result of all these factors, which may be regulated by different genes.

The influence of HLA type on drug-induced immune responses is complex, and it is interesting that HLA typing may help in the assessment of whether or not particular drug reactions are likely, especially if carried out in conjunction with genetic determinants of drug metabolism. The best example is hydralazine-related systemic lupus erythematosus (SLE) which is 10 times more frequent in DR4 patients than in the population at large (Welsh and Batchelor 1981).

More recent studies have focused on the influence of HLA type not only in truly allergic reactions but also in reactions that are considered as pseudoallergic (e.g. aspirin-induced asthma [Dekker *et al.* 1997]).

Individual differences in the immune response to specific chemicals   Genetically controlled individual differences in immunological responses to specific chemicals or groups of chemicals were found in experimental animals such as the guinea-pig (Chase 1958). They have also been shown in the immune response of mice of different strains to various antigens ranging from simple polypeptides containing as few as two or three amino acids, to large molecules, such as ovomucoid (McDevitt and Benacerraf 1969; Levine and Vaz 1970; Benacerraf and McDevitt 1972; McDevitt and Bodmer 1972). It has been shown that certain strains of mice respond to the injection of minute amounts of some of these antigens by producing high titres of reaginic (IgE) antibodies (Levine and Vaz 1970).

Studies in drug allergy in man   Genetically determined immune responses to simple chemicals or chemical groups of similar nature to those previously mentioned have not as yet been demonstrated in man. At present, the only drug allergy for which it may be possible to study these aspects in man is penicillin allergy. Although several of our penicillin-allergic patients have a family history of penicillin allergy, it could not be concluded that this was due to genetically determined specific immune response to penicillin. The main reason for this situation is the frequent occurrence in penicillin-allergic patients and their relations of allergy to a wide variety of unrelated chemicals. Among over 200 patients allergic to penicillin, however, we have seen no more than five with personal and family histories of allergy to penicillin alone.

We believed that family studies in subjects who are allergic to penicillin and in non-allergic subjects who also produce penicillin antibodies, but who do not manifest allergy (which requires a special class of antibodies of which these subjects produce little, if any), might throw some light on another interesting aspect, namely the pattern of immune response to various degradation products of the penicillin nucleus. Extensive investigations were carried out with conjugates of three metabolites that act as antigenic determinants: the 'major' determinant (the penicilloyl group); and two 'minor' determinants (the penicillenate and penicillamine groups). Using various techniques to measure the antibodies specific to these three determinants, we have not yet detected any family-specific patterns (Assem and Vickers, unpublished).

Possible influence of genetic factors in drug metabolism
Genetically determined variations in the metabolism of some drugs in turn influence the occurrence of adverse drug reactions other than allergy. Examples are prolonged apnoea after suxamethonium administration in patients with pseudocholinesterase deficiency and the polyneuritis due to isoniazid in patients who are slow inactivators of this drug. At present there is merely speculation that elements of this sort may to some extent determine the incidence, type, or manifestations of allergic drug reactions. The higher incidence of hydralazine-related SLE in slow acetylators may be considered as an example of that situation. Perhaps differences in specific and non-specific hydroxylating enzymes may also be of importance in this respect (Remmer and Schuppel 1972).

Other factors that influence the patient's response
A large number of other non-specific factors may influence the response to antigenic stimuli. These include genetic factors which operate through alterations in enzyme systems, age, sex (e.g. the higher incidence of hydralazine-related SLE in females), and perhaps nutritional factors. Epidemiological studies have shown that adverse reactions of all kinds are commoner in patients who are aged 60 years and over, and in women (Hurwitz 1969).

The occurrence of disease in organs that take part in drug metabolism may play some role in the immunological response. Epidemiological surveys did not show, however, that patients with liver or kidney disease or diabetes mellitus have a greater incidence of adverse

drug reactions (Hurwitz 1969), which suggests the possible limitations of surveys of this type.

The disease

Glandular fever and ampicillin rash

When patients with glandular fever, certain viral infections, or leukaemia are given ampicillin, many develop a skin rash which several investigators claim to be of non-allergic nature, since the allergy tests they have carried out have been negative (Knudsen 1969). There are two important points to be made here. First, ampicillin is not the only penicillin to cause a rash, though it may do so more frequently than the others. We have investigated patients with a similar rash following other penicillins including the two natural penicillins, benzylpenicillin and phenoxymethylpenicillin. Secondly, it seems more likely that the rash is due to allergy caused by an immunological abnormality induced by the disease, for other abnormalities of this kind are well known to occur in glandular fever, namely, the presence of heterophile antibodies (detected by the Paul–Bunnell test) and cold agglutinins; and the occurrence of false-positive serological tests for syphilis.

As in other infections, the virus that is thought to cause glandular fever may act as an 'adjuvant' (see below).

HIV infection

Another viral infection with an increased incidence of drug allergy (e.g. to antibiotics, a point which is of practical importance; possible desensitization is mentioned later) is the human immunodeficiency virus (HIV) (Bayard *et al.* 1992).

Adjuvant effect

In experimental work designed to induce sensitization (allergy) or potentiation of the response to an antigen in the way of increasing the amount of antibody produced, certain micro-organisms are used, such as tubercle bacilli (in complete Freund's adjuvant) and *Bordetella pertussis*. It is therefore reasonable to speculate that patients with infections due to these organisms might have a raised incidence of drug allergy.

It has been suggested that the incidence of drug allergy is higher during infection, and that, when given prophylactically, antibiotics and other chemotherapeutic agents produce allergic reactions less frequently than when they are administered during infections. This was thought to be caused by an adjuvant effect produced by bacterial infections, partly due to bacterial endotoxin (Munoz

1964). It is also possible that the tissue injury produced by infection may create more possible binding sites for haptens. The final stage of allergic reactions may also be potentiated by bacterial products. This is suggested by the finding that the injection of *B. pertussis* vaccine potentiates the toxic effects of histamine in mice (Kind 1958).

Immunological mechanisms

The four main immunological mechanisms involved in drug allergy (and in allergy in general) are shown in Table 27.1.

TABLE 27.1
Immunological mechanisms of allergic reactions
(according to Coombs and Gell classification, 1968)

Type I	Immediate-type (or anaphylactic) which is mediated by anaphylactic (reaginic) antibodies of the IgE, or possibly the IgG, class of immunoglobulins.
Type II	Autoallergy (autoimmunity), auto-sensitization being mediated by lymphocytes or antibodies.
Type III	Arthus-type, mediated by IgG, IgM, and complement 1. Typical Arthus reaction. 2. Conditions reproduced by special types of late responses to antigen challenge. 3. Immune-complex disease, serum sickness, or apparently similar syndromes.
Type IV	Delayed-type hypersensitivity (also described as cell-mediated immunity due to mediation by sensitized lymphocytes).

In the pathway of T-cell activation (mentioned above) where the MHC complex is directly involved in drug conjugation, if the MHC complex so involved is of class I, the T-cell response induced will be CD8+. This results in a delayed-type (Type IV, see above) clinical reaction. If the binding is to class II MHC, the T lymphocytes stimulated are CD4+ type (Th) and will be either Th 1, with subsequent formation of IgG antibodies, or Th 2, which result in the formation of IgE antibodies (Type I reaction, anaphylaxis). In the second pathway of T-cell activation the antigen (digested drug–protein conjugate, see above) is presented in conjunction with class-II MHC, leading almost exclusively to the stimulation of

CD4-type (Th) lymphocytes with subsequent IgG or IgE formation as described above. T cells of various subtypes secrete different arrays of cytokines which regulate or cause allergic inflammation (Umetsu and Dekruyff 1997).

It is important to stress that, apart from allergy and its underlying mechanisms, some immune responses to drugs appear to be quite harmless, for example, the symptomless formation of hapten-specific antibodies. There is evidence suggesting that this is the most common type of response to at least some, if not all, of the drugs that are capable of inducing an immunological stimulus. In certain instances these antibodies seem to inhibit the damaging influence that may be produced by the simultaneous occurrence of the other varieties of immunological responses. In these cases, the antibodies may be described as 'blocking' antibodies. This functional class of antibodies may also be induced by hyposensitization (desensitization) procedures. The best known example is the almost invariable production of non-sensitizing IgG and IgM anti-penicilloyl antibodies in patients who have received penicillin therapy. In fact, these antibodies are also found in the majority of human subjects who have not been exposed to penicillin in this way but who, presumably, have encountered penicillins present in the air or in food, particularly milk and dairy products (though this should not happen if farmers adhere to the regulations prohibiting the sale of milk from cattle treated with penicillin).

Type I (anaphylactic) reaction

This reaction deserves detailed consideration because of its acute nature, its potentially fatal outcome, and its usefulness in illustrating how the knowledge of mechanism helps both in diagnosis and treatment.

Fatal anaphylactic reactions to drugs are very rare (e.g. 10 cases were reported by the Registrar General of England and Wales in 1963; of these seven were due to penicillin). These figures may be an underestimate, for doctors are understandably reluctant to attribute a patient's death to therapy and may attribute it to disease if it is at all reasonable to do so. In the 1964–1983 survey of reported ADR in the UK, the most commonly reported causes of anaphylaxis, angioedema, and urticaria were Althesin (intravenous anaesthetic, since withdrawn), co-trimoxazole (trimethoprim–sulfamethoxazole), and the NSAID fenbufen (Griffin 1986). In a chronologically comparable way, early surveys in the USA showed that penicillin was again the most common cause of fatal anaphylactic reactions: it was implicated in 32 out of 43 anaphylactic deaths in the American Armed

Forces (Delage and Irey 1972), and it was suggested that 100–500 patients die annually from anaphylactic reactions to penicillin (Parker 1965, 1980, 1982). The incidence of minor (non-fatal) anaphylactic reactions to drugs is not known, but they are presumably much more frequent than fatal reactions. Estimates of the overall frequency of Type I reactions to the β-lactam antibiotics range from 0.7 to eight per cent, and many investigators have reported incidences over two per cent (Smith *et al.* 1966; Idsøe *et al.* 1968; Sullivan *et al.* 1981). The incidence may have declined in recent years, however, as compared with the early 1960s (Parker 1980). Other drugs have also come to prominence as causes of anaphylactic and anaphylactoid reactions (see below). In a recent 20-year study in the Netherlands (van der Klauw *et al.* 1996), analgesic drugs and NSAID were the most common cause. Amoxycillin, the most commonly used β-lactam antibiotic, was ranked in tenth place.

Anaphylactic antibodies

The anaphylactic reaction (immediate-type allergy) is the reaction mediated by certain classes of antibodies known collectively as anaphylactic (tissue-sensitizing) antibodies. Various species produce their own characteristic anaphylactic antibodies.

Various classifications are applied to these antibodies. The term 'homocytotropic' antibody was introduced by Becker and Austen (1968) to describe a specialized class of anaphylactic antibodies capable of attaching to certain target cells of the same species. Homocytotropic antibodies may further be classified into reaginic and non-reaginic. Antibodies mediating the anaphylactic reaction in man are of the reaginic type. They belong mainly to the most recently discovered γE (IgE) class of immunoglobulins. IgE antibodies are believed to have evolved as a mechanism to protect mammals against parasitic and possibly bacterial infection as well. Subversion of this system leads to allergic disease (Sutton and Gould 1993; Galli and Wershil 1996).

Non-IgE antibodies may be involved in anaphylactic reactions, particularly IgG$_4$ subclass antibodies.

Mechanism of the anaphylactic reaction

The anaphylactic reaction results from the interaction between the specific allergen and the cell-fixed anaphylactic antibodies. The cells that are particularly involved in this reaction include tissue mast cells and basophil leucocytes, and anaphylactic antibodies seem to have special affinity for these cells. The interaction between the allergen and anaphylactic antibodies fixed to these cells triggers a process which seems to involve several steps inside these cells, ultimately leading to the release of pharmacological mediators. The released mediators in turn act on certain target organs or tissues, such as vascular and bronchial smooth muscle. Thus, the reaction affects two types of cell populations; the first are 'sensitized' cells, which recognize the allergen and react to it by elaborating the pharmacological mediators, and the second are the 'effector' cells, responding to these mediators. The released mediators seem to produce their effect through 'specific' receptors on the surface of 'effector' cells, such as the bronchial smooth muscle in asthma.

In order that the antigen–antibody interaction may initiate the anaphylactic mechanism, two criteria should be fulfilled:

1. for any particular cell, sensitization requires that there should be more than one antibody molecule per cell (they indeed exist in hundreds of thousands) (Ishizaka *et al.* 1973);

2. two or more identical groups (antigenic determinants or sites) should be present in the antigen, since the main mechanism of allergen-initiated reaction is a 'bridging' process of two adjacent antibody molecules (Stanworth 1973).

Immunological concepts in Type I allergy to drugs

The aforementioned concepts have the following important consequences:

Eliciting of allergic reactions by skin and other tests

The manifestations of immediate allergic reactions cannot be produced unless both the antigen and antibodies have multiple combining groups. This explains the very frequent failure of drugs to elicit a positive skin test. This occurs in the case where the unconjugated drug is not protein-reactive, and in the case of a univalent conjugate (one haptenic residue per molecule of conjugate). On the occasions when the simple chemical itself or its derivatives react rapidly with protein, as in the case of penicillin, an immediate-type reaction may be produced.

Although a molecule bearing a single determinant (monovalent hapten) which is still capable of binding to a single antibody molecule is generally incapable of triggering an allergic reaction, it may, however, elicit a reaction under a special condition: if it has an additional chemical group that provides the possibility of a second though non-identical binding site (Raffel 1973). In contrast, contact hypersensitivity, which is an example of delayed hypersensitivity, unlike the immediate type, can be elicited frequently by the chemical itself.

Inhibition of allergic reactions by monovalent haptens

While a non-reactive chemical, or a monovalent conjugate thereof, is incapable of eliciting an allergic reaction, it can produce the opposite effect, namely, inhibition of reaction to a complete antigen, when applied simultaneously. This can be shown by inhibition of a 'direct' skin test, passive cutaneous anaphylaxis, or even of the reaction to a drug administered systemically to a patient who is allergic to this particular drug (de Weck *et al.* 1973).

The clinical applications and mechanisms of inhibition of allergic reactions by monovalent haptens, and the immunological changes observed after hyposensitization therapy will be discussed later.

Hyposensitization procedures

A patient allergic to a drug may be hyposensitized by gradually increasing the drug dosage up to the desired level, followed by repeated administration of the dose that is considered adequate. Hyposensitization can be maintained only by repeated administration of the drug, or the whole procedure should be repeated when another course of drug therapy is required (Holgate 1988).

Biochemical mechanisms and metabolic requirements of the anaphylactic reaction

It is thought that the bridging effect of antigen between adjacent antibody molecules induces configurational changes in the Fc region of the cell-fixed antibody molecule (the part of antibody attached to cell membrane), which in turn initiates a series of biochemical events inside sensitized cells (e.g. mast cells). These biochemical events (signal transduction; Razin *et al.* 1995) lead to the release or synthesis and release of various pharmacological mediators of this reaction. This process is considered to be secretory in nature. It requires calcium and energy (it can be inhibited by metabolic inhibitors which are, on the whole, toxic), but does not require oxygen. Sodium cromoglycate, the 'prophylactic' antiasthma and antiallergy drug, may be considered as the prototype of non-toxic inhibitors of the mediator-secretion process. Its action is not, however, fully understood (Foreman and Pearce 1994) and is limited because of lack of absorption after oral administration. It is only effective if applied directly: by inhalation in asthma, as an aerosol or drops in rhinitis, or as eye-drops in allergic conjunctivitis.

Pharmacological mediators of anaphylaxis

The mediators released, or formed and released, in this reaction depend on the species and tissues involved; for example, the two main mediators released from sensitized human lung tissue are histamine and slow-reacting substance of anaphylaxis (SRSA), derived from arachidonic acid, like prostaglandins. SRSA has now been

identified as mainly consisting of leukotrienes C_4 and D_4 and E_4. The list of mediators, which comprises two broad groups (pre-stored, e.g. histamine, and synthesized *de novo*, e.g. LT and other arachidonic metabolites), is expanding all the time (Austen 1997). Other candidates identified in various species are 5-hydroxytryptamine; kinins (e.g. bradykinin); thromboxanes (TX), for example, TXA_2, the main component of the so-called rabbit-aorta-contracting substance; platelet-activating factor (PAF: acetylglyceryl ether phosphorylcholine), formed in a wide range of cell types from precursor cell-membrane phospholipids through the concerted action of phospholipase A_2 and acetyl-CoA and eosinophil chemotactic factor. Mast cells (and basophil leucocytes) are also potential sources of pre-inflammatory cytokines (Galli and Wershil 1996).

Non-immunological mechanisms

Anaphylactic-like reactions

Anaphylactic-like (anaphylactoid) reactions that are not immunologically mediated may be produced by the various mechanisms listed in Table 27.2. At the cellular level (mast cell or basophil leucocyte) histamine release may be due to an idiosyncratic susceptibility to a certain chemical grouping. Physical processes may also trigger the release of histamine and other mediators; one example is the release of histamine by hyperosmolar solutions of iodinated radiocontrast media (Assem *et al.* 1983). When anaphylactoid reactions occur with drugs that are known to interact with (stimulate or block) certain receptors, for example, NMB, it is tempting to speculate that the underlying mechanism may be a receptor abnormality. Caution is needed, however, since the mechanism may still turn out to be immunological (as in the case of NMB, see below).

Several groups of drugs are capable of inducing reactions of this type, though they may also induce immunologically mediated reactions. These drugs include preanaesthetic medications, intravenous anaesthetic induction agents, iodinated radiographic contrast media, aspirin-like drugs (asthma may be induced by aspirin in 10 per cent of adults with asthma), and plasma substitutes (Assem 1977*b*; Watkins and Ward 1978; Watkins 1979; Assem 1983*a,b*; Assem *et al.* 1983; Szczeklik 1983, 1997; Quiralte *et al.* 1997). A relatively rare presentation of intolerance to NSAID (and possibly other drugs) is exercise-induced (drug-dependent) anaphylaxis (van Wijk *et al.* 1995).

In the past, a proportion of patients with the so-called 'anaphylactoid' reaction to NMB blockers were considered under this category for a variety of reasons, including: (1) they reacted on their first clinical exposure to NMB (Assem 1977*b*, 1983*b*); and (2) NMB were included among direct, 'non-immune' histamine-releasers (Paton 1957). It turned out, however, that IgE antibodies (which mediate anaphylaxis) to NMB could be detected in the serum of those patients (Baldo and Fisher 1983; Harle *et al.* 1984; see Charpin *et al.* 1983; Vervloet *et al.* 1983; Didier *et al.* 1987; see Moneret-Vautrin *et al.* 1988*a,b*; Assem and Ling 1988; Assem 1989, 1990*b*, 1992*b*). This example (see Part 2 of this chapter for further discussion of NMB) illustrates how wrong assumptions can arise.

It should be added that one of the reasons for suggesting a non-immune (IgE-independent) mechanism for the reaction to NMB was that some of the patients reacted on what appeared to be their first exposure. However, IgE antibodies were detected in some of these patients. This led to the postulation that these patients must have had exposure to chemically cross-reacting

TABLE 27.2
Mechanisms of production of drug reactions simulating manifestations of anaphylaxis

1. *Direct release of pharmacological mediators* such as histamine and 5-hydroxytryptamine:
   (a) as a process that does not normally occur: a qualitative abnormality: idiosyncrasy;
   (b) as a process that normally occurs to a much smaller extent: a quantitative abnormality: intolerance;
   (c) as a qualitative abnormality that normally occurs in other species, e.g. dextran reaction in rats, cremophor or miscellophor reaction in dogs.

2. *Direct (non-immune) activation of the complement system*

3. *Direct agonist or antagonist effects of the drug on 'target' or 'shock' organs*:
   (a) as a qualitative abnormality, e.g. bronchospasm induced by aspirin (and by other NSAID);*
   (b) as a quantitative abnormality: intolerance.

4. *Indirect effect on 'shock' organs* by interfering with the response to drugs or normal homoeostatic mechanisms, e.g. the autonomic regulatory mechanisms, balance between pathways of mediator synthesis or metabolism (lipoxygenase and cyclo-oxygenase pathways of arachidonic acid metabolism),* balance between mediators with opposite effects (bronchoconstrictor and bronchodilator prostaglandins PGD_2 and PGF_2, or cysteine leukotrienes and bronchodilator prostaglandins, mainly PGE_2).*

---

* among the possible explanations of asthma induced by NSAID (Szczeklik 1997).

compounds, presumably containing quaternary ammonium groups (QAG). Compounds containing QAG are widely distributed in nature, in the environment as well as within the body (e.g. choline-containing compounds). Speculation went as far as trying to find some link with exposure to household chemicals, biocides, and even cosmetics (Weston and Assem 1994).

The formation of circulating antibodies that produce reactions not of the classical immediate type

Examples of this in penicillin allergy are the accelerated reaction which appears 2–48 hours after the start of penicillin therapy, and the retarded reaction that occurs 3 days or more after such treatment. Another example is the drug-induced illness resembling serum sickness that may be caused by such drugs as penicillin and aspirin. Antibodies producing the Arthus reaction are also included in this category. In all these examples, the formation of immune complexes and the activation of complement takes place, thus initiating the inflammatory response or tissue damage.

Delayed-type hypersensitivity

The relation of circulating antibodies to this type of reaction is obscure, and the condition can be transferred by lymphocytes but not by serum. It has now been established that the reaction is mediated by sensitized T lymphocytes, which respond to the specific allergen (and non-specifically to certain mitogens) by producing lymphokines, which consist of a large number of protein or polypeptide substances and which are considered to be the putative soluble mediators of delayed-type hypersensitivity reactions. Among the activities of lymphokines are release of histamine and SRS (mainly leukotrienes C_4 and D_4) (Ezeamuzie and Assem 1983*a*, 1985; MacDonald 1996).

Contact sensitivity is an example of delayed hypersensitivity. The induction of contact cutaneous sensitivity occurs as a result of the conjugation of hapten with epidermal proteins. There is evidence that the ability of chemical compounds to elicit allergic contact dermatitis can be correlated with the affinity for sulphydryl-containing proteins of the skin. On subsequent exposure to the same haptens this process is repeated and the resulting conjugate elicits an allergic reaction by reacting with sensitized cells.

Autoallergy and related phenomena

The formation of hapten–protein conjugates in the body may induce marked changes in the carrier-protein molecule, depending on the degree of substitution with haptenic groups. In this way body proteins may no longer be recognized as 'self'. This may lead to the formation of a wide variety of antibodies, some of them being organ-specific (for example, antibodies against the formed elements of the blood), others not. This process (autoimmunization) may be associated with, or cause, illness (autoallergy).

The development of autoantibodies, for example red blood cell antibodies (detected by a positive Coombs test) or antinuclear antibodies, may not necessarily be associated with illness. In fact, in general, autoimmune disease (autoallergy) occurs in a minority of these patients, particularly if they have no strong disposition to such illnesses.

Drug-related systemic lupus erythematosus-like syndrome

One of the best examples that is used to illustrate the mechanisms involved in drug-induced autoallergy is the drug-related systemic lupus erythematosus syndrome (D-RSLE) (Harpey *et al.* 1972). The list of drugs capable of inducing this syndrome is shown in Table 18.2, Chapter 18.

Factors contributing to lupus induction or activation by drugs

Genetic predisposition

(a) Lupus diathesis: strong predisposition requires a weak stimulus, and *vice versa*; (b) the rate of drug metabolism, for example, slow acetylation of isoniazid and hydralazine (Perry *et al.* 1970) and of procainamide (Woosley *et al.* 1978) appears to be a predisposing factor.

Pharmacological action of the drug involved

(a) Inhibition of certain enzymes, for example, DNAase (hydralazine); (b) enhancement of formation of disulphide bonds (hydralazine) (some other factors activate rheumatoid arthritis in a similar way); (c) interference with cross-linkage of collagen and elastin (penicillamine); (d) influence on polymerization of macromolecular complexes (penicillamine); (e) antagonism of some 'physiological' protective mechanisms (e.g. antiallergy).

Possibility (e) may explain the mechanism in the case of β-blockers, particularly in view of findings indicating that catecholamines have some anti-inflammatory and antiallergy effects (predominantly due to stimulation of β-adrenoceptors). Since the antiallergy effects were not β_1 or β_2 'selective' (Assem and Schild 1971), we were not surprised to find that autoimmune phenomena such as the development of antinuclear antibodies in patients receiving β-receptor-blocking drugs were not related to the 'selectivity' of these agents in regard to the subclasses of β-receptors (β_1 and β_2) (Assem 1975, 1977a). The significance of the various autoantibodies that were found in patients with practolol 'reactions' other than SLE is still unclear.

Changes in structure or antigenicity, or both, of DNA and soluble nuclear and cytoplasmic nucleoprotein

(a) Antigenicity of photochemical products of DNA and procainamide > photo-oxidized DNA > native DNA; (b) enhancement of the antigenicity of soluble nucleoprotein by hydralazine; (c) agents that may interact with viruses: for example, penicillamine interacting with polio virus and producing the lupus syndrome in certain strains of mice and the possible interaction of some drugs with oncornavirus nucleic acid; (d) enhanced production of drug metabolites that react with autoantigen through enzyme induction.

Modulation of immune responses and allergic reactions by the autonomic nervous system

A brief summary of these concepts will be given here; for further information the reader is referred to some key reviews (Sutherland and Robison 1966; Szentivanyi 1969; Assem 1971, 1973; Barnes 1989). Most of these concepts appear to stem from work on asthma and atopy, in which the neural (autonomic) mechanisms intermingle with immune and inflammatory reactions. There is evidence to suggest that the autonomic nervous system has an influence on various immunological mechanisms, and that it may possibly modulate allergic reactions by interfering with the different steps of these reactions. Adrenergic mechanisms seem to play an important role in immediate-type and delayed-type (cell-mediated) immune reactions, as suggested by the modulatory effect of adrenergic drugs. Cholinergic mechanisms may also play some role in the regulation of immediate-type allergy, as suggested by the potentiation of antigen-induced mediator release by cholinergic drugs. Cholinergic agents also enhance the cytotoxic action of sensitized lymphocytes. Both adrenergic and cholinergic agents trigger the proliferation of, and DNA synthesis in, spleen colony-forming cells.

More recently, the inflammatory aspect of asthma was associated with additional neural mechanisms: non-adrenergic non-cholinergic mechanisms, with possible involvement of many neuropeptides. A great deal of work is required in order to assess the importance of these mechanisms.

Clinical manifestations of drug allergy

Allergic reactions to drugs produce widely variable clinical manifestations. I do not intend to give more than a brief outline of these reactions and an incomplete list of drugs causing them. Chemical compounds that constitute an industrial hazard will not be mentioned. It is important to stress that minor reactions are fairly frequent, but serious ones are rare.

Clinical manifestations of allergy to a single drug may be single or multiple, and they vary from person to person as a result of involvement of different 'target' organs. The reasons for this variability are not very clear. Of special importance is the extent of dissemination of the causative antigens, which may be influenced by the dosage and route of administration. The site at which the simple chemical undergoes metabolic processes that lead to the formation of haptenic determinants is also of importance. The localization of the reaction may also depend on the formation of organ-specific antibodies, as mentioned previously.

Anaphylaxis

Immediate reactions may be manifested by urticaria, rhinitis, bronchial asthma, angioedema, and anaphylaxis. These manifestations are the counterpart of the classical allergy to foreign protein.

Anaphylactic reactions develop within a few minutes of the administration of the offending drug, and perhaps in less than a minute in some cases. The principal manifestations are those of peripheral circulatory collapse (shock), which may be associated with one or more of the other immediate reactions, which form a broad clinical spectrum (Pumphrey and Stanworth 1996). It is important to differentiate anaphylaxis from vasovagal syncope, which may be produced by psychogenic causes, such as fear, the sight of blood, or painful stimuli. Recovery from vasovagal attacks takes place soon after lying down. The drugs and diagnostic agents that may cause anaphylactic reactions include β-lactam antibiotics (penicillins and cephalosporins), streptomycin, NMB drugs, intravenous anaesthetics, local anaesthetic agents, organic mercurials, radio-opaque iodides, plasma expanders (dextrans, polygelatin, and starch derivatives), NSAID, narcotic analgesics, preanaesthetic medications, streptokinase, heparin, vitamin K_1 oxide (reactions to injections of other vitamins such as vitamins B_1 and B_{12} have also been reported), bromsulphthalein, sodium dehydrocholate (Decholin), and demeclocycline.

It should be added that some of the above-mentioned drugs, such as radio-opaque organic iodides, NSAID, anaesthetic agents, narcotic analgesics, and plasma ex-

panders may possibly produce a reaction resembling anaphylaxis by mechanisms other than allergy. Radio-opaque organic iodides may cause angiotoxic damage and the direct release of histamine without the apparent mediation of an antigen–antibody interaction (Mann 1961; Assem et al. 1983; Genovese et al. 1996). Histamine release by these agents may be caused by hyperosmolarity or activation of the alternative pathway of the complement system (causing the generation of anaphylatoxins). This subject is discussed further in Part 2 of this chapter.

Skin manifestations

Allergic reactions to drugs are most frequently manifested by skin eruptions; these have also been reported after placebo administration (Samter and Berryman 1964). The different varieties of reactions are: urticarial, morbilliform, maculopapular, vesicular, bullous, exfoliative, and eczematous eruptions; purpura; contact dermatitis; fixed eruptions; erythema nodosum; erythema multiforme; photosensitivity; and pruritus.

Urticaria is a typical example of immediate cutaneous sensitivity (Type I, or anaphylactic; but it may be mediated by other mechanisms, e.g. Type III) while contact dermatitis is a typical manifestation of delayed-type hypersensitivity. Bullous eruptions are commonly due to the response of sensitized dermal CD8+ lymphocytes (Hertl et al. 1995; de Weck 1996), which are also found in drug-induced toxic epidermal necrolysis (TEN [Miyauchi et al. 1991]). Skin manifestations of what were previously called 'connective tissue' diseases, which are associated with (and probably caused by) autoallergy, such as lupus erythematosus, which may be induced by drugs, may be included in this list.

Certain varieties of the above reactions are produced more frequently by certain drugs. Erythema multiforme and nodosum are seen particularly in allergy to sulphonamides, barbiturates, pyrazolone derivatives, phenytoin, bromides, iodides, and troxidone. Fixed drug eruptions are most commonly due to phenolphthalein, amidopyrine, barbiturates, sulphonamides, and mepacrine. Drug-induced Stevens–Johnson syndrome is caused most frequently by barbiturates and sulphonamides. Carbamazepine may also induce this syndrome. The author has seem two severe cases due to the latter drug.

Photosensitivity occurs characteristically with sulphonamide derivatives (including those with no antibacterial activity, such as thiazide diuretics and sulphonylurea compounds), phenothiazines, tetracyclines, and non-steroidal anti-inflammatory drugs (Becker *et al.* 1996). As with many other manifestations of drug-induced disease, photosensitivity may be due to toxic or allergic reactions (Bickers 1997). The photo-excitation (by UV) of drugs or their metabolites may generate free radicals and singlet oxygen (Zhou and Moore 1997) which cause tissue damage or the formation of highly unstable and reactive haptens.

A few reports on allergy to β-adrenoceptor blocking drugs such as propranolol, practolol, and oxprenolol have been published. The skin rashes were psoriasiform, exfoliative, or urticarial eruptions, and were frequently associated with autoimmune phenomena, particularly the development of antinuclear antibodies and lupus erythematosus cells (Assem and Banks 1973; Raftery and Denman 1973; Assem 1975, 1977*a*) (see also Chapter 19).

Of all the cases of skin eruptions associated with the administration of β-adrenoceptor-blocking drugs, and reported by various authors, only eight of ours (representing 40 per cent of our series) showed direct evidence of allergy to these agents. Such evidence was obtained *in vitro* by the lymphocyte stimulation (transformation) test. This and the delayed skin response in some patients suggested a delayed-type hypersensitivity.

It is not known whether the other syndromes that have been associated with practolol administration are due to immunologically mediated reactions, but autoallergy has been suspected at least in some (see the review by Amos 1979). Various organs may be involved, particularly the skin and, more seriously, the eyes (keratoconjunctivitis sicca and its sequelae [Wright 1975; Behan *et al.* 1976]) and serous membranes, particularly the peritoneum (sclerosing peritonitis [Brown *et al.* 1974]) and the pleura (MacKay and Axford 1976). The ears (Wright 1975), the kidneys (Farr *et al.* 1975), liver (Brown *et al.* 1978), lung (Marshall *et al.* 1977), pericardium (Assem 1977*a*), and the laryngotracheal region (Assem 1977*a*) may also be affected.

An alternative (non-immune) mechanism of skin eruptions induced by long-term therapy with β-adrenoceptor-blocking drugs has been postulated by Jensen and others (1976). These authors suggested that such eruptions could be explained by a reduction in the concentration of cyclic adenosine $3',5'$-monophosphate inside epidermal cells, a mechanism that is related to the pharmacological action of these drugs.

Fever

This is one of the commonest manifestations of drug allergy in man, and many drugs, including most antibiotics and other chemotherapeutic agents, can cause fever with and without other manifestations. Pyrexia is, however, rare with some drugs, tetracycline, for instance. The underlying mechanisms have not been fully elucidated. In experimental animals drug fever may be caused by the interaction of antigen with circulating antibody (in the rabbit) or by delayed hypersensitivity (in the guinea-pig). (See the review by Cluff and Johnson [1964] for further discussion.) In the former case (circulating antibody–antigen interaction) endogenous pyrogens are produced by phagocytic leucocytes which are stimulated by the engulfment of immune complexes (Dinarello and Wolff 1978, 1982). In delayed hypersensitivity, lymphokines produced by antigen-stimulated lymphocytes seem to play some role (Chao *et al.* 1977), probably due to activation of phagocytic leucocytes.

It has now been established that the endogenous pyrogen produced by phagocytic leucocytes is 'interleukin-1' (Dinarello 1984, 1989) and that the pyrogens act by increasing arachidonate metabolites, particularly prostaglandin E_1, in the anterior hypothalamus (in the vicinity of the thermoregulatory centre) (Foreman 1994). This subject is also discussed in Chapter 29.

Serum sickness syndrome

Serum sickness is a Type III allergic reaction (Table 27.1). It is mediated by the deposition of immune complexes in small vessels, activation of immune complexes, and recruitment of granulocytes.

This syndrome may be produced by penicillin, aspirin, streptomycin, sulphonamides, and thiouracils. Like serum sickness produced by foreign serum or proteins, the disease occurs in different forms depending on the time of onset in relation to the therapeutic course. The onset of the primary form typically occurs 7–12 days after the start of therapy. The accelerated form occurs in 2 hours to 3 days. A retarded form occurs within a few weeks of drug therapy, or even after the discontinuation of therapy. The main features of this syndrome are fever, arthralgia, urticaria, and maculopapular eruptions. Lymphadenopathy, dyspnoea, wheezing, angioedema, and eosinophilia occur less frequently. The symptoms may be mild and transitory, lasting from a few hours to 4 days, or may be very serious and continue for several weeks. A variety of other complications may develop, for example, brachial plexus neuritis or other types of mononeuritis multiplex, the Guillain–Barré syndrome, optic neuritis, nephritis, carditis, and polyarteritis nodosa.

Laboratory studies may disclose albumin and hyaline casts in the urine, eosinophilia, several types of circulating antibodies and immune complexes and, rarely, plasmacytosis (Arbesman and Reisman 1971; Lowley and Frank 1988).

Neuropathy

This mainly occurs in the serum sickness syndrome. Mononeuritis and polyneuritis are thought to be due to perineural oedema. Peripheral neuritis is a fairly common manifestation of polyarteritis nodosa, in which ischaemia of the peripheral nerves seems to be the underlying mechanism. (See also Chapter 20.)

Lymphadenopathy

The enlargement of lymph nodes occurs in serum sickness. Cellular proliferation in lymph nodes and spleen may be explained by a marked antigenic stimulation. Rarely, patients receiving long-term phenytoin therapy have clinical and pathological changes highly suggestive of lymphoma (Saltzstein and Ackerman 1959; see also Chapter 26). Lymph node enlargement subsides rapidly after cessation of therapy. We reported one patient with allergy to phenylbutazone and a condition resembling Hodgkin's disease (Littlejohns et al. 1973) which disappeared after stopping this drug. A few more patients with somewhat similar clinical manifestations have been investigated in our laboratory, but lymph node biopsy which was obtained in one of them did not show the characteristics of Hodgkin's disease (Assem 1976).

Haematological manifestations

Haematological disorders induced by drugs may be due to inherited biochemical abnormalities, drug toxicity, or allergy. Some of the drugs that have been proved or suggested to be capable of producing immunological responses, and changes affecting the blood, are included in the lists given in Chapter 24. In some of these the evidence is only circumstantial and it may be hard to exclude the possibility that the reactions produced by them are manifestations of cytotoxicity or some unrevealed biochemical abnormality.

Thrombocytopenia

It has been suggested that platelet antibodies that were found in patients with thrombocytopenia due to some drugs (for example, Sedormid) were formed in response to a loose hapten–platelet complex (Ackroyd 1964). It is doubtful whether such a complex would form an adequate antigen, and it seems more likely that these haptens can react irreversibly with platelet, tissue, or plasma proteins (i.e. the antigen may not be located on platelets) by an as yet unidentified pathway. Platelet antibodies are capable of agglutinating normal platelets in vitro, in the presence of the specific hapten, and when complement is added lysis of platelets occurs. At present the mechanisms of platelet agglutination and lysis in vivo and in vitro are not well understood (Shulman 1963, 1964; Ackroyd 1964). Heparin-induced thrombocytopenia is thought to be partly immunologically mediated. Activation of platelets by IgG antibodies may occur, leading to intravascular coagulation (Warkentin 1996).

Haemolytic anaemia

Drug-induced allergic haemolytic anaemia is produced by mechanisms similar to those of thrombocytopenia (Ackroyd 1964; Petz 1985; Salama et al. 1991). Red cell antibodies seem to occur much more frequently than haemolytic reactions. It is important to remember that some of the above-mentioned drugs, such as sulphonamides and phenacetin, are also capable of causing haemolysis of cells deficient in glucose-6-phosphate dehydrogenase. Also, some of the reported instances of allergic haemolytic reactions that were apparently induced by antibiotics or other chemotherapeutic agents have been due to virus disease, particularly the myxovirus group, producing 'autosensitization' (Isacson 1967).

Leucopenia and agranulocytosis

Leucocyte agglutinins have been found in cases of agranulocytosis produced by certain drugs. These agglutinins, however, could in most cases be demonstrated only when the offending drug was given a few hours before the collection of blood for testing or, as is the case of some drugs such as sulphapyridine, by the addition of a small amount of the drug to the serum to be tested. This strongly suggests that the antigen(s) corresponding to these agglutinins is not located on the white cells.

In addition to the presence of leucocyte agglutinins in the blood of subjects with amidopyrine-induced agranulocytosis, recipients of sensitized donor blood also developed agranulocytosis (Moeschlin and Wagner 1952; Moeschlin 1958).

The relationship between antinuclear factor and leucopenia in systemic lupus erythematosus is not understood. It seems that agranulocytosis may be produced either by the removal and destruction of agglutinated white cells, or the interaction of drug, antibody, and granulocyte precursors in the bone marrow, producing maturation arrest. The onset of clinical features is usually more or less sudden, and this limits the value of routine white cell counts as a precaution.

Leucopenia or agranulocytosis due to drugs containing a thiourea group is thought to be due to 'toxicity' (an expression of idiosyncrasy in many instances) rather than to allergy. A good example of the usefulness of studies on structure–activity relationship with respect to adverse effects is the replacement of the thiourea group in metiamide (a histamine H_2-receptor antagonist that caused leucopenia) by a cyanoguanidine moiety, thus forming cimetidine, which is less likely to have that effect (Brimblecombe *et al.* 1975; but see Chapter 24).

Hypoplastic anaemia and pancytopenia

At present evidence that the hypoplastic conditions of the bone marrow that are produced by drugs are due to an immunological response is not conclusive. The induction of this condition by relatively small amounts of some drugs in some people can be explained by mechanisms other than allergy. It has been suggested that bone marrow failure may be due to unsuspected biochemical abnormality. Pharmacogenetic differences in the metabolic handling and response to drugs may underlie some of these blood dyscrasias (Spielberg 1996).

Thrombocytopenic purpura

Symmers (1962) reported several cases of thrombocytopenic purpura that were probably due to drug allergy. (Platelet disorders induced by drugs are also discussed in Chapter 24.)

Liver disease

Drug-induced hepatocellular disorders (Zimmerman and Ishak 1995) are probably not allergic: on the other hand, some cases of cholestatic jaundice probably are. This may be the case with drugs of the phenothiazine group, where jaundice may be produced after a small dose, and other phenomena that are suggestive of allergy may occur, for example, rashes, fever, blood and tissue eosinophilia, and blood dyscrasias. The inability to detect circulating antibodies in this type of reaction does not make the diagnosis of drug allergy untenable since the antigen may react with antibodies fixed to liver cells, thereby producing liver injury.

It may be that the low recurrence rate (below 40 per cent) of cholestatic jaundice when the drug is given again is evidence against the hypothesis of an allergic mechanism unless one postulates that desensitization occurs in 60 per cent of those who develop this reaction.

Latent cholestatic jaundice and, less frequently, overt jaundice may occur in association with systemic manifestations of drug allergy due to penicillin, sulphonamides, sodium aminosalicylate (PAS), and esters of the macrolide antibiotics (erythromycin and oleandomycin). Hepatitis associated with exposure to halothane is rare and the number of cases associated with enflurane is even smaller. There is doubt whether isoflurane, a more recently introduced polyhalogenated volatile anaesthetic,

can induce liver injury (Bird and Williams 1992). Methoxyflurane has been implicated in several case reports as causing hepatic necrosis and has been withdrawn. There seems to be a correlation between the proportion of the halogenated anaesthetic that is metabolized and rate of induction of liver damage. For further information the reader is referred to Chapter 13.

The absence of proper material for skin tests and the inadvisability of carrying out passive sensitization by the Prausnitz–Kustner reaction are obvious limitations to these diagnostic methods. Antituberculous drugs other than PAS, and methyldopa, may cause either a hepatitis-like condition, or cholestatic jaundice (Assem *et al.* 1969; Assem 1972*b*; Hoffbrand *et al.* 1974; Toghill *et al.* 1974). The hepatitis-like picture, which may rarely be caused by isoniazid allergy (Assem *et al.* 1969), may suggest that allergy may also account for the hepatitis caused by iproniazid, another hydrazine derivative with monoamine-oxidase-inhibiting activity.

Vasculitis and connective tissue disease

This group of reactions has far less clearly defined manifestations than the previously mentioned categories. This is due to the lack of specific organ localization. Little is understood about the underlying mechanisms, and the evidence for the involvement of immunological processes is indirect and based more on speculative assumptions than on valid criteria. Studies of this group may perhaps, however, cast some light on the pathogenesis of connective tissue diseases in general.

Lupus erythematosus-like syndrome

A clinical syndrome resembling systemic lupus erythematosus (SLE) with or without the LE-cell phenomenon, associated with treatment with various drugs (see Chapter 18), has been mentioned earlier. It is not established that this disease is due to drug allergy. Although it is reversible in the majority of cases, it may persist for years or become irreversible in some cases. It has been suggested that the drug merely unveils latent disease. In favour of this idea is the fact that some patients with so-called hydralazine-related LE have had an antecedent history suggestive of SLE (Holley 1964). The finding that some patients may have further attacks of SLE following the discontinuation of the drug is not necessarily in favour of this theory. Apart from the LE-cell phenomenon and the antinuclear factors, a positive Coombs test, and occasionally, haemolytic anaemia may be associated with the SLE syndrome.

Acute vasculitis

Acute vasculitis, predominantly affecting small vessels,

and ranging from mild cellular infiltration to acute necrosis, may be caused by drugs. The drugs most commonly implicated are penicillin, sulphonamides, and thiouracils (Symmers 1962). The clinical manifestations are petechial skin lesions, proteinuria, haematuria, and renal failure. Clinical features often include fever, dermatitis, arthralgia, oedema and, although less frequently, myositis, coronary arteritis, and gastrointestinal bleeding.

Chronic vasculitis

The prolonged administration of some drugs, such as hydrazines, thiouracils, phenytoin, sulphonamides, penicillin, and iodides, may produce polyarteritis or some other variants of chronic inflammatory vascular disease. Drug-induced vasculitis is thought to be due to antibodies directed against drug-related haptens, but this has not been proved (Roujeau and Stern 1994). Alternative explanations include direct drug toxicity and humoral or cellular immune responses against endothelial cells or other components of the vessels (McCormick 1950). Rose and Spencer (1957) doubted the aetiological relationship of drugs to polyarteritis nodosa. It is also doubtful whether the administration of drugs for short periods can produce vasculitis in which fresh lesions appear months or years after the drug has been withdrawn. It is possible, however, that acute vasculitis may become a chronic condition through some self-perpetuating mechanisms.

Polymyositis

Allergy to penicillin, and perhaps other drugs also, may be manifested by polymyositis (Parker 1965). We have encountered a patient allergic to penicillin who developed an exacerbation of the symptoms of polymyositis following a skin test with penicilloyl-polylysine.

Pulmonary manifestations

Bronchial asthma is the most common pulmonary manifestation of drug allergy. It may occur as a manifestation of systemic or local anaphylaxis (affecting respiratory airways without involvement of other systems). NSAID may induce asthma attacks, particularly in those who already had suffered from asthma. Such asthma is frequently associated with angioedema. Its mechanism is complex; some of the possible explanations are shown in Table 27.2.

Hilar lymphadenopathy and pulmonary eosinophilia occur much less frequently, and pneumonitis with pulmonary oedema is very rare. Pneumonitis may be caused by cytotoxic anticancer drugs, but may also be produced by a wide range of other drugs (Cooper *et al*. 1986). (See also Chapter 10.)

Nephropathy

Glomerulonephritis is often associated with the serum sickness syndrome or acute vasculitis due to drug allergy. Acute interstitial nephritis may probably be produced by drug allergy (Baker and Williams 1963); for drugs involved see Chapter 14. With cephalosporins the mechanism is different, since certain derivatives (e.g. cephaloridine) are nephrotoxic. Allergy to cephalosporins may, however, cause kidney disease such as interstitial nephritis (Wiles *et al*. 1979). A few cases of interstitial nephritis due to phenylbutazone have also been reported. Among the other features found in those cases were skin rashes, eosinophilia, and hepatitis. A somewhat similar syndrome due to allopurinol has also been reported (McKendrick and Geddes 1979).

Focal or diffuse glomerulonephritis, often with classic 'wire-loop' changes, is present in the kidneys in the majority of patients who die with SLE. The deposition of γ-globulin and complement on the basement membrane has been demonstrated by immunofluorescent techniques. Clinically the disease may manifest itself by acute nephritis, typical nephrotic syndrome, or varying degrees of chronic renal failure. A large number of drugs may produce the nephrotic syndrome, but allergy has not been proved in these cases. The 'nephropathy' that may be produced by phenacetin and perhaps other analgesic drugs is probably not due to allergy (but see Chapter 14).

It has been shown that the kidney may be involved in anaphylactic reactions (Assem *et al*. 1986, 1987; Abdullah and Assem 1989; see also Wiles *et al*. 1979). Mast cells have been shown in kidney tissue, in the interstitium of the cortex and outer medulla. Sensitization of kidney mast cells with IgE antibody has been demonstrated. *In vitro* experiments on sensitized human, guinea-pig, and rat kidney have shown that the most likely consequence of an anaphylactic reaction affecting the kidney is increased glomerular capillary permeability (evidence of which may be sought from urine testing for protein) and renal vasoconstriction, a phenomenon difficult to demonstrate clinically. (See also Chapter 14.)

Cardiac manifestations

Myocarditis

Myocarditis with a lymphocytic and lympho-histiocytic infiltrate may be associated with the serum sickness syndrome. It has also been reported after sulphona-mides, neoarsphenamine, iodides, penicillin, and other sensitizing drugs (Rich 1958; Burke *et al.* 1991; Garty *et al.* 1994).

Cardiac involvement in anaphylaxis

Apart from suggestive clinical reports (Bristow *et al.* 1982; Hirsh 1982; Assem and Ling 1988; Vaswani *et al.* 1996), there is strong evidence from work on isolated (*in vitro*), perfused hearts of experimental animals (Langen-dorff preparation [LP], usually perfused with buffer and not blood) that the heart, apart from being secondarily affected, may be directly involved in systemic anaphyl-axis. This phenomenon is described as 'cardiac ana-phylaxis' (CA) (Levi *et al.* 1981; Burke *et al.* 1982; Ezeamuzie and Assem 1983*b*; Levi *et al.* 1984; Assem and Ghanem 1988; Ghanem *et al.* 1988*a,b*, 1989). In the LP, gross CA is manifested by gross cardiac dysfunction occurring rapidly (1–2 min) after addition of the specific allergen to the perfusion fluid. This challenge causes concomitant release of various pharmacological me-diators (the same as mentioned before, histamine, etc.), which can readily explain the dysfunction. The develop-ment of cardiac arrhythmias (and A–V conduction block) has been associated with the effect of histamine (mainly through H_2-receptors, with a small part through H_1-receptors), which is released from tissue mast cells (also from basophil leucocytes, in the presence of blood) during the reaction, but which may also occur as a consequence of coronary vasoconstriction. Other mani-festations of CA include coronary vasoconstriction and weakened myocardial contractility, which are due to thromboxane A_2, leukotrienes C_4, D_4, and E_4 (SRSA), prostaglandin D_2 and $F_{2\alpha}$, and platelet activating factor (PAF-acether; acetylglyceryl ether phosphorylcholine, AGEPC). The cell origin of the latter group of mediators is far more varied than histamine, and includes tissue mast cells, and endothelial cells (which release PAF, Camussi *et al.* 1983); also leucocytes and mononuclear cells (including phagocytes). Platelets (*in vivo*) are also a source of PAF and thromboxane A_2. Thus, the *in vivo* reaction would be expected to involve a wider variety of mediators than the *in vitro* preparation, perfused with buffer. Some of the substances released during cardiac anaphylaxis (e.g. bradykinin and prostacyclin) protect against the development of coronary vasoconstriction and arrhythmia (Rubin and Levi 1995).

The consensus of opinion is that human heart and guinea-pig heart are similar in their response to allergen challenge and histamine (Levi *et al.* 1981, 1982), and it is reasonable to assume that the cardiac arrhythmias and changes in ECG associated with anaphylactic shock in man are partly due to a primary cardiac anaphylaxis, and not solely to the hypoxia caused by the bronchospasm or respiratory arrest common in severe anaphylaxis.

Mechanism

Mast cells have been found in heart tissues of man and experimental animals. They are located in the connec-tive tissue surrounding coronary vasculature, and in the innermost and outermost layers of cardiac tissue (sub-epicardial and subendocardial) (Ghanem *et al.* 1988*a,b*). The sensitization of cardiac mast cells with IgE mol-ecules, thus paving the way for a local reaction in the heart, has also been demonstrated both by mediator release (histamine and arachidonic acid metabolites, Marone *et al.* 1986, 1995) and by immuno-histochemical studies (Assem and Ghanem 1988; Patella *et al.* 1995).

Prevention of allergic drug reactions

Pretreatment allergy testing

The indications and limitations for 'prophylactic'/ 'predictive' testing are discussed in Part 2 of this chapter, dealing with the detection of drug allergy.

Skin testing

The predictive value of skin tests and their limitations in penicillin allergy are discussed in Part 2. There is no doubt that they provide some help in preventing allergic reactions to penicillin.

RAST tests for IgE antibodies to anaesthetics
(see Part 2)

A variety of radioallergosorbent tests (RAST) for IgE antibodies to anaesthetics, using a variety of solid-phase components, have been developed. Sepharose beads were used by some workers (Baldo and Fisher 1983; Harle *et al.* 1984; Didier *et al.* 1987; Moneret-Vautrin *et al.* 1988*a,b*). Paper RAST for anaesthetics (NMB and thiopentone) were subsequently developed by the author in conjunction with Pharmacia Ltd; these are simple and reliable, and their value was shown in patients who have had anaphylactic reactions under general anaesthesia (Assem and Ling 1988; Assem

1990*a,b*). Their value 'after the event' has paved the way for prospective 'screening' trials (before general anaesthesia), with the hope of reducing anaesthetic morbidity and mortality (Assem 1993). As yet, only a few trials have been conducted and the conclusion reached so far is that in reactions to NMB, which are the most common cause of anaphylaxis during general anaesthesia, these tests are of little value because of the relatively low specificity and relative rarity of this abnormality (Reid *et al*. 1992). In the experience of some authors (Porri *et al*. 1995) they seem to be of little value even when limited to females (who are at least four times more prone to reactions to NMB [Assem 1993*a*]). It seems that for such a screening test to be cost effective the ratio of false-positive to true-positive results should not exceed 2:1 (deduced from the estimates of Roberts 1992).

Elimination of antigenic material

Sources of antigenic material in drug preparations have been discussed earlier. It is possible to eliminate some of them.

Allergen-specific inhibition procedures

Allergic drug reactions may be inhibited prophylactically in different ways, as illustrated in Fig. 27.2.

Hapten inhibition

One of the practical outcomes of the failure of monovalent haptens to produce an allergic reaction is that if an excess of a hapten and a modest amount of an antigen are used together in challenging the sensitized cells (e.g. mast cells), the ineffective hapten, competing with the antigen, will inhibit the reaction to the antigen. The ineffectiveness of a monovalent hapten may be predicted from its chemical structure, and is indicated by the lack of a reactive group other than the single haptenic determinant. Further confirmation of this property can be obtained by work in experimental animals (Raffel 1973).

This concept of hapten inhibition has been used in the treatment of penicillin allergy, using non-reactive monovalent penicilloyl haptens, such as benzylpenicilloyl-formyl-L-lysine (BPO-Flys) (de Weck *et al*. 1973; Fig. 27.3). Failure to fulfil the criterion of non-reactivity may explain the unsuccessful cases reported by other authors (Basomba *et al*. 1978). The success of such a conjugate also depends on the relative importance of the penicilloyl determinant, compared with other determinants in the individual patient.

There have been two more recent and successful applications of the principle of hapten inhibition of anaphylactic drug reactions:

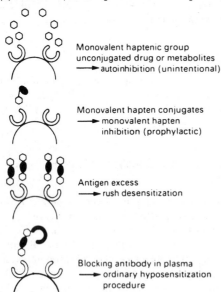

(a) Inhibition by favouring monovalent binding

Monovalent haptenic group unconjugated drug or metabolites
→ autoinhibition (unintentional)

Monovalent hapten conjugates
→ monovalent hapten inhibition (prophylactic)

Antigen excess
→ rush desensitization

Blocking antibody in plasma
→ ordinary hyposensitization procedure

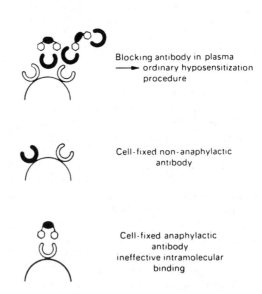

(b) Inhibition despite bivalent binding

Blocking antibody in plasma
→ ordinary hyposensitization procedure

Cell-fixed non-anaphylactic antibody

Cell-fixed anaphylactic antibody ineffective intramolecular binding

Fig. 27.2

Illustration of the various immunological mechanisms of inducing inhibition of the anaphylactic reaction to drugs, with particular reference to the nature of binding, whether monovalent or bivalent, by cell-fixed anaphylactic antibodies to the allergen.

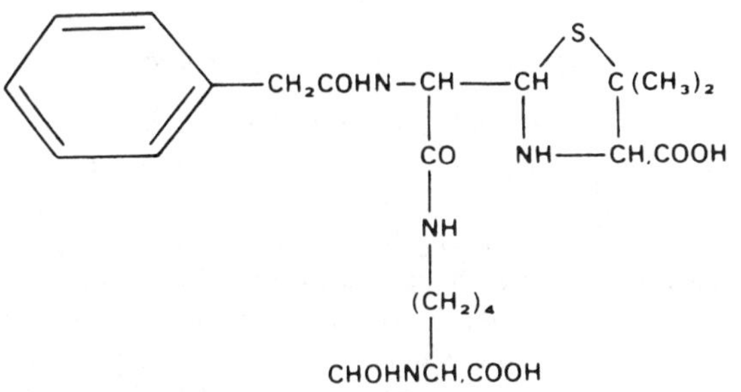

$N\alpha$-formyl-$N\varepsilon$-(α-benzylpenicilloyl)-L-lysine

FIG. 27.3

Example of a monovalent penicilloyl conjugate capable of inhibiting allergic reactions to the penicilloyl determinant, the 'major' haptenic determinant in penicillin allergy (De Weck *et al.* 1973).

1. the use of 'dextran 1' (very low molecular weight, 1 kD). The intravenous injection of 20 ml of a 15% solution of dextran 1 before the infusion of the clinical dextrans is thought to have practically eliminated the risk of severe anaphylactic reactions and fatalities related to these clinical dextrans (Lingstrom *et al.* 1988);
2. the use of monoquaternary ammonium compounds to prevent anaphylactic reactions to the bisquaternary ammonium NMB (Moneret-Vautrin *et al.* 1993).

Inhibition by antigen excess

This may occur in what is described as 'rush desensitization', in which increasing amounts of an allergen are given, eventually reaching an excess.

Spontaneous autoinhibition and hyposensitization

Since most drugs are simple chemicals, and can thus act as haptens, the bulk of a free drug, given in the usual dose, or its metabolites, may inhibit the allergic response to the small chemically conjugated fraction of the drug forming an antigen. In fact, this seems to be the way by which many allergic patients inadvertently escape reactions. Although this process may occur spontaneously, one cannot predict its occurrence.

Induction of immunological tolerance by use of a tolerogen

These methods are potentially useful in the induction of prolonged desensitization to drugs, unlike those above. Chemical modification of allergens may produce a general reduction in the immune response to these agents,

or may render them simple immunogens capable of inducing the formation of harmless antibodies, akin to those occurring frequently with certain substances, for example penicillin, as mentioned previously. Four different methods are described here as examples of a multitude of approaches that may be of potential value:

1. modification of protein allergens by conjugation with certain chemicals, for example, polyethylene glycol, may render them less allergenic, that is, reaginic (IgE) antibody production may be suppressed (Lee and Sehon 1978);
2. presentation of the hapten (in the case of drugs) as a conjugate with a carrier that is recognized by T lymphocytes as 'self'. The mechanism of tolerance here is probably the reduction in the co-operation between B and T lymphocytes in the production of hapten-specific antibodies, including those capable of inducing disease. An example of such a tolerogen is penicilloyl-isologous IgG conjugate (Borel *et al.* 1976). The induction of autoallergy might be a potential risk;
3. suppression of response to allergen by presentation of the hapten in a special way, for example, as hapten-coated liposomes (Schwenk *et al.* 1978);
4. T-cell epitopes. To downregulate the immune response, vaccines containing constructs of such epitopes (in the form of peptides) derived from the known structure of common allergenic molecules are used. Such vaccines against the common inhalant allergens are now under study (Wheeler and Drachenberg 1997). In drug allergy such an approach is not yet feasible because of the lack of knowledge about the structure of the allergenic determinants of the vast majority of drugs.

All these procedures involve taking a risk that is not justifiable, except when the underlying disease is serious and no adequate replacement for the drug in question is available. In this situation every possible measure to reduce the risk of reaction should be undertaken, by giving an appropriate cover of antiallergy drugs, by careful supervision of the patient, and by having adequate resuscitation facilities for combating acute allergic reactions.

Tests with immunologically cross-reactive agents

The best illustration of the practical value of this preventive measure can be shown in the case of cross-allergenicity between penicillin and cephalosporin derivatives (Assem and Vickers 1974), and between different neuromuscular blockers (Assem 1984*a,b*).

Prophylactic antiallergy drugs

A 'strict' example of these drugs is disodium cromoglycate, which is used mainly for allergic (atopic) asthma (for mode of action see Kay 1987; Foreman and Pearce 1994). Cromoglycate has no effect when given orally and its injection into humans is not recommended. In theory, it should prevent drug-induced asthma, particularly when immediate-type allergy is the underlying mechanism. The author had no success with it, however, when it was given to patients by inhalation prior to challenge with a test-dose of the causative drug. It is hoped that more effective drugs with this action (with no limitations on route of administration), mainly preventing the release of pharmacological mediators of immediate type allergy, will be developed in due course. They would be invaluable in prevention of potentially fatal reactions.

Catecholamines, particularly those with predominant β-receptor agonist effects, have been shown to inhibit mediator release in anaphylaxis, and to inhibit the synthesis of some mediators like histamine and SRSA (leukotrienes C_4, D_4, and E_4; see review by Assem 1973).

These drugs, or other suitable preparations, may be given as a prophylactic measure in patients with suspected or established allergy undergoing hyposensitization therapy, starting the day before, or at least a few hours before drug therapy is begun, and continuing until the danger of reaction is over.

Corticosteroids may be used prophylactically to prevent a possible reaction, by administration at least 12 hours beforehand.

Prevention of allergic reactions to penicillin

Before treatment is initiated, the doctor should ask about previous penicillin therapy and previous penicillin reactions. He should also enquire about any history of other allergic disorders, such as asthma and hay fever. The incidence of penicillin allergy in patients with such disorders, which are cited as examples of an atopic constitution, is greater than in non-atopic subjects. This history of such allergies should be considered as restricting indications for penicillin treatment to cases not manageable by other antibiotics (Levine et al. 1966; Idsøe et al. 1968; Levine and Zolov 1969). Certain other diseases seem to be associated with a raised incidence of penicillin allergy, such as glandular fever in which the incidence of skin reactions to ampicillin is said to be of the order of 90 per cent. Thus it seems logical to suggest that penicillin therapy, particularly ampicillin, should be avoided if glandular fever is suspected, even if one accepts the possibility that the rash is caused by a temporary abnormality in immune response.

Treatment of drug allergy

Acute allergic reactions/anaphylactic shock

The emergency kit should include preparations of adrenaline, an antihistamine for injection, aminophylline, and hydrocortisone hemisuccinate or methylprednisolone, and a corticosteroid aerosol. Immediate reactions are best treated with adrenaline and a parenterally administered antihistamine (but see below). In severe reactions there are many aspects of treatment that are outside the scope of this review. The following is a brief account of some of the main lines of treatment.

Adrenaline

In anaphylactic reactions adrenaline BP, 0.3–1 ml of 1:1000 solution, should be given. The route of administration is decided according to whether shock (hypotension) is present or not; intramuscular or subcutaneous injection is adequate if blood pressure shows a small change (useful in laryngeal oedema and bronchospasm). A patient in shock requires immediate treatment to restore perfusion of the brain and heart, and absorption of subcutaneous or intramuscular adrenaline is unreliable in shock. Thus, if the reaction is severe (for example, a reaction during general anaesthesia, the severity being partly due to intravenous injection of the causative agent) adrenaline at a lower concentration, 1:10 000 (100 μg per ml) or less, should be given intravenously. Hypotension is treated with a bolus injection of 4–8 μg initially; repeated if necessary, with monitoring of the ECG if possible. In cardiovascular collapse 2–4 μg per min is given, and a total of 100–500 μg may be necessary. Careful titration is necessary in order to prevent ventricular dysrhythmia (which could further add to histamine-induced dysrhythmia) and myocardial ischaemia (Sullivan 1982; Horak et al. 1983). Adrenaline is useful in counteracting bradydysrhythmia (atropine is an alternative), including bradydysrhythmia induced by histamine due to atrio-ventricular conduction block). Several makes of adrenaline emergency kit are now available (Muller et al. 1995).

Intravenous volume expansion

Fluid expansion (25–50 ml per kg) with crystalloids (Ringer–lactate solution) or colloids (5% albumin, dextran, polygelatin, or cellulose derivatives) is required to replace the loss in intravascular volume (20–37 per cent may be lost suddenly in anaphylactic reactions). Bicarbonate 0.5–1 mEq per kg is given if hypotension is prolonged or acidosis (which should be watched for) is present or likely.

Aminophylline

This drug is used mainly to treat bronchospasm; giving an initial dose of 5–6 mg per kg over 20 minutes, and following with a maintenance dose of 0.9 mg per kg per hour. Isoprenaline infusion may be needed in severe, sustained bronchospasm (disadvantages: hypotension, tachyarrhythmias, and ventricular ectopics; possible advantages: reduction of pulmonary vascular resistance [if raised], positive inotropic and chronotropic effects and dromotropic [increasing conduction velocity] effects, useful in severe bradydysrhythmia).

Antihistamines

In theory, antihistamines should be of some value, though one of their limitations is that histamine is only one of the multitude of mediators of anaphylaxis. However, their practical value has not been well established, except in acute urticarial reactions. Nevertheless, it is reasonable to give 10 mg chlorpheniramine intramuscularly. Intravenous injection of antihistamines is probably best avoided because of the risk of hypotension. Chlorpheniramine is an example of a histamine H_1-antagonist; H_2-antagonists, such as cimetidine, are of no value unless combined with H_1-antagonists. In severe anaphylaxis, combined treatment with both types of antagonist is probably better than an H_1-antagonist alone, in view of the possibility of cardiac involvement in the anaphylactic reaction (see above). Persistent hypotension, not associated with bronchospasm may also be treated with the two types of antagonist combined.

Corticosteroids

Hydrocortisone hemisuccinate 0.1–1 g, or methylprednisolone (up to 2 g) may be given intravenously in severe cases.

Rationale

The effect of corticosteroids on immediate-type allergy is surrounded by much confusion. It is true that, in order to prevent a reaction, corticosteroids have to be administered in repeated doses, starting at least 12 hours before the exposure to the causative agent. It has been shown by Church and others (1972) in sensitized rats that this treatment would prevent histamine release in local anaphylaxis induced by the intraperitoneal injection of antigen. They also have a prophylactic effect in man, causing inhibition of histamine release from mast cells, for example in skin (Greaves and Plummer 1974), and from basophil leucocytes (Assem 1985). Despite the ineffectiveness of corticosteroids 'after the event', they possess the following properties, which apart from giving them the benefit of the doubt, provide a reasonable argument in favour of their use in patients with systemic reactions:

1. corticosteroids potentiate the α-effects of catecholamines, thus, to some extent, antagonizing the effect of various substances that contribute to vasodilatation, increased vascular permeability, and oedema, which is particularly dangerous when it affects the mucous membranes of the glottis and larynx;
2. they help to restore the response to catecholamines, for example, restoration of β-receptor-mediated relaxation of bronchial smooth muscle, which is believed to contribute to their usefulness in status asthmaticus;
3. their anti-inflammatory effect may help in counteracting some manifestations of allergic reactions;
4. one expects them to suppress delayed reactions;
5. they inhibit the synthesis of some mediators of immediate-type allergy, for example, histamine and prostaglandin $F_{2\alpha}$, which play a role in immediate-type allergy and possibly in other mechanisms or types of allergy.

It should be added that, since airways obstruction produced by oedema in the larynx and glottis seems to be a source of fatalities due to drug reactions, steroid aerosols may be of value.

Supportive measures

Measures for counteracting cardiovascular collapse have to be maintained until the patient is out of danger. Specific therapeutic action should be taken and, for instance, antibiotics (preferably bactericidal) be given for prevention and treatment of infection in the case of agranulocytosis. Among the specific measures, penicillinase may be mentioned as a possible therapeutic approach in immediate reactions to penicillin particularly in the case of long-acting preparations. Its value in immediate reactions, however, has been disputed (Levine 1966).

Desensitization

If no satisfactory alternative to the offending drug is found, and if there are indications that its use is essential (for example, penicillin in bacterial endocarditis), hyposensitization should be attempted. The procedure should be carried out in hospital, in an intensive care unit so that facilities for monitoring and resuscitation are at hand. Various hyposensitization regimens, including rush desensitization (which is a practical proposition), may be used in, for example, penicillin allergy (Holgate 1988). The literature contains many papers on desensitization to several other drugs (Sullivan 1994), including co-trimoxazole (Caumes *et al.* 1997 — especially in patients with HIV infection), sulphasalazine (Holdsworth 1981) and 5-aminosalicylic acid (Lachaux *et al.* 1997). It should be stressed that maintenance of hyposensitization requires maintenance of exposure to the drug; return to the sensitized state occurs rapidly after interruption, and the whole procedure has to be repeated if further drug therapy is required. In fact, basophil histamine release (see Part 2) remains unaffected by clinical desensitization (Pienkowski *et al.* 1988). These findings suggest that the temporary tolerance to the antigen is probably due to the occupation of the allergen-binding sites of the antibody by the drug itself or its metabolites. There is no agreed regimen of prophylactic medication and antiallergy cover. Treatment may include:

1. inhibitors of mediator release or synthesis;
2. the continued use of available competitive or non-competitive antagonists to the various pharmacological mediators;
3. physiological antagonists to the actions of the pharmacological mediators, for example bronchodilators, if asthma is likely to occur.

References

Abdullah, N.A. and Assem, E-S.K. (1989). Role of thromboxane A_2 and leukotriene C_4 in the antigen-induced vasoconstriction in perfused, sensitized guinea-pig kidney. *Agents Actions* 27, 150.

Ackroyd, J.F. (1964). The diagnosis of disorders of the blood due to drug hypersensitivity caused by an immune mechanism. In *Immunological Methods*, p. 453. Blackwell, Oxford.

Amos, H.E. (1979). Immunological aspects of practolol toxicity. *Int. J. Immunopharmacol.* 1, 9.

Arbesman, C.E. and Reisman, R.E. (1971). Serum sickness and anaphylaxis. In *Immunological Disease*, Vol. II (ed. M. Samter), p. 405. Little Brown, Boston.

Assem, E-S.K. (1971). Cyclic 3',5'-adenosine monophosphate and the anaphylactic response. In *Effects of Drugs on Cellular Control Mechanisms* (ed. B.R. Rabin and R.B. Freedman), p. 259. Macmillan, London.

Assem, E-S.K. (1973). Modulation by the autonomic nervous system of immune responses and allergic reactions. *Allergol. Immunopathol.* (Suppl. 1), 117.

Assem, E-S.K. (1975). Specific immunological responses to propranolol and practolol in man. *Br. J. Clin. Pharmacol.* 2, 184.

Assem, E-S.K. (1976). Immunological and non-immunological mechanisms of some of the desirable and undesirable effects of anti-inflammatory and analgesic drugs. *Agents Actions* 6, 212.

Assem, E-S.K. (1977a). Autoimmune phenomena and autoallergy in patients treated with β-adrenoceptor blocking drugs. In *Cardiovascular Drugs*, Vol. 2 β-*Adrenoceptor Blocking Drugs* (ed. G. Avery), p. 209. Adis, Sydney.

Assem, E-S.K. (1977b). Examples of the correlation between the structure of certain groups and adverse effects mediated by immune and non-immune mechanisms (with particular reference to muscle relaxants and steroid anaesthetics). In *Drug Design and Adverse Effects* (ed. H. Bundgaard, P. Juul, and H. Kofod), p. 209. Munksgaard, Copenhagen.

Assem, E-S.K. (1983a). Reactions to general and local anaesthetics. In *Allergic Reactions to Drugs* (ed. A.L. de Weck and H. Bundgaard) *Handbook of Experimental Pharmacology*, Vol. 63, p. 259. Springer-Verlag, Berlin.

Assem, E-S.K. (1983b). Reactions to neuromuscular blocking drugs. In *Allergic Reactions to Drugs* (ed. A.L. de Weck and H. Bundgaard) *Handbook of Experimental Pharmacology*, Vol. 63, p. 299. Springer-Verlag, Berlin.

Assem, E-S.K. (1984a). Characteristics of basophil histamine release by neuromuscular blocking drugs in patients with anaphylactoid reactions. *Agents Actions* 14, 435.

Assem, E-S.K (1984b). Diagnostic and predictive test procedures in patients with life-threatening anaphylactic and anaphylactoid drug reactions. *Allergol. Immunopathol.* (Madrid) 12, 61.

Assem, E-S.K. (1985). Inhibition of histamine release from basophil leucocytes of asthmatic patients treated with corticosteroids. *Agents Actions* 16, 256.

Assem, E-S.K. (1989). Drug allergy. *Curr. Opin. Immunol.* 1, 660.

Assem, E-S.K. (1990a). Naturally occurring IgG-antibody-like substance reacting with quaternary ammonium group and neuromuscular blockers: a common finding in humans and other species. *Int. Arch. Allergy Appl. Immunol.* 91, 426.

Assem, E-S.K. (1990b). Anaphylactic anaesthetic reactions: the value of paper radioallergosorbent tests for IgE antibodies to muscle relaxants and thiopentone. *Anaesthesia* 45, 1032.

Assem, E-S.K. (1992a). Highlights of controversial issues in anaesthetic reactions. In *Allergic Reactions to Anaesthetics* (ed. E-S.K. Assem). M*onogr. Allergy* 30, 1.

Assem, E-S.K. (1992b). Anaphylactoid reactions to neuromuscular blockers: Major role of IgE antibodies and possible contribution of IgE-dependent mechanisms. In *Allergic Reactions to Anaesthetics* (ed. E-S.K. Assem). *Monogr. Allergy* 30, 24.

Assem, E-S.K. (1993). Predictive value of *in vitro* tests for the IgE-dependent and the IgE-independent anaphylactoid reactions to muscle relaxants. *Ann. Fr. Anesth. Reanim.* 12, 203.

Assem, E-S.K. and Banks, R. (1973). Practolol-induced drug eruption. *Proc. R. Soc. Med.* 66, 179.

Assem, E-S.K. and Ghanem, N.S. (1988). Demonstration of IgE-sensitized mast cells in human heart and kidney. *Int. Arch. Allergy Appl. Immunol.* 87, 101.

Assem, E-S.K. and Ling, B.Y. (1988). Fatal anaphylactic reaction to suxamethonium: new screening test suggests possible prevention. *Anaesthesia* 43, 958.

Assem, E-S.K. and Schild, H.O. (1971). Antagonism by beta-adrenoceptor blockers of the antianaphylactic effect of isoprenaline. *Br. J. Pharmacol.* 42, 620.

Assem, E-S.K. and Vickers, M.R. (1974). Tests for penicillin allergy in man. II. The immunological cross-reaction between penicillins and cephalosporins. *Immunology* 27, 255.

Assem, E-S.K., Ndoping, N., Nicholson, H., *et al.* (1969). Liver damage and isoniazid allergy. *Clin. Exp. Immunol.* 5, 439.

Assem, E-S.K., Bray, K., and Dawson, P. (1983). The release of histamine from human basophils by radiological contrast agents. *Br. J. Radiol.* 56, 647.

Assem, E-S.K., Abdullah, N.A., and Ghanem. N.S. (1986). Renal histamine: release by immune stimuli. *Agents Actions* 19, 141.

Assem, E-S.K., Abdullah, N.A., and Cowie, A.G.A. (1987). Kidney mast cells, IgE and release of inflammatory mediators capable of altering renal haemodynamics. *Int. Arch. Allergy Appl. Immunol.* 84, 212.

Austen, K.F. (1997). Diseases of immediate type hypersensitivity. In *Harrison's Principles of Internal Medicine* (14th edn) (ed. A.S. Fauci, E. Braunwald, K.J. Isselbacher, *et al.*), p. 1860. McGraw-Hill, New York.

Baker, S.B. and Williams, R.T. (1963). Acute interstitial nephritis due to drug sensitivity. *BMJ* ii, 1655.

Baldo, B.A. and Fisher, M.M. (1983). Substituted ammonium ions as allergenic determinants in allergy to muscle relaxants. *Nature* (Lond.) 306, 262.

Baldo, B.A. and Harle, D.G. (1990). Drug allergenic determinants. In *Molecular Approaches to the Study of Allergens* (ed. B.A. Baldo). *Monogr. Allergy* 30, 11.

Barnes, P.J. (1989). Neural mechanisms in airway inflammation. In *Textbook of Immunopharmacology* (ed. M.M. Dale and J.C. Foreman), p. 242. Blackwell, Oxford.

Basomba, A., Pelaez, A., VillaManzo, I.G., *et al.* (1978). Allergy to penicillin unsuccessfully treated with a haptenic inhibitor (benzylpenicilloyl-N₂-formyl-lysine, BPO-Flys). A case report. *Clin. Allergy* 8, 341.

Batchelor, F.R., Dewdney, J.M., Feinberg, J.G., *et al.* (1967). A penicilloylated protein impurity as a source of allergy to benzyl-penicillin and 6-amino-penicillanic acid. *Lancet* i, 1175.

Bayard, P.J., Berger, T.G., and Jacobson, M.A. (1992). Drug hypersensitivity reactions and human immunodeficiency virus. *J. Acquir. Immune Defic. Syndr.* 5, 1237.

BCDSP (1972). Boston Collaborative Drug Surveillance Program. Excess of ampicillin rashes associated with allopurinol or hyperuricaemia. *N. Engl. J. Med.* 386, 505.

Becker, E.L. and Austen, K.F. (1968). Anaphylaxis. In *Textbook of Immunopathology*, Vol. I (ed. P.A. Meischer and H.J. Muller-Eberhard), p. 76. Grune and Stratton, London.

Becker, L., Eberlein-Konig, B., and Przybilla, B. (1996). Phototoxity of non-steroidal anti-inflammatory drugs: *in vitro* studies with visible light. *Acta Derm. Venereol.* 76, 337.

Becker, R.M. (1960). Penicillinase treatment of penicillin reactions. *Practitioner* 184, 447.

Behan, P.O., Behan, W.H.M., Zacharias, F.J., *et al.* (1976). Immunological abnormalities in patients who had the oculomucocutaneous syndrome associated with practolol therapy. *Lancet* ii, 984.

Benacerraf, B. and McDevitt, H.O. (1972). Histocompatibility-linked immune response genes. *Science* 175, 273.

Bickers, D.R. (1997). Photosensitivity and other reactions to light. in *Harrison's Principles of Internal Medicine* (14th edn) (ed. A.S. Fauci, E. Braunwald, K.J. Isselbacher, *et al.*), p. 329. McGraw-Hill, New York.

Bird, G.L.A. and Williams, R. (1992). In *Allergic Reactions to Anaesthetics* (ed. E-S.K. Assem). *Monogr. Allergy* 30, 174.

Borel, Y., Kilham, L., Hyslop, N., *et al.* (1976). Isologous IgG-induced tolerance to benzyl penicilloyl. *Nature* 261, 49.

Brimblecombe, R.W., Duncan, W.A.M., Durant, G.J., *et al.* (1975). Cimetidine — a non-thiourea H₂-receptor antagonist. *J. Int. Med. Res.* 3, 86.

Bristow, M.R., Ginsburg, R., Kantrowitz, N.E., *et al.* (1982). Coronary spasm associated with urticaria: report of a case mimicking anaphylaxis. *Clin Cardiol.* 5, 238.

Brown, P., Baddeley, H., Read, A.E., *et al.* (1974). Sclerosing peritonitis, an unusual reaction to a β-adrenergic blocking drug (practolol). *Lancet* ii, 1477.

Brown, P.J.E., Lesna, M., Hamlyn, A.N., *et al.* (1978). Primary biliary cirrhosis after long-term practolol administration. *BMJ* i, 1591.

Burke, J.A., Levi, R., Guo, Z.-G., *et al.* (1982). Leukotrienes C₄, D₄ and E₄: effects on human and guinea-pig cardiac preparation *in vitro*. *J. Pharmacol. Exp. Ther.* 221, 235.

Burke, A.P., Saenger, J., Mullick, F. *et al.* (1991). Hypersensitivity myocarditis. *Arch. Pathol. Lab. Med.* 115, 764.

Camussi, G., Aglietta, M., Malavasi, F., *et al.* (1983). The release of platelet-activating factor from human endothelial cells in culture. *J. Immunol.* 131, 2397.

Caumes, E., Guermonprez, G., Locomte C., *et al.* (1997). Efficacy and safety of desensitization with sulphamethoxazole and trimethoprim in 48 previously hypersensitive patients infected with human immunodeficiency virus. *Arch. Dermatol.* 133, 465.

Chao, P., Francis, L., and Atkins, E. (1977). The release of an endogenous pyrogen from guinea pig leukocytes *in vitro*: a new model for investigating the role of lymphocytes in fevers induced by antigens in hosts with delayed hypersensitivity. *J. Exp. Med.* 145, 1288.

Chase, M.W. (1958). Antibodies to drugs. In *Sensitivity Reactions to Drugs* (ed. M.L. Rosenheim and R. Moulton), p. 125. Blackwell, Oxford.

Church, M.K., Collier, H.O., and James, G.W. (1972). The inhibition by dexamethasone and disodium cromoglycate of anaphylactic bronchoconstriction in the rat. *Br. J. Pharmacol.* 46, 56.

Classen, D.C., Pestotnik, S.L., Evans, S.R., *et al.* (1991). Computerised surveillance of adverse drug events in hospitalised patients. *JAMA* 266, 2847.

Cluff, L.E. and Johnson, J.E. (1964). Drug fever. *Prog. Allergy* 8, 149.

Coombs, R.R.A and Gell, P.G.H. (1968). Classification of allergic reactions responsible for clinical hypersensitivity and disease. In *Clinical Aspects of Immunology* (ed. P.G.H. Gell and R.R.A. Coombs), p. 575. Blackwell, Oxford.

Cooper, J.A.D., White D.A., and Matthay R.A. (1986). Drug-induced pulmonary disease. Part 2: Noncytotoxic drugs. *Am. Rev. Respir. Dis.* 133, 488.

Dekker, J.W., Nizanokowska, E., Schmitz-Schumann, M., *et al.* (1997). Aspirin-induced asthma and HLA-DRB1 and HLA-DPB1 prototypes. *Clin. Exp. Allergy* 27, 574.

Delage, C. and Irey, M.S. (1972). Anaphylactic deaths: a clinico-pathologic study of 43 cases. *J. Forensic Sci.* 17, 525.

de Weck, A.L. (1977). Immunological aspects of allergic reactions to drugs. In *Drug Design and Adverse Reactions* (ed. H. Bundgaard, P. Juul, and H. Tofod) Alfred Benzon Symposium X, p. 141. Munksgaard, Copenhagen.

de Weck, A.L. (1996). The European Network for Detecting and Monitoring of Drug Allergies (ENDA). *Allergy and Clinical Immunology International* 8, 105.

de Weck, A.L., Schneider, C.H., Spengler, H., *et al.* (1973). Inhibition of allergic reactions by monovalent haptens. In *Mechanisms in Allergy: Reagin-mediated Hypersensitivity* (ed. L. Goodfriend, A.H. Sehon and R.P. Orange), p. 323. Dekker, New York.

Dewdney, J.M., Maes, L., Raynaud, J.P., *et al.* (1991). Risk assessment of antibiotic residues of beta-lactams and macrolides in food products with regard to their immuno-allergic potential. *Food Chem. Toxicol.* 29, 477.

Didier, A., Cador, D., Bongrand, P., *et al.* (1987). Role of the quaternary ammonium ion determinant in allergy to muscle relaxants. *J. Allergy Clin. Immunol.* 79, 578.

Dinarello, C.A. (1984). Interleukin-1. *Rev. Infect. Dis.* 6, 51.

Dinarello, C.A. (1989). Interleukin-1. In *Textbook of Immunopharmacology* (2nd edn) (ed. M.M. Dale and J.C. Foreman). Blackwell, Oxford.

Dinarello, C.A. and Wolff, S.M. (1978). Pathogenesis of fever in man. *N. Engl. J. Med.* 298, 607.

Dinarello, C.A. and Wolff, S.M. (1982). Molecular basis of fever in humans. *Am. J. Med.* 72, 800.

Dundee, J.W. (1986). Adverse reactions to drugs and anaesthetists. *Anaesthesia*, 41, 351.

Eisen, H.N. (1959). Hypersensitivity to simple chemicals. In *Cellular and Humoral Aspects of the Hypersensitivity States* (ed. H.S. Lawrence), p. 89. Holber-Harper, New York.

Ezeamuzie, I.C. and Assem, E-S.K. (1983a). A study of histamine release from human basophils and lung mast cells by products of lymphocyte stimulation. *Agents Actions* 13, 222.

Ezeamuzie, I.C. and Assem, E.-S.K. (1983b). Effects of leukotrienes C₄ and D₄ on guinea-pig heart and the participation of SRS-A in the manifestations of guinea-pig cardiac anaphylaxis. *Agents Actions* 13, 182.

Ezeamuzie, I.C. and Assem, E-S.K. (1985). Release of slow reacting substance (SRS) from human leucocytes by lymphokine. *Int. J. Immunopharmacol.* 7, 533.

Farr, M.J., Wingate, J.P., and Shaw, J.N. (1975). Practolol and the nephrotic syndrome. *BMJ* ii, 68.

Fletcher, A.P. (1991). Spontaneous adverse drug reaction reporting vs. event monitoring: a comparison. *J.R. Soc. Med.* 84, 341.

Foreman, J.C. (1994). Pyrogenesis. In *Textbook of Immunopharmacology* 3rd edn (ed. M.M. Dale, J.C. Foreman, and T-P.D. Fan), p. 242. Blackwell, Oxford.

Foreman, J.C. and Pearce, F.L. (1994). The anti-allergic drugs. In *Textbook of Immunopharmacology* 3rd edn (ed. M.M. Dale, J.C. Foreman, and T-P.D. Fan), p. 288. Blackwell, Oxford.

Galli, S.J. and Wershil, B.K. (1996). The two faces of the mast cell. *Nature* 381, 21.

Garty, B.Z., Offer, I., Livni, E. *et al.* (1994). Erythema multiforme and hypersensitivity myocarditis caused by ampicillin. *Ann. Pharmacother.* 28,730.

Gell, P.G.H., Harington, C.R., and Michel, R. (1948). Antigenic function of simple chemical compounds: correlation of antigenicity with chemical reactivity. *Br. J. Exp. Pathol.* 29, 578.

Genovese, A., Stellato, C., Marsella, C.V., *et al.* (1996). Role of mast cells, basophils and their mediators in adverse reactions to general anaesthetics and radiocontrast media. *Int. Arch. Allergy Appl. Immunol.* 110, 13.

Ghanem, N.S., Assem, E-S.K., Leung, K.B.P., *et al.* (1988a). Guinea pig mast cells: comparative study of morphology, fixation and staining properties. *Int. Arch. Allergy Appl. Immunol.* 85, 351.

Ghanem, N.S., Assem, E-S.K., Leung, K.B.P., *et al.* (1988b). Cardiac and renal mast cells: morphology, distribution, fixation and staining properties in the guinea pig and preliminary comparison with human. *Agents Actions* 23, 123.

Greaves, M.W. and Plummer, V.M. (1974). Glucocorticoid inhibition of antigen-evoked histamine release from human skin. *Immunology* 27, 359.

Griffin, J.P. (1986). Drug induced allergic, hypersensitivity reactions. In *Iatrogenic Diseases* (3rd edn) (ed. P. D'Arcy and J.P. Griffin), p. 82. Oxford Medical Publications, Oxford.

Harle, D.G., Baldo, B.A., and Fisher, M.M. (1984). Detection of IgE antibodies to suxamethonium after anaphylactoid reactions during anaesthesia. *Lancet* i, 121.

Harpey, J.P., Caille, B., Moulias, R., *et al.* (1972). Drug allergy, and lupus-like syndrome (with special reference to penicillamine). In *Mechanisms in Drug Allergy* (ed. C.H. Dash and H.E.H. Jones), p. 51. Churchill Livingstone, Edinburgh.

Hertl, M., Jugert, F., and Merk, H.G. (1995). CD8+ dermal T cells from a sulphamethoxazole-induced bullous exanthem proliferate in response to drug-modified microsomes. *Br. J. Dermatol.* 132, 215.

Hirsh, S.A. (1982). Acute allergic reaction with coronary vasospasm. *Am. Heart J.* 10, 928.

Hoffbrand, B.I., Fry, W., and Bunton, G.L. (1974). Cholestatic jaundice due to methyldopa. *BMJ* iii, 559.

Holdsworth, C.D.(1981). Sulphasalazine desensitisation. *BMJ* 282, 110.

Holgate, S.T. (1988). Penicillin allergy: how to diagnose and when to treat. *BMJ* 296, 1213.

Holley, H.L. (1964). Drugs and the lupus diathesis. *J. Chron. Dis.* 1, 17.

Horak, A., Raine, R., Opie, L.H., *et al.* (1983). Severe myocardial ischaemia induced by intravenous adrenaline. *BMJ* 286, 519.

Hurwitz, N. (1969). Predisposing factors in adverse reactions to drugs. *BMJ* i, 536.

Idsøe, O., Guthe, T., Wilcox, R.R., *et al.* (1968). Nature and extent of penicillin side effects with particular reference to fatalities from anaphylactic shock. *Bull. WHO*, 38, 159.

Isacson, E.P. (1967). Myxoviruses and autoimmunity. *Prog. Allergy* 10, 256.

Ishizaka, T., Soto, C.S., and Ishizaka, K. (1973). Mechanisms of passive sensitization. III. Number of IgE molecules and their receptor sites on human basophil granulocytes. *J. Immunol.* 3, 500.

Jensen, H.A., Mikkelsen, H.I., Wadskov, S., *et al.* (1976). Cutaneous reactions to propranolol (Inderal). *Acta Med. Scand.* 199, 363.

Kaplan, A.P., Haak-Frendscho, M., Fauci, A., *et al.* (1985). A histamine releasing factor from activated mononuclear cells. *J. Immunol.* 135, 2027.

Kay, A.B. (1987). The mode of action of anti-allergic drugs. *Clinical Allergy* 17, 153.

Kind, L.S. (1958). The altered reactivity of mice after inoculation with *Bordetella pertussis* vaccine. *Bacteriol. Rev.* 22, 173.

Knudsen, E.T. (1969). Ampicillin and urticaria. *BMJ* i, 846.

Knudsen, E.T., Robinson, O.P.W., Croydon, E.A.P., *et al.* (1967). Cutaneous sensitivity to purified benzylpenicillin. *Lancet* i, 1184.

Knudsen, E.T., Dewdney, J.M., and Trafford, J.A.P. (1970). Reduction in incidence of ampicillin rash by purified ampicillin. *BMJ* i, 469.

Kraske, G.K., Shinaberger, J., and Klaustermeyer, V.B. (1997). Severe hypersensitivity reaction during hemodialysis. *Ann. Allergy Asthma Immunol.* 78, 21.

Lachaux, A., Leall, C., Duclaux, L.I., *et al.* (1997). Hypersensitivity to 5-aminosalicylic acid. Value of desensitization by oral route. *Arch. Pediatr.* 4, 144.

Lakshmanan, M.C., Hershey, C.O., and Breslau, D. (1986). Hospital admissions caused by iatrogenic disease. *Arch. Intern. Med*, 146, 1931.

Landsteiner, K. (1945). *The Specificity of Serological Reactions* (revised edn). Harvard University Press, Cambridge, Mass.

Laurence, D.R. and Bennett, P.N. (1992). Unwanted effects of drugs: adverse reactions. In *Clinical Pharmacology* (7th edn), p. 117. Churchill Livingstone, Edinburgh.

Lawley, T.J. and Kubota, Y. (1990). Vasculitis. *Dermatol. Clin.* 8, 681.

Lee, W.Y. and Sehon, A.H. (1978). Suppression of reaginic antibodies with modified allergens. I. Reduction in allergenicity of protein allergen by conjugation to polyethylene glycol. *Int. Arch. Allergy Appl. Immunol.* 56, 159.

Levi, R., Malm, J., Bowman, F.A., *et al.* (1981). The arrhythmogenic actions of histamine on human atrial fibres. *Circ. Res.* 49, 625.

Levi, R., Burke, J.A., Guo Z.-G., *et al.* (1984). Acetylglyceryl ether phosphorylcholine (AGEPC). A putative mediator of cardiac anaphylaxis in the guinea-pig. *Circ. Res.* 54, 117.

Levine, B.B. (1966). Immunochemical mechanisms of penicillin allergy. A haptenic model system for the study of allergic diseases of man. *N. Engl. J. Med.* 275, 1115.

Levine, B.B. and Zolov, D.M. (1969). Prediction of penicillin allergy by immunological tests. *J. Allergy* 43, 231.

Levine, B.B. and Vaz, N.M. (1970). Effect of combinations of inbred strain, antigen, and antigen dose on immune responsiveness and reagin production in the mouse. A potential mouse model for immune aspects of human atopic allergy. *Int. Arch. Allergy Appl. Immunol.* 39, 156.

Levine, B.B., Redmond, A.P., Fellner, M.J., *et al.* (1966). Penicillin allergy and the heterogeneous immune responses of many to benzylpenicillin. *J. Clin. Invest.* 45, 1895.

Lin, R.Y. (1992). A perspective on penicillin allergy. *Arch. Intern. Med.* 152, 930.

Lingstrom, K-G., Renck, H., Hedin, H., *et al.* (1988). Hapten inhibition and dextran anaphylaxis. *Anaesthesia* 43, 729.

Littlejohns, D.W., Assem, E-S.K., and Kennedy, C.T.C. (1973). Immunological evidence for two forms of allergy to pyrazolone drugs. *Rheumatol. Phys. Med.* 12, 57.

Lowley, T.J. and Frank, M.M. (1988). Immune complexes and allergic disease. In *Allergy. Principles and Practice* (ed. E. Middleton, C. Reed, E.F. Ellis, *et al.*). Mosby, St Louis.

McDevitt, H.O. and Benacerraf, B. (1969). Genetic control of specific immune responsiveness. *Adv. Immunol.* 11, 31.

McDevitt, H.O. and Bodmer, W.F. (1972). Histocompatibility antigens, immune responsiveness and susceptibility to disease. *Am. J. Med.* 52, 1.

MacKay, A.D. and Axford, A.T. (1976). Pleural effusions after practolol. *Lancet* i, 89.

McKendrick, M.W. and Geddes, A.M. (1979). Allopurinol hypersensitivity. *BMJ* i, 988.

Mann, M.R. (1961). The pharmacology of contrast media. *Proc. R. Soc. Med.* 54, 473.

Marone, G., Triggiani, M., Cirillo, R., *et al.* (1986). IgE-mediated activation of human heart *in vitro*. *Agents Actions* 18, 194.

Marone, G., de Crescenzo, G., Adt, M., *et al.* (1995). Immunological characterization and functional importance of human heart mast cells. *Immunopharmacology* 31, 1.

Marsh, D.G., Bias, W.B., Hsu, S.H., *et al.* (1973). Association between major histocompatibility (HLA) antigens and specific reaginic antibody responses in allergic man. In *Mechanisms in Allergy: Reagin-mediated Hypersensitivity* (ed. L. Goodfriend, A.H. Sehon, and R.P. Orange), p. 113. Dekker, New York.

Marshall, A.J., Barrit, D.W., Griffiths, D.A., *et al.* (1977). Respiratory disease associated with practolol therapy. *Lancet* ii, 1254.

Miyauchi, H., Hosokawa, H., Akaeda, T., *et al.* (1991). T-cell subsets in drug-induced toxic epidermal necrolysis. *Arch. Dermatol.* 127, 815.

Moeschlin, S. (1958). Agranulocytosis due to sensitivity to drugs. In *Sensitivity Reactions to Drugs* (ed. M.L. Rosenheim and R. Moulton), p. 77. Blackwell, Oxford.

Moeschlin, S. and Wagner, K. (1952). Agranulocytosis due to occurrence of leucocyte agglutinins. *Acta Haematol.* 8, 29.

Moneret-Vautrin, D.A., Gueant, J.L., Kamel, L., *et al.* (1988a). Anaphylaxis to myorelaxants: cross-sensitivity studied by radioimmunoassays compared to intradermal tests in 34 cases. *J. Allergy Clin. Immunol.* 82, 745.

Moneret-Vautrin, D.A., Laxenaire, M.C., Gueant, J.L., *et al.* (1988b). Predictive tests of the re-use of a myorelaxant, in case of anaphylaxis to myorelaxants. *N. Engl. Reg. Allergy Proc.* 9, 254.

Moneret-Vautrin, D.A., Motin, J., Mata, E., *et al.* (1993). Preventing muscle relaxant anaphylaxis. *Ann. Fr. Anesth. Reanim.* 12, 190.

Morrow, J.D., Schroeder, H.A., and Perry, H.M. Jr (1953). Studies on the control of hypertension by hyphex; toxic reactions and side effects. *Circulation* 8, 829.

Muller, U., Mosbech, H., Aberer, H., *et al.* (1995). Adrenaline for emergency kits. *Allergy* 50, 783.

Munoz, J. (1964). Effect of bacteria and bacterial products on antibody response. *Adv. Immunol.* 4, 397.

Nimmo, W.S. (1988). Reporting adverse reactions to anaesthetic drugs: a new way forward. *Anaesthesia* 43, 627.

Parker, C.W. (1965). Drug reactions. In *Immunological Diseases* (ed. M. Samter and H.L. Alexander), p. 663. Little Brown, Boston.

Parker, C.W. (1980). Drug allergy. In *Clinical Immunology* (ed. C.W. Parker), p. 1372. Saunders, Philadelphia.

Parker, C.W. (1982). Allergic reactions in man. *Pharmacol. Rev.* 34, 85.

Patella, V., Marino, I., Lamparter, B., *et al.* (1995). Human heart mast cells. Isolation, purification, ultrastructure, and immunologic characterization. *J. Immunol.* 154, 2855.

Paton, W.D.M. (1957). Histamine release by compounds of simple chemical structure. *Pharmacol. Rev.* 9, 269.

Perry, H.M., Tan, E.M., Carmody, S., *et al.* (1970). Relationship of acetyl transference activity to antinuclear antibodies and toxic symptoms in hypertensive patients treated with hydralazine. *J. Lab. Clin. Med.* 76, 114.

Pienkowski, M.M., Kazmier, W.J., and Adkinson, N.F. (1988). Basophil histamine release remains unaffected by clinical desensitization. *J. Allergy Clin. Immunol.* 82, 171.

Porri, F., Pradal, M., Rud, C., *et al.* (1995). Is systematic preoperative screening for muscle relaxant and latex allergy advisable? *Allergy* 50, 374.

Pumphrey, R.S.H. and Stanworth, S.J. (1996). The clinical spectrum of anaphylaxis in northwest England. *Clin. Exp. Allergy* 26, 1364.

Quiralte, J., Blanco, C., Castillo, R., *et al.* (1997). Anaphylactoid reactions due to nonsteroidal antiinflammatory drugs: clinical and cross-reactivity studies. *Ann. Allergy Asthma Immunol.* 78, 293.

Raffel, S. (1973). Hapten-induced anaphylactic reactions. In *Mechanisms in Allergy: Reagin-mediated Hypersensitivity* (ed. L. Goodfriend, A.H. Sehon, and R.P. Orange), p. 313. Dekker, New York.

Raftery, E.B. and Denman, A.M. (1973). Systemic lupus erythematosus induced by practolol. *BMJ* ii, 452.

Razin, E., Pecht, I., and Rivera, J. (1995). Signal transduction in the activation of mast cells and basophils. *Immunology Today* 16, 370.

Reid, M.S., Imray, J.M., and Noble, D.W. (1992). Anaesthetic allergy and prospective radioallergosorbent testing. In *Allergic Reactions to Anaesthetics* (ed. E-S.K. Assem). *Monogr. Allergy* 30, 162.

Remmel, H. and Schuppel, R. (1972). The formation of antigenic determinants. In *Hypersensitivity to Drugs*, Vol. 1 (ed. M. Samter and C.W. Parker), p. 67. Pergamon, Oxford.

Rich, A.R. (1958). Tissue reactions produced by sensitivity to drugs. In *Sensitivity Reactions to Drugs* (ed. M.L. Rosenheim and R. Moulton), p. 196. Blackwell, Oxford.

Rieder, M.J., Sear, N.H., Kanee, A., *et al.* (1991). Prominence of slow acetylator phenotype among patients with sulfonamide hypersensitivity reactions. *Clin. Pharmacol. Ther.* 49, 13.

Riley, R.J. and Leeder, J.S. (1995). *In vitro* analysis of metabolic predisposition to drug hypersensitivity reactions. *Clin. Exp. Immunol.* 99, 1.

Roberts, J.A. (1992). Allergic reactions to anaesthetics: Economic aspects of pre-operative screening. In *Allergic Reactions to Anaesthetics* (ed. E-S.K. Assem). *Monogr. Allergy* 30, 207.

Roujeau, J.C. and Stern, R.S. (1994). Severe adverse cutaneous reactions to drugs. *N. Engl. J. Med.* 331, 1272.

Rubin, L.E. and Levi, R. (1995). Protective role of bradykinin in cardiac anaphylaxis. Coronary-vasodilating and anti-arrhythmic activities mediated by autocrine/paracrine mechanisms. *Circ. Res.* 76, 434.

Salama, A., Santoso, S., and Mueller-Eckhardt, C. (1991). Antigenic determinants for the reactions of drug-dependent antibodies with blood cells. *Br. J. Haematol.* 78, 535.

Saltzstein, S.L. and Ackerman, L.V. (1959). Lymphadenopathy induced by anticonvulsant drugs and mimicking clinically and pathologically malignant lymphomas. *Cancer* 12, 164.

Samter, M. and Berryman, G.H. (1964). Drug allergy. *Ann. Rev. Pharmacol.* 4, 265.

Schwenk, R., Lee, W.Y., and Sehon, A.H. (1978). Specific suppression of anti-hapten reaginic antibody titers with hapten-coated liposomes. *J. Immunol.* 120, 1612.

Shulman, N.R. (1963). Mechanisms of blood-cell destruction in individuals sensitized to foreign antigens and its implications in autoimmunity. *Trans. Am. Assoc. Physicians* 76, 72.

Shulman, N.R. (1964). A mechanism of cell destruction in individuals sensitized to foreign antigens and its implications in autoimmunity. *Ann. Intern. Med.* 60, 506.

Simmonds, J., Hodges, S., Nicol, F., *et al.* (1978). Anaphylaxis after oral penicillin. *BMJ* ii, 1404.

Smith, J.W., Johnson, J.E., and Leighton, E.C. (1966). Studies on the epidemiology of adverse drug reactions. II. An evaluation of penicillin allergy. *N. Engl. J. Med.* 274, 998.

Spielberg, S.P. (1996). Pharmacogenetics and blood dyscrasias. *Eur. J. Haematol.* Suppl. 60, 93.

Stanworth, D.R. (ed.) (1973). Structural basis of reagin activity. In *Immediate Hypersensitivity*, p. 212. North-Holland, Amsterdam.

Stevenson, D.D., Hankammer, M.A., Mathison, D.A., *et al.* (1996). Aspirin desensitization treatment of aspirin-sensitive patients with rhinosinusitis-asthma: long-term outcomes. *J. Allergy Clin. Immunol.* 98, 751.

Stewart, G.T. (1967). Allergenic residues in penicillin. *Lancet* i, 1177.

Sullivan, T.J. (1982). Cardiac disorders in penicillin induced anaphylaxis: association with intravenous therapy. *JAMA*, 248, 2161.

Sullivan, T.J. (1994). Antigen-specific desensitization to prevent allergic reaction to drugs. *Ann. Allergy* 73, 375.

Sullivan, T.J., Wedner, H.J., Shatz, G.S., *et al.* (1981). Skin testing to detect penicillin allergy. *J. Allergy Clin. Immunol.* 68, 171.

Sutherland, E.W. and Robison, G.A. (1966). The role of cyclic 3′,5′-AMP in responses to catecholamines and other hormones. *Pharmacol. Rev.* 18, 145.

Sutton, B.J. and Gould, H.J. (1993). The human IgE network. *Nature* 366, 421.

Symmers, W.St.C. (1962). The occurrence of angiitis and other generalized diseases of connective tissues as a consequence of the administration of drugs. Symposium on drug sensitization. *Proc. R. Soc. Med.* 55, 20.

Szczeklik, A. (1983). Analgesics and non-steroidal anti-inflammatory drugs. In *Allergic Reactions to Drugs* (ed. A. de Weck and H. Bundgaard), p. 277. Springer-Verlag, Berlin.

Szczeklik, A. (1997). Mechanism of aspirin-induced asthma. *Allergy* 52, 613.

Szentivanyi, A. (1969). The beta adrenergic theory of the atopic abnormality in bronchial asthma. *J. Allergy* 42, 203.

Toghill, P.J., Smith, P.G., Benton, P., *et al.* (1974). Methyldopa liver damage. *BMJ* iii, 545.

Umetsu, D.T. and Dekruyff, H. (1997). Th1 and Th2 CD4+ cells in the pathogenesis of allergic disease. *Proc. Soc. Exp. Biol.* 215, 11.

van der Klaauw, M.M., Wilson, J.H.P., and Stricker, B.H.Ch. (1996). Drug-associated anaphylaxis: 20 years of reporting in the Netherlands (1974–1994) and review of the literature. *Clin. Exp. Allergy* 26, 1355.

van Wijk, G., de Groot, H., and Bogaard, J.M. (1995). Case report: Drug-dependent exercise-induced anaphylaxis. *Allergy* 50, 992.

Vaswani, S.K., Plack, R.H., and Norman, P.S. (1996). Acute severe urticaria and angioedema leading to myocardial infarction. *Ann. Allergy Asthma Immunol.* 77, 101.

Vervloet, D., Nizankoweska, E., Arnaud, A., *et al.* (1983). Adverse reactions to suxamethonium and other muscle relaxants under general anaesthesia. *J. Allergy Clin. Immunol.* 71, 552.

Warkentin, T.E. (1996). Heparin-induced thrombocytopenia: IgG-mediated platelet activation, platelet microparticle generation, and altered procoagulant/anticoagulant balance in the pathogenesis of thrombosis and venous limb gangrene complicating heparin-induced thrombocytopenia. *Transfus. Med. Rev.* 10, 249.

Watkins, J. (1979). Anaphylactoid reactions to intravenous substances. *Br. J. Anaesth.* 51, 51.

Watkins, J. and Ward, A.M. (eds) (1978). *Adverse Response to Intravenous Drugs.* Academic Press, London.

Welsh, K.I. and Batchelor, J.R. (1981). HLA and drug reactions. In *Drug Reactions and the Liver* (ed. M. Davis, J.M. Tredger, and R. Williams), p. 111. Pitman Medical, London.

Wendel, G.D., Stark, B.J., Jamison, R.J., *et al.* (1985). Penicillin allergy and desensitization in serious infections during pregnancy. *N. Engl. J. Med.* 312, 1229.

Wheeler, A.W. and Drachenberg, K-J. (1997). New routes and formulations for allergen-specific immunotherapy. *Allergy* 52, 602.

Wiles, C.M., Assem, E-S.K., Cohen, S.L. *et al.* (1979). Cephradine-induced interstitial nephritis. *Clin. Exp. Immunol.* 36, 342.

Woosley, R.L., Drayer, D.E., Reidenberg, M.M., *et al.* (1978). Effect of acetylator phenotype on the rate at which procainamide induces antinuclear antibodies and the lupus syndrome. *N. Engl. J. Med.* 298, 1157.

Wright, P. (1975). Untoward effects associated with practolol administration: oculomucocutaneous syndrome. *BMJ* i, 595.

Youngman, P.R., Taylor, K.M., and Wilson, J.D. (1983). Anaphylactoid reactions to neuromuscular agents: a commonly undiagnosed condition? *Lancet* ii, 597.

Zhou, W. and Moore, D.E. (1997). Photosensitizing activity of the anti-bacterial drugs sulfamethoxazole and trimethoprim. *J. Photochem. Photobiol. B.* 39, 63.

Zimmerman, H.J. and Ishak, K.G. (1995). General aspects of drug-induced liver disease. *Gastroenterol. Clin. North Am.* 24, 739.

27. Part 2 Tests for detecting drug allergy

Introduction

Before the diagnosis of an allergic drug reaction can be made, several problems have to be solved. First, one has to seek evidence of a drug reaction and to distinguish it from coincidental disease (the disease for which treatment is being given or a complication thereof, or other diseases that may be present or develop). Secondly, identification of the culprit(s) in the case of multiple therapy: this is the most frequent and difficult problem. Thirdly, allergy must be distinguished from other unwanted drug effects. Proper medical history taking, clinical findings, and investigations (proper tests) all help to achieve these goals. Identification of the drug responsible for the reaction is important for obvious reasons.

Testing for drug allergy is complicated. The second and third steps listed above, which will be discussed in detail, are largely due to: (a) the diversity of immune reactions and the problem of finding an appropriate *in vivo* test or, more importantly, an *in vitro* correlate; (b) the fact that an allergic drug reaction may be due to the drug, to any of a wide variety of degradation products (often arising *in vivo* and occasionally *in vitro*), or to impurities introduced during the preparation and storage. The possibility of immunological cross-reactions with other drugs should also be kept in mind; and (c) the lack of proper testing material, leading to false-negative results, represents one of the major limitations to the reliability of the testing procedures. Alternatively, even when positive (e.g. a wheal-and-flare response in a positive direct skin test or *in vitro* leucocyte histamine release), these tests may not necessarily indicate an allergy, since such changes may be induced in other ways, as will be explained later.

As might be expected, allergies and 'pseudoallergies' to certain drugs have been more widely investigated than others, for example, antibiotics, particularly β-lactams and co-trimoxazole, anaesthetics (general and local), analgesics, NSAID, and iodinated radio-contrast media. Consequently, in the discussion of the various investigations that follows, reference will be made mainly to these drugs.

The list of possible investigations in patients with suspected drug allergy is shown in Table 27.3. (Patch tests for investigating contact dermatitis are described in Chapter 19.)

Skin tests

Despite modern technology and the availability of alternative test procedures, including the *in vitro* tests to be described, skin testing is still widely used for the diagnosis of allergy (e.g. immediate-type allergy in asthma and hay fever). In the latter examples the matter is relatively straightforward, and the risk of testing, particularly by the prick-in method, is minimal.

Prick-in and intradermal tests

With few exceptions, in our own experience prick-in tests (with the unmodified drug) in drug allergy are comletely unreliable, and intradermal tests are used, despite a definite risk. Unlike intradermal tests for inhalant allergies, intradermal tests for drug allergy are not very reliable, even when an apparently appropriate antigen is used. This has been clearly shown by our studies in penicillin allergy (Assem and Vickers 1974a, 1975), in which skin-test false-negatives were frequently encountered.

False-positives (to intradermal testing) are of particular importance with certain drugs, for example, NMB and narcotic analgesics, particularly when high concentrations of these drugs are used (Assem 1984a, 1991; also see discussion of Routine skin testing). They are more common in this type of skin test than they are in the prick/scratch test. However, prick tests with NMB may give false-negatives, particularly with low drug concentrations (Farrell *et al.* 1988; Assem and Symons 1989; Assem 1990b, 1991).

Patch tests (McGillis *et al.* 1989; Calkin and Maibach 1993) may be used in testing for reactions other than

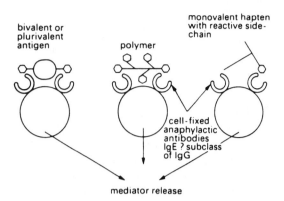

Fig. 27.4
Activation of the anaphylactic mechanism in drug allergy

TABLE 27.3
Possible investigations in patients with drug allergy

In vivo

1. Skin tests:
   (a) direct skin test;
   (b) Prausnitz–Küstner reaction.
2. Other challenge tests.

In vitro

Specific allergy tests

1. Serological studies:
   (a) detection of antibodies against different haptenic determinants;
   (b) identification of antibody classes (IgG, IgM, IgA, IgD, IgE), and subclasses (particularly of IgG_4); radioallergosorbent test for IgE antibodies*
2. Detection of tissue-sensitizing antibodies (and allergen-induced mediator release, e.g. histamine, from sensitized tissue/cells):
   (a) in serum, by passive sensitization;
   (b) cell-bound, by direct allergen challenge, e.g. leucocyte (basophil) histamine release
3. Detection of delayed-type hypersensitivity (cell-mediated immunity):
   (a) the lymphocyte transformation tests;
   (b) the macrophage migration inhibition test.
4. Other tests for antibody- or cell-mediated immunity, e.g. rosette formation by antigen-coated red cells around sensitized basophil leucocytes or lymphocytes.
5. Detection of immune complexes containing the specific hapten.

Non-specific tests for allergy

1. Total serum IgE, total leucocyte-bound IgE.
2. Indirect methods for detecting drug-specific antibodies by co-precipitation procedures, using radioisotope-labelled or unlabelled drugs:
   (a) measurement of binding to the globulin fraction of serum, using ammonium sulphate for precipitation of that fraction;
   (b) measurement of binding to serum immunoglobulins, using anti-human immunoglobulin serum for their precipitation.
3. Tests for autoantibodies, lupus erythematous cells, eosinophil count, etc.

Confirmation of anaphylactic or anaphylactoid reaction in plasma/serum:

   (a) histamine/methylhistamine;
   (b) eosinophil cationic protein;
   (c) tryptase

---

* most important

immediate-type allergy, particularly in delayed-type hypersensitivity and with agents that are capable of inducing contact dermatitis (such as local anaesthetics, Assem and Moorthy 1988).

Factors influencing the value of skin tests (with special reference to penicillin allergy)

Of all the drug allergies, penicillin allergy has been the most widely investigated; it has also been one of the most important. Therefore, we have chosen it as a model for the evaluation of skin tests as well as *in vitro* tests in drug allergy as a whole. This topic will be discussed at length here in order to elucidate several important points which are encountered in any drug allergy. The special importance of penicillin allergy and its medicolegal aspects are further discussed later in this chapter.

The importance of the testing material

The possible structural features of allergens capable of eliciting an anaphylactic reaction are shown in Fig. 27.4. There have been several reports confirming the importance of skin test material in establishing the diagnosis of penicillin allergy and predicting cases that are likely to develop anaphylactic reactions (Finke *et al.* 1965; Siegel and Levine 1965; Bierman and van Arsdel 1969; Levine and Zolov 1969).

Levine and colleagues (1967) carried out a long-term prospective study of the predictive value of immediate skin tests in 218 patients with a history of penicillin allergy. Skin tests were carried out with both benzyl-penicilloyl-polylysine and the 'minor determinants' mixture (which includes benzylpenicillin and sodium benzylpenicilloate) to determine the benzylpenicilloyl specificity and the minor haptenic determinant specificity, respectively. Positive results were obtained in only 15 per cent when the two preparations of test material were used. Penicillin alone gave a positive result in less than five per cent. These results were obtained in patients with a past history of penicillin allergy, and the incidence of positive skin tests in patients without such a history was much smaller. These results have an important bearing on the practicability of routine skin testing, which will be discussed later.

The carrier effect

It is generally believed that in order to induce an allergic response to any simple chemical such as penicillin, the drug itself or, more commonly, its metabolites must first combine, irreversibly with some large carrier molecule, such as a protein. It is therefore important to know whether the antibodies formed are specific also towards the carrier protein molecule. Levine (1962, 1963) showed that when rabbits and guinea-pigs are immunized with a benzylpenicilloyl–protein conjugate then the antibodies formed are adapted to the entire benzylpenicilloyl group, the lysine side chain, and to some adjoining structures of the immunizing carrier protein. The identification of the protein with which penicillin or its metabolites combines *in vivo* would be extremely useful since it could lead to the preparation of the correct complete antigen for use in *in vitro* diagnostic tests.

Levine and Price (1964) compared penicilloyl-polylysine (BPO:PL), penicilloyl human serum albumin (BPO:HSA), and penicilloyl human γ-globulin (BPO: HGG) as elicitors of the wheal and flare reaction in patients with a past history of penicillin allergy. They found that BPO:PL was more effective than BPO:HSA and BPO:HGG. This is probably due to the open structure of polylysine, which allows more contact between benzylpenicilloyl groups and the large antibenzylpenicilloyl combining sites than would be allowed by the more rigid structural configuration of the benzylpenicilloyl-protein conjugates.

Vickers and Assem (1974) used benzylpenicilloyl conjugates with PL, HSA, HGG, bovine serum albumin (BSA), and bovine γ-globulin (BGG), the first three being evaluated in skin tests. BPO:HSA gave positive skin tests in a slightly higher proportion of patients (seven out of 14) than with either benzylpenicillin (five out of 14) or BPO:PL (five out of 14).

Role of different haptenic determinants

As mentioned before, in allergy to any particular drug a variety of haptenic determinants are involved. The profile of sensitization to these determinants varies in different patients; hence it is important to use appropriate preparations of these determinants for allergy testing.

Skin tests in penicillin allergy with conjugates of some of the minor determinants and comparison with penicilloyl conjugate

Assem and Vickers (1975) carried out a study to assess the value of skin tests with antigens prepared from the major haptenic determinant, the benzylpenicilloyl group, and two minor determinants, the benzylpenicillenate and penicillamine groups, using human serum albumin as a carrier in all conjugates, and comparing the results with those obtained with benzylpenicillin. This study included 22 patients with established penicillin allergy; among them were the 14 patients used for the study of the previously mentioned 'carrier' effect.

No positive skin responses were obtained for any determinant in 10 control subjects. Of the 22 patients allergic to penicillin tested, 10 responded to the benzylpenicilloyl group, eight to benzylpenicillenate, and 10 to penicillamine. The BPO responses were generally greater than the benzylpenicillenate responses, and four patients responded to the benzylpenicilloyl group in the absence of a response to penicillenate and penicillamine.

Limitations

Availability of proper testing material to the non-specialist

The unmodified penicillin is the only testing material that is readily available to the doctor who is not a specialist in allergy, and even the latter may not have the proper facilities and material to detect penicillin allergy. Although penicilloyl-polylysine and minor determinant mixtures are commercially available (e.g. from the German firm Allergopharm Joachim Ganzer KG), they are used only by specialists and its wide use is inadvisable and impracticable. This imposes a great limitation on the value of skin tests as carried out in general practice. The risk involved in skin tests will be discussed later.

Other limitations of skin tests

Though the antibodies that mediate immediate-type hypersensitivity are skin-sensitizing antibodies, that is, they become 'fixed' to skin, and therefore can be detected by applying the test antigen to skin, it is still possible that other types of antibodies or subtypes of IgE and IgG_4 which are not skin-sensitizing may play a part in the allergic reaction (Levine *et al.* 1966). It is therefore not certain that potential anaphylaxis will always be detected by cutaneous testing, even when the appropriate antigen and proper techniques are employed.

It has also been shown (Assem and Vickers 1974*a,b*, 1975; Vickers and Assem 1974) that skin tests compare unfavourably with some of the *in vitro* tests (such as the lymphocyte transformation test), which will be discussed later.

The overall predictive value of skin tests

In over 150 cases, including the previously mentioned small group of patients who have undergone extensive and quantitative studies, an immediate response to benzylpenicillin was obtained in only 22 per cent of allergic patients, and 36 per cent with the best carrier. Our results contradict those of other workers in the field of penicillin allergy. Levine and Zolov (1969) state that 'skin tests were found to be valuable predictive tests for immediate (including anaphylactic) and urticarial allergic reactions to penicillin'. This comment was based on a prospective study of 218 patients with past histories of penicillin allergy on whom such tests were performed. The skin tests performed in this study used benzylpenicilloyl-polylysine and a minor determinant mixture. A further report by the Penicillin Study Group of the American Academy of Allergy (Green and Rosenblum 1971) found that whereas these reagents have a predictive accuracy of about 84 per cent in immediate reactions, test doses employing benzylpenicillin itself have an accuracy of 55 per cent. In other words, more than half of all individuals who are actually sensitive (immediate reactors) could be recognized by penicillin skin testing. The skin reaction rate was particularly high in patients who experienced penicillin reactions of the immediate type within 30 minutes.

In a more recent series of 740 patients reported by Sullivan and others (1981), skin tests were carried out with benzylpenicillin, penicilloic acid, and penicilloyl-polylysine. Sixty-three per cent of the patients gave a positive result, but the incidence of skin-test positives was inversely related to the length of time that had elapsed between clinical reactions and skin testing. The maximum incidence (93 per cent) was obtained in patients who were tested 7–12 months after reactions, while the incidence in those tested after 10 years was only 22 per cent.

Despite the marked discrepancies in the proportions of positive skin tests in patients allergic to penicillin, in the experience of different investigators, there is an overall agreement on its value, particularly in the hands of specialists, even when the results are negative (Bierman and van Arsdel 1969).

Investigation of the cross-allergenicity between penicillins and cephalosporins

In patients with suspected or proven allergy to penicillin a skin test with other penicillins should be carried out.

Although cross-reaction between different penicillins is common (because of a common ring structure), selective responses to individual penicillins do occur (due to side-chain specificity) and several papers on this aspect have recently been published (Blanca 1995a,b; Bondaruk et al. 1995; Terrados et al. 1995; Blanca et al. 1996; Sanz et al. (1996); Romano et al. 1997). Cross-reaction with cephalosporin derivatives should also be investigated. Not only will this help in deciding whether a cephalosporin derivative may be given as a replacement for penicillin in patients with penicillin allergy, but it will also help explore or confirm a suspected epitope specificity, since a cephalosporin derivative may not only share part of the ring structure, but also the side chain (Assem and Vickers 1974b; Wiles et al. 1979; Bravo et al. 1995; Sastre et al. 1996).

Medicolegal aspects

The medicolegal aspects of penicillin allergy, particularly in relation to the question of whether skin tests for penicillin allergy should be carried out as a routine, have been borne out by several cases of fatal penicillin reactions that have occurred in Malaysia and Singapore.

Fatal anaphylactic reactions to penicillin are very rare. They seem to occur in about one to two per 100 000 patients treated with penicillin (Idsøe et al. 1968), compared with an overall incidence of penicillin allergy of 0.7–10 per cent reported in different studies in different countries. The incidence of minor (non-fatal) anaphylactic reactions is estimated to be about one to five per 10 000 patient-courses of penicillin (Levine and Zolov 1969).

In a study of 151 fatal anaphylactic reactions by Idsøe and others (1968), 14 per cent of the patients had evidence of previous allergies of some kind; 70 per cent had received penicillin previously; and one-third of these had already experienced sudden allergic reactions to penicillin. In 30 per cent there was no history of previous penicillin therapy, and one should assume that these patients had been exposed to penicillin previously. This may be explained by forgetfulness by the patient, lack of records, the patient not having been told that he had had penicillin, or by 'hidden contacts' such as milk, which may contain penicillin when obtained from cattle treated with this drug.

The point at law in all these cases was, apparently, to what extent was there negligence because of failure to give a test injection? It is known from the previously mentioned work that the test is of limited value — but how limited?

Value of routine testing before penicillin therapy

A consensus of opinion, which was not possible in the past, is now emerging.

Two large clinical trials conducted in the USA (Sogn *et al*. 1992; Gadde *et al*. 1993) with the major penicillin determinant and a minor determinant mixture showed the predictive usefulness of skin tests, particularly in patients at risk. Skin tests have been recommended before starting penicillin therapy, especially for patients who have a history of sensitivity and for patients who have had any allergic disorder, but even skin tests made with diluted penicillin solution, especially intradermal tests, may present danger. A prick/scratch test is preferred. A positive test is undoubtedly significant, but a negative test does not ensure safety when the full therapeutic dose is subsequently administered.

Hazards of penicillin test injections

There is a definite risk involved in these test injections. Even minute concentrations may provoke anaphylactic reactions, such as have sometimes been experienced in connection with a skin test (Ettinger and Kaye 1964; Resnik and Shelley 1966) and after the intradermal injection of as little as 0.02 ml of a concentration of 1000 units of penicillin per ml (Berger and Eisen 1955). Rose (1953) and Driagin (1966) reported fatal anaphylactic reactions as a result of intradermal testing with penicillin. Fatal anaphylaxis may rarely follow the relatively safe scratch test (Dogliotti 1968; Novembre *et al*. 1995). In fact, an accidental scratch with a needle contaminated with traces of penicillin has been reported as provoking anaphylactic shock (Wirth 1963). These reports perhaps represent rare incidents, however, and other investigators (e.g. Levine and Zolov 1969; Sullivan *et al*. 1981; and the author) have not encountered any serious systemic reactions to skin testing.

A relatively minor risk in skin testing is antigenicity of the test material used, which may occur in non-allergic patients who may be tested either because of suspicion of allergy, or because of routine procedures. This risk is more likely when hapten–macromolecule conjugates are used. It seems logical to use conjugates with homologous proteins in order to avoid risk, and to obtain better results as pointed out previously in connection with the carrier effect. In Parker's view (1972), however, the use of hapten conjugates with homologous or autologous proteins, which would be expected to simulate those involved in drug allergy in man, appears to be of little real advantage, and their use in skin testing may produce undesirable effects, such as autosensitization. He rightly suggests the use of non-antigenic macromolecules (such as small polypeptides) as carriers for haptens in test

conjugates. Even small polypeptides, however, may be antigenic, but less so than large macromolecules.

Conclusions

1. Skin tests are not very reliable (even when carried out by a specialist) , particularly if they are performed a long time (years) after a clinical reaction. They are even less reliable in the hands of the non-specialist with no access to proper test material. The desirable range of testing material may not be available even to the specialist. It is also important to mention that potential anaphylaxis may not be detected by cutaneous testing, even when appropriate antigens and proper techniques are employed.

2. Skin and other test injections are risky, and in the allergic subject a fatal anaphylactic reaction may, albeit very rarely, follow these procedures.

3. In view of 1 and 2 (which is a weak argument) and, above all, for practical reasons, routine prospective skin testing and other *in vivo* test procedures cannot generally be advocated. They are probably not of much use in patients who have received penicillin on two or more occasions without developing adverse effects. It should be added, however, that allergy may develop in some patients who have previously received several courses of penicillin without adverse effects. As a compromise solution, these tests are indicated in selected patients:

(a) patients with a personal or family history of established or suspected allergy of any sort;

(b) where parenteral administration is planned, since any reaction may then be more serious than when the drug is given orally;

(c) if the patient has been treated with semi-synthetic penicillins, particularly by injection, or such a treatment, which carries a greater risk of allergy (Idsøe *et al*. 1968), is contemplated;

(d) patients with a suspected disease associated with a higher incidence of allergic drug reactions or immunological abnormalities, such as glandular fever, where the incidence of 'reactions' to ampicillin is said to be particularly high (Pullen *et al*. 1967). Although it is not known whether the skin test would be of value in this condition, it would perhaps help in reducing the anxiety about a possible reaction to penicillin therapy.

Indication for repeating a false-negative skin test

Negative skin tests may be obtained after a definitely allergic drug reaction. In fact this state may persist for days, weeks, or even a few months, and seems to occur particularly after severe reactions. Assem and Schild (1968) have reported an example after a severe anaphylactic reaction to penicillin. This was not surprising since temporary desensitization may follow exposure to a massive dose of allergen (see Fig. 27.2 in Part 1). It is also comparable in some respects to the occasionally dramatic improvement in some asthmatic patients following a severe reaction (unintentional) to an injection of allergen given during the course of hyposensitization therapy (McAllen *et al.* 1967). Sullivan and others (1981) have also reported a lower incidence of skin-test positives in the first 6 months after clinical reactions to penicillin, than between the seventh and twelfth months, when the incidence of positives was at its height (93 per cent).

Routine skin testing in other important allergies: anaesthesia

According to Fisher (1989) the prick test with anaesthetics (including in particular NMB, such as suxamethonium) is the simplest and cheapest and could be performed in an emergency, out of hours or prior to office anaesthesia. According to the author, these points are valid, but as stated earlier there are limitations to the value of prick testing with NMB and opioids (also see Assem 1989*b*). Though useful with suxamethonium, the test is not as reliable with other NMB, where false-positives occur frequently in normal subjects. Furthermore, false-negatives also occur with low concentration (Farrell *et al.* 1988; Assem and Symons 1989; Assem 1990*b*, 1991). Intradermal injection of high concentration, though less likely to give false-negatives, carries the risk of anaphylactic reaction (Farrell *et al.* 1988; Assem 1990*b*). The author saw a case of systemic anaphylaxis (hypotension, bronchospasm, tachycardia, skin flushing) following a negative prick test and miscalculation of the dilution of an NMB before its use in an intradermal test. These limitations point to the importance of *in vitro* testing (described in more detail below).

Alternative procedures to direct skin testing

The Prausnitz–Küstner reaction

If it is felt that a serious reaction may result from test injections, the latter should be preceded by skin scratch tests. A passive transfer by intradermal injection of serum from a sensitized donor intradermally into a normal recipient, which constitutes the Prausnitz–Küstner reaction, may prove useful when great risk is likely from a direct skin test in the patient. Nowadays, if the test is ever to be carried out, the donor serum should be tested for transferable infections, including hepatitis

B and C and human immunodeficiency virus (HIV). The currently available *in vitro* tests for Type I allergy render this test (or its safer but less sensitive replacement using a monkey as recipient [Stanworth 1973]) obsolete.

Other *in vivo* tests

Indications for *in vivo* challenge tests other than in the skin

Although the skin test is the most widely used of the tests for drug allergy, other challenge tests may be necessary. Thus, one may cite the following examples:

1. if the 'target organ' is likely to be of particular importance in connection with the route of exposure of the allergen. Thus, bronchial or nasal challenge is indicated when the allergen is inhaled, owing to contamination of the air; this may occur, and seemingly cause respiratory allergy in the form of airways obstruction (asthma) or rhinitis, in occupations such as, for example, drug manufacturing.

We have come across other examples where nurses or pharmacists developed asthmatic attacks while, or at some time after, reconstituting penicillin preparations or breaking their containers, or cleaning a drug cupboard;

2. if the manifestations of drug reactions are more or less localized in certain organs, though the drugs are given systemically either orally or by injection; for example, asthma induced by aspirin, or by intravenous anaesthetics or preanaesthetic medications;

3. if the skin test is obviously unreliable or gives non-specific reactions, as in the case of narcotic analgesics, and competitive neuromuscular blocking agents such as tubocurarine. In these instances, if *in vivo* challenge tests are at all desirable, a small test dose may be given intravenously (Assem 1977*a*);

4. a test dose may be given by the conventional route, for example, intravenously, if the skin test is negative.

The risks of *in vivo* testing cannot be overemphasized. A remarkable example was a case of fatal anaphylactic reaction that resulted from the instillation of one drop of a local anaesthetic (as a test) in the conjunctival sac of an allergic patient (Adriani 1972).

Nowadays, all such procedures should be carried out in an intensive care unit.

In vitro tests

The techniques now available, though still of limited value in the prediction of drug allergy, particularly in urgent situations, may be of great help in the management of 'cold' cases. Some of them are also restricted in the range of allergies they can detect. So until more reliable and quick methods are developed to cope with urgent situations and to cover the desired range of drugs, preventive measures will be far from satisfactory. Recent expansion has been greatest in the range of allergies that can be detected by solid-phase assays of IgE antibodies. The detection of these antibodies is valuable in the diagnosis of anaphylaxis (see radioallergosorbent test, RAST, below). There is little room for optimism, however, because there is a far greater limitation than all those mentioned above: the enormous cost (see routine testing in anaesthetic practice, below).

Serological studies

The detection of drug-specific circulating antibodies (other than IgE) proves only the occurrence of an immunological response to that particular drug, not evidence of allergy. This is best illustrated in connection with penicillin.

The usefulness of serological investigations will certainly improve when we know more about all the haptenic determinants of every allergenic drug. When this is combined with the study of the different classes of antibodies, the predictive and diagnostic value of these tests will perhaps reach a satisfactory level. Work along these lines is going on at several centres.

'When the metabolites of a drug acting as haptenic determinants have not been identified, or their synthesis and conjugation to carrier molecules is not possible, it may be possible to devise a method of circumventing this problem. An example is the generation of practolol metabolites using the rat liver mixed-function-oxidase complex *in vitro* (Amos *et al.* 1977).'

Methods of detection of the various classes of hapten-specific antibodies

The introduction of solid-phase techniques, where either the antigen or antibody is conjugated to dextran, agarose, paper, or other suitable materials, and of radioimmunoassays of many drugs (Butler 1978) has had a strong impact on methods of detecting, identifying, and quantifying antibodies to drugs and their metabolites. Older assays such as haemagglutination, precipitation, co-precipitation, and the like are rarely used now. Commercial kits for the detection of certain drug allergies by antibody measurement, using solid-phase techniques, either radioallergosorbent (RAST) or enzyme-linked immunosorbent assays (ELISA), are now available (discussed under RAST, below).

When autoimmunization is suspected, for example, in haemolytic anaemia or thrombocytopenia, tests for specific antibodies are indicated, both with regard to the drug, and the 'autoantigen'. An example of such an

exercise was initiated in relation to practolol (Assem and Banks 1973; also see Part 1 on Mechanism).

The possible assignment of different functions to different antibody classes, for example, the reaginic (skin-sensitizing) antibody producing immediate-type allergic reactions, forms the basis of a number of *in vitro* tests, which will be mentioned briefly.

In vitro tests for immediate-type drug allergy
Detection of reaginic antibodies (mainly IgE)

The description of these antibodies as reaginic preceded the discovery that they belong mainly to the IgE immunoglobulin class. This term, though outdated may still be useful because not all the tissue-sensitizing antibodies are of this class. This term is also a reminder of some the characteristics of IgE.

Almost all the initial work on these antibodies in man has been done in connection with atopy, particularly in asthma and hay fever. Application of these tests to certain drug allergies has been successful and it is reasonable to assume that in due course they will have a wider use. The most prominent feature of reaginic antibodies is their capacity to sensitize either autologous or homologous cells, which on subsequent challenge with the specific antigen will release pharmacologically active mediators, such as histamine, SRSA (leukotrienes C_4, D_4, and E_4), bradykinin, 5-hydroxytryptamine, and platelet-activating factor. These mediators of immediate allergic reactions may be estimated either by bioassays, biochemical methods with or without the use of radioisotopes, or by radioimmunological techniques, as in the case of bradykinin. The methods now available are:

1. Sensitization of tissue, for example by passive sensitization of chopped lung. Since reaginic antibodies are, in general, species-specific, human allergy may be detected by use of homologous tissue or tissue from a closely related species, such as the monkey. The use of human and monkey lung for this purpose has been reported by Assem and Schild (1968) and Assem (1972a). Other tissues or cells, for example, basophil leucocytes, may also be sensitized *in vitro*, and if these tissues are contractile (e.g. intestine or appendix), contraction of their smooth muscle may be elicited on subsequent challenge with the antigen (Schultz–Dale reaction).

2. Measurement of antigen-induced histamine release from the patient's leucocytes (Lichtenstein and Osler 1964). The leucocyte histamine-release test has been found to be very valuable, not only in the diagnosis of truly anaphylactic reactions to a wide variety of drugs but also in equally life-threatening anaphylactoid reactions (Assem and Vickers 1974a,b, 1975; Assem 1977b,

1983*a,b*, 1984*a,b*; Hirshman *et al.* 1982; Assem *et al.* 1983) which appear not to be immunologically mediated. These two 'types' of immediate reaction are clinically indistinguishable, the anaphylactoid type being identified by exclusion (lack of evidence of an immune mechanism and occurrence at first exposure). The test would not only show the release with the drug causing the clinical reaction, but generally not with others that are not structurally or pharmacologically related, but also would indicate if the patient is likely to react to related drugs that might be considered as potential alternatives. In addition, the test should also predict anaphylactoid reactions, should the need for a 'screening test' arise. It also provides a valuable tool to study the underlying abnormality and the mechanism (e.g. hyperosmolarity in the case of iodinated radiocontrast media) and characteristics of the mediator release process in the anaphylactoid reaction, for example, if the process is cytotoxic or 'secretory' in nature (Assem 1984*c*).

The release of cysteinyl leukotrienes (CLT) C_4, D_4, and E_4 from isolated leucocytes can also be used as a test (Assem 1993*b*; Mewes *et al.* 1996).

Caution against the term 'anaphylactoid' Although mediator release, for example, from basophils as in the leucocyte histamine-release test, can be triggered independently from IgE antibodies as a result of a physicochemical process (e.g. hyperosmolarity, high or low temperature, polybasic compounds, that is, effect of positive charges, or by anaphylatoxins (complement fragments C5a and C3a), it is difficult to explain most of the so-called anaphylactoid reactions and the mediator release involved. In the days before the development of tests for IgE antibodies to NMB (described below), reactions to these drugs were divided into truly anaphylactic and anaphylactoid, partly based on the history of prior exposure or its absence, and partly on whether there was evidence of an immune response to these drugs or not (Assem 1977*a,b*).

Anaphylactoid reactions to NMB, defined according to these criteria, were investigated by the leucocyte histamine-release test and were found to give a positive result (like truly anaphylactic reactions). We wanted to know what was the mechanism of histamine release in that case (loosely described as 'idiosyncratic'), and we went on to study the characteristics of histamine release (Assem 1977*b*, 1983*b*, 1984*c*). It was interesting to find that the characteristics of drug-induced histamine release from patients' leucocytes were identical to those of 'true' anaphylactic reactions (Assem 1984*c*). Histamine release could, however, be induced by the drug on its own (without any 'artificial' conjugation), which would be unusual with a simple chemical acting as hapten and not as a complete antigen. Despite this finding and the absence of any history of previous clinical exposure, we could not rule out the possibility that the reaction was truly anaphylactic (IgE-mediated). The reason for this was the demonstration that histamine release could not be elicited with compounds possessing a single quaternary ammonium group (QAG); only those with two or three QAG could release histamine — similarly to antigens, which must be at least bivalent in order to be able to elicit an anaphylactic reaction (Fig. 27.4). Therefore, it seemed possible that NMB behaved like very small antigens. Evidence to support this possibility was obtained from other *in vitro* tests. *In vitro* passive sensitization of human skin slices showed some response, drug-induced histamine release from slices that had been preincubated with patients' sera. Furthermore, patients' lymphocytes responded to the drug by increased mitosis and DNA synthesis, as shown by the increased incorporation of ^{3}H-thymidine (Assem 1983*b*).

Subsequent work has shown that most of the patients who have had anaphylactoid reactions to NMB (defined as above) had high levels of IgE antibodies to these agents (Baldo and Fisher 1983; Harle *et al.* 1984; Didier *et al.* 1987; Assem and Ling 1988; Moneret-Vautrin *et al.* 1988; Assem and Symons 1989; Assem 1990*a,b*).

3. Measurement of the release of isotopically labelled 5-hydroxytryptamine from platelets (Caspary and Comaish 1967).

The detection of immediate-type allergy by IgE tests

The discovery of IgE (see above) and the consequent introduction of IgE tests for the detection of immediate-type allergy have been two of the most important developments in the field of allergy in past years. The importance of the latter development can be seen in the light of other test procedures.

For nearly 50 years passive cutaneous transfer in man (Prausnitz–Küstner reaction, mentioned above) has been the principal indirect test for immediate-type allergy (anaphylaxis).

Before the introduction of IgE tests, all *in vivo* tests for anaphylactic antibodies in serum relied on the biological assay of these antibodies or, rather, the 'tissue-sensitizing' or 'reaginic activity' of serum, which is mediated at least in part by IgE antibodies. These tests, apart from being laborious, are available only in some research centres, and require the use of tissues from man or other primates for passive sensitization. They are qualitative, but only semi-quantitative, even when more than one dilution of the serum to be tested is used. The number of sera that can be tested in a single experiment is limited, and there are no agreed standards for assessing the 'reaginic activity' of serum. Each group of research workers may use its own reference sera, but these cannot be kept for long periods of time because of the eventual loss of activity and have to be replaced at intervals.

The measurement of allergen-specific IgE antibodies in serum by the radio-allergosorbent test (RAST, Pharmacia) (Wide *et al.* 1967) is free from some of these problems, but it has its own limitations (see discussion below). There are, however, alternative methods using, for example, an enzyme-linked immunoassay (ELISA) procedure (Voller *et al.* 1976) (see below).

Detection and measurement of allergen-specific IgE

So far, it seems that the RAST analysis, which can be carried out as originally described by Wide and others (1967, 1971) and patented by Pharmacia, or by a variety of modifications, is the best method for this type of non-biological assay of tissue-sensitizing antibodies. Other systems include the CAP FEIA assay (Pharmacia), the MAST chemiluminescent assay (CLA) (Brown *et al.* 1985), using antigen-coated cellulose threads, and 'HY.TEC EIA' (enzyme-linked immunoassay, using allergen-'coated' cellulose disks [Hycor Biomedical Inc., Kontis *et al.* 1997]). All these assays are based on the direct measurement of allergen-specific IgE, with two assumptions: (a) that tissue-sensitizing antibodies belong at least in part to the IgE class of immuno-globulins; and (b) all allergen-specific IgE antibodies are tissue-sensitizing. In the RAST analysis the allergen is conjugated to an insoluble carrier and this conjugate is used for the detection of allergen-specific IgE. The place of RAST in allergy diagnosis is difficult to assess, partly owing to technical problems. In respiratory allergy caused by inhalant allergens the results are more reliable than in food allergies (Thompson and Bird 1983).

In allergy to drugs that are simple chemicals (molecular weight less than 1000) the RAST analysis is at present of limited value, one of the main reasons being that the drug itself, or its various metabolites, which may be more important in the production of allergy, act only as haptens.

The preparation of the right hapten conjugates in an insoluble form, which is essential for the RAST procedure, is a big problem. To our knowledge the RAST analysis has so far been applied mainly (with only a very few exceptions, where it was used mainly for research purposes — see Baldo and Harle 1990) in penicillin and anaesthetic allergies (commercial kits are available). Experience with these two RAST will be discussed in detail at the end of this chapter. The HY.TEC EIA (see above) offer a wider range of 'drug-coated' disks, and their diagnostic value is under study.

Non-specific correlates of immediate-type allergy

As in the case of intrinsic asthma, where there is a possibility of an allergy to unidentifiable allergens, the use of the RAST procedure is at present out of the question for allergy to many drugs. The reason for this in these drug allergies is somewhat different: the haptenic determinants are either unknown, or methods of preparing antigens from them are not available.

The practical value of total serum IgE estimation

Many patients with suspected drug allergy present an immediate diagnostic problem requiring quick action. In these patients, skin tests, despite their potential risk and their limited value, may provide the best possible diagnostic aid. Naturally, skin tests should be avoided if the risk of a reaction is potentially high, and in patients with a widespread skin rash. Since the skin test often gives a false-negative result, due to the reasons previously explained, and a false-positive with some drugs (e.g. narcotic analgesics), the estimation of total serum IgE by the radio-immunosorbent technique (RIST), or other procedures, may provide additional diagnostic help. Kits for the RIST tests are available commercially, and results may be obtained within one day, which is not possible with other *in vitro* tests. It is of particular value where a RAST analysis is not feasible, and biological *in vitro* tests are not available. It is also of value when other *in vitro* tests are negative, or their results are either of doubtful significance, or cannot distinguish between true allergic reactions and conditions simulating allergic reactions. Examples of these situations are the direct histamine-releasing effect of some drugs (Paton 1957) and the possible effect of some drugs on other *in vitro* correlates of allergy (not necessarily those which are strict correlates of immediate-type allergy), such as the lymphocyte transformation test (LTT). Thus in the histamine release test carried out on the patients' own leucocytes, a positive result may be either due to immediate-type allergy, or to direct histamine-releasing effect, that is, where such a reaction is not mediated by anaphylactic antibodies. In the LTT several drugs may possibly inhibit the response of sensitized cells to antigen.

In all these cases, and when other allergies can be excluded (because this test is a non-specific correlate of immediate-type allergy), a positive result will confirm the diagnosis of allergy, but a negative result will not exclude it.

Reversed leucocyte anaphylaxis test

We have observed that total serum IgE may be normal in over two-thirds of patients with allergic asthma and rhinitis, and that in nearly a half leucocyte- (basophil) bound IgE was apparently higher than normal (Assem and McAllen 1970; Assem and Vickers 1972). These conclusions were based on the indirect measurement of leucocyte-bound IgE by challenging these cells with antihuman IgE serum and measuring the amount of histamine released by this treatment. The mechanism of this response is comparable to that of the antigen-induced histamine release from leucocytes sensitized with anaphylactic antibodies. The response, however, of leucocytes to anti-IgE (called 'reversed' anaphylaxis because anti-IgE takes the role of the antigen), like the total serum IgE estimation, appears to be related to the total amount of cell-bound IgE and not to the cell-bound IgE antibodies against the allergen in question. Thus, both are non-specific correlates of immediate-type allergy, but 'reversed' anaphylaxis is the more sensitive of the two tests. This is partly owing to the increased 'releasability' of histamine from the basophils of allergic patients. Immunoglobulin E (IgE) is possibly heterogeneous (e.g. in affinity to basophil or mast cell receptors) and in allergic patients it may differ from that in normal subjects (Assem and Attallah 1981).

Other in vitro *correlates of immediate-type allergy*

The basophil-degranulation test The degranulation of actively sensitized mast cells and basophil leucocytes on exposure to antigen is a correlate of immediate-type allergy. Tests for it are comparable to the previously mentioned methods in which the response of these cells is detected by measuring released pharmacological mediators. One of the drawbacks of these tests, however, is the lack of good quantitative correlation between the observed degranulation and the amount of mediator released. Apart from the relative inaccuracy of assessing the degree of degranulation, there is the inability of this technique to detect the synthesis of some mediators, for example, SRSA (leukotrienes C_4, D_4, and E_4), which is activated by antigen challenge. A new test, which also detects and measures basophil activation, employs anti-membrane antibodies (labelled with fluorescent dyes) as markers, and flow cytometry (Sabbah *et al.* 1995).

Shelley and Juhlin (1962), in an attempt to develop a useful test for reaginic antibodies, used an indirect test in the presence of non-sensitized basophils, allergic sera, and antigen. An indirect test using rabbit basophils, which are more plentiful, was described by Shelley (1961) and was used by other investigators (Katz *et al.* 1964) to study drug allergy. The reproducibility of this test has been questioned, and in view of the established species specificity of the reagins, doubt as to the relationship between the results obtained and reaginic antibodies has been expressed (Hubscher and Goodfriend 1969).

Red-cell-linked antigen–antiglobulin reaction This test, in which antiserum specific to IgE is utilized, has been used to investigate allergy to aspirin, penicillin, penicillamine, insulin, and proteolytic enzymes.

Other antihuman immunoglobulin sera may also be used in order to establish the profile of antibodies belonging to various other immunoglobulin classes (IgG, IgM, IgA, and IgD) (Steele and Coombs 1964; Devey *et al.* 1970; Wheeler 1971; Assem and Vickers 1975). There is a vague notion that the relative proportion of these antibodies to IgE antibodies may influence the outcome of an allergic reaction by inhibiting the antigen-induced response in anaphylactic sensitization, that is, by behaving as 'blocking' antibodies and interfering with the latter reaction in a number of different ways. This is thought to have some bearing on the mechanism of action of hyposensitization therapy (Assem and McAllen 1973).

Leucocyte double-layer agglutination method This test is based on rosette formation, due to immunocyto-adherence between sensitized leucocytes, particularly basophils and red blood cells coated with antigen (Fitzpatrick *et al.* 1967). The value of the leucocyte aggregation test, which is based on a somewhat similar principle, in penicillin allergy in man has been reported by Levacher *et al.* (1983).

Methods for detecting delayed-type hypersensitivity

This type of allergic reaction (Type IV in the Coombs and Gell classification [1968]), also described as cell-mediated immune response, may be detected by two main tests.

Lymphocyte transformation test

When first introduced, the lymphocyte transformation test was considered to be an *in vitro* correlate of delayed-type hypersensitivity (Coulson and Chalmers 1967). Since a positive lymphocyte transformation test may be obtained in conditions which are considered as classical examples of immediate-type allergy (Girard *et al.* 1967), this test may be made more specific for cell-mediated immunity by introducing modifications that would make it possible to assess the response of 'thymus-derived' or 'thymus-processed' lymphocytes (T lymphocytes).

This test has been applied to drug allergy by many authors. Several important points in this technique, apart from the correlation of results with the type(s) of immunological mechanism, will be discussed later.

Tests involving lymphocyte subsets

The role of CD8+ and CD4+ has been mentioned before (Hertl *et al.* 1995; Mauri-Hellweg *et al.* 1995; Zanni *et al.* 1996). These cells may be separated from the patient's peripheral blood (but occasionally from a tissue biopsy specimen) and tested with specific haptenic determinants (epitopes) prepared by chemical procedures.

Use of microsome-processed drugs in allergy testing

As mentioned before, most drugs are metabolised by cytochrome P-450-dependent enzymes. 'Microsome-processed' drugs have been used with success as testing material in the lymphocyte tests mentioned above (Hartl *et al.* 1995).

Macrophage migration inhibition test

Again, when this test was first introduced, it was thought to correlate with cell-mediated immunity (David *et al.* 1964*a*). It was also said to require both hapten and carrier for its expression, supporting the same notion (David *et al.* 1964*b*).

In this test, which is carried out by a variety of technical variations, a macrophage migration-inhibition factor (MIF) is generated by the incubation of sensitized lymphocytes with antigen (Dumonde *et al.* 1969). Two variations of this technique are (1) the use of isolated blood lymphocytes for incubation with antigen, followed by measurement of MIF (i.e. a two-stage procedure); and (2) the use of whole-blood leucocytes in a single-stage procedure.

Ortiz-Ortiz and others (1974) have shown that inhibition of leucocyte migration in patients with penicillin allergy could be passively transferred by patients' sera. This finding may be due to the liberation of MIF from activated lymphocytes, monocyte//macrophages, and possibly other sources such as the pituitary gland (Calandra and Bucala 1997). This cytokine (MIF) not only plays a pivotal role in the inflammatory response. but also has a potential regulatory role in immunologically induced disease (Lan *et al.* 1997).

Other *in vitro* tests suggested as correlates of cell-mediated immunity

Cytotoxic T lymphocyte activation   The cytotoxic activity of sensitized lymphocytes has been successfully utilized as an *in vitro* test in contact dermatitis (Deleschise and Turk 1970; Ptak *et al.* 1994).

Immunocytoadherence

When this test (a lymphocyte rosette formed between sensitized lymphocytes and antigen-coated red cells) was first introduced it was thought to correlate with cell-mediated immunity (Perrudet-Badoux and Frei 1969), but later work by Roberts and others (1971) has cast doubt on this.

Binding of labelled drugs to sensitized lymphocytes

This is another variation of the tests for demonstrating sensitized lymphocytes, which seems more likely to correlate with antibody-mediated allergy rather than cell-mediated immune reactions (Dwyer and Mackay 1970).

Methods of detecting cytotoxic antibodies

Target cells may be labelled with a suitable radioisotope, or an intracellular substance (such as an enzyme, potassium, histamine, etc) may be used as a marker to detect cell damage in the presence of specific antibody (auto-antibody) and complement. An example of the application of this technique is the detection of immunologically mediated leucopenia (Assem 1977*b*).

Detection of immune complexes

Immune complexes, representing an alternative mechanism of drug-induced immune tissue damage, may be demonstrated by different techniques. An interesting example was reported by Williams and others (1977) who found immune complexes in the serum of one patient with serum-sickness-like syndrome and jaundice, apparently due to halothane (see Chapter 11). Metabolites of halothane were associated with these complexes.

Practical experience with drug allergy testing

Relative value of different tests

The value of individual tests depends on the type of reaction (e.g. Type I or otherwise), the drug involved, and the material used in testing. Earlier studies compared a variety of *in vitro* correlates of immediate-type (Type I) allergy (e.g. Assem and co-workers 1968–1975). Table 27.4 summarizes one such comparison in 60 patients; 45 of these had penicillin allergy, and were tested with benzylpenicillin and benzylpenicilloyl polylysine, and 15 had allergy to other drugs and were tested with the unmodified drugs. Studies by other authors were mostly in agreement, for instance the lymphocyte transformation test had the highest score in sensitivity (Nyfeler and Pichler 1997).

The test of histamine release from leucocytes, which detects active sensitization, has a higher incidence of positive results than tests which are based on passive sensitization. for example, of human lung.

Tests for allergen-specific IgE antibodies (e.g. by RAST or one of the non-isotopic ELISA assays) are limited by the range of allergen disks (or other solid-phase-conjugated haptenic determinants) available commercially. These tests are simple but are probably less reliable than some biological tests, such as antigen-induced histamine release from isolated leucocytes.

TABLE 27.4
Comparison of the results of various in vitro *tests with the response to skin testing in patients with drug allergy*

	Response to skin test				Incidence in all patients tested (per cent)
	Immediate only	Delayed only	Immediate + delayed	Negative	
No. of patients	18 (30%)	4 (7%)	11 (18%)	27 (45%)	55 (33 out of 60)
% with raised serum IgE	56	25	46	19	37 (23 out of 62)
% with positive leucocyte test	70	100	100	12	56 (20 out of 36)
% with passive lung sensitization test	50	100	93	12	46 (18 out of 39)
% with positive lymphocyte stimulation test	100	100	100	66	88 (23 out of 26)

Furthermore, they detect allergen-specific IgE antibodies without testing their biological activity, and do not detect other anaphylactic antibodies (particular examples are IgG_4, and possibly other IgG subclass antibodies [Assem and Turner-Warwick 1976; Scott 1987]) which may possibly mediate immediate-type allergy, as mentioned in Part 1 of this chapter. It should be added that antibody classes other than IgE, particularly if present in great excess, may interfere with the estimation of allergen-specific IgE antibodies. There is another source of artefact, namely the presence of high levels IgE in serum, which may be non-allergic-specific in general, or may be specific to an allergen other than the one in question. The use of hydrophobic drug-solid-phase conjugates may give falsely positive cross-reactions with other hydrophobic drugs (Gueant *et al.* 1993).

The lymphocyte stimulation test gives fewer negative results than the previously mentioned *in vitro* correlates of immediate-type allergy. This is not surprising since the allergic drug reaction of most patients is likely to be due to a combination of various immunological mechanisms, Another reason is the frequent ability of the drug itself to produce lymphocyte stimulation, while in strict correlates (tests) of immediate-type allergy the use of appropriate drug conjugates is of critical value. The ability of the drug itself to stimulate the incorporation of [³H]-thymidine by the lymphocytes of allergic patients is presumably due to the formation of conjugates in the lymphocyte culture.

On the whole, the lymphocyte stimulation test offered little help in distinguishing the immunological mechanism involved in drug allergy in the majority of patients; it made little difference whether they had normal or raised IgE and whether they had a late reaction in the skin test or not.

There is a wealth of experience with certain drug allergies, such as to penicillins (which are not as important now as they were in the 1960s) and to anaesthetics. Studies of these 'model allergies' provide a useful guide in other drug allergies, and will therefore be discussed in some detail.

Penicillin allergy

In penicillin allergy the tests summarized in Table 27.4 are frequently (in about 50 per cent of cases) negative even when penicilloyl conjugates are used (see also Assem and Schild 1968) and diagnostically not superior to skin tests apart from the consideration of safety. The reason for the relatively frequent negative results even in established cases of penicillin allergy is probably the choice of an inadequate antigen. When better test reagents are used (e.g. penicilloyl conjugates to other carrier proteins), those *in vitro* tests emerge as more sensitive and reliable than skin tests (Vickers and Assem 1974). A more important improvement was obtained by using conjugates of haptenic determinants other than the penicilloyl determinant (Assem and Vickers 1975; Edwards *et al.* 1982). Tests with β-lactamase inhibitors, such as clavulanic acid (in patients who have had reactions while receiving these inhibitors) suggested that these substances did not 'specifically' contribute to the reaction (histamine release was less than with the penicillin component). They also had no significant effect on histamine release by penicilloyl conjugates (excluding the possibility of using them for inhibition of reaction).

The use of penicillin RASTs in family (general) practice has not been as useful as in specialist clinics; less than 10 per cent of primary-care patients with a supposed allergy to penicillin will have a positive RAST result (Worrall *et al.* 1994).

Anaesthetic allergies

Anaesthetic RAST

Baldo and Fisher (1983) have used the RAST test (sepharose beads used as solid phase to which the hapten was directly conjugated) in the investigation of anaphylactoid reactions of patients to NMB, some of whom were shown to have 'drug-specific' IgE antibodies although there had been no previous exposure to those drugs. These findings were of particular interest, since they suggested that allergy even to such specific drugs might be induced by prior exposure to apparently remotely related chemicals or drugs.

Paper anaesthetic RAST

Paper RAST tests for IgE antibodies to NMB and thiopentone were developed by Assem (Assem and Ling 1988; Assem and Symons 1989; Assem 1989a, 1990a,b). They were evaluated in a retrospective 18-year series of patients with 'anaphylactoid' reactions during general anaesthesia (Assem 1990b). RAST for NMB proved to be valuable and reliable, and confirmed NMB as the most common cause of the so-called anaphylactoid reaction during general anaesthesia. These reactions were, therefore, truly anaphylactic.

Comparison between various tests

Paper RAST were valuable in the preliminary investigation of anaesthetic reactions. Both skin tests and the leucocyte histamine-release test with a wide range of drug concentrations (particularly with NMB) are required in further testing of patients with positive RAST.

The leucocyte histamine-release test, however, may give positive reactions to drugs causing release of histamine that is probably not immunologically mediated but is due to a direct action of the drug. Thus some drugs, such as morphine, may induce the release of pharmacologically active substances such as histamine without the mediation of an immunological mechanism (see reviews by Lagunof and Martin 1983; White et al. 1989).

Is there a place for 'screening' for specific IgE antibodies to anaesthetics?

The case for routine screening for anaesthetic allergies is stronger than that for penicillin allergy (penicillin skin test, see above). Some anaesthetics are always given intravenously, and the incidence of reactions to these may be higher than that to penicillin. Although anaphylactic anaesthetic reactions are rare (1 in 4500 to 20 000 general anaesthetics) according to most surveys (Fisher 1975; Fisher and Baldo 1984; Vervloet 1985), they have attracted much controversy. The debate was highlighted by medicolegal arguments that followed fatal cases of anaphylaxis, the first of which was reported by Assem and Ling (1988). This patient, a 40-year-old woman, suffered cardiovascular collapse, cardiac ischaemia, and cardiac arrest during the induction of anaesthesia. A newly developed paper RAST showed a high level of IgE antibodies to the NMB given. The other two most relevant points were the absence of a history of previous anaesthesia, and manifestations that suggested the heart as the principal target of reaction. There was argument as to whether the paper RAST could be used for preoperative screening (Assem and Ling 1988; Fisher 1989; Assem 1989b).

The second case, which occurred in Scotland, raised more debate, because the sheriff suggested that, since a test (RAST for IgE antibodies to NMB and thiopentone) had then become available, anaesthetists 'should consider screening people coming onto their waiting lists for elective surgery at the initial consultation, particularly when the patient was female, had previously had suxamethonium as part of anaesthesia, and/or had shown signs of other allergy'.

Although the debate that followed was overwhelmingly against routine screening, but not against testing of patients considered at risk (Assem and Ling 1988; Brahams 1989; Noble and Yap 1989; Watkins 1989; Watkins and Milford Ward 1989; Noble 1989; Lunn 1989; Jones 1989; Fisher 1989; Assem 1989b), the general conclusion was that this question could not be addressed until there had been further evaluation of these tests, pilot prospective studies, full appraisal of the frequency of allergic reactions and their contribution to anaesthetic morbidity and mortality, consideration of cost and who will pay it and of 'cost-effectiveness', and careful consideration of medicolegal implications. Other aspects of this issue are discussed in Part 1.

Newer tests for confirming an anaphylactic or anaphylactoid reaction

The aim of the tests mentioned so far is to detect drug allergy, mainly in 'cold cases'. There is another set of blood (and sometimes urine) tests that can be applied to samples collected shortly after the 'event' to confirm a reaction or to 'monitor' it, for example, following a test dose. Sequential blood samples have to be collected, starting within minutes of the reaction, and for up to 24 hours thereafter.

Plasma/serum levels of released mediators

Five mediators/markers of reaction have been developed in the past few years:

1. histamine/methylhistamine may be measured in plasma or urine (Lorenz et al. 1981; Keyzer et al. 1985; Assem 1993a,b);
2. sulfidopeptide-leukotrienes (SLT):Urine LT4* (e.g. Oosaki et al. 1997);

3. 11-dehydrothromboxane B$_2$ (in urine, Oosaki *et al.* 1997);
4. tryptase assay in serum or plasma (Schwartz *et al.* 1989; Matsson *et al.* 1991);
5. eosinophil cationic protein* (Venge *et al.* 1988; Assem 1993*a*, 1994).

* also used in *in vitro* blood tests. SLT: a. an enzyme-linked assay, ELISA (de Weck *et al.* 1991, 1992; Furukawa *et al.* 1994; Sainte Laudy *et al.* 1997); b. radioimmunoassay (Assem 1993*a,b*).

These mediators reach peak levels in plasma/serum within one hour of an anaphylactic or anaphylactoid reaction. Histamine and tryptase are liberated from mast cells, and ECP from eosinophils, while SLT and thromboxanes are from a diversity of cells.

Measurement of complement components and activation products

See Watkins *et al.* (1978); Watkins (1987, 1990, 1992).

Further reading

de Weck, A.L. and Bundgaard, H. (eds) (1983). *Allergic Reactions to Drugs*. Springer, Heidelberg.

References

Adriani, J. (1972). Etiology and management of adverse reactions to anaesthetics. *Int. Anesthesiol. Clin.* 10, 127.

Amos, H.E., Lake, B.G., and Atkinson, H.A.C. (1977). Allergic drug reactions: an *in vitro* model using a mixed function oxidase complex to demonstrate antibodies with specificity for a practolol metabolite. *Clin. Allergy* 7, 423.

Amos, H.E., Wilson, D.V., Taussig, M.J., *et al.* (1971). Hypersensitivity reactions to acetylsalicylic acid. Detection of antibodies in human sera using acetylsalicylic acid attached to proteins through the carboxyl group. *Clin. Exp. Immunol.* 8, 563.

Assem, E-S.K. (1977*a*). Examples of the correlation between the structure of certain groups of drugs and adverse effects mediated by immune and non-immune mechanism (with particular reference to muscle relaxants and steroid anaesthetics). In *Drug Design and Adverse Effects* (ed. H. Bundgaard, P. Juul, and H. Kofod), p. 209. Munksgaard, Copenhagen.

Assem, E-S.K. (1977*b*). Leucocyte histamine release and lymphocyte transformation tests in drug reactions. *Bull. Soc. Catalana Pediatr.* 37, 183.

Assem, E-S.K. (1983*a*). Reactions to local and general anaesthetics. In *Allergic Reactions to Drugs, Handbook of Exper-*imental Pharmacology*, Vol. 63 (ed. A.L. de Weck and H. Bundgaard), p 259. Springer, Heidelberg.

Assem, E-S.K. (1983*b*). Reactions to neuromuscular blockers. In *Allergic Reactions to Drugs, Handbook of Experimental Pharmacology*, Vol. 63 (ed. A.L. de Weck and H. Bundgaard), p. 299. Springer, Heidelberg.

Assem E-S.K. (1984*a*). Allergic reactions during anaesthesia: methods of detection. In *Anaesthesia Review 2* (ed. L. Kaufman), p. 49. Churchill Livingstone, Edinburgh.

Assem, E-S.K. (1984*b*). Diagnostic and predictive test procedures in patients with life-threatening anaphylactic and anaphylactoid drug reactions. *Allergol. Immunopathol.* (Madr.) 12, 61.

Assem, E-S.K. (1984*c*). Characteristics of basophil histamine release by neuromuscular blocking drugs in patients with anaphylactoid reactions. *Agents Actions* 14, 435.

Assem, E-S.K. (1989*a*). Drug allergy. *Curr. Opin. Immunol.* 1, 660.

Assem, E-S.K. (1989*b*). Anaphylaxis. *Anaesthesia* 44, 517.

Assem, E-S.K. (1990*a*). Naturally occurring IgG-antibody-like substance reacting with quaternary ammonium groups and neuromuscular blockers: a common finding in humans and other species. *Int. Arch. Allergy Appl. Immunol.* 91, 426.

Assem, E-S.K. (1990*b*). Anaphylactic anaesthetic reactions: value of paper radioallergosorbent tests for IgE antibodies to muscle relaxants and thiopentone. *Anaesthesia* 45, 1032.

Assem, E-S.K. (1991). *In vivo* and *in vitro* tests in anaphylactic reactions to anaesthetic agents. *Agents Actions* 33, 208.

Assem, E-S.K. (1993*a*). Predictive value of *in vitro* tests for the IgE-dependent and the IgE-independent anaphylactoid reactions to muscle relaxants. *Ann. Fr. Anesth. Reanim.* 12, 203.

Assem, E-S.K. (1993*b*). Leukotriene C$_4$ release from blood cells *in vitro* in patients with anaphylactoid reactions to neuromuscular blockers. *Agents Actions* 38, C275.

Assem, E-S.K. (1994). Release of eosinophil cationic protein (ECP) in anaphylactoid anaesthetic reactions *in vivo* and *in vitro*. *Agents Actions* 41, C11.

Assem, E-S.K. and Atallah, N.A. (1981). Increased release of histamine by anti-IgE from leucocytes of asthmatic patients and possibly heterogeneity of IgE. *Clin. Allergy* 11, 367.

Assem, E-S.K and Banks, R. (1973). Practolol-induced drug eruption. *Proc. R. Soc. Med.* 66, 179.

Assem, E-S.K. and Ling, B.Y. (1988). Fatal anaphylactic reaction to suxamethonium: new screening test suggests possible prevention. *Anaesthesia* 43, 958.

Assem, E-S.K. and McAllen, M.K. (1970). Serum reagins and leucocyte response in patients with house-dust mite allergy. *BMJ* ii, 504.

Assem, E-S.K. and McAllen, M.K. (1973). Changes in challenge tests following hyposensitization with mite extract. *Clin. Allergy* 3, 161.

Assem, E-S.K. and Moorthy, A.P. (1988). Allergy to local anaesthetics: an approach to definitive diagnosis. *Br. Dent. J.* 164, 44.

Assem, E-S.K. and Schild, H.O. (1968). Detection of allergy to penicillin and other antigens by *in vitro* passive sensitization and histamine release from human and monkey lung. *BMJ* iii, 272.

Assem, E-S.K. and Symons, I.E. (1989). Anaphylaxis due to suxamethonium in a 7-year old child: a 14-year follow-up with allergy testing. *Anaesthesia* 44, 121.

Assem, E-S.K. and Turner-Warwick, M. (1976). Cytophilic antibodies in bronchopulmonary aspergillosis, aspergilloma and cryptogenic pulmonary eosinophilia. *Clin. Exp. Immunol.* 26, 67.

Assem, E-S.K. and Vickers, M.R. (1972). Serum IgE and other *in vitro* tests in drug allergy. *Clin. Allergy* 2, 325.

Assem, E-S.K. and Vickers, M.R. (1974a). Immunological response to penicillamine in penicillin-allergic patients and normal subjects. *Postgrad. Med. J.* 50, 65.

Assem, E-S.K. and Vickers, M.R. (1974b). Tests for penicillin allergy in man. II. The immunological cross-reaction between penicillins and cephalosporins. *Immunology* 27, 255.

Assem, E-S.K. and Vickers, M.R. (1975). Investigation of the response to some haptenic determination in penicillin allergy in man. *Clin. Allergy* 5, 43.

Baldo, B.A and Harle, D.G. (1990). Drug allergenic determinants. In *Molecular Approaches to the Study of Allergens* (ed. B.A. Baldo), Monographs in Allergy 28, p. 11. Karger, Basel.

Berger, A.J. and Eisen, B. (1955). Feasibility of skin testing for penicillin sensitivity. *JAMA* 159, 191.

Bierman, C.W. and van Arsdel, P.P. Jr (1969). Penicillin allergy in children: the role of immunological tests in its diagnosis. *J. Allergy* 43, 267.

Blanca, M. (1995a). Allergic reactions to penicillins. A changing world? *Allergy* 50, 777.

Blanca, M. (1995b). Allergic reactions to betalactams. *Allergy Clin. Immunol. Int.* 7, 88.

Blanca, M., Carmona, M.J., Moreno, F., *et al.* (1996). Selective immediate allergic response to penicillin V. *Allergy* 51, 961.

Bondaruk, J., Cucio-Vonlanthen, V. and Schneider, C.H. (1995). Basic aspects related to penicillin-allergy skin testing: on the variability of the hapten–paratope interaction. *Allergy* 50, 671.

Brahams, D. (1989). Fatal reaction to suxamethonium: case for screening by radioallergosorbent test? *Lancet* i, 1400.

Bravo, M.C., Ortiz, I.L., and Vazquez, R.G. (1995). Hypersensitivity to cefuroxime with good tolerance to other betalactams. *Allergy* 50, 359.

Brown, C.R., Higgins, K.W., Frazer, K., *et al.* (1985). *Clin. Chem.* 31, 1500.

Butler, V.P. (1978). The immunological assay of drugs. *Pharm. Rev.* 29, 103.

Calandra, T. and Bucala, R. (1997). Macrophage migration inhibitory factor (MIF): a glucocorticoid counter-regulator within the immune system. *Crit. Rev. Immunol.* 17, 77.

Calkin, J.M. and Maibach, H.I. (1993). Delayed hypersensitivity drug reactions diagnosed by patch testing. *Contact Dermatitis* 29, 223.

Caspary, E.A. and Comaish, J.S. (1967). Release of serotonin from human platelets in hypersensitivity states. *Nature* 214, 286.

Coombs, R.R.A. and Gell, P.G.H. (1968). Classification of allergic reactions responsible for clinical hypersensitivity and disease. In *Clinical Aspects of Immunology* (2nd edn) (ed. P.G.H. Gell and R.R.A. Coombs), p. 575. Blackwell, Oxford.

Coulson, A.S. and Chalmers, D.G. (1967). Response of human blood lymphocytes to tuberculin PPD in tissue culture. *Immunology* 12, 417.

David, J.R., Al-Askari, S., Lawrence, H.S., *et al.* (1964a). Delayed hypersensitivity *in vitro*. The specificity of inhibition of cell migration by antigens. *J. Immunol.* 93, 264.

David, J.R., Lawrence, H.S., and Thomas, L. (1964b). Delayed hypersensitivity *in vitro* III. The specificity of hapten-protein conjugates in the inhibition of cells migration. *J. Immunol.* 93, 279.

Deleschise, J. and Turk, J.L. (1970). Lymphocyte cytotoxicity: a possible *in vitro* test for contact dermatitis. *Lancet* ii, 75.

Devey, M., Sanderson, C.J., Carter, D., *et al.* (1970). IgD antibody to insulin. *Lancet* ii, 1280.

de Weck, A.L. (1971). Immunochemical mechanisms of hypersensitivity to antibiotics, solution to the penicillin allergy problem. In *New Concepts in Allergy and Clinical Immunology* (ed. U. Serafini *et al.*), p. 208. Excerpta Medica, Amsterdam.

de Weck, A.L., Furukawa, K., Dahinden, C., *et al.* (1991). A new cellular assay for the diagnosis of allergy. *Proceedings 14th ICACI*, Kyoto.

de Weck, A.L., Furukawa, K., Urwyler, A., *et al.* (1992). Sulfidoleukotriene-ELISA (SLT-ELISA) assay: A new cellular approach to the diagnosis of allergies. *Proceedings of EAACI*, Paris.

Didier, A., Cador, D., Bongrand, P., *et al.* (1987). Role of the quaternary ammonium ion determinant in allergy to muscle relaxants. *J. Allergy Clin. Immunol.* 79, 578.

Dogliotti, M. (1968). An instance of fatal reaction to the penicillin scratch test. *Dermatologica* 136, 489.

Driagin, G.B. (1966). Anaphylactic shock with fatal outcome following an intradermal test for sensitivity to penicillin. [Russian] *Terarkh* 38, 118.

Dumonde, D.C., Wolstencroft, R.A., Panayi, G.A., *et al.* (1969). Lymphokines: non-antibody mediators of cellular immunity generated by lymphocyte activation. *Nature* 224, 38.

Dwyer, J.M. and MacKay, I.R. (1970). Antigen-binding lymphocytes in human blood. *Lancet* i, 164.

Edwards, R.G.. Spachnan, D.A., and Dewdney, J.M. (1982). Development and use of three new radioallergosorbent tests in the diagnosis of penicillin allergy. *Int. Arch. Allergy Appl. Immunol.* 68, 352.

Ettinger, E. and Kaye, D. (1964). Systemic manifestations after a skin test with penicilloyl-polylysine. *N. Engl. J. Med.* 271, 1105.

Farrell, A.M., Gowland, G., McDowell, J.M., *et al.* (1988). Anaphylactoid reaction to vecuronium followed by systemic reaction to skin testing. *Anaesthesia* 43, 207.

Finke, S.R., Grieco, M.H., Connell, J.T., *et al.* (1965). Results of comparative skin test with penicilloyl-polylysine and penicillin in patients with penicillin allergy. *Am. J. Med.* 38, 71.

Fisher, M.McD. (1975). Severe histamine-mediated reactions to intravenous drugs used in anaesthesia. *Anaesth. Intens. Care* 3, 180.

Fisher, M.McD. (1989). Anaphylaxis. *Anaesthesia* 44, 516.

Fisher, M.M. and Baldo, B.A. (1984). Anaphylactoid reactions during anaesthesia. *Clin. Anaesthesiol.* 2, 677.

Fitzpatrick, M.E., Connolly, R.C., Lea, D.J., *et al.* (1967). *In vitro* detection of human reagins by double-layer leucocyte agglutination: method and controlled blind study. *Immunology* 12, 1.

Furukawa, K., Tengler, R. and de Weck, A.L. (1994). Simplified sulfidoleukotriene ELISA using LTD4-conjugated phosphatase for the study of allergen-induced leukotriene generation by isolated mononuclear cells and diluted whole blood. *J. Invest. Allergol. Clin. Immunol.* 4, 110.

Gadde, J., Spencer, M., Wheeler, B., *et al.* (1993). Clinical experience with penicillin skin testing in a large inner-city STD clinic. *JAMA* 270, 2456.

Girard, J.P., Rose, N.R., Kunz, M.L., *et al.* (1967). *In vitro* lymphocyte transformation in atopic patients: induced by antigens. *J. Allergy* 39, 65.

Green, G.R. and Rosenblum, A. (1971). Report of the penicillin study group American Academy of Allergy. *J. Allergy Clin. Immunol.* 48, 331.

Gueant, J.L., Mata, E., Masson, C., *et al.* (1993). Non-specific interactions in anti-agent IgE-RIA to anaesthetic agents. *Ann. Fr. Anesth. Réanim.* 12, 141.

Harle, D.G., Baldo, B.A., and Fisher, M.M. (1984). Detection of IgE antibodies to suxamethonium after anaphylactoid reactions during anaesthesia. *Lancet* i, 930.

Harle, D.G., Baldo, B.A., Smal, M.A., *et al.* (1986). Detection of thiopentone-reactive IgE antibodies following anaphylactoid reactions during anaesthesia. *Clin. Allergy* 16, 493.

Harle, D.G., Baldo, B.A., and Wells, J.V. (1988). Drugs as allergens: detection and combining site specificities of IgE antibodies to sulphamethoxazole. *Molecular Immunol.* 25, 1347.

Hertl, M.. Jugert, F. and Merk, H.F. (1995). CD8+ dermal T cells from a sulphamethoxazole-induced bullous exanthem proliferate in response to drug-modified liver microsomes. *Br. J. Dermatol.* 132, 215.

Hirshman, C.A., Peters, J., and Cartwright-Lee, I. (1982). Leukocyte histamine release to thiopental. *Anesthesiology* 56, 64.

Hubscher, T. and Goodfriend, L. (1969). Role of human reaginic and hemagglutinating antibodies in the indirect rabbit basophil degranulation reaction. *Int. Arch. Allergy* 35, 298.

Idsøe, O., Guthe, T., Willcox, R.P., *et al.* (1968). Nature and extent of penicillin side reactions, with particular reference to fatalities from anaphylactic shock. *Bull. WHO* 38, 159.

Jones, C.S. (1989). RAST screening for antibodies to anaesthetics. *Lancet* ii, 381.

Juhlin, L. and Wide, L. (1972). IgE antibodies and penicillin allergy. In *Mechanisms in Drug Allergy* (ed. C.H. Dash and H.E.H. Jones), p. 139. Churchill Livingstone, Edinburgh.

Katz, H.I., Gill, K.A., Baxter, D.L., *et al.* (1964). Indirect basophil degranulation test in penicillin allergy. *JAMA* 188, 351.

Keyzer, J.J., Breukelman, H., Wolthers, B.G., *et al.* (1985). Measurement of N-methylhistamine concentrations in plasma and urine during anaphylactoid reactions. *Agents Actions* 16, 76.

Knudsen, E.T., Robinson, O.P.W., Croydon, E.A., *et al.* (1967). Cutaneous sensitivity to purified benzylpenicillin. *Lancet* i, 1184.

Kontis, K.J., Chen, A., Wang, J., *et al.* (1997). Performance of a fully automated *in vitro* allergy test system. *Allergol. Immunopathol.* [Madrid] 25, 63.

Lagunoff, D. and Martin, T.W. (1983). Agents that release histamine from mast cells. *Annu. Rev. Pharmacol. Toxicol.* 23, 331.

Lan, H.Y., Bacher, M., Yang, N. *et al.* (1997). The pathogenic role of macrophage migration inhibitory factor in immunologically induced kidney disease in the rat. *J. Exp. Med.* 185, 1455.

Levacher, M., Rouveix, B., and Badenoch-Jones, P. (1983). Diagnosis of penicillin-allergy — an evaluation of the leucocyte aggregation test in man. *Clin. Allergy* 13, 21.

Levine, B.B. (1962). N(alpha-D-penicilloyl) amines as univalent hapten inhibitors of antibody dependent allergic reactions to penicillin. *J. Med. Pharm. Chem.* 5, 1025.

Levine, B.B. (1963). Studies on the dimensions of the rabbit antibenzyl-penicilloyl antibody combining sites. *J. Exp. Med.* 177, 161.

Levine, B.B. (1964). Studies on the immunological mechanisms of penicillin allergy. I. Antigenic specificities of guinea-pig skin sensitizing rabbit antibenzylpenicillin antibodies. *Immunology* 7, 527.

Levine, B.B. and Price, V.H. (1964). Studies on the immunological mechanisms of penicillin allergy. II. Antigenic specificities of allergic wheal-and-flare skin responses in patients with histories of penicillin allergy. *Immunology* 7, 542.

Levine, B.B. and Zolov, D.M. (1969). Prediction of penicillin allergy by immunological tests. *J. Allergy* 43, 231.

Levine, B.B., Redmond, A.P., Fellner, M., *et al.* (1966). Penicillin allergy and the heterogenous immune responses of man to benzylpenicillin. *J. Clin. Invest.* 45, 1895.

Levine, B.B., Redmond, A.P., Voss, H.E., *et al.* (1967). Prediction of penicillin allergy by immunological tests. *Ann. N.Y. Acad. Sci.* 145, 298.

Lichtenstein, L.M. and Osler, A.G. (1964). Studies on the mechanism of hypersensitivity phenomena. IX. Histamine release from human leukocytes by ragweed pollen antigen. *J. Exp. Med.* 120, 507.

Lorenz, W., Doenicke, A., Schoning, B., *et al.* (1981). The role of histamine in adverse reactions to intravenous agents. In *Adverse Reactions of Anaesthetic Drugs* (ed. J.A. Thornton), p. 169. Elsevier, Amsterdam.

Lunn, J.N. (1989). RAST screening for antibodies to anaesthetics. *Lancet* ii, 381.

McAllen, M., Heaf, P.J.D., and Mcinroy, P. (1967). Depot grass pollen injections in asthma: effect of repeated treatment on clinical response and measured bronchial sensitivity. *BMJ* i, 22.

McGillis, S.T., Burrall, B.A., and Huntley, A.C. (1989). Patch testing. *Clin. Rev. Allergy* 7, 441.

Matsson, P., Enander, I., Shaw, M., *et al.* (1991). Mast cell activation analysis by an immunodiagnostic assay for tryptase. *Agents Actions* 33, 218.

Mauri-Hellweg, D., Bettens, F., Mauri, D. *et al.* (1995). Activation of drug-specific $CD4^+$ and $CD8^+$ T cells in individuals allergic to sulphonamides, phenytoin and carbamazepine. *J. Immunol.* 155, 462.

Mewes, T., Riechelmann, H., and Klimek L. (1996). Increased in vitro cysteinyl leukotriene release from blood leucocytes in patients with asthma, nasal polyps, and aspirin intolerance. *Allergy* 51, 506.

Moneret-Vautrin, D.A., Gueant, J.L., Kamel, L., *et al.* (1988). Anaphylaxis to myorelaxants: cross-sensitivity studied by radioimmunoassays compared to intradermal tests in 34 cases. *J. Allergy Clin. Immunol.* 82, 745.

Newhouse, M.L., Tagg, B., Pocock, S.J., *et al.* (1970). An epidemiological study of workers producing enzyme washing powders. *Lancet* i, 689.

Noble, D.W. (1989). RAST screening for antibodies to anaesthetics. *Lancet* ii, 381.

Noble, D.W. and Yap, P.L. (1989). Screening for antibodies to anaesthetics. *BMJ* 299, 2.

Novembre, E., Bernardini, R., Bertini, G., *et al.* (1995). Skin-prick-test-induced anaphylaxis. *Allergy* 50, 511.

Nyfeler, B. and Pichler, W.J. (1997). The lymphocyte transformation test for the diagnosis of drug allergy: sensitivity and specificity. *Clin. Exp. Allergy* 27, 175.

Ortiz-Ortiz, L., Zamacona, G., Garmilla, C., *et al.* (1974). Migration inhibition test on leucocytes from patients allergic to penicillin. *J. Immunol.* 113, 993.

Oosaki, R., Mizushima, Y., Mita, H., *et al.* (1997). Urinary leukotriene E_4 and 11-dehydrothromboxane B_2 in patients with aspirin-sensitive asthma. *Allergy* 52, 470.

Parker, C.W. (1972). Practical aspects of diagnosis and treatment of patients who are hypersensitive to drugs. In *Hypersensitivity to Drugs*, Vol. 1 (ed. M. Samter and C.W. Parker), p. 367. Pergamon, Oxford.

Perrudet-Badoux, A. and Frei, P.C. (1969). On the mechanism of 'rosette' formation in human and experimental thyroiditis. *Clin. Exp. Immunol.* 5, 117.

Plautt, M., Lichtenstein, L.M., and Bloch, K.J. (1973). Failure to obtain histamine release from rat mast cells exposed to human allergic serum and specific antigen or IgE myeloma protein and anti-IgE. *J. Immunol.* 111, 1022.

Ptak, W., Friedman, A.M., and Flood, P.M. (1994). Generation of anti-hapten T cell cytotoxicity *in vivo*. Relationship to contact sensitivity and the role of contrasuppression. *Arch. Immmunol. Ther. Exp.* (Warsz.) 42, 185.

Pullen, H., Wright, N., and Murdoch, J.McC. (1967). Hypersensitivity reactions to antibacterial drugs in infectious mononucleosis. *Lancet* ii, 1176.

Resnik, S.S. and Shelley, W.B. (1966). Penicilloyl-polylysine skin test: anaphylaxis in absence of penicillin sensitivity. *JAMA* 196, 740.

Roberts, C.I., Brandriss, M.W., and Vaughan, J.H. (1971). Failure of immunocytoadherence to demonstrate delayed hypersensitivity. *J. Immunol.* 106, 1056.

Romano, A., Blanca, M., Mayorga, C., *et al.* (1997). Immediate hypersensitivity to penicillins. Studies on Italian subjects. *Allergy* 52, 89.

Rose, B. (1953). Allergic reactions to penicillin: a panel discussion *J. Allergy* 24, 383.

Sabbah, A., Lauret, M.G., and Maillard, H. (1995). Preliminary study of the basophil activation test for drug allergy using anti-membrane antibodies and flow cytometry. *Allerg. Immunol.* (Paris) 27, 274.

Sainte Laudy, J., Vallon, C., and Guerin, J.C. (1997). Importance of the leukotriene C_4 liberation test for the diagnosis of drug allergy (preliminary results). *Allerg. Immunol.* (Paris) 28, 44.

Sanz, M.L., Garcia, B.E., Prieto, I., *et al.* (1996). Specific IgE determination in the diagnosis of β-lactam allergy. *Invest. Allergol. Clin. Immunol.* 6, 89.

Sastre, J., Quijano, L-D., Novalbos, A., *et al.* (1996). Clinical cross-reactivity between amoxicillin and cephadroxil in patients allergic to amoxicillin and with good tolerance of penicillin. *Allergy* 51, 383.

Schwartz, L.B., Yunginger, J.W., Miller, J., *et al.* (1989). Time course of appearance and disappearance of human mast cell tryptase in the circulation after anaphylaxis. *J. Clin. Invest.* 83, 1551.

Scott, J.R. (1987). A review of *in-vitro* assays for IgG and IgG_4 antibodies: concept and potential applications. *N. Engl. Reg. Allergy Proc.* 385.

Shelley, W.B. (1961). New serological test for allergy in man. *Nature* 195, 1181.

Shelley, W.B. and Juhlin, L. (1962). A new test for detecting anaphylactic sensitivity. *Nature* 191, 1056.

Siegel, B.B. and Levine, B.B. (1965). Antigenic specificities of skin sensitizing antibodies in patients with immediate systemic allergic reactions to penicillin. *J. Allergy* 36, 488.

Smal, M.A., Baldo, B.A. and Harle, D.G. (1988). Drugs as allergens: the molecular basis of IgE binding to trimethoprim. *Allergy* 43,184.

Sogn, D.D., Evans, R. III, Shepherd, G.M., *et al.* (1992). Results of the National Institutes of Allergy and Infectious Diseases Collaborative Clinical Trial to test the predictive skin testing with major and minor penicillin derivatives in hospitalized adults. *Arch. Intern. Med.* 152, 1025.

Stanworth, D.R. (ed.) (1973). Molecular basis of the allergic response. In *Immediate Hypersensitivity*, p. 212. North-Holland, Amsterdam.

Steele, A.V.S. and Coombs, R.R.A. (1964). The red cell linked antigen test for incomplete antibodies to soluble proteins. *Int. Arch. Allergy* 28, 11.

Stewart, G.T. (1967). Allergenic residues in penicillin. *Lancet* ii, 1177.

Sullivan, T.J., Wedner, H.J., Shatz, G.S., *et al.* (1981). Skin testing to detect penicillin allergy. *J. Allergy Clin. Immunol.* 68, 171.

Terrados, S., Blanca, M., Garcia, J., *et al.* (1995). Nonimmediate reactions to betalactams: prevalence and role of the different penicillins. *Allergy* 50, 563.

Thompson, R.A. and Bird, I.G. (1983). How necessary are specific IgE antibody tests in asthma? *Lancet* i, 169.

Venge, R., Dahl, R., and Peterson, C.G.B. (1988). Eosinophil granule proteins in serum after allergen challenge of asthmatic patients and the effects of anti-asthmatic medication. *Int. Arch. Allergy Appl. Immun.* 87, 306.

Vervloet, D. (1985). Allergy to muscle relaxants and related compounds. *Clin. Allergy* 15, 501.

Vickers, M.R. and Assem, E-S.K. (1974). Tests for penicillin allergy in man. I. Carrier effect on response to penicilloyl conjugates. *Immunology* 26, 425.

Voller, A., Bidwell, D.E., Barlett, A., *et al.* (1976). A microplate enzyme immunoassay for toxoplasma antibody. *J. Clin. Pathol.* 29, 150.

Watkins, J. (1987). Investigation of allergic and hypersensitivity reactions to anaesthetic agents. *Br. J. Anaesth.* 59, 104.

Watkins, J. (1989). Suxamethonium anaphylaxis. *Lancet* ii, 171.

Watkins, J. (1992). Markers and mechanisms of anaphylactoid reactions. In *Allergic Reactions to Anaesthetics* (ed. E-S.K. Assem). *Monogr. Allergy* 30, 208.

Watkins, J. and Milford Ward, A. (1989). Screening for antibodies to anaesthetics. *BMJ* 299, 326.

Watkins, J., Udnoon, S., and Tausig, P.E. (1978). Mechanisms of adverse response to intravenous agents in man. In *Adverse Response to Intravenous Drugs* (ed. J. Watkins and A.M. Ward), p. 71. Academic Press, London.

Weston, A. and Assem, E-S.K. (1994). Possible link between anaphylactoid reactions to anaesthetics and chemicals in cosmetics and biocides. *Agents Actions* 41, C138.

Wheeler, A.W. (1971). A method for measuring different classes of immunoglobulins specific for the penicilloyl group. *Immunology* 21, 547.

White, M.V., Kowalski, M.L., and Kaliner, M.A. (1989). Mast cell secretagogues. In *Biochemistry of the Acute Allergic Reactions* (ed. A.I. Tauber, B.U. Wintroub, and S. Simon), p. 83. Liss, New York.

Wide, L. and Juhlin, L. (1971). Detection of penicillin allergy of immediate type by radioimmunoassay of reagins (IgE) to pencilloyl conjugates. *Clin. Allergy* 1, 171.

Wide, L., Bennich, H., and Johansson, S.G.O. (1967). Diagnosis of allergy by an *in vitro* test for allergen antibodies. *Lancet* ii, 1105.

Wiles, C.M., Assem, E-S.K., Cohen, S.L. *et al.* (1979). Cephradine-induced interstitial nephritis. *Clin. Exp. Immunol.* 36, 342.

Williams, B.D., White, N., Amlot, P.L., *et al.* (1977). Circulating immune complexes after repeated halothane anaesthesia. *Br Med. J.* ii, 159.

Wirth, L. (1963). On anaphylactic shock due to penicillin. *Milit. Med.* 128, 245.

Worrall, G.J., Hull, C., and Briffett, E. (1994). Radioallergosorbent testing for penicillin allergy in family practice. *Can. Med. Assoc. J.* 150, 37.

Youngman, P.R., Taylor, K.M., and Wilson, J.D. (1983). Anaphylactoid reactions to neuromuscular blocking agents: A commonly undiagnosed condition? *Lancet* ii, 597.

Zanni, M.P., von Greyerz, S., Schnyder, B., *et al.* (1996). T cell reactions in patients showing adverse reactions to drugs. *Inflamm. Res.* 45 (Suppl. 2), S79.

28. Toxicity of radiological contrast media

G. ANSELL

Introduction

The opacity of radiological contrast media is dependent upon the fact that they contain substances of high atomic number that absorb X-rays. Soluble contrast media are based on formulations containing iodine, which has an atomic number of 53. The soluble salts of barium (atomic number 56), are highly poisonous, and the preparations used in radiological practice therefore consist of suspensions of insoluble barium sulphate. Adverse effects of contrast media, and other complications of radiological investigations, have been comprehensively reviewed by Ansell (1996) and Ansell and others (1996). In this chapter attention will be focused on the main clinical implications of adverse reactions.

Intravascular iodinated contrast media used for urography, computed tomography, and angiography

Conventional contrast media used for excretion urography, computed tomography (CT), and angiography are water-soluble tri-iodinated derivatives of benzoic acid. The physicochemical properties of iodinated contrast media are described by Eloy and others (1991).

High-osmolar contrast media

The conventional ionic media still in current use include diatrizoate (Hypaque, Urografin, Renografin), iothalamate (Conray), and iodamide (Uromiro). In terms of toxicity, on an equiosmolar basis, there is little difference between these compounds. Modifications of the cations, using varying ratios of sodium, methylglucamine, and calcium can affect the toxicity in specific circumstances, and these are discussed in greater detail in the appropriate sections of the text.

If large doses of contrast media are administered to animals to determine the LD_{50}, a characteristic syndrome occurs (Hoppe 1959). As lethal dose levels are approached, the animals become apprehensive. Vomiting, urination, and defaecation occur, followed by muscle twitching and convulsions. At a later stage, capillary breakdown develops in the lungs, causing pulmonary haemorrhage and right heart failure.

Lower-osmolar media

A major factor in the toxicity of conventional ionic contrast media is their hypertonicity. To overcome this, ratio-3 lower-osmolar media were introduced, containing three atoms of iodine per particle in solution. There are two types of ratio-3 media. Sodium methylglucamine ioxaglate (Hexabrix), an ionic medium, is a mono-acid dimer. The non-ionic media, iopamidol (Niopam), iohexol (Omnipaque), iopromide (Ultravist), and ioversol (Optiray) are monomers. These lower-osmolar media, particularly the non-ionic media, generally cause fewer acute adverse effects. They have an appreciably increased margin of safety, but some severe reactions and deaths have occurred even with the non-ionic media. The lower-osmolar media are considerably more expensive than conventional ionic media. They were initially used in higher-risk situations (Grainger 1987) but are now more widely used, and in some countries lower-osmolar media have completely replaced conventional ionic media for intravascular use (Thomson and Dorph 1993).

Isosmolar media

Continuing development has led to the introduction of ratio-6 media such as iotrolan (Isovist) and iodixanol (Visipaque). These are non-ionic dimers which contain six atoms of iodine per particle in solution. Originally introduced for myelography, they are now being evaluated for angiography (Klow *et al.* 1993; Aspelin 1996).

Adverse reactions

In clinical use, adverse reactions to contrast media may be considered under three main categories:

1. reactions following the use of very large total doses of contrast media;
2. reactions occurring when a concentrated bolus of contrast medium has been delivered to a critical area such as the myocardium, brain, spinal cord, or kidney;
3. idiosyncratic reactions, in a susceptible patient, to a dose of contrast medium that would be harmless to most patients.

The reactions in the first two categories (Type A reactions) can be predicted to some extent from results of animal experiments, since they depend largely on the known chemotoxic effects of contrast media and on their hypertonicity. Idiosyncratic (Type B) reactions, on the other hand, are still poorly understood. Severe reactions are uncommon and death is rare, so that accumulation of data for analysis requires large-scale surveys (Ansell *et al.*1980; Shehadi and Toniolo 1980; Palmer 1989). Katayama and others (1990) and Wolf and colleagues (1991) reported surveys comparing the incidence of adverse reactions with ionic and non-ionic media.

Chemotoxic effects (Type A reactions)

Effects on the cardiovascular system

ECG changes

Routine electrocardiographic monitoring of patients undergoing excretion urography with conventional ionic contrast media has shown that significant ECG changes may occur after intravenous injection of large doses of contrast media, particularly in patients with a pre-existing abnormal ECG, coronary artery disease, or congestive heart failure. These changes were more common after bolus injections (Stadalnik *et al.* 1977). In patients with a history of angina, ischaemic ECG changes with or without chest pain have occurred following bolus injections of contrast media into the superior vena cava for digital subtraction angiography (DSA), and one patient developed ventricular fibrillation (Hesselink *et al.* 1984).

Arrhythmias have also been noted following contrast cardiac computed tomography in patients with known coronary artery disease, particularly after recent myocardial infarction (Foster and Griffin 1987).

Pulmonary oedema

In patients with incipient cardiac failure, there is particular risk of precipitating pulmonary oedema when large doses of ionic contrast media are used in high-dose urography (Ansell 1968; Davies *et al.* 1975). Pulmonary oedema may be partly due to the volume of fluid administered, but the main factor is the high osmotic load of the contrast medium. This causes withdrawal of fluid from the interstitial tissues into the intravascular compartments, with resulting hypervolaemia. The cardiotoxic and chemotoxic actions of contrast medium may also be a factor in the causation of pulmonary oedema. With sodium-containing contrast media, the high sodium load may be an aggravating factor, and low-osmolar media are preferable. Pulmonary oedema has, however, occurred in a patient with renal failure who was given iohexol (Dawson 1983).

Malins (1978) has also reported the development of pulmonary oedema following aortography under general anaesthesia, in patients with myocardial disease, and he has stressed the importance of preangiographic cardiological assessment.

Pulmonary oedema occurred in 9.3 per cent of severe reactions to conventional ionic contrast media and was a frequent feature in fatal reactions (Ansell 1996). Occasionally, increased pulmonary capillary permeability, due to anaphylactic shock, may cause a non-cardiogenic type of pulmonary oedema (Chamberlin *et al.* 1979; Soloman 1986). This may require treatment with intravenous fluids. Ioxaglate may also cause non-cardiogenic pulmonary oedema (Bouachour *et al.* 1991).

Pulmonary oedema can also be shown to occur in experimental animals, the severity being related to the dose of contrast medium and speed of injection (Måre and Violante 1983). Pretreatment with methylprednisolone at 24 hours and 30 minutes before the injection produced a significant decrease in this experimental pulmonary oedema (Måre *et al.* 1985). Iohexol caused negligible pulmonary oedema whereas ioxaglate caused a greater degree, suggesting a possible chemotoxic effect on the pulmonary capillaries (Måre *et al.* 1984).

Haemodynamic changes

In angiocardiography, large doses of concentrated contrast medium are injected very rapidly and any pre-existing cardiovascular abnormality may increase the risk of adverse effects. Fischer (1968) reviewed the complex haemodynamic changes that can take place with ionic contrast media. There may be a brief initial hypertensive phase followed by more prolonged hypotension due in part to peripheral vasodilatation and, in some cases, to depression of cardiac contractility. Alterations also occur in cardiac output and pulse rate. At the same time there are frequently transitory electrocardiographic changes, and arrhythmias may occasionally develop. In addition to its direct effect on the cardiovascular system, the hypertonicity of the contrast medium causes an increase in the serum osmolality. Extracellular fluid is drawn into the vascular compartment and the hypervolaemia resulting from haemodilution produces a rise in the left ventricular end-diastolic and left atrial pressures which may induce pulmonary oedema (Foda *et al.* 1965).

With right heart injections there may be transient pulmonary hypertension, and occasionally this is severe. Rapid injections may cause severe dyspnoea and uncontrollable bouts of coughing (Foda *et al.* 1965). The risks of pulmonary angiography are, moreover, increased in patients with pre-existing pulmonary hypertension (Mills *et al.* 1980). Blockage of the pulmonary capillaries by clumps of erythrocytes may be an important factor in causing pulmonary hypertension. It was formerly believed that this was due to aggregation of erythrocytes in the pulmonary capillaries, but Aspelin and Schmid-Schönbein (1978) suggest that the hypertonic contrast media increase the rigidity of the walls of the erythrocytes so that they are unable to pass through the pulmonary capillaries. By comparison, ioxaglate, iopamidol, and iohexol cause only minor changes in the red cell membrane (Staubli *et al.* 1982; Aspelin 1983). In patients with normal pulmonary artery pressure undergoing pulmonary angiography, iohexol caused significantly less increase in pulmonary artery pressure than diatrizoate and therefore appears safer (Tajima *et al.* 1988).

The coronary circulation is one of the critical areas where contrast media may produce vital changes. High-osmolar ionic contrast medium in the coronary circulation may cause decreased myocardial contractility, transient electrocardiographic abnormalities, arrhythmias and, in extreme cases, ventricular fibrillation. The latter is more likely to occur following injections into the right coronary artery (Levin and Gardner 1992).

The experimental work on dogs by Gensini and Di Giorgi (1964) indicated that high concentrations of sodium were toxic to the myocardium and that methylglucamine exerted a protective effect. Pure methylglucamine contrast medium was, however, subsequently found to produce an increased incidence of ventricular fibrillation when used for coronary arteriography, and it was shown that physiological quantities of sodium were desirable in the medium (Simon *et al.* 1972).

Lower-osmolar media cause fewer myocardial and haemodynamic changes (Piscione *et al.* 1991; Morris 1993) and are therefore preferred for coronary arteriography.

Thromboembolism

If non-ionic contrast media are used for coronary arteriography, adequate heparinization is important to prevent a possible higher risk of thromboembolic phenomena. A meticulous technique is imperative and blood should not be withdrawn into the injection syringe (Grollman *et al.* 1988; Hwang *et al.* 1989).

Esplugas and others (1991) found a lower incidence of thromboembolism with ioxaglate as compared with iohexol. Likewise, Grines and colleagues (1996) noted a lower incidence of ischaemic phenomena when ioxaglate was used during coronary angioplasty (see also p. 840). However, there appears to be a higher risk of vomiting (Spataro *et al.* 1987) and allergic reactions, including bronchospasm (Gertz *et al.* 1992) with ioxaglate.

Contrast nephropathy

It is now generally accepted that contrast media have a nephrotoxic potential. In a large prospective study of hospital patients, contrast media were the most common cause of drug-induced nephrotoxicity (Hou *et al.* 1983). There is a copious literature on the subject and this has recently been reviewed by Idée and others (1994) and Ansell (1996). Renal failure may be oliguric or non-oliguric and may be overlooked if follow-up is inadequate. The serum creatinine may be raised in the first 24 hours after administration of contrast medium but tends to peak between the third and seventh days. Renal failure induced by contrast media is usually reversible over a period of 2 weeks but in a few patients it may persist, requiring dialysis, or be fatal.

Risk factors

The most important risk factor for contrast nephropathy is pre-existing renal insufficiency, particularly if this is associated with insulin-dependent diabetes. Other important factors include dehydration, diuretics, low-output cardiac failure, volume of contrast medium, multiple contrast administration in azotaemic patients, and previous contrast nephropathy. Antibiotics and other nephrotoxic drugs (such as non-steroidal anti-inflammatory drugs [NSAID]) may be co-factors. Multiplicity of factors has a cumulative effect. The potential for nephrotoxicity is greater in examinations such as abdominal aortography, renal angiography, or cardioangiography.

There appears to be a small but definite increased risk of acute renal failure when intravascular contrast media are administered to patients with myelomatosis, particularly in those with additional risk factors: it is prudent to avoid contrast media in myelomatosis unless there are compelling reasons to use it.

In diabetic patients, contrast nephropathy may impair the excretion of metformin and may rarely result in fatal lactic acidosis (Jamet *et al.* 1980). The manufacturers recommend that metformin should be stopped for 48 hours before administration of intravascular contrast media and reinstated only after adequate renal function has been regained (Dachman 1995).

Pathological changes

Renal biopsy following high-dose urography has shown that histological changes similar to osmotic nephrosis may occur, but the significance of these changes is not certain (Moreau *et al.* 1975). Arteriography with diatrizoate may cause transient proteinuria and enzymuria (Nicot *et al.* 1984). Trewhella and associates (1990) demonstrated the release of vasopressin following the injection of contrast media and this may reduce renal perfusion. In animal experiments, nephrotoxicity from contrast media has been induced by sodium depletion and administration of indomethacin (Vari *et al.* 1988). Contrast media may cause aggregations of erythrocytes in the microcirculation of the rat kidney and this may reduce medullary blood flow and oxygen tension: ioxaglate caused the least aggregation (Liss 1997). Vasoconstriction by endothelin may be a co-factor in contrast nephrotoxicity, and endothelin receptor antagonists may possibly have a protective effect (Morcos *et al.* 1997).

Ionic contrast media cause an early transient rise in uric acid excretion and a marked rise in oxalate excretion at 24 hours (Gelman *et al.* 1979). This may be relevant in the causation of renal failure, particularly in urate nephropathy (Karasick and Karasick 1981). Urography in hyperuricaemic children with Burkitt's lymphoma may lead to irreversible renal failure (Mandell *et al.* 1983). Acute renal failure due to contrast media may also occur as a result of haemolysis after angiocardiography (Catterall *et al.* 1981) or in association with myoglobinuria (Winearls *et al.* 1980). When excretion urography is undertaken in the presence of renal failure, large quantities of contrast medium may remain in the circulation for several days, and extrarenal excretion may occur both through the liver (resulting in a cholecystogram) and through the small intestine. The contrast medium can, however, be removed rapidly by dialysis, and this may be necessary if a hypersensitivity reaction occurs.

Examination of the urine after intravenous urography may give rise to misleading results. The contrast medium causes an increase in the specific gravity of the urine. There may be a false-positive test for protein when the sulphosalicylic acid or nitric acid ring test is used, but the bromophenyl dye test (Albutest) is not affected. There may also be a false-positive black copper reduction reaction when a Clinitest tablet is added to the urine, thereby simulating the finding in alcaptonuria (Lee and Schoen 1966). Diatrizoate crystalluria may occur in some patients after excretion urography if the urine is cooled to room temperature. This may be confused with other types of crystalluria in routine microscopy of the urine. It is uncertain whether diatrizoate crystalluria has any relevance to contrast medium-induced renal failure (Ramsay *et al.* 1982).

Methylglucamine contrast media may interfere with the urinary estimation of catecholamines in phaeochromocytoma (McPhaul *et al.* 1984).

Experimentally, low-osmolar media show reduced nephrotoxicity but renal failure may occur even with lower-osmolar media. Rudnick and others (1995) compared the nephrotoxicity of iohexol with that of diatrizoate in a randomized multicentre study of 1196 adequately hydrated patients undergoing cardiac angiography. In patients with pre-existing renal insufficiency, contrast nephropathy (increase sCr > 1 mg per dl) occurred in four per cent of the iohexol group and 7.4 per cent of the diatrizoate group. For patients with renal insufficiency and diabetes, the incidence of contrast nephropathy was 11.8 per cent with iohexol and 27 per cent with diatrizoate. In these high-risk patients, therefore, the incidence of contrast nephropathy was approximately halved with iohexol. In non-azotaemic patients there was no significant difference in nephrotoxicity between the media: namely, diabetics 0.7 per cent and 0.6 per cent and non-diabetics nil for both media. Using a more sensitive indicator (increase sCr > 0.5 mg per dl) the incidence rates for nephrotoxicity in all groups were higher but this did not affect the significant difference in nephrotoxicity between iohexol and diatrizoate (P < 0.001).

The isosmolar non-ionic dimers iodixanol and iotrolan appear to have a similar nephrotoxic potential to that of the non-ionic monomers such as iohexol but there have been few studies of the non-ionic dimers in high-risk patients, and further evaluation is required (Deray and Jacobs 1996).

Prevention

Brezis and Epstein (1989) have summarized measures to minimize contrast nephropathy. In patients with no predisposing risk factors the danger is slight. It is important, however, to identify higher-risk groups such as patients with diabetic renal failure, severe cardiac disease with diminished renal blood flow, jaundice, pre-existing azotaemia, and multiple myeloma. The sicker the patient, the higher the risk. Contrast studies in such patients should be limited to those that are essential, weighing potential risks against expected benefits. Concomitant use of potentially nephrotoxic agents, especially NSAID, should be avoided if at all possible. Optimum correction of morbid conditions should be attempted prior to contrast administration and adequate hydration should be assured. In higher-risk patients, Rudnick and others (1995) have shown that non-ionic media such as iohexol are preferable. In patients with pre-existing azotaemia, D'Elia and colleagues (1982) recommend that the serum creatinine should be monitored at 24–48 hours after contrast administration. A persistent nephrogram or a persistent CT nephrogram may be an indicator of impending renal failure (Older *et al.* 1980; Love *et al.* 1989). With non-ionic dimers such as iodixanol, however, there may be somewhat prolonged retention of the contrast medium in the kidney without renal failure (Jakobsen *et al.* 1992). Golman and Almén (1985) suggest that clearance studies of contrast medium remaining in the plasma, after examination in susceptible patients, could give an early warning of potential nephrotoxicity in individual patients and allow appropriate remedial therapy to be started. Surgery and procedures that may be associated with renal ischaemia should be deferred to allow elimination of residual contrast medium, particularly if excretion has been slowed by impaired renal function.

Accidental overdosage in children

Deaths from cardiovascular failure with pulmonary oedema or coma, or both, have in the past been reported in a number of infants due to accidental or mistaken administration of excessive doses of conventional ionic contrast media (Ansell 1970b; McClennan *et al.* 1972; Junck and Marshall 1986). Lower-osmolar media have now generally replaced ionic media for infants. Cohen (1993) recommends that in young infants dosage should be calculated according to kilograms of body-weight rather than age, in order to avoid overdose.

Effects on the central nervous system

Hypertonic contrast media entering the cerebral circulation may alter the blood–brain barrier. Leakage across this barrier may directly damage the neural tissues, which are particularly sensitive to water-soluble contrast media. With non-ionic media there does not appear to be significant damage to the blood–brain barrier (Kendall 1996).

Lundervold and Engeset (1976), using polygraphic recordings during cerebral angiography with ionic media, found that hypotension, bradycardia, and even transient asystole might occur. These changes were more marked when the posterior cerebral arteries had been filled, suggesting that they were due to involvement of centres in the hypothalamus or brain stem. Bradycardial reactions were often followed by tachycardia and hypertension. These reflex cardiovascular changes may be more serious in patients with coronary artery disease. Focal electroencephalographic (EEG) changes may also occur on the side of the injection and, if prolonged, may be followed by evidence of neurological involvement. EEG recordings taken within a few hours after cerebral angiography may give rise to misleading localizing signs of the lesion (Binnie *et al.* 1971).

Confusional states may occur following cerebral angiography (Haley 1984). Neurological complications may also occur following aortic arch angiography (McIvor *et al.* 1987). Transient cortical blindness has been reported following *coronary* angiography (Parry *et al.* 1993).

The reduced neurotoxicity of the low-osmolar contrast media should be advantageous in cerebral angiography (Gonsette and Liesenborgh 1980). They cause less pain and discomfort and fewer EEG changes, but clinical complications due to other factors such as thromboembolism are not prevented (Nakstad *et al.* 1982; Skalpe 1988). Whereas ionic contrast media have a moderate anticoagulant effect, this is minimal with non-ionic media, and this may be a potential cause of thromboembolism (Robertson 1987). (See also p. 840)

Intravenous administration of contrast media may occasionally cause convulsions in patients who have a predisposition to epilepsy, or when very large doses are administered (Ansell 1970a). Convulsions may occur during contrast CT examinations in patients with cerebral tumours: diazepam is valuable in prophylaxis (Pagani *et al.* 1984). No convulsions occurred when iopamidol was used for CT in 169 patients with cerebral metastases (Leonardi *et al.* 1989). Benear and associates (1985) suggested that patients with thrombotic thrombocytopenic purpura may have an increased liability to contrast media convulsions.

Occasional cases of paraplegia were reported following aortography with 65% diatrizoate and 60% metrizoate (Ansell 1968). Bronchial arteriography with 70% diatrizoate has similarly been followed by paresis (Feigelson and Ravin 1965). Mishkin and others (1973) believed that the relative rarity of published reports did not reflect the true incidence of these complications. They quoted five cases notified to them during a 3-month period in 1973. There were four cases of tetraplegia (three being due to parathyroid arteriography, and one following angiography of the posterior fossa). In the fifth case, paraplegia followed attempted renal angiography.

When these neurological complications occured following angiography, the iodine content of the cerebrospinal fluid was raised. Treatment of similar cases by irrigation of the subarachnoid space with isotonic saline has given encouraging results. Systemic steroid therapy should also be started as soon as this mishap is suspected. Use of non-ionic media should eliminate this problem.

Effects on blood vessels

The intra-arterial injection of conventional contrast media results in vasodilatation and pain. This is mainly due to the hypertonicity of the media, but Lindgren (1970) has shown that chemotoxicity is also an important factor. The effect is also more marked with increasing concentrations of contrast medium. Contrast medium may also damage endothelium at the capillary level. Sodium salts appear to be more vasoactive than methylglucamine salts (Harrington and Wiedeman 1965). The local tolerance of irritant substances is, of course, much higher with intravenous injection than it is with intra-arterial injection. In a series of patients undergoing high-dose urography with methylglucamine or sodium salts of diatrizoate, however, Penry and Livingstone (1972) found that the incidence of arm pain was highest in those receiving the pure sodium media. Electron microscopy studies of the veins of rabbits showed minor endothelial changes that were related to the proportion of sodium in the diatrizoate mixture. Severe arm pain may sometimes occur after intravenous injection of 70% sodium iothalamate, and occasional cases of venous thrombosis have occurred with this and with other media (Ansell 1968; Panto and Davies 1986).

In peripheral arteriography, pain is a problem with conventional contrast media, even when they are used in low concentrations. The low-osmolar contrast media are less irritant and cause less pain. In a comparative trial by Murphy and others (1988), iohexol produced considerably less pain than methylglucamine diatrizoate, but ioxaglate (Hexabrix) caused the least pain. Isotonic non-ionic dimers appear to cause minimal discomfort.

Extravascular leakage

Extravascular leakage of hypertonic contrast media may cause a chemical cellulitis with sloughing of the soft tissues (Leung and Cheng 1980; Burd et al. 1985). With rapid injection of large doses of contrast medium for CT, the risk of extravasation is enhanced, particularly with power injection (Sistrom et al. 1991). When non-ionic contrast media have been used, conservative treatment with elevation of the limb usually resulted in resolution but careful assessment is important (Cohan et al. 1990).

Rarely, a compartment syndrome may require fasciotomy (Memolo et al. 1993). For a more detailed review see Ansell 1996 p. 249).

Effects on blood
Red cell changes
Stemerman and others (1971) described a rare case of pancytopenia due to diatrizoate, following a severe anaphylactoid reaction. More recently, repeated acute thrombocytopenia has been described following diatrizoate (Shojania 1985; Lacey et al. 1986; Chang et al. 1989). Transient benign eosinophilia may occur 24–72 hours after excretion urography. This appears to have no significance (Vincent et al. 1977).

Richards and Nulsen (1971) described severe sickling following cerebral angiography in two patients who were homozygous for sickle cell haemoglobin (SS), and McNair (1972) reported a fatality due to acute thrombosis following selective coronary arteriography. Acute haemolysis occurred in a patient with sickle-cell disease following left ventricular angiography with diatrizoate (Rao et al. 1985). In vitro experiments showed that severe sickling occurred when blood samples from SS patients were mixed with concentrations of diatrizoate above 35 per cent. This appeared to be partly due to the acidic nature of the contrast medium, and the degree of sickling was reduced but not eliminated by buffering the medium to pH 7.4. Although few cases have been described, the risk of sickling is probably greater during angiography, when relatively high concentrations of contrast medium are produced, as compared with slow intravenous injections where admixture of blood will tend to decrease the blood concentration of the contrast medium. In vitro studies indicate that the non-ionic medium iopamidol causes significantly less sickling than conventional contrast media (Rao et al. 1982).

Contrast media may cause alterations in the shape of the red cell and increased rigidity of the cell wall (Aspelin and Schmid-Schönbein 1978). These changes in the red cells also increase the microviscosity of the contrast medium–blood mixture. The greatest increase of microviscosity occurs with diatrizoate. Despite its low osmolality, metrizamide also caused a marked increase of microviscosity. The low-osmolar media ioxaglate, iopamidol, and iohexol caused a much lower increase in microviscosity and only minor change in red cell membrane and shape (Staubli et al. 1982). This shows that although osmolality is an important factor in contrast-medium toxicity it is not the only factor and the structure of the contrast medium molecule is also relevant.

When blood is aspirated into a syringe during the administration of hypertonic contrast medium, the red cells are subjected to a very high concentration of the medium. This will render them liable to subsequent haemolysis with liberation of haemoglobin and possibly other toxic substances. It is therefore preferable to avoid reinjection of the blood with the contrast medium.

Haemoglobinuria has been reported following cardioangiography with diatrizoate (Cohen *et al.* 1969).

Coagulation changes

Administration of large doses of ionic contrast media during angiography may cause hypocoagulability of the blood with inhibition of clotting and increased fibrinolytic activity. These coagulation defects may persist up to 24 hours after angiography and are believed to be due to interference with the protein factors responsible for coagulation (Stein and Hilgartner 1968). Ionic contrast media potentiate the anticoagulant action of heparin *in vitro* and this may cause problems in monitoring anticoagulant therapy (Parvez *et al.* 1982). Cardiac catheterization without injection of contrast media, on the other hand, may cause increased coagulability of the blood (Bjork 1968). Protamine sulphate causes precipitation of diatrizoate and may cause an embolus if administered through an arteriography catheter (Iannone 1975). Hexabrix is precipitated by papaverine (Pilla *et al.* 1986).

Robertson (1987) first drew attention to the possibility of clot formation which might occur when blood is aspirated into syringes containing non-ionic contrast medium and suggested that this might be a cause of thromboembolism in angiographic procedures. This observation stimulated much research and controversy, with a considerable technical literature which was reviewed by Grabowski and colleagues (1993) and Ansell (1996, p. 260). Whereas ionic contrast media have a strong anticoagulant action, non-ionic media have only a weak anticoagulant action and are therefore more permissive of thrombin generation. However, clots arising in syringes or catheters are only one source of emboli: endothelial damage and effects on platelets may also predispose to peripheral embolism. Non-ionic media appear to cause less endothelial damage than high osmolar media and have other clinical advantages. Nevertheless, when non-ionic media are used, it is essential to ensure meticulous syringe and catheter techniques. Recent *in vitro* studies by Corot and others (1996) indicate that the lower-osmolar ionic dimer ioxaglate appears to have the highest anticoagulant potential by preventing thrombin generation, and that it does not cause platelet activation. The non-ionic monomer iohexol has less anticoagulant action and, moreover, it causes major platelet activation which does not appear to be prevented by aspirin. The non-ionic dimer iodixanol has the weak-

est anticoagulant effect but it does not cause significant platelet activation (see also p. 836).

The possible significance of protein-binding by contrast media has been reviewed by Lasser (1971). There is evidence that contrast media can activate serum complement by the 'alternative pathway' and this may be one of the factors in systemic reactions (Lasser *et al.* 1980; Lasser 1989). Disseminated intravascular coagulation may, rarely, occur as a result of a severe adverse reaction to contrast medium (Zeman 1977). A fatal reaction with massive intravascular thrombosis has occurred following injection of diatrizoate in a patient with Waldenström's IgM paraproteinaemia (Burchardt *et al.* 1981).

Chemical changes

Depression of ionized calcium by chelating agents present in contrast media may affect cardiac function (Caulfield *et al.* 1975; Mallette and Gomez 1983). The diatrizoate ion also binds calcium directly whereas iopamidol does not bind calcium (Morris *et al.* 1982). The hypocalcaemia induced by contrast media may cause a transient increase in parathormone secretion (Berger *et al.* 1982). Batches of contrast medium may become contaminated by nickel during their manufacture: Leach and Sunderman (1987) found hypernickelaemia in patients undergoing coronary arteriography with Renografin 76.

Idiosyncratic (Type B) reactions

Incidence

There is probably no single factor that can explain the spectrum of idiosyncratic reactions. These range from anaphylactoid-type reactions such as urticaria, sneezing, epiphora, salivary gland enlargement, angioneurotic oedema, and bronchospasm, to the cardiovascular group with fainting, hypotensive collapse, or cardiac arrest. Other types of reaction include flushing, arm pain, nausea, vomiting, abdominal pain, paraesthesia, chest pain, dyspnoea, rigors, headache, tetany, convulsions, and coma (Ansell 1970*a*).

The incidence of reactions to ionic contrast media reported in various surveys ranged from 1 in 13 to 1 in 30 for minor reactions that required no treatment. For intermediate reactions that required some treatment but did not cause undue alarm for the patient's safety the rates varied from 1 in 57 to 1 in 130. The reported incidence of severe reactions requiring intensive treatment ranged from 1 in 1000 to 1 in 4000, while the incidence of fatal reactions varied from 1 in 15 000 to 1 in 93 000 (Ansell *et al.* 1980; Shehadi and Toniolo 1980; Hartman *et al.* 1982). Differences may be partly due to the criteria used for assessing reactions and variations in dosage. Under-reporting of reactions may also be a problem. The incidence of severe reactions reported by Katayama and others (1990) was 1 in 400 for ionic media compared with 1 in 2200 for non-ionic media. The incidence of mild, moderate, and severe reactions appeared to be reduced by a factor of 5–6 when non-ionic media were used (Palmer 1989; Katayama *et al.* 1990) but the effect on the mortality rate is still uncertain. Surprisingly, the number of notified fatal reactions does not appear to have decreased since the introduction of non-ionic media (Ansell 1996, p. 263).

Risk factors

Although some severe or even fatal reactions may occur with small doses of contrast medium, there is evidence to suggest that the incidence of severe reactions to ionic media is increased with higher doses (Ansell *et al.* 1980; Lasser *et al.* 1987). Katayama (1988) also found an increased incidence of severe and very severe reactions to ionic media with bolus injections and to a lesser extent with drip infusions. This was less apparent with non-ionic media. Older patients and those with heart disease appear to be at greater risk of severe reactions. Electrocardiographic abnormalities may occur in such patients following intravenous urography, and the incidence of these ECG changes increased with higher doses of contrast medium and with rapid injection (Stadalnik *et al.* 1977; Pfister and Hutter 1980). As previously discussed, there is also a risk of precipitating pulmonary oedema in patients with incipient congestive heart failure.

Hypotensive collapse is usually the most important feature of severe reactions. Impairment of venous return due to abdominal compression may occasionally cause hypotension, but it is probably not a major factor in most cases. With profound hypotension, there may be loss of consciousness and even convulsions. Cardiac arrhythmias may develop, or there may be transient ECG changes that may be misinterpreted as evidence of cardiac infarction. Sudden cardiac arrest may occur, but with immediate and vigorous treatment there is a reasonable prospect of recovery. Hypotensive collapse is sometimes due to vagal overactivity. These patients have bradycardia instead of the more usual tachycardia (Andrews 1976).

Patients with a history of allergy or reactions to other drugs have an increased risk of reactions to contrast media and this is particularly high in asthmatic patients, in whom the risk of a severe reaction is increased by a factor of 5 (Ansell *et al.* 1980). Bronchospasm may occur during the injection, and as little as 0.5 ml to 1 ml of contrast medium may produce a severe attack with cyanosis. β-Adrenoceptor blockers may predispose to bronchospasm. They may also increase the severity of a reaction and impair the response to treatment (Lang *et al.* 1991).

Subclinical bronchospasm can be demonstrated following the bolus injection of ionic contrast media, and this is more common in asthmatic patients. The incidence of subclinical bronchospasm is much reduced with iopamidol or iohexol and it has been suggested that these media should be used when urography is required in patients with asthma or obstructive airways disease (Dawson *et al.* 1983). Severe bronchospasm has, however, occurred in a high-risk patient with iopamidol (Ansell 1996, p. 279). Katayama (1990) found that in patients with a history of asthma, the incidence of severe and very severe reactions was 1.88 per cent using ionic media and 0.23 per cent with non-ionic media.

In patients with a previous history of a reaction to an ionic contrast medium, there is an 11-fold increased risk of a severe reaction. Approximately 40 per cent of such patients may be expected to develop a further reaction on rechallenge, but many of these repeat reactions are, of course, only minor or intermediate in type. It appears to be possible that certain ethnic groups, for example, Indians, may have a higher risk of reactions, but the reason for this is uncertain (Ansell *et al.* 1980). According to Witten and others (1973), patients with a history of 'iodism' have an increased liability to contrast medium reactions of all types. There is probably an increased risk of reactions in toxic or dehydrated patients.

Delayed reactions

Two studies (Panto and Davies 1986; McCullough *et al.* 1989) have shown that delayed reactions in the week following excretion urography are not uncommon. Approximately 12 per cent of patients reported a 'flu-like' illness resembling iodism and approximately 4.5 per cent had delayed skin rashes. These delayed skin rashes appeared to be more common with contrast media that contained methylglucamine and with non-ionic media. Symptoms suggestive of parotid enlargement were reported in between one and two per cent of patients and there was a trend to a higher incidence after non-ionic media.

Parotid gland swelling was rarely recorded following excretion urography with smaller doses of contrast media (Sussman and Miller 1956), but with the introduction of high-dose urography, and with delayed excretion due to renal failure, the condition became more frequent (Talner *et al.* 1971). It still appears, however, that it is an idiosyncratic reaction occurring in only a small proportion of patients, and it may recur in the same patient with repeated examinations. The swelling usually occur 2–4 hours after the contrast medium has been administered hours after the contrast medium has been administered and may last several days. In these delayed cases, there may be both organically bound iodine and free iodide in the saliva. Evanescent salivary gland enlargement may also occur within a few minutes of the contrast medium injection and subside over a period of a few hours (Navani *et al.* 1972). In one patient, parotid gland swelling was associated with paralysis of the facial nerve (Koch *et al.* 1969).

Armour and co-workers (1986) described a patient with transitory parotid swelling occurring shortly after contrast injection, accompanied by transitory enlargement of the pancreas noted on CT. This was associated with mild back pain.

Reports of severe skin eruptions have become more frequent since the introduction of non-ionic media but it is uncertain whether this is specifically related to the nature of the non-ionic media or whether it may be partly related to the more recent recognition of delayed reactions and the increasing use of non-ionic media. These are discussed by Ansell (1996, pp. 266–8). Exacerbation of systemic lupus erythematosus (SLE) has occurred following non-ionic media and there have been two fatal cases of Stevens–Johnson syndrome. It has been suggested that patients with SLE or on hydralazine therapy may be at particular risk from non-ionic media, but these conditions should probably be considered as contraindication to both non-ionic and ionic media. Toxic epidermal necrolysis has occurred in patients with malignant disease. Two patients with end-stage renal failure developed acute polyarthropathy.

Aldesleukin (interleukin-2) may sensitize patients to contrast media, and unusual systemic 'recall reactions' may occur if they receive contrast media several weeks later. These reactions may be severe.

In Japan and Germany during 1995 there was concern about a possible increased incidence of severe delayed reactions following intravascular use of non-ionic dimers, more particularly iotrolan; this is still under investigation (Aspelin 1996).

Miscellaneous

Transient hyperthyroidism may rarely occur following the administration of high doses of contrast medium (Shetty *et al.* 1974; Shimura *et al.* 1990). Transient hypothyroidism has been reported in infants following cardioangiography (Von Rohner *et al.* 1983).

Some reports (Chagnac *et al.* 1985; Anzola *et al.* 1986; van den Bergh *et al.* 1986) indicate that contrast media may precipitate a myasthenic crisis in patients with myasthenia gravis, particularly in those with a thymoma. This may occur with ionic or non-ionic media.

Stinchcombe and Davies (1989) reported an acute toxic myopathy starting 1 hour after intravenous urography with iopamidol. There was severe muscle pain and a raised serum creatine kinase. The condition resolved over the next 3 days. A similar case with rhabdomyolysis due to diatrizoate was reported by Carena and others (1991).

Mozley (1981) reported a fatal case of malignant hyperthermia which followed the injection of 100 ml of diatrizoate.

Weinstein and others (1985) reported a patient with a malignant VIPoma in whom iodinated contrast media caused release of vasoactive intestinal polypeptide with a marked increase in watery diarrhoea.

Prevention and treatment of reactions

Although there has been considerable research on the subject, the causes of idiosyncratic reactions to contrast media are still uncertain. The majority of these reactions appear to be pseudoallergic. There may be a number of different factors involved, including anxiety, histamine release, complement activation, and protein binding. It appears probable that there may be an immunological mechanism in at least a few contrast-media reactions. For a detailed discussion see Ansell (1996, p. 274).

Before requesting an examination involving the use of contrast medium, it is important to assess the patient's history: the radiologist should be informed of any relevant risk factors mentioned earlier. In doubtful cases, joint consultation between clinician and radiologist may be appropriate. It should be noted, however, that severe and even fatal reactions may occur in the absence of any obvious predisposing risk factors.

There is no completely reliable method of preventing contrast media reactions. Whilst the incidence of reactions is reduced with non-ionic media, cost has sometimes tended to limit their use to higher-risk patients (Grainger and Dawson 1990). In a large randomized study of patients receiving conventional ionic media, Lasser and others (1987) showed that a dose of 32 mg methylprednisolone at 12 and 2 hours before the contrast injection produced a significant reduction in the overall incidence of all grades of reaction by approximately one-third as compared with administration of placebo tablets. A single dose of methylprednisolone at 2 hours before the injection was no better than placebo. For high-risk patients, when time permits, Lasser (1988b) advocated a 3-day course of 32 mg methylprednisolone daily with the last dose 2 hours before injection of the medium. Where prolonged pretreatment is not possible, a single injection of steroid 6 hours before injection of the contrast medium might be effective. Pretreatment with corticosteroid does not, however, completely eliminate the risk of reactions. Likewise, severe reactions and deaths have also occurred after non-ionic media.

In a series of 140 patients with a previous history of moderate or severe reactions, Greenberger and Patterson (1991) attained a rate of repeat reactions as low as 0.7 per cent using a combination of non-ionic media with a prophylactic regimen of prednisolone 50 mg orally at 13, 7, and 1 hour, and diphenhydramine 50 mg orally before repeated contrast examination. In a further 41 patients in whom there was no cardiac contraindication, ephedrine 25 mg orally was added to the regimen. With this three-drug regimen there were no repeat contrast reactions.

Non-ionic media are also preferable in children and in cardiac patients. In patients with asthma it would be rational to supplement steroid prophylaxis with disodium cromoglycate.

Dawson and Sidhu (1993) questioned the added value of corticosteroid prophylaxis in high-risk patients when non-ionic media are used but Lasser and colleagues (1994) performed a carefully controlled prospective study in 1155 patients receiving non-ionic media and confirmed that a two-dose oral regimen of 32 mg methylprednisolone had a significant added protective effect.

Other prophylactic regimens that may be considered in particular circumstances include combined administration of H_1- and H_2-antagonists (Ring et al. 1985), and hyposensitization (Agardh et al. 1983). Greenberger and Patterson (1988), however, advise against the use of cimetidine in prophylaxis, and a severe reaction to contrast medium has been reported following prophylaxis with H_1 and H_2-antagonists and prednisolone (Böckmann et al. 1989).

In their survey among radiologists in the USA, Fischer and Doust (1972) showed that pretesting was unreliable in predicting the risk of a contrast medium reaction. A patient may have no reaction to a small dose of contrast medium and yet develop a fatal reaction to a larger dose (Ansell 1968). On the other hand, the test dose itself may even cause death. Shehadi (1975) concluded that pretesting was of no significant value, but the data in his paper actually showed that in patients with positive pretests, the risks of subsequent reactions were increased by a factor of 12 and there were two deaths (0.5 per cent mortality).

For ionic media, Yamaguchi and others (1991) found that a positive pretest had a predictive value of 1.2 per cent (sensitivity = 3.7 per cent). With non-ionic media, the pretest showed no predictive value. A positive pretest appears to be an indicator of increased risk, but it must be emphasized that a negative pretest does not exclude the possibility of a reaction. Yocum and others (1978) described a more refined and safer testing procedure for use in patients with a previous history of reactions to contrast medium.

Reactions are unpredictable: they may even occur de novo in patients who have previously received contrast medium without incident. Contrast media should not be injected in an isolated clinical setting (Board of the Faculty of Clinical Radiology 1996). The major modes of death are cardiovascular, respiratory, and neurological. Over 90 per cent of severe and fatal reactions commence within the first 20 minutes after injection of contrast medium. It is therefore important for the patient to be under close observation during this period so that effective treatment can be started immediately, to minimize mortality. A scheme for emergency treatment is essential (Cohan et al. 1988; Bush et al. 1991; Ansell 1996 p. 281; Board of the Faculty of Clinical Radiology 1996), with facilities to treat cardiac arrest, pulmonary oedema, respiratory impairment, etc. Treatment will depend on the clinical manifestations but, in severe reactions, intravenous steroids are usually given on an empirical basis, with oxygen administration as required. Van Sonnenberg and colleagues (1987) have shown that non-cardiogenic hypotensive shock usually responds best to fluid replacement, but vasopressors may occasionally be required. Subcutaneous adrenaline is primarily indicated for bronchospasm and other allergic type reactions, but caution is required to avoid cardiac arrhythmias. Salbutamol inhalation may be helpful in bronchospasm. Intravenous dilute adrenaline (1/10 000) may occasionally be indicated in the treatment of anaphylactic collapse, but extreme care is required. Vagal reactions may require intravenous atropine (0.6 mg). Intravenous antihistamines are useful in angioedema but they may aggravate hypotensive reactions. Chemotoxic convulsions require intravenous diazepam and oxygenation. Other manifestations may require appropriate treatment as clinically indicated.

Venography

Large doses of contrast medium may be used for peripheral venography, and the systemic effects are similar to those occurring in the investigations considered above. Albrechtsson and Ollsson (1976) drew attention to the risk of venous thrombosis following venography with conventional contrast media. This is reduced with the low-osmolar media (Albrechtsson and Ollsson 1979; Lea Thomas et al. 1982, 1984). Venography also carries an increased risk when the circulation of the leg is severely compromised. If extravasation of contrast medium occurs, this may lead to skin necrosis and gangrene (Lea Thomas 1987); this risk may be less with low-osmolar media.

Intravenous cholangiography

With the introduction of new imaging techniques there was a considerable decline in the use of intravenous cholangiography, but some institutions still considered the technique of value (Thompson *et al.* 1984; Daly *et al.* 1987; Bar-Meir *et al.* 1989). Moreover, the recent introduction of laparoscopic cholecystectomy has renewed interest in the technique (Rheuther *et al.* 1996).

Most of the literature on intravenous cholangiography relates to the use of iodipamide (Biligrafin) and ioglycamide (Biligram). These have now generally been replaced by iotroxate (Biliscopin) and iodoxamate (Cholovue, Endobil).

The range of reactions to the intravenous injection of iodipamide or ioglycamide was similar to that following the use of urographic media (see above), but reactions were frequently more severe. Other symptoms, such as liver pain or severe diarrhoea, might also occur (particularly after combined oral and intravenous media), and there were hepatotoxic reactions that appeared to be dose-related (Scholtz *et al.* 1974; Sutherland *et al.* 1977). Finby and Blasberg (1964) suggested that there was an increased incidence of toxic reactions when intravenous cholangiography was performed immediately after an oral cholecystogram. It was also suggested that the oral cholecystogram might exert a blocking action on the excretion of iodipamide. Although there has subsequently been no absolute confirmation of their findings, it is now generally considered wiser for the examinations to be separated by an interval of several days. Other drugs found to interfere with the excretion of iodipamide or ioglycamide include phenobarbitone (Nelson *et al.* 1973), oral contraceptives (Lindgren *et al.* 1974), corticosteroids (Wangermez 1975), and tolbutamide (Klumair and Pflanzer 1977).

The hypotensive action of iodipamide is increased by rapid injection (Saltzman and Sundström 1960) and the injection should always be given slowly, taking a minimum of 5 to 10 minutes. A more prolonged infusion technique over 30 minutes is preferable, and appears to reduce the incidence of reactions by a factor of two-thirds (Nilsson 1987).

The mortality rate in one survey was one in 5000 (Ansell 1970*a*). Shehadi (1975) quoted an incidence of one in 441 for severe reactions with one death in 3097 cases. Knutsen and Teisberg (1978) suggested that there may be an increased risk of severe reactions in patients with lymphoproliferative disorders.

Lalli (1984) analysed 28 deaths following intravenous cholangiography. The majority were attributed to cardiac arrest or pulmonary oedema. Although iodipamide and ioglycamide were used in smaller doses than urographic agents, they were significantly more toxic.

The dosage of contrast medium used in infusion cholangiography was the subject of debate. Cooperman and others (1968) did not find that there was any significant advantage in increasing the dose of 50% iodipamide used in the infusion from 20 ml to 40 ml. Nolan and Gibson (1970) claimed that a dose of 1 ml per kg of 50% iodipamide in an infusion provided improved visualization of the common bile duct and gall-bladder. This dose is unnecessarily high, however, and likely to increase the incidence of toxic reactions. Miller and colleagues (1969) showed that there is a transport maximum for the excretion of contrast medium through the liver and they produced diagnostic cholangiograms using as little as 3–5 ml of ioglycamide in an infusion. Moreover, the use of slow infusion techniques allows the liver to excrete the cholangiographic medium more efficiently (Whitney and Bell 1972). The value of low-dose infusion cholangiography in patients with normal liver function was confirmed by Ansell and Faux (1973) using doses of 10 ml of 50% iodipamide. When jaundice is present, results are often disappointing even with higher dose levels of iodipamide, and it is unusual for the biliary tract to be visualized when the serum bilirubin exceeds 52 μmol per litre. Ultrasound examination, transhepatic cholangiography, endoscopic retrograde cholangiopancreatography (ERCP), CT, and magnetic resonance imaging (MRI) are now the investigations of choice in jaundiced patients.

Craft and Swales (1967) reported two cases of renal failure following iodipamide administration. The risks are probably higher in patients with liver damage, who may be unduly susceptible to hypotension. Incipient renal damage may be an aggravating factor. Mudge (1971) showed that both iodipamide and oral cholecystographic media have a uricosuric action analogous to that of probenecid. He therefore advocated that all patients receiving these media should be adequately hydrated, to avoid the risk of uric acid crystalluria.

Blum and others (1984) reported a case of non-oliguric renal failure which occurred following oral cholecystography and intravenous cholangiography on the same day. Hyperuricaemia may have been an aggravating factor. Iodipamide also causes precipitation of

Bence-Jones protein and is therefore a potential cause of renal failure in myelomatosis (Lasser *et al.* 1966).

The newer intravenous cholangiographic media, iodoxamate (Cholovue, Endobil) and iotroxate (Biliscopin), are excreted more efficiently than the older media and can be used in smaller doses. They appear to be less toxic, particularly when given by infusion, but the number of cases is insufficient for adequate assessment (Nilsson 1987). These media may also cause slight or moderate alterations in liver function with intrahepatic cholestasis, iodoxamate being possibly more liable to do so than iotroxate (Dohmen *et al.* 1981).

Waldenström's monoclonal IgM paraproteinaemia is an absolute contraindication to intravenous cholangiography with ioglycamide or iodipamide, since Bauer and others (1974) have shown that these media react with the patient's plasma to cause a lethal gel-like intravascular precipitate. Other types of paraproteinaemia (IgG and mixed forms) do not appear to react with either ioglycamide or iodipamide in this fashion.

A more detailed discussion will be found in Ansell and Wilkins (1987, p. 209).

Media administered by other routes

Oral cholecystography

The most widely used oral cholecystographic media are iopanoic acid (Telepaque) and ipodate (Biloptin, Oragrafin). Diarrhoea or vomiting, or both, are not uncommon following their administration and may occasionally be severe enough to cause collapse or even to precipitate myocardial infarction in a predisposed individual. Other adverse effects include headache, dysuria, and skin rashes (Chen *et al.* 1996, p. 497).

Tishler and Gold (1969) found that a slight transient increase in serum creatinine commonly occurred following oral cholecystography, and that there might also be a false-positive sulphosalicylic acid test for protein. Bunamyodil (Orabilix) was incriminated as a cause of renal failure, and the use of large doses appeared to be a major factor (Setter *et al.* 1963). The majority of cases of renal failure following oral cholecystography have been due to this medium. Schiro and others (1971), however, reported a case of transient renal failure after the administration of 6 g of iopanoic acid. Cholecystographic media have a uricosuric action, and it is therefore important to ensure that the patient is adequately hydrated in order to avoid the risk of uric acid crystalluria (Mudge 1971). In the cases of renal failure following oral cholecystography described by Teplick and others (1965), the risk appeared to be higher in patients with liver disease. Oral cholecystographic media should not be administered in the presence of jaundice. There is commonly a slight rise in serum bilirubin following oral cholecystography, and the bromsulphthalein (BSP) retention test is also increased (Bolt *et al* 1961; Monroe and Longmore 1966). Cholecystographic media are excreted in breast milk and the examination is probably best avoided during lactation (J.A. Nelson, personal communication, 1979).

The physiological factors influencing the absorption and excretion of oral cholecystographic media have been comprehensively reviewed by Berk and others (1974, 1983). It is probable that drugs that influence liver function will affect the excretion of cholecystographic media. Experimental work in dogs by Nelson and others (1973) has shown that pretreatment with phenobarbitone increases the excretion of iopanoate in the bile, presumably as a result of enzyme induction. The excretion of iodipamide, on the other hand, is decreased by this procedure.

Because of their relatively slow excretion, oral cholecystographic media may cause elevation of serum protein-bound iodine levels for up to 3 or 4 months, but the serum butanol-extractable iodine usually returns to within normal limits in 1 month. Jacobsson and Saltzman (1971) have reviewed the effects of the various iodinated contrast media on serum iodine levels. Clinical and experimental studies suggest that the liberation of iodine from cholecystographic media may produce minor alterations of thyroid function for up to 3 months after administration, causing a slight degree of thyroid suppression in euthyroid individuals (Constantinescu *et al.* 1973) and increased hormonal synthesis in cases of thyroid adenoma (Mahlstedt and Joseph 1973). Fairhurst and Naqvi (1975) have reported two cases of frank thyrotoxicosis after oral cholecystography. Thrombocytopenic purpura may occur as a rare complication of oral cholecystography: at least five cases have been described (Hysell *et al.* 1977; Curradi *et al.* 1981; Insauti *et al.* 1983). There appears to be increased destruction of the platelets by an immunological factor in the serum that combines with the contrast medium to cause platelet lysis.

Alimentary tract

Barium sulphate

Barium sulphate is insoluble and is used in an aqueous suspension. It has usually been regarded as a relatively innocuous substance when administered in the form of a barium meal, but there have been reports of several deaths after accidental aspiration of large quantities of high-density barium used for double-contrast examinations in elderly debilitated patients with disordered swallowing, particularly when this is due to neurological causes (Chen *et al.* 1996, p. 483). Accidental inhalation of gas-forming granules of Carbex may give rise to laryngeal spasm (Mills 1990), or asthma (Griffiths and White 1994).

It is now recognized that barium examinations may rarely cause allergic reactions varying in severity from erythema or periorbital oedema to loss of consciousness with severe anaphylactic collapse and generalized urticaria. It has been suggested that this may be due to one or more of the additives used in the barium suspension, as, for example, the preservative methyl parabens (Schwartz *et al.* 1984). Gelfand and others (1985) suggested that glucagon may be responsible for some cases. In a survey of 106 reactions by Janower (1986), however, only 11 patients had received glucagon, but most reactions occurred with double-contrast techniques. Seymour and Kesack (1997) have reported another case of anaphylactic shock which occurred following a barium meal. Feczo and associates (1989) reported a fatal hypersensitivity reaction in an asthmatic patient during a barium enema. In a number of cases, allergic reactions have been attributed to latex balloon catheters (Chen *et al.* 1996, p. 496).

Thick barium may precipitate obstruction in an oesophageal stricture (Ansell and Wilkins 1987, p. 221).

Constipation is common after barium meals or barium enemas (Smith *et al.* 1988); patients should be warned of this and should be advised to take a laxative if appropriate. Barium meals should not be performed if there is any possibility of large bowel obstruction, since absorption of water in the colon may cause inspissation of the barium and may thereby convert a subacute to an acute obstruction. In elderly patients without any organic obstruction, there is still sometimes prolonged stasis of barium in the colon for 4–6 weeks after a barium meal, and lactulose appears to be useful in clearing the colon of barium in these cases (Prout *et al.* 1972). Barium retained in the appendix may rarely form an obstructing faecolith and cause acute appendicitis (Young 1958). Prolonged retention of barium may occur in the distal loop as a result of barium enemas in colostomy patients (Ansell and Wilkins 1987, p. 227). In small bowel lesions there is little risk of an obstruction being aggravated by barium, since the large amount of fluid present usually prevents inspissation, but impaction of barium has been reported in the small bowel in an infant with cystic fibrosis (Fischer and Nice 1984). Toxic dilatation of the colon

may be aggravated by a barium enema (Ansell and Wilkins 1987, p. 233).

Perforation is a rare but serious hazard of barium enema examinations. In the majority of cases reported in the literature, a self-retaining catheter had been used. Rectal biopsy preceding a barium enema may also contribute to perforation. Intraperitoneal perforation is associated with severe pain and collapse, but a large extraperitoneal perforation may initially cause few symptoms. After recovery from shock, the patient may appear deceptively well in the early stages, but unexpected deterioration and death frequently occur approximately 12 hours later (Ansell 1976, p. 339). In a series of cases with perforation following barium enema, analysed by Zheutlin and others (1952), the mortality of cases treated surgically was 47 per cent, while in patients treated conservatively it was 58 per cent. Faecal contamination of the peritoneum is an important aggravating factor, but studies by Nahrwold and others (1971) in dogs have shown that even sterile barium sulphate causes severe peritoneal irritation, with outpouring of fluid into the peritoneal cavity causing hypovolaemia. The prognosis in these animals was markedly improved by early and continued administration of large volumes of intravenous fluids. Gardiner and Miller (1973) successfully used this approach in four patients with perforation following a barium enema. Residual barium in the peritoneum eventually causes fibrogranulomatous changes and may give rise to recurrent small bowel obstruction or ureteral occlusion (Zheutlin *et al.* 1952; Herrington 1966). Barium granuloma in the rectum, due to extraperitoneal leakage, may present as an indurated ulcer or stricture resembling carcinoma (Lull *et al.* 1971)

Retroperitoneal emphysema following a double-contrast enema appears to have a less serious prognosis and may resolve with conservative therapy (Chen *et al.* 1996, p. 491).

Venous intravasation of barium may rarely occur during barium enema examinations and is usually associated with a high mortality due to pulmonary embolism of barium but occasional patients have survived (Chen *et al.* 1996, p. 493).

ECG abnormalities commonly occur during barium enema examinations, particularly in the elderly or in patients with heart disease (Eastwood 1972).

Le Frock and others (1975) showed that transient bacteraemia may occur after barium enemata. This may be important in patients with valvular disease or prostheses, or in those with immune deficiency (Hammer 1977).

Reports in the French literature suggest that a barium encephalopathy may, rarely, occur following prolonged stasis of barium in the bowel or after intraperitoneal rupture of a barium enema (Dupuy et al. 1980; Deixonne et al. 1983). Fukuda and co-workers (1989) reported a non-hepatic hyperammonaemic encephalopathy following a rectal rupture during a barium enema. They suggested that this might be due to bacterial production of ammonia.

Gastrografin

Gastrografin is a 76% aqueous solution of sodium and methylglucamine diatrizoate with 0.1% of the wetting agent Tween 80. Originally the main indication for its use was in the investigation of suspected perforation. Gastrografin has an osmolarity of 1900 milliosmols per litre, approximately six times that of normal plasma (Harris et al. 1964). This hypertonicity has a marked cathartic effect on the gastrointestinal tract. This can result in a severe hypovolaemia, which can be particularly serious in cases where the plasma volume is initially low — in, for example, dehydrated or malnourished children. Collapse may also occur in debilitated adults. Somewhat surprisingly in view of the cathartic action of Gastrografin, it appears possible that its administration postoperatively may occasionally be the cause of ileus (Davies and Williams 1971). Animal experiments suggest that administration of Gastrografin adversely affects the prognosis in intestinal ischaemia (Stordahl et al. 1989). Water-soluble contrast media may be absorbed if there has been a perforation or an area of intestinal ischaemia (Hay and Cant 1990). Hypersensitivity reactions may also occur (Ansell and Wilkins 1987, p. 227). Care should be taken to ensure that Gastrografin is not inhaled, since its hyperosmolar action may cause the onset of pulmonary oedema (Ansell 1968; Chiu and Gambach 1974).

Dilute solutions of oral Gastrografin are frequently used to opacify the bowel during abdominal CT. Miller (1997) has reported a rare anaphylactoid reaction to oral Gastrografin.

The low-osmolar media are preferable to Gastrografin for oral examination of the gastrointestinal tract. There is still some risk if they are inhaled (Gmeinwieser et al. 1990) but this is less than with Gastrografin. The adverse effects due to hypertonic media in the gastrointestinal tract are also reduced. There is less dilution of the low-osmolar media during the passage through the bowel, so that the small intestine and colon can be well visualized and they can even be used in suspected colonic obstruction in appropriate circumstances.

The hyperosmolar property of Gastrografin has been used with advantage in the non-operative treatment of uncomplicated meconium ileus: a high Gastrografin enema is administered under fluoroscopic control, and large volumes of fluid are drawn into the bowel, loosening the viscid meconium and allowing it to be passed per rectum. As with oral Gastrografin, this may cause hypovolaemia, with an increase in haematocrit and serum osmolality and a profound reduction in cardiac output. Acute hypomagnesaemia has also been reported (Godson et al. 1988). It is, therefore, important that the infant should be adequately hydrated before the procedure. Additional intravenous fluids should be administered during the examination, and the water balance should be monitored for several hours (Rowe et al. 1971). Gastrografin enemata have also been used in adults to treat chronic constipation, but a case of caecal perforation has been reported due to overdistension resulting from the hyperosmolar action of retained medium (Seltzer and Jones 1978). Inflammatory changes have been reported in the colonic mucosa following prolonged retention of a diatrizoate enema (Creteur et al. 1983).

Ross (1972) has shown that acid gastric juice causes the precipitation of diatrizoate, so that Gastrografin may, rarely, form a dense precipitate in the stomach. Gallitano and others (1976) have also reported precipitation of diatrizoate following stasis in an achlorhydric stomach. It is therefore preferable to aspirate any retained Gastrografin after the examination, when it is possible to do so. Precipitation of diatrizoate has also occurred within the intragastric balloon of a Sengstaken–Blakemore tube, preventing the tube from being withdrawn (Hugh et al. 1970).

Endoscopic and percutaneous cholangiography

Acute pancreatitis is an occasional complication of ERCP. An analysis by Hamilton and others (1983) suggested that multiple injections of contrast medium with opacification of the pancreatic duct were relevant factors. Significant quantities of contrast medium may be absorbed after ERCP and facilities should be available to treat contrast media reactions (Sable et al. 1983). Kone and colleagues (1986) reported three cases of acute renal failure related to the use of contrast medium for the purpose of percutaneous transhepatic cholangiographic examination.

Operative and T-tube cholangiography

Rarely, a fatal reaction may occur during operative cholangiography (Chen et al. 996, p. 499).

Febrile reactions may occur following T-tube cholangiography and leakage of contrast medium may cause biliary peritonitis (Chen et al. 1996, p. 499).

Bronchography

Bronchography is now rarely performed. Complications are reviewed in the fourth edition of this book.

Lymphography

The complications of lymphography have been reviewed by Macdonald (1987). Iodized oils are usually used as contrast media. They can cause iodism or allergic reactions. Allergic reactions to the patent blue-violet dye injected prior to the lymphangiogram to enable the lymphatics to be visualized may also occur. This dye causes incidental blue discolouration of the skin and urine. Extravasation of contrast medium into the skin may rarely cause a delayed dermatitis. Swelling of the limb may occur after lymphatic obstruction.

There is inevitably some degree of pulmonary oil embolism after lymphography, causing some impairment of pulmonary function. This is usually symptomless but it may be a major hazard if the patient has preexisting poor lung function. Operations and anaesthesia may be poorly tolerated in the immediate post-lymphography period. Oil embolism may also cause a chemical pneumonitis. The risk of cerebral oil embolism is increased if lymphography is performed shortly after radiotherapy to the lungs.

Mild hypothyroidism has occurred after lymphography (Heidemann et al. 1982).

Myelography, cisternography, and ventriculography

Iophendylate (Myodil, Pantopaque) an oily contrast medium, was extensively used for myelography over a period of some 30 years until the mid-1970s. Late complications due to adhesive arachnoiditis have subsequently been the subject of litigation (Craig and Macpherson 1991). Focal seizures have been reported as a late complication of intracranial iophendolate (Pascuzzi et al. 1988) and vestibular disturbances in two patients some 23 years after myelography were attributed to residual iophendylate in the internal auditory canal (Mizuno et al. 1992). More extensive information on iophendylate will be found in the fourth edition of this book.

Metrizamide (Amipaque), the first non-ionic water-soluble contrast medium, was introduced in 1977 and was widely used for intrathecal studies. The commonest adverse effects were headache, nausea, and vomiting.

These occurred more frequently in females. Rarely, there were a variety of neurological and psychiatric syndromes. Convulsions occurred in a few patients. Much of the literature on non-ionic media in myelography has been based on the use of metrizamide and it is discussed in the fourth edition of this book.

Metrizamide was replaced by the newer non-ionic media iopamidol and iohexol. These produce fewer adverse reactions than metrizamide but slight EEG changes may occur (Drayer et al. 1984; Hindmarsh et al. 1994). Mood and cognitive changes are less frequent with iopamidol or iohexol than with metrizamide (Hammeke et al. 1984; Ratcliff et al. 1986). In a comparison of iopamidol and iohexol by Davies and colleagues (1989), there was a slightly higher incidence of headache and delayed adverse effects with iopamidol. Computed tomography of the brain following iopamidol myelography shows penetration of the contrast medium into the cortex similar to that occurring with metrizamide (Drayer et al. 1983). Seizures have been reported in a very few patients following myelography with iopamidol or iohexol (Carella et al. 1982; Lipman et al. 1983; Tahta et al. 1993).

Kendall (1989) in a review of 634 paediatric myelograms drew attention to the risk of mechanical factors causing an increase in focal neurological signs of spinal cord tumours. Prolonged paraplegia has occurred as a rare complication of myelography (Bain et al. 1991). Aseptic meningitis is a recognized occasional complication of myelography (Mallat et al. 1991). A systemic anaphylactoid reaction may occur (Agildere et al. 1991).

A liberal fluid intake is believed to reduce postmyelographic complications but in a case of encephalopathy with confusion and disorientation reported by Donaghy and others (1985) there was evidence of dilutional hyponatraemia and it seemed that water intoxication might have been a contributing factor. A similar case was reported by Soriano-Soriano (1992).

Iotrolan is a new non-ionic dimer which is isotonic with cerebrospinal fluid. In a double-blind comparison with iohexol performed by Wagner and others (1994), adverse effects were broadly similar but neck pain was reduced with iotrolan.

Ionic media are approximately 10 times more neurotoxic than non-ionic, *and should never be injected intrathecally.* They are likely to cause myoclonic spasms, convulsions, and other neurological complications, which are frequently fatal. Although this has been widely recognized, many mistakes continue to occur — indeed ionic instead of non-ionic media are known to have recently been injected in over 30 patients with tragic results. The Food and Drug Administration

(USA) has recently instructed manufacturers to place a boxed label on ionic media warning against intrathecal use (Bøhn et al. 1992; Rosati et al. 1992; McLennan 1993).

Accidental intrathecal injection of ionic media should be treated by lavage of the subarachnoid space with isotonic saline (McLeery and Lewtas 1966; Tortiere et al. 1989). It would also be rational to administer a systemic corticosteroid.

If available, MRI is now generally preferable to myelography, but in selected cases myelography may still be required and may be combined with CT.

Magnetic resonance imaging and radiopharmaceuticals

Adverse reactions similar to those occurring with iodinated contrast media may result from the use of the ionic magnetic resonance contrast medium gadolineum pentolate dimeglumine (GdDTPA) (Tardy et al. 1992; Takebayashi et al. 1993) or from the non-ionic agent gadoteridol (Shellock et al. 1993).

Radiopharmaceuticals may also cause a variety of adverse reactions. These have been comprehensively reviewed by Sampson (1993). The incidence rates for such reactions are uncertain but are probably lower than those for iodinated contrast media.

References

Agardh, C-D., Arner, B., Ekholm, S., et al. (1983). Desensitisation as a means of preventing untoward reactions to ionic contrast media. Acta Radiol. [Diagn.] (Stockh.) 24, 235.

Agildere, A.M., Haliloglu, M., Cila, A., et al. 1991. Laryngeal edema following the injection of iohexol into the subarachnoid space. Neuroradiology 33, 20.

Albrechtsson, U. and Ollsson, C-G. (1976). Thrombotic side-effects of lower-limb phlebography. Lancet i, 723.

Albrechtsson, U. and Ollsson, C-G. (1979). Thrombosis following phlebography with ionic and non-ionic media. Acta Radiol. [Diagn.] (Stockh.) 20, 46.

Andrews, E.J. (1976). The vagus reaction as a possible cause of severe complications of radiological procedures. Radiology 121, 1.

Ansell, G. (1968). A national survey of radiological complications interim report. Clin. Radiol. 19, 175.

Ansell, G. (1970a). Adverse reactions to contrast agents: scope of problem. Invest. Radiol. 5, 374.

Ansell, G. (1970b). Fatal overdose of contrast medium in infants. Br. J. Radiol. 43, 395.

Ansell, G. (ed.) (1976). Complications in Diagnostic Radiology. Blackwell, Oxford.

Ansell, G. (1996) Complications of intravascular iodinated contrast media. In Complications in Diagnostic Imaging and Interventional Radiology (3rd edn) (ed. G. Ansell, M.A. Bettman, J.A. Kaufman and R.A. Wilkins), p. 245. Blackwell Science, Cambridge, Mass.

Ansell, G. and Faux, P.A. (1973). Low-dose infusion cholangiography. Clin. Radiol. 24, 95.

Ansell, G. and Wilkins, R.A. (1987). Complications in Diagnostic Imaging (2nd edn). Blackwell Scientific, Oxford.

Ansell, G., Tweedie, M.C., West, C.R., et al. (1980). The current status of reactions to intravenous contrast media. Invest. Radiol. 15 (Suppl. 6), S32.

Anzola, G.P., Capra, R., Magoni, M., et al. (1986). Myasthenic crisis during intravenous iodinated contrast injection. Ital. J. Neurol. Sci. 7, 273.

Armour, T.E., McClennan, B.L., and Glazer, H.S. (1986). Pancreatic mumps: a transient reaction to IV contrast media (case report). AJR 147, 188.

Aspelin, P. (1996). Clinical experience of the use of a non-ionic dimeric contrast medium. Europ. Radiol. 6, S23.

Aspelin, P. and Schmid-Schonbein, H. (1978). Effect of ionic and non-ionic contrast media on red cell aggregation in-vitro. Acta Radiol. [Diagn.] (Stockh.) 19, 766.

Bain, P.G., Colchester, A.C.F., and Nadarajah, D. (1991). Paraplegia after iopamidol myelography. Lancet 338, 252.

Bar-Meir, S., Ramsby, G.R., and Conn, H.O. (1989). Meglumine iodoxamate (Cholovue) in the cholangiographic visualization of the biliary tree in cirrhosis. A double blind diagnostic trial. Clin. Trials J. 26, 238.

Bauer, K., Tragi, K.H., and Bauer, G. (1974). Intravasale Denaturierung von Plasmaproteinen bei einer IgM-Paraproteinämie, ausgelöst durch ein intravenös verabreichtes lebergängiges Röntgenkontrastmittel. Wien. Klin. Wochenschr. 86, 766.

Benear, J.B., Vannata, J.B., Hosty, T.A., et al. (1985). Contrast-induced seizure associated with thrombotic thrombocytopenic purpura: case report. Arch. Intern. Med. 145, 363.

Berger, R.E., Gomez, L.S., and Mallette, L.E. (1982). Acute hypocalcaemic effects of clinical contrast media injection. AJR 138, 283.

Berk, R.N., Leopold, G.R., and Fordren, J.S. (1983). Imaging of the gallbladder. In Advances in Internal Medicine, Vol. 28, p. 387. Year Book Medical Publishers, Chicago.

Berk, R.N., Loeb, P.M., Goldberger, L.E., et al. (1974). Oral cholecystography with iopanoic acid. N. Engl. J. Med. 290, 204.

Binnie, C.D., Bernstein, D.C., Booth, A.E., et al. (1971). Clinical and electroencephalographic sequelae of carotid angiography. Acta Radiol. [Diagn.] (Stockh.) 6, 626.

Bjork, L. (1968). The effect of cardiac catheterization and angiocardiography on the coagulation activity of the blood. AJR 102, 441.

Blum, M., Liron, M., and Aviram, A. (1984). Acute renal failure following cholecystography. Am. J. Proctol. Gastroenterol. Colon. Rect. Surg. 35, 11.

Board of the Faculty of Clinical Radiology (1996). Advice on the Management of Reactions to Intravenous Contrast Media. Royal College of Radiologists, London.

Böckman, S., Bodman, K.F., and Schuster, H.P. (1989). Anaphylaktischer Schock nach Röntgenkontrastmittel trotz Prämedikation mit Ausbildung eines akuten Myokardinfarktes. *Intensivmedizin Notfallmedizin* 26, 385.

Bøhn, H.P., Reich, L., and Suljaga-Petchel, K. (1992). Inadvertent intrathecal use of ionic contrast media for myelography. *AJNR* 13, 1515.

Bolt, R.J., Dillon, R.J., and Pollard, H.M. (1961). Interference with bilirubin excretion by a gall bladder dye (Bunamiodyl). *N. Engl. J. Med.* 265, 1043.

Bouachour, G., Varache, N., Szapiro, N., *et al.* (1991). Noncardiogenic pulmonary edema resulting from intravascular administration of contrast material. *AJR* 157, 255.

Brezis, M. and Epstein M. (1989). A closer look at radiocontrast-induced nephropathy. *N. Engl. J Med.* 320, 179.

Burchardt, C.P., Flenker, H., and Schoop, H.J. (1981). Tödlicher Kontrastmittelzwischenfall bei unbehandeltem Morbus Waldenström. *Dtsch. Med. Wochenschr.* 106, 1223.

Burd, D.A.R., Santis, G., and Milward, T.M. (1985). Severe extravasation injury: an avoidable iatrogenic disaster? *BMJ* 290, 1579.

Bush, W.H. and Swanson, D.P. (1991). Acute reactions to intravascular contrast media: types, risk factors, recognition and specific treatment. *AJR* 157, 1153.

Carella, A., Federico, F., Di Cuonzo, P., *et al.* (1982). Adverse side effects of metrizamide and iopamidol in myelography. *Neuroradiology* 22, 247.

Carena, J., Magnelli, P., Puebla, M., *et al.* (1991). Rhabdomiolisis associada a medio de contrast iodido. *Medicina* (B Aires) 51, 348.

Catterall, J.R., Ferguson, R.J., and Miller, H.C. (1981). Intravascular haemolysis with acute renal failure after angiocardiography. *BMJ* 282, 779.

Caulfield, J.B., Zir, L., and Harthorne, J.W. (1975). Blood calcium levels in the presence of angiographic contrast material. *Circulation* 52, 119.

Chagnac, Y., Hadani, M., and Goldhammer, Y. (1985). Myasthenic crisis after intravenous administration of iodinated contrast agent. *Neurology* 35, 1219.

Chamberlin, W.H., Stockman, G.D., and Wray, N.P. (1979). Shock and non-cardiogenic pulmonary edema following meglumine diatrizoate for intravenous pyelography. *Am. J. Med.* 67, 684.

Chang, J.C., Lee, D., and Gross, H.M. (1989). Acute thrombocytopenia after IV administration of a radiographic contrast medium. *AJR* 152, 947.

Chen, M.Y.M., Ansell, G., and Ott, D.J. (1996). Complications of diagnostic studies of the gastrointestinal tract. In *Complications in Diagnostic Imaging and Interventional Radiology* (3rd edn) (Ed. G. Ansell, M.A. Bettman, J.A. Kaufman, and R.A. Wilkins), p. 483. Blackwell Science, Cambridge, Mass.

Chiu, C.L. and Gambach, R.R. (1974). Hypaque pulmonary edema. A case report. *Radiology* 111, 91.

Cohan, R.H., Dunnick, N.R., and Bashore, T.M. (1988). Treatment of reactions to radiographic contrast material *AJR* 151, 263.

Cohan, R.H., Dunnick, N.R., Leder, R.A., *et al.* (1990). Extravasation of nonionic radiologic contrast media: efficiency of conservative treatment. *Radiology* 176, 65.

Cohen, L.S., Kokko, J.P., and Williams, W.H. (1969). Haemolysis and haemoglobinuria following angiography. *Radiology* 92, 329.

Cohen, M.D. (1993). A review of the toxicity of nonionic contrast agents in children. *Invest. Radiol.* 28 (Suppl. 5), 587.

Constantinescu, A., Negoescu, I., Don, M., *et al.* (1973). Effects of administration of some indigenous radiologic contrast media upon the thyroid function. Clinical and experimental studies. *Rev. Roum. Endocrinol.* 10, 49.

Corot. C., Chronos, N., and Sabattier, (1996). In vitro comparison of the effects of contrast media on coagulation and platelet activation. *Blood Coagul. Fibrinolysis* 7, 602.

Cooperman, L.R., Rossiter, S.B., Reimer, G.W., *et al.* (1968). Infusion cholangiography. Thirteen years experience with 1600 cases. *AJR* 104, 880.

Craft, I.L. and Swales, J.D. (1967). Renal failure after cholangiography. *BMJ* ii, 736.

Craig, J.O.M., Macpherson, P. (1991) *A Statement on Myodil.* Royal College of Radiologists, London.

Creteur, V., Douglas, D., Galante, M., *et al.* (1983). Inflammatory colonic changes produced by contrast material. *Radiology* 147, 77.

Curradi, F., Abbritti, G., and Gray, J.M. (1981). Acute thrombocytopenia following oral cholecystography with iopanoic acid. *Clin. Toxicol.* 18, 221.

Dachman, A.H. (1995). New contraindications to intravascular iodinated contrast material. *Radiology* 197, 545.

Daly, J., Fitzgerald, T., and Simpson, C.J. (1987). Pre-operative intravenous cholangiography as an alternative to routine operative cholangiography in elective cholecystectomy. *Clin. Radiol.* 38, 161.

Davies, A.M., Evans, N., and Chandy, J. (1989). Outpatient lumbar radiculography — comparison of iopamidol and iohexol and a literature review. *Br. J. Radiol.* 62, 716.

Davies, N.P. and Williams, J.A. (1971). Tubeless vagotomy and pyloroplasty and the 'Gastrografin test'. *Am. J. Surg.* 122, 368.

Davies, P., Roberts, M.B., and Roylance, J. (1975). Acute reaction to urographic contrast media. *BMJ* ii, 434.

Dawson, P. and Sidhu, P.S. (1993). Is there a role for corticosteroid prophylaxis in patients at increased risk of reactions to intravascular contrast agents. *Clin. Radiol.* 48, 225.

Dawson, P., Pitfield, J., and Britton, J. (1983). Contrast media and bronchospasm: a study with iopamidol. *Clin. Radiol.* 34, 227.

D'Elia, J.A., Gleason, R.E., Alday, M., *et al.* (1982). Nephrotoxicity from angiographic contrast media: a prospective study. *Am. J. Med.* 72, 719.

Deixonne, B., Baumel, H., and Mauras, Y. (1983). Un cas de barytopéritoine avec atteinte neurologique intérêt du dosage du barium dans les liquides biologiques. *J. Chir.* (Paris) 120, 611.

Deray, G. and Jacobs, C. (1996). [Review] Renal tolerance of nonionic dimers. *Invest. Radiol.* 31, 372.

Dohmen, J.P.M., Lemmens, J.A.M., and Lamers, J.J.H. (1981). A double blind comparison of meglumine iotroxate

(Biliscopin) and meglumine iodoxamate (Cholovue). *Diagn. Imaging* 50, 305.

Donaghy, M., Fletcher, N.A., and Schott, G.D. (1985). Encephalopathy after iohexol myelography. *Lancet*. ii, 887.

Drayer, B.P., Allen, S., and Vassalo, C. (1984). Comparative safety of intrathecal iopamidol vs metrizamide for myelography. *Invest. Radiol.* 9 (suppl.), S 259.

Drayer, B.P., Vassalo, C., Sudilovsky, A., *et al.* (1983). A double-blind trial of iopamidol versus metrizamide for lumbosacral myelography. *J. Neurosurg.* 58, 531.

Dupuy, F., Bestagne, M.H., Rodor, F., *et al.* (1980). Encéphalopathie convulsive et sulfate de barium. *Therapie* 35, 447.

Eastwood, G.L. (1972). E.C.G. abnormalities associated with the barium enema. *JAMA* 219, 719.

Eloy, R., Corot, C., Belleville, J. (1991). Contrast media for angiography: physicochemical properties, pharmacokinetics and biocompatibility. *Clinical Materials* 7, 89–197.

Esplugas, E., Cequir, A., Jara, F., *et al.* (1991). Risk of thrombosis during coronary angioplasty with low osmolality contrast media. *Am. J. Cardiol.* 68, 1020.

Fairhurst, B.J. and Naqvi, N. (1975). Hyperthyroidism after cholecystography. *BMJ* iii, 630.

Feczo, P.J., Simms, S.S., and Bakiri, N. (1989). Fatal hypersensitivity during a barium enema. *AJR* 153, 275.

Feigelson, H.H. and Ravin, H.A. (1965). Transverse myelitis following selective bronchial arteriography. *Radiology* 85, 663.

Finby, N. and Blasberg, G. (1964). A note on the blocking of hepatic excretion during cholangiographic study. *Gastroenterology* 46, 276.

Fischer, H.W. (1968). Hemodynamic reactions to angiographic media. A survey and commentary. *Radiology* 91, 66.

Fischer, H.W. and Doust, V.L. (1972). An evaluation of pretesting in the problem of serious and fatal reactions to excretory urography. *Radiology* 103, 497.

Fischer, W.W. and Nice, C.M. (1984). Barium impaction as a cause of small bowel obstruction in an infant with cystic fibrosis. *Pediatr. Radiol.* 14, 230.

Foda, M.T., Castillo, C.A., Corliss, R.J., *et al.* (1965). The intravascular pressure response in man to contrast substance used for angiography. *Am. J. Med. Sci.* 250, 390.

Foster, C.J., Griffin, J.F. (1987). A comparison of the incidence of cardiac arrhythmias produced by two intravenous contrast media in coronary artery disease. *Clin. Radiol.* 38, 399.

Fukuda, M., Ono, I., Takemasa, T., *et al.* (1989). A fatal case with non-hepatic hyperammonemic encephalopathy following rupture of the rectum during barium enema examination. *Shashin Igaku* 44, 2217.

Gallitano, A.L., Kondi, E.S., Phillips, E., and Ferris, E. (1976). Near-fatal hemorrhage following Gastrografin studies. *Radiology* 118, 35.

Gardiner, H. and Miller, R.E. (1973). Barium peritonitis. A new therapeutic approach. *Am. J. Surg.* 125, 350.

Gelfand, D.W., Sowers, J.C., De Ponte, K.A., *et al.* (1985). Anaphylactic and allergic reactions during double control studies: is glucagon or barium suspension the allergen? *AJR* 144, 405.

Gelman, M.L., Rowe, J.W., Coggins, C.H., *et al.* (1979). Effect of an angiographic contrast medium on renal function. *Cardiovasc. Med.* 4, 313.

Gensini, G.G. and Di Giorgi, S. (1964). Myocardial toxicity of contrast agents used in angiography. *Radiology* 82, 24.

Gertz, E.W., Wisneski, J.A., Miller, R., *et al.* (1992). Adverse reactions of low osmolality contrast media during cardiac angiography: a prospective randomised multicenter study. *J. Am. Coll. Cardiol.* 19, 899.

Gmeinwieser, J., Erhardt, W., Reimann, H.J., *et al.* (1990). Side effects of water-soluble contrast agents in upper gastrointestinal tract. *Invest. Radiol.* 25, S27.

Godson, C., Ryan, M.P., and Brady, H.R. (1988). Acute hypomagnesaemia complicating the treatment of meconium ileus equivalent in cystic fibrosis. *Scand. J. Gastroenterol.* 23 (Suppl. 143), 148.

Golman, K. and Almén, T. (1985). Contrast media induced nephrotoxicity: survey and present state. *Invest. Radiol.* 20 (1 Suppl.), S 92.

Gonsette, R.E. and Liesenborgh, L. (1980). New contrast media in cerebral angiography: animal experiments and preliminary clinical studies. *Invest. Radiol.* 15 (Suppl. 6), S270.

Grabowski, E.F., Head, C., and Michelson, A.D. (1993). Nonionic contrast media, procoagulants or clotting innocents? *Invest. Radiol.* 28 (Suppl. 5), S21.

Grainger, R.G. (1987). Annotation: Radiological contrast media. *Clin. Radiol.* 38, 3.

Grainger, R.G. and Dawson, P. (1990). Low osmolar contrast media: an appraisal (editorial). *Clin. Radiol.* 42, 1.

Greenberger, P.A. and Patterson, R. (1988). Adverse reactions to radiocontrast media. *Progr. Cardiovasc. Dis.* 31, 239.

Griffiths, J. and White, P. (1994). Acute asthma precipitated by accidental inhalation of sodium bicarbonate granules (Carbex). *Clin. Radiol.* 49, 435.

Grines, C.L., Schreiber, T.C., Savas, V., *et al.* (1996). A randomised trial of low osmolar ionic versus nonionic contrast media in patients with myocardial infarction or unstable angina undergoing percutaneous transluminal coronary angioplasty. *J. Am. Coll. Cardiol.* 27, 1381.

Grollman, J.H., Liu, C.R., Astone, R.A., *et al.* (1988). Thromboembolic complications in coronary angiography associated with the use of non-ionic contrast medium. *Cathet. Cardiovasc. Diagn.* 14, 159.

Haley, E.C. (1984). Encephalopathy following arteriography: a possible toxic effect of contrast agents. *Ann. Neurol.* 15, 100.

Hamilton, I., Lintott, D.J., Rothwell, J., *et al.* (1983). Acute pancreatitis following endoscopic retrograde cholangiopancreatography. *Clin. Radiol.* 34, 543.

Hammeke, T.A., Haughton, V.M., Grogan, J.P., *et al.* (1984). A preliminary study of cognitive and affective alterations following intrathecal administration of iopamidol or metrizamide. *Invest. Radiol.* 19 (Suppl.), S 268.

Hammer, J.L. (1977). Septicaemia following barium enema. *South. Med. J.* 70, 1361.

Harrington, G.J. and Weideman, M.P. (1965). The effect of contrast media on endothelial permeability. *Radiology* 84, 1108.

Harris, P.D., Neuhauser, E.B.D., and Gerth, R. (1964). The osmotic effect of water soluble contrast media on circulating plasma volume. *AJR* 91, 694.

Hartman, G.W., Hattery, R.R., Witten, D.M., *et al.* (1982). Mortality during excretory urography: Mayo Clinic experience. *AJR* 139, 919.

Hay, M. and Cant, P.J. (1990). Case report: renal excretion of enteral Gastrografin in the absence of free intestinal perforation. *Clin. Radiol.* 41, 137.

Heidemann, P.H., Stubbe, P., Schurrnbrand, P., *et al.* (1982). Iodine-induced hypothyroidism and goitre following Lipiodol TH lymphangiography. *Eur. J. Pediatr.* 138, 82.

Herrington, J.L. (1966). Barium granuloma within the peritoneal cavity: ureteral obstruction 7 years after barium enema and colonic perforation. *Ann. Surg.* 164, 162.

Hesselink, J.R., Hayman, L.A., Chung, J.G., *et al.* (1984). Myocardial ischaemia during intravenous DSA in patients with cardiac disease. *Radiology* 153, 577.

Heydenreich, G. and Olholm Larsen, P. (1977). Iododerma after high-dose urography in an oliguric patient. *Br. J. Dermatol.* 97, 567.

Hindmarsh, T., Ekholm, S.E., Kido, D., *et al.* (1984). Lumbar myelography with iohexol and metrizamide, a double-blind clinical trial. *Acta Radiol. [Diagn.]* (Stockh.) 25, 365.

Hoffman, B., Becker, H., and Wenzel-Hora, B.I. (1987). Influence of spread and retention of iotrolan in the subarachnoid space on the side effects in myelography. *Neuroradiology* 29, 380.

Hoppe, J.O. (1959). Some pharmacological aspects of radio-opaque compounds. *Ann. N.Y. Acad. Sci.* 78, 727.

Hou, S.H., Bushinsky, D.A., Wish, J.B., *et al.* (1983). Hospital-acquired renal insufficiency: a prospective study. *Am. J. Med.* 74, 243.

Hugh, T.B., Hennessy, W.B., Gunner, W., *et al.* (1970). Precipitation of contrast medium causing impaction of Sengstaken–Blakemore oesophageal tube. *Med. J. Aust.* 1, 60.

Hwang, M.H., Piao, Z.E., Murdock, D.K., *et al.* (1989). The potential risk of thrombosis during coronary angiography using non-ionic contrast media. *Cathet. Cardiovasc. Diagn.* 16, 209.

Hysell, L.K., Hysell, J.W., and Gray, J.M. (1977). Thrombocytopenic purpura following iopanoic acid ingestion. *JAMA* 237, 361.

Iannone, L.A. (1975). Protamine–Renografin chemical embolus. *Am. Heart J.* 90, 678.

Idée, J.M., Beaufils, H., and Bonneman, B. (1994). Review. Iodinated contrast media-induced nephropathy: pathophysiology, clinical aspects and prevention. *Fundam. Clin. Pharmacol.* 8, 193.

Insauti, C.L.G., Lechin, F., and van der Digs, B. (1983). Severe thrombocytopenia following oral cholecystography. *Am. J. Hematol.* 14, 285.

Jacobsson, L. and Saltzman, G.F. (1971). Effect of iodinated roentgenographic contrast media on butanol-extractable protein-bound and total iodine in serum. *Acta Radiol. [Diagn.]* (Stockh.) 11, 310.

Jakobsen. J.Å., Lundby, B., Kristofferson, D.T., *et al.* (1992). Evaluation of renal function with delayed CT after injection of nonionic monomeric and dimeric media in healthy volunteers. *Radiology* 182, 419.

Jamet, P., Lebas de Lacour, J.Cl., Christoforou, B., *et al.* (1980). Acidose lactique mortelle après urographie intra-veineuse chez une diabétique recevant de la metformin. *Sem. Hôp.* Paris 56, 473.

Janower, M.L. (1986). Hypersensitivity reactions after barium studies of the upper and lower gastrointestinal tract. *Radiology* 161, 139.

Junck, L. and Marshall, W.H. (1986). Fatal brain edema after contrast-agent overdose. *AJNR* 7, 522.

Karasick, S. and Karasick, D. (1981). Acute urate nephropathy induced by Ticrynafen and exacerbated by urographic contrast medium. *Urol. Radiol.* 3, 51.

Katayama, H. (1988). Report of the Japanese Committee on the Safety of Contrast Media. A scientific poster session presented at the Radiological Society of North America Meeting November 1988.

Katayama, H., Yamaguchi, K., Kozuka, T., *et al.* (1990). Adverse reactions to ionic and non-ionic media. A report from the Japanese Committee on the Safety of Contrast Media. *Radiology* 175, 621.

Kendall, B. (1989). Safety aspects and tolerability of non-ionic contrast media — subarachnoid use. In *Patient Safety and Adverse Events in Contrast Media Examinations* (ed. I. Enge and J. Edgren). Excerpta Medica Medical International Congress Series 816, p. 47. Elsevier, Amsterdam.

Kendal, B. (1996). Complications of diagnostic neuroangiography. In *Complications in Diagnostic Imaging and Interventional Radiology* (3rd edn) (ed. G. Ansell, M.A. Bettman, J.A. Kaufman, and R.A. Wilkins), p. 437. Blackwell Science, Cambridge, Mass.

Klow, N.E., Levorstad, K., Berg, J., *et al.* (1993). Iodixanol in cardioangiography in patients with coronary artery disease. Tolerability, cardiac and renal effects. *Acta Radiol.* 34, 72.

Klumair, J. and Pflanzer, K. (1977). Der Einfluss oraler Antidiabetica (Sulphonylharnstoffe) auf die Ausscheidung intravenöser Gallenkontrastmittel. *Fortschr. Röntgenstr.* 126, 66.

Knutsen, K.M. and Teisberg, P. (1978). Serious adverse reactions in intravenous cholangiography (with Biligram) in lymphoproliferative disorders. *Tidskr. Nor. Laegeforen.* 98, 328.

Koch, R.L., Byl, F.M., and Firpo, J.J. (1969). Parotid swelling with facial paralysis: complication of intravenous urography. *Radiology* 92, 1043.

Kone, B.C., Watson, A.J., Gimenez, L.F., *et al.* (1986). Acute renal failure following percutaneous transhepatic cholangiography: a retrospective study. *Arch. Intern. Med.* 146, 1405.

Lacey, J., Bober-Sorcinelli, K.E., Farber, L.R., *et al.* (1986). Acute thrombocytopenia induced by parenteral radiographic contrast medium. *AJR* 146, 1298.

Lalli, A.F. (1980). Contrast media reactions: data analysis and hypothesis. *Radiology* 131, 1.

Lalli, A.F. (1984). Contrast media deaths. *Australas. Radiol.* 28, 133.

Lang, D.M., Alpern, M.B., Visintainer, P.F., *et al.* (1991). Increased risk for anaphylactoid reaction from contrast media in patients on β-adrenergic blockers or with asthma. *Ann. Intern. Med.* 115, 270.

Lasser, E.C. (1971). Metabolic basis of contrast material toxicity. Status 1971. *AJR* 113, 415.

Lasser, E.C. (1988*a*). A general and personal perspective on contrast material research. *Invest. Radiol.* 23 (Suppl. 1), S71.

Lasser, E.C. (1988*b*). Pretreatment with corticosteroids to prevent reactions to IV contrast material: overview and implications. *AJR* 150, 257.

Lasser, E.C. (1989). Allergy and allergic-like reactions in relation to contrast media. In *Patient Safety and Adverse Events in Contrast Medium Examinations* (ed. I. Enge and J. Edgren), p. 57. Elsevier, Amsterdam.

Lasser, E.C., Lang, J.H., and Zawadzki, Z.A. (1966). Contrast media/myeloma protein precipitates in urography. *JAMA* 198, 945.

Lasser, E.C., Lang, J.H., Hamblin, A.E., *et al.* (1980). Activation systems in contrast idiosyncrasy. *Invest. Radiol.* 15 (Suppl. 6), S2.

Lasser, E.C., Lang, J.H., Sovak, M., *et al.* (1977). Steroids: theoretical and experimental basis for utilization in prevention of contrast media reactions. *Radiology* 125, 1.

Lasser, E.C., Berry, C.C., Talner, L.B., *et al.* (1987). Pretreatment with corticosteroids to alleviate reactions to intravenous contrast material. *N. Engl. J. Med.* 317, 845.

Lasser, E.C., Berry, C.C., Mishkin, M.M., *et al.* (1994). Pretreatment with corticosteroids to prevent reactions to nonionic contrast media. *AJR* 162, 523.

Lea Thomas, M. (1987). Phlebography. In *Complications in Diagnostic Imaging* (2nd edn) (ed. G. Ansell and R.A. Wilkins), p. 288. Blackwell Scientific, Oxford.

Lea Thomas, M., Walters, H.L., and Briggs, G.M. (1982). A double blind comparative study of the tolerance of sodium and meglumine ioxaglate (Hexabrix) with meglumine iothalamate (Conray) in ascending phlebography of the leg. *Australas. Radiol.* 26, 288.

Lea Thomas, M., Keeling, F.P., Piaggio, R.B., *et al.* (1984). Contrast agent induced thrombophlebitis following leg phlebography: iopamidol versus meglumine iothalamate. *Br. J. Radiol.* 57, 205.

Leach, C.A. and Sunderman, F.W. (1987). Hypernickelemia following coronary arteriography caused by nickel in the radiographic contrast medium. *Ann. Clin. Lab. Sci.* 17, 137.

Lee, S. and Schoen, I. (1966). Black-copper reduction reaction simulating alcaptonuria — occurrence after intravenous urography. *N. Engl. J. Med.* 275, 266.

LeFrock, J., Ellis, C.A., Klainer, A.S., *et al.* (1975). Transient bacteraemia associated with barium enema. *Arch. Intern. Med.* 135, 835.

Leonardi, M., Lavaroni, A., Biasizzo, E., *et al.* (1989). High-dose contrast-enhanced computed tomography (CECT) with iopamidol in the detection of cerebral metastases. Tolerance of the contrast agent. *Neuroradiology* 31, 148.

Leung, P.L. and Cheng, C.Y. (1980). Extensive local necrosis following the intravenous use of X-ray contrast medium in the upper extremity. *Br. J. Radiol.* 53, 361.

Levin, D.C. and Gardiner, G.A. (1992). Coronary arteriography. In *Heart Disease. A Textbook of Cardiovascular Medicine* (ed. E. Braunwald). W.B. Saunders, Philadelphia.

Lindgren, P. (1970). Haemodynamic responses to contrast media. *Invest. Radiol.* 5, 424.

Lindgren, P., Saltzman, G.F., and Zeuchner, E. (1974). Intravenous cholecystography after peroral contraceptives. A preliminary report. *Acta Radiol. [Diagn.]* (Stockh.) 15, 217.

Lipman, J.C., Wang, A-M., Brooks, R.M., *et al.* (1983). Seizure after intrathecal administration of iopamidol. *AJNR* 9, 787.

Liss, P. (1997). Effects of contrast media on renal microcirculation. An experimental study in the rat. *Acta Radiol.* 38 (Suppl.), 409.

Love, L., Lind, J.A., and Olson, M.C. (1989). Persistent CT nephrogram: significance in the diagnosis of contrast nephropathy. *Radiology* 172, 125.

Lull, G., Bryne, P., and Sanowski, A. (1971). Barium sulfate granuloma of the rectum. A rare entity. *JAMA* 217, 1102.

Lundervold, A. and Engeset, A. (1976). Cerebral angiography. In *Complications in Diagnostic Radiology* (ed. G. Ansell), p. 151. Blackwell Scientific, Oxford.

McCleery, W.N.C. and Lewtas, N.A. (1966). Subarachnoid injection of contrast medium — a complication of vertebral angiography. *Br. J. Radiol.* 39, 122.

McClennan, B.L. (1993). Contrast media alert. *Radiology* 189, 35.

McClennan, B.L., Kassner, E.G., and Becker, J.A. (1972). Overdose at excretory urography: toxic cause of death. *Radiology* 105, 383.

McCullough, M., Davies, P., and Richardson, R. (1989). A large trial of intravenous Conray 325 and Niopam 300 to assess immediate and delayed reactions. *Br. J. Radiol.* 62, 260.

MacDonald, J.S. (1987). Lymphography. In *Complications in Diagnostic Imaging* (2nd edn) (ed. G. Ansell and R.A. Wilkins), p. 300. Blackwell Scientific, Oxford.

McIvor, J., Steiner, T.J., Perkin, G.D., *et al.* (1987). Neurological morbidity of arch and carotid arteriography: the influence of contrast medium and radiologist. *Br. J. Radiol.* 60, 117.

McNair, J.D. (1972). Selective coronary angiography. Report of a fatality in a patient with sickle cell hemoglobin. *Calif. Med.* 117, 71.

McPhaul, M., Punzi, H.A., Sandy, A., *et al.* (1984). Snuff-induced hypertension in pheochromocytoma. *JAMA* 252, 2860.

Mahlstedt, J. and Joseph, K. (1973). Decompensation of autonomous thyroid adenoma after long-term iodine intake. *Dtsch. Med. Wochenschr.* 98, 1748.

Malins, A.F. (1978). Pulmonary oedema after radiological investigation of peripheral occlusive vascular disease. Adverse reaction to contrast media. *Lancet* i, 413.

Mallat, Z., Vassa, T., Naouri, J.F., *et al.* (1991). Aseptic meningoencephalitis after myelography. *Lancet* 338, 252.

Mallette, L.E. and Gomez, L.S. (1983). Systemic hypocalcaemia after clinical injections of radiographic contrast media: amelioration by omission of calcium chelating agents. *Radiology* 147, 677.

Mandell, G.A., Swacus, J.R., Rosenstock, J., *et al.* (1983). Danger of urography in hyperuricaemic children with Burkitt's lymphoma. *J. Can. Assoc. Radiol.* 34, 273.

Måre, K. and Violante, M (1983). Pulmonary edema induced by high intravenous doses of diatrizoate in the rat. *Acta Radiol. [Diagn.]* (Stockh.) 24, 419.

Måre, K., Violante, M., and Zack, A. (1984). Contrast media induced pulmonary edema. Comparison of ionic and nonionic agents in an animal model. *Invest. Radiol.* 19, 566.

Måre, K., Violante, M., and Zack, A. (1985). Pulmonary edema following high intravenous doses of diatrizoate in the rat: effect of corticosteroid pretreatment. *Acta Radiol. [Diagn.]* (Stockh.) 26, 477.

Memolo, M., Dyer, R., and Zagonia, R.J. (1993). Extravasation injury with nonionic material. *AJR* 160, 203.

Miller, S.H. (1997). Anaphylactic reaction after oral administration of diatrizoate meglumine and diatrizoate sodium solution. *AJR* 168, 959.

Miller, G., Fuchs, W.A., and Preisig, R. (1969). Die Infusioncholangiographie in physiologischer Sicht. *Schweiz. Med. Wochenschr.* 99, 577.

Mills, J.O.M. (1990). Inhalation of Carbex. *Clin. Radiol.* 41, 69.

Mills, S.R., Jackson, D.C., Older, R.A., *et al.* (1980). The incidence, etiologies and avoidance of complications of pulmonary angiography in a large series. *Radiology* 136, 295.

Mishkin, M.M., Baum, S., and Di Chiro, G. (1973). Emergency treatment of angiography-induced paraplegia and tetraplegia. *N. Engl. J. Med.* 288, 1184.

Mizuno, M., Tsuya, Y., and Nomura, Y. (1992). Vestibular disturbance after myelography. *Oto-Rhino-Laryngol.* (Tokyo) 54, 113.

Monroe, L.S. and Longmore, W.J. (1966). Inhibition of sulfobromophthalein (BSP) conjugation with glutathione by iopanoic acid (Telepaque). *Gastroenterology* 50, 396.

Moore, R.D., Steinberg, E.P., Powe, N.R., *et al.* (1989). Frequency and determinants of adverse reactions induced by high-osmolality contrast media. *Radiology* 170, 727.

Morcos, S.K., Oldroyd, S., and Haylor, J. (1997). Contrast media induced nephrotoxicity: a new insight. *Clin. Radiol.* 52, 573.

Moreau, J.F., Droz, D., Sabto, J., *et al.* (1975). Osmotic nephrosis induced by water-soluble tri-iodinated contrast media in man. A retrospective study of 47 cases. *Radiology* 115, 329.

Morris, T.W. (1993). The phsyiologic effects of non ionic media on the heart. *Invest. Radiol.* 28 (Suppl. 5), 544.

Morris, S., Sahler, L.G., and Fischer, H.W. (1982). Calcium binding by radiopaque media. *Invest. Radiol.* 17, 501.

Mozley, P.D. (1981). Malignant hyperthermia following intravenous iodinated contrast media. Report of a fatal case. *Diagn. Gynecol. Obstet.* 3, 81.

Mudge, G.H. (1971). Uricosuric action of cholecystographic agents. A possible factor in nephrotoxicity. *N. Engl. J. Med.* 284, 929.

Murphy, G., Campbell, D.R., and Fraser, D.B. (1988). Pain in peripheral arteriography: an assessment of conventional versus ionic and non-ionic low osmolality contrast agents. *J. Canad. Assoc. Radiol.* 39: 103.

Nahrwold, D.L., Isch, J.H., Benner, R.E., *et al.* (1971). Effect of fluid administration and operation on the mortality rate in barium peritonitis. *Surgery* 70, 778.

Nakstad, P., Sortland, O., Aaserud, O., *et al.* (1982). Cerebral angiography with the non-ionic water-soluble contrast medium iohexol and meglumine-ca-metrizoate. *Neuroradiology* 23, 199.

Navani, S., Taylor, C.E., Kaufman, S.A., *et al.* (1972). Evanescent enlargement of salivary glands following tri-iodinated contrast media. *Br. J. Radiol.* 45. 19.

Nelson, J.A., Pepper, H.W., Goldberg, H.I., *et al.* (1973). Effect of phenobarbital on iodipamide and iopanoate bile excretion. *Invest. Radiol.* 8, 126.

Nicot, G.S., Merle, L.J., Charmes, J.P., *et al.* (1984). Transient glomerular proteinuria, enzymuria, and nephrototoxic reaction induced by radiocontrast media. *JAMA* 252, 2432.

Nilsson, U. (1987). Adverse reactions to iotrexate at intravenous cholangiography. *Acta Radiol.* 28, 571.

Nogrady, M.B. and Dunbar, J.S. (1968). Delayed concentration and prolonged excretion of urographic contrast medium in the first month of life. *AJR* 104, 289.

Nolan, D.J. and Gibson, M.J. (1970). Improvements in intravenous cholangiography. *Br. J. Radiol.* 43, 652.

Older, R.A., Korobkin, M., Cleeve, D.M., *et al.* (1980). Contrast-induced acute renal failure. Persistent nephrogram as clue to early detection. *AJR* 134, 339.

Pagani, J.G., Hayman, L.A., Bigelow, R.H., *et al.* (1984). Prophylactic diazepam in prevention of contrast media-induced seizures in glioma patients undergoing cerebral computed tomography. *Cancer* 54, 2200.

Palmer, F.J. (1989). The Royal Australasian College of Radiologists' (RACR) survey of reactions of intravenous ionic and non-ionic contrast media. In *Patient Safety and Adverse Events in Contrast Medium Examination.* (ed. I. Enge and J. Edgren). Excerpta Medica International Congress Series 816, p. 137. Elsevier, Amsterdam.

Panto, P.N. and Davies, P. (1986). Delayed reactions to urographic contrast media. *Br. J. Radiol.* 59, 41.

Parry, R., Ress, J., and Wilde, P. (1993). Transient cortical blindness after coronary angiography. *Br. Heart J.* 70, 563.

Parvez, R., Moncada, R., Messmore, H.L., *et al.* (1982). Ionic and non-ionic contrast media interaction with anticoagulant drugs. *Acta Radiol. [Diagn.]* (Stockh.) 23, 401.

Pascuzzi, R.M., Roos, K.L., and Scott, J.A. (1988). Chronic focal seizure disorders as a manifestation of intracranial iophendylate. *Epilepsia* 29, 294.

Pendergrass, H.P., Tondreau, R.L., Pendergrass, E.P., *et al.* (1958). Reactions associated with intravenous urography — historical and statistical review. *Radiology* 71, 1.

Penry, J.B. and Livingstone, A. (1972). A comparison of diagnostic effectiveness and vascular side-effects of various diatrizoate salts used for intravenous pyelography. *Clin. Radiol.* 23, 362.

Pfister, R.C. and Hutter, A.M., Jr (1980). Cardiac alterations during intravenous urography. *Invest. Radiol.* 15 (Suppl. 6), S239.

Pilla, T.J., Beshany, S.E., and Shields, J.B. (1986). Incompatibility of Hexabrix and papaverine. *AJR* 146, 1300.

Piscione, F., Focaccio, A., Santinelli, V., *et al.* (1990). Are ioxaglate and iopamidol equally safe and well tolerated in cardiac angiography? A randomized double-blind clinical study. *Am. Heart J.* 120, 1130.

Prout, B.J., Datta, S.B., and Wilson, T.S. (1972). Colonic retention of barium in the elderly after barium-meal examination and its treatment with lactulose. *BMJ* iv, 530.

Ramsay, A.W., Spector, M., Rodgers, A.L., *et al.* (1982). Crystalluria following excretory urography. *Br. J. Urol.* 54, 341.

Rao, A.K., Thompson, R., Durlacher, L., *et al.* (1985). Angiographic contrast agent-induced acute hemolysis in a patient with hemoglobin SC disease. *Arch. Intern. Med.* 145, 759.

Rao, V.M., Rao, A.K., Steiner, R.M., *et al.* (1982). The effect of ionic and non-ionic contrast media on the sickling phenomenon. *Radiology* 144, 291.

Ratcliff, G., Sandler, S., and Latchaw, R. (1986). Cognitive and affective changes after myelography: a comparison of metrizamide and iohexol. *AJNR* 7, 683.

Rheuther, G., Kiefer, B., and Tuchmann, A. (1996). Cholangiography before biliary surgery: single-shot MR versus intravenous cholangiography. *Radiology* 198, 561.

Richards, D. and Nulsen, F.E. (1971). Angiographic media and the sickling phenomenon. *Surg. Forum* 22, 403.

Ring, J., Rothernberger, K-H., and Clauss, W. (1985). Prevention of anaphylactoid reactions after radiographic contrast media infusion by combined H_1- and H_2-receptor antagonists: results of a prospective clinical trial. *Int. Arch. Allergy Appl. Immunol.* 78, 9.

Robertson, H.J.E. (1987). Blood clot formation in angiographic syringes containing non-ionic media. *Radiology* 162, 621.

Rosati, G., Leto di Priolo, S., and Tirone, P. (1992). Serious fatal complications after inadvertent administration of ionic water-soluble contrast media in myelography. *Eur. J. Radiol.* 15, 95.

Ross, L.S. (1972). Precipitation of meglumine diatrizoate 76% (Gastrografin) in the stomach. Observations on the insolubility of diatrizoate in the normal range of gastric acidity. *Radiology* 105, 19.

Rowe, M.I., Furst, A.H., Altman, D.H., *et al.* (1971). The neonatal response to Gastrografin enema. *Pediatrics* 48, 29.

Rudnick M.R., Goldfarb, S., Wexler, L., *et al.* (1995). Nephrotoxicity of ionic and nonionic contrast media in 1196 patients: a randomized trial. *Kidney Int.* 47, 254.

Sable, R.A., Rosenthal, W.S., and Seigle, J. (1983). Absorption of contrast medium during ERCP. *Dig. Dis. Sci.* 28, 801.

Saltzman, G.F. and Sundstrom, K-A. (1960). The influence of different contrast media for cholangiography on blood pressure and pulse rate. *Acta Radiol.* 54, 353.

Sampson, C.B. (1993). Adverse drug reactions and drug interactions with radiopharmaceuticals. *Drug Safety* 8, 280.

Schiro, J.C., Ricci, J.A., Tristan, T.A., *et al.* (1971). Transient renal insufficiency secondary to iopanoic acid. *Pennsylvania Med. J.* 74, 53.

Scholtz, F.J., Johnson, D.O., and Wise, R.E. (1974). Hepatotoxicity in cholangiography. *JAMA* 229, 1724.

Schwartz, E.E., Glick, S.N., Foggs, M.B., *et al.* (1984). Hypersensitivity reactions after barium enema examination. *AJR* 143, 937.

Seltzer, S.E. and Jones, B. (1978). Cecal perforation associated with Gastrografin enema. *AJR* 130, 997.

Setter, J.G., Maher, J.F., and Schreiner, G.E. (1963). Acute renal failure following cholecystography. *Acta Radiol.* (Stockh.) 3, 353.

Seymour, P.C. and Kesack, C.D. (1997). Anaphylactic shock during a routine upper gastrointestinal series. *AJR* 168, 957.

Shehadi, W.H. (1975). Adverse reactions to intravascularly administered contrast media: a comprehensive study based on a prospective study. *AJR* 124, 145.

Shehadi, W.H. and Toniolo, G. (1980). Adverse reactions to contrast media. A report from the Committee on safety of contrast media of the International Society of Radiology. *Radiology* 137, 299.

Shellock, F.G., Harn, H.P., Mink, J.H., *et al.* (1993). Adverse reaction to intravenous gadoteridol. *Radiology* 189, 151.

Shetty, S.P., Murthy, G.G., Shreeve, W.W., *et al.* (1974). Hyperthyroidism after pyelography. *N. Engl. J. Med.* 291, 682.

Shimura, H., Takazawa, K., Endo, T., *et al.* (1990). T_4-thyroid storm after CT scan with iodinated contrast medium. *J. Endocrinol. Invest.* 13, 73.

Shojania, M. (1985). Immune-mediated thrombocytopenia due to an iodinated contrast medium. *Can. Med. Assoc. J.* 133, 123.

Simon, A.L., Shabetai, R., Lang, J.H., *et al.* (1972). The mechanism of production of ventricular fibrillation in coronary angiography. *AJR* 114, 810.

Sistrom, C.L., Gay, S.B., and Peffley, R.N. (1991). Extravasation of iopamidol and iohexol during contrast-enhanced CT: report of 28 cases. *Radiology* 180, 707.

Skalpe, I.C. (1988). Complications in cerebral angiography with iohexol (Omnipaque) and meglumine metrizoate (Isopaque Cerebral). *Neuroradiology* 30, 69.

Slasky. B.S. (1981). Acute renal failure, contrast media, and computer tomography. *Urology* 28, 309.

Smith, H.J., Jones, K., and Hunter, T.B. (1988). What happens to patients after upper and lower gastrointestinal tract barium studies? *Invest. Radiol.* 23, 822.

Soloman, D.R. (1986). Anaphylactoid reaction and non-cardiac pulmonary edema following intravascular administration of contrast media. *Am. J. Emerg. Med.* 4, 146.

Soriano-Soriano, C., Jimenez-Jimenez, F.J., Egido-Herero, J.A., *et al.* (1992). Acute encephalopathy following myelography with iohexol. *Acta Neurol.* 14, 127.

Spataro, R.F., Katzberg, R.W., Fischer, H.W., *et al.* (1987). High-dose clinical urography with the low- osmolality contrast agent Hexabrix: comparison with a conventional contrast agent. *Radiology* 162, 9.

Stadalnik, R.C., Vera, Z., DaSilva, O., *et al.* (1977). Electrocardiographic response to intravenous urography: prospective evaluation of 275 patients. *AJR* 129, 825.

Staubli, M., Braunschweig, J., and Tillman, U. (1982). Changes in the rheological properties of blood as induced by sodium/meglumine ioxaglate as compared with sodium/meglumine diatrizoate and metrizamide. *Acta Radiol. [Diagn.]* (Stockh.) 23, 401.

Stein, H.L. and Hilgartner, M.W. (1968). Alteration of coagulation mechanism of blood by contrast media. *AJR* 104, 458.

Stemerman, M., Goldstein, M.L., and Schulman, P.L. (1971). Pancytopenia associated with diatrizoate. *N.Y. State J. Med.* 11, 1220.

Stinchcombe, S.J. and Davies, P. (1989). Acute toxic myopathy: a delayed adverse effect of intravenous urography with iopamidol 370. *Br. J. Radiol.* 62, 949.

Stordahl, A., Haider, T., and Laerum, F. (1989). Acute lethality after enteral administration of contrast media in anaesthetised rats with intestinal ischaemia. *Acta Radiol. [Diagn.]* (Stockh.) 30, 213.

Sussman, R.M. and Miller, J. (1956). Iodide mumps after intravenous urography. *N. Engl. J. Med.* 255, 433.

Sutherland, L.R., Edwards, L.A., Medline, A., *et al.* (1977). Meglumine iodipamide (Cholografin) hepatotoxicity. *Ann. Intern. Med.* 86, 437.

Tahta, K., Özgent, T., Berker, M., *et al.* (1993). Status epilepticus following iohexol myelography. *Neuroradiology* 35, 322.

Tajima, H., Kumazaki, T., Tajima, N., *et al.* (1988). Effect of iohexol and diatrizoate on pulmonary arterial pressure following pulmonary angiography. A clinical comparison in man. *Acta Radiol. [Diagn.]* (Stockh.) 29, 487.

Takebayashi, S., Sugiyama, M., Magase, M. (1993). Severe adverse reaction to IV gadopentate dimeglumine. *AJR* 160, 659.

Talner, L.B., Lang, J.H., Brasch, R.C., *et al.* (1971). Elevated salivary iodine and salivary gland enlargement due to iodinated contrast media. *AJR* 112, 380.

Tardy, B., Guy, C., Barbral, G., *et al.* (1992). Anaphylactic shock induced by intravenous gadopentate dimeglumine. *Lancet* 339, 494.

Tartiere, J., Gerard, J-L., Peny, J., *et al.* (1989). Acute treatment after accidental intrathecal injection of hypertonic contrast medium. *Anesthesiology* 71, 169.

Tejler, L., Almen, T., and Holtas, S. (1977). Proteinuria following nephroangiography, 1. Clinical experiences. *Acta Radiol. [Diagn.]* (Stockh.) 18, 634.

Teplick, R.M. and Sanen, F.J. (1965). Acute renal failure following oral cholecystography. *Acta Radiol.* (Stockh.) 3, 353.

Thompson, G.J.L., Simpson, C.J., and Hansell, D.T. (1984). The early diagnosis of acute gallbladder disease: the accuracy of overnight eight-hour infusion cholangiography. *Br. J. Radiol.* 57, 685.

Thompson, W.M., Mills, S.R., Bates, M., *et al.* (1983). Pulmonary angiography with iopamidol and Renografin 76 in normal and pulmonary hypertensive dogs. *Acta Radiol. [Diagn.]* (Stockh.) 24, 425.

Thomson, H.S. and Dorph, S. (1993). High-osmolar and low-osmolar contrast media. An update on frequency of adverse drug reactions [Review article]. *Acta Radiol.* 34, 205.

Tishler, J.M. and Gold, R. (1969). A clinical trial of oral cholecystographic agents: Telepaque, Sodium Oragrafin and Calcium Oragrafin. *J. Can. Assoc. Radiol.* 20, 102.

Trewhella, M., Dawson, P., Forsling, M., *et al.* (1990). Vasopressin release in response to intravenously injected contrast media. *Br. J. Radiol.* 63, 97.

van den Bergh, P., Kelly, J.J., Carter, B., *et al.*(1986). Intravascular contrast media and neuromuscular junction disorders. *Ann. Neurol.* 19, 206.

van Sonnenberg, E., Neff, C.C., and Pfister, R.C. (1987). Life-threatening reactions to contrast media administration: comparison of pharmacologic and fluid therapy. *Radiology* 162, 15.

Vari, R.C., Laksmi, A., Natarajan, L.A., *et al.* (1988). Induction, prevention and mechanisms of contrast-media-induced acute renal failure. *Kidney Int.* 33, 699.

Vincent, M.E., Gerzof, S.G., and Robbins, A.H. (1977). Benign transient eosinophilia following intravenous urography. *JAMA* 237, 2629.

Von Rohner, G., Rautenberg, H.W., and Höffner, B. (1983). Transiente Hypothyreose bei Saüglingen nach Röntgencontrastmitteln. *Röntgenpraxis* 36, 301.

Wagner, A., Jensen, C., Saebye, A., *et al.* (1994). A prospective comparison of iotrolan and iohexol in lumbar myelography. *Acta Radiol.* 35, 182.

Wangermez, J. (1975). La prévention des accidents par la cholangiographie-perfusion. Comparaison entre les corticoïdes et l'acide tranéxamique. *J. Radiol. Electrol.* 56, 142.

Weinstein, G.S., O'Doriso, T.M., and Joehl, R.J. (1985). Exacerbation of diarrhoea after iodinated contrast agents in a patient with a VIPoma. *Digest. Dis. Sci.* 30, 588.

Whitney, B. and Bell, G.D. (1972). Simple bolus injection or slow infusion for intravenous cholangiography? Measurement of iodipamide (Biligrafin) excretion using a rhesus monkey model. *Br. J. Radiol.* 45, 891.

Winearls, C.G., Ledingham, J.G.G., and Dixon, A.J. (1980). Acute renal failure precipitated by radiographic contrast medium in a patient with rhabdomyolysis. *BMJ* 281, 1603.

Witten, D.M., Hirsch, F.D., and Hartman, G.W. (1973). Acute reactions to urographic contrast medium. Incidence, clinical characteristics and relationship to history of hypersensitivity states. *AJR* 119, 832.

Wolf, G.L., Mishkin, M.M., Roux, S.G., *et al.* (1991). Ionic contrast agents, ionic agents combined with steroids and nonionic agents. *Invest. Radiol.* 26, 404.

Yamaguchi, K., Katayama, H., Takashima, T., *et al.* (1991). Prediction of severe adverse reaction to ionic and nonionic contrast media in Japan: evaluation of pretesting. A report from the Japanese Committee on Safety of Contrast Media. *Invest. Radiol.* 178, 363.

Yocum, M.W., Heller, A.M., and Abels, R.I. (1978). Efficacy of intravenous pretesting and antihistamine prophylaxis in radio-contrast media-sensitive patients. *J. Allergy Clin. Immunol.* 62, 309.

Young, M.O. (1958). Acute appendicitis following retention of barium in the appendix. *Arch. Surg.* 77, 1011.

Zeman, R.K. (1977). Disseminated intravascular coagulation following intravenous pyelography. *Invest. Radiol.* 12, 203.

Zheutlin, N., Lasser, E.C., and Rigler, L.G. (1952). Clinical studies on the effect of barium in the peritoneal cavity following rupture of the colon. *Surgery* 32, 967.

29. Disorders of temperature regulation

K. WOODHOUSE

Normal body temperature control

Human body temperature is controlled within a narrow range. Normally, a circadian rhythm occurs with a relative peak in the late afternoon and early evening and a trough in the early hours of the morning (Bernheim *et al*. 1979). A variety of physiological and behavioural mechanisms have evolved to maintain thermoregulation. For example, if we feel cold, the behavioural response is to put on an extra sweater or light the fire; the physiological responses include vasoconstriction to reduce heat loss and shivering to generate heat. By contrast, a perception of heat results in shedding of clothes, vasodilatation, and sweating (Bernheim *et al*. 1979).

Fever

Practically all drugs can cause fever under certain circumstances — certainly adverse drug reactions should always be considered in patients with obscure or unexplained pyrexia.

Production of fever

The usual mechanism by which fever is brought about in infective and inflammatory illnesses is probably by the generation of endogenous pyrogen (Atkins and Bodel 1979). A variety of cells, including polymorphs, monocytes, Kupffer cells, and alveolar macrophages are capable of producing these compounds after appropriate stimulation by, for example, antigen/antibody reaction (Atkins and Bodel 1971) or by exposure to bacterial endotoxin (Rawlins and Cranston 1972).

Endogenous pyrogen has been shown to affect cells in the preoptic region of the hypothalamus (Cooper *et al*. 1967); it causes fever by increasing the firing rates of temperature-sensitive neurones in this 'thermoregulatory centre', thus increasing the hypothalamic temperature 'set point'. It seems that several intermediaries are involved in this series of events, including prostaglandins and other arachidonic acid metabolites (Laburn *et al*. 1977) and brain monoamines such as noradrenaline and serotonin (Feldberg and Myers 1963; Atkins and Bodel 1979).

Classification of drug-induced fever

Drugs may induce fever by a variety of mechanisms including:
1. acting as a direct or indirect pyrogen or by causing inflammation or tissue damage;
2. causing pyrogen release as part of their pharmacological action;
3. altering thermoregulation by central, peripheral, or metabolic means;
4. inducing hypersensitivity reactions;
5. causing immunosuppression;
6. as a result of patient idiosyncrasy.

Fever as a result of inflammation, tissue damage, or pyrogenic activity

Many drugs cause a local inflammatory phlebitis following intravenous infusion, with resultant fever. These include hypertonic fluids, amphotericin (Seabury 1961), and a variety of antibiotics, such as erythromycin, vancomycin, and cephalosporins (Berger *et al*. 1976). A more serious local reaction is the development of a sterile abscess, again resulting in fever. This may occur following intramuscular injections of drugs such as paraldehyde, quinine, pentazocine (Parks *et al*. 1971), diclofenac (Ali and Mathias 1991), and aurothioglucose (Sowa 1993).

Local inflammatory responses and associated fever are also frequent following vaccine administration. Pneumococcal vaccine is a good example (Uhl *et al*. 1978; Honkanen *et al*. 1996). Regarding the more commonly used vaccines in children, it is quite difficult to obtain accurate figures for the incidence of febrile reactions. As early as 1945, Sako (1945) observed systemic reactions with fever following pertussis vaccination in 7.1 per cent of subjects. More recently, higher fever than 38°C has been reported in 44 per cent of children given diphtheria/pertussis/tetanus toxoid/poliomyelitis vaccine (Ipp *et al.* 1987). The use of paracetamol as a prophylactic antipyretic has been recommended (Ipp *et al.* 1987).

Some drugs appear to have a systemic pyrogenic action. Fever is a feature of the cytokine-release syndrome induced by the immunosuppressant muromonab-C D3 (OKT3), usually when the first dose is given (Abdallah *et al.* 1996; Diasio and LoBuglio 1996). In some instances, particularly with agents derived from microorganisms, this is likely to be due to contamination with bacterial or other pyrogens; examples include colaspase (asparaginase) (Ekert *et al.* 1972) and amphotericin (Seabury and Dascomb 1958). Certainly, purification of amphotericin significantly reduced the occurrence of febrile reactions to it (Groel 1963; Tynes *et al.* 1963).

Other drugs may, however, be exogenous pyrogens themselves. Bleomycin administered systemically or into a body cavity is certainly pyrogenic (Dinarello *et al.* 1973), fever of up to 41°C occurring in 40–60 per cent of patients within 2–6 hours after the first intravenous dose (Dollery 1991), and it has been suggested that at least part of this action may be due to the drug rather than contaminants; similarly, interferon, administered either intramuscularly (Scott *et al.* 1981) or intrathecally (Ruutiainen *et al.* 1983), almost invariably causes a temperature rise. This drug is a biological product, and it has been suggested that the fever is due to contaminants; even highly purified preparations, however, cause fever and it is likely that interferon is inherently pyrogenic (Scott *et al.* 1981).

Fever due to pyrogen release as part of pharmacological action

The intended action of drugs can itself directly or indirectly induce fever. Perhaps the best example of this is the Jarisch–Herxheimer reaction, which may occur in some patients treated with penicillins for syphilis. Endotoxin is released from dead spirochaetes, resulting in fever 6–8 hours after starting therapy; this is often accompanied by rash, rigors, myalgia, and malaise (Gelfand *et al.* 1976).

In addition, several types of malignant cells, for example, those of acute leukaemia, histiocytic lymphoma, and Hodgkin's disease, can secrete endogenous pyrogen, resulting in fever as part of the disease process (Bernheim *et al.* 1979; Atkins and Bodel 1971). Treatment of the disease by chemotherapy may theoretically

result in cell death, release of further pyrogen, and subsequent fever (Bodel *et al.* 1980), although it must be said that most fevers in patients with cancer who receive chemotherapy are due to intercurrent infections.

In the case of streptokinase, a drug which is frequently pyrogenic, at least some of the fever may be due to the release of unspecified metabolites during thrombolysis (Kakkar *et al.* 1969). It is unlikely to be due to contamination with bacterial endotoxin or other agents, as the fever generally begins 14–20 hours into treatment, peaking at 24–36 hours. A febrile response to endotoxin would be expected to begin within 1–2 hours of starting therapy.

Fever due to altered thermoregulation

Drugs may theoretically modify thermoregulation in several ways: (a) centrally, (b) peripherally, and (c) by affecting metabolism and heat production. In practice, central effects are probably most important. Although drugs with anticholinergic properties such as atropine, antihistamines, and tricyclic antidepressants can decrease sweating, and sympathomimetics such as amphetamines can produce vasoconstriction, the fever they produce in overdose (Judge and Dumard 1953; Jordan and Hempson 1960; Noble and Matthew 1969; Mikolich *et al.* 1975) is due at least in part to central rather than these peripheral actions.

Experimental evidence for central thermomodulatory effects of some drugs is strong: catecholamines, serotonin, anticholinergics, and prostaglandins have all been shown to give temperature rises in various species of experimental animals when injected intraventricularly (Hellon 1975; Cranston 1979). Hyperthermia followed the intracisternal injection of papaverine during craniotomy for an intracranial aneurysm (McLoughlin 1997).

Tricyclic antidepressant overdose is frequently associated with fever (Noble and Matthews 1969), and this may well be due to increased concentrations of catecholamines in the synaptic cleft. Intraventricular administration of the tricyclic desipramine in rats results in brisk fever, even when given in small doses (Cranston *et al.* 1972). Similarly, monoamine oxidase inhibitors can result in dramatic fever when taken in overdose, or when taken with tricyclics (Simmons *et al.* 1970). Phenoxybenzamine has been suggested for control of fever in cases in which several antidepressants have been taken in overdose, as it also controls the associated hypertension (Simmons *et al.* 1970).

Atropine is another agent that frequently gives rise to fever when taken in overdose: in up to 20 per cent of such cases the patient is febrile (Shader and Greenblatt 1971). Oxybutynin, an antimuscarinic agent with effects similar to those of atropine, has caused heatstroke with hyper-thermia is a 76-year-old man (Adubofour *et al.* 1996). This effect is, once more, likely to be partially centrally mediated, although decreased sweating may be an as-sociated factor. The use of dopamine-blocking agents in combination with anticholinergics may also result in hyperpyrexia, even in therapeutic dosage; this has oc-curred in patients receiving benztropine together with trifluoperazine, haloperidol, or chlorpromazine, and in patients taking benztropine with chlorprothixene and chlorpromazine (Westlake and Rastegar 1973). This interaction can sometimes pose therapeutic problems, as patients with anticholinergic poisoning are often dis-turbed and hallucinated. Use of neuroleptics to control these symptoms will obviously worsen the situation. Benzodiazepines should probably be used in these cir-cumstances, and fever reduced by skin cooling.

Fever is part of the serotonin syndrome (Kudo *et al.* 1997), which is discussed Chapter 20.

Other agents may also produce fever partly by central effects. For example, pyrexia is not uncommon when prostaglandins are used to induce termination of preg-nancy, either by the intra-amniotic or intravenous route (Fraser and Brash 1974), and it is known that intra-ventricular administration of prostaglandins in exper-imental animals is pyrogenic (Milton and Wendlandt 1971). Similarly, injection of H_2-blockers into the third ventricle of chickens causes fever, while injection of H_2-agonists produces a temperature fall (Nistico *et al.* 1978). Conceivably, some of the rare cases of fever caused by cimetidine could be due to this mechanism, although this seems doubtful, as this drug does not cross the blood–brain barrier in significant amounts.

Fever as part of hypersensitivity reactions

There is no doubt that fever is a prominent clinical feature of hypersensitivity (allergic) drug reactions. A drug fever, initially low-grade and subsequently increas-ing, will often start within 7–10 days of drug adminis-tration. It will normally persist as long as the drug is given, but will subside rapidly on discontinuation. Re-challenge will result in recurrence of fever within hours.

Fever may often be the first sign of a hypersensitivity reaction: in a study of 68 cases of drug allergy, of which 31 were fatal, fever was an early feature in almost one-third (Cluff and Johnson 1964). Similarly, in a review of 38 patients with phenytoin hypersensitivity, fever was a prominent feature in 14 cases and the only sign of a reaction in one (Haruda 1979). It is impractical to discuss all drugs that may induce a hypersensitivity reaction, but in several instances fever may be the most prominent feature of the event.

Antituberculous drugs

Fever is a common feature of adverse reactions to anti-tuberculous drugs. In a large study of 1744 cases of tuberculosis treated with various combinations of anti-tuberculous drugs, it was found that adverse reactions occurred in 10.3 per cent of those treated with strepto-mycin, of which 26.8 per cent were associated with fever; in 8.8 per cent of those treated with *p*-aminosalicylic aid (PAS), of which 43.3 per cent were associated with fever; and in 1.3 per cent of those given isoniazid, of which 59 per cent were febrile (Berte *et al.* 1964). Fever also occurs in patients taking rifampicin and, interestingly, is more frequent in those given the drug intermittently rather than continuously, in keeping with a hypersen-sitivity reaction (Zierski 1973).

Antibacterials

Febrile reactions to antibiotics do occur, but are the major feature of only a small number of cases, being more common in association with other manifestations of allergy such as rash and abnormal liver function. In a study of 2877 patients admitted to hospital and given antibiotics it was found that overall 5.4 per cent of patients developed an adverse reaction of some kind, but in only nine individuals was fever the only or the most prominent feature, three of whom had received penicil-lin, three cephalothin, and one each ampicillin, oxa-cillin, and tetracycline (Caldwell and Cluff 1974). From a 13-month study of 43 adult patients with cystic fibrosis who received 13 differen antibacterials, alone or in combination, it was concluded that in those patients who developed fever it was due to piperacillin rather than to any of the other antibacterials given to the patients (Mallon *et al.* 1997). Minocycline has caused a marked rise in temperature in three patients, who also developed fatigue, polyarthritis, and livedo reticularis (Elkayam *et al.* 1996).

Methyldopa

Fever with methyldopa is well described (Furhoff 1978) and seems to occur in up to three per cent of those given the drug. It is the most common adverse reaction associ-ated with methyldopa — of 308 reports in the 1960s and 1970s in Sweden, 166 were of febrile reactions. There appears to be a slight preponderance (60 per cent) of women (Furhoff 1978). Many cases are associated with hepatitis and abnormal liver function tests, reflecting the hypersensitivity nature of the reactions (Klein and Kaminsky 1973; Chopra *et al.* 1996).

Miscellaneous drugs

Fever during phenytoin treatment is not uncommon and has been mentioned above; it is frequently simply part of a symptom complex that may include rashes, the Stevens–Johnson syndrome, adenopathy, hepatitis, and blood dyscrasia (Stanley and Fallon-Pellici 1978; Haruda 1979; Chopra *et al.* 1996).

Procainamide is another drug that can induce fever as a major symptom of an adverse drug reaction (Hey *et al.* 1965). Transient eosinophilia may occur. Febrile responses to procainamide tend to occur within the first 2–18 days of treatment; the response is probably independent of the subsequent risk of developing the lupus syndrome (Hey *et al.* 1965).

By contrast, those who develop an early febrile reaction to hydralazine may well be rather more likely to develop lupus subsequently (Perry 1973).

Angiotensin-converting-enzyme inhibitors, such as captopril, may cause fever (Hoorntje *et al.* 1979).

In some cases it is probable that febrile reactions associated with drug hypersensitivity may not be due to the drug *per se*, but to contaminants. For example, antibiotics or egg proteins found in some vaccine products may result in hypersensitivity reactions (see above), and the abnormal constituents present in some preparations of L-tryptophan have been responsible for the eosinophilia–myalgia syndrome (see Chapter 20).

Fever in immunosuppressed patients

A detailed description of this problem is beyond the scope of this chapter. Patients, however, who are immunocompromised by treatment, be it as a result of cancer chemotherapy or an idiosyncratic reaction, are clearly at risk of opportunistic infection, often with associated fever. This problem is dealt with elsewhere in this book (Chapter 25).

Fever as a result of patient idiosyncrasy

Glucose 6-phosphate dehydrogenase deficiency

This enzyme deficiency, dealt with in greater detail elsewhere (see Chapters 5 and 24), is an inherited defect of red cell metabolism (Gross *et al.* 1958). When exposed to a variety of drugs such patients may develop a brisk haemolysis (Carson *et al.* 1956), and this reaction, as with most haemolytic reactions, may be accompanied by a febrile illness.

Malignant hyperthermia

This condition is one of the most dramatic complications of anaesthesia. It was first described by Saidman and Colleagues (1964), and may occur after exposure to a variety of anaesthetic agents, notably halothane and suxamethonium (Noble *et al.* 1973), although it has been reported with nitrous oxide (Ellis *et al.* 1974), cyclopropane (Lips *et al.* 1982), tubocurarine (Britt *et al.*

1974), isoflurane (McGuire and Easy 1990), and even during epidural anaesthesia with lignocaine and bupivacaine (Kilmanek *et al.* 1976). The syndrome comprises a rapid rise in body temperature (of at least 2°C per hour and up to 1°C every 5–10 minutes), accompanied by some or all of the following: rigidity, hyperventilation, cyanosis, acidosis, hyperphosphataemia, and hyperglycaemia. Initial hyperkalaemia and hypercalcaemia may be followed by hypokalaemia and hypocalcaemia. If the patient is not treated, the temperature may rise to over 42–43°C, and the mortality is 60–70 per cent (Britt and Kalow 1968).

The frequency of malignant hyperpyrexia has been estimated to be appoximately 1 case per 50 000–100 000 anaesthetics in adults, and 1 per 15 000 in children. In some reported cases resting creatine phosphokinase and aldolase levels may be elevated (Isaacs and Barlow 1970); but this is by no means invariable. A more accurate prediction of risk can be made by demonstrating, *in vitro*, that muscle strips obtained by biopsy show, by sustained contraction, an increased sensitivity to a variety of agents, including halothane, caffeine, potassium, and temperature change (Moulds and Denborough 1974*a,b*). The most widely used *in vitro* test is the caffeine–halothane contraction test (CHCT).

Early studies (Denborough *et al.* 1973) demonstrated some histological changes in some subjects with this disease. These comprised the presence of cores in 55 per cent of Type 1 muscle fibres — 'central core disease'. Similar findings had been described in muscle fibres from Landrace pigs, which also show a susceptibility to develop malignant hyperpyrexia.

The porcine equivalent of MH has been designated the porcine stress syndrome, and this has proven a most useful model in which to study human MH. The underlying biochemical defect appears to be an unregulated release of calcium ions from the sarcoplasmic reticulum into the myoplasm of skeletal muscle cells (Iazzo *et al.* 1988). Early genetic studies had indicated that a locus for MH was present on chromosome 19q12-13.2 in human families (McCarthy *et al.* 1990). Additionally, the gene for the skeletal muscle sarcoplasmic reticulum calcium release channel RYR1 (ryanodine receptor) was also localized to the same region, and was suggested as a candidate gene responsible for MH (McKenzie *et al.* 1990). An RYR1 mutation (Arg614Cys) has been shown to be the cause of porcine MH. This mutation has also been found in 5–10 per cent of human MH families (MacLennan and Phillips 1992; Deufel *et al.* 1995). Subsequently, several mutations of the RYRl site have been shown to be related to MH susceptibility; Arg163Cys, Gly248Arg, Gly341Arg, Ile403Met,

Tyr522Ser, Gly2433Arg, Arg2434His, and Cys35Arg (Gillard *et al.* 1992; Quane *et al.* 1993, 1994*a,b*; Zhang *et al.* 1993; Keating *et al.* 1994; Phillips *et al.* 1994; Lynch *et al.* 1997).

Various treatment strategies have been adopted and supportive measures, including artificial ventilation and cooling, treatment of acidosis, and attention to electrolyte balance, are crucial. Of pharmacological treatments, procaine (Harrison 1971), procainamide (Noble *et al.* 1973), and dexamethasone (Ellis *et al.* 1974) have all been advocated. The most effective treatment, however, is undoubtedly intravenous dantrolene sodium. Repeated doses of 1 mg per kg are given at 5 to 10-minute intervals until the syndrome is controlled. A total of 2–3 mg per kg is usually sufficient in humans, but in susceptible pigs up to 10 mg per kg has been given (Hall 1980). This drug should always be immediately available during anaesthesia (Hall 1980).

This subject is also discussed in Chapter 20.

Neuroleptic malignant syndrome (NMS)

A syndrome of uncontrolled heat reaction, similar to malignant hyperpyrexia but in general slightly less dramatic, has been reported following the administration of neuroleptic drugs. The clinical picture comprises hyperthermia, muscle rigidity, fluctuating consciousness, and autonomic disturbances, such as tachycardia, labile blood pressure, incontinence, dyspnoea, and sweating.

NMS tends to occur after physical exhaustion or dehydration, or both, and has been described with haloperidol, thiothixene, and piperazine phenothiazines. The likelihood is that it can be precipitated by most neuroleptics. The syndrome may persist for 5–10 days after discontinuing the drug, much longer if depot preparations have been used. Mortality may approach 20 per cent (Caroff 1980). A case in which hypothyroidism was suspected to have predisposed to the syndrome, induced by thioridazine and haloperidol, has been reported (Moore *et al.* 1990).

It may well be that dopamine receptor modulation is an important factor in the pathogenesis of this condition. The author has seen at least two patients with a similar, but milder, clinical picture following abrupt withdrawal of levodopa.

Unlike MH it would appear that NMS is probably not related to mutations at the RYR1 locus. Miyatake *et al.* (1996) investigated six mutations in this gene in 10 NMS patients, using a single-strand confirmation polymorphism analysis (SSCP), and they found no evidence of an association between NMS and mutations at the RYR1 gene.

This subject is also discussed in Chapter 20.

Hypothermia

Hypothermia is usually defined by the presence of a deep body temperature, measured by reliable means, of less than 35°C (Keatinge 1987). Approximately three per cent of patients admitted to British hospitals in winter have body temperatures below this level. The majority are elderly, and in most cases, the hypothermia is secondary either to disease, such as stroke or pneumonia, or to drugs (Keatinge 1987). Elderly survivors of accidental hypothermia have been shown to have impaired thermoregulatory reflexes (Collins *et al.* 1977), and in these patients, drugs that further impair thermoregulation, level of consciousness, or central thermoregulatory control, may cause hypothermia. Barbiturates, neuroleptics, and alcohol are common culprits (Caird and Scott 1986; Keatinge 1987). The condition may occur even with relatively small doses in susceptible patients — hypothermia has been reported after as little as a single dose of 5 mg nitrazepam, given to a woman in an environmental temperature of 27°C (Impallomeni and Ezzat 1976). Severe hypothermia has followed intravenous administration of amphotericin B in a patient with HIV infection (Barlows *et al.* 1996). Mild hypothermia developed in three children treated with azithromycin for pyogenic infections (Kavukçu *et al.* 1997).

Concurrent disease may also be a precipitating factor; for example, a single dose of chlorpromazine has produced hypothermia in a hypothyroid patient (Mitchell *et al.* 1959), and certainly benzodiazepines and neuroleptics should be avoided in such patients. Bromocriptine has been held responsible for recurrent falls in temperature (to as low as 35.5°C) in a 59-year-old man suffering from Parkinson's disease (Pfeffer 1990). In addition to direct effects on thermoregulation, drugs may produce the condition by inducing illnesses that are themselves associated with hypothermia, and low body temperatures are not infrequent in those with lactic acidosis induced by phenformin (Assan *et al.* 1975), and have also been reported in drug-induced hypoglycaemia (Carter 1976). Hypothermia is notoriously common in cases of drug overdosage, and patients with barbiturate or alcohol poisoning, especially if found in cold environments, are frequently very cold (Keatinge 1987).

Drugs affecting cutaneous vasoconstriction can also cause a marked fall in core temperature: thus, any drug blocking sympathetic function will prevent vasoconstriction, increase heat loss, and encourage the development of hypothermia. This was clearly shown in the case of the ganglion-blocker hexamethonium (Hamilton *et al.* 1954), although this is now largely of historical interest. Prazosin, however, is still widely used, and this drug also appears capable of causing hypothermia (de Leeuw and Birkenhäger 1980), although central mechanisms are likely to be involved as well. Falls in body temperature are also well recognized by anaesthetists, and this is likely to be due to impairment of both peripheral and central thermoregulatory reflexes. The problem is likely to occur at the extremes of age, being particularly important in the neonate. In normal adult patients, heat loss is unlikely to be serious if the ambient temperature is kept over 21°C (Carrie and Simpson 1988). The shivering common after halothane anaesthesia does not seem to be universely associated with significant falls in temperature, and may be part of a generalized muscular reaction (Carrie and Simpson 1988).

Finally, hypothermia may follow the intravenous infusion of large quantities of cold blood or other cold infusion fluids. This is a particular problem in babies (Hey et al. 1969), but problems may arise in adults (Boyan 1964), and local cooling of the heart, with resultant arrhythmias, may occur. Use of cold peritoneal dialysis fluid may also result in a fall in core temperature.

The treatment of drug-induced hypothermia follows the same lines as accidental hypothermia of any cause: supportive measures are essential, with attention to fluid and electrolyte balance, glucose homoeostasis, together with gradual rewarming (Keatinge 1987).

Classification of reactions

It is not always possible to classify disorders of thermal regulation as Type A or B reactions. Some reactions, however, such as those caused by drugs with pyrogenic activity, are clearly Type A, whereas others are clearly Type B, a result of patient idiosyncrasy, for example, malignant hyperpyrexia of anaesthesia. In many cases multiple mechanisms may well operate.

References

Abdallah, K.A., David-Neto, E., Centeno, J.R., et al. (1996). Reversal of OKT3-related shivering and chest tightness by intravenous meperidine. *Transplantation* 62, 145.

Adubofour, K.O., Kajiwara, G.T., Goldberg, C.H., et al. (1996). Oxybutynin-induced heatstroke in an elderly patient. *Ann. Pharmacother.* 30, 144.

Ali, M.T. and Mathias I.M. (1991). Continued problems with diclofenac. *Anaesthesia* 46, 1089.

Assan, R., Heulin, C., Girard, J.R., et al. (1975). Phenformin induced lactic acidosis in diabetic patients. *Diabetes* 24, 791.

Atkins, E. and Bodel, P. (1971). Role of leucocytes in fever. In *Pyrogen and Fever* (ed. G. Wostenholme and J. Birch). Churchill Livingstone, Edinburgh.

Atkins, E. and Bodel, P. (1979). Clinical fever: its history, manifestations and pathogenesis. *Fed. Proc.* 38, 57.

Barlows, T.G.III., Luber, A.D., Jacobs, R.A., et alt. (1996). Hypothermia following the intravenous administration of amphotericin B. *Clin. Infect. Dis.* 23, 1187.

Berger, S., Ernst, E.C., and Barza, M. (1976). Comparative incidence of phlebitis due to buffered cephalothin, cephopirin and cephamandole. *Antimicrob. Agents Chemother.* 9, 575.

Bernheim, H.A., Block, L.H., and Atkins, E. (1979). Fever: pathogenesis, pathophysiology and purpose. *Ann. Intern. Med.* 91, 261.

Berte, S.J., Dimase, J.D., and Christianson, C.S. (1964). Isoniazid, para-aminosalicylic acid and streptomycin intolerance in 1744 patients. *Annu. Rev. Respir. Dis.* 90, 598.

Bodel, E., Ralph, P., Wenc, K., et al. (1980). Endogenous pyrogen production by Hodgkin's disease and human histiocytic lymphoma cell lives in vitro. *J. Clin. Invest.* 65, 514.

Boyan, C.P. (1964). Cold or warmed blood for massive transfusions? *Am. Surg.* 160, 282.

Britt, B.A. (ed.) (1987). Dantrolene, an update. In *Malignant Hyperthermia*, p. 325. Martinus Nijhoff Press, Amsterdam.

Britt, B.A. and Kalow, W. (1968). Hyperrigidity and hyperthermia associated with anaesthesia. *Ann. N.Y. Acad. Sci.* 151, 947.

Britt, B.A., Locher, W.G., and Kalow, W. (1969). Hereditary aspects of malignant hyperthermia. *Can. Anaesth. Soc. J.* 16, 89.

Britt, B.A., Webb, G.E., and Leduc, C. (1974). Malignant hyperthermia induced by curare. *Can. Anaesth. Soc. J.* 21, 371.

Caird, F.I. and Scott, P.J.W. (1986). *Drug Induced Diseases In the Elderly*. Elsevier, Amsterdam.

Caldwell, J.R. and Cluff, L.E. (1974). Adverse reactions to antimicrobial agents. *JAMA* 230, 77.

Caroff, S.N. (1980). The neuroleptic malignant syndrome. *J. Clin. Psychiatry* 41, 79.

Carrie, L.E.S. and Simpson, P.J. (1988) *Understanding Anaesthesia*, p. 257. Heinemann, London.

Carter, W.P. (1976). Drug induced hypoglycaemia and hypothermia. *J. Maine Med. Assoc.* 67, 272.

Chopra, S., Levell, N.J., Cowley, G., et al. (1996). Systemic corticosteroids in the phenytoin hypersensitivity syndrome. *Br. J. Dermatol.* 134, 1109.

Cluff, L.E. and Johnson, J.E. (1964). Drug fever. *Prog. Allergy* 8, 149.

Collins, S.K.J., Dove, C., and Exton-Smith, A.N. (1977). Accidental hypothermia and compromised temperature homoeostasis in the elderly. *BMJ* i, 353.

Cooper, K.E., Cranston, W.I., and Honour, A.J. (1967). Observations on the site and mode of action of pyrogens in the rabbit brain. *J. Physiol.* (Lond.) 191, 325.

Cranston, W.I. (1979). Central mechanisms of fever. *Fed. Proc.* 38, 49.

Cranston, W.I., Hellon, R.F., Luff, R.H., et al. (1972). Hypothalamic endogenous noradrenaline and thermoregulation in the cat and rabbit. *J. Physiol.* (Lond.) 223, 59.

De Leeuw, P.W. and Birkenhäger, W.H. (1980). Hypothermia: a possible side effect of prazosin. *Br. Med. J.* 281, 1187.

Denborough, M.A., Bennett, X., and Anderson, R. McD. (1973). Central core disease and malignant hyperpyrexia. *BMJ* i, 272.

Deufel, T., Sudbrack, R., Feist, Y., *et al.* (1995). Discordance, in a malignant hyperthermia pedigree, between *in vitro* contracture-test phenotypes and haplotypes for the MHS 1 region on chromosome 19q12-13.2, comprising the C1840T transition in the RYR1 gene. *Am. J. Hum. Genet.* 56, 1334.

Diasio, R.B. and LoBuglio, A.F. (1996). Immunomodulators: Immunosuppressive agents. In *Goodman and Gilman's The Pharmacological Basis of Therapeutics* (9th edn) (ed. J.G. Hardman, L.E. Limbird, P.G. Molinoff, and R.W. Ruddon), p. 1303. McGraw Hill, London.

Dinarello, G.A., Ward, S.B., and Wolff, S.M. (1973). Pyrogenic properties of bleomycin. *Cancer Chemother. Rep.* 57, 393.

Dollery, C. (ed.) (1991). Bleomycin. In *Therapeutic Drugs*, p. 399. Edinburgh, Churchill Livingstone, Edinburgh.

Ekert, H., Colebatch, J.H., and Matthews, R.N. (1972). Short courses of cytosine arabinoside and L-asparaginase in children with acute leukemia. *Cancer* 30, 643.

Elkayam, O., Yaron, M., and Caspi, D. (1996). Minocycline induced arthritis associated with fever, livedo reticularis, and pANCA. *Ann. Rheum. Dis.* 55, 769.

Ellis, F.R., Clarke, I.M.C., Appleyard, T.N., *et al.* (1974). Malignant hyperpyrexia induced by nitrous oxide and treated with dexamethasone. *BMJ* iv, 270.

Feldberg, W. and Myers, R.D. (1963). A new concept of temperature regulation by amines in the hypothalamus. *Nature* 200, 1325.

Fraser, I.S. and Brash, I.H. (1974). Comparison of extra and intra-amniotic prostaglandins for therapeutic abortion. *Obstet. Gynecol.* 43, 97.

Furhoff, A.K. (1978). Adverse reactions with methyldopa — a decade's reports. *Acta Med. Scand.* 203, 425.

Gelfand, J.A., Elin, R.J., Berry, F.W., *et al.* (1976). Endotoxaemia associated with the Jarisch–Herxheimer reaction. *N. Engl. J. Med.* 295, 211.

Gillard, E.F., Otsu, K., Fujii, J., *et al.* (1992). Polymorphisms and deduced amino acid substitutions in the coding sequence of the ryanodine receptor (RYR1) gene in individuals with malignant hyperthermia. *Genomics* 13, 1247.

Groel, J.T. (1963). Amphotericin B reactions. *Am. Rev. Respir. Dis.* 88, 565.

Hall, G.M. (1980). Dantrolene and the treatment of malignant hyperthermia. *Br. J. Anaesth.* 52, 847.

Hamilton, M., Henley, K.S., and Morrison, B. (1954). Changes in peripheral circulation and body temperature after hexamethonium bromide. *Clin. Sci.* 13, 225.

Harrison, G.G. (1971). Anaesthetic-induced malignant hyperpyrexia: a suggested method of treatment. *BMJ* iii, 454.

Haruda, F. (1979). Phenytoin sensitivity: 39 cases. *Neurology* 29, 1480.

Hayward, J.N. and Boshell, B.R. (1957). Paraldehyde intoxication with metabolic acidosis. Report of two cases, experimental data and a critical review of the literature. *Am. J. Med.* 23, 965.

Hellon, R.F. (1975). Monoamines, pyrogens and cations: their action on central control of body temperature. *Pharmacol. Rev.* 26, 289.

Hey, E.B., Makous, N., and van der Veer, J.B. (1965). Fever and chills as a reaction to procainamide hydrochloride therapy. *Arch. Intern. Med.* 116, 544.

Hey, E.N., Kohlinsky, S., and O'Connel, B. (1969). Heat loss from babies during exchange transfusion. *Lancet* i, 335.

Honkanen, P.O., Keistinen, T., and Kiveld, S-L. (1996). Reactions following administration of influenza vaccine alone or with pneumococcal vaccine in the elderly. *Arch. Intern. Med.* 156, 205.

Hoorntje, S.J., Weening, J.J., Kallenberg, C.G.M., *et al.* (1979). Serum sickness-like syndrome with membranous glomerulopathy in a patient on captopril. *Lancet* ii, 1297.

Iaizzo, P.A., Klein, W., and Lehmann-Horn, F. (1988). Fura-2 detected myoplasmic calcium and its correlation with contracture force in skeletal muscle from normal and malignant hyperthermia susceptible pigs. *Pflügers Arch.* 411, 648.

Impallomeni, M. and Ezzat, R. (1976). Hypothermia associated with nitrazepam administration. *BMJ* i, 223.

Ipp, M.M., Gold, R., Greenberg, S., *et al.* (1987). Acetaminophen prophylaxis of adverse reactions following vaccination of infants with diphtheria–pertussis–tetanus toxoid/polio vaccine. *Pediatr. Infect. Dis.* 6, 721.

Isaacs, H. and Barlow, M.B. (1970). Malignant hyperpyrexia during anaesthesia: a possible association with subclinical myopathy. *BMJ* i, 275.

Jordan, S.C. and Hampson, F. (1960). Amphetamine poisoning associated with hyperpyrexia. *BMJ* ii, 844.

Judge, D.J. and Dumard, K.W. (1953). Diphenhydramine (Benadryl) and tripelennamine (Pyribenzamine) intoxication in children. *Am. J. Dis. Child.* 85, 545.

Kakkar, V.V., Franc, C., O'Shea, M.J., *et al.* (1969). Treatment of deep venous thrombosis with streptokinase. *Br. J. Surg.* 56, 178.

Kavukçu, S., Uuz, A., and Aydin, A. (1997). Hypothermia from azithromycin. *J. Toxicol. Clin. Toxicol.* 35, 225.

Keating, K.E., Quane, K.A., Manning, B.M., *et al.* (1994). Detection of a novel RYR1 mutation in four malignant hyperthermia pedigrees. *Hum. Mol. Genet.* 3, 1855.

Keatinge, W.R. (1987). Cold and drowning. In *Oxford Textbook of Medicine* (ed. D.J. Weatherall, J.G.G. Ledingham, and D.A. Warrell), p. 6.95. Oxford University Press.

Kilmanek, J., Majewski, W., and Walenick, K. (1976). A case of malignant hyperthermia during epidural anaesthesia. *Anaesth. Resusc. Intens. Ther.* 4, 143.

King, J.O., Denborough, M.A., and Zapf, P.W. (1972). Inheritance of malignant hyperpyrexia. *Lancet*, i, 365.

Klein, H.O. and Kaminsky, N. (1973). Methyldopa fever: recurrence of symptoms with resumption of therapy. *N.Y. State J. Med.* 73, 448.

Kudo, K., Sasaki, I., Tsuchiyama, K., *et al.* (1997). Serotonin syndrome during clomipramine monotherapy: comparison of two diagnostic criteria. *Psychiatr. Clin. Neurosci.* 51, 43.

Laburn, H., Mitchell, D., and Rosendorff, C. (1977). Effects of prostaglandin antagonism on sodium arachidonate fever in rabbits. *J. Physiol.* (Lond.) 267, 559.

Lips, F.J., Newland, M., and Dutton, G. (1982). Malignant hyperthermia triggered by cyclopropane during caesarian section. *Anesthesiology* 56, 144.

Lynch, P.J., Krivosic-Horber, R., Reyford, H., *et al.* (1997). Identification of heterozygous and homozygous individuals with the novel RYRl mutation Cys35Arg in a large kindred. *Anesthesiology* 86, 620.

McCarthy, T.V., Healy, J.M.S., Heffron, J.J.A., *et al.* (1990). Localisation of the malignant hyperthermia susceptibility locus to human chromosome 19q12-13.2. *Nature* 343, 562.

McGuire, N. and Easy, W.R. (1990). Malignant hyperthermia during isoflurane anaesthesia. *Anaesthesia* 45, 124.

Mackenzie, A.E., Korneluk, R.G., Zorzato, F., *et al.* (1990). The human ryanodine receptor gene, its mapping to 19q13.1, placement in a chromosome 19 linkage group, and exclusion as the gene causing myotonic dystrophy. *Am. J. Hum. Genet.* 46, 1082.

MacLennan, D.H. and Phillips, M.S. (1992). Malignant hyperthermia. *Science* 256, 789.

Mikolich, J.R., Paulson, C.W., and Cross, C.J. (1975). Acute anticholinergic syndrome due to jimson seed ingestion. Clinical and laboratory observations in six cases. *Ann. Intern. Med.* 83, 321.

Milton, A.S. and Wendlandt, S. (1971). Effects on body temperature of prostaglandins of the A, E and F series on injection into the third ventricle of anaesthetised cats and rabbits. *J. Physiol.* (Lond.) 218, 325.

Mitchell, J.R.A., Surridge, D.H.C., and Willison, R.G. (1959). Hypothermia after chlorpromazine in myxoedema psychosis. *BMJ* ii, 932.

Miyatake, R., Iwahashi, K., Matsushita, M., *et al.* (1996). No association between the neuroleptic malignant syndrome and mutations in the RYRl gene associated malignant hyperthermia. *J. Neurol. Sci.* 143, 161.

Moore, A.P., Macfarlane, I.A., and Blumhardt, L.D. (1990). Neuroleptic malignant syndrome and hypothyroidism. *J. Neurol. Neurosurg. Psychiatry* 53, 517.

Moulds, R.F.W. and Denborough, M.A. (1974*a*). Biochemical basis of malignant hyperpyrexia. *BMJ* ii, 241.

Moulds, R.F.W. and Denborough, M.A. (1974*b*). Identification of susceptibility to malignant hyperpyrexia. *BMJ* ii, 245.

Nistico, G., Rotiroti, D., De Sarro, A., *et al.* (1978). Mechanism of cimetidine-induced fever. *Lancet* ii, 265.

Noble, J. and Matthew, H. (1969). Acute poisoning by tricyclic antidepressants: clinical features and management of 100 patients. *Clin. Toxicol.* 2, 403.

Noble, W.H., McKee, D., and Gates, B. (1973). Malignant hyperthermia with rigidity successfully treated with procainamide. *Anesthesiology* 39, 450.

Parks, D.L., Perry, H.O., and Muller, S.A. (1971). Cutaneous complications of pentazocine injections. *Arch. Dermatol.* 104, 231.

Perry, H.M. (1973). Late toxicity to hydralazine resembling systemic lupus erythematosus or rheumatoid arthritis. *Am. J. Med.* 54, 58.

Pfeffer, R.F. (1990). Bromocriptine-induced hypothermia. *Neurology* 40, 383.

Phillips, M.S., Khanna, V.K., DeLeon, S., *et al.* (1994). The substitution of Arg for Gly2433 in the human skeletal muscle ryanodine receptor is associated with malignant hyperthermia. *Hum. Mol. Genet.* 3, 2181.

Quane, K.A., Healy, J.M.S., Keating, K.E., *et al.* (1993). Mutations in the ryanodine receptor gene in central core disease and malignant hyperthermia. *Nat. Genet.* 5, 1.

Quane, K.A., Keating, K.E., Manning, B.M., *et al.* (1994*a*). Detection of a novel common mutation in the ryanodine receptor gene in malignant hyperthermia: Implications for diagnosis and heterogeneity studies. *Hum. Mol. Genet.* 3, 471.

Quane, K.A., Keating, K.E., Healy, J.M.S., *et al.* (1994*b*). Mutation screening of the RYRl gene in malignant hyperthermia: Detection of a novel Tyr to Ser mutation in a pedigree with associated central cores. *Genomics* 23, 236.

Rawlins, M.D. and Cranston, W.I. (1972). Clinical studies on the pathogenesis of fever. In *The Pharmacology of Thermoregulation*, p. 264. Symposium, San Francisco.

Ruutiainen, J., Panelius, M., and Cantell, K. (1983). Toxic effects of interferon administered intrathecally. *BMJ* 280, 940.

Saidman, L.J., Havard, E.S., and Eger, E.I. (1964). Hyperthermia during anaesthesia. *JAMA* 190, 1029.

Sako, W. (1945). Immunisation against pertussis with alum precipitated vaccine. *JAMA* 127, 379.

Scott, G.M., Secher, D.S., Flowers, D., *et al.* (1981). Toxicity of interferon. *BMJ* 282, 1345.

Seabury, J.H. (1961). Experience with amphotericin B. *Chemotherapia* 3, 81.

Seabury, J.H. and Dascomb, H.E. (1958). Experience with amphotericin B for the treatment of systemic mycoses. *Arch. Intern. Med.* 102, 960.

Shader, R.I. and Greenblatt, D.J. (1971). Uses and toxicity of belladonna alkaloids and synthetic anticholinergics. *Sem. Psychiatr.* 3, 449.

Simmons, A.V., Carr, D., and Ross, E.J. (1970). Case of self-poisoning with multiple antidepressant drugs. *Lancet* i, 214.

Sowa, J.M. (1993). Sterile oily abscess from gold therapy. *Arthritis Rheum.* 36, 1632.

Stanley, J. and Fallon-Pellici, V. (1978). Phenytoin hypersensitivity reaction. *Arch. Dermatol.* 114, 1350.

Tynes, B.S., Otz, J.P., Bennett, I.J.E., *et al.* (1963). Reducing amphotericin B reactions. A double blind study. *Am. Rev. Respir. Dis.* 87, 264.

Uhl, G., Farber, J., Moench, T., *et al.* (1978). Febrile reactions to pneumococcal vaccine. *N. Engl. J. Med.* 299, 1318.

Wallerstein, R.O. and Aggeler, P.M. (1964). Acute hemolytic anaemia. *Am. J. Med.* 37, 92.

Westlake, R.J. and Rastegar, A. (1973). Hyperpyrexia from drug combination. *JAMA* 225, 1250.

WHO (1973). Pharmacogenetics. *WHO Tech. Rep. Ser.* 524.

Zhang, Y., Chen, H.S., Khanna, V.K., *et al.* (1993). A mutation in the human ryanodine receptor gene associated with central core disease. *Nat. Genet.* 5, 46.

Zierski, M. (1973). Side effects under intermittent rifampicin: a general review. *Bull. Un. Int. Tuberc.* 48, 119.

30. Obstetrical and gynaecological disorders

S. M. CALVERT and J. O. DRIFE

Introduction

Many drugs used in obstetrics and gynaecology have adverse reactions that cause unwanted obstetrical and gynaecological disorders. A number of drugs used for other conditions can also have adverse effects resulting particularly in gynaecological symptoms. Drugs specifically affecting the fetus are discussed in Chapter 7.

Gynaecological disorders

Amenorrhoea and galactorrhoea

This subject is dealt with in the chapter on Endocrine Disorders (Chapter 15).

Menstrual disturbance

Menstrual disturbance is caused by a number of drugs, most of which cause irregular, rather than heavy, bleeding.

Hormonal preparations

Progestogen-only contraceptives frequently cause abnormal bleeding patterns. Broome and Fotherby (1990) report their clinical experience with the progestogen-only pill (POP). Out of 324 POP users, 77 discontinued the pill because of bleeding disturbances. Less than 40 per cent of their patients using the POP for more than 6 months had regular menstrual cycles, although the number of short cycles tended to decrease as time went on. In a review of POP and bleeding disturbances, Kovacs (1996) confirmed that menstrual disturbance is the commonest quoted reason for the discontinuation of the POP (up to 25 per cent of users). He also commented that the mechanism of action of the POP on the endometrium is poorly understood and unpredictable.

Depot medroxyprogesterone acetate (Depo-Provera) is a 3-monthly injection providing excellent contraception. It tends to cause irregular spotting and bleeding in the months after the first injection, but most women develop oligomenorrhoea or amenorrhoea after subsequent injections (Nelson 1996).

The Norplant subdermal progestogen-only contraceptive (levonorgestrel-loaded rods) also provides highly effective contraception. Fan and Sujuan (1996) reported an analysis of menstrual diary recordings of 306 patients. There was an increase in the total number of days of bleeding, with bleeding being irregular and prolonged. The number of days of spotting reduced after 6–12 months of use and the overall cumulative termination rate for menstrual problems was only 13 per cent.

Biswas and colleagues (1996) found a similar frequency of bleeding problems with Norplant-2, a second-generation implant system.

Over recent years a levonorgestrel-loaded intrauterine contraceptive device (IUCD) has been in widespread use. Spotting and irregular scanty bleeding were the most frequent menstrual complaints in users of this IUCD in a study by Sivin and Stern (1994). The incidence of these complaints markedly diminished after the first year of use, with the vast majority of patients becoming amenorrhoeic or oligomenorrhoeic. In a similar study, Andersson and co-workers (1994) found that termination rates for spotting and irregular bleeding were similar in users of levonorgestrel-loaded coils and copper-loaded coils, but that there were significantly fewer terminations for heavy bleeding in those using the levonorgestrel IUCD. They also confirmed the increasing likelihood of amenorrhoea with time.

Mainwaring and others (1995) studied bleeding patterns in women using Norplant, Depo-Provera, or a POP. Depo-Provera resulted in fewer total days of blood loss than either of the two other methods of contraception.

Breakthrough bleeding or spotting (i.e. intermenstrual bleeding) is also seen with the combined oral contraceptive pill, occurring in 33–66 per cent of patients in one study (Droegemueller *et al.* 1989). Often it is due to poor compliance and missed pills, but Droegemueller and colleagues (1989) showed that the incidence of abnormal bleeding varied according to drug formulation.

In patients being prescribed any hormone-based contraceptive, counselling about the menstrual side effects is important especially in those who are to use progestogen-only preparations.

Other drugs

Spironolactone when used in hirsute women caused metrorrhagia (irregular intermenstrual bleeding) in 56 per cent of women (Helfer *et al.* 1988), but the incidence diminished when the dose of spironolactone was reduced. The mechanism by which spironolactone induces metrorrhagia is not clear but alterations in the serum progesterone levels, and chronic anovulation, may be responsible. Helfer and colleagues recommend that idiopathic hirsutism be treated with a maximum dose of 50 mg spironolactone twice daily on days 4–21 of the menstrual cycle.

Bleeding is the most serious complication of warfarin usage, being increasingly likely the higher the International Normalised Ratio (INR). In the Italian Study on Complications of Oral Anticoagulant Therapy (ISC-OAT Study — Palareti *et al.* 1996) 16 out of 1184 women had abnormal uterine bleeding, although these were classed as only minor bleeding episodes. While the bleeding may have been provoked by warfarin, it may have unmasked an underlying pathological change and cannot be ignored.

Endometrial abnormalities

Oestrogen

Oestrogen causes endometrial proliferation during the normal menstrual cycle. Progesterone induces secretory changes in the endometrium. If conception does not take place, the endometrium is shed during menstruation, so protecting the endometrium from continued proliferation, a withdrawal of both oestrogen and progesterone being required for this to occur. Persistent proliferation can lead to hyperplastic and ultimately malignant change within the endometrium. It is for these reasons that women with an intact uterus are advised to use combined (oestrogen amd progestogen) hormone replacement therapy (HRT) rather than unopposed oestrogen. Evidence has built up about the effect of HRT on the risk of the development of endometrial cancer. In the first epidemiological study of sufficient

size, Persson and colleagues (1989) showed a two- to threefold risk of developing endometrial cancer with unopposed oestrogen HRT. They report that the addition of progestogens either removes the increased risk or delays its onset.

This topic is further discussed in the chapter on Neoplastic Disease (Chapter 26).

Tamoxifen

Tamoxifen is a synthetic, non-steroidal antioestrogenic drug with some oestrogenic properties. It is used as palliative therapy for advanced breast cancer and as adjuvant therapy for earlier stage disease in both premenopausal and postmenopausal women. Over recent years there have been many reports and studies on the effect of tamoxifen on the endometrium, particularly in postmenopausal women.

Dew and Eden (1995), for example, report six cases of the endometrial effects of tamoxifen, including the development of cystic hyperplasia of the endometrium, benign endometrial polyps, and endometrial cancer. Lahti and colleagues (1993) reported a significantly increased number of polyps in asymptomatic women taking tamoxifen compared with controls. Ismail (1994) found that a greater number of tamoxifen-treated patients undergoing surgery for abnormal bleeding had endometrial polyps (both simple and atypical) and endometrial hyperplasia compared with matched controls. An excess of atypical hyperplasia in women taking tamoxifen was found by Kedar and co-workers (1994). Ugwumadu and colleagues (1993) report a case of tamoxifen-induced adenomyomatous endometrial polyp and adenomyosis.

Little is known about the malignant potential of these polyps, but there is increasing evidence of an association between endometrial carcinoma and tamoxifen use. Ismail (1994) comments on the finding of a number of polyp-cancers among his relatively small series of patients and suggests that endometrial polypogenesis may form an intermediate stage between simple endometrial hyperplasia and endometrial malignancy. Fornander and others (1989) found a relative risk of developing endometrial cancer of 6.4 after 5 years' use. Several other authors have also found an increased risk of endometrial cancer in tamoxifen-treated patients (relative risk 1.3–7.5 — see review by Daniel *et al.* 1996). Soltan and Hutcheson (1997) reported a case of concurrent endometrial carcinoma, fallopian tube carcinoma, and a benign serous cystadenoma in a patient on tamoxifen. They suggested that the possibility of this patient having developed multiple-organ pelvic tumours for reasons that were not related to tamoxifen use was remote.

The mechanism by which tamoxifen exerts its effects on the endometrium is not yet clear, but it seems likely to be due to its agonist properties, especially in the low-oestrogenic postmenopausal state. Ugwumadu and colleagues (1993) speculated that there might be more than one population of oestrogen receptors responding to tamoxifen, allowing both atrophic and proliferative changes, or that growth sites might have lost their sensitivity to the antioestrogenic effects of tamoxifen.

Neven (1993), while recognizing the possible link between tamoxifen and the development of endometrial lesions, raised the possibility of other confounding factors such as obesity. Excess body fat is linked to an increase in oestrogen-receptor-positive breast cancer, and is also important in relation to endogenous oestrogen production.

In the previously discussed study by Fornander and colleagues (1989), the dose of tamoxifen used was 40 mg daily. A reduced dose of tamoxifen may therefore be advisable. However, Jose and others (1995) reported a case of endometrial carcinoma developing on a dose of 20 mg tamoxifen daily. Ismail (1994) suggested that the total cumulative dose might be important, all his cases of malignancy having received more than 35 g of tamoxifen. In Fornander's study (1989), patients receiving treatment for only 2 years did not appear to be at increased risk whereas those using tamoxifen for 5 years were. This might well have been related to the total dose of tamoxifen received or the length of time during which the endometrium was exposed to the drug.

Several authors have speculated whether the concurrent use of a progestogen might have a protective effect on the endometrium (Neven 1993; Dew and Eden 1995; Daniel *et al.* 1996), but this has yet to be proven. Its effect on the breast cancer for which the tamoxifen was prescribed is also unclear.

Because of the risks of pathological endometrial changes developing in patients on tamoxifen, abnormal vaginal bleeding should be investigated promptly. It may also be advisable to perform routine periodic endometrial biopsies or pelvic ultrasound scans in postmenopausal women taking tamoxifen, especially as it is impossible to predict those patients at particular risk of developing endometrial abnormalities (Cohen *et al.* 1993).

Daniel and colleagues (1996) say, however, that despite the apparent increased risk of endometrial cancer in breast cancer patients receiving tamoxifen, the net benefit outweighs the risk. Further research is needed

into the effects of tamoxifen, including optimum dose and duration.

While most cancers reportedly caused by tamoxifen are adenocarcinomas, others have been reported. Cases of uterine stromal sarcoma (Beer *et al.* 1994), leiomyosarcoma (McCluggage *et al.* 1996), and a malignant mixed Müllerian tumour (Clarke 1993) have all been reported following tamoxifen treatment. A number of unusual types of tumour, including clear-cell tumours and leiomyosarcomas, were also found by Silva and colleagues (1994), although they recognized that the development of these might have been unrelated to tamoxifen usage. Further evidence is needed to establish a link between tamoxifen and these rarer uterine cancers.

Fibroids (leiomyomata)

Leiomyomata are benign smooth-muscle tumours that occur commonly in the uterus (where they are called fibroids), although they can rarely occur in other sites such as the lung or retroperitoneal space. It is traditionally taught that fibroids are oestrogen dependent, growing during the reproductive years and often becoming smaller after the menopause (Vollenhoven *et al.* 1990). HRT has been shown to increase the size of uterine fibroids (Sener *et al.* 1996), as well as apparently causing the development of a retroperitoneal leiomyoma (Dixon and Vyas 1997). Although the main culprit in HRT may be oestrogen, there is some evidence that progesterone may have a role in the development of fibroids (Vollenhoven *et al.* 1990; Rein *et al.* 1995). A recent case report by Harrison-Woolrych and Robinson (1995) would appear to confirm this. They noted massive enlargement of a fibroid in a patient being treated for metastatic carcinoma of the breast with high-dose progestogen (megestrol acetate), the size of the fibroid reducing on withdrawal of the progestogen.

Tamoxifen is frequently used in patients with breast cancer, having been shown to improve survival. Increasingly, adverse endometrial effects of tamoxifen are being reported (see above). There is also some suggestion that tamoxifen administration can induce the growth of fibroids: Kang and colleagues (1996) reported a 73-year-old patient who developed large fibroids after taking tamoxifen. In this patient with low endogenous oestrogen levels, it might have been the agonist properties of tamoxifen exerting their effect on the fibroids.

Of note is evidence from Parazzini and colleagues (1992) which showed that there was no increased risk of developing fibroids with the use of the combined oral contraceptive pill.

Further research is needed to determine the role of both oestrogen and progesterone, and their antagonists, in the development of fibroids. In the meantime, patients known to have fibroids should be warned that HRT may cause the latter to increase in size.

Endometriosis

Endometriosis is a condition in which endometrial-type tissue becomes implanted in sites other than the uterus, most commonly on the pelvic peritoneal surfaces and the ovaries. There are several theories as to its cause (such as retrograde menstruation or coelomic metaplasia), but no theory explains all the ectopic sites at which endometriosis has been reported. Cyclical ovarian activity causes the ectopic endometrium to bleed, resulting in inflammation and scarring. Treatment options are therefore aimed at abolishing the normal menstrual cycle using, for example, danazol or gonadotrophin-releasing-hormone agonists.

There is considerable debate as to whether HRT causes endometriosis *de novo*, or has an effect on pre-existing disease. Goh and Hall (1992) reported a case of severe endometriosis developing in a patient taking cyclical combined therapy, but they acknowledged that postmenopausal endometriosis is uncommon. There have been suggestions that oestrogen HRT should be opposed with a progestogen in patients who are known to have endometriosis, even after hysterectomy, in order to prevent the persistence of the disease. However, Sutton (1990) considered it safe to use oestrogen replacement therapy alone in patients who had undergone hysterectomy and bilateral oöphorectomy for endometriosis, and did not advise the addition of progesterone.

Svigos (1990) suggested that the use of clomiphene citrate for the treatment of anovulatory infertility may cause the development of endometriosis, and speculated that this might be the reason for poor pregnancy rates despite resumption of normal ovulation.

Ovarian abnormalities

Ovarian cysts

Ovarian cysts are a relatively common finding in premenopausal women; many are simple cysts resulting from cyclical ovarian activity, others are caused by drugs.

Tayob and others (1985) demonstrated the increased frequency of functional ovarian cysts in women using progestogen-only oral contraception (POP) compared with a control group of women not exposed to hormones. Of 12 patients using POP who developed cysts,

seven complained of symptoms, although most cysts resolved spontaneously. Broome and colleagues (1995) showed an increased incidence of enlarged follicles or cysts in women using POP, most of which were asymptomatic and transient.

The levonorgestrel ($20 \mu g$ per day)-loaded intra-uterine contraceptive device (IUCD) has also been shown to increase the incidence of ovarian follicular enlargement or cysts when compared with a group of copper IUCD users, presumably reflecting the systemic effects of levonorgestrel (Sivin and Stern 1994).

Norplant users also have been shown to have a higher rate of ovarian cysts, probably as a result of disordered folliculogenesis. Shaaban and others (1993) showed that nearly 46% of long-term users of Norplant had excessive follicular enlargement, but these rarely exceeded 50 mm in diameter and most disappeared within a short time.

Clomiphene citrate therapy for induction of ovulation has been reported to cause ovarian cysts which in one case resulted in bilateral adnexal torsion (Bider *et al.* 1991).

Hochner-Celnikier and colleagues (1995) reported five cases of premenopausal women who developed ovarian cysts while taking tamoxifen; indeed, Shushan and colleagues (1996) reported that ovarian cysts are a common adverse effect of tamoxifen therapy, most cysts disappearing after withdrawal of the drug. The reason for the development of these cysts is unclear. It has been suggested that it might be due to the rise in gonadotrophin levels brought about by a fall in circulating oestrogen. This may be true for premenopausal women, but it does not seem as plausible an explanation in those past the menopause in whom there is no change in oestradiol level with tamoxifen usage (Shushan *et al.* 1996).

Ovarian hyperstimulation syndrome

Ovarian hyperstimulation syndrome (OHSS) is an iatrogenic complication of ovulation induction. It varies in severity, in its most severe form being characterized by massive ovarian enlargement, ascites, pleural effusion, oliguria, and thromboembolic events. The pathophysiology of OHSS is not clear. Increased capillary permeability, perhaps brought about by prostaglandins or histamine, or by activation of the renin–angiotensin system (Rizk 1994), has been suggested as the primary event.

OHSS is most commonly seen after superovulation for *in vitro* fertilization, and the incidence of moderate to severe disease varies from 0.6 to 14% of cases (Rizk 1994). It is commoner in conception cycles (Haning *et al.*

1983) and amongst patients with polycystic ovarian disease (MacDougall *et al.* 1992; Rizk and Smitz 1992). The combined use of gonadotrophin-releasing-hormone antagonists and human menopausal gonadotrophin (HMG) results in an increased incidence of OHSS compared with HMG alone (but with a greater pregnancy rate) (Ron-el *et al.* 1991). Attempts at preventing OHSS may be made by close monitoring of follicle development and oestradiol levels, and in selected patients withholding the administration of human chorionic gonadotrophin (HCG), or by cryopreserving the embryos (which can then be transferred at a later date) (Tiitinen *et al.* 1995).

Ovulation induction using either HMG or pure urinary follicle-stimulating hormone (uFSH) is also associated with OHSS. Mild disease is seen in up to 23% of patients and severe disease in up to 3.5% of cases (Rizk 1994). Patients with polycystic ovarian syndrome are at most risk. Some authors suggest that the use of uFSH rather than HMG in these patients is associated with lower rates of OHSS (Raj *et al.* 1977; Dale *et al.* 1992), but others are not so convinced (Check *et al.* 1985). In patients with polycystic ovarian syndrome great care is needed with very careful ultrasound and biochemical monitoring. If the development of OHSS is thought likely, it may be prevented by the withholding of HCG.

Clomiphene citrate has been associated with mild OHSS but has only rarely been reported to cause severe disease (Roland 1970; Morgan *et al.* 1983).

Ovarian cancer

Concern has been voiced in recent years about the risk of ovarian cancer in patients who have received treatment for infertility.

Whittemore and others (1992), in an analysis of case–control studies, found that women who had used fertility drugs had three times the risk of developing ovarian cancer of non-users with no infertility problem. They suggested that the infertility itself plays a minor role in this increased risk and that the fertility drugs are responsible for most of the increase in risk. A further study (Rossing *et al.* 1994) found an increase in ovarian cancer and borderline tumours in women exposed to clomiphene for more than 12 cycles. However, in another study, Venn and colleagues (1995), failed to show any rise in ovarian cancer rates in patients undergoing *in vitro* fertilization.

In a response to the Whittemore paper, the International Federation of Fertility Societies organized a task force (Cohen 1993) which critically analysed the evidence presented in this study. They concluded that although a causal link between fertility drugs and ovarian cancer could not be excluded, it clearly had not been demonstrated. This finding was echoed in a review of the literature by Bristow and Karlan (1996) who stated that currently available data in the literature suggests an association between ovulation induction and ovarian cancer, but does not necessarily indicate a causal link.

A more recent paper (Unkila-Kallio *et al.* 1997) reports the cases of 11 women with ovarian cancer with a known period of infertility, nine of whom had had ovulation induction by clomiphene citrate or gonadotrophin. Four patients had received clomiphene for more than 12 cycles. While their figures support a causative effect of fertility drugs in the initiation of ovarian cancer, they advise caution in the interpretation, as it is still not clear what proportion of the increased risk of cancer is due to infertility or nulliparity itself. The protective effect of any pregnancy achieved through fertility treatment must be taken into account as well.

Until further studies have elucidated the absolute risk, care must be taken in fertility practice. It is recommended that clomiphene be used for a maximum of 12 cycles.

Vaginal/vulval symptoms

Adverse drug reactions uncommonly cause vaginal disorders. Probably the commonest complaint is the occurrence of vaginal candidiasis (thrush) after completion of a course of a broad-spectrum antibiotic. Antibiotic administration is a well-known risk factor for the development of *Candida albicans* vaginitis (Monif 1985) due to the reduction in normal vaginal bacteria, particularly lactobacilli, which usually prevent candidal overgrowth. In a study by Bluestein and colleagues (1991), of 74 women prescribed antibiotics, 24 developed vaginal thrush. Sobel (1985) states that virtually no antibiotic is immune from this frequent complication; agents such as tetracycline, ampicillin, and cephalosporins appear to be the commonest offenders.

Vaginal and vulval soreness, itching, or burning is occasionally seen in patients using oestrogen cream for the treatment of urogenital atrophy.

Vaginal dryness is a common complaint in patients on gonadotrophin-releasing-hormone agonists (e.g. goserelin, nafarelin, buserelin, leuprorelin) as an effect of hypo-oestrogenism (Kennedy *et al.* 1990).

A rare condition, vaginitis emphysematosa, has been reported in a patient taking cyclosporin after a renal transplant (Tjugum *et al.* 1986). This condition is characterized by multiple gas-filled cystic lesions within the vagina and it is thought that there may be an underlying immune aetiology.

Another rare adverse effect on the vagina was reported by King and Horowitz (1993). A 37-year-old patient developed vaginal and vulval anaesthesia after commencing fluoxetine for a depressive illness. Her vaginal symptoms gradually resolved on withdrawing the drug. The authors did not offer any explanation for this reaction.

Drug-induced premenstrual syndrome

The premenstrual syndrome (PMS) is a cyclical condition characterized by the development of various premenstrual symptoms which resolve at the onset of menses. Its cause is not entirely clear but progesterone appears to play a role.

Exogenous progestogens can induce PMS-like symptoms. In a study on progestogen intolerance, Smith and colleagues (1994) questioned 52 women taking cyclical progestogens. The commonest symptoms (occurring in 13 to 18 patients) were bloating, painful breasts, mood swings, fatigue, depression, irritability, skin disorders, weight gain, anxiety, and general aches and pains. They found that different progestogens tended to cause different symptom complexes, a fact which may be useful in managing women who experience symptoms of progestogen intolerance. Norethisterone was more likely to cause pain-complex symptoms, while dydrogesterone produced more adverse effects on concentration and mood.

Broome and Fotherby (1990) found three patients out of 358 progesterone-only pill users who complained specifically of premenstrual tension, and 23 others who complained of bloating, weight gain, depression, or tiredness, as well as 40 women who complained of breast tenderness or discomfort. Similar symptoms have also been reported in patients using depot medroxyprogesterone acetate (Depo-Provera) (Nelson 1996) and the levonorgestrel-loaded intrauterine contraceptive device (Andersson et al. 1994), although symptoms often lessen with time.

Breast disease

Breast pain

Progesterone increases ductal cell proliferation and vascular and lymphatic congestion in the breast, which may result in mastalgia (Nelson 1996). Patients taking cyclical progestogen in combined HRT often complain of breast tenderness or swelling when they start the progesterone phase. Sixteen out of 52 women taking cyclical progesterone complained of painful breasts (Smith et al. 1994).

Many patients using progesterone-only contraceptives complain of breast discomfort, tenderness, swelling, or pain. Broome and Fotherby (1990) found that out of 358 progesterone-only pill (POP) users, 77 reported adverse effects, of which breast tenderness was the commonest (occuring in 40 women). Breast tenderness or swelling was found in 2.9 per cent of patients using depot medroxyprogesterone acetate (Depo-Provera), but the mastalgia tended to improve with time (Nelson 1996). Breast tenderness was also given as a reason for termination of use of the levonorgestrel intrauterine device in some patients in a study by Andersson and colleagues (1994).

Breast tenderness has been reported in patients receiving cyclosporin for ocular disorders (Palestine et al. 1984). Three patients (one male, two female) out of 26 complained of breast tenderness but it was not significant enough to discontinue treatment and resolved within 1–2 months. The mechanism for its occurrence is not clear.

Breast cancer

Concern has been expressed about the risk of breast cancer in women on hormone replacement therapy. In a recent paper the Collaborative Group on Hormonal Factors in Breast Cancer (CGHFBC) (1997) found that the risk of breast cancer was increased in women using HRT and more so with greater duration of use. The effect was reduced after cessation of HRT and had largely disappeared after about 5 years. Colditz and colleagues (1995) found a similarly increased risk and also noted that the addition of a progestogen did not protect against it. Patients who wish to take HRT need to be aware of the facts and be advised of their individual potential risks and benefits.

There are also concerns over the increased risk of developing breast cancer with the use of the combined contraceptive pill. Although the results of some studies are conflicting, more recent data does suggest that long-term use of the combined pill may have a significant effect on breast cancer incidence (Brooks et al. 1992).

There have also been worries about the effect of depot medroxyprogesterone acetate (Depo-Provera) on the incidence of breast cancer. In an analysis of two case–control studies, Skegg and colleagues (1995) found an increased risk of breast cancer in recent or current users of Depo-Provera, but no increase in risk in those who had used it 5 years or more previously. A causal link is not established and Skegg suggests that the increased risk could be due to enhanced detection in this group of women, or accelerated growth of pre-existing tumours. This subject is also discussed in the chapter on Neoplastic Disease (Chapter 26).

Obstetrical disorders

Ectopic pregnancy

Ectopic pregnancies are pregnancies implanting in a site other than the uterus, most commonly the fallopian tube. Several case reports and studies have suggested an increased incidence of ectopic pregnancy in patients having ovulation induction with clomiphene (see review by Venn and Lumley 1994).

Heterotopic pregnancy is the coexistence of an intra-uterine pregnancy and an ectopic gestation. In spontaneous conceptions the incidence of this has been reported to be between about 1 in 30 000 pregnancies (Reece *et al.* 1983). However, the incidence in pregnancies conceived by either ovulation induction or assisted reproduction is much higher (possibly as high as 1 in 100 pregnancies), although the reasons for this are not clear. With *in vitro* fertilization, the technique of embryo transfer may be relevant. In gamete or zygote intrafallopian transfer it is likely that one or more embryos remain in the fallopian tube, perhaps as a result of poor tubal function, while another migrates into the uterus.

It is not understood, however, why patients conceiving with clomiphene citrate and/or gonadotrophins (FSH/LH) have a higher incidence of ectopic or heterotopic pregnancy. Possible theories include the antioestrogenic effect of clomiphene or the effect of sex steroids on tubal function (Tal *et al.* 1996). De Muylder and colleagues (1994) reported a case of a heterotopic ovarian pregnancy in a patient given clomiphene, the cause of which cannot readily be explained by poor tubal function. It may simply be that multiple ovulation alone increases the risk of ectopic and heterotopic gestations (Venn and Lumley 1994).

The progesterone-only pill has also been linked to an increased chance of ectopic gestation. Netter (1996) suggested that it creates a state of permanent oestrogenicity with luteal insufficiency that disturbs tubal function.

Multiple pregnancy

Twin pregnancies resulting from spontaneous conceptions account for in the order of 1 in 80 births. The incidence of multiple births is, however, rising due to the increase in the use of ovulation induction and assisted-reproduction techniques. Clomiphene is the simplest drug used for ovulation induction and is associated with an increased multiple-birth rate, most commonly as twins, which can be explained by the effect of clomiphene on the maturation of one or more ovarian follicles

and oöcytes (Venn and Lumley 1994). Using more sophisticated methods of ovulation induction (such as preparations of the gonadotrophins, FSH, and LH) high numbers of multiple pregnancies have been reported, often with frequent higher-order multiples such as quadruplets or quintuplets (Evans *et al.* 1995). Patients undergoing ovulation-induction programmes need to be carefully monitored to ensure that, where multiple follicles are developing, fertilization is not allowed to occur.

With *in vitro* techniques, two or three embryos are commonly transferred into the uterus, resulting in an increase in twin and triplet pregnancies, but Human Fertilisation and Embryology Authority guidelines no longer permit the transfer of larger numbers of embryos.

Patients undergoing any form of ovulation induction or assisted conception need to be aware of the risk of conceiving a multiple pregnancy.

Uterine rupture

Uterine rupture is a rare occurrence (estimated by Plauche *et al.* (1984) to be approximately 4–5/10 000 deliveries). The risk is increased in multiparous patients, in induced labours, and in the presence of a uterine scar (either from a caesarean section or a myomectomy, or possibly the site of traumatic uterine perforation at the time of a previous uterine curettage).

The use of oxytocin (Syntocinon) for augmentation of a poorly progressing labour is common practice in most hospitals in the UK. Its use in nulliparous patients is generally safe and effective, but caution should be exercised in multiparous women. Several case reports have demonstrated the association of uterine rupture of the unscarred uterus in multiparous patients with the use of oxytocin (Sweeten *et al.* 1995; Miller *et al.* 1997). The thinner, previously distended myometrium seems to be at greater risk when contractions of greater strength and frequency are generated by the use of oxytocin.

The use of oxytocin has also been associated with the rupture of a scarred uterus following a previous Caesarean section (demonstrated in a case–control study by Leung *et al.* 1993). It appears that rupture is more likely when oxytocin is used for augmentation of poor progress than when used for induction of labour. Therefore, a thorough assessment of the patient is required before using oxytocin to augment labour in multiparae or those who have had a previous Caesarean section.

Induction of labour is commonly achieved with intra-vaginal prostaglandin and this has also been associated with an increased incidence of uterine rupture. The use of prostaglandins brings about cervical ripening and often initiates labour. Frequent mild contractions are

often a feature of prostaglandin use and hyperstimulation has been reported (Nuutila and Kajanoja 1996).
Both prostaglandin E_1 (misoprostol) and E_2 (Prostin)
have been associated with uterine rupture (Azem *et al.*
1993; Bennett 1997). Both these authors once again
suggest that multiparae are most at risk. Nordin (1993)
demonstrates another high-risk group: women with a
scarred uterus. Care should be taken when using prostaglandins to induce labour in these patients.

Mid-trimester termination of pregnancy is now usually
brought about by the use of intravaginal prostaglandins.
More recently it has become common practice to give a
dose of mifepristone (a progesterone antagonist) 36–48
hours before the prostaglandin. This seems to shorten
the induction-to-abortion interval (Rodger and Baird
1990). The use of mifepristone and a prostaglandin
(either misoprostol or gemeprost) has been reported to
have caused uterine rupture (Norman 1995; Phillips *et al.*
1996). It is recommended that any woman who has not
aborted 24 hours after the prostaglandin was started
should be carefully reviewed (Thong *et al.* 1995). Once
again, patients undergoing second-trimester termination who have had a previous Caesarean section are at
greater risk of uterine rupture (Chapman *et al.* 1996).

References

Andersson, K., Odlind, V., and Rybo, G. (1994). Levonor-
gestrel-releasing and copper-releasing (Nova T) IUDs during five years of use: A randomized comparative trial.
Contraception 49, 56.

Azem, F., Jaffa, A., Lessing, J.B., *et al.* (1993). Uterine rupture
with the use of a low-dose vaginal PGE2 tablet. *Acta Obstet.
Gynecol. Scand.* 72, 316.

Beer, T.W., Buchanan, R., and Buckley, C.H. (1994). Uterine
stromal sarcoma following tamoxifen treatment. *J. Clin.
Pathol.* 48, 596.

Bennett, B.B. (1997). Uterine rupture during induction of
labour at term with intravaginal misoprostol. *Obstet.
Gynecol.* 89, 832.

Bider, D., Goldenberg, M., Ben-Rafael, Z., *et al.* (1991).
Bilateral adnexal torsion after clomiphene citrate therapy.
Hum. Reprod. 6, 1443.

Biswas, A., Leong, W.P., Ratnam, S.S., *et al.* (1996). Menstrual
bleeding patterns in Norplant-2 implant users. *Contraception* 54, 91.

Bluestein, D., Rutledge, C., and Lumsden, I. (1991). Predicting the occurrence of antibiotic-induced candidial vaginitis
(AICV). *Fam. Pract. Res. J.* 11, 319.

Bristow, R.E. and Karlan, B.Y. (1996). Ovulation induction,
infertility and ovarian cancer risk. *Fertil. Steril.* 66, 499.

Brooks, M.D., Fraser, S.C.A., Ebbs, S.R., *et al.* (1992). Malignant disease of the breast. In *Gynaecology* (ed. R. Shaw, P.

Souter, and S. Stanton), p. 493. Churchill Livingstone,
Edinburgh.

Broome, M., Clayton, J. and Fotherby, K. (1995). Enlarged
follicles in women using oral contraceptives. *Contraception*
52, 13.

Broome, M. and Fotherby, K. (1990). Clinical experience with
the progestogen-only pill. *Contraception* 45, 489.

Chapman, S.J., Crispens, M., Owen, J., *et al.* (1996). Complications of midtrimester pregnancy termination: the effect of
prior cesarean delivery. *Am. J. Obstet. Gynecol.* 175, 889.

Check, J.H., Wu, C-H., Gocial, B., *et al.* (1985). Severe ovarian
hyperstimulation syndrome from treatment with urinary
follicle-stimulating hormone: two cases. *Fertil. Steril.* 43,
317.

Clarke, M. (1993). Uterine malignant mixed mullarian tumour
in a patient on long-term tamoxifen therapy for breast
cancer. *Gynecol. Oncol.* 51, 411.

Cohen, I., Rosen, D., Shapira, J., *et al.* (1993). Endometrial
changes in postmenopausal women treated with tamoxifen
for breast cancer. *Br. J. Obstet. Gynaecol.* 100, 567.

Cohen, J. International Federation of Fertility Societies.
(1993). Fertility drugs and ovarian cancer. *Fertil. Steril.* 60,
406.

Colditz, G.A., Hankinson, S.E., Hunter, D.J., *et al.* (1995).
The use of estrogens and progestins and the risk of breast
cancer in postmenopausal women. *N. Engl. J. Med.* 332,
1589.

Collaborative Group on Hormonal Factors in Breast Cancer.
(1997). Breast cancer and hormone replacement therapy:
collaborative reanalysis of data from 51 epidemiological
studies of 5205 women with breast cancer and 108 411
women without breast cancer. *Lancet* 350, 1047.

Dale, P.O., Tanbo, T., Haug, E., *et al.* (1992). Polycystic ovary
syndrome: low-dose follicle stimulating hormone administration is a safe stimulation regimen even in previous hyper-
responsive patients. *Hum. Reprod.* 7, 1085.

Daniel, Y., Inbar, M., Bar-Am, A., *et al.* (1996). The effects of
tamoxifen treatment on the endometrium. *Fertil. Steril.* 65,
1083.

De Muylder, X., De Loecker, P., and Campo, R. (1994).
Heterotopic pregnancy after clomiphene ovulation induction. *Eur. J. Obstet. Gynecol. Reprod. Biol.* 53, 65.

Dew, J.E. and Eden, J.A. (1995). Gynaecological complications of women treated with tamoxifen for breast cancer.
Aust. N.Z. J. Obstet. Gynaecol. 35, 198.

Dixon, J.C. and Vyas, S.K. (1997). Retroperitoneal leiomyoma
presenting after hormone replacement therapy. *J. Obstet.
Gynaecol.* 17, 592.

Droegemueller, W., Rao Katta, L., Bright, T.G., *et al.* (1989).
Triphasic randomised clinical trial: comparative frequency
of intermenstrual bleeding. *Am. J. Obstet. Gynecol.* 161,
1407.

Evans, M.I., Littmann, L., St. Louis, L., *et al.* (1995). Evolving
patterns of iatrogenic multifetal pregnancy generation: Implications for aggressiveness of infertility treatments. *Am. J.
Obstet. Gynecol.* 172, 1750.

Fan, M. and Sujuan, G. (1996). Menstrual bleeding patterns in Chinese women using the Norplant subdermal system. *Hum. Reprod.* 11 (Suppl. 2), 14.

Fornander, T., Cedermark, B., Mattsson, A., *et al.* (1989). Adjuvant tamoxifen in early breast cancer: occurrence of new primary cancers. *Lancet* i, 117.

Goh, J.T.W.and Hall, B.A. (1992). Postmenopausal endometrioma and hormonal replacement therapy. *Aust. N.Z. J. Obstet. Gynaecol.* 32, 384.

Haning, R.V., Austin, C.W., Carlson, I.H., *et al.* (1983). Plasma estradiol is superior to ultrasound and urinary estriol glucuronide as a predictor of ovarian hyperstimulation during induction of ovulation with menotropins. *Fertil. Steril.* 40, 31.

Harrison-Woolrych, M. and Robinson, R. (1995). Fibroid growth in response to high-dose progestogen. *Fertil. Steril.* 64, 191.

Helfer, E.L., Miller, J.L., and Rose, L.I. (1988). Side-effects of spironolactone therapy in the hirsute woman. *J. Clin. Endocrinol. Metab.* 66, 208.

Hochner-Celnikier, D., Anteby, E., and Yagel, S. (1995). Ovarian cysts in tamoxifen-treated women with breast cancer — a managment dilemma. *Am. J. Obstet. Gynecol.* 172, 1323.

Ismail, S.M. (1994). Pathology of endometrium treated with tamoxifen. *J. Clin. Pathol.* 47, 827.

Jose, R., Kekre, A., George, S., *et al.* (1995). Endometrial carcinoma in a tamoxifen-treated breast cancer patient. *Aust. N.Z. J. Obstet. Gynaecol.* 35, 201.

Kang, B.S., Baxi, L., and Heller, D. (1996). Tamoxifen-induced growth of leiomyomas. A case report. *J. Reprod. Med.* 41, 119.

Kedar, R.P., Bourne, T.H., Powles, T.J., *et al.* (1994). Effects of tamoxifen on uterus and ovaries of postmenopausal women in a randomised breast cancer prevention trial. *Lancet* 343, 1318.

Kennedy, S.H., Williams, I.A., Brodribb, J., *et al.* (1990). A comparison of naferilin acetate and danazol in the treatment of endometriosis. *Fertil. Steril.* 53, 998.

King, V.L., Jr and Horowitz, I.R. (1993). Vaginal anaesthesia associated with fluoxetine use. *Am. J. Psychiatry* 150, 984.

Kovacs, G. (1996). Progestogen-only pills and bleeding disturbances. *Hum. Reprod.* 11 (Suppl. 2), 20.

Lahti, E., Blanco, G., Kauppila, A., *et al.* (1993). Endometrial changes in postmenopausal breast cancer patients receiving tamoxifen. *Obstet. Gynecol.* 81, 660.

Leung, A.S., Farmer, R.M., Leung, E.K., *et al.* (1993). Risk factors associated with uterine rupture during trial of labour after cesarean delivery: a case-control study. *Am. J. Obstet. Gynecol.* 168, 1358.

MacDougall, M.J., Tan, S.L., and Jacobs, H.S. (1992). In-vitro fertilisation and the ovarian hyperstimulation syndrome. *Hum. Reprod.* 7, 597.

Mainwaring, R., Hales, H.A., Stevenson, K., *et al.* (1995). Metabolic parameter, bleeding and weight changes in U.S. women using progestin-only contraceptive. *Contraception* 51, 149.

McCluggage, W.G., Varma, M., Weir, P., *et al.* (1996). Uterine leiomyosarcoma in a patient receiving tamoxifen therapy. *Acta Obstet. Gynecol. Scand.* 75, 593.

Miller, D.A., Goodwin, T.M., Gherman, R.B., *et al.* (1997). Intrapartum rupture of the unscarred uterus. *Obstet. Gynecol.* 89, 671.

Monif, G.R.G. (1985). Classification and pathogenesis of vulvovaginal candidiasis. *Am. J. Obstet. Gynecol.* 152, 955.

Morgan, H., Paredes, R.A. and Lachelin, G.C. (1983). Severe ovarian hyperstimulation after clomiphene citrate in a hypothyroid patient. *Br. J. Obstet. Gynaecol.* 90, 977.

Nelson, A.L. (1996). Counselling issues and the management of side-effects for women using depot medroxyprogesterone acetate. *J. Reprod. Med.* 41, 391.

Netter, A. (1996). Ectopic pregnancies in subjects on progestin-only pills. *Fertil. Steril.* 65, 1078.

Neven, P. (1993). Tamoxifen and endometrial lesions. *Lancet* 342, 452.

Nordin, A.J. (1993). Lower segment uterine scar rupture during induction of labour with vaginal prostaglandin E_2. *Postgrad. Med. J.* 69, 592.

Norman, J.E. (1995). Uterine rupture during therapeutic abortion in the second trimester using mifepristone and prostaglandin. *Br. J. Obstet. Gynaecol.* 102, 332.

Nuutila, M. and Kajanoja, P. (1996). Local administration of prostaglandin E_2 for cervical ripening and labour induction: the appropriate route and dose. *Acta Obstet. Gynecol. Scand.* 75, 135.

Palareti, G., Leali, N., Coccheri, S., *et al.* on behalf of the Italian Study on Complications of Oral Anticoagulant Therapy. (1996). Bleeding complications of oral anticoagulant treatment: an inception-cohort, prospective collaborative study (ISCOAT). *Lancet* 348, 423.

Palestine, A.G., Nussenblatt, R.B., and Chan, C. (1984). Side effects of systemic cyclosporine in patients not undergoing transplantation. *Am. J. Med.* 77, 652.

Parazzini, F., Negri, E., La Vecchia, C., *et al.* (1992). Oral contraceptive use and risk of uterine fibroids. *Obstet. Gynecol.* 79, 430.

Persson, I., Adami, H., Bergkvist, L., *et al.* (1989). Risk of endometrial cancer after treatment with oestrogens alone or in conjunction with progesterone: results of a prospective study. *BMJ* 298, 147.

Phillips, K., Berry, C., and Mathers, A.M. (1996). Uterine rupture during second trimester termination of pregnancy using mifepristone and a prostaglandin. *Eur. J. Obstet. Gynecol. Reprod. Biol.* 65, 175.

Plauche, W.C., Von Almen, W., and Muller, R. (1984). Catastrophic uterine rupture. *Obstet. Gynecol.* 64, 792.

Raj, S.G., Berger, M.J., Grimes, E.M., *et al.* (1977). The use of gonadotrophins for the induction of ovulation in women with polycystic disease. *Fertil. Steril.* 28, 1280.

Reece, E.A., Petrie, R.H., Sirmans, M.F., *et al.* (1983). Combined intrauterine and extrauterine gestations: a review. *Am. J. Obstet. Gynecol.* 146, 323.

Rein, M.S., Barbieri, R.L., and Friedman, A.J. (1995). Progesterone: A critical role in the pathogenesis of uterine myomas. *Am. J. Obstet. Gynecol.* 172, 14.

Rizk, B. (1994). Ovarian hyperstimulation syndrome. In *Progress in Obstetrics and Gynaecology*, Vol. 11 (ed. J. Studd), p. 311. Churchill Livingstone, London.

Rizk, B. and Smitz, J. (1992). Ovarian hyperstimulation syndrome after superovulation using GnRH agonists for IVF and related procedures. *Hum. Reprod.* 7, 320.

Rodger, M.W. and Baird, D.T. (1990). Pretreatment with mifepristone (RU486) reduces the interval between prostaglandin administration and expulsion in second trimester abortion. *Br. J. Obstet. Gynaecol.* 97, 41.

Roland, M. (1970). Problems of ovulation induction with clomiphene citrate with a report of a case of ovarian hyperstimulation. *Obstet. Gynecol.* 35, 55.

Ron-el, R., Herman, A., Golan, A., *et al.* (1991). Gonadotrophins and combined gonadotrophin-releasing hormone agonist/gonadotrophin protocols in a randomised prospective study. *Fertil. Steril.* 55, 574.

Rossing, M.A., Daling, J.R., Weiss, N.S., *et al.* (1994). Ovarian tumours in a cohort of infertile women. *N. Engl. J. Med.* 331, 771.

Sener, A.B., Seckin, N.C., Ozmen, S., *et al.* (1996). The effects of hormone replacement therapy on uterine fibroids in postmenopausal women. *Fertil. Steril.* 65, 354.

Shaaban, M.M., Segal, S., Salem, H.T., *et al.* (1993). Sonographic assessment of ovarian and endometrial changes during long-term Norplant use and their correlation with hormone levels. *Fertil. Steril.* 59, 998.

Shushan, A., Peretz, T., Uziely, B., *et al.* (1996). Ovarian cysts in premenopausal and postmenopausal tamoxifen-treated women with breast cancer. *Am. J. Obstet. Gynecol.* 174, 141.

Silva, E.G., Tornos, C.S., and Follen-Mitchell, M. (1994). Malignant neoplasms of the uterine corpus in patients treated for breast carcinoma: the effects of tamoxifen. *Int. J. Gynecol. Pathol.* 13, 248.

Sivin, I. and Stern, J. (1994). Health during prolonged use of levonorgestrel 20 μg/d and the Copper TCu 380Ag intrauterine contraceptive devices: a multicenter study. *Fertil. Steril.* 61, 70.

Skegg, D.C.G., Noonan, E.A., Paul, C., *et al.* (1995). Depot medroxyprogesterone acetate and breast cancer. *JAMA* 273, 799.

Smith, R.N.J., Holland, E.F.N., and Studd, J.W.W. (1994). The symptomatology of progestogen intolerance. *Maturitas* 18, 87.

Sobel, J.D. (1985). Epidemiology and pathogenesis of recurrent vulvovaginal candidiasis. *Am. J. Obstet. Gynecol.* 152, 924.

Soltan, A.S. and Hutcheson, R.B. (1997). A case of concurrent endometrial carcinoma, fallopian tube carcinoma and a benign right ovarian serous cystadenoma with tamoxifen therapy. *J. Obstet. Gynaecol.* 17, 596.

Sutton, C. (1990). The treatment of endometriosis. In *Progress in Obstetrics and Gynaecology*, Vol. 8 (ed. J. Studd), p.251. Churchill Livingstone, London.

Svigos, J.M. (1990). Endometriosis and clomiphene citrate. *Lancet* 335, 475.

Sweeten, K.M., Graves, W.K., and Athanassiou, A. (1995). Spontaneous rupture of the unscarred uterus. *Am. J. Obstet. Gynecol.* 172, 1851.

Tal, J., Haddad, S., Gordon, N., *et al.* (1996). Heterotopic pregnancy after ovulation induction and assisted reproductive technologies: a literature review from 1971 to 1993. *Fertil. Steril.* 66, 1.

Tayob, Y., Adams, J., Jacobs, H.S., *et al.* (1985). Ultrasound demonstration of increased frequency of functional ovarian cysts in women using progestogen-only oral contraception. *Br. J. Obstet. Gynaecol.* 92, 1003.

Thong, K.J., Lynch, P., and Baird, D.T. (1995). Uterine rupture during therapeutic abortion in the second trimester using mifepristone and prostaglandin. *Br. J. Obstet. Gynaecol.* 102, 844.

Tiitinen, A., Husa, L-M., Tulppala, M., *et al.* (1995). The effect of cryopreservation in prevention of ovarian hyperstimulation syndrome. *Br. J. Obstet. Gynaecol.* 102, 326.

Tjugum, J., Jonassen, F., and Olsson, J-H. (1986). Vaginitis emphysematosa in a renal transplant patient. *Acta Obstet. Gynecol. Scand.* 65, 377.

Ugwumadu, A.H.N., Bower, D., and Kin-Hoi Ho, P. (1993). Tamoxifen induced adenomyosis and adenomyomatous endometrial polyp. *Br. J. Obstet. Gynaecol.* 100, 386.

Unkila-Kallio, L., Leminen, A., Tiitinen, A., *et al.* (1997). Malignant tumours of the ovary or the breast in association with infertility: a report of thirteen cases. *Acta Obstet. Gynecol. Scand.* 76, 177.

Venn, A. and Lumley, J. (1994). Clomiphene citrate and pregnancy outcome. *Aust. N.Z. J. Obstet. Gynaecol.* 34, 56.

Venn, A., Watson, L., Lumley, J., *et al.* (1995). Breast and ovarian cancer incidence after infertility and in vitro fertilisation. *Lancet* 346, 995.

Vollenhoven, B.J., Lawrence, A.S., and Healy, D.L. (1990). Uterine fibroids: a clinical review. *Br. J. Obstet. Gynaecol.* 97, 285.

Whittemore, A.S., Harris, R., Itnyre, J., and the Collaborative Ovarian Cancer Group. (1992). Characteristics relating to ovarian cancer risk: collaborative analysis of 12 US case-control studies. *Am. J. Epidemiol.* 136, 1184.

31. Drug-induced sexual dysfunction and infertility

D.N. BATEMAN

Introduction

It is conventional to divide adverse effects of drugs on the reproductive system into those that impair sexual drive (libido), those that impair functional performance, and those that produce infertility. In practice, most of the published literature in this area relates to male sexual dysfunction. There is some information to suggest that female sexual function may be equally disturbed by drugs, but the magnitude of these effects has been more difficult to quantify in women.

Drug-induced sexual dysfunction

Human sexual function is dependent upon two factors: libido, or sexual desire, and physiological function.

Libido is influenced by reproductive hormones and the emotional physical health of the individual, together with the availability, interest, and attractiveness of sexual partners (Korenman 1983; Smith and Talbert 1986). Testosterone is necessary for normal sexual arousal, probably in both men and women; and in men testosterone deficiency is associated with impotence. Hyperprolactinaemia may be associated with a reduction in serum testosterone and impotence. Returning testosterone levels to normal in patients with hyperprolactinaemia does not always restore potency (Krane *et al.* 1989).

The physiological mechanisms of sexual responsiveness are divided into four phases in men and women. In the first, the excitement of arousal phase, the phase of congestion results in either an erection in men or, in women, swelling of the vagina, labia minora, and clitoris. Pathways involved in control of erection, and the corresponding female changes, include sympathetic activity, with sympathetic activation responsible for

detumescence; parasympathetic activation, which is erectile; and non-adrenergic, non-cholinergic pathways, probably principally involving nitric oxide, which is also erectile. Other receptors that have been implicated in erectile function include histamine H_1-receptors, H_2-receptors, which cause relaxation, and 5-HT receptors, which appear to activate contraction of the corpora cavernosa and smooth muscle of the penis. In men, erection occurs when the smooth muscle of the arteries and corpora of the penis are relaxed, and the erectile tissue fills with blood at arterial pressure. The drainage of the penis is impaired by physical compression related to local pressure. Appropriate erectile function is therefore determined by adequate neurological control, adequate arterial flow, and appropriate penile drainage, and a blocking mechanism. The nerve pathways involved in these functions include in particular spinal cord roots S2–S5 via the pudendal nerve. Efferent parasympathetic impulses pass via the nervi erigentes to produce vasoconstriction (Duncan and Bateman 1993).

Changes in blood supply in the female occur principally in the lower vaginal vault, the labia minora, and the clitoris. In women, the pathways and vascular influences are therefore analogous to those affecting the penis. However, the responses appear to take more time to develop, the changes in vascular function produce less rigidity, and the lubrication that occurs in the vagina is thought to be analogous to a 'sweating' phenomenon, since there appear to be no mucus-secreting glands in the vaginal wall (Stevenson and Umstead 1984).

The plateau or lubrication phase involves secretion of mucus in both male and female. In the male, the secretions are produced from Cowper's gland, the glands of Littré, and the prostate. These secretions, together with sperm, constitute semen. In the female Bartholin's and Skene's glands are involved in the secretion of a limited amount of mucoid lubricants. As women age, there is a relationship between the capacity to produce this lubricating material and falling oestrogen levels.

In the third (orgasmic) phase the physiology in men and women is no longer analogous. In men, the orgasmic phase is divided into emission and ejaculation. Sympathetic reflexes from the thoracolumbar region of the spinal cord (T12–L3) stimulate α-adrenoceptors and result in the contraction of the smooth muscle of the prostate, seminal vesicles, vas deferens, and ampulla. Afferent impulses are transmitted through the pudendal nerve to the sacral portion of spinal cord (S2–S4) and return as a reflex arc to the pelvis and perineal musculature. This results in a tonic–clonic contraction of the bulbocavernosus muscles, which receive innervation from the sympathetic nerves, together with a sympathetic-mediated contraction of the vas deferens and seminal vesicles. These processes result in ejaculation of seminal fluid. Under some circumstances, closure of the urethra at the bladder neck does not occur appropriately and semen may pass backwards into the bladder (retrograde ejaculation).

In women, there is no counterpart of ejaculation but contraction of the pelvic and perineal musculature occurs. The contraction is believed to be mediated by reflex mechanisms, through pathways probably similar to those in the male. In both men and women, orgasm is associated with sympathetic outflow and results in tachycardia, increased respiration, and sweating.

A final refractory phase occurs in the period following orgasm. In this phase the male temporarily cannot repeat intercourse. The phase is generally thought to be absent in the female but is not important in the development of drug-induced sexual dysfunction in either sex.

Perhaps because of the more physically obvious effect in men, drug-induced sexual dysfunction has been more commonly reported in men than women. Evaluation of adverse effects of drugs and sexual function is complicated by the fact that many drugs that have been associated with effects on sexual activity are given for disorders which may themselves be associated with impaired sexual function. Prominent examples are the association between sexual problems in men and the effects of antihypertensive and psychiatric therapies. Even without treatment, impotence is more common in hypertensive patients than in an age-matched control group (Bulpitt *et al.* 1976). The incidence of sexual dysfunction in untreated psychiatric patients has been reported to be as high as 70 per cent, depending on the types of patients studied (Beck 1976; Beaumont 1978; Lief 1979; Nestoros and Lehmann 1979). The prevalence of sexual dysfunction in populations of unwell patients is likely to be higher than the accepted prevalence within the normal population (Slag *et al.* 1983). Further complications are the decline in sexual performance with age (Felstein 1980; Bancroft 1982) and the effects of alcohol and smoking. The knowledge that drugs may interfere with sexual performance may itself be a factor in patients' perception of drug effects.

Single case reports are particularly difficult to assess even if a causal relationship seems plausible. Often adequate baseline (pretreatment) information is lacking and positive rechallenge may reflect either the pharmacological action of a drug or anticipatory stress. Ideally, therefore, control studies are necessary to establish causal relationships and they are the only valid way to assess accurately the incidence of sexual adverse effects with particular drugs. As with all studies of this nature the methodology used will influence the results. Underreporting of sexual adverse events is common, but a higher incidence will be obtained by using a detailed check-list or specific questions than if open-ended questions are used. Similarly, spontaneous reporting by patients of sexual adverse effects is extremely low. The use of appropriate control groups is therefore important. Matching for effects of disease, drug, age, smoking, and alcohol are crucial factors in this equation. In practice, very few reported studies have considered smoking or alcohol consumption in their analyses.

A final issue encountered in some of the published literature is the failure of authors to use clear definitions. The term impotence is used variously to include failure of erection or problems with ejaculatory function, and it may be difficult for the reader to determine either the effect the drug is having or to postulate pharmacological mechanisms. Actions of all drugs may be central, through effects on libido, or peripheral by direct interactions with physiological processes.

Drugs causing sexual dysfunction

The majority of drug effects on sexual function are mediated through Type A reactions. They are generally predicable or at least explainable on the basis of known pharmacology. They also tend to be dose related. It may, however, be difficult to establish in an individual patient whether the mechanism of an adverse event is central or peripheral, the effect of the disease being treated, or the anxiety produced by diagnosis.

Antihypertensive drugs

The prevalence of both impotence and ejaculatory disorders is significantly greater in treated hypertensive patients than in matched controls (Bulpitt and Dollery 1973; Bulpitt *et al.* 1976; Hogan *et al.* 1980; Medical

Research Council Working Party 1981). One problem with the older studies is that the types of drugs used were different from those in use today. Nevertheless, in the study by Bulpitt and others (1976) 25 per cent of patients reported impotence on therapy as compared with 17 per cent untreated hypertensives and seven per cent of normotensive controls. Ejaculatory failure was also documented in 25 per cent of treated patients, as compared with seven per cent of untreated patients and zero among normotensive controls. Later studies (Bulpitt *et al.* 1989) have suggested the rates of impotence will depend on the type of drug used to treat hypertension. Not surprisingly, adrenergic-blocking agents, less frequently used nowadays, were associated with higher rates of impotence and ejaculatory failure (Bulpitt and Dollery 1973). The centrally acting α-agonist clonidine, and methyldopa, which lowers blood pressure by a similar mechanism, also have caused loss of libido, impotence, and ejaculatory failure (Newman and Salerno 1974; Alexander and Evans 1975; Hogan *et al.* 1980; Taylor *et al.* 1981). The precise mechanisms of these effects are uncertain; postulated routes include increases in prolactin (which is not always found); sedative and depressant effects of methyldopa and clonidine; and, potentially, effects resulting from reduced sympathetic outflow.

β-Adrenoceptor blockers

Effects of β-blockers on sexual dysfunction relate in part to their physical structure and pharmacological properties. It would appear that those which are more lipid soluble, for example, propranolol, are more likely to be implicated in reports of adverse effects on sexual function than more water-soluble compounds such as atenolol. Early studies on β-blockers tended to be with the older drugs, and thus there is evidence that propranolol is associated with impotence, the rate being reported in the Medical Research Council study in 1981 (MRC Working Party 1981) as 14 per cent of patients after 12 weeks of therapy. Other workers confirm this association (Warren and Warren 1977; Burnette and Chahine 1979; Hogan *et al.* 1980). Rates of between 10 and 15 per cent impotence are generally reported, as compared with a nine per cent rate in control patients in the MRC study, for example. The precise mechanism of the effect of the β-blockers is debated. Propranolol has additional effects on $5HT_{1A}$ receptors as well as on β-receptors. This may explain why propranolol seems to have been more prone to these effects than is atenolol. Nevertheless, there are individual reports in adverse drug reaction databases, such as the CSM yellow-card database, implicating other β-blockers.

The effects of β-blockers on female sexual function are less well defined. Although Buffum (1982) reported decreased libido in association with propranolol, among 9837 hypertensive patients described in the same study receiving nadolol, another (water-soluble) β-blocker, there were only 30 reports of unspecified sexual dysfunction in recipients. This study did not indicate the relative sex ratio of the patients and therefore it is uncertain what the sex of the affected patients was. In a study involving atenolol, chlorthalidone, and placebo, the rates of complaints of sexual dysfunction were 19.8 per cent with atenolol, 17.6 per cent with chlorthalidone, and 14.5 per cent with placebo (Wassertheil-Smoller *et al.* 1991). The combined α and β-adrenoceptor antagonist labetalol in men appears to affect ejaculation rather than erection, presumably due to the α-adrenergic antagonist effects acting at the bladder neck, causing retrograde ejaculation. In laboratory studies, erection in volunteers was not affected but delayed ejaculation was affected in a dose-related manner (Riley *et al.* 1982). In a study in women the effects of labetalol were reduced vaginal lubrication, in comparison with propranolol and placebo. In the same study the rise in blood pressure at orgasm was reduced by labetalol but not significantly by propranolol. The interpretation of this data is difficult but it would suggest that labetalol might have some adverse effects on sexual function in women (Riley and Riley 1981).

Pure α-adrenergic antagonists also seem to produce failure of ejaculation. This is commonly reported with phenoxybenzamine (Kedia and Perski 1981), and also with indoramin (Pentland *et al.* 1981), but may be less common with the newer agents such as prazosin (Stessman and Ben-Ishay 1980).

Diuretics

Thiazide diuretics were recognized to cause impotence in the MRC trial (MRC Working Party 1981), with an incidence of 16 per cent at 12 weeks. Subsequent studies suggested that the incidence was lower than this (Grimm *et al.* 1985; Helgeland *et al.* 1986). Chang *et al.* (1991) demonstrated a two- to sixfold higher rate of sexual dysfunction in patients taking diuretics than in those taking placebo.

In women, decreased libido and decreased vaginal lubrication had been reported (Semmens and Semmens 1978; Moss and Procci 1982; Wartman 1983; Stevenson and Umstead 1984). In one study comparing atenolol, chlorthalidone, and placebo the effects of weight-reduction regimens appeared to affect the incidence of sexual problems in women receiving chlorthalidone (Wassertheil-Smoller *et al.* 1991): 24 per cent of women who followed their usual diet reported sexual problems compared with five per cent who were on a weight-reducing programme (P=0.03). It seems unlikely the diuretic was responsible for this difference, which probably reflected issues such as body image.

While early investigators suggested that the impaired sexual function secondary to diuretics was related to volume loss or hypokalaemia, it is much more likely that these effects relate to the effects of thiazides on smooth muscle (Soyka and Mattison 1981). This effect on smooth muscle is likely to compromise vasoconstriction, essential for erection in men, and may also be responsible for the alteration of vaginal lubrication reported in women in some studies.

Spironolactone is a competitive aldosterone antagonist but because of its steroid structure probably has androgenic effects. It causes gynaecomastia, decreased libido, and erectile failure in between four and 30 per cent of patients. The incidence of sexual dysfunction increases when the drug is given in combination with other drugs (Williams et al. 1987; Bulpitt et al. 1989). Testosterone is thought to have a role in maintenance of libido, and spironolactone appears to inhibit the binding of dihydrotestosterone. In women it has been reported to be associated with altered vaginal lubrication and decreased libido. In higher doses, spironolactone produces menstrual irregularity (Spark and Melby 1968), and at doses of 100–200 mg a day six of nine women developed amenorrhoea, though normal menstruation returned within 2 months of stopping therapy (Levity 1970). Although neither of these studies was placebo controlled, they do suggest an important effect of spironolactone. At very high doses (>450 mg per day) spironolactone will produce infertility, but this is much higher than the doses now used in clinical practice.

Calcium antagonists

Calcium antagonists seem in general to cause less problems with sexual function than do β-blockers or diuretics (Marley and Curran 1989); the most commonly studied has been nifedipine. In one study (Dombrowski et al. 1995) it was reported that verapamil produced hyperprolactinaemia in a patient who was impotent. When verapamil was discontinued the prolactin returned to normal. What evidence there is suggests that nifedipine is also less likely to cause sexual dysfunction in women (Duncan and Bateman 1993).

ACE inhibitors

A large study reporting data on over 30 000 patients (Schoernberger et al. 1990) suggested that captopril is relatively free of adverse effects on sexual function. In this study, women who were switched from thiazide diuretics and β-blockers to captopril reported improved sexual function, whereas there was no change in those who were switched from calcium antagonists.

Psychotropic drugs

Assessing sexual dysfunction in patients with psychiatric illness is obviously a problem. The underlying condition being treated, particularly in the case of depression, is likely to alter sexual behaviour. In schizophrenic patients, sexual activity may be reduced or occasionally increased, but in general loss of libido is a feature, particularly in patients with negative symptoms. It is therefore difficult to assess accurately the effects of drugs on libido, since as the illness improves so does this aspect of it. These drugs, however, have actions that impair functional components of sexual behaviour.

Antidepressants

Antidepressant drugs come in three categories: classic tricyclic antidepressants, monoamine-oxidase inhibitors (MAOI), and serotonin-reuptake inhibitors (SSRI). Tricyclic antidepressants have a range of pharmacological activities including anticholinergic properties. They are well recognized to cause impotence (Segraves 1982; Mitchell and Popkin 1983; Segraves 1982). One other important feature of these agents is that they cause delayed or retrograde ejaculation. This is probably a reflection of their α-adrenoceptor antagonist activity. Monoamine-oxidase inhibitors similarly cause impotence and ejaculatory failure. Interestingly, both these types of antidepressants have been used successfully to treat premature ejaculation (Mitchell and Popkin 1983). In women, reduced orgasm has been reported with a range of tricyclic antidepressants including imipramine, clomipramine, and amoxapine. In a patient reported by Sovner (1983) substitution of desipramine for imipramine restored normal orgasm. This suggests that this effect of tricyclics is related to their α-antagonist activity, since desipramine does not possess this property. It may also be that this adverse effect relates to the property of imipramine to block the reuptake of serotonin, an action which is less evident in desipramine.

The SSRI group of antidepressant drugs has also been associated with sexual dysfunction. Thus fluoxetine has been associated with failure of orgasm in both men and women (Kline 1989; Lydiard and George 1989). In one study fluoxetine was associated with impotence in 8.3 per cent of patients (Herman et al. 1990), but this compares favourably with rates of up to 30 per cent reported with MAOI (Remick et al. 1989). Doogan (1991) reported that the SSRI sertraline was associated with a 16.5 per cent incidence of sexual dysfunction. Other workers suggested that the lowest incidence of sexual dysfunction caused by this group of drugs occurs with fluvoxamine rather than paroxetine or sertraline (Brock and Lue 1993).

In summary, all antidepressants seem to impair sexual dysfunction. New antidepressants are clearly not free from this adverse effect, although the frequency may differ between different agents.

Antipsychotic drugs

Classical antipsychotic phenothiazines such as chlorpromazine and thioridazine have a wide variety of pharmacological effects including their antidopaminergic effect, the cause of their antipsychotic activity, anticholinergic effects, and α-adrenoceptor antagonist activity. These drugs cause both impotence and ejaculatory dysfunction (Mitchell and Popkin 1982). Thioridazine appears particularly likely to cause sexual dysfunction: one study in the 1970s (Kotin *et al.* 1976) suggested it was present in 60 per cent of patients receiving thioridazine. In this study, the incidence was 25 per cent in patients taking other psychotic drugs. More selective antipsychotics, such as haloperidol and pimozide, are said to cause fewer problems with sexual function, but there is a well-documented case report of impotence with pimozide (Ananth 1982) and with sulpiride (Weizman *et al.* 1985).

The effect of drugs such as antipsychotics (and the antiandrogenic H$_2$-receptor antagonist cimetidine) on sperm function in hyperprolactinaemic patients was investigated by Okada and colleagues (Okada *et al.* 1996). Among 264 men with reduced sperm function attending an infertility clinic, 15 patients were identified as having persistent hyperprolactinaemia. Of these, six were taking cimetidine and six psychiatric medication. When the drugs were stopped, serum prolactin returned to normal, but sperm function did not appear to improve.

As with the antihypertensive drugs, the influence of antipsychotic medication on female sexual dysfunction has been less well examined. However, there are case reports of impaired orgasm with thioridazine and with trifluoperazine (Degan 1982; Shen and Park 1982).

Lithium has occasionally been reported to produce changes in sexual function, including impotence and decreased libido (Blay *et al.* 1982; Kristensen and Jørgensen 1987; Ghadirian *et al.* 1992). The magnitude of these effects in patients who have been treated for a manic depressive disorder, in which hypersexuality may be a feature of the disease, is obviously a problem.

Anxiolytic drugs, in particular benzodiazepines, seem to have little effect on sexual function. The drugs are sedative, and this obviously may be a factor in reducing sexual activity, and Riley and Riley (1986) suggest that benzodiazepines have inhibited orgasm in female volunteers. In contrast, withdrawal of benzodiazepines has been reported to increase sexual activity (Nutt *et al.* 1986). In one report (Othmer and Othmer 1987), the anxiolytic buspirone was reported to improve sexual function in anxious patients and the improvement did not seem to correlate with changes in anxiety.

Cimetidine

Cimetidine is an H$_2$-antagonist which also has antiandrogenic activity. It has been associated with both gynaecomastia and impotence. These effects appear dose related in that, when the drug was used at high dose for treatment of gastric hypersecretory states, gynaecomastia and impotence occurred in 11 and nine of 22 patients respectively (Jensen *et al.* 1983). The effects of cimetidine are reversible. In most patients receiving therapy for peptic ulcer disease, the incidence of sexual dysfunction is low. In some patients who developed gynaecomastia and impotence on cimetidine, substitution with ranitidine resulted in improvement in symptoms (Peden and Wormsley 1982; Jensen *et al.* 1983). These effects are not generally seen with other H$_2$-antagonists although case reports of sexual dysfunction have been reported with both ranitidine and famotidine (*The Medical Letter* 1987). Whether cimetidine has effects on libido in women is unclear but, as an antiandrogen, it might be expected to do so occasionally.

Anticonvulsants

Male epileptics treated with a variety of anticonvulsant regimens have been reported to have reduced sexual activity and impotence (Christiansen *et al.* 1975; Toone *et al.* 1983). One postulated mechanism is an induction of hormone metabolism caused by enzyme-inducing anticonvulsants. Free testosterone levels fall and sex-hormone-binding globulins are increased in patients on these drugs (Toone *et al.* 1983; MacPhee *et al.* 1988). Sodium valproate, which lacks enzyme-inducing activity, does not affect sex hormone levels or seem to interfere with sexual function (MacPhee *et al.* 1988). Similar comments probably also apply to other new anticonvulsants, although there do not appear to have been any systematic studies.

Sex hormones

Anabolic steroids, corticosteroids, and oestrogens all suppress the hypothalamo–pituitary axis (Wilson and Griffin 1980). All these agents seem to reduce gonadotrophic hormone release and hence there is a fall in the circulating level of testosterone. The antiandrogen cyproterone acetate may produce impotence, it also reduces sexual arousal, a condition for which it is sometimes used. The effects are dose related. LRH analogues used in the management of prostatic carcinoma also reduce testosterone levels and may therefore produce impotence (*The Lancet* 1983).

Sexual problems are reported in women taking oral contraceptives. They have been attributed to the progesterone component of the pill but this is not clearly established. Loss of libido, however, may be associated with the use of oral contraceptives.

Ketoconazole and related compounds

Ketoconazole and other antifungals of the same group inhibit gonadal and adrenal synthesis of androgens and reduce plasma testosterone levels (Allen *et al.* 1983; Pont *et al.* 1992). Loss of libido, gynaecomastia, and impotence have been reported occasionally in men treated with ketoconazole (Schurmeyer and Nieschlag 1982).

Drugs of abuse

Cigarette smoking is associated with impotence, probably because of its association with atherosclerotic vascular disease (Nakagawa *et al.* 1990). In animal studies, smoking produced an impairment in the erectile mechanism (Juenemann *et al.* 1987) and similar findings have been reported in man (Shabsigh *et al.* 1988).

Excess alcohol intake is known to affect all phases of human sexual response (Miller and Gold 1988). At low doses this inhibition may be associated with increased libido; at higher doses, however, the CNS depressant effects result in the reverse. Chronic alcoholism results in liver dysfunction and may be associated with decreased testosterone and increased oestrogen levels, together with alcoholic polyneuropathy. All these may produce impotence. A survey of patients enrolled in an alcohol detoxification programme suggested that 75 per cent had had sexual dysfunction in the preceding 6 months and the majority of these (66 per cent) were still complaining of problems up to 9 months after treatment had been completed (Fahrner 1987).

Long-term use of opiates such as methadone, morphine, and heroin has been reported to cause reduced libido and impotence. Sexual activity is said to return to normal during periods of abstinence (Mendelson and Mello 1982). Opiates suppress pituitary LH secretion and produce a fall in serum testosterone. These effects are temporary, and probably dose related.

Cocaine, which is increasingly used as a drug of abuse, has been reported both to increase and to inhibit sexual performance (Smith *et al.* 1984). Marijuana and other cannabinoids may reduce testosterone levels and reduce erectile function (Brock and Lue 1993). At low doses there are reports of sexual enhancement, with opposite effects following long-term high-level use (Buffum 1982). Testosterone levels are increased following administration of tetrahydrocannabinol in mice (Dalterio *et al.* 1981) and this may be one postulated mechanism for the effects of cannabis as a stimulant of sexual activity.

Other drugs

A large number of other drugs have been associated with impaired sexual function, but it is difficult to know whether these reports are of genuine associations. Thus, there are occasional reports of impotence with non-steroidal anti-inflammatory drugs (Wei and Hood 1980; Miller *et al.* 1989); bromocriptine has been reported to cause impotence in men with Parkinson's disease (Cleeves and Findley 1987); etretinate has been reported to cause erectile dysfunction in men and loss of libido associated with menstrual disturbance in women (Halkier-Sørensen 1987). Hyperprolactinaemia occurs with metoclopramide, and reduced libido and impotence have been reported with this drug (Berlin 1986).

Priapism

Drugs which prevent detumescence in men may result in priapism. This has been ascribed to α-antagonist activity, preventing constriction of the blood vessels supplying erectile tissue. Whether this is the only receptor mechanism involved is unclear; thus, anticholinergic drugs have been reported to reverse priapism induced by phenothiazines (Banos *et al.* 1989). Priapism has been attributed to phenothiazines, trazodone, prazosin, labetalol, phenelzine, guanethidine, hydralazine, nifedipine, and anticoagulants (see Bhalla *et al.* 1979; Law *et al.* 1980; Yeragani and Gershon 1987; Rayner *et al.* 1988; Banos *et al.* 1989).

Infertility

Cytotoxic drugs

Drugs affecting fertility may do so either by a direct action on gonadal function, or indirectly by the inhibition of pituitary secretion of gonadotrophins. Cytotoxic drugs are the most commonly used agents that are associated with infertility. The effects of these drugs may depend on the age of the patient, whether pre- or postpubertal. In addition, the effects on men and women seem to differ.

In adult men, cytotoxic drugs predominantly affect the germinal epithelium, producing reductions in sperm count and secondary elevation of plasma FSH (Schilsky *et al.* 1980). It seems likely that the alkylating agents are more toxic to testes than are some other groups of cytotoxic drugs. Cyclophosphamide and chlorambucil both produce azoöspermia when used as single agents (Callis *et al.* 1980; Schilsky *et al.* 1980). The extent of damage and the likelihood of recovery depend on dose and duration of treatment. Irreversible effects can be seen with both these drugs, but recovery has been reported up to a year or more after treatment has been stopped. In treatment of Hodgkin's disease, azoöspermia is common (Chapman *et al.* 1981; Whitehead *et al.* 1982). This may persist in over 80 per cent of patients, but recovery has been reported and is likely to occur more frequently in patients who are aged under 30 when treated (Waxman 1983). Newer regimens for management of Hodgkin's disease may be less toxic (Kreuser *et al.* 1987). Most male patients who are to undergo intensive chemotherapy should, if they wish to have children, be advised to have sperm taken for preservation before they start treatment.

Methotrexate is thought to be less toxic than the alkylating agents but still causes a reduction in sperm count. When used in the treatment of psoriasis, doses used are much smaller, though even here reversible reductions in sperm counts have been reported (Sussman and Leonard 1980).

In women, cytotoxic drugs acting on the ovary produce loss of primordial follicles with failure of ovulation and endocrine functions. This results in oligomenorrhoea or amenorrhoea with loss of libido, and menopausal symptoms (Shalet 1980). Alkylating agents are, as in men, the most toxic. Again the effects are age related, presumably relating to the numbers of follicles available at the time of treatment (Chapman 1982). There is some evidence that ovarian damage may be progressive after treatment is finished (Chapman *et al.* 1979). It should be stressed that not all cytotoxic drug therapies and regimens adversely effect ovarian function; thus, in a survey of patients who had had chemotherapy for chorion carcinoma, Rustin and co-workers (1984) showed that 187 of 217 women who wished to conceive after therapy had at least one live birth. These patients had received methotrexate and 37 who had a live infant had also received cyclophosphamide. In the survey, the patients who had the most drugs seemed to have less chance of pregnancy.

In children, the effects on boys and girls are also somewhat different. The ovaries of prepubertal girls seem relatively resistant to cytotoxic drugs because follicular activity is low before puberty. As would be expected, there is a dose–response relationship, and if the drugs are given in high enough dosage gonadal damage may be produced. The long-term effects of ovarian damage in childhood are unclear. In boys testicular damage has been demonstrated by testicular biopsy (Lendon *et al.* 1978; Shalet 1980). Cyclophosphamide and cytarabine seem to produce the most damage. Although effects in pubertal boys may be greater, sperm counts were reduced in boys who had received therapy with cyclophosphamide or chlorambucil before puberty (Shalet 1980). The effects are dose related, and the dose used in the management of the nephrotic syndrome in children appears to have only minor effects, and probably does not normally produce infertility (Trompeter *et al.* 1981). Alkylating agents appear to have a greater propensity to induce testicular damage than other agents, such as vincristine and vinblastine (Aubier *et al.* 1987).

Sulphasalazine

Azoöspermia and infertility are well-recognized complications in men receiving treatment with sulphasalazine for inflammatory bowel disease (Birnie *et al.* 1981). This effect is usually reversible, and sperm counts return to normal within about 2–3 months of stopping therapy. Semen analysis shows a decrease in sperm density, poor sperm motility, and abnormal morphology (Toovey *et al.* 1981; Hudson 1982). The effects on sperm function seem to derive from the sulphapyridine component of the sulphasalazine. Return to normal fertility has been reported in patients in whom sulphasalazine was replaced by mesalazine (Cann and Holdsworth 1984; Riley and Riley 1986). Other sulphonamides do not appear to affect fertility, either in experimental animals or in man. It has therefore been suggested that the pyridine component of the sulphapyridine molecule is the likely toxic agent. Another possibility is that the effects are due to the antifolate effects of the drug (Hudson *et al.* 1982).

There are case reports of other antimicrobials affecting fertility, but in general the studies have not been controlled and are difficult to assess. Transient depression of sperm count has been reported with nitrofurantoin (Yunda and Kushniruk 1974). A reduction in sperm count was also reported in 14 of a series of 40 patients treated with co-trimoxazole (Murdia *et al.* 1978) but more recent work has not confirmed the observation. These drugs are usually used only for short periods of time unless being used to treat patients with the acquired immune deficiency syndrome.

Hormones

Production of normal semen and ovulation are controlled by gonadotrophin release. High doses of testosterone, such as are used by body builders, will suppress LH secretion and produce infertility. This is likely to be reversible. Hormonal oral contraceptives work by this mechanism.

Other drugs

While a few drugs have been shown to inhibit sperm motility *in vitro*, the significance of the findings is uncertain, since the concentrations *in vivo* are generally far less than those employed experimentally, and there is no really convincing evidence that these effects are clinically important.

References

Alexander, W.D. and Evans, J.I. (1975). Side effects of methyldopa. *BMJ* 2, 501.

Allen, J.M., Kerle, D.J., Ware, H., *et al.* (1983). Combined treatment with ketoconazole and luteinising hormone releasing hormone analogue; a novel approach to resistant progressive prostatic cancer. *BMJ* 287, 1766.

Ananth, J. (1982). Impotence due to pimozide. *Am. J. Psychiatry* 139, 1374.

Aubier, F., Flamant, F., Brauner, R., *et al.* (1987). Male gonadal function after chemotherapy for solid tumours in childhood. *J. Clin. Oncol.* 7, 403.

Bancroft, J. (1982). Erectile impotence — psyche or soma? *Int. J. Androl.* 5, 353.

Banos, J.E., Bosch, F., and Farre, M. (1989). Drug-induced priapism. *Med. Toxicol.* 4, 46.

Beaumont, G. (1978). Sexual side-effects of psychotropic drugs. *Br. J. Clin. Pract.* (Symposium Suppl.) 4, 45.

Beck, A.T. (1976). *Depression: Clinical, Experimental and Therapeutic Aspects.* Harper and Row, New York.

Berlin, R.G. (1986). Metoclopramide-induced reversible impotence. *West J. Med.* 144, 359.

Bhalla, AK., Hoffbrand, B.I., Phatak, P.S., *et al.* (1979). Prazosin and priapism. *BMJ* 2, 115.

Birnie, G.G., McLeod, T.I.F., and Watkinson, G. (1981). Incidence of sulphasalazine-induced male infertility. *Gut* 22, 425.

Blay, S.L., Ferraz, M.P.T., and Calil, H.M. (1982). Lithium-induced male sexual impairment: two case reports. *J. Clin. Psychiatry* 43, 497.

Brock, G.B. and Lue, T.F. (1993). Drug-induced male sexual dysfunction — an update. *Drug Saf.* 8, 414.

Buffum, J. (1982). Pharmacosexology: the effects of drugs on sexual function. A review. *J. Psychoactive Drugs* 14, 5.

Bulpitt, C.J. and Dollery, C.T. (1973). Side effects of hypotensive agents evaluated by a self-administered questionnaire. *BMJ* 3, 485.

Bulpitt, C.J., Dollery, C.T., and Carne, S. (1976). Change in symptoms of hypertensive patients after referral to hospital clinic. *Br. Heart J.* 38, 121.

Bulpitt, C.J., Beevers, G., Butler, A., *et al.* (1989). The effects of anti-hypertensive drugs on sexual function in men and women: a report from the DHSS Hypertension Care Computing Project. *J. Hum. Hypertens.* 3, 53.

Burnett, W.C. and Chahine, R.A. (1979). Sexual dysfunction as a complication of propranolol therapy in men. *Cardiovasc. Med.* 5, 811.

Callis, L., Nieto, J., Vila, A., *et al.* (1980). Chlorambucil treatment in minimal lesion nephrotic syndrome: a reappraisal of its gonadal toxicity. *J. Pediatr.* 97, 653.

Cann, P.A. and Holdsworth, C.D. (1984). Reversal of male infertility on changing treatment from sulphasalazine to 5-aminosalicylic acid. *Lancet* ii, 1119.

Chang, S.W., Fine, R., Siegel, D., *et al.* (1991). The impact of diuretic therapy on reported sexual function. *Arch. Intern. Med.* 151, 2402.

Chapman, R.M. (1982). Effect of cytotoxic therapy on sexuality and gonadal function. *Sem. Oncol.* 9, 84.

Chapman, R.M., Sutcliffe, S.B., and Malpas, J.S. (1979). Cytotoxic-induced ovarian failure in women with Hodgkin's disease. *JAMA* 242, 1877.

Chapman, R.M., Sutcliffe, S.B., and Malpas, J.S. (1981). Male gonadal dysfunction in Hodgkin's disease. *JAMA* 245, 1323.

Christiansen, P., Deigaard, J., and Lund, M. (1975). Potens, fertilitet og konshormonudskillelse hos yngre mandlige epilepsilidene. *Ugeskr. Laeger* 137, 2402.

Cleeves, L. and Findley, L.J. (1987). Bromocriptine-induced impotence in Parkinson's disease. *BMJ* 295, 367.

Dalterio, S., Bartke, A., and Mayfield, D. (1981). 9-Tetrahydrocannabinol increases plasma testosterone concentrations in mice. *Science* 213, 581.

Degan, K. (1982). Sexual dysfunction in women using major tranquillisers. *Psychosomatics* 23, 959.

Dombrowski, R.C., Romeo, J.H., and Aron, D.C. (1995). Verapamil-induced hyperprolactinemia complicated by a pituitary incidentaloma. *Ann. Pharmacother.* 29, 999.

Doogan, D.P. (1991). Toleration and safety of sertraline: experience wordlwide. *Int. Clin. Psychopharmacol.* 6 (Suppl. 2), 47.

Duncan, L. and Bateman, D.N. (1993). Sexual function in women — do anti-hypertensive drugs have an impact? *Drug Saf.* 8, 225.

Fahrner, E.M. (1987). Sexual dysfunction in male alcohol addicts: prevalence and treatment. *Arch. Sex. Behav.* 16, 247.

Felstein, I. (1980). Sexual function in the elderly. *Clin. Obstet. Gynecol.* 7, 401.

Ghadirian, A.M., Annable, L., and Belanger, M.C. (1992). Lithium, benzodiazepines and sexual function in bipolar patients. *Am. J. Psychiatry* 149, 801.

Grimm, R.H., Cohen, J.D., and McFate Smith, W. (1985). Hypertension management in the Multiple Risk Factor Intervention Trial (MRFIT). *Arch. Intern. Med.* 145, 1191.

Halkier-Sørensen, L. (1987). Menstrual changes in a patient treated with etretinate. *Lancet* ii, 636.

Helgeland, A., Strommen, R., Hagelund, C.H., *et al.* (1986). Enalapril, atenolol and hydrochlorothiazide in mild to moderate hypertension. *Lancet.* i, 872.

Herman, J.B., Brotman, A.W., Pollack, M.H., *et al.* (1990). Fluoxetine induced sexual dysfunction. *J. Clin. Psychiatry* 51, 25.

Hogan, M.J., Wallin, J.D., and Baer, R.M. (1980). Antihypertensive therapy and male sexual dysfunction. *Psychosomatics* 21, 234.

Hudson, E., Dore, C., Sowter, C., *et al.* (1982). Sperm size in patients with inflammatory bowel disease on sulphasalazine therapy. *Fertil. Steril.* 38, 77.

Jensen, R.T., Collen, M.J., Pandol, S.J., *et al.* (1983). Cimetidine-induced impotence and breast changes in patients with gastric hypersecretory states. *N. Engl. J. Med.* 308, 883.

Juenemann, K-P., Lue, T.F., Benowitz, N.L., *et al.* (1987). Effect of cigarette smoking on penile erection. *J Urol.* 138, 438.

Kedia, K.R. and Persky, L. (1981). Effect of phenoxybenzamine on sexual function in man. *Urology* 18, 620.

Kline, M.D. (1989). Fluoxetine and anorgasmia. *Am. J. Psychiatry* 146, 804.

Korenman, S.G. (1983). Clinical assessment of drug-induced impairment of sexual function. *Chest* 83 (Suppl.).

Kotin, J., Wilbert, D.E., Verburg, D., *et al.* (1976). Thioridazine and sexual dysfunction. *Am. J. Psychiatry* 133, 82.

Krane, R.J., Goldstein, I., and de Tejada, I.S. (1989). Impotence. *N. Engl. J. Med.* 321, 1648.

Kreuser, E.D., Xiros, N., and Hetzel, W.D. (1987). Reproductive and endocrine gonadal capacity in patients treated with COPP chemotherapy for Hodgkin's disease. *J. Cancer Res. Clin. Oncol.* 113, 260.

Kristensen, E. and Jørgensen, P. (1987). Sexual function in lithium-treated manic depressive patients. *Pharmacopsychiatry* 20, 165.

The Lancet. (1983). New treatment for prostatic cancer. *Lancet* ii, 438.

Law, M.R., Copland, R.F.P., Armistead, J.G., *et al.* (1980). Labetalol and priapism. *BMJ* 1, 115.

Lendon, M., Hann, I.M., Palmer, M.K., *et al.* (1978). Testicular histology after combination chemotherapy in childhood for acute lymphoblastic leukaemia. *Lancet* ii, 439.

Levity, J.I. (1970). Spironolactone therapy and amenorrhoea. *JAMA* 130, 2014.

Lief, H.I. (1979). Sexual survey No 5: current thinking on sex and depression. *Med. Asp. Hum. Sex.* 11, 22.

Lydiard, R.B. and George, M.S. (1989). Fluoxetine-related anorgasmy. *South. Med. J.* 81, 933.

MacPhee, G.J.A., Larkin, J.G., Butler, E., *et al.* (1988). Circulating hormones and pituitary responsiveness in young epileptic men receiving longterm antiepileptic medication. *Epilepsia* 29, 468.

Marley, J.E. and Curram, J.B. (1989). General practice data derived tolerability assessment of antihypertensive drugs. *J. Int. Med. Res.* 17, 473.

The Medical Letter (1987). Drugs that cause sexual dysfunction. *Medical Letter* 29, 65.

Medical Research Council Working Party (1981). Adverse reactions to bendrofluazide and propranolol for the treatment of mild hypertension. *Lancet* ii, 539.

Mendelson, J.H. and Mello, N.K. (1982). Hormones and psychosexual development in young men following chronic heroin use. *Neurobehav. Toxicol. Teratol.* 4, 441.

Miller, N.S. and Gold, M.S. (1988). The human sexual response and alcohol and drugs. *J. Subst. Abuse Treat.* 5, 171.

Miller, L.G., Rogers, J.C., and Swee, D.E. (1989). Indomethacin-associated sexual dysfunction. *J. Fam. Pract.* 29, 210.

Mitchell, J.E. and Popkin, M.K. (1982). Antipsychotic drug therapy and sexual dysfunction in men. *Am. J. Psychiatry* 139, 633.

Mitchell, J.E. and Popkin, M.K. (1983). Antidepressant drug therapy and sexual dysfunction in men: a review. *J. Clin. Psychopharmacol.* 3, 76.

Moss, H.B. and Procci, W.R. (1982). Sexual dysfunction associated with oral antihypertensive medication: A critical survey of the literature. *Gen. Hosp. Psychiatry* 4, 121.

Murdia, A., Mathur, V., Kothari, L.K., *et al.* (1978). Sulpha–trimethoprim combinations and male infertility. *Lancet* ii, 375.

Nalagawa, S., Watanabe, H.O., and Nakao, M. (1990). Sexual behaviour in Japanese males relating to area, occupation, smoking, drinking and eating habits. *Andrologia* 22, 21.

Nestoros, J.N. and Lehmann, H.E. (1979). Neuroleptics and male sexual dysfunction. *Int. Drug Ther. Newsletter* 14, 21.

Newman, R.J. and Salerno, H.R. (1974). Sexual dysfunction due to methyldopa. *BMJ* 4, 106.

Nutt, D., Hackman, A., and Hawton, K. (1986). Increased sexual function in benzodiazepine withdrawal. *Lancet* ii, 1101.

Okada, H., Iwamoto, T., Fujioka, H., *et al.* (1996). Hyperprolactinaemia among infertile patients and its effects on sperm functions. *Andrologia* 28, 197.

Othmer, E. and Othmer, S.C. (1987). Effect of buspirone on sexual dysfunction in patients with generalised anxiety disorder. *J. Clin. Psychiatry* 48, 201.

Peden, N.R. and Wormsley, K.G. (1982). Effect of cimetidine on gonadal function. *Br. J. Clin. Pharmacol.* 14, 565.

Pentland, B., Anderson, D.A., and Critchley, J.A.J. (1981). Failure of ejaculation with indoramin. *BMJ* 284, 1433.

Pont, A., Williams, P.L., Loose, D.S., *et al.* (1982). Ketoconazole blocks adrenal steroid synthesis. *Ann. Intern. Med.* 97, 370.

Rayner, H.C., May, S., and Walls, J. (1988). Penile erection due to nifedipine. *BMJ* 296, 137.

Remick, R.A., Froese, C., and Keller, F.D. (1989). Common side effects associated with monoamine oxidase inhibitors. *Prog. Neuropsychopharmacol. Biol. Psychiatry* 13, 497.

Riley, A.J. and Riley, E.J. (1981). The effect of labetalol and propranolol on the pressor response to sexual arousal in women. *Br. J. Clin. Pharmacol.* 12, 341.

Riley, A.J. and Riley, E.J. (1986). Cyproheptadine and antidepressant-induced anorgasmia. *Br. J. Psychiatry* 148, 217.

Riley, A.J., Riley, E.J., and Davies, H.J. (1982). A method for monitoring drug effects on male sexual response: the effect of single dose labetalol. *Br. J. Clin. Pharmacol.* 14, 695.

Riley, S.A., Lecarpentier, J., Mani, T., *et al.* (1987). Sulphasalazine induced seminal abnormalities in ulcerative colitis: results of mesalazine substitution. *Gut* 38, 1008.

Rustin, G.J.S., Booth, M., Dent, J., *et al.* (1984). Pregnancy after cytotoxic chemotherapy for gestational trophoblastic tumours. *BMJ* 288, 103.

Schilsky, R.L., Lewis, B.J., Sherins, R.J., *et al.* (1980). Gonadal dysfunction in patients receiving chemotherapy for cancer. *Ann. Intern. Med.* 93, 109.

Schoenberger, J.A., Testa, M., Ross, A.D., *et al.* (1990). Efficacy, safety, and quality-of-life assessment of captopril antihypertensive therapy in clinical practice. *Arch. Intern. Med.* 150, 301.

Schurmeyer, T. and Nieschlag, E. (1982). Ketoconazole-induced drop in serum and saliva testosterone. *Lancet* ii, 1098.

Segraves, R.T. (1982). Male sexual dysfunction and psychoactive drug use. *Postgrad. Med.* 71, 227.

Semmens, J.P. and Semmens, F.J. (1978). Inadequate vaginal lubrication. *Medical Aspects of Human Sexuality* 12, 58.

Shabsigh, R., Fishman, I.J., and Scott, F.B. (1988). Evaluations of erectile impotence. *Urology* 32, 83.

Shalet, S.M. (1980). Effects of cancer chemotherapy on gonadal function of patients. *Cancer Treat. Rev.* 7, 141.

Shen, W.W. and Park, S. (1982). Thioridazine-induced inhibition of female orgasm. *Psychiat. J. Univ. Ottawa* 7, 249.

Slag, M.F., Morley, J.E., Elson, M.K., *et al.* (1983). Impotence in medical clinic outpatients. *JAMA* 249, 1736.

Smith, D.E., Wesson, D.R., and Apter-Marsh, M. (1984). Cocaine and alcohol induced sexual dysfunction in patients with addictive disease. *J. Psychoactive Drugs* 16, 359.

Smith, P.J. and Talbert, R.L. (1986). Sexual dysfunction with anti-hypertensive and antipsychotic agents. *Clin. Pharm.* 5, 373.

Soyka, L.F. and Mattison, D.R. (1981). Prescription drugs that affect male sexual function. *Drug Therapy* 11, 60.

Spark, R.F., and Melby, J.C. (1968). Aldosteronism in hypertension. The spironolactone response test. *Ann. Intern. Med.* 69, 685.

Stessman, J. and Ben-Ishay, D. (1980). Chlorthalidone-induced impotence. *BMJ* 281, 714.

Stevenson, J.G. and Umstead, G.S. (1984). Sexual dysfunction due to anti-hypertensive agents. *DICP* 18, 113.

Sussman, A. and Leonard, J.M. (1980). Psoriasis, methotrexate and oligospermia. *Arch. Dermatol.* 116, 215.

Taylor, R.G., Crisp, A.J., Hoffbrand, B.I., *et al.* (1981). Plasma sex hormone concentrations in men with hypertension treated with methyldopa and/or propranolol. *Postgrad. Med. J.* 57, 425.

Toone, B.K., Wheeler, M., Nanjee, M., *et al.* (1983). Sex hormones, sexual activity and plasma anticonvulsant levels in male epileptics. *J. Neurol. Neurosurg. Psychiatry* 46, 824.

Toovey, S., Hudson, E., Hendry, W.F., *et al.* (1981). Sulphasalazine and male infertility: reversibility and a possible mechanism. *Gut* 22, 445.

Trompeter, R.S., Evans, P.R., and Barratt, T.M. (1981). Gonadal function in boys with steroid-responsive nephrotic syndrome treated with cyclophosphamide for short periods. *Lancet* i, 1177.

Wartman, S.A. (1983). Sexual side effects of antihypertensive drugs: treatment strategies and strictures. *Postgrad. Med.* 73, 133.

Warren, S.C. and Warren, S.G. (1977). Propranolol and sexual impotence. *Ann. Intern. Med.* 86, 112.

Wassertheil-Smoller, S., Blanfox, M.D., Oberman, A., *et al.* (1991). Effect of antihypertensives on sexual function and quality of life: the TAIM Study. *Ann. Intern. Med.* 114, 613.

Waxman, J. (1983). Chemotherapy and the adult gonad: a review. *J. R. Soc. Med.* 76, 144.

Wei, J. and Hood, J.C. (1980). Naproxen and ejaculatory dysfunction. *Ann. Intern. Med.* 93, 933.

Weizman, A., Maoz, B., Treves, I., *et al.* (1985). Sulpiride-induced hyperprolactinaemia and impotence in male psychiatric out-patients. *Prog. Neuropsychopharmacol. Biol. Psychiatry* 9, 193.

Whitehead, E., Shalet, S.M., Morris Jones, P.H., *et al.* (1982). Gonadal function after combination chemotherapy for Hodgkin's disease in childhood. *Arch. Dis. Child.* 47, 287.

Williams, G.H., Croog, S.H., Levine, S., *et al.* (1987). Impact of antihypertensive therapy on quality of life: effect of hydrochlorothiazide. *J. Hypertens.* 5, S29.

Wilson, J.D. and Griffin, J.E. (1980). The use and misuse of androgens. *Metabolism* 29, 1278.

Yeragani, V.K. and Gershon, S. (1987). Priapism related to phenelzine therapy. *N. Engl. J. Med.* 317, 117.

Yunda, I.F. and Kushniruk, Y.I. (1974). Effect of nitrofurantoin preparations on spermatogenesis. *Bull. Exp. Biol. Med.* 77, 534.

32. Masking effects of drugs

C. J. DAVIES and D. M. DAVIES

Definition

Masking occurs when drug therapy alters the clinical symptoms or signs of a disease, and possibly also its radiological appearances and laboratory test findings, without curing it, so that correct diagnosis is delayed or prevented — sometimes with serious consequences. Some of the examples given here may appear to be of historical interest only, but in fact they are by no means unknown today.

Abdominal disorders

The longest recognized example of drug masking is the effect of morphine in patients with abdominal emergencies or intracranial lesions (see below). Of the former, a distinguished surgeon (Cope 1921) wrote eloquently: 'Morphine puts an efficient screen in front of the symptoms . . . the fire burns but is not visible . . . it is possible for the patient to die happy in the belief that he is on the road to recovery, and in some cases the medical attendant may for some time be induced to share the delusive hope.'

Later, the advent of the antibacterial drugs brought many problems of this kind, which have been summarized (Davies 1979) as follows: 'The arrival of the sulphonamides and antibiotics brought new masking hazards. When treated with these drugs, some abdominal disorders lost their classical symptoms and signs. Because of rapid and impressive cures in a few cases, too much was expected of the new drugs; and, lulled into an unjustified sense of security, some doctors became blasé when dealing with abdominal emergencies, taking less care in their observation of the case and with their diagnosis. Worse, they supposed that conditions for which surgical intervention had hitherto been regarded as mandatory could now be cured by drugs. In consequence, appendices, gall bladders, and obstructed portions of the gut perforated and intra-abdominal abscesses and peritonitis followed, often with quite atypical symptoms and signs.'

Adrenal corticosteroids, by suppressing some elements of the inflammatory response, have masking effects similar to those of the antibacterials — for example, abolishing the symptoms and signs of diverticulitis (Corder 1987).

Antacids have also been implicated in drug masking. Mineral antacids may relieve symptoms of gastric carcinoma for a while, though they are unlikely to prevent correct diagnosis when the case has been investigated endoscopically or radiologically, but the same is not true of acid-suppressant drugs, and cases in which malignant gastric ulcers healed during treatment with the H_2-receptor blocking agent cimetidine have been reported (Taylor et al. 1978), and Murray and colleagues (1978) observed a similar effect of this drug on an ulcerating lymphoma of the stomach.

In severe gut infections the use of such potent antidiarrhoeal drugs as codeine phosphate, co-phenotrope (diphenoxylate with atropine), and loperamide may suppress diarrhoea initially, so delaying recognition of blood and mucus in the stools, which indicate the serious nature of the disorder; and continued treatment with these drugs in serious infections of this type can lead to the dangerous complications of ileus or toxic megacolon. When diarrhoea is accompanied by systemic symptoms and signs — severe malaise and fever — or has followed oral antibacterial therapy, it is unwise to administer powerful antidiarrhoeal agents.

Epidural anaesthesia during labour may mask the initial symptoms and signs of ruptured uterus.

Neurological disorders

The dangers of morphine in patients with a head injury were well described by Bagley (1945): 'It promotes sleep indistinguishable from coma, it depresses further an already embarrassed respiratory centre, and its miotic effect modifies the localizing value of pupillary signs.'

The symptoms and signs of meningitis or of a developing brain abscess have on occasion been masked by antibacterial treatment of much less serious infections, such as pharyngitis, sinusitis, or otitis media.

It is now well known that folic acid when given alone in pernicious anaemia or another vitamin B_{12} deficiency disease can correct the blood changes but will not prevent, and indeed may precipitate, subacute combined degeneration of the spinal cord.

Psychiatric disorders

A not uncommon medical mistake is to oversedate patients, particularly if elderly, who are confused, restless, and noisy, when the mental disorder has been caused, or at least aggravated, by an over-full bladder or colon. Heavy sedation merely induces stupor in which the patient rests uneasily while these organs continue to distend; and if a phenothiazine is used, particularly chlorpromazine intravenously, hypotension can occur and may result in cerebral ischaemia or thrombosis, so aggravating the situation.

Confusion and restlessness can also be due to hypoxia, which may go unrecognized if symptoms are suppressed by sedatives; and appropriate treatment may not then be given or may be delayed.

In a seriously depressed patient who appears on superficial examination to be suffering only from anxiety, treatment with a sedative or tranquillizer may relieve anxiety symptoms without affecting the depressive component of the illness and correct diagnosis may be delayed, sometimes with disastrous consequences. Even psychiatrists may on occasion mask the true diagnosis by their use of drugs; thus a patient suspected of being schizophrenic may be treated with a phenothiazine which controls some of the features of the illness, and only when severe depression makes its appearance is it realized that the correct diagnosis is one of manic-depressive psychosis.

Respiratory disorders

When antibacterial drugs were introduced the aetiology of pleural effusion became more difficult to establish, for when one of these drugs had been given at the onset of the illness no longer was an apparently sterile effusion containing mainly lymphocytes virtually diagnostic of post-primary tuberculosis in a young patient.

Empyema may be overlooked when pneumonia seems to have responded satisfactorily to antibacterial therapy.

Endocrine and metabolic disorders

Sedatives and tranquillizers may mask the early symptoms, suggestive of anxiety, of a phaeochromocytoma, while the headaches and peripheral vasoconstriction that sometimes occur in this condition have been relieved by antimigraine drugs and vasodilators respectively.

Most cases of hypothyroidism are due to primary thyroid failure, but very occasionally the disorder is the result of pituitary disease with multiple hormone deficiency. If this is unrecognized and the patient is treated only with thyroxine, an adrenal crisis may be precipitated. This has been known for very many years, but reminders still appear to be necessary (Naghmi 1996; *British National Formulary* 1997). The same situation can arise when hypothyroidism due to autoimmune thyroiditis is treated with thyroxine when an accompanying subclinical adrenal insufficiency, caused by the same autoimmune disturbance, is unrecognized (Soest and Müller-Lissner 1996).

Adrenal corticosteroids have an inhibitory effect on the pituitary–adrenal axis, causing deficiency of the endogenous adrenal hormones, for which they provide a substitute that is usually adequate until the body is put under severe stress by some serious acute illness or major surgical operation, when acute adrenal insufficiency can occur and complicate and confuse diagnosis.

Non-selective β-adrenoceptor blockers, such as propranolol, can induce hypoglycaemia and delay recovery from this complication in either diabetic or non-diabetic patients. Both selective and non-selective agents can mask the warning signs and symptoms of hypoglycaemia, except sweating. The subject is discussed in more detail in Chapter 16.

In diabetic patients taking insulin or oral hypoglycaemic drugs, general anaesthesia will obviously eliminate the behavioural abnormalities, will mask the pupillary signs, and, if muscle relaxants have been administered, abolish the muscular rigidity and tremor and the extensor plantar responses that are found in severe hypoglycaemia. Sweating and tachycardia still occur but are not specific, since they may have other causes. Consequently, blood glucose concentrations should be checked during long operations in patients considered to be at risk of hypoglycaemia.

Other disorders

The non-steroidal anti-inflammatory drugs can relieve arthralgia in the early stages of such collagen diseases as systemic lupus erythematosus and so delay correct diagnosis and more effective treatment. The more powerful of these drugs are also capable of alleviating the symptoms of temporal arteritis and polymyalgia rheumatica but, unlike corticosteroids, they have no effect on the underlying pathological process, so that such disastrous events as retinal arterial occlusion can still occur in a symptom-free patient. Indomethacin is known to have masked the signs of osteomyelitis in a patient with rheumatoid arthritis.

Phenylbutazone was once a popular remedy for superficial thrombophlebitis. It is no longer used in the United Kingdom for this purpose, but this may not be true of other parts of the world. Successful relief of a single attack of thrombophlebitis may tempt the doctor to repeat the treatment if the disease recurs, and he may forget that recurrent attacks (perhaps even an isolated attack) can be a sign of occult neoplastic disease.

A somewhat different type of drug masking arises when a drug successfully alleviates symptoms initially and then appears to become less effective. At this point the doctor may, not unreasonably, think that the most appropriate action is to increase the dose, and not think of the alternative explanation — namely, that the drug itself has produced damage that has now become responsible for similar symptoms. An example is a case encountered by us in which painful polyarthritis, most marked in the hips, was associated with systemic lupus erythematosus. The joint pains responded for a while to oral corticosteroids but then recurred with increasing severity. Repeat radiographs now revealed that the patient had developed bilateral aseptic necrosis of the femoral head, presumably induced by the steroid therapy.

Anticoagulants can both unmask an unsuspected disease and at the same time mask it — by providing a plausible but erroneous explanation for the revealing sign. It is sometimes assumed that bleeding in patients taking anticoagulants merely indicates an excessive anticoagulant effect, but bleeding may be a manifestation of a serious occult lesion: in a study of 220 episodes of haemorrhage during anticoagulant therapy, Roos and Van Joost (1965) found that 64 per cent of the affected patients had an underlying abnormality — a tumour, ulcer, or stone — as a cause of the bleeding.

Haemofiltration for acute renal failure will lower the patient's body temperature, as also will the infusion of large volumes of unwarmed blood or intravenous or intraperitoneal fluids. This effect can delay detection of the pyrexial response to an infection.

Radiographic and laboratory investigations

Antibacterial therapy can modify the usual radiographic appearances of certain disorders, so that in some cases they mimic other diseases. Thus, partly resolved myelitis may take on the appearance of Paget's disease, cortical hyperostosis, osteoid osteoma, or fibrous dysplasia (Bose 1959a, b). Even the characteristic pictures of neoplastic disease can alter during antibacterial therapy, suggesting regression of the lesion and an alternative diagnosis. The radiographic changes most commonly affected in this way are those of bronchial carcinoma, but cases have been encountered in which the appearances of osteogenic sarcoma and myeloma changed significantly during treatment with an antibacterial drug.

A most unusual kind of drug masking has been observed in which prolonged low-dose treatment with co-trimoxazole (trimethoprim with sulphamethoxazole) induced an alteration in bacterial metabolism resulting in negative laboratory cultures despite continuing infection in the patient. The case is described in more detail on page 760.

Very many other laboratory test results can be affected by drug therapy, sometimes causing diagnostic confusion and unnecessary investigations. This subject is dealt with in detail in Chapter 17.

References

Bagley, C., Jr. (1945). In *Textbook of Surgery* (ed. F. Christopher), W.B. Saunders, London.

Bose, K.S. (1959a). Observations on the changes of pattern in chronic pyogenic osteomyelitis following inadequate administration of penicillin. *J. Indian Med. Assoc.* 32, 271.

Bose, K.S. (1959b). Atypical osteomyelitis following inadequate antibiotic therapy: its similarity with fibrous dysplasia. *J. Indian Med. Assoc.* 33, 464.

British National Formulary No. 33 (1997). Thyroxine. British Medical Association and Royal Pharmaceutical Society of Great Britain, London.

Cope, Z. (1921). *The Early Diagnosis of the Acute Abdomen.* Oxford University Press, London.

Corder, A. (1987). Steroids, non-steroidal anti-inflammatory drugs, and serious septic complications of diverticular disease. *BMJ* 195, 1238.

Davies, D.M. (1979). Hazards of drug masking. In *Topics in Therapeutics* (ed. D.M. Davies and M.D. Rawlins), p. 120. Pitman Medical, Tunbridge Wells.

Murray, C., Chapman, R., Isaacson, P., et al. (1978). Cimetidine and malignant gastric ulcer. *Lancet* i, 1092.

Naghmi, R. (1996). Acute adrenal insufficiency. *Medicine Digest* 22 (1), 6.

Roos, J. and Van Joost, H.E. (1965). The cause of bleeding during anticoagulant treatment. *Acta Med. Scand.* 178, 129.

Soest, R. and Müller-Lissner, S. (1996). Clinical manifestation of adrenal cortical insufficiency during thyroid hormone substitution. *Dtsch. Med. Wochenschr.* 121, 406.

Taylor, R.H., Menzies-Gow, N., Lovell, D., et al. (1978) Misleading response of malignant gastric ulcer tpo cimetidine. *Lancet* i, 968.

interactions of clinical importance

M. PIRMOHAMED and M. L'E. ORME

Introduction

Information about drugs continues to increase exponentially. The number of reported drug interactions is rising continually and it becomes increasingly difficult to keep abreast of developments in the subject, and to sort out the clinically irrelevant interactions from those that are clinically important.

The potential for drug interaction is continually present. In most developed countries there are two to three thousand single chemical entities available for prescription and in many cases these are deliberately marketed in combination, so that the number of marketed products (including the combination products) may be in excess of ten thousand. In addition to prescription-only medicines (POM), there is a wide range of drugs available 'over the counter' (Honig and Gillespie 1995). These may not be thought of by the patient as drugs, and the prescribing physician may be unaware that the patient is taking them. Over the last few years some foodstuffs, most notably grapefruit juice, have also attracted attention as a source of possible adverse interactions with drugs.

Prevalence of drug interactions

Many patients take several drugs concurrently, so the potential for drug interactions is very considerable, and it is perhaps surprising that adverse drug interactions are not more common. Early studies showed that patients who are admitted to hospital are on average taking four or five drugs at the same time and one in five patients receives 10 or more during a hospital stay (Crooks and Moir 1974). One patient described by Prescott was given 41 drugs during a single admission (Prescott 1973); another in the USA received more than 50 in a 24-hour period (Koch-Weser 1973). Polypharmacy is not restricted to the elderly but is also increasingly common in younger patients with chronic diseases such as AIDS, where patients often take 10 or more drugs, increasing the chances of interactions (Bayard et al. 1992).

It is difficult to provide accurate estimates of the prevalence of drug interactions mainly because various studies have used different criteria for definition (particularly in distinguishing between clinically significant and non-significant interactions). This has led to widely discordant figures; it is thought that between six and 30 per cent of all adverse drug reactions are due to drug interactions. For example, the Boston Collaborative Drug Surveillance program (BCDSP) looked at about 10 000 patients exposed to nearly 84 000 drugs (BCDSP 1972). Out of 3600 adverse drug reactions reported, only 234 (6.5 per cent) were attributable to drug interactions. A more recent study in Australia found that 4.4 per cent of all adverse drug reactions which resulted in hospital admission were due to interactions (Stanton et al. 1994). In contrast, in a study of patients on medical wards, 22 per cent of adverse reactions to drugs were due to drug interactions (Borda et al. 1968). In a nursing home population, Blaschke and colleagues (1981) found that 19 per cent of patients were receiving drugs known to interact, while in an outpatient population the figure was 23 per cent (Stanaszek and Franklin 1978). The importance of distinguishing between clinically significant and non-significant interactions in studies has been highlighted by a study in a general practice setting in Australia (Paulet et al. 1982): in 428 prescriptions examined, 2400 drug-drug combinations were identified but only 37 possible interactions were detected, and none was thought to be of clinical significance. When interpreting studies investigating the prevalence of drug interactions, it is also important to remember that interactions are not recognized by many doctors, and even when they are, they are often not reported.

Despite the problems in estimating the exact incidence of interactions, there is good evidence to show that certain patients may be at increased risk.

TABLE 33.1
Drugs at particular risk of interaction

Effect	Drugs involved
Saturable hepatic metabolism	ethanol phenytoin theophylline
Patient dependent on prophylactic effect	cyclosporin glucocorticoids oral contraceptives
Drug has steep dose–response curve	chlorpropamide verapamil
Drug has narrow therapeutic range	digoxin lithium warfarin
Drug has major toxic effects	aminoglycosides cytotoxic drugs digoxin lithium monoamine oxidase inhibitors

For example, the elderly are at particular risk of adverse drug interactions, and the risk also increases as the number of drugs given concurrently rises (Smith *et al.* 1966; Law and Chalmers 1976; D'Arcy 1982). Other groups of patients at particular risk of adverse drug interactions include those on long-term therapy for chronic diseases, such as Addison's disease, AIDS, epilepsy, diabetes, hepatic or renal disease, transplantation recipients, and those with more than one prescribing doctor (Brodie and Feely 1988); also patients in intensive care and patients undergoing complicated surgical procedures (Zarowitz *et al.* 1985; May *et al.* 1987; Beers *et al.* 1990). Certain drug groups are also more likely to be involved in interactions, either because of the nature of the drug, or because the drug has a narrow therapeutic index (Table 33.1).

Clinical importance of drug interactions

Many textbooks of clinical pharmacology and pharmacy contain long lists of drug interactions of doubtful clinical importance. Why should this be?

1. Many drug interactions are first described in animal studies, often when doses of the drugs used have been much greater than those used clinically. The disposition of many drugs differs between species, and thus drug interactions observed in an animal study *in vivo* may not be encountered in man. Sometimes the opposite is true: rifampicin is a potent inducer of P-450 enzymes in man, but much less potent in rats and guinea-pigs, which are used in screening studies (Oesch *et al.* 1996).

2. Drug interactions are often described initially in *in vitro* studies, either in an isolated tissue or in a test tube. Protein-binding interactions that occur *in vitro* rarely occur in clinical practice (MacKichan 1989). Indeed, it is quite hard to find a clinically relevant drug interaction solely due to displacement from protein binding (as opposed to displacement plus inhibition of metabolism). Particular examples are drug interactions with non-steroidal anti-inflammatory drugs (NSAID), many of which were thought to be due to protein-binding displacement. It has taken a lot of effort and experimental time to show that NSAID do not, in general, cause significant displacement of protein-bound drugs in man (Orme 1986).

3. Some drug interactions are described initially after a single case in man. The first, positive report may be confirmed in later studies. Difficulties arise when further investigation fails to demonstrate a significant interaction. This may be because the interpretation of the initial case was mistaken, or the interaction occurs only rarely, or the systematic studies have been insufficiently sensitive to detect it. For the one patient affected, however, it may be important. In order to establish the true frequency of the interaction it might be necessary to study a large number of subjects — perhaps several hundred — and this would clearly not be possible. This is a real problem, for example, with the oral contraceptives, and the debate over their interactions with broad-spectrum antibiotics (Back and Orme 1990) (see also below).

Definition of 'drug interaction'

In the literature there is considerable confusion over what is or is not a drug interaction. Usually, concern over drug interactions only arises when an adverse event is caused. Some drug interactions, however, are beneficial for the patient; and, indeed, two drugs may deliberately be given together for their combined effects (e.g. levodopa and carbidopa). Even though this aspect of drug interactions is not of prime concern for this book, we shall look at it briefly later in this chapter.

Some drug interactions are reported in the literature when only an additive effect is noted. Thus, the combination of phenobarbitone and alcohol will lead to more sedation than either drug alone; glucocorticoids will compound the hypokalaemia caused by thiazide diuretics. These are the expected results of two drugs having additive effects on a pharmacological endpoint and will not be considered further. A true drug

TABLE 33.2
Mechanisms of drug interactions

Pharmaceutical interactions
Occurring outside the patient (e.g. in infusion bottle or syringe)

Pharmacokinetic interactions
Absorption: during passage of drug from the gastrointestinal tract to the blood stream.
Distribution: during the passage of drug to its site of action (e.g. protein-binding displacement).
Metabolism: during the biotransformation of a drug (enzyme inhibition or induction).
Excretion: during excretion from the body, primarily via the kidneys.

Pharmacodynamic interactions
Synergistic: two drugs prescribed together produce a greater effect than the sum of their individual effects.
Antagonistic: one of two drugs prescribed together significantly reduces the effect of the other.

---

interaction is one where the pharmacological outcome is not just a direct result of their two individual effects. Thus, synergism may occur where the combined effect of two drugs is considerably greater than the sum of their individual effects. Alternatively, antagonism may result when one drug largely prevents the effect of another.

Mechanisms of drug interactions

Table 33.2 lists the mechanisms commonly involved in drug interactions. These are usually divided into three types: first, pharmaceutical interactions which occur outside the body; secondly, pharmacokinetic interactions where one one drug affects the absorption, distribution, metabolism, or excretion of another; and thirdly, pharmacodynamic intereactions where one drug interferes with the mechanism of action of another drug or affects physiological control processes. This approach to drug interactions is useful, since an understanding of the mechanism behind any particular interaction can help to predict likely interactions with new drugs. Thus an enzyme inducing agent, such as rifampicin or phenytoin, is likely to induce the metabolism of many drugs that are oxidized or conjugated in the liver and so diminish their therapeutic effect.

We now consider each of the mechanisms in turn before looking at some of the drug groups for which drug interactions seem to be especially relevant.

Pharmaceutical interactions

It is often forgotten in the hurly-burly of clinical work that drugs may interact even before they are even administered to the patient, whether orally or parenterally. Any oral drug formulation may contain up to 25 ingredients and may comprise, in addition to the drug itself, binders, fillers (e.g. lactose), colouring and tasting substances, and several other excipients. During development, much effort will have been devoted to ensuring that none of these substances interact with the drug itself, and the stability and purity of the formulation will have been checked over prolonged periods of time and under various adverse storage conditions (e.g. low or high temperature, high humidity).

It is with parenteral mixtures that the clinician has to be particularly careful, and guidance will usually be given by the pharmacists. Additions of one drug to another in an intravenous infusion or syringe should always be avoided if possible. This subject has been reviewed elsewhere (Smith 1984) and there is a 750-page pharmaceutical textbook devoted entirely to this subject (Trissel 1996). Problems particularly arise if other drugs are added to an infusion of heparin, penicillin, hydrocortisone, or theophylline.

The following drugs are physically incompatible with heparin: amikacin, amiodarone, diazepam, droperidol, erythromycin, gentamicin, kanamycin, morphine, pentazocine, pethidine, polymyxin, and promethazine; and if one of these is added to a heparin infusion a precipitate forms within 5–10 minutes.

Aminophylline is incompatible in solution with chlorpromazine and other phenothiazines, such as promazine and prochlorperazine, dobutamine, pentazocine, pethidine, and some tetracycline salts. As stated earlier, good clinical practice dictates that no more than one drug should be placed in an infusion bottle or syringe. If it is vital to give two drugs by intravenous injection simultaneously, further advice should be sought. It may be appropriate, if venous access is difficult, to give one drug by injection into the side arm of a running infusion containing the second drug.

Pharmacokinetic interactions

Drug interactions during absorption

Many such interactions have been studied and, as mentioned earlier, not all of them are relevant. Some that have employed a static *in vitro* system have shown what appear to be significant interactions, while others involving an *in vivo* system have shown only minor changes. This subject has been reviewed by Welling (1984) and by Gugler and Allgayer (1990).

It is always going to be difficult to assess the clinical significance of this type of interaction because of the contrast between kinetic and dynamic effects. It may be relatively easy to show, for example, that an aluminium hydroxide antacid reduces the bioavailability of keto-profen from 78.3 per cent to 60.9 per cent (Ismail *et al.* 1987) when studied in healthy volunteers. To show the clinical significance of this in patients, however, is likely to be much more difficult. A statistically significant reduction in the bioavailability of warfarin caused by cholestyramine (Robinson *et al.* 1971) is likely to be much more significant clinically than an apparently greater reduction in the bioavailability of penicillin when given with neomycin (Cheng and White 1962). Warfarin clearly has a low therapeutic index while penicillin has the opposite property.

Drugs may interact during absorption by a variety of mechanisms.

Effect on gastrointestinal motility

Drugs are mainly absorbed from the upper small intestine, the surface area of which greatly exceeds that of the stomach. Thus, a drug that affects gastric emptying might be expected to delay the absorption of other drugs (Nimmo 1976; Greiff and Rowbotham 1994). In practice this happens, but the amount of drug absorbed is not greatly affected by changes in the gastric emptying rate. Thus metoclopramide, by increasing the rate of gastric emptying, increases the rate of absorption of para-cetamol (Nimmo *et al.* 1973) as well as other drugs such as levodopa and lithium (see Welling 1984). The interaction between metoclopramide and paracetamol is used therapeutically in patients with migraine to speed the onset of the analgesic action of paracetamol. Cisapride, a gastrointestinal prokinetic agent, may have effects which are similar to metoclopramide. For example, it has been shown to increase the maximum concentration of diazepam by 17 per cent, which may be clinically significant in certain patients (Bateman 1986). In the reverse direction, drugs with anticholinergic properties such as tricyclic antidepressants and opioids, inhibit gastric emptying and may slow the rate of absorption (but often not the quantity absorbed) of concomitantly administered drugs (Greiff and Rowbotham 1994). This type of interaction is usually of little clinical significance.

Luminal effects

Drug absorption interactions may also take place in the lumen of the gut when one drug may bind chemically or physically to another. Table 33.3 lists those drugs for which such interactions are thought to be of clinical relevance.

TABLE 33.3
Clinically significant drug interactions occurring during drug absorption

1. *Via changes in gastrointestinal motility*
   (a) Metoclopramide — enhances the rate of absorption of:
       lithium
       levodopa
       paracetamol
   (b) Cisapride enhances the rate of absorption of:
       diazepam

2. *Via effects in the lumen of the gut*
   (a) Antacids — reduce the absorption of:
       captopril
       ciprofloxacin
       tetracyclines
   (b) Cholestyramine — reduces the absorption of:
       digoxin
       thyroxine
       warfarin
   (c) Tetracycline — reduces the absorption of:
       iron salts (both drugs show poor absorption)
   (d) Charcoal — reduces the absorption of:
       carbamazepine
       phenobarbitone

3. *Via damage to gastrointestinal mucosa*
   Cytotoxic drugs reduce the absorption of:
       phenytoin
       verapamil

Antacids

There is a large literature on drug interactions with antacids and the subject has been extensively reviewed (Gugler and Allgayer 1990; Sadowski 1994). The main groups of drugs for which such interactions have been described include antibiotics, β-adrenoceptor-blocking drugs, captopril, digoxin, H_2-antagonists, iron salts, NSAID, and theophylline. The literature is often confusing. Thus, the absorption of diflunisal appears to be reduced by aluminium hydroxide but enhanced by magnesium hydroxide (Verbeeck *et al.* 1979; Tobert *et al.* 1981). Undoubtedly, the interaction between tetracyclines and antacids is significant, since tetracycline forms insoluble chelates with divalent and trivalent ions (Neuvonen 1976), and the absorption of tetracyclines is reduced by 80 per cent by aluminium- and magnesium-containing antacids. Chelate formation is also responsible for the reduced absorption of the quinolone antibiotics ciprofloxacin and ofloxacin when given with either aluminium- and/or magnesium-containing antacids (Höffken *et al.* 1985; Lode 1988) or ferrous salts (Polk *et al.* 1989). The interaction can be prevented if the antibiotic is not given until at least 6 hours after the antacid (Sadowski 1994). Elevation of gastric pH is another mechanism by which antacids can affect absorption. Thus, absorption of captopril can be significantly reduced (42 per cent reduction in the area-under-the-curve) by simultaneous administration of an aluminium–magnesium antacid although this is less than the reduction (56 per cent) seen with eating (Mäntylä *et al.* 1984). Certain antacids such as sodium bicarbonate may affect urinary excretion of drugs by increasing urinary pH. For example, a change in urinary pH from 6.5 to 7 by sodium bicarbonate was enough to decrease urinary quinidine excretion by 50 per cent with a consequent prolongation in the QT interval (Gerhardt *et al.* 1969). It is likely that other antacid interactions are only rarely of clinical significance.

Anion-exchange resins — cholestyramine

This agent is an anion-exchange resin that binds cholesterol and bile acids in the gut and prevents their reabsorption. In addition to binding bile acids, it also binds other antacid drugs that may be administered at the same time. This resin has been shown to reduce the absorption of warfarin (Robinson *et al.* 1971), thyroxine (Northcutt *et al.* 1969), and antibacterials such as sulphamethoxazole (Parsons and Paddock 1975). Other anion exchange resins such as colestipol may also impair drug absorption (Kauffman and Azarnoff 1973) but the problem seems less than with cholestyramine. The solution is, however, relatively simple. A 2-hour gap should be left between taking cholestyramine and taking other drugs, preferably giving the other drug first. Then no interaction is likely to be seen (Welling 1984).

Tetracycline

It has already been pointed out that antacids prevent the absorption of tetracycline (Neuvonen 1976). Tetracycline, however, may chelate other ions — in particular iron salts, with resultant poor absorption of the iron (Neuvonen 1976). This is in fact a double interaction, since both tetracycline and the iron will be poorly absorbed. Again the interaction can be prevented by giving the iron either 3 hours before or 2 hours after the tetracycline (Gothioni *et al.* 1972).

Activated charcoal

This agent has been implicated in reducing the absorption of certain drugs. Neuvonen and Elonen (1980) showed that it could reduce the absorption of phenobarbitone, phenylbutazone, and carbamazepine by up to 95 per cent. In practice, activated charcoal in sufficient quantity to have this effect is used clinically only in patients who have taken overdoses to prevent absorption and to interfere with enterohepatic and entero–enteral circulations of various drugs (Pond *et al.* 1984; Boldy *et al.* 1987).

Damage to gastrointestinal tract

The absorption of some drugs may be reduced due to damage of the small intestine and this is most likely to be seen with cytotoxic therapy. The absorption of phenytoin (Fincham and Schottelius 1979) and verapamil (Kuhlmann *et al.* 1985) has been shown to be reduced by 20–35 per cent in patients taking cytotoxic drugs such as methotrexate, carmustine, or vinblastine for the treatment of malignant disease. The reduced absorption was accompanied by evidence of loss of therapeutic effect. It is likely that this is an aspect of drug interactions that is under-reported.

Other mechanisms of drug interaction during the absorption process have been reported, mainly involving alteration of bowel flora and thus interfering with the deconjugation of drugs and the enterohepatic circulation. This will be discussed at more length during consideration of drugs interacting with oral contraceptive steroids.

Drug interaction during distribution of drugs

Once a drug is absorbed into the body it is then distributed to its site of action, and during this process it may interact with another drug. In practice the main source of these interactions is displacement from protein-binding sites. While basic drugs are largely bound to acid α_1-glycoprotein in plasma, acidic drugs are bound to albumin. There are several distinct sites to which drugs are bound on the albumin molecule (e.g. the warfarin site, the diazepam site). If other drugs that bind to the same sites are taken, then competition for the binding site occurs and the first drug may be displaced to circulate free (or unbound) in the plasma. This interaction is readily demonstrated *in vitro* for many drugs, and since the unbound drug is the part that produces the pharmacological effect, it is perhaps natural to assume that enhanced pharmacological effects will occur. The protein-binding-displacement interactions have, however, come under closer and closer scrutiny over the last 15–20 years (Sellers 1979; McElnay and D'Arcy 1983), with the conclusion that most are of doubtful clinical importance. Nevertheless, many textbooks still perpetuate the largely mythical view that protein-binding interactions are of considerable clinical significance. Phenylbutazone was recognized to potentiate the anticoagulant effect of warfarin as long ago as 1959 (Nordoy 1959). Further clinical reports confirmed this within a few years and Solomon and colleagues (1968) showed that, *in vitro*, phenylbutazone displaced warfarin from its protein-binding site. It was perhaps natural to link the two as cause and effect, and since many other NSAID also displaced warfarin from protein-binding sites on albumin it was assumed that any NSAID would enhance the anticoagulant effect of warfarin. It has taken many years to show the true mechanism of this interaction and that most NSAID do not have adverse pharmacokinetic interactions with anticoagulants such as warfarin. The interaction between phenylbutazone and warfarin is due to a stereoselective inhibition of the metabolism of warfarin (Sellers 1984). Warfarin as currently marketed consists of a racemic mixture of two enantiomers, R-warfarin and S-warfarin, S-warfarin being five times as potent as R-warfarin. Phenylbutazone inhibits the metabolism of S-warfarin and induces that of R-warfarin, as shown in Figure 33.1. Thus, in the presence of phenylbutazone, there is no overall change in the kinetics of racemic warfarin, but a greater proportion of warfarin in plasma is the more potent S-form (Lewis *et al.* 1974; O'Reilly *et al.* 1987). Drugs like indomethacin (Vessell *et al.* 1975), naproxen (Jain *et al.* 1979), and diclofenac (Krzywanek and Breddin 1977) do not increase the anticoagulant effect of warfarin. Care, however, is still needed when NSAID are given to patients on warfarin, because of their tendency to cause gastric ulceration

and affect platelet function by inhibiting cyclo-oxygenase, both of which increase the likelihood of gastrointestinal bleeding.

Current evidence suggests that, for most drugs, if a displacement interaction occurs, then the free concentration of the displaced drug will rise temporarily, but metabolism and distribution will return the free concentration to its previous level and the time this takes will be primarily dependent on the half-life of the displaced drug (MacKichan 1989). The biological significance of the temporary rise in free concentration is not clear but is unlikely to be very much on its own. The total (i.e. free plus bound) concentration of the displaced drug in plasma will fall and this may be of significance if total concentration is being measured for the purpose of therapeutic drug monitoring. This suggests that for drugs where the metabolism or excretion is not inhibited, protein-binding-displacement interactions are therefore of no clinical significance (MacKichan 1989). If, however, the metabolism or excretion of the displaced drug is inhibited at the same time (restrictive clearance), then an interaction will be seen. A typical example is that of methotrexate and NSAID, which is discussed in greater detail below.

Drug interactions occurring during metabolism

Many of the clinically relevant drug interactions occur because of alterations in the rate of metabolism of the drug concerned. Most drugs now used in clinical practice are lipid-soluble and cannot be eliminated as such because they will be reabsorbed across the renal tubule. Metabolic processes convert the lipid-soluble drug to more water-soluble products that can be excreted in the urine or bile. There are two main types of drug metabolic process: phase I reactions involving oxidation, hydrolysis, or reduction; and phase II reactions, which are synthetic reactions involving conjugation of the drug (or its phase I product) with, for example, glucuronic acid, sulphate, or glycine. Products of phase II reactions are nearly always pharmacologically inactive, but phase I products are often active either therapeutically or toxicologically (Garattini 1985). The rate of drug metabolism varies widely between individuals and is determined by both genetic and environmental factors. There are many factors that can affect the rate (or route) of drug metabolism (see Chapter 5), and one of the most important is the concomitant administration of other drugs.

The rate of drug metabolism may be increased by the process of enzyme induction, in which the enzyme inducer increases the velocity of the drug metabolic

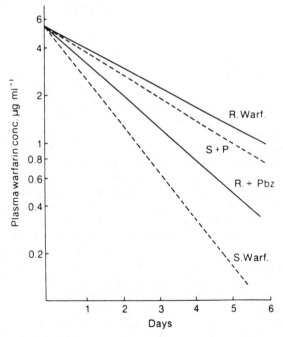

FIG. 33.1

Plasma warfarin concentration decay over a 6-day period after the oral administration of *R*-warfarin and *S*-warfarin to human volunteers before (R. Warf./S. Warf.) and after phenylbutazone (R+P/S+P) 100 mg t.i.d. for 10 days.
(Reproduced by kind permission of the authors and of the editor of the *Journal of Clinical Investigation* [1974] 53, 1607.)

TABLE 33.4
Cytochrome P-450 isozymes involved in the metabolism of drugs and xenobiotics

P-450 isoform	Substrates	Inducers	Inhibitors
CYP1A2	Clozapine Theophylline	Cigarette smoke Omeprazole	Ciprofloxacin Furafylline
CYP2A6	Halothane Methoxyflurane	Phenytoin Rifampicin	Tranylcypromine
CYP2C9	Diclofenac Tolbutamide Warfarin	Barbiturates Rifampicin	Sulphaphenazole
CYP2C19	Citalopram Diazepam Ompeprazole	Rifampicin	Tranylcypromine
CYP2D6	Codeine Haloperidol Metoprolol Nortriptyline	not inducible	Quinidine
CYP2E1	Enflurane Halothane Paracetamol	Alcohol (chronic use)	Disulfiram
CYP3A4	Amiodarone Carbamazepine Cyclosporin Terfenadine	Carbamazepine Gluocorticoids Phenytoin Rifampicin	Erythromycin Ketoconazole
CYP4A1	Testosterone	Clofibrate	

Only a few inhibitors/inducers are mentioned for each P-450 isoform

TABLE 33.5
Drugs known to inhibit human drug metabolism and cause significant drug interactions

Antibacterial compounds	Chloramphenicol Ciproflxacin Erythromycin Isoniazid Metronidazole Sulphonamides
Antifungal drugs	Fluconazole Itraconazole Ketoconazole
Cardiovascular drugs	Amiodarone Diltiazem Quinidine Verapamil
Central nervous system drugs	Fluoxetine Fluvoxamine Paroxetine Sertraline Sodium valproate
Gastrointestinal drugs	Cimetidine Lansoprazole Omeprazole
Rheumatological drugs	Allopurinol Azapropazone Phenylbutazone
Other	Disulfiram Ethanol (acute) Indinavir Ritonavir Saquinavir

reaction. There is a long list of enzyme inducers that have been detected in animal studies but relatively few are known in man. Table 33.4 lists those inducers known to cause problems in man, and the relevant P-450 isoforms that they affect.

The rate of drug metabolism may be reduced by drugs that usually compete for the enzyme site although, rarely, the inhibiting drug may bind to the enzyme site and either inactivate or destroy it. Table 33.5 lists those drugs that are known to inhibit drug metabolism in man and to cause significant interactions. This area has been reviewed extensively elsewhere (Park and Breckenridge 1981; Park et al. 1995, 1996).

The field of drug metabolism has advanced considerably in the last few years. The main enzymes responsible for drug oxidation are the cytochrome P-450 enzymes. It is now clear that there are many different isoforms of the P-450 enzymes (Boobis and Davies 1984; Bronsen 1990). A classification based on gene sequence homology has therefore been developed in order to overcome the confusion in nomenclature which arose as a result of the discovery of these multiple forms (Nebert et al. 1989). Thus, 74 major families have now been designated (labelled CYP1, CYP2, etc.) each of which contains genes of at least 40 per cent sequence homology. Within

each family, several subfamilies (CYP1A, CYP1B, etc.) can reside provided that the genes within these subfamilies show at least 55 per cent homology. The final Arabaic numeral in the classification (CYP1A1, CYP1A2 etc.) designates a unique isozyme (theoretically 100 per cent homology, but with a three per cent allowance for natural mutations). This system, which is updated periodically (Nebert et al. 1989, 1991; Nelson et al. 1993, 1996), has provided a robust and serviceable framework for the growth of knowledge in P-450 research. With respect to man, it is only necessary to focus on four main families as shown in Table 33.4. Each family contains a relatively small number of subfamilies with a cluster of individual isozymes in each. The importance of these isozymes of P-450 for drug interactions is that both enzyme inducers and enzyme inhibitors are likely to be selective in the range of isozymes they affect (Table 33.4).

Enzyme induction

The process of enzyme induction requires new protein synthesis, so its maximum effect is not seen for 2–3 weeks after starting an enzyme-inducing agent; similarly, the effect may take some weeks to wear off when the inducing drug is stopped. Rifampicin is unusual in this regard in having a more rapid onset and offset (Park and Breckenridge 1981). Two days' treatment of nasal carriage of meningococci with rifampicin will induce the metabolism of other drugs therapy (e.g. oral contraceptive steroids — see below). Enzyme induction usually results in the reduction of the pharmacological effect of the induced drug but where the metabolites are active the reverse may occur.

Oral anticoagulants

The hypoprothrombinaemic effect of oral anticoagulants such as warfarin is reduced by enzyme-inducing agents such as carbamazepine, barbiturates, and rifampicin. The mechanism involves induction of the P-450 isoform CYP2C9 (Goldstein and DeMorais 1994), which is largely responsible for the metabolism of warfarin. These interactions have been known for some years and several reviews have been written (Koch-Weser and Sellers 1971; Macleod and Sellers 1976; Serlin and Breckenridge 1983). An occasional patient will need, say, both warfarin and carbamazepine and particular care with anticoagulant control will then be needed.

Corticosteroids

Enzyme-inducing agents enhance the metabolic clearance of corticosteroids such as hydrocortisone (Werk *et al.* 1964), prednisolone (Petereit and Meikle 1977), and dexamethasone (Haque *et al.* 1972) by causing induction of CYP3A4. Thus enzyme-inducing agents given to corticosteroid-dependent patients may induce respiratory problems in those with asthma (Brooks *et al.* 1972), worsen disease control in patients with rheumatoid arthritis (Brooks *et al.* 1976), and lead to deterioration in renal allograft function, or failure of patients with the nephrotic syndrome to improve (see McInnes and Brodie 1988). Patients with Addison's disease may need increased dosage of corticosteroids to prevent relapse (Edwards *et al.* 1974).

Clinicians need to be aware that if enzyme-inducing agents are given to patients taking corticosteroids, an increase in dosage will be needed, with a corresponding reduction when the agent is stopped.

Oral contraceptive steroids

Combined oral contraceptive preparations and progestogen-only preparations lose their contraceptive effect when taken together with an enzyme-inducing agent (Back and Orme 1990). This aspect of drug interaction will be covered separately later in this chapter.

Cyclosporin

Cyclosporin undergoes extensive metabolism by CYP3A4 in man, and both organ toxicity and immunosuppressive activity appear to be related to cyclosporin concentrations in blood (Canafax and Ascher 1983). Enzyme-inducing agents, such as phenytoin, lower cyclosporin concentrations in blood (see Figure 33.2) by inducing CYP3A4 (Freeman *et al.* 1984; Nation *et al.* 1990).

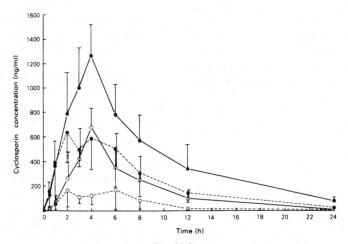

FIG. 33.2

Cyclosporin concentrations measured by high-pressure liquid chromatography before (——) and after (– – –) administration of phenytoin (300–400 mg daily) to six volunteers taking cyclosporin. Concentrations are shown both in whole blood (○) and in serum (●).

(Reproduced by kind permission of the authors and of the editor of the *British Journal of Clinical Pharmacology* [1984] 18, 887.)

Paracetamol

Paracetamol is relatively non-toxic when taken in therapeutic dosage. In overdosage, however, it leads to hepatic-necrosis which can be fatal. Bioactivation of paracetamol by CYP1A2, CYP2E1, and CYP3A4 (Pirmohamed *et al.* 1994) to a toxic quinoneimine metabolite is thought to be responsible for the hepatic damage. It has been shown that patients who are chronic abusers of alcohol (which leads to induction of CYP2E1) (Black and Raucy 1986; Bray *et al.* 1991), and those on anticonvulsants (Bray *et al.* 1992) such as phenytoin and carbamazepine (which induce CYP3A4) may develop hepatotoxicity at lower paracetamol dosage than those not taking an enzyme inducer. Therefore, treatment with *N*-acetyl-cysteine in these patients should be commenced at lower plasma paracetamol levels than are used for other patients (Bray 1993). It is also important to note that in alcohol abusers hepatic injury has been reported at doses of paracetamol which are generally considered to be non-toxic (Zimmerman and Maddrey 1995; Schiødt *et al.* 1997).

Theophylline

Theophylline has a low therapeutic index, and its elimination depends largely on metabolism by CYP1A2 and CYP3A4 (Tjia *et al.* 1996). This being so, it is not surprising that drug interactions with theophylline are clinically very important, and the subject has been reviewed extensively (Jonkman and Upton 1984). The elimination of theophylline is so markedly enhanced (through induction of CYP3A4) by phenytoin (Marquis *et al.* 1982) and phenobarbitone (Landay *et al.* 1978) that dosage increments of 30–40 per cent are required to keep the plasma concentration within the therapeutic range. Rifampicin also increases theophylline metabolic clearance and lowers the plasma concentration (Hauser *et al.* 1983). The polycyclic aromatic hydrocarbons in tobacco smoke can induce the P-450 isoform CYP1A2, and thereby the metabolism of theophylline; the inducing effect may persist for 2–3 months after quitting smoking (Hunt *et al.* 1976).

Enzyme inhibition

Enzyme inhibition is potentially more important in terms of drug interactions than enzyme induction. The speed of onset is usually more rapid, being determined largely by the half life of the inhibited drug. Thus for drugs with a short half-life, the effect may be seen within 24 hours of the administration of the inhibiting agent. Table 33.4 lists drugs inhibiting specific P-450 isoforms while Table 33.5 provides a more comprehensive list of

enzyme inhibitors which have been responsible for clinically significant drug interactions.

Drugs with metabolism sensitive to enzyme inhibition

Oral anticoagulants   The metabolism of warfarin is, as discussed above, inhibited by phenylbutazone, with potentially disastrous effects (Lewis *et al.* 1974). A number of other drugs, such as dextropropoxyphene, metronidazole, miconazole, omeprazole, sulphonamides, and tamoxifen, have been reported to inhibit the metabolism of warfarin (McInnes and Brodie 1988; Harder and Thurmann 1996). These interactions are only rarely of clinical significance. Cimetidine has been shown to inhibit the metabolism of S-warfarin (Toon *et al.* 1987), with enhanced anticoagulant effects. The H_2-antagonists ranitidine, famotidine, and nizatidine, by contrast, do not inhibit warfarin metabolism (O'Reilly 1984).

Cyclosporin   The metabolism of cyclosporin by CYP3A4 is inhibited by ketoconazole, erythromycin, and diltiazem (Ferguson *et al.* 1982; Ptachcinski *et al.* 1985; McInnes and Brodie 1988) and cyclosporin toxicity may then result. Recently, grapefruit juice has also been shown to inhibit cyclosporin metabolism (Yee *et al.* 1995); this is discussed in greater detail below. It is interesting to note that concomitant use of ketoconazole (First *et al.* 1989), diltiazem (Jones *et al.* 1997), or grapefruit juice (Yee *et al.* 1995), with careful monitoring of cyclosporin plasma concentrations, has been advocated by certain transplant units in order to allow a reduction in cyclosporin dosage, and hence cost.

Theophylline   Inhibition of theophylline metabolism is likely to lead to severe adverse effects, particularly cardiac arrhythmias and convulsions. Several drugs inhibit theophylline metabolism (Jonkman and Upton 1984), including allopurinol and propranolol. However, the three most important drugs in this respect are cimetidine, erythromycin, and ciprofloxacin.

Cimetidine reduces the clearance of theophylline by 30–50 per cent (Jackson *et al.* 1981; Breen *et al.* 1982; Jonkman and Upton 1984). This is a potentially fatal interaction, and cimetidine may often be given to patients taking theophylline because of the gastric upset the latter tends to cause. Although ranitidine is less likely to cause inhibition of theophylline metabolism, it is not entirely devoid of this effect (Kirch *et al.* 1984).

Erythromycin is another drug likely to be given concurrently with theophylline that has been shown to inhibit the metabolism of theophylline by inhibiting CYP3A4. Not all studies have shown this convincingly, and it appears that erythromycin needs to be given for several days before the effect is seen (Jonkman and Upton 1984). The clearance of theophylline is reduced by between 10 and 25 per cent by treatment with erythromycin for 5–7 days, and the dose of theophylline should be reduced accordingly (Branigan *et al.* 1981; May *et al.* 1982).

Ciprofloxacin raises concentrations of theophylline, almost certainly by inhibiting its metabolism by CYP1A2 (Maesen *et al.* 1984).

Phenytoin   The enzyme responsible for metabolising phenytoin, CYP2C9, is saturable at phenytoin concentrations above 10–15 mg per litre (Kutt 1971). CYP2C9 is inhibited by a number of drugs, including allopurinol, amiodarone, azapropazone, chloramphenicol, cimetidine, isoniazid, metronidazole, omeprazole, sulphonamides, and sodium valproate (Rodin *et al.* 1981; Nation *et al.* 1990). No particular drug is especially likely to do this and care should always be taken when prescribing an additional drug to a patient already receiving phenytoin.

Carbamazepine   The metabolism of carbamazepine is inhibited by sodium valproate (MacPhee *et al.* 1988). This is due to inhibition of microsomal epoxide hydrolase (Kerr *et al.* 1989), and leads not only to dose-dependent neurological adverse effects, but possibly also to an increased risk of teratogenicity (Kaneko *et al.* 1988). Significant interactions (by inhibition of P-450) have been reported with chloramphenicol, cimetidine, erythromycin, isoniazid, dextropropoxyphene and sulphonamides (Vasko 1990), although many of these are now mainly of historical interest. However, occasional problems are still seen in this area, as reported by MacPhee and co-workers, who showed that verapamil and diltiazem, by acting as competitive inhibitors of CYP3A4, inhibited the metabolism of carbamazepine with an increase of 50 per cent in the plasma concentration and consequent neurotoxic sequelae. An alternative calcium antagonist, nifedipine, had no such effect (Brodie and MacPhee 1986; MacPhee *et al.* 1986).

Inhibiting drugs

Amiodarone   Warfarin metabolism is inhibited by amiodarone (Watt *et al.* 1985) and this affects both *R*- and *S*-warfarin enantiomers (O'Reilly *et al.* 1987). Amiodarone also inhibits the metabolism of phenytoin and probably also that of quinidine and flecainide. Interactions with other drugs, such as digoxin and calcium-channel-blocking drugs, are important but may not be due to enzyme inhibition (Lesko 1989).

Cimetidine   Cimetidine inhibits the cytochrome P-450 enzymes in a non-selective fashion by binding to their haem moiety. In addition to inhibiting the metabolism of warfarin (Serlin *et al.* 1979), theophylline (Jackson *et al.* 1981), phenytoin (Nation *et al.* 1990) and

carbamazepine (Vasko 1990), cimetidine has been shown to inhibit the metabolism of such drugs as chlormethiazole, diazepam, labetalol, and propranolol (Gerber *et al.* 1985). In the case of these last four drugs, it is unlikely that significant clinical problems will be caused. Ranitidine is, in general, viewed as having no effect on drug metabolism, but there are some reported examples of it causing enzyme inhibition involving notably, fentanyl, metoprolol, and nifedipine, but the clinical significance of these is unclear (Kirch *et al.* 1984).

Ethanol   Although chronic ethanol consumption may cause enzyme induction, acute alcohol ingestion has been shown to inhibit drug metabolism. In general, ethanol levels need to be fairly high, and many studies in which blood ethanol levels have been maintained at 800–1500 mg per litre have shown inhibition of the metabolism of such drugs as diazepam, chlordiazepoxide, and lorazepam (Sellers *et al.* 1980). The clearance of drugs, such as diazepam, that undergo oxidation is affected to a greater extent than those, such as lorazepam, that undergo conjugation (Desmond *et al.* 1980; Hoyumpa *et al.* 1981). It is unlikely that any effects will be seen with social drinking but elimination of drugs following an overdose is likely to be slower if alcohol has also been consumed to excess. Interestingly, excess alcohol protects against liver damage in patients taking an overdose of paracetamol since the P-450 pathway which produces the toxic metabolite is inhibited (Banda and Quart 1982). As stated above, chronic alcohol ingestion, conversely, makes paracetamol hepatotoxicity worse by enzyme induction. In addition to a pharmacokinetic element, with centrally acting drugs, such as benzodiazepines, there is also a pharmacodynamic element, the combination of the two producing increased sedation (Fraser 1997). This is a particular problem in the elderly where it may lead to falls and impairment of driving (Adams 1995).

Allopurinol   Allopurinol is recognized as a weak inhibitor of P-450 enzymes in man (Vessell *et al.* 1970). Its clinical relevance in this regard, however, is very minor. There is no effect on theophylline metabolism (Jonkman and Upton 1984) and there is little evidence of any interaction between allopurinol and phenytoin (Nation *et al.* 1990). Allopurinol is important, however, by virtue of its inhibition of xanthine oxidase. Certain cytotoxic drugs, such as azathioprine or its metabolite 6-mercaptopurine, are partly metabolised by xanthine oxidase, and if this enzyme is inhibited by allopurinol the clinical effects of the cytotoxic drugs are enhanced, with haemolysis or bone marrow suppression (Bacon *et al.* 1981).

The dosage of azathioprine must be reduced by 75 per cent when allopurinol therapy is started concomitantly.

Drug interactions during excretion

We have already noted that most drugs are lipid-soluble and hence need to be metabolised to make them soluble enough in water to be excreted. As a result, few drugs are sufficiently water-soluble to be excreted unchanged. Interactions during excretion are described for digoxin, lithium, and methotrexate, and these are described elsewhere in this chapter. The effect of diuretics and NSAID leads to a rise in lithium concentration, and methotrexate clearance is reduced by NSAID. The renal tubular system is able both actively to secrete and passively to reabsorb a number of drugs. There are separate active transport systems for acidic and basic drugs in the proximal tubule, and competition for the active transport systems can be expected to occur between drugs secreted by the acidic system and those secreted by the basic system. Table 33.6 lists the drugs secreted by these systems, but the best known interactions are the beneficial interactions between probenecid and penicillin (Kampmann *et al.* 1972) and probenecid and indomethacin (Baber *et al.* 1978).

Pharmacodynamic interactions

Pharmacodynamic interactions are less readily classified than those due to changes in pharmacokinetics, but in general, they can be divided into synergistic and antagonistic interactions. Table 33.7 lists some of the more common examples. In some cases the interaction is due to effects at the receptor, but in other cases the interaction is due to an effect on biochemical or physiological mechanisms.

Direct receptor effects

Clearly the agonists at a particular receptor (e.g. a β-adrenoceptor) will interact with antagonists at that receptor but this is entirely expected and requires no further discussion. Spironolactone prevents the healing effects of carbenoxolone on gastric ulcer; and, in turn, carbenoxolone competitively antagonizes the renal effects of spironolactone — both effects probably occurring through an action at the aldosterone receptor (Doll *et al.* 1968).

The hypoprothrombinaemic effects of warfarin are potentiated by clofibrate, quinidine, and dextrothyroxine; and in each case it is proposed that the mechanism is

TABLE 33.6
*Acidic and basic drugs actively transported
into the renal tubular lumen*

Acidic	Basic
Aciclovir	Amiloride
Bumetanide	Cimetidine
Cephalosporins	Ethambutol
Frusemide	Procainamide
Indomethacin	Ranitidine
Penicillins	
Phenobarbitone	
Probenecid	
Salicylates	
Sulphonamides	
Thiazide diuretics	

TABLE 33.7
*Examples of synergistic and antagonistic
pharmacodynamic interactions*

Interacting drugs	Pharmacological effect
Synergistic interactions	
alcohol and benzodiazepines	increased sedation
NSAID and warfarin	increased risk of bleeding
ACE inhibitors and potassium-sparing diuretics	hyperkalaemia
verapamil and β-adrenoceptor antagonists	bradycardia and asystole
Antagonistic interactions	
thiazides and oral hypoglycaemic agents	hyperglycaemia
penicillins and tetracycline	reduced penicillin efficacy
NSAID and antihypertensive drugs	poor BP control
tricyclic antidepressants and adrenergic-neurone antagonists	poor BP control
digoxin and frusemide	hypokalaemia and digoxin toxicity

an increased affinity of warfarin for its putative receptor site (Solomon and Schrogie 1967; Starr and Petrie 1972).

Indirect receptor effects

A number of pharmacodynamic interactions are considered separately, later in the chapter. These include interactions involving monoamine oxidase inhibitors, interactions between NSAID and diuretics, and between NSAID and antihypertensive drugs.

β-Adrenoceptor antagonists and hypoglycaemic agents

In patients treated with insulin or oral hypoglycaemic agents, the use of β-blockers can produce hypoglycaemia (Reveno and Rosenbaum 1968). In addition, the recognition of hypoglycaemia by a patient may be impaired by β-blockers because of the lack of the usual warning symptoms. Propranolol reduces glycogen breakdown and delays the rise in blood glucose after hypoglycaemia (Davidson *et al.* 1976), while cardioselective drugs such as atenolol have no such effects (Davidson *et al.* 1976). In patients taking propranolol, the hypoglycaemic reaction is associated with a bradycardia rather than the usual tachycardia. In those taking selective β-blockers, such as metoprolol, the heart rate rises and there is little change in blood pressure (Davidson *et al.* 1976). Patients taking insulin or oral hypoglycaemic drugs are thus best advised to take a selective, rather than a non-selective agent, if a drug of this kind is indicated.

β-Adrenoceptor antagonists and other cardioactive drugs

The combination of β-blockers and verapamil has been recognized for some years as deleterious (Krikler and Spurell 1974). Not only is there a combination of the negative inotropic effects of both drugs, resulting in heart failure, but hypotension, atrioventricular block, and asystole have been noted. Other antiarrhythmic agents given concurrently with β-blockers can also produce adverse effects — notably heart failure and hypotension — and examples include nifedipine (Robson and Vishwanath 1982), disopyramide (Gelipter and Hazell 1980), and lignocaine (Graham *et al.* 1981).

Pharmacodynamic interactions have also been reported with other antiarrhythmic drugs. For example, combining amiodarone (a class III antiarrhythmic) with class I agents such as flecainide (Jung *et al.* 1993) or propafenone (Figa *et al.* 1994) can prolong the QT interval and lead to life-threatening arrhythmias.

Spironolactone and potassium chloride

The combination of spironolactone, with its potassium-retaining effect, and potassium chloride is to be avoided, since it has led to hyperkalaemic paralysis and death (McInnes and Ramsay 1987). Indeed, no potassium-retaining diuretic (including triamterene and amiloride) should be given with potassium chloride. In a study by the Boston Collaborative Drug Surveillance Program, hyperkalaemia attributable to spironolactone was found in 5.7 per cent of medical patients not receiving potassium salts, while in patients with renal failure also taking potassium salts the figure rose to 42 per cent (Greenblat and Koch-Weser 1973). The combination of potassium and a potassium-sparing diuretic should always be

avoided. Angiotensin-converting-enzyme inhibitors, such as captopril, can also cause a dangerous rise in the serum potassium concentration and problems have arisen when spironolactone was given to patients taking such a preparation (Heel *et al.* 1980).

Drug interactions with specific drug groups

Oral contraceptive steroids (OC)

Oral contraceptive steroids are used by some 2 million women in the United Kingdom and by perhaps 60′ million women worldwide. Since there has been a trend to lower the dose of steroids in the preparations over the last 10–15 years, drug interactions have assumed a greater importance than previously.

Effect of contraceptive steroids on other drugs

OC do have effects on the metabolism of other drugs, but in general these are of minor importance. OC may inhibit the metabolism of drugs metabolised by P-450 enzymes. For example, the clearance of diazepam was reduced by 40 per cent when OC were given (Abernethy *et al.* 1982). Similarly, the clearance of caffeine, metoprolol, prednisolone, and theophylline is reduced in OC users, but the changes are relatively small compared with the interindividual variations that are seen in drug metabolism (Back and Orme 1990). Oral contraceptives are reported to enhance the effect of antidepressants and of warfarin, but these changes are not of clinical significance (Breckenridge *et al.* 1979). For drugs metabolised by conjugation (e.g. temazepam), the clearance is enhanced by about 50 per cent (Stoehr *et al.* 1984).

One interesting interaction concerns cyclosporin and ethinyloestradiol, both of which are metabolised primarily by the same cytochrome P-450 isoform (CYP3A4) (Bronsen 1990). In a woman treated with cyclosporin, the plasma concentrations rose when the oral contraceptive was started, and this may have been because of competitive inhibition of CYP3A4 (Deray *et al.* 1987).

Effect of other drugs on OC steroids

Antituberculous drugs

Reimers and Jezek described contraceptive failure in 1971 in women taking antituberculous drugs with their OC. It was quickly realized that the enzyme-inducing agent rifampicin was responsible, and a number of other reports have since appeared (Orme *et al.* 1983). Studies showed that rifampicin induced the metabolism both of

TABLE 33.8

Anticonvulsants and antibiotics implicated in cases of contraceptive failure in women taking OC

Anticonvulsants	No. of reports
Carbamazepine	6
Ethosuximide	4
Phenobarbitone	20
Phenytoin	25
Primidone	7
Sodium valproate	1
Cephalosporins	2
Co-trimoxazole	5
Erythromycin	2
Metronidazole	3
Penicillins	32
Tetracyclines	12
Trimethoprim	2
Others	5

The data come from reports to the Committee on Safety of Medicines in the United Kingdom received between 1968 and 1984 (see Back *et al.* 1988).

ethinyloestradiol (Back *et al.* 1980a) and of the progestogens (Back *et al.* 1979) by inducing CYP3A4 (Guengerich 1988). From a clinical point of view, the degree of induction by rifampicin (up to four- or fivefold), the interindividual variation in induction, and the 6-month courses of rifampicin that are usually given, together mean that women taking rifampicin should not rely on OC for their contraception. This also applies, as mentioned earlier, even to women taking rifampicin only

for 2 days to kill nasal meningococci. They should use alternative contraceptive precautions during treatment and for one month after the course of rifampicin is finished.

Anticonvulsants

A wide variety of anticonvulsants has been reported to cause contraceptive failure when given to women taking OC (Coulam and Annegers 1979; Orme *et al.* 1983). Table 33.8 lists those anticonvulsants that have been implicated in reports to the Committee on Safety of Medicines (CSM) in the UK between 1968 and 1984 (Back *et al.* 1988). Kinetic data are relatively sparse in this field, but phenobarbitone has been shown to cause a fall in the blood level of ethinyloestradiol, presumably by enzyme induction (Back *et al.* 1980b). The interaction between ethinyloestradiol and phenobarbitone is shown in Figure 33.3. Similarly, carbamazepine and phenytoin have been shown to reduce the plasma concentration of both ethinyloestradiol and progestogens in women taking single doses of OC (Crawford *et al.* 1990). The degree of change seen in these studies is quite sufficient to cause contraceptive failure, but it is now possible to achieve contraceptive control by using a higher dose OC preparation. The patients should be started on a 50 μg ethinyloestradiol preparation, and if breakthrough bleeding occurs into the second cycle of use, the dose can be increased to 80 μg (or if necessary to 100 μg). Breakthrough bleeding is a reasonable clinical sign of relative oestrogen deficiency. Even though more steroid

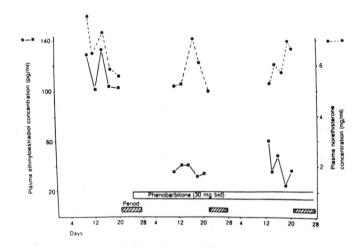

FIG. 33.3

Plasma ethinyloestradiol (■——■) and norethisterone (●---●) concentrations in a patient during a control cycle of oral contraceptive steroid use and during two subsequent cycles of use when the patient was treated with phenobarbitone 30 mg twice daily.

(Reproduced by kind permission of the authors and of the editor of *Contraception* [1980] 22, 495.)

metabolites will be produced, there is no evidence that these have any pharmacological activity. Alternatively, a standard dose of OC can be used if sodium valproate is used as the anticonvulsant, since this anticonvulsant does not interact with OC (Crawford *et al.* 1986).

Antibiotics

Broad-spectrum antibiotics have been implicated in causing contraceptive failure in women taking OC. There are a number of individual case reports in the literature, involving tetracycline, ampicillin, and erythromycin (Orme *et al.* 1983) and 63 pregnancies were reported to the CSM between 1968 and 1984 in women taking antibiotics with their OC preparation (Back *et al.* 1988). The antibiotics implicated are shown in Table 33.8. In a study of pill method failures recorded in reliable pill takers over a 4-year period, Sparrow (1987) in New Zealand found that antibiotics were implicated in 23 per cent of the 163 cases noted. Systematic studies with broad-spectrum antibiotics have, however, shown no evidence of any interaction between these antibiotics and OC. Such antibiotics include ampicillin (Friedman *et al.* 1980; Joshi *et al.* 1980; Back *et al.* 1982), co-trimoxazole (Grimmer *et al.* 1983), tetracycline, and erythromycin (Orme and Back 1986). Indeed, co-trimoxazole significantly increased the blood levels of ethinyloestradiol and made the OC significantly more effective as judged by a fall in FSH levels. This makes the CSM data in Table 33.8 even harder to understand.

The proposed mechanism involves the enterohepatic circulation of ethinyloestradiol, which is conjugated with sulphate and with glucuronide in the gut wall and liver respectively. These conjugates are excreted in the bile and when they reach the colon they are hydrolysed by gut bacteria (primarily *Clostridia* spp.) to liberate unchanged ethinyloestradiol, which is then reabsorbed into the body. Broad-spectrum antibiotics reduce dramatically the ability of faecal micro-organisms to hydrolyse ethinyloestradiol (Chapman 1981), and thus ethinyloestradiol conjugates would be expected to be lost in the faeces with a resultant fall in circulating ethinyloestradiol concentrations. Most data sheets currently recommend that alternative contraceptive precautions should be taken if a broad-spectrum antibiotic is given to a woman taking OC. In addition, a number of medicolegal cases involving this interaction have been settled out of court, it being the legal view that, as this is an pharmacologically plausible — though not yet proven —interaction, a practitioner would be negligent were he or she not to heed the advice given in the Summary of Product Characteristics. It is likely that this is a rare interaction: the enterohepatic circulation of ethinyl-

oestradiol is probably of very minor importance in most people, as judged from data from women with ileostomies (Grimmer *et al.* 1986).

Drug interactions with NSAID

Drug interactions with NSAID are becoming increasingly important, particularly as the use of NSAID continues to increase. The clinically relevant interactions of NSAID with anticoagulants have been covered above. Many other interactions with NSAID have been described (see Webster 1985; Orme 1986; Miners 1989; Verbeeck 1990). The important ones are shown in Table 33.9; those with antacids, digoxin, and between NSAID

TABLE 33.9
Clinically important drug interactions with NSAID

Antihypertensive drugs	loss of BP control
Lithium	lithium toxicity
Loop diuretics	fluid retention
Methotrexate	methotrexate toxicity
Oral anticoagulants	haemorrhage
Phenytoin	phenytoin toxicity
Thiazide diuretics	loss of BP control

probably have little clinical relevance. One important interaction that involves kinetics is the interaction between NSAID (particularly salicylates) and methotrexate. The renal clearance of methotrexate is reduced by 30–50 per cent if such drugs are given together, and deaths have resulted from this interaction (Singh *et al.* 1986, Thyss *et al.* 1986). If NSAID are given to patients taking methotrexate for the treatment of malignancy, the dose of methotrexate should be halved and the patient closely monitored for adverse effects, particularly bone marrow suppression. A clinically important interaction is much less likely when NSAID are used with low-dose methotrexate (i.e. less than 20 mg per week), although care should still be exercised in patients with impaired renal function (Brouwers and Desmet 1994).

Pharmacodynamic interactions with NSAID are increasingly being reported, particularly with diuretics and antihypertensive drugs.

Loop diuretics

The diuretic effect of many drugs is impaired by NSAID. This interaction was first observed between aspirin and spironolactone, but is now chiefly noted with loop diuretics. The reports have primarily involved indomethacin, which has been shown to blunt the diuretic response to frusemide (Patak *et al.* 1975) and to bumetanide (Pedrinelli *et al.* 1980). NSAID are known to cause salt and water retention, but the mechanism is almost certainly more complicated than this. The renal clearance of frusemide is reduced by indomethacin (Smith *et al.* 1979) but it is likely that the mechanism chiefly involves renal prostaglandins. Prostaglandin E$_2$ is important as a renal vasodilator and becomes particularly relevant in disease states (as opposed to the normal healthy state). Other NSAID such as flurbiprofen (Symmons *et al.* 1983), ibuprofen, and naproxen (Yeung Laiwah and Mactier 1981) also inhibit the diuretic effect of frusemide. Interestingly, this action of thiazides is not impaired by indomethacin even though the hypotensive effect is reduced (Favre *et al.* 1983). It is increasingly common to see patients whose heart failure has deteriorated in spite of increased doses of frusemide, not infrequently because of the concurrent use of an NSAID.

Antihypertensive drugs

Indomethacin was first reported to antagonize the hypotensive effect of β-adrenoceptor antagonists by Durao and co-workers in 1977. Since then the interaction has been confirmed in controlled studies (Watkins *et al.* 1980; Wing *et al.* 1981). Figure 33.4 shows the effect on blood pressure of giving indomethacin to patients taking bendrofluazide or propranolol (Watkins *et al.* 1980). Indomethacin has also been shown to reduce the hypotensive effect of other antihypertensive drugs, such as captopril (Silberbauer *et al.* 1982) and the calcium-channel blocker felodipine (Morgan and Anderson 1993). There are relatively few data concerning other NSAID, but it does seem to be a class effect rather than

restricted to indomethacin, since flurbiprofen has also been shown to inhibit the hypotensive effect of propranolol but not that of atenolol (Webster *et al.* 1983). The effect of NSAID seems to be due to inhibition of renal prostaglandin production, and patients with pre-existing low renal renin activity, i.e. negroes and the elderly, seem to be the most susceptible (Morgan and Anderson 1993). It is possible that adaptation may occur in the long-term with blood pressure returning to baseline, although there have been few long-term studies to test this hypothesis (Weinblatt 1989).

Drug interactions with monoamine oxidase inhibitors

Monoamine oxidase inhibitors (MAOI) are effective antidepressant drugs but are now little used because of their dangerous interactions with food and with other drugs. Nevertheless, some psychiatrists use them regularly and feel that, in the right patient, they are more effective than other antidepressant drugs. MAOI achieve their effect by inhibiting the intraneuronal enzyme monoamine oxidase and, as a result, noradrenaline breakdown in the adrenergic nerve ending is much reduced. This leads to the nerve ending having large stores of noradrenaline ready for release into the synaptic cleft in response to either a neuronal discharge or an indirectly acting amine. The action of the directly acting amine noradrenaline is not affected by MAOI, but the hypertensive effects of adrenaline are potentiated by

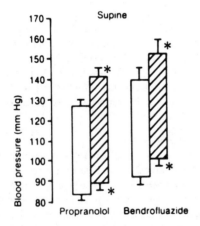
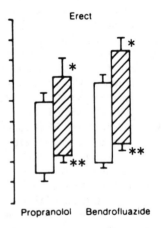

FIG. 33.4

Effect on supine and erect blood pressures of adding either indomethacin (hatched bars) 100 mg daily for 3 weeks, or placebo (open bars) to hypertensive patients receiving treatment with bendrofluazide (n=5) or propranolol (n=8). ★ P<0.05   ★★ P<0.01
(Reproduced with permission of the authors and the editor of the *British Medical Journal* [1980] 281, 702.)

some MAOI (see Chapter 9) to a degree that, while not harmful to healthy patients, may be a hazard to those with cardiovascular disease.

The main indirectly acting amines include amphetamine, tyramine, phenylpropanolamine, and phenylephrine (the latter two also have direct effects on α-receptors). Tyramine is normally present in foodstuffs (e.g. cheese and red wine) and is metabolised in the gut wall to inactive metabolites, so does not enter the bloodstream. The enzyme responsible for this metabolic step, however, is monoamine oxidase and in patients taking MAOI, such as phenelzine or tranylcypromine, the tyramine will be absorbed intact. Amines such as phenylephrine and phenylpropanolamine are present in many cough and cold cures and are readily available over the counter in pharmacies. Thus the ingestion of tyramine (in food) or phenylpropranolamine can lead to a massive release of noradrenaline from adrenergic nerve endings and a syndrome of sympathetic overactivity results with hypertension, headache, excitement, hyperpyrexia, and cardiac arrhythmias (Tollefson 1983). Subarachnoid haemorrhage and death have resulted, and all patients taking MAOI should be instructed explicitly about these problems. Termination of this effect depends upon new enzyme synthesis once the MAOI is stopped, and thus precautions need to continue for 3 weeks after the MAOI has been stopped. The problem is encountered with non-selective MAOI. It does not, however, occur with the more selective (Type B) MAOI, such as selegiline when this drug is given in the doses used for Parkinson's disease (5–10 mg daily), though it has been suspected of having caused tyramine-induced hypertension when given in the larger doses (20 mg daily) sometimes given for depression (McGrath *et al.* 1989).

MAOI also interact with other drugs, such as pethidine and tricyclic antidepressants. The danger of these interactions has been underestimated in recent years. It is now clear that, for the antidepressants at least, the drugs that block noradrenaline reuptake are relatively safe (e.g. imipramine, trimipramine). The danger comes particularly with the use of drugs that selectively block the reuptake of serotonin such as clomipramine and fluoxetine (Lader 1990). The combination of MAOI and inhibitors of serotonin reuptake is potentially lethal. The basis of this pharmacodynamic interaction is thought to be an increase in serotonin levels within the CNS, and is clinically manifest as mental status changes, hyperthermia, rigidity, and autonomic instability. It has been recommended that at least 5 weeks should elapse between the discontinuation of fluoxetine and the initiation of an MAOI (Finley 1994).

TABLE 33.10
Clinically significant interactions with SSRI

SSRI	Interacting drug
Fluoxetine	tricyclic antidepressants
	MAOI
	phenytoin
	haloperidol
	carbamazepine
Fluvoxamine	tricyclic antidepressants
	MAOI
	warfarin
	phenytoin
	theophylline
	clozapine
Paroxetine	tricyclic antidepressants
	MAOI
Sertraline	tricyclic antidepressants
	MAOI

(Adapted from Finley 1994)

Drug interactions with selective serotonin reuptake inhibitors (SSRI)

Selective serotonin reuptake inhibitors are a relatively new class of antidepressants which have been shown to interact with a wide range of drugs. *In vitro* and *in vivo* studies have shown that the basis for the interactions in most cases is their ability to inhibit the P-450 enzymes (Devane 1994; Mitchell 1994; Preskorn and Magnus 1994). It is interesting to note that the different SSRI currently available, despite having similar pharmacological properties and therapeutic efficacy, vary in their ability to inhibit the different P-450 isoforms (Park *et al.* 1995). For example, paroxetine is the most potent SSRI in inhibiting CYP2D6, followed in descending order by fluoxetine, sertraline, and fluvoxamine (Crewe *et al.* 1992). In contrast, fluvoxamine is a more potent inhibitor of CYP1A2 and CYP2C9 than the other SSRI (Devane *et al.* 1997; Schmider *et al.* 1997). Table 33.10 lists the clinically significant interactions that have been reported with the different SSRI. The interaction with tricyclic antidepressants (which are metabolised by CYP2D6) has attracted the most attention (Finley 1994). Fluoxetine has been reported to increase tricyclic concentrations by 350 per cent, and can in some cases precipitate neurotoxicity (Preskorn *et al.* 1994). The combination of tricyclic antidepressants and SSRI should therefore be used with caution, if at all. Of the different SSRI, citalopram is the least likely to inhibit the P-450 enzymes.

Drug interactions with non-sedating antihistamines

Astemizole and terfenadine, both non-sedating antihistamines, have been reported to cause life-threatening cardiac arrhythmias (Rankin 1997). Attention has primarily focused on terfenadine, which is the more widely used. Terfenadine is a pro-drug that is converted to a carboxylic acid metabolite by CYP3A4 (Pirmohamed *et al.* 1994). It cannot normally be detected in the plasma after standard doses, unless its metabolism has been inhibited, as can occur with various drugs including ketoconazole, itraconazole, erythromycin, and clarithromycin (Ament *et al.* 1997). Grapefruit juice also inhibits the metabolism of terfenadine (Benton *et al.* 1996; Honig *et al.* 1996). When any of these drugs are given together with terfenadine, the elevated plasma terfenadine concentration leads to prolongation of the QT interval, which in turn, may lead to the polymorphic ventricular tachycardia termed *torsade de pointes* (Rankin 1997). Both terfenadine and astemizole block the ventricular potassium channels, particularly the rapidly activating component of the delayed rectifier, which increases the duration of the action potential and the QT interval (Salata *et al.* 1995). Because of the risk of arrhythmias with terfenadine, the legal status of the drug has recently been changed, so that it is now only available on prescription in the UK (Rankin 1997). Its active metabolite, fexofenadine, which does not affect potassium channels (Woosley *et al.* 1993), has recently been marketed as a drug in its own right.

Drug interactions with protease inhibitors

The protease inhibitors (saquinavir, ritonavir, indinavir, nelfinavir) are a group of promising new anti-HIV compounds which, by inhibiting the retroviral aspartyl protease, cause the production of immature non-infectious virions, thus interrupting viral spread (Debouck 1992). These drugs are metabolised by P-450 enzymes, in particular CYP3A4, but also, to a lesser extent, CYP2C9 and CYP2D6 (Eagling *et al.* 1997). Their involvement in drug interactions is usually a consequence of either the induction or inhibition of CYP3A4.

Protease inhibitors will often be co-prescribed with drugs known to induce CYP3A4 such as rifampicin (for the treatment of tuberculosis), rifabutin (for the treatment of *Mycobacterium avium* complex), and anticonvulsants. This would be expected to increase the metabolism of the protease inhibitors, reduce their bioavailability, and impair their anti-HIV effect (Barry *et al.* 1997).

Protease inhibitors also act as enzyme inhibitors, with ritonavir being the most potent. This may lead to clinically significant interactions, not only with drugs metabolised by CYP3A4 but also drugs metabolised by other P-450 isoforms. For example, a recent case report demonstrated that saquinavir inhibits CYP3A4-mediated

metabolism of midazolam, resulting in prolonged sedation and respiratory depression (Merry *et al.* 1997*b*). Concomitant administration of ritonavir with rifabutin results not only in the induction of ritonavir metabolism, but also inhibition of rifabutin metabolism, producing a fourfold increase in the area under the rifabutin plasma concentration-time curve (Barry *et al.* 1997). This increases the risk of rifabutin-induced uveitis, so alternative antimycobacterial therapy should be considered in patients taking ritonavir. Inhibition of the metabolism of desipramine (CYP2D6) and tolbutamide (CYP2C9) by ritonavir has also been demonstrated (Kumar *et al.* 1996). Given the necessity for using combination therapy in HIV disease, more than one protease inhibitor may be used simultaneously in some patients. Co-administration of ritonavir with saquinavir in patients with advanced HIV disease produced a 16-fold increase in the peak plasma concentration and a 21-fold increase in the area under the saquinavir plasma concentration–time curve (Merry *et al.* 1997*a*). This is a potentially beneficial interaction, since the increased bioavailability of saquinavir may result in enhanced antiviral activity and allow reduction of its dose. With the likely increase in the use of protease inhibitors over the next few years, it is probable that many new, clinically significant interactions will be reported. Given our knowledge of the pharmacology and metabolism of the protease inhibitors, and that of concomitantly administered drugs, it should be possible to anticipate, and thus avoid or minimize most of the interactions.

Drug interactions with grapefruit juice

Grapefruit juice, when administered with certain drugs, increases their bioavailability, and either enhances their pharmacodynamic effects or leads to toxicity (Ameer and Weintraub 1997). This is because one or more as yet unidentified components of grapefruit juice can inhibit CYP3A4 in the gut, and therefore affect the metabolism of drugs such as cyclosporin, midazolam, and terfenadine (Lown *et al.* 1997). It has in fact been suggested that grapefruit juice could be used to increase the bioavailability of cyclosporin A and allow a reduction in its dose, and thus cut the cost of using this expensive drug (Yee *et al.* 1995).

Drug interactions with digoxin

There are many interactions with digoxin (Rodin and Johnson 1988; Magnani and Malini 1995), which often have both pharmacodynamic and pharmacokinetic elements. Although most are of little clinical significance, there are many which are important, and can be easily avoided. For example, diuretic-induced hypokalaemia, which increases the risk of digoxin-induced cardiotoxicity (Steiness and Olesen 1976), can be avoided by careful monitoring of serum potassium concentration.

The absorption of digoxin is incomplete, and earlier formulations showed marked interindividual variation in absorption. Modern formulations do not have the same problems to any significant degree; thus many of the drugs that have been believed in the past to have reduced the absorption of digoxin can be regarded as of historical interest only. Cholestyramine and, to a lesser extent, colestipol reduce the absorption of digoxin, but these interactions can be easily avoided by giving the two drugs at least 2 hours apart (Rodin and Johnson 1988).

Quinidine raises plasma digoxin concentrations two- to threefold in 90 per cent of patients (Pedersen et al. 1980). The mechanism is complicated, and involves a combination of a decrease in the volume of distribution of digoxin by 40 per cent, and decreases of up to 50 per cent in its renal and 65 per cent in its non-renal clearances (Doering 1979). The interaction is clinically important and leads to adverse effects (especially cardiotoxicity) which are more marked in elderly patients (Walker et al. 1983). In many countries (e.g. the UK), however, quinidine is rarely used as an antiarrhythmic agent and thus the interaction is rarely a problem. Similar interactions have also been reported with other cardiovascular drugs. For example, verapamil can increase plasma digoxin concentrations by as much as 200 per cent by decreasing its renal and non-renal clearances (Johnson et al. 1987). Nifedipine (Hutt et al. 1986), and possibly diltiazem (Rameis et al. 1984), but not the new dihydropyridine calcium-channel blocker amlodipine (Schwartz 1988), can also interact with digoxin.

Amiodarone, which may be co-prescribed with digoxin, can increase digoxin concentration by up to 100 per cent by reducing both renal and non-renal clearances (Oetgen et al. 1984). Toxicity may be avoided by reducing digoxin concentration by 50 per cent prior to starting amiodarone (Magnani and Malini 1995). Flecainide (Weeks et al. 1986) and propafenone (Calvo et al. 1989), class Ic antiarrhythmic agents, also increase serum digoxin concentrations.

Drug interactions with lithium

Thiazide treatment is associated with a reduction of about 25 per cent in lithium clearance (Peterson et al. 1974) and a similar change is seen with loop diuretics (Kerry et al. 1980). During long-term diuretic therapy there is increased proximal tubular excretion of sodium and this increases lithium reabsorption. Serum concentrations of lithium will rise by about 30 per cent, leading to toxicity unless the dose is reduced.

NSAID also interact with lithium, probably by decreasing its renal clearance, with a consequent increase in its plasma concentration. This interaction has been described with several NSAID (Verbeeck 1990), notably indomethacin, ibuprofen (Ragheb et al. 1980), and diclofenac (Reimann and Frölich 1980). If patients taking lithium are given NSAID, then the dose of lithium should be decreased by 25 per cent and its plasma concentration monitored.

Drug interactions between anticancer drugs

Combination therapy with anticancer drugs is very common, so interactions are to be expected. This is a specialized field and the reader is referred to the review by Balis (1986) for further information. We have already noted the problems that may arise when allopurinol is given to patients on azathioprine or mercaptopurine (Bacon et al. 1981), and the reduced renal clearance of methotrexate caused by NSAID (Thyss et al. 1986). Both interactions are potentially very harmful.

Beneficial drug interactions

Drugs are often given together for their beneficial effect in combination. We have come across a number of such examples so far, including probenecid with penicillin or with indomethacin, and levodopa with carbidopa (a peripheral decarboxylase inhibitor). In general, the combination of drugs in the treatment of hypertension is additive rather than synergistic (Lam and Shepherd 1990). Other examples of beneficial interactions are shown in Table 33.11.

Over the last 5 years or so, the concept of using P-450 enzyme inhibitors to prevent drug toxicity has been suggested. This requires that a drug should cause toxicity through its metabolite, the formation of which is catalysed by a biochemically and pharmacologically characterized enzyme for which an enzyme inhibitor is available. The best example is the concomitant administration of cimetidine with dapsone. The hydroxylamine metabolite of the latter causes methaemoglobinaemia; studies in volunteers (Coleman et al. 1990) and in patients with dermatitis herpetiformis (Coleman et al. 1992; Rhodes et al. 1995) have shown that concomitant administration of cimetidine decreases methaemoglobinaemia and thus increases the tolerability of dapsone. The use of disulfiram, a CYP2E1 inhibitor (Table 33.4) before halothane anaesthesia has also been suggested as a way of preventing halothane hepatitis (Kharasch et al. 1996).

TABLE 33.11
Examples of beneficial interactions

Salbutamol with theophylline
β-Adrenoceptor antagonists with antianginal and antihypertensive drugs
Levodopa with decarboxylase inhibitors
Levodopa/decarboxylase inhibitors with anticholinergic drugs
Sulphonylureas with biguanides
Thrombolytic drugs with aspirin
Heparin with aspirin
Opioid analgesics with phenothiazines
Thiazide or loop diuretics with potassium-sparing diuretics
Cimetidine with dapsone

Conclusions

Drug interactions are an important facet of therapy and as we have seen they can lead either to loss of the therapeutic effect or to adverse effects. Some generalizations are possible. First, a knowledge of the mechanism involved allows us to understand the interaction and, one hopes, anticipate similar problems in the future when new but similar drugs appear on the market. Secondly, there are certain areas of drug therapy in which interactions are more likely, either because of the nature of the drugs (e.g. cytotoxic drugs) or because the drug has a low therapeutic index (Table 33.1). Thirdly, certain patients are more susceptible to adverse drug interactions and the reasons for this have been discussed. A consideration of these points should make adverse drug interactions less likely.

References

Abernethy, D.R., Greenblatt, D.J., Divoll, M., *et al.* (1982). Impairment of diazepam metabolism by low dose estrogen-containing oral contraceptive steroids. *N. Engl. J. Med.* 306, 791.

Adams, W.L. (1995). Potential for adverse drug-alcohol interactions among retirement community residents. *J. Am. Geriatr. Soc.* 43, 1021.

Ameer, B. and Weintraub, R.A. (1997). Drug interactions with grapefruit juice. *Clin. Pharmacokinet.* 33, 103.

Ament, P.W. and Paterson, A. (1997). Drug interactions with the nonsedating antihistamines. *American Family Physician* 56, 223.

Baber, N.S., Halliday, L., Sibeon, R.G., *et al.* (1978). The interaction between indomethacin and probenecid. A clinical and pharmacokinetic study. *Clin. Pharmacol. Ther.* 24, 298.

Back, D.J. and Orme, M.L'E. (1990). Pharmacokinetic drug interactions with oral contraceptives. *Clin. Pharmacokinet.* 18, 472.

Back, D.J., Breckenridge, A.M., Crawford, F.E., *et al.* (1979). The effect of rifampicin on norethisterone pharmacokinetics. *Eur. J. Clin. Pharmacol.* 15, 193.

Back, D.J., Breckenridge, A.M., Crawford, F.E., *et al.* (1980*a*). The effect of rifampicin on the pharmacokinetics of ethinyloestradiol in women. *Contraception* 21, 135.

Back, D.J., Bates, M., Bowden, A., *et al.* (1980*b*). The interaction of phenobarbital and other anticonvulsants with oral contraceptive steroid therapy. *Contraception* 22, 495.

Back, D.J., Breckenridge, A.M., MacIver, M., *et al.* (1982). The effects of ampicillin on oral contraceptive steroids in women. *Br. J. Clin. Pharmacol.* 14, 43.

Back, D.J., Grimmer, S.F.M., Orme, M.L'E., *et al.* (1988). Evaluation of Committee on Safety of Medicines Yellow Card reports on oral contraceptive-drug interactions. *Br. J. Clin. Pharmacol.* 25, 527.

Bacon, B.R., Treuhaft, W.H., and Goodman, A.M. (1981). Azathioprine-induced pancytopenia. *Arch. Intern. Med.* 141, 223.

Balis, F.M. (1986). Pharmacokinetic drug interactions of commonly used anticancer drugs. *Clin. Pharmacokinet.* 11, 223.

Banda, P.W. and Quart, B.D. (1982). The effect of mild alcohol consumption on metabolism of acetaminophen in man. *Res. Commun. Chem. Pathol. Pharmacol.* 38, 57.

Barry, M., Gibbons, S., Back, D., *et al.* (1997). Protease inhibitors in patients with HIV disease — Clinically important pharmacokinetic considerations. *Clin. Pharmacokinet.* 32, 194.

Bateman, D.N. (1986). The action of cisapride on gastric-emptying and the pharmacodynamics and pharmacokinetics of oral diazepam. *Eur. J. Clin. Pharmacol.* 30, 205.

Bayard, P.J., Berger, T.G., and Jacobson, M.A. (1992). Drug hypersensitivity reactions and human immunodeficiency virus disease. *J. Acquir. Immune Defic. Syndr.* 5, 1237.

BCDSP (Boston Collaborative Drug Surveillance Program) (1972). Adverse Drug Interactions, *JAMA* 220, 1238.

Beers, M.H., Storrie, M., and Lee, G. (1990). Potential adverse drug interactions in the emergency room. *Ann. Intern. Med.* 112, 61.

Benton, R.E., Honig, P.K., Zamani, K., *et al.* (1996). Grapefruit juice alters terfenadine pharmacokinetics resulting in prolongation of repolarization on the electrocardiogram. *Clin. Pharmacol. Ther.* 59, 383.

Black, M. and Raucy, J. (1986). Acetaminophen, alcohol, and cytochrome P-450. *Ann. Intern. Med.* 104, 427.

Blaschke, T.F., Cohen, S.N., and Tatro, D.S. (1981). Drug–drug interactions and aging. In *Clinical Pharmacology in the Aged Patient* (ed. L.F. Jarvik, D.J. Greenblatt, and D.D. Harman), p. 11. Raven Press, New York.

Boldy, D.A.R., Heath, A., Ruddock, S., *et al.* (1987). Activated-charcoal for carbamazepine poisoning. *Lancet* i, 1027.

Boobis, A.R. and Davies, D.S. (1984). Human cytochromes P-450. *Xenobiotica* 14, 151.

Borda, I.T., Sloane, D., and Jick, H. (1968). Assessment of adverse reactions within a drug surveillance program. *JAMA* 205, 645.

Branigan, T.A., Robbins, R.A., Cady, W.J., *et al.* (1981). The effects of erythromycin on the absorption and disposition kinetics of theophylline. *Eur. J. Clin. Pharmacol.* 21, 115.

Bray, G.P. (1993). Liver failure induced by paracetamol. *BMJ* 306, 157.

Bray, G.P., Mowat, C., Muir, D.F., *et al.* (1991). The effect of chronic alcohol intake on prognosis and outcome in paracetamol overdose. *Hum. Exp. Toxicol.* 10, 435.

Bray, G.P., Harrison, P.M., O'Grady, J.G., *et al.* (1992). Long-term anticonvulsant therapy worsens outcome in paracetamol-induced fulminant hepatic failure. *Hum. Exp. Toxicol.* 11, 265.

Breckenridge, A.M., Back, D.J., and Orme, M.L'E. (1979). Interactions between oral contraceptives and other drugs. *Pharmacol. Ther.* 7, 617.

Breen, K.J., Bury, R., Desmond, P.V., *et al.* (1982). Effects of cimetidine and ranitidine on hepatic drug metabolism. *Clin. Pharmacol. Ther.* 31, 297.

Brodie, M.J. and Feely, J. (1988). Adverse drug interactions. *BMJ* 296, 845.

Brodie, M.J. and MacPhee, G.J.A. (1986). Carbamazepine neurotoxicity precipitated by diltiazem. *BMJ* 292, 1170.

Bronsen, K. (1990). Recent developments in hepatic drug oxidation: Implications for clinical pharmacokinetics. *Clin. Pharmacokinet.* 18, 220.

Brooks, P.M., Buchanan, W.W., Grove, M., *et al.* (1976). Effects of enzyme-induction on metabolism of prednisolone: clinical and laboratory study. *Ann. Rheum. Dis.* 35, 339.

Brooks, S.M., Werk, E.E., Ackerman, S.J., *et al.* (1972). Adverse effects of phenobarbital on corticosteroid metabolism in patients with bronchial asthma. *N. Engl. J. Med.* 286, 1125.

Brouwers, J.R.B. and de Smet, P.A.G. (1994). Pharmacokinetic-pharmacodynamic drug interactions with nonsteroidal antiinflammatory drugs. *Clin. Pharmacokinet.* 27, 462.

Calvo, M.V., Martinsuarez, A., Luengo, C.M., *et al.* (1989). Interaction between digoxin and propafenone. *Therapeutic Drug Monitoring* 11, 10.

Canafax, D.M. and Ascher, N.I. (1983). Cyclosporine immunosuppression. *Clin. Pharm.* 2, 515.

Chapman, C.R. (1981). *Absorption and Metabolism of Steroid Prodrugs.* Ph.D. thesis, University of Liverpool.

Cheng, S.H. and White, A. (1962). Effect of orally administered neomycin on the absorption of penicillin V. *N. Engl. J. Med.* 267, 1296.

Coleman, M.D., Scott, A.K., Breckenridge, A.M., *et al.* (1990). The use of cimetidine as a selective inhibitor of dapsone *N*-hydroxylation in man. *Br. J. Clin. Pharmacol.* 30, 761.

Coleman, M.D., Rhodes, L.E., Scott, A.K., *et al.* (1992). The use of cimetidine to reduce dose-dependent methaemoglobinaemia in dermatitis herpetiformis patients. *Br. J. Clin. Pharmacol.* 34, 244.

Coulam, C.B. and Annegers, J.F. (1979). Do anticonvulsants reduce the efficacy of oral contraceptives? *Epilepsia* 20, 519.

Crawford, P., Chadwick, D., Cleland, J., *et al.* (1986). The lack of effect of sodium valproate on the pharmacokinetics of oral contraceptive steroids. *Contraception* 33, 23.

Crawford, P., Chadwick, D., Martin, C., *et al.* (1990). The interaction of phenytoin and carbamazepine with oral contraceptive steroids. *Br. J. Clin. Pharmacol.* 30, 892.

Crewe, H.K., Lennard, M.S., Tucker, G.T., *et al.* (1992). The effect of selective serotonin reuptake inhibitors on cytochrome-P4502D6 (CYP2D6) activity in human liver microsomes. *Br. J. Clin. Pharmacol.* 34, 262.

Crooks, J. and Moir, D.C. (1974). The detection of drug interaction in a hospital environment. In *Clinical Effects of Interaction between Drugs* (ed. L.E. Cluff and J.C. Petrie), p. 255. Excerpta Medica, Amsterdam.

D'Arcy P.F. (1982). Drug reactions and interactions in the elderly patient. *Drug. Intell. Clin. Pharm.* 16, 925.

Davidson, N. McD., Corral, R.J.M., Shaw, T.D.R., *et al.* (1976). Observations in man of hypoglycaemia during selective and non-selective beta blockade. *Scot. Med. J.* 22, 69.

Debouck, C. (1992). The HIV-1 protease as a therapeutic target for AIDS. *AIDS Res. Hum. Retroviruses* 8, 153.

Deray, G., Le Hoang, P., Cacoub, P., *et al.* (1987). Oral contraceptive interaction with cyclosporin. *Lancet* ii, 158.

Desmond, P.V., Patwardhan, R.V., Schenker, S., *et al.* (1980). Short-term ethanol administration impairs the elimination of chlordiazepoxide in man. *Eur. J. Clin. Pharmacol.* 18, 275.

Devane, C.L. (1994). Pharmacokinetics of the newer antidepressants — clinical relevance. *Am. J. Med.* 97, S13.

Devane, C.L., Markowitz, J.S., Hardesty, S.J., *et al.* (1997). Fluvoxamine-induced theophylline toxicity. *Am. J. Psychiatry* 154, 1317.

Doering, W. (1979). Quinidine-digoxin interaction: pharmacokinetics, underlying mechanism and clinical implications. *N. Engl. J. Med.* 301, 400.

Doll, R., Langman, M.J.S., and Shawdon, H.H. (1968). Treatment of gastric ulcer with carbenoxolone — antagonistic effect of spironolactone. *Gut* 9, 42.

Durao, V., Prata, M.M., and Goncalves, L.M.P. (1977). Modification of antihypertensive effect of beta-adrenoceptor blocking agents by inhibition of endogenous prostaglandin synthesis. *Lancet* ii, 1005.

Eagling, V.A., Back, D.J., and Barry, M.G. (1997). Differential inhibition of cytochrome P450 isoforms by the protease inhibitors, ritonavir, saquinavir and indinavir. *Br. J. Clin. Pharmacol.* 44, 190.

Edwards, D.M., Courtenay-Evans, R.J., Galley, J.M., *et al.* (1974). Changes in cortisol metabolism following rifampicin therapy. *Lancet* ii, 549.

Favre, L., Glasson, Ph., Riondel, A., *et al.* (1983). Interaction of diuretics and non-steroidal anti-inflammatory drugs in man. *Clin. Sci.* 64, 407.

Ferguson, R.M., Sutherland, D.E.R., Simmons, R.L., *et al.* (1982). Ketoconazole, cyclosporin metabolism and renal transplantation. *Lancet* ii, 882.

Figa, F.H., Gow, R.M., Hamilton, R.M., *et al.* (1994). Clinical efficacy and safety of intravenous amiodarone in infants and children. *Am. J. Cardiol.* 74, 573.

Finley, P.R. (1994). Selective serotonin reuptake inhibitors — pharmacological profiles and potential therapeutic distinctions. *Ann. Pharmacother.* 28, 1359.

First, M.R., Schroeder, T.J., Weiskittel, P., *et al.* (1989). Concomitant administration of cyclosporin and ketoconazole in renal-transplant recipients. *Lancet* ii, 1198.

Fincham, R.W. and Schottelius, D.D. (1979). Decreased phenytoin levels in antineoplastic therapy. *Ther. Drug Monit.* 1, 277.

Fraser, A.G. (1997). Pharmacokinetic interactions between alcohol and other drugs. *Clin. Pharmacokinet.* 33, 79.

Freedman, M.D. and Olatidoye, A.G. (1994). Clinically significant drug-interactions with the oral anticoagulants. *Drug Saf.* 10, 381.

Freeman, D.J., Laupacis, A., Keown, P.A., *et al.* (1984). Evaluation of cyclosporin-phenytoin interaction with observations on cyclosporin metabolites. *Br. J. Clin. Pharmacol.* 18, 887.

Freis, E.D. (1984). Veterans administration cooperative study on nadolol as monotherapy and in combination with a diuretic. *Am. Heart J.* 108, 1087.

Friedman, C.I., Huneke, A.L., Kim, M.H., *et al.* (1980). The effect of ampicillin on oral contraceptive effectiveness. *Obstet. Gynecol.* 55, 33.

Garattini, S. (1985). Active drug metabolites. An overview. *Clin. Pharmacokinet.* 10, 216.

Gelipter, D. and Hazell, M. (1980). Interaction between disopyramide and practolol. *BMJ* 280, 52.

Gerber, M.C., Tejwani, G.A., Gerber, N., *et al.* (1985). Drug interactions with cimetidine: an update. *Pharmacol. Ther.* 27, 353.

Gerhardt, R.E., Knouss, R.F., and Thyrum, P.T. (1969). Quinidine excretion in aciduria and alkaluria. *Ann. Intern. Med.* 71, 927.

Goldstein, J.A. and Demorais, S.M.F. (1994). Biochemistry and molecular-biology of the human CYP2C subfamily. *Pharmacogenetics* 4, 285.

Gothioni, G., Neuvonen, P.J., Mattila, M., *et al.* (1972). Iron-tetracycline interaction: Effect of time interval between the drugs. *Acta Med. Scand.* 191, 409.

Graham, C.F., Turner, W.N., and Jones, J.K. (1981). Lidocaine-propranolol interactions. *N. Engl. J. Med.* 304, 1301.

Greenblatt, D.J. and Koch-Weser, J. (1973). Adverse reactions to spironolactone: a report from the Boston Collaborative Drug Surveillance Program. *Clin. Pharmacol. Ther.* 14, 136.

Greiff, J.M.C. and Rowbotham, D. (1994). Pharmacokinetic drug-interactions with gastrointestinal motility modifying agents. *Clin. Pharmacokinet.* 27, 447.

Grimmer, M., Allen, W.L., Back, D.J., *et al.* (1983). The effect of cotrimoxazole on oral contraceptive steroids in women. *Contraception* 28, 53.

Grimmer, S.F.M., Back, D.J., Orme, M.L'E., *et al.* (1986). The bioavailability of ethinyloestradiol and levonorgestrel in patients with an ileostomy. *Contraception* 33, 51.

Guengerich, F.R. (1988). Oxidation of 17α-ethinyl-estradiol by human liver cytochrome P450. *Molec. Pharmacol.* 33, 500.

Gugler, R. and Allgayer, H. (1990). Effect of antacids on the clinical pharmacokinetics of drugs. An update. *Clin. Pharmacokinet.* 18, 210.

Haque, N., Thrasher, K., Werk, E.E., *et al.* (1972). Studies on dexamethasone metabolism in man: Effect of diphenylhydantoin. *J. Clin. Endocrinol. Metab.* 34, 44.

Harder, S. and Thurmann, P. (1996). Clinically important drug-interactions with anticoagulants — an update. *Clin. Pharmacokinet.* 30, 416.

Hauser, A.R., Lee, C., Teague, R.B., *et al.* (1983). The effect of rifampicin on theophylline disposition. *Clin. Pharmacol. Ther.* 33, 254.

Heel, R.C., Brogden, R.N., Speight, T.M., *et al.* (1980). Captopril — a preliminary review of its pharmacological properties and therapeutic efficacy. *Drugs* 20, 409.

Heubel, F. and Netter, K.F. (1979). Atypical inducing properties of rifampicin. *Biochem. Pharmacol.* 28, 3373.

Höffken, G., Borner, K., Glatzel, P.D., *et al.* (1985). Reduced enteral absorption of ciprofloxacin in the presence of antacids. *Eur. J. Clin. Microbiol.* 33, 345.

Honig, P.K. and Gillespie, B.K. (1995). Drug-interactions between prescribed and over-the-counter medication. *Drug Saf.* 13, 296.

Honig, P.K., Wortham, D.C., Lazarev, A., *et al.* (1996). Grapefruit juice alters the systemic bioavailability and cardiac repolarization of terfenadine in poor metabolizers of terfenadine. *J. Clin. Pharmacol.* 36, 345.

Hoyumpa, A.M., Patwardhan, R.V., Schenker, S., *et al.* (1981). Effect of short-term ethanol administration on lorazepam clearance. *Hepatology* 1, 47.

Hunt, S.N., Jusko, W.J., and Yurchak, A.M. (1976). Effect of smoking on theophylline disposition. *Clin. Pharmacol. Ther.* 19, 546.

Hutt, H.J., Kirch, W., Dylewicz, P., *et al.* (1986). Dose-dependence of the nifedipine digoxin interaction. *Arch. Toxicol.* S9, 209.

Jackson, J.E., Powell, J.R., Wandell, M., *et al.* (1981). Cimetidine decreases theophylline clearance. *Am. Rev. Respir. Dis.* 123, 615.

Jain, A., McMahon, F.G., Slattery, J.T., *et al.* (1979). Effect of naproxen on steady-state serum concentration and anticoagulant activity of warfarin. *Clin. Pharmacol. Ther.* 25, 61.

Johnson, B.F., Wilson, J., Marwaha, R., *et al.* (1987). The comparative effects of verapamil and a new dihydropyridine calcium channel blocker on digoxin pharmacokinetics. *Clin. Pharmacol. Ther.* 42, 66.

Jones, T.E., Morris, R.G., and Mathew, T.H. (1997). Diltiazem-cyclosporin pharmacokinetic interaction — dose–response relationship. *Br. J. Clin. Pharmacol.* 44, 499.

Jonkman, J.H.G. and Upton, R.A. (1984). Pharmacokinetic drug interactions with theophylline. *Clin. Pharmacokinet.* 9, 309.

Joshi, J.V., Joshi, U.M., Sankhali, G.M., *et al.* (1980). A study of the interaction of low dose combination oral contraceptive with ampicillin and metronidazole. *Contraception* 22, 643-652.

Jung, W., Mlezko, R., Manz, M., *et al.* (1993). Efficacy and safety of combination therapy with amiodarone and type I agents for treatment of inducible ventricular tachycardia. *PACE* 16, 778.

Kampmann, J., Hansen, J.M., Siersbaek-Nielsen, K., *et al.* (1972). Effect of some drugs on penicillin half life in blood. *Clin. Pharmacol. Ther.* 13, 516.

Kaneko, S., Otani, K., Fukushima, Y., *et al.* (1988). Teratogenicity of antiepileptic drugs: analysis of possible risk factors. *Epilepsia* 29, 459.

Kauffman, R.E. and Azarnoff, D.L. (1973). Effect of colestipol on gastrointestinal absorption of chlorothiazide in man. *Clin. Pharmacol. Ther.* 14, 886.

Kerr, B.M., Rettie, A.E., Eddy, C., *et al.* (1989). Inhibition of human liver microsomal epoxide hydrolase by valproate and valpromide: *in vitro/in vivo* correlation. *Clin. Pharmacol. Ther.* 46, 82.

Kerry, R.J., Ludlow, J.M., and Owen, G. (1980). Diuretics are dangerous with lithium. *BMJ* 281, 371.

Kharasch, E.D., Hankins, D., Mautz, D., *et al.* (1996). Identification of the enzyme responsible for oxidative halothane metabolism — implications for prevention of halothane hepatitis. *Lancet* 347, 1367.

Kirch, W., Hoensch, H., and Janisch, H.D. (1984). Interactions and non-interactions with ranitidine. *Clin. Pharmacokinet.* 9, 493.

Koch-Weser, J. (1973). Drug interactions in cardiovascular therapy. *Am. Heart J.* 90, 93.

Koch-Weser, J. and Sellers, E.M. (1971). Drug interactions with coumarin anticoagulants. *N. Engl. J. Med.* 285, 487, 547.

Krikler, D.M. and Spurrell, R.A.J. (1974). Verapamil in the treatment of paroxysmal supraventricular tachycardia. *Postgrad. Med. J.* 50, 447.

Krzywanek, H.J. and Breddin, K. (1977). Beeinflusst Diclofenac die orale Antikoagulantinstherapie und die Plätchenaggregation?.;'. *Medizin. Welt.* 28, 1843.

Kuhlmann, J., Woodcock, B., Wilke, J., *et al.* (1985). Verapamil plasma concentrations during treatment with cytostatic drugs. *J. Cardiovasc. Pharmacol.* 7, 1003.

Kumar, G.N., Rodrigues, A.D., Buko, A.M., *et al.* (1996). Cytochrome P450-mediated metabolism of the HIV-1 protease inhibitor ritonavir (ABT-538) in human liver microsomes. *J. Pharmacol. Exper. Ther.* 277, 423.

Kutt, H. (1971). Biochemical and genetic factors regulating dilantin metabolism in man. *Ann. N.Y. Acad. Sci.* 179, 704.

Lader, M.H. (1990). Interactions that matter — monoamine oxidase inhibitors. *Prescribers' Journal* 30, 48.

Lam, Y.W.F. and Shepherd, A.M.M. (1990). Drug interactions in hypertensive patients. Pharmacokinetic, pharmacodynamic and genetic considerations. *Clin. Pharmacokinet.* 18, 295.

Landay, R.A., Gonzalez, M.A., and Taylor, J.C. (1978). Effect of phenobarbital on theophylline disposition. *J. Allergy Clin. Immunol.* 62, 27.

Law, R. and Chalmers, C. (1976). Medicines and elderly people. A general practice survey. *BMJ* i, 565.

Lesko, L.J. (1989). Pharmacokinetic drug interactions with amiodarone. *Clin. Pharmacokinet.* 17, 130.

Lewis, R.J., Trager, W.F., Chan, K.K., *et al.* (1974). Warfarin. Stereochemical aspects of its metabolism and the interaction with phenylbutazone. *J. Clin. Invest.* 53, 1607.

Lode, H. (1988). Drug interactions with quinolones. *Rev. Infect. Dis.* 10 (Suppl. 1), 132.

Lown, K.S., Bailey, D.G., Fontana, R.J., *et al.* (1997). Grapefruit juice increases felodipine oral availability in humans by decreasing intestinal CYP3A protein expression. *J. Clin. Invest.* 99, 2545.

McElnay, J.C. and D'Arcy, P.F. (1983). Protein binding displacement interactions and their clinical importance. *Drugs* 25, 495.

McGrath, P.J., Stewart, J.W., and Quitkin, F.M. (1989). A possible L-deprenyl-induced hypertension reaction. *J. Psychopharmacol.* 9, 110.

McInnes, G.T. and Brodie, M.J. (1988). Drug interactions that matter. A critical reappraisal. *Drugs* 36, 83.

McInnes, G.T. and Ramsay, L.E. (1987). Pharmacology and clinical use of antimineralocorticoids. In *Pharmacology and Clinical Uses of Inhibitors of Hormone Secretion and Action* (ed. M. Furr and A. Wakeling), p. 233. Baillière Tindall, London.

MacKichan, J.J. (1989). Protein binding drug displacement interactions: fact or fiction. *Clin. Pharmacokinet.* 16, 65.

Macleod, S.M. and Sellers, E.M. (1976). Pharmacodynamic and pharmacokinetic drug interactions with coumarin anticoagulants. *Drugs* 11, 461.

MacPhee, G.J.A., McInnes, G.T., Thompson, G.G., *et al.* (1986). Verapamil potentiates carbamazepine neurotoxicity: a clinically important inhibitory interaction. *Lancet* i, 700.

MacPhee, G.J.A., Mitchell, J.R., Wiseman, L., *et al.* (1988). Effect of sodium valproate on carbamazepine disposition and psychomotor profile in man. *Br. J. Clin. Pharmacol.* 25, 59.

Maesen, F.P., Teengs, J.P., Baur, C., *et al.* (1984). Quinolones and raisd plasma concentrations of theophylline. *Lancet*, ii, 530.

Magnani, B. and Malini, P.L. (1995). Cardiac glycosides — drug interactions of clinical significance. *Drug Saf.* 12, 97.

Mäntylä, R., Männistö, P.T., Vuorela, A., *et al.* (1984). Impairment of captopril bioavailability by concomitant food and antacid intake. *Int. J. Clin. Pharm. Ther. Toxicol.* 33, 626.

Marquis, J-F., Carruthers, S.G., Spence, J.D., *et al.* (1982). Phenytoin–theophylline interactions. *N. Engl. J. Med.* 307, 1189.

May, D.C., Jarboe, C.H., Ellenburg, D.T., *et al.* (1982). The effects of erythromycin on theophylline elimination in normal males. *J. Clin. Pharmacol* 22, 125.

May, J.R., DiPiro, J.T., and Sisley, J.F. (1987). Drug interactions in surgical patients. *Am. J. Surg.* 153, 327.

Merry, C., Barry, M.G., Mulcahy, F., *et al.* (1997a). Saquinavir pharmacokinetics alone and in combination with ritonavir in HIV-infected patients. *AIDS* 11, F29.

Merry, C., Mulcahy, F., Barry, M., *et al.* (1997b). Saquinavir interaction with midazolam: Pharmacokinetic considerations when prescribing protease inhibitors for patients with HIV disease. *AIDS* 11, 268.

Miners, J.O. (1989). Drug interactions involving aspirin (acetylsalicylic acid) and salicylic acid. *Clin. Pharmacokinet.* 17, 327.

Mitchell, P.B. (1994). Selective serotonin reuptake inhibitors — adverse-effects, toxicity and interactions. *Adverse Drug React. Toxicol. Rev.* 13, 121.

Morgan, T. and Anderson, A. (1993). Interaction of indomethacin with felodipine and enalapril. *J. Hypertens.* 11, S338.

Nation, R.L., Evans, A.M., and Milne, R.W. (1990). Pharmacokinetic drug interactions with phenytoin. *Clin. Pharmacokinet.* 18, 37, and 131.

Nebert, D.W., Nelson, D.R., Adesnik, M., *et al.* (1989). The P450 gene superfamily. Update on the naming of new genes and nomenclature of chromosomal loci. *DNA* 8, 1.

Nebert, D.W., Nelson, D.R., Coon, M.J., *et al.* (1991). The P450 superfamily: update on new sequences, gene mapping, and recommended nomenclature. *DNA Cell Biol.* 10, 1.

Nelson, D.R., Kamataki, T., Waxman, D.J., *et al.* (1993). The P450 superfamily — update on new sequences, gene-mapping, accession numbers, early trivial names of enzymes, and nomenclature. *DNA Cell Biol.* 12, 1.

Nelson, D.R., Koymans, L., Kamataki, T., *et al.* (1996). P450 superfamily: update of new sequences, gene mapping, accession numbers and nomenclature. *Pharmacogenetics* 6, 1.

Nemeroff, C.B., Devane, C.L., and Pollock, B.G. (1996). Newer antidepressants and the cytochrome P450 system. *Am. J. Psychiatry* 153, 311.

Neuvonen, P.J. (1976). Interactions with the absorption of tetracyclines. *Drugs* 11, 45.

Neuvonen, P.J. and Elonen, E. (1980). Effect of activated charcoal on absorption and elimination of phenobarbitone, carbamazepine and phenylbutazone in man. *Eur. J. Clin. Pharmacol.* 17, 51.

Nimmo, J., Heading, R.C., Tothill, P., *et al.* (1973). Pharmacological evaluation of gastric emptying: Effects of propantheline and metoclopramide on paracetamol absorption. *BMJ* i, 587.

Nimmo, W.S. (1976). Drugs, disease and gastric emptying. *Clin. Pharmacokinet.* 1, 189.

Nordoy, S. (1959). Combined treatment with phenylbutazone and anticoagulants. *Tidskr. Nor. Laegefor.* 79, 143.

Northcutt, R.C., Stiel, J.N., Hollifield, J.W., *et al.* (1969). The influence of cholestyramine on thyroxine absorption. *JAMA* 208, 1857.

Oesch, F., Arand, M., Benedetti, M.S., *et al.* (1996). Inducing properties of rifampicin and rifabutin for selected enzyme-activities of the cytochrome-P-450 and UDP-glucuronosyltransferase superfamilies in female rat-liver. *J. Antimicrob. Chemother.* 37, 1111.

Oetgen, W.J., Sobol, S.M., Tri, T.B., *et al.* (1984). Amiodarone–digoxin interaction. Clinical and experimental observations. *Chest* 86, 79.

O'Reilly, R.A. (1984). Comparative interaction of cimetidine and ranitidine with racemic warfarin in man. *Arch. Intern. Med.* 144, 989.

O'Reilly, R.A., Trager, W.F., Rettie, A.E., *et al.* (1987). Interaction of amiodarone with racemic warfarin and its separated enantiomorphs in humans. *Clin. Pharmacol. Ther.* 42, 290.

Orme, M.L'E. (1986). Drug interactions. In *Therapeutics in Rheumatology* (ed. J.M.H. Moll, H.A. Bird, and A. Rushton), p. 87. Chapman and Hall, London.

Orme, M.L'E. and Back, D.J. (1986). Interactions between oral contraceptive steroids and broad spectrum antibiotics. *Clin. Exp. Dermatol.* 11, 327.

Orme, M., Back, D.J., and Breckenridge, A.M. (1983). Clinical pharmacokinetics of oral contraceptive steroids. *Clin. Pharmacokinet.* 8, 95.

Park, B.K. and Breckenridge, A.M. (1981). Clinical implications of enzyme induction and enzyme inhibition. *Clin. Pharmacokinet.* 6, 1.

Park, B.K., Pirmohamed, M., and Kitteringham, N.R. (1995). The role of cytochrome P450 enzymes in hepatic and extrahepatic human drug toxicity. *Pharmacol. Ther.* 68, 385.

Park, B.K., Kitteringham, N.R., Pirmohamed, M., *et al.* (1996). Relevance of induction of human drug-metabolizing enzymes: pharmacological and toxicological implications. *Br. J. Clin. Pharmacol.* 41, 477.

Parsons, R.L. and Paddock, G.M. (1975). Absorption of two antibacterial drugs, cephalexin and cotrimoxazole, in malabsorption syndromes. *J. Antimicrob. Chemother.* 1 (Suppl.), 59.

Patak, R.V., Mookerjee, B.K., Bentzel, C.J., *et al.*. (1975). Antagonism of the effects of furosemide by indomethacin in normal and hypertensive man. *Prostaglandins* 10, 649.

Paulet, N., Bury, P.C., Needleman, M., *et al.* (1982). Drug interactions. A study and evaluation of their incidence in Victoria. *Med. J. Aust.* 1, 80.

Pedersen, K.E., Hastrup, J. and Hvidt, S. (1980). The effect of quinidine on digoxin kinetics in cardiac patients. *Acta Med. Scand.* 207, 291.

Pedrinelli, R., Magagni, A., Arzilli, F., *et al.* (1980). Influence of indomethacin on the natriuretic and renin-stimulating effect of bumetanide in essential hypertension. *Clin. Pharmacol. Ther.* 28, 722.

Petereit, L.B. and Meikle, A.W. (1977). Effectiveness of prednisolone during phenytoin therapy. *Clin. Pharmacol. Ther.* 22, 912.

Peterson, V., Hvidt, S., Thomsen, K., *et al.* (1974). Effect of prolonged thiazide treatment on renal lithium clearance. *BMJ* iii, 143.

Pirmohamed, M., Kitteringham, N.R., and Park, B.K. (1994). The role of active metabolites in drug toxicity. *Drug Saf.* 11, 114.

Polk, R.E., Healy, D.P., Sahai, J., *et al.* (1989). Effect of ferrous sulfate and multivitamins with zinc on absorption of ciprofloxacin in normal volunteers. *Antimicrob. Agents Chemother.* 33, 1841.

Pond, S.M., Olson, K.R., Osterloh, J.D., *et al.* (1984). Randomized study of the treatment of phenobarbital overdose with repeated doses of activated-charcoal. *JAMA* 251, 3104.

Prescott, L.F. (1973). Clinically important drug interactions. *Drugs* 5, 161.

Preskorn, S.H. and Magnus, R.D. (1994). Inhibition of hepatic P-450 isoenzymes by serotonin selective reuptake inhibitors

— *in vitro* and *in vivo* findings and their implications for patient-care. *Psychopharmacology Bull.* 30, 251.

Preskorn, S.H., Alderman, J., Chung, M., *et al.* (1994). Pharmacokinetics of desipramine coadministered with sertraline or fluoxetine. *J. Clin. Psychopharmacol.* 14, 90.

Ptachcinski, R.J., Carpenter, B.J., Burckart, G.J., *et al.* (1985). Effect of erythromycin on cyclosporin levels. *N. Engl. J. Med.* 313, 1416.

Ragheb, M., Ban, T.A., Buchanan, D., *et al.* (1980). Interaction of indomethacin and ibuprofen with lithium in manic patients under a steady state lithium level. *J. Clin. Psychiatry* 41, 397.

Rameis, H., Magometschnigg, D., and Ganzinger, U. (1984). The diltiazem–digoxin interaction. *Clin. Pharmacol. Ther.* 36, 183.

Rankin, A.C. (1997). Non-sedating antihistamines and cardiac arrhythmia. *Lancet* 350, 1115.

Rau, S.E., Bend, J.R., Arnold, J.M.O., *et al.* (1997). Grapefruit juice terfenadine single-dose interaction: Magnitude, mechanism, and relevance. *Clin. Pharmacol. Ther.* 61, 401.

Reimann, I.W. and Frölich, J.C. (1980). Effect of diclofenac on lithium kinetics. *Clin. Pharmacol. Ther.* 30, 348.

Reimers, D. and Jezek, A. (1971). Rifampicin und andere Antituberkulostatika bei gleichzeitiger oraler Kontrazeption. *Prax. Klin. Pneumonol.* 25, 255.

Reveno, W.S. and Rosenbaum, H. (1968). Propranolol and hypoglycaemia. *Lancet* i, 920.

Rhodes, L.E., Tingle, M.D., Park, B.K., *et al.* (1995). Cimetidine improves the therapeutic toxic ratio of dapsone in patients on chronic dapsone therapy. *Br. J. Dermatol.* 132, 257.

Robinson, D.S., Benjamin, D.M., and McCormack, J.J. (1971). Interaction of warfarin and non systemic gastrointestinal drugs. *Clin. Pharmacol. Ther.* 12, 491.

Robson, R.H. and Vishwanath, M.C. (1982). Nifedipine and beta blockade as a cause of heart failure. *BMJ* 284, 104.

Rodin, E.A., De Sousa, G., Haidukewych, D., *et al.* (1981). Dissociation between free and bound phenytoin levels in the presence of valproate sodium. *Arch. Neurol.* 38, 240.

Rodin, S.M. and Johnson, B.F. (1988). Pharmacokinetic drug interactions with digoxin. *Clin. Pharmacokinet.* 15, 227.

Sadowski, D.C. (1994). Drug interactions with antacids — mechanisms and clinical significance. *Drug Saf.* 11, 395.

Salata, J.J., Jurkiewicz, N.K., and Wallace, A.A., *et al.* (1995). Cardiac electrophysiological actions of the histamine h-1-receptor antagonists astemizole and terfenadine compared with chlorpheniramine and pyrilamine. *Circ. Res.* 76, 110.

Schiødt, F.V., Rochling, F.A., Casey, D.L., *et al.* (1997). Acetaminophen toxicity in an urban county hospital. *N. Engl. J. Med.* 337, 1112.

Schmider, J., Greenblatt, D.J., von Moltke, L.L., *et al.* (1997). Inhibition of CYP2C9 by selective serotonin reuptake inhibitors in vitro: studies of phenytoin *p*-hydroxylation. *Br. J. Clin. Pharmacol.* 44, 495.

Schwartz, J.B. (1988). Effects of amlodipine on steady-state digoxin concentrations and renal digoxin clearance. *J. Cardiovasc. Pharmacol.* 12, 1.

Sellers, E.M. (1979). Plasma protein displacement interactions are rarely of clinical significance. *Pharmacology* 18, 225.

Sellers, E.M. (1984). Drug displacement interactions: a case study of the phenylbutazone–warfarin interaction. In *Drug Protein Binding* (ed. M. Reidenberg), p. 257. Praeger Publishers, New York.

Sellers, E.M., Naranjo, C.A., Giles, H.G., *et al.* (1980). Intravenous diazepam and oral ethanol interaction. *Clin. Pharmacol. Ther.* 28, 638.

Serlin, M.J. and Breckenridge, A.M. (1983). Drug interactions with warfarin. *Drugs* 25, 610.

Serlin, M.J., Sibeon, R.G., Mossman, S., *et al.* (1979). Cimetidine: interaction with oral anticoagulants in man. *Lancet* ii, 317.

Serlin, M.J., Sibeon, R.G., and Breckenridge, A.M. (1981). Lack of effect of ranitidine on warfarin action. *Br. J. Clin. Pharmacol.* 12, 791.

Silberbauer, K., Stanek, B., and Templ, H. (1982). Acute hypotensive effect of captopril in man is modified by prostaglandin synthesis inhibition. *Br. J. Clin. Pharmacol.* 14 (Suppl. 2), 87S.

Singh, R.R., Malaviya, A.N., and Pandey, J.N. (1986). Fatal interaction between methotrexate and naproxen. *Lancet* i, 1390.

Smith, D.E., Brater, D.C., Lin, E.T., *et al.* (1979). Attenuation of furosemide's diuretic effect by indomethacin: pharmacokinetic evaluation. *J. Pharmacokinet. Biopharm.* 7, 265.

Smith, J.W., Seidl, L.G., and Cluff, L.E. (1966). Studies on the epidemiology of adverse drug reactions. V. Clinical factors influencing susceptibility. *Ann. Intern. Med.* 65, 629.

Smith, M. (1984). Drug interactions involving infusion therapy. In *Clinically Important Adverse Drug Interactions. Vol. 2 Nervous System, Endocrine System and Infusion Therapy* (ed. J.C. Petrie), p. 329. Elsevier, Amsterdam.

Solomon, H.M. and Schrogie, J.J. (1967). Change in receptor site affinity: a proposed explanation for the potentiating effect of D-thyroxine on the anticoagulant response to warfarin. *Clin. Pharmacol. Ther.* 2, 797.

Solomon, H.M., Schrogie, J.J., and Williams, D. (1968). The displacement of phenylbutazone 14C and warfarin 14C from human albumin by various drugs and fatty acids. *Biochem. Pharmacol.* 17, 143.

Sparrow, M.J. (1987). Pill method failures. *N.Z. Med. J.* 100, 102.

Stanaszek, W.F. and Franklin, C.E. (1978). Survey of potential drug interaction incidence in an outpatient clinic population. *Hosp. Pharm.* 13, 255.

Stanton, L.A., Peterson, G.M., Rumble, R.H., *et al.* (1994). Drug-related admissions to an Australian hospital. *J. Clin. Pharm. Ther.* 19, 341.

Starr, K.F. and Petrie, J.C. (1972). Drug interactions in patients on long term oral anticoagulant and antihypertensive adrenergic neurone blocking drugs. *BMJ* iv, 133.

Steiness, E. and Olesen, K.H. (1976). Cardiac arrhythmias induced by hypokalaemia and potassium loss during maintenance digoxin therapy. *Br. Heart J.* 38, 167.

Stoehr, G.P., Kroboth, P.D., Juhl, R.P., *et al.* (1984). Effect of oral contraceptives on triazolam, temazepam, alprazolam, and lorazepam kinetics. *Clin. Pharmacol. Ther.* 36, 683.

Symmons, D.P.M., Kendall, M.J., Rees, J.A., *et al.* (1983). The effect of flurbiprofen on the response to frusemide in healthy volunteers. *Int. J. Clin. Pharmacol. Ther. Toxicol.* 21, 350.

Thyss, A., Milano, G., Kubar, J., *et al.* (1986). Clinical and pharmacokinetic evidence of a life-threatening interaction between methotrexate and ketoprofen. *Lancet* i, 256.

Tjia, J.F., Colbert, J., and Back, D.J. (1996). Theophylline metabolism in human liver microsomes — inhibition studies. *J. Pharmacol. Exp. Ther.* 276, 912.

Tobert, J.A., De Schepper, P., Tjandramaga, T.B., *et al.* (1981). Effects of antacids on the bioavailability of diflunisal in the fasting and postprandial states. *Clin. Pharmacol. Ther.* 30, 385.

Tollefson, G.D. (1983). Monoamine oxidase inhibitors: a review. *J. Clin. Psychiatry* 44, 280.

Toon, S., Hopkins, K.J., Garstang, F.M., *et al.* (1987). Comparative effects of ranitidine and cimetidine on the pharmacokinetics and pharmacodynamics of warfarin in man. *Eur. J. Clin. Pharmacol.* 32, 165.

Trissel, L.A. (1996). *Handbook on Injectable Drugs* (9th edn). American Society of Hospital Pharmacists, Washington, U.S.A.

Van Cleef, G.F., Fisher, E.J., and Polk, R.E. (1997). Drug interaction potential with inhibitors of HIV protease. *Pharmacotherapy* 17, 774.

Vasko, M.R. (1990). Drug interactions. In *Rational Therapeutics* (ed. R.L. Williams, D.C. Brater, and J. Mordenti), p. 175. Marcel Dekker, New York.

Verbeeck, R.K. (1990). Pharmacokinetic drug interactions with non steroidal anti inflammatory drugs. *Clin. Pharmacokinet.* 19, 44.

Verbeeck, R., Tjandramaga, T.B., Mullie, A., *et al.* (1979). Effect of aluminium hydroxide on diflunisal absorption. *Br. J. Clin. Pharmacol.* 7, 519.

Vessell, E.S., Passananti, G.T., and Greene, F.E. (1970). Impairment of drug metabolism in man by allopurinol and nortriptyline. *N. Engl. J. Med.* 283, 1484.

Vessell, E.S., Passananti, G.T., and Johnson, A.O. (1975). Failure of indomethacin and warfarin to interact in normal human volunteers. *J. Clin. Pharmacol* 15, 486.

Walker, A.M., Cody, R.J., and Greenblatt, D.J. (1983). Drug toxicity in patients receiving digoxin and quinidine. *Am. Heart J.* 105, 1025.

Watkins, J., Abbott, E.C., Hensby, C.N., *et al.* (1980). Attenuation of hypotensive effect of propranolol and thiazide diuretics by indomethacin. *BMJ* 281, 702.

Watt, A.H., Stephens, M.R., Buss, D.C., *et al.* (1985). Amiodarone reduces plasma warfarin clearance in man. *Br. J. Clin. Pharmacol.* 20, 707.

Webster, J. (1985). Interactions of NSAIDs with diuretics and beta blockers. Mechanisms and implications. *Drugs* 30, 32.

Webster, J., Hawksworth, G.M., McLean, I., *et al.* (1983). Attenuation of the antihypertensive effect of single doses of propranolol and atenolol by flurbiprofen. *Proc. 2nd World Conf. Clin. Pharmacol. Ther.*, Abstract No. 2.

Weeks, C.E., Conard, G.J., Kvam, D.C., *et al.* (1986). The effect of flecainide acetate, a new antiarrhythmic, on plasma digoxin levels. *J. Clin. Pharmacol* 26, 27.

Weinblatt, M.E. (1989). Drug interactions with nonsteroidal antiinflammatory drugs (NSAIDs). *Scand. J. Rheumatol.* S83, 7.

Welling, P. (1984). Interactions affecting drug absorption. *Clin. Pharmacokinet.* 9, 404.

Werk, E.E., McGee, J., and Sholiton, L.J. (1964). Effect of diphenylhydantoin on cortisol metabolism in man. *J. Clin. Invest.* 43, 1824.

Wing, L.M.H., Bune, A.J.C., Chalmers, J.P., *et al.* (1981). The effects of indomethacin in treated hypertensive patients. *Clin. Exp. Pharmacol. Physiol.* 8, 537.

Woosley, R.L., Chen, Y.W., Freiman, J.P., *et al.* (1993). Mechanism of the cardiotoxic actions of terfenadine. *JAMA* 269, 1532.

Yee, G.C., Stanley, D.L., Pessa, L.J., *et al.* (1995). Effect of grapefruit juice on blood cyclosporin concentration. *Lancet* 345, 955.

Yeung Laiwah, A.C. and Mactier, R.A. (1981). Antagonistic effect of non-steroidal anti inflammatory drugs on frusemide induced diuresis in cardiac failure. *BMJ* 283, 714.

Zarowitz, B., Conway, W., and Popvich, J. (1985). Adverse interactions of drugs in critical care patients. *Henry Ford Hosp. Med. J.* 33, 48.

Zimmerman, H.J. and Maddrey, W.C. (1995). Acetaminophen (paracetamol) hepatotoxicity with regular intake of alcohol: analysis of instances of therapeutic misadventure. *Hepatology* 22, 767.

34. Medicolegal aspects and implications

R. E. FERNER

Introduction

Adverse drug reactions by definition cause harm, and patients who are harmed may seek legal redress. In that way, civil actions for damages, and even criminal charges, can in some circumstances be brought by those who have suffered from adverse effects. More rarely, adverse drug effects can alter behaviour so that patients commit criminal acts that they would not otherwise have done. Rarer still are the instances of adverse reactions that lead a patient to believe that a criminal act has been committed, when in fact it has not. The adverse reaction may in either event be advanced as a defence to the crime. This chapter deals with some of these matters.

The application of English law in a particular case is guided by previous judgments in similar cases. Some examples are quoted. Relevant monographs and reviews include Dukes and Swartz (1988), Leahy Taylor (1988), Jones (1991), Kennedy and Grubb (1994), Ferner (1996a), and Norman (1996). The interested reader will find in these works more details of legal cases cited here.

Negligence

Negligence is a tort, a civil wrong for which one party (the plaintiff) can claim damages from another (the defendant).

A person is negligent if he or she owes a duty of care to another, but fails to show sufficient care, and, as a direct and reasonably foreseeable consequence, the second person suffers harm.

Negligence and the doctor

Doctors owe their patients a duty of care, and must therefore take reasonable steps to see that their patients do not come to harm as a result of their actions or inactions. The standard which has to be met has been defined by the Courts.

Bolam v. Friern Hospital Management Committee [1957]
'Negligence means failing to act in accordance with the standards of reasonably competent medical men at the time.' In other words, a doctor does not have to be the best possible doctor in order to avoid being negligent. In fact, if he or she has acted in the way that a responsible body of comparable practitioners would have done, then there is no negligence, even if some other comparable practitioners would have acted differently.

This judgment is the basis of the 'Bolam test': are there other reasonable doctors (of the same specialty) who would have chosen to follow the same course of action as a defendant? If so, the defendant is not negligent. A more recent case suggests that the cause of action must 'rightly' be accepted as proper. Unsafe practices can sometimes become the norm: an example is the practice that was common at the time that the *Herald of Free Enterprise* sank for the masters of similar ferries to leave port before both sets of bow doors were closed. Even though many masters followed this practice, that did not exonerate Captain Lewry of the *Herald*.

The question of whether a reasonable body of responsible practitioners would have behaved like the defendant is usually answered by hearing evidence from expert witnesses (see below).

Whether a particular course of action is judged to be reasonable depends on the circumstances of the individual case. For example, it would no doubt be reasonable to administer direct-current shock without an anaesthetic in an attempt to cardiovert a patient in ventricular fibrillation who had suffered a cardiac arrest, but quite inappropriate to do so if the patient had atrial fibrillation and was conscious.

The doctor has also to take into account the special characteristics of each patient before using a drug treatment. This means that there is a duty to be aware of relevant characteristics, and to discover whether they are present. Obvious examples include: allergy to the proposed drug or to related drugs; current treatment which might interact with the drug; and a medical condition that might predispose to adverse effects. Several cases unfortunately emphasize these points.

Chin Keow v. Government of Malaysia [1967]
A patient was allergic to penicillin, and had a medical card marked 'allergic to penicillin'. A doctor, without enquiring of the patient or consulting the card, injected procaine penicillin, and the patient died within an hour from an allergic reaction. It was held to be a clear case of negligence.

Anonymous (Ferner and Whittington 1994)
A man developed gout and his general practitioner prescribed the non-steroidal anti-inflammatory drug azapropazone, which is also mildly uricosuric. The patient happened also to be taking warfarin, as the general practitioner should have known or established. Azapropazone can interact with warfarin and enhance its anticoagulant effect (see Chapter 33). That happened in this case, and the patient suffered a massive gastrointestinal haemorrhage and died.

Anonymous (Ferner 1995)
A woman was diagnosed as hypertensive at a Well Woman Clinic, and her general practitioner saw her and, failing to take note of her history of asthma, prescribed propranolol. The patient took one capsule, developed status asthmaticus, and died (see Chapter 10). The case was settled out of court for a substantial sum.

A doctor is not negligent simply because the patient does not recover as a result of treatment. It is in the way of things that some diseases cannot be treated successfully, and that some patients fail to recover in spite of appropriate treatment. Sometimes, however, things go so badly wrongcc that negligence appears on the face of it to be the only likely explanation. It is said in such circumstances that '*res ipsa loquitur*': the thing speaks for itself. The defendant then has to prove that there was no negligence, whereas normally the plantiff has to prove that there was.

Cassidy v. Ministry of Health [1951]
A man who suffered from Dupuytren's contracture involving the third and fourth fingers of his left hand was operated on. The hand became useless. If the plaintiff had to prove that some particular doctor or nurse was negligent, he would not be able to do so. But he was not put to that impossible task: he says, 'I went into hospital to be cured of two stiff fingers. I have come out of hospital with four stiff fingers, and my hand is useless. That should not have happened if due care had been used. Explain it if you can.'

The defendant can sometimes rise to the challenge to explain.

Roe v. Ministry of Health [1954]
The plaintiff was one of two patients who underwent spinal anaesthesia and suffered permanent paralysis. The glass ampoules containing anaesthetic solution had been stored in phenol solution. It was subsequently discovered that phenol had leaked through microscopic cracks into the anaesthetic solution and caused spinal cord damage. At the time of the operations, it was not known that this could occur, nor was it reasonably foreseeable. 'Doctors, like the rest of us, have to learn by experience; and experience often teaches the hard way. Something goes wrong and shows up a weakness and then it is put right.' There was no negligence.

The case of *Roe v. Ministry of Health* emphasizes the need to judge whether there was negligence by the standards at the time of the acts or omissions, not by the standards at the time of trial.

Evolving standards

It is often difficult to say exactly when standards change, and this is particularly the case with adverse reactions. One or a few isolated case reports may ultimately be attributed to chance associations, although they may also be a strong indicator that something is amiss. Thalidomide embryopathy is an example of the latter phenomenon (see Chapter 7). When warnings are widely published, then competent practitioners should be aware of them, and failure to heed them is correspondingly serious.

Examples of wide publication in the United Kingdom might be inclusion in the data sheet or Summary of Product Characteristics (found in the *ABPI Data Sheet Compendium*), or the *British National Formulary,* or the Medicines Control Agency publication *Current Problems in Pharmacovigilance*. In the United States, the *Physician's Desk Reference* is the equivalent of the *Data Sheet Compendium*.

Dukes and Swartz (1988) suggest:
'a)   The physician should have ready knowledge of all significant risks associated with the drugs which he uses every day . . .
'b)   For the drugs which he uses only exceptionally (and as regards uncommon and minor risks of those which he uses regularly) the physician should have corresponding data to hand so that he can refresh his memory.'

The doctor also has a duty to impart relevant information to the patient, so that the patient can decide whether to accept advice on treatment, and what action to take if problems occur. Examples of possible negligence include:

– failure to warn of a common adverse effect;
– failure to warn of a rare but serious adverse effect;
– failure to warn of interactions (e.g. between warfarin and other drugs);
– failure to explain the importance of warning symptoms (e.g. a sore throat while taking carbimazole); and
– failure to warn of danger to others (e.g. an unborn child, if the patient is a woman of childbearing age).

Anonymous (Gwynne 1984)

A patient with pulmonary tuberculosis was treated with rifampicin, isoniazid, and ethambutol. After about 8 months of treatment, the patient developed retinopathy which was due to the ethambutol (see Chapter 21). The patient said he had never been warned of possible damage to his eyesight. The doctor maintained that he had warned the patient at the start of treatment and at each subsequent visit. There was no record in the notes to this effect.

The judge decided (on the balance of probabilities) that no warning had been given, and that the doctor had been negligent. The Medical Defence Union commented as follows:

'There is little doubt that had the defendant doctor made even the briefest of notes on the clinical records that warnings had been given and repeated, he would not have been found negligent.'

There has in the past been a patronizing reluctance to burden patients with worries about their treatment. The more modern practice of telling patients about adverse effects might be deleterious if it deterred patients from taking medicines which were likely to do them good. Worse still, telling patients about adverse effects might lead to them experiencing those very adverse effects. Fortunately, published research on this subject fails to show any increase in the incidence of adverse effects in patients warned of their possible occurrence (Lamb *et al.* 1994).

Actual cause

Having demonstrated that a practitioner has fallen below the standard to be expected at the relevant time, a plaintiff will then have to establish that the practitioner's failing was the cause of harm. The legal test is that the harm would not have happened *but for* the defendant's failing.

Robinson v. The Post Office [1974]

A man was given a test dose of antitetanus vaccine, but the doctor giving it waited only one minute before deciding there was no allergic reaction and administering the rest of the dose. It was standard practice to wait 30 minutes. Over a week later, the patient developed an allergic encephalitis from the vaccine, which caused brain damage.

The test dose is designed to test for immediate-type hypersensitivity. Encephalitis is a delayed-type hypersensitivity reaction, and such a reaction would not have been apparent even if the doctor had waited 30 minutes. Although the doctor failed to carry out the test to the expected standard, that was not the cause of the subsequent harm, and there was no liability for damages.

The problem of causation (the legal problem of deciding the cause of harm) is particularly difficult with adverse drug reactions, since it depends both on the general problem of showing that the drug can cause the reaction, and on the specific question of whether the drug caused the harm in this patient.

Establishing whether the following statements hold can help in a particular case:

- the defendant has been harmed;
- the defendant has been exposed to the drug or medicine;
- the exposure took place before the harm ascribed to the medicine occurred;
- the time between exposure and harm was neither so long nor so short that the exposure could not have accounted for the harm;
- the extent of exposure (the dose) was sufficient to cause the harm;
- where the harm is temporary, it remits after the exposure ceases ('dechallenge');
- where the harm is temporary, it recurs after the exposure recommences ('rechallenge');
- the harm is known to occur with the medicine in question; and
- there is no better explanation for the harm than exposure to the medicine.

Karch *et al.* (1976) found wide variation in expert opinion on whether cases of illness were caused by drugs. This should worry the lawyers (and perhaps their experts).

The doctor has a duty to consider harm to the patient, but also to others. An example is the possible harm that can come to a fetus as a result of drugs prescribed to the mother (see Chapter 6). In England, the Congenital Disabilities Act (Civil Liability) 1976 gives a statutory right for a liveborn child, disabled as a consequence of some person's fault, to bring a civil action. Both the doctor and the drug manufacturer owe a duty of care under this Act. The Act does not allow a child to bring an action against its mother (except for injuries in motor accidents). It is a defence to have given medical treatment to the parent in accordance with prevailing medical opinion.

Examples where a doctor would be liable are: treatment of a woman of childbearing age with an oral retinoid such as etretinate, without taking heed as to whether she might be pregnant or become so; and similar treatment without any warning to her of the consequences for the fetus.

Negligence and the drug manufacturer

The manufacturer of a product can be liable if his negligence causes the user harm. The relationship was defined in a classic English case.

Donoghue v. Stephenson [1932]

A woman drank part of a bottle of lemonade and developed gastroenteritis. A decomposing snail was found at the bottom of the bottle. The judge held that the manufacturer of the lemonade was liable to pay damages. 'You must take reasonable care to avoid acts or omissions which you can reasonably foresee would be likely to injure your neighbour.'

'Your neighbour' was defined as any person who is so closely and directly affected that you should think of them when considering who is likely to be affected by your act. A patient certainly falls into this category, viewed from the perspective of the drug manufacturer (and of the company marketing the drug if it is manufactured by someone else).

There are usually serious impediments to showing that a company was liable for the adverse effects of its products. There is a presumption that the licensing authority has examined the question of the products quality, efficacy, and safety, and been satisfied that it is of a sufficiently high standard for the intended use. In use, adverse effects may become apparent, but they are rarely established with certainty for some time. There is often considerable debate about the link between cause and effect. This was a stumbling block in the actions brought against Burroughs Wellcome for damages in children with neurological difficulties after pertussis vaccine: it proved impossible to show 'on the balance of probabilities' that pertussis vaccine caused irreversible brain damage.

If a link between a drug and an adverse effect can be demonstrated, there is then the problem of showing that a generally recognized adverse effect has been the cause of injury in a specific case. An example of problems of this type is the series of actions ('class actions') alleging damage from chronic prescription of benzodiazepines, leading to addiction. Withdrawal symptoms from the drugs so closely resembled the conditions for which the drugs are usually prescribed that it was generally impossible in any individual to say that the symptoms were the result of the drug, and the class action was abandoned.

Actions against manufacturers can, however, succeed on other grounds. If testing is faulty or inadequate, the manufacturer can be held liable.

Stanilon [1958]
'Stanilon' was an oral antiseptic made in France and marketed for use against boils. The active ingredient was an organotin compound, diiodoethyltin. Toxicity testing had been undertaken with a single batch of capsules intended to contain a dose of 50 mg each, but containing in fact only 3 mg each, as the result of a pharmaceutical error. This low dose failed to cause toxic symptoms. The marketed capsules contained 15 mg of drug each. That dose was sufficient to cause organotin poisoning, and 102 patients died as a result. The pharmacist responsible was imprisoned, and his company was held liable for damages by a French court.

Kenneth Best v. Wellcome Foundation [1992]
This is an Irish case in which a baby boy was vaccinated with diphtheria, tetanus, and polio vaccine and suffered fits that night and subsequently. He remained gravely mentally retarded. The pertussis component of the vaccine, manufactured by Burroughs Wellcome, was made in Britain. It was tested in accordance with the prevailing British standards, and additional tests were also made. The vaccine passed the British tests, but failed a test (used in the United States) specifying the maximum potency, and also failed an additional test, not demanded by authorities in Britain or the United States, called the mouse weight gain test. No reason for these results was found, and the vaccine was released for use.

It was held that Wellcome was negligent to allow the vaccine to be released when it had failed to pass the tests it had decided to use, even though it was not obliged by statute to use them. The Appeal Court was satisfied as to causation, and damages were awarded against the Wellcome Foundation.

Adequate information

The manufacturer (or the company marketing the drug if it is manufactured by someone else) also has to ensure that the user is informed, directly or through the doctor (the 'learned intermediary'), of potential adverse effects. In deciding whether a warning is adequate, a court would take into account the severity of the possible effect, the number of users who were in danger from it, and the likelihood of it occurring.

Lesser v. Farb and Smith Kline & French Laboratories [1971]
In this American case, a 30-year-old woman was treated for depression with trifluoperazine and developed parkinsonism (see Chapter 20). The plaintiff contended that the information in the *Physician's Desk Reference* (the United States equivalent of the *ABPI Data Sheet Compendium*) was misleading, and the package insert implied that the adverse effects of trifluoperazine were rare and easily reversible: this was contradicted by reports in the medical literature over the preceding 10 years. The manufacturer was held partly to blame for the harm to the patient.

The manufacturer or marketer cannot rely on doctors discovering from other sources that certain products are liable to cause adverse reactions.

Davidson v. Connaught Laboratories [1980]
In a Canadian case where a doctor gave rabies vaccine made by the defendant, and the plaintiff suffered neurological damage, the company was held to have provided inadequate information: there was no mention of myelitis, neuritis, paralysis, or death. (The case failed, since the plaintiff had been warned of these things by another doctor, and because the warnings would not have altered the first doctor's decision to give the vaccine).

In addition to actions for negligence, the manufacturer of a medicinal product may be strictly liable under the Consumer Protection Act 1987 if his product is defective, that is, if it is less safe than the reasonable user has a right to expect. There is no need to prove negligence. A defence would be that, at the time his product was supplied, the state of scientific knowledge was such that he could not reasonably have been able to predict or discover the defect.

Negligence and the Licensing Authority

In the United Kingdom, the Medicines Act of 1968 established the system for approving medicinal products. Before granting a marketing authorization (product licence), the Licensing Authority has to satisfy itself as to the safety, efficacy, and quality of a product for its intended use. It is an open question whether the Licensing Authority would be held to owe a duty of care to members of the public in granting a licence (Jones 1991). The Licensing Authority has, from time to time, been sued as part of a wider action. The Opren (benoxaprofen) and Merital (nomifensine) litigation are examples. However, the position of the Authority as defendant has not been formally considered.

The status of the marketing authorization (product licence) in determining how a doctor should act has been discussed (Mather and Kelly 1995; Ferner 1996*b*). In principle, the authorization is merely a permit to give the manufacturer or distributor the right to make medicinal claims for a specific product within the terms of the authorization. These stipulate the indications for the product. When a doctor prescribes, he or she is not constrained by the terms of the authorization, but must take careful note of the responsibility to prescribe reasonably when deviating from the terms of the authorization.

There are difficulties in applying this approach uniformly, since the manufacturer or distributor can ask for the terms of the authorization to be as broad or as narrow as he wishes. In particular, he does not have to have an authorization which is identical to that of a rival manufacturer of an identical product. The situation is further confused by the lack of published summaries of product characteristics ('data sheets') for generic products. A doctor who writes a prescription using the approved name rather than a trade name cannot easily know the terms of the authorization for the specific product that the pharmacist will dispense.

There are other structural difficulties with the system, since the authorization necessarily omits discussion of the use of the product in groups in whom the manufacturer has not tested it. This commonly means children and pregnant women, in whom therapeutics is made correspondingly more difficult and onerous for the prescriber. The golden rule is that a prescription is reasonable if a responsible body of prescribers (of the same specialty) would have done the same thing: the Bolam test, described above.

Criminal negligence, manslaughter, and murder

Negligence is usually a matter for the civil courts. However, in some circumstances, doctors (and others) can be so reckless as to whether they cause harm, that they are guilty of a criminal act. In the present context, if a doctor is so reckless in the treatment of a patient that the patient dies, then he or she can face a charge of manslaughter.

R. v. Sullman and Prentice [1993]
A young boy was treated for leukaemia with cycles of chemotherapy. He was due for treatment with intravenous vincristine and intrathecal methotrexate. A senior house officer supervised the house physician in performing the lumbar puncture, while a nurse drew up the drugs. The vincristine was inadvertently given intrathecally, and caused a fatal arachnoiditis. The doctors were charged with manslaughter; they were acquitted on appeal.

R. v. Alam (Evening Mail — Birmingham 3 March 1994)
A general practitioner performed a circumcision on a young boy in his surgery, and then gave an intramuscular analgesic. The boy went home, but suffered a respiratory arrest and died. The analgesic was diamorphine. The doctor was charged with manslaughter and pleaded guilty.

Mens rea

A person can only be convicted of certain crimes if a specific intent existed at the time of the crime. For example, a person can only be convicted of murder if his or her intention was to cause death or serious injury. Without that intent ('*mens rea*') the accused is not guilty of murder.

R. v. Khan and Khan (The Guardian 2 July 1997)
Two drug dealers enticed a 16-year-old prostitute to their house. They gave her abnormally pure heroin (diamorphine) and she suffered the classical adverse effect of respiratory depression. The drug dealers did nothing, and the girl died. They were acquitted of murder because it could not be proved that their intention in giving her heroin was to cause her serious harm, but were convicted of manslaughter because they were reckless as to whether she lived or died.

If the doctor intends to use a drug to cause the death of a patient, or to do serious harm, and the patient dies as a consequence, then that is murder.

R. v. Cox [1993]
A consultant rheumatologist had for many years cared diligently for a patient crippled by rheumatoid arthritis. She was terminally ill and in great pain, and implored him to relieve her of her misery. He administered an intravenous

dose of potassium chloride sufficient to kill her, and she died shortly afterwards. This was the doctor's intention. The prosecution alleged attempted murder, probably because the patient was so near death that the cause of her demise was uncertain. The doctor was convicted.

Most British doctors avoid these serious difficulties by relying on the doctrine of dual effects (Quill *et al.* 1997). Where a patient is terminally ill, and the main aim of treatment is to relieve suffering, then the use of a drug to secure this effect is justified even if its adverse effects are serious and can be lethal. The widespread and humane use of diamorphine in terminal care is supported (implicitly) by this doctrine.

Adverse reactions and the actions of the patient

The actions of a patient can be modified by adverse effects of the drugs used in treatment. This is particularly, but far from exclusively, true of drugs used to treat psychiatric disorders.

A person has to be able to formulate an intent in order to commit murder.

Anonymous (Milne 1979)
A man suffering from depression was treated with maprotiline (an atypical tricyclic antidepressant), Mandrax (a mixture of methaqualone and diphenhydramine), and lorazepam. One night he killed his widowed mother. He had no memory of what happened. He was charged with murder.

An electroencephalogram showed the features of temporal lobe epilepsy, although there was no prior history of this. The events were consistent with a temporal lobe fit. Maprotiline can lower the seizure threshold and unmask epilepsy in those predisposed to it but not previously manifesting it. The man was acquitted.

An exception to the rule of intent is where voluntary intoxication leads to an abnormal state of mind during which a crime is committed.

R v. Tandy [1989]
An alcoholic woman drank nearly the whole of a bottle of vodka and then strangled her 11-year-old daughter. She was convicted of murder. A legal debate ensued in the Court of Appeal as to whether she was voluntarily intoxicated, or whether she was involuntarily intoxicated because her alcoholism was a form of brain damage. Her conviction was upheld.

The courts have considered in detail the meaning of voluntary intoxication.

R. v. Hardie [1985]
A man was charged with offences of criminal damage. Before the alleged offence he had taken about five diazepam tablets belonging to another person, 'to calm his nerves'. The Court of Appeal held that diazepam was 'wholly differ-

ent in kind from drugs which are liable to cause unpredictability or aggressiveness . . .'. There was no reason to suppose that the defendant knew that diazepam could alter the perceived risks of his actions, or that as an adverse effect it might indeed cause unpredictable or aggressive behaviour, and so none to suppose that this was voluntary self-intoxication. The conviction was quashed.

R. v. Lipman [1970]
A man took lysergide (LSD) and while under its influence was overcome by a hallucination that he was being attacked by snakes at the centre of the Earth. In fighting with the imaginary snakes, the accused killed his girlfriend and was charged with manslaughter. In his defence it was said that he was intoxicated. However, since no specific intent is required in manslaughter, this was held to be irrelevant, and he was convicted.

A number of drugs, including benzodiazepines and anabolic steroids, can cause aggression as an adverse effect. A longer list of drugs can induce hallucination or psychosis when prescribed in therapeutic dosage (see Chapter 23). Some drugs, notably benzodiazepines and opioids, may cause psychotic reactions on withdrawal. All of these drugs may be considered when trying to explain irrational, bizarre, or uncharacteristic behaviour. This is usually of importance in criminal trials, but can be relevant in civil matters (such as deciding whether a person was fit to draft a will).

Imagined crimes

Drugs can on rare occasions so alter the patient's perception of the world that he believes a crime has taken place even though it has not.

Anonymous (Brahams 1990a,b)
A young student began to hyperventilate and went to the emergency room of a (Canadian) hospital, where her treatment included intravenous diazepam. She alleged that the physician who attended to her had sexually assaulted her while she was still sedated. He gave evidence that he had asked the patient to 'squeeze [two of his fingers] hard', and she had misinterpreted this request. He was acquitted at trial, but nonetheless suffered professional sanctions.

Anonymous (Mitchell 1995)
A young woman had some teeth extracted under general anaesthetic, and the consultant anaesthetist present inserted a diclofenac suppository during anaesthesia for postoperative pain relief. The anaesthetist told the woman after she woke that he had inserted the suppository. Later, the woman noted a vaginal discharge, and went to the police thinking that she had been sexually assaulted. The suppository had been placed inadvertently in the vagina, not the rectum. This was doubly unfortunate, because it led to the police involvement and it later led to a hearing before the General Medical Council in which the anaesthetist was

found to have inserted the suppository without prior valid consent and thus to have assaulted his patient.

Expert witnesses and adverse reactions

In the United States, an expert witness is one who is 'qualified as an expert by knowledge, skill, experience, training, or education' (Hood 1994).

The role of expert evidence has recently been much debated in the United States in the wake of a decision in the following case.

Daubert v. Merrell Dow Pharmaceuticals (Bertin and Hefinin 1994).

This was one of a series of cases regarding Bendectin (dicyclomine — Debendox in the United Kingdom — a drug used to treat nausea in pregnancy) and its alleged relationship to birth defects in the babies born to mothers who had taken it. The plaintiff's experts relied on animal studies, arguments from chemical structures, and a novel and unpublished re-examination of epidemiological data. The defendant's experts reviewed only published epidemiological data to show that there was no substantial evidence of an association between Bendectin and birth defects.

The judge in the Daubert case refused to admit the unpublished re-analysis of the epidemiological data, using the principle that 'it was not sufficiently established to have general acceptance in the field to which it belonged.' The case went to the Supreme Court of the United States. The Supreme Court reversed the lower court's decision, and rejected the 'general acceptance' test. Instead, the Court advised 'a preliminary assessment of whether the reasoning or methodology underlying the testimony is scientifically valid and of whether that reasoning or methodology properly can be applied to the facts in issue.'

The *Daubert* ruling places a greater burden on the Court to examine expert testimony, but problems associated with scientific uncertainty are likely to plague legal fact-finding and dispute resolution as long as the the law sometimes asks science to provide answers that do not exist (Bertin and Hefinin 1994).

Summary

There is a risk of harm from adverse effects of any drug treatment. Those responsible for prescribing the treatment have a duty to warn the patient of the risks and to keep them as low as possible. Others involved with the manufacture, distribution, provision, and administration of the drug have parallel duties. Failure to carry out these duties invites the bringing of a civil action for damages, or, on rare occasion, a criminal action. From time to time, adverse effects alter the state of mind of an accused person, or of an alleged victim of crime. Such effects can be of considerable medicolegal importance.

Acknowledgement

The author is very grateful to Dr Elizabeth Driver, of Cameron McKenna, Solicitors, for her helpful comments.

References

Bertin, J.E. and Hefinin, M.S. (1994). Science, law, and the search for truth in the courtroom: Lessons from Daubert v. Merrell Dow. *J. Law, Medicine, Ethics* 22, 6.

Brahams, D. (1990a). Benzodiazepines and sexual fantasies. *Lancet* 335, 157.

Brahams, D. (1990b). Benzodiazepine sex fantasies — acquittal of dentist. *Lancet* 335, 403.

Dukes, M.N.G. and Swartz, B. (1988). *Responsibility for Drug-induced Injury*. Elsevier, Amsterdam.

Ferner, R.E. (1995). More errors in prescribing and giving medicines. *J. Medical Defence Union* 11, 80.

Ferner, R.E. (1996a). *Forensic Pharmacology. Medicines, Mayhem, and Malpractice*. Oxford University Press.

Ferner, R.E. (1996b). Prescribing licensed medicines for unlicensed indications. *Prescribers J.* 36, 73.

Ferner, R.E. and Whittington, R.M. (1994). Coroner's cases of death due to errors in prescribing or giving medicines or to adverse reactions: Birmingham 1986–1991. *J. R. Soc. Med.* 87, 145.

Gwynne, A.L. (ed.) (1984). *Cautionary Tales*. The Medical Defence Union, London.

Hood, R.D. (1994). Some considerations for the expert witness in cases involving birth defects. *Reprod. Toxicol.* 8, 269.

Jones, M. A. (1991). *Medical Negligence*. London, Sweet and Maxwell.

Karch, F.E., Smith, C.L., Krezner, B., *et al.* (1976). Adverse drug reactions — a matter of opinion. *Clin. Pharmacol. Therap.* 19, 489.

Kennedy, I. and Grubb, A. (1994). *Medical Law: Text with Materials* (2nd edn). Butterworth, London.

Lamb, G.C., Green, S.S., and Heron, J. (1994). Can physicians warn patients of potential side effects without fear of causing those side effects? *Arch. Intern. Med.* 154, 2753.

Leahy Taylor, J. (1981). Medicolegal aspects and implications. In *Textbook of Adverse Drug Reactions* (2nd edn) (ed. D.M. Davies). Oxford University Press.

Mather, C.M.P. and O'Kelly, S.W. (1995). Unlicensed drug administration. *Anaesthesia* 50, 189.

Milne, H. B. (1979) Epileptic homicide. *Br. J. Psych.* 134, 547.

Norman, E. (1996). Legal considerations. In Ferner, R.E. (1996a) op. cit.

Quill, T.E., Dresser, R., and Brock, D.W. (1997). The rule of double effect — a critique of its role in end-of-life decision making. *N Engl. J. Med.* 337, 1768.

Index

A

Butyrophenones (see also individual drugs)
causing
dyskinesias, 248, 596, 597, 598
galactorrhoea, 394
hypoglycaemia, 423
psychiatric disorders, 700
xerostomia, 661

C

Cadmium causing
acidosis, respiratory, 443, 446
metabolic, 443, 446
effect on zinc, 476
Fanconi syndrome, 446
Caeruloplasmin, drugs affecting, 486
Caffeine causing
acidosis, respiratory, 448
cardiac arrhythmias, 131, 133
cardiac ischaemia, 150
chromosome damage 76
effect on
cholinesterase, 493
lactate dehydrogenase tests, 490
headache (withdrawal) 594
hyperglycaemia, 414
hypokalaemia, 459
malignant hyperthermia 56
psychiatric disorders, 686, 695, 699
tremor, 599
Caffeine–propanolamine causing
hypertension, 169
Calcification, ectopic, drugs causing, 546
Calcipotriol causing
hypercalcaemia, 461, 462
Calcitonin causing hypocalcaemia, 461
Calcium antagonists (see also individual
drugs)
and cancer, 784
causing
cardiac arrhythmias, 130–1
cardiac depression, 145
effect on catecholamine tests, 390
flushing, 569
galactorrhoea, 394
gingival changes, 240, 241–2
gynaecomastia, 393
hypercalcaemia, 461
hyperglycaemia, 414
hypo-oxaluria, 483
myalgia, 610
liver damage, 298
psychiatric disorders, 676, 682, 691, 692,
702
sexual dysfunction, 878
taste disorders, 660
Calcium salts causing
acidosis, metabolic, 446
constipation, 266
effect on cryptosporidial infection, 767
hypoglycaemia, 423
hypo-oxaluria, 483
Calomel causing drug reactions, 2
Camphor causing oral ulceration, 236
Cancer (see also Leukaemia)
causing adverse reactions, 51–2

drugs studied, suspected, or implicated
265, 361, 572, 741–2, 778–85, 866,
869, 870
Candidiasis
and oral contraceptives, 766
drugs inducing or aggravating,
260, 572, 658, 663, 766–7
Cannabis causing
chromosome damage, 75
gynaecomastia, 393
psychiatric disorders, 675, 680–1, 689–90,
693, 694, 695
seizures, 594
sexual dysfunction, 880
Capgras syndrome caused by lithium, 691
Capreomycin causing ototoxicity, 644
Caproxamine causing effect on
plasma protein tests, 483, 484
Captopril causing
acidosis, metabolic, 447
agranulocytosis, 736
arthralgia/arthritis, 548
bronchospasm, 211
bullous eruption, 571
cough, 211
effect on
aldosterone, 389
angiotensin-converting enzyme, 493
creatine kinase, 489
γ-glutamyl transferase, 492
zinc, 475
exanthematous eruption, 568
facial oedema, 250
fetal/neonatal disorders, 93
fever, 860
gynaecomastia, 393
hypoglycaemia, 420
hyponatraemia, 451, 454
lichenoid eruption, 573
liver damage, 280, 297–8, 308
neuropathy, peripheral, 606
psychiatric disorders, 687, 702
renal damage, 341, 354, 355
salivation, 661
sexual dysfunction, 878
stomatitis, 236
taste disorders, 249, 660
thromboembolism, 186
zinc deficiency, 475
Carbachol causing
bronchoconstriction, 211
lacrimation, 630
psychiatric disorders, 700
Carbamates causing neuromuscular block,
608
Carbamazepine causing
agranulocytosis, 736
allergy, 800
anaemia (red cell aplasia), 736
asthma, 213
cardiac arrhythmias, 136–7
chromosome damage, 72
dyskinesias, 248, 597
effect on
aspartate aminotransferase, 490
caeruloplasmin, 486
eye movements, 636–7
immunoglobulins, 758, 761
lipids, 430
prealbumin, 484
retinol-binding protein, 484
sex-hormone-binding globulin, 485

staphylococcal infection, 761
thyroxine-binding globulin, 485
vasopressin, 396
encephalopathy, 588
erythema multiforme, 236, 575
erythroderma, 568
exanthematous eruption, 568
fetal/neonatal disorders, 98
fixed drug eruption, 572
folate deficiency, 497
hypersensitivity syndrome, 568
hypertension, 178
hyponatraemia, 451
lichenoid eruption, 573
liver damage, 293, 307, 311
lupus erythematosus, 552, 553
osteoporosis, 466
pancreatitis, 267
porphyria, 478
pseudolymphoma, 572
psychiatric disorders, 674, 685, 687, 693,
696, 699–700
renal damage, 348, 350
seizures, 591
thrombocytopenia, 737
thromboembolism, 186
Carbenicillin causing
alkalosis, metabolic, 449
chromosome damage, 70
effect on
creatine kinase, 489
plasma protein tests, 483
hypokalaemia, 460
renal damage, 350
seizures, 592
taste disorders, 659
thrombocytopenia, 737
Carbenoxolone causing
effect on
aldosterone, 389
creatine kinase, 488
hypertension, 172
hypokalaemia, 458, 460
muscle damage, 352, 353
myoglobinuria, 352, 353
myopathy, 613
renal damage, 350
Carbex — see X-ray contrast media
Carbimazole causing
agranulocytosis, 736
anaemia, aplastic, 734
arthralgia/arthritis, 548
effect on
creatine kinase, 542
hypothyroidism, 383
thyroid hormones and tests, 383
fetal/neonatal disorders, 102
liver damage, 299
muscle damage, 542
myalgia, 542, 610
taste disorders, 249
Carbohydrates causing
acidosis, respiratory, 442
Carbon dioxide causing anosmia, 659
Carbon disulphide causing anosmia, 659
Carbon monoxide causing chorea, 599
Carbonic anhydrase inhibitors causing
acidosis, metabolic, 443
Carboplatin causing
anaemia aplastic, 734
hypomagnesaemia, 473
hyponatraemia, 451
liver damage, 312

Chlorhexidine causing
  methaemoglobinaemia, 54
  oral discolouration, 239
  ototoxicity, 643
  salivary gland disorders, 247
  stomatitis, 235
  taste disorders, 660
2-Chlorodeoxyadenosine causing
  neuropathy peripheral, 603
Chloroform
  and carcinogenicity, 30
  causing
    cardiac depression, 145
    deaths, 2
    malignant hyperthermia, 616
    neuroleptic malignant syndrome, 600,
      601
    oral ulceration, 236
    seizures, 593
p-Chlorophenylalanine, causing
  effect on 5-HIAA tests, 398
Chloroquine
  aggravating psoriasis, 573
  and fetal/neonatal disorders, 91
  causing
    abscesses, 764
    agranulocytosis, 736
    corneal opacities, 632
    dyskinesias, 596
    effect on
      amylase, 492–3
      eye muscles, 637
      eyebrow/eyelash pigmentation, 630
    fetal/neonatal disorders, 655
    fixed drug eruption, 567
    gastric haemorrhage, 262
    hypoglycaemia, 422
    hypokalaemia, 459
    lichenoid eruptions, 238, 573
    muscle damage, 543
    myopathy, 615
    nail changes, 571
    neuromuscular block, 51, 608, 610
    neuropathy, peripheral, 604, 606
    oral
      lichen planus, 238
      pigmentation, 238
      ulceration, 660
    ototoxicity, 651
    peptic ulceration, 262
    pigmentation, 576
    psychiatric disorders, 677, 687, 691, 692
    retinopathy, 634–5
    seizures, 592
    thrombocytopenia, 737
Chloroquinoxaline causing hypoglycaemia,
  423
Chlorothiazide causing agranulocytosis, 736
Chlorpheniramine causing
  fetal/neonatal disorders 86
  psychiatric disorders, 672, 701
  thrombocytopenia, 737
Chlorphentermine and pulmonary
  hypertension 34
Chlorpromazine causing
  agranulocytosis, 736
  anaemia, aplastic, 734
  bladder dysfunction, 362
  cardiac arrhythmias, 126
  cataract, 633
  chromosome damage, 72
  corneal opacities, 632

drug masking, 886
dyskinesias, 248
effect on
  cholinesterase, 493
  growth hormone, 395
  haptoglobin tests, 486
  immunglobulins, 487
  phaeochromocytoma, 176
  thyroid hormone, 384
  TRH/TSH, 382
erythematous eruption, 568
fetal/neonatal disorders, 99
fever, 859
galactorrhoea, 394
hypothermia, 861
hypothyroidism, 385
lens opacities, 633
liver damage, 295–6, 307, 311
lupus erythematosus, 356, 552, 553
muscle damage, 542
nail changes, 571
pigmentation, 576
  oral, 238
  eyelid, 630
photosensitivity, 569
pigmentation
  eyelid, 630
  skin, 576
psychiatric disorders, 672, 680, 684
renal damage, 356
sexual dysfunction, 879
vitamin B_2 deficiency, 494
Chlorpropamide causing
  agranulocytosis, 736
  alcohol flushing, 57–8
  anaemia, aplastic, 734
  anaemia, aplastic (red cell aplasia), 736
  effect on vasopressin, 396
  erythema multiforme, 236
  hyponatraemia, 451, 453
  liver damage, 299, 307, 311
  neuromuscular block, 51
  neuropathy, orofacial, 248
  oral lichen planus, 237
  porphyria, 478
  pseudomembranous colitis, 762
  pulmonary eosinophilia, 215
  purpura, 754
  thrombocytopenia, 737
Chlorpropamide–alcohol flushing, 569
Chlorprothixene causing
  fever, 859
  hypouricaemia, 482
  lupus erythematosus, 552, 553
  dyskinesias, 596
Chlorthalidone
  and
    lupus erythematosus, 552, 553
    sexual dysfunction, 877–8
  causing
    agranulocytosis, 736
    effect on zinc, 476
    hyperglycaemia, 414
    hypokalaemia, 459
    muscle damage, 353
    myoglobinuria, 353
    myopathy, 613
    pancreatitis, 266
    pseudoporphyria, 479
    thrombocytopenia, 737
Chlorzoxazone causing
  dyskinesias, 598

myopathy, 611
neuromuscular block, 608
neuropathy, peripheral, 606
seizures, 593
Cholangiography — see X-ray contrast
  media
Cholebrin — see X-ray contrast media
Cholelithiasis — see Gallstones
Cholera and antacids, 762
Cholesterol embolism, drugs causing,
  185
Cholestyramine causing
  acidosis, metabolic, 443, 444
  anosmia, 659
  constipation, 266
  effect on serum folate, 498
  hypo-oxaluria, 483
  malabsorption, 263, 264
  vitamin deficiency
    vitamin A, 499
    vitamin B_{12}, 264, 496
    vitamin D, 499
    vitamin E, 500
    vitamin K, 501
Cholinergic syndrome, drugs causing
  671, 672
Cholinergics (see also invidual drugs)
  causing
    bronchospasm, 211
    effect on
      amylase, 492
      vision, 633
    lacrimation, 630
    miosis, 633
    salivation, 661
Cholinesterase, drugs affecting, 493
Cholovue — see X-ray contrast media
Chorea — see Dyskinesias
Chorionic gonadotrophin causing
  chromosome damage, 73
  gynaecomastia, 392, 393
Chromosome damage
  detection, 65–8
  drugs studied, suspected, or implicated,
    69–76
  measurements, 76–7
  mechanisms, 77
  nature, 65
  significance, 68–9
  tests, 65–8
Cianidanol causing
  haemoglobinuria, 353
  renal damage, 353
Cibenzoline causing hypoglycaemia,
  421
Cilazapril causing
  effect on lipids, 428
  hypouricaemia, 482
Cimetidine
  aggravating Sjögren's syndrome, 247
  and
    diarrhoea caused by *Campylobacter*,
      759, 762
    fetal/neonatal disorders, 85–6
  causing
    agranulocytosis, 736
    arthralgia/arthritis, 548
    cardiac arrhythmias, 136–7
    chorea, 598
    coma, 587
    drug masking, 885

D

E

G

J

K

L

M

Mexiletine causing
  cardiac
    arrhythmias, 126
    depression, 142, 143
  effect on
    aspartate aminotransferase, 491
  hypotension, 183
  psychiatric disorders, 676, 691
  seizures, 593
Mezlocillin causing renal damage, 350
Mianserin causing
  facial oedema, 250
  hyperglycaemia, 414
  liver damage, 295
  psychiatric disorders, 699
  seizures, 593
  thrombocytopenia, 737
Miconazole causing
  effect on creatine kinase, 489
  hyponatraemia, 454
Micromelia, drugs causing, 3
Mifepristone causing
  effect on ACTH, 388
  uterine rupture, 872
Milk, cows', causing hypercalcaemia, 461
Milk–alkali syndrome causing
  alkalosis, metabolic, 449
  hypercalcaemia, 357, 461–2
  osteosclerosis, 546
  renal calculi, 357
Milrinone and cardiomyotoxicity, 139
Minocycline causing
  cardiac pigmentation, 152
  fever, 859
  liver damage, 290, 308
  lupus erythematosus, 552, 553
  nail changes, 571
  oral discolouration, 238
  ototoxicity, 644, 646–7
  peripheral ischaemia, 179
  skin pigmentation, 576
  renal damage, 348, 350
  vasculitis, 574
Minoxidil
  and lupus erythematosus, 552, 553
  causing
    effect on catecholamine tests, 390
    erythema multiforme, 236
    fetal/neonatal disorders, 93
    hirsuties, 571
    hypertension (withdrawal), 170
    myalgia, 611
    pericardial disease, 153
    thrombocytopenia, 737
Miosis, drugs causing, 633
Misonidazole causing
  neuropathy, peripheral, 606
  ototoxicity, 652
Misoprostol causing
  alkalosis metabolic, 446
  fetal/neonatal disorders, 86
Mithramycin causing
  hypocalcaemia, 461
  hypokalaemia, 458, 460
  liver damage, 304
  skin pigmentation, 576
Mitomycin causing
  anaemia, aplastic, 734
  chromosome damage, 65, 66
  corneal ulceration, 632–3
  liver damage, 312
  pneumonitis, 216

pulmonary oedema, 205
  renal damage, 348, 350
  stomatitis, 660
Mitotane causing effect on
  cortisol-binding globulin, 484
  sex-hormone-binding globulin, 485
  thyroxine-binding globulin, 485
Mitoxantrone causing
  anaemia, aplastic, 734
  hypomagnesaemia, 474
  nail changes, 571
Mizoribine causing chromosome damage, 71
Moclobemide causing
  psychiatric disorders, 699
Molgramostim causing hypothyroidism, 385
Mono-octanoin causing pulmonary oedema,
    205
Morazone causing
  nicotinic acid deficiency, 495
Morphine
  age effects, 14
  causing
    acidosis, respiratory, 442
    bronchospasm, 209
    drug masking, 885–6
    effect on
      gastrointestinal motility, 261
      phaeochromocytoma, 176
    miosis, 633
    porphyrinuria, 479
    psychiatric disorders, 674, 685, 691, 700
    reactivation of herpes simplex, 765
    respiratory depression, 209, 442
    sexual dysfunction, 880
    thrombocytopenia, 737
Mouth, allergic reactions, 234–5
Mouth washes causing
  black hairy tongue, 240
  stomatitis, 235
MPTP causing dyskinesias, 597
Mucormycosis, drugs aggravating or
  inducing, 767
Muromonab-CT3 (OKT3) causing
  effect on
    cytomegalovirus infections, 765
    Epstein–Barr virus infection, 765
  encephalopathy, 588
  fever, 858
  thromboembolism, 186
Muscinol, effect on growth hormone, 395
Muscle damage (fibrosis, necrosis,
  rhabdomyolysis)
  drugs causing, 352–3, 542–3, 610
Muscle relaxants causing
  acidosis, respiratory, 442
  malignant hyperthermia, 56, 860
  respiratory depression, 442
Muscle weakness, ocular, drugs causing, 637
Mustine causing
  cancer, 778
  cataract, 632
  contact dermatitis, 580
  effect on phagocytes, 759
  fetal/neonatal disorders, 100
  leukaemia, 782, 783, 784
  nail changes. 571
  neuropathy, peripheral, 604
  ototoxicity, 651
  pigmentation, 576
  sexual dysfunction, 391, 392
Myalgia
  drugs causing, 52, 541–5, 611, 613

in electrolyte deficiency, 541
in myopathy, 541
in retroperitoneal fibrosis, 541
Myelomatosis, dangers with
  X-ray contrast media, 836, 845
Myoclonus, drugs causing, 848
Myoglobinaemia/myoglobinuria (see also
  Muscle damage)
  drugs causing, 352–3, 543, 837
Myopathy
  causing myalgia, 541
  drugs causing, 610–15, 842
Myositis (see also Eosinophilia–myalgia
  syndrome)
  drugs causing, 613
Myotonia, drugs aggravating or causing, 615

N

Nabumetone causing psychiatric disorders,
  702
Nabuphine causing psychiatric disorders, 685
Nadolol
  and alopecia, 570
  causing
    effect on
      lipids, 428
      thyroxine-binding globulin, 485
    psychiatric disorders, 682
    sexual dysfunction, 877
Nafcillin causing
  hypokalaemia, 460
  renal damage, 350
Naftidrofuryl causing hyperoxaluria, 482
Nail changes, drugs causing, 571
Nalidixic acid
  and lupus erythematosus, 552, 553
  causing
    acidosis
      lactic, 425, 445, 446
      metabolic, 443
    anaemia, haemolytic, 739
    arthralgia/arthritis, 548
    effect on VMA tests, 390
    hyperglycaemia, 415
    intracranial hypertension, 595, 636
    neuropathy, orofacial, 248
    papilloedema, 595, 636
    photosensitivity, 569
    pseudoporphyria, 479
    seizures, 592
Nalmefene causing hyperglycaemia, 414
Nalorphine causing
  effect on growth hormone, 395
  hypertension, 178
  psychiatric disorders, 692
Naloxone causing
  hyperglycaemia, 414
  hypertension, 178
  psychiatric disorders, 692
  pulmonary oedema, 205
Nandrolone causing
  effect on
    aspartate aminotransferase, 491
  gynaecomastia, 392
  psychiatric disorders, 683

O

Q

S

T

U

V

W

Y

Z